AACN's Clinical Reference for Critical-Care Nursing

AACN's Clinical Reference for Critical-Care Nursing

Marguerite Rodgers Kinney, RN, DNSc, FAAN
Professor of Nursing
School of Nursing
University of Alabama at Birmingham
Birmingham, Alabama

Donna Rogers Packa, RN, DSN
Professor of Nursing and
Associate Dean for Academic Affairs
University of Mississippi School of Nursing
Jackson, Mississippi

Sandra Byars Dunbar, RN, DSN, FAAN
Associate Professor and
Coordinator of Critical Care Nursing
Nell Hodgson Woodruff School of Nursing
Emory University
Atlanta, Georgia

Third edition

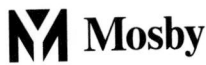 Mosby

St. Louis Baltimore Boston Chicago London Philadelphia Sydney Toronto

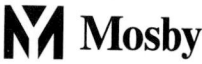 **Mosby**

Dedicated to Publishing Excellence

Publisher: Alison Miller
Editor: Theresa Van Schaik
Developmental Editor: Jeanne Rowland
Project Supervisor: Barbara Bowes Merritt
Editing and Production: The Bookmakers, Incorporated
Designer: David Zielinski

Notice

As new medical and nursing research and clinical experience broaden our knowledge, changes in treatment and drug therapy are required. The editors and the publisher of this work have made every effort to ensure that the drug dosage schedules herein are accurate and in accord with the standards accepted at the time of publication. Readers are advised, however, to check the product information sheet included in the package of each drug they plan to administer to be certain that changes have not been made in the recommended dose or in the contraindications for administration. This recommendation is of particular importance in regard to new or infrequently used drugs.

THIRD EDITION

Printed in the United States of America

Mosby–Year Book, Inc.
11830 Westline Industrial Drive
St. Louis, Missouri 63146

Library of Congress Cataloging-in-Publication Data

AACN's clinical reference for critical-care nursing   /   [edited by]
    Marguerite Rodgers Kinney,   Donna R. Packa,   Sandra Byars Dunbar—
3rd ed.
        p.   cm.
    Includes bibliographical references and index.
    ISBN 0-8016-6452-7
        1. Intensive care nursing.   I. Kinney, Marguerite Rodgers.
    II. Packa, Donna Rogers.   III. Dunbar, Sandra Byars.
        [DNLM: 1. Critical Care—nurses' instruction.   WY   154   A112   1993]
    RT120.I5A18   1993
    610.73′61—dc20
    DNLM/DLC
    for Library of Congress   92-48549
                                                                      CIP

93   94   95   96   97   GW/VH   9   8   7   6   5   4   3   2   1

About the Editors

MARGUERITE KINNEY is professor and coordinator of cardiovascular nursing at the University of Alabama at Birmingham. She is a former president of the American Association of Critical-Care Nurses and is a fellow of the American Academy of Nursing and a member of Sigma Theta Tau, the international honor society in nursing.

Dr. Kinney was born in Tuscaloosa, Alabama, and has lived all her life in the South. She received both the bachelor of science and the master of science in nursing from the University of Alabama and the doctor of nursing science from the Catholic University of America. Her research has been in the area of patient teaching, energy expenditure, nursing diagnosis, and quality of life.

DONNA PACKA is professor of nursing and Associate Dean for Academic Affairs at The University of Mississippi School of Nursing. Dr. Packa received her bachelor of science in nursing from Murray State University in Murray, Kentucky. She received the master of science in nursing and doctor of science in nursing degrees from the University of Alabama at Birmingham. Dr. Packa has served as a reviewer for *Focus on Critical Care* and was a member of the editorial board for *Heart & Lung*. She currently serves as a reviewer for the *American Journal of Critical Care*. Her research has examined quality of life in patients with chronic cardiac disease, caring behaviors of critical care nurses, and caring and noncaring behaviors of nurse managers.

SANDRA DUNBAR is associate professor and coordinator of critical care nursing in the Adult Health Program, Nell Hodgson Woodruff School of Nursing, Emory University in Atlanta, Georgia. She received the bachelor of science in nursing from the Florida State University in Tallahassee, master of nursing from the University of Florida, Gainesville, and was awarded the doctor of science in nursing from the University of Alabama at Birmingham. Her research has examined the effects of patient education after acute myocardial infarction, needs of families of critically ill patients, patient and family coping with treatment for life-threatening dysrhythmias, and chronobiological applications in nursing. Dr. Dunbar is a fellow of the American Academy of Nursing and has served as president of the American Association of Critical-Care Nurses.

Contributors

Thomas S. Ahrens, RN, DNSc, CCRN
Clinical Specialist, Critical Care
Barnes Hospital
St. Louis, Missouri
Chapters 27-30

Charold L. Baer, RN, PhD, FCCM, CCRN
Professor and Chair
Department of Adult Health and Illness
School of Nursing
Oregon Health Sciences University
Portland, Oregon
Chapters 8, 9, 34-36

Anne E. Belcher, RN, PhD
Associate Professor
School of Nursing
University of Maryland
Baltimore, Maryland
Chapter 16

Mary-Michael Brown, RN, MS, CCRN
Nursing Coordinator Cardiovascular Surgical Unit
Georgetown University Hospital
Washington, D.C.
Chapter 26

Alice E. Davis, RN, PhD, CCRN, CNRN
Assistant Professor, Adult Critical Care
Nell Hodgson Woodruff School of Nursing
Emory University
Atlanta, Georgia
Chapter 55

Mary Ann DiMola, RN, MA
Director of Corporate Education
St. Vincent's Health Group
Jacksonville, Florida
Chapter 53

Jeanne E. Doyle, RN, BSN
Executive Director of the Society of Peripheral
Vascular Nursing
Boston University Medical Center
The University Hospital
Boston, Massachusetts
Chapter 25

Janice A. Drass, RN, BSN, CDE*
Senior Clinical Nurse
National Institutes of Health
Clinical Center Nursing Department
Bethesda, Maryland
Chapter 39

Sandra B. Dunbar, RN, DSN, FAAN
Associate Professor and Coordinator of Critical
Care Nursing
Nell Hodgson Woodruff School of Nursing
Emory University
Atlanta, Georgia
Chapters 1, 17

Janet S. Eagan, RN, MSN
Clinical Instructor
Boston University Medical Center
The University Hospital
Boston, Massachusetts
Chapter 21

Dorrie K. Fontaine, RN, DNSc, CCRN
Associate Professor and Coordinator
Trauma/Critical Care Nursing
School of Nursing
University of Maryland
Baltimore, Maryland
Chapter 13

Maurene A. Harvey, RN, MPH, CCRN, FCCM
Nurse Educator
Consultants in Critical Care, Inc.
Glendale, California
Chapter 56

*The opinions expressed herein are those of the authors and do not necessarily reflect those of the National Institutes of Health, USPHS, U.S. Department of Health and Human Services, or Veterans Administrations.

Barbara J. Holtzclaw, RN, PhD, FAAN
Director of Research
Hugh Roy Cullen Professor of Nursing
School of Nursing
The University of Texas Health Science Center at
San Antonio
San Antonio, Texas
Chapter 14

Mary Ann House-Fancher, RN, MSN, CCRN
Associate Professor
School of Nursing
University of Florida
Gainesville, Florida
Chapter 59

Molly Johantgen, RN, MSN
Critical Care Specialist
The Christ Hospital
Cincinnati, Ohio
Chapters 23, 25

Marguerite Rodgers Kinney, RN, DNSc, FAAN
Professor of Nursing
School of Nursing
University of Alabama at Birmingham
Birmingham, Alabama
Chapter 1

Karin T. Kirchhoff, RN, PhD, FAAN
Professor, College of Nursing
University of Utah
Director of Nursing Research
Department of Nursing
University of Utah Hospital
Salt Lake City, Utah
Chapter 3

Catherine Nuss Kotecki, RN, MS
Staff Nurse
Our Lady of Lourdes
Camden, New Jersey
Chapter 15

Joanne M. Krumberger, RN, MSN, CCRN
Critical Care Clinical Nurse Specialist
Milwaukee Veterans Administration Medical Center
Milwaukee, Wisconsin
Chapters 49, 50, 51

Diane Panton Lapsley, RN, MS, CS
Cardiovascular Clinical Nurse Specialist
West Roxbury Veterans Administration Medical Center
West Roxbury, Massachusetts
Chapter 24

Beverley J. Leyerle, RN, MPH, CCRN
Department of Surgery
Cedars-Sinai Medical Center
Los Angeles, California
Chapter 4

Teresa Choate Loriaux, RN, MSN, CDE
Managing Editor, *The Endocrinologist*
Portland, Oregon
Chapters 37-39

Anne M. McCoy, RN, MSN, CCRN
Critical Care Specialist
H. Lee Moffitt Cancer Center and Research Institute
Tampa, Florida
Chapter 48

Rhonda M. McLain, RN, MN, CCRN
Clinical Nurse Specialist, Critical Care/Emergency
Services
Northlake Regional Medical Center
Atlanta, Georgia
Chapter 17

Aline Mierzejewski, RN, BSN, CCRN
Critical Care Patient Care Manager
H. Lee Moffitt Cancer Center and Research Institute
Tampa, Florida
Chapter 48

Pamela H. Mitchell, RN, PhD, ARNP, CNRN, FAAN
Professor of Physiological Nursing
University of Washington
Seattle, Washington
Chapters 18, 31-33

Anne M. Morrissey, BSN, MS, CCRN
Nurse Manager
Cardiac Catheterization Laboratory
Boston University Medical Center
The University Hospital
Boston, Massachusetts
Chapter 22

Glenda Nelson, RN, BSN
Staff Development Coordinator
DePaul Health Center
Bridgeton, Missouri
Chapter 27

Cynthia O'Sullivan, RN, MSN
Nurse Manager
Surgical Intensive Care Unit
Boston University Medical Center
The University Hospital
Boston, Massachusetts
Chapter 26

Donna Rogers Packa, RN, DSN
Professor of Nursing and
Associate Dean for Academic Affairs
University of Mississippi School of Nursing
Jackson, Mississippi
Chapter 1

Suzanne S. Prevost, RN, MSN, CCRN
Assistant Professor
Northwestern State University
Shreveport, Louisiana
Chapter 19

Kathleen A. Puntillo, RN, DNSc
Associate Professor of Nursing
Sonoma State University
Rohnert Park, California
Chapter 12

Julia Ann Purcell, RN, MN, CCRN
Clinical Nurse Specialist, Cardiology
Emory University Hospital
Atlanta, Georgia
Chapter 10

Juanita Reigle, RN, MSN, CCRN
Practitioner-Teacher
University of Virginia Health Sciences Center
Charlottesville, Virginia
Chapter 2

Cindy Hylton Rushton, RNC, MSN, FAAN
Clinical Nurse Specialist in Ethics
The Johns Hopkins Children's Center
Baltimore, Maryland
Chapter 2

Deborah L. Scherger, RN, CSPI
Charge Nurse
Rocky Mountain Poison and Drug Center
Denver, Colorado
Chapter 58

M. Michael Shabot, MD, FACS
Department of Surgery
Cedars-Sinai Medical Center
Los Angeles, California
Chapter 4

Claire E. Sommargren, RN, BSN, CCRN
Critical Care Staff Nurse
Instructor, Nursing Education Department
Dominican Santa Cruz Hospital
Santa Cruz, California
Chapter 5

Rae Nadine Smith, RN, MS
Clinical Nurse Specialist
President, Medical Communications and Associates
Salt Lake City, Utah
Chapter 4

Susan L. Smith, RN, MN
Clinical Nurse Specialist (Liver Transplantation)
Emory University Hospital
Atlanta, Georgia
Chapter 57

Ruth Stanley, PharmD
Clinical Pharmacy Specialist
Department of Veterans Affairs
Birmingham Veterans Administration Medical Center
Birmingham, Alabama
Drug Appendix

Susan L. Stewart, RN, MS, CCRN
Staff Nurse
Ellis Hospital
Schenectady, New York
Chapter 26

Nancy A. Stotts, MN, EdD
Associate Professor
University of California, San Francisco
San Francisco, California
Chapters 52, 54

Debra Tribett, RN, MS, CCRN
Critical Care Nurse Consultant
Edgewater, Maryland
Chapters 40-47

Nancie Urban, RN, MSN, CCRN
Cardiovascular Clinical Nurse Specialist
Waukesha Memorial Hospital
Waukesha, Wisconsin
Chapter 6

Carolyn D. Viall, RN, MSN, CNSN
Clinical Specialist
Caremark, Inc.
Cleveland, Ohio
Chapter 11

Joan Vitello-Cicciu, RN, MSN, CCRN, CS
Surgical Critical Care Clinical Specialist
Boston University Medical Center
The University Hospital
Boston, Massachusetts
Chapters 20-26

Gayle R. Whitman, RN, MSN
Director, Cardiothoracic Nursing
Cleveland Clinic Hospital
Cleveland, Ohio
Chapter 7

James B. Winkler, RN, MA
The Matrix Group
Jacksonville, Florida
Chapter 53

Jill A. Wooten, RN, BSN
Quality Assurance Coordinator
Home Health Agency of Chapel Hill
Chapel Hill, North Carolina
Chapter 53

Kathleen M. Wruk, RN, MHS
Managing Director
Rocky Mountain Poison and Drug Center
Denver, Colorado
Chapter 58

Reviewers

June C. Abbey, RN, PhD, FAAN
Vanderbilt University School of Nursing
Nashville, Tennessee

David S. Castelan, RN, BS, CCRN
Temple City, California

John Clochesy, RN, MS, CN, FCCM
Case Western Reserve University
Cleveland, Ohio

Pam Davis, RN, MN, CCRN
Emory University
Atlanta, Georgia

Margaret Doherty, RN, MS
Marin General Hospital
Kentfield, California

Maryellen K. Dye, RN, MSN
Hershey Medical Center
Hershey, Pennsylvania

Richard Eastman, MD
National Institutes of Health
Bethesda, Maryland

Roberta S. Erickson, RN, PhD
Oregon Health Sciences University
Portland, Oregon

Marcus Foreman, RN, PhD
University of Illinois, Chicago
Chicago, Illinois

Jan Foster, RN, MSN, CCRN
The University of Texas
M.D. Anderson Cancer Center
Houston, Texas

Dyrie M. Francis, RN, MSN, CCRN
Mercy Hospital
Miramar, Florida

Divina Grossman, RN, PhD
Florida International University
Miami, Florida

Marge Hamilton, RN, MSN
Camden County College
Blackwood, New Jersey

Mairead Hickey, RN, EdD
Brigham and Women's Hospital
Boston, Massachusetts

Ann Hoher, RN, MSN, CCRN, CS
St. Mary's Hospital
Rochester, Minnesota

Rosemary Lee, RN, MSN, CCRN, CNS
Cedars Medical Center
Miami, Florida

D. Lynn Loriaux, MD, PhD
Oregon Health Sciences University
Portland, Oregon

Susan McMillan, RN, PhD
University of South Florida
Tampa, Florida

Lorna Schumann, RN, PhD, CCRN
Post Falls, Idaho

Sharon A. Siegelski, RN, MS
H. Lee Moffitt Cancer Center and Research Institute
Tampa, Florida

Allen Spanier, MD, FRCS(C), CSPQ
McGill University
Montreal, Quebec

Mary Tesler, RN, MS
University of California, San Francisco
San Francisco, California

Ann B. Townsend, RN, BSN
Cardiology Associates
Cherry Hill, New Jersey

Rita Vargo, RN, MSN, CCRN
Cleveland Clinic Foundation
Cleveland, Ohio

Cheryl L. Wooten, RN, MSN
Scripps Memorial Hospital
LaJolla, California

Foreword

As we enter the twenty-first century, the needs of critically ill patients will be more complex and the critical care environment more technologically sophisticated than ever before. Preparing for the future will require commitment from practitioners to acquire the knowledge and develop the competencies to assure their ability to optimally contribute to a health care system that is driven by the needs of patients

Critical Care Patient of the Future

As life expectancy increases, there will be more demand for care of the elderly with critical illnesses. The impact of immunological and genetic advances in the treatment of disease will present new issues and challenges when caring for patients. The acuity level of critically ill patients will be higher, requiring a 25% increase in the required hours of professional nursing care over the next decade. Patient and family involvement in health care decisions and the knowledge required to make those decisions will be greater than ever.

Critical Care Environment of the Future

The complexity of the critical care environment in the future will continue to increase. Technological advances will push the limits of how we currently support patients. New cardiac, pulmonary, and renal assist devices will provide vital support when organs fail, allowing patients to survive previously fatal illnesses. Noninvasive methods for assessment and monitoring of critically ill patients will significantly reduce iatrogenic complications which are prevalent today.

The interface of bedside technologies with clinical information systems will expand the automated control of cardiopulmonary function. Cardiopulmonary stability and optimal organ functioning will be enhanced as continuous physiological data (e.g., arterial blood gases, potassium and glucose levels) are interpreted by computers and sophisticated algorithms will guide pharmacological and mechanical ventilator inverventions automatically.

Critical Care Practitioners of the Future

Critical care practitioners of the future will have greater autonomy, decision making capabilities, and more responsibility for the coordination of the patient experience. These changes, coupled with the environmental changes in critical care, will require integrated thinking. As practitioners care for patients and their families, the ability to consider various perspectives— physiological, psychological, emotional, social, organizational—will be pivotal to achieving optimal patient outcomes. Practitioners working in an interdependent manner, with a patient needs–driven framework, will be able to make their optimal contribution.

Preparing for the Future

High levels of knowledge acquisition will be required to meet the increasingly complex needs of the critically ill patient across the life span. Knowledge is a fundamental component of competent, caring nursing practice. It is essential to understand the phenomenon of the critical illness experience if practitioners are to make their optimal contribution to patient care. *AACN's Clinical Reference for Critical-Care Nursing*, 3rd ed., provides an in-depth, knowledge source for critical care nurses as they prepare for the future. Each edition of the text has updated and expanded information and issues of importance to critical care practitioners. The authors have succeeded in providing current, essential information about the disease entities which lead to critical illness, and the therapeutic management and technologies associated with critical care. The emphasis on research-based nursing interventions abounds throughout the text. Most importantly, the authors have shared with the reader a sense of how the illness experience impacts the patient and family and the profound impact that humanistic nursing care can have on meeting the needs of the critically ill.

Marianne Chulay, RN, DNSc
Clinical Nurse Specialist
Critical Care Nursing
Clinical Center, National Institutes of Health
Bethesda, Maryland
President, American Association of Critical-Care Nurses
(1992-1993)

Contents

PART ONE

Conceptual Foundations for Critical Care Nursing Practice

1

Introduction to Critical Care Nursing

Marguerite R. Kinney

Donna R. Packa

Sandra B. Dunbar

The evolution of critical care units in the general hospitals of the United States is a contemporary phenomenon, but the concept of critical care nursing is not new. Florence Nightingale recognized the importance of placing wounded soldiers who were the sickest in locations where they would receive careful surveillance from the attending nurses.[1] Louisa May Alcott wrote that during the Civil War she held her watch over the sickest and most helpless soldiers.[2] And so it seems that vigilance has played an important role in shaping our view of critical care nursing. But is vigilance sufficient to describe critical care nursing and to differentiate it from other nursing practice specialties?

Hawken[3] analyzed definitions of critical care nursing found in current texts and concluded that none of the proposed definitions clearly differentiated critical care nursing from other specialties. She asked: Does critical care encompass a concept, population, group of services, or environment? What is the role, scope, and focus of critical care?

Documents from the American Association of Critical-Care Nurses (AACN) address critical care nursing as a concept. Building on the American Nurses' Association's (ANA) definition of nursing,[4] the AACN defines critical care nursing as that specialty within nursing which deals with human responses to life-threatening problems.[5] A federal panel emphasizes a population group by stating that "critical care encompassed all patients whose conditions were totally unstable, totally nursing dependent, requiring sophisticated technologies and thus requiring many hours of care per patient."[6] A definition emerging from a forum sponsored by the Foundation for Critical Care encompasses services and environment as well as population group. Participants in the forum defined critical care as "the immediate care of patients with either illness or injury that threatens life or significant disability. It also includes care of patients, at high risk of critical events, who require monitoring in an intensive care (ICU) setting. Quality critical care is that which maximizes the possibility of full recovery or, alternatively, minimizes pain and suffering."[7] A final definition, also emerging from a national conference, emphasizes concept and services. Pioneers in the field of critical care proposed that critical care is directed toward acute, life-threatening illnesses or injuries that are reversible by medical intervention and require minute-to-minute observation and diagnosis as well as rapid therapy to reverse physiological derangements.[8]

SCOPE OF CRITICAL CARE NURSING PRACTICE

Recognizing the limitations inherent in any brief and concise definition of critical care nursing, AACN elaborates on its definition through a description of the scope of critical care nursing practice.[9] The scope is defined by the dynamic interaction of the critically ill patient, the critical care nurse, and the critical care environment (Figure 1-1). Critical care nursing is goal directed and endeavors to ensure effective interaction of these three requisite elements to bring about competent nursing practice and optimal patient outcomes within an environment supportive of both. The framework within which critical care nursing is practiced is based on a scientific body of knowledge, the application of that knowledge through the nursing process, and multidisciplinary collaboration in the care of the patient.

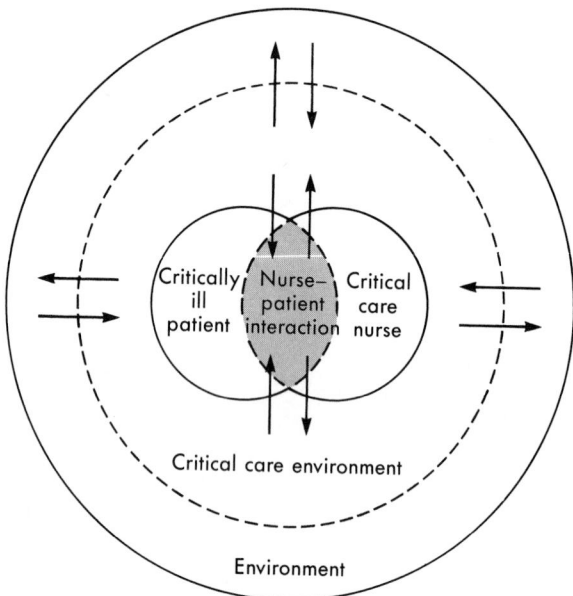

Figure 1-1   The scope of critical care nursing.

From American Association of Critical-Care Nurses. (1986). *AACN scope of practice.* Newport Beach, CA: Author.

The Critically Ill Patient

The scope of critical care nursing recognizes the centrality of the critically ill patient who has life-threatening problems or is at high risk for developing such problems. Because of the illness, the patient requires constant and intensive multidisciplinary assessment and intervention to restore stability, prevent complications, and achieve and maintain optimal responses.

In recognition of critically ill patients' primary need for restoration of physiological stability, the critical care nurse coordinates interventions directed at resolving life-threatening problems. Nursing activities also focus on support of the patient's adaptation, restoration of health, and preservation of the patient's rights, including the right to refuse treatment to the extent permitted by law, or to die. Inherent in the patient's response to critical illness is the need to maintain psychological, emotional, and social integrity. The familiarity, comfort, and support provided by social relationships can enhance effective coping. Therefore, the concept of the critically ill patient includes the interaction and influence of the patient's family or significant other(s).

The Critical Care Nurse

The critical care nurse is a licensed professional who is responsible for ensuring that all critically ill patients receive optimal care. Basic to accomplishing this goal is individual professional accountability

through adherence to standards of nursing care of the critically ill and through a commitment to act in accordance with ethical principles.

Critical care nursing practice encompasses the diagnosis and treatment of a patient's responses to life-threatening health problems. The critical care nurse is the one constant in the critical care environment and is responsible for coordination of the care delivered by many different health care providers. With the nursing process as a framework, the critical care nurse uses independent and collaborative interventions to restore stability, prevent complications, and achieve and maintain optimal patient responses. Independent nursing interventions are those actions which are in the unique realm of nursing and include manipulation of the environment, teaching, counseling, and initiating referrals. Collaborative nursing interventions are actions determined through multidisciplinary collaboration. Underlying the application of these interventions is a holistic approach that expresses human warmth and caring. This art, in conjunction with the science of critical care nursing, is essential to the interaction between the critical care nurse and critically ill patient in attaining optimal outcomes.

Because the critical care environment is constantly changing, the critical care nurse must respond effectively to the demands created by this environment for the broad application of knowledge. Essential for maintaining competency in critical care nursing is a commitment to ongoing education concurrent with an expanding base of experience.

Education and preparation for critical care nursing should be consistent with standards for critical care nursing education and practice. The AACN's *Education Standards for Critical-Care Nursing*[10] specify goals for providing high-quality critical care education. The text includes structure standards, which identify those features that must be in place for a successful educational program or activity to occur, as well as process standards, which include all stages of an educational program.

The Critical Care Environment

The critical care environment can be viewed from three perspectives. On one level the critical care environment is defined by those conditions and circumstances surrounding the direct interaction between the critical care nurse and the critically ill patient. The immediate environment must constantly support this interaction to achieve desired patient outcomes. Adequate resources, in the form of readily available emergency equipment, needed supplies, effective support systems for managing emergent patient situations, and measures for ensuring the patient's safety, are requisites. The framework for nursing practice in this setting is provided by standards for nursing care of the critically ill.

The institution or setting within which critically ill patients receive care represents another element of the critical care environment. At this level, the critical care management and administrative structure ensure effective care delivery systems for differing populations of critically ill patients through provision of adequate human, material, and financial resources; through required quality systems; and through maintenance of standards of nursing care of the critically ill.

Additional elements contributing to effective care delivery include participatory decision making, collaborative practice, and educational preparation for critical care nursing. Participatory decision making provides for nursing input into decisions affecting the nurse–patient interaction. The Joint Commission on Accreditation of Healthcare Organizations (JCAHO) acknowledges the importance of participatory decision making by requiring a multidisciplinary approach with input from both nursing and medicine.[11] The National Commission on Nursing has supported collaboration by proposing that nurse administrators have authority equal to that of medical leaders within institutions.[12] A consensus conference on critical care medicine held at the National Institutes of Health in 1983 recommended that "organizational structures should promote and require that nurses and physicians work together as colleagues at all levels—especially the medical director and nursing director."[13] These groups based their recommendations for collaboration on demonstrated positive experiences and common sense.

A collaborative practice model facilitates multidisciplinary problem solving and ethical decision making. An important study published in 1986 by Knaus and colleagues[14] of 5,000 patients in 13 tertiary care facilities sought to determine factors that accounted for differences between predicted and actual death rates. Examination of the data revealed that differences could *not* be attributed to the patient's physiological status, to the degree of sophistication of available technology, or to whether the facility was a teaching institution. Rather, differences in patient outcome were related to the degree of interaction and communication between nurses and physicians. The researchers concluded that involvement and interaction of critical care personnel can influence the outcome of critical illness. A further positive influence of multidisciplinary collaboration was noted by Baggs and colleagues,[15] who studied the amount of collaboration reported by nurses and residents relative to transfer decisions from the MICU. After controlling

for severity of patient illness, the amount of collaboration reported by nurses was found to be a significant predictor of negative patient outcome. As reported collaboration increased, there was a decrease in the incidence of negative outcomes as measured by readmission to the MICU or death. These studies offer hard data in support of collaboration between physicians and nurses that should not be ignored.

EVALUATION OF CRITICAL CARE

Interwoven like threads throughout the scope of the critical care nursing statement are concepts of structure, process, and outcome which are basic elements in the evaluation of quality care.[16] *Structure* refers to the system in which care is delivered or the resources used in the delivery of care. The broadest perspective of the environment encompasses a global view of those factors that have an impact on the provision of care to the critically ill patient. Monitoring of legal, regulatory, social, economic, and political trends is necessary to promote early recognition of the potential implications for critical care nursing and to provide a basis for a timely response.

Activities that constitute care are the *process*, and these activities take two forms: technical and interpersonal. For more than two decades the activities that constitute care have been labeled "the nursing process," which includes assessment, diagnosis, planning, intervention, and evaluation. Although recently this process has been criticized[17] as being reductionistic and restrictive for nursing practice, it does guide nurses to assess biological, psychological, and social dimensions of their patients and to plan and implement interventions based on the assessment. The process also has an evaluative component. Finally, *outcomes* are the end results for the patient or the desired consequences of patient-centered care. Several important factors have contributed to the present era of assessment and accountability, described by Relman as "the third revolution in medical care."[18] These factors include the need for cost containment, a renewed sense of competition, and concerns about the effectiveness and appropriateness of clinical practice.[19]

AACN first published *Standards for Nursing Care of the Critically Ill*[20] in 1981, setting forth the structure and process standards important for measuring quality patient care. These standards were updated in 1989.[21] In 1990 the circle of evaluation was completed with the release of AACN's *Outcome Standards for Nursing Care of the Critically Ill.*[22]

The Quality of Care Nursing Diagnosis Model (Figure 1-2) takes into account structures, process, and outcomes.[22] The straight lines at level 1 designate theorized relationships between the concepts of structure, process, and outcome. At level 2 arrows indicate

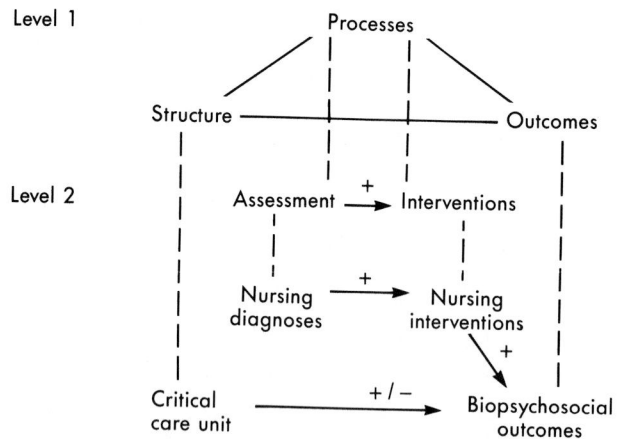

Level 1

Level 2

(NOTE: + = positive outcome; +/− = positive or negative outcome)

Figure 1-2 Quality of care nursing diagnosis model.
From American Association of Critical-Care Nurses. (1990). *Outcome standards for nursing care of the critically ill* (p. 8). Laguna Niguel, CA: Author.

causal relationships. A positive sign indicates that a positive relationship has been theorized while a negative sign indicates that a negative relationship has been theorized. The structure is the critical care unit. Process is both assessment (used to make nursing diagnoses) and interventions (used to implement the specific nursing activities related to the nursing diagnoses).[23] Outcomes are labeled biopsychosocial outcomes and relate to physiological and psychosocial improvement. For example, in the critical care unit, nursing diagnoses lead to nursing interventions, and nursing interventions then lead to biopsychosocial outcomes. The critical care environment may influence patient outcomes directly, regardless of nursing interventions that may or may not be performed. The line between the critical care unit and patient outcomes indicates this possibility. For example, preexisting conditions, the many health care professionals involved in care, and environmental factors also may have an effect on the patient's recovery, despite appropriate nursing interventions. Although it is theorized that diagnosing the problem and implementing nursing interventions to treat the problem will have a positive effect on patient outcomes, intervention research in nursing is limited.

CRITICAL CARE NURSING RESEARCH

In 1991, AACN convened a national panel of 50 critical care nurse experts to identify and prioritize research topics for critical care nursing. Using real-time interactive computer technology to achieve consensus, the panel identified priorities for clinical practice research and for research on the context within which critical care nursing takes place, that is, the

structure for care. The priorities for *clinical practice research* are:

Techniques to optimize pulmonary functioning and prevent pulmonary complications

Weaning of mechanically ventilated patients

Effect of nursing activities/interventions on hemodynamic parameters

Nutritional support modalities and patient outcomes

Interventions to prevent infection

Pain assessment and pain management techniques

Accuracy and precision of invasive and noninvasive monitoring devices

Effect of nursing activities, environmental stimuli, and human interactions on intracranial and cerebral perfusion pressure

Data from these studies will expand opportunities for testing the relationships theorized in the Quality of Care Nursing Diagnosis Model.

Priorities for research on the *context within which critical care nursing takes place* are:

Incorporation of research findings into critical care nursing practice

Levels of nursing competence (e.g., certification) and the effect on patient outcomes

Occupational hazards (e.g., HIV, noise, substance abuse, premature delivery)

Ethical issues related to initiation, maintenance, and withdrawal of life support technology (e.g., living wills)

Patient care delivery models for critical care

Collaboration and communication among health care professionals

Role of critical care nurses in decisions regarding resuscitation status of critically ill patients

Data generated from this collection of studies will reveal environmental influences that may have positive or negative influences on physiological and psychosocial recovery.

Establishing outcomes based on nursing interventions and identifying criteria to be used in evaluating patient outcomes promotes autonomy and accountability in nursing practice. It is desirable that every critically ill patient be cared for by a critical care nurse, but this level of care is not always available. Thus, nursing activities may be delegated to supporting personnel[24] but only after careful consideration of a number of factors. What is the potential for harm to the patient, including infection, hemorrhage, hypoxemia, nerve damage, psychosocial distress, and others? Before delegating a nursing activity, the critical care nurse must assess the risk the activity poses for an individual patient. What is the complexity of a nursing activity? The greater the complexity, the less desirable it is to delegate an activity. What problem solving is required and what innovation is needed? Adapting a nursing activity and evaluating its outcome are the responsibilities of the registered nurse. When a patient's response to an activity is unpredictable or unknown, delegation of the activity is not advised. To what extent will patient interaction be diminished by delegation of the nursing activity? It is undesirable to delegate activities to the extent that the time the critical care nurse spends with a patient or family is curtailed and the nurse's ability to effectively plan, coordinate, and evaluate care is restricted. In summary, it is inappropriate to delegate nursing activities that comprise the core of the nursing process and require specialized knowledge, judgment, and skill. These activities include initial patient assessment or intervention, formulating nursing diagnoses, establishing goals of care, developing a nursing care plan, and evaluating a patient's progress toward goal achievement. Use of support personnel should never interfere with the implementation of AACN's *Standards for Nursing Care of the Critically Ill* or *Outcome Standards for Nursing Care of the Critically Ill.*

SIGNIFICANCE OF CRITICAL CARE NURSING

A critical illness or injury is a significant event in the lives of individuals and their loved ones. Critical care nurses have a unique opportunity to share in these events and to bring their special knowledge and skills to the caring encounter. Although it is difficult to define critical care nursing precisely, evidence indicates that patients view critical care nursing as a special blending of vigilance, healing, and mutuality.[25] These behaviors are reflected in the statement from the 1983 Consensus Conference on Critical Care Medicine which noted that "nurses are the key element in critical care. The continual presence and judgment of the professional nurse positively influence patient care outcomes."[13]

REFERENCES

1. Nightingale, F. (1859). *Notes on nursing*. London: Harrison & Sons.
2. Alcott, L. M. (1963). *Hospital sketches* (p. 47). Boston: James Redpath.
3. Hawken, P. L. (1990). Response to AACN position statements: The education perspective. In B. J. Daly, & J. Boller (Eds.), *Critical care in the nursing curriculum* (pp. 1-8). Laguna Niguel, CA: AACN.
4. American Nurses' Association. (1980). *Nursing: A social policy statement*. Kansas City, MO: Author.
5. American Association of Critical-Care Nurses. (1984). *Definition of critical care nursing* (AACN position statement). Newport Beach, CA: Author.
6. U.S. Department of Health and Human Services. (1988). *Sixth report to the president and congress on the status of health personnel in the United States* (Report No. HRS-P-OD-88-1, pp. 10-64). Washington, DC: U.S. Government Printing Office.
7. Foundation for Critical Care. (1990). *Critical minutes, 1*(2), 1-4: Author.
8. Kinney, M. R. (1987). Critical care: Needed more than ever before. *Focus on Critical Care, 14*(5), 7.
9. American Association of Critical-Care Nurses. (1986). *AACN scope of practice*. Newport Beach, CA: Author.
10. Alspach, J. G., Bell, J., Canobbio, M. M., et al. (Eds.). (1986). *Education standards for critical-care nursing*. St. Louis: Mosby.
11. Joint Commission on Accreditation of Healthcare Organizations. (1991). *Accreditation manual for hospitals*. Chicago: Author.
12. National Commission on Nursing. (1983). *Summary report and recommendation*. Chicago: Author.
13. National Institutes of Health Consensus Conference. (1983). Critical care medicine. *Journal of the American Medical Association. 250*, 798-804.
14. Knaus, W., Draper, E., Wagner, D., et al. (1986). An evaluation of outcome from intensive care in major medical centers. *Annals of Internal Medicine, 104*, 410-418.
15. Baggs, J., Ryan, S., Phelps, C., et al. (1992). The association between interdisciplinary collaboration and patient outcomes in a medical intensive care unit. *Heart Lung, 21*, 18-24.
16. Donabedian, A. (1966). Evaluating the quality of medical care. *Milbank Memorial Fund Quarterly, 83*, 323-325.
17. Nagle, L. M., & Mitchel, G. J. (1991). Theoretic diversity: Evolving paradigmatic issues in research and practice. *Advances in Nursing Science, 14*, 17-25.
18. Relman, A. S. (1988). Assessment and accountability: The third revolution in medical care. *New England Journal of Medicine, 319*, 1220-1222.
19. Epstein, A. M. (1990). The outcomes movement—will it get us where we want to go? *New England Journal of Medicine, 323*, 266-270.
20. American Association of Critical-Care Nurses. (1981). *Standards for nursing care of the critically ill*. Reston, VA: Reston Publishing.
21. American Association of Critical-Care Nurses. (1989). *Standards for nursing care of the critically ill* (2nd ed.). Norwalk, CT: Appleton & Lange.
22. American Association of Critical-Care Nurses. (1990). *Outcome standards for nursing care of the critically ill*. Laguna Niguel, CA: Author.
23. Block, D. (1975). Evaluation of nursing care in terms of process and outcome. *Nursing Research, 24*, 256-263.
24. American Association of Critical-Care Nurses. (1990). *Delegation of nursing and nonnursing activities in critical care: A framework for decision making*. Laguna Niguel, CA: Author.
25. Burfitt, S., Greiner, D., Miers, L. J., et al. (1992). Professional nurse caring as perceived by critically ill patients: A phenomenologic study. Unpublished manuscript.

2

Ethical Issues in Critical Care

Cindy Hylton Rushton

Juanita Reigle

THE ROLE OF NURSES IN ETHICAL DECISION MAKING

Nurses are sometimes reluctant to offer moral or ethical advice to patients or to become involved in discussions about ethical issues. Traditionally, the analysis of moral problems has been directed to physicians, and nurses have been marginalized and often excluded from moral or ethical decision making. However, nurses comprise the largest number of health care professionals, maintain the closet contact with patients and families, and frequently are most familiar with the patient's values, concerns, and needs. The uniqueness of the nurse–patient relationship tends to encourage patients and families to discuss their understanding and interpretation of their situation. Failure of the nurse to engage in these discussions and analyses leads to inadequate and incomplete evaluation of the issues.

The traditional values of nursing reflected the status of women at an earlier time. In the 19th and early 20th centuries, nurses were expected to uphold the reputation of the physician and not to question authority. The concept of the obedient nurse was advanced during the training of students with the expectation of total loyalty to the hospital and physician.[1]

The more contemporary values of advocacy, accountability, and individualized, patient-centered care flourished in the 1960s. The 1976 revision of the American Nurses' Association's (ANA) *Code for Nurses*, reproduced in Appendix 2A, reflects these changing values by shifting the obligation of the nurse away from the physician and toward the patient.[2] The primary value emphasized in the *Code* is respect for human dignity and patient self-determination.

Underlying these contemporary values is a fundamental belief in holistic care. Nurses realize that health cannot be guaranteed by curing an illness and that the goal of nursing is not the eradication of disease. Rather, the goal is to enable the patient, family, and significant others to adjust to changes in health.

Nursing actions are directed toward maximizing the control exerted by the patient and family. In this way, the nurse advances the patient's sense of personhood, self-worth, and dignity. This ideology is based on such humanistic criteria as quality of life or coping ability, rather than a disease classification approach.

Political involvement and collaborative relationships are two emerging values in nursing. The personal and professional satisfaction of nurses in their work is associated significantly with their relationships with physicians.[3] The situational nature of nursing practice and the complexity of the health care environment require close interaction and honest communication between physicians and nurses. The impetus for collaborative practice must come from both professions and must be supported by institutional policies.

The ANA *Code for Nurses* represents the formal code of ethics of the nursing profession. It expresses the moral values and beliefs of the profession and represents to the public the covenant that nursing makes with society. It is organized into eleven primary statements which address the interests and concerns of the profession. Included in the primary statements are discussions regarding the patient's right to self-determination, the nurse's responsibility to protect the patient against the incompetent practice of other health care professionals, and the nurse's obligation to maintain professional competence. The accompanying interpretive statements amplify the values and obligations set forth in the tenets.

Many changes have been incorporated into the *Code* over the past 40 years, reflecting the dynamic nature of nursing practice. Despite the changes, the *Code* has consistently focused on the health care environment in which care to the patient is delivered. Rather than outlining the rights of the nurse, the *Code* emphasizes the responsibilities of the individual nurse and of the nursing profession. Furthermore, the ANA has developed related documents and position statements that further delineate nursing's role in ethical issues. Several of these are presented in the appendix of this chapter.

To supplement the general ANA *Code for Nurses*, nursing specialty organizations also provide ethical guidance. The American Association of Critical-Care Nurses (AACN) supports the nurse's involvement in ethical decision making and outlines the nurse's moral responsibilities in several position statements and related documents.[4,5] These publications highlight the moral obligations and duties of critical care nurses and provide guidance to the nurse involved in ethical dilemmas arising in clinical practice.

A number of models of ethical decision making may provide guidance to nurses facing a moral issue.[6,7,8,9] Traditionally such models are based on an approach whereby ethical principles are applied to resolve moral quandaries, that is, a "principle-based" approach. However, it is important to recognize that nursing is dominated by a care orientation in addition to the moral claims, duties, and rights described by other traditions. The perspective of care is an essential, valuable dimension of moral deliberation that nurses should recognize and foster. From a care orientation, nurses see moral judgments as emotional, contextual, and based on the special circumstances of the situation; the uniqueness of individuals and particular dynamics of their relationships are endorsed as essential components of moral decision making.

A care orientation in the interpretation of moral issues is not without risks or controversy.[10,11] Traditional bioethical theories have emphasized impartiality and rational application of particular principles and rules. Moral reasoning, which involves empathy, acknowledges vulnerability, and emphasizes connectedness and responsiveness, has been viewed as illegitimate and irrational. In addition, the ethic of care is a feminist contribution to ethical theory, and its critics assert that practice of such an ethic reinforces the stereotypical roles that women have fought to overcome.[10] In other words, the oppression of women may be perpetuated by encouraging empathy and compassion.[11]

The application of an ethic that may potentiate the subjugation and suppression of women is disquieting to a profession whose members are predominantly women. Much of nursing's history reveals a continuing struggle to move beyond the traditional, oppressive nurse–physician relationship and become more independent of medicine. The ethic of care, however, does not compel or involve self-sacrifice or submission.[10] Conceivably, change can be effected by reconceptualizing the values and qualities of nurturance, attentiveness, and compassion rather than entirely rejecting the care orientation. Moreover, adopting a care orientation does not preclude the application of traditional theories and principles to

ethical questions. Rather, the care orientation may guide nurses in applying ethical principles in particular situations and thereby may inform the process for decision making.[12]

The ethical issues that confront nurses may be considerably different from those facing physicians. Nurses have a variety of responsibilities and allegiances that contribute to the scope and nature of the ethical issues encountered. These responsibilities are complicated by the fact that nurses perform both independent nursing actions and dependent nursing functions. Despite these barriers, nurses are now asserting their voices in the moral domain. Concerns about situations that hamper the delivery of high quality patient care, such as inadequate staffing, unsafe practices, insufficient salaries, long hours, and lack of recognition and acceptance of the nurse's judgment and knowledge are being discussed openly.[1]

Nurses bring to the decision making process a unique awareness of the dynamics of the situation. The education and experience of nurses prepare them to view the patient and family holistically and as a unit with multiple needs. Nursing humanizes health care by contributing the qualities of imagination, compassion, and inspiration to an environment submerged in science and technology. The nursing perspective is increasingly necessary for effective resolution of ethical issues.

ADVOCACY

Historically, advocacy has been a dominant theme in nursing. The nurse's primary role as patient advocate is central to the ANA *Code for Nurses*[2]. A position statement of the AACN has affirmed the role of the critical care nurse as patient advocate. This statement, which is reproduced in Appendix 2B, provides important guidance for nursing behaviors in patient advocacy. It affirms the nurse's obligation to respect the patient's right to autonomous, informed decision making; to respect the values, beliefs, and rights of the patient; to intervene on behalf of the patient; to support the patient's decisions; to intercede for patients unable to speak for themselves; to assist in the decision-making process; to act as a liaison; to represent the patient's choices; and to monitor and safeguard the quality of patient care.[4] Clearly, being an advocate is an important professional activity for nurses.

Definition

To be effective advocates, nurses need to clearly understand what it means to be an advocate. An advocate is generally defined as one who pleads another's cause. Advocacy applied to nursing has been defined as helping to maintain individuality and humanism while providing expert nursing care.[13]

Behaviors essential to the advocacy role include developing nursing approaches based on scientific knowledge and ethical standards; promoting patient well-being through physical, emotional, spiritual, and psychosocial interventions; promoting continuity of care; facilitating communication; minimizing environmental stressors; protecting patient interests; and meeting family needs.[13]

Advocacy generally implies acting to safeguard and advance the interests of another. It is not acting in the place of someone else; it is assisting patients or their surrogates to make informed choices and to act in their best interest. Advocacy should not be confused with "rescuing" someone. Nurses can, however, become confused about the boundaries of their advocacy role. Instead of acting *with* the patient, they adopt a paternalistic approach that undermines a patient's authority to act for himself or herself. That is, they begin to make decisions *for* the patient instead of *with* the patient. The appropriate advocacy role for nurses involves advising, sharing specific information, and offering recommendations to enable patients to make their own decisions. Despite attempts to characterize the nurse's role as patient advocate and consistent affirmation of that role, much confusion surrounds the scope of the nurse advocate role and methods for consistently implementing it.

Embedded in an understanding of the nurse advocate role is an appreciation of the moral responsibilities that accompany assumption of the role. By virtue of their socially sanctioned role in health care, nurses have specific moral obligations or duties toward their patients. Unlike physicians nurses are not generally chosen by the patient. Patients accept our ministrations as part of the overall package of health care when they are in need. It has been suggested that the moral obligations of nurses arise from a fiduciary relationship, that is, a relationship built on trust. This fiduciary relationship is valuable only because of public confidence and support.

According to Leah Curtin, "the proposed ideal of advocacy is based upon our common humanity, our common needs, and our common human rights."[14] This commonality with patients is the basis for the nurse–patient relationship. Recognizing and sharing a common destiny with patients allows nurses to view each person as a unique, unified individual who is both interrelated with and interdependent on others. Furthermore, Curtin suggests that it is our commitment to maintaining our integrity as persons that underscores our commitment to advocacy, particularly when patients are unable to speak for themselves.[14]

Models of Nurse Advocacy

A variety of models of advocacy have been advanced for nursing practice, including guardian of patient rights,[15] preserver of patient values,[16] the respect for persons model,[17] and social advocacy.[18] Each model emphasizes several dimensions of the nurse's advocacy role and provides useful guidance in discharging the corresponding obligations of the role.

Care as a Model for Nurse Advocacy

One useful model for nurse advocacy is care. Advocacy is a logical extension of the care ethic. From the care perspective advocacy is predicated on virtues and notions of care rather than on principles that emphasize individual rights and justice. It does not consist merely of upholding the patient's right to self-determination by appealing to rights alone. Advocacy based on care gives attention to the special circumstances and context of the specific situation in which moral action occurs instead of merely considering the patient's interests and preferences in isolation. Such a model supports the nurse's efforts to assist patients or their families to find unique meaning or purpose in their living or their dying and to assist them in realizing goals that promote a meaningful life or death.

Intimacy is a crucial dimension of the care perspective, and advocacy is based on a trusting relationship between the patient and nurse or other health care provider. Care as a model for advocacy implies that the nurse must be engaged in a relationship with the patient to appreciate his or her unique values and life goals. Much of what nurses do for and with patients is very personal. Their sustained relationship and interaction with the patient allows them to feel patients' pain, suffering, happiness, successes, and disappointments. They are able to see a patient's journey in an "up front and personal" way.

The values and expectations involved in certain roles and relationships are seen as primary from this vantage point. Thus, being an advocate involves appreciating the relationships that are significant to the patient and understanding how those relationships affect his or her care. At times it may lead advocates to enlarge their conception of what it means to respect the patient so as to include considerations about the interests of others that are essential to the patient's well-being.

Advocacy based on care also emphasizes not only the interconnections of patients with others but also the interrelationships of the members of the health care team. It recognizes that nurses work collaboratively with physicians and others to advance patients' interests and goals. In fact, successful advocacy demands reciprocal interaction and communication among all who are involved in the care of a patient. It also recognizes that nurses (as well as their colleagues) have obligations to patients and families, to other members of the health care team, to the institutions where they practice, to society, and to themselves. To be effective advocates, nurses must be familiar with the values and philosophy of the unit and the institution. They must know the nursing, medical, and administrative hierarchy and how to work successfully within the system.

In some instances, advocacy may require nurses to intervene when a decision is clearly not in the patient's best interest. Nurses are often the first to recognize these situations and can either initiate direct action to address the issues or report these situations to persons who can effect change in the organization.

Barriers to Nurse Advocacy

Nurses have a legitimate moral responsibility to advocate on behalf of patients and their families. Why, then, are there also instances of ineffective or nonexistent advocacy by nurses? Consider some of the potential barriers: poor communication, unequal power or authority, misinformation or lack of information, inadequate professional socialization, unclear professional/personal boundaries, unclear understanding of the advocacy role, conflicting interests or loyalties, scarce human and material resources, and failure to engage in the moral discourse.

Advocacy can also be jeopardized by a nurse's overinvolvement or underinvolvement. When nurses remain detached from their patients and families they lack an important avenue for effective advocacy. Failure to know the patient and to engage in the moral discourse short-circuits a nurse's advocacy. In such instances, nurses see themselves as uninvolved in decision making and therefore not culpable for the decisions of others. By not engaging in the moral discourse, they are able to criticize the actions of others without themselves being accountable for the decision or its implementation. Noninvolvement provides an excuse to blame others; in doing so nurses shirk their role in the patient's care. The unengaged observer risks becoming a "moral coward." To be effective advocates, nurses must be willing to share in the experiences of patients, families, and colleagues and the decisions they make.

In contrast, nurses may lose sight of their professional boundaries and become overidentified with the patient or family. By doing so they jeopardize their ability to maintain a therapeutic relationship and effective advocacy. When nurses interpret their advocacy role to include being a friend of the patient and family, effective advocacy is jeopardized.

Risks of Advocacy

Advocacy is not a benign endeavor. Advocating for and supporting the basic values, rights, and beliefs of the critically ill patient is not without controversy or conflict. Nurses may find themselves in conflict with the patient, the patient's family, the health care team, or the institution in which they work. Often advocacy is jeopardized by conflicting interpretations of patients' interests. In some cases nurses have been accused of insubordination and have suffered loss of reputation, license, friends, and self-esteem. Those who act alone and without the benefit of an organized problem-solving process seem to be at higher risk of such outcomes.

The personal integrity of nurses may also be jeopardized as they attempt to discharge their advocacy responsibilities. Nurses may be party to carrying out a course of treatment that they believe is contrary to the patient's best interest without an opportunity to express their concerns or discomfort. For example, a nurse may be required to provide innovative therapies such as extracorporeal membrane oxygenation (ECMO) beyond the usual treatment parameters for the sake of a scientific protocol rather than any measurable benefit in patient outcome. In such instances it may be clear that the benefits to be realized by the patient have been exhausted and that the continuation of the therapy is causing family and caregivers considerable anguish. At this juncture many nurses experience profound moral distress.[19] Moreover, nurses may be asked to engage in activities that are morally reprehensible to them, such as repeatedly resuscitating a patient terminally ill with cancer or providing medically futile therapy to a patient at the insistence of the family. The result is a loss of personal and professional integrity, particularly if such instances are recurring and are not satisfactorily resolved.

Another closely related risk of advocacy involves the suffering that caregivers experience through their caring. By the nature of their relationship with the patient and family over time, nurses develop a unique connectedness that creates opportunities for recognizing suffering and responding compassionately to it. Nurses describe intense emotions in response to the circumstances in which they find themselves. Many describe feelings of compassion toward their patients and the plight they must endure. Their patients suffer the indignity of being seriously ill, damage to their self-image, useless depletion of their financial resources, the stress of loved ones who desperately hope for their recovery, and anxiety resulting from an overwhelming sense of powerlessness in a situation beyond their control. And nurses suffer because they understand and identify with these patient responses.[20]

Nurses who participate in end-of-life decisions or who carry out the decisions of others experience a variety of conflicts: between different moral positions; between competing obligations and their corresponding responsibilities to patients, families, colleagues, institutions, or themselves; and conflicts that can place their moral integrity in jeopardy. These conflicts culminate not only in the suffering of patients and their families but also in personal suffering for the nurse.[20]

Nurses who engage in advocacy activities are often unsure about the level of risk they should assume on behalf of their patients. Generally, when intervening will promote the patient's well-being, prevent harm, or advance the patient's interests, there is a general duty toward advocacy.[21] In some situations, however, advocacy may place the nurse at risk. According to the ANA, the duty to advocate depends on the level of risk to the nurse.[22] If there is significant risk to the nurse that can be minimized, there is an obligation to advocate. When risks are significant and the nurse could be harmed because the risks cannot be minimized, certain risks do not have to be assumed by the nurse. "Accepting personal risk which exceeds the limits of duty is not morally obligatory; it is a moral option."[22] The ANA statement on risk versus responsibility provides nurses with guidance for distinguishing when a risk implies a moral duty in contrast to a moral option. According to the ANA statement, advocacy is indicated if:

> 1) The patient is at significant risk of harm or damage if the nurse does not assist the patient, 2) the nurse's intervention or care is directly relevant to preventing harm, 3) the nurse's care will probably prevent harm, loss, or damage to the patient, or 4) the benefit to the patient outweighs any harm the nurse may incur and does not present more than minimal risk to the health care provider.[22]

Nurses must be mindful, however, that the degree of risk to them is directly influenced by the norms and culture of the organization in which they practice.[21] Nurses must weigh the risks of advocacy with the potential benefits to determine their individual threshold for action.

Strategies to Support Advocacy

Risks of advocacy can be reduced by understanding the advocacy role, using a systematic decision-making process, clarifying values, appropriately enlisting the support of others, working within the organizational framework, being educated about the nature of ethical issues, and using appropriate communication skills. Advocacy can also be enhanced by developing trusting, therapeutic relationships with patients and families, fostering a care delivery model that supports continuity of care, addressing caregiver suffering, and being accountable for one's actions and recognizing the accountability of others for their actions. Nurses, physicians, and administrators must share responsibility for formulating policies that support the role of the nurse as patient advocate. Advocacy is facilitated by collaborative practice, mechanisms for dispute resolution, bioethics committees with adequate and appropriate nursing representation, and an environment that encourages nurses to bring ethical issues to the forefront.

If each participant in the moral community (composed of health care professionals from different disciplines) is able to appreciate the moral obligations of others, then we have made a significant step toward fulfilling our collective obligation to be patient advocates. Nurses are in a crucial position to create a climate that is respectful of the needs and preferences of patients or their surrogates. Nurses have tremendous power within their organizations to create an atmosphere that supports individual differences and preferences and promotes shared decision making. Moreover, nurses must be the catalysts for creating an environment where advocacy is expected and rewarded rather than punished and suppressed.

MORAL FRAMEWORK FOR ETHICAL DECISION MAKING

Shared Decision Making

A morally defensible framework for ethical decision making by competent adults is based on a framework of shared decision making.[23,24] Such a framework gives priority to promotion of patient well-being and a respect for patient self-determination. Choices among treatment options should promote the well-being of individuals according to their unique goals, values, and preferences. Decisions are shared between a patient and the professionals who render health care. The health care professionals offer expert knowledge, recommendations, and advice about medically accepted and available options, and the patient decides which option will best promote his or her life goals and values.[24] To comprehend the values that influence a patient's choice of action, the nurse must appreciate the context of that patient's life, including the family system and the patient's cultural, religious, and spiritual affiliations and preferences.[25]

Ethical Principles

Respect for Autonomy

This tradition of shared decision making is based on a recognition of the importance of the ethical principles of respect for persons and the derivative principle of autonomy. Americans traditionally believe that patients have a right to make important decisions about the course of their lives. One aspect of this right is patients' right to control what happens to their bodies. That right implies that such decisions as whether to use life-sustaining treatment should, in the final analysis, be theirs. This right is often referred to as the patient's right to self-determination or autonomy. *Autonomy* means that a decision about treatment options requires a choice by the patient who has decision-making capacity. Contemporary nursing strongly affirms the patient's right to self-determination in relation to treatment decisions. These decisions should not occur in isolation but within the context of a collaborative relationship between the patient and members of the health care team.

When patients lack capacity to choose for themselves, someone else must represent their particular values and preferences. Generally family members act as surrogates unless the individual or the court has previously designated someone else.[23,24] The surrogate seeks to make choices based on the patient's previously expressed directives, knowledge of his or her unique preferences and values, or as a reasonable person in the patient's circumstances would.[23] The surrogate acts on the patient's behalf to intepret the treatment options that will advance the patient's interests, goals, and preferences. Likewise a framework based on collaboration and shared decisions can be extended to surrogates who make decisions on behalf of their loved ones.[24]

In the critical care environment, however, members of the health care team may extend their concern for protecting the patient from difficult decisions, future guilt, and remorse by acting paternalistically. In this case we may feel obliged to decide *for* the patient instead of *with* the patient. In this situation the premises from which the framework for shared decision making is derived are violated. The scale for decision making is tipped in favor of the preferences of the professional, not of the patient. There may be instances in which paternalism is justified, but such occasions are limited. Critical care professionals must be sensitive to such risks. Instead of adopting a professionally dominated, unilateral, paternalistic approach, they should seek to safeguard and uphold the spirit of shared decision making.

Beneficence and Nonmaleficence

Another important element in shared decision making is the principle of beneficence and its corollary, nonmaleficence. Patient well-being is of prime importance when determining the appropriateness of certain treatments. This principle means that patient benefit outweighs patient burden. The obligation to promote good for the patient is basic to the relationship between health care professionals and patients and is affirmed by the ANA *Code for Nurses.*[2]

Each individual, including health care professionals, evaluates differently the benefits and burdens of

a treatment and the life it offers. Consequently, the obligation to promote a patient's good involves identifying the benefits and burdens of the treatment from that patient's perspective. Once the preferences and values of the patient are known, the question becomes: Do the burdens of the treatment outweigh the associated benefits *from the patient's perspective*? If the answer is yes, it is ethically acceptable to withhold or withdraw the treatment.

Alternatively, if the treatment provides more benefits than burdens from the patient's perspective, treatment should be provided. In the critical care setting there is often significant uncertainty about the potential benefits and burdens associated with treatments. Generally, when it is unclear whether the benefits or burdens are greater, it is appropriate to err on the side of life and provide the treatment until there is compelling evidence to the contrary. It is helpful to look for ways to maximize certainty by acquiring additional information or assessing the preferences of the patient and the meaning assigned to different burdens. Health care professionals must be careful not to hide behind uncertainty as a rationalization for excessive treatment.

Sanctity of Human Life

One of the foremost values in society and in the health care arena is sanctity of human life. This moral value places the burden of proof on those who would shorten life or fail to forestall death. Regard for this principle guards against the erosion of respect for life in our society and helps to protect the interests of vulnerable populations. Still, it is only a presumption and one of many values that must be weighed in analyzing what is in the best interest of the patient. This value should not be viewed as an imperative that precludes reasoned deliberation and decision making. Consideration must be given not only to how long a life lasts but to how a life gets lived. Medicine and nursing are concerned primarily with enhancing, or at least not diminishing, the quality of people's lives. Medicine can prolong life, but never indefinitely; it mainly affects the comfort or ease with which a life is lived.

Justice

The principle of justice pertains to an individual patient's access to an adequate level of health care and to the distribution of available health care resources. The *Code for Nurses* focuses on the delivery of care with respect for human dignity, which is not to be defined in terms of personal attributes, socioeconomic status, or the nature of an illness. The implications of this position for critical care nurses are profound. This provision requires that a criterion

must be identified to act in the patient's behalf. Many states have statutory provisions that delineate strategies for identifying a surrogate decision-maker. Generally, a family member is most familiar with the patient's preferences and most concerned about the patient's welfare. The nurse should encourage family involvement in identifying the individual who can advocate the patient's interests.

Ideally, the surrogate decision-maker is familiar with the patient's wishes and can use this knowledge to determine how the patient would have reacted to the situation. If, however, the patient's goals, beliefs, and preferences are not known, the surrogate decision-maker relies on the best interest standard to guide decision making. Applying this standard, the surrogate decision-maker bases the choice of treatment on what would be in the patient's best interest. In other words, the surrogate weighs the benefits and burdens of each proposed treatment and chooses a course that protects the patient's welfare.[24]

Neither the best interest standard nor the doctrine of substituted judgment are problem free, and the most reliable evidence is obtained directly from the patient. Therefore, the nurse has a responsibility to initiate early and open discussions about personal choices and preferences surrounding treatment and end-of-life care. Because these discussions often evoke strong emotions, the subject is often avoided. Evading this clinical encounter does not serve the patient's interests and impedes the decision-making process when the patient loses capacity.

Living wills and other oral and written statements are not absolute. They are considered as evidence of patient preferences and should be evaluated within the context of good decision making. As with any situation, unless the professional can produce compelling evidence contrary to the expressed preferences of the patient, the nurse's obligation is to generally support the patient's decision. If there are compelling reasons to disregard the expressed preferences of the patient or surrogate, professionals should seek proper institutional review and in some cases judicial review and notify the individual or surrogate of the rationale for not following the directive.

Informed Consent

The requirement for consent is often perplexing because of the rapidly changing condition of the patient, the need for invasive therapies, the emotional distress experienced by patients, and families' lack of time to deliberate over treatment options.

To achieve informed consent in the legal sense several requirements must be met: (1) information relevant to the decision must be disclosed, (2) consent must be given voluntarily without duress or fraud,

and (3) the patient or designated surrogate must have the legal capacity to make the decision. In other words, the patient has sufficient and accurate information to make an informed choice and is free of undue influence (internal or external) in making or acting upon that choice. To have legal capacity, the patient or designated surrogate must be of an age legally authorized to give consent *and* must not have been determined by a court to lack mental capacity for making decisions about medical care.

These legal principles are based on an ethical concern for autonomy. To many, informed consent is merely a formality whereby relevant information is disclosed by the physician and either oral or written authorization by the patient or legal surrogate is obtained and witnessed. However, Faden and Beauchamp suggest that a more stringent standard is morally required; such a standard emphasizes assuring that the decision-maker has an *understanding* of what is at stake without subtle or overt coercion, manipulation, or undue persuasion.[28] In this case the professional must take steps to assist the decision-maker to fully appreciate the scope of the decision, treatment options, and possible alternatives; confirm the decision-maker's understanding; and consciously seek to reduce subtle or overt manipulation of vulnerable decision-makers.[28] Nurses and physicians should therefore be mindful of the potential obstacles to informed consent. They should strive to maintain the highest ethical standards despite the ease with which patients or their surrogates may defer to the professional's judgment during a life-threatening situation. Moreover, such an approach shifts the focus of the endeavor from the completion of a form to the process whereby true consent occurs.

To be fully informed, patients must receive information which is accurate, sufficient, and comprehensible. *Accuracy* is interpreted to mean *complete*, without deception, and within the limits of what is currently known or believed to be true. The *gray areas* of scientific knowledge should be labeled as such, and *opinion*, even informed opinion, should be openly acknowledged. Patients or their surrogates should be told of the uncertainties surrounding certain treatments and informed when poorly tested treatments or those of marginal benefit are being considered. Accuracy encompasses a complete range of treatment options, including no treatment, and disclosure of the risks and benefits of each option.

There are two standards by which one can measure the sufficiency of information. The first standard is the profession-oriented position, which defines sufficiency in terms of what the *professional* feels the patient should know. As patient-oriented professionals, however, nurses reject this position in favor of one that defines sufficiency from the patient's point of view.[29] The law also requires a patient-oriented measure of sufficiency.

The second standard of sufficiency requires that the patient or surrogate be given all the material information a *reasonable person* would need to know to make a decision under similar circumstances.[24] The materiality standard is viewed, at law, as an objective test that is evaluated after the fact by a judge or jury. To meet the materiality standard, the professional must consider what a reasonable person with characteristics of this particular patient would want and need to know to choose among the available treatment options. Thus, the patient or surrogate must be given all the material information made necessary by the patient's life situation or personal attributes such as gender, age, or occupationally related data. Additionally, information known to be of importance to the patient, even if it is not of statistical significance to the case, should also be disclosed. For instance, a patient who is a Jehovah's Witness should be told if a blood transfusion may be necessary during a surgical procedure.

When professionals must consider the informational needs of those who may seem less advantaged, as in the case of poor, elderly, or retarded persons, it is common to conclude that less information is desired or needed. Both ethics and law would caution against such a conclusion. The more invasive or risky the procedure, or the more affecting the consequences, the more important it is to consult with others who can inform the professional of factors that may be important in decisions made by a patient possessing certain characteristics.

For a patient to be informed, he or she must comprehend the information. Information is comprehensible when it is conveyed in the language of the patient. The language of the patient may be aural or visual, English or another language, formal or colloquial, medically technical or simple, or any combination of these characteristics. The vehicle used, such as one-to-one discussion, film, booklet, or group education, should be one customarily employed by the patient when seeking counsel or advice.[30]

When the patient is fully informed but the pressure of the situation (whether personal or professional pressure) weighs heavily upon decision making, consent may not be considered freely given, though in some instances it may be regarded as implied. *Implied consent* is based on the actions of the individual patient. For example, an individual who voluntarily submits to a routine medical examination is implying consent for routine treatment. However, consent is implied only if the individual has some understanding of the treatment and the risks associated with the

procedure. Implied consent should not be presumed if the procedure or treatment is complex and the individual is unlikely to understand its potential risks or consequences. Therefore, the complexity of procedures and treatments in critical care units precludes implied consent.[31] Consent that is freely given has not been swayed by habit, impulse, irrationality, coercion, duress, fraud, deceit, or undue influence. It is not uncommon that the very mission of the critical care unit leads patients and professionals alike toward preordained decisions, making consent a foregone conclusion. Thus, the critical care environment may itself be a strong deterrent to free consent. In the critical care setting, there may be instances in which the boundaries between experimental and standard medical treatment become blurred. Misconceptions of this kind create inconsistent expectations regarding the rigor of the consent process and add to ethical unrest. Nurses must continually analyze the clinical and scientific data themselves and initiate open and ongoing discussions with members of the health care team to clarify misconceptions and establish consistent standards for obtaining consent.

Two approaches to consent in critical care merit attention here. With the first approach, consent to all ordinary care within the unit is implied by the patient's presence. That is, a reasonable person is admitted to the critical care unit to receive all the benefits the unit can offer, and there is no need to obtain consent for procedures performed within the unit unless the procedure is experimental or otherwise out of the ordinary. In contrast, if consideration is given to withholding all or most medical treatment or to writing a "do not resuscitate" decision, then the patient may also reasonably be considered for transfer from the unit since the patient's condition cannot benefit from critical care interventions.

With the second approach, the patient's presence in the critical care unit is determined more by technology or convenience, and the patient's consent must be constantly reevaluated with the help of surrogate decision-makers, if necessary. In this approach, decisions to withhold treatment, especially selected treatments, may or may not be accompanied by decisions to transfer the patient from the unit. Transfer decisions may be made on the basis of factors such as cost reimbursement, physician preference, or bed space in the general nursing units. Such an approach is consistent with the model of shared decision making that undergirds the moral framework for making decisions.

Concern about costly, nonconsensual treatment of disproportionate benefit to the patient has been increasing. Demands by patients or surrogates for marginally beneficial or futile treatments are also of concern. It is possible that legally and perhaps ethically, consent in critical care will move toward a combination of the two approaches. Justification and implementation of such changes, however, must include opportunities for ongoing ethical and legal debate and dialogue among health care providers and consumers of critical care interventions.

The issue of coercion, while important, is less a concern in critical care than is the patient's ability to make a reasoned choice when burdened by biologic disequilibrium. Can the patient whose electrolytes are askew, whose body is wreaked with pain, whose mentation is clouded by drugs truly give free consent? Our inclination is to say no, but maybe is the better answer. Pain, drugs, or physiological imbalance do not automatically preclude a patient from making a free decision. When the patient's capacity to participate in decisions is intermittent or limited by biological disequilibrium, critical care nurses should attempt to restore capacity by correcting or minimizing the effects of such factors, for example, by relieving pain, correcting metabolic abnormalities, or allowing for uninterrupted rest. Knowledge of the patient and a thorough assessment are keys to evaluating such factors. Thus, informed consent moves full circle. The professional must know the patient to know if consent is freely given.

No discussion of informed consent is complete without discussion of who is legally accountable for informing the patient or surrogate about proposed medical or nursing interventions. The general rule in law is that the professional selecting the treatment option or intervention is the one who supplies the information and is accountable for accuracy, sufficiency, and comprehensibility of the information. If a physician attempts to inform a patient about nursing intervention options, the physician is accountable for knowing the current standards of nursing practice, the research findings, and the risks and benefits of each option. Similarly, nurses are held accountable for information possessed by the treating physician if the nurse takes on the duty of informing the patient about medical treatment options. It is consistent with respect for human dignity for nurses to insist upon the patient's right to receive information from the person who has control over the treatment option and access to the most complete information about that option. The responsibility for obtaining consent generally rests with the physician. However, nurses have an important responsibility to ensure that the consent process is carried out appropriately.

Some centers use standardized consent protocols to ensure that all pertinent points are covered during the consent process. These practices help to assure that during a crisis situation the physician obtaining consent does not omit important points. However, such protocols should not replace efforts to ensure adequate understanding and communication. During the consent process it is essential that patients or their surrogates be allowed and assisted to discuss their values and concerns and to inquire about potential risks and burdens that they consider meaningful. The critical care nurse may be involved in assuring that adequate information is provided, responding to questions raised by patients or surrogates, and gathering evidence of proper informed consent such as witnessing a signature or verifying oral consent over the telephone. Nurses must be mindful that patients or their surrogates may withdraw their consent at any time. If such expressions are made, immediate action must be taken to convey the information to other members of the health care team.

Confidentiality and Privacy

It is not unusual for certain members of our society to be particularly vulnerable to breaches of confidentiality. Victims of sexual assault, patients with AIDS, and women seeking abortions frequently have confidential information disclosed in a careless or casual manner. Inadvertent disclosure of personal information may result in psychological or physical harm to the patient. The patient's medical record as well as all conversations with the patient should be treated as confidential.

The concept of confidentiality is fundamental to the moral integrity of the nursing profession. *Confidentiality* refers to the nondisclosure of information received from a patient. *Privacy* refers to a right to be left alone, a right, in a sense, to have secrets.[32] In health care, privacy incorporates the right to control who can invade one's body and to expose oneself even to medically prescribed display. The right to privacy includes the right to decide to withhold or discontinue life-sustaining measures. The nurse–patient relationship is based on mutual respect and trust. The *Code for Nurses* outlines the nurse's responsibility to protect the patient's confidentiality and privacy.[2] The ethical standard of confidentiality obliges health care professionals to refrain from disclosing information of a private, personal nature without the expressed consent of the patient. Neither marital, family, nor significant other relationships alone overcome the confidential nature of medical information. Thus, nurses are legally constrained in their communication with obviously intimate family or friends of the patient. The nurse can advance the patient's interests by openly discussing the limits of confidentiality with the patient and disclosing only the minimum amount of information necessary. Administrators and health care providers should develop policies that protect patients' interests and require health care professionals to report any unauthorized disclosure of information received in confidence.[31]

Moral Values

The values that underlie the concept of confidentiality and privacy include fidelity, respect for persons, and nonmaleficence. *Fidelity* refers to faithfulness in relationships and to keeping promises. The nurse–patient relationship is based on mutual respect, trust, and loyalty. Patients expect nurses to treat sensitive information confidentially, and when this trust is broken the relationship is also broken. Moreover, patients may be harmed by inappropriate disclosure of medical or social information. Adherence to the concepts of confidentiality and privacy is strongly upheld in the *Code for Nurses*.[2]

In some situations, the duty to protect confidential information may conflict with the duty to disclose information. Child abuse, for example, must be disclosed according to state statutes. Such disclosures are not considered unauthorized, and clinicians are protected by law when reporting this information. When confidential information must be reported or potential harm to a third party may be prevented by disclosure, the nurse encourages the patient to disclose the information directly.

END-OF-LIFE DECISIONS

The Nurse's Role

Cases involving the continuation or withdrawal of life-sustaining treatments are frequently encountered in the critical care setting. Caring for patients at this time in their lives raises unique ethical questions and poses a challenge for critical care nurses. A nurse's professional duty to benefit patients and promote life often conflicts with responsibilities to prevent and remove harm. Although the issues are complex, the critical care nurse is often the pivotal person to facilitate decision making and support the patient and family during this difficult process.

Nurses as members of the health care team and as patient advocates have an important role in resolving end-of-life issues. The nurse participates in determining when withholding or withdrawing certain treatments is appropriate for the patient. Because of the unique relationship between nurses and their patients, nurses are often in an ideal situation to express patient preferences and advocate on their behalf with other members of the health care team. Advocacy may also involve assisting patients and their families to interpret and understand information crucial for good decision making and to articulate their values and preferences. In addition, nurses often help implement a decision to forego certain treatments. Great emotional intensity surrounds decisions to withhold or withdraw treatments. Nurses who participate in such decisions need an atmosphere of mutual support when terminating treatments. Nurses must collaborate with all participants to create an environment where optimal communication, deliberation, and decision making can occur.

Discussions about foregoing life-sustaining treatment often begin with the issue of cardiopulmonary resuscitation (CPR). In many institutions, CPR is treated as an entitlement of all patients, without regard for appropriateness in specific situations. When discussions arise about withholding CPR and writing "do not resuscitate" (DNR) decisions, families may feel the health care team is "giving up" on their loved one. Instead, the suitability of CPR and the probable unsuccessful outcome of this intervention should be explained to the family. An emphasis on comfort and care will alleviate the family's feelings of abandonment.

Institutions should have policies describing documentation of discussions surrounding the issue of DNR. A DNR decision should be clearly written by the attending physician and should be reviewed routinely, particularly when changes in the patient's condition occur. *Slow codes*, *chemical codes*, and other variations of DNR decisions often reflect inadequate or incomplete discussions with the family or patient, and further exploration into treatment decisions is imperative.

Court decisions have affirmed that the paramount value is to be placed on the patient's expressed desire regarding life-sustaining treatment and that it is of great importance to provide comfort measures when all medical intervention is discontinued.[33] The *Code* underscores this point in its statement that:

> The measures nurses take to care for the dying client and the client's family emphasize human contact . . . they enable the client to live with as much physical, emotional, and spiritual comfort as possible, and they maximize the values the client has treasured.[2]

The values a patient has affirmed in life may include such values as what has been called "dying with dignity," which may involve deciding to forego life-sustaining treatment.

The President's Commission has made it clear that, in its estimation, patients have a moral and a legal right to refuse either the initiation or continuation of life-sustaining treatment. The Commission writes:

> Neither criminal nor civil law—if properly interpreted and applied . . . forces patients to undergo procedures that will increase their suffering when they wish to avoid this by forgoing life sustaining treatment.[24]

Failure to respect the competent patient's desire to

have life-sustaining treatment withheld or withdrawn may result in liability for unconsented touching of the patient (battery), invasion of privacy, and/or failure to meet the standard of reasonably prudent, competent nursing practice (negligence). State statutes and regulations should be consulted to determine whether the legislature or licensing agency has client advocacy as a criterion for competent nursing practice and whether state statutes specifically address such issues (see Appendix 2D).

Traditional Distinctions Surrounding End-of-life Care

Ordinary versus Extraordinary

Traditionally, treatments were required if they were considered ordinary and were not obligatory if they were extraordinary. Ordinary treatments were usual, widely available, and not burdensome. Extraordinary treatments were burdensome, expensive, unusual, and often invasive. This distinction has blurred over the years, and what was once considered extraordinary, such as hemodialysis or mechanical ventilation, is now thought of as ordinary. Decisions to withhold or withdraw treatments should not be argued on such tenuous grounds.

Withholding versus Withdrawing Therapies

Cases involving questions of forgoing treatment often include some element of discomfort with withdrawing therapies that have already been started or with not beginning additional therapies. The literature of bioethics contains a great deal of debate about the distinction between withdrawing and withholding a therapy. Generally, it is agreed that any justification for initiating a treatment is also valid justification for withdrawing a treatment,[34] that is, the continued provision of a therapy or the initiation of a particular therapy will not benefit the patient, or would be disproportionately burdensome, or both. This position is upheld in AACN's position statement on withholding or withdrawing life-sustaining treatment (see Appendix 2E).[5] This distinction is, however, sometimes confusing in the clinical setting. Great significance may be associated with withdrawing certain therapies, thus creating a great deal of emotional and ethical turmoil.

Despite consensus among philosophers and legal scholars, clinicians find that emotionally there is a great difference between stopping and not starting a therapy. Often professionals will comment that once a therapy has been initiated, it is unethical to stop it. Their discomfort may be fueled by the direct relationship between their actions and an often dramatic change in the patient's condition. For example, when the ventilator is removed from a patient with end stage COPD, the consequences of respiratory collapse and death occur quickly. In contrast, if that same patient develops *Candida* sepsis and antifungal agents are not provided, the decline in condition is less dramatic. Slow deterioration rather than an immediate death may occur. In both cases the outcome is the same, only the timing and circumstances of death have been altered. If a systematic and fully reasoned decision-making process is followed, with clear identification of patient goals, this distinction becomes clearer.

For many, it is the discomfort associated with their role in orchestrating death or changing the dying trajectory that makes them uneasy about foregoing treatment. Health care professionals use very powerful tools to treat disease and prevent death, and they take seriously the power society has entrusted in them. Although such a responsibility is great, health care professionals must not fall prey to being moral cowards when the burdens of treatment clearly outweigh the benefits for the patient. Health care professionals are equally as responsible for prolonging suffering as they are for failing to intervene.

Balancing Benefits and Burdens

Patient well-being is of prime importance when determining the appropriateness of certain treatments. Will a given life-sustaining treatment promote the patient's good? Answering this question in the critical care setting is often difficult because a number of competing interests clash. A conflict of values between the patient, family, and health care team members may occur, or the patient's goals may conflict with technological capabilities or research goals. Competing economic interests may also be present. Nurses and other health care providers must remember that technology can sustain life but there must be a net benefit to the patient. Health care professionals are *not* obligated to use a technology just because it is available. They must take responsibility not only for using technology but for using it responsibly, by considering the harms and burdens associated with its use from the patient's perspective.

Moreover, extending life is usually but not always good. Some argue that biological existence is necessary for other interests to be advanced and that therefore life must be prolonged whenever possible. However, a patient's life may be full of pain or suffering, and the patient may prefer to forego the treatment even though it may shorten life. Affirming the patient's worth does not mean that it is acceptable to treat a patient beyond the limits of his or her wishes, or beyond the point of benefit; to do so is a violation of a traditional moral norm of nursing. Ethically, to go beyond these limits constitutes *vitalism*: the preservation of human biological life at any cost simply because it is human biological life. Vitalism is morally unacceptable in nursing because it is perceived as a violation of the dignity of the individual, or more succinctly, as harm.[35] In settings where an all-out effort is made to sustain life, professionals must not be swept along by their own capabilities into vitalism.

Nurses who may be party to doing more harm than good by using life-sustaining technologies struggle with the ambiguity of these decisions. Even though nurses generally do not have the central decision-making responsibility for an action, each nurse must individually evaluate the situation to assess the net benefit and degree of harm that may occur. The nurse must then weigh important moral values, evaluate possible course of action, and recognize the moral significance of his or her actions.[36] Moreover, nurses must communicate their views and concerns and assume an active role in the decision-making process.

Foregoing Artificially Provided Hydration and Nutrition

Decisions to forego artificially provided nutrition and hydration are particularly troubling to nurses. Providing nourishment to vulnerable individuals is inextricably tied to expressions of care and compassion. It is often troubling to nurses to withdraw a technology that is seen as basic and esssential. Critical care nurses view artificial feeding as a simple technology, barely invasive, and more beneficial than burdensome to most patients. Nevertheless, artificially provided nutrition and hydration may provide no benefit to the patient and, in fact, may be harmful.[37] Aspiration pneumonia, infections, pulmonary edema, mental confusion, and nausea are several complications of artificially provided nutrition and hydration. Moreover, the extension of a terminal process may prolong suffering and impede a dignified death.

Although considerable debate surrounds the provision of artificial hydration and nutrition, some professionals view these measures as medical therapies that can be withheld or withdrawn. As such, they should be instituted or foregone according to a reasoned process of deliberation about the benefits and burdens to the patient. As with all other interventions, the expected benefits should outweigh the accompanying burdens. Nurses are justified in honoring the preferences of competent patients and following the written directives of previously competent patients regarding the provision of hydration and nutrition. (See Appendix 2F.) Such action is supported by the *Code for Nurses*, the nurse's role as patient advocate, and the ethical principle of respect for persons.

Futility

Generally, the concept of *futility* refers to an intervention that does not benefit the patient, one that will not achieve the intended result. If a treatment achieves no physiological or psychological benefit to the patient, there is no obligation to provide it. However, there is considerable debate in the literature and among clinicians about the definition of futility. Like many other terms used in clinical practice such as DNR, futility is liberally interpreted and conveys a variety of subtle differences.

Some authors have suggested that distinguishing an effect from a benefit will aid in our understanding of the term.[38,39] Many interventions can produce an *effect* on the patient's anatomy, physiology, or chemistry without a *benefit* to the patient. In contrast, a benefit can be understood as an improvement of the patient's prognosis, or as the maintenance or enhancement of the patient's comfort, well-being, or general state of health.[38] As Youngner suggests, we often understand benefit in terms of a treatment's physiological effect. However, if such an intervention is not placed in the context of the patient's overall condition and goals, it may be effective but of no benefit to the patient: it will not alter the natural course of the patient's disease or enhance the quality of his or her existence in a meaningful way.[39] Still, defining the threshold for a futile or useless treatment remains difficult. Are there legitimate criteria for defining effectiveness?

The way in which one defines futility is necessarily subjective. To address this concern, some authors suggest using a probability calculation of benefit based on an individual or collective experience with similar cases.[38] Experienced clinicians often rely on empirical data regarding the probable success of a given intervention or treatment protocol. Although absolute precision in such predictions is impossible, educated predictions about the efficacy of certain treatments can often be made. From this vantage point, futile treatments are those that will not accomplish the intended physiological result.[38]

Difficulties with such an approach occur. What is the threshold for making such distinctions? Is this case significantly similar to other cases? Does the concept of futility apply if the proposed treatments are not useless but have low efficacy? Individual answers will differ. Probability assessments are not neutral. Statistical misinterpretations occur. The methods may be used inappropriately to attach numbers to intuitive feelings. Clearly, a decision to count a therapy as futile will be shaped by the decision-maker's views of human nature and scientific data, as well as by moral convictions. It seems too simplistic to assume that the problem can be solved by scientific data alone. We must recognize the limitations of any quantitative measure of probable outcome such as a severity of illness scoring system. Although useful in some situations, a statistical regression model that accounts for the full range of variables that influence outcome has yet to be developed.

Others suggest that determining futility should involve the patient's unique determination of benefit and burden by incorporating human factors other than hard data into the equation.[40] Such distinctions allow consideration of the unique meaning a patient attaches to his or her present and future life and that individual's unique interpretation of which benefits are meaningful. Such qualitative dimensions of futility can be measured according to whether the patient will survive in a state that has sufficient quality of life to permit a claim that the treatment will benefit the patient. Knowing the patient's values and preferences helps caregivers determine whether this particular therapy will contribute to the shared goals for the patient.

A problem with the qualitative approach is the lack of mechanisms for determining the standards and processes for making judgments. Qualitative distinctions depend on some kind of social consensus about acceptable quality of life or fair allocation of health care resources. Some have interpreted the whole futility debate as a question of resource allocation and cost/benefit analysis. Such concerns raise questions about whether it is always necessary to use every available technology to treat every patient who needs or wants it. What is the proper end of our care: should it always be to extend life for as long as possible or should it be to achieve some measure of meaningful life, however defined? Moreover, such discussions often raise questions about who should determine futility, the patient or the physician and health care team? May patients demand futile treatments or should patients merely be notified by their physicians that a treatment will not be provided? At present there is no consensus about the scope of respect that is required to maintain a model of shared decision making when questions of futility arise.

Defining futility, like defining other dimensions of care, is inexact. It can create conflict for both patients and caregivers, particularly when treatment goals are unclear. Critical care professionals should actively engage in an ongoing dialogue about the definition of futility and its proper role in determining the scope of care to be provided.

Euthanasia

Currently, in the United States the issue of euthanasia concerns allowing patients to die, for example, by foregoing life-sustaining treatment rather than actively bringing death about, as by lethal injection. Intentionally terminating the life of another for compassionate reasons is referred to as *active euthanasia*, or *"mercy killing."* Proponents of active euthanasia argue that individuals should not be sentenced to lives of irreversible and intolerable suffering, and that it is sometimes more benevolent and humane to help suffering persons die.

Opponents of euthanasia argue that unbearable suffering would not occur if pain-relieving medications and procedures were used adequately.[41] Some opponents argue that, although active euthanasia may not be intrinsically wrong, the risks of abuse outweigh the potential value. Many persons believe that harm will come to vulnerable individuals, such as the physically disabled or mentally impaired, if euthanasia is legalized.[42] Physicians and nurses are also concerned that if euthanasia is legalized, patients will become distrustful of health professionals and relationships between health professionals and patients will deteriorate.

Arguments against active euthanasia are rooted in the principle of *nonmaleficence*. The professional codes of both medicine and nursing forbid killing and regard active euthanasia as incompatible with the values and goals of the professions.[43] Society permits health professionals to treat severe pain at the end of life with amounts of medication that may depress respiration and hasten death. However, the consequence of death is unintended, and nurses have a moral duty to alleviate pain. The fact that death is a foreseeable consequence, albeit an unintended consequence, does not equate to active euthanasia. (See Appendix 2G.)

JUSTICE AND ALLOCATION OF RESOURCES

Issues involving the distribution of health care resources arise at two levels. The macroallocation level involves the share of societal resources allocated to specific societal goods. Within health care, the term *macroallocation* refers to the division of a resource such as money among several services such as transplantation programs, critical care, or outpatient services.[34,43]

The term *microallocation* is applied to the individual level and decisions that determine the distribution of a specific resource. Critical care nurses participate in microallocation decisions when determining which patient needs the greatest amount of nursing care. Microallocation issues arise because resources are limited and all who are in need therefore cannot receive given resources.

The ethical principles of beneficence and justice are central to issues of resource allocation and rationing. The principle of *beneficence* requires the nurse to help others and to promote good. This principle may be realized on two levels: the patient level and the societal level.[34] Each perspective advocates a different view concerning the allocation of limited resources.

On the patient level, the nurse fulfills the duty of beneficence by allocating resources on the basis of individual patient needs. Therefore, scarce resources are distributed to those with immediate needs and without regard to the needs of potential patients or the community at large.

Realizing beneficence at the societal level involves allocating resources on the basis of the needs of society and considering the greatest good for the entire community. The focus shifts from crisis care and doing good for the individual patient to preventive care and actions that benefit society.

At the bedside, the critical care nurse often makes allocation decisions based on duty to the individual patient. Until a more comprehensive plan to distribute scarce health care resources in the United States is developed, patient-centered beneficence will control the direction of health care allocation.

When applied to allocation issues, the principle of justice preserves fairness and equality. Resources must be distributed in a manner which promotes public good and acknowledges that each individual has an equal opportunity to achieve health. The principle of justice is fundamental to issues of equal access and a decent minimum of health care.[34,43] The just distribution of critical care goods and services is a particularly thorny ethical issue. A variety of principles have been proposed for the just distribution of resources, including (1) fairness, (2) greatest need, (3) probability of benefit, and (4) ability to pay.[34]

Many believe that justice is best explicated in terms of fairness.[34] The principle of justice as fairness requires some kind of equal opportunity or access to a good or service. A broader view of fairness requires equal access to some basic level of care by all.[34] It is argued that health care is a basic good because good health provides the opportunity for other goods to be pursued, and the relief of pain, suffering, and disability is valuable in itself.[24] But providing equal access to everyone is expensive. Human needs are limitless, even though resources are never unlimited and society as well as individuals must always make choices about how to allocate resources. Therefore, dollars spent on expensive critical care interventions are not available to provide a basic level of care to greater numbers of individuals. The question is raised whether certain interventions provide enough benefit to warrant consideration as a basic form of care. If so, equal access to them by all persons who could potentially benefit from them is required despite the high costs.

As with other scarce resources, providing critical care interventions to all who may benefit may be impractical and prohibitive because of cost. Society may decide that providing certain critical care services as a basic minimum standard of care is too expensive because more basic care would have to be foregone. This view may lead some to question whether such interventions should be offered to anyone since it is impossible to provide the service to all.

Alternatively, to maximize use of limited resources society may decide that certain critical care technologies should be restricted but not eliminated. Even though the technology does offer substantial benefit to some, and the research itself is a valuable step toward future benefits, if such technologies are to be provided to some but not all, fair methods of distributing them among eligible persons must be devised.

Currently, the allocation of critical care services is based on a determination of greatest need and an assessment of the probability of a positive outcome. In the future, as the demand for critical care services increases and availability remains limited, pressure will increase to use criteria like quality of life and social worth. Society must confront the tension between allocation schemes and concerns about discrimination on the basis of disability.

If full equality in the allocation of critical care services is to be achieved, each eligible patient would have to have a fair chance of receiving treatment regardless of geographic location. Realistically, some critical care services cannot be provided in every locale. However, regional access may be regarded as the minimum standard to assure equal access. When resources are scarce and outcomes involve life or death, some method of ordering based on randomization, lottery, or queueing is often imposed.[34] At the individual level this means that critical services may be allocated on a first-come, first-served basis that allows all candidates who reach a critical care center to have equal access to the therapy.

ETHICAL ISSUES IN PROFESSIONAL PRACTICE
Confronting Unsafe Practice

Nurses working in critical care settings may identify situations in which the competence, skill, and propriety of decisions and actions of others may be called into question. Unsafe practices may be caused by incompetence, complacency, laziness, lack of informed consent, human error, lack of current knowledge or skill, emotional distress, stress, physical illness, or substance abuse.[21] When such instances are identified, nurses often struggle to respond in an ethically justifiable manner.

The ANA *Code for Nurses* addresses the nurse's professional responsibility to confront unsafe practice: "The nurse acts to safeguard the client and public when health care and safety are affected by incompetent, unethical, or illegal practice by any person." The interpretive statements explain further that "as an advocate for the client, the nurse must be alert to and take appropriate action regarding any instances of incompetent, unethical or illegal practice by any member of the health care team or the health care system, or any action on the part of others that places the rights or best interests of the client in jeopardy."[2]

In addition to ethical standards, state and federal laws mandate that nurses and other health care professionals report incompetent practice. Generally, regulations governing nursing practice require that all violations of the state's nurse practice act be reported to the appropriate authorities. Failure to report incompetent practice may be considered professional misconduct, leading to disciplinary action by the licensing board. Despite mandatory reporting laws in some states, there is wide variation among states in addressing such instances and in the effectiveness of reporting mechanisms.[21]

Hospitals are also responsible for reporting unsafe practice. Regulations issued by regulatory or accrediting agencies, such as the Joint Commission on Accreditation of Healthcare Organizations (JCAHO), mandate that hospitals be accountable for maintaining various professionals including nurses.[44] Evidence of the institution's compliance with such standards is generally defined in written policies and procedures related to professional conduct and practice. High-risk occurences, for example, may be documented by incident reports or memoranda of concern. Hospital policies must also include mechanisms for investigating infractions and define a disciplinary procedure when allegations of incompetent or unsafe practice are substantiated.[21]

Allowing unsafe situations to proceed does not relieve the nurse of the moral obligation to report unsafe practices. In fact, nurses are actually cooperating or acting as accomplices in the situation if they fail to report it. For example, a nurse identifies that a drug dosage is beyond the level recommended for patient safety and brings it to the attention of the prescribing physician. The physician responds by stating that he or she is aware of recommendations but wants this dose to be given immediately. Even if the nurse refrains from performing an unsafe or unethical practice, his or her conscience may not be relieved if another is allowed to carry it out. The ANA *Code* clearly states that "neither physician's orders nor the employing agency's policies relieve the nurse of accountability for actions taken and judgments made."[2] Hence, despite a nurse's values and the fears of retaliation, reprisal, or ostracism, there is a clear duty to act.

When nurses identify instances of unsafe practice, the nursing environment must be such that it supports nurses who respond to their ethical duty, and there must be institutional mechanisms or processes for handling ethical and legal concerns. Any mechanism must be safe, effective, and expeditious. It is demoralizing to attempt to right a grievous or persistent wrong to a patient, only to face a cumbersome or obstructive process that impedes moral action. Ideally, in addition to standard reporting procedures, emergency procedures should also be in place for addressing situations in which the nurse believes that patient welfare is in imminent jeopardy. The process should also include a mechanism for giving feedback about the progress and resolution of the investigation.

It is prudent to implement strategies to facilitate a fair and systematic investigation of the problem. A plan should be developed to safeguard patient well-being while the allegations are being investigated. Throughout an investigation of possible unsafe practices, confidentiality must be strictly maintained for the protection of all parties involved. Allegations of unsafe practice have the potential to damage reputations and careers and must be approached with utmost care. Before making such allegations, nurses should systematically examine the situation to determine whether reporting is warranted. Levine-Ariff and Groh suggest a process and key questions for assessing a potentially unsafe practice.[21]

1. *Verify the facts.* Before allegations of unsafe practice are made, the facts surrounding the incident should be independently verified. Verify your perceptions and information by going directly to the individuals involved. Avoid heresay and unsubstantiated opinions held by others. Recognize that individuals' perceptions can quickly be regarded as fact when passed on in reports or through conversations. Make sure that your discomfort is not a result of your own lack of knowledge or experience.

2. *Fully assess the situation.* Key questions to consider include:
   - Is the practice truly incompetent, illegal, or unethical, or is it a practice with which you do not agree? For example, there are many techniques for performing certain procedures. Use of an alternative technique is not necessarily an unsafe practice.
   - Would an uninvolved panel of experts view the practice as acceptable? Is this something that any other prudent practitioner would do under similar circumstances? Is it within the scope of the "community standard of practice"?
   - Has a patient or other person been harmed? Or does the potential for harm exist? Patient safety and well-being is of primary concern. If patients are in actual or potential danger, the nurse must

act immediately to protect their welfare. The amount of harm to the patient is the primary consideration regardless of the degree of competency, intentions, or uncaring attitude of the practitioner.[45]

- What degree of harm has been caused? The greater the harms, the greater the nurse's obligation to intervene to protect the patient.
- If the outcome had been different, would the conduct seem acceptable? Sometimes there are situations when the outcome is unfavorable regardless of the skill or competency of the professionals involved. Determine whether you are reacting to a practice that, although it might be considered unorthodox, is not unsafe, and that if the outcome had been favorable, would be lauded as innovative.[21]
- Is this a pattern of behavior or an isolated incident? For example, individuals with substance abuse problems often begin to demonstrate a pattern of behaviors that result in multiple errors. Each individual behavior may not seem significant, but the behaviors taken collectively can indicate a serious problem. Perhaps the problem has been identified, but the person is unwilling or unable to face the problem and seek treatment.[21]

3. *Determine the level of risk to the nurse.* A nurse must also determine risks associated with different courses of action, including personal, professional, moral, legal, and social ramifications. After examining these risks, a nurse must determine how much risk he or she should endure on behalf of patients or groups of patients. A nurse may face great risks in reporting unsafe practice. Although nurses are not obligated to undertake more than their fair share of risks and sacrifices, determining a fair level of risk is difficult. Nurses must recognize that each individual will establish his or her own threshold for acceptable risks and sacrifices and, therefore, there may be considerable variation among individual nurses.[45]

After considering these issues and deciding a practice is unsafe and the level of risk to the nurse is reasonable, the nurse must develop a plan of action. Generally, a nurse should make the concerns known to those involved in the questionable practice. If the response is unsatisfactory, the nurse must bring the issue to the attention of the management and follow institutional guidelines and policies for reporting such occurrences. Each institution should have policies and procedures that define expectations about professional behavior and patient care. Procedures must delineate the organizational channels to be used to resolve conflict, report unsafe practices, and challenge

decisions made by others. In addition, each institution should have standards of care that define the minimum level of care that every patient should always receive. Mechanisms for monitoring the extent of compliance to these standards should be established, including quality assurance and nursing representation on hospital and medical staff committees.[21]

Reporting outside the institution should be a rare occurrence. Such reporting should be considered only after all other avenues have been exhausted. If, however, there is no solution within the organization, a nurse may consider going outside the organization to report unsafe practices. Reporting outside the institution often involves state licensing boards or agencies that conduct periodic inspections of institutions. Before deciding to "blow the whistle," nurses should carefully assess the internal and external environment, clarify personal values, consider personal and professional consequences, clarify moral issues, determine the legal issues, and realistically determine the chance for success.[21]

Regardless of a nurse's conviction that instances of unsafe practice should be reported, doing so ultimately requires courage and a supportive environment. Nurses should collaborate with administrators and colleagues to develop a system that minimizes the occurrence of unsafe practices and includes appropriate polices and procedures, standards of care, and continuing education about reporting unsafe practices. In addition, support systems such as employee assistance programs that provide confidential counseling and referral services must be developed.[21]

CREATING AN ENVIRONMENT FOR OPTIMAL DECISION MAKING

If nurses are to act ethically, they must practice in an environment that fosters and supports open communication, tolerates diversity, and promotes optimal decision making through reasoned analysis and deliberation. Nurses must be involved in all levels of decision making. A collaborative nurse–physician relationship enhances communication and provides avenues for clarifying patient goals and treatment plans, and for resolving conflicts when they occur. Support systems that include ongoing professional education, values clarification, psychosocial counseling, clearly defined institutional policies, and mechanisms for dispute resolution are essential ingredients of such an environment. Moreover, critical care nurses must also be familiar with professional standards, institutional and external resources, legal and public policy guidelines in their state, and current ethical thinking regarding the issues they face.

Open, ongoing communication among all members of the team is crucial for optimal functioning.

Periodic team meetings or patient care conferences to clarify patient and therapeutic goals, discuss ethical concerns, and develop plans of care are advantageous. Such meetings can also be useful before initiating innovative treatments for patients whose clinical course is unusual or complex. The indications for the therapy can be clarified, the potential benefits and burdens for a patient assessed, and the criteria for continuing or discontinuing the therapy defined. Often these cases generate much distress when treatment goals are unclear and health care professionals differ in their perceptions of benefit to the patient. Potential conflict should be recognized and addressed by ongoing evaluation and discussion of the patient's progress.[46]

Nurses must collaborate with other health care providers and leaders to create an environment conducive to the examination and discussion of ethical questions. Multidisciplinary ethics rounds can provide an important forum for analyzing and deliberating about the ethical dimensions of individual cases, prospectively or retrospectively. Moral discourse is a valuable way to identify and clarify where the points of moral disagreement reside.

A process for resolving ethical disputes including review by institutional ethics committees is a valuable safeguard. Ideally, institutional ethics committees should be multidisciplinary and should include nurses who provide direct patient care and nurses who assume other roles. Such inclusion will represent the unique ethical obligations of nurses and provide them with opportunities for advocacy on behalf of their patients. When moral disagreements occur, efforts must be made to obtain the most current factual information regarding the points of controversy. Participants should agree on a common framework to guide discussion, develop a common understanding of the language used for concepts or definitions, and engage in a balanced discussion of different viewpoints.[34]

In addition, it is essential that institutions have in place policies that address processes for diagnosing death by neurological criteria (brain death); requesting and donating organs and tissues; foregoing treatment, including resuscitation and artificial hydration and nutrition; assessing patients' decision-making capacity; designating surrogates; and executing advance directives. It is also advantageous to develop professional safeguards that define the scope of professional responsibility to participate in ethically unsatisfactory situations, mechanisms to transfer care to another equally qualified nurse, and mechanisms for judicial review when appropriate. Nurses must also participate on institutional review boards (IRBs) to review research proposals and to evaluate the impact of new technologies on nursing practice.[46]

Nurses must be familiar with state statutes governing nursing practice and patient care. In general, it is customary to find that law and ethics are mutually supportive.[47] In some uncommon instances, however, the demands of ethics exceed and conflict with the demands of the law. In such cases, the nurse must choose whether to violate legal or ethical precepts. Such decisions are not easily made. When a nurse chooses in favor of ethical obligation over the obligation of the law, it should be done from an informed position. That is, the consequences of such an action should be known before the decision is made.

REFERENCES

1. Donahue, M. P. (1985). *Nursing: The finest art*. St. Louis: Mosby–Year Book.
2. American Nurses' Association. (1985). *Code for nurses with interpretive statements*. Kansas City, MO: The Association.
3. Benner, P. (1984). *From novice to expert: Excellence and power in clinical nursing practice*. Menlo Park, CA: Addison-Wesley.
4. American Association of Critical-Care Nurses. (1989). *The role of the critical care nurse as patient advocate*. Aliso Viejo, CA: AACN.
5. American Association of Critical-Care Nurses. (1990). *Withholding and/or withdrawing treatment*. Aliso Viejo, CA: AACN.
6. Aroskar, M. A. (1980). Anatomy of an ethical dilemma: The practice. *American Journal of Nursing, 80,* 661-663.
7. Curtin, L. (1978). A proposed model for critical ethical analysis. *Nursing Forum, 17,* 12-17.
8. Murphy, M. B., & Murphy, J. (1976). Making ethical decisions systematically. *Nursing 76, 6,* 13-15.
9. Uustal, D. (1985). *Values and ethics in nursing: From theory to practice*. East Greenwich, RI: Educational Resources in Nursing and Wholistic Health.
10. Klein, J. T. (1991). Transforming ethical theory. *APA Newsletter on Feminism and Philosophy, 90*(2), 92-96.
11. Sichel, B. A. (1991). Different strains and strands: Feminist contributions to ethical theory. *APA Newsletter on Feminism and Philosophy, 90*(2), 86-92.
12. Carse, A. (1991). The voice of care: Implications for bioethical education. *Journal of Medicine and Philosophy, 16,* 5-28.
13. Smith, C. (1979). A decade of patient advocacy. *Heart Lung, 8,* 926-928.
14. Curtin, L. (1986). The nurse as advocate: a philosophical foundation for nursing. In P. I. Chinn (Ed.), *Ethical issues in nursing* (pp. 11-20). Rockville, MD: Aspen.
15. Winslow, G. (1984). From loyalty to advocacy: A new metaphor for nursing. *Hastings Center Report, 14,* 32-40.

16. Gadow, S. (1980). Existential advocacy: philosophical foundations of nursing. In S. Spicker, & S. Gadow (Eds.), *Nursing images and ideals: Opening dialogue with the humanities.* New York: Springer.

17. Murphy, C. P. (1983). Models of the nurse–patient relationship. In C. P. Murphy, & H. Hunter (Eds.), *Ethical problems in the nurse–patient relationship.* Boston: Allyn & Bacon.

18. Fowler, M. D. (1989). Social advocacy. *Heart Lung, 18,* 97-99.

19. Wilkinson, J. M. (1987/88). Moral distress in nursing practice: experience and effect. *Nursing Forum, 23*(1), 16-29.

20. Rushton, C. H. (1992). Caregiver suffering in critical care nursing. *Heart Lung, 21,* 303-306.

21. Levine-Ariff, J., & Groh, D. (1990). *Creating an ethical environment.* Baltimore: Williams & Wilkins.

22. American Nurses' Association. (1986). *Statement regarding risk versus responsibility in providing nursing care.* Kansas City, MO: ANA.

23. The Hastings Center. (1987). *Guidelines on the termination of life-sustaining treatment and the care of the dying.* Bloomington: Indiana University Press.

24. President's Commission for the Study of Ethical Problems in Medicine and Biomedical and Behavioral Research. (1983). *Deciding to forego life-sustaining treatment.* Washington, DC: U.S. Government Printing Office.

25. Grodin, M., & Burton, L. A. (1988). Context and process in medical ethics: The contribution of family-systems theory. *Family Systems Medicine, 6,* 435.

26. Doukas, D. J., & McCullough, L. B. (1991). The values history: The evaluation of patient's values and advance directives. *Journal of Family Practice, 32,* 145-153.

27. Patient Self Determination Act of 1990, P.L. 101-508 (1990).

28. Faden, R. R., & Beauchamp, T. L. (1986). *A history and theory of informed consent.* New York: Oxford University Press.

29. American Nurses' Association. (1980). *Nursing: A social policy statement.* Kansas City, MO: ANA.

30. Fowler, M. D. (1986). T'aint cricket: ethical comments on patient informedness. *Heart Lung, 15,* 414-415.

31. White, M. L. (1991). Confidentiality and privacy. In J. C. Fletcher (Ed.), *Introduction to clinical ethics and health care law.* Charlottesville, VA: The Center for Biomedical Ethics.

32. Oran, D. (1975). *Law Dictionary for non-lawyers.* St. Paul, MN: West Publishing.

33. *Barber v. Superior Court,* Cal App. 3d, 1985.

34. Beauchamp, T. L., & Childress, J. F. (1989). *Principles of biomedical ethics* (3rd ed.). New York: Oxford University Press.

35. McCormick, R. A. (1974). To save or let die: The dilemma of modern medicine. *JAMA, 229,* 172-176.

36. Davis, A. J. (1987). The boundaries of intervention: issues in the noninfliction of harm. In M. D. Fowler, & J. Levine-Ariff, (Eds.), *Ethics at the bedside.* Philadelphia: Lippincott.

37. Lynn, J., & Childress, J. F. (1983). Must patients always be given food and water? *Hastings Center Report, 13,* 17-21.

38. Schneiderman, L. J., Jecker, N. S., & Jonsen, A. R. (1990). Medical futility: Its meaning and ethical implications. *Annals of Internal Medicine, 112,* 949-954.

39. Youngner, S. (1988). Who defines futility? *JAMA, 260,* 2094-2095.

40. Lantos, J. D., Singer, P. A., Walker, R. M., et al. (1989). The illusion of futility in clinical practice. *American Journal of Medicine, 87,* 81-84.

41. Fowler, M. D. (1988). On killing patients. *Heart Lung, 17,* 322-323.

42. Seigler, M. *Washington Post,* October 4, 1988.

43. Reigle, J. (1989). Resource allocation issues in critical care nursing. *Nursing Clinics of North America, 24,* 1009-1015.

44. Joint Commission on Accreditation of Healthcare Organizations. (1992). *Accreditation manual for hospitals.* Oakbrook Terrace, IL: JCAHO.

45. Jameton, A. (1984). *Nursing practice: The ethical issues.* Englewood Cliffs, NJ: Prentice-Hall.

46. Rushton, C. H. (1988). Ethical decision making in critical care: Part 2. Strategies for nurse preparation. *Pediatric Nursing, 14,* 497-501.

47. Fowler, M. D., & Chaney, E. A. (1983). Ethics and law in nursing: Reconcilable differences. Unpublished manuscript.

2-A

American Nurses' Association Code for Nurses

PREAMBLE

The Code for Nurses is based on belief about the nature of individuals, nursing, health, and society. Recipients and providers of nursing services are viewed as individuals and groups who possess basic rights and responsibilities, and whose values and circumstances command respect at all times. Nursing encompasses the promotion and restoration of health, the prevention of illness, and the alleviation of suffering. The statements of the Code and their interpretation provide guidance for conduct and relationships in carrying out nursing responsibilities consistent with the ethical obligations of the profession and quality in nursing care.

CODE FOR NURSES

1. The nurse provides services with respect for human dignity and the uniqueness of the client unrestricted by consideration of social or economic status, personal attributes, or the nature of health problems.
2. The nurse safeguards the client's right to privacy by judiciously protecting information of a confidential nature.
3. The nurse acts to safeguard the client and the public when health care and safety are affected by the incompetent, unethical, or illegal practice of any person.
4. The nurse assumes responsibility and accountability for individual nursing judgments and action.
5. The nurse maintains competence in nursing.
6. The nurse exercises informed judgment and uses individual competence and qualifications as criteria in seeking consultation, accepting responsibilities, and delegating nursing activities to others.
7. The nurse participates in activities that contribute to the ongoing development of the profession's body of knowledge.
8. The nurse participates in the profession's efforts to implement and improve standards of nursing.
9. The nurse participates in the profession's efforts to establish and maintain conditions of employment conducive to high-quality nursing care.
10. The nurse participates in the profession's effort to protect the public from misinformation and misrepresentation and to maintain the integrity of nursing.
11. The nurse collaborates with members of the health professions and other citizens in promoting community and national efforts to meet the health needs of the public.

From American Nurses' Association. (1985). *Code for nurses with interpretive statements.* Kansas City, MO: ANA.

$$\boxed{\textbf{2-B}}$$

Role of the Critical Care Nurse as Patient Advocate

THE AMERICAN ASSOCIATION of Critical-Care Nurses believes that patient advocacy is an integral component of critical care nursing practice. Therefore, definitions of advocacy and the behaviors that typify advocacy are essential.

WHEREAS, the *Code for Nurses* (American Nurses' Association, 1985) requires that nurses safeguard the patient and the public when health care and safety are affected by the incompetent, unethical, or illegal practice of any person, and

WHEREAS, many definitions of advocacy exist, and

WHEREAS, critical care nurses are confronted with situations that require them to act immediately on the patient's behalf, and

WHEREAS, personal and professional risks are associated with being a patient advocate, and

WHEREAS, state nurse practice acts may require the nurse to be a patient advocate, and

WHEREAS, the process of informed consent mandates that the patient or the patient's surrogate be informed fully and give consent freely, and

WHEREAS, the continuum of advocacy is not limited to the individual but may extend to societal concerns,

THEREFORE, BE IT RESOLVED THAT the American Association of Critical-Care Nurses believes the critical care nurse is a patient advocate,

AND THAT the American Association of Critical-Care Nurses defines advocacy as respecting and supporting the basic values, rights, and beliefs of the critically ill patient.

BE IT FURTHER RESOLVED THAT the American Association of Critical-Care Nurses believes that as a patient advocate, the critical care nurse shall do the following:

1. Respect and support the right of the patient or the patient's designated surrogate to autonomous informed decision making.
2. Intervene when the best interest of the patient is in question.
3. Help the patient obtain necessary care.
4. Respect the values, beliefs, and rights of the patient.
5. Provide education and support to help the patient or the patient's designated surrogate make decisions.
6. Represent the patient in accordance with the patient's choices.
7. Support the decisions of the patient or the patient's designated surrogate or transfer care to an equally qualified critical care nurse.
8. Intercede for patients who cannot speak for themselves in situations that require immediate action.
9. Monitor and safeguard the quality of care the patient receives.
10. Act as liaison between the patient, the patient's family, and health care professionals.

BE IT RESOLVED THAT the American Association of Critical-Care Nurses recognizes that health care institutions are instrumental in providing an environment in which patient advocacy is expected and supported.

ALSO, BE IT FURTHER RESOLVED THAT as patient advocate, critical care nurses initiate and promote actions to improve the health care of the critically ill through social change.

REFERENCE

American Nurses' Association. (1985). *Code for nurses with interpretive statements.* Kansas City, MO: Author.

From American Association of Critical-Care Nurses. (1989). *Position statement: Role of the critical care nurse as patient advocate.* Aliso Viejo, CA: AACN.

2-C

American Nurses' Association Position Statement on Nursing and the Patient Self-Determination Act

Summary: The American Nurses' Association (ANA) believes that nurses should play a primary role in implementation of the Patient Self-Determination Act, passed as part of the Omnibus Budget Reconciliation Act of 1990. It is the responsibility of nurses to facilitate informed decision-making for patients making choices about end-of-life care. The nurse's role in education, research, patient care and advocacy is critical to implementation of the Patient Self-Determination Act within all health care settings.

The Patient Self-Determination Act, passed as part of the Omnibus Budget Reconciliation Act of 1990, becomes effective December 1, 1991. The federal law applies to all health care institutions receiving Medicare or Medicaid funds and requires that all individuals receiving medical care must be given written information about their rights under state law to make decisions about medical care, including the right to accept or refuse medical or surgical treatment. Individuals must also be given information about their rights to formulate advance directives such as living wills and durable powers of attorney for health care. Patients must be made aware of their rights to make decisions about these issues upon admission (in the case of hospitals or skilled nursing facilities), enrollment (in the case of health maintenance organizations), on first receipt of care (in the case of hospices) or before the patient comes under an agency's care (in the case of home health personal care agencies).

ANA supports the patient's right to self-determination and believes that nurses will and must play a primary role in implementation of the law. Ideally, decisions about advance directives should be made by the patient with the family and the primary care provider prior to admission. The formation of advance directives is an important decision and will inevitably involve nurses who are the most omnipresent professionals in health care facilities. It is imperative that the decision making that will fall to patients and their families as they make choices about end-of-life care be facilitated by nurses.

- Each nurse should know the laws of the state in which she/he is practicing pertaining to advance directives, and should be familiar with the strengths and limitations of the various forms of advance directive.
- The nurse is one of several health care professionals who has a responsibility for ensuring that the advance care directives initiated by the patient are current and reflective of the patient's choices. Facilitating self-determination of patients with respect to end-of-life decisions is a process that includes evaluating changes in the patient's perspective and health state.
- The nurse has a responsibility to facilitate informed decision making, including but not limited to advance directives.
- ANA recommends that these questions about advance directives be part of the nursing admission assessment: Do you have basic information about advance care directives including living wills and durable power of attorney? Do you wish to initiate an advance care directive? If you have already prepared an advance care directive, can you provide it now? Have you discussed your end-of-life choices with your family and/or designated surrogate and health care team workers?
- The role of the nurse is critical in implementation of the Patient Self-Determination Act and includes public education, research, patient care, advocacy, education of the profession and inservice education of other health care providers.

From American Nurses' Association. (1991). *Position statement on nursing and the patient self-determination act.* Kansas City, MO: ANA.

INTERPRETIVE STATEMENT
WHAT'S AN ADVANCE MEDICAL DIRECTIVE?

Advance medical directives are of two types: treatment directives, often referred to as "living wills," and appointment directives, often referred to as "power of attorney" or "health proxies."

A LIVING WILL—states what medical treatment you choose to omit or refuse in the event that you are unable to make those decisions yourself and are terminally ill.

A DURABLE POWER OF ATTORNEY FOR HEALTH CARE—appoints a proxy - usually a relative or trusted friend to make medical decisions on your behalf if you can no longer decide for yourself. It has broader applications than a living will and can apply to any illness or injury that could leave you incapacitated.

An advance directive does not need to be written, reviewed or signed by an attorney. It must be witnessed by two people (in many states witnesses may not be your heirs, relatives or physicians).

An advance directive applies only if you are unable to make you own decisions because you are incapacitated or if, in the opinion of two physicians, you are otherwise unable to make decisions for yourself. It can be changed or canceled at any time.

An advance directive is intended to help others make decisions for you. It may be as simple or as complex as you feel necessary. For example, a simple statement indicating that in the case of an incurable illness or catastrophic injury you do not wish to be kept alive by artificial means such as CPR, artifical respiration or tube-feeding is an advance directive.

A copy of the advance directive should be given to your family, physician and anyone you designate as a proxy. In addition, you should bring a copy of it with you if you are admitted to a hospital or nursing home.

The Patient Self-Determination Act (PSDA), effective December 1, 1991, **does not require** patients to have or fill out an advance directive. It does require hospitals and other health care organizations to tell patients that they have the right to do so in accordance with existing state law. PSDA is not applicable in federal facilities such as Veteran's Administration Hospitals that do not receive Medicare or Medicaid funds.

Additional Resources

National

Choice in Dying
250 West 57th St.
New York, NY 10107
212/246-6973

Alzheimers Association
70 East Lake St., Suite 600
Chicago, IL 60601
1-800-621-0379

AARP Legal Counsel for the Elderly
1909 K St., NW
Washington, DC 20049
202/833-6720

Association for Death Education & Counseling
638 Prospect Ave.
Hartford, CT 06105
203/232-4825

American Bar Association
1800 M St., NW, South Lobby
Washington, DC 20036
202/331-2200

Children of Aging Parents
2761 Trenton Rd.
Levittown, PA 19056
215/945-6900

State Resources

Information and advice regarding the law in your state may be obtained from the following:
State Department of Health
State Office on Aging
State or Regional Hospital Association
State Bar Association
University Centers on Aging

Effective Date: November 18, 1991
Status: New position statement
Originated by: Task Force on End-of-Life Decisions
Adopted by: ANA Board of Directors
Related Past Action: 1. Code for Nurses with Interpretive Statements, 1985
                         2. Guidelines on Withdrawing or Withholding Food and Fluid, 1988

$$\boxed{\textbf{2-D}}$$

American Nurses' Association Position Statement on Nursing Care and Do-Not-Resuscitate Decisions

Summary: Nurses bear a large responsibility at the time a patient experiences cardiac arrest for either initiating resuscitation or ensuring that unwanted attempts to resuscitate do not occur. Nurses face ethical dilemmas concerning confusing or conflicting DNR orders and this statement includes specific recommendations for the resolution of some of these dilemmas.

Although cardiopulmonary resuscitation has been used effectively since the 1960s (Kouwenhoven et al., 1960), the widespread use and possible overuse of this technique and the presumption that it should be used on all patients has been a subject of recent debate (U.S. Congress, 1987). The ways in which do-not-resuscitate (DNR) decisions are made and implemented continues to be a source of confusion and contention in the delivery of nursing care (Stenberg, 1988; MacIntosh, 1989). Practices regarding DNR decision-making and record-keeping vary from one health care institution to the next (Lo, 1991). There is a range of thinking about the nurse's participation in DNR decision-making. At some hospitals, the DNR policies actually indicate that the nurse is not to inquire about or initiate any discussion regarding extraordinary procedures with the patient; as this is perceived as the sole responsibility of the physician. Others have argued that nurses have a central role in DNR decision-making and have the competence and relevant authority to write DNR orders (Yarling, McElmurray, 1983).

Nurses are actively involved in the decision-making about resuscitation and bear a large responsibility at the time a patient experiences cardiac arrest for either initiating resuscitation or ensuring that unwanted attempts to resuscitate do not occur (Stenberg, 1988). Nurses commonly face the following types of dilemmas concerning confusing or conflicting DNR orders:

1. Interpreting DNR orders especially in circumstances in which a "no code" order has been qualified as in "chemical code only," "or resuscitate but do not intubate" etc.;
2. Interpreting DNR orders in which there is some attempt to demonstrate or mimic a response, perhaps for the benefit of family members, that stops short of a full resuscitation effort as in "slow code" or "show code";
3. DNR orders that are not accompanied by progress notes in the medical record indicating how the decision was made;
4. DNR orders that accompany patients from one facility to another with no periodic review or conversely DNR orders that are time-limited and therefore not in effect when a patient transfers from one facility to another;
5. Concerns about stigmatizing patients with DNR orders through the use of special symbols on armbands, etc.; and
6. Concerns about abandonment of other types of needed care for patients who are designated as DNR.

In view of the confusion and complexity that continue to surround DNR decisions and their implementation, ANA makes the following recommendations:

1. The choices and values of the competent patient should always be given highest priority, even when these wishes conflict with those of health care providers and families;
2. In the case of the incompetent or never competent patient, any existing advance directives or the decisions of surrogate decision-makers acting in the patient's best interest should be determinative;

From American Nurses' Association. (1992). *Position statement on nursing care and do-not-resuscitate decisions.* Washington, DC: ANA.

3. The DNR decision should always be a subject of explicit discussion among the patient, the family (one or more significant others as identified by the patient), any designated surrogate decision maker acting in the patient's best interest and the health care team and include consideration of the efficacy and desirability of CPR, a balancing of benefits and burdens to patients and therapeutic goals;

4. Nurses need to be aware of and have an active role in developing DNR policies within the institutions where they work;

5. DNR orders must be clearly documented, reviewed and updated periodically to reflect changes in the patient's condition (JCAHO, 1992);

6. A DNR order is separate from other aspects of a patient's care and there should be no implied or actual abandonment of other types of care for patients with DNR orders, which should continue to be evaluated on a burdens versus benefits basis;

7. Nurses have a duty to educate patients and their families about all types of termination of treatment decisions and should encourage patients and their families to think about these decisions before admission to health care facilities;

8. Nurses have a responsibility to educate patients and their families about various forms of advance directives such as living wills, durable power of attorney, etc. (Omnibus, 1990);

9. There should be clear mechanisms in place within each health care facility (preferably, the use of an interdisciplinary ethics committee with nurse members) for the resolution of disputes among health care professionals or among patients, families and health care professionals concerning DNR orders, and

10. If it is the nurse's personal belief that her moral integrity is compromised by her professional responsibility to carry out a particular DNR order, she should transfer the responsibility for the patient's care to another nurse.

The appropriate use of DNR orders can prevent suffering for many patients who choose not to extend their lives after experiencing cardiac arrest. As the primary continuous health care provider in health care facilities, the nurse must be involved in the planning as well as the implementation of resuscitation decisions. Clear DNR policies at the institutional level which include the basic features that ANA recommends, will enable nurses to effectively participate in this crucial aspect of patient care.

REFERENCES

American Nurses' Association, *Code for Nurses with Interpretive Statements,* Kansas City, Missouri: ANA, 1985.

Council on Ethical and Judicial Affairs, American Medical Association, "Guidelines for the Appropriate Use of Do-Not-Resuscitate Orders," *Journal of the American Medical Association,* April 10, 1991, Vol. 266, No. 14, pp. 1868-1871.

The Hastings Center, *Guidelines on the Termination of Life-Sustaining Treatment and the Care of the Dying,* New York: The Hastings Center, 1987.

Joint Commission on the Accreditation of Healthcare Organizations, "Nursing Care Standards," *Accreditation Manual for Hospitals,* Oak Bluffs Terrace, Illinois: 1992.

Kouwenhoven, WB; Jude, JR, Knickerbocker, GG, "Closed-chest cardiac massage," *JAMA,* 1960, 179:84-97.

Lo, Bernard, "Unanswered Questions About DNR Orders," (editorial), *Journal of the American Medical Association,* April 10, 1991, Vol. 265, No. 14, pp. 1874-1876.

MacIntosh, Janice. "Ethics and an ethical dilemma: to resuscitate or not." *Canadian Critical Care Nursing Journal,* 1989 Mar/Apr 6(1):20-22.

Miles, S.H.; Moldow, D.G., "Hospital Policies on Limiting Medical Treatment," *Archives of Internal Medicine* 144:1841-1843, 1984.

Mozdzierz, G.J.; Schlesinger, S.E., "Do-Not-Resuscitate Policies in Midwest Hospitals: A Five-State Survey," *Health Services Research* 20:949-960, 1986.

Omnibus Budget Reconciliation Act of 1990, Public Law 101-508, sec. 4207 and 4751.

Stenberg, M.J. "The responsible powerless": nurses and decisions about resuscitation, *Journal of Cardiovascular Nursing,* 1988 Nov; 3(1):47-56.

U.S. Congress, Office of Technology Assessment, *Institutional Protocols for Decisions About Life-Sustaining Treatments*, Special Report OTA-BA-389 (Washington, DC: U.S. Government Printing Office, July 1988).

U.S. Congress, Office of Technology Assessment, *Life-Sustaining Technologies and the Elderly*, OTA-BA-306 (Washington, DC: U.S. Government Printing Office, July 1987).

Yarling, R; McElmurray, B. "Nurses' Role in DNR Orders: A Clinical Policy Proposal in Nursing Ethics," *Advances in Nursing Science*, 5(4), July 1, 1983, 1-12.

Effective Date: April 2, 1992
Status: New Position Statement
Originated by: Task Force on Nurse's Role in End-of-Life Decisions
Adopted by: ANA Board of Directors, April 2, 1992
Related Past Action: 1. Code for Nurses with Interpretive Statements, 1985

2-E

Withholding and/or Withdrawing Life-Sustaining Treatment

ADVANCES IN HEALTHCARE technology have dramatically increased the ability to prolong life. Because of these advances, ethical and legal dilemmas arise when complex therapy is instituted to sustain vital functions, even when there is no hope of reversing the disease processes.

The American Association of Critical-Care Nurses recognizes that critical care nurses have a significant role in supporting a patient's preferences and beliefs about ending treatments of this type.

THEREFORE, AACN resolves that when choices about withholding and/or withdrawing life-sustaining treatments are being considered, critical care nurses should collaborate with individual patients or their surrogates, phsyicians and other healthcare providers. This should happen in an atmosphere that promotes reasoned deliberation and communication of a patient's preferences and best interests.

To support this resolution, AACN believes that the following elements are essential for nursing practice:
- Critical care nurses will participate in ongoing assessment of a patient's ability to make decisions about their own healthcare.
- Critical care nurses will participate in discussions exploring the patient's beliefs about end-of-life care at the earliest appropriate time. The best time for discussions and decision-making about withholding and/or withdrawal of life-sustaining treatment is before entry into the healthcare system.
- When patients cannot make decisions for themselves, their preferences may be determined from advanced directives (such as living wills or durable power of attorney for health care), previous spoken or written information and personal lifestyle.
- Critical care nurses, as patient advocates, will initiate and promote the decision-making process and assure that nursing care goals are consistent with patient preferences or best interests.
- In the event that life-sustaining treatment is withheld or withdrawn, critical care nurses will participate in planning, implementing, and evaluating supportive care. Supportive care includes providing comfort, hygiene, safe surroundings and emotional support for patients and the family.

Thus, AACN believes that healthcare institutions must have policies that direct a process to withhold and/or withdraw life-sustaining treatment. These policies should include:
- A process for ongoing review of treatment goals and interventions. The scope of the care the patient will receive should be specified in writing.
- A process for designating a surrogate when the patient does not have decision-making capacity.
- A process for dispute resolution among patients, surrogates, and health care team members when there is disagreement about the decision-making process.
- A process for transferring care of a patient to another qualified critical care nurse, when a decision to withhold and/or withdraw life-sustaining treatment conflicts with the nurse's personal beliefs and values.

This position on withholding and/or withdrawing life-sustaining treatment is based on these beliefs and ethical principles:
1. Individuals have a moral and legal right and responsibility to make decisions about their healthcare and the use of life-sustaining treatment.
2. There is no moral or legal difference between withholding and withdrawing treatment. Considerations that justify not initiating treatment also justify withdrawing treatment.
3. A person's capacity to make decisions is shown by their ability to: understand relevant information, reason, and deliberate about choices, reflect on information according to their individual values and preferences, and communicate their decision to healthcare providers.
4. The process for decision-making on behalf of incapacitated patients should be directed by the established standards of substituted judgment or best interests.

From American Association of Critical-Care Nurses. (1990). *Position statement: Withholding or withdrawing life-sustaining treatment.* Laguna Niguel, CA: AACN.

DEFINITIONS

Advance Directives: A document in which a person gives advance directions about medical care or designates who should make medical decisions on their behalf if they should lose decision-making capacity. There are two types of advance directives; treatment directives, such as living wills, and proxy directives, such as durable power of attorney for health care.

Best Interest Standard: This standard gives priority to the protection of the patient's welfare. In these cases the designated surrogate tries to make a choice on the patient's behalf that seeks to implement what is in the patient's best interests by reference to more objective, societally shared criteria.

Substituted Judgment: The doctrine of substituted judgment requires that the surrogate attempt to reach the decision that the incapacitated person would make if he/she were able to choose. This standard preserves the patient's interest in self-determination.

Bibliography

American Association of Critical-Care Nurses (1989). *Role of the critical care nurse as a patient advocate.* Newport Beach, CA: Author.

American Nurses' Association (1985). *Code for nurses with interpretive statements.* Kansas City, MO: Author.

President's Commission for the Study of Ethical Problems in Medicine and Biomedical and Behavioral Research (March 1983). Washington, DC: Government Printing Office.

The Hastings Center (1987). *Guidelines on the termination of life-sustaining treatment and the care of the dying.* Briarcliff Manor, NY: Author.

2-F

American Nurses' Association Position Statement on Foregoing Artificial Nutrition and Hydration

Summary: The American Nurses' Association (ANA) believes that, the decision to withhold artificial nutrition and hydration should be made by the patient or surrogate with the health care team. The nurse continues to provide expert care to patients who are no longer receiving artificial nutrition and hydration.

Food and water, the act of feeding and the act of providing fluids, are concepts and actions closely tied to our basic beliefs regarding care and are fundamentally tied to our membership in the human community. Many of our social encounters, developmental memories, and human interactions center around events involving food and drink. The rich symbolism of feeding is intimately linked to caring, symbolizing compassion, nurturance, and commitment. Caring is a characteristic central to the profession of nursing. A key component of nursing care is the assessment and management of the nutritional needs of patients throughout the lifespan from birth to death.

Artificial nutrition and hydration should be distinguished from the provision of food and water. Food and water provided to patients by mouth is the usual means of providing nurtition to patients. There are, however, situations in which nutrition can only be provided by artificial means. The provision of nourishment and hydration by artificial means (i.e., through tubes inserted into the stomach, intestine, or blood vessel) is qualitatively different from merely assisting with feeding.

- Like all other intervention, artificially provided hydration and nutrition may or may not be justified. It should be instituted or foregone only after a process of reasoned decision making focused upon estimates of benefits and burdens to the patient. For example, a neurological assessment of the patient completed by a physician is an important feature of estimating burdens and benefits. The burdens vary with the particulars of the patient, the substances to be delivered, the mode of delivery, and the anticipated outcome. Ethical difficulties arise when it is unclear whether food and fluid are more beneficial or harmful. Since they are essential for life, this uncertainty leads to questions about whether life, under certain circumstances, might be a greater harm than death. As in all other interventions, the anticipated benefits must outweigh the anticipated burdens for the intervention to be justified.

- Outcomes such as weight gain, increased caloric intake or changes in laboratory test results do not themselves serve as adequate justification for this intervention. Such changes in the absence of any relation to overall well-being of the patient as a person, are not persuasive reasons to begin or continue to provide artificial nutrition or hydration.

Since competent, reflective adults are generally in the best position to evaluate various harms and benefits to themselves in the context of their own values, life projects, and tolerance of pain, their acceptance or refusal of food and fluid should be respected. This ethical judgment is now well established through legal precedent affirming the right of competent patients to refuse treatment, including nutrition and hydration (Nelson, 1986; Grant, Forsythe, 1987; Cruzan, 1990). In cases where a patient is unable to make his wishes known, or is unable to evaluate the benefits and harms of refusing artificial nutrition and hydration, the decision of a surrogate should be relied upon. A surrogate decision maker, preferably designated by the patient, is one who makes decisions in the best interest of the patient and without self interest.

- It is morally, as well as legally, permissible for nurses to honor the refusal of food and fluid by competent patients in their care. *The Code for Nurses with Interpretive Statements,* the historical evolution of nurses' professional responsibilities as patient advocates, and the general moral principle of respect for persons as ends in themselves rather than means, support this view.

From American Nurses' Association. (1992). *Position statement on foregoing artificial nutrition and hydration.* Washington, DC: ANA.

- Dying patients, whether at home or in institutions, typically have a decline in appetite and refuse even their favorite foods. Caretakers unaware of this phenomenon and concerned to maintain "proper nutrition" may need to understand that such a decline is normal and that efforts to ensure "good nutrition" are unnecessary and can be inappropriate (Schmitz, 1991).

- Advance directives such as living wills or the legal assignment of durable power of attorney are indications of choices and values and should be followed. Thus, advance directives, including those involving artificial nutrition and hydration should be followed (Omnibus, 1990).

- In circumstances in which the patient never has been competent (including infants, children, many mentally disabled persons, and the never competent mentally ill), the patient's surrogate in collaboration with the health care team decides whether the provision of artificial nutrition and hydration is in the patient's best interest.

- When artificial nutrition is foregone, the nurse continues to provide high quality care, minimize discomfort, (mouth care, skin care, ice chips) and promote patient dignity. The nurse demonstrates caring by continuing to provide expert care: pain control, skin care, personal hygiene, privacy and compassionate touch.

- The nurse needs to provide support and education to the family members of patients who are no longer receiving nutrition and hydration about the process of dying and provision of comfort measures.

    Health care institutions should have policies that direct a process for decision making regarding foregoing artificial nutrition and hydration.

- Such policies should include a process for the resolution of disputes among patient's surrogates, and health care team members when there is disagreement.

- A process for transferring care of a patient to another qualified nurse, when a decision to forego artificial nutrition and hydration conflicts with the nurse's own personal beliefs and values, should be in place in each institution.

REFERENCES

American Nurses' Association, *Code for Nurses with Interpretive Statements*, Kansas City, Missouri: ANA, 1985.

Brophy v. New England Sinai Hospital Inc., Amicus Curiae Brief, American Academy of Neurology, 1989.

Cruzan v. Director, Missouri Department of Health 58 U.S.L.W. 4916 (25 June 1990).

Grant, E.R. and Forsythe, C., "A Plight of the Last Friend: Legal Issues for Physicians and Nurses in Providing Nutrition and Hydration," *Issues in Law and Medicine*, Vol. 2, No. 4, January, 1987, pp. 279-299.

Nelson, L.J., "The Law, Professional Responsibility and Decisions to Forego Treatment," *Quality Review Bulletin*, Joint Commission on Accreditation of Hospitals, January, 1986.

Omnibus Budget Reconciliation Act of 1990, Public Law 101-508, Sec. 4207 and 4751.

Schmitz, P., "The Process of Dying with and without Feeding and Fluids by Tube," *Law Medicine and Health Care*, Vol. 19:1-2, Spring, Summer, 1991, pp. 23-26.

Additional Reading

Billings, J.B., "Comfort Measures for the Terminally Ill—Is Dehydration Painful?," *Journal of the American Geriatrics Society*, Vo. 33 (11), September, 1985, pp. 808-810.

Carper, B., "The ethics of caring," In P. Chinn (Ed.), *Ethical Issues in Nursing*. Rockville, MD: Aspen Publications, 1986.

Cranford, R.E., "The persistent vegetative state: The medical reality. Getting the facts straight," *Hastings Center Report*, 18 (1), 1988, pp. 27-32.

Gadow, S. "Covenant without cure: Letting go and holding on in chronic illness," in *The Ethics of Care and Ethics of Cure*, In J. Watson and M.A. Ray (eds), New York: National League of Nursing, 1989.

Hastings Center, *Guidelines on the termination of life-sustaining treatment and the care of the dying,* New York: 1987.

Lynn, J. and Childress, J.F., "Must patients always be given food and water?" *Hastings Center Report,* 13 (5), 17-21, 1983.

Miles, S.H. and August, A., "Courts, gender and the right to die," *Law, Medicine and Health Care,* 18 (1-2) 85-95, 1990.

Mumma, C., "Withholding nutrition: A nursing perspective," *Nursing Administration Quarterly,* 10, 31-38, 1986.

Paris, J.J., "When the Burdens of Feeding Outweigh the Benefits," *Hastings Center Report,* 16 (1) 30-32, 1986.

President's Commission for Study of Ethical Problems in Medicine and Biomedical and Behavioral Research, *Deciding to forego life-sustaining treatment: Ethical, medical, and legal issues in treatment decisions,* Washington, DC: U.S. Government Printing Office, March 1983.

U.S. Congress, Office of Technology Assessment, *Life Sustaining Technologies and the Elderly,* Washington, DC: Government Printing Office, 1988.

Wurzbach, M.E., "The dilemma of withholding or withdrawing nutrition," *Image,* 22 (4), 226-230, 1990.

Zerwekh, J.V., "The dehydration question," *Nursing 83,* 13, 47-51, 1983.

Effective Date:	April 2, 1992
Status:	New Position Statement
Originated by:	Task Force on Nurse's Role in End-of-Life Decisions
Adopted by:	ANA Board of Directors, April 2, 1992
Related Past Action:	1. Code for Nurses with Interpretive Statements, 1985
	2. Guidelines on Withdrawing or Withholding Food and Fluid, 1998

$$\boxed{\textbf{2-G}}$$

American Nurses' Association Position Statement on Promotion of Comfort and Relief of Pain in Dying Patients

Summary: Nurses should not hesitate to use full and effective doses of pain medication for the proper management of pain in the dying patient. The increasing titration of medication to achieve adequate symptom control, even at the expense of life, thus hastening death secondarily, is ethically justified.

Nursing has been defined as the diagnosis and treatment of human responses to actual or potential health problems (American Nurses' Association, 1980). When the patient is in the terminal stage of life when cure or prolongation of life in individuals with serious health problems is no longer possible, the focus of nursing is on the individual's response to dying. Diagnosis and treatment then focuses on the promotion of comfort which becomes the primary goal of nursing care.

One of the major concerns of dying patients and their families is the fear of intractable pain during the dying process. Indeed, overwhelming pain can cause sleeplessness, loss of morale, fatigue, irritability, restlessness, withdrawal, and other serious problems for the dying patient (Spross, 1985, Amenta, 1988, Eland, 1989, Melzack, 1990). Nurses play an extremely important role in the assessment of symptoms and the control of pain in dying patients because they often have the most frequent and continuous patient contact. In planning nursing care of dying patients, "the patient has a right to have pain recognized as a problem, and pain relief perceived by the health care team as a need." (Spross, McGuire, Schmitt, 1990).

The assessment and management of pain should be based on a thorough understanding of the individual patient's personality, culture and ethnicity, coping style and emotional, physical and spiritual needs, and on an understanding of the pathophysiology of the disease state (Dalton & Fenerstein, 1988). The main goal of nursing intervention for dying patients should be maximizing comfort through adequate management of pain and discomfort as this is consistent with the expressed desires of the patient. Toward that end, the patient should have whatever medication, in whatever dosage, and by whatever route is needed to control the level of pain as perceived by the patient (Wanzer et al., 1989).

Careful titration of pain medication is essential to promote comfort in dying patients. The proper dose is "the dose that is sufficient to reduce pain and suffering" (Wanzer et al., 1989). Tolerance to pain medications often develops in patients after repeated and prolonged use. Thus, both adults and children may require very high doses of medication to maintain adequate pain control. These doses may exceed the usual recommended dosages of the particular drug for patients of similar age and weight (Eland, 1989, Foley, 1989, Inturrisi, 1989, Schmitt, 1990).

While it is well known that pain medications often have sedative or respiratory depressant side effects, this should not be an overriding consideration in their use for dying patients as long as such use is consistent with the patient's wishes. The increasing titration of medication to achieve adequate symptom control, even at the expense of maintaining life or hastening death secondarily, is ethically justified. The nurse assumes responsibility and accountability for individual nursing judgments and actions (American Nurses' Association, 1985). Nurses should not hesitate to use full and effective doses of pain medication for the proper management of pain in the dying patient.

From American Nurses' Association. (1991). *Position statement on promotion of comfort and relief of pain in dying patients.* Kansas City, MO: ANA.

REFERENCES

Amenta, M., & Bohnet, N.L. (Eds.) (1986). "Palliative care nursing." New York, Little, Brown and Company.

American Nurses' Association (1980). *Nursing: A Social Policy Statement.* Kansas City, MO: the American Nurses' Association.

American Nurses' Association (1985). *Code for Nurses with Interpretive Statements.* Kansas City, MO: the Association.

Dalton, J.A. & Fernerstein, M. (1988). Biobehavioral factors in cancer pain. *Pain,* 33, 137-147.

Eland, J.M. (1989). "Pharmacologic Management of Pain." In B. Martin (Ed.) *Pediatric Hospice Care: What Helps.* Children's Hospital of Los Angeles.

Foley, K. (1989). Controversies in cancer pain: Medical perspectives. *Cancer,* 63 (supplement), 2257-2265.

Inturrisi, C.E. (1989). Management of cancer pain: Pharmacology and principles of management. *Cancer,* 11, 2308-2320.

Melzack, R. (1990). The tragedy of needless pain. *Scientific American,* 262, 27-33.

Schecter, N.L., Altman, A., Weisman, S. (1990). "Report of the Consensus Conference on the Management of Pain in Childhood Cancer." 86(5), 813-834.

Spross, J.A., McGuire, D.B., Schmitt, R.N. (1990). Oncology Nursing Society Position Paper on Cancer Pain, Part 1. *Oncology Nursing Forum,* 17(4), 595-606.

Spross, J.A., McGuire, D.B., Schmitt, R.N. (1990b). Oncology Nursing Society Position Paper on Cancer Pain, Part II., *Oncology Nursing Forum,* 17, 751-760.

Spross, J.A., (1985). Cancer pain and suffering: Clinical lessons from life, literature, and legend, *Oncology Nursing Forum,* 12, 23-31.

Twycross, R.G., & Fairfield, S. (1982). Pain in far-advanced cancer. *Pain,* 14, 303-310.

Wanzer, S.H., et al. (1989). The physician's responsibility toward hopelessly ill patients: A second look. *New England Journal of Medicine,* 320, 884-849.

Bibliography

American Pain Society Subcommittee on Quality Assurance Standards (1990). Standards for Monitoring Quality of Analgesic Treatment of Acute Pain and Cancer Pain. *Oncology Nursing Forum,* 17, 952-954.

Benedict, S. (1989). The Suffering Associated with Lung Cancer. *Cancer Nursing,* 12, 34-40.

Beyer, J.E., & Levin, C.R. (1987). Issues and Advances in Pain Control in Children. *Nursing Clinics of North America,* 22, 661-676.

Eland, J. (1988). Pharmacologic Management of Acute and Chronic Pain. *Issues in Comprehensive Pediatric Nursing,* 11, 93-111.

Fagerhuth, S., & Strauss, A. (1977). *The Politics of Pain Management,* San Francisco, CA: Addison-Wesley Publishing Company.

Foster, R., & Hester, N. (1990). The relationship between pain ratings and pharmacologic interventions for children in pain. In D.C. Tyler & E.J. Krane (Eds.) *Advances in Pain Research and Therapy,* Vol. 15, (pp. 31-36). New York: Raven Press.

Hester, N., Foster, R., & Beyer, J. (1990). Clinical Judgement in Assessing Children's Pain. In Watt-Watson & M. Donovan (Eds.), *Pain Management for Nurses.* Toronto: B.C. Decker.

Jay, S., Elliott, C., & Varni, J. (1986). Acute and Chronic Pain in Adults and Children with Cancer. *Journal of Consulting and Clinical Psychology,* 54, 601-607.

McCaffery, M., & Beebe, A. (1989). *Pain: A Clinical Manual for Nursing Practice.* St. Louis, Mo: The C.B. Mosby Company.

McGuire, D.B., & Harbro, C.H., (Eds). *Cancer Pain Management.* Orlando, FL: Grune & Stratton.

Miser, A., & Miser, S. (1989). The Treatment of Cancer Pain in Children. *Pediatric Clinics of North America,* 36, 979-999.

Miser, A.W. (1990). *Evaluation and Management of Pain in Children with Cancer.* In D.C. Tyler, E.J. Krane (Eds.) *Advances in Pain Research and Therapy: Pediatric Pain.* Vol. 15. NY: Raven Press.

Effective Date:	September 5, 1991
Status:	New position statement
Originated by:	Task Force on the Nurse's Role in End-of-Life Decisions
Adopted by:	ANA Board of Directors
Related Past Action:	1. Code for Nurses with Interpretive Statements, 1985
	2. Position Statement on Nurses' Participation in Capital Punishment, 1988

3

Critical Care Nursing Research

Karin T. Kirchhoff

Critical care nursing has grown substantially since the inception of intensive care units in the late 1960s. The focus of critical care nursing research has broadened from an almost exclusive interest in cardiovascular disease to the psychological and physiological aspects of any critical illness. The purpose of this chapter is to (1) identify the forces that have influenced critical care research in the past and are likely to continue, (2) trace the evolution of critical care research through past research and research summaries, and (3) describe the impact of the American Association of Critical-Care Nurses (AACN) and the National Center for Nursing Research on the evolution of critical care nursing research (both past and present). The future of critical care research is projected. In the past all of these influences have been viewed as separate threads without much interaction. They are now increasingly seen as interrelated, shaping each other synergistically.

FORCES SHAPING CRITICAL CARE RESEARCH

Emphasis on Outcomes

Major national bodies, involved in accreditation of health care facilities, such as the Joint Commission on Accreditation of Healthcare Organizations (JCAHO), and in reimbursement of health care costs, such as Medicare/Medicaid, have recently changed the focus of their evaluation activities from process to outcomes. It is no longer sufficient to provide evidence that the needed resources are available and that the appropriate activities occurred. There is now additional pressure to provide evidence that expected outcomes were achieved. With such a large financial incentive at stake, health care organizations are trying to assure that desired outcomes do indeed occur. In addition, available information about health care facilities includes more than their resources such as number of beds or types of services. The federal government now publishes outcome data such as hospital-specific mortality statistics for Medicare patients. Critical care research will need a greater emphasis on outcomes, and programs of research in hospitals or in critical care will be evaluated in terms of their impact on patient and nursing outcomes.

Health Care Economics

A second dynamic force affecting hospitals is the change in their financial picture. Patients admitted to hospitals have a higher acuity at admission, and more procedures occur on an outpatient basis. While new diseases and new technologies have increased the complexity of patient care, reimbursement for this care has decreased. Hospitals have found themselves in financial difficulty, and the total number of hospitals in the United States has been decreasing, especially in rural areas. The complexion of hospital beds is changing; in the near future, entire hospitals will contain intensive care beds instead of having critically ill patients only in intensive care units. The rising acuity of the critically ill increases the complexity of available research subjects; patients with an uncomplicated first myocardial infarction and no other medical conditions are either not placed in critical care units or are there for a very short time. The human resources needed to conduct such research are now diminished because of increasing demands on the time of personnel.

Nurse Vacancy Rates

The third dynamic force, the nursing shortage, has been continually present but has changed in status and presentation. The situation is viewed as a demand problem, not a supply problem. Most recently, the number of nurses has not dramatically increased, yet the nursing vacancy rates in hospitals have dropped. Vacancy rates are calculated by dividing the number of open full-time equivalents (FTEs) by the number of budgeted FTEs. Consequently the vacancy rate is sensitive to a decrease in budgeted positions, which in turn is affected by the hospital's overall financial status. Some hospitals have not hired additional nurses, and a few have even decreased their rosters. The adjustment in the demand is at least partially explained by the rise in nurses' wages during the shortage. Higher wages have increased total labor costs even as hospitals are facing shortfalls from lower reimbursement. All of these changes will reduce the amount of budgeted indirect time nurses can use to conduct research or to apply research findings.

Federal Funding

Another dynamic force affecting critical care nursing research is the decrease in federal funding available for it. A paradox exists. While federal funding for nursing research was housed within the Division of Nursing, $0.5 million was received in contrast to $5 million appropriated in 1985. In 1986, with the move of federal funding to the National Institutes of Health (NIH), the National Center for Nursing Research (NCNR) had a $19 million budget. In 1991, that budget was $40 million. Meanwhile, the percentage of proposals eventually receiving funding has dropped precipitously. The ratio of the number of funded proposals divided by the number of submitted proposals is called the success rate. In 1987, the success rate of research program grants at NCNR was 30%. In 1991, the average success rate for NIH was 25%; for the NCNR it was 12%. The increase in proposals submitted has been greater than any increase in appropriations to the NCNR.

Bergstrom suggested some alternatives in light of these statistics.[1] She recommended that funding beyond the annual NIH increase is needed to support NCNR. Because of attempts to balance the federal budget and the reluctance to provide dramatic increases in the NIH budget, individual scientists and nursing organizations must seek alternative resources. Bergstrom recommended multidisciplinary research and practice teams to expand options for accomplishing objectives. Also, scientists may need to consider methods for stretching research dollars. The proposed institute status for NCNR may be associated with a better success rate.

In considering sources of funding other than NCNR, the agencies' priorities need to be considered. A new federal agency, the Agency for Health Care Policy and Research (AHCPR), has been developed with three areas of research: (1) medical effectiveness—patient outcome research, (2) database development, and (3) research on dissemination methods. The private foundation funding the most dollars

in health care research is the Robert Wood Johnson Foundation. In its publication, *Advances*, the foundation listed three new priorities: (1) access to care, (2) complex chronic illness across the continuum, and (3) substance abuse. Critical care nurses will need to consider how to compete for these funds.

All of these forces act on the clinical facilities in which critical care research is conducted and upon the resources necessary for conducting clinical research. These forces must be considered in future planning.

HISTORY OF CRITICAL CARE RESEARCH
Reviews of Research

One method of examining past accomplishments in critical care research is to consider a series of summaries of research provided by critical care researchers. In an early review article, Kinney studied the scientific basis for critical care nursing practice from 1972 to 1982.[2] She reviewed *Heart & Lung, Nursing Research*, and the *Proceedings of the National Teaching Institute*, and classified studies by problems of nursing practice (tasks and technology) and modalities of patient care (care and comfort, prevention of trauma, promotion of recovery, health appraisal and education, and coordination of care). She recommended a sustained effort in a topical area, replication of studies, a need for an increase in reliable and valid instruments, and clinical trials.

Lindsey reviewed research for clinical practice from 1970 to 1981 that used physiologic variables.[3] She reviewed *Communicating Nursing Research, Nursing Research, Research in Nursing and Health, Western Journal of Nursing Research, Cancer Research*, and *Heart & Lung*. She classified studies by individual, individual's environment, and clinical nursing therapeutics. She found that very few studies focused on similar phenomena and there was little evidence of confirmation or refutation of findings. Lindsey suggested that students in master's programs should conduct replication studies. She identified shortcomings similar to those found in previous reviews. Additional problems described included the variety of phenomena studied, subjects' having a variety of conditions or being studied at a variety of times in the illness trajectory, and concerns about the differences between clinical significance and statistical significance.

Dracup summarized empirical studies reported between 1975 and 1985.[4] She used computer searches that were augmented by manual searches and indexes and organized the issues by structure of the critical care units, process of nursing and outcomes of critical care, and ethical dilemmas. By using this broader search technique, rather than a review of selected nursing journals, she found that the studies of delivery of nursing care were conducted by researchers from a variety of disciplines. Yet, in some areas, nurse researchers were quite absent, so that the reported studies lacked a nursing perspective. For example, the large body of knowledge on patient outcomes reflected medicine's orientation toward cure. She saw little information about the effect of nursing care in the ICU on patient survival, quality of life, and health maintenance. She found the shortcomings of the studies to be decreasing with more carefully designed studies, multicentered studies, and attention to the reliability and validity of instruments.

Some problems continued. Studies still utilized a single unit, usually the coronary care unit, lacked randomization, and were primarily descriptive. Dracup recommended that future research in critical care use experimental studies to evaluate the effectiveness of nursing interventions on physical and psychological outcomes. She stressed the need for formulation and testing of appropriate theory, and the need for research in ethics.

Keller summarized cardiovascular nursing research from 1969 to 1988 in *Progress in Cardiovascular Nursing.*[5] She critiqued several reviews of cardiovascular nursing research. The first review she considered was written by Foster, Kloner, and Stengrevics, who summarized cardiovascular nursing research by surveying *Nursing Research, Heart & Lung, Patient Counseling and Health Education,* and *Cardiovascular Nursing* from 1970 to 1981.[6] They found only two review articles, one on psychological responses to open heart surgery and one on coronary precautions. They concluded that only a few investigators have followed a single line of inquiry, such as cardiac rehabilitation, suctioning, placement of nitroglycerine ointment, and hemodynamic monitoring. The most frequently studied subjects were patients with myocardial infarction (n = 22), and the most frequently studied topic was nursing procedures (n = 18). These reviewers were concerned because sample sizes were small, studies were descriptive, and no further study was undertaken after the first report. They recommended replication, the continuation of research efforts, the encouragement of research efforts in practice settings, collaboration between clinical and academic nurses in research, and a focus of studies on the most significant nursing problems.

Also summarized by Keller were reports by Kinney, Yarcheski, and Packa and Norris.[5,7,8,9] Kinney summarized the research presented as abstracts at the American Heart Association's Scientific Sessions from 1972 to 1983 and categorized those studies in eight themes.

Yarcheski summarized cardiovascular nursing research published in *Nursing Research, Research in Nursing and Health, Western Journal of Nursing Research,* and *Heart & Lung* from 1960 to 1985. She conceptually categorized the studies within the four characteristics essential to the development of a scientific base for practice: research by members of the discipline, relevance to practice, theoretical basis, and methodologic soundness. She found that in 59 studies there had been a substantial increase in the number of studies reported by nurses, the focus of research had shifted from acute to long-term aspects of patient care, the strategy employed by researchers was a research-then-theory approach, and the methodology employed by nurse researchers had become more complex.

Packa and Norris reviewed the same journals from 1982 to 1985.[9] They concluded that the designs in the reviewed studies were predominantly descriptive and that conceptualization was almost nonexistent in that only three research reports named a conceptual framework.

In addition to examining prior reviews, Keller surveyed several additional journals from 1985 to 1988.[5] She found that the volume of cardiovascular research published from 1985 to 1988 had doubled in comparison to that of the previous four years. Although she found increases in sample sizes, the sampling method was still that of convenience. The methods of design and analysis used reflected increasing complexity. Keller found a relative increase in the use of conceptualization to guide the research compared to that found by Packa and Norris. She categorized the studies around nine themes: health-related behaviors, activity, invasive pressure monitoring techniques, families, patient adherence, patient education, stress, anxiety and coping, and perception of care. In light of the ANA Cabinet of Nursing Research Priorities and those of NCNR, Keller noted that one priority, that of technology dependency and its effect on patients and families, has received little attention despite the need for research.[10]

Cowan reviewed cardiovascular research from 1977 through 1987.[11] She categorized 138 studies into (1) individual adaptation to coronary artery disease, (2) family adaptation to coronary artery disease, (3) environments: supporting and nonsupporting, and (4) clinical therapeutics. She also found that most of the studies were diverse, yielding fragmentary contributions to nursing knowledge. Her recommendations include studies on quality of life, prevention of cardiovascular disease, the interaction of physiological and behavioral responses, and family adaptation to crises of cardiovascular disease.

VanCott and colleagues analyzed critical care nursing practice research published from 1979 to 1988.[12] They reviewed *Heart & Lung* and five general nursing research journals to identify nursing practice research. They found a significant increase in the number of nursing practice research reports published in the second half of the decade as compared to the first half of the decade. More than half of the articles (57%) were intervention oriented.

Historical Documents in Critical Care Research

AACN has produced a number of documents that reflect the importance of research to the organization. In 1984, a document on ethics in critical care research was published. Recognizing that research conducted in critical care units directly or indirectly affects the practice of critical care nursing, the role of the critical care nurse was delineated in this document.[13]

AACN also published *Standards of Nursing Care of the Critically Ill*.[14] Comprehensive Standard IV states: "The plan of nursing care shall be implemented according to the priority of identified problems/needs." The supporting Standard IVd states, "The critical-care nurse shall integrate current scientific knowledge with technical and psychomotor competency." This statement strongly supports the use of research in clinical practice.

The mission statement of AACN in 1981 and reiterated in 1991 lists three values. The second value states: "Research is needed to develop a scientific basis for critical-care nursing practice and to achieve a broad understanding of the role and impact of critical-care nurses on patient outcomes." The updated mission and value statement for 1991-1992 contains this same value.[15]

Outcome Standards for Nursing Care of the Critically Ill includes strong statements about the use of outcome standards by the researcher.[16] Two major uses for the outcome standards are (1) to cite research-based interventions that are appropriate for dissemination and (2) to use and provide direction for the testing of untested interventions: " . . . research is needed that examines changes that occur in patients' health status as a result of nursing action." All of these documents provide evidence of the long-time commitment and support for research in critical care nursing that AACN has evidenced.

AACN's Role

The first Research Committee of AACN was established in the late 1970s. The role of this committee was to begin the major research activities of the organization. Under its guidance, the scientific sessions of the National Teaching Institute (NTI) were initiated; abstracts were solicited, reviewed, and accepted for the NTI. To assist with research utilization this committee either abstracted or compiled abstracts of current research applicable to critical care nursing, leading to several publications.

Concerns about which questions in critical care nursing required the most attention resulted in the development of the Delphi study of priorities in critical care research, later published by Lewandowski and Kositsky.[17] Although some studies have been conducted on these priorities, further research is needed before the findings can be applied to clinical practice. Unless results are similar and confidence can be held across a number of studies, practice should not be changed and more research on the same topic should be encouraged. Funk found 38 studies published on the top 15 priorities when 11 journals were assessed for publications from 1983 through 1987.[18] The number of studies per priority ranged from none to eight. In November 1991, AACN held a consensus conference on research priorities. Using Likert and magnitude estimation scaling, research priorities were set by a panel of 50 expert critical care nurses. Priorities for clinical practice research and research on the context within which critical care nursing takes place can be found in Appendix 3A.

Subsequent research committees undertook the initiation of distinguished research lecturers as an integral part of the NTI, and offered awards for the completion of high-quality studies. The grants program, sponsored by AACN with assistance from corporate sponsors, is noteworthy, especially in light of the proportional decrease in federal funding. The three research grants available are the Critical Care Research Grant (up to $15,000), the Mentorship Grant (up to $5,000), the Translating Research into Practice Grant (up to $6,000), and the Hewlett-Packard/AACN Critical Care Nursing Research Grant ($30,000).

To assess the impact of critical care nursing on patient outcomes, AACN sponsored a demonstration unit at Overlake General Hospital in Seattle, Washington.[19] The NCNR has subsequently funded a larger, multisite replication of the findings from this single demonstration unit.

Another notable effort of AACN was the sponsoring of national study groups. In proposing such an idea the Research Committee wanted to sponsor pilot work on a problem facing critical care nurses that would be studied by several investigators. When the topic of suctioning was selected, the discussion was about the isolated studies done up to that point, the frequency of use of suctioning in all different critical care units, the patient populations and age groups studied thus far, and the potential danger to patients when suctioning is not done correctly. AACN facilitated the first national study group by funding its meetings and awarding pilot money to strengthen the development of subsequent research proposals. This group received $1.5 million to study suctioning, using common outcome measures in different patient populations. These grants ended in Spring 1990, and the researchers presented a symposium of their results at the 1990 National Teaching Institute. Also, three of the members received additional funding through 1994-1995.

A Second National Study Group was formed in the fall of 1990. The focus of this group is patient outcomes in critical care nursing. A Third National Study Group was announced in the spring of 1992 and will address weaning of mechanically ventilated patients.

A large project requiring the cooperation of many critical care nurses was the Thunder Project. The research committee developed a data collection protocol examining the use of heparin in arterial lines. This research project was conducted in 239 hospital-approved sites, coordinated by the national office. Findings will be available in early 1993.

AACN is being viewed across the country as a role model for specialty organizations, particularly in light of its promotion of research. The organization has funded studies for the conduct of research as well as for the application of research findings. Outstanding research has been rewarded. Examples include the IVAC award and the Distinguished Research Lecturer at the NTI. AACN has been innovative in both funding and rewarding research while maintaining a base in practice, thus successfully blending the two.

CURRENT PUBLISHED RESEARCH

To review the present status of critical care research the author searched single publications in addition to the previously cited reviews between January 1989 to March 1991 in preparation for the first Critical-Care Nursing Research Conference. The MEDLINE search strategy used the terms *critical care* and *research* as the medical subject headings (MESH) and as text words. The "explode" strategy was used for maximum intake. An interesting issue emerged in classifying the selected titles: the definition of critical care. For example, the term *critically ill* might be used in an abstract, but the study was about AIDS patients or patients receiving bone marrow transplantation.

Defining Critical Care

Critically ill patients are not always in the critical care unit, especially with the recent development of bone marrow units and oncology units with sophisticated treatment and diagnostic facilities. Some labor and delivery units are designating a few beds as critical care beds. If critical care is defined by the patients studied and where they usually receive care, then a quandary exists in that AIDS patients are sometimes critically ill and in ICUs, but they do not *usually* receive their care there.

Should a study be classified as critical care only if a critical care unit is the setting of the data collection, or could the study be considered for inclusion if the results of the conducted research are applicable to critical care but data were collected in a different setting? Perhaps critical care research is defined by the variables under study. For example, is critical care research limited to physiological variables? Major psychosocial issues require study as well. Therefore, critical care research could be broadly defined as studies relevant for critical care practice rather than limited only to those that occur in a critical care setting. These questions will be relevant when authors attempt to summarize critical care research without limiting the search to journals publishing critical care articles; reliability in inclusion or exclusion of studies will be hampered.

The titles obtained in the search were reviewed as well as the printed abstracts. The topics reported are only those that involve a study or, at least, an evaluation process.

Recently Published Topics

Organizational Studies

These studies focused on the critical care unit rather than on a specific clinical intervention. Study topics were the cost of nursing excellence in critical care; the report of the demonstration unit; hardiness, stress, and burnout; and a special care unit for chronically critically ill patients.[19,20,21,22]

Therapeutics

The topics of these studies were specific nursing interventions, such as positioning, exercise, ingestion of cold fluids, pulmonary artery measurements, the use of heparin in intravascular lines, the temperature of injectate for hemodynamic measurements, the use of pulse oximetry, meeting psychological needs of patients, and the measurement of nocturnal sleep patterns in trauma patients.[23-31] Additionally, issues of prevention were addressed for unintentional extubation and pressure ulcers.[32,33] The assessment of cardiac pain and the use of intuition were also topics studied.[34,35]

Families

The study of families in critical care seems to be of great interest. Two studies on needs and a review article of studies were published from 1976 to 1990.[36,37,38] Also identified were nursing interventions for families of cardiac surgical patients, two studies on family support groups, and a family intervention program in the medical intensive care unit.[39,40,41,42]

A recently published review of critical care research reported on 129 articles published between 1979 and 1988.[12] *Heart & Lung* produced 87% of the sample, although five other research journals were searched. Although the majority of the topics were addressed in only one study, several areas were identified as having potential for meta-analysis: cardiac output, the effects of positioning on pulmonary artery pressures, oxygenation during suctioning, and cardiac teaching. Concerns about the lack of replication and small sample sizes continue. The authors found clear and appropriate results and an increase in the number of studies, especially those testing interventions.

Funding for Critical Care Research

In February 1991 Dr. Mary Lucas, Chief, Acute and Chronic Illness, NCNR, NIH, reviewed the research funded by NCNR and NIH. Studies directly related to critical care were on the topics of suctioning, confusion, cardiovascular stress, cardiovascular patients, transplantation, and the operation of critical care units. Studies funded by NCNR but less directly related to critical care were studies of pediatric pain; physiologic studies (where the information might later be used in the critical care unit); organizational studies; a single exploratory center grant that focused on critical care; and nursing procedures that could be used in critical care settings.

A search was conducted of other NIH institutes and centers other than NCNR to find studies that directly related to critical care. Topics found were preferences for care, caregivers' sleep loss, diagnostics–therapeutics, and preparation for coronary artery bypass grafting.

NIH is obviously only one funding agency, but with the establishment of NCNR within NIH it is an important resource for nursing research. Other funding agencies, such as the Agency for Health Care Policy Research, the Veterans Administration, and the National Institute of Mental Health, might be alternative avenues for funding at the federal level. National foundations and professional organizations, as well as the local chapters of these organizations, are additional sources of funds for studies that require external resources. One of the advantages in conducting research in critical care is the ready availability of equipment, patients, and personnel.

THE FUTURE

Strategies for Conducting Research

To promote the conduct of research in the future, AACN has provided assistance with the training required to conduct research by providing preconference research sessions planned by the Research Committee. Additional strategies are research courses and advanced education for critical care nurses. The development of a user-friendly research book, such as Mateo and Kirchhoff's *Conducting and Using Research in the Clinical Setting*, provides guidance for nurses who have not had the full spectrum of research training.[43]

Other sources of funding need to be developed and used by nurse researchers in critical care. Perhaps more interaction with companies that make the products used in the research or with foundations that have not sponsored health care research would augment the funding provided at the federal level. AACN has developed a targeted research program to promote corporate funding of research that is linked to the particular corporation and to national priorities for critical care research.

The Nurse Researchers Employed in Clinical Settings group is another avenue to be tapped as a resource for consultation. The 1991 mailing list for this group contains almost 150 names of nurse researchers employed in clinical settings. Although few of them have a critical care background, they would be able to assist with the methodology for critical care research.

Strategies for Applying Research

With an increase in research publications, number of journals, and number of research meetings, concern about the use of research findings has increased. How can these studies be summarized in a meaningful way and then translated into practice?

AACN's response to this challenge is seen in the grants program. One of the grants is specifically tied to translating research into practice. The research sessions at the National Teaching Institute and the poster sessions provide opportunities for critical care nurses to dialogue with critical care researchers about their research. Questions about the study and its applicability to practice can occur in this environment.

AACN-sponsored publications are good avenues

for the dissemination of research. Examples are the *AACN Nursing Scan in Critical Care*, *The American Journal of Critical Care*, *AACN Clinical Issues in Critical Care Nursing*, and *Critical Care Nurse*.

Another strategy that needs to be employed is the publication of research review articles in the research journals. For example, the literature review in a master's thesis might be worthy of a separate publication if it integrates the literature well and has recommendations for practice. The research summarized in a grant proposal is sometimes worthy of publication by itself, especially when it includes directions for practice and additional research. The strategy of providing research summaries helps staff nurses who do not have the resources to conduct the computer search, copy the articles, review, critique, summarize, and then draw conclusions for practice.

A number of hospital committees can make use of research findings. The quality assurance committee might use research or research reviews to assist in standardizing nursing care protocols and expected outcomes. The policy and procedures committee or the standards committee could take advantage of similar publications for setting the care standards in an institution.

Another mechanism for assisting in research utilization is the journal club. This club can take on many different complexions. For example, in a coronary care unit the latest issue of a cardiovascular nursing journal could be used, or in a department-wide group all of the research on "noise in hospitals" could be reviewed. How the group is structured and which literature is reviewed will determine the potential outcome of the group. When all of the research on a selected topic is reviewed, critiqued, and summarized by a journal club composed of members who feel comfortable in that function, direction for changes in practice can be decided upon, and those responsible for making the change can be identified. Other positive outcomes might be the sensitization of the group to problems throughout the hospital even if they do not have clear solutions, and the stimulation of sharing some of the latest research findings with peers.

A number of articles have been written to facilitate the conduct of research in critical care. Investigators of a funded critical care study detailed suggestions to improve studies from the selection of the research topic through data collection. They included copies of the protocol sheet and a data collection sheet.[44] Since the number of subjects in ICUs is small, the advantages of multisite research are evident. Dibble, Bostom-Ezrati, and Rizzuto offered suggestions for addressing the special issues that arise in these studies.[45] Gaining approval and support, sample size, data collection, pilot work, and unanticipated problems were discussed. Bringing the study to closure and disseminating the findings at the cooperating institutions are the final steps.

Often, bedside equipment is used to collect data. Attention to the reliability of the instruments and the data collection procedures is critical.[46,47]

The relationship has been weak among the forces affecting hospitals and more specifically critical care units; the funding possibilities of NIH, AACN, and others; and the outcomes of critical care research. In the future these separate threads will exert a stronger effect on each other. NCNR's request to all professional nursing groups for prioritization of research needs has stimulated much activity. The emphasis on outcomes has influenced NCNR as well as AACN to focus efforts in this area. The interrelationships will necessarily be stronger in the future, and that will be positive.

REFERENCES

1. Bergstrom, N. (1991). Message from the chairperson. *Council of Nurse Researchers, American Nurses' Association* (newsletter), *18*(1), 2.
2. Kinney, M.R. (1984). The scientific basis for critical care nursing practice: 1972 to 1982. *Heart Lung, 13,* 116-123.
3. Lindsey, A. M. (1985). Research for clinical practice: Physiological phenomena. *Heart Lung, 13,* 496-507.
4. Dracup, K. (1987). Critical care nursing. In J. J. Fitzpatrick, & R. L. Taunton (Eds.), *Annual review of nursing research,* vol. 5. New York: Springer.
5. Keller, C. (1990). Cardiovascular nursing research review: 1969 to 1988. *Progress in Cardiovascular Nursing, 5*(1), 26-33.
6. Foster, S. B., Kloner, J. A., & Stengrevics, S. S. (1984). Cardiovascular nursing research: past, present, and future. *Heart Lung, 13,* 111-116.
7. Kinney, M. R. (1985). Trends in cardiovascular nursing research: 1972-83. *Cardiovascular Nursing, 21*(5), 25-30.
8. Yarcheski, A. (1986). Trends in cardiovascular nursing research: an analysis. *Journal of Cardiovascular Nursing, 1*(1), 67-76.
9. Packa, D. R., & Norris, B. W. (1987). Conceptualization in cardiovascular nursing research. *Cardiovascular Nursing, 23,* 125-129.
10. American Nurses' Association (ANA) Cabinet of Nursing Research. (1985). *Directions for nursing research: Toward the twenty-first century.* Kansas City, MO: ANA.
11. Cowan, M. (1990). Cardiovascular nursing research. In J. J. Fitzpatrick, R. L. Tauton, & J. Q. Benoliel (Eds.), *Annual review of nursing research.* New York: Springer.
12. VanCott, M. L., Tittle, M. B., Moody, L. E., et al. (1991). Analysis of a decade of critical care nursing practice research: 1979 to 1988. *Heart Lung, 20,* 394-397.
13. American Association of Critical-Care Nurses (AACN). (1984). *AACN position statement: Ethics in critical care research.* Newport Beach, CA: AACN.
14. American Association of Critical-Care Nurses (AACN) Standards Committee. (1989). *Standards for nursing care of the critically ill* (2nd ed.). Reston, VA: Reston Publishing.
15. American Association of Critical-Care Nurses (AACN). *AACN mission statement.* Laguna Niguel, CA: AACN.
16. American Association of Critical-Care Nurses (AACN). (1990). *Outcome standards for nursing care of the critically ill.* Laguna Niguel, CA: AACN.
17. Lewandowski, L. A., & Kositsky, A. M. (1983). Research priorities for critical care nursing: A study by the American Association of Critical-Care Nurses. *Heart Lung, 12,* 35-44.
18. Funk, M. (1989). Research priorities in critical care nursing. *Focus on Critical Care, 16,* 135-138.
19. Mitchell, P. H., Armstrong, S., Simpson, T. F., et al. (1989). American Association of Critical-Care Nurses demonstration project: Profile of excellence in critical care nursing. *Heart Lung, 18,* 219-237.
20. Armstrong, S., Simpson, T., Nield, M., et al. (1991). The cost of nursing excellence in critical care. *Journal of Nursing Administration, 21*(2), 27-34.
21. Topf, M. (1989). Personality hardiness, occupational stress, and burnout in critical care nurses. *Research in Nursing and Health, 12,* 179-186.
22. Daly, B. J., Rudy, E. B., Thompson, K. S., et al. (1991). Development of a special care unit for chronically critically ill patients. *Heart Lung, 20,* 45-51.
23. Tidwell, S. L., Ryan, W. J., Osguthorpe, S. G., et al. (1990). Effects of position changes on mixed venous oxygen saturation in patients after coronary revascularization. *Heart Lung, 19,* 574-578.
24. Burek, K. A., Kirscht, J., & Topol, E. J. (1989). Exercise capacity in patients 3 days after acute, uncomplicated myocardial infarction. *Heart Lung, 18,* 575-580.
25. Haughey, B. P. (1990). Ingestion of cold fluids: related to onset of arrhythmias? *Critical Care Nurse, 10,* 98-110.
26. Dolter, K. J. (1989). Increasing reliability and validity of pulmonary artery measurements. *Dimensions of Critical Care Nursing, 8,* 193-191.
27. Bolgiano, C. S., Subramaniam, P. T., Montanari, J. M., et al. (1990). The effect of two concentrations of heparin on arterial catheter patency. *Critical Care Nurse, 10,* 47-57.
28. Groom, L., Elliott, M., & Frisch, S. (1990). Injectate temperature: Effects on thermodilution CO measurements. *Critical Care Nurse, 10,* 112-120.
29. Peters, K., Caulfield, A., Schultz, P., et al. (1990). Increasing clinical use of pulse oximetry. *Dimensions of Critical Care Nursing, 9,* 107-111.
30. Turnock, C. (1989). A study into the views of intensive care nurses on the psychological needs of their patients. *Intensive Care Nursing, 5,* 159-166.
31. Fontaine, D. K. (1989). Measurement of nocturnal sleep patterns in trauma patients. *Heart Lung, 18,* 402-410.
32. Pesiri, A. J., Stewart, K., Kobe, E., (1990). Protocol for prevention of unintentional extubation. *Critical Care Nursing Quarterly, 12*(4), 87-90.
33. Glavis, C., & Barbour, S. (1990). Pressure ulcer prevention in critical care: State of the art. *AACN Clinical Issues, 1,* 602-613.
34. Guyton-Simmons, J., & Mattoon, M. (1991). Analysis of strategies in the management of coronary patients' pain. *Dimensions of Critical Care Nursing, 10*(1), 21-27.
35. Rew, L. (1990). Intuition in critical care nursing practice. *Dimensions of Critical Care Nursing, 9*(1), 30-37.
36. Coutu-Wakulczyk, G., & Chartier, L. (1990). French validation of the critical care family needs inventory. *Heart Lung, 19,* 192-196.

37. Forrester, D. A., Murphy, P. A., Price, D. M., et al. (1990). Critical care family needs: Nurse–family member confederate pairs. *Heart Lung, 19,* 655-661.

38. Hickey, M. (1990). What are the needs of families of critically ill patients? A review of the literature since 1976. *Heart Lung, 19,* 401-415.

39. Ward, C. R., Constancia, P. E., & Kern, L. (1990). Nursing interventions for families of cardiac surgery patients. *Cardiovascular Nursing 5*(1), 34-42.

40. Halm, M. A. (1990). Effects of support groups on anxiety of family members during critical illness. *Heart Lung, 19,* 62-71.

41. Sabo, K. A., Kraay, C., Rudy, E., et al. (1989). ICU family support group sessions: Family members' perceived benefits. *Applied Nursing Research 2,* 82-89.

42. Cray, L. (1989). A collaborative project: Initiating a family intervention. *Focus on Critical Care, 16,* 213-218.

43. Mateo, M. A., & Kirchhoff, K. T. (1991). *Conducting and using research in the clinical setting.* Baltimore: Williams & Wilkins.

44. Tyler, D. O., Clark, A. P., Winslow, E. H., et al. (1990). Strategies for conducting clinical nursing research in critical care. *Critical Care Nursing Quarterly, 12*(4), 30-38.

45. Dibble, S. L., Bostrom-Ezrati, J., & Rizzuto, C. R. (1990). Developing multisite research in critical care. *Dimensions of Critical Care Nursing, 9*(4), 236-242.

46. Engstrom, J. L. (1988). Assessment of the reliability of physical measures. *Research in Nursing and Health, 11,* 383-389.

47. Gift, A. G., & Soeken, K. L. (1988). Assessment of physiologic instruments. *Heart Lung, 17,* 128-133.

3-A

AACN Research Priorities

Priorities for clinical practice research in critical care nursing are:

- Techniques to optimize pulmonary functioning and prevent pulmonary complications
- Weaning of mechanically ventilated patients
- Effect of nursing activities/interventions on hemodynamic parameters
- Techniques for real-time monitoring of tissue perfusion and oxygenation
- Nutritional support modalities and patient outcomes
- Interventions to prevent infection
- Pain assessment and pain management techniques
- Accuracy and precision of invasive and noninvasive monitoring devices
- Effect of nursing activities, environmental stimuli and human interactions on intracranial and cerebral perfusion pressure

Priorities for research on the context within which critical care nursing takes place are:

- Incorporation of research findings into critical care nursing practice
- Levels of nursing competence (e.g., certification) and the effect on patient outcomes
- Occupational hazards (e.g., HIV, noise, substance abuse, premature delivery)
- Ethical issues related to initiation, maintenance and withdrawal of life support technology (e.g., living wills)
- Patient care delivery models for critical care
- Collaboration and communication among health care professionals
- Role of critical care nurses in decisions regarding resuscitation status of critically ill patients

From American Association of Critical-Care Nurses. (1992). *AACN Research Priorities*. Aliso Viejo, CA: AACN.

4

Instrumentation

Rae Nadine Smith

Beverley J. Leyerle

M. Michael Shabot

Today's critical care environment is continually evolving through medical, diagnostic, and technological advances. These advances require that health care professionals serve as sophisticated users of devices that support the critically ill patient or assist in his or her care. The goal of this chapter is to provide a review of technical devices and computer systems for the critical care environment. The use of computer-based instrumentation has dramatically increased since publication of the second edition of this text, and the trend appears to be toward increasing computerization. We therefore begin this chapter with an expanded section on the clinical uses of computer techology. Specific types of instrumentation commonly used in today's critical care environment are then discussed. Cardiac monitoring and cardiac management are described in Chapter 10 and Chapters 20-26.

Over the course of a day, critical care nurses measure several hundred parameters on each critically ill patient using a myriad of devices and instruments. Clinicians spend enormous amounts of time in collecting this information and transcribing it into the medical record. Much of this information is collected from devices that are run by microprocessors. For example, a simple infusion pump can be programmed to deliver a specified volume (rate), track volume delivery from a predefined total volume, and sound an alarm for line occlusion. They can be programmed for secondary infusion of piggyback medications, resuming prior parameters upon completion. The nurse or clinician reads the number appropriate to the infusion of the intravenous solution from the front panel of the infusion pump, transcribing these data into the medical record. Since these pumps are microprocessor based, it seems they are not being used to the fullest potential.

In non–health care industries, computers perform routine, tedious, time-consuming, clerical tasks. The questions arise: "Why are microprocessor-based medical devices not doing these tasks for the nurse?" The collection, retrieval, interpretation, and analysis of data are the very tasks for which computers were developed. Through the use of a "host" computer, many of the sophisticated devices described in this chapter can be made to interface (to "talk" to each other), freeing the nurse from tedious clerical tasks while providing more time for bedside care.

A host computer, interfacing with the myriad of technical devices at the bedside, can deliver patient information at the point of care, the bedside. The computer becomes the focus of data collection, retrieval, interpretation, and display. Hundreds of parameters are funneled into the computer and presented to the end user in the most useful form. Derived hemodynamic parameters such as cardiac index and systemic vascular resistance, hemodynamic profiling, and arterial blood gas parameters associated with intrapulmonary shunting are only a few examples of the value of today's instrumentation.

Critical care nursing is defined as the diagnosis and management of human responses in patients with life-threatening illness.[1] Access to, interpretation, and understanding of a wide range of physiological variables are intrinsic to this function. Since instrumentation must be used to acquire data often and accurately, a basic understanding of the instrumentation is as important to today's critical care nurses as an understanding of the measured physiology.

COMPUTER APPLICATIONS IN CRITICAL CARE

Computer Terms and Functions

A computer can be thought of as a functional unit or device capable of performing computations and logic operations. It can be made up of one or more components that function together; this is what is commonly referred to as the *hardware*. However, hardware is incapable of doing anything useful by itself. The computer needs a series of instructions that completely control its function. These instructions are referred to as *software*.

Microprocessors are computers whose functional elements have been reduced to microscopic size; however, their power is equivalent to the largest computers of just a few years ago. The use of microprocessors has changed the way new equipment is designed. The fact that a particular piece of equipment contains a microcomputer may not be obvious to the user. Computers are now incorporated in most biomedical equipment providing increased functionality, flexibility, and complexity.

In the critical care environment, a multitude of devices are microprocessor driven, including bedside physiological monitors, intraaortic balloon pumps, urimeters and infusion pumps, to name a few. Since these devices are microprocessor based, they foster connectivity to each other or to larger "host" computers. The advantage of this type of connectivity is that data collection, correlation, and display can be performed by a computer system rather than a nurse. In many ICUs, the computer has become an important adjunct to patient management and has moved the nurse back to the bedside and away from tedious clerical and charting tasks.

Host computers are known by many names, including clinical information systems, bedside information systems, patient data management systems, patient care systems, point-of-care systems, medical information systems, bedside charting systems, and patient charting systems. Despite differences in name, their objectives and functions are quite similar. Clinical information systems (CISs) automatically acquire, display, and report crucial patient information. These systems automate data collection from bedside devices, such as patient monitors, infusion pumps, and ventilators, as well as from ancillary systems, such as laboratory information computers. CISs automatically update information as conditions change. By capturing data electronically, the CISs minimize manual data transcription and allows clinicians to spend less time on manual documentation (Figure 4-1). These systems make critical ICU information more accurate, timely, and accessible.

CISs work at the point of care, providing information where and when it is needed. These systems are usually flexible, allowing users to access information in the format that is most appropriate for their work. With a CIS, authorized hospital personnel can also use their workstations or terminal to retrieve information for clinical, administrative, educational, and research purposes.[2]

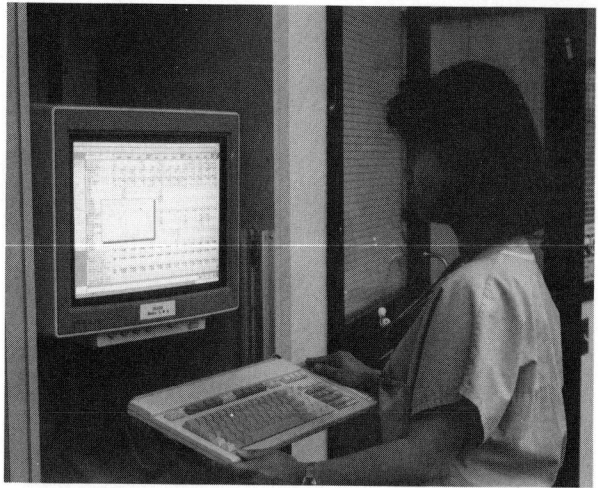

Figure 4-1 A critical care nurse reviewing data entry using a Hewlett-Packard CareVue 9000 bedside terminal. Courtesy of Cedars-Sinai Medical Center, Los Angeles, California.

The computerized critical care environment was introduced by Weil in 1966.[3] In the beginning this technology lacked many of the features found today. Early computer systems often required large quantities of space, energy, and money and were only programmed to perform a few functions. Because of the size and cost of maintenance, few institutions could justify the cost-benefit ratio. However, in the past 25 years computer technology has advanced to the point where computers are relatively inexpensive, compact, and portable; they can perform sophisticated analysis and sorting with rapid digital display of information on high-resolution bedside screens.[4]

These advances in computer hardware and software have ushered in an era in which computers can assist clinicians with the diagnostic and decision-support aspects of patient care. Critical care nurses are provided with a completely new tool for planning of care. In many ICUs the pen has become obsolete. Today's nurses can "chart" using several computer techniques. The exact mode of data entry is unique to each CIS and tailored to the needs of the environment. Computer-generated choice list, touch screens, trackballs, mice, light pens, and even voice input (Figure 4-2) are options in available systems.

Clinical Use of Computer Technology in Critical Care

Computers streamline the charting process by providing patient flowsheets, medical records, progress notes, care plans, physicians' orders, and other information previously available only on paper. For administrators, these systems provide operational data needed to run an efficient health care business. Automated medical records can be the basis for qual-

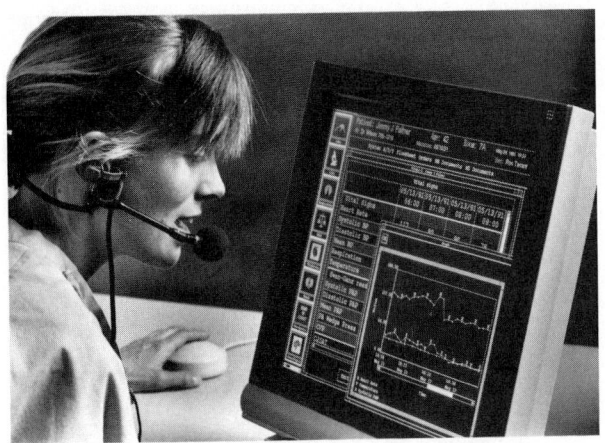

Figure 4-2 Sunquest's critical care information system, the IntelliCare system, allows input from an optional voice recognition module.

Courtesy of Sunquest Information Systems, Inc., Tucson, Arizona.

ity assurance audits and resource management for assessment of patient outcome.[2]

Data Acquisition

The critically ill patient in today's ICU challenges nurses and physicians in areas of skill and clinical judgment. Their ability to provide optimum care relies on availability of real-time information for effective, timely decision making and ordering of appropriate therapies.[5,6]

Bedside device interfaces to a CIS provide the unique focal point for the acquisition, confirmation, and retrieval of real-time data. The major data sources for computerized information systems are physiological (bedside monitors), clinical laboratory, blood gas analysis, pharmacy, admitting department, radiology department, multiphasic screening centers, catheterization laboratory, infectious disease department, metabolic support services, medical records, and the patient medical history.[6] Use of computer interfaces allows the CIS to query or receive systematic and reliable data from other computers or devices on a regular basis. The CIS collects the raw data, organizes it into logical data sets and presents the data to the clinician in a visually meaningful way.

Dasta, in 1990, described the computer as "the ultimate slave to the clinician."[4] The ease by which data can be collected and displayed for nurse or physician review by a CIS cannot be rivaled by a manual system. In the past, nurses and physicians have spent enormous amounts of time attempting to gather and make sense out of separate pieces of information. Clinical information systems take information polled from bedside devices and present this information in context with clinical laboratory results, blood gas values, and calculations performed automatically for de-

rived hemodynamic variables such as systemic vascular resistance, left ventricular stroke work, oxygen consumption, and pulmonary shunt fraction.

The information available for CISs can be reviewed on high resolution screens in a variety of formats. The most common format is a tabular display of data, which can be rapidly scanned to determine patient progress or to review significant physiological events.[5] Values that are outside acceptable physiological ranges can be highlighted by the use of color or symbols. Information thus displayed allows for immediate identification of trends such as rising capillary wedge pressures, falling systemic resistance, or adverse responses to therapeutic interventions (Figure 4-3).

Another useful format for data display is graphical display, which shows specific sets of data in a visual, pictorial fashion. For example, Figure 4-4 is a serial display of a patient's left ventricular stroke work index (LVSWI) against the pulmonary capillary wedge pressure (PCWP). The data points are displayed as an overlay to the normal Starling curve for left ventricular function. The ability of the CIS to zoom in on a specific window of time can provide a visual, readily understandable picture of the patient's response to therapeutic interventions.

Data acquired from a number of bedside devices and its use directly influence the management and care of an ICU patient. However, the development of device interfaces and connections to a CIS is not as easy as it seems. Until recently most device interfaces were "home grown" connections. Such interfaces are labor intensive in development and usually applicable only to one device and one CIS. It has become apparent in the CIS environment that there is a tremendous need for a communications standard for transfer of information from bedside medical devices to clinical information systems. In 1984, a committee of the Institute of Electrical and Electronic Engineers was organized to develop standards for a Medical Information Bus (MIB), which is described later in this chapter. This committee has drafted a set of standards that will permit connecting disparate devices to a network, allowing for rapid communication between devices and the CIS.[4]

Electronic Flowsheets

In a noncomputerized ICU, nurses spend up to 40% of their time performing clerical tasks and communicating patient information to other caregivers.[7] In the course of a day, nurses collect and record several thousand data points per patient. The manual collection and recording of information of this volume is not only time consuming and fraught with potential error but takes time away from the delivery of direct patient care.

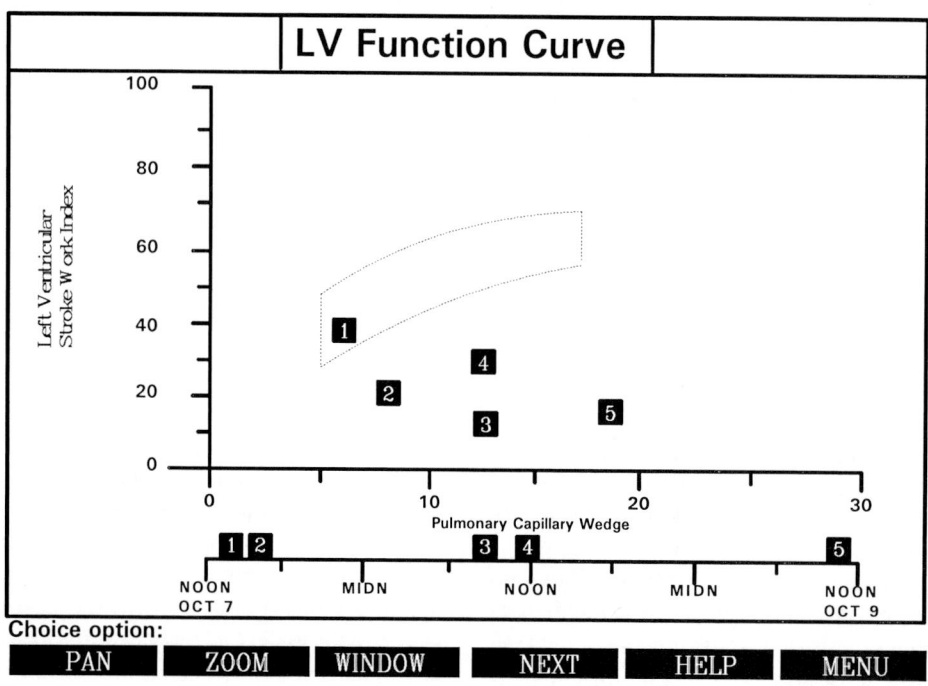

		FLOWSHEET (q1hr)	25Sep91 0800	0900	1000	1100	25Sep91 1200	1300	1400	1500	25Sep91 1600
QUICK LOOK	V	Temperature	98.5	98.6	98.4	98.2	98.6	98.6	98.6	98.6	98.4
	I	Temp Site	Bladder	Bladder	Bladder	Bladder	Bladder	Bladder	Bladder	Bladder	Bladder
VITALS GRAPH	T	Core Blood Temp	36.9	36.9	36.7	37.0	36.8	36.8	36.7	36.8	36.7
	A	Heart Rate	73	62	73	65	69	59	64	77	61
	L	Rhythm 1	Sinus	Sinus	Sinus	Sinus	Sinus	Sinus	Sinus	Sinus	PAC's
LABS	S	Rhythm 2						S Brady	S Brady	Sinus	S Brady
		Resp Rate	0	18	24	26	21	14	16	20	14
		Cuff BP									
VENT DATA		NIBP	79	138/ 80	145/ 78	147/ 71	140/ 76	127/ 66	144/ 78	158/ 79	138/ 67	144/ 73
		Art BP	80	137/ 76	141/ 81	134/ 80	133/ 77	136/ 76	138/ 76	134/ 79	129/ 75	132/ 68
VITALS HEMODY	H	PA	11	23/ 12	25/ 14	21/ 8	26/ 12	22/ 6	22/ 9	17/ 9	13/ 5	20/ 9
	E	PCW			11			6				11
	M	PAD-PCW			3			0				-2
INTAKE OUTPUT	O	RA/CVP	5	8	10	7	8	5	5	3	3	4
		CO			7.46			7.85				7.52
NURSE MISC		CI			3.81			4.01				3.84
		SI			52.2			68.0				63.0
		SVRI			1889			1615				1937
NEURO DETAIL		PVRI			139.9			106.3				34.7
		LVSWI			71.0			79.5				83.1
VASC DETAIL		O2AVI			575.3							
		VO2I										
		Qs/Qt										
PtCARE GRID		Dopamine mcq/kq/min	2.0	2.0	2.0	2.0	2.0	2.0	2.0	2.0	2.0	2.0
	R	Tube										
SYSTEM ASSESS	E	O2 Source			CoolMt	CoolMt	CoolMt	CoolMt	CoolMt	Prongs	Prongs	Prongs
	S	FiO2 %				50	35	35	35			
	P	O2 Flow Rate								4	4	4
LINE ASSESS		TcSaO2	98	99	97	98	98	98	98	97	98	100
		End Tidal CO2										
	A	FiO2		0.40		0.50	0.35					
	B	O2 L/m									4	
	G	pHa		7.41		7.40	7.42				7.42	
		PaO2		151		188	129				134	
		PaCO2		37		40	40				41	

Figure 4-3 Tabular display with abnormal physiological parameters.

Figure 4-4 Left ventricular function curve.

The traditional folded, multipaged flowchart used in most ICUs requires the transcription of selected information, (such as blood pressure, heart rate, temperature, and hemodynamic parameters), into small designated areas or boxes on a standardized form, repeatedly throughout the shift. Manual records are often cumbersome, illegible, and restricted to the review of a single individual.[4] Information entered into the manual record is also subject to transcription er-

ror. For example, a potassium level of 3.5 mEq/L could be accidentally transcribed as 5.3 mEq/L. Inappropriate medical management based on this transcription error could negatively influence patient outcome.

Computerization of the medical record integrates nurse-validated bedside data with clinical laboratory data, pharmacotherapy, radiological interpretation, and other therapies providing a comprehensive record that can be used at several workstations simultaneously. The medical record becomes manageable and legible. The reliability of information extracted from the computer and formatted for the medical record is markedly enhanced as compared with manual methods.[5]

With the introduction of the computer-generated medical record, nurse charting time has been reduced by an estimated 50%.[8] According to Tolbert, if 40% of a nurse's time is spent in the management of patient information, automation of the medical record reduces this time by 50%.[7] For example, a nurse who had spent 3.2 hours of an 8-hour shift in information management now spends 1.6 hours performing the same tasks. The actual time saving may even be greater, since a portion of time was previously spent in communicating information. Less communication is required when the medical record is accessible and used effectively by many users simultaneously.

Traditionally the medical record had a single purpose: providing a legal record of patient activities during a single hospital stay. With the transition of manual recording of patient events to computerization of the same information, CIS data that was used solely for direct patient care can now be tapped for other uses beyond the bedside.[9] Data can be transferred from the medical record into a multipatient database. Physiological data, severity of illness, and nursing interventions can be viewed in the context of patient outcomes and nursing productivity, thus providing management with valuable information about cost-effective and medically effective patient care practices.

Decision Support Systems

CIS-generated *decision support* has been defined as the use of a computer as an adjunct to patient care, always available to the clinician to assist in the application of decision support logic as patient data are entered by care providers. The CIS thus acts as an expert partner capable of assisting with decision making throughout the care and management of the critically ill patient.

The amount of data presented to the nurse or physician in an ICU is enormous, making it difficult to assimilate and comprehend. A decision support system helps turn *data* into clinically useful *information*. For example, a CIS could be programmed to prompt the nurse to evaluate the patient's physical status on the basis of a particular assessment or physiological parameter obtained elsewhere in the nursing process. The CIS could thus assist nurses in identifying interventions that would prevent adverse events.

Nurses are taking an active role in defining decision support systems. The field of nursing informatics is evolving as an interactive, synergistic effort combining nursing practice with the computerization of the nursing process. According to Hannah: "Computers are the ideal medium by which to integrate patient data and the nursing process with standardized care plans. The goal of nursing informatics is to guide the design, use, management, and evaluation of computer systems that will meet the needs of nurses."[10] Decision support systems should be used to extend the nurse's decision-making processes, not to replace the human component of nursing decision making.[11] Appropriate nursing care decisions are based upon a fundamental knowledge base and use of the nursing process.

Clinical Alerts

Nursing clinical alerts function on the premise that alerting the nurse to the potential for error improves the quality of care and outcome for the patient. *Clinical alerts* are automated notices of life-threatening conditions as they are received by the CIS. For example, a particular laboratory value, such as a serum potassium of 2.8 mEq/L, may be so abnormal that it is considered a "critical" or "panic" value. Rather than simply recording this result as abnormal when it is transmitted from the laboratory, a CIS can be programmed to highlight the critical or "panic" value as a function of decision support alerts on the patient's display.

Nursing can define parameters by which specific nursing interventions must be undertaken. For example, the tubing and dressing on intravenous lines are usually changed at predetermined intervals, often specified by a policy and procedures manual. A CIS could be programmed to alert nurses at the appropriate time for a specific patient.

Another example of a nursing alert can make use of prior medical records. For a patient who has a history of confusion and falls, the CIS can prompt the nurse to evaluate the patient and institute appropriate measures to prevent recurrences. Such a simple intervention can mean shortened lengths of stay and major cost savings to the institution, not to mention averting the potentially deleterious effect a fall would have on the patient.

Management Tools

The CIS data used in patient care and in the generation of the legal medical record are of a kind familiar to clinicians, whether in computerized or manual form. The use of the same data for patient classification and prediction of outcome, including survival, may be less familiar.

Numerous patient classification systems and scoring systems have been described elsewhere, including the Therapeutic Intervention Scoring System (TISS), the Acute Physiology and Chronic Health Evaluation

Physiological Variables Used by Simplified Acute Physiology Score (SAPS)

Age	Hematocrit
Body temperature	White blood count (WBC)
Heart rate	
Systolic blood pressure	Serum glucose
Urinary output	Serum potassium
Blood urea nitrogen (BUN)	Serum sodium
	Serum bicarbonate
Spontaneous respiratory rate or ventilation or CPAP	Glasgow Coma Score

Partial Listing of Procedures and Interventions Identified by Therapeutic Intervention Scoring System (TISS)*

Admission	Plan of care revision
Discharge	Arterial pressure catheter
Pulmonary artery catheter	Central venous pressure catheter
Intracranial pressure catheter	Oxygen source (Ambu, ventilator)
Atrial deparrhythmias	Ventricular arrhythmias
Code blue event	Vasoactive IV drugs
Antiarrhythmic IV drugs	Miscellaneous IV drugs
Taking vital signs	Performing PA measurements
Performing cardiac outputs	Performing neurological checks
Blood gases	Blood transfusions
IV bottles hung	Hyperalimentation bottles hung
Enteral feeding bottles	Hemodialysis
Chest tubes	GI drainage tubes
Wound irrigations	Bedside glucose checks
Transfers for tests	Seizure episodes
Weight measurements	

*The therapeutic intervention scoring system (TISS) classifies the severity of illness by quantifying the number of therapeutic interventions performed by the critical care nurse. The more critical the patient, the more therapeutic interventions performed, requiring more nursing time. TISS totals the number of interventions for the previous 24 hours and calculates a TISS based upon a score of one to four per intervention.

III (APACHE III), the Simplified Acute Physiology Score (SAPS), and the Computerized Intensity-Intervention Score (CIIS).[12-19] This discussion is confined to the method by which such information can be extracted from a CIS.

The common denominator for all classification or scoring systems is measurement of certain physiological variables. An electronic chart permits routine queries about physiological parameters and interventions as documented by nurses, physicians, and clinical and blood gas laboratories, as well as other clinical and demographic data. Each variable can be identified, counted, scored, and weighted according to an algorithm unique to the scoring system. For example, APACHE III uses 12 variables plus age and previous health status, whereas SAPS evaluates 14 variables and TISS identifies 76 independent nursing interventions. Possible physiological variables and interventions for inclusion in a scoring system are listed in the boxes on this page. The time and resources required to extract this kind of detailed chart data make these systems extremely labor intensive in a noncomputerized environment.[12,13,14,15] A CIS can extract these scoring parameters reliably and automatically. One example of a computerized scoring system is the CIIS,[17] a combination of SAPS and TISS scores extracted from a computerized medical record.

Each of these systems aims to provide a common standard by which intensive care can be evaluated in terms of outcome and effectiveness. For the first time, computers have provided a method for comparing patient outcomes between ICUs within an institution, among ICUs and hospitals in the community or a much wider scope, nationally, and even internationally.[16,20] However, patient classification and scoring systems are fraught with problems similar to those relating to development of device interfaces. A universally accepted standard is needed. True comparisons between ICU facilities will be realized only when

patient classification systems and resources are standardized.[21]

The CIS provides management with an additional advantage: the capacity to analyze data collected by the computer system into a medical database. Managers can access the database to perform statistical analyses on past utilization history, to make predictions on staffing needs, for resource utilization, and to gauge the potential effects of quality assurance programs. The latter function warrants additional discussion.

Quality Assurance

Most hospital quality assurance (QA) and resource management (RM) departments have yet to tap the power of computerized CIS. The CIS provides an economical and reliable means by which to gather four types of QA data for quality and utilization analyses. In 1990, Weissman and associates[21], described these areas as (1) general statistics, (2) specific indicators, (3) occurrence screening, and (4) targeted reviews. Most QA and RM departments rely on a qualified staff to extract the required data manually by performing random chart audits. This process is tedious, time consuming, and extremely costly. Electronic chart audits performed by CIS are not only faster, but *every* chart can be audited against standards for efficiency and quality of care. The availability of information from all charts reviewed daily provides hospitals with a powerful tool for aggressively maintaining or improving areas of performance that directly affect patient outcome and survival.

In the late 1980s, several regulatory agencies such as the Health Care Financing Authority (HCFA) and the Joint Commission for Accreditation of Healthcare Organizations (JCAHO) changed their focus from "process orientation" to "outcome orientation." These agencies requested more detailed information about outcomes, including trends. These requirements cannot be met solely by manual or electronic chart reviews. Only data objectively extracted from the electronic record by a comprehensive CIS, together with available demographic, outcome, and financial data, can answer requests of this type.

Autoextraction of data by CIS provides a unique trade-off for the hours previously spent by QA and RM nurses culling data from charts. The time saved can now be channeled into timely analysis and reporting of meaningful indicators.

A recent QA study was undertaken by an ICU to determine whether patients receiving intravenous (IV) alimentation in the perioperative period were experiencing problems with glucose control. It is well documented that perioperative disturbances in endogenous catecholamine and glucocorticoid metabolism impair the body's ability to handle a glucose load. The question posed was "Would it be better to forgo nutritional support in the perioperative period than to risk wide fluctuations in serum glucose?" In a manual system, a study of this magnitude would require the review of hundreds or thousands of charts. However, in this case a definitive answer was obtained with simple queries to the CIS and the laboratory information system. These queries allowed for the correlation of each patient's IV alimentation status with laboratory glucose results.

For a 6-month period, a total of 4,985 serum glucose values for 1,189 consecutive patients were found. Of the 4,985 serum glucose values reported, only 48 (0.96%) were found to be in the critically abnormal range of more than 400 mg/dl or less than than 40 mg/dl (Figure 4-5). Nearly all the critical values represented hyperglycemia, as shown in the Table 4-1. Although the incidence of hyperglycemia was greatest in patients receiving perioperative IV nutrition, these episodes were transient. No detrimental effects occurred that would support discontinuation of nutrition prior to surgery.

The question posed in this QA study—whether to continue to provide intravenous hyperalimentation in the perioperative period or to withhold it—was answered in a matter of a few hours. The resulting de-

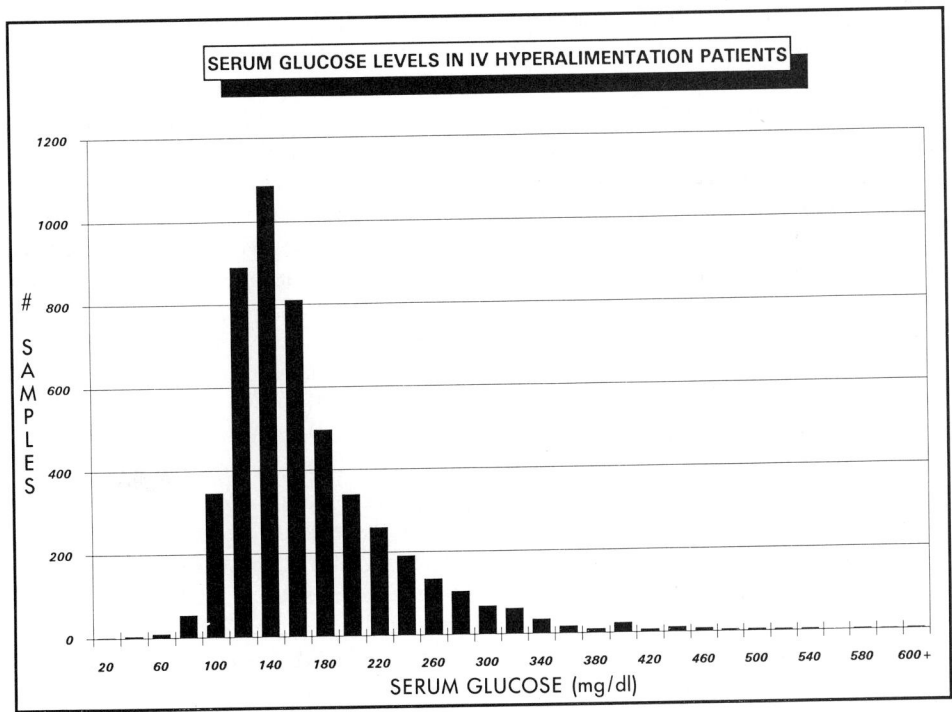

Figure 4-5   Histogram of 4,985 serum glucose levels for 1,189 patients included in the IV-TPN Quality Control Monitor.

TABLE 4-1   **Incidence of Critically Abnormal Glucose Values in Representative Quality Assurance Study**

	No. Patients	No. Glucose Values	Serum Glucose >400 mg/dl (%)	Serum Glucose <40 mg/dl (%)
IV nutrition	89	996	17 (1.7)	0 (0.0)
No IV nutrition	1,040	3,989	28 (0.7)	3 (0.1)
p value			0.003	ns

cision could be promptly implemented to influence both patient care management and cost in a positive manner.

There are many aspects of ICU care that can and should be evaluated through the QA and RM process. However, if these aspects are unmeasurable or difficult to ascertain, QA and RM programs cannot be effective. A comprehensive CIS is extremely valuable to both management and the ICU staff as it automatically gathers crucially needed data in an environment otherwise poorly suited for administrative data collection.

Future Applications

The application of computer technology in day-to-day patient care places hitherto undreamt-of power and resources at the bedside. Bedside physiological data, severity of illness, nursing interventions, decision support, and actual patient outcome can be synergistically integrated into the delivery of patient care.

Nursing Research

CIS provides a valuable medium for nursing research. The establishment of relational databases, decision-support trees, nursing documentation, and care plans allows access to information that would previously have been collected manually. Data can now be extracted from a dynamic reference population to answer such questions as whether "routine" nursing care has an impact on the patient outcome.

Limited nursing resources together with cost containment measures, necessitate that the nursing profession define which nursing activities most positively influence patient care within the briefest possible timeframe. CIS can provide this information. As Ozbolt and associates[22] have noted, nursing, unlike medicine, has no generally accepted taxonomies of nursing diagnoses, nursing objectives, or nursing interventions: "Nurses have been unable either to identify the data that would be critical indicators of each diagnosis, or to trace logical pathways from data to diagnoses." The CIS could help to bridge this gap through bedside research that would directly affect clinical practice.

The end users of CISs are making inroads into this area of the nursing process. By means of decision-support trees, nursing alerts, and the online application of the nursing process, CISs provide the framework by which research can be performed as part of daily patient care. The capability of the nurse to compare nursing interventions, with known outcomes for patients of like populations, can assist in the selection of appropriate and optimal interventions. Time spent performing unnecessary routine tasks or interventions with proven lack of efficacy in similar circumstances can be eliminated. The delivery of effective patient care can be driven by actual patient outcomes.

An example of a standardized practice that proved to be of little value to patient outcome was the 5-minute frequency of measuring vital signs in patients receiving vasopressive agents. When the therapeutic use of nitroprusside was first introduced, the package insert dictated the taking of blood pressure every 5 minutes. This monitoring frequency soon became an institutional standard of practice. When technologic advances brought reliable invasive measurement with continuous visual display of blood pressure, few institutions altered their monitoring policy. Nurses were still required to check blood pressure every 5 minutes for patients receiving nitroprusside. An intelligent look at invasive monitoring was required to realize the advantage it offered in saving nurses' time. Similarly, the advantages that CIS offers must be evaluated by clinical nursing research.

Medical Information Bus

The Medical Information Bus (MIB) is a formal standards effort organized under the auspices of the Engineering and Biology in Medicine Society (EMBS) of the Institute of Electronic and Electrical Engineers (IEEE). In 1984, these groups initiated an MIB Committee to produce a common hardware and software standard for the connection of bedside devices to data management and monitoring systems. This effort was necessitated by today's critical care environment. A critically ill patient in the ICU is usually surrounded by equipment: a ventilator; a physiological monitor that captures the heart rate, blood pressure, respira-

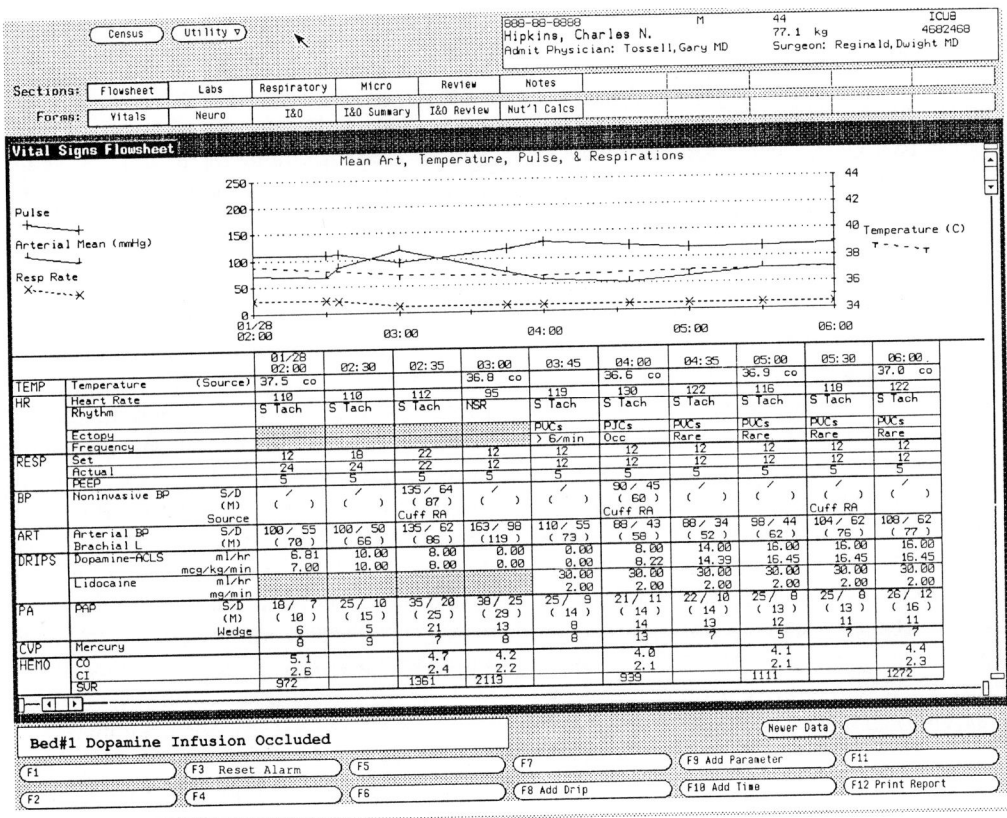

Figure 4-6 Demonstration of the medical information bus remote alarm state. Infusion has become occluded, and the infusion device has sensed the occlusion and is broadcasting the alarm state on the patient display.

tory rate, and hemodynamic parameters from invasive catheters; a pulse oximeter, several infusion pumps; collection devices for urine, chest tube, and gastric output; and perhaps an intraaortic balloon pump. Each of these devices saves the clinician time in some way. However, as these devices have become more commonplace and functionally complex, they have added to the burden of documentation.

The MIB will provide a vendor-independent method of connecting bedside devices to host computer systems. With automatic acquisition of data from bedside equipment, the nurse will need only to verify information presented on the computer screen instead of reading it from each piece of equipment and transcribing it into a computer. Verification of the data is not only faster, but the data has been collected and presented to the user in a more accurate manner that decreases the potential for transcription errors.

Another MIB benefit is the ability to capture and transmit device-state and alarm information. Prompt response to an alarm in current systems is delayed first by determining at which bed the alarm is occurring and then by determining which device is in alarm. The MIB can capture the alarm state of a device and transmit this and other clinically relevant informa-

tion. The nurse can be given a specific message such as "BED #1 DOPAMINE INFUSION OCCLUDED" (Figure 4-6). The nurse can then go directly to the patient's bedside and resolve the problem quickly.

Continued advances in medicine and technology create a fertile environment in which the use of the MIB will grow and become increasingly sophisticated. One advanced use of the MIB currently in the research phase is the ability to do closed-loop infusions. First described by Sheppard and associates in 1973,[23] this therapeutic approach allows the titration and delivery of a medication based on an algorithm and specific monitored parameters. The usual example is the administration of a vasodilating drug based upon the mean arterial pressure (MAP). Once the desired range for the MAP has been defined by the clinician, the arterial line monitor feeds back the MAP via the MIB to the infusion pump and the pump titrates the drug accordingly. This application has far-reaching implications for the care of hemodynamically unstable patients.

Evolving Technology

Several potential benefits of CIS have not yet been realized by users. Most CISs are networked to data-producing systems such as the clinical laboratory, the blood gas laboratory, and many ICU measuring devices, but automatic access to the outcome data in other hospital computers is not generally available. It will not be long before CIS users require that all systems be fully networked so that automatic analyses of severity-adjusted outcome can be carried on in the background. Severity data for a given time period—biweekly, monthly, quarterly, or yearly—can then be automatically compared to all available outcome criteria, rapidly producing both routine reports and non-routine alerts. Such CISs will provide earlier warning for adverse events and trends than are provided by current manual QA methods. Full use of the capabilities within a comprehensive CIS will provide more medically effective and cost-effective ICU care.

Although many believe that the principal benefit of a CIS to the ICU is the maintenance of a well-organized, legible patient care flowsheet, the CIS user believes that this represents only the most superficial level of CIS function. CISs can be programmed to automatically provide a second level of function in the daily measurement of severity of illness and intensity of interventions. Acuity measurements and intervention scoring have proven to be invaluable in the daily management of a busy ICU, including triage of patients into and out of the unit and allocation of caregiver resources.[19] A third level of ICU data management, is the use of CIS-derived analyses to evaluate long term outcomes. The ongoing mass of severity and intensity data, when combined with such information as mortality and nosocomial infection rates, is a powerful tool in assessing quality of care and modifying a clinical practice accordingly.

PARAMETER ACQUISITION INSTRUMENTATION

Invasive Monitoring

For selected patients, the precise information needed to assist in diagnosis, to define therapy, and to evaluate the patient's response to selected therapy is best obtained through continuous invasive monitoring. Physiological pressure measurements include arterial, venous, pulmonary artery, intracranial, spinal, gastrointestinal, urinary bladder, esophageal, intrauterine, intracompartmental, and interstitial pressures. Other parameters obtained via invasive measurements include blood gases and flow. Invasive monitoring indicates procedures that require penetration of the skin, such as placement of an arterial cannula, a pulmonary artery catheter, or an intracranial pressure measurement device. Some pressures measured, for example, pulmonary artery (PA), pulmonary capillary wedge (PCW), central venous (CVP), left atrial (LAP), and intracranial (ICP), are not readily detectable using noninvasive techniques.

The first report of direct arterial measurement was by Lambert and Wood in 1947. Ryder published on ICP monitoring in 1952, and in 1970 Swan and Ganz introduced the flow-directed, balloon-tipped pulmonary artery catheter. Invasive procedures are now widely used to complement and supplement noninvasive forms of assessment, such as history taking, physical examination, pulse oximetry, and ECG monitoring. Invasive techniques provide the quickest, most accurate physiological data. Eliminating the need for frequent, intermittent manual measurements, such as vital signs and blood gas samplings, permits more time to be devoted to other aspects of caring for the critically ill patient. In the hands of skilled personnel, the insertion and maintenance of invasive lines to obtain accurate and continuous data provide less risk to the patient than the alternative of intermittent, estimated data. These procedures can be done with a high degree of safety and are well tolerated by the seriously ill patient.

Basic Pressure System

A frequently used system for the continuous measurement of physiological pressure consists of a cannula or catheter connected to a transducer via a system of stopcocks and tubing. The area between the patient's blood or cerebral spinal fluid (CSF) and the diaphragm of the transducer is filled with solution to transmit the pressure from the patient to the monitor:

Cannula → Stopcock → Pressure Tubing →
Transducer → Monitor

An understanding of the basic principles of transducers and amplifiers will facilitate the setting up and use of any type of monitoring equipment for any type of pressure measurement.

Transducers

A transducer is a device that converts one form of energy into another. It may be defined as a device used to change a varying pressure into a proportionately varying signal that can be displayed on an oscilloscope, meter, and/or recorder. In blood pressure monitoring, a transducer converts physiological pressure to an electric signal that can be displayed on a monitor. There are many types of transducers in use for both invasive and noninvasive hemodynamic pressure monitoring. Most transducers are isolated, protecting patients against inadvertent shock and equipment failure.

The following information is designed as a guide for the selection and use of reusable and disposable transducers in the critical care environment.

Reusable Transducers

A wide variety of reusable transducers is available. Solid-state technology has produced smaller, more durable transducers that can resist severe impact shock, electrical damage from electrocautery and defibrillation, and higher levels of overpressurization. These improvements have made transducers more compatible with the critical care environment, in which transducers may be dropped, caught in siderails, overpressurized by syringes, or subjected to the high-voltage discharge of defibrillators and electrosurgical instruments. A variety of reusable transducers are available.

The small, lightweight, solid-state miniature transducer, often having a shorter cable than is found in the standard-size transducers, is frequently preferred for direct patient mounting. Transducer holders designed for patient mounting, usually with Velcro straps, are available.

Catheter-tip transducers provide high-fidelity measurements of pressure, sound, and velocity. Pressures and sounds associated with heart valve closure, swallowing, bladder function, and digestion can be recorded simultaneously. They are used primarily for research. Their major clinical application is in the cardiac catheterization laboratory. Catheter-tip pressure transducers are available in a variety of configurations, ranging in size from 4F to 8F, with one to six pressure sensors per catheter; velocity sensors; electrodes for stimulating, recording biopotentials, or measuring electrical impedance; and with various lumens for slow or high-speed injection, fluid sampling, and external pressure monitoring. Advances in semiconductor technology have improved stability and durability of these highly specialized transducers. After careful cleaning, most reusable transducers may be sterilized with ethylene oxide gas or glutaraldehyde solution.

Disposable Transducers

Disposable accurate, small, lightweight, rugged, and inexpensive transducers have eliminated many of the problems associated with reuse of transducers in the critical care setting. They are pretested, precalibrated, and presterilized, minimizing the risk of cross-contamination. Preassembly reduces the risk of contamination associated with component assembly and saves valuable set-up time. Most disposable transducer setups are designed for either automatic self-filling or rapid manual filling. It is recommended that the disposable transducers be changed with the monitoring line, usually every 48 hours. Patient transfer is facilitated by not having to keep track of the transducer or change transducers for monitoring compatibility. Since transducer cleaning, sterilization, repair, and replacement are eliminated, many hospitals find disposable transducers more cost-effective.

The majority of disposable transducers are based on semiconductor technology. The patient's physio-

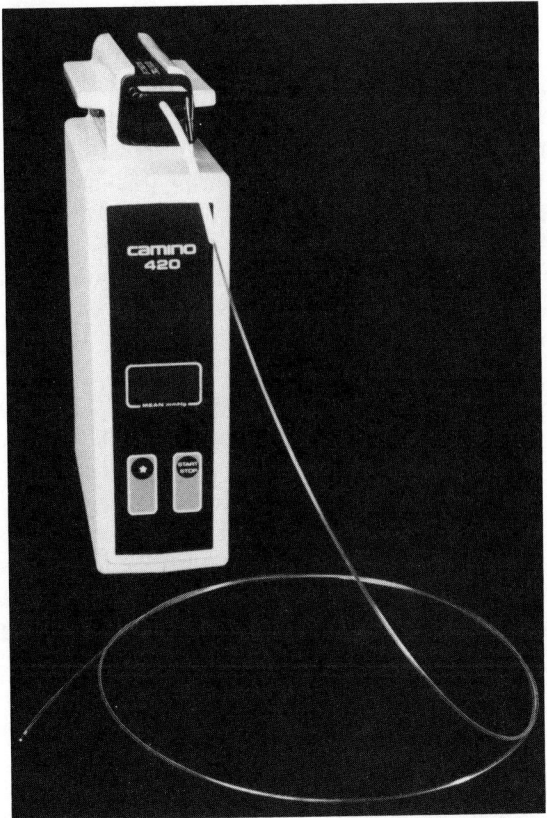

Figure 4-7 Fiberoptic transducer catheter and digital pressure monitor, used primarily for ICP monitoring. Courtesy of Camino Laboratories.

logical pressure is transmitted to the external transducer sensor via a fluid-filled catheter system. The fiberoptic transducer, located at the tip of a catheter, eliminates the need for a fluid-filled system. The fiberoptic system consists of a fiberoptic catheter attached to a digital pressure monitor with an optional waveform display. Fiberoptic catheters are used primarily for monitoring intracranial pressures (Figure 4-7).

When selecting either a reusable or disposable transducer, manufacturer specifications should be reviewed for pressure ranges (usually −50 to 350 mmHg), overpressure tolerance, nonlinearity and hysteresis (accuracy), electrical isolation, thermal coefficients (temperature stability), light stability, and monitor compatibility.

Monitoring Kits

A wide variety of disposable presterilized, preassembled kits are available for both reusable and disposable transducers. They reduce the risk of contamination during assembly as well as set-up time. Kits should be evaluated for their effect on dynamic response as well as for safety characteristics of the connectors and continuous flush devices.

Interface Adaptor Cables

All transducers require specific cables to make the monitor and the transducer compatible. With disposable transducers, the cable usually stays with the monitor when the transducer is disconnected. The cables should have labels indicating the name of the monitor manufacturer and model type. Active electronic cables provide monitor–transducer compatibility by compensating for the high-output impedance of the transducer element. Use of an incorrect cable can lead to errors in pressure readings.

Pressure Amplifiers

The pressure amplifier or module in the monitor enlarges or amplifies the signal being transmitted from the patient via the transducer. Although widely diverse in appearance, all amplifiers perform the same basic functions. These consist of the following:

1. *Display*: Digital or analog meters display systolic, diastolic, and/or mean pressure, usually in millimeters of mercury.
2. *Alarm controls*: A means of selecting the highest and lowest acceptable range for the pressure being monitored.
3. *Alarms*: Audible and visual alarms indicate when a pressure change is above or below the range set on the meter.
4. *Balance (zero) control*: A means of adjusting the transducer to a zero reading at atmospheric pressure.
5. *Calibration control*: A means of adjusting the amplifier, oscilloscope, and/or recorder to read the same pressure the transducer is receiving. Some monitors are precalibrated; others incorporate electronic calibration or calibration (cal) factors.
6. *Gain control (sensitivity)*: A means of controlling the accuracy and size of the pressure displayed. For example, since pulmonary artery pressures are considerably lower than systemic arterial pressures, it is necessary to enlarge the waveform so that important waveform variations are easily visualized. This is done by changing the range switch on the amplifier to enlarge the signal being received. Frequently used gains are 0 to 250 or 300 mmHg for arterial blood pressure, 0 to 60 or 90 mmHg for pulmonary artery and intracranial pressures, and -5 to $+20$ or 30 mmHg for central venous pressures. Most monitors have an autoranging function that automatically selects the appropriate gain for the pressure being monitored.

Balancing and Calibration

All transducers must be balanced (zeroed) before and during pressure measurements. A balanced transducer gives a reading of zero (± 1 mmHg). Since physiological pressures are relative to atmospheric pressures, the transducer must be balanced at atmospheric pressure. This is done by referencing (venting) the diaphragm of the transducer to air while it is balanced via the amplifier. The level of the vascular pressure transducer system that is vented to air (e.g., stopcock port) should be at the patient's fourth intercostal midaxillary (right atrial) level. For every 1 inch of discrepancy between heart level and transducer level, there will be an error of approximately 2 mmHg.

Prior to balancing, a fluid-filled transducer should be attached to the monitor with the power turned on for the time recommended by the manufacturer, usually 1 to 5 minutes. Transducers in use for blood pressure measurement should be balanced approximately every 8 hours. Transducers in use for low-range pressures, such as pulmonary artery and intracranial pressure, should be balanced approximately every 2 to 4 hours. In addition, they should be rebalanced when they are repositioned, if the pressure reading is in question, or if there is a loss of power. Some monitoring systems feature zero balancing storage, making it possible to hold the zero for some time after power loss.

Once the transducer is balanced, most systems require calibration. Calibration refers to adjusting the monitor to display the pressure being exerted on the transducer. Most monitors now use a combination electronic balance and calibration system. Since the most accurate form of calibration is by mercury sphygmomanometer, all monitors should periodically be checked with this system.

Dynamic Response Testing

Dynamic response is a significant factor in the accuracy of physiological pressure readings. Dynamic response is the ability of a monitoring system to accurately reproduce the patient's pressure signal on the monitor. It is affected by the interdependent parameters of compliance or elasticity, fluid mass, and resistance or friction. To assess dynamic response, it is necessary to evaluate the natural frequency and damping coefficient. Although all components of a pressure-monitoring system affect response, in the clinical setting the fluid-filled catheter system between the patient and the transducer is the aspect most likely to affect the accuracy of the pressure measurements. The presence and degree of pressure measurement distortion can be determined by dynamic response testing. In the critical care setting, this is usually done with a continuous flush device and is often referred to as a "square-wave test" (Figure 4-8). Activation of a fast flush valve provides an alteration in the pressure waveform trace that can be used to identify waveform distortion caused by overdamped and under-

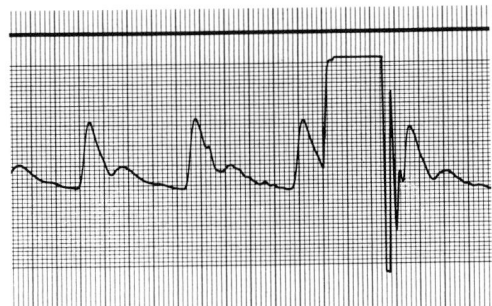

Figure 4-8 "Square-wave test" illustrating optimal dynamic response with accurate waveform. Note that the "square-wave" extends sharply below the baseline with minimal ringing and returns quickly to the arterial pressure waveform. Providing the monitoring system is correctly balanced and calibrated, this "square-wave test" indicates correct set-up with accurate systolic and diastolic pressure readings.

damped signals. Natural frequency and damping coefficients can be calculated. Measures such as eliminating air bubbles and reducing the compliance of line components can eliminate the false low systolic and false high diastolic pressure reading inaccuracies secondary to overdamping, while the use of variable damping devices can reduce the false high systolic readings associated with underdamping.

To optimize dynamic response, the monitoring system should be as simple as possible, contain the least compliant components available, have minimal connecting tubing, and be air-free. For accurate pressure measurement, the monitoring system should be periodically balanced and calibrated, with dynamic response testing used to ensure optimal dynamic response.

Direct (Invasive) Vascular Pressure Measurements

Central Venous Pressure (CVP)

Central venous pressure (CVP) is the pressure of blood in the right atrium or vena cava. During opening of the tricuspid valve, right ventricular pressures are reflected, providing measurements of right ventricular end-diastolic pressures (RVEDP). The CVP may be measured via the proximal port of a pulmonary artery catheter or via a catheter placed into the jugular, subclavian, or antecubital vein (median basilic or lateral cephalic) and advanced into the superior vena cava. Either percutaneous or cutdown insertion techniques may be used.

Central venous pressure measurements are useful for detecting changes in the right side of the heart. The CVP falls when the volume of blood returning to the heart is reduced, as with bleeding, dehydration, drug-induced vasodilation, or vigorous diuresis. El-

evated CVP may be seen with right ventricular failure, cardiac tamponade, a vasoconstrictive state, tricuspid stenosis or insufficiency, or a state of increased blood volume such as overtransfusion or overhydration. Used in conjunction with other clinical data, the CVP may provide important patient management information.

The right atrial waveform consists of A, C, and V waves, indicating atrial systole, valve closure, and ventricular systole, respectively. For continuous readings with a closed system, the CVP line may be set up the same as an arterial line.

Both short- and long-term central venous catheters (CVCs) are available in single and multilumen configurations. For short-term catheters (4 to 6 weeks), antiseptic coatings and antimicrobial cuffs have demonstrated prophylaxis against *Candida*, gram-positive and gram-negative bacteria and methacillin-resistant *Staphylococcus aureus*.

Left Atrial Pressure (LAP)

This measurement is usually associated with cardiovascular surgery and requires surgical placement of the catheter directly into the left atrium. Left ventricular end diastolic pressure (LVEDP) is measured. Although it is important to keep air out of all vascular lines, this requirement is critical with the LAP line. Air on this side of the circulation may interrupt blood flow in the coronary arteries and cerebral vasculature. This is a short-term line and is not routinely fast-flushed or used for obtaining blood samples.

The waveform consists of an A wave (atrial systole), a C wave (valvular closure), and a V wave (ventricular systole).

Pulmonary Artery and Pulmonary Capillary Wedge Pressures

Pressures within the pulmonary artery generated by contraction of the right ventricle to pump blood through the lungs reflect left ventricular function. With the Swan-Ganz technique, either pulmonary artery (PA) or mean pulmonary capillary wedge (PCW) pressure may be obtained by inserting a flow-directed, balloon-tipped catheter via a large vein through the right side of the heart and into a branch of the pulmonary artery.

Before 1970, left heart function could be directly measured only in the cardiac catheterization laboratory. Use of the pulmonary artery catheter for diagnosis was supplemented by its use for monitoring after Drs. Swan and Ganz developed the flow-directed, balloon-tipped catheter. Ordinarily, this procedure is now done without fluoroscopy at the bedside, with the position of the catheter being determined by the pressure waveforms.

Indications for pulmonary artery pressure measurements include:

1. Cardiac problems
2. Intravascular volume control
3. Pulmonary problems
4. Cardiac output determinations
5. Mixed venous blood samples
6. $S\bar{v}O_2$ monitoring
7. Temporary pacing

Pulmonary artery catheters are available in a wide variety of configurations. Capabilities include direct-pressure monitoring from the right atrium, right ventricle, and pulmonary artery; cardiac output via thermodilution; continuous mixed venous oxygen saturation monitoring; and insertion of temporary pacing leads. The style and size of catheter used depend upon the type of patient being monitored. For the adult patient, the four- or five-lumen 7 or 8 French catheter is most frequently used. This enables the measurement of right atrial (CVP), PA, and PCW pressures with intermittent cardiac output determinations via thermodilution and continuous $S\bar{v}O_2$.

Before insertion, the transducer system is set up as described in regard to arterial blood pressure using as short a length of pressure tubing as possible. Sterile technique is used in filling all pressure lumens with flush solution, usually mildly heparinized. The balloon is submerged in solution and inflated to test its symmetry and integrity. Tiny air bubbles can be detected if the balloon is defective.

The catheter is inserted via the internal or external jugular, subclavian, antecubital (median basilic or lateral cephalic), or femoral vein. The catheter is then advanced through the right atrium. Respiratory fluctuations in the waveform may be detected at this time. A large excursion in the right atrial waveform may be demonstrated by having the patient cough. The balloon may be inflated in the atrium (usually) or immediately after the flow of blood has propelled it through the tricuspid valve into the right ventricle. Although room air is usually used for balloon inflation, carbon dioxide should be used if a right-to-left shunt or septal defect is known or suspected. The solubility of carbon dioxide in blood minimizes the risk of air emboli entering the systemic circulation. As soon as the catheter enters the right ventricle, the balloon should be at full inflation to reduce stimulation of the ventricular wall during insertion. The circulation of blood through the heart will then float the catheter through the pulmonary valve into the pulmonary artery, advancing it until the balloon wedges in a distal branch of the pulmonary artery. Once it is determined that the catheter is correctly placed, an x-ray should be taken to confirm catheter-tip location, and the catheter should be sutured into

place. As with an arterial line, the pulmonary artery line should be continually monitored.

It is very important that the critical care nurse be thoroughly familiar with pulmonary artery pressure waveforms, since these waveforms are used to determine the positioning of the catheter in the heart (Figure 4-9). It should be kept in mind that patients with chronic lung disease or ischemic heart disease often have pressures considerably higher than the normal range.

Right Atrial (RA) Pressure

Right atrial (RA) pressure reflects right ventricular (RA) pressure. It consists of three positive and three negative waves, or descents. The positive waves are A, C, and V. The A wave indicates right atrial systole. The C wave is caused by movement of the closed tricuspid valve during atrial diastole; the V wave is caused by atrial diastole. The negative waves are X, X′, and Y, with the X indicating relaxation, X′ atrioventricular movement, and Y passive right atrial emptying.

Right Ventricular (RV) Pressure. The ventricular waveform is demonstrated by a rapid rise representing isovolumetric contraction, followed by opening of the pulmonary valve with blood ejected from the RV into the pulmonary artery. With closure of the pulmonary valve, right ventricular pressure falls rapidly. The tricuspid valve opens with passive filling of the right ventricle from the right atrium.

Pulmonary Artery (PA) Pressure. Pulmonary artery (PA) systolic pressure represents right ventricular contraction; PA diastolic pressure reflects resistance to flow by small arterioles and pulmonary capillaries. When there is no pulmonary vascular obstruction, PA diastolic pressure is approximately the same as PCW pressure. A positive difference of 6 mmHg or more between PCW pressure and pulmonary diastole pressure indicates the presence of obstructive vascular disease in the lungs, such as pulmonary fibrosis, pulmonary embolus, or cor pulmonale. Therefore, a patient's PCW and PA diastolic pressure need to be correlated before it can be assumed that the PA diastolic pressure is providing an accurate reflection of pulmonary venous pressure, PCW, LAP, or left ventricular end-diastolic pressure (LVEDP). Pulmonary artery pressures are expressed in terms of systolic, diastolic, and mean pressures. A normal pulmonary artery pressure is 25/10 with a mean of 15 mmHg; a normal pulmonary capillary wedge pressure is in the range of 8 to 12 mmHg.

Pulmonary Capillary Wedge (PCW) Pressure. The pulmonary capillary wedge pressure obtained when the inflated catheter balloon occludes a branch of the pulmonary artery indicates (1) the presence and de-

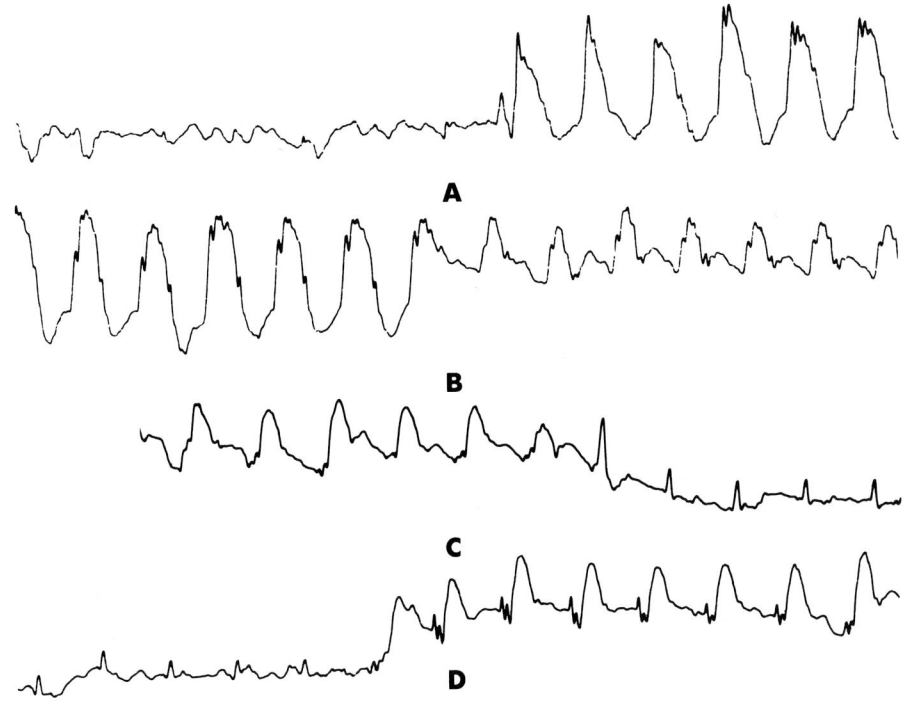

Figure 4-9 Waveforms during insertion of pulmonary artery catheter. *A,* Right atrium to right ventricle. *B,* Right ventricle to pulmonary artery. *C,* Pulmonary artery to pulmonary capillary wedge. *D,* Pulmonary capillary wedge to pulmonary artery.

gree of pulmonary congestion and (2) the performance of the left ventricle via mean left atrial and mean left ventricular diastolic pressure (in the absence of mitral valve disease). A normal PCW with a normal cardiac output indicates satisfactory ventricular performance.

The PCW waveform consists of A and V waves. The A wave indicates left atrial contraction during left ventricular relaxation. The V wave reflects left atrial relaxation during left ventricular contraction. A "giant V" wave can indicate mitral regurgitation. For maintenance of PA lines, it is essential to be able to differentiate between PA and PCW waveforms (see Figure 4-9).

Risks Associated with Vascular Lines

The three major risks associated with invasive vascular pressure monitoring are hemorrhage, thrombosis with emboli, and infections. These complications can be kept to a minimum when patients are under the care of a skilled critical care team with adequate instrumentation.

1. Bleeding back is the most obvious and most acute problem. The pressure of the systemic arterial system can cause rapid exsanguination through the 18- or 20-gauge cannula commonly used for arterial lines. Bleeding back is controlled by main-

taining the flush solution in a closed system at a pressure greater than the patient's systolic pressure. Any leak within the system, such as disconnected tubing or a stopcock in the wrong position, will cause bleeding back. It is essential that the alarm limits be set correctly and used to notify staff immediately of this complication.

2. Thrombus formation with the risk of emboli can be minimized by continuously flushing the vascular line with a mildly heparinized solution. The development of thrombus will cause dampening of the waveform and initiate an alarm condition.

3. To prevent infection, sterile techniques must be used for the insertion and maintenance of invasive lines. Disposable diaphragm domes are strictly for one-patient use. The resterilization and reuse of these disposable domes have resulted in death secondary to sepsis. The use of preassembled, sterile, disposable monitoring kits and premixed flush solution is recommended.

4. Evidence of infection at the cannulation site is an indication for cannula removal.
   See Table 4-2.
   Risks associated with pulmonary artery pressure monitoring include thrombosis, emboli, perforation of the pulmonary artery, pulmonary infarction, intracardiac knotting of the catheter, ventricular ar-

TABLE 4-2   Troubleshooting Invasive Lines

Problem	Cause	Intervention
Overdamping of waveform (usually results in false low systolic and false high diastolic readings)		
A. Bleeding back	Patient's pressure has become higher than counteracting pressure of flush solution.	If continual flush device is being used, counteracting pressure (i.e., pressure bag) should be at 300 mmHg.
	Loose connection in the system.	Check that all connections between patient and transducer are secure.
	Incorrect stopcock position.	Check stopcock positions. Flush line and check for a good waveform.
B. Air bubbles	Loose connection in system.	Check to be certain all connections are secure.
	Cracked stopcock, continuous flush device, or pressure tubing.	Change continuous flush device, pressure tubing, or stopcock with visible signs of damage.
	Pulling air into system during fast flushing with continuous flush device.	When using fast flush valve, watch drip chamber and control amount of valve pressure to prevent turbulence in drip chamber. Flush out all air bubbles between diaphragm of transducer and patient.
C. Clotting	Inadequate flush solution.	Adjust drip rate to 3 to 6 minidrops per minute (3 to 6 ml/hr). Flush using fast flush valve of continuous flush device. (If waveform remains damped, aspirate with a syringe. Do not reinject any aspirated blood, since it may include clots.)
Transducer will not balance	Damaged transducer.	Try another transducer.
	Transducer may be connected to wrong amplifier.	Check the amplifier connection.
	Broken amplifier.	Change amplifiers.
Drifting	Insufficient warm-up time.	Allow recommended time for transducer warm-up with power on.
	Air vents in cable may be kinked or compressed.	Make certain cable is not compressed.
False low reading	Overdamped signal.	Eliminate air bubbles and compliant system components.
	Transducer not balanced correctly. Positioned above pressure source.	Place transducer at heart level for vascular pressures and level of foramen of Monro for ICP, and rezero with transducer vented to air.
	Calibration incorrect.	Repeat balancing and calibration procedures.
False high reading	Underdamped signal.	Variable damping device.
	Transducer not balanced correctly. Positioned below pressure source.	Rebalance. For each foot of discrepancy between transducer and pressure source, there is an error of approximately 25 mmHg.
	Flush solution being administered too rapidly. A maximal continual flush during pressure measurement is 6 to 8 ml/hr.	Slow continual flush to 3 to 6 ml/hr.
	Air in the system.	Remove all air. At times, air in system will amplify pressure signal.

TABLE 4-2   **Troubleshooting Invasive Lines—cont'd**

Problem	Cause	Intervention
Cuff blood pressure different from direct blood pressure	Direct pressure is more accurate, particularly in hypotensive patients. Transducer pressure usually reads higher than cuff pressure.	None.
	Transducer measures systolic and diastolic from same heartbeat, whereas with cuff pressures systolic is taken from one beat and diastolic from another.	
	Low cardiac output and peripheral vasoconstriction make it difficult to hear indirect pressure.	
No waveform on oscilloscope	Transducer connected incorrectly.	Make certain transducer is securely connected and appropriate amplifier connector is used.
	Incorrect trace position.	Reposition trace.
	Cannula against vessel wall.	Reposition cannula.
	Incorrect gain setting.	Check to see that amplifier is not set on too low a gain.
	Damaged transducer.	Try another transducer.
	Broken amplifier.	Change amplifiers.
	Transducer not open to patient's pressure.	Check positions of stopcocks.
	Broken oscilloscope.	Replace oscilloscope.
Loss of ICP waveform	Occlusion of intracranial pressure measurement device.	Flush intracranial catheter or SA screw as directed by physician.
	Bent or broken fiberoptic catheter.	Replace fiberoptic catheter.
	Air between transducer diaphragm and pressure source.	Disconnect transducer and eliminate air from system.
Correlation of pressure readings taken with a water manometer to that taken with a transducer	Water manometers measure in cmH_2O, amplifiers usually display in mmHg.	Conversion: 1 mmHg = 1.36 cmH_2O.
Erratic or noisy traces	If a nonisolated transducer (exposed metal case) is in use, it may be secondary to electrical noise such as electrocautery.	Use an isolated transducer.
Erratic or noisy traces (continued)	May mean that moisture has entered the back of the transducer via venting tubes in cable.	Use a different transducer on patient. Check cable for evidence of cracks. If cracked, have it repaired.
		Moisture may be removed from transducer by:
		a. Placing transducer through aeration cycle of a gas sterilizing chamber.
		b. Several days at room temperature (not in use).
	Patient's movement.	Limit patient's movement. Use solid-state transducers.
Frequent damping of waveform	The cannula may have lodged against a vessel wall.	A slight alteration in position of cannula will sometimes resolve this.
	A clot may be forming.	This may be indicated by the ability to flush but not aspirate the line.
	Air may be trapped between transducer diaphragm and dome.	Follow manufacturer's instructions for debubbling.

rhythmias, sepsis, and balloon rupture. The risk can be minimized by careful insertion and maintenance of the PA line.

Air emboli can result from the direct injection of air into the proximal or distal ports and/or balloon rupture. The latex balloon tends to absorb lipoprotein from the blood, causing it to lose elasticity, thereby increasing the risk of balloon rupture. Fragments of the balloon may become emboli. Ideally, the catheter should be removed from the patient and discarded after approximately 48 hours.

PA catheters tend to be thrombinogenic. Continuous flushing of a heparinized solution through both distal and proximal lumens will aid in preventing thrombus formation. The development of thrombus at the lumens will be demonstrated as a damped waveform. Syringe flushing of the lumens may cause thrombotic emboli.

PA catheters may spontaneously advance into a wedge position without the balloon being inflated. If this occurs, it will be demonstrated on the monitor by a change in waveform from PA to wedge, a change in the mean pressure reading, and a drop in PA diastolic pressure. Leaving the balloon inflated for periods any longer than necessary for obtaining wedge readings may lead to pulmonary infarction.

Arrhythmias are often associated with catheter insertion and are resolved by correct placement or removal of the catheter. Should the catheter fall back into the right ventricle from the PA, ventricular tachycardia may occur. The ECG should be monitored during insertion and maintenance of the line to indicate arrhythmias. Pneumothorax and damage to the brachial plexus by direct trauma or bleeding have been reported with catheter insertions via the subclavian or internal jugular veins.

The frequency of wedge measurement should be limited to avoid trauma to the pulmonary artery vessel wall. In addition, care should be taken not to "over-wedge" the catheter. During balloon inflation, the oscilloscope should be watched. As soon as the waveform converts from a PA to a PCW pattern, inflation should be stopped and the volume used to inflate the balloon noted. This procedure minimizes trauma to the vessel and prevents false high or low pressure reading caused by overinflation of the balloon.

Direct and Indirect Blood Pressure Measurement

Systemic arterial blood presure, the force that perfuses the entire body with blood, is the cardiovascular parameter most commonly monitored. On an individual basis, variations in blood pressure (BP) may be caused by alterations in body posture; emotional or painful stimuli; muscular, cerebral, or gastrointestinal activity; environmental factors such as noise; and the use of tobacco, coffee, or other drugs with direct or neurally mediated vasomotor properties.

Blood pressure may be measured invasively (directly) or noninvasively (indirectly) to provide information on circulatory status and interaction between the heart and arterial system. Disparities routinely exist between direct and indirect blood pressure measurements, with indirect methods usually underestimating systolic pressure and over- or underestimating diastolic pressures. Henneman and Henneman state that "the relationship between blood pressure and blood flow, particularly in critically ill patients, suggests that it is unreasonable to expect that pressures obtained by direct monitoring methods will be the same as those derived by indirect methods that are flow dependent."[27] As noninvasive blood pressure has become more common and more sophisticated, many clinicians have tried to determine the accuracy of noninvasive devices by direct comparison with invasive systems.[28,29,30] It is not possible to include a full discussion of all factors that cause discrepancies between direct and indirect measurements, but it is important that clinicians practicing in areas where accurate blood pressures are an important part of determining patient management understand why these discrepancies occur. This requires a basic understanding of the effects of cardiovascular physiology, pathophysiology, and technology in both invasive and noninvasive pressure measurements.

A wide variety of invasive and noninvasive blood pressure devices are available. In selecting a device, it is important to consider why the blood pressure is being measured and what other parameters, such as arterial blood gas measurements, are required. For example, if a blood pressure device is being selected for use primarily with unstable patients who tend to have low blood pressure and require frequent blood sampling, one will probably want to use an invasive system that can measure pressure accurately in any range while providing access to arterial blood. For patients who are more apt to have pressures within the range of accuracy offered by noninvasive systems, and with infrequent need for access to arterial blood, a noninvasive device that offers decreased risk and cost would probably be more suitable. Other factors to consider are accuracy, ease of setup and use, troubleshooting, reliability, and durability, as well as the instructional support system provided by the manufacturer.

Variables that affect the accuracy of invasive blood pressure measurements include the dynamic response of the system (compliance, fluid mass, resistance), hydrostatic pressure, location of the arterial catheter, and patient-induced resonance. Variables that affect waveform interpretation and accuracy of noninvasive blood pressure measurements include cuff size and application; method of cuff inflation and deflation (step or linear); patient–transducer interface; distribution of tissue pressure; the technique used to determine mean arterial pressure, systole, and diastole; and the accuracy of trending.

Direct Systemic Arterial Blood Pressure

In critically ill hypertensive or hypotensive patients, alterations in cardiac output and peripheral vasoconstriction, combined with the inherent errors of the indirect method, cause measurement errors that could seriously distort blood pressure data. Such incorrect data could lead to inappropriate diagnosis and management. Indications for direct or invasive systemic arterial blood pressure monitoring include:

1. *Hypotension:* It is not always possible to obtain blood pressures indirectly in a patient in shock. Obviously the patient still has a pressure at this critical stage, and it is very important to be able to ascertain the pressure accurately. When the patient has a low stroke volume and a low cardiac output with excessive peripheral vasoconstriction, Korotkoff sounds may not be heard at all.

2. *Derived parameters:* The combining of arterial blood pressure values with other bedside parameters to develop hemodynamic profiles facilitates optimal, patient-specific therapeutic intervention.

3. *Vasoactive drug therapy:* The administration of drugs that markedly lower or raise blood pressure, such as sodium nitroprusside or dopamine, requires continual monitoring of pressure for safe, effective regulation.

4. *Blood sampling:* The need for frequent blood samples for measurement of PaO_2, $PaCO_2$, pH, and other parameters is a major indication for an arterial line. The placement of an arterial cannula leads to fewer complications than repeated needle punctures of an artery.

5. *Neurological conditions:* In patients with increased intracranial pressure (IICP), or the potential to develop it, measures are taken to maintain cerebral perfusion pressures (mean arterial pressure minus mean intracranial pressure) of at least 50 mmHg. In the patient with stroke, maintaining the mean arterial pressure at a level above 60 to 70 mmHg is believed to be helpful in preventing the loss of autoregulation mechanisms in areas of focal cerebral ischemia. Patients with acute cervical cord injuries are often hypotensive. An increase in blood pressure may be a sign that abnormal pressure is being exerted on the spinal cord. For example, a postoperative laminectomy patient may develop increased pressure on the cord from bleeding.

Catheter Insertion. The direct measurement of systolic, diastolic, and mean arterial blood pressure is usually done by cannulating the radial, brachial, or femoral arteries. Ordinarily, after suitable preparation of the skin, the cannula is placed percutaneously and sutured in place. Occasionally an arterial cutdown is required. Systemic arterial pressure may also be obtained via catheterization of the central aorta or the axillary or superficial temporal arteries.

Although the radial artery is small and anatomically unstable, it usually has good collateral circulation. It is routinely used for short-term (less than 24 hours) monitoring of patients after cardiac surgery. The patient's palmar arch should be assessed prior to insertion of the radial line. This can be done by using the Allen test, as described in the box below, a Doppler ultrasound device, or both. Prior to insertion of a radial line, the patient's wrist is restrained in a position of mild hyperextension to avoid kinking the cannula. A kinked cannula interferes with infusion of the continual flush solution.

An alternative insertion site is the brachial artery. This vessel is larger and more anatomically stable than the radial artery, with less collateral circulation. For patients requiring long-term monitoring or for the restless patient, the femoral artery is frequently used. This is a large, anatomically stable artery with minimal collateral circulation. Location of the arterial cannula affects both contour and values of arterial pressures. For example, systolic pressure obtained in the femoral artery may be 25 to 50 mmHg higher than pressure in the radial or brachial arteries. Little variation occurs in diastolic pressures.

Waveform. A normal arterial waveform consists of a sharp ascent during systole with a gradual descent

---

Allen Test Procedure

1. Simultaneously compress both the ulnar and radial arteries and open and close the hand to promote exsanguination. This takes approximately 1 minute.
2. Following release of one artery, usually the ulnar, there should be a blushing (reactive hyperemia) of the extended hand within 5 seconds.

This reactive hyperemia due to capillary refilling indicates adequate circulation to the hand. If blanching occurs, it is evidence of inadequate palmar arch circulation. A radial artery cannula placed in such a patient could lead to the complication of ischemia of the hand. A false-positive Allen test may occur with hyperextension of the fingers or wrist.

during diastole (Figure 4-10). The downstroke has a dicrotic notch, indicating closure of the aortic valve. The more distal the cannula is from the aorta, the sharper the upstroke and the less defined the dicrotic notch. The ascent during systole correlates with electrical depolarization of the ventricles as demonstrated in the ECG by the QRS complex. Delay between the QRS and systolic ascent can be caused by many factors. One of these is the distance between the cannulated vessel and the left ventricle. For example, more lag time will be noted between the QRS and the upstroke of the waveform if the cannula is in the femoral artery rather than in the central aorta. The dicrotic notch correlates with the T wave documenting the end of ventricular repolarization. Cardiac dysrhythmias can be reflected in alterations in the arterial pressure waveform (Figure 4-11). Other causes of waveform variations are the patient's clinical state, certain drugs, cardiac output, and vascular resistance,

as well as artificial pacemakers and artifacts in the monitoring system. Infrequently, inspirations and expirations affect the overall waveform pattern, particularly in the dehydrated patient (Figure 4-12).

Bedside Setup. A variety of satisfactory systems is available for direct blood pressure measurement. The components are usually preassembled in a sterile kit. The use of a monitoring kit and premixed heparin flush solution reduces the risk of setup contamination. Recent studies indicate that 0.9% sodium chloride may be as effective as heparinized saline in maintaining patency of intermittent flush devices.[31]

After the system has been connected to the patient's vascular catheter, it is flushed by activating the fast flush valve, and the waveform is checked for any sign of over- or underdamping. The minidrop rate should be verified at 3 to 6 minidrops per minute (3 to 6 ml/hr) and the pressure infusor at 300 mmHg.

Noninvasive Blood Pressure Measurement

Noninvasive blood pressure (NIBP) devices, available for both intermittent and continuous blood pressure monitoring, may be classified as manual or automatic.

Manual Techniques

Auscultation. The most common manual noninvasive method of obtaining a blood pressure is the auscultatory technique, using a standard sphygmomanometer and stethoscope. This method is based on Korotkoff sounds, the tapping sounds that become audible as the occluding pressure in the blood pressure cuff declines, allowing blood to pass through the artery under the cuff. The accuracy of this standard procedure is affected by the equipment, cuff size, technique, impedance of peripheral blood flow, high pe-

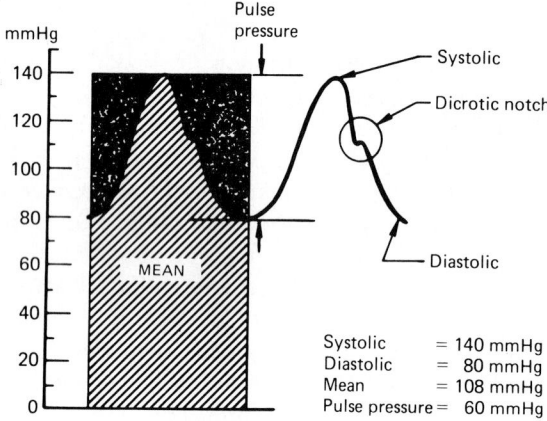

Figure 4-10 Typical arterial pressure waveform.

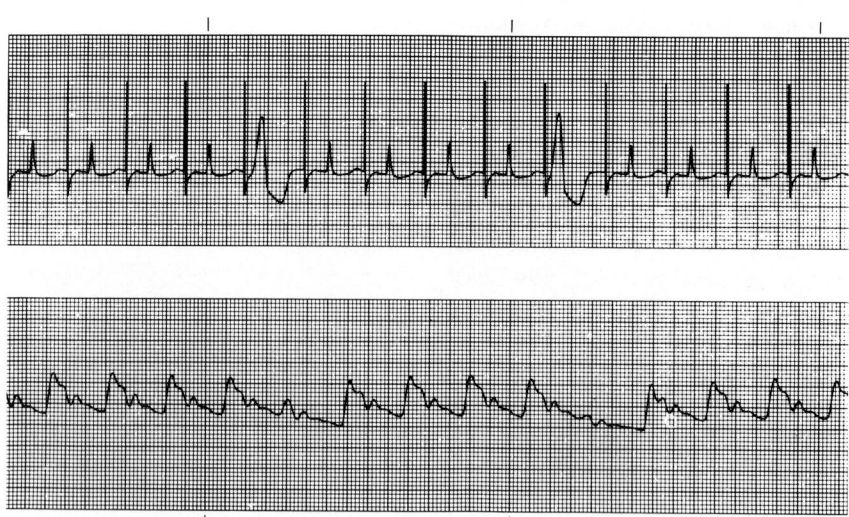

Figure 4-11 Effect of PVC on arterial pressure waveform demonstrating decreased stroke volume (paper speed 25 mm/sec).

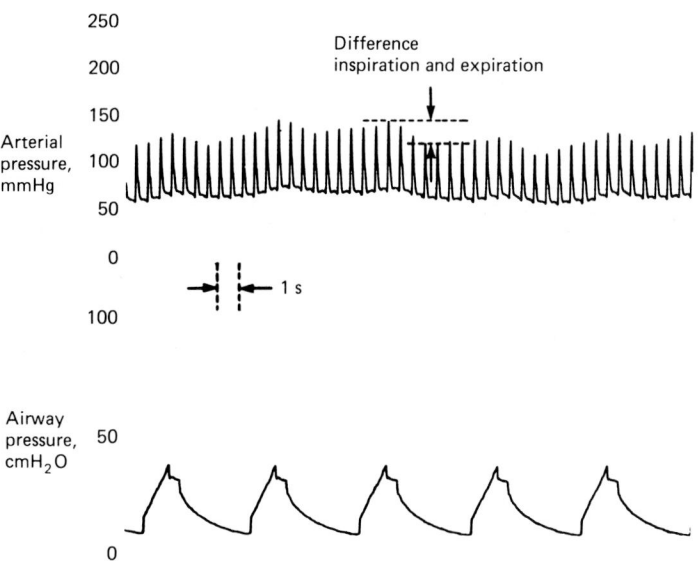

Figure 4-12 Effect of airway pressure on arterial pressure (paper speed 5 mm/sec).

ripheral vascular resistance, patients receiving axillary infusions of vasopressors, obesity, and severe peripheral edema.

Palpation. The manual palpation technique is similar to auscultation but is not dependent on blood flow and does not require the generation of Korotkoff sounds. As the cuff is deflated to just below the systolic level, a spurt of blood passes through the brachial artery under the cuff. At the peak of systole, a weak pulse can be felt at the wrist by palpating the radial artery.

Automatic Techniques

During the last few years, a variety of automatic noninvasive blood pressure measurement techniques have been introduced. It should be remembered that with noninvasive devices that employ inflation and deflation of pressure cuffs, factors that affect the accuracy of standard manual sphygmomanometers systems still apply. For example, the correct cuff width is 120% to 150% of the diameter of the extremity being measured. The cuff bladder should be one half to two thirds of the extremity circumference, with the cuff snugly applied but not occlusive. When the cuff is too large, false low measurements are obtained, whereas false high measurements are seen with cuffs that are too small. To improve accuracy, color-coded sizes of bladderless cuffs are now available.

Oscillometric Method. The most common automatic, noninvasive method of obtaining intermittent blood pressure measurements is the oscillometric method (Figure 4-13). This method, available since 1976, is used when the need for frequent blood pressure determinations is expected to be relatively brief

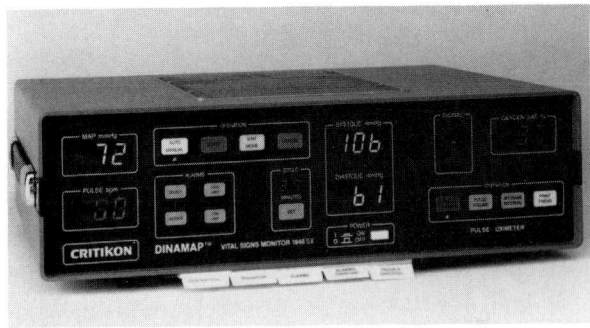

Figure 4-13 Noninvasive Blood Pressure (NIBP). Automatic, oscillometric, noninvasive blood pressure monitor with pulse oximeter. DINAMAP Blood Pressure Monitor with OXYTRAK Pulse Oximeter. Courtesy of CRITIKON.

and the need for arterial blood sampling is expected to be minimal or absent. The oscillometric method uses a double air bladder enclosed in a cuff and applied in the conventional way. The proximal bladder is inflated to occlude blood flow while residual air is maintained in the distal bladder. Systolic blood pressure is indicated at the point where pulsations are first detected, mean arterial pressure at the point where maximum oscillations occur, and diastolic pressure at the point where oscillations disappear. The values are digitally displayed. Although oscillometric devices may be set to obtain very frequent blood pressure determinations (such as one per minute), this may cause tissue ischemia with discomfort and pain experienced by the patient.

Oscillometric systems are available as stand-alone monitors or as combination monitors with pulse ox-

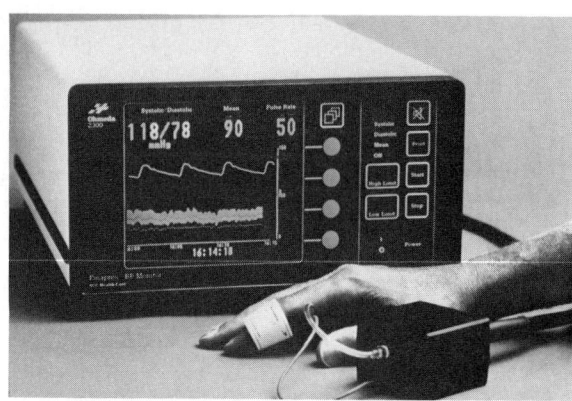

Figure 4-14 Continuous Noninvasive Blood Pressure (CNIBP). A small blood pressure cuff is placed around a finger and inflated to a pressure that equals the pressure in the artery, until the artery is just about to collapse. The arterial diameter under the cuff varies with changes in intra-arterial pressure. The cuff pressure changes to the same degree as the intraarterial pressure, maintainig a dynamic, constant pressure difference over the arterial wall known as the transmural pressure. Based on the Penaz method, a photoplethysmograph continuously measures the arterial diameter under the cuff, providing calibrated, continuous, automatic blood pressure measurements with a calibrated blood pressure waveform.
Finapres System, Courtesy of Ohmeda.

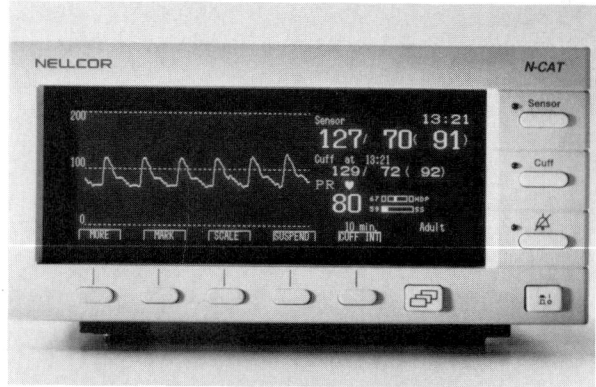

Figure 4-15 Continuous Noninvasive Blood Pressure (CNIBP). With this continuous, arterial tonometry technique, an array of very small doazoelectric pressure transducers strapped over the wrist measure the pressure change (amplitude) in the radial artery. The pulse pressure is calibrated to a standard oscillometric measurement obtained from a brachial artery oscillometric cuff that is an integral part of this continuous BP measurement monitoring system. Systolic, diastolic, and mean arterial pressures are measured with a display of the arterial waveform and real time trending.
N-CAT, Courtesy of Nellcor.

imetry, ECG, temperature and invasive pressure. Many noninvasive blood pressure devices incorporate use of the oscillometric method of blood pressure determination by cuff. For example, one system combines radial artery tonometry (transducer array) with intermittent oscillometric cuff measurements to provide arterial waveforms and real-time trending between intermittent oscillometric measurements.

Doppler (Acoustic) Method. Two methods are used in currently available devices. One detects motion of the blood vessel wall; the other method detects blood flow. The blood flow detection technique may be used during low flow, hypotensive states for spot checks to magnify the Korotkoff sounds.

Continuous Method. New blood pressure monitoring technologies make it possible to obtain accurate, continuous, noninvasive, arterial blood pressure measurements with waveform documentation (Figures 4-14 and 4-15). To determine system accuracy and appropriate clinical applications, an understanding of the methods and the variables affecting them is essential. Noninvasive techniques available at present include tonometry/oscillometry, pulse wave velocity measurement/oximetry, pulse pressure calibration, and the Penaz method which consists of a photoelectric plethysmograph mounted in an inflatable cuff and an electropneumatic transducer that controls air pressure in the cuff by a servosystem.

Cardiac Output/Cardiac Index (CO/CI)

Cardiac output, expressed in liters per minute, is the amount of blood pumped by the heart. It is the product of heart rate and stoke volume (the amount of blood ejected with each heartbeat). *Cardiac index* is the cardiac output per square meter of body surface area (height and weight). A small person requires less circulating blood and, therefore, less cardiac output than a larger person. By calculating the cardiac output and then computing the cardiac index according to the individual's height and weight, a more specific and useful measurement is available.

The intermittent measurement of cardiac output is essential to determine a patient's response to drugs that affect the heart and the blood vessels. With the aid of cardiac output measurements, a patient's response to a given therapeutic program can be recognized and alternative methods of therapy selected if the response is not satisfactory.

Techniques

Both invasive and noninvasive techniques are available for the measurement of cardiac output. Although there has been a slight increase in the use of noninvasive methods, application in critical care has been limited by the level of skill and experience required to use these expensive, somewhat complex devices and the difficulty of interpreting data expressed in bioimpedance terms. One noninvasive method of determining cardiac output is by changes in thoracic electrical impedance. An alternating current applied to the chest determines impedance changes caused by alterations in the distribution of blood within the chest during systole and diastole. Impedance changes are related directly to changes in cardiac stroke volume. Stroke volume is calculated by formulas that include body temperature, distance between electrodes, hematocrit, and left ventricular ejection time. Since cardiac output equals heart rate times stroke volume, the calculated stroke volume is multiplied by the heart rate to determine cardiac output noninvasively. Correlations between this and other noninvasive methods and invasively measured cardiac output have been variable.[29,32] Additional studies are being done to determine the accuracy and limitations of this noninvasive method.

The most suitable procedure and the one most commonly used to determine cardiac output on the critically ill patient is thermodilution, an invasive technique. The technique was introduced by Fegler in 1954 but did not become clinically applicable until the development of the balloon-tipped, flow-directed catheter by Swan and Ganz in 1970. A multilumen, multipurpose balloon-tipped catheter is inserted into the vena cava through the right side of the heart and into the patient's pulmonary artery. A bolus of cool solution, either D_5W or normal saline, is injected into the right atrium via the proximal port of the catheter. As venous mixing occurs, primarily in the right ventricle, the temperature of the injectate is altered. A thermistor bead (small thermometer) located near the tip of the catheter, which is in the pulmonary artery, measures the change in the temperature of the blood caused by the injection. A cardiac output computer, using the amount of temperature change that has occurred between the injection into the right atrium and the flow through the pulmonary artery, calculates the cardiac output in liters per minute. Using the patient's height, weight, and cardiac output, the cardiac index is determined.

This procedure requires:
1. A flow-directed thermodilution catheter
2. A monitoring system
3. Injectate (saline, D_5W)
4. A thermodilution cardiac output computer, preferably with recorder

A balloon-tipped, flow-directed catheter is prepared for insertion. This includes testing the integrity of the balloon under solution, testing the thermistor by attaching it to the cardiac output computer, filling all lumens with heparinized flush solution, and attaching the catheter to the monitoring system. The catheter must be kept sterile during these procedures.

The minimal requirements for a safe system for the insertion of the catheter into the pulmonary artery include a two-channel oscilloscope, an ECG amplifier, and at least one pressure amplifier and transducer. The transducer set-up is similar to that of an arterial line. The only difference is that the catheter is attached to the transducer system and filled before insertion. In this way the pressure waveforms can be used to identify the location of the catheter tip within the heart during and after insertion.

For measuring cardiac output, room temperature injectate is usually preferable to iced injectate. It provides more accurate cardiac output measurements because less heat absorption occurs during injection and it is easier to prepare with less risk of contamination. Because of the proximity of the pulmonary artery to the lungs, there are times when a greater temperature differential between the blood and the injectate is necessary. Conditions that usually necessitate the use of iced injectate include cardiac output greater than 10 L/min, dilated cardiomyopathy, patients receiving mechanical ventilation, and patients with erratic respiratory patterns such as Cheyne-Stokes.

A variety of injectate delivery systems is available. It has been noted that closed injectate systems are cost-effective and significantly decrease the incidence of contamination.

Cardiac Output/Cardiac Index Computers and Catheters

Computers are available in modular, stand-alone, and combination monitoring configurations. A large variety of multilumen, multifunction PA catheters are also available. Ideally, the computer should be able to display cardiac output in liters per minute, and the temperature of the patient and the injectate in degrees Celsius or Fahrenheit.

The computer should have a test cycle so that the accuracy of the instrument can be verified before the procedure is begun on the patient. Alarms may indicate a low battery, faulty catheter, broken interface cable, or incorrect injectate temperature or volume. The computer is corrected for the size of the catheter being used, the number of centimeters inserted, whether iced or room temperature injectate is used, and the warming of the injectate by the patient's body temperature (computation constant).

Cardiac output systems are now available for the assessment of both right and left heart performance. One such combination monitor is the ejection fraction cardiac output computer. When used with a volumetric thermodilution catheter with intracardiac electrodes (right ventricular and PA), the monitor obtains right ventricular (RV) function parameters in addition to cardiac output and index. Right ventricular parameters obtained include RV ejection fraction, a prime determinant of left ventricular preload; RV stroke volume; RV end-diastolic volume; heart rate indices; and RV end-systolic volume. Indications for these measurements include increased pulmonary vascular resistance (PEEP, sepsis, pulmonary embolus, disease), right or left ventricular dysfunction, volume disturbances (burns, fluid imbalance), and major cardiothoracic surgical procedures.

Thermal Curve

Usually a 5 mm/sec recorder is used to record the thermal curve (Figure 4-16). The curve is very useful in determining the accuracy of the cardiac output measurements. Many CO monitors now display the curve on the oscilloscope. Ordinarily, a series of four injections is done, with the first being discarded. If room temperature injectate is used, the bolus is injected into the proximal right atrial port at 1-minute intervals. For iced injectate, 1½-minute intervals are used. Three measurements are made to allow for normal variations in the patient's heart rate and stroke volume. If one cardiac output value is significantly different from the others, the cause may be determined by evaluation of the thermal curve. An inverse correlation exists between the area under the curve and the patient's cardiac output. In other words, the greater the area under the curve, the lower the cardiac output. Fluctuations in the baseline of the curve may be the result of respiratory irregularities.

Guidelines

1. Prior to measurement, the position of the catheter in the pulmonary artery should be determined to ensure that the thermistor is not lodged against a vessel wall. This can be done by inflating the balloon and determining exactly the volume required to convert the PA waveform into a PCW. If less than 75% of maximum balloon volume is required, the catheter is too far advanced in the pulmonary artery for correct cardiac output determination, although it may be satisfactory for routine monitoring of PA and PCW.
2. Prior to the first measurement, the right atrial lumen is flushed with the same temperature and volume of injectate to be used for the following injections. Wait 1 minute if using room temperature injectate and 1½ minutes after iced. The maximum injection volume for a 7 French catheter is 10 ml; for a 5 French, 5 ml.
3. Make certain the volumes in the syringes are the same and inject as rapidly and smoothly as possible at the 1- or 1½-minute intervals for a series of three measurements.
4. Low or erratic measurements may be due to lodg-

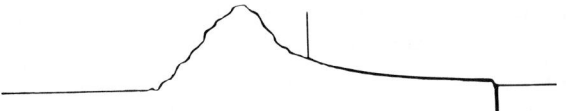

Figure 4-16   Cardiac output thermal curve trace (paper speed 5 mm/sec).

ing of the thermistor against a vessel wall or thrombus formation over the thermistor bead.
5. When possible, all IV solution should be reduced to keep-open rates for 3 to 5 minutes prior to and during the cardiac output determinations.

Respiratory and Blood Gas Monitoring

Overview of O_2/CO_2 Transport

Since the cardiopulmonary system must maintain a balance between oxygen delivery ($\dot{D}O_2$) and oxygen consumption ($\dot{V}O_2$) to sustain life, the continuous assessment of cardiopulmonary function is an important component of critical care.[33] Clinical assessment of cardiopulmonary function is aided by the use of bedside arterial blood gas measurements (ABGs) and bedside monitors designed to measure SpO_2, $S\bar{v}O_2$, $ETCO_2$ and rSO_2.[34-41] The delivery of oxygen (O_2) to the tissue is dependent on three variables: (1) the amount of functional hemoglobin in the blood, (2) the saturation of the hemoglobin with oxygen, and (3) the delivery of the saturated hemoglobin molecule, known as oxyhemoglobin, to the tissue. Clinically, oxygen and carbon dioxide tensions, acid–base balance, and the amount of hemoglobin in the arterial blood are determined by obtaining an arterial blood sample; the amount of hemoglobin saturated with oxygen is determined from an arterial blood sample (SaO_2) or by a pulse oximeter (SpO_2) and the delivery of oxygenated blood to the tissue level is determined by obtaining a cardiac output measurement. Approximately 98% to 99% of the oxygen transported to tissue is bonded to hemoglobin and measured as saturation (SaO_2, SpO_2, $S\bar{v}O_2$). The remaining 1% to 2% of oxygen is dissolved in plasma and measured as oxygen tension (PaO_2, PvO_2). This small amount of oxygen dissolved in plasma affects the oxygen saturation of hemoglobin.

In the normal adult, one liter of blood carries approximately 200 ml of oxygen. Therefore, with a normal cardiac output of 5 L per minute, as much as one liter of oxygen is delivered to the tissue per minute. At the tissue level, when oxygen delivery is adequate, the amount of oxygen consumed equals the amount of oxygen demanded or required. Normal body tissue consumes approximately 250 ml of the 1,000 ml of oxygen delivered by arterial blood per minute, with the remaining 750 milliliters being returned by venous blood to the right side of the heart. In the right ventricle, the venous blood returned to the right atrium by the inferior vena cava and superior vena cava mixes, passing into the pulmonary artery as mixed venous blood. Clinically, the amount of hemoglobin saturated with oxygen in the mixed venous blood is determined from a pulmonary artery blood sample or by pulmonary artery oximetry ($S\bar{v}O_2$).

As the mixed venous blood passes through the lungs for reoxygenation, CO_2 is released. CO_2 measurements may be obtained from blood samples, or by capnography ($ETCO_2$). Noninvasive measurements of regional saturation of the hemoglobin in the brain are obtained by a cerebral oximeter (rSO_2). A detailed description of each of these blood gas monitoring technologies follows.

Bedside Arterial Blood Gas Analysis (ABGs)

Arterial blood gas (ABG) measurements provide information on the adequacy of oxygenation, ventilation, and acid–base balance. They are indicated in patients when abnormalities in pH, $PaCO_2$, and PaO_2 are anticipated and are useful in determining whether observed symptoms are caused by the original disorder or by the patient's compensatory efforts. Alterations in arterial blood gases may be caused by abnormal gas exchange mechanisms including hypoventilation, impaired diffusion, shunting, and ventilation–perfusion inequality.

Until recently, blood gas samples were routinely sent to a laboratory for analysis. Portable, microprocessor-based systems with rechargeable battery packs and integral printers to provide hard copies of measured and calculated values are now available for intermittent bedside blood gas analysis on patients with arterial catheters (Figure 4-17). These precalibrated, easy-to-use systems provide rapid availability of blood gas data while reducing the risk of exposure to patient blood.

For continuous intraarterial blood gas monitoring, an optical sensor, or optode, may be placed through a 20-gauge arterial catheter, extending slightly beyond the tip of the catheter. Using a Y-site, arterial pressure waveforms may still be monitored and arterial blood samples obtained with the optode in place. By a method based on fiberoptic spectroscopy (similar to the method used in fiberoptic pulmonary artery or intracranial pressure systems), light is used to monitor chemical changes in the body. The sensor can monitor PaO_2, $PaCO_2$, and pH for up to 96 hours. Periodic calibrations are required in this system to compensate for "drift" (erroneous readings). "Drift" may be caused by the formation of fibrin or thrombus

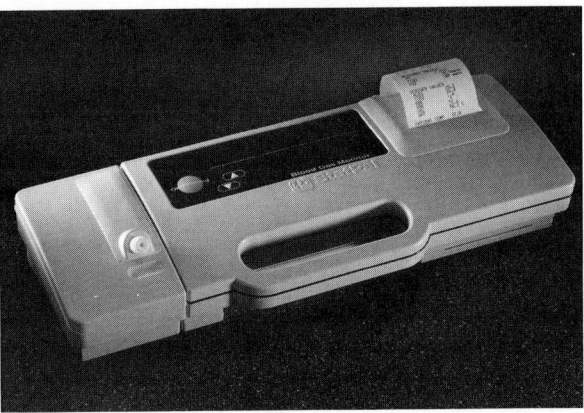

Figure 4-17 Portable bedside blood gas analysis system. A sample of arterial blood is injected into a disposable, precalibrated sensor module. Within 60 seconds, pH, PO_2, and $PaCO_2$ are displayed, with measured and calculated parameters available as a printout.
StatPal II, Courtesy of PPG Industries, Inc.

on the catheter, or by damage to the fiberoptic catheter or an electronic change in the system.

Oximetry

Oximeters measure blood oxygen saturation by quantitating the difference in color of blood caused by either absorption or reflection of light by oxygenated hemoglobin (oxyhemoglobin, HbO_2) and reduced hemoglobin (deoxyhemoglobin, Hb). Four types of oximetry are used with critically ill patients: (1) intermittent laboratory determinations of the oxygen saturation levels in both arterial and venous blood samples (CO-oximetry), (2) noninvasive, continuous monitoring of the arterial saturation of hemoglobin (pulse oximetry, SpO_2), (3) invasive, continuous determinations of mixed venous oxygen saturations (pulmonary artery oximetry, $S\bar{v}O_2$) and (4) cerebral oximetry (rSO_2).

CO-oximetry. Blood gases may be analyzed by laboratory co-oximeters, sometimes referred to as carbon monoxide oximeters. These instruments use a multiple-wavelength technique to determine fractional saturation. They measure all hemoglobins, including dysfunctional hemoglobins such as methemoglobin (MetHb) and the carboxyhemoglobin (COHb) that results from carbon monoxide (CO), as seen with smokers. Bedside pulse oximeters have a two-wavelength technique, using red and infrared light to determine the functional saturation. Bedside functional saturations provide information on the ratio of oxygenated (HbO_2) to reduced or deoxygenated hemoglobin (Hb). Laboratory CO-oximeter fractional saturations provide information on the ratio of oxygenated hemoglobin to all hemoglobins. It is important to remember that readings obtained by laboratory CO-oximeters will not be exactly the same as readings obtained by pulse (arterial) and pulmonary artery (venous) oximetry.

Pulse Oximeter:
$$SpO_2 = \frac{HbO_2}{HbO_2 + Hb}$$

CO-Oximeter:
$$SaO_2 = \frac{HbO_2}{HbO_2 + Hb + COHb + MetHb}$$

Pulse Oximetry (SpO_2). A pulse oximeter is a device that provides noninvasive measurements of the percentage of oxygen saturation of hemoglobin in arterial blood. It indicates the relative concentrations of oxyhemoglobin and reduced or deoxyhemoglobin by quantifying the amount of light transmitted through the blood and tissue. The amount of arterial saturation (SaO_2) measured by pulse oximetry is identified as SpO_2.

The interface between the adult, pediatric, and neonatal patient and the monitor is provided by a variety of sensors or probes. These are available in both disposable and reusable configurations. Short- and long-term SpO_2 monitoring may be done from the fingers, toes, hands, feet, forehead, ears, or the bridge of the nose. Pulse oximeters are available as modular components of central monitoring systems, as stand-alone instruments, and in combination monitors (Figure 4-18).

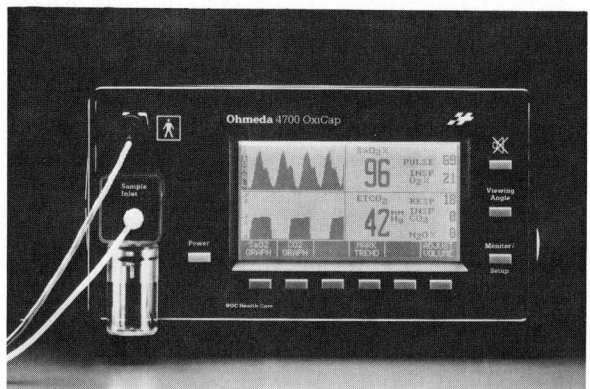

Figure 4-18 Example of a combination monitor used for simultaneously assessing oxygenation and ventilation, while providing an indication of changes in arterial pressure and perfusion. It continuously monitors SaO_2, inspired O_2, and pulse rate with an arterial waveform. The continuous capnography reading is accompanied by a CO_2 waveform, respiratory rate, and inspired CO_2. Both real time and end-tidal CO_2 trends are displayed.
OxiCap, Courtesy of Ohmeda.

Theory. The measurement of arterial oxygen saturation by pulse oximetry is based on two technologies, optical plethysmography and spectrophotometry. When a sensor or probe is placed on the patient, for example on the finger, pulsatile arterial blood flow is detected by optical plethysmography, a technique that displays a waveform from pulsatile blood. The arterial hemoglobin saturation is measured by spectrophotometry, a technique that quantifies the amount of transmitted light. The sensor contains two light emitters that shine red and infrared light through the pulsatile arterial blood and tissues, in this example a finger, to a photodetector on the opposite side of the finger. The photodetector measures the amount of red and infrared light not absorbed by the blood, bone, and tissue in the finger and converts it into a reading indicating the percentage of arterial hemoglobin saturated with oxygen.

Troubleshooting. For pulse oximetry (SpO_2) readings to be accurate, it is important to remember that pulse oximetry technology is based on the following assumptions:
1. Pulses are arterial.
2. All light emitted by the sensor passes through pulsatile vascular beds.
3. There is an adequate functional hemoglobin concentration in the arterial blood.
4. No extraneous dyes are present.

This means that correct sensor and probe application is essential, and that SpO_2 readings will be affected in patients who have dysfunctional hemoglobins, such as carboxyhemoglobin with carbon monoxide poisoning, or in patients who have had diagnostic studies involving dye injection.

Application. Pulse oximetry (SpO_2) readings provide information on the amount of oxygen available for delivery to the tissues. A normal arterial oxygen saturation (SaO_2, SpO_2) at sea level is 95%. The percentage decreases as altitude increases. For example, a normal SaO_2 at an altitude of 5,000 feet is 92%. By detecting hypoxemia, a deficiency of O_2 in arterial blood, the SpO_2 warns of hypoxia, inadequate oxygen at the tissue level. A sudden change in the SpO_2 reading provides an early warning of alterations in O_2 delivery, warning of the need to assess the patient immediately. For example, a drop in SpO_2 occurs when the patient is not receiving adequate O_2, as seen with a ventilator disconnection; when there is interference with oxygenation, as during endotracheal suctioning; or when there is interference with the delivery of oxygenated blood to the tissue level, as with decreased cardiac output during acute myocardial infarction.

Pulmonary Artery Oximetry (S$\bar{v}O_2$). Mixed venous oxygen saturation (S$\bar{v}O_2$) measurements, obtained via an invasive pulmonary artery catheter, provide a means of assessing how well the body's compensatory mechanisms have responded to assure that oxygen supply meets oxygen demand. Whereas SpO_2 measurements provide information on the overall adequacy of the delivery of oxygenated blood to the tissues, $S\bar{v}O_2$ measurements provide information on the overall adequacy of tissue oxygenation.

The interface between the patient and the monitor is provided by a balloon-tipped, flow-directed, fluid-filled fiberoptic catheter positioned in the mixed venous blood in the pulmonary artery. In addition to obtaining $S\bar{v}O_2$ measurements, this catheter is usually used for hemodynamic monitoring of pulmonary artery and wedge pressures and measurements of cardiac output and cardiac index by the thermodilution method.

Theory. A fiberoptic bundle in the pulmonary artery (PA) catheter transmits light to and from red blood cells flowing past the distal tip of the catheter. By means of reflection spectrophotometry, the relative intensity or color of reflected light is analyzed and converted into a reading indicating the amount of venous hemoglobin saturated with oxygen.

Troubleshooting. For venous oximetry ($S\bar{v}O_2$) readings to be accurate, the light and sensors in the tip of the PA catheter must "see" flowing mixed venous blood. This means that the PA catheter must be positioned in the pulmonary artery so that the tip is not against the vessel wall; not in an area of stagnant blood flow, as seen with balloon or spontaneous wedging; and not covered by a clot or debris. The accuracy of the readings is also affected by high and low (less than 25%) hematocrit values and by calibration errors.

Application. Venous oximetry ($S\bar{v}O_2$) provides information on the overall adequacy of tissue oxygenation. Readings in the normal range of 60% to 80% usually indicate a balance between oxygen supply and oxygen demand. An $S\bar{v}O_2$ that decreases by at least 10% from the previous measurement, a reading of less than 60%, or both indicate decreased oxygen delivery ($\dot{D}O_2$), as documented by the pulse oximeter, or increased O_2 consumption ($\dot{V}O_2$). With low $S\bar{v}O_2$ readings, clinical interventions are based on increasing the amount of oxygen delivered, decreasing the amount of oxygen demanded or consumed at the tissue level, or both.

Cerebral Oximetry (rSO_2). A cerebral oximeter provides noninvasive measurements of regional oxygen saturation (rSO_2) of the hemoglobin in the brain. Brain oximetry is used to indicate the risk of cerebral hypoxemia or ischemia in adult patients. Like other types of oximeters currently in use, the cerebral oximeter displays real-time saturation and trend data

and provides printouts. The interface between the adult patient and the monitor is provided by a disposable sensor. The sensor should not be placed over a sinus or a hematoma.

Theory. The measurement of cerebral oxygen saturation is based on infrared optical spectroscopy. Infrared light can penetrate several centimeters through scalp, skull, and cranial contents.

Application. The region and depth of the brain being measured is determined by placement of the light source and sensors on the scalp. Since the intracranial microvasculature is composed of approximately 75% venous, 20% arterial, and 5% capillary blood, cerebral oxygen saturation readings differ from arterial oximetry (SpO_2) values. Whereas a normal SpO_2 reading is approximately 95%, a normal rSO_2 reading is approximately 73%. Readings are not affected by low blood pressure, hypothermia, or cardiac arrest.[42]

Capnography ($ETCO_2$, $PETCO_2$). Capnography is the noninvasive, continuous measurement and graphical display of the carbon dioxide concentration, or partial pressure, at the patient's airway. It provides a means of evaluating "the overall balance between production of CO_2, transport of CO_2, regional changes in ventilation, changes in total alveolar ventilation, and problems with the ventilatory circuit."[39] A normal, stable capnogram (waveform) indicates an equilibrium between carbon dioxide production and transport and alveolar ventilation. A healthy adult at rest produces CO_2 at 200 ml/min.

The interface between the patient and the monitor varies according to the type of monitor (mainstream or sidestream) and whether or not the patient is intubated. With intubated patients, gas samples are obtained directly from the airway. For nonintubated patients, expired gas samples may be obtained with specially designed nasal prongs. Although these look similar to prongs used for O_2 administration, one of the prongs is used only for obtaining CO_2 samples from one of the nares. Capnography monitors are available in modular, stand-alone, and combination monitoring configurations.

Theory. The measurement of exhaled CO_2 by capnography is based on infrared absorption spectroscopy. The amount of red light absorbed by a sample of the CO_2 exhaled by the patient during the ventilatory cycle is converted into a graphical wavelength display of inhaled and exhaled CO_2, with a numeric reading in mmHg.

Troubleshooting. A common misconception is that the end-tidal PCO_2 ($PETCO_2$) measured by capnography is the same as arterial PCO_2 ($PaCO_2$). The difference between $PETCO_2$ measurements and $PaCO_2$ measurements in blood gases reflects the amount of dead space ventilation and is referred to as a gradient. In persons with normal lung function, the exhaled PET_{CO_2} is usually 1 to 5 mmHg less than the arterial blood Pa_{CO_2}. The gradient, or difference between the two values, increases in patients with lung disease, probably because of changes in ventilation or perfusion. The accuracy of the readings is dependent on good sampling techniques. Moisture and debris, such as secretions, in exhaled gas samples tend to make the capnograph inaccurate or nonfunctional.

Carbon dioxide waveforms may be difficult to interpret in the ICU because of: (1) marked changes in breath-to-breath tidal volume during spontaneous ventilation; (2) changes in CO_2 production with changes in metabolic rate, and (3) changes in dead space/tidal volume ratio.

Application. A normal end-tidal CO_2 (end-exhalation) reading is approximately 38 mmHg. Carbon dioxide production is increased with fever and sepsis and decreased by hypothermia, muscular relaxation, and increased depth of anesthesia. Changes in CO_2 dynamics may indicate the onset of ventilatory acidosis and aid in the clinical assessment of a patient being weaned from ventilatory support.

Pulmonary Monitoring

Significant advances have occurred in bedside respiratory monitoring. The continuous measurement of respiratory mechanics in the critically ill patient can provide indications of pending respiratory failure, evaluate the effectiveness of bronchodilator therapy on airway resistance or intrinsic PEEP, and facilitate information for efficient ventilator management and timely weaning.[43] Pulmonary mechanics monitoring of the acute care patient provides continuous measurement of flow, airway, and esophageal pressures (Figures 4-19 and 4-20).

Work of Breathing. Respiratory work of breathing measures patient effort during mechanical ventilation. It may be used for spontaneous or for assisted, patient-initiated breaths. Normal work of breathing is 0.45 to 0.65 joules per liter (J/L). Ventilator dependence is probable if work of breathing exceeds 0.75 joules per liter. Successful weaning is likely when work is less than 0.70 J/L.

Intrinsic PEEP. During mechanical ventilation, air trapped in the alveoli at positive end-expiration (PEEP) can increase the risk of barotrauma, compromise cardiac output, and lead to difficulty in ventilator weaning. Monitoring of esophageal and airway pressures in conjunction with flow provides continuous assessment of intrinsic PEEP. Intrinsic PEEP may be caused by high ventilator rate settings; shallow, rapid breathing; obstructed airways; occluded or incorrectly sized endotracheal tubes; and increased patient/ventilator circuit resistance (Figure 4-21).

Some ventilators incorporate components or may be adapted to interface with a computer system to provide graphical and digital pulmonary data. Hand-held pulmonary function/ventilation monitors are available to monitor extubation parameters such as respiration rate (RR), tidal volume (TV), minute volume (MV), and forced exhalation parameters such as forced vital capacity (FVC) and peak flow. Critical care applications include preextubation evaluation and ventilator weaning measurements.

Respiratory Rate/Apnea. Respiratory rate may be continuously monitored by means of the principle of impedance pneumography. Two electrodes are placed on the patient's chest, approximately midaxillary at

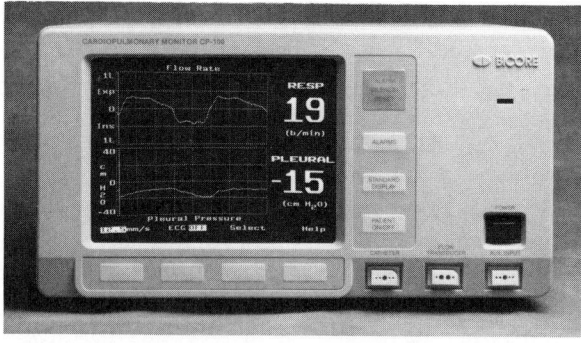

Figure 4-19 Cardiopulmonary Monitor for the continuous measurement of respiratory mechanics including work of breathing, respiratory drive, and pulmonary mechanics.

Courtesy of Bicore Monitoring Systems.

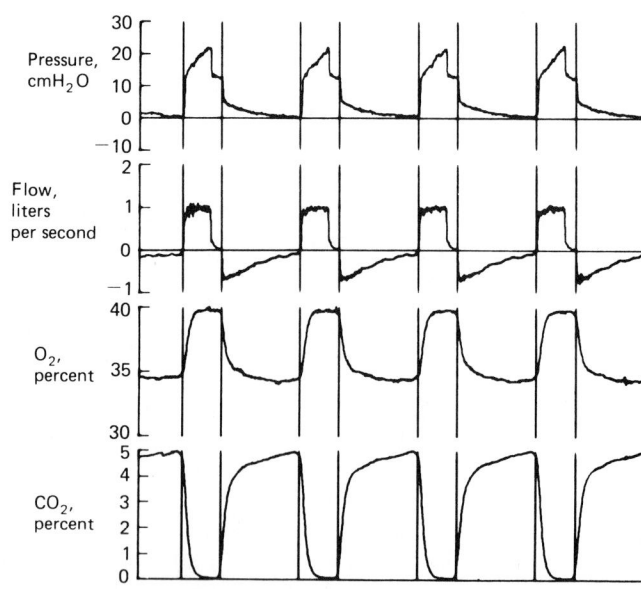

Figure 4-20 Computer-acquired respiratory waveforms.

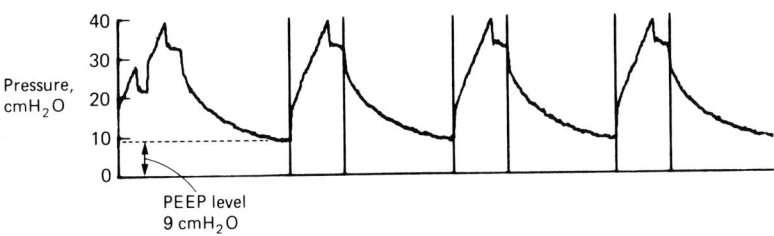

Figure 4-21 Airway pressure with PEEP.

the level of maximal chest excursion. An ECG signal may also be obtained. A respiratory amplifier displays the respiratory rate, and a respiratory waveform may be displayed on an oscilloscope and/or recorder. Amplifiers with audible alarms are available which indicate periods of apnea as well as respiratory rate. Impedance apnea monitors are available in combination with a pulse oximeter, providing respiratory rate, oxygen saturation, and heart rate data. Impedance chest wall monitoring is available with many ICU cardiac monitors. Apnea monitors are particularly valuable for infants. Indications in adult patients include advanced age, severe COPD, and extensive surgery.

This type of respiratory monitoring is based upon the relationship between the tidal volume and thoracic electrical impedance. As the patient breathes, the changing volume of air in the lungs alters the thoracic impedance (resistance to the electrical signal through the thorax). Thoracic impedance increases during inhalation and decreases during exhalation.

Technique and location of electrode placement are very important. Many monitors indicate if the electrodes have been adequately applied for respiratory rate monitoring. Frequently, the level of the electrodes must be changed when mechanical ventilation is initiated or terminated. The sensitivity of the amplifier may need to be adjusted if the depth of the patient's respirations changes.

Verification of Alterations

As with all instrumentation, alterations in readings need to be correlated with the patient's clinical condition and when possible, confirmed with alternative technologies. For example, SpO$_2$ and S$\overline{v}$O$_2$ oximetry readings may be verified by blood sample analysis. It is important to remember that readings obtained by laboratory CO-oximeters will not be exactly the same as readings obtained by pulse and venous oximetry. In the critically ill patient, there is often an imbalance between the amount of oxygen delivered to the tissues and the amount of oxygen required to meet tissue needs. Bedside blood gas monitoring technologies are useful in assisting the clinician in quickly and accurately identifying oxygen supply–demand imbalances

and assessing the effectiveness of the therapeutic interventions used during management of critical illness. A variety of stand-alone, component, and combined bedside blood gas monitors are commercially available.

Intracranial Pressure Monitoring

In patients with existing or potential neurologic deficit, intracranial pressure (ICP) monitoring provides a method for assessing change and helps to direct care including ventilatory support, positioning, the use of positive end-expiratory pressure (PEEP), and drug therapy. When used in conjunction with clinical assessment and other invasive and noninvasive assessment techniques, such as magnetic resonance imaging (MRI), CT scanning, emission tomography (SPET, PET), and evoked potentials, ICP monitoring has significantly aided in the diagnosis, treatment, and prognosis of patients with a potential for developing increased intracranial pressure (intracranial hypertension). The correlation of ICP measurements with other assessment techniques frequently reduces the time required for accurate diagnosis, increases the time available for treatment, provides continual feedback on response to selected treatments, and assists with prognosis. The continuous monitoring of intracranial pressure, first reported by Guillaume and Janny in 1951, is now routinely used in the management of severe head injury, coma-producing subarachnoid hemorrhage, hydrocephalus, encephalitis, space-occupying mass lesion and intracranial infection, and also after hypoxic or ischemic insults to the brain.[44]

The proven value of ICP monitoring and the need for an accurate, reliable, and simple method of measurement has led to the development of numerous devices and techniques.[45] There are basically four techniques for measuring ICP: (1) intraventricular, (2) subarachnoid (subdural), (3) epidural (extradural), and (4) intraparenchymal (intracerebral) (Figure 4-22). All four methods require strict aseptic technique during insertion and maintenance. A continuous flush device is contraindicated in all ICP monitoring techniques. The usual duration for ICP monitoring is 3 to 5 days. The diagnostic and therapeutic benefits of

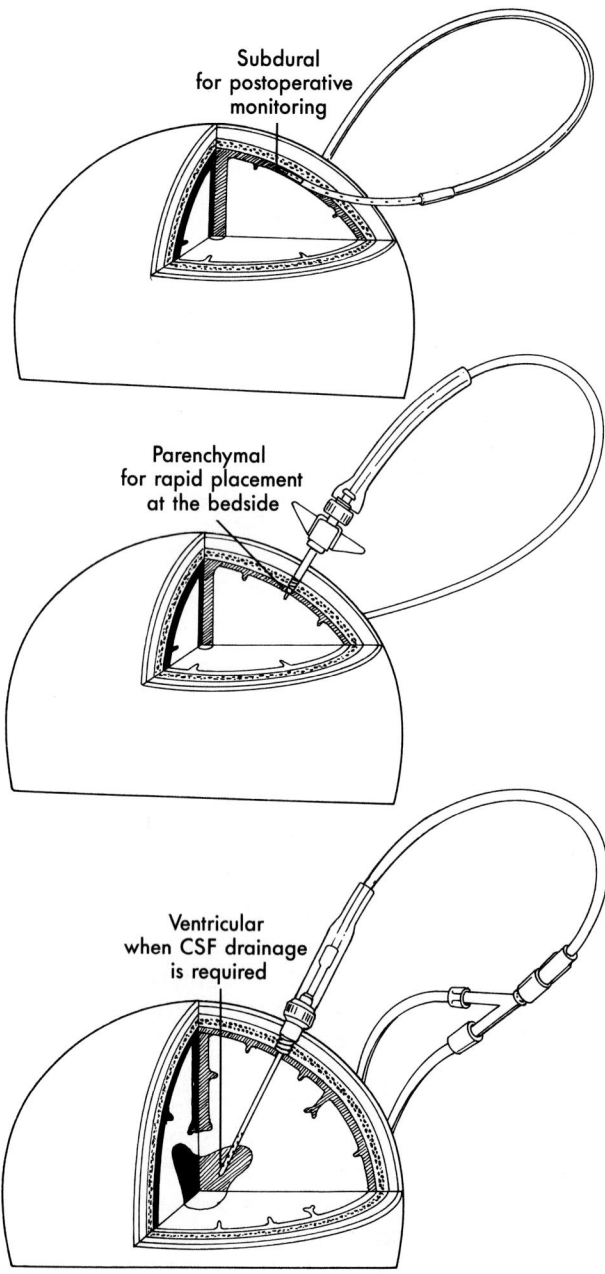

Figure 4-22 Fiberoptic techniques for ICP monitoring. Courtesy of Camino Laboratories.

ICP monitoring far outweigh the minimal risk. ICP measurements usually provide an indication of changes in ICP dynamics before such changes are clinically evident, facilitating the initiation of measures to reduce increased intracranial pressure. Therapies used to normalize ICP and maintain adequate cerebral perfusion include the use of hyperventilation to reduce intracerebral blood volume; CSF drainage to reduce intracerebral CSF volume; a variety of pharmacological agents to induce diuresis, sedation, or paralysis; and surgery.

Ranges and Waveforms

Range. Intracranial pressure is routinely monitored as mean pressure, although systolic and diastolic pressures should be noted. Because there is a linear relationship between pulse pressure and ICP, pulse pressure may be used to estimate intracranial elastance, particularly in the patient with cerebral vasoparalysis.

Normal ICP ranges between 0 and 10 mmHg, with an upper limit of 15 mmHg. The ICP may rise to the level of the mean arterial pressure (MAP), particularly during coughing or straining. In a person with normal compensatory mechanisms, these pressure fluctuations are well tolerated. Acutely ill patients however, may demonstrate symptoms associated with increased intracranial pressures in the range of 20 to 25 mmHg. Although protocols vary, measures to reduce ICP are usually initiated if the patient shows neurological deterioration, such as a score of 7 or less on the Glasgow Coma Scale or an ICP of 15 mmHg or greater. Controlling and decreasing ICP is a means of maintaining cerebral oxygenation via adequate cerebral blood flow.

Waveforms. The ICP waveforms provide an index of ICP dynamics. The appearance of ICP waveforms varies according to the technique of measurement being used and the patient's pathological condition. Hemodynamic and respiratory oscillations can be observed in ICP traces (Figure 4-23). Sometimes the waveforms closely resemble arterial pressure waveforms; at other times they resemble CVP waveforms. To varying degrees, oscillations corresponding to the arterial pulsations are seen. At times, a small "a" wave is superimposed on diastole, reflecting right atrial pressure. Alterations in arterial driving force, disturbance of venous outflow, and cerebral vasodilation have been correlated with changes in waveform appearances.

In patients with an ICP of less than 20 mmHg, a slower waveform, synchronous with respiration and caused by changes in intrathoracic pressure, can be seen. Some patients exhibit waveform variations referred to as A, B, and C waves.

A waves, also known as *plateau waves*, are spontaneous, rapid increases of pressure between 50 and 200 mmHg, occurring at variable intervals. They tend to occur in patients with moderate elevations of ICP, last 5 to 20 minutes, and fall spontaneously. The plateau waves are usually accompanied by a tempo-

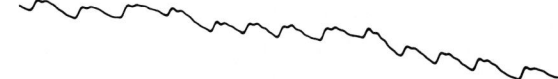

Figure 4-23 Intracranial pressure waveform illustrating hemodynamic and respiratory oscillations.

> ### Advantages and Disadvantages of Intraventricular Pressure Measurement
>
> **ADVANTAGES**
> - Direct measurement of pressure from the CSF
> - Access for CSF drainage or sampling
> - Access for determining volume pressure responses (VPR)
> - Access for instillation of drug
>
> **DISADVANTAGES**
> - Need to puncture the brain
> - Difficulty in locating the lateral ventricle following midline shifting of the ventricle or collapse of the ventricle as a normal compensatory mechanism for increases in pressure
> - Blockage of the catheter by fluid components or the ventricle wall
> - Risks of intracranial hemorrhage and infection. During opening of the dura and puncturing of the ventricle there is a slight risk (<2%) of an intracranial hemorrhage. The risk of infection, related to the duration of monitoring, and frequency of opening the system to the atmosphere, is reported between less than 1% up to 6%. An increased infection rate is associated with catheters in place for more than 5 days[46]

rary increase in neurologic deficit. Although the mechanism of A waves has not been firmly established, they are believed to indicate decreased intracranial compliance, and measures should be used to prevent their occurrence. They may occur with an increase in blood volume accompanied by decrease in blood flow. The sudden reversal of high pressure may be caused by increased CSF absorption with reduction of CSF pressure. Falls in central perfusion pressure with intact autoregulation and low intracranial compliance have been correlated with the initiating plateau waves. Plateau waves may be set off by a stimulus to vasodilation or by nonspecific stimuli such as hypo- or hyperventilation, pain, and aroused mental activities.

B waves are small, sharp, rhythmic waves with pressures up to 50 mmHg, occurring at a frequency of 0.5 per minute to 2.0 per minute. They correspond to changes in respiration, providing clues to periodic respiration related to poor cerebral compliance or pulmonary dysfunction. B waves are often seen with Cheyne-Stokes respirations. At times, they occur in patients with normal ICP and no papilledema. They may be secondary to oscillations of cerebral blood volume.

C waves, also known as Traube-Hering-Mayer waves, are small, rhythmic waves with pressures up to 20 mmHg, occurring at a rate of approximately 6

per minute. They are related to the blood pressure. Like A waves, they indicate severe intracranial compression, with limited remaining volume residual within the intracranial space.

Cerebral Perfusion Pressure (CPP)

Cerebral perfusion pressure (CPP) is the blood pressure gradient across the brain and is the effective pressure by which the brain is perfused. CPP provides a clinical estimate of cerebral circulation. It is calculated by subtracting the mean ICP from the mean systemic arterial pressure (MAP): CPP = MAP − ICP. To provide an adequate blood supply and, therefore, oxygen delivery to the brain, a cerebral perfusion pressure of at least 60 mmHg is required. Cerebral blood flow may totally cease at pressures somewhat above zero.

Intracranial Pressure Monitoring Methods

Intraventricular Technique. The intraventricular technique of ICP measurement was first reported in 1951 and remains the most frequently used method. It requires the placement of a catheter into the lateral ventricle. A twist-drill hole, or small burr hole, is placed 2.5 cm from the midline and 1.5 cm in front of the coronal suture, usually on the nondominant side. A ventriculostomy catheter is inserted through the cerebrum into the anterior horn of the lateral ventricle. On occasion, the occipital horn is used. Connected to the ventricular catheter by a stopcock or pressure tubing is a pressure transducer. Sterile saline or Ringer's lactate solution is used to provide the fluid column between the CSF and diaphragm of the transducer.

A miniature transducer may be positioned directly on the patient's head. Alternatively, a standard-size transducer is mounted at the bedside, with the venting port positioned at the level of the foramen of Monro. External landmarks for this position are the edge of the brow or the tragus of the ear. For every 1 inch of discrepancy between the level of the transducer and the pressure source, there is an error of approximately 2 mmHg.

A disposable fiberoptic transducer-tipped catheter may be placed in the ventricle. This eliminates the need for the fluid column required with external transducers. A Y-connector at the proximal end of the catheter facilitates attachment to the monitor and a CSF drainage system. The advantages and disadvantages are listed in the box above.

Subarachnoid Technique. The measurement of ICP by means of a subarachnoid screw or bolt was first reported in 1973. The screw device is inserted through a twist-drill hole and extends into the subdural or subarachnoid space. Although the cerebrum is not penetrated, pressures, as with the intraventricular technique, are measured directly from the CSF. A transducer filled with saline or Ringer's lactate solution may be fastened directly to a stopcock on the screw or connected by pressure tubing. As with any technique for monitoring ICP, a continuous flush device is contraindicated. An alternative technique for monitoring subarachnoid pressure is the subarachnoid (subdural) catheter or the ribbon-shaped cup catheter, available in both adult and pediatric sizes. The subarachnoid catheter is usually inserted through a twist-drill hole and opened dura, then tunneled subcutaneously. The disposable fiberoptic transducer is introduced through a small subarachnoid–subdural bolt, with the catheter extending just beyond the tip of the bolt. The catheter is usually used in conjunction with a craniotomy procedure and is inserted through a subcutaneous tunnel and burr hole. Volume pressure responses have been determined with these techniques. Subarachnoid pressures usually correlate well with intraventricular pressures.

The advantages of subarachnoid techniques include (1) direct pressure measurement from CSF, (2) no need to penetrate the cerebrum to locate the ventricle, (3) access for determining volume pressure responses, (4) access for CSF drainage and sampling, and (5) relative ease of insertion. Its disadvantages include a risk of complications comparable to those associated with intraventricular technique and the need for a closed skull. Greater difficulty in VPR studies and with CSF drainage than ventricular catheters may be experienced. Blockage of the measuring device and/or underestimation of ICP during episodes of elevated ICP may possibly occur.

Epidural Technique. The epidural technique for ICP measurement involves placement of an epidural device such as a balloon with radioisotopes, a radio transmitter, or a fiberoptic or pneumatic transducer between the skull and the dura. Some researchers believe that dural compression and surface tension, as well as thickening of the dura during prolonged monitoring, tend to cause inaccuracies in the pressure readings. Although subarachnoid and intraventricular pressures correlate well with each other, there have been inconsistent correlations between direct CSF pressure and pressure measurement using various epidural techniques.

The epidural technique is less invasive than others and permits the use of selected transducers for anterior fontanelle monitoring. However, it provides a questionable reflection of CSF pressure. With high ICPs, epidural pressures may considerably overread ventricular pressures. Response time is slow. Many systems are unable to pick up transient peaks caused by Valsalva maneuvers and respiratory changes. It provides no route for CSF drainage and sampling,

and volume pressure responses are not obtainable. Some systems cannot be zeroed and calibrated after measurement is initiated. Transducer placement may be difficult. The transducer must touch but not indent the dura and must be parallel to, or coplanar with, the dura. If the dura is stretched, the pressure recording will be affected by dural compliance.

Intraparenchymal Technique. The development of disposable fiberoptic transducer–tipped catheters and the improvement of catheter-tipped microtransducers has made intracerebral (intraparenchymal) pressure monitoring possible.[47,48] The intraparenchymatous technique provides a means of obtaining ICP recordings in patients with compressed and dislocated ventricles. The catheter is inserted through a small subarachnoid bolt and, after puncture of the dura and coagulation of the arachnoid membranes, advanced several centimeters into the white matter of the brain. Brain tissue pressures correlate well with ventricular pressures.

Since the sensitivity and linearity of the fiberoptic transducer–tipped catheter are precalibrated, it is not necessary to balance the transducer after insertion. The mean ICP is continuously displayed on a portable monitor that interfaces with a standard monitoring system for oscilloscopic display and print out of ICP waveforms and values. The advantages and disadvantages are listed in the box below.

Posterior Fossa Monitoring

Procedures for ICP monitoring and therapeutic drainage of CSF are usually done in the supratentorial compartment of the intracranial cavity. There is little

---

Advantages and Disadvantages of Intraparenchymal ICP Monitoring

ADVANTAGES
- Accurate: correlates well with ventricular pressures
- Ease of insertion
- Eliminates fluid coupling, flushing, leveling, and debubbling
- Minimizes artifact, leaks, drift, and infection
- Eliminates effect of hydrostatic pressure on readings
- No need to balance after insertion
- No calibration required

DISADVANTAGES
- Catheter breakage with bending, tension or rough manipulation
- No route for CSF drainage and sampling
- Inability to zero or calibrate after insertion
- Requires dedicated equipment

difference in pressure between the normal infra-tentorial and supratentorial compartments. There have been questions, however, about whether supratentorial monitoring accurately reflects changes in the posterior fossa during certain conditions such as surgery. The risk of damage to critical structures within the posterior fossa and potential complications, including cerebrospinal fluid leak, cranial nerve palsies, and brain-stem irritation with resulting autonomic dysfunctions have been a deterent to the use of posterior fossa monitoring. A preliminary report has documented successful intracranial pressure monitoring with direct therapeutic drainage from the posterior fossa in patients requiring posterior fossa surgery.[49] Postoperative posterior fossa (infratentorial) recordings were found to be 50% higher than supratentorial space measurements within the first 12 hours and 10% to 15% higher during the next 12 hours. The infratentorial and supratentorial compartments had equilibrated within 48 hours. No monitoring complications were reported.

The advantage of posterior fossa monitoring would be direct measurement from infratentorial surgical site. Disadvantages are a possible increase in risk and the need for surgical placement.

Telemetry Technique

Telemetry systems are available for use with both epidural and intraventricular devices. They are designed to reduce the risk of infection during long-term monitoring of patients with hydrocephalus and some metabolic encephalopathies, and of patients with brain tumors who are undergoing chemotherapy.

Troubleshooting

When a fiberoptic ICP monitoring system is being used, it is important to prevent kinking or bending of the fiberoptic catheter. With fluid-filled ICP monitoring systems, it is important to remember that a continuous flush system is not used. These systems are occasionally flushed with a small amount of fluid (for example, 0.25 ml of sterile saline without preservative) as directed by a physician. Other than flushing techniques, troubleshooting procedures are similar to those used with vascular lines (Table 4-2). The systems must be aseptically set up and maintained and correctly calibrated. Fluid-filled systems must be correctly positioned, balanced, and kept air free.

Risks and Complications

As with all procedures, the benefits of ICP monitoring must be weighed against the associated risks and complications. The risks associated with ICP monitoring are related to the type of device used and its location, the degree of invasiveness, the susceptibility of the patient to infection, restriction of patient movement, and monitoring errors. Complications reported with ICP monitoring include infection, hematomas, seizures, cerebral puncture, cranial nerve palsies, and CSF leaks.[49] The incidence of ICP-related complications has been quoted between 1.1% and 7.7%.[46]

Computer-processed EEG Monitoring

Computer-processed EEG monitoring is a noninvasive method of continuously monitoring brain activity. Unlike conventional diagnostic EEG monitoring, this technology is relatively easy to set up and use. Raw EEG data are processed, compressed, and displayed in a color format that makes significant trends in the oxygenation and perfusion of the patient's brain easy to detect. The technique is of value in detecting cerebral ischemia caused by conditions such as hypoxemia, hypotension, or impaired circulation. Interpretation by neurologists or EEG technicians is seldom, if ever, necessary.

Portable EEG systems have proved useful in operating rooms, recovery rooms, and for selected ICU patients. The interface between the patient and the monitor is provided by pregelled, disposable adhesive electrodes. In the operating room, EEG monitors are used to show changes in the EEG caused by anesthetic agents. In the ICU, continuous EEG techniques have been used to monitor brain activity during barbiturate coma, to document seizure activity, and to assist in prognosis. Ischemic episodes are indicated by a decrease in high-frequency activity followed by a loss of power and amplitude in the EEG signal. Most EEG monitors provide a printed copy of the trends displayed on the screen. Some have the capability of concurrent analysis and display of somatosensory-evoked potentials.

Temperature

A variety of peripheral and core techniques are available for the measurement of temperature, an important vital sign in the critically ill. These techniques include electronic thermometers with disposable probe covers, glass/mercury thermometers, liquid crystal skin strips, esophageal thermometers, pulmonary artery catheters, tympanic membrane infrared probe thermometers, and urinary bladder thermistor catheters.[50,51,52]

Peripheral temperatures, measured at the mouth, skin or axilla, may be affected by ingested food, fluids, and medication; talking, smoking, and mouth breathing; probe tip contact with tissue; exercise; and environmental temperatures. For oral temperatures taken with the electronic thermometers, the probe tip should be placed under and to the side of the tongue so that the probe tip is in the sublingual pocket near the sublingual artery. The patient's lips should be closed around the disposable probe cover and the probe held in place during the procedure. Since skin temperature is a function of peripheral circulation, it is affected by changes in peripheral vascular activity. Liquid crystal adhesive strips, usually placed on the forehead, change color at different temperatures, providing a numerical reading within 30 seconds. Sterile, disposable temperature probes are available for skin surface monitoring. Not all temperature probes are interchangeable. The caregiver is responsible for determining that the probe being used is the one specified by the manufacturer of the thermometer or the hypo/hyperthermia unit being used.

Core temperatures are less influenced by external factors and more accurately reflect the mean temperature of vital organs. High core temperatures have been associated with high metabolic demands due to sepsis and metabolic acidosis. A high core temperature may contraindicate ventilator weaning. Core body temperatures may be measured from the esophagus, rectum, tympanic membrane, pulmonary artery, or urinary bladder. Multifunction esophageal catheters with thermistors measure core temperatures while functioning as nasogastric tubes. Sterile, disposable esophageal and rectal probes are available for monitoring hyper/hypothermia. For rectal temperatures taken with electronic thermometers with disposable probe covers, the rectal probe is inserted approximately 1 cm, tilted to come into contact with the tissue, and held in place during the procedure. Continuous monitoring of rectal temperatures, done with probes inserted more deeply, has been associated with bowel wall perforation.

For the bedside measurement of core body temperatures in ICU patients, tympanic membrane infrared probes (auditory canal thermometer, tympanic thermometer), pulmonary artery thermistor catheters (thermodilution catheters), and urinary bladder thermistor catheters have become increasingly popular. The tympanic thermometer with disposable probe cover, resembling an otoscope, is inserted into the auditory canal. The auditory canal infrared probe measures infrared energy emitted primarily from the tympanic membrane, providing a reading within 3 seconds. Measurements should be taken from an ear exposed to air. Devices are available which, in addition to displaying core temperature, can be calibrated to display simulated oral and rectal temperatures.

Pulmonary artery catheters that determine cardiac output measurements by the thermodilution technique have thermistors for measuring pulmonary artery blood temperatures. They provide continuous measurements of the chest blood core temperature. Urinary bladder catheters are available with thermistors that float in the urine within the bladder, providing a monitored display of abdominal urine core temperatures. Variations in temperature readings according to the method used have been reported.[51,52]

Several microprocessor-controlled systems with patient safety systems, including high temperature alarms, are available for cooling and heating patients. In addition to the widely used hyper/hypothermia blanket systems, localized cold therapy systems designed to reduce edema and accelerate the healing process of damaged tissue are available. A variety of small pads, some configured for areas such as the knee, hip, or shoulder, may be applied to surgical incisions or areas of traumatic injury. Although orthopedic–neurological injuries and procedures are the most common use, localized cold therapy is also employed for patients who have had urologic, obstetric–gynecologic, and general surgical procedures.

Convective air warming systems, consisting of a microprocessor-controlled system with alarms and an inflated warming tube, provide a continuous flow of heated air to the peripheral areas of the body. Most commonly used with postoperative patients, systems are available that do not interfere with patient assessment and maintenance of support systems such as IVs and other tubing.[50]

THERAPEUTIC INSTRUMENTATION
Vascular Access Devices (VAD)

With increases in patient acuity, decreases in length of hospital stay, and advances in intravenous technology, vascular access devices have changed.[53] Because of the frequency of needlesticks and associated risks of occupationally acquired infection, many intravenous catheters and blood sampling systems now incorporate methods for limiting the risk of needlestick during use and disposal.[54,55] The IV catheters most commonly seen in critical care are: peripheral, midline, peripherally inserted central catheter (PICC), central venous catheter (CVC), pulmonary artery catheters and implantable VADs. Catheter maintenance varies according to catheter type.[56] Transparent adhesive dressings are most commonly used with the various venous lines.

Short *peripheral catheters* are for short-term access (48 to 72 hours) to peripheral veins. Examples include the *Angiocath,* JELCO, *Insyte,* and *butterfly* types.

Midline devices such as the *Landmark,* are over-the-needle, hydrophilic venous access devices specifically designed for intermediate-term therapies (1 to 6 weeks), such as intravenous antibiotics. The catheter is usually placed in the cephalic or brachial vein,

1 or 2 inches above or below the antecubital fossa, and advanced up to 7 inches. This catheter position provides better hemodilution of medications than short peripheral catheters. Fluoroscopic confirmation is not required. Hydration of the catheter occurs within approximately 30 minutes, with the catheter becoming softer and expanding two gauge sizes in diameter. Aseptic mechanical phlebitis and chemical phlebitis have occurred with this catheter.[57]

Central venous catheters may be *single- or multilumen.* They are made from a variety of materials and are available for both short-term and long-term use. Examples include the *Hickman, Broviac,* and *Groshong* catheters. For patients requiring more than one intravenous treatment, these vascular access devices reduce the number of venipunctures required as well as a number of IV sites.[53,58] To reduce the risk of nosocomial, device-related bacteremia or septicemia, short-term central venous catheters (4 to 6 weeks) are available with antiseptic surfaces and antimicrobial cuffs. They are inserted through the subclavian, internal jugular, brachial, or (rarely) femoral vein. Long-term (years) catheters are placed centrally, frequently with a tunneling technique. Fluoroscopic or x-ray confirmation is required to confirm correct tip location in the superior vena cava above the junction of the right atrium and parallel to the vessel wall. Short-term central venous catheters, often called central venous pressure (CVP) catheters, may be used to monitor right heart pressures. Single- and multi-lumen catheters are used for chemotherapy, blood sampling, transfusions, medications, fluids, and total parenteral nutrition (TPN). The majority of drugs can be given concurrently with multilumen catheters. One study did show precipitation when phenytoin and TPN were administered through a double-lumen catheter. No precipitation was noted when the same drugs were administered via a triple lumen catheter.[59]

Central venous catheters require meticulous maintenance. Because of the tip location in the superior vena cava and, in some cases the use of multiple lumens and frequent accessing, patients with catheters in place have a higher risk of morbidity and mortality than those with other VAD: 80% to 90% of nosocomial bloodstream infections related to intravascular devices occur with central venous catheters.[24,26]

Long-line, *peripherally inserted central catheters* (PICC) are inserted percutaneously into a vein in the arm, usually the brachial vein, with the tip advanced to the axillary, subclavian, or brachiocephalic vein or the superior vena cava.[60] Fluoroscopic confirmation of catheter position in the superior vena cava is required. These moderate- to long-term single- or double-lumen catheters, available in several lengths and gauges, are designed for use with chemotherapy,

blood sampling, transfusions, medications, fluid therapy, and TPN. They can remain in place for several months. Examples include the *Intrasil, Per-Q-Cath,* and *Cook* catheters.

Implantable VAD are surgically implanted devices that provide central venous access via a Huber needle. The major indication is for long-term, intermittent administration of drugs and fluids. Examples are the *Port-A-Cath* and *Mediport* devices.

Balloon tipped, flow-directed, multilumen, *pulmonary artery* (Swan-Ganz) *catheters* are inserted percutaneously via venous cutdown through the right side of the heart and into either branch of the pulmonary artery. Pressure waveforms are monitored continuously during insertion to determine catheter location. X-ray is required for confirmation of tip placement in a branch of the pulmonary artery. These devices are for short-term use, with removal recommended within 72 hours of insertion. A variety of catheter sizes and configurations are available for specialized functions. These include PA pressures, right and left heart function, pacing, blood sampling, mixed venous oximetry ($S\bar{v}O_2$), RV ejection fractions, fluid administration, and obtaining cardiac output via thermodilution.

Infusion Pumps

As intravenous therapy has become more varied and complex, the number and complexity of the devices used to administer these drug and fluid therapies has also increased. In critical care applications the simple rate controller, which is similar in principle to IV infusion by gravity adjusted by a roller clamp with the addition of an alarm, is not always adequate. For many patients, a programmable volumetric infusion pump or syringe pump capable of exerting pressure to overcome resistance to infusion is required for delivering IV therapy.[61]

The volumetric pump functions on the principle of direct volume replacement at a controlled rate, providing a more accurate volume and rate of infusion. During fluid administration the pump exerts pressure within a specified range to overcome the resistance caused by factors such as small catheters, viscous solutions, and high counteracting physiological pressures (increased vascular resistance, coughing, crying, seizure activity). Pump pressure is listed in pounds per square inch: 51.7 mmHg equals 1 lb/in². Some pumps are capable of ranges approximating gravity (~25 mmHg/foot) and exert up to 20 lb/in² (1,043 mmHg) before the pump reaches an occlusion pressure that automatically stops the infusion. A wide variety of infusion pumps are currently used for many applications. Volumetric pumps are available with fixed pressure limits (preset by manufacturer), variable pressure limits, disposable cassettes, safety features and alarms, user prompting for setup and troubleshooting, and a choice of AC power or battery operation. In selecting the appropriate infusion pump, the clinical application has to be considered. Specialized pumps are available for multidrug therapy, pain management medication with bolus capability, high rate fluid administration, intermittent dose administration, chemotherapy, and TPN with taper. Other pump features to consider are the incremental rate adjustments, accuracy and consistency of flow, adjustable occlusion pressures, ease of programming, delivery system for secondary medications, and safety features and alarms (e.g., risk of uncontrolled flow, infiltration detection, air detection, disconnect, automatic KVO rate).

For ambulatory patients, small, computerized, ambulatory infusion pumps are available with programs for pain management, chemotherapy, and administration of drugs or fluids (Figure 4-24) as well as TPN. Different models can provide continuous or intermittent drug delivery; may be patient- or clinician-activated; and have audible and visual alarms to alert the user to low battery, depleted battery, low reservoir volume, system error, high pressure, and so on. The interval and amount of patient-activated pain management doses can be programmed and the number of patient-activated doses actually administered reported, as well as the total amount of drug delivered from an individual reservoir. Optional three-level electronic lockout functions can be adjusted by the clinician to meet the needs of the individual patient. For example, if the patient is concerned about accidentally pushing the incorrect key, the pump can be locked to prevent any change in the program, with the medication cassette reservoir locked for drug security. If, however, the patient is comfortable with programming the pump, the lock level can be adjusted

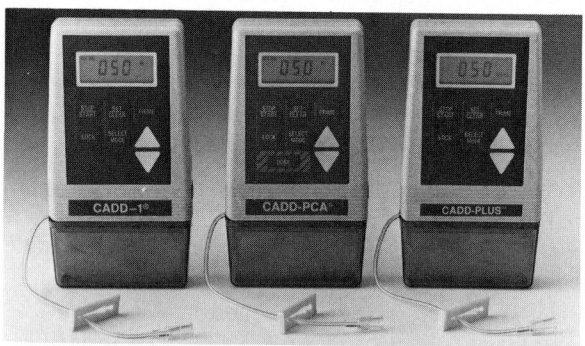

Figure 4-24 Ambulatory infusion pumps for pain management, chemotherapy, and drug administration. CADD-1; PCA; PLUS Infusion Pumps.
Courtesy of Pharmacia Deltec Inc., St. Paul, Minnesota.

to provide total patient programming, including changing of medication cassettes, IV fluid bags, and TPN. The pumps may be used with disposable batteries, AC power, or rechargeable batteries and come with accessories such as backpacks designed to hold bags of TPN or IV fluids, as well as small packs that fit onto a belt and allow easy access to controls and function display. The critical care nurse may be responsible for educating patients regarding the use of these pumps.

Closed-loop Infusion: The programmable pumps discussed above are sometimes referred to as open-loop or manually controlled systems. The next generation of infusion devices are closed-loop or automatic systems. Whereas the infusion pumps now in common use are controlled by the user, the next generation of computer-controlled pumps will be part of a system that, after initial programming, are actually controlled by the patient's physiological responses as discussed earlier in the section on computer applications. For example, when a patient is receiving a vasoactive drug such as sodium nitroprusside to control blood pressure, the amount of the drug being administered is automatically adjusted or titrated in response to the patient's changes in blood pressure. The automatic system is based on parameters initially programmed in by the clinician and can, of course, be converted by the clinician to a manual system or reprogrammed at any time. Closed-loop systems, sometimes referred to as servo-controlled or feedback controlled systems, are still in the developmental stage for certain uses.[62]

Autotransfusion

Autotransfusion is the collection, filtration, and reinfusion of the patient's own (autologous) blood. When guidelines established by the American Association of Blood Banks are followed, autologous blood is the safest type of blood for transfusion.[63] A major advantage of autotransfusion is the elimination of the risk of the transmission of donor-related diseases such as hepatitis, AIDS (acquired immune deficiency syndrome), or syphilis. Other advantages include elimination of transfusion reactions, reduction of religious objections, cost-effectiveness, availability, and superior blood quality. Autologous blood contains viable platelets and normal levels of 2,3-DPG (diphosphoglycerate), essential to adequate tissue oxygenation. In contrast, platelets in homologous (bank) blood become nonviable within 24 hours and lose all 2,3 DPG within 10 days. In addition, unlike homologous bank blood, various clotting factors remain near normal in autologous blood.

A variety of autologous blood transfusion systems is available for whole blood autotransfusion and component (washed or processed) autotransfusion. Regional anticoagulants such as CPD (citrate-phosphate-dextrose), ACD (acid-phosphate-dextrose), and sometimes heparin are used with most autotransfusion systems. The most commonly used regional anticoagulant is CPD, the same anticoagulant used in homologous blood. The citrate chelates calcium, preventing the blood from coagulating, with the phosphate and dextrose providing metabolic support of the blood. Systemic heparinization is often prescribed for surgical patients receiving intraoperative autotransfusion. Heparin prevents clotting by interfering with the information of thromboplastin and thrombin.

Whole blood autotransfusion is most frequently used in *emergency trauma* situations and during postoperative management after cardiovascular surgery. Whole blood systems are easier to set up and use than the cell washer–processor systems used most commonly in operating rooms and blood banks. Indications for emergency autotransfusion include hemothorax (most common application) and primary injuries of the lungs, liver, chest wall, heart, pulmonary vessels, spleen, kidneys, inferior vena cava, and iliac, portal, and subclavian veins.

In *elective surgery* for patients with rare blood types, for procedures in which massive blood loss is anticipated, for patients in whom immunization may present a complication, and for those who refuse homologous blood, predeposit phlebotomy may be used. One or more units of autologous blood are collected prior to an elective surgical procedure for reinfusion as needed during or after the surgery.

For intraoperative use the hemodilution method is used primarily with open heart surgery. One or two units of autologous blood are collected, usually in the operating room just prior to the surgical procedure, with concomitant replacement by crystalloid or colloid solution. The whole blood is reinfused postoperatively.

Intraoperative autotransfusion has been used most frequently for pooled blood collected from a body cavity during thoracic and cardiovascular procedures. It has also been used for orthopedic, gynecologic, general, and neurosurgical procedures. A cell washer–processor is often used to reduce anticoagulated whole blood to washed red blood cells for reinfusion. Specially trained operators are required for cell washer–processor autologous blood systems. These centrifuge devices separate plasma from red blood cells, removing debris, irrigating solutions, activated factors, anticoagulants, and free hemoglobin. Enteric contamination is reduced but not eliminated by cell washing. The red blood cells are resuspended in normal saline prior to reinfusion.[64]

Postoperative chest drainage–autotransfusion systems are used to collect shed mediastinal blood via chest tubes after cardiac surgery. Multipurpose systems combine standard water-seal chest drainage with a system for collecting, filtering, and reinfusing autologous blood. The autologous blood may be reinfused as whole blood or washed blood.

Contraindications

The use of autotransfusion is usually contraindicated in the presence of blood contamination by bacteria, infestation, bile, urine, malignant cells, amniotic fluid, or gastrointestinal fluids; in the presence of a substance not intended for intravenous use (e.g., topical hemostatic agents); and in coagulopathies and excessive hemolysis such as that found in injuries more than 6 hours old. Although orthopedic surgery was often considered a contraindication for the use of autotransfusion, systems specifically designed for use with orthopedic patients are now available. The type of autotransfusion system used depends on the patient and the application.

Risks

Although autologous techniques have proved safe and effective and no major complications have been reported with equipment currently available, certain risks are associated with autotransfusion procedures. These include hemolysis, sepsis, air and particulate emboli, coagulation, thrombocytopenia, and citrate toxicity. Hemolysis, the primary effect of autotransfusion systems on blood, causes a reduction in hematocrit, an increase in serum and urine hemoglobin, and accumulation of erythrocyte debris. Today's autotransfusion systems are designed to reduce damage to blood cells during collection. A microaggregate (microemboli) filter is routinely used during the infusion of autologous blood. Unwashed blood should be reinfused within 4 to 6 hours from initial collection.

Autologous blood transfusion has proved to be a safe, effective method for reducing the risks associated with homologous blood transfusion in selected patients. It may be life-saving for rapidly bleeding patients or those with rare blood types.

Intravascular Gas Exchanger (IVOX)

The IVOX, an intravenous mechanical blood oxygen–carbon dioxide exchange device that augments O_2/CO_2 gas transfer, was first implanted into a human recipient in 1990. It is used to support patients whose lungs no longer have the ability to completely satisfy the body's need for oxygen and the elimination of carbon dioxide. The temporary lung-assist device is used in combination with a ventilator for up to 14 days in patients with severe but yet reversible respiratory failure to prevent life-threatening hypoxemia or hypercarbia. The underlying hypothesis is that sending oxygenated blood to the pulmonary vascular bed may improve the performance of the natural lungs and ease the burden on lungs that need time to rest and heal. The IVOX device is undergoing clinical trials as this text is written. Preliminary findings indicated that it is a viable new method for managing critically ill ICU patients with severe, potentially reversible, acute respiratory failure.[65]

Indications for the device include: (1) acute respiratory failure due to etiologies such as near drowning, smoke inhalation, trauma, and pneumonia; and (2) adult respiratory distress syndrome (ARDS) as seen with direct lung injury (pulmonary contusion, pneumonia, pulmonary aspiration, exposure to high partial pressures of oxygen) or an extrathoracic injury (pancreatitis, near drowning, disseminated intravascular coagulation, multiple long bone fractures, massive trauma, hypertransfusion, and sepsis).

The IVOX is a miniaturized, hollow-fiber oxygenator that is placed in the inferior vena cava (Figure 4-25). It exchanges oxygen and carbon dioxide in venous blood before the blood reaches the lungs. A bundle of hollow, thromboresistant-coated fibers carries oxygen from an external tank to the blood. Oxygen in the molecular form passes through the fiber walls into the oxygen-poor blood. At the same time, carbon dioxide, found in relatively high concentrations in venous blood, passes through the hollow fiber wall and is pulled out by the external suction pump. Initial studies indicate that up to approximately one third of the metabolic demand may be provided by IVOX. Although similar in theory to extracorporeal oxygenators used during open heart surgery, it has only about 20% of the surface area. The extensive monitoring required by extracorporeal membrane oxygenation (ECMO) and extracorporeal CO_2 removal (ECCO$_2$R) is not required. No significant complications or unfavorable sequelae attributed to IVOX use have so far been encountered in ongoing clinical tests or trials with ARDS patients. Evidence of significant clinical benefit was observed in a majority of patients and in computer models. It is hoped that IVOX will reduce the high mortality rates associated with acute respiratory failure, and shorten the duration of mechanical ventilation. The IVOX is not available for general use in the United States at this time.

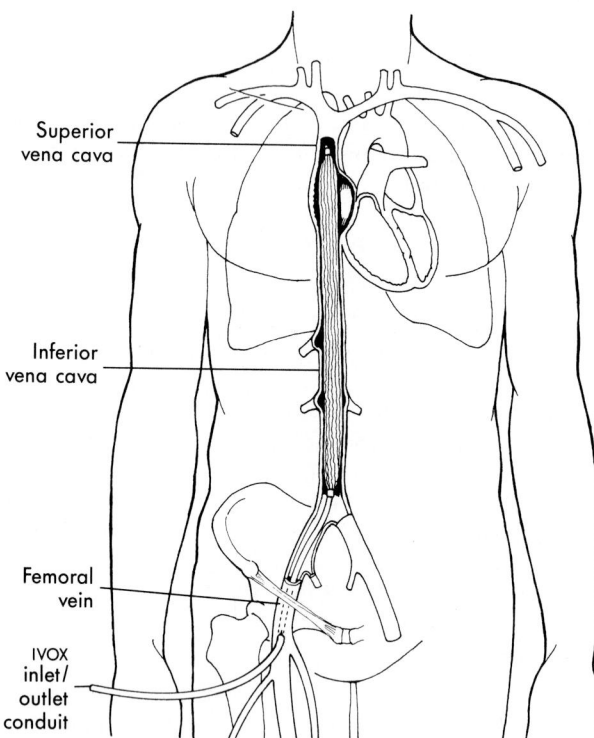

Superior
vena cava

Inferior
vena cava

Femoral
vein

IVOX
inlet/
outlet
conduit

Figure 4-25   IVOX Intravascular Oxygenator placed via the femoral vein into the vena cava.
Courtesy of CardioPulmonics.

REFERENCES

1. American Association of Critical-Care Nurses. (1984). *Definition of critical care nursing.* Newport Beach, CA: Author.
2. Kramer, M. R. (1990). *Choosing a clinical information system: A blueprint for your success.* Waltham, MA: Hewlett-Packard Company.
3. Shabot, M. M. (1985). Software for computers and calculators in critical care medicine. *Software in Healthcare,* Feb./Mar., 26-39.
4. Dasta, J. F. (1990). Computers in critical care: Opportunities and challenges. *The Annals of Pharmacotherapy, DICP,* Nov. (24), 1084-1092.
5. Leyerle, B. J., LoBue, M., Shabot, M. M., et al. (1988). The PDMS as a focal point for distributed patient data. *International Journal of Clinical Monitoring and Computing,* 5,155-161.
6. Gardner, R. M., West, B. J., Pryor, A., et al. (1982). Computer-based ICU data acquisition as an aid to clinical decision-making. *Critical Care Medicine,* 10(12), 823-830.
7. Tolbert, S. H., & Pertuz, A. E. (1971). Study shows how computerization affects nursing activities in ICU. *Hospitals, JAHA,* 51(9), 79-83.
8. Dorenfest, S. E. (1987). Review of PDMS in the surgical intensive care units. Sheldon Dorenfest and Associates, Chicago (private communication).
9. Leyerle, B. J., LoBue, M., & Shabot, M. M. (1990). Integrated computerized databases for medical data management beyond the bedside. *International Journal of Clinical Monitoring and Computing,* 7, 83-89.
10. Hannah, K. J. (1988). Classification of decision-sup-

port systems. In M. J. Ball, K. J. Hannah, U. Gerdin, et al. (Eds.), *Nursing informatics: Where caring and technology meet* (pp. 260-266). New York: Springer-Verlag.

11. Brennan, P. T. (1988). Modeling for decision support. In M. J. Ball, K. J. Hannah, U. Gerdin, et al. (Eds.), *Nursing informatics: Where caring and technology meet* (pp. 267-273). New York: Springer-Verlag.

12. Knaus, W. A., Draper, E., Wagner, D., et al. (1989). APACHE III—Study design: Analytic plan to evaluation of severity and outcome. *Critical Care Medicine, 17,* 5176-5180.

13. Cullen, D. J., Civetta, J. M., Briggs, B. A., et al. (1974). Therapeutic intervention scoring system: A method for quantitative comparison of patient care. *Critical Care Medicine, 2,* 57-60.

14. Le Gall, J. R., Loriat, P., Alperovitch, A., et al. (1984). A simplified acute physiology score for ICU patients. *Critical Care Medicine, 12,* 975-977.

15. Keene, A. R. & Cullen, D. J. (1983). Therapeutic intervention scoring system: Update 1983. *Critical Care Medicine, 11,* 1-3.

16. Knaus, W. A., Draper, E., Wagner, D. P., et al. (1986). An evaluation of outcome from intensive care in major medical centers. *Annals of Internal Medicine, 104,* 410-418.

17. Shabot, M. M. (1987). Automatic extraction of intensity intervention scores from a computerized surgical ICU flowsheet. *American Journal of Surgery, 154,* 72.

18. Shabot, M. M., Leyerle, B. J., LoBue, M., et al. (1988). First day intensity-intervention score predicts ICU and in-hospital deaths. *Critical Care Medicine, 16,* 412.

19. Shabot, M. M., LoBue, M., & Leyerle, B. J. (1987). Use of automatic computerized intensity-intervention scores to measure the appropriateness of ICU utilization. *Symposium for Computer Application in Medical Care Proceedings, 11,* 671.

20. The French Multicenter Group of ICU Research. (1989). Factors related to outcome in intensive care: French multicenter study. *Critical Care Medicine, 17,* 490.

21. Weissman, C., Mossel, P., Haimet, S., et al. (1990). Integration of quality assurance activities into a computerized patient data management system in an intensive care unit. *Quarterly Review Bulletin,* November, 398-403.

22. Ozbolt, J., Abrahaim, I. L., Schaltz, S., et al. (1990). Nursing information systems. In E. H. Shortliff, & L. E. Perravit. (Eds.), *Medical informatics—computer applications in health care* (pp. 244-272). New York: Addison-Wesley.

23. Sheppard, L. C., Kouchoukos, N. T., & Kirklin, J. W. (1973). The digital computer in surgical intensive care automation. *Computer, 6,* 29-34.

24. Maki, D. G. (1988). An attachable silver-impregnated cuff for prevention of infection with central venous catheters: A prospective randomized multicenter trial. *American Journal of Medicine, 85,* 307-314.

25. Flowers, R. H., Schwenzer, K. J., Kopel, R. F., et al. (1989). Efficacy of an attachable subcutaneous cuff for the prevention of intravascular catheter-related infection: A randomized controlled trial. *JAMA, 261*(6), 878-883.

26. Corona, M. L., & Durbin, C. G. (1990). Infections related to central venous catheters. *Mayo Clinic Proceedings, 65,* 979-986.

27. Henneman, E. A., & Henneman, P. L. (1989). Intricacies of blood pressure measurement: Reexamining the rituals. *Heart Lung, 18*(3), 263-272.

28. Bruner, J. M. R., Krenis, L. J., Kunsman, J. M., et al. (1981). Comparison of direct and indirect method of measuring arterial blood pressure. *Medical Instrumentation, 15,* 11-21, 97-101, 182-188.

29. Durbin, C. G., Jr. (1990). Noninvasive hemodynamic monitoring. *Respiratory Care, 35*(7), 709-716.

30. Rutten, A. J. (1986). A comparative study of the measurement of mean arterial pressure using automatic oscillometers, arterial cannulation, and auscultation. *Anaesthesia Intensive Care, 14,* 58-65.

31. Ashton, J., Gibson, V., & Summers, S. (1990). Effects of heparin versus saline solution on intermittent infusion device irrigation. *Heart Lung, 19*(6), 608-612.

32. Woo, M. A., Hamilton, M., Stevenson, L., et al. (1991). Comparison of thermodilution and transthoracic electrical bioimpedance cardiac outputs. *Heart Lung, 20*(4), 357-362.

33. Carpenter, K. D. (1991). Oxygen transport in the blood. *Critical Care Nurse, 11*(9), 20-33.

34. Callaham, M., & Barton, C. (1990). Prediction of outcome of cardiopulmonary resuscitation from end-tidal carbon dioxide concentration. *Critical Care Medicine, 18*(4), 358-362.

35. Shapiro, B. A., & Cane, R. D. (1989). Blood gas monitoring: Yesterday, today, and tomorrow. *Critical Care Medicine, 17*(6), 573-581.

36. Zaloga, G. P., Hill, T. R., Strickland, R. A., et al. (1989). Bedside blood gas and electrolyte monitoring in critically ill patients. *Critical Care Medicine, 17*(9), 920-925.

37. Szaflarski, N. L. (1989). Use of pulse oximetry in critically ill adults. *Heart Lung, 18*(5), 444-454.

38. White, K. M. (1990). The physiologic basis for continuous mixed venous oxygen saturation monitoring. *Heart Lung, 19*(5, Pt. 2), 548-551.

39. Nelson, L. D. (1990). Real-time monitoring of gas exchange. In J. L. Vincent (Ed.), *Update in intensive care and emergency medicine.* New York: Springer-Verlag.

40. Chopin, C., Fesard, P., Mangaluboyl, J., et al. (1990). Use of capnography in diagnosis of pulmonary embolism during acute respiratory failure of chronic obstructive pulmonary disease. *Critical Care Medicine, 18*(4), 353-357.

41. Szaflarski, N. L., & Cohen, N. H. (1991). Use of capnography in critically ill adults. *Heart Lung, 20*(4), 363-374.

42. McCormick, P., Melville, S., Goetting, M. G., et al. (1991). Noninvasive cerebral optical spectroscopy for

monitoring cerebral oxygen delivery and hemodynamics. *Critical Care Medicine, 19*(1), 89-97.

43. Knebel, A. R. (1991). Weaning from mechanical ventilation: Current controversies. *Heart Lung, 20*(4), 321-334.

44. Smith, R. N. (1990). Intracranial pressure monitoring. In C. M. Hudak (Ed.), *Critical care nursing* (5th ed.) (pp. 537-556). Philadelphia: Lippincott.

45. Allen, R. (1988). Intracranial pressure: A review of clinical problems, measurement techniques and monitoring methods. *Journal of Medical Engineering and Technology, 10,* 299-315.

46. Franges, E. Z., & Beideman, M. E. (1988). Infections related to intracranial pressure monitoring. *Journal of Neuroscience Nursing, 20,* 94-103.

47. Sundbarg, G., Nordstrom, C. H., Messeter, K., et al. (1987). A comparison of intraparenchymatous and intraventricular pressure recording in clinical practice. *Journal of Neurosurgery, 67,* 841-844.

48. Barker, E. (1990). Avoiding increased intracranial pressure. *Nursing 90, 20*(5), 64Q-64RR.

49. Rosenwasser, R. H., Kleiner, L. I., Krzeminski, J. P., et al. (1989). Intracranial pressure monitoring in the posterior fossa: A preliminary report. *Journal of Neurosurgery, 71,* 503-505.

50. Lennon, R. L., et al. (1990). Evaluation of a forced-air system for warming hypothermic postoperative patients. *Anesthesia and Analgesia, 70,* 424-427.

51. Earp, J. K., & Finlayson, D. (1991). Relationship between urinary bladder and pulmonary artery temperature: A preliminary study. *Heart Lung, 20*(3), 265-270.

52. Nierman, D. M. (1991). Core temperature measurement in the intensive care unit. *Critical Care Medicine, 19*(6), 818-823.

53. Viall, C. D. (1990). Your complete guide to central venous catheters. *Nursing 90, 20*(2), 34-41.

54. Jagger, J., Hunt, E. H., & Pearson, R. D. (1988). Rates of needle-stick injury caused by various devices in a university hospital. *New England Journal of Medicine, 319*(5), 284-288.

55. Jagger, J., et al. (1990). Estimated cost of needlestick injuries for six major needle devices. *Infection Control and Hospital Epidemiology, 11*(11), 584-588.

56. Holder, C., & Alexander, J. (1990). A new and improved guide to IV therapy. *American Journal of Nursing,* February, 43-47.

57. Fontaine, P. J. (1991). Performance of a new softening expanding midline catheter in home intravenous therapy patients. *Journal of Intravenous Nursing, 14*(2), 91-99.

58. Thomason, S. S. (1991). Using a Groshong central venous catheter. *Nursing 91, 21*(10), 58-60.

59. Collins, J. L., & Lutz, R. J. (1991). In vitro study of simultaneous infusion of incompatible drugs in multilumen catheters. *Heart Lung, 20*(3), 271-277.

60. Rountree, D. (1991). The PIC catheter: A different approach. *American Journal of Nursing,* August, 22-28.

61. Millam, D. A. (1990). Controlling the flow: Electronic infusion devices. *Nursing 90, 20*(8), 65-68.

62. Bednarski, P., Siclari, T., Voigt, A., et al. (1990). Use of a computerized closed-loop sodium nitroprusside titration system for antihypertensive treatment after open heart surgery. *Critical Care Medicine, 18*(10), 1061-1065.

63. Committee on Standards, American Association of Blood Banks. (1991). *Standards for Blood Banks and Transfusion* (14th ed.) (Section L).

64. Smith, R. N. (1990). Autologous blood transfusion. In C. M. Hudak (Ed.), *Critical care nursing* (5th ed.) (pp. 216-223). Philadelphia: Lippincott.

65. Mortensen, J. D., Berry, G., & Winters, S. (1990). IVOX: An intracorporeal device for temporary augmentation of blood gas transfer in subjects with acute respiratory insufficiency. *Cardiac Chronicle, 4*(4), 1-6.

5

Environmental Hazards

Claire E. Sommargren

Potential health and safety hazards in hospitals have been the focus of increased attention in recent years, and nowhere in the hospital environment is there a greater variety and concentration of these problems than in the critical care unit. A large proportion of these hazards are the direct result of scientific and technological advances in the diagnosis and treatment of disease.

The best defense against exposure to health and safety risks for critical care nurses is a current knowledge of existing hazards and effective preventive strategies. This is not as simple as it sounds, however, because innovations in equipment and procedures occur almost daily.

Hazards are easier to identify if the nurse is familiar with a classification framework for them. Health and safety hazards within the critical care environment can generally be grouped into five major categories: biological, chemical, ergonomic, physical, and psychological (Table 5-1).[1]

Although specific protective strategies for each type of occupational hazard can be identified, other, more general control principles can be applied to a broad range of environmental risks. Perhaps the most important of these measures is staff education. This can be accomplished through orientation and inservice education programs, independent study, and review of current literature.

The periodic walk-through inspection, a standard method used by occupational health professionals for identifying problems, can be adapted for use by critical care nurses as well. It consists of walking through the unit, following the flow of activity, while noting any potential or actual hazards. These should be reported immediately to the appropriate hospital department. The walk-through inspection is an excellent way for nurses to apply their observational skills to assessing the work environment.

Once a hazard has been identified, measures can be taken to prevent or reduce exposure of individuals.

These measures may include substitution, engineering controls, work practice modification, administrative controls, and personal protective equipment (Table 5-2).

It is impossible to eliminate all occupational hazards in the critical care unit. An optimal level of safety should be the goal. This can be accomplished through a strong employee health and safety program established in cooperation with the critical care staff, administration, infection control personnel, and employee health professionals.

BIOLOGICAL HAZARDS

Biological hazards are those presented by a variety of living organisms that can be transmitted from the patient to the nurse: bacteria, viruses, and parasites. Transmission to the nurse usually occurs through the contact or airborne routes. Contact transmission can be either direct or indirect. It can occur directly by respiratory droplets, by the percutaneous or mucous membrane routes, or by the oral–fecal route. Indirect contact transmission occurs through contact with contaminated inanimate objects. Airborne transmission can occur when organisms travel in microscopic airborne particles called droplet nuclei, which can spread over long distances within a space on normal air currents. In the general community, vehicle-borne transmission, that is, by contaminated food or water, and vector-borne transmission, by insects, may occur. However, these routes are not significant in the transfer of biological hazards to nurses.

When an infectious agent is transmitted from a source to a host, one of several conditions occurs, depending on the susceptibility of the host. The host may become colonized by the agent, that is, the organism may grow and reproduce but does not invade the body's tissues. On the other hand, the microbe may gain entry into the body and cause infection to occur. If clinical signs and symptoms occur, this is called infectious disease. It is the person who is col-

TABLE 5-1   Potential Occupational Hazards for Critical Care Nurses

Category	Examples
Biological Hazards: Transmission of living organisms, such as bacteria, viruses, and parasites	Human immunodeficiency virus (HIV)
	Hepatitis A virus
	Hepatitis B virus
	Hepatitis C virus
	Hepatitis D virus
	Mycobacterium tuberculosis
	Herpes viruses:
	Herpes simplex virus
	Cytomegalovirus
	Varicella zoster virus
	Neisseria meningitidis
	Intestinal pathogens
	Sarcoptes scabiei
Chemical Hazards: Exposure to natural or synthetic chemical substances	Soaps
	Solvents
	Cleaning agents:
	Glutaraldehyde
	Household bleach
	Formaldehyde
	Compressed gases
	Waste anesthetic gases
	Pharmacological agents:
	Antineoplastic agents
	Ribavirin
	Pentamidine
Ergonomic Hazards: Injury from poor matching of the job, the environment, and the worker	Work station hazards
	Manual lifting
Physical Hazards: The transfer of physical energy from the environment to the individual	Radiant energy:
	Visible light
	Ionizing radiation
	Lasers
	Electricity
	Noise
	Stress
	Shift work
	Violence:
	Physical violence
	Verbal abuse
Psychological Hazards: Psychological stressors that can lead to adverse physical, emotional, or behavioral effects	

TABLE 5-2   Control Methods for Environmental Hazards

Method	Examples
Substitution: Replacement of a potentially harmful agent, device, or procedure with one that is less hazardous	Changing the type of soap because of occurrences of dermatitis
	Using a needleless system to deliver IV medications, instead of a standard system with needle
Engineering Controls: Modification of a device or environment to reduce workers' exposure to hazards	Installing a ventilation system that will provide an appropriate rate of air exchange
	Installing puncture-resistant containers for used needles in patient care areas
Work Practice Modification: Implementation of a plan of action to change personnel behaviors that may put themselves or others at risk for exposure to hazards	Presentation of an educational program that outlines the proper method of disposing of needles and other sharp instruments
	Reinforcing the concept that nurses should request assistance when lifting heavy patients
Personal Protective Equipment: Equipment used to place a physical barrier between the worker and a hazard	Using protective eyewear while a surgical laser is in use
	Using gloves when handling body fluids containing blood
Administrative Controls: Removal of a worker from a situation or environment to reduce the worker's exposure to a hazard	Adjusting a nurse's schedule to eliminate rotating shifts, because of documented negative health effects
	Reassigning of a pregnant nurse to avoid her exposure to ribavirin

onized, or asymptomatically infected, who presents the greatest danger to nurses. If potential infectiousness is not recognized, caregivers may not take protective measures.

Although a wide variety of microbes is present in the critical care environment, most do not present a risk of transmission to the nurse with a normally functioning immune system. In addition, studies have shown that the pregnant nurse is at no greater risk for acquiring infection than the nonpregnant nurse.[2] However, because some infectious agents may have negative health effects on the fetus or neonate, nurses of childbearing age should be particularly diligent in incorporating appropriate infection control measures into their daily practice.

The biological hazards of greatest concern to critical care nurses include the bloodborne pathogens, human immunodeficiency virus (HIV) and hepatitis B virus; the herpes viruses; and *Mycobacterium tuberculosis*. Other pathogens, such as *Neisseria meningitidis* and intestinal pathogens, may also pose a threat, but their transmission to caregivers occurs infrequently.[3]

Protection against some infectious diseases, including rubella (German measles), rubeola (measles), and hepatitis B, can be effectively accomplished by vaccination. The Centers for Disease Control (CDC) of the United States Public Health Service recommends that all health care workers having contact with patients have documentation of immunity to rubeola and rubella, either by medical history or vaccination.[4] In addition, the CDC recommends that all medical personnel at risk for exposure to hepatitis B virus, including critical care nurses, become immunized.[5] The Occupational Safety and Health Administration (OSHA) has mandated that such vaccination be made reasonably available to these employees and that the cost be borne by the employer.[6]

Several simple measures can afford the nurse significant protection from biological hazards. Potentially harmful microorganisms can be effectively removed from the skin by thorough hand washing. The nurse may also reduce risk of exposure by covering the infectious agent's port of exit or entry with such equipment as surgical dressings, masks, gloves, or protective eyewear.

Another important principle in preventing the transmission of infectious agents to nurses concerns the preservation of an intact skin barrier. The skin on the hands is vulnerable to drying and cracking, especially when the hands are washed frequently. Liberal use of moisturizing lotion after washing can help to counteract the drying effect of soaps. The cuticle area on the perimeter of the fingernail must be kept intact to prevent infection. Activities that may damage this area, such as biting or vigorous manicure, should be avoided.

Of particular concern are injuries to the hands by sharp objects such as needles and instruments. Bloodborne pathogens, including human immunodeficiency virus and hepatitis B virus, can be transmitted to the nurse in this manner. The nurse may also be exposed to toxic pharmacological agents, such as antineoplastic drugs, by needle-stick injury. The incidence of such injury is not known, but it is a daily occurrence in most hospitals. One difficulty in estimating the frequency of needle-stick injury is the problem of underreporting. In one study of medical house staff, 70% of such incidents were found to be unreported.[7]

The incidence of needle-stick and sharp-object injuries can be reduced by educating all personnel at risk about the proper handling of needles and "sharps," using needle-proof containers to hold used equipment, and eliminating the practice of recapping or breaking used needles. Needle disposal containers should be emptied when two-thirds to three-quarters full. In one study, 8.4% of needle-stick injuries were found to be caused by used needles protruding from disposal containers.[8] Many new devices, such as needle-less injectors and needle guards, are being introduced to help reduce the incidence of needle-stick injury.

The role of ongoing education in the reduction of exposure to biological hazards cannot be overemphasized. Periodic updated inservice educational offerings on infection control issues and continuous reinforcement of protective techniques are essential to a preventive program. The critical care and infection control departments must work as a team to prevent transmission of infectious disease to the nursing staff.

Human Immunodeficiency Virus and Hepatitis B Virus

Because of their similar modes of transmission and control strategies, hepatitis B virus (HBV) and human immunodeficiency virus (HIV) are discussed together. They are both bloodborne pathogens that can be transmitted in the health care setting by introduction of infective secretions via the percutaneous and permucosal routes. In the community, transmission may also take place at birth, through sexual contact, or by the use of contaminated needles.

Blood and body fluids containing visible blood are the chief sources of infection, but semen, vaginal secretions, body tissues, cerebrospinal fluid, pleural fluid, pericardial fluid, synovial fluid, peritoneal fluids, amniotic fluid, and saliva in dental procedures may also present the risk of transmission. Materials such as feces, urine, nasal secretions, sputum, sweat, tears, and vomitus that do not contain visible blood do not present a risk for transmission of HIV and HBV in the health care setting.[9]

Although HIV and HBV share almost identical modes of transmission, the risk of nurses acquiring HBV infection is far greater than that for HIV infection. It has been estimated that after needlestick injury, the risk for disease with an HBV-contaminated needle is 6% to 30%, whereas the risk with an HIV-contaminated needle is less than 1%.[10] This difference has been generally attributed to the fact that concentration of virus in blood and body fluids is far higher in HBV infection than in HIV infection.

Hepatitis B is an infectious process of the liver caused by the HBV virus. It is usually characterized by malaise, anorexia, nausea, vomiting, abdominal pain, and jaundice. The results of infection can range from asymptomatic infection to fulminant, fatal hepatitis, with a reported case-fatality rate of approximately 1.4%.[11] Sequelae of HBV infection include asymptomatic carriage of the virus, chronic persistent hepatitis, cirrhosis, and primary hepatocellular carcinoma.

Adults who become infected with HBV have a 6% to 10% chance of becoming chronic HBV carriers.[5] The danger that these asymptomatic, and often unknown and unsuspected, carriers present to health care workers is underscored by the CDC's estimate that there are presently 750,000 to 1,000,000 infectious carriers of HBV in the United States.[11]

HBV infection is estimated to occur in 300,000 persons per year in the United States. This includes 6,000 to 8,000 cases among health care workers.[5] Past studies have demonstrated that 15% to 30% of health care workers with frequent exposure to blood may show serological evidence of past or present HBV infection.[4]

To protect themselves, critical care nurses should become immunized against HBV. As mentioned earlier, a safe and effective vaccine against HBV has been in use since 1982. The CDC has recommended that health care workers ideally be immunized during their training and before their first occupational exposure to blood.[12]

Infection with HIV causes defects in the body's immune system. Although a flu-like syndrome may occur soon after infection, most often there are no symptoms for several months or years. Initial symptoms, which may include weight loss and lymphadenopathy, progress to the onset of opportunistic infections and neoplasms. HIV is the causative agent of acquired immunodeficiency syndrome (AIDS), a progressive and ultimately fatal illness that has been defined by specific criteria by the CDC.[13]

The occurrence of AIDS was first reported in the United States in 1981. In the following 10 years, 179,000 cases have been reported to public health departments, and 63% of these persons have died. HIV infection is now among the leading causes of death in men and women less than 45 years of age, and in children between 1 and 5 years of age.[14] As HIV infection affects more diverse segments of the population, critical care nurses must bear in mind that, as is the case with HBV infection, many HIV-infected persons may remain asymptomatic and unrecognized for years. No vaccine protecting against HIV currently exists.

One of the most effective control strategies to prevent exposure to HIV and HBV is the implementation of universal precautions, by which the blood and certain body fluids of *all* persons are considered to be potentially infectious. First proposed by the CDC in 1987[15] and updated in 1988,[9] universal precautions have been accepted as standard practice by health care institutions throughout the country. These precautions include guidelines regarding the use of barrier devices (gloves, masks, protective eyewear), handwashing, prevention of needle-stick and sharp-object injuries, protective mouthpieces for resuscitation, and the management of significant exposures to HIV. OSHA has mandated the use of universal precautions, as well as other exposure control measures, in its standard on Occupational Exposure to Bloodborne Pathogens.[6]

Critical care nurses are at significant risk for acquiring transmitted bloodborne pathogens, and they should be well-versed in universal precautions. Any percutaneous or mucous membrane exposure to blood or other body fluids, or any prolonged exposure of the skin (especially nonintact skin) to blood, should be reported immediately to the employee health service and infection control department so that appropriate management of the exposure may be implemented without delay.

Other Hepatitis Viruses

Hepatitis A Virus

Hepatitis A virus (HAV) causes an illness that is clinically indistinguishable from other forms of hepatitis. However, unlike HBV, HAV is transmitted through fecal contamination and oral ingestion. Outbreaks have been caused by contamination of food and water. Children with HAV infection may be asymptomatic, and the severity of symptoms increases with age. HAV has a case-fatality rate of 0.6%. HAV infection does not result in a chronic carrier state.

HAV transmission can be controlled by using gloves when contact with feces is anticipated, washing hands thoroughly after contact with feces or articles contaminated with feces, and avoiding eating in patient care areas. Nosocomial transmission of HAV to nurses is not common.

Hepatitis C Virus

Until recently, viral hepatitis not classified as HBV or HAV was classified under a general heading of non-A, non-B hepatitis. In May 1990 it became possible through serological tests to identify hepatitis C virus (HCV), which is transmitted via the parenteral route. HCV is believed to be the major etiological agent in bloodborne non-A, non-B hepatitis.[16] HCV presents a potential risk of transmission to critical care nurses in the same manner as HBV, and control methods are identical to those for HBV. So far there is no evidence of HCV being transmitted by casual contact. Research studies are continuing in an attempt to determine other possible routes of transmission.

Hepatitis D Virus

Hepatitis D virus (HDV) has also recently been identified. It appears to cause infection only in the presence of HBV, either as a coinfection during acute hepatitis B, or as a superinfection in chronic HBV carriers. Both coinfection and superinfection with HDV may cause fulminant hepatitis. Since HDV infection occurs only with HBV, preventive methods for HBV will also control transmission of HDV.

Mycobacterium Tuberculosis

The transmission of *Mycobacterium tuberculosis* (MTB) has been recognized as an occupational hazard for health care workers for many years. However, there has been renewed interest in this infectious agent in recent years because of its prevalence among immunocompromised patients and recent immigrants to the United States from less developed countries.

Mycobacterium tuberculosis is designated as an acid-fast bacterium (AFB) because of distinctive laboratory staining characteristics. It can cause disease in many organs and structures of the body, but when discussed in terms of occupational hazards for nurses, the focus is primarily on pulmonary or laryngeal tuberculosis.

This bacterium is transmitted by the airborne route from the lungs of an infected patient to the lungs of the nurse. The bacterium exits from the infected person in the form of droplet nuclei, microscopic particles produced when the person coughs, speaks, or sneezes. These droplet nuclei travel on air currents for long distances within a building.

Symptoms of active pulmonary tuberculosis include fever, night sweats, cough, and weight loss. However, the greatest threat of transmission to the nurse arises from the patient in whom tuberculosis is unsuspected, particularly if the patient has an active cough or is intubated.

Methods used to detect MTB infection include the tuberculin skin test, which is useful in detecting infection in persons without signs of active disease; the chest x-ray; and bacteriology smear and culture of at least three sputum specimens on different days.

It is of concern, however, that MTB infection is sometimes difficult to diagnose, particularly in patients who are also infected with HIV. In the general population, 20% to 50% of persons with pulmonary tuberculosis may have negative sputum smears.[17] In addition, sputum smears from HIV-infected persons with pulmonary tuberculosis are less likely to document acid-fast bacteria than those from persons with normal immune systems. Patients infected with HIV may also have impaired response to the tuberculin skin test and atypical radiological findings in the presence of MTB infection.

Because of the emergence of multi-drug-resistant MTB strains that are resistant to one or more of the common antituberculosis agents, patients receiving antituberculosis drugs should not automatically be assumed to be noninfectious. Any patient with symptoms consistent with tuberculosis should be investigated for MTB infection. The patient should be considered infectious until either infection is ruled out or satisfactory clinical response to antituberculosis drugs has been demonstrated.

Transmission of MTB can be controlled by reducing the spread of infectious droplet nuclei into the air circulation. No single measure completely eliminates the hazard, but a combination of methods may reduce risk substantially. Patients who are able to do so should be instructed to cover all coughs and sneezes with a tissue. With patients who cannot cooperate or are intubated, caregivers should wear a well-fitting surgical mask or particulate respirator. The CDC has issued clear guidelines on precautions against MTB, including isolated ventilation systems and air filters, the use of masks and particulate respirators, decontamination of equipment, and surveillance of personnel for tuberculosis transmission.[17]

Herpesviruses

Virtually every person has been exposed to one or more of the herpesviruses before reaching adulthood. These viruses may cause infection in several parts of the body, most commonly the oral or genital mucous membranes, the cuticle of the fingernail, and the nervous system. Herpesviruses affecting critical care nurses include herpes simplex virus, cytomegalovirus, and herpes zoster virus.

Herpes Simplex Virus

Herpes simplex virus (HSV) is most commonly known as the virus causing vesicular lesions of the oral and genital mucous membranes. It is also the causative agent of herpetic whitlow, an infection of the cuticle area around the fingernail. The virus may lie dormant in the tissues after primary infection, becoming reactivated at some future time to again produce lesions.

Herpes simplex virus is transmitted from patient to nurse through contact with oral, respiratory, or cervical secretions, or contact with herpetic lesions. Control of HSV is easily accomplished by (1) wearing gloves *on both hands* whenever contact with oral or respiratory secretions, such as with suctioning, mouth care, or the taping of endotracheal tubes, is anticipated; (2) wearing gloves when contact with herpetic lesions, cervical secretions, or vaginal mucosa is likely; and (3) thorough hand washing after any direct patient care.

Cytomegalovirus

Cytomegalovirus (CMV) is another virus that causes a primary infection and then may be reactivated to again cause symptoms at a later time. First exposure to CMV usually occurs during childhood. Infants, children, and immunosuppressed patients are the major reservoirs of CMV in hospitals. The mode of transmission is believed to be direct contact with persons excreting CMV or contact with their respiratory secretions, urine, feces, semen, or cervical secretions. Studies have revealed frequent transmission of CMV from children attending day-care centers to their parents and to day-care personnel,[18,19] but increased risk of transmission from patients to hospital personnel has not been demonstrated.[20,21]

Cytomegalovirus infection is usually asymptomatic, or it may cause a mild flu-like syndrome. The major concern regarding CMV is the occurrence of primary infection, or reactivation of previous infection, during pregnancy. Such infection has the potential for causing damage to the fetus, ranging from mild hearing impairment to microcephaly. Cytomegalovirus is the most commonly occuring congenital infection.

Transmission of CMV to the nurse can be effectively controlled by hand washing after contact with patients or with urine, respiratory secretions, or other body fluids. Gloves should be worn if such contact is anticipated. Nurses should refrain from kissing infant and toddler patients.

Varicella Zoster Virus

Varicella zoster virus (VZV) is the causative agent of two distinct illnesses: varicella (chickenpox) and herpes zoster (shingles). Varicella usually occurs as a mild childhood disease, and 90% of adults have immunity by having had either varicella or asymptomatic infection. Symptoms include mild fever, malaise, and a vesicular rash. These symptoms may be more severe in adults and immunosuppressed persons, and serious sequelae such as pneumonia may occur. Varicella causes approximately 100 deaths per year in the United States.[22]

Varicella is transmitted chiefly by the airborne route but also by direct contact with vesicular or mucous membrane secretions. Transmission can take place when the source person is in the prodromal phase of the disease, before the rash appears.

Varicella zoster virus is also responsible for herpes zoster. This condition is believed to be caused by the reactivation of VZV that has been dormant in the body. It is characterized by vesicular lesions along the path of a peripheral nerve. Herpes zoster is not likely to be transmitted from person to person. However, the causative agent, VZV, can be transmitted by direct contact with the vesicular fluid of herpes zoster, possibly resulting in varicella in the nonimmune person.

The nosocomial transmission of VZV is of primary concern for those nurses having no history of either varicella or herpes zoster and a negative serological test for antibodies to VZV. These individuals must avoid any contact with patients with VZV infection. Should contact inadvertently occur, as in the prodromal stage, such personnel should be restricted from direct patient care for the duration of the incubation period (10-21 days). Caregivers who develop varicella are considered infective and must be restricted from work until all of the lesions are dried and crusted.

Sarcoptes Scabiei

Scabies is a condition caused by a parasitic mite, *Sarcoptes scabiei,* which is transmitted by skin-to-skin contact and burrows under the host's skin to lay its eggs. This causes intense itching and skin eruptions, and burrows are often visible on the skin. Affected areas may include the arms, axillae, hands, wrists, thighs, genitalia, and the area beneath the breasts.

Initial treatment with a scabicide, repeated in 7 to 10 days, eliminates the mite. The patient should be considered noninfective after the first treatment. The nurse should wear gown and gloves during direct patient contact if immediate treatment is not possible.

CHEMICAL HAZARDS

Critical care nurses work with chemical substances every day. Exposure to some of these agents may present a potential risk for negative health effects. Chemical hazards include such obviously dangerous substances as antineoplastic drugs and formaldehyde. However, seemingly innocuous materials such as hand soaps, benzoin, and isopropyl alcohol can also cause negative health effects.

Since 1988, the Federal Hazard Communications Standard has required that hospitals provide specific information to their employees regarding potentially hazardous substances. Material Safety Data Sheets (MSDS), which are required by law to be kept in the workplace, identify the hazardous chemical substances present in the critical care unit. The MSDS contain basic information about each substance, including its physical properties, routes of exposure, health effects, and recommendations for cleanup of accidental spills. Nurses should periodically review the MSDS on their unit to become familiar with potential risks that may be faced frequently.

Negative health effects may occur soon after exposure to a chemical hazard. These acute effects may include such symptoms as skin eruption, headache, and nausea. On the other hand, adverse effects may be chronic in nature, not presenting until years after exposure. Examples of such chronic effects are cancer, genetic defects, and lung disease.

Inhalation of a chemical substance provides the most rapid and significant route of entry into the bloodstream. Compounds may also be absorbed through the skin after direct contact, or may be inadvertently ingested during eating, smoking, or applying makeup with contaminated hands.

Soaps

Soaps can cause drying, chapping, cracking, and inflammation of the skin. Sensitization to soaps may occur after days, weeks, or years of use, causing severe allergic skin reaction after exposure.

The use of moisturizing lotion after hand washing may help eliminate drying and chapping, thereby aiding in the maintenance of an intact skin barrier. If an allergic reaction occurs, the nurse should try to identify the chemical ingredient responsible for the sensitivity and substitute an alternative product that does not contain this agent.

Solvents

Solvents are compounds that can dissolve other compounds. In the critical care unit, common solvents are isopropyl alcohol, benzoin, and acetone. Solvents can enter the body by inhalation and skin absorption.

Exposure to solvents can produce a variety of central nervous system symptoms including fatigue, headache, drowsiness or insomnia, vertigo, impaired memory, concentration problems, mood changes, and feelings of exhilaration.[23] Skin exposure can also cause drying and irritation of the affected area.

Exposure can be prevented by wearing gloves when handling solvents and by avoiding the inhalation of vapors. Solvents, like all chemical substances, should be kept in tightly capped containers that are clearly labeled to indicate their contents.

Cleaning Agents

Glutaraldehyde

Glutaraldehyde and related compounds are cleaning agents commonly used in critical care units. Exposure via inhalation or skin contact may cause lightheadedness, nausea, chest tightness, and irritation of the skin, eyes, and respiratory system. Although long-term health effects are not yet well documented, animal studies have shown glutaraldehyde exposure to be associated with fetotoxicity, DNA damage, and mutagenicity.[24] Glutaraldehyde should be used only as directed and only in well-ventilated areas.

Bleach

Household bleach, commonly used as a disinfectant, can cause skin, eye, and respiratory irritation. Care should be taken to avoid splashing into the eyes. Gloves should be worn to prevent skin contact, and inhalation of mist from spray bottles must be avoided.

Formaldehyde

Of particular concern to critical care nurses is exposure to formaldehyde, a caustic substance used as a cold sterilant. It is most commonly used in laboratories and central supply areas but may be seen in critical care units as a sterilant for dialysis equipment.

Formaldehyde exposure may occur by direct contact or inhalation. Splashes to the eye can cause corneal damage and severe injury. Skin contact commonly leads to dermatitis and, if the contact is chronic softening and discoloration of the fingernails.

Negative health effects resulting from the inhalation of formaldehyde vary in severity according to the concentration of the formaldehyde vapors and the frequency of exposure. Low concentrations cause eye and respiratory irritation. More concentrated exposures may cause chest tightness, tachycardia, coughing, and a sensation of pressure in the head. Very high concentrations may cause pneumonitis, pulmonary edema, and death. Nurses who have repeated exposures may become sensitized and experience eye irritation, upper respiratory symptoms, or asthmatic reactions when exposed to levels that do not cause symptoms in others. Formaldehyde odor is not a reliable indicator of its presence because even short periods of exposure decrease a person's ability to smell it.[24]

Animal studies have demonstrated formaldehyde's mutagenic and carcinogenic properties. The National Institute for Occupational Safety and Health (NIOSH) considers formaldehyde to be a potential carcinogen in the workplace.[25]

Control strategies for exposure to formaldehyde have been recommended by NIOSH.[25] These focus on the prevention of exposure and include environmental monitoring, personal protective equipment, medical monitoring, and engineering controls.

Compressed Gases

Compressed gases used in critical care units include oxygen, and less commonly, helium and carbon dioxide. Most oxygen in hospitals is stored in a central location and distributed through a system of pipes to patient care areas, but cylinders continue to be used during patient transport.

Any cylinder of compressed gas can pose a safety hazard because the gas has been compressed inside the cylinder until it is almost liquid. If the cylinder is heated, the gas will expand, and continued heating and expansion of the gas will lead to explosion of the cylinder. It is therefore essential that compressed gas cylinders be stored away from sources of heat or extremes in temperature.

Cylinders should always be secured in racks. A

freestanding cylinder may fall over and break, causing the sudden release of pressure. Particular attention should be paid to securing oxygen cylinders to beds or stretchers during transport to prevent them from rolling to the floor.

Oxygen can also present a fire hazard. Although it is not a flammable gas, it does support and accelerate combustion. Open flames and smoking should never be allowed in an area where oxygen is in use.

Waste Anesthetic Gases

The effects of exposure to waste anesthetic gases among operating room personnel have been well studied during the past 20 years. In this setting, the main source of exposure is leakage from anesthesia equipment. However, critical care nurses may also be exposed to waste anesthetic gases as they are exhaled by postoperative patients.

Acute effects of exposure to waste anesthetic gases include fatigue, irritability, drowsiness, depression, headache, nausea, and impaired coordination and judgment.[26] Long-term studies have suggested an increased incidence of liver and kidney disease, cancer, and adverse reproductive effects.[26,27] Further, it has been documented that even low levels of exposure can cause toxic effects.[28]

Nurses should avoid close contact with the air exhaled by postoperative patients. If acute symptoms occur, the nurse should leave the area as soon as possible. Adequate ventilation and air exchange in patient rooms are the best control methods in the prevention of exposure. Repeated reports of acute toxic symptoms may warrant investigation of the adequacy of air exchange in patient care areas.

Pharmacological Agents

One class of drugs, antineoplastic agents, has been well studied and is known to be potentially hazardous to nurses. However, little research has been conducted on the short- and long-term effects of other pharmacological agents that are encountered daily. It is therefore wise to treat all drugs as potential chemical hazards and to limit occupational exposure to these substances as much as possible. This can be accomplished by avoiding the inhalation of drug dust or aerosolized droplets, preventing direct skin contact with drugs, wiping up all spills immediately, washing hands thoroughly after preparing and administering medications, and refraining from eating or drinking in areas where medications are stored, prepared, or administered.

The importance of these precautions is underscored by recent concerns about potential negative health effects of two commonly used medications,

ribavirin and pentamidine, which are discussed in this section.

Antineoplastic Agents

Antineoplastic, or cytotoxic, drugs are those used in the treatment of cancer. They work by interfering with the structure or metabolism of malignant cells, thereby preventing their growth and development. More than 30 antineoplastic agents are currently in use, and many of these have been shown to have the potential for causing negative health effects.

Accidental exposure can occur by inhalation of the aerosolized agent during preparation, or by direct skin absorption as a result of spills or by contact with the urine of patients receiving antineoplastic agents. In addition, these agents can be ingested if hands or surfaces are contaminated with these substances.

Acute effects include vertigo, nausea, headache, skin or mucous membrane reactions, and allergic reactions. Some agents can cause severe tissue necrosis upon direct contact or accidental needlestick injury. Numerous studies involving both human and animal subjects have suggested serious chronic effects including mutagenicity, embryotoxicity, carcinogenicity, and teratogenicity.[29]

Because of the risks involved in handling antineoplastic agents, OSHA has issued clear guidelines regarding the necessary equipment, preparation, administration, handling, and disposal of these substances.[30] Only nurses who have received special education and training, and who are thoroughly familiar with the OSHA guidelines, should handle or administer antineoplastic drugs.

Ribavirin

Ribavirin is an antiviral agent used in the treatment of severe respiratory syncytial virus (RSV) infections in children. It is administered by the aerosol route, allowing much of the drug to be released into the environment, where it can be inhaled by caregivers, precipitate in the delivery equipment, and accumulate on surfaces and bed linens. In addition, the patient's respiratory secretions may contain the drug.[31]

Exposure to aerosolized ribavirin can cause eye irritation in persons wearing contact lenses, coughing, and throat irritation. Persons with underlying respiratory conditions may develop wheezing and shortness of breath. Of even greater concern are data regarding possible mutagenic properties of the drug, and studies are currently investigating the possibility of carcinogenicity. Animal studies have demonstrated evidence of testicular atrophy and teratogenic and embryolethal effects, although there have been no reports of birth defects in humans to date.[32]

Control strategies focus on reducing the release of ribavirin into the environment and minimizing caregivers' contact with the substance. These strategies include the use of specially designed delivery equipment and scavenging systems. The patient receiving the drug should be placed in a private room with static or negative air pressure, with the door closed at all times. A sign indicating the presence of ribavirin and its hazards should be posted outside the patient's room to make staff, and visitors, aware of the risks.

It is currently recommended that gown, gloves, and hair and shoe covers be worn by persons entering the room, although data are inconclusive regarding the effectiveness of these measures in reducing exposure. In addition, persons who wear contact lenses should wear goggles. Studies indicate that surgical and dust masks are ineffective in preventing exposure to ribavirin. A respirator must be worn if exposure to aerosolized ribavirin is unavoidable.[33]

Because of the degree of potential reproductive risk, it is recommended that women who are pregnant or likely to become pregnant be informed of the health hazards involved and make an informed choice about whether or not to care for persons receiving ribavirin. Persons with respiratory conditions should minimize their contact with ribavirin. It is recommended that alternative work assignments be made available to those who believe they are at risk.[33]

Pentamidine

Pentamidine is a drug used to prevent *Pneumocystis carinii* infection in persons infected with HIV. Exposure to aerosolized pentamidine may cause coughing and wheezing in both patients receiving treatment and their caregivers, particularly those with a history of smoking or asthma. The safety of pentamidine exposure during pregnancy has not yet been established.

Exposure to pentamidine should be minimized or eliminated. Special filters for nebulizer equipment, when properly used, can significantly decrease the amount of pentamidine released into the environment.

Pentamidine can also play a role in exposing nurses to a biologic hazard. Because it causes profuse coughing, it can play a role in the airborne transmission of *Mycobacterium tuberculosis* from patient to nurse. The CDC has recommended that all patients be screened for active tuberculosis before aerosolized pentamidine treatment is begun. Pentamidine treatments for a patient with suspected or confirmed active tuberculosis must be administered in a room specifically designed to minimize the airborne spread of *M. tuberculosis*. Personnel entering this room during treatments must further protect themselves by wearing a particulate respirator.[17]

ERGONOMIC HAZARDS

Ergonomics is the science that deals with the relationship between the worker, the kind of work being performed, and the workspace in which the work is done. In an ergonomically correct environment, the flow of work is smooth and without obstruction. Physical and psychological stress, which occur with any work, are kept at a minimal level. This is the ideal workplace, but unfortunately few critical care units fit this description.

Ergonomic hazards exist when there is a mismatch between the worker, the environment, and the task at hand. Such hazards can pose both acute and chronic negative health effects for critical care nurses. Acute effects include muscle sprains and strains, lacerations, and contusions. Chronic effects may include chronic low back pain, joint disorders, and psychological stress.

Work Station Hazards

The work station is the space in which a certain set of tasks is to be performed. Improper design or misguided work practices can lead to a number of work station hazards.

Work stations in the critical care unit, such as patient care rooms, nurses' stations, and utility rooms, should be designed to provide clear traffic patterns, conveniently located equipment, and easy access to the work being done. In reality, patient care areas are frequently too small or of poor design. As a result, nurses practice within a maze of equipment and must assume awkward working positions. Wall-mounted equipment, such as cardiac monitors, may be too high for access by shorter persons, or sufficiently low to present the danger of head injury to tall personnel. Uneven floors can present the potential for falls.

Some work station hazards may be caused not by poor design but rather by improper work practices of personnel. Equipment left in hallways may block traffic patterns, increasing physical stress when patients or emergency equipment need to be moved quickly. Heavy boxes or equipment stored on high shelves may lead to soft tissue injury and muscle strain. Falls may occur if spilled liquids are not cleaned up promptly, or if unstable chairs, rather than sturdy step stools, are used to reach equipment that is too high.

Although injuries caused by work station hazards are frequently of an acute nature, symptoms may be insidious in onset and cumulative. A flaw in work station design should be suspected when there are frequent or repeated reports of staff injury.

The goal of assuring a safe and healthful workplace can be achieved by critically examining the work environment. Any ergonomic problems should be reported promptly. Some deficiencies can be corrected only by major remodeling, but many are easily remedied by minor ergonomic measures or modification of work practices.

Manual Lifting

Despite the development of sophisticated patient care devices, manual lifting continues to be an essential part of nursing practice. In addition to positioning and lifting patients, nurses frequently must move beds and heavy equipment. The result, all too often, is musculoskeletal injury, and the lower back is most commonly the site of such injury.

Back injuries account for almost half of all compensation claims among hospital workers in the United States.[24] Despite these statistics, back injuries among nurses are believed to be significantly underreported. In one study, 41% of a sample of nurses working in a large hospital had experienced back pain within the previous 6 months, yet only 4% had filed workers' compensation claims.[34]

The onset of back pain may occur either gradually or suddenly after prolonged sitting or standing, or can be precipitated by lifting, bending, or twisting. Often, working in an awkward position, particularly forward flexion, may cause the onset of back pain. The discomfort can range from mild to severe and may be constant or intermittent. It may be accompanied by secondary muscle spasm, which sometimes causes the back to lock in a oblique or forward-flexed position. Sciatica, back pain that radiates down the leg, usually indicates a condition arising in an intervertebral disk. It may be accompanied by numbness or tingling in the affected foot.

Although the exact pathophysiology of nonspecific low back pain is largely unknown, it is generally believed to be caused by changes in the spine that occur with the aging process. After age 25, degenerative changes in both the vertebrae and the intervertebral disks may make the spine less resistant to workloads and thus more vulnerable to injury.[35]

Many factors play a part in the high rate of back injury among nurses. Patient care involves frequent lifting of heavy loads, bending, twisting, and extended forward reaches. The human form is bulky and inefficiently shaped for being lifted. Work is often performed in awkward positions, and uncooperative patients may increase the workload by resisting movement. The risk for back injury is further increased in emergency situations involving the sudden collapse of a patient or the need for immediate, unanticipated lifting.

In the past, literature on the prevention of back injury has emphasized the role of personal actions on the part of the nurse, such as exercise and body mechanics. Although there is much to be said for personal fitness and good work practices, the results of research studies have not clearly shown whether such measures actually help prevent back injury.[36] A more balanced approach takes into account several factors. The combination of an ergonomically well designed workspace, control of work demands, and adherence to specific work practices may play a major role in the prevention of lower back injury.

The layout of the patient care area should allow good access to the patient, reducing the need to reach or twist. The nurse should get as close as possible to a load, such as a patient or object, before attempting to move or lift it. Work surfaces and equipment should be adjustable in height so that patient care can be performed at a level that will reduce or eliminate bending of the trunk of the body. If work must be done in a lowered position, kneeling will place less stress on the lumbar muscles than bending or squatting.

Perhaps the most important principle to remember in preventing injury to the back is that of matching the workload to human capability. Critical care nurses must realize that no matter how correct their technique, they are risking back injury if the workload capability of the musculoskeletal structure is exceeded. An object that is 35% of a person's body weight is considered excessively heavy,[37] and should not be lifted without assistance. This means that a nurse who weighs 130 pounds should not attempt to lift, without help, any workload or patient that weighs more than 45½ pounds. This assistance can be in the form of other personnel or mechanical lift or transfer devices. Adequate staffing is an essential part of a back injury prevention program.

Any work-related musculoskeletal injury should be reported to the employee health department without delay. This not only assures proper treatment of the injury but also allows a realistic assessment of the scope of ergonomic problems that may exist within the institution. Timely modification of these problems may prevent future injuries among nursing staff, thereby ultimately reducing the hospital's compensation costs.

PHYSICAL HAZARDS

Physical hazards are those that involve the transfer of physical energy to the nurse; they are associated primarily with the "machinery" of critical care. Included in this category are radiation, electricity, and noise.

Radiant Energy Hazards

Electromagnetic radiation, or radiant energy, exists in various forms. Some kinds of radiant energy, such as x-rays, have become commonplace in critical care nursing. Others, such as radiowaves and gamma rays, are not as familiar.

The different types of radiant energy all lie within the electromagnetic spectrum according to their particular wavelengths (Figure 5-1). Wavelength is expressed in nanometers (nm). One nm is equal to one billionth of a meter.

Human beings are exposed to the full spectrum of electromagnetic radiation every day. Sunlight and cosmic rays are natural sources of radiant energy. Some man-made sources are cardiac monitors, microwave ovens, and x-ray equipment. The different types of radiant energy produce distinct physiological effects. Some are beneficial and necessary for life, but others are harmful; these are known as physical hazards. Radiant energy hazards common in the critical care unit are visible light, ionizing radiation, and lasers.

Visible Light

Visible light is that which can be seen by the human eye. Incandescent and fluorescent lighting fixtures are sources of visible light in the critical care unit. Excessively harsh, glaring lights can cause eye fatigue and headaches. Unshielded or unfiltered fluorescent lights, particularly when positioned at eye level, are a common source of problems. No long-term health effects have been documented.

Discomfort produced by inappropriate lighting can be eliminated by the use of filters or shields, or by repositioning lighting fixtures to eliminate glare. For

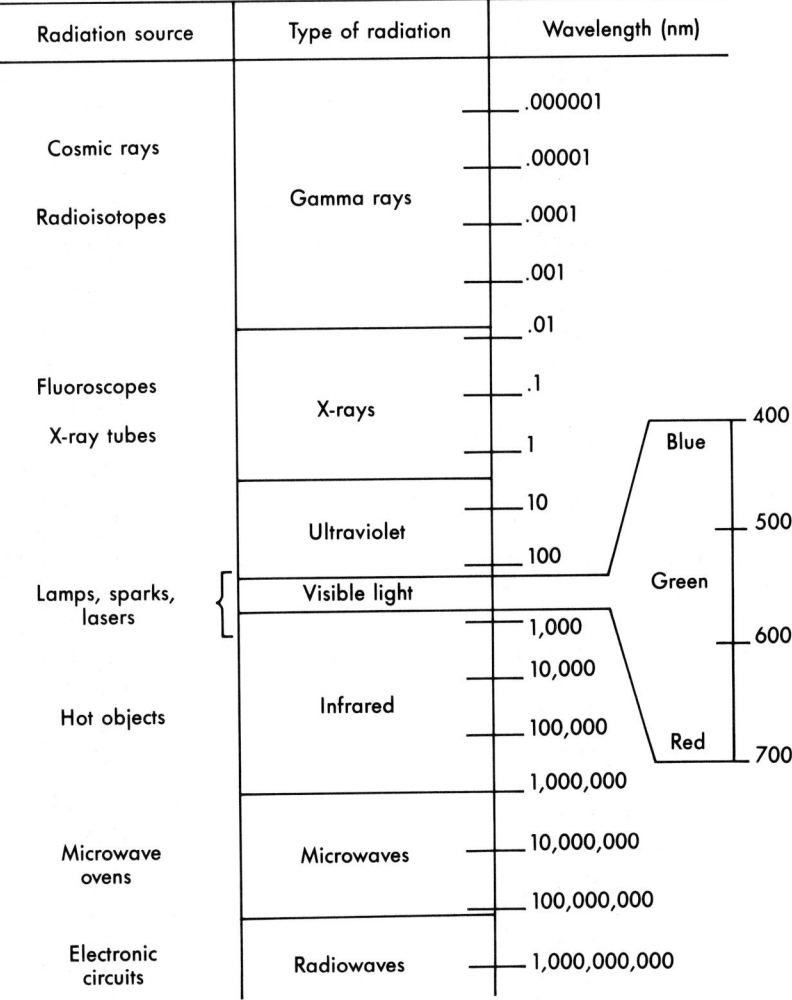

Figure 5-1   Spectrum of electromagnetic radiation.

the physical and psychological comfort of both staff and patients, provision should be made for adjusting to lower lighting levels at night.

Ionizing Radiation

Ionizing radiation is a type of electromagnetic radiation that has shorter wavelengths than visible light. Both x-rays and gamma rays are types of ionizing radiation. Sources of ionizing radiation in the critical care unit are x-rays done in patient care areas, fluoroscopy equipment, and patients who have received diagnostic radioactive materials.

Because of its energy level, ionizing radiation is capable of injuring human cells by disrupting the atomic structure of component molecules. Changes in genetic structure, alteration in metabolism, and abnormalities of cell division can result from exposure to ionizing radiation. Cells that divide rapidly, such as those of the gonads, blood-forming tissues, skin, and eye lenses, are most dramatically affected.

Brief exposure to high doses of ionizing radiation can cause acute radiation syndrome (radiation sickness), bone marrow depression, cerebral edema, and death. However, when ionizing radiation as a hazard for critical care nurses is being discussed, it is exposure to low doses over a long time that is of concern. The effects of radiation exposure are cumulative, and resultant health problems may not appear until years after exposure. Chronic effects of ionizing radiation include cancer, lung and kidney fibrosis, cataracts, sterility, and aplastic anemia. Exposure of the fetus can lead to congenital abnormalities, mental retardation, and fetal death.

The National Council on Radiation Protection and Measurements (NCRP) has established maximum permissible dose (MPD) limits for persons with and without occupational exposure. The quantity of irradiation incurred by an exposed person is expressed in units called rems. The current MPD for workers in radiology departments is 5 rems/year. Nurses outside radiology departments are permitted to accrue 0.5 rems/year. Workers who are exposed to 1.25 rems/year or greater must wear a film badge to monitor exposure.[38]

The exact amount of radiation exposure that will cause biologic damage is unknown, but any exposure is believed to involve some risk. Therefore, nurses should avoid all occupational radiation exposure. Recent studies support earlier evidence that even low levels of radiation are more hazardous than previously believed. Recently, a panel of international experts on ionizing radiation recommended a significant reduction in existing permissible dose limits for radiation.[39]

The exposure of critical care nurses to ionizing radiation can be eliminated if specific control strategies are employed. As a first measure, all diagnostic x-rays should be performed in the radiology department where proper engineering controls, such as lead shielding, are in place. Portable x-rays should be used only when there is no alternative.

If portable x-rays or fluoroscopy must be used, the nurse should stay as far away as possible from the source of radiation. A minimum distance of 10 feet has been recommended.[40] If the nurse must remain closer than 10 feet, a lead apron covering front and back must be used to shield against exposure to radiation. For longer exposures, such as during angiography, thyroid shields and lead goggles should be worn.[24] If the hands must be near the radiation source, such as when restraining or positioning the patient, lead gloves should be worn. No part of the body should ever be directly exposed to ionizing radiation.

Because the dose of radiation is directly proportional to the length of time of exposure, nurses should minimize the time of exposure to an ionizing radiation source as much as possible, even when protective lead garments are used.

All persons who operate radiology equipment, including fluoroscopy equipment, should do so only after receiving thorough training. Educational programs should include the proper use and maintenance of protective lead garments. Lead aprons, gloves, and thyroid shields must be stored without folding or creasing. If care is not taken, the lead will develop holes and cracks that will allow the passage of ionizing radiation. Lead garments should be checked at least annually for integrity.

Another source of ionizing radiation is the body substances of persons who have received radioactive materials during diagnostic procedures. The urine, feces, and other body substances are considered to be radioactive for up to 24 hours after the test. Waterproof gloves should be used to prevent contact when disposing of these substances. Most diagnostic procedures involve small doses of radioactive materials with very short half-lives, and contact with the patient presents no radiation hazard.

Lasers

Lasers produce a form of radiant energy that is focused and intense. The very high energy density of laser light makes it useful in surgery for cutting, ablation, and cauterization. However, lasers are being used more frequently outside of the surgical suite for procedures such as endoscopy, and may be seen in the critical care unit.

Laser light occurs in the form of a well-defined

beam of very concentrated light. This beam is of a specific wavelength, again expressed in nm, and of narrow spectral range. The light that is emitted from the laser may fall in different places on the electromagnetic spectrum, both visible and invisible. (See Figure 5-1.)

Because of their high energy output, lasers can pose hazards to personnel. The manufacture, labeling, and approved uses for laser devices are regulated by the Center for Devices and Radiological Health (CDRH), of the U.S. Food and Drug Administration. A number of other organizations have also issued guidelines.

The American National Standards Institute (ANSI) has published standards for the safe use of lasers in health care,[41] and these standards are recognized by OSHA. ANSI has also devised a classification system based on the intensity of the laser beam:[41]

Class I lasers: used mostly in laboratories, have minimal power, present no significant risk, and require no special labeling or precautions.

Class II lasers: used in procedures as aiming beams for invisible laser beams and cause no harm with brief viewing, although prolonged viewing may produce chronic, degenerative eye damage.

Class III lasers: commonly used in ophthalmology procedures, have moderate power, and can injure the eye if viewed directly, or indirectly by reflection.

Class IV lasers: high-powered lasers commonly used in hospitals. They can cause ocular injury, burns, and fires, either from direct contact with the laser beam or from reflected radiation.

Most lasers used for medical purposes belong to class III or IV and are capable of causing moderate to serious injury to the eyes and skin. These lasers may also present potential biological risk from the smoke, safety risk from combustion of flammable materials, or electrical hazard from the high voltage power supply required by the devices. Nurses should be present during laser procedures only if they have completed a laser education program that includes information on safe operation, hazards, and control strategies. Whenever a laser is in use, a warning sign, specifying that protective eyewear is required, must be posted outside the room.

Precautions must be taken to prevent reflection of the laser beam, since it can pose as much danger as direct contact. All reflective or shiny objects, including jewelry and mirrors, must be removed from the room, and nonreflective instruments must be used.

The part of the body most vulnerable to injury from laser light is the eye. Damage, which can lead to partial or total blindness of the affected eye, can be caused by contact of either a direct or a reflected laser beam with the eye. Ocular injury can be prevented by wearing protective eyewear whenever a laser is in use. Goggles must be specifically matched to the wavelength of the type of laser being used. ANSI standards recommend a program of ophthalmological medical surveillance for personnel routinely working with lasers.

Laser beam exposure of the skin can cause mild to serious burns. Protective coverings should be used if the hands are near the laser's target field area.

Lasers can cause fires by igniting dry drapes, bedclothes, and other materials. The danger is further intensified in an oxygen-enriched environment. All flammable materials in the target area should be moistened with sterile water. Flammable substances, such as alcohol, should be removed from the target area.

Laser smoke plumes have always been regarded as objectionable, because of an unpleasant odor and eye irritation. Since 1975, however, studies have suggested that viable bacterial or viral agents may be present in the plume, presenting the possibility of transmission to exposed persons. Smoke evacuation systems must always be used during laser procedures, and masks, preferably special laser masks, should be worn for additional protection.[42]

Electrical Hazards

Electricity is an occupational hazard frequently encountered in the critical care unit. Virtually all electronic and mechanical patient care devices are powered by electricity. To protect themselves and their patients against this potential hazard, nurses need a basic understanding of electrical principles.

Electrical current is the continual flow of electrons along a conductive path. For these electrons to flow from one point to another, there must be a voltage difference between the two points. This voltage difference is generated at the power plant and is carried via power lines to access points, which are the familiar three-holed electrical outlets. The slot on the top right of the outlet is the charged or hot line, the slot on the top left is the neutral line, and the round hole at the bottom is the ground line. The electrical current flows from the charged line, through the device plugged into the outlet, and then out through the neutral line. The device is powered when the electrical current flows through it.

Ideally, the electrical current is completely contained within the circuit as described above. However, this is not always the case, and some current may leak into the device itself. The function of the third, round hole, or ground line, in the electrical outlet is to take this stray current harmlessly away from the appliance.

Unfortunately, there can be a flaw either in the device or in the ground line itself, allowing electrical charge to accumulate within the device and pose the danger of electrical shock.

A conductor is any material that allows electrons to flow freely. Examples of good conductors are water and metal. The human body can also conduct electrical current, although not as efficiently as water or metal. For this reason, a person can inadvertently act as a conductive path for electrical current if a circuit is completed between a faulty piece of equipment and a good ground, such as plumbing or another piece of electrically powered equipment. The result of this situation is electrical shock.

Health effects of electrical shock can range from a tingling sensation to burns of varying severity, cardiac dysrhythmias, and death. If the level of electrical current is beyond the "let go range," involuntary contraction of the muscles of the hands and arms prevents the victim from letting go of the source of electrical shock. This may progress to exhaustion, paralysis of the respiratory muscles, respiratory failure, and death.[43]

Any discussions of electrical hazards that face critical care nurses must include hazards to the patient. Many patients in the critical care unit are considered to be "electrically sensitive," that is, they have in place some device, such as a central intravenous line or pacemaker wire, that can provide a pathway allowing electrical current to travel directly to the myocardium. Such patients can develop life-threatening dysrhythmias when very low levels of electrical current, hardly perceptible to an individual with an intact skin barrier, are introduced via a direct cardiac pathway. This is known as *cardiac microshock*.

The electrically sensitive patient can be protected by a few simple measures. Rubber gloves should be worn whenever handling the external end of catheters or wires positioned in the heart. All conductive parts of a pacemaker system should be covered with rubber gloves or moistureproof dressings. The nurse should not touch the patient and an electrical device at the same time. Finally, if the nurse or patient feels a tingling sensation when touching a surface, biomedical engineering personnel should be called promptly to investigate the source.

Prevention of exposure to electrical hazards can be accomplished in part by a strong biomedical engineering program, which includes periodic maintenance of all electrical devices, safety testing of new equipment before it is put into service, and regular testing of all electrical wiring and wall outlets. OSHA has adopted the National Electrical Code (NEC)[44] as a standard to ensure an electrically safe environment. In addition to the NEC, hospitals are subject to state and local regulations regarding electrical safety.

Critical care nurses must be able to recognize electrical hazards before an untoward incident. Any faulty equipment should be taken out of service, clearly tagged as defective, and reported to the biomedical engineering department. Electrical hazards include damaged equipment such as a plug or cord that is cracked, frayed, or becomes warm during use; an electrical outlet that is cracked or loose; separation of a plug from its cord; and an electrical device that has been dropped or had liquid spilled into it, makes unusual noises or odors, or smokes during use.

Inadequately grounded equipment, including any device with a two-pronged plug or a plug with a bent or broken grounding pin, can also present the risk of shock. "Cheaters" (ungrounded adaptors) should never be used. Electrical devices owned by patients or personnel should not be allowed in patient care areas because of unverified grounding.

Some electrical hazards can be avoided by proper work practices of personnel. To avoid separation of the cord and plug, the plug should be removed from the wall receptacle by firmly grasping the plug, not the cord, and pulling straight out. Wall receptacles should never be overloaded by using mutliple-outlet adaptors, which can be a serious fire hazard. During defibrillation, all personnel must stand clear of the patient, bed, and bedclothes. A dry environment, including bedclothes, floors, and other surfaces, must be maintained around electrical equipment. Electrical devices should not be touched with wet hands.

Noise

Noise is any unwanted or unpleasant sound. Noise is perceived when sound waves, vibrations in the air, are conducted via the ear. Noise can been classified as continuous or impulsive. *Continuous noise* is maintained at a constant level with little variation, whereas *impulsive noise* is intense and of short duration, occurring at regular or irregular intervals. A critical care unit is likely to contain the continuous background noise of ventilators or bubbling chest suction equipment, punctuated at irregular intervals by impulsive noises such as monitor alarms and ringing telephones.

Sound can be described in terms of three characteristics: loudness, frequency, and amplitude. Loudness is a subjective perception of sound, and there is no way to measure it. Frequency, or pitch, can be measured in cycles per second (Hertz or Hz). Amplitude, or intensity, can be measured in decibels (dB). The decibel scale is logarithmic rather than linear, so that when a sound increases by 10 dB, it increases ten times in intensity.

The U.S. Environmental Protection Agency (EPA) has defined sound levels greater than 40 dB during the day, and 35 dB at night as "noise" in the hospital setting.[45] Background noise in critical care units has been measured at the 60 dB range, while intermittent noise may be as high as 90 dB.[46] Standards now exist for continuous noise but not for impulsive noise. Measurement techniques for a combination of continuous and impulsive noise, which is the pattern in most critical care units, do not exist at this time.

Noise levels in critical care units are probably not high enough to cause hearing loss, but other potential health effects are of concern. A general stress reaction can occur in exposed persons, leading to physiological changes in the cardiovascular, endocrine, and neurological systems.[24] One study demonstrated noise levels in nursing units to be high enough to reduce productivity.[47] In addition, excessive noise can hamper communications and the ability to concentrate on critical job functions. Research into the long-term effects of exposure to noise has been inconclusive.

Most noise in the critical care unit can be reduced or eliminated quite easily. Personnel can help control noise levels by keeping doors closed, keeping conversations to a minimum, attending to patient call lights and monitor alarms promptly, and setting the volume on alarms and telephone ringers as low as practical. Modification of equipment, such as adjusting mechanisms so that doors cannot slam, lubricating wheels on carts, and locating noisy equipment such as computer printers only on sturdy surfaces with adequate cushioning, can significantly decrease noise levels. Quietness of operation should be considered as an important feature in purchasing new patient care equipment. If noise continues to be a problem, further strategies might include using movable acoustical screens, installing sound-absorbing materials on walls, floors, or ceilings, and re-routing traffic patterns.

PSYCHOLOGICAL HAZARDS

Psychological hazards are environmental stressors in the critical care unit that may lead to emotional, behavioral, or physical symptoms. Although exposure to some of these stressors can be significantly reduced or eliminated, many are unavoidable elements of critical care nursing practice. Critical care nurses should become familiar with effective control strategies for the psychological hazards they may face every day.

Stress

All practicing critical care nurses know what occupational stress is, and have probably experienced it frequently. Stress has been described as psychological discomfort caused when a person's coping abilities are exceeded.[48] Stress is certainly not unique to critical care nursing, but the demands that are faced in critical care units undoubtedly place staff in a position of high risk for exposure.

Frequently, a situation may be very stressful to one nurse but not to a colleague. Whether a person perceives a situation as stressful depends on many factors, including personality, family and social relationships, past experiences, interpersonal skills, and health status. Occupational stress in the critical care unit can arise from a number of stimuli, including physical characteristics of the unit, caring for seriously ill or dying patients, interpersonal conflicts, dissatisfaction with unit management, perceived inadequacy of skills or knowledge, and life events outside of the work site.[49]

In the physical environment of the critical care unit, inadequate supplies, malfunctioning equipment, noise, glaring lights, and crowded work stations can cause, or escalate, psychological discomfort among personnel.

Caring for unstable or dying patients and their families is the daily work of critical care nursing. The need to deal frequently with complex therapies, emergency interventions, emotional situations, and ethical controversies may increase stress.

Interpersonal conflicts may involve other members of the nursing staff, managers, physicians, or other hospital departments. Conflicts can arise because of personality, ineffective leadership, poor communications, and disagreement over treatment.

Problems with unit management, including inadequate staffing, inappropriate admissions, floating to other units, heavy workload, and shift rotation, are frequent sources of job stress.

Critical care nurses may become psychologically taxed when they feel that they do not have the knowledge and skills necessary to meet the demands of their job. This feeling can result from inadequate orientation or insufficient instruction when new patient care equipment or procedures are introduced.

Persons may be more susceptible to work-related stress when responsibilities of family, school, or finances have already strained their psychological resources.

Response to occupational stress may be manifested in physical, emotional, or behavioral symptoms. Physical signs are related to the "fight or flight" reaction to stress: elevated blood pressure, muscle tension, and an increase in pulse and respirations. Prolonged exposure may bring about headaches, gastrointestinal disturbances, increased susceptibility to illness, insomnia, and alteration in appetite. Behavioral symptoms may include decreased productivity, decline in work performance, increase in accident and error rate, a rise in absenteeism, inability to concentrate, and lethargy. Emotional changes, including depression, negativism, irritability, withdrawal, emotional outbursts, and hostility may also be exhibited.[50,51,52] Studies of other professions exposed to job stress have revealed an increased risk for peptic ulcers and hypertension, but the long-term health effects of occupational stress among critical care nurses are largely unstudied and unknown.[53] Critical care nurses must learn to recognize that these symptoms may be caused by exposure to excessive stress. Once the cause is known, appropriate control strategies can be put into place.

Whenever possible, the source of stress should be eliminated. The physical environment should be assessed for stressors and corrective actions initiated. Administrative mechanisms should ensure adequate supplies and prompt repair of broken equipment. Efforts should be made to secure adequate staffing and realistic workloads. Stress related to shift work may be alleviated by allowing staff more control in designing work schedules.

Educational programs should address the changing demands for knowledge and skills placed upon critical care nurses. They should include timely orientation to new patient care equipment. Programming can assist nurses in acquiring communication and conflict resolution skills. Efforts should be made to develop within the critical care unit a culture of peer and managerial support for staff, and mechanisms for providing staff with control of their practice.

Other techniques that have been useful in reducing stress include balancing work with social and recreational activities, regular physical exercise, good nutrition, and relaxation techniques. Critical care nurses experiencing significant job stress can be helped through an employee assistance program that incorporates psychological counseling. Such a program should be readily accessible to the staff.

Shift Work

If patients are to be provided with nursing care around the clock, shift work is unavoidable. Numerous studies have shown shift work, particularly night and rotating shifts, to produce a number of short-term physical and psychological effects. These include chronic fatigue, gastrointestinal disturbances, anorexia, and peptic ulcer.[54] Shift workers sleep fewer total hours and less soundly than non-shift workers. The ability to complete complex cognitive tasks may decline, and the rate of both accidents and errors may rise.[55] Shift workers generally interact less frequently with family, friends, and other support groups. Psychological symptoms may include depression, withdrawal, irritability, and anxiety. Although some studies have demonstrated an association between shift work and cardiovascular risk factors,[56]

relatively little is known about the long-term health effects of shift work.[55]

Negative health effects of shift work are thought to be related to the disruption of the normal biologic, or circadian, rhythm of the body. When individuals follow a normal diurnal pattern of work and sleep, that is, working during the day and sleeping at night, their circadian rhythm is the same on the days they work and on days off. The body's circadian "clock" is synchronized to a diurnal schedule.

Persons working the night shift on a regular basis may become synchronized to a nocturnal pattern, that is, the opposite sleep/wake pattern. Consistency of this pattern on work days and days off is the key to maintaining a synchronized biological clock. Many night shift and rotating shift workers, however, must revert to a diurnal pattern on their days off for business and social reasons. This prevents their circadian clocks from becoming synchronized in a regular pattern. Rotating shift workers face the greatest difficulty because their sleep/wake patterns change each time their shifts change.

The simplest way to alleviate the negative effects of shift work is for the worker to choose a shift, such as night shift, and maintain the same nocturnal sleep/wake pattern on days off. If rotating shifts are unavoidable, then it is better to be on each shift for a 3- to 4-week block of time. With this pattern, the circadian clock is synchronized most of the time. Rapid rotation of shifts should be considered only when there is no alternative. If this is the case, the preferred pattern is clockwise rotation, that is, day to evening to night shift.[56]

Some individuals, approximately 20% of the population, cannot physically tolerate the circadian desynchronization of shift work.[57] Certain underlying medical problems, such as diabetes, gastrointestinal disorders, sleep disturbances, epilepsy, and emotional instability, may become worse with abnormal sleep/wake cycles. In addition, it is believed that age may increase susceptibility to the problems associated with disrupted circadian rhythms.[57]

Violence

Violence is the use, or threatened use, of physical force with the intent to injure or damage a person or object. Critical care nurses may be exposed to some form of violence in the course of their practice, including assault, battery, or verbal abuse.

Physical Violence

The term *assault* refers to the threatened use of physical force, or an unsuccessful attempt at causing physical injury. *Battery* is the actual use of physical force with the intent to injure. Nurses may be the object of such physical violence in the workplace from patients, visitors, or other persons who have entered the hospital building.

Physical violence may produce a number of symptoms in exposed persons. These can, understandably, include fear, anger, increased startle response, and muscle tension. Other common responses are depression, communication difficulties, gastrointestinal symptoms, insomnia, and headaches.[58]

It is believed that violence is significantly underreported by nurses. The reasons for this are unclear but are thought to involve the fear that the incident will be viewed as having been provoked by the nurse or as having been caused by a failure on the nurse's part. The nurse may also be unwilling to become involved in a cumbersome reporting mechanism.[59]

Violence is generally preceded by recognizable escalating stages. Nurses can protect themselves by learning to recognize when the potential for violence is building and then to initiate specific verbal and behavioral techniques to prevent overt violence.[60]

When the violent person is a patient, medication may be useful in averting violent behavior. Subduing a violent patient should never be attempted without adequate personnel. Nurses should learn to recognize when such help is necessary and should know how to summon emergency assistance in their institution.

Verbal Abuse

Verbal abuse is a form of psychological violence that can have serious emotional and behavioral effects. It has been defined as "any communication a nurse perceives to be a harsh, condemnatory attack upon herself, professionally or personally."[61] The nurse may be the target of verbal abuse from patients or their families, physicians, supervisors, or peers. In many cases, the abuser may use verbal abuse as means of coping with a stressful situation.

A recent study showed that nurses are abused verbally approximately once a week, most often by physicians. This was shown to have a significant negative impact on nurses' performance and behavior. Documented responses included emotional trauma, distraction, decreased morale, physical illness, a decline in job satisfaction, increased errors, decreased productivity, and increased staff turnover.[62]

Strong managerial and peer support is essential in reducing the incidence and impact of verbal abuse. Educational programs focusing on negotiation, communication, conflict resolution, and assertiveness can assist nurses in successfully diffusing abusive behavior. The nursing staff should respond consistently and professionally to incidents of verbal abuse. These measures, backed by an administrative policy and procedure for handling such situations, can help convey that verbal abuse is not an accepted form of communication.

DIRECTIONS FOR RESEARCH

The health and safety of health care workers has been the focus of increased attention in recent years. Much research has been done on topics associated with the hospital environment. It becomes quite evident, however, after reading this chapter, that there are many gaps in our knowledge about occupational hazards in critical care.

Back injury is one of the most common occupational injuries among nurses, yet research on its occurrence in the nursing population has been sparse. Existing guidelines on manual lifting focus on the lifting of boxes and bales, not human bodies.

Little is known about long-term effects of chronic low-dosage exposure to some chemical substances, including glutaraldehyde, formaldehyde, waste anesthetic gases, ribavirin, and other pharmacologic agents such as antibiotics.

Studies are needed to explore the long-term consequences of shift work and exposure to workplace stress. Research must continue to investigate the hazards that laser plumes may pose to caregivers.

Critical care nurses are exposed to a wide variety of environmental hazards in the workplace. Regulatory agencies and institutions work diligently to formulate guidelines and standards to protect health care workers. Hospital administrators are increasingly aware of their obligation to provide a workplace that is safe. The ultimate responsibility for maintaining health and well-being, however, lies with each individual nurse.

Critical care nurses must learn about the occupational hazards they face and the ways in which they can protect themselves. They must learn to ask the right questions to get the answers they need to reduce the incidence of work-related illness and injury.

An overview of the most common environmental hazards in the critical care unit has been presented. At the end of the chapter is a list of governmental and professional organizations involved in the health and safety of health care workers. These organizations can be excellent resources to assist critical care nurses in ensuring a safe and healthful workplace.

REFERENCES

1. Sommargren, C., Carlisle, P., Heacock, N., et al. (1989). *AACN handbook on occupational hazards for the critical care nurse.* Newport Beach, CA: American Association of Critical-Care Nurses.
2. Valenti, W. (1986). Infection control and the pregnant health care worker. *American Journal of Infection Control,* 14(1), 20-27.
3. Sommargren, C. (1990). Occupational safety. In J. Spicer, & M. Robinson (Eds.), *Managing the environment in critical care nursing* (pp. 120-138). Baltimore: Williams & Wilkins.
4. Centers for Disease Control. (1991). Update on adult

immunization: Recommendations of the Immunization Practices Advisory Committee (ACIP). *Morbidity and Mortality Weekly Report, 40*(RR-12), 1-52.

5. Centers for Disease Control. (1990). Public health burden of vaccine-preventable diseases among adults: Standards for adult immunization practice. *Morbidity and Mortality Weekly Report, 39*(41), 725-729.

6. Occupational Safety and Health Administration. (1991). 29 CFR Part 1910.1030, Occupational exposure to bloodborne pathogens; Final rule. *Federal Register, 56*(235), 64004-64182.

7. Mangione, C., Gerberding, J., & Cummings, S. (1991). Occupational exposure to HIV: Frequency and rates of underreporting of percutaneous and mucocutaneous exposures by medical housestaff. *American Journal of Medicine, 90*, 85-90.

8. Neuberger, J., Harris, J., Kundin, W., et al. (1984). Incidence of needle-stick injuries in hospital personnel: Implications for prevention. *American Journal of Infection Control, 12*(3), 171-176.

9. Centers for Disease Control. (1988). Update: Universal precautions for prevention of transmission of human immunodeficiency virus, hepatitis B virus, and other bloodborne pathogens in health-care settings. *Morbidity and Mortality Weekly Report, 37*(24), 377-382, 387-388.

10. Department of Labor/Department of Health and Human Services. (1987). *Joint advisory notice: Protection against occupational exposure to hepatitis B virus (HBV) and human immunodeficiency virus (HIV).* Washington, DC: Author.

11. Centers for Disease Control. (1990). Protection against viral hepatitis: Recommendations of the Immunization Practices Advisory Committee (ACIP). *Morbidity and Mortality Weekly Report, 39*(RR-2), 1-23.

12. Centers for Disease Control. (1991). Hepatitis B virus: A comprehensive strategy for eliminating transmission in the United States through universal childhood vaccination: Recommendation of the Immunization Practices Advisory Committee (ACIP). *Morbidity and Mortality Weekly Report, 40*(RR-13), 1-25.

13. Centers for Disease Control. (1987). Revision of the CDC surveillance case definition for acquired immunodeficiency syndrome. *Morbidity and Mortality Weekly Report, 36*(Suppl 1S):3S-15S.

14. Centers for Disease Control. (1991). Update: acquired immunodeficiency syndrome—United States, 1981-1990. *Morbidity and Mortality Weekly Report, 40*(22), 358-363, 369.

15. Centers for Disease Control. (1987). Recommendations for prevention of HIV transmission in health-care settings. *Morbidity and Mortality Weekly Report, 36*(Suppl 2S), 3S-18S.

16. Centers for Disease Control. (1991). Public Health Service inter-agency guidelines for screening donors of blood, plasma, organs, tissues, and semen for evidence of hepatitis B and hepatitis C. *Morbidity and Mortality Weekly Report, 40*(RR-4), 1-17.

17. Centers for Disease Control. (1990). Guidelines for preventing the transmission of tuberculosis in health-

care settings, with special focus on HIV-related issues. *Morbidity and Mortality Weekly Report, 39*(RR-17), 1-29.

18. Pass, R., Hutto, C., Ricks, R., et al. (1986). Increased rate of cytomegalovirus infection among parents of children attending day-care centers. *New England Journal of Medicine, 314*, 1414-1418.

19. Adler, S. (1989). Cytomegalovirus and child day care: Evidence for an increased infection rate among day care workers. *New England Journal of Medicine, 321*, 1290-1296.

20. Balcarek, K., Bagley, R., Cloud, G., et al. (1990). Cytomegalovirus infection among employees of a children's hospital. *Journal of the American Medical Association, 263*(6), 840-844.

21. Lipscomb, J., Linneman, C., Hurst, P., et al. (1984). Prevalence of cytomegalovirus antibody in nursing personnel. *Infection Control, 5*(11), 513-518.

22. Ivey, F., & Gerner, H. (1987). Adults do get chicken pox. *American Journal of Nursing, 87*(12), 1658-1659.

23. Baker, E., & Fine, L. (1986). Solvent neurotoxicity: The current evidence. *Journal of Occupational Medicine, 28*(2), 126-129.

24. National Institute for Occupational Safety and Health. (1988). *Guidelines for protecting the safety and health of health care workers.* Cincinnati, OH: DHHS (NIOSH) Publication No. 88-119.

25. National Institute for Occupational Safety and Health. (1981). *Current intelligence bulletin 34—Evidence on the carcinogenicity of formaldehyde.* Cincinnati, OH: DHHS (NIOSH) Publication No. 81-111.

26. National Institute for Occupational Safety and Health. (1977). *Criteria for a recommended standard: Occupational exposure to waste anesthetic gases and vapors.* Cincinnati, OH: DHHS (NIOSH) Publication No. 77-140.

27. Cohen, E. (1981). *Anesthetic exposure in the workplace.* Littleton, MA: PSG Publishing.

28. Rogers, B. (1986). Exposure to waste anesthetic gases. *American Association of Occupational Health Nurses Journal, 34*(12), 574-579.

29. Rogers, B. (1987). Health hazards to personnel handling antineoplastic agents. *Occupational Medicine: State of the Art Reviews, 2*(3), 513-516.

30. Yodaiken, R. (1986). *Work practice guidelines for personnel dealing with cytotoxic (antineoplastic) drugs.* Washington, DC: Office of Occupational Medicine, Directorate of Technical Support, Occupational Safety and Health Administration.

31. Prows, C. (1989). Ribavirin's risks in reproduction—how great are they? *Maternal Child Nursing, 14*(6), 400-404.

32. Centers for Disease Control. (1988). Assessing exposures of health-care personnel to aerosols of ribavirin—California. *Morbidity and Mortality Weekly Report, 37*, 560-563.

33. California Department of Health Services. (1990). *HESIS hazard alert: Ribavirin.* Berkeley, CA: Author.

34. Harber, P., Billet, E., Gutowski, M., et al. (1985). Occupational low-back pain in hospital nurses. *Journal*

of Occupational Medicine, 27(7), 518-524.

35. Snook, S., Fine, L., & Silverstein, A. (1988). Musculoskeletal disorders. In B. Levy, & D. Wegman (Eds.), *Occupational health: Recognizing and preventing work-related disease.* Boston: Little, Brown.

36. Harber, P., Billet, E., Vojtecky, M., et al. (1988). Nurses' beliefs about cause and prevention of occupational back pain. *Journal of Occupational Medicine, 30*(10), 797-800.

37. Owen, B. (1980). How to avoid that aching back. *American Journal of Nursing, 80*(5),894-897.

38. U.S. Nuclear Regulatory Commission. (1984). *United States nuclear regulatory commission rules and regulations (Title 10, Chapter 1, Code of federal regulations—energy. Part 20, Standards for protection against radiation).* Washington, DC: Author.

39. Bureau of National Affairs, Inc. (1990). International panel recommends reduction in radiation dose limit. *Occupational Safety and Health Reporter, 20*(4), 125-126.

40. Hale, J. (1988). *A radiation safety primer for hospital nursing staff.* Philadelphia: Hospital of the University of Pennsylvania, Department of Radiology.

41. American National Standards Institute. (1988). *American national standard for the safe use of lasers in health care facilities.* Toledo, OH: Laser Institute of America.

42. Ball, K. (1990). *Lasers—the perioperative challenge.* St. Louis: Mosby.

43. Mylrea, D., & O'Neal, L. (1976). Electricity and electrical safety in the hospital. *Nursing 76, 6*(1), 52-59.

44. National Fire Protection Association. (1983). *National fire codes: Vol. 6 and 7.* Quincy, MA: Author.

45. U.S. Environmental Protection Agency. (1974). *Information on levels of environmental noise requisite to protect public health and welfare with an adequate margin of safety.* Report No. 550-9-74-004. Washington, DC: Author.

46. Hilton, A. (1987). The hospital racket: How noisy is your unit? *American Journal of Nursing, 87*(1),59-61.

47. Seidlitz, P. (1981). Excessive noise levels detrimental to patients, staff. *Hospital Progress, 62*(2), 54-56, 64.

48. Topf, M. (1989). Personality hardiness, occupational stress, and burnout in critical care nurses. *Research in Nursing and Health, 12,* 179-186.

49. Steffen, S. (1980). Perceptions of stress: 1800 nurses tell their stories. In K. Claus, & J. Bailey (Eds.), *Living with stress and promoting well-being.* St. Louis: C.V. Mosby.

50. Marks, L., & Reed, J. (1984). Stress: Part 2. The challenge of making stress a positive force. *AAOHN Update Series, 1*(10).

51. Lewis, D., & Robinson, J. (1986). Assessment of coping strategies of ICU nurses in response to stress. *Critical Care Nurse, 6*(6), 38-43.

52. Bailey, J. (1980). Job stress and other stress-related problems. In K. Claus, & J. Bailey (Eds.), *Living with stress and promoting well-being.* St. Louis: C.V. Mosby.

53. Norbeck, J. (1985). Coping with stress in critical care nursing: Research findings. *Focus on Critical Care, 12*(5), 36-39.

54. Gordon, N., Cleary, P., Parker, C., et al. (1986). The prevalence and health impact of shiftwork. *American Journal of Public Health, 76*(10), 1225-1228.

55. Czeisler, C., Moore-Edge, M., & Coleman, R. (1983). Resetting circadian clocks: Applications to sleep disorders and occupational health. In C. Guilleminault, & E. Lugaresi (Eds.), *Sleep—wake disorders: Natural history, epidemiology, and long-term evolution.* New York: Raven.

56. Jung, F. (1986). Shiftwork: Its effect on health performance and well-being. *American Association of Occupational Health Nurses Journal, 34*(4), 161-164.

57. LaDou, J. (1982). Health effects of shift work. *Western Journal of Medicine, 137*(6), 525-530.

58. Lenehan, G., & Turner, S. (1984). Treatment of staff victims of violence. In J. Turner (Ed.), *Violence in the medical care setting: A survival guide.* Rockville, MD: Aspen.

59. Engel, F., & Marsh, S. (1986). Helping the employee victim of violence in hospitals. *Hospital and Community Psychiatry, 37*(2), 159-162.

60. Kurlowicz, L. (1990). Violence in the emergency department. *American Journal of Nursing, 90*(9), 35-39.

61. Cox, H. (1991). Verbal abuse nationwide: Part 1. Oppressed group behavior. *Nursing Management, 22*(2), 32-35.

62. Cox, H. (1991). Verbal abuse nationwide: Part 2. Impact and modifications. *Nursing Management, 22*(3), 66-69.

RESOURCE AGENCIES AND ASSOCIATIONS

Occupational Safety and Health Administration (OSHA), Department of Labor, 200 Constitution Avenue NW, Washington, DC 20210. OSHA ensures compliance of employers with the provisions of the Occupational Health and Safety Act. It conducts workplace inspections and provides information on current standards in response to requests. Twenty-three states, Puerto Rico, and the U.S. Virgin Islands have their own OSHA programs. The remainder of the United States is regulated by Federal OSHA standards. Regional offices are located in 10 major cities throughout the United States.

National Institute for Occupational Safety and Health (NIOSH), 4676 Columbia Parkway, Cincinnati, OH 45226, (513) 533-8287. NIOSH conducts research, develops recommendations regarding occupational hazards for OSHA, and investigates workplace hazards as requested by workers and employers. NIOSH maintains regional offices in Boston, Atlanta, and Denver.

Centers for Disease Control (CDC), U.S. Department of Health and Human Services, Public Health Service, Atlanta, GA 30333. The CDC collects statistics and publishes guidelines for infectious diseases and hospital infection control programs.

American Association of Occupational Health Nurses (AAOHN), 3500 Piedmont Road NE, Atlanta, GA 30305. AAOHN is a professional and educational organization of registered nurses interested in occupational health issues.

Association of Hospital Employee Health Professionals (AHEHP), 1722 J Street, Sacramento, CA 95814. AHEHP is a professional organization involved with health and safety issues in hospitals.

Association for Practitioners in Infection Control (APIC), 505 East Hawley Street, Mundelein, IL 60060, (312) 949-6052. APIC is an organization of health care professionals interested in infectious diseases and hospital infection control programs.

Nurses Environmental Health Watch, Inc. (NEHW), 33 Columbus Avenue, Somerville, MA 02143. NEHW is an organization involved with the education of nurses and the public about environmental and occupational health concerns.

6

Patient Responses to the Environment

Nancie Urban

The critical care environment is notorious for its extremes of technology. Indeed, few other specialties within the health care system impose as much "high-tech" as the intensive care unit. This technology provides innumerable advantages in the treatment of disease and the saving of lives, but it has also been the focus of criticism. Dehumanization, perhaps the most noted of these criticisms, may present the greatest challenge to a patient's ability to cope with the critical care experience.

The many machines, devices, and interventions inherent in the critical care unit are the obvious source of claims that critical care is technical to the point of being dehumanizing. The technology of the critical care unit presents a unique challenge to the health care team as well. Nurses in particular must direct a great deal of attention to the machinery, devices, and complex treatment protocols required in the care of the critically ill. In addition, the sheer number of caregivers, specialists, and technicians may cause fragmented care that further compounds the potentially dehumanizing nature of critical care. In other words, the technology of the critical care unit includes both the machines and the personnel. Since the machines are unable to alter their function according to individual patient needs, the critical care nurse becomes the essential force in integrating the technology and the entire health care team with preservation of the humanity of the patient.

The presence of technology without compensatory "high touch" has been associated with rejection of technology.[1] Unfortunately, rejection of technology is not an easy option in the critical care unit. Although some patients may choose to refuse life-supporting technology, many find themselves recipients of all the critical care unit has to offer before other options are considered. In addition, personnel who are perceived by patients to be cold and efficient rather than warm and caring may increase patients' stress and compromise their ability to cope with their illness or the critical care environment. The critical care nurse truly plays the essential role in providing the "high touch" that can balance the "high-tech" of the critical care environment.

This chapter describes the effects of the critical care environment on patients and nursing interventions that may support patients' ability to cope with the critical care experience.

COPING WITH THE CRITICAL CARE EXPERIENCE

Introduction to the health care system can be an intimidating experience for an individual. Consider the effect of entering an unfamiliar building that was designed for efficiency rather than comfort. Add to this being deprived of one's clothing and personal valuables; the endless repetition of questions, many of which are of a highly personal nature; and severely limited contact with familiar persons and objects. Under such circumstances claims of dehumanization, feelings of threatened personal dignity, and potential inability to cope are not surprising.

Needs of the Critically Ill

Human needs have been defined as conditions to be fulfilled to maintain life or well-being that encompass physical, psychological, and sociocultural aspects.[2] Human needs may change with the person or the situation but always involve all three components in a highly integrated fashion.

The critically ill patient may be thought of as having both physical needs and "person" or human needs (Figure 6-1). Critically ill persons have physical needs, first of all, to survive and recover. They also express the need to recover with a minimum of suffering.[2] Person needs include the need to be seen as an indi-

117

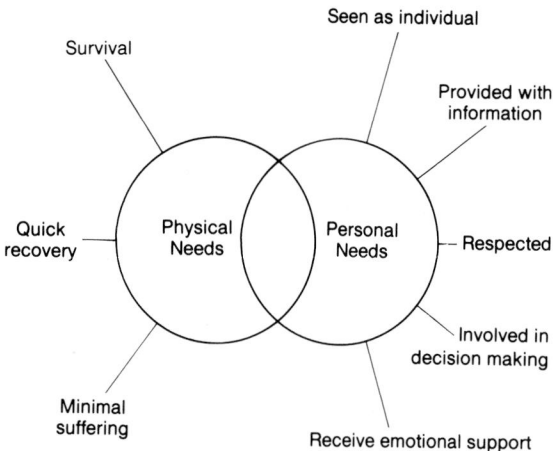

Figure 6-1 Dual needs of the critically ill.

TABLE 6-1 Types of Coping and Associated Behaviors

Coping Type	Associated Behavior
Responses that modify the situation	Negotiation Providing discipline Giving or receiving advice
Responses that alter or control the meaning of a problem	Neutralizing responses Rationalization Selective shutting out Positive comparisons Denial
Responses that help manage stress after it has occurred	Passive acceptance Withdrawal Magical thinking Hopefulness Avoidance of worry Relaxation

vidual, to be respected, to be provided information, to be involved in decision making regarding care, and to receive emotional support. All of these needs must be considered in context with the cultural background of patients and their families as well. A highly interactive process among patient, family, and staff is required for successful fulfillment of the dual needs of the critically ill. Without full attention to both sets of needs, critically ill patients are placed at a physiological as well as at a psychological disadvantage.

The critically ill are often viewed as being highly dependent because of the unstable nature of their situation. In addition, life-threatening illness may prompt a focus on physical needs to the exclusion of other needs. Often comatose, heavily medicated, or otherwise unable to directly participate in decision making regarding their care, the critically ill may be at higher risk of having their person needs overlooked. Such an imbalance between the physical and person needs has been associated with the traditional medical model of western health care.[3] While successful in the basic treatment of diseases, the mind–body dualism of this approach is often dissatisfying to the patient. The holistic approach of treating both physical and person needs is not only more satisfying to the patient but may yield greater success in the overall recovery.[4] As a result, putting the person needs of the patient aside is not only discourteous but may be unethical and even unscientific.

Individual Coping Styles

A critical care experience is undoubtedly a tremendous challenge to an individual's ability to cope. The physical stressors of critical illness coupled with the psychological strain of the illness and the critical care environment can easily overwhelm even the most hardy individual.

Pearlin and Schooler define coping as the way a person responds to things to avoid being harmed by life's strains.[5] They describe three different types of coping with associated behaviors as described in Table 6-1.

A more detailed definition of coping is put forth by Lazarus and Folkman as "the constantly changing cognitive and behavioral efforts to manage specific external and/or internal forces that are appraised as taxing or exceeding the resources of the person."[6] This perspective views coping as a process rather than as a single act. In addition, these authors define psychological stress as "a particular relationship between the person and the environment that is appraised by the person as taxing or exceeding his or her resources and endangering his or her well-being."[6] Both definitions are based on the premise that people are capable of conscious appraisal of their situation. Automatic reactions such as unconscious defense mechanisms would not apply from this perspective. In addition, Lazarus and Folkman make no distinction between coping efforts that are effective in eliminating the stressors and those that are not. As a result, coping may be viewed as managing the stress or stressor rather than eliminating or overcoming the source of stress. Actions or responses that effectively manage the stress or the individual's response to a stressor would be seen as evidence of successful coping. The critical care environment presents significant risk of inducing the state of "endangered well-being" described by Lazarus and Folkman. But though the physiological stress of a critical illness cannot be minimized, a person's ability to evaluate and interpret the experience cognitively will have a significant impact on that person's coping response.

A number of personal characteristics have been associated with positive coping behaviors and outcomes. Hardiness, or a high degree of internal control, as well as commitment and responsiveness to challenge contribute to a positive self-view.[7] Closeness and commitment in relationships are also seen as very positive forces.[5] Numerous authors cite the characteristic of flexibility as a key asset.[5,8,9,10] Self-consciousness and attention to internal cues are considered precursors to active coping. Without these characteristics, individuals may not recognize critical cues related to stressful events and, consequently, may not seek information that would assist them in coping.[11]

Figley has summarized several factors that influence an individual's ability to cope in an emergency situation.[12] These factors include previous experience in a similar situation, personal hardiness, an ability to concentrate under pressure, and an internal locus of control. In addition, situational factors of individual ability to communicate with other victims, ability to ignore the degree to which the experience may be humiliating or degrading, and the sense of helplessness to influence or stop the situation are noted as significant. Inasmuch as a critical illness might be considered an emergency, these factors deserve careful consideration by critical care nurses in their assessment of patients' coping ability.

Building on the work of Lazarus, Thoits describes two specific methods of coping that include both behavioral and cognitive components.[13] *Problem-focused coping* includes direct action on the environment or on the self to alter the circumstances that are perceived as threatening. The behavioral actions may include leaving the situation, replacing disturbing aspects of the situation with more acceptable aspects, or inventing new solutions to the existing stressors. Cognitively, the individual may reinterpret the circumstances so that they are perceived as less threatening.

Emotion-focused coping consists of attempts by the individual to control undesirable feelings caused by a stressful situation. Behaviorally, use of mood- or perception-altering drugs or techniques such as biofeedback may be employed. Avoidance or seeking reassurance may also be attempted. Cognitively, an individual may reinterpret or relabel negative feelings as something more positive or socially acceptable.

Clearly, coping is a multidimensional process that varies according to the individual's perception of the situation, personal resources, and other demands. Equally clear is the fact that the critical care experience creates a level of stress that presents maximum challenge to patients' ability to cope. Consequently, a careful assessment of patient coping ability is an important component of nursing care for the critically ill. The most important aspect of this assessment is to ask patients how they have coped with stress in the past. If a patient has had a previous critical care experience, specific questions about how that experience was handled could yield valuable information in anticipating current needs. If the patient is not a reliable source, the family or significant others may provide essential insight to help the nurse interpret the patient's behavior accurately and to plan patient-focused care. Equally important is identification of the patient's primary support system. Often this will be a spouse or other family member, but regardless of who the support may be, the nurse must focus on fostering the patient's access to it.

Nursing Management

Ineffective patient coping presents a serious threat to the physical as well as the psychological recovery of critically ill patients. Outcomes and interventions for the management of this serious nursing diagnosis as described in *AACN's Outcome Standards for Nursing Care of the Critically Ill* are presented later in the chapter.[14] Encouraging the patient to use formerly successful coping strategies and fostering contact with the patient's support system are among the most important of the interventions noted. Controlling the external environment is also an important strategy and one that is almost exclusively within the realm of nursing.

IMPACT OF THE CRITICAL CARE ENVIRONMENT

The tremendously technical nature of the critical care environment exposes the patient to many abnormal stimuli. At the center of this situation is the potential for almost total loss of privacy and very little preservation of the patient's dignity unless explicit plans are implemented to preserve both. Critical care units with curtains rarely drawn between the beds, together with assessments and treatments that often involve exposing the bodies of patients, set the stage for loss of privacy that would be considered unbelievable in other contexts. These and other aspects of the critical care environment, summarized in Table 6-2, have both a physical and a psychological impact on the patient. In addition, lack of privacy means that patients can view activities occurring at other patients' bedsides. Negative patient responses such as increased heart rate, dysrhythmias, and self-reports of increased anxiety have been documented in a study of CCU patients who observed procedures performed on other patients.[15]

TABLE 6-2 **Physical and Psychological Impact of the Critical Care Environment on the Critically Ill Patient**

Physical Impact	Psychological Impact
Crowding	Lack of privacy
Lighting	Sensory overload
Odors	Sensory monotony
Noise	Sensory deprivation
Painful	Isolation
touch	Sleep deprivation

Physical Environment

Most critical care units have an element of crowding. Open-style units with only curtains between the beds often appear crowded, especially as additional equipment is brought in. Even in units with individual cubicles, crowding can be a problem. Supplemental equipment and lack of windows, regardless of the basic design of the unit, can cause patient, family, and staff to feel crowded. The result is a violation of territoriality: the need of all individuals for a personally determined minimum amount of space between themselves and others or objects around them. Violation of that space causes a magnification effect on the stress perceived by patients.[16] In an already stressful environment with physical stressors also in play, aspects such as crowding compound the negative effect.

Lighting is another major stressor in the critical care environment. The bright overhead lights necessary for procedures and assessments can have a deleterious effect on the patient. Bright lights shining directly overhead may actually be painful to patients. The elderly are particularly susceptible to the glare from bright overhead lights. Many also have diminished visual acuity, and often have difficulty adjusting to the typical ICU lighting.[17] In addition, constant lighting around the clock interrupts natural sleep/wake cycles and contributes to sleep deprivation in critically ill patients. Appropriate amounts of uninterrupted sleep are essential to psychological integrity.[18] Sleep has also been shown to influence ability to respond to physical stressors in an adaptive way and to promote healing.[19]

Odors in the critical care environment may also distress patients, especially if the odors are coming from themselves. The issue of odors has been cited frequently in studies conducted to determine patient stressors related to the critical care environment.[19] Aside from the unpleasant nature of many odors, some odors may be a source of fear more than embarrassment to patients such as when the odor cannot

be identified or is related to a pathological condition rather than to normal body functions.

Noise is one of the most significant problems in the critical care environment. Noise levels measured at less than 40 dB permit rest and sleep. Noise levels in the average critical care unit range from 45 to 85 dB.[20] Considering that those who are ill are less tolerant of any noise, elevated levels of noise take on even greater significance. In the many studies of the level of noise from machinery and activity in critical care units, several interesting findings emerge. The constant low, rhythmic noise from a ventilator, for example, has been found to be less bothersome to patients than was anticipated.[19] In fact, constant low-pitched noise that becomes part of the background may have a soothing or filtering effect, screening patients from more bothersome sounds. The noises reportedly most disturbing to patients are high-pitched, loud, or unexpected.[19] Another unpleasant quality is noise that increases in intensity or is likely to persist rather than noise that decreases in intensity or is of very short duration.[19] The elderly are especially vulnerable to sleep disturbance from excessive or disruptive noise.[17] In persons already at higher risk for sensory disruption, sleep deprivation due to noise is an unnecessary additional hazard. Most significant, however, is the finding that the noises perceived by the patients to be the most disturbing are those that are produced by the staff. Conversation and loud laughter are disturbing to patients, causing them to worry that they are the focus of staff comments.[21]

Touch is another reality of the critical care unit that may be perceived negatively. In this context, touch that results in pain or an invasion of privacy is the issue. Indeed, the critically ill have to be touched in ways that could be perceived as unpleasant or threatening so that they can be provided with needed intervention and care. Even the simple act of turning a patient may cause pain in certain situations. The need to touch patients in performing procedures cannot be avoided, but such touching need not occur without warning nor lack appropriate prior explanation. In addition, critically ill children have been reported to be particularly sensitive to tactile stimulation, often overreacting to stimuli such as room temperature, dressings, and any form of touch.[22]

Psychological Environment

A complex psychological environment also exists within the critical care unit and in conjunction with the physical environment, has a major impact on patients. The illness of the patient alone may provoke severe psychological as well as physical demands. In addition, the invasion of privacy discussed earlier as an element of the physical environment may also psychologically impair patients by threatening their dignity, self-esteem, and self-concept. Preservation of these factors is as necessary to the well-being of the patient as is the patient's physical recovery.

Sensory overload of abnormal stimuli is prevalent in critical care units. Disturbances such as beeping monitors, alarms, ringing telephones, suction equipment, ventilators, and constant interruptions combine to bombard patients constantly with stimuli that are quite unlike what they are accustomed to. When combined with a lowered ability to tolerate stressors brought about by the illness itself, an overload of abnormal stimuli may overwhelm patients. In addition, the repetitive nature of many of these stimuli may lead to sensory monotony. The result may be an environment that begins to assume a reality all its own for patients.

Sensory deprivation of familiar stimuli serves as the alternate to sensory overload in the psychological environment of the critical care unit. Sometimes overridden by technological overload and other times simply absent, familiar sights, sounds, and smells may become distant memories to the critically ill. Critically ill patients have reported the deprivation of simple human touch as most significant.[22] Critically ill children appear to be especially vulnerable to loss of normal stimuli. Signs and symptoms of adverse effects include lower pain threshold, decreased verbalization, shortened attention span, claustrophobia, and misconceptions regarding time.[23] In addition, extensive monitoring may result in almost total restraint of patients of all ages and may compound the overwhelming psychological impact of the critical care environment.

Similarly to sensory deprivation, isolation presents a serious situation in critical care. One might wonder how anyone could feel isolated in a critical care unit that normally bustles with activity and patient interruptions 24 hours a day. The isolation, however, is a product of separation from family, familiar surroundings, and social activity as well as the physical illness, pain, and alien environment. Rigid, severely restricted visiting rules compound the problem by limiting contact between the patients and their significant others. There can be little wonder that patients may begin to feel cast adrift in a terrible nightmare. Recognizing that patients are important members of their family units and may desperately crave the comfort and reassurance that the presence of their family often brings is a key step in minimizing this negative consequence of critical care.[24]

Sleep deprivation is another aspect of the psychological environment of the critical care unit that has been studied and reported extensively in the literature. Associated with both physical and psychological well-being and recovery, adequate uninterrupted sleep is essential to healthy individuals and is especially important to the critically ill.[25] Ability to cope with and recover from critical illness may be severely compromised by sleep deprivation.[26] Yet environmental conditions in the critical care unit often impose a degree of sleep deprivation that is unequaled by any other area in the health care system. While understandable in terms of the amount of continuous care that critically ill patients require, sleep deprivation must be avoided in order to preserve the mind and spirit of the patient as well as to promote physical healing.

PATIENT RESPONSES

Many critically ill patients appear to tolerate the critical care experience remarkably well. Other patients, however, may experience suffering that transcends that caused by their illness. Even unconscious or paralyzed patients who are unable to demonstrate obvious signs of psychological strain may nonetheless be experiencing great distress.[27] Patients' responses to the critical care environment are summarized in the box below.

Fear and Anxiety

Two common responses to the critical care experience are *fear* and *anxiety*. Fear may be of death, pain, or potential disability. Fear is a relatively concrete feeling that is focused on a particular situation or event. In contrast, anxiety is a more vague feeling of apprehension or uneasiness that may not have a specific source.[28] Fear of the critical care environment in combination with fear related to the illness is a frequent source of anxiety. Even though patients may feel offended by the invasion of privacy, painful procedures, restraints, and the like, they also have an acute sense of their need for the care and the caregivers. The dichotomy of feeling anger or fear about the care that is being provided, yet at the same time recognizing the need for the care and the care providers may underlie the anxiety so many critically ill patients experience.

Patient Responses to the Critical Care Environment

Fear
Anxiety
Sleep pattern disturbance
Depression
Powerlessness
Spiritual distress
Pain intolerance
ICU psychosis

Sleep Pattern Disturbance

Sleep pattern disturbance is a patient response to the critical care environment that may become a precurser for additional coping problems. Studies have shown that with lights, sounds, and activity constant 24 hours a day in the ICU, patients rarely have an opportunity to sleep at night.[29] In addition, interruptions timed at approximately every 20 minutes make completion of a normal, 90-minute sleep cycle impossible. This problem poses a particularly high risk for the elderly critical care patient because the aging process disrupts normal sleep cycles and REM sleep patterns under even the best conditions.[30] (See Chapter 13 for a more in-depth discussion of sleep deprivation.)

Depression

Depression is an all too common response to the critical care experience. Behaviors including lack of motivation, withdrawal, tearfulness, and avoidance of eye contact may signal a patient who has become depressed. Patients who are depressed may also become anorexic, further complicating their recovery by inadequate nutrition. Sleep disturbances, either insomnia or increased sleep and lethargy, may also be symptoms of depression. Feelings of worthlessness, helplessness, despair, or threatened self-esteem may worsen depression. Finally, depression may be accompanied by dependency behavior that may frustrate the most dedicated efforts to rehabilitate the patient.

Powerlessness

Powerlessness is a particularly difficult problem. When patients decide that there is nothing they can do to influence the outcome of their situation, powerlessness exists.[31] Powerlessness is associated with disinterest in events and activities associated with care, extreme lack of motivation, and an "I don't care" attitude that may severely hinder recovery and rehabilitation. Individuals who normally are in control or power positions in their daily lives may be at special risk for powerlessness when placed in the extremely dependent role of the critically ill patient. Anyone, however, may develop a sense of being out of control when subjected to the exceptionally structured environment of the critical care unit with its extremely competent, "in charge" personnel.

Spiritual Distress

Some practitioners consider spiritual distress to be a "neglected crisis" since this problem may be avoided or misinterpreted by staff.[32] Critical illness may certainly provoke spiritual questioning and conflict in patients and their families. Spiritual distress may be based on formal religious beliefs or on beliefs associated with a more general value system. In any case, unless the staff are secure in their personal beliefs and values, recognizing and dealing with this response can be difficult. Spiritual distress must be clarified, however, so that appropriate interventions may be instituted. Referral to another member of the staff, a consultant, or a chaplain is recommended in situations where the primary caregivers are uncomfortable or have insufficient time to devote to resolving this serious psychologic problem. Lack of specific attention to this response may complicate the patient's ability to cope with the experiences in the critical care unit.

Pain

Pain is often a major problem for both patients and staff in the critical care unit. Research has demonstrated that patients in critical care units appear to have heightened pain perception.[19] Increased perception of pain is also associated with anxiety and environmental stressors such as noise. In any case, pain management becomes an essential priority in critical care. A component of such pain management may include environmental alterations such as noise control and measures to reduce fear and anxiety.

ICU Psychosis

ICU psychosis, or altered sensory perception, deserves special attention in any discussion of patients' responses to critical care. Influenced by both the illness and the environment, an episode of psychosis is a distressing occurrence for the patient, family, and staff.[33] Identifying the specific cause of ICU psychosis is very difficult as it includes both physical and psychological factors. The illness itself may be a major factor. In addition, factors such as electrolyte imbalance, oxygenation deficits, fever, and pain will influence the patient's perceptions and behavior. The alien and unfamiliar nature of the environment with its seemingly bizarre machines and noises also serves as a cause. The need for physical restraint may further provoke paranoid feelings. The culmination of all the sensory overload coupled with sleep deprivation often leads to overtly psychotic reactions in patients.

Signs and symptoms of ICU psychosis often begin with perceptual distortions that are very patient-specific. Examples of such distortions include perceiving a speckled pattern on ceiling tiles as insects, interpreting the blowing sounds of an airflow system as rain or running water, or mistaking an intraaortic balloon pump positioned at the foot of a bed for an animal.

Disorientation, especially to time and place, commonly occurs. Day and night quickly blend and blur as lights remain on and procedures are carried out at regular intervals 24 hours a day. In addition, units without windows compound the inability of patients to maintain orientation to time. Disorientation to place is also common. When asked where they are, disoriented patients may reply "home," perhaps out of wishful thinking; "here with you," perhaps as a means to avoid admitting they really cannot recall where they are; or "hell," perhaps the most accurate description of what their experience must seem to be.

Actual hallucinations may also occur with ICU psychosis. Ranging from amusing to terrorizing, hallucinations warrant careful assessment. At times, patients may realize that what they see is not actually there. Unfortunately, this realization may not dispel the hallucination. More often, patients believe their hallucinations to be real. Swift intervention is especially important for hallucinations that are frightening.

Overt paranoia further complicates the problem of ICU psychosis. Many of the procedures and activities that are necessary in the care of the critically ill may provide a fertile basis for paranoid thoughts. This reality adds to the difficulty in correcting this problem. Paranoia may also be directed at family members, or patients may involve family members in their paranoid behavior. This situation requires extremely sensitive intervention to protect patients and their family members from feelings of guilt or distrust of the staff.

Restlessness and outright combativeness are frequent behavioral components of ICU psychosis. Combativeness may require the use of restraints to protect both the patient and the staff. Use of restraints, however, may accent the patient's paranoid fears. Sedation is usually necessary. The best treatment, of course, is to institute interventions to prevent the psychosis from occurring in the first place. Essential interventions include fostering adequate sleep, providing structured contact with familiar stimuli such as family members or favorite television programs, and controlling pain. Fortunately, ICU psychosis is temporary and usually resolves within 48 hours of transfer out of the ICU, assuming that transfer is a reasonable option.[34]

NURSING MANAGEMENT

Protecting patients from ill effects of the critical care environment is a significant responsibility of the nurse. Who is better able to manage this important aspect of a patient's care than the health care professional who is at the bedside 24 hours a day? Accomplishing this worthy goal presents many unique challenges.

Nursing interventions that may be effective in managing some of the specific patient responses discussed in the previous section are shown in the sections that follow. Taken from *AACN's Outcome Standards for Nursing Care of the Critically Ill*, the abbreviated care plans include expected outcomes.[14] Discussion of interventions for sleep pattern disturbance can be found in Chapter 13.

■ **NURSING DIAGNOSIS**
  Ineffective patient coping.

OUTCOME STANDARD AND CRITERIA
  Coping is effective as evidenced by:
- Participation in decisions regarding health
- Support from social network
- Physical limitations acknowledged
- Sleep/wake pattern normal for person and unit activity
- Decrease in fear, anger, withdrawal, or other maladaptive coping behaviors

NURSING INTERVENTIONS
- Eliminate or modify causes of ineffective coping
- Assist problem solving by reducing concerns into small parts
- Plan for contact with significant others
- Support adaptive coping responses
- Adjust environmental stimuli per patient needs
- Assist in identification of available resources
- Encourage expression of feelings
- Keep patient informed of health status
- Teach relaxation techniques

■ **NURSING DIAGNOSIS**
  Fear.

OUTCOME STANDARD AND CRITERIA
  Fear is absent or reduced as evidenced by:
- Statement that fear is absent or reduced
- Absence or reduction in signs of fear

NURSING INTERVENTIONS
- Eliminate or modify cause of fear if possible
- Diminish impact of fear by establishing alternative approaches (e.g., consistent daily routine)
- Adapt the environment to counteract fear (e.g., leave lights on, provide familiar objects)
- Convey empathic understanding
- Promote presence of comforting significant others
- Teach patient fear management techniques
- Monitor patient participation in decision making

■ **NURSING DIAGNOSIS**
  Anxiety.

OUTCOME STANDARD AND CRITERIA
  Anxiety is absent or reduced as evidenced by:
- Statement that anxiety is absent or reduced
- Absence or reduction in signs of anxiety

NURSING INTERVENTIONS
- Eliminate or modify the causes of the anxiety if possible
- Support existing coping mechanisms

- Speak slowly and calmly
- Convey empathic understanding
- Promote presence of comforting significant others
- Focus on the present
- Remove excessive stimulation
- Occupy patient with simple, repetitive task
- Guide patient through relaxation techniques
- Anticipate concerns and reinforce orientation to environment
- Give concise directions
- Provide honest information
- Schedule medication in anticipation of anxious moments

■ **NURSING DIAGNOSIS**
Depression.

OUTCOME STANDARD AND CRITERIA
Depression is absent or reduced as evidenced by:
- Statement that depression is absent or reduced
- Absence or reduction in signs of depression

NURSING INTERVENTIONS
- Eliminate or modify causes if possible
- Convey empathic understanding
- Promote presence of comforting significant others
- Provide honest information with emphasis on positive aspects
- Identify realistic goals with patient
- Measure progress in small increments with emphasis on each level of accomplishment
- Use humor as appropriate
- Consider medication as appropriate

■ **NURSING DIAGNOSIS**
Powerlessness.

OUTCOME STANDARD AND CRITERIA
Sense of control is perceived as evidenced by:
- Expression of control over situation or events
- Participation in activities of daily living
- Participation in decision making

NURSING INTERVENTIONS
- Eliminate or modify cause if possible
- Provide control or choices whenever possible
- Identify where patient retains control despite current losses
- Involve patient and family in care
- Convey empathic understanding
- Promote presence of comforting significant others
- Provide frequent updates on progress toward therapeutic goals

■ **NURSING DIAGNOSIS**
Spiritual distress.

OUTCOME STANDARD AND CRITERIA
Spiritual distress is absent or reduced as evidenced by:
- Expression of satisfaction with meaning and purpose of current situation
- Absence or reduction of conflict between religious beliefs and prescribed health care regimen

NURSING INTERVENTIONS
- Listen as patient talks about value system or religious values
- Assist patient to live life fully in the present by focusing on joy, hope, and progress
- Respect and acknowledge the patient's religious beliefs
- Refer to clergy as appropriate
- Provide support to patient and family when conflicts between beliefs and recommended care occur
- Assist with prayer as requested
- Provide privacy for reflection or spiritual expression
- Assist with spiritual reading as requested
- Identify previous sources of spiritual strength
- Respect presence of religious objects, music, or television programs
- Provide for safety/comfort within the context of acceptable religious beliefs and practices

■ **NURSING DIAGNOSIS**
Pain.

OUTCOME STANDARD AND CRITERIA
Pain is absent or controlled as evidenced by:
- Statement that pain has been relieved
- Signs of pain absent
- Vital signs within normal ranges
- Body relaxed

NURSING INTERVENTIONS
- Eliminate or modify causes if possible
- Tailor pain management program to patient
- Position to facilitate pain relief
- Handle patient gently
- Use external techniques or devices as appropriate (e.g., heat, cold, massage, TENS)
- Schedule medication for maximum coverage of pain control
- Warn patient before any potentially painful procedure
- Provide support during painful procedures
- Use distraction techniques to help manage pain
- Guide through relaxation methods
- Teach patient relaxation methods

■ **NURSING DIAGNOSIS**
Altered sensory perception.

OUTCOME STANDARD AND CRITERIA
Appropriate response to sensory stimuli as evidenced by:
- Orientation to person, place, time
- Accurate description of environment

NURSING INTERVENTIONS
- Eliminate or modify causes if possible
- Provide frequent reorientation to time and place
- Provide meaningful sensory stimulation (e.g., clock, calendar, window, TV)
- Enhance function of impaired senses (e.g., glasses, hearing aid)

- Enhance use of other senses to compensate for impaired senses (e.g., verbal descriptions for visually impaired)
- Schedule care to minimize sleep interruptions
- Provide adequate lighting with adjustments for day–night cycles
- Promote presence of reassuring significant others and/or familiar objects
- Orient patient to environment, equipment, and sounds as needed

In addition to the specific nursing care just outlined, several general approaches listed in the box to the right may be used to help patients cope with the critical care experience. These are very simple strategies that typically yield tremendous rewards.

First, and perhaps foremost, patients should be treated with the respect due any individual. Addressing patients by their appropriate title and family name, especially when the patient is an adult, is important. Many individuals consider a stranger addressing them by their first name disrespectful, even when that familiarity is intended to put them at ease. These same individuals as patients may not state that they do not wish to be addressed by their first name. In fact, when asked if their first name may be used, they may say yes out of fear that they will alienate the nurse if they refuse. An unsolicited invitation to use the patient's first name is the best indication that a first-name basis is acceptable to the patient. Exceptions include patients who may be comatose or otherwise neurologically impaired and therefore may be inclined to respond to their more familiar first name rather than their family name.

Another primary aspect of nursing intervention is to preserve a patient's privacy and dignity. Such intervention may present a difficult challenge in the critical care unit, especially when the patient requires extensive monitoring and support. Suddenly appearing at the bedside may startle a patient and may certainly be viewed as an invasion of basic privacy. Strategies to optimize a patient's privacy include knocking before entering the patient's room or cubicle. If there is nothing to knock on, an announcement of one's presence may be substituted. Also, assessment and procedures can be conducted so that as little of the patient's body is exposed as possible, and judicious use of curtains and doors should become commonplace. Keeping the patient informed of all activities, regardless of how minor they may be, also adds to a patient's self-respect and privacy.

Conversation that does not include the patient should be strictly avoided at the bedside. Whether such conversation is related to the patient or is simply a personal exchange between caregivers, it is inappropriate. Such conversation serves to reduce the status of the patient to that of an object. It is rude at

> ## Nursing Management to Support Effective Coping with the Critical Care Environment
>
> Address respectfully
> Acknowledge feelings and emotions
> Preserve privacy
> Control bedside conversation
> Offer choices
> Encourage participation
> Maintain independent identity
> Control noise
> Allow adequate sleep
> Structure activities
> Use comforting touch liberally
> Facilitate family contact

the very least and may contribute to paranoia or feelings of worthlessness and powerlessness at the worst. This is not to say that personal conversation should never occur at the bedside. When the patient is included, general conversation may provide a pleasant distraction from the otherwise stressful environment of the critical care unit. Conversation may be easier to control among the nursing staff than among other members of the health care team. A tactful reminder usually serves to keep everyone on track without unnecessary embarrassment for anyone.

Offering patients choices, no matter how trivial, helps them maintain a sense of control and may be instrumental in averting feelings of powerlessness. Encouraging participation in decision making and care as much as is realistic based on the patient's ability is another strategy. Critically ill patients are very sensitive to the preferences of their caregivers. Dependency is fostered in patients in subtle as well as direct ways.[35] Involving patients in their care as much as possible minimizes this effect.

In a somewhat similar vein, helping the patient maintain a sense of identity separate from the critical care unit may also have empowering value. Adoption of the sick role may be especially dangerous for the patient who becomes a long-term resident in the critical care unit. Directing the family to bring in personal items from home such as family photographs, pictures drawn by young members of the family, or a favorite pillow all help to maintain a sense of connection to home for the patient. In addition, coordinating care so that the patient may be taken outside the unit for a short time may yield extremely positive results. Strategies such as these also help patients to maintain a sense of hope that they are still a part of the world and that they may yet recover. Any intervention that supports a sense of hope in the patient is worth whatever effort is required because, without hope, recovery may be impossible.[36]

Controlling noise is another environmental intervention that can yield important results. Minimizing the amount of equipment in the patient's room will help reduce noise. This intervention will also help reduce the sense of crowding and violated personal territory that patients often experience in critical care. If there are doors to each patient's area, keeping them closed whenever possible is an important intervention. Carpeting in the corridors also helps reduce the noise of unit traffic. Turning off all equipment that is not in use (especially suction equipment, which can be particularly noisy) is another successful strategy. Making sure that patients have been oriented to the unit's sounds, especially alarms, is important so that they are not unnecessarily frightened by them. Turning the audio pulse monitors down, if not off, positioning ventilators so that the exit valve points away from the patient's head, and refilling infusion pumps before they alarm are just a few additional interventions that can be accomplished with relative ease if they are planned.

Providing adequate opportunities for uninterrupted sleep is an essential nursing intervention (see Chapter 13). Control of noise and lights is usually an essential aspect of this intervention. Sleep research unanimously supports the conclusion that adequate sleep is essential for physical and psychological survival.[37] The minimum amount of time needed to complete a sleep cycle is 90 minutes to 2 hours. Planning care to allow 2-hour periods of uninterrupted sleep, especially during the night hours, may have a remarkable effect on preventing ICU psychosis and promoting a patient's recovery.

Structuring activity in the critical care unit may aid in protecting patients from adverse effects of the critical care environment. Scheduling therapeutic activities such as assessments, bathing, physical therapy, and treatments so that adequate rest can be obtained by patients is an important component of such structure. Radio and television, commonly used to help patients maintain a sense of connection to the outside world, are also best used in a structured manner. Most important, music and program selections must be based on patient preferences rather than those of the care providers. In addition, continuous playing of the radio or television 24 hours a day should be avoided so that day–night orientation is not compromised.

Touch may also be used as a nursing intervention to manage a patient's responses to the critical care environment. When critically ill and extensively monitored, a patient may begin to feel like an untouchable object. The need to touch patients for the purpose of assessments and procedures may compound their feelings of dehumanization. A gentle touch, intended to provide comfort rather than specific therapy, reinforces patients' sense of themselves as worthy of human attention and concern.[38] Families should also be encouraged to touch the patient regardless of the amount of technological intervention that may be involved in the patient's care. Lowering the side rails so that family members can reach the patient, offering a chair so that they can make themselves more comfortable, and giving permission for them to touch the patient are simple, yet effective, methods for facilitating the positive use of touch by the patient's family. The many tubes, wires, and machines may intimidate family members and cause them to hesitate to touch the patient. Clearing a path to the patient and encouraging physical contact between family and patient provide a source of touch that may become the patient's primary tie to a sense of humanity.

Maintaining relationships between patients and their families is a final area of nursing intervention designed to help patients weather the critical care experience. Visiting opportunities need to be planned individually to accommodate familial and cultural variances as well as the clinical situation. Contact with family provides a source of normal stimuli, support, and comfort. Facilitating family visits may be the key intervention in preventing the feeling of isolation that critically ill patients may develop. Reported by patients and family members alike, the need for contact is significant and may have considerable impact on patient responses to the critical care experience.[23]

Nursing interventions to minimize adverse patient responses to the critical care environment involve both awareness of those responses and a willingness to take necessary action.[39] Passive acceptance of the potentially dehumanizing aspects of the critical care environment is not acceptable, and, hopefully, not common. Nurses must be willing to alter the "routines" on behalf of the patient when appropriate. At times, active advocacy on behalf of the patient may be required to protect the patient from unnecessary physical and psychological strain from the critical care environment. These goals may be difficult to achieve at times, especially when the patient is extremely unstable and requires extraordinary physical support. The benefits of successful implementation of a plan of care that meets both the physical and psychological needs of the patient, however, are quality nursing care and optimum patient outcomes.

TRANSFER ANXIETY

Despite the unpleasant nature of being hospitalized in the critical care unit, many patients are anxious and even fearful about being transferred from the area. The constant monitoring and presence of the staff may give a sense of security. Also, the extremely intensive nature of care in the critical care unit often facilitates a high level of trust in the nurse–patient relationship. Transfer to the stepdown unit means less supervision and the need to get to know new staff. Both of these factors may diminish the patient's trust in the staff during the initial transfer period. In addition, the time of transfer may be the first time that family members consider it safe enough to leave the hospital for a short time. The patient's support system may then be depleted at a sensitive time.[40]

Nursing interventions that prevent, control, or reduce transfer anxiety begin with the awareness that transfer is a time of stress for the patient. Studies of coronary care patients have revealed that the stress of transfer has adverse physiological effects such as increased heart rate, increased blood pressure, and increased risk of cardiac dysrhythmias.[41] Preparation for transfer is most successful when it is structured and includes allowing patients opportunities to ventilate their feelings, portraying the transfer as a positive sign of recovery, identifying the patient's individual learning needs regarding the transfer, preparing the patient in advance of the transfer so that it does not come as a surprise, and showing trust in the expertise of the nurses on the transfer unit.[42] Facilitation of the transfer process requires a skillful approach that is carefully structured so that the patient can be separated from the intense environment of the critical care unit without unnecessary concern or anxiety.

REFERENCES

1. Naisbitt, J. (1982). *Megatrends*. New York: Warner Books.
2. Bergman, R. (1983). Understanding the patient in all his human needs. *Journal of Advanced Nursing, 8,* 185-190.
3. Garrett, S., & Garrett, B. (1982). Humaneness and health. *Topics in Clinical Nursing, 3*(1), 7-12.
4. Friedman, H., & DiMatteo, M. (1979). Health care as an interpersonal process. *Journal of Social Issues, 35*(1), 1-11.
5. Pearlin, L. I., & Schooler, C. (1978). The structure of coping. *Journal of Health and Social Behavior, 19,* 2-21.
6. Lazarus, R. S., & Folkman, S. (1984). *Stress, appraisal, and coping.* New York: Springer.
7. Kobosa, S. C., Maddi, S., & Kahn, S. (1982). Hardiness and health: A prospective study. *Journal of Personality and Social Psychology, 1,* 168-177.
8. Murphy, L. B. (1974). Coping, vulnerability and resilience in childhood. In G. V. Coelho, D. A. Hamburg, & J. E. Adams (Eds.), *Coping and adaptation* (pp. 69-100). New York: Basic Books.
9. Dimsdale, J. E. (1978). Coping—every man's war. *American Journal of Psychotherapy, 32,* 402-413.
10. Fife, B. L. (1985). A model for predicting the adaptation of families to medical crisis: An analysis of role integration. *Image: the Journal of Nursing Scholarship, 17,* 108-112.
11. Suls, J., & Fletcher, B. (1985). Self-attention, life stress, and illness: A prospective study. *Psychosomatic Medicine, 47,* 469-481.
12. Figley, C. R. (1983). Catastrophes: An overview of family reactions. In C. R. Figley, & H. I. McCubbin (Eds.), *Stress and the family II: Coping with catastrophe* (pp. 3-20). New York: Brunner Mazel.
13. Thoits, P. (1986). Social support as coping assistance. *Journal of Consulting and Clinical Psychology, 54*(4), 416-423.
14. Kuhn, R. (1990). *AACN's Outcome Standards for Nursing Care of the Critically Ill.* Laguna Niguel, CA: American Association of Critical-Care Nurses.
15. Vanson, R., Katz, B., & Krekeler, K. (1980). Stress effects on patients in critical care units from procedures performed on others. *Heart Lung, 9*(3), 494-497.
16. Gowan, N. (1979). The perceptual world of the intensive care unit: An overview of some environmental considerations in the helping relationship. *Heart Lung, 8*(2), 340-344.
17. Williams, M. (1989). Physical environment of the intensive care unit and elderly patients. *Critical Care Quarterly, 12*(1), 52-60.
18. Helton, M., Gordon, S., & Nunnery, S. (1980). The correlation between sleep deprivation and intensive care unit syndrome. *Heart Lung, 9*(3), 464-468.
19. Baker, C. (1983). Sensory overload and noise in the ICU: Sources of environmental stress. *Critical Care Quarterly, 7*(1), 66-80.
20. Hilton, A. (1985). Noise in acute patient care areas. *Research in Nursing and Health, 8,* 283-291.
21. Hansell, H. (1984). The behavioral effects of noise on man: The patient with ICU psychosis. *Heart Lung, 13*(1), 59-65.
22. MacKellaig, J. (1986). A study of physiological effects of intensive care with particular emphasis on patients in isolation. *Intensive Care Nursing, 2,* 176-185.
23. Betz, C. (1982). Sensory disturbances among children in the ICU. *Dimensions of Critical Care Nursing, 1*(3), 145-151.
24. Boykoff, S. (1986). Visitation needs reported by patients with cardiac disease and their families. *Heart Lung, 15*(6), 573-578.
25. Brewer, M. (1986). To sleep or not to sleep: The consequences of sleep deprivation. *Critical Care Nurse, 5*(6), 35-40.
26. Beglinger, J. (1983). Coping tasks in critical care. *Dimensions of Critical Care Nursing, 2*(2), 80-89.
27. Dootson, S. (1990). Sensory imbalance and sleep loss. *Nursing Times, 86*(35), 26-29.
28. Carpenito, L. (1987). *Nursing diagnosis: Application to clinical practice* (2nd ed.). Philadelphia: Lippincott.
29. Hilton, B. (1976). Quantity and quality of patient's sleep and sleep disturbing factors in a respiratory intensive care unit. *Advanced Nursing, 1,* 453-468.
30. Kartman, J. (1985). Sleep and the elderly critical care patient. *Critical Care Nurse, 5*(6), 52-56.

31. Miller, J. (1983). *Coping with chronic illness: Overcoming powerlessness.* Philadelphia: Davis.

32. Ryan, J. (1984). The neglected crisis. *American Journal of Nursing, 84,* 1257-1258.

33. Kleck, H. (1983). ICU syndrome: Onset, manifestations, treatment, stressors, and prevention. *Critical Care Quarterly, 6*(1), 21-28.

34. Easton, C., & MacKenzie, F. (1988). Sensory-perceptual alterations: Delirium in the intensive care unit. *Heart Lung, 17*(3), 229-235.

35. Griffin, J. (1982). Forced dependency in the critically ill. *Dimensions of Critical Care Nursing, 1*(6), 350-352.

36. Ramlow, M. (1984). Hope. *Focus on Critical Care, 9*(5), 10.

37. Fisher, M., & Moxham, P. (1979). ICU syndrome. *Critical Care Nurse, 4*(3), 39-45.

38. McGuire, M. (1983). A touch in the dark. *Critical Care Nurse, 3*(5), 53-56.

39. Carter, S. (1983). Rehumanizing the nursing role: A question of love. *Topics in Clinical Nursing, 5*(10), 11-17.

40. Schwartz, L., & Brenner, Z. (1979). Critical care unit transfer: Reducing patient stress through nursing interventions. *Heart Lung, 8*(3), 540-546.

41. Toth, J. (1980). Effect of structured preparation for transfer on patient anxiety on leaving coronary care unit. *Nursing Research, 29*(1), 28-34.

42. Poe, C. (1982). Minimizing stress of transfer responses. *Dimensions of Critical Care Nursing, 1*(6), 364-374.

43. Curtin, L. (1984). Nursing: High-touch in a high-tech world. *Nursing Management, 15*(7), 7-8.

44. Lambert, V., & Lambert, C. (1991). Behavioral responses to the critical care environment. In M. Shekleton, & K. Litwack (Eds.), *Critical care nursing of the surgical patient.* Philadelphia: Saunders.

PART THREE

Phenomena of Concern in Critical Care Nursing Practice

7

Shock

Gayle R. Whitman

Maintenance of adequate tissue perfusion is a basic and essential function for the survival of any living cell, organ, or system. In the critical care setting maintaining this basic function frequently becomes the major activity and primary goal. Shock, or inadequate tissue perfusion, is often blatant, as in cases of severe cardiogenic shock or hemorrhage. On the other hand, it can also be a less obvious or silent process, such as is seen in early septic shock. Therapy to maintain tissue perfusion may be singular, involving only volume replacement, or complex, involving volume replacement, pharmacological manipulation, and mechanical supports. In all these instances the role of the critical care nurse is paramount. As the consistent presence at the patient's bedside, the critical care nurse will most frequently identify subtle or acutely overt assessment parameters that indicate the development of shock. In addition, the nurse plans, implements, and evaluates appropriate nursing interventions to limit the effects of inadequate perfusion while concurrently collaborating with the physician in implementing medical therapies to reverse the shock state. To perform these functions effectively it

is essential that the critical care nurse recognize and understand these processes. This chapter describes the alterations that occur in shock, from the cellular to the systemic level, and delineates the appropriate interventions for preventing, limiting, or reversing inadequate perfusion.

CELLULAR AND SUBCELLULAR ANATOMY AND PHYSIOLOGY

All types of cells are not exactly alike in structure and function, but they possess to varying degrees some similarities. Typically, a cell consists of two major components: the nucleus and the cytoplasm (Figure 7-1). The *nucleus* is the control center of the cell. It is responsible for reproduction and for controlling the many chemical reactions that occur throughout the cell. The nucleus is situated in the middle of the cell, surrounded by cytoplasm and encapsulated by the nuclear membrane. This *nuclear membrane* consists of two layers made of lipids, carbohydrates, and proteins. It has large pores that facilitate the flux of fluid and particles between the nucleus and the cytoplasm. The nucleus contains large amounts of de-

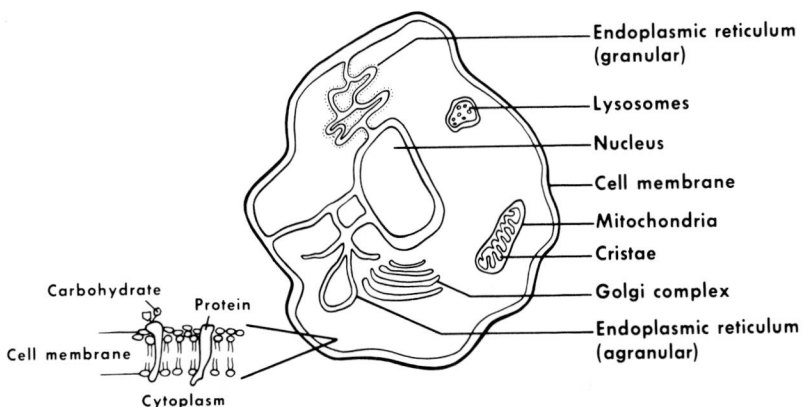

Figure 7-1 Schematic representation of a typical cell and its organelles. Section of the cell membrane (lower left) depicting protein and carbohydrate portions which extend from the membrane and serve as receptor sites for various agents.

oxyribonucleic acid (DNA) in the form of genes. The genes determine the function and activities that occur in the cytoplasm of the cell and actively engage in replication.

Surrounding the nucleus floats the *cytoplasm*. Within the cytoplasm there are numerous highly organized physical structures called *organelles*. The major organelles of the cell include the mitochondria, the endoplasmic reticulum, the Golgi complex, the lysosomes, and the peroxisomes. The *mitochondria* are considered the powerhouses of the cell since they are responsible for producing energy from the nutrients and oxygen that the cell receives from the capillary circulation. The number of mitochondria per cell varies among types of cells, depending upon the amount of energy each cell needs. Under normal circumstances, the mitochondria can produce 95% of the body's energy needs via aerobic metabolism. The mitochondria accomplish this by converting glucose into energy via the process of glycolysis. With this process 1 mol of glucose in the presence of oxygen can synthesize 36 mol of adenosine triphosphate (ATP) (Figure 7-2). Adenosine triphosphate is a high-energy phosphate that readily releases a phosphate radical and then forms adenosine diphosphate (ADP). During this process, it also releases energy, and it is this energy that drives the numerous cellular processes. Conversely, ADP can easily recombine with a phosphate group to form another ATP so that constant energy sources are available. Under anaerobic conditions, that is, without oxygen, 1 mol of glucose can synthesize only 3 mol of ATP. Therefore, any process that limits cellular oxygen delivery affects energy production.

Structurally, the mitochondrial walls consist of an outer and an inner membrane. On the inner membrane are numerous infoldings which form shelves, or cristae, where oxidative enzymes responsible for ATP production are stored.

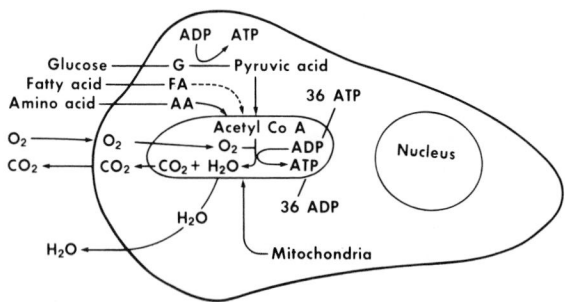

Figure 7-2 Formation by the mitochondria of adenosine triphosphate.

Adapted from Guyton, A. (1991). *Textbook of medicine physiology* (8th ed.). Philadelphia: Saunders.

Another organelle, the *endoplasmic reticulum* (ER), is a network of tubular structures which connects with the nuclear membrane and then extends into the cytoplasm. The ER transports substances from one part of the cell to another. Portions of the ER have ribosomes attached to them and appear granular. These are referred to as the *granular endoplasmic reticulum*. The ribosomes contain ribonucleic acid (RNA) and play a major function in the synthesis of protein. The portion of the ER without attached ribosomes is called the *smooth* or *agranular ER*. This structure plays a role in lipid synthesis. The smooth ER can also control glycogen breakdown when glycogen is used for energy, and can detoxify substances such as drugs, since it also stores enzymes.

The *Golgi complex* appears similar to the agranular ER. It consists of four or more stacked layers of flat, thin vesicles near the nucleus. This complex works closely with the ER, processing substances such as proteins after the ER synthesizes them. These processed substances then are packaged in vesicles which are released from the Golgi complex. They either extrude their protein contents outside the cell or they fuse their contents to structures inside the cell. Many vesicles fuse with the cell membranes or walls of the mitochondria and thereby replenish those structures with new proteins.

In addition, the Golgi complex synthesizes fructose and galactose and causes saccharide polymers such as hyaluronic acid and chondroctin sulfate to be formed. These latter substances are major components of the interstitial spaces where they serve as filler or gel between collagen fibers and the cells.

Finally, the last major structures to be considered are the *lysosome* and *peroxisome*, which serve as intracellular digestive systems. The lysosome has a double lipid membrane that encapsulates various hydrolytic enzymes. These enzymes are capable of splitting an organic compound into two or more parts. Normally, the lysosomes engulf unwanted substances such as dead cells or damaged substances, and their enzymes digest and thereby remove them. Lysosomes also contain bactericidal agents that can kill phagocytized bacteria before they cause cellular damage. Specifically, these agents include *lysozyme,* which dissolves bacterial membranes; *lysoferrin,* which binds iron and other metals needed for bacterial growth; and acids with a pH less than 4.0. Peroxisomes, which are similar to lysosomes in structure, contain oxidases. Several of these oxidases are capable of producing hydrogen peroxide, which can poison bacterial metabolic systems. It has also been shown to have a direct effect on the functioning and activity of the excitation/contraction coupling system in the cardiac muscle.[1] Although lysosomes and peroxisomes are effective and remarkable assets to the cell when the cell is functioning optimally, under certain pathological conditions they can rupture their membranes and spill these same contents internally. Internal cellular destruction then ensues and the cell autolyses.

All these organelles and the cytoplasm are also encapsulated by a bilayer cellular membrane consisting of lipids, proteins, and carbohydrates (see Figure 7-1). The lipid components of the cell membrane are arranged in two straight rows on top of each other. This lipid bilayer makes the cell almost impermeable to water and to water-soluble substances such as glucose, ions, urea, and others. On the other hand, fat-soluble substances such as oxygen and carbon dioxide can penetrate this portion of the membrane.

The proteins in the membrane are intermittently scattered throughout the lipids and largely serve two functions. First, because they are wedged between the lipids, they can provide structural pathways or pores through which water and water-soluble substances, especially ions, can diffuse between intracellular and extracellular fluids. In addition, some reside entirely on the inside of the membrane and act almost exclusively as enzymes. The carbohydrates are most often found on the outside of the membrane. There they play a role in the immune system and serve as receptor substances for hormones such as epinephrine and nor-epinephrine (catecholamines).

Molecular Transport

If the cell is to live and grow, it must be able to bring nutrients and oxygen through the cell membrane. The three major processes by which this is accomplished are diffusion, active transport, and endocytosis. *Diffusion* is the movement of particles from the side of the membrane where its concentration is high to the side where it is low. As previously mentioned, some particles can diffuse through the pores or pathways created by the wedged proteins in the cellular membrane, and some easily diffuse through the lipid portions. Another method of diffusion is *facilitated diffusion*. In this instance, a particle diffuses or moves through the lipid portion of the cell membrane by combining first with a carrier substance. In tandem, the carrier substance and the particle cross the membrane and enter the cell. This is the mechanism by which glucose enters the cell.

Active transport similarly involves moving a particle attached to a carrier from one side of the membrane to the other. Active transport, however, occurs from an area of low concentration to an area of high concentration. Facilitated diffusion can move particles only in the direction of higher to lower concentrations. In active transport, this uphill action is powered by energy in the form of adenosine triphos-

phate (ATP). This energy is delivered to the cell membrane from the cytoplasm. Several substances use this method of entry into the cell. The most common are sodium, potassium, calcium, hydrogen, urate and chloride ions, amino acids, and various sugars.

The most important ionic active transport system is the sodium–potassium pump (Na^+/K^+ pump) or sodium pump. Present in all cells, the sodium pump serves to pump sodium out of the cell and into the extracellular fluid and to bring potassium from the extracellular fluid into the intracellular fluid. The carrier substance for this activity is sodium–potassium ATPase. This ATPase can bind sodium and potassium and can split ATP molecules to use their energy for active transport. The active transport process is initiated inside the cell and requires intracellular ATP to carry out its actions. Therefore, any deficit in cellular ATP production will seriously affect this ionic pump as well as many functions.

Another process that can serve to transport particles into the cell is the process of *endocytosis*. With endocytosis, the cellular membrane actually engulfs the extracellular fluid and its contents or particulate. Once inside the cell, the materials are digested and destroyed. Both phagocytosis and pinocytosis are mechanisms of endocytosis. In *phagocytosis,* large particles, bacteria, and other cells or particles of degenerating tissue are removed. *Pinocytosis* is the ingestion of minute quantities of extracellular fluid and dissolved substances. Phagocytosis will occur when objects that have an electropositive charge contact the cell membrane. Most natural substances in the extracellular fluid are negatively charged. Foreign material and damaged tissues are specially prepared by antibodies via a process of *opsonization* so that they are positively charged, making them ideal candidates for phagocytosis. Pinocytosis occurs in the same manner when substances such as electrolytes and proteins contact the membrane. Once inside the cell, lysosomes attach to the substances and begin to hydrolyze them into amino acids, glucose, fatty acids, phosphates, and other chemicals.

In addition to these transport functions, the cell membrane plays an important role in many chemical pathways. One that becomes particularly important in shock is the process related to adrenergic receptor reactions. Figure 7-3 schematically depicts the series of reactions that originate at the cell membrane level, cascade into the cell, and lead to enhanced myocardial contractility. On the surface of cell membranes are many receptor sites that can ultimately elicit different responses. In this situation, the receptor site is an alpha 1 receptor site which, once activated, should improve muscle contraction. Once an agonist (a substance that elicits a response) binds with this site,

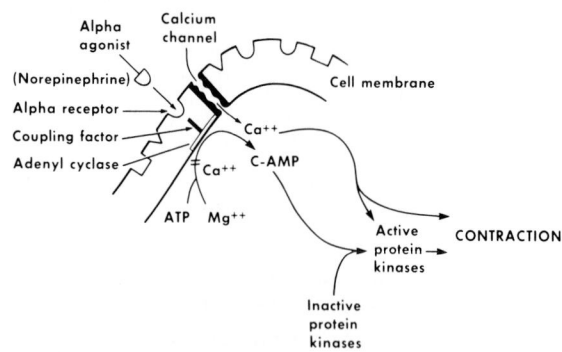

Figure 7-3   Triggering of the contraction process by an alpha agonist via a cell membrane receptor site.

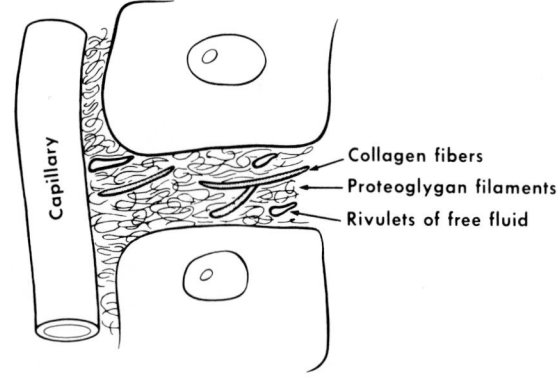

Figure 7-4   Structure of the interstitium, consisting of proteonglycan filaments and collagen bundles.

Adapted from Guyton, A. (1991). *Textbook of medical physiology* (8th ed.). Philadelphia: Saunders.

adenyl cyclase is activated. Adenyl cyclase is an enzyme embedded in the cellular membrane. A coupling factor, a G protein, is also believed to be present in the cell membrane to facilitate the interaction between the agonist and adenyl cyclase. Once adenyl cyclase is activated, ATP in the presence of magnesium is converted to 3',5-cyclic adenosine monophosphate (cyclic AMP, or cAMP). Cyclic AMP can be deactivated by an enzyme called phosphodiesterase or it can remain active and convert inactive protein kinase into active protein kinase. This ultimately leads to an enhancement of a number of calcium-dependent processes that improve muscle contraction. This mechanism is discussed later in the chapter, but it is highlighted here to illustrate another major function of the cell membrane. Integrity of the cell membrane is of paramount importance in maintaining structural and metabolic functions of the cell.

The interstitium provides a connection between the cells. One sixth of the body's tissue is interstitium. The interstitium consists of two major solid structures: *collagen fiber bundles* and *proteoglycan filaments* (Figure 7-4). These proteoglycan filaments synthesized from products made in the Golgi complex are very thin. When combined with the interstitial fluid, they form a gel between the cells. This gel prevents fluid in the body from rapidly moving to dependent segments after any positional change, and it also helps prevent microorganisms from rapidly gaining access to the body. Fluid moves through the interstitium mostly by diffusion. Scattered throughout the interstitium are rivulets of free fluid. As fluid accumulates in the interstitial bed it first expands the gel 30% to 50%. Further expansion beyond this point is not possible; excess fluid then accumulates in the rivulets. Once in the rivulets the fluid is very mobile. Clinically, this results in pitting edema. Pitting edema can be elicited by pressing on an edematous area for a few seconds and seeing the creation of an inden-

tation in the skin. This indentation usually disappears a few seconds later. This indentation and subsequent disappearance reflects the mobility of the fluid in the rivulets.

Capillary and Fluid Dynamics

As was mentioned earlier, oxygen and nutrients make their way to the cells via the capillary system. The capillary system is so extensive that cells are generally no farther away from a capillary than 30 microns (μm). The structure of a typical capillary network is depicted in Figure 7-5. Arterioles continuously surrounded by smooth muscle fibers gradually develop into metarterioles which are only intermittently surrounded by smooth muscle fibers. These smooth muscle fibers, which are responsible for the expansion and contraction of the diameter of these vessels, are controlled by the sympathetic nervous system. Sympathetic stimulation causes vasoconstriction and thereby alters the volume of these vessels and thus the volume of blood in the peripheral circulation. Because of the amount of smooth muscle encapsulating the arteriole, the diameter of the arteriole can be altered to a greater extent than the metarteriole, and therefore arteriolar vasoconstriction has a greater impact on the circulatory status.

Between the metarterioles and the capillaries there is a junction known as the *precapillary sphincter*. This sphincter, which consists of a band of smooth muscle fibers surrounding the capillary, regulates the flow of blood to the capillary. Neither the capillaries nor the sphincters have sympathetic fibers attached to them to assist them in constricting; however, under normal circumstances these sphincters and the smooth muscle of the metarteriole intermittently contract and relax on their own 5 to 10 times a minute. This opening

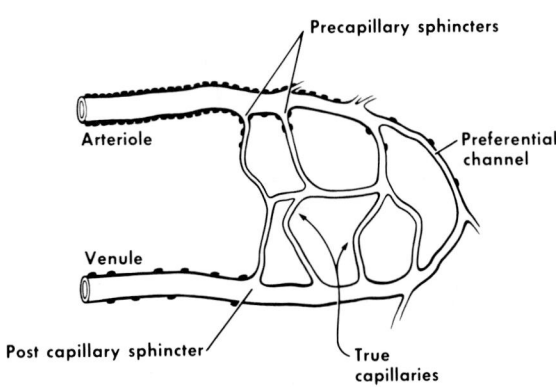

Figure 7-5 Typical capillary network depicting arterioles, metarterioles, capillaries, venules, and veins.

Adapted from Guyton, A. (1991). *Textbook of medical physiology* (8th ed.). Philadelphia: Saunders.

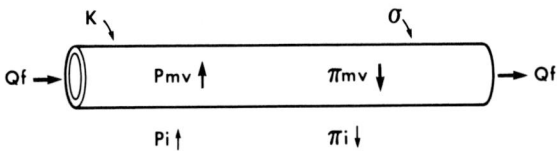

Figure 7-6 Starling's equation governing the effect of forces on the capillary.

the following equation and in Figure 7-6.

$$Qf = K(Pmv - Pi) - K\sigma\,(\pi mv - \pi i)$$

in which

Qf = Net transvascular flow of fluid through the vessel.

K = Capillary filtration coefficient. This value varies from one type of tissue to another and refers to that tissue's particular permeability. The permeability of brain tissue, for example, is significantly less than that in the intestine, and therefore movement of substances across the capillaries in the brain is limited.

Pmv = Microvascular or capillary hydrostatic pressure. This is the fluid pressure in the capillary which favors outward flow of fluid across the capillary membrane.

Pi = Interstitial hydrostatic pressure. This refers to fluid pressure in the interstitium which favors movement of fluid into the capillary and out of the interstitium.

σ = Protein reflection coefficient. This coefficient relates to the size of protein molecules which would be able to sieve through the membrane.

πmv = Serum protein osmotic pressure. This force tends to draw fluid into the capillary and out of the interstitium.

πi = Interstitial protein osmotic pressure. This refers to the pressure which favors movement of fluid out of the capillary and into the interstitium.

and closing of the sphincters is referred to as *vasomotion.* It is controlled by autoregulation. That is, when the tissue oxygenation level is low, the sphincter relaxes and blood enters the capillary. As that area becomes adequately oxygenated, that sphincter will close and another will open in an area of inadequate oxygenation. Blood flow to the capillaries then is not continuous but intermittent. There are two types of capillaries, the *preferential channels,* which are relatively large, and the *true capillaries,* which are small. The walls of the capillaries themselves consist of only one layer of endothelial cells. Small intercellular clefts or slitlike pores lie between adjacent endothelial cells. In addition, some have *fenestrae,* large openings in the middle. Substances can pass back and forth between the capillary and the interstitium, either through the capillary membrane by diffusion or pinocytosis, or across the intercellular clefts or fenestrae by diffusion.

Finally, as blood exits the capillaries, it returns to the venules. As can be seen by the diagram, the venules also are surrounded intermittently by smooth muscle fiber. This muscle allows them also to contract. Even though there is less smooth muscle available on the venules for contraction, contraction can be quite strong, since the pressure the venules are working against, the venous pressure, is lower than the arteriolar pressure.

In addition to their role as carriers of nutrients and oxygen, the capillaries are crucial to maintaining a balanced movement of fluid between themselves and the interstitial spaces. Although the movement of this fluid is accomplished by the process of diffusion, this movement is controlled by certain forces inside the capillary and in the interstitial spaces. These forces and their relationship to each other are illustrated in

Under normal circumstances, there is a tremendous amount of movement and flux of fluid and substances across the capillary membrane. However, with these forces operating, normally there is little net difference in movement of fluid in and out of the capillary. Any net increase in movement out of the capillary and into the interstitium is then removed from the interstitium by the lymphatic system and is ultimately returned to the vascular bed. As you will see later in the chapter, a major alteration of any of these forces or an alteration in capillary wall integrity, such as occurs in permeability leaks, can lead to significant symptoms.

PATHOPHYSIOLOGY OF SHOCK

Generally, shock has been defined as a state that develops when there is inadequate tissue perfusion. And certainly in the case of cardiogenic shock or hemorrhagic shock, this is true. However, in hyperdynamic stages of septic shock, xenon studies have shown that the blood flow to the capillaries may be greater than normal.[2] The major problem in this situation appears to be an inability of the cell to appropriately extract and utilize substrates and oxygen from that delivered blood. Therefore, shock more appropriately should be considered as a pathophysiological abnormality in which there is inadequate blood flow to vital organs and/or the inability of the tissues or individual cell to metabolize nutrients normally. The clinical syndrome of shock and its sequelae result from sustained, inadequate tissue perfusion and utilization which then leads to alterations in tissue metabolism, structure, and function at the subcellular, cellular, and systems levels.[2,3,4]

Cellular Responses to Shock

The general sequence of events that occurs in the cell during shock is well documented.[2,5,6] It is depicted in Figure 7-7. The decrease in oxygenation reduces the cell membrane potential and alters membrane permeability. Consequently, both structural and metabolic processes are affected. The sodium pump begins to fail, thus altering transport processes. Potassium effluxes out of the cell, and intracellular sodium and water increase. As sodium accumulates in the cell, the Na^+/K^+-ATPase pump is stimulated to work faster. This increases the consumption of ATP and forces the mitochondria to increase production. However, with inadequate oxygen delivery, this production quickly slows. As ATP production decreases and damage to the cell membrane occurs, cAMP production declines. As indicated earlier, cAMP plays a crucial role in catecholamine function, calcium regulation, and numerous other cellular processes. In order to form, cAMP needs the presence of ATP and adenyl cyclase.

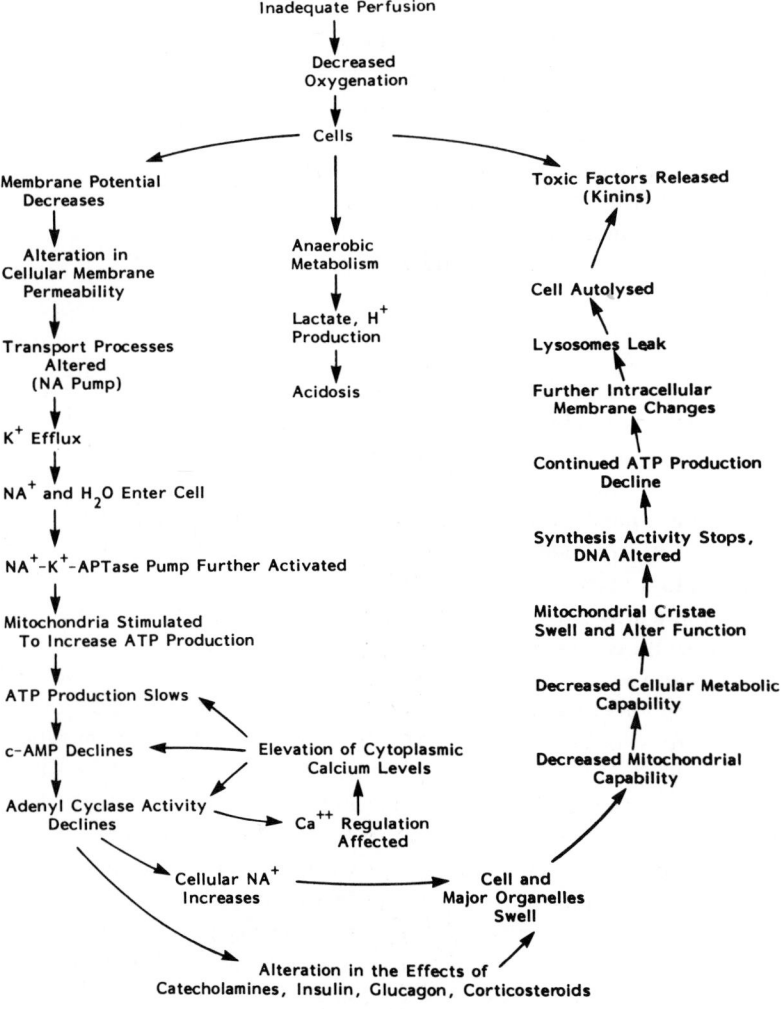

Figure 7-7 Effects of inadequate perfusion at the cellular level.

Adapted from Chaudry, I. D. (1983). Cellular mechanisms in shock and ischemia and their correction. *American Journal of Physiology, 245,* R117.

Normally, adenyl cyclase is attached to the cell membrane, readily available to assist in the transformation of cAMP. With a loss of ATP and a breakdown in the cellular wall, cAMP is decreased, and the reactions it initiates are diminished.

Calcium fluxes develop, and calcium regulation is compromised. Normally the mitochondria contain significant supplies of calcium. As ATP continues to convert to ADP, free phosphates accumulate in the cytoplasm. This causes the mitochondria to lose their calcium supply. Also, with impairment of the cell membrane, calcium leaves the extracellular fluid and enters the cell. All these actions create an elevation of the cytoplasmic Ca^{2+} levels, and this appears to inhibit the mitochondria from releasing ATP into the cytoplasm. High cytoplasmic calcium also interferes with the adenyl cyclase in the cell membrane, thereby decreasing the production of cAMP. As mentioned earlier, this affects the cell's response to adrenergic agents.

At this stage, not only does the cell itself swell but the major organelles such as the ER, the mitochondria, and the cell membrane also swell. Protein synthesis and ion pumps begin to halt their actions. As the cristae and the inner mitochondrial membranes swell, only minimal ATP synthesis can occur since now the structures responsible for production are destroyed. At this point, if perfusion is reinstituted the cell can still recover; however, if not halted at this point, anaerobic glycolysis continues to take over, and lactic and pyruvic acid production continue to increase. Ultimate cellular survival becomes less and less likely.

At this point the lysosomes begin to leak and release their hydrolases, enzymes that initiate internal digestion of the remaining cellular contents. Ultimately these enzymes will assist in the destruction of neighboring cells. The proteolytic enzymes from the lysosomes are particularly active and can convert inactive kininogens into active kinins. One of these kinins is *bradykinin*, which is a potent vasodilator responsible for skin flushing, which can develop particularly in septic shock. Bradykinin is also linked with the ability to increase capillary permeability.

The rate of progression through this entire series of events varies from cell to cell. Skeletal muscle cells and smooth cells move very slowly through this process, perhaps because these cells have a high capacity for anaerobic metabolism. Even if circulation is reestablished before the cell autolyses, the cells do not immediately return to their correct size. It takes time for the edema to resolve and, consequently, further damage, injury, and perhaps death can result from the ischemia induced by the edematous environment. In addition, it has recently become apparent that the restoration of oxygen to cells and tissues can trigger further cellular damage. This process known as *reperfusion injury* occurs when large quantities of superoxide radicals and hydrogen peroxide are produced during reoxygenation. These substances are capable of eliciting severe cellular damage.[7]

Systemic Responses to Shock

The previous section described the sequential responses of individual cells to inadequate perfusion. As inadequate perfusion persists and significant numbers of cells are affected, organ systems begin to malfunction and clinically perceptible signs and symptoms begin to appear. At this point hypoxemia, hypotension, and acidosis begin to activate some of the body's compensatory mechanisms.

One of the first mechanisms to be activated is the sympathetic nervous system. Falls in arterial pressure are quickly sensed by the baroreceptors in the aorta and the carotid sinus. Once stimulated, these receptors send impulses to the vasomotor center in the medulla. Consequently, the vasomotor center signals the sympathetic nerve fibers throughout the body to discharge norepinephrine from their endings. This discharge causes vasoconstriction of the arteriolar beds, thereby raising arterial pressure. In addition, the adrenal medulla is sympathetically stimulated by the vasomotor center to release both epinephrine and norepinephrine into the bloodstream. In this manner, even cells not attached to sympathetic fibers, such as the metarterioles, are exposed to the vasoconstrictor effects of these hormones.

In early stages of shock, blood is shunted away from organs that tolerate ischemia well, such as the skeletal muscles, fat, and skin. In these areas, arterioles contract and shunt blood away from the capillaries and through arteriovenous fistulas into the venous system. In organs that cannot tolerate lack of oxygen, such as the heart and brain, the arterioles remain open and the true capillaries still receive their blood flow.[8] As shock progresses this mechanism fails. The arteriolar and precapillary sphincters require sufficient energy in the form of ATP to maintain a vasoconstrictive state. As energy dissipates, the sphincters relax and blood then flows into these organs and sequesters. Sludging of the blood in these capillary beds occurs, and the microcirculation becomes blocked. Metabolic waste products, microaggregates of platelets, white blood cells, and clots accumulate, further enhancing sludging and contributing to the development of metabolic acidosis. Arachidonic acid metabolites such as thromboxane A_2 and prostacylin are also thought to be important in the events that occur in the microcirculation. Serum levels of these substances are high in severe shock. Thromboxane

A_2 is produced by white blood cells, platelets, and parenchymal tissues of the kidneys and lungs. It is a potent platelet aggregator and a vasoconstrictor. Prostacyclin is produced by the vascular endothelium and is a potent anti–platelet aggregator and a vasodilator. These two substances normally counterbalance each other and maintain homeostasis. However, in severe hypovolemic and septic shock the actions of thromboxane A_2 seem to dominate. This might contribute significantly to the clotting and sludging in the microcirculation typical of these states.[9]

As was noted above, epinephrine is important in the body's response to shock. In addition to its effect on the vascular bed it enhances myocardial contractility and increases blood levels of glucose. It accomplishes the latter by increasing the breakdown of glycogen, by increasing gluconeogenesis from amino acids and lactate, and by inhibiting the secretion of insulin. Epinephrine also increases serum levels of free fatty acids by stimulating lipolysis. All these activities help supply the body with readily available energy sources to maintain metabolic functions. Serum levels of the glucocorticoids, cortisone and cortisol, also rise in early stages of shock. They, as epinephrine, play a role in producing glucose and free fatty acids. Additionally, glucocorticoids have a mild inotropic effect on the myocardium and may assist in stabilizing subcellular, cellular, and endothelial membranes.

A fall in arterial pressure near the aortic and carotid bodies can also initiate a respiratory compensatory response. If the fall in arterial pressure decreases oxygen concentration to the receptors, the respiratory rate rises. This is a mechanism by which the body increases oxygenation.

Another compensatory mechanism is the formation of angiotensin, another powerful vasoconstrictor. When the juxtaglomerular apparatus in the nephron senses a fall in arterial pressure or sodium concentration, it releases renin. Renin cleaves renin substrate into angiotensin I. Angiotensin I is converted into angiotensin II in the lungs, and this stimulates the adrenal cortex to synthesize and release aldosterone. Aldosterone allows the kidney to save sodium and water and to excrete potassium and hydrogen. This provides the body with a mechanism to maintain or retain volume. In addition, angiotensin II causes marked constriction of the peripheral arterioles and a moderate constriction of the veins, thus assisting in increasing systemic blood pressure.

The formation of *antidiuretic hormone* (ADH), or *vasopressin,* is also a component of the body's compensatory plan. Vasopressin is the body's most potent vasoconstrictor substance. It is formed in the hypothalamus and secreted by the posterior pituitary in response to a decreased blood pressure and an in-

creased osmolality. Vasopressin is released as early as 15 minutes following an insult.[10] The fall in blood pressure activates the baroreceptors that stimulate the hypothalamus and posterior pituitary to synthesize and release ADH. The osmolality directly affects the hypothalamus. If the osmoreceptors detect a dilute osmolality, then ADH is inhibited; if the osmolality is high, then ADH is secreted. Also, in shock states a loss of 10% of the person's blood volume can create a moderate release of ADH. Loss of blood volume is detected by low-pressure receptors in the atria. Other factors responsible for an increase in ADH production are trauma, pain, anxiety, morphine, tranquilizers, and some anesthetic agents. The action of ADH is both direct and indirect. Vasopressin has a direct vasoconstrictor effect on blood vessels and can thereby increase systemic vascular resistance. Additionally, it indirectly augments venous return and cardiac output by stimulating the distal renal tubules to reabsorb water.

The reverse stress relaxation response of the circulatory system also plays a compensatory role. This mechanism allows blood vessels, once volume has been lost, to constrict around the remaining blood volume so that the volume left will more adequately fill the circulation. This mechanism assists in returning blood to the myocardium. Other mechanisms that assist in returning volume to the vascular bed and then ultimately to the myocardium include the absorption of fluid from the intestines and from the interstitium.

All the previously identified mechanisms are initiated at the peripheral level via baroreceptors, chemoreceptors, or low-pressure receptors. One last powerful response remains in the central nervous system and this is referred to as the *CNS ischemic response.* This response is elicited when the vasomotor cells begin to experience ischemia and high levels of high carbon dioxide and lactic acid, usually when arterial pressure falls below 50 mmHg. This stimulation elicits a sympathetic drive that can raise the arterial pressure by 15 to 20 mmHg.

Associated Problems

As the effects of shock persist, specific organ systems begin to develop clinical syndromes in response to their ischemic states. Inadequate perfusion leads to a decreased removal of waste products and metabolites in the cell's immediate environment, since the normal function of circulation is not only to perfuse and bring in oxygen and nutrients but also to carry away metabolic waste products. As these waste products accumulate, they can depress the reticuloendothelial system (RES). Under normal circumstances this system plays an important role in phagocytosis and removal of waste products. The exact cause of RES dysfunction is not known; however, it has been reported that it may be associated with dysfunction of the opsonization process. As stated earlier, this is a process whereby foreign or waste materials are acted upon by antibodies which make them positively charged. Positively charged materials are targets for phagocytosis, and without this marking process these substances will not be identified as removable.[11] There is a strong correlation between the degree of RES dysfunction and mortality.[12]

The pulmonary system can be affected tremendously by shock. Pulmonary edema states can develop as the forces in the capillary fluid dynamics equation are altered. In patients with cardiogenic shock, a cardiac or hydrostatic pulmonary edema can develop. In this situation, as the left ventricle fails and left ventricular volumes and pressures rise, pulmonary pressures also rise. Capillary or microvascular hydrostatic pressure in the lung rise in turn, and fluid begins to

leak out into the interstitial spaces. If the increase is moderate, the lymphatics drain the excess fluid. However, as transudation of this fluid approaches 200 ml per hour, the lymphatics are no longer able to keep pace with the fluid removal, and interstitial pulmonary edema develops[13] (Figure 7-8A). As the capillary hydrostatic pressure increases further, fluid begins to accumulate in the alveoli, leading to the development of alveolar edema (Figure 7-8B). The mainstay of therapy for these types of pulmonary edema is aimed at fluid removal, either with diuretics or by improving myocardial contractility.

Another type of pulmonary sequela that can develop in shock states is permeability pulmonary edema. There are generally two types of this pulmonary edema. The first, *noncardiac edema* (NCE), develops when there is damage to the capillary endothelium (Figure 7-8C). This damage allows colloid to leak across the capillary and lie in the interstitium. In this fashion, the interstitial protein osmotic pres-

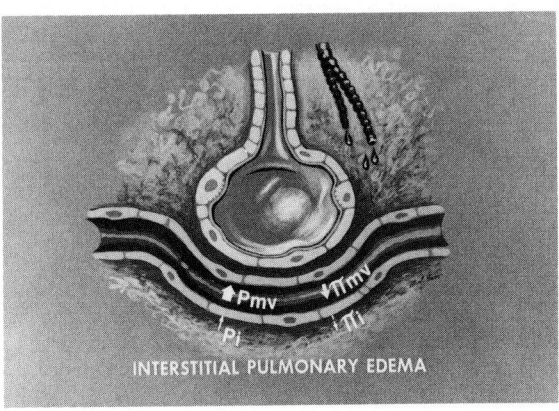

A

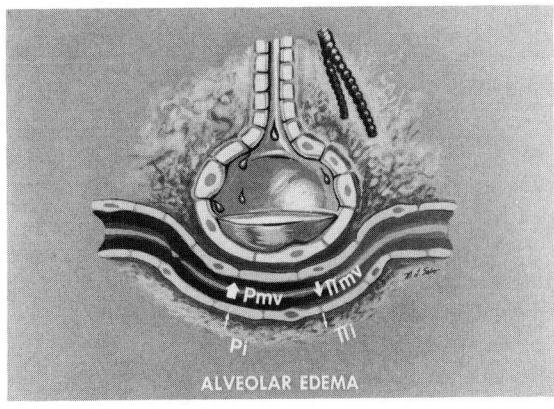

B

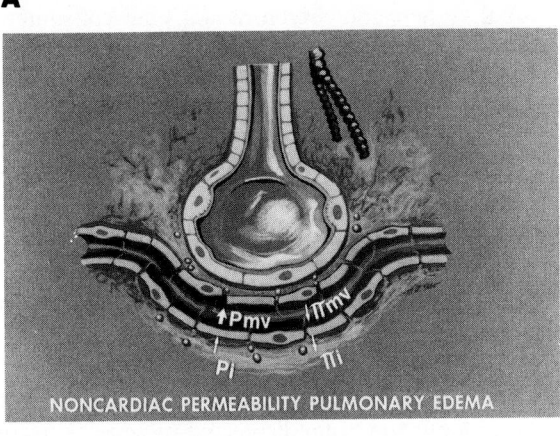

C

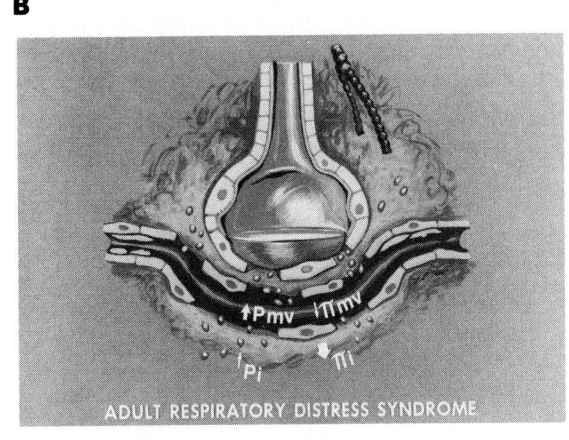

D

Figure 7-8   *A,* Alveolar and pulmonary capillary changes associated with interstitial pulmonary edema. The lymphatics can no longer remove fluid rapidly enough, and it accumulates in the interstitial space. *B,* Alveolar and capillary changes with alveolar edema. Fluid is now sequestering in both the interstitium and the alveoli. *C,* Alveolar and capillary changes seen in noncardiac edema. Capillary endothelial cells are disrupted. *D,* Alveolar and capillary changes seen in adult respiratory distress syndrome. Alveolar epithelial and capillary endothelial cells are disrupted.

sure is altered, thus favoring fluid sequestering in the interstitium. The precipitating factors in this endothelial damage can be ischemic damage to the lung parenchyma itself or the effects of toxic factors. Noncardiac permeability pulmonary edema develops into adult respiratory distress syndrome (ARDS) when the permeability damage involves both capillary endothelium and alveolar epithelial structures (Figure 7-8D). In this situation, the leakage and cellular disruption are so great that colloid leaks into both the interstitium and the alveoli. This tremendously alters the normal fluid equation and favors fluid accumulation in both the interstitium and alveoli. Adult respiratory distress syndrome develops when there is a massive insult to the cells, either a severe ischemic insult from low-flow states or more commonly an exposure to toxic substances which are released in septic shock.

Disseminated intravascular coagulopathy (DIC) is another associated problem that can develop as a consequence of inadequate perfusion states. Under normal circumstances the processes of thrombosis (clot formation) and fibrinolysis (clot digestion) occur at a localized site of an injury and ultimately prevent hemorrhage. In DIC, these processes occur generally throughout the microcirculation and cause extensive hemorrhage. In the setting of inadequate tissue perfusion, DIC is most likely to be triggered by infectious agents, massive tissue trauma, or burns. These processes serve as the initiators of this clot formation/clot digestion cycle. In the clot formation process, thrombin is generated from prothrombin. In the circulation, thrombin cleaves fibrinogen to form insoluble fibrin clots. These fibrin clots deposited in the microcirculation lead to tissue ischemia and contribute to the consumption of platelets and other clotting factors such as fibrinogen, prothrombin, and factors V, VIII, and XIII. The clot dissolution, process or fibrinolysis, digests fibrinogen, fibrin, and factors II, V, VIII, and XIII. In addition, fibrin degradation products are formed after fibrinogen and the newly formed fibrin monomers are split by plasmin. These fibrin degradation products are potent anticoagulants. These factors—the consumption or digestion of platelets and clotting factors, the fibrinolytic or clot dissolution activity of plasmin, and the anticoagulant properties of fibrin degradation products—contribute to the systemic bleeding and hemorrhage problems seen clinically with DIC.

Management of DIC involves corrective treatment of the underlying triggering event, replacement of clotting factors, and heparin therapy[14,15] (Chapters 42 and 56). Replacement component therapy generally includes platelet units to replace platelets; fresh frozen plasma to replace factors V, VIII, and XIII; and cryo-precipitate to replace fibrinogen and factor VIII. The use of heparin therapy remains controversial as there exist no controlled studies which support its efficacy.[16]

Prerenal and acute renal failure are common sequelae of shock states. With a slight or moderate decrease in cardiac output, the kidney compensates as discussed earlier by conserving sodium and water and by shunting its blood flow from the cortical nephrons to the sodium-saving juxtaglomerular ones. Urine produced during this stage is low in volume and is concentrated. With the restoration of perfusion, the kidney will most often quickly resume normal functioning. However, with severe and prolonged falls in cardiac output the renal parenchymal cells become damaged and acute tubular necrosis develops. It should also be pointed out that, in addition to ischemia, other factors contribute to the development of acute renal failure. Some of these factors include tubular obstruction, glomerular ultrafiltration, back diffusion, decreased glomerular permeability coefficient, persistent fibrin deposits in the glomerular capillary, and changes in intracellular biochemistry.[17]

Hepatic complications seen in hypoperfusion states include centrolobular necrosis, enlarged Kupffer cells, and fatty infiltrates. These processes lead to alterations in hepatic functions such that transaminase and bilirubin levels rise and albumin and prothrombin production falls. Gastrointestinal problems also develop as erosions and ulcerations in the stomach and enteritis develop. These alterations are believed to be caused by back diffusion of hydrogen ions across the mucosa and maldistribution of blood flow to the mucosa due to low flow. The mucosa is primarily affected since it performs most of the work for the gastrointestinal system and therefore is a high consumer of oxygen. As nutrition to the mucosa is curtailed, the mucosal barrier becomes impaired and microorganisms and endotoxins can now move easily into the systemic circulation resulting in bacteremia and septic shock.[10] Additionally, Mallory-Weiss syndrome can be produced by shock. This syndrome consists of longitudinal lacerations of the gastric mucosa below the esophagus and is frequently associated with hemorrhage. Major bleeding from these areas can be avoided by increasing the gastric pH with antacids or drugs.[18]

Generally, the last organ to be damaged by the shock state is the brain. Protected by several cerebral compensatory mechanisms, blood flow to the brain is preserved when all other vessels are constricted. The final pathway for neuronal injury varies according to the etiology of the insult. Specifically, abrupt anoxic injury will develop subsequent to a cardiopulmonary arrest; ischemic injury follows hypovolemic shock, and inflammatory/metabolic insults result from septic shock.[19] Regardless of etiology, all these pathways lead to neuronal damage. Clinically the patient gradually declines from restless and agitated states to somnolence and coma. Evaluation of the extent of permanent CNS damage may be difficult to ascertain since other depressive factors such as acidosis and other metabolic derangements may be present concurrently, and/or the patient may have residual drug effects from analgesics or narcotics.

Stages of Shock

In general, shock can be divided into three stages: compensated, decompensated, and irreversible.[20,21] *Compensated,* or nonprogressive, *shock* is the stage during which the severity of the shock and the intensity of the compensatory mechanisms are such that the vital organs remain adequately perfused and full recovery is possible. *Decompensated,* or progressive, *shock* is the stage during which the severity of the shock or the inadequacy or failure of the compensatory mechanisms is such that the vital organs are hypoperfused. In this progressive stage the shock becomes steadily worse until death. In hypovolemic shock, for example, a moderate loss of blood volume from an external hemorrhage may trigger the previously described compensatory mechanisms, and adequate perfusion to vital organs is maintained. If, however, volume loss continues without replacement, the patient might additionally develop myocardial ischemia from poor coronary artery filling, leading to eventual decompensation. Effective treatments would be aimed at supporting the compensatory mechanisms and remedying the underlying problem. *Irreversible shock* occurs when the extent of the shock is so severe that no type of therapy will be adequate to save the person's life.

ETIOLOGIES OF ALTERED TISSUE PERFUSION

Generally, there are four major types of shock: hypovolemic, cardiogenic, distributive, and obstructive. Each of these types has specific mechanisms whereby tissue perfusion is altered. In *hypovolemic shock,* inadequate volume causes a decrease in tissue perfusion, whereas in *cardiogenic shock* an inadequate pump causes a decrease in tissue perfusion. Maldistribution of the circulation and obstruction to the distribution of the circulation are the major factors interfering with tissue perfusion in *distributive* and *obstructive shock.*

Hypovolemic Shock

Hypovolemic shock develops when blood volume is insufficient to fill the intravascular space.[22] This occurs in states associated with obvious or direct volume losses and in states associated with indirect volume losses. Direct losses occur with external hemorrhage, diarrhea, vomiting, massive diuresis, and loss of plasma from skin lesions or exposed burn areas. Direct losses are for the most part easily identifiable and can to some extent be quantified. Indirect losses are less measurable and can be caused by situations in which sequestering of fluids occurs in third spaces. For example, this can be seen in patients with cirrhosis who sequester fluid in the peritoneal cavity. Interstitial tissue spaces can also serve as reservoirs of fluid, particularly when there is an alteration in capillary permeability or when there is a fall in colloidal osmotic pressure. In intestinal obstruction there is a tendency for fluid to mobilize from the intestinal capillaries and fill the lumen of the intestine, thereby creating an intravascular deficit. Internal hemorrhages such as a hemothorax, hemorrhagic pancreatitis, a ruptured spleen, or long bone fractures also lead to hypovolemic shock. Lastly, severe salt depletion, Addisonian crisis, and hypopituitarism can also serve as causes of hypovolemic shock.[23,24]

Generally, there are three stages of hypovolemic shock: mild, moderate, and severe.[25] Depending on the severity and the rate of the volume loss, the patient may progress through these stages very slowly or very rapidly. In the mild stage, the patient generally experiences a blood volume deficit ranging from 0% to 10% or approximately 50 ml.

This volume deficit creates a reduction in venous return and cardiac output which is sensed by the baroreceptors. The autonomic nervous system is activated and the subsequent increase in sympathetic constriction of the vasculature and the increase in myocardial contractility maintain arterial pressure and cardiac output. Secretion of vasopressin, renin, and aldosterone also begins at this point. Blood flow is shunted away from the skin, fat, and skeletal tissues, and the patient may begin to appear pale. The first phase of the transcapillary refill mechanism becomes activated when the sympathetic nervous system constricts the precapillary sphincters, the postcapillary sphincters, and the small veins. With this, the capillary hydrostatic pressure decreases and fluid moves from the interstitium into the capillary. The ultimate rate of transcapillary refill can be as high as 1 liter an hour. Since the large fenestrae in the capillary are normally closed at this time, minimal protein moves into the circulation with this volume.[26] Because of the activation of all these mechanisms the patient remains relatively if not totally asymptomatic during this mild stage of hypovolemic shock. In general, the relationship between cardiac output and acute volume loss is not a straight line but rather a curved one (Figure 7-9). The curve represents the protective effects of the

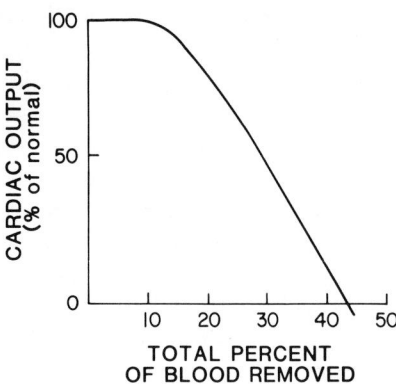

Figure 7-9 The effect of blood volume removal on cardiac output.

compensatory mechanisms. Major deteriorations in cardiac output generally occur with volume losses exceeding 25% to 30%. Without the protective effects of the sympathetic reflexes, death would occur with only a 15% to 20% loss of blood volume.

Almost concurrently, as the first stage is activated, the second phase of transcapillary refill begins to additionally assist in volume restoration.[27] In the initial phase, fluid moved from the interstitium into the intravascular compartment. This created an increase in capillary hydrostatic pressure and a subsequent dilution in plasma protein concentration. The falling interstitial hydrostatic pressure and the rising interstitial oncotic pressure allow protein to mobilize from the interstitium and invade the vascular space. In addition, the elevated interstitial oncotic pressure facilitates movement of fluid from intracellular sites to interstitial lodgings.[28] The end result is continued restitution of volume losses. Albumin synthesis has been reported to increase by 12% to 75% after hemorrhage.[29] However, the magnitude of protein returned to the vascular bed shortly after the onset of hemorrhage indicates that the source of albumin is more likely to be preformed albumin mobilized from the interstitium rather than newly formed albumin.

In moderate hypovolemic shock, cardiac output and arterial pressure fall significantly, and blood volume is reduced by 15% to 20%. There is intense arteriolar vasoconstriction and diminished blood flow to the liver, pancreas, kidneys, and gastrointestinal tract. In this stage there is also a general venoconstriction which assists in increasing venous return to the general circulation. The intense adrenergic discharge that occurs causes tachycardia, tachypnea, cutaneous vasoconstriction, pallor, diaphoresis, piloerection, apprehension, and restlessness. Synthesis of replacement blood components occurs but cannot keep pace with massive losses. Platelets and poly-

morphonuclear leukocytes are the elements most quickly mobilized. Plasma proteins are restored at various rates, and red cells take the longest to form.

In severe hypovolemic shock, the blood volume deficit exceeds 25%, and small additional losses create major falls in cardiac output, blood pressure, and tissue perfusion. At this point, all the compensatory mechanisms are functioning at maximum capacity, and even the brain and the myocardium now are subject to a fall in perfusion. The patient becomes confused, anxious, agitated, obtunded, and comatose. Metabolic alterations now become very evident. Hyperglycemia develops as glucose is mobilized. Lipids are also mobilized, and lactate levels rise. Severe lactic acidosis and oliguria develop, and mixed venous oxygen tension is low.

At this point, the precapillary sphincters may lose their spasm while the postcapillary sphincters remain constricted. This allows capillary hydrostatic pressure to elevate and facilitates loss of volume and protein into the interstitial spaces. If the shock state persists, cellular death from severe organ vasoconstriction occurs.

The goal of therapy in hypovolemic shock is to restore adequate intravascular volume as quickly as possible. This can be accomplished most readily by the infusion of replacement solutions and by the use of external devices. These therapies are discussed in detail in a later section.

Cardiogenic Shock

Cardiogenic shock occurs when the myocardium cannot function as a pump to maintain adequate tissue perfusion. The direct cause is a severe impairment of ventricular pumping function. However, other mechanisms such as hypovolemia and vasomotor, metabolic, or microcirculatory dysfunction may contribute to progressive cardiovascular deterioration. The highest incidence of cardiogenic shock occurs in patients who have atherosclerotic heart disease in which either a massive singular myocardial infarction or multiple small myocardial infarctions have destroyed 40% to 50% of the left ventricular myocardium. Cardiogenic shock may also develop if the infarction creates mechanical problems such as mitral regurgitation from a papillary muscle rupture or if a ventricular septal defect due to an intraventricular septal infarction is created. Additionally, patients with end-stage cardiomyopathies may also develop cardiogenic shock.

A transient cardiogenic shock sometimes develops after cardiac surgery in which the myocardium is depressed following hypothermia, cardioplegic arrest, and surgical incisions. And lastly, dysrhythmias can

Etiologies of Cardiogenic Shock

Acute myocardial infarction
    Loss of 40% to 50% of critical myocardial mass
    Mechanical complications
    Perforated intraventricular septum
    Papillary muscle rupture or dysfunction
    Cardiac rupture
    Ventricular aneurysm
Cardiomyopathies (end-stage)
    Congestive
        Alcoholic, hypertensive, ischemic, myocarditis,
          amyloid, idiopathic
    Hypertrophic
    Restrictive
Valvular heart disease
    Severe valvular stenosis
    Acute valvular regurgitation
Postoperative low cardiac output syndrome
Dysrhythmias

be responsible for this shock state. A listing of etiologies of cardiogenic shock is given in the box above. Regardless of the etiology, the end result is a cardiac output insufficient to meet tissue needs. As already explained, the initial problem is an impairment of ventricular pumping action. This creates a reduction in stroke volume and cardiac output. If this fall in cardiac output is not compensated by an increase in vascular resistance, the mean arterial pressure will fall. This will further compromise the ventricle since coronary artery blood flow is in part determined by aortic pressure. A fall in aortic root diastolic pressure will lead to a fall in coronary artery blood flow. If the compensatory mechanisms are working, the systemic vascular resistance will rise in an attempt to maintain mean arterial pressure. Concurrently, the sympathetic nervous system activates the release of catecholamines. This release may have a detrimental effect as well. It increases the afterload or the resistance against which the ventricle must contract to eject volume. In addition, the sympathetic drive increases ventricular contractility, which might also potentiate myocardial ischemia and, hence, failure.

The left ventricular end-diastolic volume and pressure continue to rise so long as the ventricle fails to eject adequate volumes. This increase leads to distention of the ventricular cavity, which further increases afterload and also can limit filling of endocardial coronary arteries, thereby creating endocardial ischemia. The elevated left ventricular end-diastolic pressure is passively transmitted to the pulmonary veins and the

pulmonary bed. The resultant increase in pulmonary venous pressure can lead to the development of pulmonary edema. Arterial hypoxemia is related to this pulmonary venous congestion, and hypoxia and concurrent acidosis lead to an elevated pulmonary artery pressure. Right ventricular failure can also develop. Additionally, a right ventricular infarction can occur isolated from this left ventricular event if right ventricular coronary artery disease is present.

Although the hypovolemic patient is best described in phases, hemodynamic subset classifications are most commonly used to describe a patient's progressing into or recovering from cardiogenic shock. Figure 7-10 depicts a hemodynamic subset classification in which the cardiac index is compared to the pulmonary capillary wedge pressure (PCWP). Patients in class A have a cardiac index greater than 2.2 L/min/m^2 and normal to low pulmonary capillary wedge pressures. This class is generally reflective of patients who have experienced small myocardial infarcts. Mortality in this group is generally 10%. Class B is characterized by patients with a cardiac index lower than 2.2 L/min/m^2 and pulmonary capillary wedge pressures lower than 18 mmHg. This class represents patients who are relatively hypovolemic. Mortality in this group is usually 30% to 50%. In class C, cardiac indexes are greater than 2.2 L/min/m^2, and the wedge pressures are elevated. This group is generally hypervolemic and also experiences a mortality of 30% to 50%. Finally, class D patients present with a cardiac index lower than 2.2 L/min/m^2 and elevated filling pressures. Mortality in this group can be as high as 90% as the patient moves to the lower right portion of that class. The majority of patients with cardiogenic shock can be categorized as class D.

The generally agreed-upon index for cardiogenic shock is a cardiac index of less than 1.8 L/min/m^2 in a patient with adequate volume load. Therefore, if the cardiac index is less than 1.8 and the PCWP is less than 18 mmHg, the etiology of the shock state is perhaps more hypovolemic than cardiogenic. Using this method of classification as a background, therapeutic modalities for the cardiogenic shock patient

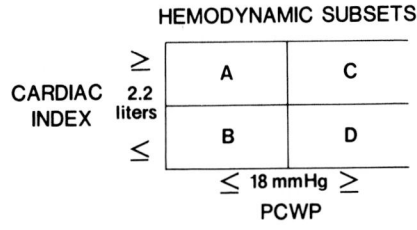

Figure 7-10 Hemodynamic subset classification.

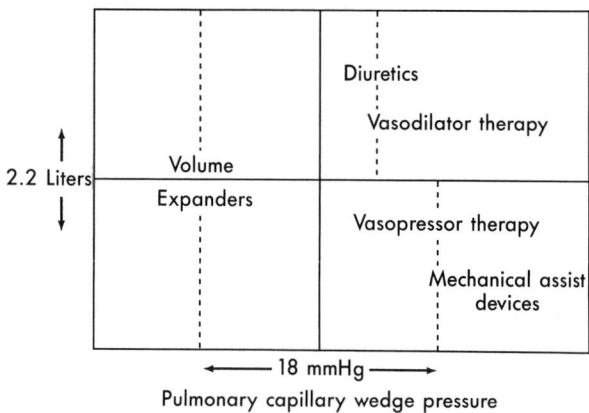

Figure 7-11 Treatment modalities commonly associated with the hemodynamic subset classifications.

can be sequentially delineated for the classes (Figure 7-11). Specific therapies are discussed later in this chapter.

Obstructive Shock

Obstructive shock develops when there is a physical obstruction to flow somewhere in the circulatory system. This can develop with pulmonary embolisms, dissecting aortic aneurysms, pericardial tamponade, atrial myxoma, tension pneumothorax, or a ruptured hemidiaphragm with evisceration of abdominal contents into the thoracic cavity. These events impair venous return because of the high pressures surrounding the right atrium. With tension pneumothorax and a ruptured hemidiaphragm, venous return is impaired because the great veins are compressed as they enter the chest. Clinically, with the exception of the distended neck veins, these patients resemble those in hypovolemic shock. Ultimate treatments for these patients are largely surgical.

Distributive Shock

The term *distributive shock* refers to states in which there is an abnormal distribution of the intravascular volume. Septic, anaphylactic, and neurogenic shock all fall in this classification. In septic shock, the abnormal distribution of intravascular volume is due to the massive vasodilation related to the response to microorganisms and their by-products. Before describing the specific pathophysiological changes associated with septic shock, it is helpful to view septic shock from the perspective of a clinical continuum which gradually progresses through the stages of septicemia: preshock, hyperdynamic shock, hypodynamic shock, and multiple system organ failure.[31] The progression through these phases depends on the types and number of organisms, the treatment-related factors to which the host is exposed, and the risk factors inherent in the host.[31,32]

Inherent risk factors for sepsis within the host include chronic diseases such as cardiac, pulmonary, renal, or hepatic disease; immune disorders; diabetes mellitus or alcoholism; malnutrition; debilitation; pregnancy; or extremes of age. Inadequate myocardial, respiratory, endocrine, immune, or renal function limits the host's ability to cope with the numerous stresses associated with septic shock. In hepatic disease, the ability of the host's Kupffer cells to phagocytize bacteria is altered. This factor is also present in hosts with a history of alcoholism. In addition, these patients are also generally malnourished. The risk of a ruptured ectopic pregnancy or an incomplete septic abortion serves to make pregnancy a risk factor. Age extremes—hosts under the age of 1 and over 65 years of age—are also placed at high risk due to developmental changes in immune systems.

Treatment-related factors associated with a high risk of septic shock are also quite numerous. Invasive devices such as intravascular or intracavity catheters or drains serve as ideal portals for microorganisms to gain access to a host. Some surgical procedures, such as genitourinary procedures, place the host at a higher risk because they may introduce microorganisms. Also, in recent years immunosuppression has developed into a significant risk factor. Use of irradiation or cytotoxic drug therapy for neoplastic disease and the growing use of immunosuppressive agents in transplant patient populations have generated a whole new group of patients whose immune systems have been iatrogenically suppressed. These hosts are susceptible not only to typically virulent bacteria but also to many normal flora. Finally, widespread use of antibiotics has led to the development of multiresistant organisms, organisms resistant to currently available antibiotics. The major causative organisms in septic shock are gram-negative bacteria, which are responsible for two thirds of all cases of septic shock.[33] Additionally, gram-positive bacteria, viruses, fungi, and rickettsiae are also causative agents.

When bacteria invade an organism and die, they release substances embedded in their walls. These substances have varying deleterious effects on specific tissues and organs. Gram-positive bacteria release substances known as exotoxins which have minimal effects on tissues. Gram-negative bacteria, on the other hand, release substances known as endotoxins. Septic shock resulting from gram-negative organisms is also known as endotoxic shock. Endotoxins are lipopolysaccharides embedded in the cell walls of gram-negative bacteria. When released in the circulation, they can activate numerous protein systems and other chemical mediators that can create major deleterious effects.[34]

The specific protein systems that are activated are the complement, clotting, kinin, and renin–angiotensin systems. The specific initiators of these systems are not known yet. However, the microorganism itself, certain immune cells, or a leukocyte endogenous mediator (LEM) which is released after phagocytosis of the organism have all been considered initiators. Under normal situations the complement system, a system of nine different enzyme precursors, attacks invading agents and initiates local tissue reactions that protect against damage by the microorganism. Although the complement system is usually a protective mechanism, its effects are so systemic and widespread that major problems develop in septic shock. Specifically, activation of complement increases release of C5a and C3a, proteins known as anaphylatoxins. C5a enhances neutrophil aggregation. This aggregation can lead to microembolization and ultimately to tissue ischemia. Additionally, as neutrophils aggregate they can cause endothelial cell damage that can lead to peripheral vascular insufficiency. Activation of complement also leads to increased production of platelets, leukocytes, and mast cells, thereby stimulating the release of histamine, prostaglandins, bradykinin, and serotonin, all vasoactive mediators. Again, under normal circumstances and on small levels, these substances cause a beneficial vasodilation and increased capillary permeability. This vasodilation increases blood flow to locally damaged tissue and assists in fighting the infection. The increased capillary permeability allows the area to wall itself off from the rest of the tissue so that microorganisms do not travel as far.[20] In sepsis, however, this process is occurring throughout the body, and massive vasodilation and widespread capillary permeability can be disastrous. The last sequela of complement system activation is myocardial depression, which is largely seen in the hypodynamic stage of septic shock.

The clotting system is also activated by endotoxin, which stimulates Hageman factor (factor XII). This initiates the development of multiple fibrin clots, which impair blood flow and consequently perfusion. This inappropriate clotting and resultant consumption of clotting factors can cause disseminated intravascular coagulation (DIC) (Chapter 42). Factor XII also stimulates the conversion of inactive kinins to active kinins, specifically bradykinin and serotonin, which are potent vasodilators that can also tremendously alter capillary permeability.

The production of renin and consequently angiotensin is mediated by microorganisms. Activation of the renin–angiotensin system creates the release of epinephrine, norephinephrine, and aldosterone; con-sequently, sympathetic drive is increased, myocardial contractility improved, and sodium and water retained.

Other chemical mediators that are activated by various stimuli include histamine, prostaglandins, leukotrienes, tumor necrosis factor (TNF), myocardial depressant factor (MDF), and leukocyte endogenous mediator (LEM).[35,36,37] Histamine, released by the mast cells, causes capillary permeability, vasodilation, and myocardial depression. The prostaglandin thromboxane A_2, produced by platelets, is a potent platelet aggregator. Prostaglandin E_2 is also released in septic shock and is associated with pulmonary vasoconstriction in animals in septic shock.[34] 2-Prostacyclin (PGI_2), another prostaglandin, decreases in septic shock. A lack of PGI_2 leads to thrombogenesis and peripheral vascular insufficiency since its normal role is as a vasodilator and an antiplatelet aggregator. Leukotrienes increase vascular permeability, edema, and bronchoconstriction and also assist in neutrophil aggregation. Tumor necrosis factor (TNF) is released from macrophages; it modulates and amplifies immune responses to infection. In animals, myocardial depressant factor (MDF) is released from the pancreas after periods of hypoperfusion. More recently, a correlation between the presence of a circulation MDF and a decrease in ejection fraction in a group of patients with septic shock has been found.[38] In addition to depressing cardiac function, MDF also inhibits phagocytosis and causes splanchnic vasoconstriction.[39] Studies have also indicated that depressed myocardial function may be partially attributed to an attenuation of calcium sequestration in the sarcoplasmic reticulum; this could reduce the efficiency of the excitation–contraction coupling mechanism.[40]

The last chain of events activated by microorganisms is the leukocyte endogenous mediator system. In conjunction with endogenous pyrogen and lymphocyte activating factor, LEM creates endorphin release; an increase in protein catabolism of skeletal muscle; glucagon and insulin release from the pancreas; an alteration in heat regulation by the hypothalamus; an increase in amino acid uptake; hepatic synthesis of acute phase reactants such as the alpha and beta globulins, fibrinogen, and polysaccharides; and increased release of neutrophils from the bone marrow. Also, endorphins are believed to induce hypotension and myocardial depression in septic shock and hemorrhagic shock.

As indicated earlier, the stages of septic shock include septicemia, preshock, hyperdynamic and hypodynamic shock, and multisystem organ failure. In the first stage, septicemia, the host reactions and system changes already described are initiated. The sympathetic nervous system is activated, and the patient experiences tachycardia, an increased cardiac output, and an increased respiratory rate. In the preshock phase, the patient's systemic vascular resistance is decreased, the cardiac index is increased, and the mean arterial pressure remains nearly normal. As the patient proceeds to the next stage, a hypotensive event is triggered by a fall in the cardiac index to normal values and a decrease in systemic vascular resistance. The myocardium fails to compensate for the fall in systemic vascular resistance. After that, a return of the cardiac index to higher levels and significant increases in systemic vascular resistance achieve only minor arterial pressure elevations.[41] This hypotensive event initiates the hyperdynamic stage consisting of significant peripheral vasodilation, a low systemic vascular resistance, and increased or normal cardiac output/cardiac index and hypotension. The next phase is the hypodynamic phase in which the cardiac output and index are very low, the systemic vascular resistance is elevated, and there is inadequate tissue perfusion and profound hypotension. The contractility of the myocardium is directly affected further by MDF, hypoxemia, acidosis, and endotoxins, leading to an even greater fall in cardiac output. The sympathetic nervous system activates, and tremendous vasoconstriction develops in an attempt to maintain perfusion. However, tissue ischemia increases. Vasoconstriction coupled with the previous and concurrent vasodilation create a capillary environment where there is slow, sluggish flow and inadequate oxygenation. Sludging of blood in such an environment is conducive to microemboli formation and clotting malfunctions, and thus DIC.

The patient gradually slips into the next and last stage, multisystem organ failure. Mizock[32] details three phases to this stage. In phase one, the patient experiences septicemia, respiratory failure, and hypoxemia. Hepatic dysfunction begins to manifest itself in phase two, and the patient experiences a reduced serum albumin and is jaundiced. Mizock also states that coma, anemia, stress ulcers, inadequate wound healing, and anergy to skin test antigens are present. Finally, in phase three, the patient proceeds to biventricular failure, pulmonary edema, atelectasis, and pneumonia. If treatment is not successful, the patient then finally expires with coagulopathy, refractory hypotension, and asystole. Treatments for septic shock can include volume replacement, pharmacological therapy, and mechanical assistance (Chapter 56).

Neurogenic shock is also a form of distributive shock. As with septic shock, the physiological change is related to abnormal distribution of volume due to vasodilation. The major cause of neurogenic shock is loss of vasomotor tone. This can develop after deep general anesthesia or spinal anesthesia, especially when spinal anesthesia extends up the spinal column. Damage to the basal regions of the brain or prolonged medullary ischemia can also cause vasomotor collapse.

In *anaphylactic shock*, another type of distributive shock, an antigen–antibody reaction is the initiating event. This reaction can cause direct damage to the adjacent vascular walls and also cause cells throughout the body to release histamine and histamine-like substances. This results in tremendous vasodilation with resultant hypotension and increased capillary permeability with loss of fluid into the interstitial space (Chapter 45).

DATA ACQUISITION

As was stated in the beginning of this chapter, it is the critical care nurse's responsibility to constantly assess and identify the subtle and blatant findings and parameter changes indicative of inadequate tissue perfusion. Both subjective and objective data should be gathered and analyzed. Some findings will be consistently present regardless of the etiology of inadequate perfusion. However, in some instances assessment parameters are quite helpful in establishing a diagnosis, as their values vary depending on the etiology of inadequate perfusion. The following section describes such assessment parameters, and Table 7-1 summarizes assessment findings that can vary with different etiologies and stages of shock.

Subjective Data

In the early stages of shock the patient may be adequately alert and awake to report various symptoms which are significant. *Thirst*, a conscious desire for water, is a common complaint in both hypovolemic and cardiogenic shock. In hypovolemic patients, thirst is usually expressed when there has been a 10% loss of blood volume. Patients with a low cardiac output from congestive heart failure also develop an intense thirst. It is theorized that this thirst is created by the presence of excessive amounts of angiotensin II which stimulates a neural center under the third ventricle of the brain.[20]

Nausea, the conscious recognition of a subconscious excitation of the medulla close to the vomiting center, is another subjective symptom. Sequestering of fluid in the gastrointestinal tract as is seen in some types of hypovolemic and cardiogenic shock can cause an irritative impulse to be transmitted to the medulla. *Apprehension, anxiety,* and *fear* are also described by patients in early shock stages and are related to elevated serum levels of catecholamines and to hypoxemia. Initial peripheral vasoconstriction will also lead to subjective symptoms of being *cold*. Finally, *syncope*

TABLE 7-1 Assessment Parameters for Selected Stages and Types of Shock

	Cardiogenic		Hypovolemic		Distributive		Obstructive	
SUBJECTIVE								
Thirst	↑		↑					
Nausea	↑		↑					
Anxiety	↑		↑		↑		↑	
OBJECTIVE								
Heart rate	↑/↑	↑↓	↑	↑	↑	↑↓	↑	↑
Dysrhythmias	↑↑	↑↑↑		↑	—	↑↑	—	↑
Temperature								
Core	↑	↑	—	—	↑↑↑	↑↑	—	—
Skin	↓	↓	—	↑	↑	↓	—	↓
BLOOD PRESSURE								
Mean arterial pressure	—	↓	—	↓	↑/—	↓	—	↓
Pulse pressure	↓	—	↓	—	—	↓	↓	↓
Diastolic	—	↓	—	↓	↓	↓/—	—	↓
Systolic	↓	↓	↓	↓	↓	↓	↓	↓
HEMODYNAMIC PARAMETERS								
Right atrial pressure	↓/—	↑↑	↓	↓↓	↓	↑	↑	↑↑
PAP	↑	↑↑	↓	↑↑	↓	↑	↑/—	↑/—
PCWP	↑	↑↑	↓	↑↑	↓	↑↑↓	↓	↓
SVR	↑	↑↑↑	—	↑↑↑	↓↓	↑↑↑	—	↓↓↓
CO/CI	↓	↑↑↑	↓	↑↑↑	↑↑	↓↓↓	↓	↓↓↓
S̄vo₂	↓	↓↓↓	—	↓↓	↑/—	↓↓↓	—/↓	↓
RESPIRATORY PARAMETERS								
Tachypnea	↓	↑↑	↑	↑	↑	↑↑	↑	↑
Rales/rhonchi	↑	↑↑	—	—	↑	↑↑	↑/—	↑/—
Chest x-ray changes	↑	↑↑	—	—	↑	↑↑	↑/—	↑/—
ACID–BASE FINDINGS								
Respiratory alkalosis	↑		↑		↑		↑	
Metabolic acidosis		↑		↑		↑↑		↑
	DECOMPENSATED	COMPENSATED	LATE	EARLY	DECOMPENSATED	COMPENSATED	DECOMPENSATED	COMPENSATED

upon changing positions, particularly from supine to upright positions, may be a reflection of a hypovolemic state.

Objective Data

Heart Rate

Generally, patients will experience a sinus tachycardia of 110 to 120 beats per minute or as high as 200 beats per minute as the myocardium attempts to compensate for the low cardiac output through a rate increase. One exception to this may occur in patients with cardiogenic shock secondary to an infarct of the inferior or posterior myocardial wall. In this situation, ischemic stimulation of cholinergic ganglia at the posterior margin of the AV node may reflexively produce sinus bradycardia or heart block. Excessively high heart rates (greater than 150 beats per minute) can lead to a fall in cardiac output and a higher incidence of ischemic dysrhythmias. Dysrhythmias, such as conduction defects or supraventricular or ventricular dysrhythmias, are most commonly seen in patients experiencing cardiogenic shock; however, in the presence of severe acidosis or hypoxia, premature ventricular contractions (PVC) may be commonplace. Additionally, the release of histamine in septic shock has been demonstrated to cause AV conduction abnormalities and ventricular dysrhythmias.[42] S₃ and/or S₄ heart sounds will develop as the myocardium itself fails. This occurs most frequently in cardiogenic shock but can also develop in the end stages of distributive shock. In cardiogenic shock, cardiac murmurs such as the holosystolic murmur of a ventricular septal defect or mitral regurgitation may develop in the presence of these structural abnormalities. A transient functional mitral regurgitant murmur can similarly develop with excessive volume loading.

Ischemic changes on the electrocardiogram can occur, particularly in patients with underlying coronary artery disease. However, ST segment elevations and subendocardial ischemic changes have been documented in patients without ischemic heart disease during both septic and hemorrhagic shock. These were presumably caused by severe anemia or by a decrease in coronary perfusion pressure.[43]

Severe muscle weakness and fatigue are two of the earliest symptoms of shock. These result from the decreased supply of nutrients to the muscles and are evidenced when the patient attempts any activity from ambulation to breathing.

Skin Color and Temperature

Because of the extensive vasoconstriction associated with inadequate perfusion, the patient's skin color is generally pale, except in the hyperdynamic septic state, in which it is generally reddened and moist. As perfusion becomes tremendously compromised, mottling and cyanosis develop. Piloerection (goose bumps) occurs as a means of reducing loss of body heat. The skin is cool to the touch.

The measurement of the temperature gradient between the ventral surface of the great toe and ambient room temperature has demonstrated that parameter to be a good predictor of survival in patients in hypovolemic, septic, and cardiogenic shock. Specifically, studies demonstrate that patients who survived circulatory shock had increases in the toe minus ambient room temperature gradient of more than 4° C. Patients with a gradient less than 3° C for a 12-hour period generally died of their low-flow state. Monitoring the toe temperature and toe gradient difference to room air can help in quantifying the subjective assessment of skin temperature, and also in assessing the value of the therapeutic actions undertaken.[44]

Rectal, oral, and core temperatures are generally within normal limits or are slightly below normal because of metabolic slowing and initial vasodilation. The body therefore tends to cool especially if the skin is exposed. Exceptions to this occur in sepsis where, particularly with gram-negative endotoxin release, the hypothalamus is stimulated and temperatures can rise to the levels of 38.3° to 40.5° C (101° to 105° F). Slight temperature elevations can develop in cardiogenic shock. This is a consequence of the tissue damage associated with myocardial infarction. Mild hypothermia may develop in some cases of distributive shock, particularly in the presence of gram-positive organisms.

Blood Pressure

Monitoring blood pressures in these patients is a critical activity. Cuff blood pressures are generally inadequate due to the severe vasoconstriction and low stroke volumes these patients generate. For these reasons, the Korotkoff sounds are barely audible and difficult to discern. Cuff blood pressures can underestimate the true arterial pressure by an average of 15 mmHg and occasionally by as much as 100 mmHg. Therefore, intraarterial pressure monitoring is required.

Three components of the arterial pressure should be monitored and evaluated: the pulse pressure, the diastolic pressure, and the systolic pressure. The pulse pressure is the difference between the systolic and diastolic pressures and primarily reflects the stroke volume and resistance to blood flow in the aorta and its major branches. Changes in the pulse pressure reflect stroke volume changes. For example, if a blood pressure changes from 100/60 to 90/70, and thus the pulse pressure falls from 40 to 20 mmHg, the stroke volume will be decreased by 50%.[4] Diastolic pressure is most reflective of the amount of vasoconstriction present, particularly in the arterioles. And, finally, systolic pressure is determined by these other two pressures. In all cases of shock, the mean arterial pressure falls either slowly or precipitously. However, the pattern of alterations viewed in these other three components varies according to the etiology of the inadequate perfusion state.

In the compensated stages of cardiogenic or hypovolemic shock the systolic pressure may fall slightly, but the diastolic pressure will remain constant or will perhaps increase owing to vasoconstriction. This allows the pulse pressure to narrow, and this may be the first significant change that occurs in the blood pressure measurement. As the patient moves into the decompensated stage, both systolic and diastolic pressures will fall, and the pulse pressure will then remain constant. In distributive shock another pattern develops. With vasodilation, both systolic and diastolic pressures fall, and thus the pulse pressure remains constant. During late stages when vasoconstriction develops, the diastolic pressure is affected slightly and may remain constant or slow its decline. This then allows the pulse pressure to narrow slightly.

Hemodynamic Parameters

Monitoring of hemodynamic parameters is essential for the accurate diagnosis and treatment of shock states. Commonly monitored parameters include the central venous pressure (CVP), the pulmonary artery pressure (PAP), the pulmonary capillary wedge pressure (PCWP), and mixed venous oxygen saturation ($S\bar{v}O_2$). Normal values for these parameters are as follows:

CVP	3-11 mmHg
PAP	
Pulmonary artery systolic pressure (PAS)	20-30 mmHg
Pulmonary artery diastolic pressure (PAD)	10-15 mmHg
Pulmonary artery mean pressure (PAM)	10-20 mmHg
PCWP	4-12 mmHg
$S\bar{v}O_2$	60% to 80%

In addition, derived parameters such as the systemic vascular resistance (SVR), the pulmonary vascular resistance (PVR), and the cardiac index (CI) are also monitored. Normal values for these parameters are as follows:

SVR	800-1,300 $dyn/sec/cm^{-5}$
PVR	80-240 $dyn/sec/cm^{-5}$
CO	5-8 L/min
CI	2.5-3.5 $L/min/m^2$

In cardiogenic shock, the majority of the hemodynamic alterations are manifested by the parameters that reflect the function of the left ventricle. Specifically, the PCWP becomes elevated as the left ventricle loses its contractility and blood sequesters in the left ventricle and left atrium, then passively fills the pulmonary tree. Since most infarctions involve the left ventricle as opposed to the right ventricle, the CVP, the main indicator of right heart function, is not affected. If, however, right heart failure or biventricular failure develops, then the CVP becomes elevated. Pulmonary artery systolic and diastolic pressures generally remain in their normal ranges. Cardiac output/cardiac index is diminished, and SVR is elevated due to the sympathetic drive which develops. PVR is generally unaffected until significant pulmonary changes develop, and $S\bar{v}O_2$ is low as oxygen delivery falls in the tissues.

In hypovolemic shock, all parameters are diminished. The CVP is low because of inadequate filling of the right heart. Additionally, the PCWP and PAP pressures are low because of inadequate volume. The cardiac output and cardiac index are within lower than normal ranges, the SVR remains normal or slightly elevated owing to vasconstriction, and the $S\bar{v}O_2$ is low.

With distributive shock several changes develop. In the hyperdynamic state, since the patient is experiencing vasodilation and fluid is sequestering peripherally, the filling pressures are initially low. The SVR is low also because of the massive vasodilation the patient experiences. Cardiac output is exceptionally elevated, perhaps as a compensatory response to deliver blood to a peripheral bed where there is diffuse shunting. Consequently, the $S\bar{v}O_2$ is also elevated as unused oxygen is returned in the venous system. As hypodynamic shock develops, the cardiac output and index fall, and the SVR rises as the patient vessels constrict. The right and left heart filling pressures now rise as the vascular bed constricts and the myocardium fails. With obstructive shock, the cardiac output is low since blood cannot pass easily into the left heart because the pulmonary bed or the right-sided inflow tracts are obstructed. The CVP is elevated by this obstruction while the PCWP is normal or in lower ranges.

Respiratory Changes

As with other organ systems, the rate and intensity of respiratory changes a patient experiences in a shock state vary with the severity of that state. For example, in cardiogenic shock following a massive myocardial infarction the respiratory alterations that develop are rapid and acute. In slowly evolving poor perfusion states the symptoms also evolve slowly. Earlier, the physiological changes associated with interstitial and alveolar pulmonary edema were described. Generally, it is these two types of pulmonary problems that the patient in cardiogenic shock develops. With interstitial edema the patient develops dyspnea and tachypnea. The tidal volume remains the same, but the minute ventilation increases. Slight wheezing may develop, and fine to moderate moist rales or crackles can be auscultated. The chest film generally demonstrates some lymphatic enlargement, and Kerley B lines are present. Arterial blood gas assays generally exhibit slight alkalosis and slight arterial hypoxemia.

The foregoing symptoms reflect the accumulation of fluid in the interstitial spaces between the alveoli and therefore are not dramatic clinically. However, once alveolar edema develops, dramatic signs and symptoms appear. Severe dyspnea develops as the fluid in the alveoli inhibits gas exchange. Intubation and mechanical ventilation are generally required at this point. Coarse gurgles and wheezing are heard throughout the chest. The chest x-ray is characterized by diffuse haziness. Blood-tinged sputum is present. This sputum has a low protein content, specifically, less than 60% of the plasma protein concentration. This last finding can be important when a differential diagnosis between hydrostatic edema and permeability edema is necessary. In permeability edema the ratio is greater than 60%; that is, pulmonary secretions approach serum plasma composition. Therefore, a permeability leak must be present in the alveoli to allow this admixture. In alveolar edema, the alveolus is intact and there is no sieving of protein into the sputum.[45,46]

In distributive shock, particularly the septic type, in which the initiating problem is not volume but rather toxic substances, the clinical picture of permeability edema is more likely to arise. With this entity, tachypnea and increased minute ventilation develop. Sequestering of fluids in the interstitium and alveoli is generally not present so that rales and rhonchi may or may not be significant. However, as capillary endothelial and alveolar epithelial cells are damaged, hypoxemia develops rapidly, and mechanical assistance is required. Refractory hypoxemia is frequently present with ARDS. This term refers to the inability to improve arterial oxygenation despite increases in the percentage of delivered inspired oxygen. Lung compliance is decreased as evidenced by increases in plateau inspiratory pressures via the mechanical ventilation circuit. Chest x-ray findings demonstrate diffuse haziness, and the cardiac silhouette is normal. The plasma protein content, as mentioned earlier, is usually greater than 60%.

Physical respiratory findings in hypovolemic and obstructive shock are generally nonspecific since the pulmonary bed is not generally a major focus in their etiologies.

Arterial Blood Gases and Acid–Base Changes

Because of the previously mentioned hyperventilation, blood gas measurements obtained in early stages of shock generally reflect adequate arterial oxygenation and a respiratory alkalosis. As the shock progresses, a slight to moderate arterial hypoxemia develops as oxygen delivery begins to fall. The exception to this occurs in hypovolemic shock; the arterial oxygenation may remain within the normal limits because of a decreased amount of blood in the lung. In this case the ventilation/perfusion ratio increases, and thus better pulmonary compliance and function are present.

As lactate and hydrogen ions accumulate in shock, a metabolic acidosis develops. This causes the patient to hyperventilate further as a compensatory measure. If the $PaCO_2$ is driven below 25 mmHg this severe hypocapnea may itself cause hemodynamic impairment.

Metabolic alkalosis generally does not occur in patients in shock. However, on occasion it may develop in patients receiving high doses of antacids or in those undergoing removal of large quantities of gastric secretions. When metabolic alkalosis is present the degree of metabolic acidosis present is masked and underappreciated. This may later prove problem-

atic as the severe acidosis may become almost refractory to treatment.

If the shock state is not improved the metabolic acidosis will increase. Additionally, a respiratory acidosis will develop as the patient gradually loses the ability to excrete carbon dioxide as the number of functional pulmonary capillaries decreases. Gradually the $PaCO_2$ rises and reaches levels above normal. In the final stages of shock the blood gases demonstrate a combined metabolic and respiratory acidosis with an elevated $PaCO_2$, a low bicarbonate, and a very low pH.[41]

Hematological Parameters

Thrombocytopenia (platelet levels less than 150,000-250,000/ml) can develop in septic shock as platelets sequester in the capillary and pulmonary beds. Early in sepsis, leukopenia (WBC levels less than 5,000/ml) may be present due to white blood cell aggregation. This is generally followed by leukocytosis as a WBC response is elicited by the septic focus. Additionally, as disseminated intravascular coagulation evolves coagulation abnormalities develop. Fibrin degradation products (FDPs) and prothrombin times increase as clotting factors are consumed and fibrinogen levels fall as a result of clotting in the capillaries.

Measurement of arterial lactate levels has recently become a common practice in caring for shock patients. An indicator of anaerobic metabolism, lactate levels greater than 2 mmol/L indicate a shock state. Increases in lactate levels from 2 to 8 mmol/L are associated with a decrease in survival from 90% to 10%. Monitoring the trends of this level, however, is more beneficial than following isolated values.[47,48] Falling lactate values indicate an improvement in perfusion. Serum glucose levels also fluctuate in sepsis with hyperglycemia developing early in sepsis and hypoglycemia occurring when glucose stores become incapable of meeting metabolic demands.

Urine Output and Composition

Within the context of shock states the renal system is not viewed as a vital organ but as a peripheral organ. Therefore, regardless of the type of shock, the kidney is immediately affected by hypoperfusion and provides signs and symptoms of severity of the hypoperfusion. Generally there is a good correlation between the amount of renal blood flow and the amount of urine output. Since renal blood flow depends on cardiac output, any alterations in cardiac output greatly influence urinary output. Therefore, if cardiac output falls precipitously, there is a concurrent precipitous fall in urine output. With a moderate or gradual fall in cardiac output the composition of the urine output may change prior to changes in urinary volume, and alterations in certain serum and urine laboratory values will occur. With a moderate fall in cardiac output the renal arterioles constrict and blood flow is shunted from the cortical nephrons of the kidney to the juxtaglomerular nephrons. In addition, the renin–angiotensin–aldosterone system discussed earlier is activated. This system also allows the body to conserve sodium.

The end result of these effects is sodium retention assisting in volume conservation, a mechanism by which the body increases its currently low cardiac output. Consequently, the volume of urine produced may fall slightly and its composition will change. In relation to the volume, the kidney will still produce volumes greater than 400 ml a day. Volumes less than this amount or less than 0.5 ml per kilogram per hour are generally considered oliguric levels. However, the urine composition will be low in sodium, generally less than 20 mmol/L. Additionally, the specific gravity will be greater than 1.015 and the urine/serum osmolality ratio will be greater than 1.5.

All these values indicate that the nephrons are still functional and are trying to compensate for the inadequate perfusion. Serum levels of urea nitrogen rise during this stage owing its back diffusion across the nephron; however, serum creatinine levels remain within normal ranges since the nephron still remains capable of clearing this metabolic end product. The end result is a blood urea nitrogen/creatinine ratio of greater than 10:1. This state is generally referred to as a prerenal state or a prerenal failure state.

As the fall in perfusion to the kidney persists, and the renal parenchyma itself becomes damaged, acute tubular necrosis ensues. In this state, urine output falls to anuric levels. Because the nephron can no longer continue with its functions, urine sodium levels rise to levels greater than 30 mmol/L as sodium traverses the nephron untouched, and specific gravities fall to levels equal to 1.010. This latter value reflects the kidney's inability to concentrate urine. Additionally, the urine/serum osmolality ratio approaches a level less than 1:5. Blood urea nitrogen (BUN) and creatinine ratios remain in a 10:1 ratio since urea nitrogen continues to be reabsorbed and creatinine is no longer cleared.[4,49]

Consciousness Level

The patient's level of consciousness can range from mildly confused to comatose. Initially, anxious behavior may be present due to slight hypoxemia and the catecholamine drive the patient experiences. Gradually, as cardiac output and cerebral perfusion fall, lethargy and confusion develop. With severe hypoperfusion and metabolic alterations, unresponsiveness and coma develop.

Gastrointestinal Findings

As cardiac output falls, blood flow is gradually shunted to areas of high priority and away from other organs. The gastrointestinal system falls into the category of non-highly prioritized systems and as such can become ischemic. The low flow leads initially to changes in gastrointestinal function consisting of hyperperistalsis followed by diminished motility. If alert, the patient may complain of nausea. Bowel sounds become hypoactive and the abdomen may become distended, particularly if third spacing is occurring in this area. Insertion of a nasogastric tube may be required to assist in the removal of gastric secretions that cannot move adequately through the intestinal system. Ulcerations may develop and Hematest-positive gastric contents may be present. If this inadequate perfusion persists, an ischemic gut can develop. This can further compound the shock state as fluid sequesters in the area and the metabolic acidosis worsens. Animal studies have demonstrated that enteral nutritional support can restore intestinal microvascular blood flow better than parenteral nutrition in sepsis. This enhanced blood flow may contribute to improved maintenance of mucosal integrity. Additional investigation is required before clinical application of this finding is implemented.[50]

MEDICAL MANAGEMENT
Position

In all types of shock positioning the patient to facilitate ventilation and to prevent skin breakdown is vital. Optimally, this involves having the patient sit in an upright position which allows the diaphragm to fall and the chest to expand maximally. In addition, frequent position changes to avoid pressure ulcers from developing would be desirable. However, most often the patient's tenuous hemodynamic status makes these positions unachievable, and the supine position with the head of the bed elevated 20° to 30° is perhaps the most optimal position the patient can tolerate. In this event, turning the patient from side to side is also desirable. If a full side-lying position cannot be achieved, even slight elevation of the shoulders or rotation of the hip with a single pillow will help improve local tissue perfusion. Heel and elbow protectors are also beneficial.

The idea of altering a patient's position to improve hemodynamic values remains controversial. Placing a patient in Trendelenburg's position with the legs elevated higher than the torso probably does little to improve cardiac output in the shock state. This elevation may increase pressure in the veins and venules but does so at the expense of the myocardium, which now experiences a greater afterload.[51] However, in a hypovolemic patient with a healthy myocardium, this maneuver may be transiently beneficial until volume replacement has been accomplished.

Positioning a patient in obstructive shock can be very critical. An atrial myxoma, for example, while partially attached to the atrial wall, may also have a mobile portion that can move to obstruct either the pulmonary veins or the mitral valve orifice. When this occurs, immediate cardiac decompensation follows. In this situation, the nurse at the bedside needs to be aware that this phenomenon can occur and then must decide which position provides the patient with the best hemodynamic response.

Pneumatic Antishock Garment (PASG)

The PASG suit is an inflatable trouser consisting of an abdominal compartment and two separate lower-extremity compartments. Each compartment has its own inflating and pressure-relief valve. The suit exerts titratable external pressure on the abdomen and lower extremities. The external counterpulsation created by inflation has several beneficial effects. The redistribution of venous blood flow from the abdomen and lower extremities to organs above the diaphragm creates an autotransfusion effect, and a redistribution of 750 to 1,000 ml can be appreciated. Autotransfusion is accompanied by an increase in central venous pressure and in both aortic and carotid flow and pressure with a concomitant decrease in femoral flow and pressure. Systemic vascular resistance, arterial blood pressure, and stroke volume are increased. However, cardiac output is unchanged because of a consequent decrease in heart rate. The bradycardia is a result of depressor reflex stimulation secondary to increased aorta and carotid sinus arterial pressures. Other concomitant physiological effects include an increased venous return to the lungs with a corresponding increase in pulmonary wedge pressure and also mild lactic acidosis related to a diminished lower-extremity blood flow. A decrease in respiratory excursion due to abdominal compression may also create acidosis.

Clinical indications for use of the PASG include hypovolemic and neurogenic shock, intraabdominal hemorrhage, hemorrhage of any portion of the body encircled by the device, and femoral and pelvic fracture splinting. Bleeding is decreased through an external tamponade effect from the direct pressure being exerted and through internal pressure. The external compression is transmitted to the internal vasculature with a resulting increase in intraperitoneal pressure.

Nursing care of the patient includes vigilance to hemodynamic changes related to volume needs and to the pressure readings of the suit compartments. The latter are assessed to ensure adequate suit inflation. As the suit may depress respiratory excursion, continued respiratory assessment, including monitoring of breathing patterns, arterial blood gases, tidal volume, and vital capacity, is essential. Pressure on the abdominal organs may cause emesis as well as defecation and/or urination, and therefore a nasogastric tube and Foley catheter should be in place.

Removal of the suit is determined by the attainment of a normovolemic and hemodynamic state. Deflation is achieved gradually, 5 mmHg at a time. Venous access must be maintained and on-site volume replacement must be available. A drop in systolic blood pressure automatically stops the deflation process until restoration of blood pressure is achieved and sustained. After successful deflation the suit should be left in place for at least 12 hours before it is removed.[52,53]

Volume Replacement

Volume replacement to some extent is essential in any type of shock. Generally, this procedure is carried out to correct relative or absolute hypovolemia and restore an adequate intravascular volume to establish hemodynamic stability necessary for optimum tissue perfusion, and to maintain the oxygen-carrying capacity of the intravascular volume.[54] The amount of volume replaced is individually determined; however, some general rules of thumb exist. Table 7-2 describes steps that Weil and Rackow recommend for volume resuscitation.[55] The needed type of volume is related to the type of intravascular deficit the patient experiences. Specific replacement fluids are described in the next section and in Table 7-3.

Crystalloids

Crystalloids are solutions that consist of dextrose in water or electrolytes dissolved in water. Since electrolytes are freely permeable to the vascular membrane, infusion of electrolytes helps expand in both plasma fluid volume and interstitial fluid volume. Interstitial volume expansion can be a disadvantage in clinical situations in which intravascular fluid volume expansion is the primary need. Specifically, an approximate amount of only one fourth of infused saline solutions remains in the vascular space. The other 75% rapidly diffuses into the interstitial space. Therefore, a patient may have double or triple the amount of crystalloids infused as compared to colloids in order to obtain the same degree of plasma expansion.[56] In patients with altered capillary permeability this leakage into the interstitial space is even greater.

TABLE 7-2   Fluid Challenge Protocol

Step I

Observe baseline readings of CVP or PCWP for 10 min

Step II

If CVP value	Then rate of fluid infusion
Less than 12 cmH$_2$O	20 ml/hr
Between 12 and 18 cmH$_2$O	10 ml/hr
Greater than 18 cmH$_2$O	5 ml/hr
If PCWP value	Then rate of fluid infusion
Less than 12 mmHg	20 ml/hr
Between 12-18 mmHg	10 ml/hr
Greater than 18 mmHg	5 ml/hr

Step III

Infuse fluid for 10 min

If CVP increases more than 5 cmH$_2$O

If PCWP increases more than 7 mmHg

} Stop infusion

Step IV

At end of 10 min

If CVP increases by 2 cmH$_2$O or less

If PCWP increases by 3 mmHg or less

} Repeat challenge

If CVP increases by 2 to 5 cmH$_2$O

If PCWP increases by 3 to 7 mmHg

} Discontinue infusion

Step V

Observe patient for 10 min

If CVP falls to within 2 cmH$_2$O of initial value

If PCWP falls to within 3 mmHg of initial value

} Resume challenge

If CVP does not fall to within 2 cmH$_2$O of initial value

If PCWP does not fall to within 3 mmHg of initial value

} Discontinue challenge

Adapted from Weil, M. H., & Rackow, E. C. (1984). A guide to volume repletion. *Emergency Medicine 16*, 101-110.

Therefore, crystalloids are not the agent of choice when permeability problems are suspected or present. Another disadvantage associated with crystalloids is that patients given crystalloid fluids tend to easily and perhaps prematurely develop peripheral edema. This peripheral edema is frequently identified as an indication of fluid overload and consequently crystalloid resuscitation is halted before adequate vascular volume is actually achieved.[57]

Normal saline, as an isotonic solution, is an excellent solution to replace extracellular body fluid. It increases plasma volume, but it can dilute extracellular calcium and potassium, causing hypokalemia, hypernatremia, and metabolic acidosis. Serum electrolyte values should be checked frequently during saline infusion. Normal saline solution is an ideal solution to use in patients with hypovolemic shock when the red blood cell mass is adequate. Because of its high sodium content, it is generally not used in patients with cardiogenic shock.

Lactated Ringer's solution is also used to replace body fluid and serves to buffer acidosis since the lactate it contains is converted to bicarbonate in the liver. Also used in hypovolemic states, this fluid is avoided in cardiac patients because of the sodium load. In addition, it should be used carefully in low-flow states since it can increase lactic acidosis. Simple Ringer's solution, however, can be given to patients with hypoperfusion since it contains no lactate. It also replaces body fluid and electrolytes but should be used cautiously in cardiogenic shock patients.

Half normal saline or 0.45% saline solution is also used to raise total fluid volume. Its infusion dilutes plasma proteins and electrolytes, and it readily moves into the interstitial and intracellular areas and leads to edema. However, this solution and dextrose with 0.2% sodium chloride, because of their relatively low sodium content, are perhaps the best agents for volume replacement in patients with significant cardiac problems. Dextrose 5% and water (D$_5$W), also referred to as free water, evenly distributes itself throughout the entire body. For this reason, it is an excellent agent to use for the treatment of dehydration. Caution needs to be used in administration of D$_5$W since it will also dilute the serum levels of electrolytes when given in sufficient quantities.

Colloids

In contrast to crystalloids, colloids are relatively impermeable to the vascular membrane. They determine the oncotic or colloidal osmotic pressure that maintains the balance of water between the interstitial spaces and the intravascular space. Both natural and synthetic colloids are commercially available. The most abundant natural colloid is albumin. Normally,

TABLE 7-3 **Volume Replacement Solutions and Their Ingredients**

CRYSTALLOIDS

Normal saline	0.9% sodium chloride in water	Sodium	154 mEq/L
		Chloride	154 mEq/L
		Osmolality	308 mEq/L
Lactated Ringer's	0.9% sodium chloride in water with electrolytes and buffers	Sodium	130 mEq/L
		Potassium	4 mEq/L
		Calcium	2.7 mEq/L
		Chloride	107 mEq/L
		Lactate	27 mEq/L
		pH	6.5
Ringer's solution	0.9% sodium chloride in water with potassium and calcium	Sodium	147 mEq/L
		Potassium	4 mEq/L
		Calcium	5 mEq/L
		Chloride	156 mEq/L
Half normal saline	0.45% sodium chloride in water	Sodium	77 mEq/L
		Chloride	77 mEq/L
5% Dextrose in water (D₅W)	5% dextrose		

COLLOIDS

5% Albumin (Albumisol)	Aqueous fraction of pooled plasma prepared from whole blood in buffered nomal saline 250- and 500-ml bottles	Albumin	50 g/L
		Sodium	130 to 160 mEq/L
		Potassium	300 mosm/L
		Osmolality	
		Osmotic pressure	20 mmHg
		pH	6.4 to 7.4
25% Albumin (salt-poor)	25-, 50-, and 100-ml bottles	Albumin	240 g/L
		Globulins	10 g/L
		Sodium	130 to 160 mEq/L
		Osmolality	1,500 mosm/L
		pH	6.4 to 7.4
Dextran			
Low-molecular-weight dextran (LMWD)	500-ml bottles, 10% dextran in normal saline or D₅M	Glucose polysaccharide molecules with an average molecular weight of 40,000	
High-molecular-weight dextran (HMWD)	500-ml bottles, 6% dextran in normal saline or D₅M	Glucose polysaccharide molecules with an average molecular weight of 70,000	
Hetastarch	500-ml bottles, 6% solution of a synthetic polymer of hydroxethyl starch in normal saline	Branched chain hydroxyethyl starch prepared from amylopectin	
		Sodium	154 mEq/L
		Chloride	154 mEq/L
		Osmolality	310 mosm/L
		Colloid osmotic pressure	30-35 mmHg

albumin is a major agent in the retention of fluid in the vascular space. With a molecular weight of 68,000, albumin is primarily responsible for the plasma oncotic pressure. Commercially, albumin is available in 5% and 25% solutions. It is an excellent agent to give when the goal is to increase the plasma colloid osmotic pressure and thus plasma volume. It is particularly useful in hypovolemic shock with protein losses as is seen following burns. For every milliliter of 5% albumin infused, the plasma volume expands 1 ml.[58] And for every 25 g of 25% albumin infused, the plasma volume increases by 400 ml.[58,59]

In hypovolemic states, albumin infusions have also demonstrated their ability to bring serum albumin to normal levels. However, some studies have indicated that albumin resuscitation can decrease the other plasma proteins such as immunoglobulins. The clinical significance of these data is as yet unclear.[60]

Dextran is a synthetic agent that consists of several sizes of linear glucose polymers. Dextran is fractionated into low-molecular-weight dextran (LMWD) and high-molecular-weight dextran (HMWD). LMWD has a molecular weight around 40,000, making it similar in that respect to albumin. Its half-life is approximately 2 hours, and it has plasma-expanding capabilities of 1.5 times its volume. High-molecular-weight dextran has a molecular weight of 70,000 and a half-life of 12 hours. Both agents are useful when there is a need to rapidly expand the plasma volume. Both agents are also associated with coagulation problems and may cause bleeding in patients as they decrease platelet adhesiveness and dilute clotting factors such as fibrinogen. Therefore, dextran may not be the ideal replacement fluid in hemorrhage since it may exacerbate the problem. Dextrans can also interfere with blood grouping when administered in large volumes. Most recently a 7.5% sodium chloride in 6% dextran 70 solution has demonstrated its effectiveness as a volume replacement fluid in hypotensive trauma patients.[61]

Hetastarch is a hydroxethyl starch that has an average molecular weight of 69,000. Since it is similar to albumin in molecular weight it has generally the same volume-expansion characteristics. However, its effects can last up to 36 hours. Studies have demonstrated it to be as effective in increasing blood pressure, cardiac output, and tissue perfusion as 5% albumin.[59,62] In addition, it can increase colloidal osmotic pressure to levels three times higher in hypovolemic patients than 5% albumin or normal saline solution.[63] Hetastarch has been shown to increase serum amylase levels since it combines with amylase during the degradation process. Since the half-life of hetastarch is so long, levels of the attached amylase also become elevated. Glucose levels also rise following infusion of hetastarch because glucose is a byproduct of hetastarch's degradation process. If dilution of clotting factors occurs from excessive infusion of hetastarch, clotting parameters such as the prothrombin time, partial thromboplastin time, and platelet count will be affected.

Blood and Blood Products

The use of whole blood as a replacement agent is generally restricted to hypovolemic shock states associated with hemorrhage or in situations where the hemoglobin is less than 12 g/100 ml and the hematocrit is less than 30%.[55] Whole blood less than 24 hours old is preferable since older stored blood contains fewer clotting factors and more cellular debris, potassium, citrate, and other waste products. Additionally, stored blood is deficient in 2,3-diphosphoglycerate (2,3-DPG), and this deficiency enhances the affinity of hemoglobin for oxygen and consequently decreases oxygen release to the tissues. If banked blood is given, calcium also needs to be administered since the citrate in banked blood binds with calcium and thereby decreases circulating levels of ionized calcium. With massive transfusion, this loss of ionized

calcium can seriously affect myocardial contractility. All efforts are made to cross-match the recipient and donor blood prior to transfusion. However, in the severely hypovolemic trauma patient when time is limited, it has been demonstrated that type-specific non-cross-matched blood is safe to administer and more rapidly available.[64]

Packed red cells are also used as replacement agents when the hematocrit is less than 30% and the red cell mass needs to be increased to improve the oxygen-carrying capacity of the blood. The advantage of packed cells over whole blood is that less infused volume is required to deliver the red cell mass, and fewer metabolic waste products are infused. This makes packed cell infusion an attractive alternative for cardiogenic shock patients. Disadvantages center on the high viscosity of the cells, which makes them difficult to infuse, and their lack of coagulation factors so that other blood components may be necessary to replace those components. Fresh frozen plasma contains plasma proteins, clotting factors, and plasma and is used to replace clotting factors and restore plasma volume in hypovolemic shock.

The need for fresh frozen plasma can be assessed by the results of the prothrombin time (PT), partial thromboplastin time (PTT), and fibrinogen levels. The PTT is a measure of the intrinsic pathway while the PT measures the extrinsic pathway. If either is abnormal, fresh frozen plasma is indicated. Plasma needs to be administered as soon as it is thawed so that deterioration of its clotting factors is limited. Plasma does not contain platelets, so that if thrombocytopenia is identified as the cause of hemorrhage, platelet units need to be transfused.

Cryoprecipitate is another blood component that can be used to control coagulopathies. It contains all the clotting elements of fresh frozen plasma except platelets. Its advantage is that it requires only 20 ml of volume to deliver equivalent factors compared to fresh frozen plasma's 200 ml of volume. Therefore, cryoprecipitate is ideal for patients in congestive heart failure. It is also especially rich in factor VIII and fibrinogen and is most frequently given following fluid resuscitation in which a dilutional coagulopathy has developed. Studies have also demonstrated that cryoprecipitate may assist in restoring opsonic activity after injury and may be valuable in septic shock.[64]

Artificial Blood

In this category there are generally two different types of agents, both of which are currently undergoing investigation and are as yet not part of conventional volume replacement therapies. These agents are stroma-free hemoglobin and artificial red cells. *Stroma-free hemoglobin* is hemoglobin stripped of all its cell membrane elements. It is obtained from outdated human red blood cells and has a significant capacity for carrying oxygen. *Artificial red cells,* or synthetic erythrocytes, are formed by encapsulating concentrated hemoglobin solutions in microcapsules. In animal studies these microcapsules have been shown to have the same oxygen and carbon dioxide–carrying capacity as real erythrocytes.[65,66] Again, while currently not part of the conventional treatment plan, these agents hold considerable promise.

Pharmacological Interventions

For the most part the goals of pharmacological therapy in shock are the same regardless of the type of shock. In all types of shock there is first a need to increase perfusion to vital organs, to limit or decrease the amount of myocardial demand this vital organ perfusion requires, and to decrease pulmonary congestion. In addition, increasing peripheral organ perfusion is also a goal.[67] In cardiogenic shock, these goals are achieved by surgical, mechanical, or pharmacological support. In hypovolemic shock, these goals are achieved by volume replacement for the most part, but in severe states or in end stages, pharmacological support is necessary. And in septic shock, volume manipulation and pharmacological agents are the major therapies. The next section briefly describes agents used in shock.

Vasopressors and Inotropes

Numerous vasopressors and inotropes can be used to improve blood flow to vital organs. They most often accomplish this by their beta-adrenergic activity which increases myocardial contractility, and their alpha-adrenergic effects, which allow them to vasoconstrict peripheral organs. Other pathways for their effects also exist, however. The pathways that lead to enhanced contractility are illustrated in Figure 7-12, and the effects of frequently used drugs are detailed in Table 7-4. Whatever the mechanism of action, the end result of these effects is improved flow to vital organs, decreased flow to peripheral organs, and an increase in myocardial workload and hence oxygen consumption due to the increased contractility and increase in afterload. In the shock state, these effects may be briefly appropriate, but peripheral organ ischemia needs to be reversed as soon as possible.

Dopamine hydrochloride (Intropin) is perhaps the most common vasopressor. As an inotrope, it increases cardiac contractility through its beta-adrenergic receptor activity. However, in addition, at low doses of 1 to 2 µg per kilogram per minute, its actions are exerted on the peripheral bed dopaminergic receptor sites in the renal and mesenteric areas. Dopamine's action is to dilate these vessels selectively to assist in improving blood flow to them despite the low cardiac output. In shock states this role is very critical because the renal beds, being viewed as nonvital organs, become constricted early in shock. Dopamine continues to serve as a vasodilator to the peripheral beds when the dose is increased to 2 to 4 µg per kilogram per minute. However, as doses exceed 6 µg per kilogram per minute, its effects on the peripheral beds become progressively more vasocon-

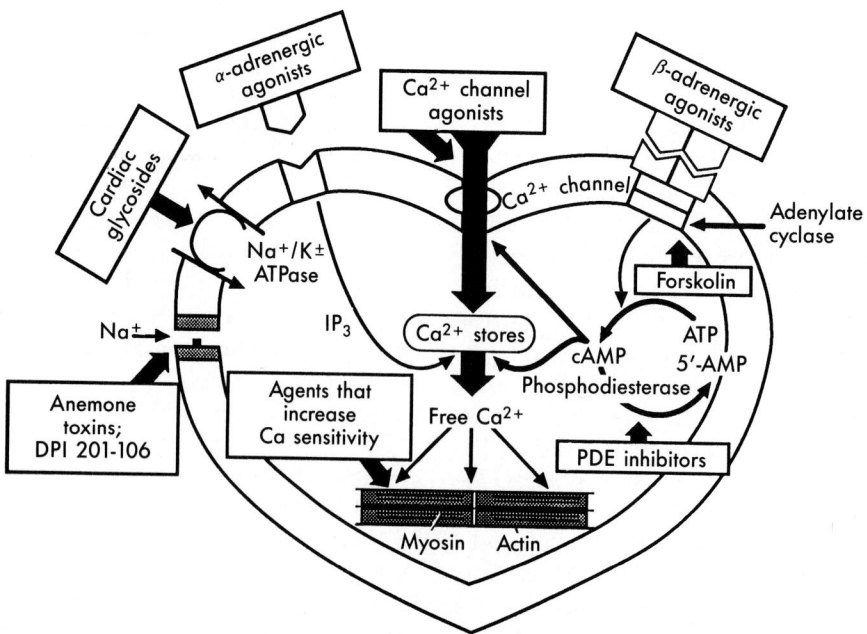

Figure 7-12   Schematic representation of the various pathways leading to enhanced contractility.
Adapted, with permission, from Wetzel, B., & Havel, N. (1988). *Trends in pharmacological science—TIPS Reviews.* Essex: Elsevier Science Publishing.

TABLE 7-4   Relative Mechanisms of Action and Effects of Commonly Used Vasopressors and Inotropes

	Mechanism of Action			Effects		
	Alpha	Beta$_1$	Other	Cardiac Output	Heart Rate	Systemic Vascular Resistance
Dopamine	+ + +	+ + +		+ + +	+ +	+
Dobutamine	+	+ + +		+ + +	+ (+ + +)	+
Isoproterenol	−	+ + +		+ + +	+ + +	− −
Norepinephrine	+ + +	+ + +		+ + +	+ +	+ + +
Epinephrine	+ + +	−		+ + +	+ +	+ + +
Amrinone	−	−	Phophodiesterase III inhibitor	+ + +	+	− −
Phenylephrine	+ + +	−		+ + +	+	+ + +
Methoxamine	+ + +	−		+ + +	+	+ + +
Glucagon	−	−	Adenyl cyclase activator			
Prenalterol		+ +		+ +	+	−
Dopexamine		+ +		+ + +	+ +	−
Pimobendan			Ca^{2+} sensitizer	+ +	−	−

strictive as both arterioles and veins constrict. At these doses, dopamine is similar to other vasopressors.[68]

Dobutamine hydrochloride (Dobutrex) is a synthetic catecholamine that acts on the beta-adrenergic receptors and thus enhances contractility. It is an ideal agent to use in any stage of cardiogenic shock and in late distributive shock. When dobutamine is administered in doses greater than 10 to 15 μg per kilogram per minute tachycardia may become a problem. This may create myocardial ischemia in patients with failing ventricles and may necessitate a change in vasopressors or additional lowering of systemic vascular resistance.[69,70]

Isoproterenol hydrochloride (Isuprel) is a beta agonist that can enhance contractility but also serves as a chronotropic agent. It is useful in shock states when bradycardia is present. It is also useful in situations of elevated pulmonary vascular resistance because it can lower this resistance. The major disadvantage of this drug is its tendency to create supraventricular and ventricular tachyarrhythmias. In cardiogenic shock, this could facilitate the extension of a myocardial infarction.

Norepinephrine (Levophed) in doses less than 0.02 to 0.2 μg per kilogram per minute creates a moderate yet significant increase in contractility due to its beta-adrenergic receptor effects. At doses exceeding 0.3 μg per kilogram per minute, it becomes a strong peripheral arteriolar and venous constrictor due to its alpha effects and is an ideal agent for severe shock in which significant peripheral vasodilatation is present. The increase in systemic vascular resistance that norepinephrine creates, however, can severely impair left ventricular ejection, particularly in cardiogenic or septic shock patients where the myocardium is already failing dramatically. Careful titration to avoid this effect is essential.[71]

In theory, norepinephrine is an ideal agent to administer in late stages of septic shock, when the goal is to increase systemic vascular resistance. In the clinical setting, however, it is frequently ineffective in this endeavor as are other alpha agents. Chernow[72] has demonstrated that, in sepsis, the number of alpha receptors which would normally elicit constriction of the vascular beds appear to be down-regulated or decreased. In addition, as Figure 7-13 illustrates, there is evidence that in sepsis the calcium channel in the cell closes, and the other receptors inhibit the alpha receptors from functioning. Specifically, high prostacyclin levels activate the PGI$_2$ receptors and turn off the alpha receptors, and the circulating endorphins activate their receptors, turning off more alpha receptors. These cellular events then lead to the clinical situation where massive doses of norepinephrine or other catecholamines are infused but the systemic vascular resistance remains static. However, Chernow has also demonstrated that infusion of an experimental calcium agonist can open the calcium channel and can improve blood pressure by bypassing the adrenergic pathway and working directly on the cellular contractile process. This laboratory finding has tremendous relevance for future investigations and explains the ineffectiveness of some protocols in septic shock.

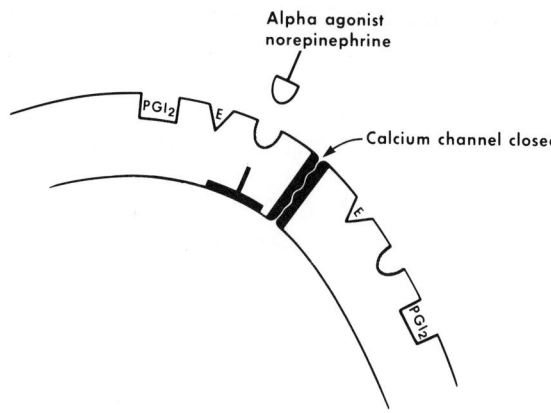

Figure 7-13 Blockade of various receptor sites in endotoxic shock with consequent disruption of the metabolic pathways which produce muscle contraction.

Epinephrine as a beta-adrenergic agent also elicits a strong inotropic response. In low doses it decreases systemic vascular resistance, and in high doses it increases vascular resistance. As with some of the other agents described, the positive inotropic effects of this agent are negated once systemic vascular resistance becomes elevated enough to stress or impede left ventricular function. Once this occurs the shock state worsens. Therefore, most of these agents are used concurrently with vasodilators to achieve the optimum hemodynamic effects.

Phenylephrine hydrochloride (Neo-Synephrine) is a pressor agent that accomplishes its effects without any beta-adrenergic action. It is a pure alpha-adrenergic drug and consequently raises blood pressure by constricting the peripheral beds. Methoxamine hydrochloride (Vasoxyl) is also an alpha-adrenergic stimulator that causes significant vasoconstriction.[73,74]

Amrinone lactate, classified as a phosphodiesterase III inhibitor, is a nonglycoside, nonadrenergic cardiotonic agent. By inhibiting the enzyme phosphodiesterase, amrinone enhances the availability of cyclic AMP, which is a major factor in cardiac contractility. Amrinone is generally administered by giving an initial intravenous loading dose (0.75-1.5 mg/kg) and then maintained by a continuous infusion at a rate of 5 to 20 mg per kg per minute.[75]

In addition to these commonly used agents there are other inotropes that increase contractility. Hypertonic solutions of glucose, insulin, and potassium (GIK) have been shown to improve hemodynamic parameters in bacterial shock. The exact mechanism for this outcome is not known, but it is believed that the result is related to the ability of the solution to decrease myocardial cellular edema, enhance the excitation–contraction coupling process, and improve the energy balance, particularly in depressed left ventricles.[76]

Glucagon is another weak inotropic agent that has some limited usefulness. Glucagon activates adenyl cyclase without using the beta receptor, and via this mechanism can increase contractility. Because of this, glucagon has been found to be effective in shock states when beta-adrenergic blockade is present.[77,78]

Prenalterol is a beta agonist agent with selective inotropic effects, fewer chronotropic effects, and minimal peripheral actions. It has shown some effectiveness in the treatment of patients with cardiogenic shock following an acute myocardial infarction.[77] Dopexamine is a synthetic catecholamine with mild beta agonist activity and systemic and renal vasodilator effects. Consequently, it increases cardiac output and lowers systemic vascular resistance and has been demonstrated to be effective in early stages of cardiac failure.[79] A newer category of inotropes are the calcium sensitizing agents. The general actions of these agents are to increase the sensitivity of troponin to calcium activation and hence to increase contractility. Clinical trials with one of these agents, pimobendan, has demonstrated satisfactory early effects in treating cardiac failure.[80]

Calcium was identified earlier in this chapter as a critical element in the excitation–contraction mechanism of the myocardium and other muscles. Because of this inotropic effect, replacement and administration of calcium during treatment of the shock patient is essential. Particularly after infusion of whole blood, calcium may need to be administered since the citrate in banked blood binds with calcium. This makes calcium unavailable for metabolic processes such as contraction. Additionally, administration of calcium may be necessary following hemorrhagic and septic shock, as evidence indicates that there is a fall in ionized calcium levels in these conditions.[81,82]

Vasodilators

In the previous section it was stated that the primary goal of pharmacological therapy is to increase vital organ perfusion and concurrently to limit or decrease the myocardium's workload as much as possible and limit pulmonary congestion. Vasodilators produce these latter two effects by dilating the veins and arterioles to different extents. By dilating the veins and venules, venous capacitance is increased, and this decreases preload, thereby diminishing pulmonary congestion. By dilating the arterioles, the systemic vascular resistance is lowered, and this decreases impedance to left ventricular ejection. Consequently, myocardial oxygen consumption is lessened. In addition, coronary artery dilators can be administered to assist in increasing the supply of oxygen to the myocardium. Specific agents responsible for these actions include nitroprusside (Nipride), phentolamine (Regitine), and nitroglycerin (Tridil).

Nitroprusside is a potent, rapidly reversible peripheral vasodilator that rapidly reduces systemic vascular resistance by its actions on both the peripheral venous and arterial beds. It is administered via a continuous infusion, and therefore its effects can be titrated and controlled. Phentolamine is an alpha-adrenergic blocking agent that also serves as a direct relaxant of vascular smooth muscle. It reduces preload and afterload by relaxing both the arterial and venous beds; however, its actions are predominantly arterial. Nitroglycerin primarily acts as a venous dilator. It increases venous capacitance but has also been demonstrated to increase blood flow in the coronary artery collateral vessels.[83,84] Morphine sulfate can also be used as a vasodilator. As a powerful venodilator, it can reduce preload and can also reduce myocardial oxygen consumption. Morphine can also block sympathetic stimulation and this assists in decreasing afterload.

Vasodilators are not always used in shock, but they can be excellent adjunct agents in decreasing elevated vascular resistances and preloads. Most commonly, they are employed in cardiogenic and late-stage septic shock.

Antidysrhythmic Agents

Particularly in cardiogenic and septic shock, dysrhythmia management may become necessary. Dysrhythmias generally develop from injury to the myocardium as can be seen in acute infarctions, or develop in response to hypoxia and acidosis. The first hallmark, then, of dysrhythmia management dictates that adequate oxygenation and acid–base balance be present. If so, other agents may be effective (see also Chapter 10 and the Appendix). For treatment of bradycardia, atropine or isoproterenol can be used. Insertion of a temporary transvenous pacemaker may also be required to treat a persistent bradycardia. Supraventricular tachydysrhythmias also develop, particularly when the atria become distended with excessive volume. Atrial fibrillation, flutter, and tachycardia can be treated with digoxin, verapamil, esmolol, adenosine or propranolol. These agents are used with caution in cardiogenic or late-stage septic shock since they accomplish their intended effects by depressing contractility or increasing myocardial oxygen demand. Ventricular tachydysrhythmias and premature beats can be treated with lidocaine, procainamide, or bretylium. Both lidocaine and procainamide may also depress contractility and bretylium may potentiate the hypotension of shock, so caution should also be used with these agents.

Beta-adrenergic blocking agents, such as propranolol, have been shown to be effective in preventing myocardial hypoxic damage and limiting the effects of ischemia that develop from sympathetic drive. It has also been suggested that they can prevent myocardial necrosis in some patients who would have otherwise developed an infarction.[85] These agents should not be administered to prevent infarct extension if bradycardia or hypotension exist, because these agents will only exacerbate these problems and cardiogenic shock will develop.[86]

Corticosteroids

Currently, the evidence for the use of high dose corticosteroids in early stages of septic and traumatic shock is equivocal. The hypothesized beneficial effects of steroid therapy include reduced cellular permeability; interference with leukocyte degranulation and prostaglandin synthesis; inhibition of adrenocorticotrophic hormone (ADH), endorphins, and interleukin-1 release; and exertion of an anticoagulant effect. However, at present, clinical studies consistently continue to provide conflicting evidence about the achievement of these outcomes.[87,88,89]

Diuretics and Renal Replacement Therapies

Diuretics are also valuable adjunctive agents in shock states. They are particularly helpful in maintaining patency of the renal tubules and reducing preload, thereby helping to diminish pulmonary congestion. Caution should be used in their administration since they can be nephrotoxic and can produce acute tubular necrosis. This usually occurs when they are administered during episodes of low cardiac output where they then have a long residence time in the nephron. In this situation, they are chemically irritating to renal cells and cause disruption. Commonly used agents include furosemide (Lasix), bumetadine (Bumex), and ethacrynic acid (Edecrin). Mannitol, an osmotic diuretic, can also be used in the presence of normovolemia and adequate left ventricular function. Vasodilators, such as dopamine at low doses, can be used to dilate the renal vessels thus overcoming their vasoconstricted state.

More recently, several continuous renal replacement therapies (CRRT) have been demonstrated as effective, hemodynamically stable methods of removing both excessive fluid and solutes in oliguria.[90,91,92] Three methods of CRRT are currently available for use in acute renal failure: slow continuous ultrafiltration (SCUF), continuous arteriovenous hemofiltration (CAVH), and continuous arteriovenous hemodialysis (CAVHD). Figure 7-14 depicts these systems. All three systems use a ultrafiltration membrane that is attached to a vascular access such as a shunt. Blood

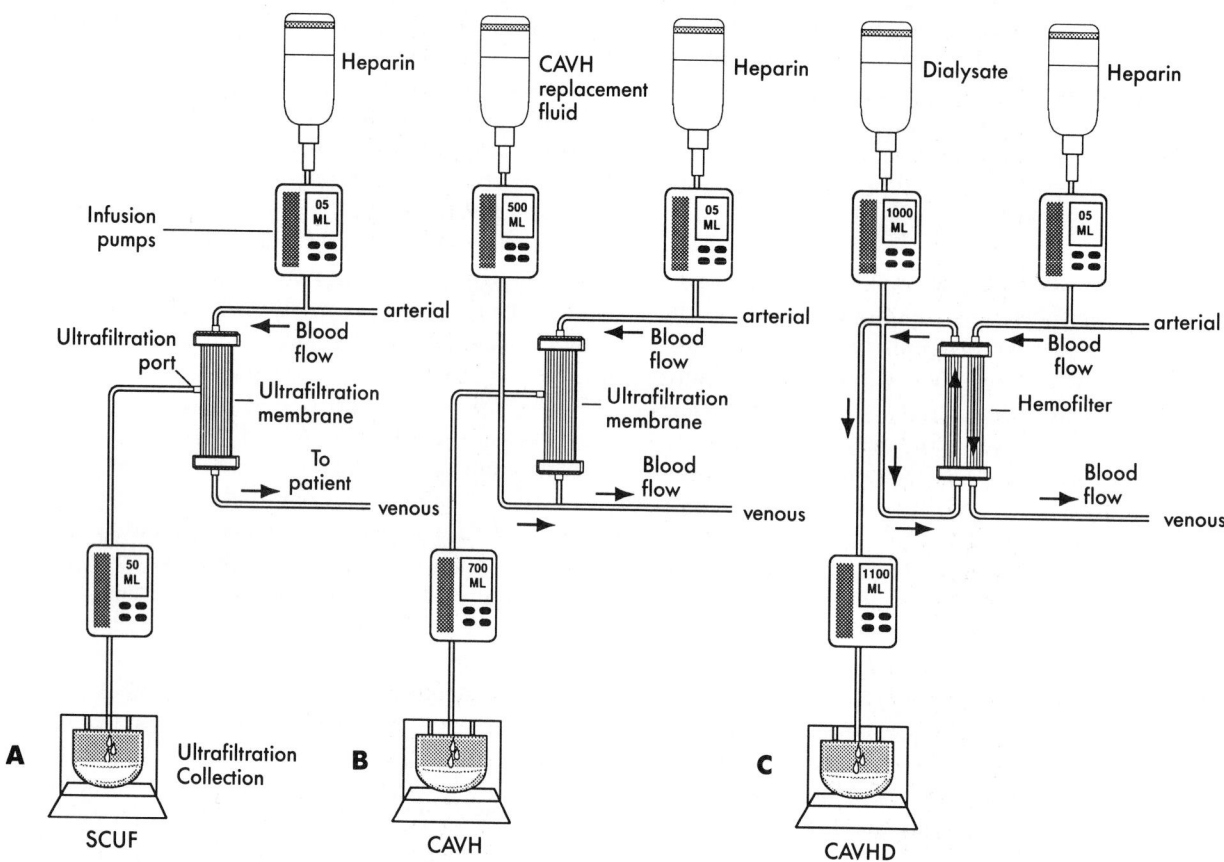

Figure 7-14   Schematic representation of *A,* slow continuous ultrafiltration (SCUF), *B,* continuous arteriovenous hemofiltration (CAVH), and *C,* continuous arteriovenous hemofiltration and dialysis (CAVHD).

flows from the arterial side through the ultrafiltration membrane and returns via the venous port. Heparin is infused via the arterial port to prevent clotting in the membrane. The ultrafiltration membrane has a sieving capability that allows plasma water and solutes to pass through it and exit via an outflow port. Generally, infusion pumps are attached to this port to regulate the fluid removal. Slow continuous ultrafiltration is the simplest method of hemofiltration. Its primary goal is the removal of volume which is accomplished by convective removal of plasma water and some solutes. Ultrafiltration removal rates generally range from 200 to 300 ml per hour. This technique is well suited for patients with cardiogenic shock with mild renal insufficiency for whom fluid removal is the only requirement.

When moderate fluid and solute removal is required, CAVH is the recommended therapy. To accomplish this, large volumes of fluid exchanges are required to remove toxic solutes such as urea and potassium. As is depicted in Figure 7-14*B,* large volumes of CAVH replacement solution are infused via the venous port while equally large amounts of fluid

are removed from the ultrafiltrate port. This balancing of fluid avoids volume overloads. Additionally, by removing more volume than is infused, a negative fluid balance can be achieved. Since the volume infused is free of potassium, urea, and other toxic solutes contained in the removed volume, this technique gradually reduces the toxic solute concentration by dilution. When aggressive and extensive removal of solute in addition to fluid is required as is seen in severe sepsis, CAVHD is used. This system closely mirrors dialysis except that it is done on a continuous basis. As Figure 7-14*C* illustrates, the basic system is the same with a hemofilter attached to an arteriovenous access site and with the arterial port receiving heparin. The hemofilter is somewhat different. In this therapy, peritoneal dialysate or a custom dialysate is infused into the hemofilter only, countercurrent to the patient's blood flow. The dialysate infusion rate is 1,000 ml per hour. Solutes are removed according to their concentration gradient. Generally patients with blood urea nitrogen levels greater than 100 mg/dl require CAVHD. These forms of CRRT can continue for days to weeks at a time and allow large volumes of vasoactive agents, nutritional fluids, or antibiotics to be infused without worsening the patient's volume or toxic solute status.

Antibiotics

Ideally, antibiotic therapy should not be prescribed until the infecting organisms have been identified. However, in severe cases of septic shock, prescription of antibiotics may be based on the most likely infecting organisms. For example, if the infection is thought to be hospital-acquired and occurs in a non-immunosuppressed patient (neutrophil count greater than 1,000 per mm^3), an aminoglycoside and a third-generation cephalosporin are recommended. If, however, the patient is immunosuppressed (neutrophil count less than 1,000 per mm^3), an aminoglycoside for gram-negative bacteria coverage and a penicillin agent such as nafcillan or piperacillin for gram-positive bacteria coverage are recommended.[93,94]

Heparin

Low-dose heparin therapy may be required in patients who develop disseminated intravascular coagulation as a consequence of septic shock. It is intended to limit microcoagulation. The recommended dosage is generally 50 to 100 units per kilogram by intravenous bolus with lower doses given if the platelet count is less than 100,000 m^3. Indications for the use of heparin are otherwise quite limited; they include deep venous thrombosis and pulmonary embolism, or other arterial thrombosis. If heparin is administered, concurrent replacement with fibrinogen, clotting factors, and platelets also needs to occur so that a major hemorrhage does not ensue from the heparin therapy.[94] Most recently, gabexate mesilate, tranexamic acid, and low molecular weight heparin have shown equal or improved outcomes as compared with heparin in clinical trials measuring treatments of DIC.[95,96,97]

Other Agents

Other therapeutic avenues for the treatment of shock have been addressed. From an immunological perspective, the use of a human antiserum to the endotoxin core of gram-negative bacteria originally appeared to improve survival in gram-negative bacteremia.[98] However, a more recent trial using anti-J5 hyperimmune intravenous immunoglobulins failed to demonstrate a reduced mortality.[99] It has been mentioned previously that thromboxane A$_2$ is implicated in the genesis of endotoxic shock. Investigations with dazoxiben, a thromboxane synthetase inhibitor, indicate that it can lower plasma thromboxane levels in patients with sepsis and adult respiratory distress syndrome. Although it lowered thromboxane levels, however, dazoxiben did not alter the clinical course in the patients studied.[100] Prostacylin may also have a beneficial effect on tissue perfusion due to its ability to inhibit white cell and platelet activation and thereby reduce the severity of tissue damage.[101]

Naloxone hydrochloride (Narcan) has also entered the arena of controversial drugs used to treat shock. An opiate receptor antagonist, naloxone has been shown in some cases to reverse the hypotension in hypovolemic, endotoxemic, and spinal shock caused by endorphins and other endogenous opiates. However, not all investigators achieved the same positive results with naloxone, and further studies are needed to determine its ultimate efficacy.[102,103]

Diphenhydramine (Benadryl) can also be given to patients in septic shock. When given at the beginning of the hyperdynamic phase, it can block histamine release. Aspirin, ibuprofen (Motrin), and indomethacin (Indocin) given to block the synthesis of leukotrienes are also being investigated. This helps diminish pulmonary vasoconstriction. Additional agents that require clinical evaluation include antibodies to neutrophil receptor sites and TNF, anti-C5a antibodies, anti–arachidonic acid metabolite agents, oxygen free radical scavengers, ATP/MgCl$_2$, thyrotropin releasing factor, and calcium agonists that bypass the adrenergic receptor.[104,105,106]

Correction of Acid–Base Abnormalities

The majority of acid–base abnormalities that develop in shock improve spontaneously once adequate ventilation and perfusion are achieved. In hypovolemic shock, however, there may be a transient increase in acidosis following initial volume resuscitation. This develops because of the washout of lactic acid from the tissues that occurs when perfusion dramatically improves as it frequently does in hypovolemic shock. If severe metabolic acidosis persists, then therapy should be initiated to reverse the imbalance. Acidosis can go uncorrected until pH reaches 7.15 or less; evidence indicates that myocardial depression does not develop until the pH is 6.9.[94] Once correction is required, the agent of choice is sodium bicarbonate. Overcorrection should be avoided because the incidence of supraventricular tachycardia increases with a pH higher than 7.5.[107]

Circulatory Assist Devices

Several circulatory assist devices can be used to stabilize patients in shock: the external counterpulsation device, the intraaortic balloon pump (IABP), the Hemopump, and the external right and left ventricular assist devices (RVAD, LVAD). The external counterpulsation system is similar to the pneumatic antishock garment. The difference lies in the fact that with external counterpulsation, the suit will inflate and deflate in conjunction with the cardiac cycle. Specifically, during diastole the system is pressurized, thereby increasing coronary blood flow. During systole, it deflates to avoid increasing the afterload. It is usually only placed on the patient four times daily for 50 to 120 minutes. Its efficacy is best seen in patients with cardiogenic shock in class A or B of the hemodynamic subset classification.[108,109]

The intraaortic balloon pump (IABP) is a sausage-shaped balloon mounted on a catheter which is inserted most often through the femoral artery and is then placed distal to the left subclavian artery in the descending thoracic aorta. The action of the balloon is to inflate during systole (Figure 7-15). Inflation allows blood to be pushed retrograde into the aortic root. This increases coronary artery blood supply and hence oxygenation. Deflation of the balloon just prior to systolic ejection creates a negative intraaortic pressure and therefore decreases afterload. By these actions of increasing coronary artery blood flow and decreasing afterload, the total work of the heart is reduced. Intraaortic balloon pumping is most commonly used in patients with cardiogenic shock. However, it can also assist in the hypodynamic stage of septic shock to support a failing myocardium while antibiotics and other activities are employed to control the sepsis.[110,111,112]

The Hemopump consists of an arterial cannula that is inserted through the femoral artery and is advanced upward toward the aortic arch and past the aortic valve into the left ventricle. Blood is lifted out of the left ventricle and ejected into the aorta via an axial flow pump located on the distal portion of the cannula positioned in the descending thoracic aorta. This pumping mechanism is capable of generating nonpulsatile continuous blood flow of rates ranging from 0.5 L to 3.5 L/min/m². The Hemopump is used most often in patients with cardiogenic shock. It has been associated with 50% survival rates.[113,114]

The last type of circulatory assist device is the external ventricular assist device. These devices are indicated for use in patients with markedly impaired ventricular failure unresponsive to pharmacological or IABP support. It is also used in patients with end-stage cardiac disease who are waiting transplantation and who are deteriorating. These devices vary in their specific designs, but their techniques generally consist of removing blood via cannulas from the left atrium or ventricle and reinfusing it into the aortic root, or removing blood from the right atrium or ventricle and infusing it into the pulmonary artery. This technique bypasses the ventricle and consequently requires no ventricular contraction. Blood flow in these systems can be either pulsatile or nonpulsatile and is maintained by roller, centrifugal, or pneumatically powered drive systems.[115,116,117,118]

All the systems described are temporary. They are discontinued or the patient is weaned from them as improvement is noted.

NURSING MANAGEMENT: CASE STUDY

Mrs. W. is a 54-year-old white female who, while attending her daughter's wedding reception, developed shortness of breath and left-sided shoulder and chest discomfort. Upon arrival in the emergency room, her cuff blood pressure was 80/58; heart rate was sinus tachycardia at 120 beats per minute; respiratory rate was 34 breaths per minute; S3 and S4 heart sounds were heard; the ECG showed ST changes in leads I and aVL; the chest film revealed a normal cardiac silhouette and clear lung fields; and fine moist rales were present in the lower lobes. Arterial blood gases were pH = 7.50, PaO_2 = 85, $PaCO_2$ = 30. Her skin was cool and clammy, and peripheral pulses were weak.

An initial diagnosis of a lateral wall myocardial infarction was established, and Mrs. W. was transferred to the coronary care unit, where a pulmonary artery flow–directed catheter was inserted. The thermodilution cardiac output was 4.5 L/min with a cardiac index of 2.2 L/min/m². Pulmonary capillary wedge pressure was 14 mmHg, and right atrial pressure was 9 mmHg. Systemic vascular resistance was 1,500 dyn/sec/cm⁻⁵. An indwelling Foley catheter was inserted, and the hourly urine output was 20ml. Concurrent therapy with supplemental oxygen ad-

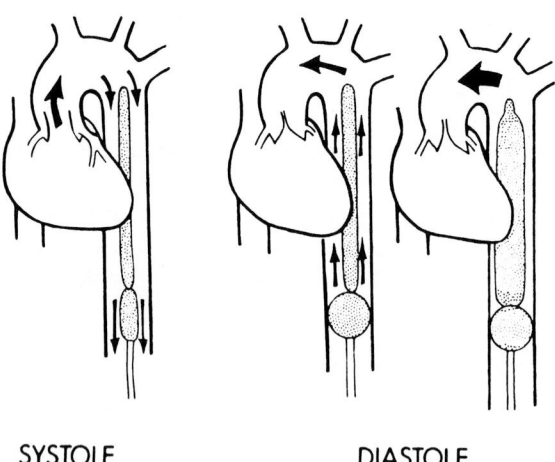

SYSTOLE   DIASTOLE

Figure 7-15 Schematic representation of the intraaortic balloon catheter in systole and diastole.

ministration, volume loading, dobutamine, nitroglycerine, and nitroprusside infusions was initiated, and over the next hour the cardiac index rose to 2.5 L/min/m², the PCWP rose to 16 mmHg, and the right atrial pressure to 12 mmHg. The systemic vascular resistance fell to 1,280 dyn/sec/cm⁻⁵. Urine output increased to 50 ml per hour. Appropriate nursing diagnosis and specific interventions for cardiogenic shock are described below.

■ NURSING DIAGNOSIS

Decreased cardiac output, related to decreased contractility from myocardial infarction, myocardial structure abnormalities, and conduction system disturbances and dysrhythmias.

OUTCOME STANDARD AND CRITERIA

The patient will exhibit signs of adequate cardiac output and contractility as evidenced by:
- Normal CO/CI: CO = 5 L/min, CI = 2.5–3.5 L/min/m²
- Warm vasodilated extremities
- Adequate peripheral pulses
- Adequate urinary output: 0.5 ml per kilogram per hour
- Absence of further ECG changes
- Absence of dysrhythmias or presence of a hemodynamically stable dysrhythmia
- Normal sensorium

NURSING INTERVENTIONS

- Identify and describe factors that can further alter contractility after a myocardial infarction (see box on p. 145 for etiologies of cardiogenic shock). Specifically, in this patient with a lateral wall infarction, rupture or dysfunction of the chordae tendineae or the papillary muscle can develop, creating mitral regurgitation. Premature ventricular contractions or other ventricular dysrhythmias may develop and further limit cardiac output since damage is located in the ventricle. Atrial dysrhythmias are less likely to occur but may develop, particularly following mitral regurgitation as the left atrium is stretched from the regurgitant flow.
- Monitor, assess, and record signs and symptoms of decreased contractility and increased cardiogenic shock.
  Decreased CO/CI: CO less than 5 L/min or CI less than 2.2 L/min/m².
  Hypotension: Systolic blood pressure less than 80 mmHg and/or MAP less than 60 mmHg.
  Elevated SVR: SVR greater than 1,300 dyn/sec/cm⁻⁵.
  Elevated left ventricular filling pressures: PCWP greater than 18 mmHg.
  Urinary output less than 30 ml/hr or less than 0.5 ml per kilogram per hour.

Presence or development of S_3 and S_4 heart sounds.
Presence or development of a new murmur; with lateral wall infarction, papillary muscle rupture is common, thereby creating mitral regurgitation and consequently a holosystolic murmur.
Jugular venous distention; this will develop when biventricular failure occurs.
Increase in quality and extent of rales; this can indicate a worsening pulmonary function and development of pulmonary edema.
Tachycardia: heart rate greater than 110 beats per minute.
Cold, clammy skin.
Decreased peripheral pulses.
Decreased level of consciousness.
Presence of a pulsus alternans on the arterial tracing. This is a pattern of alternating high and low arterial pressure waves. It is a classic sign of left ventricular failure and reflects a myocardium that has limited reserve and hence alternating capabilities for contraction.
Hypoxemia and acidosis.
Presence of new ECG changes or development of dysrhythmias.
Fall in $S\bar{v}O_2$ readings.
- Implement strategies according to either the physician's prescriptions or standing unit policies to improve myocardial contractility.
  Identify commonly used pharmacological drugs that improve contractility. Identify their routes of administration, actions, and dosages. These drugs can include:
  Dopamine
  Dobutamine
  Amrinone
  Isoproterenol
  Norepinephrine
  Epinephrine
  Digoxin
  Glucagon
  Calcium chloride
  Oxygen
  Sodium bicarbonate
  Administer pharmacological agents at doses specified by physician's prescriptions and titrate them when appropriate to achieve parameters determined by physician. Usual parameters might include an MAP greater than 60 mmHg and/or a CI greater than 2.5 L/min/m². During administration of these vasopressors and inotropic agents the nurse should perform the following:
  Observe MAP every 2 to 3 minutes when active titration of vasoactive drugs is being done.
  Record MAP every 15 minutes or more fre-

quently to adequately reflect patient's clinical course.

Observe for new or increased dysrhythmias or ECG changes that might indicate further myocardial ischemia from too much inotropic drive.

Monitor filling pressures for hypervolemic parameters. The presence of v waves on the PCWP tracing could indicate regurgitant blood flow back across mitral valve. This regurgitant flow can occur following rupture of papillary muscle or can develop if ventricle is distended sufficiently to prevent mitral valve cusps from approximating during closure, and consequently regurgitation occurs.

Obtain CO/CI parameters per physician prescriptions or unit routines.

- Implement strategies according to either physician's prescriptions or standing unit policies to decrease afterload or reverse systemic vasoconstriction.

Identify commonly used pharmacological drugs that decrease vasoconstriction. Identify their routes of administration, actions, and dosages. These drugs can include:
Sodium nitroprusside
Phentolamine
Nitroglycerine

Administer pharmacological agents at dosages specified by physician's prescriptions and titrate them when appropriate to achieve parameters determined by physician. Usual parameters might include: lower the SVR to levels less than 1,300 $dyn/sec/cm^{-5}$ and maintain MAP greater than 80 mmHg.

Observe MAP every 2 to 3 minutes during active titration of these agents.

Record MAP every 15 minutes to provide a record that adequately reflects patient's response to these therapies.

Observe the monitored filling pressures every 2 to 3 minutes, i.e., right atrial pressure or pulmonary artery diastolic pressure.

Record filling pressures every 15 minutes to adequately capture patient's responses. Observe for hypovolemia due to vasodilator effects of drugs.

If severe hypovolemia and hypotension develop, immediately decrease or discontinue vasodilator.

Avoid MAP pressures less than 60 mmHg since at levels lower than this coronary blood supply can become diminished and further ischemia or infarction could ensue.

■ **NURSING DIAGNOSIS**

Impaired gas exchange, related to acute alterations in tissue perfusion.

OUTCOME STANDARD AND CRITERIA

Gas exchange is adequate as evidenced by:
- Adequate respiratory rate and rhythm
- Adequate color
- Absence of adventitious sounds
- Presence of normal breath sounds
- Normal chest x-ray
- Adequate arterial blood gas values:
  PaO_2 = to 100 mmHg with FiO_2 at 0.40
  $PaCO_2$ = 35 to 45 mmHg
  pH = 7.35 to 7.45
- Adequate neurological status

NURSING INTERVENTIONS

- Identify and describe mechanisms or factors that contribute to impairment of gas exchange in association with inadequate tissue perfusion states (see Associated Problems section). Hydrostatic pulmonary edema such as interstitial or alveolar edema is most likely to occur after a myocardial infarction or in cardiogenic shock. These edemas develop from inadequacy of the left ventricle to maintain adequate stroke volumes. Consequently, left ventricular end-diastolic pressure and volume rise, creating fluid sequestration in pulmonary bed.

- Monitor, assess, and record signs and symptoms of hydrostatic edema.

Inadequate rate, rhythm, and depth of respiration.

Inadequate arterial blood gases, particularly mild to moderate hypoxemia and respiratory alkalosis.

Presence of abnormal breath sounds, particularly crackles or wheezes, as fluid entrapment narrows airways and causes wheezes and accumulation in alveoli of fluid precipitates. Absence of breath sounds may indicate a pneumothorax, a potential complication associated with high levels of positive end-expiratory pressure.

Abnormal chest film, specifically lymphatic enlargement, presence of Kerley B lines, and diffuse haziness.

Presence of excessive bronchial secretions with low protein/serum protein ratios.

- Implement strategies according to either physician's prescriptions or standing unit policies to maintain adequate gas exchange.

Position patient to facilitate optimum expansion of lungs. Most frequently this is achieved in upright, supine position so that diaphragm is lowered. However, severe hypotension often prevents this position and a 30° to 40° supine head elevation is all that can be achieved. If patient is intubated, lateral recumbent positions can be used. Repositioning every hour is advisable to prevent atelectasis and areas of poor ventilation from developing. If unilateral lung involvement exists, rotate between "good"-lung-down and supine positions.

Assist with maintaining or initiating adequate oxygenation therapies: nasal oxygen to endotracheal intubation.

Perform suctioning procedures as necessary. In patients with known coronary artery ischemia, constant observation of ECG is essential to assure rapid identification of abnormalities with subsequent immediate discontinuation of suctioning and reoxygenation. Limit suctioning duration to less than 15 seconds.

Provide information and care to reduce patient's anxiety and fear.

Frequently remind patient that ventilator has taken over the work of breathing but that this is only temporary.

Provide patient with a method of communicating: paper and pencil or alphabet board.

If patient is on controlled ventilation, assess if patient is out of phase with ventilator and supply reassurance and sedation as necessary. Breathing against or out of phase with ventilator can increase myocardial workload and jeopardize a recovering myocardium.

Over the next 4 hours, Mrs. W. became progressively more short of breath and again experienced chest discomfort. Her crackles became progressively more coarse, and a v wave was discerned on her PCWP tracing. A holosystolic murmur was heard over her apex, and she began to have frequent premature ventricular contractions. Arterial blood gases now were pH = 7.59, PaO_2 = 65, $PaCO_2$ = 25. She was intubated and placed on mechanical ventilation. The cardiac index was 1.9 L/min/m², the systemic vascular resistance was 1,800 dyn/sec/cm⁻⁵, and the PCWP was 32 mmHg. Vasoactive drugs were appropriately increased, and Mrs. W. was taken to the cardiac catheterization laboratory. A left-sided catheterization study was performed, which revealed mitral regurgitation, 80% occlusion of the left anterior descending artery, total occlusion of the high lateral circumflex vessel, and 50% occlusion of the low lateral circumflex artery. The right coronary artery was open, and the ventriculogram demonstrated hypokinesis of the anterior and lateral walls. No dyskinetic or akinetic areas were found. The patient was taken to the operating room where a mitral valve replacement was performed and myocardial revascularization was performed on the left anterior descending and lower circumflex vessel. Her postoperative course was unremarkable except for occasional premature ventricular contractions for which she was given procainamide. She was discharged 10 days after surgery.

Approximately 4 weeks later, Mrs. W. was brought to the emergency room by her son, who stated that she had had a seizure at home that morning and ever since was confused and lethargic. On admission her temperature was 105° F (40.5° C), she was experiencing shaking chills, cuff blood pressure was 106/60, heart rate was 120 beats per minute, surgical incisions were intact and revealed no obvious sites of infection, and valve sounds were clear and intact. She was admitted to the critical care unit and a pulmonary artery flow–directed catheter was inserted. Specific values were as follows: RAP = 3 mmHg; PAS = 25 mmHg; PAD = 8 mmHg; PCWP = 7 mmHg; CO = 9 L/min; CI = 3.6 L/min/m²; and SVR = 800 dyn/sec/cm⁻⁵. An arterial line was inserted, and MAP was 62 mmHg. At this point, admission laboratory data returned to reveal her hemoglobin and hematocrit to be 12.0 g/100 ml and 34% and the WBC to be 500 per milliliter. Her leukopenia was thought to be related to her procainamide therapy. Blood, sputum, and urine cultures were obtained. Mrs. W. was placed in reverse isolation, and the procainamide was discontinued. Because of the low filling and arterial pressures, volume replacement with crystalloid and colloid solutions was initiated. Within a 2-hour period the RAP was 7 mmHg and the PCWP was 10 mmHg. The MAP remained at 60 mmHg and the CI fell to 2.5 L/min/m². Dobutamine was initiated for inotropic support and low dose dopamine was started when the urinary output fell to 20 ml per hour. Intubation and mechanical ventilation were instituted as the patient continued to be tachypneic and arterial blood gases demonstrated a PaO_2 of 69 with a non-rebreathing mask on with an oxygen flow of 60%. The MAP continued to fall to 50 mmHg, the cardiac index fell to 1.9 L/min/m², and the SVR rose to 1,800 dyn/sec/cm⁻⁵. The rate of the dobutamine infusion was increased and shortly after, an infusion of norepinephrine was initiated when no response was achieved. A small-dose infusion of phentolamine was also started in an attempt to decrease the systemic vascular resistance and facilitate cardiac output. Specific culture reports were as yet not available so broad-spectrum antibiotics were started. Appropriate nursing diagnosis and actions related to septic shock are listed on p. 168.

■ **NURSING DIAGNOSIS**

Fluid volume deficit, related to massive vasodilation.

OUTCOME STANDARD AND CRITERIA

Fluid volume deficit is adequate as evidenced by:

- Adequate CO/CI: CO = 5 L/min, CI = 2.5-3.5 L/min/m²
- Adequate filling pressures: RAP = 7 mmHg, PCWP = 10-12 mmHg
- Normotension
- Absence of physical signs and symptoms of hypovolemia or hypervolemia
- Adequate electrolyte, hematological, and coagulation profiles
- Adequate urinary output: 0.5 ml per kilogram per hour
- Normal skin turgor and moist mucous membranes

NURSING INTERVENTIONS

- Identify and describe factors of mechanisms that contribute to alterations in volume status associated with shock. In hyperdynamic stages of septic shock significant vasodilation develops, and a relative hypovolemia appears. This is treated with aggressive volume replacement. Careful assessment must take place during the replacement process since if sepsis continues and worsens, patient will gradually or abruptly develop vasoconstriction. Consequently, within 1 hour the nurse may be dealing with a hypovolemic patient and then a hypervolemic patient.
- Monitor, assess, and record signs and symptoms of hypovolemia and hypervolemia:

  CO/CI outside normal parameters.

  Filling pressures above or below normal parameters.

  Alterations in hemodynamic wave configurations. In hypovolemic patients fluctuations in baseline of right atrial pressure occur with inspiration and expiration. Also, in hypovolemic states the arterial wave configuration is characterized by a slow upstroke, a prolonged peak, and a dicrotic notch that is less than one third the height of the curve. (In hypervolemic patients a *v* wave on the PCWP trace indicates regurgitant flow across mitral valve. This can occur with structural damage to mitral valve or as a functional consequence in which excessive dilation of ventricle from volume overload causes mitral valve cusps to fail to approximate, and hence there is regurgitation. Since in this case the patient has had a valve replacement, these above factors do not apply. However, in sepsis there is always a concern that valvular endocarditis can occur, which creates the possibility of erosion around the valve ring which can produce regurgitation.)

  Alterations in skin turgor. In hypervolemic patients pitting edema develops, whereas in hypovolemic situations skin turgor is diminished and tenting occurs. *Tenting* refers to the ability to pinch the skin upwards and have it remain in that position

for a few seconds. Capillary refill is not a useful predictor for mild-to-moderate hypovolemia in adults.[119]

Tachycardia: Tachycardia occurs in both hypo- and hypervolemic states.

Alterations in peripheral pulses. In hypovolemia, weak, thready, easily obliterated pulses are present, in hypervolemia full and bounding pulses are the rule.

Alterations in breath sounds. Hydrostatic pulmonary edema can commonly occur with overaggressive volume replacement.

- Implement strategies according to either physician's prescriptions or standing unit policies to assist in controlling volume status.

  Identify therapies and agents commonly used to control volume status. Recognize specific side effects and specific procedures for administering these agents:

  Crystalloid solutions

  Colloids

  Blood products

  Administer preceding agents per physician's prescriptions or unit routines. During administration observe for signs of hypovolemia or hypervolemia and perform the following:

  Monitor MAP and heart rate consistently and record every 15 minutes. Observe for signs of myocardial ischemia.

  Monitor filling pressures consistently. The pulmonary artery systolic and pulmonary artery diastolic pressures can be constantly displayed since volume is not given through these lines. Their values should be documented every 15 minutes during periods of aggressive fluid replacement. If the right atrial port is not used for fluid administration it should also be monitored constantly. If it is used for volume infusion, parameter recordings should still be obtained every 30 minutes. In patients with known poor left ventricular function, values should be obtained between each 100 to 200 ml of volume infused.

  Obtain CO/CI as needed.

  Monitor and assess for signs of hypovolemia and hypervolemia.

  Monitor and assess electrolyte, hematological, and coagulation parameters.

  Carefully label, verify, and record all fluid administered.

  Observe for development of adverse reactions and record appropriately.

  Monitor and record hourly urinary outputs, nasogastric drainage, or any other measurable output loss.

Calculate and record fluid intake as a cumulative and ongoing process following infusion of every 100 to 200 ml of volume.

The pH was progressively becoming more acidotic and sodium bicarbonate was given. Ventilation was increased and a FiO_2 of 100% with 10 cm of PEEP was required to maintain a PaO_2 of 75 mmHg. An infusion of epinephrine was added and the MAP continued to fall to 39 mmHg; the cardiac index was 0.9 L/min/m² and the systemic vascular resistance was 2,300 dyn/sec/cm⁻⁵. A percutaneous intraaortic balloon pump catheter was inserted, and pumping was initiated. The patient stabilized with a MAP of 40 mmHg and a cardiac index of 1.0 L/min/m² for the next 30 minutes. Gradually over the next 8 hours her MAP returned to 70 mmHg; CI increased to 2.4 L/min/m² and SVR returned to 1,700 dyn/sec/cm⁻⁵. With the patient stabilized, an extensive physical examination revealed a small perirectal abscess from a hemorrhoid. Within 72 hours, the intraaortic balloon and the vasoactive pharmacological support were discontinued. Mrs. W.'s pulmonary function gradually improved and she was extubated 1 week later. Discharge from the hospital occurred 2 weeks later.

REFERENCES

1. Manson, N. H., & Hess, M. L. (1983). Interaction of oxygen free radicals and cardiac sarcoplasmic reticulum: Proposed role in the pathogenesis of endotoxin shock. *Circulatory Shock, 10,* 205-213.
2. Duff, J. H. (1976). Cardiovascular changes in sepsis. *Heart Lung, 5,* 722.
3. MacLean, L. D. (1985). Shock. A century of progress. *Annals of Surgery, 201,* 407-414.
4. Wilson, R. F. (1980). The pathophysiology of shock. *Intensive Care Medicine, 6,* 89-100.
5. Ledingham, I. M. (1989). Cell therapy in shock. *Resuscitation, 18,* S85-S99.
6. Chaudry, I., Ohkawa, M., Clemens, M. G., et al. (1983). Alterations in electron transport and cellular metabolism with shock and trauma. In A. Lefler, & W. Schumer (Eds.), *Molecular and cellular aspects of shock and trauma.* New York: Liss.
7. Granger, D. N., Hollwarth, M. E., & Parks, D. A. (1986). Ischaemia–reperfusion injury: Role of oxygen-derived free radicals. *Acta Physiology Scandinavia, 548,* 47-63.
8. Messmer, K., & Kreimeier, U. (1989). Microcirculatory therapy in shock. *Resuscitation, 18,* S51-S61.
9. Lefer, A. (1984). Role of prostaglandins and thromboxanes in shock states. In A. Altura, A. Lefer, & W. Schumer (Eds.), *Handbook of shock and trauma* (pp. 355-376). New York: Raven.
10. Wilson, M. F., Brachett, D. J., Tompkins, P., et al. (1981). Elevated plasma vasopressor during endotoxin and *E. coli* shock. *Advances in Shock Research, 6,* 15-26.
11. Saba, T. M., & Jaffe, E. (1980). Plasma fibronectin opsonic glycoprotein: Its synthesis by vascular endothelial cells and role in cardiopulmonary integrity after trauma as related in RES function. *American Journal of Medicine, 68,* 577-594.
12. Altura, B. (1980). Reticuloendothelial system and neuro-endocrine stimulation in shock therapy. *Advances in Shock Research, 3,* 3-25.
13. Staub, N. C. (1974). Pulmonary edema. *Physiology Review, 54,* 3-25.
14. Carter, A. J. (1985-1986). Disseminated intravascular coagulation. In M. C. Brain, & C. McCullock (Eds.), *Current therapy in hematology oncology.* St. Louis: Mosby.
15. Snyder, E. L. (Ed.). (1983). *Blood transfusion therapy. A physician's handbook.* Arlington, VA: American Association of Blood Banks.
16. Feinstein, D. I. (1982). Diagnosis and management of disseminated intravascular coagulation: The role of heparin therapy. *Blood, 60,* 284-287.
17. Rasmussen, H., & Ibels, L. (1982). Acute renal failure: multivariate analysis of causes and risk factors. *American Journal of Medicine, 73,* 211-218.
18. Riede, V., Sandritter, W., & Mittermayer, C. (1981). Circulatory shock: A review. *Pathology, 13,* 299-311.
19. Hotter, A. (1989). The pathophysiology of shock brain. *Critical Care Nursing Clinics of North America, 1,* 123-130.
20. Guyton, A. C. (1991). *Textbook of medical physiology* (8th ed.). Philadelphia: Saunders.
21. Wells, S. (1982). Nursing care of patients in shock: Part 3. Evaluating the patient. *American Journal of Nursing, 82,* 1723-1746.
22. Meyers, K., & Hickey, M. (1988). Nursing management of hypovolemic shock. *Critical Care Nursing Quarterly, 11,* 57-67.
23. Billhardt, R., & Rosenbush, S. (1986). Cardiogenic and hypovolemic shock. *Medical Clinics of North America, 70,* 853-876.
24. Houston, M. C., Thompson, W. L., & Robertson, D. (1984). Shock: Diagnosis and management. *Archives of Internal Medicine, 144,* 1433-1439.
25. Collins, J. (1982). The pathophysiology of hemorrhagic shock. In J. Collins (Ed.), *Massive transfusion in surgery and trauma* (pp. 5-29). New York: Liss.
26. Casley-Smith, J. R. (1976). The functioning and interrelationship of blood capillaries and lymphatics. *Experientia, 32,* 1-12.
27. Drucker, W. R., Christopher, D. J., Chadwick, M. D., et al. (1981). Transcapillary refill in hemorrhage and shock. *Archives of Surgery, 116,* 1344-1353.
28. Pirkle, J. C., & Gann, D. S. (1976). Expansion of interstitial fluid is required for full restitution of blood volume after hemorrhage. *Journal of Trauma, 16,* 937-947.
29. Grossman, J., Yalow, A. A., & Wiston, R. E. (1960). Albumin degradation and synthesis influenced by hydrocortisone, corticotropin and infection. *Surgical Forum, 9,* 528-550.
30. Gafford, F., & Ayers, S. (1985). Shock associated with myocardial infarction: Pathophysiology, diag-

nosis, treatment and prevention. In H. McIntosh (Ed.), *Baylor College of Medicine Cardiology Series: Vol. 8* (pp. 6-27). Princeton, NJ: Cardiology Series.

31. Rice, V. (1991). Shock, a clinical syndrome: An update: Part 4. Nursing care of the shock patient. *Critical Care Nurse, 11,* 28-40.

32. Mizock, B. (1983). Septic shock, a metabolic perspective. *Archives of Internal Medicine, 144,* 579-585.

33. Cowley, R. A., & Trump, B. F. (1982). *Pathophysiology of shock, anoxia and ischemia.* Baltimore: Williams & Wilkins.

34. Morrison, D., & Ryan, J. L. (1987). Endotoxins and disease mechanisms. *Annual Review of Medicine, 38,* 417-432.

35. Wilson, M. F., & Brackett, D. J. (1983). Release of vasoactive hormones and circulatory changes in shock. *Circulatory Shock, 11,* 225-234.

36. Tracey, K. J., Lowry, S. F., & Cerami, A. (1987). Physiological responses to cachectin. In: Tumour necrosis factor and related cytoxins. *CIBA Foundation Symposiums, 131,* 88-108.

37. Littleton, M. (1988). Prostaglandins and leukotrienes as mediators of shock and trauma. *Critical Care Nursing Quarterly, 11,* 11-20.

38. Parker, M., Shelhamer, J., & Bacharach, S. (1984). Profound but reversible myocardial depression in patients with septic shock. *Annals of Internal Medicine, 100,* 483-490.

39. DeSantes, D., Phillips, P., Spath, M. A., et al. (1981). Delayed appearance of circulating myocardial depressant factor in burn patients. *Annals of Emergency Medicine, 10,* 22-24.

40. Littleton, M. (1988). Pathophysiology and assessment of sepsis and septic shock. *Critical Care Nursing Quarterly, 11,* 30-47.

41. Abraham, E., Bland, R., & Cobo, J. (1984). Sequential cardiorespiratory patterns associated with outcome in septic shock. *Chest, 85,* 75-79.

42. Trzeciakowski, J. P., & Leu, R. (1982). Reduction of ventricular fibrillation threshold by histamine: Resolution into separate H_1 and H_2 components. *Journal of Pharmacology and Experimental Therapies, 223,* 774-783.

43. Terradellas, J. B., Bellot, J. F., Saris, A. B., et al. (1982). Acute and transient ST segment elevation during bacterial shock in seven patients without apparent heart disease. *Chest, 81,* 444-448.

44. Henning, R. J., Weiner, F., Valdes, S., et al. (1979). Measurement of toe temperature for assessing the severity of acute circulatory failure. *Surgery, Gynecology and Obstetrics, 149,* 1-7.

45. Carlson, R. W., Schaeffer, R. C., Michaels, S. G., et al. (1979). Pulmonary edema fluid. *Circulation, 50,* 1161-1166.

46. Fein, A., Grossman, R. F., & Jones, J. G. (1979). The value of edema fluid protein measured in patients with pulmonary edema. *American Journal of Medicine, 67,* 32-37.

47. Rackow, E. C., & Weil, M. H. (1990). Physiology of blood flow and oxygen utilization by peripheral tissue in circulating shock. *Clinical Chemistry, 36*(8B), 1544-1546.

48. Vincent, J. L., & DuFaye, P. (1983). Serial lactate determination during circulatory shock. *Critical Care Medicine, 11,* 449-451.

49. Lucas, C. E., Rector, F. E., Werner, M., et al. (1973). Altered renal homeostasis with acute sepsis. *Archives of Surgery, 106,* 444-449.

50. Gosche, J., Garrison, N., Harris, P., et al. (1990). Absorptive hyperemia restores intestinal blood flow during *Escherichia coli* sepsis in the rat. *Archives of Surgery, 125,* 1573-1576.

51. Sibbald, W. J. (1979). The Trendelenburg position: Hemodynamic effects in hypotensive and normotensive patients. *Critical Care Medicine, 7,* 218-228.

52. McSwain, N. E. (1988). Pneumatic antishock garment: State of the art 1988. *Annals of Emergency Medicine, 17,* 506-525.

53. Slye, D. A. (1990). The physiologic responses to the use of a pneumatic antishock garment (PASG) in the care of the patient experiencing shock. *Orthopaedic Nursing, 9,* 43-52.

54. Rice, V. (1984). Shock management: Part 1. Fluid volume replacement. *Critical Care Nurse, 4,* 69-82.

55. Weil, M. H., & Rackow, E. C. (1984). A guide to volume repletion. *Emergency Medicine, 16,* 101-110.

56. Ross, A. D., & Angaram, D. M. (1984). Colloids versus crystalloids—a continuing controversy. *Drug Intelligence and Clinical Pharmacy, 18,* 202-212.

57. Shine, K. I., Kuhn, M., Young, L. S., et al. (1980). Aspects of the management of shock. *Annals of Internal Medicine, 93,* 723-734.

58. Collins, J. A., Murawski, K., & Shafer, A. W. (1982). Massive transfusion in surgery and trauma. *Progress in Clinical and Biological Research, 108,* 31-35.

59. Kuhn, M. (1991). Colloids vs crystalloids. *Critical Care Nurse, 11,* 46-51.

60. Faillace, D. F., Ledgerwood, A. M., & Lucas, C. E. (1982). Immunoglobulin changes after varied resuscitation regimens. *Journal of Trauma, 22,* 1-5.

61. Maningas, P. A., Mattox, K., Pepe, P., et al. (1989). Hypertonic saline-dextran solutions for the prehospital management of traumatic hypotension. *American Journal of Surgery, 157,* 528-533.

62. Puri, V. K. (1983). Resuscitation in hypovolemia and shock: A prospective study of hydroxyethyl starch and albumin. *Critical Care Medicine, 11,* 518-523.

63. Haupt, M. T., & Rackow, E. C. (1982). Colloid osmotic pressure and fluid resuscitation with hetastarch, albumin and saline solutions. *Critical Care Medicine, 10,* 159-162.

64. Newman, P. N., Ramsay, G., & Ledingham, I. M. (1986). Cryoprecipitate replacement of fibronectin in septic shock. *Intensive Care Medicine, 12,* 188.

65. Rudowski, W. (1990). Modern oxygen carriers: State of the art 1990. *Materia Medica Polona, 1,* 3-7.

66. Keipert, D. E., Minkovitz, J., & Chang, I. M. S. (1985). Crosslinked stroma-free polyhemoglobin as a

potential blood substitute. *International Journal of Artificial Organs, 5,* 383-385.

67. Wells, S. (1982). Nursing care of patients in shock: Part 1. Pharmacotherapy. *American Journal of Nursing, 82,* 943-964.

68. Richard, C., Recome, J. L., & Remalko, A. (1983). Combined hemodynamic effects of dopamine and dobutamine in cardiogenic shock. *Circulation, 67,* 620-626.

69. Rackow, E. C. (1984). Of shock and vasoactive drugs. *Emergency Medicine, 8,* 115-123.

70. Edwards, J., Brown, C., Nightingale, P., et al. (1989). Use of survivors' cardiorespiratory values as therapeutic goals in septic shock. *Critical Care Medicine, 17,* 1098-1103.

71. Desjars, P., Pinaud, M., Potel, G., et al. (1987). A reappraisal of norepinephrine therapy in human septic shock. *Critical Care Medicine, 15,* 134-137.

72. Chernow, B., & Roth, B. L. (1986). Pharmacologic manipulation of the peripheral vasculature in shock: Clinical and experimental approaches. *Medicine, 13,* 566-570.

73. Rice, V. (1991). Shock, a clinical syndrome: An update: Part 3. Therapeutic management. *Critical Care Nurse, 11,* 34-39.

74. Boyd, J. L., Stanford, G. G., & Chernow, B. (1989). The pharmacotherapy of septic shock. *Critical Care Clinics, 5,* 133-150.

75. LeJemtel, T. H., Keung, E., Sonnenblick, E. H., et al. (1979). Amrinone: A new non-glycosidic, non-adrenergic cardiotonic agent effective in the treatment of intractable myocardial failure in man. *Circulation, 59,* 1098-1104.

76. Bronsveld, W., Van den Bos, G. C., & Thijs, L. G. (1985). Use of glucose-insulin-potassium (GIK) in human septic shock. *Critical Care Medicine, 13,* 566-570.

77. Sanders, M., Kostis, J., & Frishman, W. (1989). The use of inotropic agents in acute and chronic congestive heart failure. *Medical Clinics of North America, 73,* 283-314.

78. Chernow, B. (1988). Glucagon: A potentially important hormone in circulatory shock. *Perspectives in Shock Research, 264,* 284-293.

79. Sonntag, H., Henning, H., & Yoshimine, K. (1990). Cardiovascular and renal haemodynamic effects of dopexamine: comparison with dopamine. *British Journal of Anaesthesiology, 65,* 380-387.

80. Remme, W. J., Wiesfeld, A. C., Look, M. P., et al. (1989). Hemodynamic effects of intravenous pimobendan in patients with left ventricular dysfunction. *Journal of Cardiovascular Pharmacology, 14*(Suppl. II), S41-S44.

81. Woo, P., Carpenter, M. A., & Trunkey, D. D. (1979). Ionized calcium: The effect of septic shock in the human. *Journal of Surgical Research, 26,* 605-611.

82. Harrigan, C., Lucas, C. E., & Ledgewood, A. M. (1983). Significance of hypocalcemia following hypovolemic shock. *Journal of Trauma, 23,* 488-493.

83. Chiariello, M. (1976). Comparison between the effects of nitroprusside and nitroglycerin on ischemic injury during acute myocardial infarction. *Circulation, 54,* 766-772.

84. Cerra, F., Hassett, J., & Siegel, J. (1978). Vasodilator therapy in clinical sepsis with low-output syndromes. *Journal of Surgical Research, 25,* 180-183.

85. Peter, T., Norris, R. M., Clark, E. D., et al. (1978). Reduction of enzyme levels by propranolol after acute myocardial infarction. *Circulation, 57,* 1091-1099.

86. Geddes, J. S., Adgey, A. A., & Pantridge, J. F. (1980). Prevention of cardiogenic shock. *American Heart Journal, 99,* 243-254.

87. Nicholson, D. (1989). Review of corticosteroid treatment in sepsis and septic shock. *Critical Care Clinics, 5,* 151-155.

88. Bone, R. C., Fisher, C. J., & Clemmer, J. P. (1987). A controlled clinical trial of high dose methyl-prednisolone in the treatment of severe sepsis and septic shock. *New England Journal of Medicine, 317,* 653.

89. The Veterans Administration System Cooperative Study Group. (1987). Effect of high-dose glucocorticoid therapy on mortality in patients with clinical signs of systemic sepsis. *New England Journal of Medicine, 317,* 659.

90. Price, C. (1991). Continuous renal replacement therapy: The treatment of choice for acute renal failure. *ANNA Journal, 18,* 239-244.

91. Warnholtz, A., Slater, A. D., & Golper, T. A. (1991). Continuous arteriovenous hemofiltration in the critically ill patient. *Journal of the Kentucky Medical Association, 89,* 111-114.

92. Paganini, E. P. (1986). *Acute continuous renal replacement therapy.* Boston: Martinus Nijhoff.

93. Roach, A. C. (1990). Antibiotic therapy in septic shock. *Critical Care Nursing Clinics of North America, 2,* 179-186.

94. Hanson, G. (1988). Management of patients with shock and sepsis. *Blood Reviews, 2,* 134-139.

95. Umeki, S., Adachi, M., Watanabe, M., et al. (1988). Gabexate as a therapy for disseminated intravascular coagulation. *Archives of Internal Medicine, 148,* 1409-1412.

96. Takada, A., Takada, Y., Mori, T., et al. (1990). Prevention of severe bleeding by tranexamic acid in a patient with disseminated intravascular coagulation. *Thrombosis Research, 58,* 101-108.

97. Oguma, Y., Sakuragawa, N., Maki, M., et al. (1991). Clinical effect of low molecular weight heparin on DIC: A multicenter cooperative study in Japan. *Thrombosis Research, 59,* 37-49.

98. Baumgartner, J. D., Glaucer, M. P., & McCutchan, J. A. (1985). Prevention of gram-negative shock and death in surgical patients by antibody to endotoxin core glycolipid. *Lancet, 11,* 59-63.

99. Baumgartner, J. D., & Glauser, M. P. (1987). Immunotherapy of life-threatening gram-negative infections: Facts and controversies. In J. L. Vincent, & L. G. Thijs (Eds.), *Update in intensive care and emergency medicine: Vol. 4. Septic shock European view* (pp. 248-259). Berlin: Springer-Verlag.

100. Reines, H. D., Halushka, P. V., Olanoff, L. S., et al. (1985). Dazoxiben in human sepsis and adult respiratory distress syndrome. *Clinical Pharmacology Therapy, 37,* 391-396.

101. Bihari, D. J., & Tinker, J. (1988). The therapeutic value of vasodilator prostaglandins in multiple organ failure associated with sepsis. *Intensive Care Medicine, 15,* 2-7.

102. Rock, P., Silverman, H., Plump, D., et al. (1985). Efficacy and safety of naloxone in septic shock. *Critical Care Medicine, 13,* 28-33.

103. Bonnet, F., Bilaine, J., & Lhoste, F. (1985). Naloxane therapy in human septic shock. *Critical Care Medicine, 13,* 972-975.

104. Miyazaki, M., Okuda, C., & Mizobe, T. (1989). Pathophysiology of circulatory shock: An overview. *Magnesium, 8,* 163-178.

105. Aderka, D. (1991). Role of tumor necrosis factor in the pathogenesis of intravascular coagulopathy of sepsis: Potential new therapeutic implications. *Israel Journal of Medicine Sciences, 27,* 52-60.

106. Dinarello, C. A. (1991). The proinflammatory cytokines interleukin-1 and tumor necrosis factor and treatment of the septic shock syndrome. *Journal of Infectious Disease, 163,* 1177-1184.

107. Ream, A. K., & Fogdall, R. P. (1982). *Acute cardiovascular management: Anesthesia and intensive care.* Philadelphia: Lippincott.

108. Soroff, H. S. (1974). External counterpulsation: Management of cardiogenic shock after myocardial infarction. *Journal of the American Medical Association, 229,* 1441-1445.

109. Amsterdam, E. A. (1980). Clinical assessment of external pressure circulatory assistance in acute myocardial infarction. *American Journal of Cardiology, 45,* 349-353.

110. Alcan, K., Stertzer, S., & Wallsh, E. (1984). Current status of intra-aortic balloon counterpulsation in critical care cardiology. *Critical Care Medicine, 12,* 489-493.

111. Pennington, D. (1989). Emergency management of cardiogenic shock. *Circulation, 79,* I149-I151.

112. Raper, R., & Fisher, M. M. (1988). Profound reversible myocardial depression after anaphylaxis. *Lancet, 560,* 386-389.

113. Rutan, P. M., Rountree, W. D., & Myers, K. K. (1989). Initial experience with the hemopump. *Critical Care Nursing Clinics of North America, 1,* 527-534.

114. Johnson, D. (1989). Hemopump regulatory update. *Nimbus News, 1,* 1.

115. Rose, D. M., Connolly, M., & Cunningham, J. (1989). Technique and results with a roller pump left and right heart assist device. *Annals of Thoracic Surgery, 47,* 124-130.

116. Marchetta, S., & Stennis, E. (1988). Ventricular assist devices: Applications for critical care. *Journal of Cardiovascular Nursing, 2,* 39-46.

117. Miller, K., & Pitz, K. (1989). Symbion acute ventricular assist device: Nursing challenge. *Critical Care Nurse, 8,* 143-151.

118. Icenogel, T. B., Williams, R. J., & Smith, R. G. (1989). Extracorporeal pulsatile biventricular support after cardiac transplantation. *Annals of Thoracic Surgery, 47,* 614-621.

119. Schriger, D. (1991). Capillary refill—is it a useful predictor of hypovolemic states? *Annals of Emergency Medicine, 20,* 601-605.

8

Fluid and Electrolyte Balance

Charold L. Baer

The life of every individual depends on the maintenance of a stable internal environment. That internal environment is composed of water, electrolytes, and metabolic end products. In a normal, healthy person, the internal environment is regulated and maintained by a variety of physiological functions. However, when a person experiences a critical illness due to an acute or chronic pathological condition, the normal homeostatic mechanisms of the body are often not sufficient to maintain a stable internal environment. As a result, alterations in the internal environment occur and directly affect the individual's physiological functioning, physical appearance, and behavior. Indeed, these alterations may be severe enough to precipitate the individual's death. Therefore, it is essential that the patient receive supportive care from the health care team during this period of instability.

All members of the health care team play important supportive roles in the patient's care during this time, but much of the responsibility resides with the nurse because of proximity and the amount of time spent with the individual. Because the nurse has the most frequent, consistent, and extensive contact with the patient, he or she can quickly detect changes in patterns of function or behavior. The nurse's responsibilities in relation to alterations in a patient's internal environment include (1) monitoring, (2) interpreting, (3) reporting and recording, (4) intervening, and (5) evaluating. Figure 8-1 illustrates this relationship.

As depicted in Figure 8-1, the nurse's responsibilities are implemented in response to the external manifestations exhibited by the individual because of the alterations in the internal environment. The nurse functions in a systematic manner that begins with *monitoring*. This includes observing the patient as well as assessing all laboratory and technological data. Monitoring is followed by *interpreting*, which involves using one's knowledge of the individual's history, physiology, and pathophysiology to determine if the information gained from monitoring is

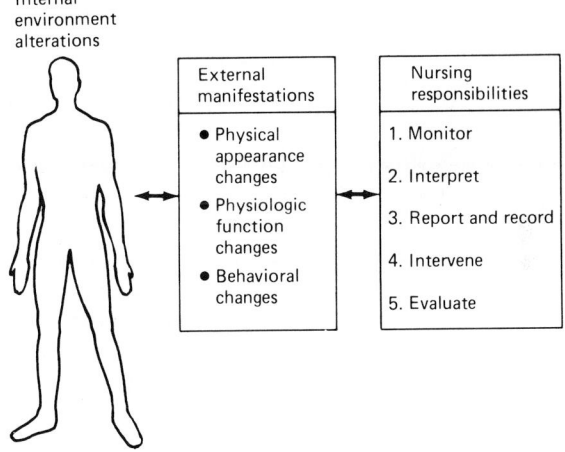

Figure 8-1 Nursing responsibilities related to alterations in an individual's internal environment.

normal or abnormal for the patient and to what degree. Then the information is *reported* and *recorded*. This responsibility is important because in order to provide quality care, periodic assessments of the patient must be documented as well as conveyed to the physician.

The next responsibility of the nurse is *intervening*. Intervening is the essence of health care, whether it is based on nursing or medical prescriptions. Intervening means *action*, and it is action that makes the impact on the individual's health state. A nurse could monitor, interpret, report, and record forever, but unless there is action taken on the basis of those functions, the patient's condition may continue to deteriorate. All action, however, must be based on sufficient data because to intervene inappropriately could also threaten the individual's stability.

The final responsibility of the nurse is to *evaluate* the results of the intervention on the basis of the desired patient outcomes or, in other words, to find out if the actions taken altered the individual's health state.

These five responsibilities or functions, performed at periodic intervals as determined by the health state of the patient, provide the framework for delivering nursing care.

The implementation of these nursing responsibilities has a significant impact on the care of the patient with an altered internal environment. To perform these responsibilities, the nurse must have a basic comprehension of the components of the internal environment. This discussion is designed to provide information prerequisite to that understanding.

DISTRIBUTION OF BODY FLUIDS
Total Body Water

The total body water of an adult is approximately 60% of the total body weight in kilograms. This percentage varies according to the muscle mass, amount of body fat, and age of the individual. Since muscles contain a high proportion of water, someone with a large muscle mass would have a higher percentage of total body water than someone with less muscle mass. Fat contains less water than lean tissues, so individuals with more body fat tend to have a lower percentage of total body water. These two facts explain why females have lower percentages of total body water than males. Age also affects the percentage of total body water; as a person ages, the percentage decreases. Therefore, a lean, young adult male would theoretically have the highest percentage of total body water, while an obese, elderly female would have the lowest.

Amounts and Distribution

The total body water of an individual is distributed into several different compartments. The two principal compartments are the intracellular and extracellular fluid spaces. The *intracellular fluid space* includes all the water contained within the cells, including the red blood cells, which are also designated as part of the intravascular fluid. The *extracellular fluid space* includes the water contained in several smaller fluid compartments. Among these compartments are the interstitial, plasma, transcellular, bone, and connective tissue spaces. Of these fluid spaces, the interstitial and plasma spaces contain functional, or accessible, extracellular fluid, while the transcellular (pleural, peritoneal, joint, and cerebrospinal fluid spaces), bone, and connective tissue spaces contain nonfunctional, or nonaccessible, extracellular fluid. Each of these fluid compartments or spaces contains a percentage of the individual's total body water. Figure 8-2 illustrates the distribution of the total body water throughout the compartments by percentage of body weight for a normal, healthy adult male. It also indicates that there is an additional fluid compartment, the *intravascular space,* that contains both ex-

TABLE 8-1 Distribution of Total Body Water per Compartment in Percentage of Body Weight and Liter Volume for a Normal, Healthy Adult Male and Female

Compartment	70-kg Male		60-kg Female	
	% Body Weight	Volume, L	% Body Weight	Volume, L
Intracellular	32.5	23	27.5	17
Red blood cells	3	2	3	2
Other cells	29.5	21	24.5	15
Extracellular	27.5	19	27.5	17
Interstitial	12.5	9	12.5	7
Plasma	4.5	3	4.5	3
Transcellular	1.5	1	1.5	1
Bone	4.5	3	4.5	3
Connective tissue	4.5	3	4.5	3
Intravascular*	7.5	5	7.5	5
Red blood cells	3	2	3	2
Plasma	4.5	3	4.5	3

* Combination of intracellular and extracellular fluid.

tracellular and intracellular fluid. The percentages of body water shown in Figure 8-2 are translated into liter volumes for a normal, healthy 70-kg male and 60-kg female in Table 8-1.

ELECTROLYTE COMPOSITION OF BODY FLUIDS

An individual's internal environment does not consist merely of water; it also contains numerous electrolytes. These electrolytes are essential to a variety of physiological functions. The specific physiological functions in which each electrolyte participates are delineated in the discussion of each electrolyte later in this chapter. The electrolytes are present in different amounts in the major fluid compartments of the body. Table 8-2 presents the approximate amount of each of the electrolytes in the major fluid compartments.

OSMOLALITY, OSMOLARITY, AND TONICITY

The distribution of body fluids in the different compartments depends primarily on the osmotic pressure that exists in those spaces. This osmotic pressure is referred to as the osmolality, osmolarity, or tonicity of the fluid in the space.

Definitions

Osmolality is the concentration of solute, expressed in terms of the number of particles per liter

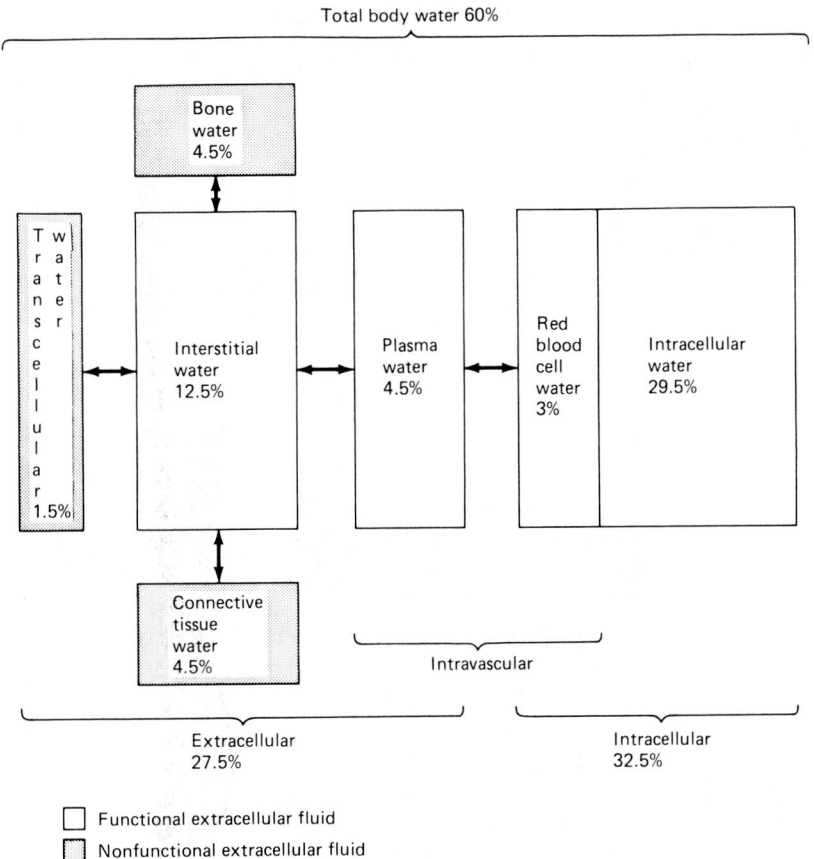

Figure 8-2   The distribution of total body water by compartment according to the percentage of body weight for a normal healthy adult male.

TABLE 8-2   Approximate Electrolyte Composition of the Major Fluid Compartments of the Body in Milliequivalents per Liter

Ions	Plasma	Interstitial Fluid	Intracellular Fluid
Cations			
Na	142	145	10
K	4.5	4	135
Ca	5	3	10
Mg	2.5	2	25
Totals	154	154	180
Anions			
Cl	104	115	5
HCO$_3$	24	27	10
HPO$_4$	2	2	100
SO$_4$	1	1	5
Organic acid	6	7	10
Protein	17	2	50
Totals	154	154	180

of *solvent. Osmolarity* is the concentration of solute, expressed in terms of the number of particles per liter of *solution. Tonicity* describes the comparison of the osmolality or osmolarity of one solution to another. If solution A has a higher osmolality than solution B, solution A is described as being hypertonic to solution B. Solution B, on the other hand, is hypotonic to solution A, because solution B has a lower osmolality. If both solutions were of equal osmolality, they would be described as being isotonic to each other. Such is the case with the body fluids of the normal individual.

Osmolality and osmolarity concentration measurements are so similar in dilute solutions, such as the body fluids, that they are often used interchangeably. The two measurements are not obtained by the same method, however, and the laboratory should specify which measurement is being reported. In most cases, the laboratories use a freezing-point method of determining concentration that measures osmolality. Hence, the term *osmolality* tends to be used more frequently when discussing the concentration of body fluids.

Osmolality and osmolarity are both measured in milliosmoles. A milliosmole is $\frac{1}{1,000}$ of an osmole. An osmole, the unit for measuring osmotic pressure, is equal to the number of particles in 1 g molecular weight of a dissolved, nondiffusible, nonionizable substance. The normal osmolality of extracellular and intracellular body fluids is approximately 280 to 295 mosm/L.

Regulation

The osmolality of body fluids is regulated by the osmoreceptor–antidiuretic hormone system and thirst. The osmoreceptor–antidiuretic hormone system involves the functions of the hypothalamus, neurohypophysis, antidiuretic hormone, and renal tubules, while thirst is primarily associated with the hypothalamus.

The Osmoreceptor–Antidiuretic Hormone System

The osmoreceptor–antidiuretic hormone system responds to alterations in the osmolality of the body fluids of as little as 1% to 2%. The response begins with the osmoreceptors that regulate the release of antidiuretic hormone. The osmoreceptors are specialized neurons located in or near the supraoptic nuclei of the anterior hypothalamus. These neurons contain fluid chambers filled with intracellular fluid that continuously emit nerve impulses. The fluid chambers respond specifically to changes in the extracellular fluid concentration, with sodium being the most effective stimulant. When the osmolality of the extracellular fluid decreases, making it hypotonic to the fluid in the chambers, water enters the fluid chambers to establish equilibrium between the two fluids. The influx of water forces the fluid chambers to swell, leading to a decreased rate of impulse discharge. This means that fewer impulses are transmitted from the osmoreceptors in the supraoptic nuclei through the pituitary stalk to the neurohypophysis to promote the release of antidiuretic hormone. Thus, as illustrated in Figure 8-3, less antidiuretic hormone is secreted.

When the extracellular fluid osmolality increases, the reverse of the process occurs. The increase in osmolality creates extracellular fluid that is hypertonic to the fluid in the chambers. Water then leaves the fluid chambers and flows into the extracellular fluid, shifting the system toward equilibrium. This outflow of water results in a shrinking of the fluid chambers and an increase in the rate of impulse discharge to the neurohypophysis. The net effect, as shown in Figure 8-4, is an increased secretion of antidiuretic hormone.

Antidiuretic hormone is synthesized in the supraoptic and paraventricular nuclei of the hypothalamus and stored as granules in the posterior pituitary.

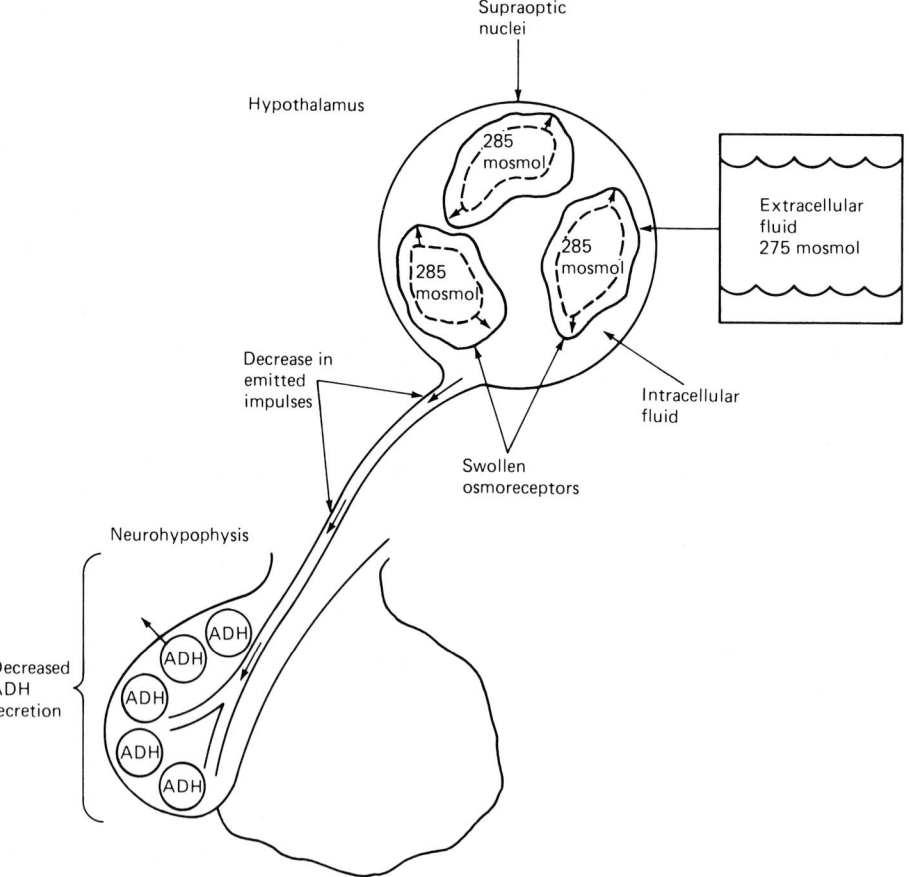

Figure 8-3   The osmoreceptor–antidiuretic hormone system response to decreased extracellular fluid osmolality.

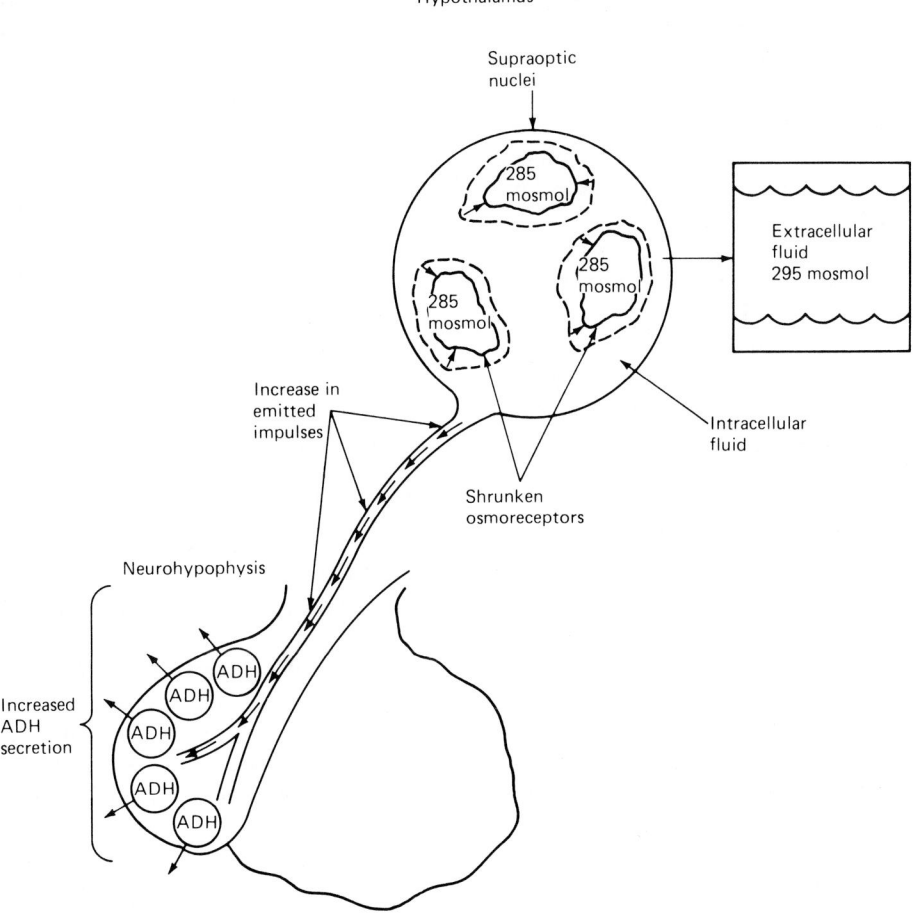

Figure 8-4   The osmoreceptor–antidiuretic hormone system response to increased extracellular fluid osmolality.

It is secreted into the blood according to the rate of impulses transmitted from the osmoreceptors to the neurohypophysis. Once it is in the blood, it circulates to the kidneys and acts on the distal tubules and collecting ducts to increase water reabsorption. Thus, the more antidiuretic hormone secreted, the more water reabsorbed.

In summary, the osmoreceptor–antidiuretic hormone system responds to a decrease in extracellular fluid osmolality by decreasing the secretion of antidiuretic hormone, resulting in less water reabsorption, more water excretion, and a return of the osmolality to normal. Conversely, the system reacts to an increase in extracellular fluid osmolality by increasing the secretion of antidiuretic hormone, resulting in more water reabsorption, less water excretion, and a return of the osmolality to normal.

Thirst

Thirst, the primary regulator of water intake, is also an important mechanism in regulating the osmolality of body fluids. The hypothalamus contains a thirst center that slightly overlaps the osmoreceptor area. Thirst is stimulated by the effect of intracellular dehydration on the neurons in the thirst center. It is inhibited by the act of drinking and by fullness of the gastrointestinal tract. These two states excite peripheral sensory receptors that transmit impulses to the thirst center to decrease the thirst. Thus, the thirst mechanism is actually inhibited *before* the intracellular dehydration is alleviated. This is a protective feedback mechanism to prevent voluntary water intoxication.

Calculating Osmolality Values

The most accurate method for determining osmolality is direct measurement. Plasma osmolality can be quickly and accurately measured by determining its freezing point, since the freezing point of a solution decreases in direct proportion to its osmolality. If the plasma osmolality has not been measured, however, it can still be calculated or estimated using other serum laboratory values. It has been found that in normal plasma, the osmotic coefficients and other solute concentrations cancel each other in such a manner that the sodium concentration multiplied by two equals the plasma osmolality. The plasma osmolality, however, is also significantly influenced by glucose and urea, so they must be included in the calculation. In order to include glucose and urea in a formula for determining plasma osmolality, their values must be converted to milliosmoles. A simplified formula for including sodium, glucose, and urea in the calculation of plasma osmolality is:

$$2 \text{ Na (mEq/L)} + \frac{\text{Glucose (mg/100 ml)}}{18}$$
$$+ \frac{\text{BUN (mg/100 ml)}}{3}$$
$$= \text{serum osmolality (mosm/L)}$$

The formula would be applied in the following manner:

Individual's serum laboratory values:

$$\text{Na} = 140 \text{ meq/L}$$

$$\text{Glucose} = 90 \text{ mg/100 ml}$$

$$\text{BUN} = 18 \text{ mg/100 ml}$$

$$2(140) + \frac{90}{18} + \frac{18}{3} = \text{serum osmolality (mosm/L)}$$

$$280 + 5 + 6 = 291 \text{ mosm/L}$$

This calculated value would provide a close approximation of the actual serum osmolality.

TRANSPORT PROCESSES

The processes involved in the transport of fluids and electrolytes include osmosis, diffusion, active transport, filtration, pinocytosis, and phagocytosis. Each of these processes affects the movement of fluids and electrolytes in a specific way.

Osmosis

Osmosis is a process that results from the kinetic motion of molecules in solution on either side of a semipermeable membrane. The motion of the molecules is such that water will pass through the membrane to the side that has the greater concentration of nondiffusible substances. This process results in a movement toward establishing equilibrium between the concentration of the solutions on either side of the membrane.

Osmosis can be negated by applying a pressure gradient across the semipermeable membrane in a direction opposite to that of the water flow. The amount of pressure required to negate osmosis is called the *osmotic pressure* of the solution.

Diffusion

Diffusion is the net movement of a given substance from one point to another due to the random kinetic motions of its molecules. Molecules diffuse from areas of higher concentration to areas of lower concentration. The net effect of this continuous kinetic movement is the establishment of an equal concentration of the substance throughout the medium, be it liquid, solid, or gas.

The rate at which diffusion occurs is determined by (1) the concentration gradient, (2) the cross-sectional area of the container or chamber, (3) the temperature of the solution, (4) the molecular weight of the molecules, and (5) the distance the molecules have to travel. The greater the concentration gradient, cross-sectional area, and temperature, the greater the diffusion rate. The greater the molecular weight and distance, the lower the diffusion rate.

Active Transport

The process of moving a substance against a concentration, electrical or pressure gradient is called *active transport*. In active transport, energy must be expended to move the substance against the gradient across the cell membrane. The energy that is expended probably comes from the adenosine triphosphate that is available in large quantities just inside the cell membrane.

Filtration

Filtration is the process of moving water and dissolved substances through a permeable membrane from an area of higher pressure to an area of lower pressure. In the sense described here, filtration results from the hydrostatic pressure produced by the pumping action of the heart. Filtration is opposed by the oncotic pressure created by proteins in the solution.

Pinocytosis and Phagocytosis

Pinocytosis and phagocytosis are transport processes that move substances across cell membranes by invagination and ingestion. Pinocytosis is the process of transporting primarily proteins and strong electrolyte solutions by invagination. Invagination functions in the following manner: (1) Molecules in the extracellular fluid approach the surface of a cell. (2) Absorption causes the molecules to adhere to the cell surface. (3) The molecules alter the surface tension of the cell membrane. (4) The cell membrane folds inward, pulling the adhering molecules with it. (5) The outer edges of the cell membrane then rejoin to form a continuous cell wall. (6) The result is a cell with a pinocytic vesicle incorporated within its walls. Pinocytosis seems to be the only way of transporting proteins through the cell membrane.

Phagocytosis is the process of transporting large particles of selected matter by cellular ingestion. Ingestion occurs in the same sequence of steps as invagination. The only difference is that a phagocytic vesicle is formed rather than a pinocytic vesicle. Phagocytosis is an efficient method of eradicating selected matter such as bacteria, other cells, and degenerating tissue. In order for matter to be selected for phagocytosis, it must have the following characteristics: (1) a rough, irregular surface; (2) an electropositive surface charge; and (3) the ability to adhere to the phagocytic cell. This third characteristic is enhanced by the antibodies called *opsonins* that combine with the particles.

FLUID AND ELECTROLYTE REQUIREMENTS

In discussing the daily fluid and electrolyte requirements for the normal adult, the following must be considered: (1) the average daily fluid intake and output, and (2) the composition of specific body fluids.

Average Daily Fluid Intake and Output

The average daily fluid intake and output volumes are reflections of the net fluid gains and losses of the body from all sources. Table 8-3 provides a list of the sources and ranges of the volumes for those gains and losses. It is significant to note that in the healthy adult who is in a state of dynamic equilibrium, the volumes of the gains and losses are equal.

Composition of Specific Body Fluids

Each of the specific fluids in the body has its own composition. Table 8-4 presents an analysis of the body fluids in terms of their major cations, anions, and water compositions.

Alterations in Fluid and Electrolyte Requirements

Healthy adults deal with alterations in the water and electrolyte composition of their body fluids by the normal process of ingestion. They eat and drink the appropriate foods and fluids to maintain the equilibrium of their internal environment. However, when adults experience dysfunction, they often cannot cope

TABLE 8-3   Average Adult Daily Fluid Intake and Output

Intake		Output	
Source	Volume, ml	Source	Volume, ml
Water from fluids	500–1,700	Urine	800–1,600
Water from food	800–1,000	Vapor from lungs and skin	600–1,200
Water from oxidation	200–300	Feces	100–200
Total	1,500–3,000	Total	1,500–3,000

TABLE 8-4   Water and Electrolyte Composition of Selected Body Fluids

Body Fluid	Na, mEq/L	K, mEq/L	Cl, mEq/L	HCO_3, mEq/L	Water, ml/day
Cerebrospinal fluid	140	3.3	130	24	500
Sweat	45	5	60	—	500
Saliva	40	20	30	30	1,500
Gastric juice	60	10	85	—	2,500
Bile	150	5	100	40	500
Pancreatic juice	140	5	75	120	700
Small bowel fluid	110	5	105	20	3,000
Normal feces	10	10	15	—	100
Loose feces	80	30	60	—	3,000+
Urine	90	80	90	—	1,500

with the alterations in their internal environment and require professional assistance. In the process of receiving this assistance, they often develop additional changes in the water and electrolyte composition of their body fluids. As a result, they may experience a variety of undesirable physiological, psychological, and behavioral changes due to the alterations.

The alterations individuals experience are due to varying levels of the following substances in the body: water, sodium, potassium, calcium, magnesium, chloride, phosphates, sulfates, proteins, and organic acids. The remainder of this chapter discusses the functions, regulation, and variances of each of these substances. The variances for most of the substances are presented in terms of the following framework: definition, etiology, clinical assessment parameters, laboratory assessment data, clinical and nursing implications, and treatment.

WATER
Functions

The functions of water in the body are (1) to provide the internal medium for cell metabolism, (2) to transport nutrients and waste products, (3) to participate in chemical and metabolic processes, (4) to provide a lubricant for moving parts, and (5) to participate in the regulation of body heat.

Regulation

The regulation of body water is accomplished by the complex action and interaction of the following: the renal concentration and dilution of urine, circulating angiotensin II, antidiuretic hormone, and thirst.

Renal Concentration of Urine

The kidneys produce a concentrated urine by conserving body water while excreting solute. The concentration process occurs primarily through the countercurrent mechanism that takes place within the renal medullary interstitium. It is composed of two processes: countercurrent multiplication and countercurrent exchange.

The countercurrent multiplication process occurs in the loop of Henle and is the mechanism that enables the body to excrete urine that has an osmolality higher than that of serum. The process facilitates this phenomenon by creating hypertonic medullary interstitial fluid from the generation of multiplying osmotic gradients through the active transport of sodium and chloride from the impermeable ascending limb of the loop of Henle.

The countercurrent exchange process is the maintenance component of the countercurrent mechanism. This process involves the vasa recta, blood vessels that are looped around the tubules in the renal medullary interstitium. The vasa recta minimize the loss of solute from the interstitium by passive diffusion, thus maintaining the osmotic gradients necessary for the countercurrent multiplication process.

Both of these processes involved in the countercurrent mechanism are significantly affected by the secretion of antidiuretic hormone. Antidiuretic hormone increases the permeability of the renal collecting ducts to water, which assists in producing an osmotically concentrated urine. Antidiuretic hormone also assists in maintaining the hypertonic medullary interstitium by decreasing the rate of blood flow through the vasa recta of the medulla.

Renal Dilution of Urine

The ability of the kidney to affect body water by excreting excessive water in dilute urine is dependent upon two mechanisms. The first mechanism is the active transport of sodium and chloride from the impermeable ascending limb of the loop of Henle. This mechanism results in a glomerular filtrate that is hypotonic to the plasma. The second mechanism is the decreased reabsorption of water that occurs in the collecting ducts due to their decreased permeability. The result of this mechanism is that the filtrate remains hypotonic and a dilute urine is excreted.

Circulating Angiotensin II

Circulating angiotensin II affects body water by increasing the passive reabsorption of water to increase the total volume. Angiotensin II is the potent vasoconstrictor produced via the renin–angiotensin system in response to a real or perceived decrease in arterial pressure or extracellular fluid volume, or an alteration in the renal intratubular sodium load. Angiotensin II not only promotes vasoconstriction but also stimulates the suprarenal cortex to secrete al-

dosterone. Aldosterone facilitates the active reabsorption of sodium, passive reabsorption of water, and active secretion of potassium in the renal tubules. The net effect of these processes is an increase in body water.

Antidiuretic Hormone and Thirst

The effects of antidiuretic hormone and thirst on body water are to conserve and replace it. The mechanisms by which antidiuretic hormone and thirst achieve their results were outlined previously in the discussion regarding osmolality.

Variances

The variances or imbalances associated with body water are hypervolemia and hypovolemia. These labels indicate expansion and contraction of body water, but they do not indicate what type of expansion or contraction has occurred. To provide that information, the expansion or contraction would need to be further categorized as isosmotic, hyperosmotic, or hyposmotic in relation to normal plasma. This additional categorization would assist the health care personnel in understanding the imbalance more completely. For example, an isosmotic contraction would indicate that the individual had lost equal amounts of solute and water. A hyposmotic expansion would indicate that the individual had gained more water than solute in the process of achieving the imbalance. Obviously, applying this additional classification to the individual's health state necessitates understanding the etiology of the existing imbalance.

Hypervolemia

Definition and Etiology

Hypervolemia is an excess in extracellular fluid volume. It has many specific causes, but the following three general factors seem to be common to all: (1) increased sodium and water levels due to retention, or excessive intake, or both; (2) decreased renal excretion of water and sodium; and (3) decreased mobilization of fluid within the intravascular space.

Some specific causes of an excess in extracellular fluid volume are excessive ingestion or intravenous infusion of sodium chloride, renal dysfunction, inappropriate secretion of antidiuretic hormone, excessive use of adrenal cortical hormone therapy, hyperaldosteronism, hypoproteinemia, cirrhosis, and cardiac dysfunction.

Data Acquisition

Physical Assessment. Clinically, an individual experiencing hypervolemia might exhibit any combination of the following signs and symptoms: acute weight gain, usually in excess of 5% of the total body weight; systemic, peripheral edema that may be pitting in nature; puffy eyelids; ascites; increased central venous pressure; hypertension; bounding pulse; dyspnea; and moist rales in the lungs.

Based on these signs and symptoms, the nurse would focus on the following clinical parameters to assess an individual for the presence of hypervolemia: body weight, skin turgor and elasticity, central venous pressure, blood pressure, pulse, respiratory patterns, lung auscultation, cardiac auscultation, and in some cases abdominal girth and neck vein distension.

Diagnostic Procedures. Data obtained from laboratory testing of blood and urine samples can provide the nurse with valuable information in assessing an individual's internal environment. To interpret the data reported, the nurse must know the normal values for those items tested. Each institution has its own set of standardized normal values that have been calibrated and calculated according to the specific equipment used, but in most cases the normal values tend to be very similar. Table 8-5 presents the normal values for selected substances, frequently tested for in the blood, and Table 8-6 presents normal values for selected substances frequently tested for in the urine.

Laboratory assessment data may be of dubious assistance in determining the presence of excessive extracellular fluid volume, particularly if the imbalance is isotonic. However, the following changes are often present: decreased serum values for hematocrit, hemoglobin, and red blood cell counts; and decreased urine values for sodium and specific gravity. Depending upon the etiology of the imbalance, there may also be an increase or a decrease in the serum sodium and an increase in the serum blood urea nitrogen and creatinine values.

TABLE 8-5 Normal Values for Selected Serum Laboratory Tests

Item	Normal Values*
Sodium	136-146 mEq/L
Potassium	3.5-5.5 mEq/L
Chloride	96-106 mEq/L
BUN	9-20 mg/100 ml
Creatinine	0.7-1.5 mg/100 ml
Calcium	8.5-10.5 mg/100 ml
Phosphorus	2.0-4.5 mg/100 ml
Carbon dioxide combining power	24-28 mEq/L
Magnesium	1.6-2.2 mEq/L
Osmolality	280-295 mosm/kg H_2O
Hematocrit	40% to 50%
Hemoglobin	12-16 g/100 ml

* Values given are eclectic and for adults.

TABLE 8-6 Normal Values for Selected Urine Laboratory Tests

Item	Normal Values*
Amount	1,200-1,500 ml
Specific gravity	1.003-1.030
pH	5.0-8.0
Creatinine	1.0-1.6 g/24-hour period
Osmolality	50-1,200 mosm/kg H_2O
Sodium	50-130 mEq/L
Potassium	20-70 mEq/L
Chloride	50-130 mEq/L
Calcium	5-12 mEq/L
Phosphorus	1 g/24-hour period
Magnesium	2-18 mEq/L

* Values given are eclectic and for adults.

Medical and Nursing Management

The primary clinical implication of hypervolemia for the individual is that it could result in pulmonary edema, a life-threatening complication.

The nursing implications of hypervolemia include performing both monitoring functions and therapeutic interventions. The specific monitoring functions are (1) to measure all intake and output precisely; (2) to maintain accurate records of all intake and output; (3) to obtain accurate daily weights; (4) to monitor all vital signs frequently; and (5) to observe for peripheral dependent, systemic, and pulmonary edema.

Therapeutic interventions include (1) providing only those fluids and foods that are consistent with the restrictions; (2) administering prescribed diuretics appropriately; and (3) infusing intravenous fluids (if prescribed) at a constant, appropriate rate. Excessive extracellular fluid volume is usually treated by eradicating or dealing therapeutically with the causative factors and decreasing the excess volume. Decreasing the excess volume often involves using diuretics, fluid and sodium restrictions, and in some cases, dialysis therapy.

Edema

Edema is often associated with hypervolemia. However, edema, can, and does, accompany other imbalances as well as many pathological conditions. Indeed, edema is such a common occurrence that it warrants further discussion.

Definition and Etiology

Edema is an excessive accumulation of interstitial fluid. It may be either localized or generalized. Localized edema results from either the activation of the inflammatory process or the decreased physiological

TABLE 8-7 **Factors Influencing Edema Formation**

Factor	Clinical Examples
Sustained increase in capillary pressure	Dependent venous stasis Thrombophlebitis
Decreased plasma oncotic pressure	Starvation–catabolic states Nephrotic syndrome
Decreased tissue pressure	Malnutrition Glucocorticosteroid therapy
Increased capillary permeability	Burns Infection
Lymphatic obstruction	Neoplasms Burns
Dilation of precapillary sphincters	Insect toxins Inflammation

ability to remove interstitial fluid from a specific area of the body. Generalized edema results from clinical dysfunction in a primary body system responsible for transporting or regulating fluids and electrolytes. Such body systems include the cardiovascular, renal, lymphatic, endocrine, hepatic, gastrointestinal, respiratory, and neurological systems. In others words, pathologic dysfunctions in any body system can potentially lead to the formation of edema.

Edema can result from a variety of causes. However, each cause seems to have its origin in one or more of the six influencing factors listed in Table 8-7.

Data Acquisition

Physical Assessment. Clinically, assessment of an edematous individual focuses on the following parameters: (1) the presence and degree of edema; (2) the location and distribution of edema; (3) the color, integrity, turgor, elasticity, sensitivity, and temperature of the skin; (4) the presence and degree of neck vein distention; (5) body weight; (6) vital signs; and (7) the presence and degree of discomfort (particularly in dependent body parts).

Diagnostic Procedures. The laboratory data most helpful in assessing an individual in terms of edema are serum and urine protein and sodium values. The amounts of these substances vary according to the cause of the edema, but the usual pattern is that of hypoproteinemia, hypoalbuminemia, proteinuria, albuminuria, and hyponaturia. The serum sodium level varies so greatly depending on the cause that it is difficult to identify any specific pattern that is associated with edema. It is accurate to say, however, that in some cases of edema, the serum sodium is altered significantly enough to require frequent monitoring.

Medical and Nursing Management

Edema can have several clinical implications for an individual, some of which are very hazardous to well-being. The significance of edema is dependent upon its location, severity, and mobility. Certainly severe, painful edema of dependent extremities is significant, but not as significant as mild or moderate cerebral or pulmonary edema. Generalized edema can pose problems, but those problems can be vastly intensified if the edema is mobilized and large shifts of fluid from the interstitial to the intravascular space occur.

Many of the nursing implications associated with edema are similar to those previously discussed in relation to hypervolemia, especially the monitoring functions. Included in those monitoring functions are (1) monitoring and recording intake and output accurately, (2) assessing the status of edematous tissues, (3) obtaining precise daily measurements of weight, (4) monitoring vital signs and laboratory data periodically, and (5) assessing for changes in venous pressure.

Therapeutic nursing interventions that might be used with an individual with edema include (1) providing only fluids and foods consistent with the prescribed restrictions; (2) administering diuretics and other medications as prescribed; (3) providing meticulous skin care to prevent the breakdown of edematous tissues; (4) maintaining bed rest or a decreased level of activity appropriate to the degree of edema; and (5) promoting comfort in edematous extremities by elevating them, repositioning them carefully and frequently, and ensuring the appropriate use of constrictive and nonconstrictive clothing, coverings, or bandages on them.

The treatment of edema is based on four general principles. Those principles are (1) to treat the underlying primary disease or pathological condition responsible for the edema, (2) to restrict the amount of salt and water intake according to the needs of the patient, (3) to promote the mobilization of edema fluid, and (4) to promote excretion of edema fluid. Adherence to these treatment principles usually results in a decrease in, if not total resolution of, the edema.

Hypovolemia

Definition and Etiology

Hypovolemia is a deficit in extracellular fluid volume. Extracellular fluid volume deficit occurs as a result of any one of the following three abnormal physiological processes: (1) excessive loss of fluids and electrolytes, (2) decreased intake of fluids and electrolytes, and (3) shifts of fluid and electrolytes into nonaccessible areas such as third spaces.

The process of losing excessive amounts of fluids and electrolytes seems to be the underlying mechanism in most etiologies of hypovolemia. The most common reasons for such losses are vomiting, gastrointestinal suction, diarrhea, draining fistulas or wounds, systemic infection, profuse diaphoresis, burns, and excessive use of diuretics.

The two causes of hypovolemia due to a decreased intake of fluids and electrolytes are (1) coma, an inability to swallow, or any other state in which it is physically impossible for the individual to ingest substances; and (2) the absence or unavailability of fluids and electrolytes.

The process of "third spacing," or the shifting of extracellular fluid into cavities where it accumulates and is physiologically inaccessible for use by the body, is another underlying mechanism for hypovolemia. Clinical examples of third spacing include ascites, peritonitis, intestinal obstruction, burns, and pancreatitis.

Data Acquisition

Physical Assessment. An individual with an extracellular fluid volume deficit will exhibit any number of the following clinical signs and symptoms: acute weight loss, usually in excess of 5% of the total body weight; dry skin and mucous membranes; decreased skin turgor and elasticity; longitudinal wrinkling or furrows of the tongue; subnormal body temperature; lassitude or fatigue; oliguria or in a few cases anuria; thirst; decreased postural systolic blood pressure; decreased tension or turgor of the eyeball; decreased venous pressure; increased pulse rate; and decreased perspiration. Of all of these parameters, body weight is considered by many to be the most important indicator of a person's fluid balance. In fact, body weight has been used to roughly categorize degrees of extracellular fluid volume deficit. Table 8-8 presents one such categorization.

Diagnostic Procedures. The laboratory data that are the most useful in assessing an individual for hypovolemia include serum hemoglobin, hematocrit, red blood cell count, and BUN levels; and urine sodium, chloride, and specific gravity values. The urine/serum osmolality ratio also provides valuable assessment data, as can the serum sodium if the cause of the imbalance is considered. The pattern of these values exhibited by an individual experiencing hypovolemia includes increased serum values for hematocrit, hemoglobin, red blood cell count, and blood urea nitrogen; decreased urine values for sodium and chloride; increased urinary specific gravity; increased urine/serum osmolality ratio; and variable serum sodium values depending on the etiology of the imbalance.

The importance of including urine values in assessing an individual for hypovolemia should be emphasized. Many clinicians believe that the urine values may provide the earliest signs of hypovolemia. The parameters most frequently cited as guidelines for determining if the specific urine values are indicative of hypovolemia are a sodium content less than 20 mEq/L, a specific gravity greater than 1.026, and a urine/serum osmolality ratio greater than 2.

Medical and Nursing Management

The clinical significance of hypovolemia for a patient is that there are insufficient body fluids to carry out the normal physiological and metabolic processes necessary to sustain life. Of course, the more severe the imbalance the greater the threat to the patient's well-being.

Nursing monitoring functions related to hypovolemia include (1) obtaining accurate daily weights; (2) measuring and recording *all* intake and output accurately; (3) assessing vital signs, venous pressure, and laboratory data periodically; (4) frequently measuring expanded third-space areas, such as the abdomen; (5) assessing the status of the skin and mucous membranes periodically; and (6) continually evaluating the individual's overall energy level.

Nursing interventions used with an individual with hypovolemia are (1) to administer intravenous replacement fluids precisely at a constant rate; (2) to ensure that all fluids administered to the individual, including irrigation solutions, are of the appropriate electrolyte balance; (3) to provide frequent oral hygiene to maintain the integrity and hydration state of the mucous membranes; and (4) to provide skin care to decrease breakdown and promote integrity.

The treatment of hypovolemia has two components. The first component is to treat or correct the primary cause of the imbalance. The second component is to replace lost fluids and electrolytes.

Replacement therapy is usually instituted according to a trilevel approach. The first level is based on an assessment of the individual's renal status. If there is a question about the adequacy of the individual's

---

TABLE 8-8 **Degrees of Extracellular Fluid Volume Deficit According to Percentage Loss of Total Body Weight**

Degree of Extracellular Fluid Volume Deficit	Loss of Total Body Weight, %
Mild	2-5
Moderate	6-10
Severe	11-15
Fatal	>15

renal function, a hydrating solution is given to challenge the renal system and promote function. This hydrating solution is usually composed of water, carbohydrate (in the form of 5% dextrose), sodium, and chloride. Once the presence of adequate renal function has been established, replacement therapy moves to the second level.

The second level of replacement therapy can be initiated as soon as it has been determined that renal function is adequate. Thus, in some cases, the first-level replacement can be omitted, and replacement therapy actually begins with second-level solutions. Second-level solutions are balanced solutions designed to supply water, calories, and electrolytes in sufficient quantities to meet the maintenance needs of the body as well as to correct existing deficits. These solutions are composed of physiological proportionate amounts of water, carbohydrate, sodium, potassium, magnesium, chloride, phosphate, and lactate. These balanced solutions are often called *all-purpose* solutions and are used frequently in fluid replacement therapy.

Third-level replacement therapy is aimed at replacing specific, concurrent, or ongoing water and electrolyte losses. This level of therapy involves using solutions individually prescribed to replace specific fluid and electrolyte losses, such as those created by gastrointestinal suction or fistula drainage. These solutions are composed of water, carbohydrate, and varying amounts of specific electrolytes selected to meet the needs of the patient. It is not uncommon in replacement therapy to see both balanced solutions and specifically created solutions used concurrently to achieve and maintain proper balance.

SODIUM

Functions

Sodium, the major cation of extracellular fluid, has four general functions in the body. Those functions are (1) to promote the normal distribution and volume of fluids in the body by creating and maintaining the normal osmolality of those fluids; (2) to enhance the transcellular movement of substances by altering cell permeability; (3) to promote normal neuromuscular irritability by enhancing the conduction and transmission of electrochemical impulses; and (4) to contribute to the regulation of acid–base balance by exchanging with selected cations such as potassium and hydrogen, and combining with certain anions such as chloride and bicarbonate.

Regulation

The renal system, in concert with other mechanisms, has primary responsibility for regulating the reabsorption and excretion of sodium. Approxi-

mately 99% of the total filtered load of sodium is reabsorbed by various parts of the nephron, leaving only about 1% to be excreted in the urine. Of the 99% that is reabsorbed, about 70% is actively reabsorbed in the proximal tubule, 20% is passively reabsorbed in the loop of Henle, 8% is actively reabsorbed in the distal tubule, and about 1% is actively reabsorbed in the collecting duct. This reabsorption and excretion of sodium is influenced by several factors, many of which are related to maintaining an effective arterial blood volume. Those influencing factors include glomerulotubular balance, aldosterone, third factor, the redistribution of renal blood flow, peritubular capillary oncotic pressure, the serum sodium concentration, catecholamines, and prostaglandins.

Glomerulotubular Balance

Glomerulotubular balance is the phenomenon of having the rate of tubular sodium reabsorption change in the same direction as the filtered load of sodium because of alterations in the glomerular filtration rate. This mechanism prevents the loss of large amounts of sodium that would result from increases in the glomerular filtration rate.

Aldosterone

Aldosterone is a mineralocorticoid hormone that is secreted through the activation of the renin-angiotensin system in response to a real or perceived decrease in effective arterial volume. Aldosterone acts on the distal renal tubule to promote increased sodium and water reabsorption and potassium excretion.

Third Factor

"Third factor" is thought to be a natriuretic regulatory mechanism that increases the renal excretion of sodium in the presence of saline volume expansion. The factor is thought to function independently of aldosterone and glomerular filtration rate in regulating sodium excretion. Research continues to be conducted on third factor to determine its precise physiological nature and composition.

Redistribution of Renal Blood Flow

The redistribution of renal blood flow occurs as a result of a reduction in effective arterial volume sufficient enough to decrease the total blood flow to the kidneys. In such a situation, blood is shunted from the cortical nephrons to the juxtamedullary nephrons. The juxtamedullary nephrons, with their long loops of Henle, tend to retain more sodium for reabsorption than do the cortical nephrons. Thus, this selective perfusion of the juxtamedullary nephrons promotes the increased reabsorption of sodium.

Peritubular Capillary Oncotic Pressure

The peritubular capillaries regulate sodium reabsorption and excretion according to the amount of oncotic pressure in them. An increased protein concentration (usually resulting from a volume and/or sodium deficit), which increases the oncotic pressure, promotes the reabsorption of sodium and water from the nephron. This process assists in returning the peritubular capillary oncotic pressure to normal.

Serum Sodium Concentration

Serum sodium levels seem to influence sodium reabsorption and excretion, but the exact mechanism for this influence is not known. However, it is known that hyponatremia promotes, and hypernatremia inhibits, sodium reabsorption by the renal tubules.

Catecholamines

Catecholamines are thought to enhance sodium reabsorption, but again, the mechanism for this action is not clearly understood. There seem to be differing opinions as to whether the effect of the catecholamines is direct or indirect in relation to sodium reabsorption.

Prostaglandins

The role of prostaglandins in the regulation of sodium is controversial. It seems that certain prostaglandins may have a natriuretic effect, but the mechanism for that effect is not yet clear. Further research is required on prostaglandins, as well as other factors, before all of the mechanisms involved in sodium regulation are precisely comprehended.

Variances

The variances or imbalances related to sodium are hypernatremia and hyponatremia. It should be noted, however, that serum sodium levels cannot be assessed in isolation. When serum sodium levels are assessed, it is sodium concentration that is being measured, and concentration should not be evaluated without considering fluid volume. Indeed, the variances in serum sodium can occur in conjunction with euvolemia, hypovolemia, or hypervolemia. Thus, serum sodium and fluid volume should be assessed concurrently. Such as assessment, then, makes it possible to determine, for example, if an increased serum sodium level is actually due to hypernatremia, or if it is merely a reflection of hypovolemia. In the latter instance, the serum sodium level is not indicative of total body sodium, which might be normal. Rather, it is indicative of having the same amount of sodium present in less fluid volume. With this caution in mind, the discussion concerning hypernatremia and hyponatremia can proceed.

Hypernatremia

Definition and Etiology

Hypernatremia is an excess of sodium in the extracellular fluid. Hypernatremia can result from two types of causes: (1) those that promote either the loss of water in excess of sodium loss or the inadequate replacement of water; and (2) those that facilitate sodium retention or excess. Examples of the first type are decreased water intake, the inability to swallow, unconsciousness, the unavailability of fluids, vomiting, diarrhea, diabetes insipidus, osmotic diuresis, fever, heat stroke, high environmental temperatures, hyperventilation, and dialysis therapy. Examples of the second type are excessive ingestion or infusion of sodium chloride, ingestion of seawater, acidosis, renal dysfunction, primary hyperaldosteronism, excessive use of corticosteroid therapy, and neurological lesions.

Data Acquisition

Physical Assessment. The hypernatremic individual usually exhibits many of the following signs and symptoms: dry, sticky mucous membranes; a rough, dry tongue; flushed, dry skin; increased tissue turgor; thirst; decreased lacrimation; elevated body temperature; tachycardia; oliguria; lethargy; central nervous system irritability; muscular rigidity and weakness; tremors; seizures; and coma.

Diagnostic Procedures. The laboratory values that provide the most data for assessing a patient for hypernatremia are serum sodium and chloride, and urine sodium, chloride, osmolality, and specific gravity. The levels of those values that provide a general pattern consistent with hypernatremia are the following: a serum sodium greater than 146 mEq/L, a serum chloride greater than 106 mEq/L, a urine sodium less than 50 mEq/L, a urine chloride less than 50 mEq/L, a urine osmolality of greater than 800 mosm/L, and a urine specific gravity greater than 1.030.

Medical and Nursing Management

Hypernatremia can result in serious clinical difficulties for an individual. Probably the most significant problems are those related to the central nervous system and neuromuscular functioning. Certainly it is easy to visualize the effects of muscular hyperirritability, seizures, and coma on one's health state. Such problems are definitely a threat to well-being and necessitate appropriate nursing support.

The nursing support related to hypernatremia includes the following monitoring functions: (1) assessing the skin turgor, temperature, color, and moisture; (2) assessing the moisture of the tongue and mucous membranes; (3) obtaining precise daily weights; (4) measuring and recording intake and output accurately; (5) monitoring vital signs and laboratory values periodically; (6) assessing muscle movement; and probably the most important function, (7) frequently assessing the neurological status and level of consciousness.

Nursing interventions that provide support for the hypernatremic patient are: (1) providing fluids and foods consistent with the prescribed restrictions; (2) maintaining skin integrity through the use of meticulous hygienic measures, moisturizing agents, and frequent repositioning; (3) maintaining the integrity of the oral cavity with frequent oral care employing a variety of nondehydrating agents; (4) promoting comfort by decreasing thirst using a variety of creative measures; (5) instituting seizure precautions; and (6) providing for the patient's general, overall environmental safety.

The treatment for hypernatremia revolves around treating the cause and correcting the imbalance. The ideal form of treatment is to address the primary disorder that perpetuates the imbalance, and whenever possible, this is done. The second part of the treatment, correcting the imbalance, is based on the nature of the etiology. The general criteria for therapeutic intervention are: (1) if the imbalance is due to a loss of extracellular fluid, intravenous isotonic saline solution will be administered to correct the imbalance; and (2) if the imbalance is due to a sodium excess, the individual's daily sodium intake will be restricted to anywhere from 0.5 g to 2 g, and intravenous 5% dextrose and water will be given to replace the intracellular fluid deficit created by the hypernatremia. More specific therapeutic guidelines are presented in Table 8-9.

Hyponatremia

Definition and Etiology

Hyponatremia is a deficit of sodium in the extracellular fluid. It has two types of causes: (1) those that produce dilutional extracellular fluid expansion, and (2) those that result in a deficit of sodium. The causes of dilutional hyponatremia are excessive ingestion or infusion of electrolyte-free solutions, excessive use of tap water enemas, irrigation of gastrointestinal tubes with electrolyte-free solutions, renal dysfunction, inappropriate secretion of antidiuretic hormone, cirrhosis, congestive heart failure, and hyperglycemia. (In the case of hyperglycemia, it has been estimated that each 100 mg/100 ml increase in the glucose concentration above normal results in sufficient extracellular fluid volume expansion to decrease the serum sodium concentration by about 1.6 mEq/L.)

A deficit of sodium is caused by inadequate ingestion of dietary sodium, infusions of solutions that are sodium-deficient, salt-wasting renal dysfunction, potent diuretic therapy, adrenal insufficiency, severe vomiting, severe diarrhea, excessive perspiration, gastrointestinal suction, potassium depletion, burns, "third spacing," and severe malnutrition.

Data Acquisition

Physical Assessment. An individual experiencing hyponatremia may exhibit any combination of the following signs and symptoms: fatigue, muscle weakness, lethargy, confusion, headache, tremors, hyperreflexia, convulsions, coma, apprehension, anorexia, nausea, vomiting, abdominal cramps, diarrhea, and oliguria. As with hypernatremia, the neurologic signs and symptoms of hyponatremia seem to be the most

---

TABLE 8-9   Guidelines for Treating Hypernatremia

Volume Status	Urine Osmolality	Urine Na$^+$	Treatment
Hypovolemia	Hypertonic	<10 mEq/L	Isotonic saline IV followed by hypotonic saline IV or oral water
Hypovolemia or euvolemia	Isotonic or hypotonic	>20 mEq/L	Isotonic saline IV followed by hypotonic saline IV or oral water
Hypovolemia or euvolemia	Hypotonic, isotonic, or hypertonic	Variable (usually >20 mEq/L)	Water replacement as hypotonic IV fluid or oral water
Hypovolemia or euvolemia	Hypertonic	Variable (usually >20 mEq/L)	Water replacement as hypotonic IV fluid or oral water
Hypervolemia or euvolemia	Isotonic or hypertonic	>20 mEq/L (usually much greater)	Water replacement as hypotonic IV fluid or oral water and diuretics

clinically significant. However, because the neurological signs and symptoms are so similar in the two conditions, they offer little help in differentiating between the two states. Therefore, the gastrointestinal signs and symptoms may be more discriminating, even if clinically less significant, in identifying hyponatremia.

Diagnostic Procedures. Hyponatremia can be identified from an assessment of the following laboratory data: serum sodium and chloride, and urine sodium, osmolality, and specific gravity. The general pattern characteristic of hyponatremia is a serum sodium less than 136 mEq/L; a serum chloride less than 96 mEq/L; a variable urine sodium, usually less than 20 mEq/L; a urine osmolality less than 300 mosm/L; and a urine specific gravity less than 1.010.

Medical and Nursing Management

Clinically, hyponatremia can be a life-threatening imbalance, depending on its severity. The hazards to the patient stem from the effects of the imbalance on the central nervous system. These effects, ranging from mere confusion to convulsions and coma, certainly represent a threat to the individual's health state. These effects, however, usually do not occur unless the serum sodium falls below 120 mEq/L.

Nursing monitoring functions that are performed in relation to hyponatremia include (1) assessing levels of consciousness and central nervous system functioning frequently, (2) assessing muscle strength and energy levels periodically, (3) obtaining precise daily weights, (4) measuring and recording intake and output accurately, and (5) monitoring vital signs and laboratory data at intervals.

Nursing interventions that would be performed for an individual with hyponatremia are (1) giving foods and fluids high in sodium content as prescribed; (2) maintaining fluid restrictions as prescribed (interventions 1 and 2 are *not* done in concert, since the first

aims at replacement therapy and the second at returning a diluted, expanded extracellular fluid volume to normal); (3) instituting seizure precautions; (4) promoting the conservation of energy by limiting activity; (5) establishing a physical environment conducive to maintaining the individual's safety and orientation; and (6) promoting overall comfort by using creative pain-relieving methods and administering medications as prescribed.

The treatment of hyponatremia depends, of course, on its etiology. The first goal of therapy is to treat the cause or primary disorder responsible for the imbalance. The second goal is to treat the imbalance. The general parameters for therapeutic intervention are: (1) if the imbalance is the result of a dilutional expansion of the extracellular fluid, treatment will consist of restricting the fluid intake (and in some cases administering diuretics); and (2) if the imbalance is due to sodium loss, replacement therapy in the form of oral preparations, dietary provisions, or hypertonic or isotonic saline infusions will be instituted. More specific therapeutic guidelines are presented in Table 8-10.

POTASSIUM
Functions

Potassium, the major cation of the intracellular fluid, has several important physiological functions in the body. Those functions include (1) creating and maintaining the osmotic pressure of the intracellular fluid, (2) maintaining the transmembrane electrical potential difference between the extracellular and intracellular spaces that regulates neuromuscular excitability and is necessary for muscle contraction, (3) participating in the maintenance of acid–base balance, (4) enhancing the synthesis of protein, and (5) participating in the metabolism of carbohydrates and synthesis of glycogen.

TABLE 8-10 **Guidelines for Treating Hyponatremia**

Volume Status	Urine Osmolality	Urine Na$^+$	Treatment
Hypovolemia	Hypertonic	<10 mEq/L	Isotonic saline IV
Hypovolemia	Hypotonic, isotonic, or hypertonic	>20 mEq/L	Isotonic saline IV, possibly accompanied by moderate water restriction
Euvolemia	Hypertonic	>20 mEq/L	Fluid restriction, possibly accompanied by salt replacement and/or diuretics
Hypervolemia	Hypertonic	<10 mEq/L	Fluid restriction
Hypervolemia	Isotonic or hypertonic	>20 mEq/L	Fluid restriction

Regulation

Potassium is regulated primarily by the renal system. Although some potassium is lost in perspiration and the feces, the kidneys remain the foremost organ for its excretion and reabsorption. The renal handling of potassium begins at the glomerulus where it is filtered. Of that filtered load of potassium, about 70% is actively reabsorbed in the proximal tubule, 20% is passively reabsorbed in the loop of Henle, and the remaining 10% is delivered to the distal tubule. Further active reabsorption can occur in the distal tubule and collecting duct, depending on the level of potassium in the body. The *principal* activity of the distal tubule, however, is the active or passive secretion of potassium. This distal tubular secretion, the main regulator of renal potassium excretion, is influenced by the following factors: aldosterone, the amount of sodium delivered to the distal tubule, hydrogen ion secretion, the presence of nonreabsorbable anions, urine flow rates, potassium intake, and diuretic therapy.

Aldosterone

Aldosterone, a mineralocorticoid hormone, increases potassium excretion through two highly interrelated mechanisms. The first mechanism is related to the increased permeability of the distal tubular luminal membrane to potassium and sodium. This change in permeability enhances the diffusion of potassium out of the tubular cell into the lumen where it can be excreted. It also enhances the entry of sodium from the lumen into the tubular cell, thereby facilitating active sodium reabsorption. The increase in sodium reabsorption increases the transmembrane potential difference in the distal tubule, which facilitates the passive diffusion of potassium into the lumen for excretion.

The second mechanism of aldosterone is related to an increased concentration of potassium in the tubular cell. Aldosterone stimulates the peritubular uptake of potassium, thereby increasing the concentration in the tubular cell. This increase in concentration enhances the passive diffusion of potassium into the lumen where it can be excreted.

Sodium Delivery to the Distal Tubule

The effect of the concentration of distal tubular sodium on potassium excretion has been mentioned in the discussion on aldosterone. When increased concentrations of sodium are delivered to the distal tubule, the amount of sodium that is reabsorbed is increased. The increased reabsorption of sodium creates an increase in the transmembrane potential difference which facilitates the passive diffusion of potassium into the tubular lumen where it can be excreted. Thus,

the end result is an increase in urinary potassium excretion.

Hydrogen Ion Secretion

The secretion of distal tubular potassium is influenced by the rate of hydrogen ion secretion. In acute acidotic conditions, there is an extracellular to intracellular shift of hydrogen ions and an intracellular to extracellular shift of potassium. The lower intracellular concentration of potassium in the distal tubular cells decreases the electrical and chemical gradients that enhance the passive secretion of potassium into the lumen. This results in a decreased renal secretion and excretion of potassium, accompanied by a preferential obligatory secretion of hydrogen ions that is facilitated by the increase in the intracellular concentration of hydrogen ions. Of course, the reverse of this process occurs in alkalotic states, and there is an increased urinary excretion of potassium.

Nonreabsorbable Anions

Nonreabsorbable anions, such as phosphate, sulfate and bicarbonate, are those anions that cannot accompany reabsorbed sodium as easily as chloride does. When levels of these anions in the distal tubular fluid are elevated, the negative transmembrane electrical gradient is increased as sodium is reabsorbed, resulting in a greater diffusion of potassium into the lumen. Thus, this mechanism increases the urinary excretion of potassium.

Urine Flow Rates

Urine flow rates seem to have some correlation with urinary potassium secretion and excretion rates. When urine flow increases, so does potassium secretion and excretion. Likewise, when urine flow decreases, there is also a decrease in the urinary secretion and excretion of potassium. The mechanisms responsible for these variations seem to be the increased sodium concentration that accompanies the urine flow to the distal tubule and the decreased reabsorption of potassium that results from the low potassium concentration of the luminal fluid. Both of these factors contribute to the increased urinary excretion rates of potassium in the presence of high urine flow rates.

Potassium Intake

An increase in the extracellular concentration of potassium due to increased intake increases the urinary secretion and excretion rate of potassium. The effect of an increased extracellular potassium concentration on the rate of urinary secretion and excretion of potassium results from its participation in the following processes: (1) the production of a higher tubular luminal concentration of potassium, (2) the stimulation of increased aldosterone secretion, (3) the production of an increased transmembrane potential difference at the distal tubular cell, and (4) the stimulation of sodium-potassium-adenosine triphosphatase secretion which increases the rate of potassium flow across the peritubular cell membranes.

Diuretic Therapy

Most of the pharmacological agents that produce diuresis are kaliuretic and cause increased urinary losses of potassium. The mechanisms by which they produce this effect vary according to the specific diuretic employed. However, most of them function by either increasing the urinary flow rate, decreasing potassium reabsorption, increasing sodium delivery to the distal tubule, or altering the transmembrane potential.

The variances associated with potassium are hyperkalemia and hypokalemia.

Hyperkalemia

Definition and Etiology

Hyperkalemia is an excess of potassium in the extracellular fluid. The etiologies of hyperkalemia can be classified into three general categories based on the mechanism by which they produce the excess in potassium. Those categories are decreased renal excretion, translocation from the cells, and increased intake. Those etiologies that result in hyperkalemia because of a decreased renal excretion include renal dysfunction, adrenocortical insufficiencies such as Addison's disease and hyporeninemic hypoaldosteronism, and the use of potassium-sparing diuretics such as spironolactone or triamterene.

Those etiologies that result in hyperkalemia because of the translocation of potassium from the intracellular to the extracellular fluid space include severe catabolism, burns, rhabdomyolysis, acute acidosis, intravascular hemolysis, and hyperkalemic familial periodic paralysis.

Hyperkalemia can also be caused by the excessive intake of potassium, usually in the form of intravenous infusion or the oral ingestion of medications or food substances that are high in potassium. This etiology, however, is rarely the cause of hyperkalemia if the individual has normal renal function. This is because in most instances it is difficult to exceed the renal capacity for excreting potassium, so even additional loads of potassium are easily excreted. The renal excretion capacity can be exceeded, however, by large bolus intravenous infusions of potassium.

In addition to all the above causes of hyperkalemia, there are other changes that occur in the body that produce a false hyperkalemia. Pseudohyperkalemia can result from the following: increased leukocyte or thrombocyte counts; the hemolysis of drawn blood samples, sometimes due to using a very small-gauge needle, and using a tourniquet to assist in drawing blood samples.

Data Acquisition

Physical Assessment. Most of the clinical signs and symptoms of hyperkalemia are related to the neuromuscular, cardiac, and gastrointestinal systems. Those signs and symptoms as exhibited by the hyperkalemic individual include mental confusion, neuromuscular hyperexcitability, weakness, paresthesia, ascending flaccid paralysis, cardiac dysfunction (as described below), cardiac arrest, abdominal distention, diarrhea, intestinal colic, and oliguria (which is more a reflection of the etiology than an effect of the imbalance).

The cardiac dysfunction that occurs in response to hyperkalemia seems to follow a distinct pattern. The earliest signs of dysfunction are seen on the electrocardiogram in the form of tall, peaked, tented T waves and a depressed ST segment. As the imbalance progresses, the P waves decrease in amplitude and the PR interval is prolonged. Then atrial asystole occurs with a widened QRS complex that eventually merges with the T wave forming the sine wave characteristic of hyperkalemia. Dysrhythmia, fibrillation, and cardiac arrest can occur at any time during the foregoing sequence of events, depending on the severity of the hyperkalemia and its rapidity of progression.

Diagnostic Procedures. The laboratory value that is most useful in assessing an individual for hyperkalemia is the serum potassium. A serum potassium level greater than 5.5 mEq/L is indicative of hyperkalemia.

The urinary potassium value may provide additional data. However, this value will vary depending on the etiology of the imbalance and, thus, may be more reflective of the specific etiology than of the existence or magnitude of the imbalance.

Medical and Nursing Management

The clinical significance of hyperkalemia is based on its profound effect on the neuromuscular and cardiac systems. Certainly nothing could be worse for a patient than paralysis or cardiac arrest.

The nursing implications associated with hyperkalemia include monitoring or assessing the following: (1) rate, rhythm, and characteristics of the pulse (with or without a cardiac monitor); (2) level of consciousness and orientation; (3) muscle strength, sensation, and movement; (4) characteristics of the abdomen; (5) characteristics of the feces; (6) laboratory values; and (7) urinary output.

Also included in the nursing implications of hyperkalemia are the following interventions: (1) providing only those foods and fluids that are consistent with the prescribed potassium restriction; (2) administering medications as prescribed; (3) establishing a safe physical environment for the individual; (4) providing stimuli appropriate for enhancing orientation; (5) instituting limited active or passive range of motion exercises; (6) assisting with the normal activities of daily living; and (7) providing meticulous skin care at the rectal orifice.

The treatment of hyperkalemia focuses on eliminating the primary cause and correcting the imbalance. Measures for correcting the imbalance are aimed at (1) reducing potassium intake, (2) antagonizing the membrane effect of hyperkalemia, (3) shifting the potassium intracellularly, and (4) increasing the excretion of potassium.

Reducing the potassium intake is accomplished by restricting the amounts of potassium ingested in dietary substances or medications and/or infused in intravenous solutions. The usual daily restriction of potassium is about 40 mEq, but this amount can vary according to the specific needs of the individual.

The agents most frequently used to antagonize the effect of hyperkalemia on the cell membrane are calcium salts, such as calcium chloride, or hypertonic sodium salts, such as sodium chloride or sodium bicarbonate. Although these agents may be very successful in treating severe cases of hyperkalemia quickly (because they are effective within 1 to 5 minutes after administration), they are also therapeutically very transient and last only 30 minutes. Furthermore, they have no effect on either serum or total body potassium levels.

Infusions of glucose and insulin or sodium bicarbonate will correct hyperkalemia by facilitating the shift of potassium into the cell. For example, when 1 g of glucose is converted to glycogen, approximately 3.6 mEq/L of potassium are retained intracellularly. The glucose and insulin therapy becomes effective about 10 to 15 minutes after infusion, but the sodium bicarbonate requires about an hour. Both agents produce only a temporary correction of the imbalance that is perhaps 2 to 4 hours in duration. Both agents will decrease the serum potassium level but have no effect on total body potassium.

The increased excretion of potassium is effected through the use of sodium chloride infusions, cation exchange resins, diuretics, and dialysis. Sodium chloride infusions are effective within 1 hour but do not last very long. The infusions reduce the serum potassium level but have only a slight effect on the total body potassium. Cation exchange resins, diuretics, and dialysis are effective within minutes to hours and last longer than the other types of therapies mentioned. All three methods are effective in decreasing both the serum and total body potassium levels.

Hypokalemia

Definition and Etiology

Hypokalemia is a deficit of potassium in the extracellular fluid. It results from the following five categories of causes: (1) an increased intracellular shift of potassium, (2) decreased potassium intake, (3) increased gastrointestinal potassium loss, (4) excessive renal potassium loss, and (5) excessive integumentary potassium loss.

Specific etiologies that cause hypokalemia by enhancing the intracellular shift of potassium are acute alkalosis, the intravenous infusion of glucose and insulin, and familial hypokalemic periodic paralysis.

The etiologies associated with a decreased intake are the inability to physically ingest fluids or foods, the unavailability of food or fluids, the infusion of large quantities of potassium-free intravenous solutions, and the prolonged ingestion of diets deficient in potassium.

Increasing the gastrointestinal loss of potassium is the mechanism by which the following etiologies cause hypokalemia: vomiting, fistulas, malabsorption, diarrhea, inflammatory bowel disease, laxative abuse, and ureterosigmoidostomies.

Etiologies that induce hypokalemia by increasing the renal excretion of potassium include diuretic therapy, renal tubular acidosis, chronic interstitial nephritis, primary and secondary hyperaldosteronism, Cushing's syndrome, adrenal steroid therapy, the excessive ingestion of mineralocorticoid-like substances such as licorice, and diabetic ketoacidosis.

The loss of potassium through the integument in the form of excessive perspiration also causes hypokalemia. This etiology is most frequently observed in individuals who exercise or work intensely in hot climates.

Data Acquisition

Physical Assessment. The clinical manifestations of hypokalemia are evident in almost every system of the body. This imbalance seems to produce signs and symptoms in the neuromuscular, cardiovascular, respiratory, gastrointestinal, endocrine, and renal systems. Table 8-11 summarizes the signs and symptoms of hypokalemia that are observed in those body systems.

Diagnostic Procedures. The most significant laboratory values used in assessing an individual for hypokalemia are the serum values for potassium, bicarbonate, and pH. A serum potassium of less than 3.5 mEq/L and an elevated plasma bicarbonate and pH are indicative of hypokalemia.

Other laboratory values that provide additional

TABLE 8-11   **Signs and Symptoms of Hypokalemia According to Body Systems**

System	Signs and Symptoms
Neuromuscular	Drowsiness, confusion, apathy, irritability, coma, muscle weaknesses, paresthesias, muscle pain, muscle cramps, muscle tenderness, hyporeflexia, tetany, paralysis
Cardiovascular	Weak pulse; bradycardia; ECG changes, including a depressed ST segment; flattened, inverted T waves; and U waves
Respiratory	Muscle weakness, hypoventilation
Gastrointestinal	Nausea, vomiting, anorexia, abdominal distention, abdominal cramps, paralytic ileus
Endocrine	Polydipsia, hyperglycemia, and in some cases negative nitrogen balance
Renal	Polyuria, nocturia

information in assessing for hypokalemia are the urine osmolality, pH, potassium, and phosphate. The levels of those urine values that are consistent with hypokalemia are a decreased osmolality, a decreased pH, a normal potassium (within the first 3 weeks of the imbalance, then it decreases), and an increased phosphate.

Medical and Nursing Management

Hypokalemia presents many clinical problems for the individual. The most significant of those problems are the apnea, cardiac dysrhythmias, muscle paralysis, and paralytic ileus that may develop as the hypokalemia progresses in severity. With the possibility of such severe alterations occurring, the implications for nursing support are critical.

Nursing support includes the following monitoring functions: (1) assessing the rate, rhythm, and characteristics of the respirations and the pulse (with or without a cardiac monitor); (2) monitoring all other vital signs; (3) assessing the level of consciousness frequently; (4) evaluating muscle strength, movement, and sensation; (5) assessing the characteristics of the abdomen; (6) monitoring bowel sounds; (7) measuring and recording intake and output accurately; and (8) monitoring the appropriate laboratory values.

Nursing support for the patient with hypokalemia includes the following interventions: (1) administering oral or intravenous potassium preparations carefully and as prescribed; (2) positioning the individual to facilitate adequate respirations; (3) providing ap-

propriate stimuli to promote orientation; (4) establishing a safe physical environment for the individual; (5) providing creative comfort measures; and (6) assisting the individual with the normal activities of daily living.

The treatment of hypokalemia involves eliminating the cause, if possible, and correcting the imbalance. The preferred method for correcting hypokalemia is to replace the deficit orally with high-potassium foods or potassium supplements. (When liquid potassium preparations are given, they should be well diluted to decrease gastrointestinal irritation.) Using this method of replacement therapy decreases the likelihood of creating a rebound hyperkalemia.

Intravenous administration of potassium chloride is usually used to replace acute potassium deficits. The potassium chloride is infused into a peripheral vein usually at a rate of 10 to 20 mEq/hr using a concentration of 40 mEq/L. This rate and concentration ensures that the deficit will be slowly but adequately corrected with minimum risk to the individual.

CALCIUM

Functions

Calcium, an important, abundant cation in the body, is involved in a variety of physiological functions. Included among those functions are the following: (1) participating in bone formation and metabolism; (2) influencing neural transmission and function; (3) initiating muscle contraction; (4) participating as a coenzyme in blood coagulation and activation of the complement system; (5) influencing cardiac action potential; (6) participating in the regulation of many enzyme systems; (7) influencing the secretion of exocrine and endocrine glands; and (8) preserving the functional integrity of cellular membranes.

Regulation

Serum calcium is regulated primarily by exchange between the extracellular fluid and the intestines, bones, and kidneys. Figure 8-5 illustrates these regulatory relationships and indicates their relative importance by the size of the arrows. These exchanges, or relationships, are influenced by a variety of hormonal and other factors as summarized in Table 8-12.

Intestines

The intestines absorb from 25% to 70% of the dietary calcium ingested. The efficiency of this absorption seems to vary inversely with the amount of calcium ingested. The absorption process is enhanced by vitamin D, parathyroid hormone, and growth hormone. It is inhibited by thyrocalcitonin and glucocorticoid hormones.

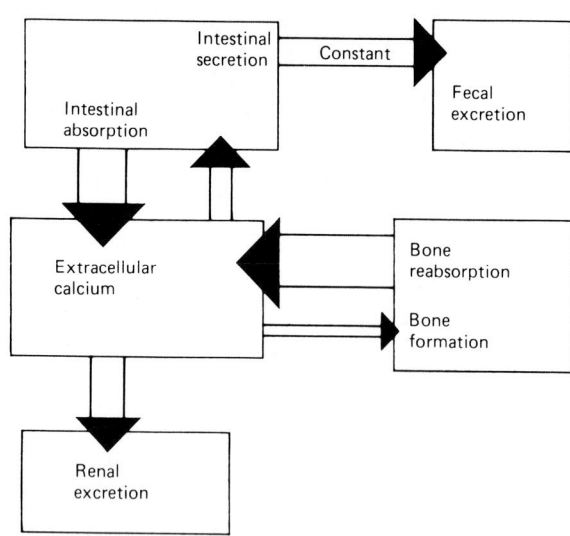

Figure 8-5 Mechanisms for regulating extracellular calcium (arrow size indicates relative importance).

In addition to supplying the body with essential calcium by the absorption process, the intestines also secrete calcium, which is excreted (along with the unabsorbed calcium) in the feces. The intestinal secretion of calcium seems to be constant in terms of amount and is not dependent upon the quantity ingested.

Bones

The movement of calcium to and from the bones contributes significantly to maintaining a normal extracellular ionized calcium concentration. Although it seems that the rates of bone formation (calcium deposition) and bone resorption (calcium release) participate in the exchange process equally, that is not the case. Bone resorption appears to be the principal process involved in the exchange and thus compensates for lowered serum calcium levels. Bone resorption is stimulated by vitamin D, parathyroid hormone, thyroid hormone, prostaglandins, and acidosis. It is inhibited by thyrocalcitonin, glucocorticoid hormones, androgen, estrogen, hyperphosphatemia, and alkalosis.

Kidneys

The renal system regulates calcium by maintaining a balance between intake and output. The renal regulation of calcium is mainly excretory and varies according to dietary intake. Of the filtered calcium load, about 55% is reabsorbed in the proximal tubule, about 30% is reabsorbed in the loop of Henle, and about 12% is reabsorbed in the distal tubule. The remaining 3% is excreted by the kidneys. The renal excretion of calcium is increased by the following:

increased effective arterial pressure, most diuretics, hypercalcemia, hypophosphatemia, thyrocalcitonin, growth hormone, thyroid hormone, glucocorticoids, and acidosis. Those factors that decrease the renal excretion of calcium include decreased effective arterial volume, thiazide diuretics, hypocalcemia, hyperphosphatemia, vitamin D, parathyroid hormone, and alkalosis.

The variances associated with calcium are hypercalcemia and hypocalcemia.

Hypercalcemia

Definition and Etiology

Hypercalcemia is an excess of calcium in the extracellular fluid. It can be related to a variety of etiologies, the most common of which is malignant tumors. Other causes are vitamin D intoxication, hyperparathyroidism, hypophosphatasia, hyperproteinemia, hyperthyroidism, adrenal insufficiency, renal dysfunction, immobilization, thiazide diuretics, milk–alkali syndrome, sarcoidosis, tuberculosis, idiopathic infantile hypercalcemia, and vitamin A intoxication.

Data Acquisition

Physical Assessment. The clinical signs and symptoms that may accompany hypercalcemia include fatigue, muscle weakness, muscle hypotonicity, drowsiness, lethargy, disorientation, loss of memory, depression, stupor, coma, deep bone pain, anorexia, nausea, vomiting, constipation, thirst, polyuria, renal stones, and cardiac dysrhythmia, which can progress to cardiac arrest. (Hypercalcemia is evidenced on the electrocardiogram by a shortened QT interval.)

Diagnostic Procedures. In assessing an individual for hypercalcemia, the following values provide important data: serum calcium, urine calcium, urine osmolality, and urine specific gravity. The pattern characteristic of hypercalcemia is a serum calcium greater than 10.5 mg/100 ml, an increased urine calcium, a decreased urine osmolality, and a decreased urine specific gravity. Remember that serum calcium must be evaluated in terms of serum albumin, and for every 1.0 mg/100 ml change in albumin from the norm of 4.0 mg/100 ml, there is a corresponding change of 0.8 mg/100 ml in the serum calcium.

Medical and Nursing Management

The clinical implications of hypercalcemia are very significant for the individual. Not only can this imbalance precipitate in cardiac arrest, but it can also lead to renal dysfunction, central nervous system depression, pain, and pathological fractures.

The implications for nursing include performing the following monitoring functions: (1) assessing the

TABLE 8-12 Factors Influencing Calcium Regulation

Regulating System	Stimulating Factor	Inhibiting Factor
Intestinal (absorption)	Vitamin D Parathyroid hormone Growth hormone	Thyrocalcitonin Glucocorticoid hormones
Skeletal (bone resorption)	Vitamin D Parathyroid hormone Thyroid hormone Prostaglandins Acidosis	Thyrocalcitonin Glucocorticoid hormones Androgen Estrogen Hyperphosphatemia Alkalosis
Renal (excretion)	Increased arterial pressure Most diuretics Hypercalcemia Hypophosphatemia Thyrocalcitonin Growth hormone Thyroid hormone Glucocorticoid hormones Acidosis	Decreased arterial pressure Thiazide diuretics Hypocalcemia Hyperphosphatemia Vitamin D Parathyroid hormone Alkalosis

rate, rhythm, and characteristics of the pulse; (2) evaluating the level of consciousness frequently; (3) monitoring muscle movement, strength, and tone; (4) assessing bowel sounds; (5) measuring and recording intake and output accurately; (6) obtaining a daily weight; (7) straining and monitoring the urine for stones; and (8) monitoring all appropriate laboratory data.

Nursing interventions performed with a hypercalcemic individual are (1) to encourage frequent ambulation whenever appropriate; (2) to institute active and passive range of motion exercises; (3) to provide appropriate stimuli to increase the patient's level of orientation; (4) to provide a safe physical environment for the individual; (5) to encourage acid–ash fluids such as cranberry or prune juice; (6) to encourage an increased oral intake of fluids; (7) to administer medications as prescribed; (8) to provide foods and fluids that are consistent with the dietary restrictions, if any are prescribed; and (9) to institute extra safety precautions and provide for gentle movement of the individual.

As with all other types of imbalances, the treatment of hypercalcemia involves treating the underlying cause and correcting the imbalance. Thus, whenever possible, an attempt is made to deal with the etiology as soon as it is feasible.

Hypercalcemia can be corrected by a variety of therapeutic methods. One of the first methods employed is the administration of saline infusions. These infusions not only hydrate the individual but also dilute the extracellular calcium concentration and in-

crease the renal excretion of calcium through the sodium diuresis. Diuretics are also given to increase the renal excretion of calcium. Other forms of treatment include administering the following: sodium bicarbonate to induce alkalosis and reduce the ionized calcium fraction; phosphate to inhibit the resorption of bone; glucocorticoids to inhibit calcium absorption and shift the extracellular calcium intracellularly; mithramycin, indomethacin, or calcitonin to decrease bone resorption; ethylenediaminetetraacetic acid (EDTA) to lower the serum calcium by chelation; and dialysis therapy to deplete the serum calcium.

Hypocalcemia

Definition and Etiology

Hypocalcemia is a deficit of calcium in the extracellular fluid. It is caused by the following: hypoproteinemia; idiopathic, surgical, or pseudohypoparathyroidism; renal dysfunction; hyperphosphatemia; vitamin D deficiency; magnesium deficiency; acute pancreatitis; inadequate dietary intake; intestinal malabsorption; alkalosis; excessive administration of citrated blood; massive subcutaneous infections; osteomalacia; and malignant neoplasms, especially those with bone metastases.

Data Acquisition

Physical Assessment. The person experiencing hypocalcemia exhibits a variety of signs and symptoms, the majority of which are neuromuscular. Clinical signs and symptoms of hypocalcemia include numbness and tingling of the extremities, circumoral tingling, muscle cramps, tetany, positive Chvostek's and Trousseau's signs, epileptiform seizures, laryngeal stridor, carpopedal spasms, hyperreflexia, mental depression, psychoses, cardiac arrest, abdominal cramps, nausea and vomiting, diarrhea, cataracts, keratitis, dry skin, brittle nails, alopecia, coagulation dysfunction (rarely occurs), and pathological fractures. If the individual is being assessed by means of a cardiac monitor, the electrocardiogram will reflect a lengthened ST segment and a prolonged QT interval, which are characteristic of hypocalcemia.

Diagnostic Procedures. The serum calcium is the most helpful of all the laboratory data for determining hypocalcemia. A serum calcium value less than 8.5 mg/100 ml is indicative of hypocalcemia.

Medical and Nursing Management

Clinically, hypocalcemia presents many hazards to the patient's health state and normal ability to function. The neuromuscular effects of hypocalcemia alone constitute major problems for the individual. Add to those effects the cardiovascular and gastrointestinal effects, and the patient, indeed, becomes severely compromised and in need of supportive care from the nurse.

Supportive nursing care for an individual experiencing hypocalcemia includes performing the following monitoring functions: (1) assessing neuromuscular function frequently; (2) monitoring rate, rhythm, and characteristics of the pulse; (3) evaluating the rate, pattern, and characteristics of the respirations; (4) checking Chvostek's sign periodically (this involves percussing the facial nerve in the area of the face just anterior to the auricle of the ear. If this percussion elicits a unilateral twitching of the facial muscles, including the eyelid and lips, it indicates hypocalcemia.); (5) testing Trousseau's sign periodically (this involves occluding the blood supply to an extremity to produce ischemia. Usually this sign is tested by applying a tourniquet, or inflating a blood pressure cuff around the upper extremity for 3 or 4 minutes. If the induced ischemia precipitates carpopedal spasms, it indicates hypocalcemia.); (6) assessing the individual's mental status; (7) monitoring the characteristics of the feces; (8) assessing visual acuity and the characteristics of the eyeballs; (9) evaluating the intactness of the skeletal system; (10) assessing the characteristics of the skin, nails, and hair; and (11) monitoring the serum calcium values and the electrocardiograms.

The intervening functions that are performed with the hypocalcemic individual are (1) providing a safe physical environment for the patient; (2) instituting seizure precautions; (3) providing an environment with decreased, but appropriate amounts of stimuli;

(4) administering prescribed medications appropriately; (5) providing foods that are high in calcium and low in phosphorus, if prescribed; (6) providing meticulous hygienic care for the skin, nails, and hair; and (7) implementing a variety of nursing comfort measures to deal with the gastrointestinal effects.

Hypocalcemia is treated by dealing with the underlying cause, if possible, and correcting the imbalance. The therapy used to correct the imbalance differs, depending on whether the imbalance is acute or chronic. Acute hypocalcemic imbalances are usually treated with intravenous infusions of calcium chloride, calcium gluconate, or calcium gluceptate. (The individual receiving digitalis is monitored extremely closely during these infusions because calcium increases the sensitivity of the heart to digitalis and thus may precipitate digitalis toxicity.)

Chronic calcium depletion is effectively treated by the following methods: administering daily doses of oral calcium preparations, such as calcium lactate, calcium gluconate, or calcium carbonate; administering daily doses of oral vitamin D preparations; increasing dietary intake of calcium through the use of foods high in calcium content; and restricting the dietary intake of foods high in phosphorus content.

MAGNESIUM
Functions

The functions of magnesium in the physiological processes of the body include the following: participating as a coenzyme in transphosphorylation reactions that result in a release of energy; activating other enzyme systems and thus influencing carbohydrate metabolism, protein synthesis, and nucleic acid synthesis and metabolism; acting as a mediator at the myoneural junction; activating adenosine triphosphatase; acting as a mediator of neural transmission in the central nervous system; influencing the transport of sodium and potassium across cell membranes; acting as a structural element of bone; and influencing the secretion of parathyroid hormone.

Regulation

The extracellular concentration of magnesium is regulated by intestinal absorption and secretion, an exchange process between bone and the extracellular fluid, and renal excretion.

Intestinal Absorption and Secretion

Approximately 30% to 40% of the magnesium ingested is absorbed by the intestines, primarily the small intestines. The efficiency of this absorption varies inversely with the amount of dietary magnesium ingested. The absorption process seems to be enhanced by parathyroid hormone and vitamin D and inhibited by thyrocalcitonin.

There appears to be some intestinal secretion of magnesium, but it is minimal.

Exchange between Bone and Extracellular Fluid

The exchange of magnesiuim between bone and the extracellular fluid seems to contribute minimally to the regulation of extracellular magnesium concentration. The factors that govern this exchange process are elusive and have yet to be defined.

Renal Excretion

The renal excretion of magnesium is the primary determinant of magnesium balance in the body. Reabsorption of magnesium occurs in all parts of the tubule but more so in the ascending limb of the loop of Henle. This reabsorption is regulated by the tubular maximal capacity which seems to be equal to the filtered load of magnesium that is present at normal plasma concentrations of magnesium. Therefore, even small increases in extracellular magnesium surpass the tubular maximal reabsorption capacity and increase the renal excretion of magnesium. Factors other than hypermagnesemia that increase the renal excretion of magnesium include extracellular fluid volume expansion, especially with saline solutions; diuretic agents including osmotic diuretics; renal vasodilation; hypercalcemia and hypercalciuria; thyrocalcitonin; alcohol ingestion; thyroid hormone; growth hormone; increased sodium intake; acute metabolic acidosis; chronic mineralocorticoid effect; and phosphate depletion. Factors that decrease the renal excretion of magnesium are hypomagnesemia, parathyroid hormone, and decreased extracellular fluid volume.

The variances associated with magnesium balance are hypermagnesemia and hypomagnesemia.

Hypermagnesemia

Definition and Etiology

Hypermagnesemia is an excess of magnesium in the extracellular fluid. It occurs rather infrequently because of the renal system's capacity to excrete large quantities in excess of normal. Therefore, the primary etiology of hypermagnesemia is renal failure. Other factors that can cause hypermagnesemia include adrenal insufficiency, shock, hypothermia, and an increased intake of magnesium. An increased intake of magnesium may result from excesses in any of the following that contain it: infusions of intravenous solutions, intramuscular injections, oral laxatives, or enemas.

Data Acquisition

Physical Assessment. The clinical signs and symptoms of hypermagnesemia depend on the severity of the imbalance. Mild hypermagnesemia may occur without clinically observable signs and symptoms. As the severity of hypermagnesemia increases, however, many signs and symptoms are observed, increasing in severity as magnesium levels rise. Table 8-13 pre-

TABLE 8-13 **Signs and Symptoms of Different Levels of Hypermagnesemia According to Body System**

Serum Magnesium Level, mEq/L	Body System	Signs and Symptoms
2.2 to 3.0	None	None
3.1 to 5.0	Vascular	Hypotension
	Gastrointestinal	Nausea
		Vomiting
		Thirst
	Nervous	Depressed deep tendon reflexes
	Integumentary	Flushing
5.1 to 7.0	Nervous	Drowsiness
		Depression
7.1 to 10.0	Nervous	Loss of deep tendon reflexes
	Muscular	Weakness
	Cardiac	Sinus bradycardia
		Prolonged PR interval
		Prolonged QT interval
10.1 to 15.0	Respiratory	Hypoventilation
	Muscular	Paralysis
	Nervous	Coma
15.1 to 20.0	Cardiac	Arrest
	Respiratory	Apnea

sents a correlation of serum magnesium levels with signs and symptoms according to body system.

Diagnostic Procedures. The serum magnesium level is the most significant laboratory value used in assessing an individual for hypermagnesemia. A serum magnesium value greater than 2.2 mEq/L indicates hypermagnesemia even though it may not be clinically observable.

Medical and Nursing Management

Clinically, the effects of hypermagnesemia are not hazardous to the individual until the serum magnesium level rises to four or five times its normal value. At that point, the condition threatens not only the patient's ability to function but even the ability to survive.

The nursing care of the individual experiencing hypermagnesemia includes the following monitoring functions: (1) assessing the rate, rhythm or pattern, and characteristics of all vital signs; (2) assessing the level of consciousness frequently; (3) evaluating muscular strength and function periodically; (4) monitoring neurologic responses; (5) monitoring renal output frequently; (6) assessing gastrointestinal function; and (7) monitoring serum magnesium values and the electrocardiogram.

Nursing interventions performed with the hypermagnesemic patient are (1) administering the prescribed medications appropriately; (2) providing a safe physical environment for the individual; (3) providing appropriate stimuli for maintaining orientation; (4) positioning the person appropriately to facilitate adequate respirations; (5) maintaining bed rest and a decreased activity level as appropriate; (6) instituting active and passive range of motion exercises; and (7) providing nursing comfort measures appropriate for dealing with the gastrointestinal signs and symptoms.

Goals for the treatment of hypermagnesemia are to correct the underlying disorder, counteract its harmful effects, and increase renal excretion. Correcting the underlying disorder is easy if the hypermagnesemia is due to excessive intake. However, it may be impossible to treat or stop the underlying cause if it is renal failure.

The harmful effects of hypermagnesemia can be effectively counteracted by infusing intravenous calcium preparations because the calcium ion antagonizes the action of the magnesium ion on the neuromuscular junction.

Increasing the renal excretion of magnesium can be accomplished in the presence of normal renal function by expanding the extracellular fluid volume with saline solution, administering diuretics, or both. If renal dysfunction is present, dialysis therapy will effectively remove the increased serum levels of magnesium.

Hypomagnesemia

Definition and Etiology

Hypomagnesemia is a deficit of magnesium in the extracellular fluid. The etiologies of hypomagnesemia can be classified according to the following five categories: (1) decreased intake, (2) decreased intestinal absorption, (3) excessive loss of body fluids, (4) excessive loss in the urine, and (5) miscellaneous factors.

Those etiologies of hypomagnesemia that are included in the category of decreased intake are prolonged intravenous therapy using magnesium-free solutions, protein-calorie malnutrition, and starvation.

The category of etiologies that result in hypomagnesemia due to decreased intestinal absorption include malabsorption syndrome such as nontropical sprue, surgical resection of the small bowel, and hereditary intestinal defects in magnesium absorption.

The etiologies of hypomagnesemia that are classified in the category of excessive loss of body fluids are intestinal biliary fistulas, abuse of enemas and nonmagnesium laxatives, prolonged use of nasogastric suctioning, and severe diarrhea, such as that which accompanies ulcerative colitis.

The category of etiologies that produce hypomagnesemia due to excessive magnesium loss in the urine include chronic alcoholism; diuretic therapy; primary hyperaldosteronism; the diuretic phase of acute renal failure; hypercalcemia, particularly in association with primary hyperparathyroidism, malignancies, and vitamin D intoxication; hyperthyroidism; phosphate deficiency; renal tubular acidosis; diabetic ketoacidosis; chronic renal failure with magnesium wasting; idiopathic renal magnesium wasting; cardiac glycosides; and aminoglycosides.

The last category of etiologies of hypomagnesium is the group of miscellaneous causes that include acute pancreatitis, hypoparathyroidism, idiopathic hypomagnesemia, inappropriate secretion of antidiuretic hormone, burns, and multiple transfusions with citrated blood.

Data Acquisition

Physical Assessment. The clinical signs and symptoms of hypomagnesemia are very similar to those seen with hypocalcemia. The hypomagnesemic individual will exhibit any combination of the following signs and symptoms: muscle fasciculation; muscle weakness; coarse, flapping tremors; ataxia; vertigo; paresthesias; positive Chvostek's and Trousseau's signs; generalized tetany; generalized muscle spasticity; spontaneous carpopedal spasms; seizures; apathy; confusion; irritability; psychoses; depression; nystagmus; hypertension; cardiac dysfunction; dysphagia; anorexia; and nausea.

If the patient is being assessed by means of a cardiac monitor, the electrocardiogram will reflect the following changes: a prolonged QT interval, broadened T waves of decreased amplitude, and an occasional shortened ST segment.

Diagnostic Procedures. The laboratory values used to assess an individual for hypomagnesemia are the serum magnesium, calcium, and potassium, and the urine magnesium and calcium. The levels of these values that are characteristic of hypomagnesemia are a serum magnesium of less than 1.6 mEq/L, a decreased serum calcium and potassium, and a decreased urine magnesium and calcium.

Medical and Nursing Management

The clinical implications of hypomagnesemia are significant because of the extensive involvement of the neuromuscular system. Having that particular body system so compromised certainly places the patient at risk.

The implications of hypomagnesemia for the nursing care of the individual require that the following monitoring functions be performed: (1) assess neurological function frequently; (2) monitor the level of consciousness periodically; (3) assess muscle strength and movement; (4) check Chvostek's and Trousseau's signs; (5) assess gastrointestinal function; (6) monitor the rate, rhythm, and characteristics of the pulse; (7) monitor all other vital signs, and (8) assess the appropriate laboratory values periodically.

The nursing interventions performed with the hypomagnesemic patient include (1) instituting seizure precautions, (2) providing a safe physical environment for the individual, (3) maintaining bed rest or limited activity as appropriate, (4) instituting active and passive range of motion exercises as appropriate, (5) providing appropriate stimuli for maintaining orientation, and (6) providing nursing comfort measures to deal with the gastrointestinal effects.

As with all the other imbalances, the treatment of hypomagnesemia is aimed at halting the primary cause and correcting the imbalance. The imbalance is usually corrected by administering either intravenous infusions of magnesium sulfate or magnesium chloride, or intramuscular injections of magnesium sulfate. The replacement therapy usually consists of administering 10 to 40 mEq of magnesium daily until the serum magnesium level returns to normal. Dietary substances and oral magnesium preparations can also be used as replacement therapy, particularly in cases of mild hypomagnesemia. It should be noted, however, that intestinal absorption of oral magnesium preparations is extremely variable, thus necessitating continuous monitoring of the individual's serum magnesium level.

CHLORIDE

Functions

The functions of chloride in the body are to assist in maintaining the osmotic pressure of the extracellular fluid, to participate in maintaining water balance, to participate in normal gastric digestion by providing an acid medium through the production of hydrochloric acid, and to assist in maintaining acid–base balance.

Regulation

Extracellular chloride concentration is regulated primarily by the renal system. This regulation is dependent upon aldosterone secretion and the acid–base balance of the body fluids.

In general, the renal handling of chloride is very similar to that of sodium, primarily because the two ions are coupled in many of the reabsorption, secretion, and transport processes, thus maintaining electrical neutrality. In most instances, then, chloride ion movement is passive and depends on active sodium transport. There are, however, two sites in the tubular system where this dependent relationship does not exist. The first site is the proximal tubule, where chloride reabsorption and excretion are dependent upon hydrogen ion secretion rather than on sodium transport. Thus, the degree of proximal tubular acidification determines the amount of chloride that is reabsorbed and excreted. The nature of this relationship is such that an increase in hydrogen ion secretion in the proximal tubule results in a compensatory increase in chloride excretion in response to an increase in bicarbonate reabsorption.

The second site is in the loop of Henle, where chloride ion transport may be more active than passive. Consequently, chloride movement is less dependent on sodium transport in this portion of the tubule.

The influence of aldosterone in the regulation of chloride is secondary to its effect on sodium and water reabsorption. As was previously discussed, aldosterone acts on the distal tubule and collecting duct to increase the reabsorption of sodium. As the sodium is actively reabsorbed, water and chloride are passively reabsorbed along with it. As a result, there is increased reabsorption of sodium, chloride, and water.

The variances in the balance of extracellular chloride are hyperchloremia and hypochloremia.

Hyperchloremia

Definition and Etiology

Hyperchloremia is an excess of chloride in the extracellular fluid. Hyperchloremia is caused by the following: excessive intake of chloride, usually in the form of medications; renal tubular acidosis; ureterosigmoidostomy; and increased salt intake, especially if there is an associated decrease in the extracellular fluid volume.

If the chloride increase is not accompanied by a proportional increase in sodium, hyperchloremia acidosis can result because of decreased hydrogen ion secretion in the proximal tubule.

Data Acquisition

Physical Assessment. The individual experiencing hyperchloremia that is disproportionate to the hypernatremia exhibits the following signs and symptoms: muscle weakness, decreased level of consciousness, and deep, rapid respirations. The person experiencing hyperchloremia that is proportionate to the hypernatremia will exhibit signs and symptoms that are reflective of either the increased sodium concentration or the decreased fluid volume. (The signs and symptoms of both of those imbalances have been previously delineated.)

Diagnostic Procedures. The laboratory values that provide the most data for assessing a patient in terms of hyperchloremia include the following: serum chloride, sodium, bicarbonate, and pH; and urine pH and specific gravity. The pattern of these values that is consistent with hyperchloremia is a serum chloride greater than 106 mEq/L, an increased serum sodium, a decreased serum bicarbonate and pH, an increased urine pH, and a decreased urine specific gravity. The changes in serum pH and bicarbonate and urine pH are reflective, of course, of the hyperchloremic acidosis rather than hyperchloremia accompanied by a proportionate hypernatremia.

Medical and Nursing Management

The clinical implications of hyperchloremia are related to the acidotic, hypernatremic, and hypovolemic conditions that may accompany it. This array of imbalances, which will significantly interfere with internal physiological processes, will create threats to the individual's well-being.

The implications of hyperchloremia for providing nursing care for the individual include monitoring and intervening functions related to all the mentioned imbalances. Since the nursing behaviors related to the hypovolemic and hypernatremic individual have been previously delineated, they will not be repeated, and only those actions specific for caring for the patient's hyperchloremia imbalance are discussed.

Monitoring functions performed with individuals experiencing hyperchloremia include (1) assessing the level of consciousness frequently; (2) monitoring the rate, rhythm, and characteristics of the respirations; (3) evaluating muscle strength; (4) monitoring appropriate laboratory values; and (5) monitoring all other vital signs.

The intervening nursing functions performed with hyperchloremic individuals are (1) to provide a safe physical environment for the patient; (2) to position the individual appropriately to facilitate adequate respirations; (3) to provide adequate, appropriate stimuli to promote orientation; (4) to maintain an activity level consistent with his or her muscle strength; (5) to administer fluids and/or medications as prescribed by the physician; and (6) to restrict chloride intake if consistent with the plan of care.

The treatment of hyperchloremia usually involves a combination of the following therapies: treating the primary underlying cause; administering or encouraging fluids to dilute the serum chloride; administering sodium bicarbonate; and, in some cases, administering diuretics.

Hypochloremia

Definition and Etiology

Hypochloremia is a deficit of chloride in the extracellular fluid. It is caused by the following: excessive loss of gastric secretions, usually due to vomiting or nasogastric suctioning; excessive secretion or administration of adrenocorticoid hormones; decreased intake, usually seen with severely salt-restricted diets; and, in some cases, rigorous use of diuretic therapy.

Hypochloremia is usually associated with hyponatremia, and if the loss of the two ions is proportional, the serum pH will remain virtually unchanged. However, if the chloride loss is disproportionately higher than the sodium loss, a hypochloremic alkalosis may result.

Data Acquisition

Physical Assessment. The hypochloremic individual with chloride loss disproportionate to the sodium loss exhibits the following signs and symptoms: muscle weakness; tetany; agitation; irritability; and slow, shallow respirations. An individual with hypochloremia that has resulted from proportionate losses of chloride and sodium exhibits the signs and symptoms characteristic of hyponatremia, hypovolemia, or both. Those signs and symptoms have been previously discussed.

Diagnostic Procedure. The laboratory values that provide the most data in determining hypochloremia in the individual are the following: serum chloride, sodium, bicarbonate, and pH. The pattern characteristic of hypochloremia is a serum chloride less than 96 mEq/L, a decreased serum sodium, and increased serum bicarbonate and pH values.

Medical and Nursing Management

The clinical implications for the hypochloremic patient are most definitely related to the alkalosis, hyponatremia, and hypervolemia that may accompany the hypochloremia. The interrelationship of those imbalances in an individual certainly jeopardizes well-being and necessitates supportive nursing measures.

The monitoring and intervening nursing behaviors implemented with individuals experiencing hyponatremia and hypervolemia have been previously discussed. Therefore, only those nursing behaviors that directly relate to the care of the hypochloremic individual are discussed at this time.

Monitoring functions performed in caring for an individual experiencing hypochloremia include (1) assessing the level of consciousness; (2) monitoring the rate, rhythm, and characteristics of the respirations; (3) evaluating all other vital signs; (4) assessing muscle strength and movement; (5) measuring and recording intake and output accurately; and (6) monitoring appropriate laboratory values.

Intervening functions performed with the hypochloremic patient are (1) to provide a safe physical environment for the individual; (2) to provide a quiet environment with decreased stimuli to minimize agitation; (3) to limit activity in accordance with muscle strength; (4) to provide foods and fluids high in chloride if appropriate; and (5) to administer prescribed medications correctly.

The treatment of hypochloremia includes treating the primary underlying cause and correcting the imbalance. The imbalance is usually corrected by replacing the lost chloride with sodium chloride, potassium chloride, or ammonium chloride. Replacement therapy usually involves replacing three fourths of the imbalance with sodium chloride and one fourth with potassium chloride. Ammonium chloride is used in place of potassium chloride if the serum potassium concentration is already elevated.

PHOSPHATE

Functions

The functions of the anion phosphate in the body are (1) participating as a structural element of bone; (2) influencing the production of energy sources by the red blood cells that are necessary for oxygen delivery; (3) participating in the metabolism of carbohydrates, lipids, and nucleic acids; (4) acting as the major urinary buffer in the formation of titratable acid; (5) participating in oxidative phosphorylation; (6) influencing the absorption of glucose and glycerol in the intestines; and (7) maintaining the structural integrity of the cell wall.

Regulation

The extracellular concentration of phosphate is regulated by the following four mechanisms: intestinal absorption, exchanges between bone and extracellular fluids, exchanges between the intracellular and extracellular fluid, and renal excretion.

Intestinal Absorption

Of all the dietary phosphate ingested, approximately 70% is absorbed in the jejunum, and the remaining 30% is excreted in the feces. The intestinal absorption of phosphate is increased by parathyroid hormone and vitamin D and decreased by thyrocalcitonin and binding by calcium or antacids.

Bone and Extracellular Fluid Exchange

The regulation of extracellular phosphate by exchange between bone and extracellular fluid depends primarily upon a similar exchange process that occurs as part of calcium homeostasis. When calcium is resorbed or released from bone, phosphate accompanies it. Likewise, when calcium is deposited in bone, phosphate is also deposited. The more active of the two exchange processes in regulating extracellular phosphate concentration is bone resorption. Bone resorption is increased by parathyroid hormone and vitamin D and decreased by thyrocalcitonin.

Intracellular and Extracellular Fluid Exchange

The concentration of phosphate in the extracellular fluid is also influenced by the exchange of phosphate ions between the intracellular and extracellular fluids. The rate of this exchange is dependent upon the rate of glycolysis that occurs in the cell. When glycolysis occurs, phosphate shifts into the cell. Thus, an increase in glycolysis would increase the phosphate shift into the cell, and a decrease in glycolysis would increase the shift of phosphate out of the cell. The factors that would facilitate glycolysis and thus phosphate shift into the cell include acute alkalosis and the administration of glucose, insulin, or epinephrine. Acute acidosis is one factor that would increase the shift of phosphate out of the cell, probably due to tissue hypoxia with its accompanying increase in ATP degradation.

Renal Excretion

The renal regulation of phosphate is excretory in nature. The renal excretion of phosphate is dependent primarily upon parathyroid hormone and the serum concentration of phosphate. These two factors affect renal excretion by determining the amount and rate at which phosphate can be reabsorbed by the kidney.

About 70% of the filtered phosphate is reabsorbed in the proximal tubule and 25% in the distal tubule. This reabsorption is dependent upon the tubular maximal reabsorptive capacity that is established by parathyroid hormone.

The renal excretion of phosphate is increased by the following factors: parathyroid hormone, acute fluid volume expansion, hyperphosphatemia, thyrocalcitonin, metabolic acidosis, hypokalemia, and diuretics that function by acting on the proximal tubule. The renal excretion of phosphate is decreased by vitamin D, growth hormone, hypophosphatemia, and a decrease in fluid volume.

The variances or imbalances that occur in relation to phosphate are hyperphosphatemia and hypophosphatemia.

Hyperphosphatemia

Definition and Etiology

Hyperphosphatemia is an excess of phosphate in the extracellular fluid. It is caused by the following: renal dysfunction (probably the most common cause), hypoparathyroidism, pseudohypoparathyroidism, hyperthyroidism, excessive ingestion or infusion of phosphate salts, catabolic states, neoplastic diseases, and overingestion of vitamin D metabolites.

Data Acquisition

Physical Assessment. An inverse relationship exists between phosphate and calcium in the extracellular fluid. Therefore, a hyperphosphatemic condition is accompanied by hypocalcemia. This relationship accounts for the fact that the clinical signs and symptoms of the hyperphosphatemic individual are indeed the same as those seen in the hypocalcemic individual. Those signs and symptoms have been previously delineated and will not be repeated. It should be noted, however, that the primary effect of hypocalcemia on the individual is in relation to the neuromuscular system.

Diagnostic Procedures. The laboratory values used to assess the individual in relation to hyperphosphatemia are the serum phosphorus and calcium values. The pattern characteristic of hyperphosphatemia is a serum phosphorus greater than 4.5 mg/100 ml and a decreased serum calcium.

Medical and Nursing Management

Since the clinical manifestations of hyperphosphatemia are the same as those accompanying hypocalcemia, it is logical that the clinical implications and nursing behaviors are also the same. Those implica-

tions and behaviors have been previously discussed in relation to hypocalcemia.

The treatment of hyperphosphatemia is aimed at eliminating the cause and correcting the imbalance. The imbalance can be corrected by the following methods: restricting the intake of phosphate; administering intestinal phosphate-binding agents, such as aluminum hydroxide gel; administering diuretics if renal function is present; and implementing dialysis therapy if renal dysfunction is present.

Hypophosphatemia

Definition and Etiology

Hypophosphatemia is a deficit of phosphate in the extracellular fluid. The following are causes of hypophosphatemia: primary and secondary hyperparathyroidism; primary renal tubular defects in phosphate reabsorption; states of chronic metabolic acidosis, as seen with renal tubular acidosis and ureterosigmoidostomies; hypokalemia; extracellular fluid volume expansion; administration of phosphate binders; vomiting; malabsorption; starvation; prolonged use of phosphate-free intravenous solutions; abnormalities in vitamin D metabolism, as in vitamin D–associated rickets; alcohol withdrawal; the recovery phase of diabetic ketoacidosis; the administration of agents designed to increase glycolysis; severe burns; and the recovery phase of malnutrition.

Data Acquisition

Physical Assessment. The clinical signs and symptoms exhibited by a hypophosphatemic individual are, of course, direct manifestations of the biochemical changes produced by the imbalance. Those biochemical changes are significant, not only to the individual's functioning but also to the nurse's understanding of the associated clinical signs and symptoms. Therefore, those biochemical changes are summarized according to body system in the box on p. 201.

The resulting clinical signs and symptoms exhibited by the hypophosphatemic patient are: irritability, confusion, disorientation, seizures, coma, anisocoria, ptosis, nystagmus, muscle weakness, paresthesias, tremors, ataxia, ballism, dysrhythmia, hyperventilation, anorexia, nausea, vomiting, bruising, bone pain, pathological fractures, and arthralgias. If the imbalance is prolonged, there may be additional clinical signs and symptoms exhibited in relation to platelet dysfunction and decreased white blood cell phagocytic activity.

Diagnostic Procedures

The most significant laboratory value used in assessing an individual for hypophosphatemia is the

Biochemical Changes Accompanying Hypophosphatemia According to Body System

CENTRAL NERVOUS
Hypoxia
Abnormal conduction velocity

NEUROMUSCULAR
Rhabdomyolysis
Increased CPK
Decreased transmembrane resting potential gradient

HEMATOLOGICAL
Red cell rigidity
Hemolysis
Decreased 2,3,-DPG resulting in tissue hypoxia
Decreased phagocytosis
Decreased chemotaxis
Platelet destruction
Shift of the hemoglobin dissociation curve

CARDIOVASCULAR
Decreased electrical conduction
Decreased mechanical function

RESPIRATORY
Decreased ATP, creating fatigue

GASTROINTESTINAL
Increased calcium absorption

HEPATIC
Hepatic dysfunction due to decreased oxygen

SKELETAL
Increased calcium resorption
Decreased osteoid calcification

RENAL
Hypercalciuria
Hypophosphaturia
Decreased H^+ ion excretion
Decreased tubular reabsorption of HCO_3 and glucose
Increased synthesis of vitamin D
Bicarbonaturia

serum phosphorus. A serum phosphorus less than 2 mg/100 ml is consistent with hypophosphatemia. Urine laboratory values may provide additional assessment data because hypophosphatemia seems to result in hypercalciuria, hypophosphaturia, bicarbonaturia, and decreased hydrogen ion excretion.

Medical and Nursing Management

The clinical implications of hypophosphatemia for the individual are certainly threatening to well-being. The most significant implications of hypophosphatemia for the patient seem to be related to its effects on the central nervous and neuromuscular systems. These effects decrease the individual's ability to carry out the activities of daily living, as well as to partic-ipate in health care. Thus, he or she requires nursing support.

Monitoring functions that are a part of nursing support include (1) assessing muscle strength, (2) evaluating the individual's level of consciousness, (3) monitoring for signs of associated hypercalcemia, (4) assessing the individual's comfort level, (5) observing for signs of decreased clotting or decreased inflammatory response, (6) monitoring intake, (7) monitoring all vital signs, and (8) monitoring appropriate laboratory values.

The intervening functions performed in hypophosphatemia are: (1) assisting with the activities of daily living; (2) providing activity in accordance with muscle strength; (3) instituting active and passive range of motion exercises; (4) providing stimuli appropriate for maintaining orientation; (5) establishing a safe physical environment for the individual; (6) providing food and fluids high in phosphate, if appropriate; (7) presenting small amounts of food and fluids at intervals in an appetizing manner; (8) providing nursing comfort measures; and (9) administering medications as prescribed.

Hypophosphatemia is usually treated by dealing with the primary underlying cause and replacing the lost phosphate. The replacement therapy may be implemented using either oral or intravenous phosphate preparations or, in cases of mild imbalance, dietary substances.

SULFATE
Functions

The functions of sulfate in the body are to participate in the synthesis of sulfated mucopolysaccharides for the cartilage and bone matrix, to influence the synthesis of heparin and the mucoprotein secretions of the gastrointestinal tract, and to detoxify drugs and foreign compounds in the liver.

Regulation

The concentration of sulfate in the extracellular fluid seems to be regulated by intake, the rate of release by metabolic degradation, and renal excretion. The exact mechanisms for these regulating processes are not known. The variances in sulfate balance in the body seem to be clinically insignificant.

PROTEIN
Functions

The primary functions of protein in the body are (1) to provide colloid osmotic pressure for regulating fluid volume, (2) to participate in enzyme processes, (3) to influence the development of natural and acquired immunity, (4) to participate in the regulation of acid–base balance, (5) to participate in blood coagulation, and (6) to influence the production of hormones and some vitamins.

Regulation

The concentration of extracellular protein is regulated by the following factors: dietary intake, the rate of formation by the liver, and the rate of use by the tissues. The variance in protein balance that has clinical significance for the individual is hypoproteinemia.

Hypoproteinemia

Definition and Etiology

Hypoproteinemia is a deficit of protein in the extracellular fluid. Hypoproteinemia is caused by the following: inadequate dietary intake; hemorrhage; severe prolonged infection; gastrointestinal disorders that inhibit absorption, such as obstruction or fistulas; fractures; medical disorders and surgical procedures that produce catabolic states; hypokalemia; and prolonged illness, especially when accompanied by fluid imbalances.

Data Acquisition

Physical Assessment. The individual experiencing hypoproteinemia exhibits the following signs and symptoms: weight loss, muscle wasting, decreased muscle tone, fatigue, mental and emotional depression, anorexia, nausea, vomiting, decreased wound healing, decreased immunity or resistance to infection, and edema.

Diagnostic Procedures. The laboratory value that provides the most significant data for assessing an individual in relation to hypoproteinemia is the serum albumin. A serum albumin value of less than 4 g/100 ml is consistent with hypoproteinemia. Other laboratory values that may provide additional data, if iron intake has been adequate, are hemoglobin, hematocrit, and red blood cell count. Decreased values for those three items, in the presence of adequate iron intake, are consistent with hypoproteinemia.

Medical and Nursing Management

The clinical implications of hypoproteinemia for the individual are very significant. Without adequate protein, the individual does not heal or resist infection well. Thus, he or she is predisposed to developing life-threatening complications such as septicemia.

The implications of hypoproteinemia for providing nursing care for the patient indicate that the following monitoring behaviors be performed: (1) monitoring protein intake frequently; (2) obtaining precise daily weights; (3) assessing muscle strength and movement; (4) assessing level of consciousness periodically; (5) monitoring gastrointestinal functioning; (6) assessing skin integrity, texture, and turgor; (7) monitoring vi-

tal signs; and (8) monitoring appropriate laboratory values.

Intervening behaviors performed in hypoproteinemia are (1) providing a physical environment that decreases exposure to bacterial contamination, (2) maintaining a limited activity level consistent with the person's muscle strength, (3) instituting active and passive range of motion exercises, (4) assisting with the activities of daily living, (5) providing stimuli appropriate to maintain orientation, (6) providing meticulous skin care, (7) instituting nursing comfort measures to deal with the gastrointestinal effects, (8) using creative nursing measures to decrease mental depression, and (9) providing high-protein foods and fluids as prescribed.

Hypoproteinemia is treated by dealing with the underlying cause and correcting the imbalance. The imbalance is usually corrected by providing a high-protein diet balanced with adequate calories, vitamins, and minerals; using high-protein oral supplements; or infusing proteins and amino acids parenterally. In some cases, the high-protein oral intake is given via a nasogastric tube if the individual has difficulty taking nourishment.

ORGANIC ACIDS

Organic acids, such as pyruvic acid and lactic acid, which are produced as a result of carbohydrate metabolism, are present in small amounts in the extracellular fluid. Normally, these fixed, nonvolatile acids are clinically not significant for the individual because they are buffered and excreted by the kidneys. When they are produced in abnormal quantities, they result in a change in the acid–base balance of the body. Thus, the clinical significance of having abnormal quantities of organic acids in the extracellular fluid will be discussed in Chapter 9.

CRITICAL CARE IMPLICATIONS

This chapter has discussed the regulation and assessment of fluid and electrolyte balance. The critical care nurse is constantly making decisions about patient care based on this information. In conducting an assessment of a patient, the critical care nurse proceeds by beginning with the highest priority substance for the individual. In general, the critical care nurse would assess the patient in the following order: fluid volume, acid–base balance, potassium, calcium, sodium, chloride, magnesium, and phosphate. Certainly, this order might change depending on the specific history and presenting behaviors of the individual, but all areas would be included in the assessment. To assist the critical care nurse in performing this assessment, the signs and symptoms of each imbalance have been summarized according to body systems in the box on pp. 203-206.

Signs and Symptoms of Fluid and Electrolyte and Acid–Base Imbalances According to Body Systems

HYPERVOLEMIA

Cardiovascular System
  Weight gain
  Systemic edema
  Ascites
  ↑ CVP
  Hypertension
  Bounding pulse

Respiratory System
  Dyspnea
  Moist rales

Integumentary System
  Puffy eyelids

HYPOVOLEMIA

Central Nervous System
  Lassitude

Neuromuscular System
  Fatigue

Cardiovascular System
  Weight loss
  ↓ Postural BP
  ↑ Pulse
  ↓ Venous pressure

Gastrointestinal System
  Thirst

Integumentary System
  Dry skin
  Dry mucous membranes
  ↓ Skin turgor
  ↓ Elasticity
  Furrowed tongue
  ↓ Temperature
  ↓ Eyeball turgor
  ↓ Perspiration

Renal System
  Oliguria

METABOLIC ACIDOSIS

Central Nervous System
  Headache
  Drowsiness
  ↓ Mentation
  Confusion
  Coma
  Seizures

Neuromuscular System
  Fatigue

Cardiovascular System
  Hypotension
  Hypoxia
  Dysrhythmia

Respiratory System
  Kussmaul respirations

Gastrointestinal System
  Anorexia
  Nausea
  Vomiting

Integumentary System
  Tissue hypoxia

METABOLIC ALKALOSIS

Central Nervous System
  Seizures
  Belligerence
  Confusion
  Stupor
  Coma

Neuromuscular System
  Irritability
  Tetany

Cardiovascular System
  Dysrhythmia

Respiratory System
  Hypoventilation

Gastrointestinal System
  Nausea
  Vomiting
  Diarrhea

RESPIRATORY ACIDOSIS

Central Nervous System
  ↓ Mentation
  Apprehension
  Restlessness
  Headache
  Drowsiness
  Disorientation
  Coma

Neuromuscular System
  Fatigue
  Muscle weakness
  Flapping tremors
  Uncoordination
  ↓ Reflexes

Cardiovascular System
  Tachycardia

Respiratory System
  Hypoventilation
  Dyspnea

Integumentary System
  Cyanosis

Continued.

Signs and Symptoms of Fluid and Electrolyte and Acid–Base Imbalances According to Body Systems—cont'd

RESPIRATORY ALKALOSIS

Central Nervous System
Vertigo
Syncope
Nervousness
Seizures
↓ Mentation
Confusion
Anxiety

Neuromuscular System
Paresthesias
Muscle cramps
Tetany
↓ Psychomotor function

Cardiovascular System
Dysrhythmia
Hypotension

Respiratory System
Dyspnea
Hyperventilation

Integumentary System
Perioral paresthesia

HYPERKALEMIA

Central Nervous System
Confusion

Neuromuscular System
Hyperexcitability
Muscle weakness
Paresthesias
Flaccid paralysis

Cardiovascular System
Dysfunction
Arrest

Gastrointestinal System
Distention
Diarrhea
Intestinal colic

HYPOKALEMIA

Central Nervous System
Drowsiness
Confusion
Apathy
Coma

Neuromuscular System
Irritability
Muscle weakness
Paresthesias
Muscle pain
Muscle cramps
Muscle tenderness
Hyporeflexia
Tetany
Paralysis

Cardiovascular System
Weak pulse
Bradycardia

Respiratory System
Weakness
Hypoventilation

Gastrointestinal System
Nausea
Vomiting
Anorexia
Distention
Cramps
Paralytic ileus
Polydipsia
Hyperglycemia
Negative nitrogen balance

Renal System
Polyuria
Nocturia

HYPERCALCEMIA

Central Nervous System
Drowsiness
Lethargy
Disorientation
Loss of memory
Depression
Stupor
Coma

Neuromuscular System
Fatigue
Muscle weakness
Hypotonicity

Cardiovascular System
Dysrhythmia
Arrest

Gastrointestinal System
Anorexia
Nausea
Vomiting
Constipation
Thirst

Skeletal System
Deep bone pain

Renal System
Polyuria
Calculi

HYPOCALCEMIA

Central Nervous System
Seizures
Depression
Psychoses

Signs and Symptoms of Fluid and Electrolyte and Acid–Base Imbalances According to Body Systems—cont'd

Neuromuscular System
  Paresthesias
  Muscle cramps
  Tetany
  Positive Chvostek's sign
  Positive Trousseau's sign
  Carpopedal spasms
  Hyperreflexia

Cardiovascular System
  Arrest

Respiratory System
  Laryngeal stridor

Gastrointestinal System
  Cramps
  Nausea
  Vomiting
  Diarrhea

Integumentary System
  Circumoral paresthesia
  Cataracts
  Keratitis
  Dry skin
  Brittle nails
  Alopecia

Skeletal System
  Pathological fractures

HYPERNATREMIA
Central Nervous System
  Lethargy
  Irritability
  Seizures
  Coma

Neuromuscular System
  Muscular rigidity
  Muscular weakness
  Tremors

Cardiovascular System
  Tachycardia

Gastrointestinal System
  Thirst

Integumentary System
  Dry, sticky mucous membranes
  Rough, dry tongue
  Flushed, dry skin
  ↑ Turgor
  ↓ Lacrimation
  ↑ Temperature

Renal System
  Oliguria

HYPONATREMIA
Central Nervous System
  Lethargy
  Confusion
  Headache
  Seizures
  Coma
  Apprehension

Neuromuscular System
  Fatigue
  Muscle weakness
  Tremors
  Hyperreflexia

Gastrointestinal System
  Anorexia
  Nausea
  Vomiting
  Cramps
  Diarrhea

Renal System
  Oliguria

HYPERCHLOREMIA
Central Nervous System
  ↓ Level of consciousness

Neuromuscular System
  Muscle weakness

Respiratory System
  Deep and rapid respirations

HYPOCHLOREMIA
Central Nervous System
  Agitation
  Irritability

Neuromuscular System
  Muscle weakness
  Tetany

Respiratory System
  Slow and shallow respirations

HYPERMAGNESEMIA
Central Nervous System
  Drowsiness
  Depression
  Coma

Neuromuscular System
  ↓ Deep reflexes
  Loss of deep reflexes
  Muscle weakness
  Paralysis

Cardiovascular System
  Hypotension
  Bradycardia
  Arrest

Continued.

Signs and Symptoms of Fluid and Electrolyte and Acid–Base Imbalances According to Body Systems—cont'd

Respiratory System
  Hypoventilation
  Apnea

Gastrointestinal System
  Nausea
  Vomiting
  Thirst

Integumentary System
  Flushing

HYPOMAGNESEMIA

Central Nervous System
  Seizures
  Apathy
  Confusion
  Irritability
  Psychoses
  Depression

Neuromuscular System
  Muscle fasciculation
  Muscle weakness
  Flapping tremors
  Positive Chvostek's sign
  Positive Trousseau's sign
  Tetany
  Muscle spasticity
  Carpopedal spasms
  Nystagmus
  Paresthesias

Cardiovascular System
  Hypertension
  Dysfunction

Gastrointestinal System
  Anorexia
  Nausea
  Dysphagia

HYPERPHOSPHATEMIA

Central Nervous System
  Seizures
  Depression
  Psychoses

Neuromuscular System
  Paresthesias
  Muscle cramps
  Tetany
  Positive Chvostek's sign
  Positive Trousseau's sign
  Carpopedal spasms
  Hyperreflexia

Cardiovascular System
  Arrest

Respiratory System
  Laryngeal stridor

Gastrointestinal System
  Cramps
  Nausea
  Vomiting
  Diarrhea

Integumentary System
  Circumoral paresthesia
  Cataracts
  Keratitis
  Dry skin
  Brittle nails
  Alopecia

Skeletal System
  Pathologic fractures

HYPOPHOSPHATEMIA

Central Nervous System
  Irritability
  Confusion
  Disorientation
  Seizures
  Coma
  Anisocoria
  Ptosis
  Nystagmus

Neuromuscular System
  Muscle weakness
  Paresthesias
  Tremors
  Ataxia
  Ballism

Cardiovascular System
  Dysrhythmia

Respiratory System
  Hyperventilation

Gastrointestinal System
  Anorexia
  Nausea
  Vomiting

Integumentary System
  Bruising

Skeletal System
  Bone pain
  Pathological fractures
  Arthralgias

BIBLIOGRAPHY

Aberman, A. (1982). The ins and outs of fluids and electrolytes. *Emergency Medicine, 14,* 121, 123-124, 127.

Andersson, B. (1978). Regulation of water intake. *Physiological Reviews, 58,* 582-602.

Arieff, A. I., & DeFronzo, R. A. (1985). *Fluid, electrolyte and acid–base disorders* (Vol. 1). New York: Churchill Livingstone.

Calhoun, K. A. (1990). Serum potassium concentration abnormalities. *Critical Care Nursing Quarterly, 13*(3), 34-38.

Carroll, H. J., & Oh, M. S. (1989). *Water, electrolyte and acid–base metabolism: Diagnosis and management* (2nd ed.). Philadelphia: Lippincott.

Chambers, S. K. (1987). Metabolic bone disorders: Imbalances of calcium and phosphorus. *Nursing Clinics of North America, 22*(4), 861-872.

Chenevey, B. (1987). Overview of fluids and electrolytes. *Nursing Clinics of North America, 22*(4), 749-759.

Collins R. D. (1983). *Illustrated manual of fluids and electrolyte disorders* (2nd ed.). Philadelphia: Lippincott.

Conner, C. S. (1984). Hypophosphatemia. *Drug Intelligence and Clinical Pharmacy, 18*(7/8), 595.

DeRubertis, F. R. (1984). Hypercalcemia and hypocalcemia. *Topics in Emergency Medicine, 5*(5), 64-73.

Felver, L. (1980). Understanding the electrolyte maze. *American Journal of Nursing, 80,* 1591-1595.

Felver, L., & Pendarvis, J. H. (1989). Electrolyte imbalances: Intraoperative risk factors. *AORN Journal, 49*(4), 992-1006.

Folk-Lighty, M. (1984). Solving the puzzles of patient's fluid imbalances. *Nursing 84, 14*(2), 39-41.

Gelderman, J. M., Goodman, S. L., & Cohen, D. B. (1979). Magnesium—the forgotten electrolyte, *JACEP, 8*(5), 204-208.

Graves, L. (1990). Disorders of calcium, phosphorus, and magnesium. *Critical Care Nursing Quarterly, 13*(3), 3-13.

Guyton, A. C. (1991). *Textbook of medical physiology* (8th ed.). Philadelphia: Saunders.

Humes, H. D., Narins, R. G., & Brenner, B. M. (1979). Disorders of water balance. *Hospital Practice, 4*(3), 133-145.

Isley, W. L. (1990). Serum sodium concentration abnormalities. *Critical Care Nursing Quarterly, 13*(3), 82-88.

Janson, C., Birnbaum, G., & Baker, F. J., II. (1983). Hypophosphatemia. *Annals of Emergency Medicine, 12*(2), 107-116.

Jones, D. H. (1991). Fluid therapy in the PACU. *Critical Care Nursing Clinics of North America, 3*(1), 109-120.

Keyes, J. L. (1985). *Fluid, electrolyte, and acid base regulation.* Monterey: Wadsworth Health Sciences Division.

Klahr, S. (1978). *Differential diagnosis: Renal and electrolyte disorders.* New York: Arco.

Koch, S. M., & Taylor, R. W. (1992). Chloride ion in intensive care and medicine. *Critical Care Medicine, 20*(2), 227-240.

Massry, S. G. (1978). The clinical pathophysiology of magnesium. *Contributions to Nephrology, 14,* 64-73.

Mathewson, M. (1989). Intravenous therapy. *Critical Care Nurse, 9*(2), 21-36.

Maxwell, M. H., & Kleeman, C. R. (1987). *Clinical disorders of fluid and electrolyte metabolism* (4th ed.). New York: McGraw-Hill.

McFadden, E. A., & Zaloga, G. P. (1983). Calcium regulation. *Critical Care Quarterly, 6*(3), 12-21.

McGeown, M. G. (1983). *Critical management of electrolyte disorders.* Boston: Martinus Nijhoff.

Menzel, L. K. (1980). Clinical problems of electrolyte balance. *Nursing Clinics of North America, 15*(3), 559-576.

Menzel, L. K. (1980). Clinical problems of fluid balance. *Nursing Clinics of North America, 15*(3), 549-558.

Metheny, N. M. (1992). *Fluid and electrolyte balance: Nursing considerations* (2nd ed.). Philadelphia: Lippincott.

Metheny, N., & Snively, W. D. (1983). *Nursing handbook of fluid balance* (4th ed.). Philadelphia: Lippincott.

Narins, R. G. (1979). A practical approach to managing hyponatremia. *Consultant, 19*(2), 25-29, 34-35.

Otrakji, J. (1983). Disorders of potassium metabolism. *Topics in Emergency Medicine, 5*(2), 53-57.

Poyss, A. S. (1987). Assessment and nursing diagnosis in fluid and electrolyte disorders. *Nursing Clinics of North America, 22*(4), 773-783.

Quinlan, M. (1983). Would you recognize this dangerous electrolyte imbalance? *RN, 46*(3), 50-55.

Rice, V. (1983). Magnesium, calcium, and phosphate imbalances; their clinical significance. *Critical Care Nurse, 3*(3), 90-112.

Rice, V. (1984). Shock management: Part 1. Fluid volume replacement. *Critical Care Nurse, 4*(6), 69-82.

Rose, B. D. (1989). *Clinical physiology of acid–base and electrolyte disorders* (3rd ed.). New York: McGraw-Hill.

Ross, A. D., & Angaram, D. M. (1984). Colloids vs. crystalloids—a continuing controversy. *Drug Intelligence and Clinical Pharmacy, 18*(3), 202-212.

Schrier, R. (1992). *Renal and electrolyte disorders* (4th ed.). Boston: Little, Brown.

Sneid, D. (1983). Hypercalcemia. *Topics in Emergency Medicine, 5*(2), 8-17.

Thomas, A. G. (1983). Disorders of sodium metabolism. *Topics in Emergency Medicine, 5*(2), 46-52.

Vander, A. J. (1991). *Renal physiology* (4th ed.). New York: McGraw-Hill.

Verbalis, J. G., & Robinson, A. G. (1984). Hypernatremia and hyponatremia. *Topics in Emergency Medicine, 5*(4), 79-89.

Weil, M. H., & Rackow, E. C. (1984). A guide to volume repletion. *Emergency Medicine, 16*(8), 100-105, 108-110.

Yarnell, R. P., & Craig, M. P. (1991). Detecting hypomagnesemia. *Nursing 91, 21*(7), 55-57.

Zaloga, G. P. (1992). Hypocalcemia in critically ill patients. *Critical Care Medicine, 20*(2), 251-262.

Zaloga, G. P., & Chernow, B. (1983). Magnesium metabolism in critical illness. *Critical Care Quarterly, 6*(3), 22-27.

Zaloga, G. P., & Rainey, T. G. (1986). Hypocalcemia in the critically ill: When to suspect and what to do. *The Journal of Critical Illness, (4)*, 12-23.

Zeluff, G. W., Suki, W. N., & Jackson, D. (1978). Hypokalemia—cause and treatment. *Heart Lung, 7(5)*, 854-860.

Zeluff G. W., Suki, W. N., & Jackson, D. (1980). Hypercalcemia—etiology, manifestations, and management. *Heart Lung, 9(1)*, 146-151.

9

Acid–Base Balance

Charold L. Baer

Acids and bases are essential to the body not only for their participation in physiological processes, but also for helping to maintain a stable environment to facilitate those processes. The physiological processes and associated chemical reactions of the body occur in a stable, slightly alkaline environment. When the normal balance of that environment is disturbed through an increase or decrease in hydrogen ions, those processes and reactions may be accelerated, deterred, or totally inhibited. Thus, a change in the pH of the internal environment can affect the entire body. As a result, the individual will require nursing and medical support during the period of instability to sustain life and regain normal function. Appropriate nursing support cannot be provided unless the nurse is able accurately to assess, plan, implement, and evaluate care for the patient. This discussion provides information basic to the nurse's comprehension of the components of acid–base balance and imbalance in order to facilitate the provision of appropriate nursing support for the individual.

FUNCTIONS

The acid–base balance of body fluids or, more specifically, the pH of the internal environment, is an essential component of metabolism. Variations in pH will produce significant deviations in metabolic function by altering blood flow, secondary messengers and/or cellular structure, electrolytes, proteins, and gradients. For example, as the pH rises, the following metabolic changes occur: (1) lactate production increases; (2) insulin-induced glycolysis increases; (3) Krebs cycle oxidations in the muscles and renal cortex decrease; (4) gluconeogenesis in the renal cortex decreases; (5) the 2,3-diphosphoglycerate concentration in the red blood cell falls, with a corresponding left shift in the oxyhemoglobin dissociation curve; (6) vascular tone decreases; and (7) circulating catecholamines have a stronger effect. A decrease in pH will create the following changes: (1) decreased lactate production; (2) decreased conversion of inactive phosphorylase B to active phosphorylase A; (3) decreased quantities of liver glycogen; (4) increased Krebs cycle oxidations in the muscles and renal cortex; (5) increased gluconeogenesis in the renal cortex; (6) decreased glycolysis; (7) decreased lipolysis; (8) increased pulmonary vascular resistance; (9) increased pulmonary blood flow; (10) decreased threshold levels for ventricular fibrillation; (11) decreased cardiac sensitivity to catecholamines; (12) an increased 2,3-diphosphoglycerate concentration in the red blood cell, with a corresponding right shift in the oxyhemoglobin dissociation curve; (13) decreased peripheral resistance; (14) decreased mesenteric blood flow; (15) decreased pulmonary macrophage function; (16) decreased granulocyte function; (17) decreased immune responses; (18) decreased insulin secretion and binding to receptors; and (19) decreased pancreatic amylase secretion. In addition, variations in pH will also influence the transmembrane movement of certain substrates such as serine and alanine, and hepatic processes such as acetate oxidation, glycogen synthesis, and glutamine metabolism.

REGULATION

The hydrogen ion concentration, or pH, of body fluids is maintained and regulated by the following three mechanisms: the body fluid buffers, the respiratory system, and the renal system. These mechanisms act by buffering hydrogen ions to prevent not only increases in hydrogen ion concentration, which would result in acidosis, but also decreases in hydrogen ion concentration, which would result in alkalosis.

Body Fluid Buffer System

The body fluid buffer system is composed of buffer pairs consisting of a weak acid and its conjugate base, a salt of that weak acid. Table 9-1 presents the composition and approximate amounts of those buffer pairs in the body. As is depicted in Table 9-1, the carbonic acid–sodium bicarbonate pair is the primary

TABLE 9-1   **Composition of the Body Fluid Buffer System**

Buffer Pairs		% Contributed to Total Buffering
Weak Acid	**Conjugate Base**	
Carbonic acid (H_2CO_3)	Sodium bicarbonate ($NaHCO_3$)	53
Hemoglobin (Hb)	Potassium hemoglobinate (KHb)	35
Oxyhemoglobin ($HHbO_2$)	Potassium oxyhemoglobinate ($KHbO_2$)	
Plasma protein (HPr)	Proteinate (NaPr)	7
Acid organic phosphate ($NaRHPO_4$)	Alkaline organic phosphate (Na_2RPO_4)	3
Acid inorganic phosphate (NaH_2PO_4)	Alkaline inorganic phosphate (Na_2HPO_4)	2

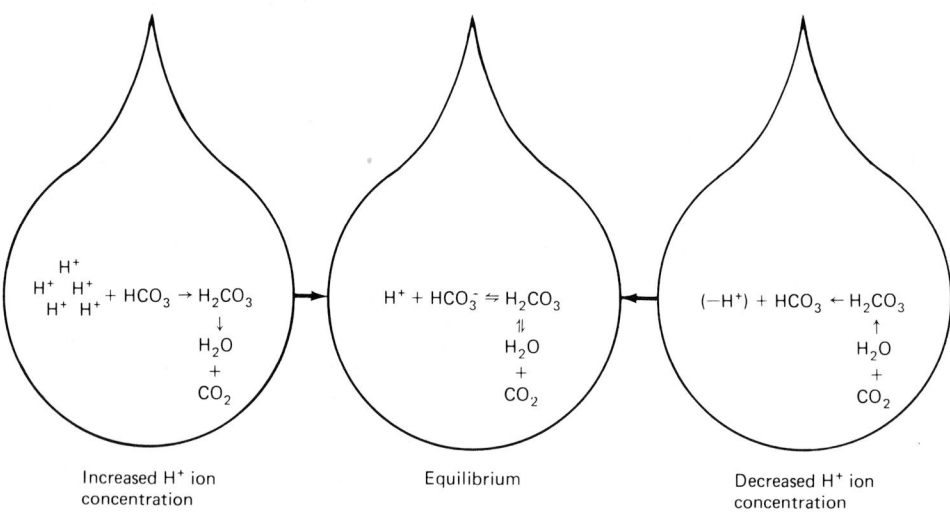

Figure 9-1   Regulation of hydrogen ion concentration by the body fluid buffer system using the carbonic acid–bicarbonate pair.

constituent of the body fluid buffer system. Figure 9-1 uses the carbonic acid–bicarbonate buffer pair to illustrate how the body fluid buffer system functions.

The body fluid buffer system reacts within a fraction of a second to prevent changes in hydrogen ion concentration in the body fluids. Because of its fast action, it is often called the first line of defense against acid–base imbalances.

Respiratory System

The respiratory system regulates hydrogen ion concentration in the body fluids by altering the amount of carbon dioxide available for forming carbonic acid. This alteration in the amount of available carbon dioxide is governed by the respiratory control center in the medulla which varies the rate and depth of ventilation according to the carbon dioxide concentration. The response to an increase in carbon dioxide concentration is an increase in the rate and depth of ventilation. Thus, the carbon dioxide concentration in the alveoli is decreased and less is available for forming carbonic acid. The reciprocal of this process

occurs when there is a decrease in carbon dioxide concentration in the alveoli. Figure 9-2 illustrates these respiratory processes for regulating hydrogen ion concentration in the body fluids.

The respiratory system usually responds to changes in hydrogen ion concentration within 1 to 3 minutes to prevent imbalances from occurring.

Renal System

The renal system regulates the hydrogen ion concentration in body fluids through the following five processes: (1) hydrogen ion secretion; (2) sodium reabsorption; (3) bicarbonate reabsorption; (4) excretion of titratable acids, or acidification of phosphate salts; and (5) ammonia synthesis. Figure 9-3 depicts these processes.

The renal system requires hours to days to respond to changes in hydrogen ion concentration and thus is the slowest, although the most effective, regulatory method.

The variances or imbalances associated with acid–base changes are metabolic acidosis, metabolic al-

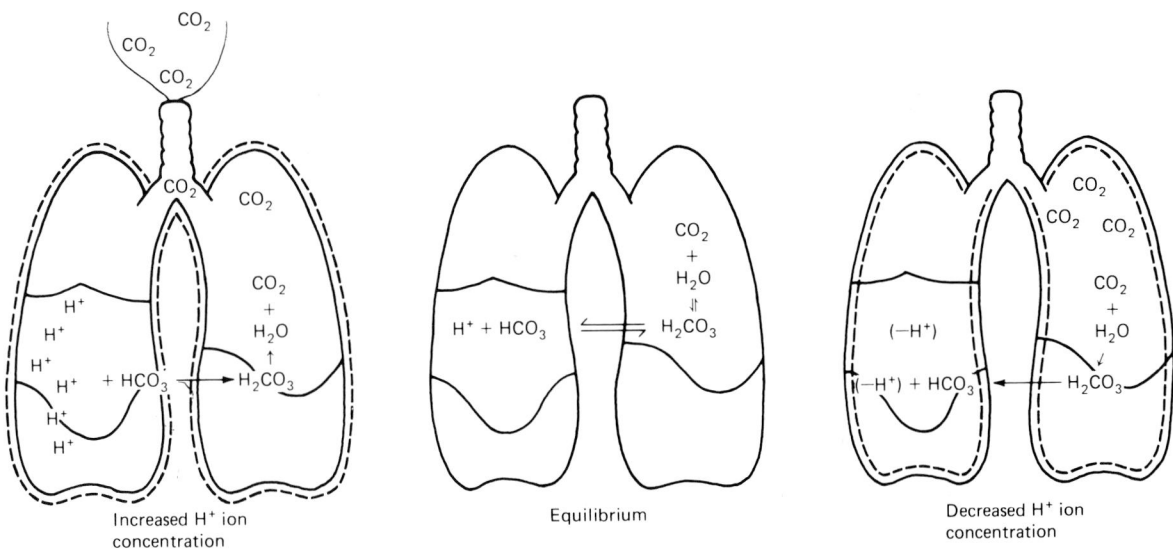

Figure 9-2   Regulation of hydrogen ion concentration by the respiratory system.

kalosis, respiratory acidosis, and respiratory alkalosis. Steps for interpreting blood gas values are given in the box on p. 213.

METABOLIC ACIDOSIS

Definition and Etiology

Metabolic acidosis is a deficit of bicarbonate in the extracellular fluid. It is related to two categories of etiologies: causes that produce a loss of bicarbonate from the body, or causes that produce increased amounts of nonvolatile acids in the body.

Those etiologies that produce a loss of bicarbonate from the body result in hyperchloremic acidosis with a normal anion gap. That means that the individual's serum sodium value minus the sum of the chloride and bicarbonate values equals a value that falls within the normal range for the anion gap of 8 to 16 mEq/L. In other words, the formula for calculating the anion gap is:

$$\text{Anion gap} = Na^+ - (Cl^- + HCO_3)$$

When the formula is applied to those etiologies that produce increased amounts of nonvolatile acids in the body, the result is an increase in the anion gap.

Those etiologies that produce a loss of bicarbonate from the body include renal tubular acidosis; use of carbonic anhydrase inhibitors; extracellular fluid volume expansion; hyperalimentation; administration of chloride-containing acids, such as hydrochloric acid or ammonium chloride; diarrhea; draining fistulas of the pancreas or small bowel; ureterosigmoidostomy; ileal conduit; and the use of anion exchange resins, such as cholestyramine.

Those etiologies that produce metabolic acidosis by increasing the amount of acid in the body, creating a normochloremic acidosis, are renal failure, diabetic ketoacidosis, lactic acidosis, starvation, ethanol intoxication, tissue hypoxia, paraldehyde intoxication, salicylate intoxication, methanol intoxication, and high-fat diets.

Data Acquisition

Physical Assessment

The individual experiencing metabolic acidosis exhibits a combination of the following signs and symptoms: headache, fatigue, drowsiness, decreased mental function, confusion, coma, seizures, hypotension, tissue hypoxia, cardiac dysrhythmia, Kussmaul respirations, anorexia, nausea, and vomiting.

Diagnostic Procedures

The laboratory values that provide the most significant data for assessing the acid–base balance of an individual are the blood gas values. Table 9-2 presents the normal values for both arterial and mixed venous blood gas samples. In addition to the blood gas values, selected serum and urine values also provide significant assessment data.

The pattern of laboratory values that is characteristic of metabolic acidosis is a pH lower than 7.37, a bicarbonate level less than 22 mEq/L, a base excess less than −2, a decreased P_{CO_2}, an increased serum potassium; and usually a decreased urine pH that may vary depending on the etiology.

Medical and Nursing Management

The clinical implications of metabolic acidosis for the patient are significant because the body does not tolerate changes in hydrogen ion concentration in the internal environment very well. Such changes will ac-

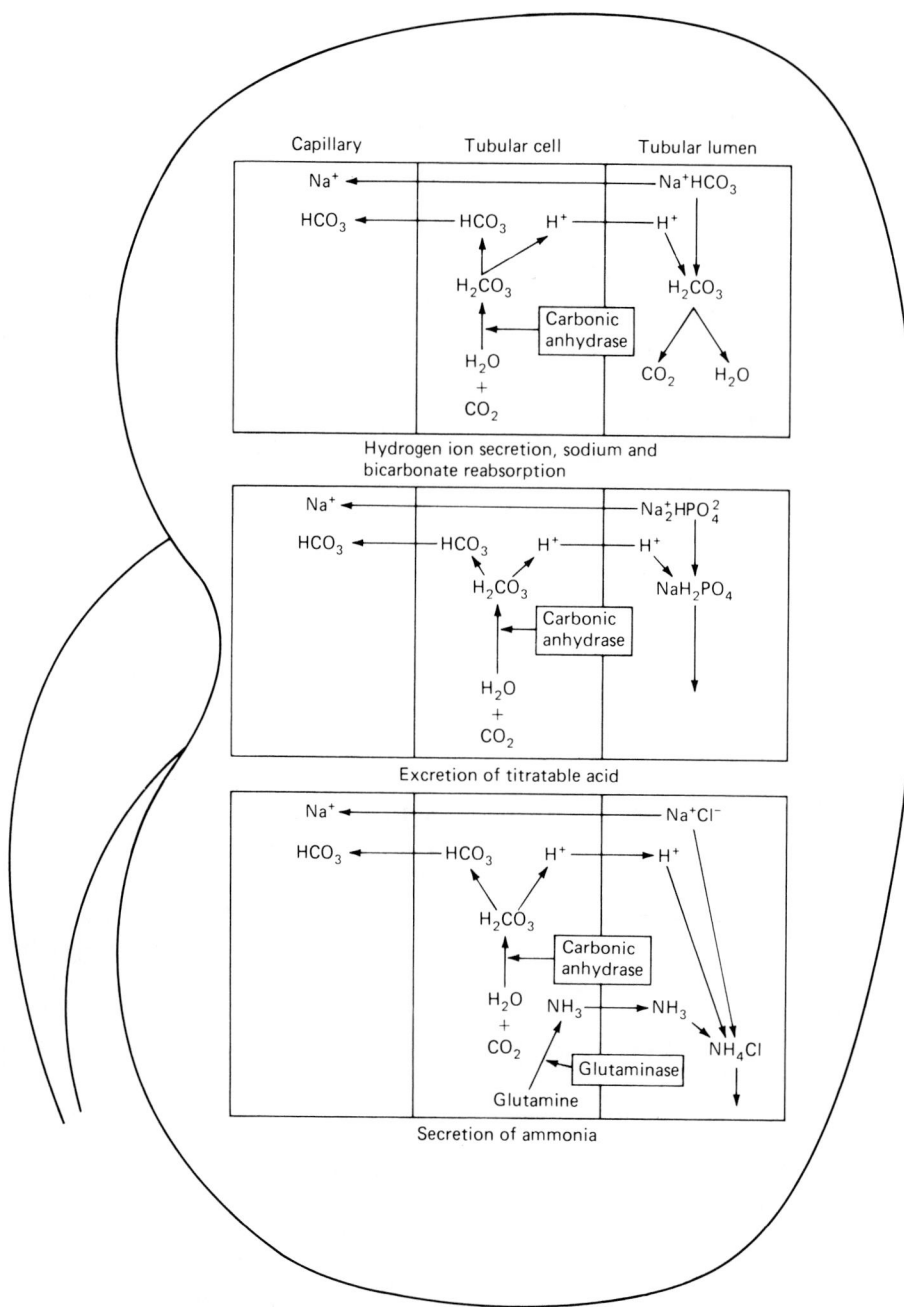

Figure 9-3 Regulation of hydrogen ion concentration by the renal system.

celerate, deter, or inhibit various metabolic processes, creating greater hazards to the individual's health state. However, the most threatening change that occurs with severe acidosis is cardiovascular collapse due to arteriolar dilation and decreased cardiac contractility. This change obviously can lead to the patient's death.

The nursing monitoring functions performed when an individual experiences metabolic acidosis include (1) assessing the level of consciousness periodically; (2) evaluating overall muscle strength; (3) assessing

the rate, rhythm, pattern, and characteristics of all vital signs, especially the pulse and respirations; (4) monitoring the color and temperature of the skin as a means of determining tissue perfusion status; (5) assessing gastrointestinal functioning; (6) measuring and recording intake and output meticulously; (7) obtaining accurate daily weights; (8) assessing the comfort level frequently; (9) assessing for signs of hyperkalemia; and (10) monitoring appropriate laboratory values periodically.

Nursing interventions that are performed for the

Steps for Interpreting Blood Gas Values

1. Assess the pH and determine if it is increased, indicating alkalosis; decreased, indicating acidosis; or normal, indicating no imbalance.
2. Assess the Pco_2 and decide if it is increased, decreased, or normal.
3. Assess the HCO_3 and decide if it is increased, decreased, or normal.
4. If there is an imbalance, determine whether it is respiratory or metabolic. Remember the Pco_2 is the acid, respiratory component of acid–base balance and HCO_3 is the base, metabolic component.
5. Assess the Po_2 and O_2 saturation and determine if they are increased, decreased, or normal.
6. Determine the type of nursing interventions necessary to assist the patient in coping with the acid–base imbalance.

TABLE 9-2   Normal Blood Gas Values

Substance Measured	Arterial Blood	Mixed Venous Blood
pH	7.37 to 7.43 (7.35 to 7.45)*	7.33 to 7.39 (7.31 to 7.41)*
Po_2	80 to 100 mmHg	35 to 40 mmHg
O_2 saturation	95% to 97%	70% to 75%
Pco_2	37 to 43 mmHg (35 to 45 mmHg)*	41 to 51 mmHg
HCO_3	22 to 26 mEq/L	22 to 26 mEq/L
BE (base excess)	+2 to −2	+2 to −2

* The more liberal range is gaining wider acceptance as being the norm.

patient with metabolic acidosis are (1) administering fluids and medications as prescribed, (2) instituting seizure precautions, (3) maintaining bed rest and instituting active and passive range of motion exercises, (4) assisting the individual in assuming a position to facilitate respirations, (5) providing stimuli appropriate to maintaining orientation, (6) providing nursing comfort measures to deal with the gastrointestinal effects, (7) providing frequent oral hygiene using nondrying agents, and (8) establishing a safe physical environment for the individual.

The treatment of metabolic acidosis is aimed at dealing with the underlying cause. Thus, the therapy used will vary according to the etiology. However, if the acidosis is severe, it is important to replace the lost bicarbonate while treating the underlying cause. The general rule is to replace the bicarbonate loss slowly with an appropriate alkali over several hours. It is also suggested in this case that a slight undercorrection be achieved to prevent a rebound metabolic alkalosis from occurring.

METABOLIC ALKALOSIS

Definition and Etiology

Metabolic alkalosis is an excess of bicarbonate in the extracellular fluid. It is caused by the following: vomiting; gastrointestinal suctioning; diarrhea (if it has a high chloride content); diuretic therapy; laxative abuse; cystic fibrosis; primary and secondary hyperaldosteronism; Cushing's syndrome; licorice abuse; excessive ingestion of bicarbonate, or other alkalinizing salts; hypokalemia; and hypercalcemia.

Data Acquisition

Physical Assessment

Metabolic alkalosis is exhibited clinically in an individual by a combination of the following signs and symptoms: increased neuromuscular irritability, tetany, seizures, belligerence, confusion, stupor, coma, hypoventilation, cardiac dysrhythmia, nausea, vomiting, and diarrhea.

Diagnostic Procedures

The laboratory data used to assess an individual for metabolic alkalosis are provided primarily by the blood gas values, but selected serum and urine values can also be of assistance. The pattern of laboratory values characteristic of metabolic alkalosis is a pH greater than 7.43; a bicarbonate greater than 26 mEq/L; a base excess greater than +2; an increased Pco_2; a decreased serum chloride; a decreased serum potassium; a decreased serum calcium; and a decreased urine chloride, the degree of which depends on the etiology. If the etiology of the metabolic alkalosis is associated with extracellular fluid volume depletion, the patient exhibits a urinary chloride of less than 10 mEq/L. If the etiology is related to extracellular fluid volume expansion, the urinary chloride is greater than 20 mEq/L.

Medical and Nursing Management

The clinical significance of metabolic alkalosis for a patient is related to the neuromuscular and respiratory effects of the imbalance. The hyperirritability of the central nervous system and the compensatory hypoventilation represent definite risks to a person's well-being.

The nursing monitoring functions performed when an individual experiences metabolic alkalosis include (1) assessing the level of consciousness; (2) evaluating neuromuscular function periodically; (3) monitoring muscle strength and movement; (4) assessing the rate, rhythm, pattern, and characteristics of all vital signs, especially respirations; (5) measuring and recording intake and output accurately; (6) obtaining precise measurement of daily weights; (7) assessing the characteristics of the feces; (8) monitoring Chvostek's and Trousseau's signs for hypocalcemia; and (9) monitoring appropriate laboratory values periodically.

The intervening functions that are part of the nursing care performed for patients with metabolic alkalosis are (1) establishing a safe physical environment, (2) instituting seizure precautions, (3) providing stimuli appropriate to maintaining orientation, (4) assisting the individual with the activities of daily living, (5) providing nursing comfort measures to deal with the gastrointestinal effects of the imbalance, and (6) administering fluids and medications as prescribed.

The treatment of metabolic alkalosis involves eliminating the primary cause and correcting the imbalance. Correcting the imbalance is accomplished by a four-level therapeutic approach. This therapeutic approach includes (1) replacing any extracellular fluid volume deficit with saline; (2) administering chloride (in the form of ammonium chloride or arginine hydrochloride if the sodium chloride in the saline solution is not sufficient to replace the lost anion); (3) correcting the potassium depletion with potassium chloride; and (4) increasing the excretion of bicarbonate by using carbonic anhydrase–inhibiting diuretics, or, in instances of renal dysfunction, by dialysis therapy.

RESPIRATORY ACIDOSIS

Definition and Etiology

Respiratory acidosis is an excess of carbonic acid in the extracellular fluid. It is caused by etiologies that create hypoventilation and result in the retention of carbon dioxide in the body. Those etiologies are categorized according to the mechanisms responsible for creating the hypoventilation. There are five categories of etiologies that result in respiratory acidosis: (1) airway obstructions, (2) depressants of the respiratory center, (3) defects in the nerves and muscles of respiration, (4) lung diseases, and (5) thoracic cage disorders. Table 9-3 presents specific examples for each of the categories of etiologies of respiratory acidosis.

Data Acquisition

Physical Assessment

The individual experiencing respiratory acidosis exhibits many of the following signs and symptoms: dull, slow mental responses; apprehension; restlessness; headache; drowsiness; disorientation; coma; tachycardia; hypoventilation; dyspnea; fatigue; weakness; flapping tremors; uncoordination; and decreased reflexes. Cyanosis due to hypoxia is also present as a very late sign of respiratory acidosis.

TABLE 9-3 Specific Etiologies of Respiratory Acidosis

Category	Examples
Airway obstructions	Aspiration
	Foreign bodies
	Pulmonary embolus
	Severe bronchospasms
	Pulmonary edema
	Laryngeal edema
Depressants of the respiratory center	Sedatives
	Chronic narcotic abuse
	Metabolic alkalosis
	General anesthesia
	Increased intracranial pressure
	Medullary tumors
	Meningitis
	Vertebral artery embolism or thrombosis
Defects in the nerves and muscles of respiration	Myasthenia gravis
	Guillain-Barré syndrome
	Poliomyelitis
	Botulism
	Spinal cord injury
	Paralysis associated with hypo- or hyperkalemia
Lung diseases	Chronic obstructive pulmonary disease
	Smoke inhalation
	Pneumonia
	Atelectasis
	Asthma
	Interstitial lung disease
	Bronchitis
	Bronchiectasis
Thoracic cage disorders	Flail chest
	Pneumothorax
	Pickwickian syndrome
	Ankylosing spondylitis

Diagnostic Procedures

The blood gas values provide the most significant laboratory data for assessing an individual for respiratory acidosis. However, there are some serum and urine values that can provide additional assessment data. The characteristic pattern of values exhibited by patients experiencing respiratory acidosis is a pH less than 7.37, a PCO_2 greater than 43 to 45 mmHg, a normal to increased bicarbonate, a normal to decreased PO_2, a normal to increased serum potassium, and a decreased urine pH.

Medical and Nursing Management

The clinical significance of respiratory acidosis for a patient is related not only to the effects of the acidosis on the body but also to the effects of the accompanying hypoxia. Without sufficient oxygen, the human organism cannot survive. Thus, this imbalance indeed represents a crisis and requires nursing support in the form of monitoring and intervening functions.

The monitoring functions performed for a patient experiencing respiratory acidosis include (1) assessing skin color, temperature, and moistness for signs of hypoxia; (2) monitoring the rate, rhythm, pattern, and characteristics of all vital signs; (3) assessing the level of consciousness frequently; (4) evaluating muscle strength, coordination, and movement; (5) assessing the individual's comfort level; and (6) monitoring all appropriate laboratory values at intervals.

The intervening functions performed for the individual with respiratory acidosis are (1) providing a safe physical environment; (2) maintaining a decreased activity level consistent with the level of hypoxia, (3) assisting the patient with all activities of daily living, (4) providing a quiet environment with enough stimuli to maintain orientation, (5) providing emotional support and reassurance, (6) assisting the individual to assume a position that facilitates adequate respirations, (7) instituting preventive pulmonary maintenance therapies to increase the removal of carbon dioxide by the lungs (turning, coughing, deep breathing, suctioning, resistance breathing), (8) administering oxygen when appropriate and as prescribed, and (9) administering fluids and medications if prescribed.

The goal for treating respiratory acidosis is to reestablish effective ventilation for the individual. In some instances this may require creating an artificial airway and/or using mechanical ventilation until the primary etiology can be treated. Bicarbonate and oxygen may be administered concurrently with efforts to treat the cause in an attempt to correct or lessen the immediate effects of the imbalance.

RESPIRATORY ALKALOSIS
Definition and Etiology

Respiratory alkalosis is a deficit of carbonic acid in the extracellular fluid. It is caused by etiologies that produce hyperventilation and a decrease of carbon dioxide in the body. Those etiologies include alcoholic intoxication, anemia, gram-negative sepsis, meningitis, encephalitis, head trauma, brain lesions, congestive heart failure, exercise, fever, cirrhosis, paraldehyde intoxication, pulmonary fibrosis, hypoxia, thyrotoxicosis, mechanical hyperventilation, salicylate intoxication, anxiety, hysteria, and voluntary hyperpnea.

Data Acquisition
Physical Assessment

The individual experiencing respiratory alkalosis exhibits a combination of the following signs and symptoms: breathlessness, vertigo, syncope, nervousness, paresthesias of the extremities, perioral paresthesia, muscle cramps and tetany, seizures, decreased mental function, confusion, decreased psychomotor performance, anxiety, hyperventilation, cardiac dysrhythmia, and hypotension.

Diagnostic Procedures

The blood gas values are the most significant laboratory data used in assessing an individual for respiratory alkalosis. The characteristic pattern is a pH greater than 7.43, a P_{CO_2} less than 37 mmHg, and a decreased bicarbonate.

Medical and Nursing Management

The clinical significance of respiratory alkalosis for a patient is related to the neuromuscular effects it produces. Those effects make it impossible for a person to function and carry out the normal activities of daily living. The individual may also develop life-threatening seizures as a result of the respiratory alkalosis.

The nursing monitoring functions performed when a patient experiences respiratory alkalosis include (1) assessing the level of consciousness frequently; (2) monitoring the rate, rhythm, pattern, and characteristics of all vital signs; (3) monitoring sensation in the extremities and perioral area; (4) assessing muscle movement and strength; and (5) monitoring all appropriate laboratory data.

The intervening functions performed for an individual experiencing respiratory alkalosis are (1) establishing a safe physical environment for the individual; (2) maintaining an activity level appropriate to the degree of weakness, vertigo, and syncope; (3) instituting seizure precautions; (4) providing sufficient stimuli to maintain orientation; (5) assisting the individual in performing activities of daily living; (6) providing emotional support and reassurance; (7) instituting nursing measures to assist in decreasing hyperventilation and increasing carbon dioxide (such as teaching breathing exercises or having the individual breathe in and out of a paper bag, thus rebreathing carbon dioxide); and (8) administering medications as prescribed.

The treatment of respiratory alkalosis is aimed at dealing with the underlying cause. However, when it is not possible to eradicate the cause, sedation, administration of 3% to 5% carbon dioxide, and breathing exercises are used to correct the imbalance.

CRITICAL CARE IMPLICATIONS

This chapter has discussed the regulation and assessment of acid–base balance. The information contained in this chapter is continuously utilized by clinicians as they make decisions about patient care.

Because of the importance of acid–base balance in maintaining a stable internal environment for the individual, the content of this discussion assumes high priority for the critical care nurse. In fact, acid–base balance is second only to fluid balance in priority in relation to patient care. Thus, the critical care nurse must be well acquainted with this information and ready to apply it in all instances. To assist the nurse in making such applications, the signs and symptoms of each acid–base imbalance have been summarized according to body systems in the box on pp. 203-206. The acid–base imbalances appear there in priority order and follow the fluid volume imbalances.

BIBLIOGRAPHY

Aberman, A. (1984). An update on diabetic ketoacidosis. *Emergency Medicine, 16*(3), 90, 92-93, 97-98.

Brenner, M. & Welliver, J. (1990). Pulmonary and acid-base assessment. *Nursing Clinics of North America, 25*(4), 761-770.

Clausen, J. L., & Murray, K. M. (1985). Clinical applications of arterial blood gases: How much accuracy do we need? *Journal of Medical Technology, 2*(1), 19-21.

Cohen, J. J., & Kassirer, J. P. (1982). *Acid–base.* Boston: Little, Brown.

Flenly, D. C. (1982). Blood gas and acid–base interpretation. *Respiratory Care, 27*(3), 311-317.

Flomenbaum, N. (1984). Acid–base disturbances. *Emergency Medicine 16*(3), 59-61, 65-66, 71-72, 77-78, 81-86, 88-89.

Glass, L. B., & Jenkins, C. A. (1983). The ups and downs of serum pH. *Nursing 83, 13*(9), 34-41.

Greenberg, A. (1984). Common emergencies of acid–base balance. *Topics in Emergency Medicine, 5*(4), 1-16.

Greene, D. A. (1984). Diabetic ketoacidosis. *Topics in Emergency Medicine, 5*(4) 17-32.

Grogono, A. W. (1986). Acid–base balance. *International Anesthesiology Clinics, 24*(1), 11-20.

Guyton, A. C. (1991). *Textbook of medical physiology* (8th ed.). Philadelphia: Saunders.

Hricik, D. E., & Kassirer, J. P. (1983). Understanding and using the anion gap. *Consultant, 23*(7), 130-134, 143.

Janusek, L. W. (1984). Metabolic acidosis: Physiology, signs and symptoms, *Nursing 84, 14*(7), 44-45.

Keyes, J. L. (1985). *Fluid, electrolyte, and acid–base regulation.* Monterey: Wadsworth Health Sciences Division.

Kurtzman, N. A., Arruda, J. A. L., & Westenfelder, C. (1978). Renal regulation of acid–base homeostasis. *Contributions to Nephrology, 14*, 1-13.

Mathewson, M., & Mathewson, R. E. (1987). Establishing acid–base balance. *Critical Care Nurse, 7*(5) 77-85.

Maxwell, M. H., & Kleeman, C. R. (1987). *Clinical disorders of fluid and electrolyte metabolism* (4th ed.). New York: McGraw-Hill.

Miller, W. C. (1984). The ABCs of blood gases. *Emergency Medicine, 16*(3), 37-38, 43-45, 48, 51-52, 54-56.

Moore, V. B. (1979). Analyzing the ABG analysis. *Nursing 79, 9*(9), 28-33.

Neff, J. A. (1984). Acid–base balance: A tool for rapid evaluation. *Journal of Emergency Nursing, 10*(6), 322-324.

Perkins, C., & Bralley, H. K. (1983). Metabolic alkalosis. *Nursing 83, 13*(1), 57.

Porter, R., & Lawrenson, G. (1982). *Ciba Foundation symposium 87—Metabolic acidosis.* London: Pitman.

Rice, V. (1987). Acid–base derangements in the patient with cardiac arrest. *Focus on Critical Care, 14*(6), 53-61.

Ryou, K. (1981). Interpretation of acid–base status. *Journal of the American Medical Technologists, 43*, 61-65.

Schrier, R. (1992). *Renal and electrolyte disorders* (4th ed.). Boston: Little, Brown.

Shapiro, B. A. (1991). *Clinical application of respiratory care* (4th ed.). St. Louis: Mosby–Year Book.

Taylor, D. L. (1984). Respiratory acidosis—physiology, signs, and symptoms, *Nursing 84, 14*(10), 44-45.

Vander, A. J. (1991). *Renal physiology* (4th ed.). New York: McGraw-Hill.

York, K. (1987). The lung and fluid–electrolyte and acid–base imbalances. *Nursing Clinics of North America, 22*(4), 805-815.

York, K., & Moddeman, G. (1989). Arterial blood gases. *AORN Journal, 49*(5), 1308-1317.

10

Cardiac Electrical Activity

Julia Ann Purcell

Function of the heart muscle is dependent on an interaction between an electrical stimulus and a mechanical response. The importance of the electrical activity of the heart, therefore, cannot be overstated. This chapter is devoted to describing the propagation of the electrical stimulus; explaining the measurement of cardiac electrical activity in the clinical setting; and discussing the cause, identification, and treatment of common electrical abnormalities.

Electrophysiology

Transmembrane Potential

Within intracellular and extracellular fluids are concentrations of electrolytes normally totaling about 155 mEq/L of positively charged ions (cations) and negatively charged ions (anions). Usually, excess numbers of cations accumulate along the outside surface of the cell membrane, while excess numbers of anions accumulate along the inside of the membrane, resulting in a *transmembrane potential*. The internal environment of the atrial and ventricular myocardial cells measures about -90 millivolts (mV) as compared with the outside. The cell is said to be *polarized* when the internal environment is negative compared to the outside.

Development of Potential

The two electrolytes most involved in the physics of transmembrane potentials are sodium and potassium. The intracellular concentration of potassium is approximately 140 mEq/L while the extracellular concentration normally ranges between 3.5 and 4.5 mEq/L. Conversely, the intracellular sodium concentration is approximately 10 mEq/L; the extracellular sodium concentration is approximately 140 mEq/L. The concentration gradient for potassium favors movement from the inside to the outside of the cell. Sodium is favored to move intracellularly along its concentration gradient.

Calculation of the resting transmembrane potential is based on the potential for diffusion across the cell membrane as a result of ionic concentration and electrical gradients. As potassium diffuses out of the cell along its concentration gradient, it leaves behind large numbers of negatively charged proteins, organic phosphates, and other anions which are too large to diffuse through the cell membrane. The internal concentration of nondiffusible anions is approximately 150 mEq/L; the external concentration is approximately 5 mEq/L. Thus, the internal environment of the cell becomes increasingly negative, while the extracellular environment becomes increasingly positive. The positive charges line up outside the cell membrane, attracted by the internal negativity. A balance is reached when the concentration gradient for potassium efflux is equalized by the internal attraction of the negative ions for those remaining positive ions. The actual calculation of -90 mV is based on the Nernst equation, which states that a cation gradient favoring outward movement causes internal negativity, while an anion gradient in the reverse direction also causes internal electronegativity.

When the extracellular potassium concentration increases, the resting transmembrane potential can become more negative. The electrical gradient remains unchanged, but the concentration gradient for potassium diminishes; therefore, the transmembrane potential could exceed the normal negativity of -90 mV (hyperpolarization).

The role of other ions in the development of transmembrane potential is a relatively passive one. The next most abundant anion is chloride, which has an extracellular concentration of approximately 100 mEq/L and an intracellular concentration of about 4 mEq/L. This distribution is maintained by the electrical gradient within the cell which repels the negative chloride ion. Magnesium, a cation with an intracellular concentration of 58 mEq/L and a very low extracellular concentration, follows a diffusion pattern similar to that of potassium, while calcium has a relatively low concentration both intra- and extracellularly. The major role of calcium and magnesium is thought to be the alteration of membrane permeability to other ions.

The Action Potential

Any stimulus that increases the permeability of the membrane to sodium so that a critical threshold is reached will generate an *action potential*. The cardiac action potential is a graphic representation of the rapid and abrupt pulselike changes in the membrane potential (Figure 10-1). The electrical potential, measured in mV, is indicated along the vertical axis of the graph. Time, measured in milliseconds (ms), is indicated along the horizontal axis. The action potential consists of three to five phases, labeled as phase 0 through phase 4. Each phase represents a particular electrical event or combination of electrical events. The events, the duration of the events and action potential, and the transmembrane potential vary with the type of cardiac cell being measured. Figure 10-1A depicts an action potential representative of a normal ventricular muscle cell. The cardiac action potential of the sinus node is illustrated in Figure 10-1B.

Depolarization (Phase 0)

Once the internal negativity decreases from its resting potential of approximately -90 mV to -60 mV or the threshold potential (TP in Figure 10-1A), a very rapid loss of negativity and positive overshoot to about $+30$ mV occurs, and the fiber is *depolarized*. This rapid change in potential is identified as *phase 0* on the cardiac action potential.

The basis for the very rapid change in the permeability of the membrane is unknown. Guyton postulated that certain channels or pores exist for the passage of sodium which, during resting potential, are obstructed through calcium binding to proteins in the membrane.[1] Because calcium is a cation, sodium is repelled and cannot pass through. Following excitation of the membrane, the calcium ions are somehow dislodged from their binding sites, and sodium rapidly diffuses into the cell. Others have theorized the existence of actual activation gates which open to allow sodium passage during phase 0 of the action potential, and inactivation gates which inhibit the fast sodium current later on in the depolarization of the muscle fiber.

The resting membrane potential is a critical determinant in depolarization. A reduction in the negativity of the resting potential can lead to inexcitability of the fiber even if the concentration for sodium is normal. The inactivation process for the sodium channels, then, is extremely important because the fast sodium channels are not thought to function properly unless the membrane is returned to the normal resting potential. Once an action potential has been generated, the fast sodium channels cannot be activated again until the membrane has been returned to near resting potential, thus preventing sustained muscle contraction.

Once the peak of the positive overshoot is approached within the membrane, the rapid sodium influx has diminished considerably. This happens for at least two reasons: (1) the increase in positivity inside the membrane begins to repel further influx of sodium; and (2) the inactivation process blocks the fast sodium channels, perhaps through binding with calcium or by means of the inactivation gates.

Early Repolarization (Phase 1)

Once rapid sodium influx is terminated, a brief phase of repolarization occurs. This early repolarization is identified as *phase 1* and results from a rapid but brief influx of the anion chloride and an efflux

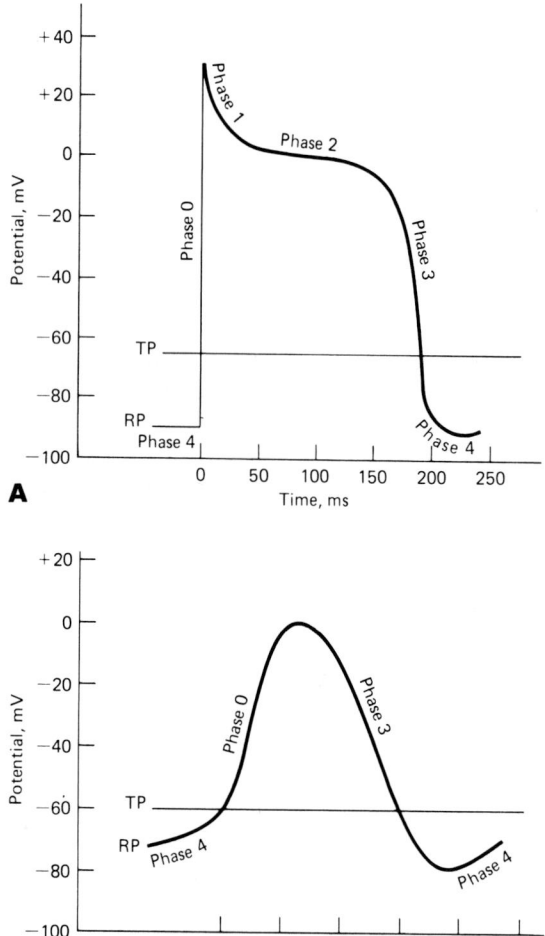

Figure 10-1 Transmembrane potentials (TMP) from two types of cells. *A*, TMP from ordinary myocardial muscle fibers. *B*, TMP from the SA node which is representative of myocardial cells capable of automaticity. See text for discussion.

Adapted from Hurst, J. W., Logue, R. B., Schlant, R. C., et al. (Eds.). (1990). *The heart, arteries, and veins* (7th ed.). New York: McGraw-Hill.

of potassium. During this phase the transmembrane potential is reduced to approximately 0 mV.

The Plateau (Phase 2)

Myocardial cells have a longer *plateau (phase 2)* of the action potential than do skeletal muscle cells. There seems to be a slow inward sodium current that is different from the rapid influx of sodium during phase 0. In addition, there is a slow calcium inward current that is instrumental in myocardial contractility. Apparently, both ions are carried by the same inward channel.

The concentration gradient is unchanged for potassium, thereby promoting an outward current of potassium that would bring about rapid repolarization of the fiber. During phase 2, however, the permeability of the membrane for potassium decreases, thereby decreasing potassium conductance (anomalous rectification). Consequently, the fiber is able to sustain contraction.

Repolarization (Phase 3)

Return of the membrane to resting potential in *phase 3 (repolarization)* is accomplished almost entirely by potassium efflux along its concentration gradient. Also, the slow inward currents of sodium and potassium are inactivated. With the rapid outward movement of potassium, the cell becomes increasingly negative until resting potential is restored.

Active Transport of Sodium and Potassium (Phase 4)

Maintenance of the resting potential is clearly dependent on potassium. However, sodium has a concentration gradient favoring inward movement. During the resting state *(phase 4)* of the action potential, the membrane is 50 to 100 times less permeable to sodium than to potassium. Even so, some sodium does leak into the cell during the resting state. Were the sodium allowed to build up within the cell, resting potential would soon be dissipated. The sodium pump is in constant operation to actively transport sodium to the extracellular fluid against its concentration gradient. An active transport pump also functions to bring potassium into the cell against its concentration gradient. The sodium and potassium pumps require energy to function and can become inhibited by medication such as digitalis and perhaps also by ischemia. The effect of inhibition of the potassium pump is the same as inhibition of the sodium active transport mechanism: loss of internal electronegativity.

Excitability

When cardiac tissue is capable of being depolarized by a stimulus, it is said to be *excitable*. Although the degree of excitability depends on many factors, at any given physiological state it is related to the phase of the cardiac cycle. During phase 4, the excitability of the cardiac cell is at a maximum. Beginning at phase 0 and continuing to approximately the midpoint of phase 3, the cell is in a period of *absolute* or *effective refractoriness*, and excitability is zero (ARP, ERP on Figure 10-2). No stimulus, regardless of magnitude, will produce a response. The period from the midpoint of phase 3 extending to just before the beginning of phase 4 is known as the *relative refractory period* (RRP on Figure 10-2). The fiber is capable of generating an action potential, but only if the stimulus is stronger than that which would be required during phase 4. During a brief period following phase 3 and ending when the fiber returns to its resting potential, known as the *supernormal period* and shown as SNP on Figure 10-2, a stimulus slightly less than normal can cause a propagated action potential. Generally, the later in phase 3 that stimulation occurs, the greater the amplitude and velocity of conduction. However, the action potential that results from excitation during the supernormal period is not unusually large; rather, the action potential is usually reduced in amplitude due to the slow recovery of the sodium channels.

The basis for the refractory periods probably resides with the inactivation of the fast sodium currents occurring in repolarization; thus, the closer the membrane is to resting potential when excited, the more fast sodium channels will be reactivated. The duration of the refractory period varies according to the type of action potential, whether a fast or slow response, and probably according to other factors as well. In cells characterized by the slow response, the effective

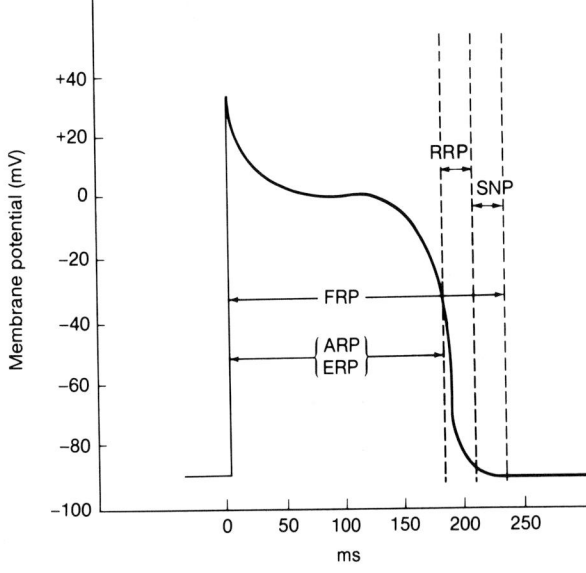

Figure 10-2 Relative excitability during the cardiac action potential. FRP = full refractory period. See text for discussion.

refractory periods are longer than in the normal myocardial fiber. The absolute refractory periods can continue well beyond phase 3, and the relative refractory period continues into phase 4. Impulses that arrive somewhat early in phase 4 are conducted very slowly, even though the membrane is at resting potential and fully repolarized.

Automaticity

Certain specialized fibers within the myocardium possess the property of *automaticity;* that is, they attain threshold in the absence of any external stimulus. These automatic, or pacemaker, cells lie primarily within the sinoatrial (SA) node, the atrioventricular (AV) junction, and the Purkinje network of the cardiac conduction system. A comparison of the action potential of an automatic myocardial fiber (see Figure 10-1B) with that of a normal ventricular myocardial fiber (see Figure 10-1A) shows the following: The resting potential of the sinus node automatic cells can be seen to be much slower and less negative; the phase 0 upstroke is more sluggish; and the amplitude of the action potential is not as great as that of a ventricular myocardial fiber—there is little or no positive overshoot within the action potential of the automatic cell. In addition, the automatic cell is capable of diastolic depolarization. During phase 4 of the sinoatrial (SA) node fiber, the membrane does not maintain a constant resting potential as do ventricular myocardial fibers, and diastolic depolarization brings the membrane to threshold, eliciting an action potential. Generally, these properties are limited to automatic cells; however, under certain conditions such as ischemia, the action potential of other cells may shift to assume some of the properties of the pacemaker or "slow" action potential by a rise in threshold potential from −90 mV to leads of approximately −60 mV. It is apparent that conduction in tissue responding with a "slow" action potential would be characterized by a decreased conduction velocity, a property that can increase the potential for conduction block.

The ionic basis of the slow-response action potential parallels phase 2 of the ventricular myocardial fiber or fast-response cell. The positive overshoot does not occur within the slow-response cell, presumably because there is no rapid influx of sodium. For all practical purposes, then, there is no corollary of phase 1 or phase 2 within the slow-response cell; the slow inward currents for sodium and calcium account for the slow positive upstroke of phase 0 in Figure 10-1B.

Action Potential Propagation

Since the myocardium is surrounded by intracellular and extracellular fluids that are replete with electrolytes, the myocardial fibers are surrounded by excellent conductors of electricity. With stimulation of the fiber, the positive charges flow inward, thus attracting negative ions to the external surface. Because current flows from higher to lower potential, the external flow is in the direction of right to left (from positive to negative), while intracellularly it flows from left to right (Figure 10-3). At any given point in the process of activation there is a boundary that separates the depolarized and polarized zones. It is these differences in potential that are measured by the lead systems of the electrocardiograph. During the period in which depolarization has been completed and the muscle sustains activation, there is no difference in electrical potential and, therefore, no current to be measured by the electrocardiograph.

The velocity of conduction across the muscle is dependent on the difference in potential between the activated and resting muscle. The greater the magnitude of the action potential and the faster the positive overshoot occurs, the more rapidly conduction occurs. When the resting potential becomes more positive, such as in ischemic tissue or with premature beats, the velocity of conduction diminishes.

The impulse, once initiated, is propagated in all directions until depolarization of the entire myocardium has been effected; this is known as the "all-or-nothing law." The impulse spreads from one muscle fiber to the next with no additional stimulation until the wave of excitation reaches a point where there is insufficient voltage to attain threshold potential. The heart behaves as a single cell, a functional syncytium.

Automatic pacemaker cells, or those cells which are characterized by the slow response, possess a much slower speed of conduction. The greater vulnerability of the slow response fibers to block has already been mentioned. In addition, these fibers are unable to conduct at rapid rates. The velocity of conduction may differ according to the direction of conduction (whether antegrade or retrograde) in the slow-response fibers. The basis of reentry exists in the frequency with which a slow-response fiber can conduct an impulse in one direction but block it in the opposite direction.

Normal Electrical Conduction

The SA Node

At the junction of the superior vena cava and the right atrium lies the normal pacemaker of the heart, the *sinoatrial (SA) node.* The node is approximately 10 to 20 mm long, 3 to 4 mm wide, and 2 mm thick. The functional organization of the sinus node is probably such that several groups of sinus node cells undergo pacemaker activity simultaneously and without interference from each other. The obvious benefit is that in the event of failure in the excitation of one

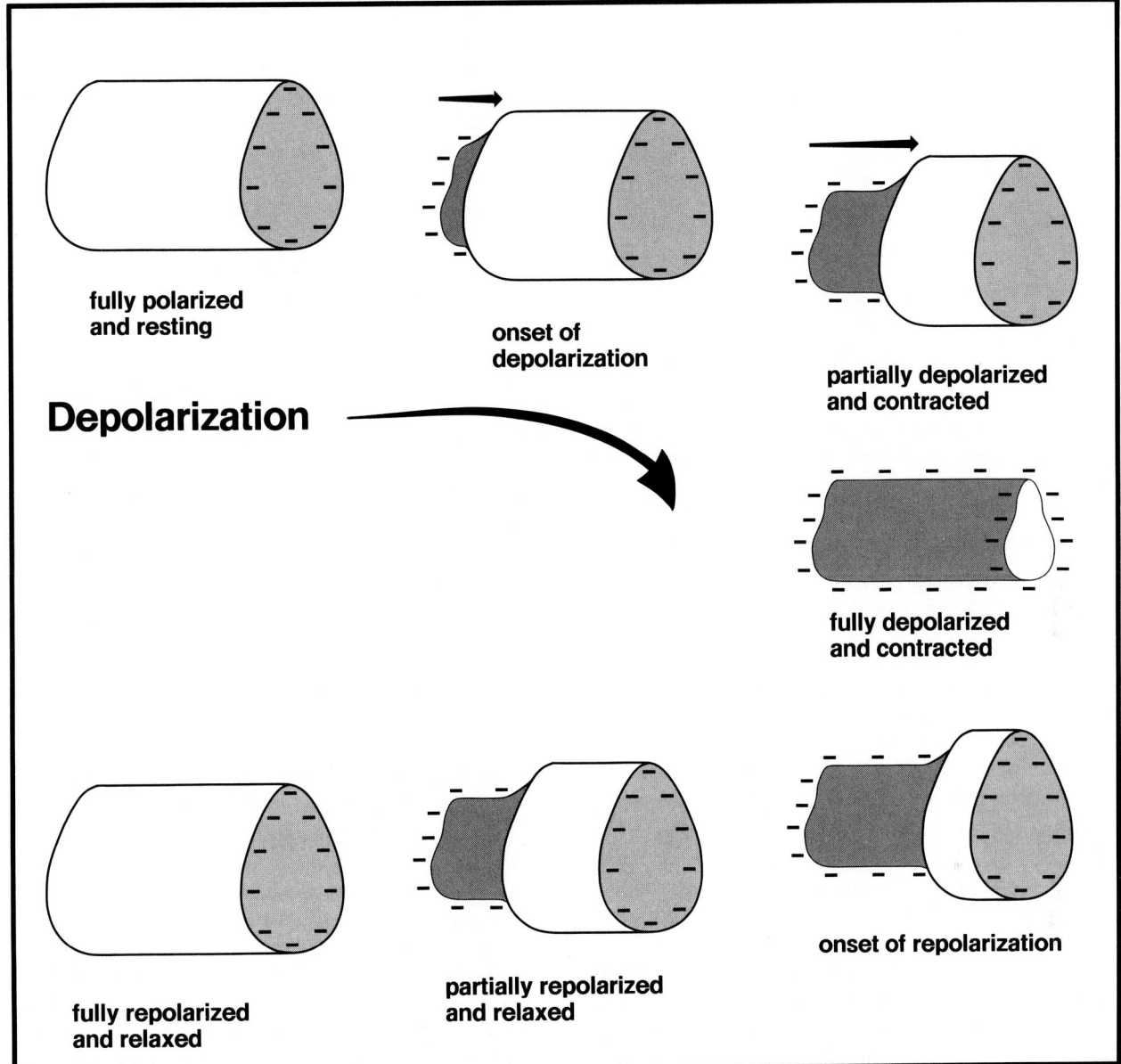

**fully polarized
and resting**

**onset of
depolarization**

**partially depolarized
and contracted**

Depolarization

**fully depolarized
and contracted**

**fully repolarized
and relaxed**

**partially repolarized
and relaxed**

onset of repolarization

Figure 10-3   Depolarization and repolarization of a muscle fiber. See text for description.
From Huszar, R. J. (1988). *Basic dysrhythmias.* St. Louis: Mosby–Year Book.

group of cells, another is available with little change in rate. Pathological conditions involving the SA node are frequently related to its anatomic position or blood supply. Because the node is superficial, lying scarcely a millimeter beneath the pericardium, it is subject to diseases affecting the superficial tissues, for example, pericarditis.

Because the major function of the SA node is to serve as pacemaker of the heart, its action potential is typical of a slow-response cell (Figure 10-4). The property that determines this role as pacemaker is that of diastolic depolarization. In addition, the SA node has a low resting membrane potential in com-

parison to other myocardial fibers. The cause of the low resting potential is thought to be a very high sodium conductance within the sinus membranes. In-activation of the potassium current during phase 4, together with early opening of the slow sodium and calcium channels, is presumably the basis of diastolic depolarization.

The frequency of discharge of the SA node is ordinarily determined through control of the sympathetic and parasympathetic nervous systems. With an increase in sympathetic stimulation, norepinephrine is released from the nerve endings to increase the heart rate as well as to increase cardiac excitability and

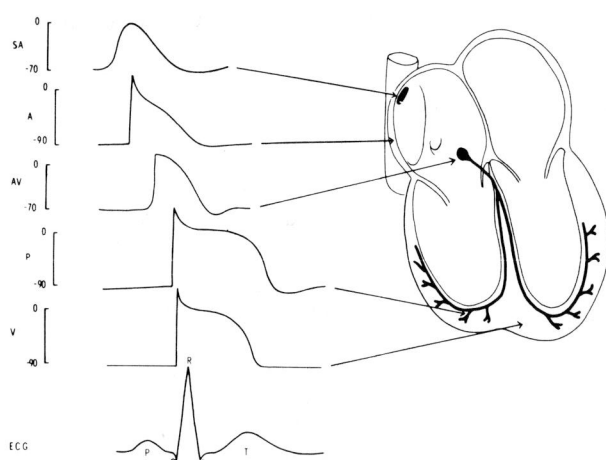

Figure 10-4 Comparison of action potentials in differing myocardial tissue. Sinoatrial (SA) pacemaker cells possess phase 4 spontaneous depolarization, a slow upstroke in phase 0, poorly differentiated phases 1 and 2, and a well-developed repolarization in phase 3. Atrial muscle cells (A) are characterized by a rapid upstroke in phase 1, with a well-developed positive overshoot and a relatively long phase 3. Phases 2 and 3 are difficult to differentiate. Atrioventricular cells (AV) may possess a period of hyperpolarization at the end of phase 3 and do not appear to possess true phase 4 diastolic depolarization. The Purkinje cells (P) possess an extremely rapid upstroke in phase 1 and a lengthy phase 2, and they appear to demonstrate phase 4 depolarization. Ventricular cells (V) have a much shorter repolarization phase (phase 2) than Purkinje cells and do not possess diastolic depolarization.

Adapted from Hurst, J. W., Logue, R. B., Schlant, R. C., et al. (Eds.). (1990). *The heart, arteries, and veins* (7th ed.). New York: McGraw-Hill.

contractility. The effect of norepinephrine lies in its ability to increase membrane permeability to sodium which, in the sinus node, causes an increase in the velocity of reduction in membrane potential to threshold, thereby increasing the heart rate. Stimulation of the parasympathetic system causes release of acetylcholine at the vagal nerve endings. Acetylcholine produces the opposite effect of norepinephrine on the heart: It decreases the rate of discharge at the SA node and decreases the rate of conduction of the impulse from the atria to the ventricles. When stimulated by acetylcholine, the cardiac fibers become extremely permeable to potassium so that very rapid efflux of potassium occurs within the cell. This results in hyperpolarization of the fiber because its resting potential is more negative than normal and, therefore, less excitable.

Another effect of vagal stimulation on the SA node resulting from the decrease in rate can be escape beats from lower pacemakers within the conduction system; if the reduction in sinus discharge continues, the lower pacemaker takes over at a slower rate than that of the sinus node. Normally the intrinsic rate of sinus discharge is between 60 and 100 impulses per minute, with a minimum range of 40 to 50 and a maximum of 200 to 220 impulses per minute.

Atrial Conduction

From the SA node, the impulse is immediately conducted through the atria and to the AV node via the internodal pathways. The sinus node fibers are continuous with the atrial fibers; thus the impulse spreads in a wavelike pattern in all directions, reaching the distal portions of the atria in about 0.08 second. The atrial action potential is illustrated in Figure 10-4. It is difficult to differentiate phase 2 from phase 3; repolarization (phase 3) is also prolonged.

AV Conduction

The action potential within the AV node region (N) is similar to that of the SA node (see Figure 10-4). The resting potential is less than in the ordinary myocardial fiber, and the refractory period extends beyond phase 4. There may be a period of hyperpolarization at the end of phase 3, followed by a return to a stable resting potential. Cells within this area are not thought to demonstrate true diastolic depolarization. The AV node exhibits the property of decremental conduction; that is, impulses are blocked that would be conducted in other areas of the heart, and should the atria depolarize at a high rate, only a portion of the impulses are normally conducted through the AV node. The major goal of decremental conduction is to prevent the ventricles from contracting before adequate filling occurs.

The effects of norepinephrine and sympathetic stimulation upon the AV node consist of increasing excitability within the potential pacemakers of the AV junction as well as an increase in conduction time. Parasympathetic stimulation, as previously mentioned, can either lengthen conduction time from the node to the ventricle, or cause partial or even complete blockage of atrial impulses within the node and result in junctional escape rhythms. The intrinsic rate within the junction is approximately 40 to 60 impulses per minute.

Transmission through the Purkinje System

The *Purkinje system* has the major task of rapidly and synchronously conducting the wave of excitation to the ventricular myocardial fibers. As noted in Figure 10-4, the action potential of the Purkinje fiber has a very rapid upstroke as well as a prolonged plateau phase (phase 2). The Purkinje action potential also demonstrates spontaneous diastolic depolarization.

In addition to its primary function as an extremely rapid conductor of the atrial impulse to the ventricles, the Purkinje system has two other fundamental properties. The first relates to the very long repolarization phase mentioned above. Figure 10-5 compares the refractory periods of the specialized conducting system. The shaded areas at the bottom represent refractory periods; it is apparent that the areas with the greatest refractory periods are the AV node and the distal Purkinje fibers (DPFs). The DPF are also called *gate cells* in recognition of their role in protecting the ventricles from premature beats which may be conducted by the AV node but are blocked by the gate cells because of their long refractory period. This mechanism is especially effective at slow heart rates. As the heart rate increases, the refractory period within the gate cells decreases. Within the AV node, however, the absolute refractory period remains unchanged and can even increase with very rapid rates; thus, the AV node assumes the role of the Purkinje gate cells in tachycardia.

The Purkinje system also can function as the heart's pacemaker. Though the action potential does not exhibit the classic slow response of the other automatic cells, the pacemaker function of the Purkinje fibers is evident through diastolic depolarization and can become manifest through escape rhythms or in assumption of the role of pacemaker of the heart in severe conduction disturbances, as in complete heart block. The intrinsic rate of the Purkinje system is usually less than 40 impulses per minute.

ELECTROCARDIOGRAPHY

Purpose

The electrocardiogram (ECG) gives essential information regarding variations in rate and rhythm of the heart, effects of altered electrolyte concentrations, the electrical orientation of the heart as influenced by anatomical factors, and the influence of certain drugs such as digitalis. The electrocardiogram gives no direct information regarding the contractile state or mechanical performance of the heart.

Lead System

An electrocardiograph is essentially a modification of the galvanometer, in that there are two terminals: one connected to a positive electrode and one connected to a negative electrode. When the two electrodes are placed at different points in an electrical field, a lead is formed; the axis of that lead is described by joining the two sites with a hypothetical line.

Bipolar leads record the potential between a positive and a negative electrode which are placed within the area of electrical potential. A unipolar lead gives information about the variation in potential taking

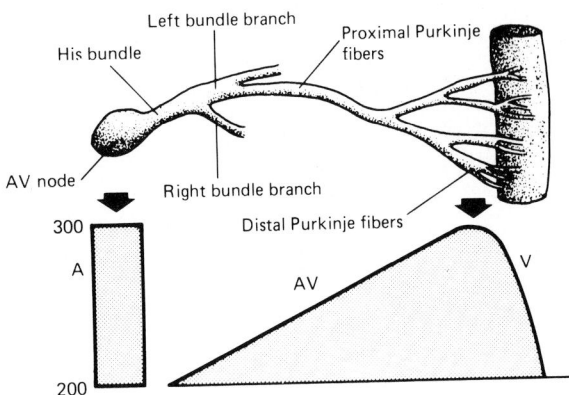

Figure 10-5 Refractory periods within the heart. Represented in the upper diagram is the conduction system: the AV node, His bundle, left and right bundle branches, and the conduction tissue connecting junctional and ventricular conducting tissue, which is divided into the proximal Purkinje fibers and distal Purkinje fibers. The shaded areas are representative of refractory periods, the ordinate being 200 to 300 ms. The arrows emphasize peak refractory periods in the AV node and distal Purkinje network. See text for further details.

place underneath a single exploring electrode. It records the difference between an indifferent electrode (which is at zero potential) and the exploring electrode (positive).

Figure 10-6 represents a ventricular muscle strip which is connected to a unipolar lead. Exploring electrodes, which are attached to a recorder, are placed at three points on the muscle strip: on the endocardium, on the epicardium, and at the midportion of the strip. The direction of depolarization in the normal ventricle extends from endocardium to epicardium; the reverse is true for the direction of repolarization.

In the polarized or resting state, depicted in section *A* of Figure 10-6, there is no difference in potential and, therefore, no activity to be measured. With excitation, the epicardial lead inscribes an upstroke because it faces the positive side of the advancing electric charge. As a wave of depolarization arrives at the electrode, depicted in sections *C* and *D*, the peak of the deflection occurs and the muscle strip is completely depolarized; the deflection then returns very suddenly to baseline. The conventional description of the first positive deflection in ventricular activation is the *R wave*. Briefly following the R wave is a short period in which the muscle remains activated and at the same potential. This period in which no change in potential occurs (isoelectric period) is called the *ST segment*. With repolarization, the negative charge precedes the positive and travels to the endocardial

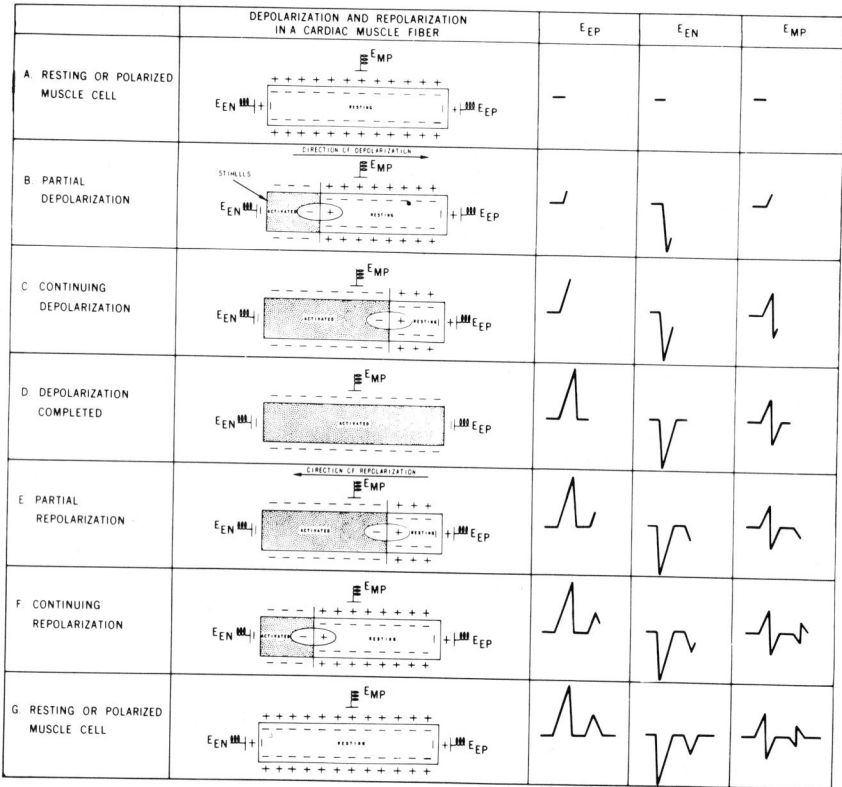

	DEPOLARIZATION AND REPOLARIZATION IN A CARDIAC MUSCLE FIBER	E$_{EP}$	E$_{EN}$	E$_{MP}$
A. RESTING OR POLARIZED MUSCLE CELL		—	—	—
B. PARTIAL DEPOLARIZATION				
C. CONTINUING DEPOLARIZATION				
D. DEPOLARIZATION COMPLETED				
E. PARTIAL REPOLARIZATION				
F. CONTINUING REPOLARIZATION				
G. RESTING OR POLARIZED MUSCLE CELL				

Figure 10-6   The potentials recorded by unipolar leads during depolarization and repolarization of a cardiac muscle fiber. E$_{EP}$, epicardial lead; E$_{EN}$, endocardial lead; E$_{MP}$, a lead at the midpoint of the muscle strip. See text for further description.

From Friedman, H. H. (1985). *Diagnostic electrocardiography and vectorcardiography.* New York: McGraw-Hill.

end of the muscle. When the charge faces the positive exploring electrode, an upright deflection, the *T wave*, is inscribed. So long as repolarization and depolarization take place in opposite directions, the R and T waves are recorded in the same direction.

In the endocardial lead, the electrode faces the negative side of the charges; therefore, an initial negative deflection, the *Q wave*, is inscribed. The peak of the activation occurs rapidly and closer to the beginning of the wave of current where the electrode is closest to the negative charge. As the wave moves away from the electrode to complete activation of the muscle, the deflection returns gradually to the baseline. This ventricular deflection is termed the *QS wave*. Because repolarization occurs in the reverse direction and the negative charge faces the electrode, an inverted T wave is recorded.

When the exploring electrode is equidistant from the ends of the muscle, first a positive deflection occurs; as the wave of excitation passes the electrode (Figure 10-6C), maximum amplitude is reached and the deflection becomes negative as the charge moves away from the electrode. A biphasic complex, which is termed an *RS waveform,* is recorded. The T wave produced is also biphasic.

Relationship between Lead Axis and Amplitude

The magnitude of the waveforms is greatest when the direction of electrical forces lies parallel to the lead axis. This is shown in Figure 10-7 in which various leads are noted with broken lines in a hexaxial reference system. Note that when electrical forces are parallel to a lead (in this case the horizontal lead), the deflection is of greatest magnitude (Figure 10-7, arrow A). If the forces are directed toward, but not parallel to the lead axis, the deflection diminishes in magnitude (Figure 10-7, arrows B and C). Finally, if the direction of the forces is perpendicular to the lead axis, the deflection may be small, isoelectric, or equiphasic (Figure 10-7, arrow D). When forces are directed away from the positive electrode of a lead, the deflection is negative; however, the relationship regarding magnitude remains the same (Figure 10-7, arrow E).

Einthoven Triangle

The basis of modern electrocardiography resides in the system devised by William Einthoven. His hypothesis assumes that the heart lies in the center of an equilateral triangle, the apices of which are the right and left shoulders and pubic region; and that

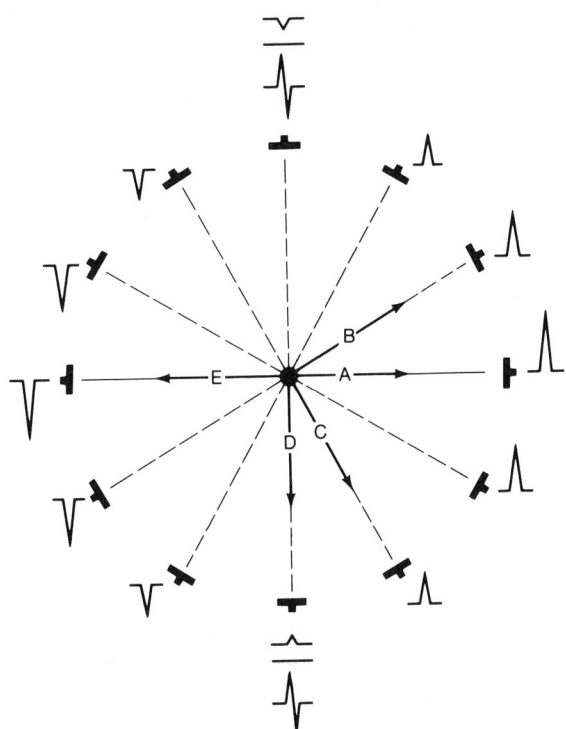

Figure 10-7 Various QRS complexes during depolarization of a muscle strip plotted in a hexaxial reference frame. See text for discussion.

Adapted from Chung, E. K. (1985). *Electrocardiography: Practical applications with vectorial principles.* Norwalk, CT: Appleton-Century-Crofts.

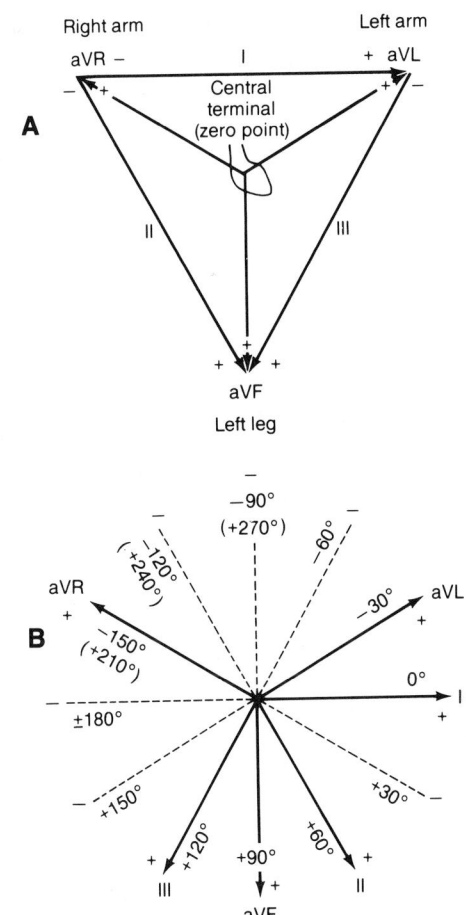

Figure 10-8 Einthoven's triangle and hexaxial reference system. *A,* Einthoven's equilateral triangle showing the axes of bipolar standard limb leads I, II, and III. Superimposed on the triangle are the axes of the unipolar limb leads. The heart is at the center or zero point. *B,* The axes of the standard and augmented limb leads are combined to form the hexaxial reference system, a modified version of Einthoven's triangle. See text for a more detailed description.

the body fluids act as a volume conductor so that the standard limb leads record differences in potential between the apices of the triangle. The conventional limb leads are (1) *lead I,* recording the differences in potential between the negative right (RA) and positive left (LA) arms; (2) *lead II,* recording the differences between the negative RA and positive left leg (LL); and (3) *lead III,* measuring the variations between the left arm (negative) and left leg (positive) (Figure 10-8*A*). The standard limb leads are such that in most persons the electrical recordings of the three leads produce positive deflections.

Unipolar leads recorded from the right arm (VR), left arm (VL), and left leg (VF) are based on the theory that the indifferent electrode located at the central terminal maintains zero potential throughout the cardiac cycle (see Figure 10-8*A*). By comparing the potential of an exploring electrode with that of the central terminal, it is evident that only the variation of potential under the exploring electrode is recorded. Because the deflections that are measured are very small, augmentation of their amplitude is performed so that these leads are designated as *aVR, aVL,* and *aVF.* These leads together with the three bipolar leads

describe the electrical forces along the frontal plane.

Modification of Einthoven's triangle such that the center point of the three bipolar leads is superimposed on the central terminal of the three unipolar leads produces a hexaxial reference system (Figure 10-8*B*). The lines of the reference system create twelve 30° angles which together total 360° or a full circle. The angles above the lead I axis or the horizontal axis are identified with minus signs, that is, −30° to −150°, and the angles below the lead I axis are labeled with positive signs (+30° to +150°). The positive and negative ends of the lead I axis are labeled as 0° and ±180°, respectively. The hexaxial reference system is useful in determining the electrical axis of depolarization and repolarization forces.

TABLE 10-1 Placement of Positive and Negative Electrodes for Each of the 12 Leads of an Electrocardiogram

Lead	+ Electrode	− Electrode
I	Left arm	Right arm
II	Left leg	Right arm
III	Left leg	Left arm
aVR	Right arm	
aVL	Left arm	
aVF	Left leg	
V_1	4th intercostal space, right sternal border	
V_2	4th intercostal space, left sternal border	
V_3	Midway between V_2 and V_4	
V_4	5th intercostal space, midclavicular line	
V_5	5th intercostal space, anterior axillary line	
V_6	5th intercostal space, midaxillary line	

Precordial Leads

There are six precordial leads identified on the electrocardiogram as V_1 through V_6. These leads are unipolar in that they utilize a positive electrode and an indifferent electrode with zero potential. By convention the six precordial electrodes are placed as noted in Table 10-1. Occasionally, additional precordial leads are recorded from the right precordium. Common examples are V_3R and V_4R which provide another viewpoint over the right chest. These chest leads all depict the electrical forces of the heart in the horizontal or transverse plane.

When looking at the deflections of the QRS complexes in the precordial leads, the observer will note that the magnitude of the R wave progresses from V_1 or V_2 to V_6 (Figure 10-9). This normal occurrence is due to the way the ventricles are depolarized. The papillary muscles and interventricular septum are activated first, except for a small section near the base of the septum (Figure 10-9, phase 1). Because the initial wave of depolarization is oriented to the right and superiorly, a small R wave is recorded in the right

VENTRICULAR DEPOLARIZATION IN THE NORMAL HEART

SEQUENCE OF VENTRICULAR ACTIVATION

PHASE 1 INITIAL SEPTAL ACTIVATION. (0.01 SEC)

PHASE 2 CONTINUED ACTIVATION OF SEPTUM AND ACTIVATION OF APICO-ANTERIOR PORTIONS OF RIGHT AND LEFT VENTRICLES. (0.02 SEC)

PHASE 3 COMPLETION OF SEPTAL ACTIVATION AND ACTIVATION OF MOST, IF NOT ALL, OF RIGHT VENTRICLE AND MOST OF LEFT VENTRICLE. (0.04-0.06 SEC)

PHASE 4 ACTIVATION OF POSTEROBASAL REGION OF LEFT VENTRICLE, BASE OF SEPTUM AND BASE OF RIGHT VENTRICLE. (0.06-0.08 SEC)

QRS COMPLEXES IN THE PRECORDIAL LEADS

VENTRICULAR ACTIVATION VECTORS IN THE TRANSVERSE PLANE

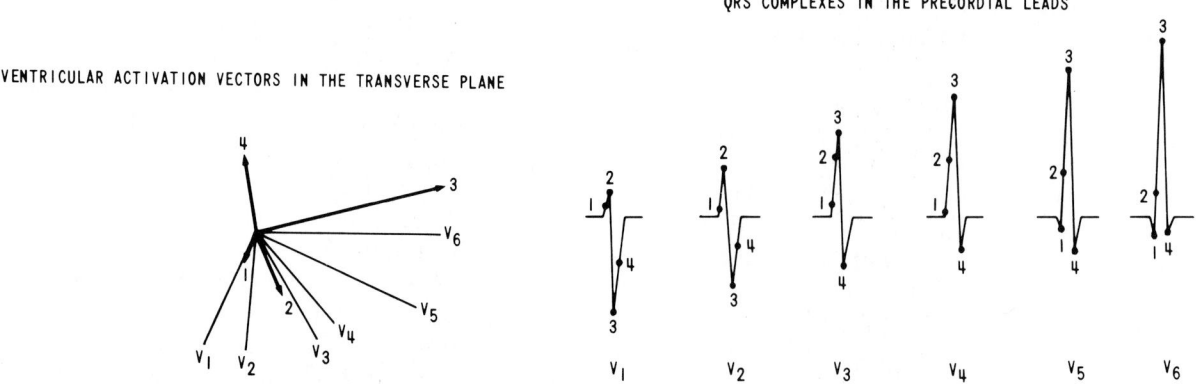

Figure 10-9 Schematic representation of ventricular depolarization in the normal heart. See text for description.
From Friedman, H. H. (1985). *Diagnostic electrocardiography and vectorcardiography.* New York: McGraw-Hill.

precordial leads (usually in both V_1 and V_2 but sometimes only in V_2) and a small Q wave is recorded from the left precordium (V_5 and V_6).

The activation spreads from endocardium to epicardium and over both the right and left ventricles (Figure 10-9, phase 2). Because the left ventricle is greater in mass and, therefore, greater in electrical potential, it determines the direction, polarity, and magnitude (vector) of the QRS as anterior and leftward and inscribes a positive R wave in most ECG leads. During the third phase, most of both ventricles are depolarized, and again, the left ventricle overpowers the right ventricular waveform. Because this phase has considerable amplitude and is oriented leftward and posteriorly, a deep S wave is recorded in the right precordial leads, while tall R waves are recorded in the left precordial leads. V_3 and V_4 are considered transitional leads, representing the end of phase 3. Activation of the posterobasal region of the left ventricle, the base of the septum, and the base of the right ventricle occurs during phase 4. The upstroke of the S wave in the right precordial leads (V_1 and V_2) and the downstroke of the R wave and a small S wave in the left precordial leads (V_4 through V_6) are inscribed on the electrocardiogram.

Monitoring Leads

Since the ECG electrodes attached to the arms and legs record all electrical events, that is, the action potentials of skeletal muscle cells during extremity movements, it is not practical to obtain routine and continuous recordings of the heart's electrical activity in this manner. Consequently, modifications of the standard limb and precordial leads are used. Electrode placement for the monitor limb leads is similar to the standard placement except that the left and right shoulder or subclavicular areas and the lower left quadrant of the abdomen are used for electrode placement (Figure 10-10A).

Using five ECG electrodes on the chest, bedside monitors with two or more channels for ECG monitoring are commonly programmed to include monitor lead II and a modified chest lead (MCL). In the case of MCL_1, the precordial V_1 lead is simulated by placing the positive electrode in the standard V_1 position, the negative electrode just below the left midclavicle, and the ground electrode below the right midclavicle (Figure 10-10B). Other precordial leads can be simulated in a similar manner; MCL_6 is the most common and has the positive electrode placed in the standard V_6 position.

Waves, Complexes, and Intervals

The electrical activity of the entire heart is inscribed on the ECG as a series of waveforms, each of which

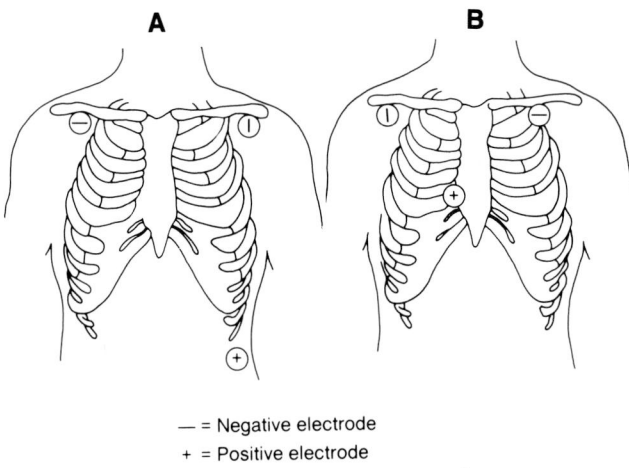

A　　　　　　　　**B**

— = Negative electrode
+ = Positive electrode
I = Indifferent or ground electrode

Figure 10-10　Electrode placement for routine monitoring. *A,* Electrode placement for monitoring lead II. *B,* Electrode placement for MCL_1.

represents a particular electrical event in the cardiac cycle. The waveforms are identified by the letters P, Q, R, S, T, and U (Figure 10-11).

P Wave

Atrial depolarization is represented on the ECG by the *P wave.* The duration of atrial depolarization is less than 0.11 second in normal hearts. The height of the P wave is normally less than 3 mm. The waveform should be upright and symmetrically rounded in leads I, II, aVF, and V_4 through V_6 (see Figure 10-11) and inverted in lead aVR. It may be diphasic, flat, or inverted in leads III, V_1, and V_2, but the negative component should not be excessively deep or wide. If the P wave is peaked or notched, it is abnormal and indicates abnormal depolarization of one or both atria secondary to chamber enlargement or conduction defect.

QRS Complex

The *QRS complex* represents ventricular depolarization. The *Q wave* is the first negative deflection after the P wave; it may or may not be present, depending on the given lead being monitored; and it reflects normal ventricular activity. The *R wave* is the first positive deflection after the P wave. The negative deflection after the R wave is the *S wave* (see Figure 10-11). This complex is by convention identified with all three letters, but it is possible that more or fewer of the waveforms will be inscribed. For example, when no positive deflection occurs, a QS wave exists. If more than one R or S is inscribed, the second is indicated by a prime (') and is called R prime (R') or S prime (S'). When it is necessary to describe each portion of the complex specifically,

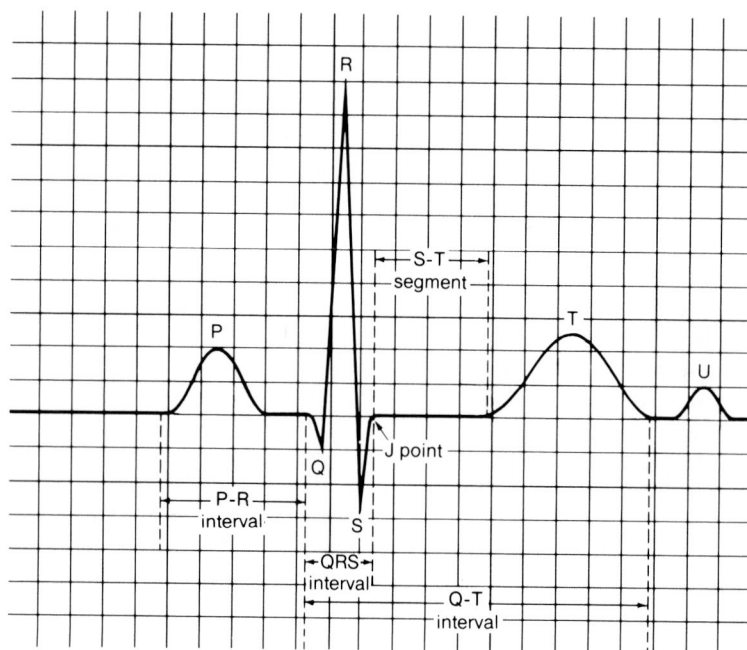

Figure 10-11   Electrocardiographic complexes and intervals representative of lead II.

lower- and uppercase letters are used to denote the relative sizes of the components, that is q or Q, r or R, and s or S.

ST Segment

The isoelectric line following the QRS complex and ending with the start of the T wave is the *ST segment* (see Figure 10-11). As noted earlier, this represents the period after ventricular depolarization when there is no change in electrical potential. The junction between the end of the QRS complex and the beginning of the ST segment is referred to as the *J point* (see Figure 10-11). Normally the ST segment begins flat on the baseline (isoelectric) and curves gently and imperceptibly into the proximal limb of the T wave. However, it may be elevated up to 1 mm in the limb leads or 2 mm in some precordial leads. It is normally not depressed more than 0.50 mm. If it is excessively elevated or depressed, pathological conditions such as myocardial injury should be considered.

T Wave

The *T wave* represents the recovery phase after ventricular depolarization (see Figure 10-11). This deflection should be upright in leads I, II, and V_3 to V_6 and inverted in lead aVR. In leads III, aVL, V_1, and V_2 the direction of the deflection is variable. The T wave is normally slightly rounded and slightly asymmetric. Sharply pointed or grossly notched T waves should be considered suspicious. The height of the T wave is normally less than 5 mm in the limb leads and less than 10 mm in the precordial leads. T waves

may be diminished, elevated, or inverted due to drugs, electrolyte imbalance, ischemia, or injury. The last one half to one third of the T wave is often referred to as the vulnerable period. An electrical stimulus during this portion of the T wave may precipitate a serious ventricular dysrhythmia.

U Wave

A small and usually positive deflection immediately following the T wave and preceding the P wave is the *U wave* (see Figure 10-11). The exact cause of this deflection is unknown, but it is thought to be the result of the slow repolarization of the intraventricular conduction system. Frequently the U wave is so small that it is unidentifiable. It may be visualized best in lead V_3. If a prominent U wave is noted, one should rule out hypokalemia. It is of interest to note that most ventricular extrasystoles occur at about the same time as the U wave in the cardiac cycle.

PR Interval

The period from the beginning of the P wave to the beginning of the QRS complex is the *PR interval* (see Figure 10-11). This portion of the cardiac cycle represents the time required for the original impulse to travel from the SA node through the atria and the AV node to the bundle branches. The duration of the PR interval is normally between 0.12 and 0.20 second. A delay in the PR interval (PR greater than 0.20 second) indicates a conduction delay through the AV node or depressed conduction secondary to drug therapy such as digitalis. A shortened PR interval indicates an abnormal conduction pathway that allows the impulse to bypass the AV node and cause early ventricular stimulation.

QRS Width

The *QRS width* is that period required to depolarize the ventricles (see Figure 10-11). Normally this interval is between 0.06 and 0.10 second. Prolongation up to 0.12 second indicates an interventricular conduction defect and prolongation equal to or greater than 0.12 second is indicative of complete block in a bundle branch. Consequently, the ventricles are depolarized abnormally. Causes of a prolonged QRS width are ischemia or injury of the conduction system, premature systoles from the atria which depolarize aberrantly through the ventricles, and ventricular extrasystoles.

QT Interval

Measuring from the beginning of the QRS complex to the end of the T wave, one obtains the duration of the *QT interval,* which represents the entirety of ventricular electrical systole (see Figure 10-11). This portion of the cardiac cycle varies with the heart rate, being shorter in rapid rates and longer in slower heart rates. Calculation of the QT interval is accomplished using the formula

$$\text{QT calculation} = \frac{\text{QT (measured)}}{\sqrt{\text{RR interval(s)}}}$$

and is indicated on the ECG as the QT_c. When the heart rate is 60 to 100 beats per minute, any QT interval greater than one half of the preceding RR interval is considered to be abnormally long as well as any QT_c greater than 0.42 second.

Critical care nurses should be familiar with and use the formula for calculating the QT interval when analyzing ECGs because individuals with prolonged QT intervals are predisposed to reentrant dysrhythmias. Causes of QT interval prolongation include myocarditis secondary to congestive heart failure, ischemic heart disease, or rheumatic fever; cerebrovascular disease; and electrolyte disturbance, particularly hypocalcemia. Drug therapy with quinidine, disopyramide, and amiodarone may prolong the QT interval as may hypothermia or stringent dieting.

The QT interval may also be abnormally short. Digitalis therapy, hypercalcemia, and potassium intoxication may cause short QT intervals. Unfortunately though, the lower limit of normal for the QT interval is not well defined.

Heart Rate and Rhythm Determination

Standard ECG paper is made up of a series of 1-mm squares from which both voltage and time can be measured (Figure 10-12). Each group of five small squares is marked by a darker line. Voltage is measured along the vertical axis of the graph. At normal standardization, every 10 mm of stylus excursion is equal to 1 mV (1 mm = 0.1 mV). Time is measured along the horizontal axis, and at normal recording speed of 25 mm/sec each millimeter equals 0.04 second (40 ms) and 5 mm or one large square equals 0.20 second (200 ms). Thus, at the normal speed, 1,500 small and 300 large squares pass through the recorder each minute.

Heart Rate Calculation

A number of methods are available for calculating the heart rate on the ECG. The first options are used for regular rhythms. The last one described should be used when the cardiac rhythm is irregular, but it can also be used for regular rhythms to obtain a general estimate.

If the cardiac rhythm is regular, that is, the RR interval is constant, and heart rate can be determined

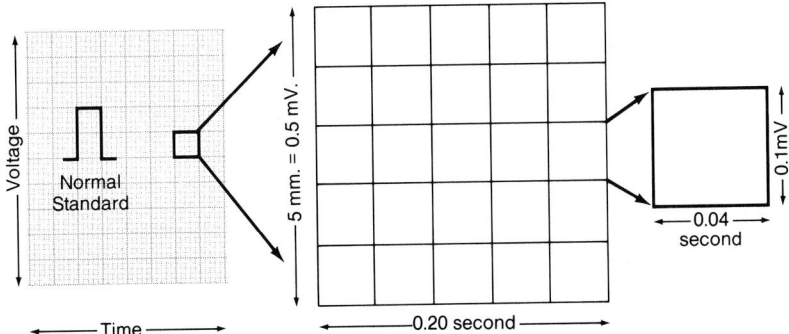

Figure 10-12   Standard ECG paper. ECG paper is a graph divided into millimeter squares. Time is measured on the horizontal axis with each small square equal to 0.04 second (at 25 mm/sec paper speed) and each large square equal to 0.20 second. Note the time markers at the top of the paper indicating a 3-second interval. Markers are usually located at 2- or 3-second intervals. Voltage is measured on the vertical axis of the graph. At normal standardization (1 mV), each small square is equal to 0.1 mV.

quickly and quite accurately by dividing the number of large squares per minute, 300, by the number of large squares between two consecutive R waves. For example, if the RR interval is three large squares, the heart rate is 100 (300 ÷ 3 = 100). Figure 10-13A illustrates this method of heart rate determination and gives the heart rate for six different RR intervals.

Unfortunately, not all RR intervals can be measured by whole large squares. Frequently, the RR interval is composed of a number of both large and small squares. Figure 10-13B illustrates such a circumstance. In this example the RR interval is composed of four large and two small squares, and the heart rate is 69 beats per minute. This rate is determined by dividing the total number of horizontal small squares on the ECG paper (1,500) by the number of small squares in the RR interval. In Figure 10-13B, 1,500 ÷ 22 = 69/minute. Note also the scale inscribed on Figure 10-11B for calculating the rate

of the P waves. "Start" signifies the initial marker placed at the onset of the P wave. The user estimates the atrial rate where the onset of the next P crosses the scale, that is less than 75 but more than 60.

When the heart rate is irregular, the foregoing methods do not yield accurate rates. Consequently, an alternative method must be used. In this method, the number of cardiac cycles (RR intervals) in a 6-second period (30 large squares = 6 seconds) is counted and multiplied by 10. This method is made easier because ECG paper used at 25 mm/sec speed is usually marked off in 3-second sections by vertical lines at the top of the paper. Figure 10-14 illustrates this method of calculating heart rate.

Rhythm Determination

The regularity of the cardiac rhythm is important to assess because it provides information regarding the site of the electrical stimulus, the function of that

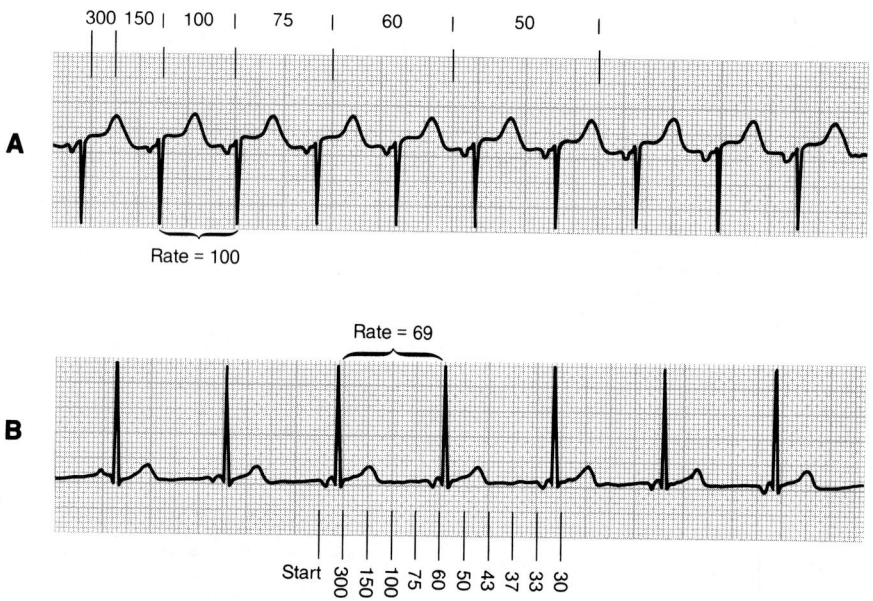

Figure 10-13 Rapid heart rate determination. *A*, Divide 300 by the number of large squares between R waves. In this example the rate is about 100. Rates for six RR intervals are shown. *B*, When the RR interval is not equal to a large square interval but falls between the large square markers, the rate can be calculated as described in the text. The rate for this rhythm strip is 69. Values for small squares between various large square markers are shown.

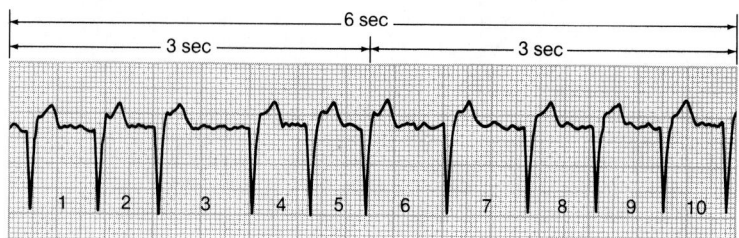

Figure 10-14 Measurement of heart rate per minute by counting number of cardiac cycles in a 6-second interval and multiplying by 10. In this example, there are 10 cycles per 6 seconds, resulting in a rate of 100 (10 × 10 = 100).

site, and whether more than one site is influencing the cardiac cycle. The easiest way to make this assessment is to measure the RR (or PP) intervals and determine if they are constant in length. This can be done with calipers or with marks made on a piece of paper. The rhythm is said to be regular if the length of the shortest and longest RR (or PP) intervals varies by less than 0.16 second. If the intervals vary by more than 0.16 second, the rhythm is irregular and should be further assessed for a pattern of irregularity. The rhythm may be regularly irregular, thus showing a definite pattern, or it may be totally erratic.

Electrical Axis Determination

The axis of a lead can be divided into a positive and negative portion by a perpendicular line through its center. Figure 10-8B illustrates the axis in degrees and the positive and negative poles of the frontal plane bipolar and unipolar leads. The frontal plane is defined by two axes, the left and right axis, or lead I, and the superior and inferior axis, or lead aVF. Leads I and aVF divide the frontal plane into four quadrants (Figure 10-15). The *left superior* quadrant is circumscribed by the negative pole of lead aVF and the positive pole of lead I whereas the *left inferior* quadrant is circumscribed by the positive pole of both leads I and aVF. The positive pole of lead aVF and the negative pole of lead I are the borders for the *right inferior* quadrant. The *right superior* quadrant is bordered by the negative pole of leads I and aVF.

When determining the electrical axis in the frontal plane, one identifies the direction of the sum of the electrical forces (vectors) of one cardiac cycle. Two rules, the *quadrant rule* and the *perpendicular rule,* assist in identifying the electrical axis of the P wave,

the QRS complex, and the T wave. For the purposes of this discussion, the determination of only the QRS axis will be described. The axis of the P and T waves are determined following the same format.

The *quadrant rule* localizes the mean QRS vector to one of the four frontal plane quadrants. The specific quadrant is identified by looking at the direction of the QRS deflections in leads I and aVF. If the QRS in lead I is predominantly positive, but in lead aVF it is predominantly negative, the mean vector points somewhere in the left superior quadrant, or 0° to −90°. If, however, the QRS deflection is positive in both leads I and aVF, the mean vector lies within the left inferior quadrant, or 0° to +90°. When the QRS deflection is negative in lead I and positive in aVF, the mean vector is directed toward the right inferior quadrant, or +90° to ±180°. The right superior quadrant, −90° to ±180°, is the location of the mean vector when the QRS deflection is negative in leads I and aVF.

The *perpendicular rule* localizes the mean QRS vector in degrees. This rule states that the mean QRS vector lies perpendicular to the axis of the lead with the most equiphasic complex (equally positive and negative QRS deflection) and in the previously identified quadrant. Therefore, to determine the degree of the QRS axis, the lead with the most equiphasic or isoelectric QRS is identified. Next, the lead perpendicular to the first lead is identified. (It is useful to note that leads perpendicular to each other are I and aVF, II and aVL, and III and aVR.) Finally, note the degrees of the axis of the perpendicular lead in the quadrant selected with the quadrant rule.

The steps to follow, then, for determining the electrical axis of the QRS are:

1. Examine lead I and determine if the forces are directed to the right or to the left. If the QRS in lead I is positive, the vector is to the left. If the QRS in lead I is negative, the vector is to the right.
2. Examine lead aVF and determine if the forces are directed inferiorly or superiorly. The QRS in lead aVF will be positive if the vector is inferior, and negative if the vector is superior.
3. After identifying where the information gained in steps 1 and 2 overlap, one identifies the general direction of the QRS vector.
4. Locate the most equiphasic or isoelectric QRS from leads I through aVF and identify that lead.
5. Identify the lead perpendicular to the lead selected in step 4. This lead should have the greatest amplitude. If it does not, repeat step 4 to ensure correct lead identification.
6. Identify the degrees of the axis of the lead in step 5. Remember to select the pole of the lead which lies in the quadrant identified in step 3.

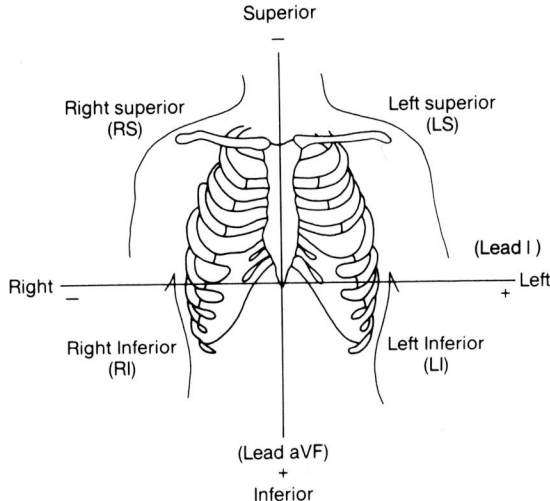

Figure 10-15 Quadrants of the frontal plane. Leads I and aVF divide the frontal plane into four quadrants: left superior (LS), left inferior (LI), right inferior (RI), and right superior (RS). See text for further discussion.

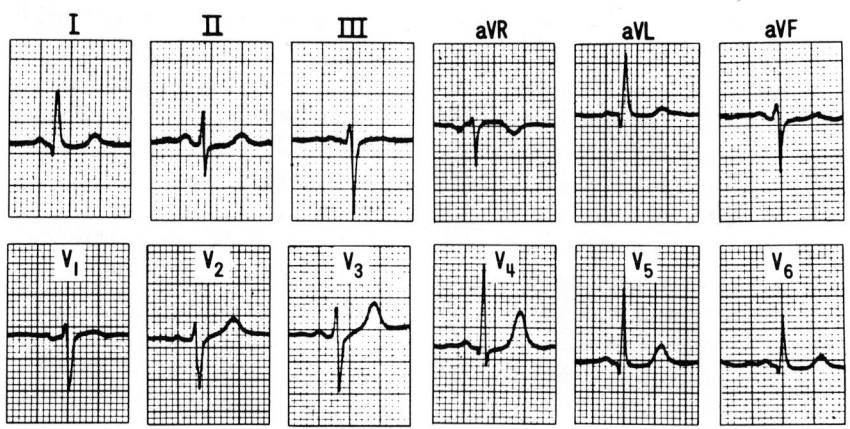

Figure 10-16   A normal electrocardiogram from an elderly woman. The QRS in lead I is positively deflected, indicating the forces are directed to the left. The electrical forces in aVF are directed superiorly (the QRS is a negative deflection). Therefore, the mean axis is in the left superior quadrant. The QRS in lead II is the most equiphasic, indicating that the mean forces are directed parallel to lead aVL, the lead perpendicular to lead II. Lead II in the left superior quadrant is at −30°. Consequently, the mean QRS axis for this ECG is −30°.

From Friedman, H. H. (1985). *Diagnostic electrocardiography and vectorcardiography.* New York: McGraw-Hill.

Review Figure 10-16 for an example of how these steps are used to identify the QRS axis for the frontal plane leads of the ECG.

In a normal ECG, the electrical axis of the QRS in the frontal plane leads should be between −30° and +100°. The mean QRS vector normally shifts leftward as an individual ages. If the axis falls outside the boundaries of normal, it is said to have rotated or deviated to the right (clockwise shift) or to the left (counterclockwise shift).

Left axis deviation (LAD) exists when the frontal plane QRS axis is −30° or more superior. A number of clinical conditions or circumstances may cause this deviation. Some of the causes include: (1) mechanical shifts secondary to respiratory expiration or a high diaphragm from pregnancy, ascites, or abdominal tumors; (2) left anterior hemiblock or left bundle branch block; (3) left ventricular hypertrophy; (4) congenital lesions such as endocardial cushion defect and several other cyanotic and acyanotic defects; (5) Wolff-Parkinson-White syndrome; (6) emphysema; (7) hyperkalemia; and (8) ventricular ectopic rhythms.[2] *Extreme* or *marked left axis deviation* exists when the QRS axis is −45° or more superior. Usually, marked LAD is due to left anterior hemiblock, but pure inferior wall myocardial infarction without left anterior hemiblock may also be a cause.

When the QRS axis is rotated clockwise to +100° or more, *right axis deviation* (RAD) exists. Causes of RAD include (1) mechanical shifts secondary to inspiration or emphysema, (2) right ventricular hypertrophy, (3) right bundle branch block, (4) left posterior hemiblock, (5) dextrocardia, (6) ventricular ectopic rhythms, and (7) Wolff-Parkinson-White syndrome.[2]

When the electrical axis falls within the right superior quadrant the frontal axis is said to be *indeterminant.* The reason for this is that without a vectorcardiogram, it is impossible to know whether the forces were directed to this area by extreme right axis deviation or extreme left axis deviation. The clinical situation may provide some clues.

It should be noted that it is possible to determine the mean vector in the horizontal plane. In this situation a different hexaxial reference system, the precordial hexaxial system, is used. Directions on this reference system are right, left, anterior, and posterior. A discussion of the method for determining the horizontal QRS axis is beyond the scope of this chapter.

Normal 12-Lead Electrocardiogram

Systematic Review of the ECG

To determine if the ECG is normal or abnormal a systematic review is recommended. A number of formats are available, and one should be selected and used consistently for all ECG analyses. The format suggested by Marriott is used in this chapter.[2]

The first step in ECG analysis involves rhythm assessment. Examine both the PP and RR intervals for regularity. If one or both are irregular, is there a pattern to the rhythm or is it completely erratic? Is there a relationship between the two rhythms? Next, the rates of both atrial and ventricular depolarization are determined. Methods for determining rate were discussed previously.

Once the rhythm and rate have been determined, close inspection of each wave, complex, and interval should follow. Begin by inspecting each P wave, noting the direction of the deflection, the amplitude, the width, whether it is diphasic, and the presence or absence of notching and peaking. Of course it is also important to note the absence of any P waves. The axis of the P wave may also be identified.

Follow P wave inspection with measurement of the PR interval. Consider if all intervals are the same or if they vary. Also note whether the measurement obtained is within normal limits. Proceed to evaluate the QRS width. Next, measure the QT interval, taking care not to measure a QU interval by mistake. Calculate the QT.

After measuring the PR, QRS, and QT intervals, analyze the QRS complex. First, measure the amplitude in the various leads, noting excessive or low voltage. Then look for Q waves. Note the leads in which they are present. Measure the depth and width. Determine the frontal plane electrical axis for the QRS. Note whether there is deviation to either the right or the left. Next, look at the relative prominence of the component waves in the precordial leads. Is there a normal R wave progression? In which lead does the deflection of the complex pass through transition (change from a predominantly negative to a predominantly positive waveform)? While examining the precordial leads, note the timing of the *intrinsicoid deflection*. This deflection is measured from the beginning of the QRS complex to the point on the isoelectric line which would be intersected by an imaginary perpendicular line from the peak of the R wave (Figure 10-17). A delay in the intrinsicoid deflection generally indicates ventricular enlargement or a block of the ventricular conduction system. Last, examine the general configuration of the total complex, noting the presence and location of any slurs or notches.

After the examination of the QRS, assess for ST segment elevation or depression and note the leads where any changes are observed. Look for any abnormal sharp angles or notches.

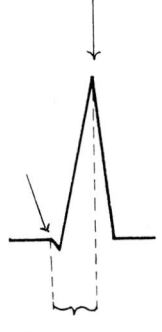

0.05 sec or more

Figure 10-17 The intrinsicoid deflection (time from the beginning of the QRS complex to the peak of the R wave) measured horizontally.

From Conover, M. B. (1992). *Understanding electrocardiography* (6th ed.). St. Louis: Mosby–Year Book.

The direction, shape, and height of the T wave are assessed next. Remember that sharply pointed or grossly notched T waves are abnormal and should be assessed further for the possible cause. The mean vector of the T wave may be identified if desired. Look for U waves next. Lead V_3 may provide the best view.

Once the ECG has been examined and information analyzed, various interpretations may be made. The cause of abnormalities can be identified many times by comparing findings to the ECG criteria for specific clinical situations and previous ECGs. The critical care nurse must know which ECG findings to report and when to report that information.

Criteria for a Normal ECG

Table 10-2 lists the criteria that need to be present for an ECG to be interpreted as normal. Figure 10-18 is an example of a normal ECG.

ABNORMALITIES OF ELECTRICAL ACTIVITY

The electrocardiogram may be altered by a number of anatomical and physiological conditions including electrolyte imbalance, ischemia, and chamber enlargement. In addition, effects of drug therapy may alter the ECG. Changes in the ECG which these conditions create may include alterations in voltage, electrical axis, rate, rhythm, and timing of intervals. Following is a discussion of some of the more common abnormalities of electrical activity.

Dysrhythmias

When considering cardiac rhythm disturbances (dysrhythmias) it is important to bear in mind the relationship between heart rate and cardiac output. Stroke volume (SV) and heart rate (HR) determine cardiac output. Consequently, if the heart rate is excessively slow, the cardiac output will be reduced unless there is a sufficient increase in stroke volume to offset the effect. Conversely, if there is an increase in the heart rate, cardiac output will rise, assuming there is not a concurrent drop in stroke volume. At very rapid rates it is likely that cardiac output will fall because the ventricular diastolic filling time is reduced, thereby reducing the stroke volume. Therefore, monitoring for and understanding cardiac rhythm disturbances is crucial in the critical care environment.

Genesis of Dysrhythmias

Abnormalities in cardiac rhythm are a consequence of disturbances in electrical impulse formation, impulse conduction, or a combination of formation and conduction. The three mechanisms of disturbance in impulse formation are the result of (1) normal automaticity, (2) abnormal automaticity, or (3) triggered activity. Mechanisms that cause disturbances

TABLE 10-2   **Criteria for a Normal Electrocardiogram**

Component	Criteria
Rhythm	Atrial and ventricular rhythms are the same.
	RR and PP intervals vary less than 0.16 sec.
Rate	Atrial and ventricular rates are equal and between 60 and 100 cycles per minute.
P wave	Present; only one P for every QRS.
Direction of deflection	Upright in leads I, II, aVF, and V_{4-6}; inverted in aVR; and may be diphasic, flat, or inverted in leads III, V_1, and V_2.
Amplitude	<3.0 mm.
Width	1.5 to 2.5 mm (0.06 to 0.10 sec).
Shape	Gently rounded without notches or peaks.
Axis	0° to +90°.
PR interval	0.12 to 0.20 sec (adults); 0.11 to 0.18 sec (infants and children).
QRS interval	0.06 to 0.10 sec.
QT interval	<half the preceding RR interval in normal rates.
	$QT_c \geq 0.39$ sec in males and 0.42 sec in females.
QRS complex	Follows each P wave.
Q waves	Width: ≤0.039 sec.
	Depth: If present, up to 1-2 mm deep in I, aVL, aVF, V_5, and V_6. Deep QS or Qr in aVR and possibly in III, V_1, and V_2.
Amplitude	>5 mm and <25 mm in limb leads; 5 to 30 mm in V_1 and V_6; 7 to 30 mm in V_2 and V_5; 9 to 30 mm in V_3 and V_4.
R progression	Progressive rise in R wave amplitude from V_1 or V_2 to V_6.
Axis	−30° to +100° in frontal plane.
Transition	V_3 or V_4.
Intrinsicoid deflection	≤0.02 sec in V_1; ≤0.04 sec in V_6.
ST segment	Isoelectric, but may be elevated ≤1 mm in limb leads and ≤2 mm in some precordial leads.
	Not depressed more than 0.05 mm.
	Curves gently into proximal limb of T wave.
T wave	
Direction	Upright in I, II, and V_{3-6}; inverted in aVR; and varies in III, aVL, aVF, V_1, and V_2.
Shape	Slightly rounded and asymmetric.
Height	≤5 mm in limb leads; ≤10 mm in precordial leads.
Axis	Left and inferior.
U wave	
Direction	Upright.
Amplitude	0.33 mm in precordial leads (average); 2.5 mm (maximum).
Width	≤0.24 sec.

in impulse conduction include (1) decremental conduction, (2) inhomogeneous conduction, (3) supernormal conduction, (4) concealed conduction, and (5) unidirectional block with or without reentry. A brief discussion of some of these mechanisms is warranted. However, for a more in-depth presentation of the genesis of dysrhythmias, the reader is directed to current electrocardiography texts.

Normal Automaticity. The mechanism of automaticity was described earlier in this chapter. The sinus node normally initiates the cardiac rhythm because its cells spontaneously depolarize and reach threshold potential faster than do the pacemaker cells of other areas of the heart. The rate of spontaneous depolarization in the sinus node is influenced by the balance between the sympathetic and parasympa-

thetic autonomic effects, temperature and metabolic activity of the pacemaker cells, and the effect of electrolyte and pH changes on the heart. Consequently, if the autonomic balance or the environment of the sinus node cells is altered, the rate of impulse formation is changed. If the rate of phase 4 depolarization is increased in pacemaker cells other than those in the sinus node, for example the junction or ventricles, the automaticity of those sites is said to be *enhanced*. Extrasystoles or tachycardias may result. Conversely, if the rate of spontaneous depolarization of the sinus node is decreased, bradycardia or escape rhythms result.

Abnormal Automaticity. When conditions are suitable, cells that do not normally have automaticity may depolarize spontaneously during phase 4. The

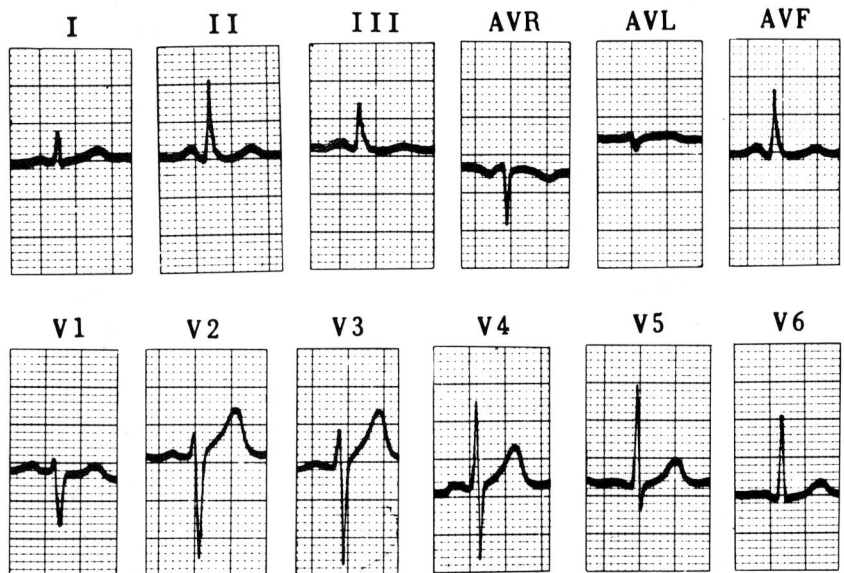

Figure 10-18   A normal electrocardiogram. Follow the format discussed in the text to systematically interpret the ECG.
From Friedman, H. H. (1985). *Diagnostic electrocardiography and vectorcardiography.* New York: McGraw-Hill.

automaticity in these sites may be depressed by acetylcholine and encouraged by catecholamines. However, the abnormal automaticity may not suppress faster pacemakers and may in fact be accelerated by overdrive pacing.

Triggered Activity.   The term *triggered activity* refers to ectopic firing, often repetitive, that occurs in the absence of enhanced automaticity and is not sustained by reentrant conduction. It results from afterdepolarizations, either early or late, that are of a magnitude great enough to reach threshold potential. The role of this mechanism in the creation of clinically observed dysrhythmias is still unclear.

Unidirectional Block with Reentry.   Reentrant circuits or loops may be established when an initiating impulse, from either the SA node or an ectopic site, encounters an area of slow conduction that is long enough to delay the impulse passing through until the rest of the myocardium is nonrefractory. An area of unidirectional conduction inhibits or blocks impulse propagation in one direction but permits the impulse to pass through from the opposite direction, allowing it to restimulate the repolarized tissue. Figure 10-19 illustrates a reentrant loop which in this instance is located in the Purkinje fibers of the ventricles. However, reentrant circuits with one-way block may appear in the SA node, the atria, the AV junction, or the ventricles. Accessory pathways may serve as one branch of a reentry loop.

Classification of Dysrhythmias

There are several ways to classify cardiac dysrhythmias. It is useful to classify them according to whether they result from disturbances in impulse for-

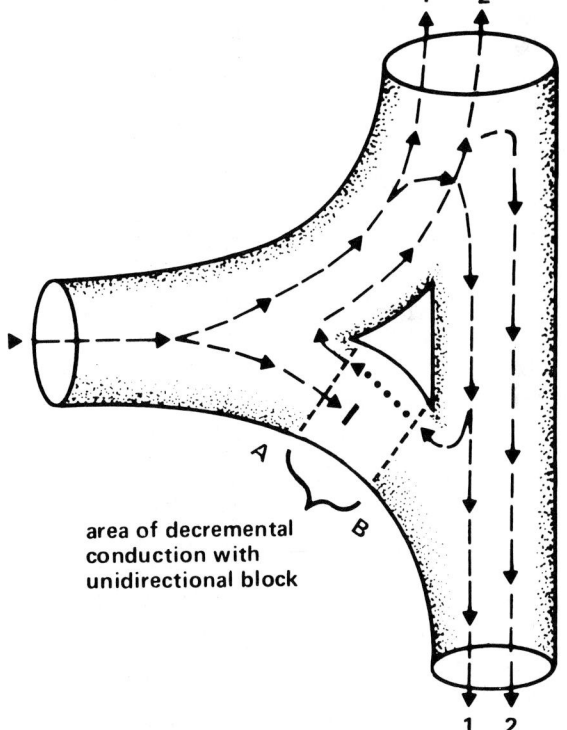

Figure 10-19   Reentry at the point of impingement of a Purkinje fiber on the ventricular myocardium. A region of decremental conduction with unidirectional block (A-B) blocks antegrade conduction of the normal impulse (1) but allows this impulse to traverse the depressed region in the retrograde direction (dotted line) after a delay. This retrograde impulse reenters the myocardium proximal to the region of decremental conduction after the proximal tissue has recovered from the normal impulse, thereby allowing the retrograde impulse to initiate a premature systole (2).
From Katz, A. M. (1977). *Physiology of the heart.* New York: Raven.

mation, impulse conduction, or a combination of these. However, in the clinical setting dysrhythmias are more commonly classified by rate (tachycardias or bradycardias), by site of origin (sinus node, atria, junction, or ventricles), or by a combination of systems. For the purposes of this text, a combination of systems is used but the site of origin is the predominant classifying characteristic.

Sinus Node Dysrhythmias

Disturbances in either impulse formation or impulse conduction in the SA node result in sinus node dysrhythmias. These rhythm disturbances are characterized by a P wave of sinus origin and a constant and normal PR interval. However, the configuration of the P wave, the rate of impulse formation, and the regularity of the cycle may be abnormal depending upon the given rhythm disturbance. The following discussion of sinus dysrhythmias includes sinus bradycardia, sinus tachycardia, sinus arrhythmia, wandering atrial pacemaker, sinus arrest, and sinoatrial block.

Sinus Bradycardia. *Sinus bradycardia* is a rhythm originating in the sinus node but at a slower than normal rate (less than 60 beats per minute). Figure 10-20 is a rhythm strip depicting sinus bradycardia. Note that all aspects of the electrocardiographic recording are normal except for the rate. The usual rate of sinus bradycardia is from 45 to 59 beats per minute, but it may be lower.

Sinus bradycardia may coexist with sinus arrhythmia but does not always do so. The rhythm must be distinguished from sinus arrest, SA block, AV junctional escape rhythm, idioventricular rhythm, and atrial fibrillation or flutter with AV block.

Sinus bradycardia is common in healthy young adults, especially those with well-conditioned cardiovascular systems, and in the elderly, particularly during periods of sleep or awakening. Altered automaticity secondary to increased parasympathetic influence is the usual cause of spontaneous sinus bradycardia. Several pharmacological agents, such as reserpine, methyldopa, guanethidine, digitalis, beta blockers, and calcium channel blockers may slow the sinus rate.

Symptoms from sinus bradycardia generally do not occur unless the rate is very slow or the rhythm appears in the presence of cardiac disease. Generally this rhythm disturbance requires no therapy; however, if the rate is markedly low, creating a reduction in cardiac output, sympathomimetic drugs such as atropine, isoproterenol, or epinephrine may be administered. If the rhythm fails to respond to drug treatment, pacemaker therapy may be needed.

Sinus Tachycardia. A sinus rhythm with a rate in excess of 100 beats per minute is characteristic of *sinus tachycardia*. Rates between 101 and 160 beats per minute are usual, but rates up to 180 beats per minute may be found in young adults during exercise. All other criteria for normal sinus rhythm are present (Figure 10-21). However, with the increase in rate may come other electrocardiographic changes, such as ST segment or T wave alterations and prominent or inverted U waves. The PR interval may be short-

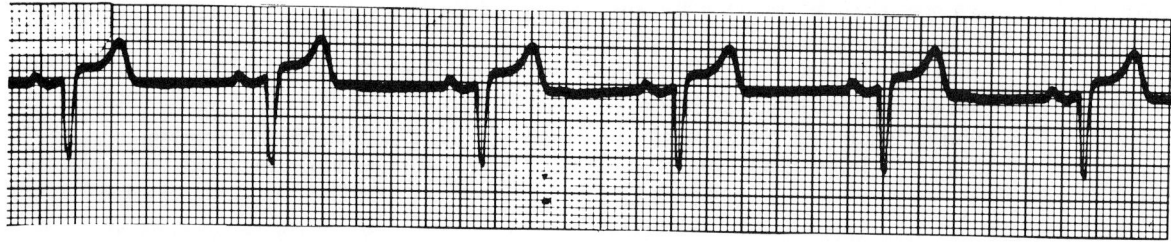

Figure 10-20   Sinus bradycardia. This rhythm strip was recorded from lead MCL₁. The heart rate is 52 beats per minute. The PR, the QRS, and the QT intervals are normal. The configuration of the QRS complex, the 1- to 2-mm ST segment elevation, and the T wave are normal for this lead.

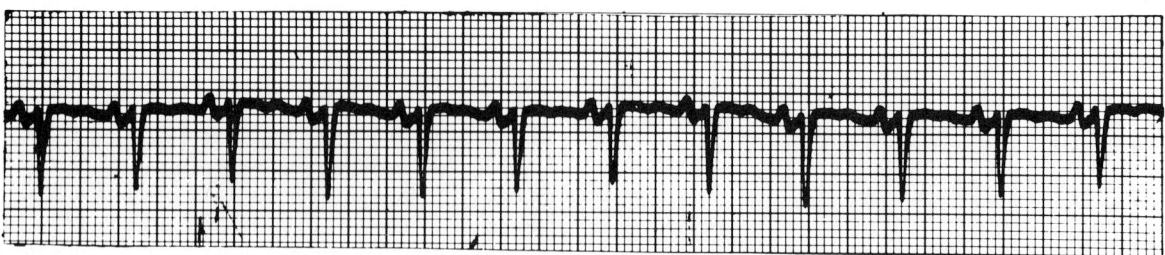

Figure 10-21   Sinus tachycardia. The heart rate of this rhythm strip, recorded from lead MCL₁, is 120 beats per minute. Other measurements are normal for a sinus rhythm.

ened, and the P wave voltage may be increased. Occasionally the PR interval is increased.

Sinus tachycardia is often observed in healthy persons after physical exercise; emotional stress; ingestion of coffee, tea, or alcohol; or smoking a cigarette. The rhythm may result from administration of sympathomimetic agents such as epinephrine and isoproterenol, or parasympatholytic agents such as atropine. Individuals with congestive heart failure, shock, acute rheumatic fever, pulmonary embolism, acute myocardial infarction, malignancy, or chronic lung diseases may exhibit an associated sinus tachycardia. It is also likely to be noted in individuals with an elevated temperature. The clinical significance of sinus tachycardia relates to the underlying cause of the rhythm.

This dysrhythmia generally does not produce symptoms. However, some individuals may complain of palpitations, restlessness, and anxiety while the rhythm is occurring, particularly if it is very rapid and persists for a long time. A functional systolic murmur may be heard at either the base or apex of the heart during a rapid sinus tachycardia when the rhythm is associated with a high cardiac output state.

Treatment for sinus tachycardia is generally aimed at the underlying disease. Of course, the patient's hemodynamic status should be monitored to detect early signs of cardiac output deficits secondary to the tachycardia. In healthy individuals the rhythm generally returns to normal without therapy once the causative factor is eliminated.

Sinus Arrhythmia. When the PP (or RR) cycles of a sinus rhythm vary by 0.16 second or more, the disturbance is identified as *sinus arrhythmia* (Figure 10-22). As with sinus bradycardia and sinus tachycardia, all other features of the rhythm usually meet the criteria for a normal sinus rhythm, although frequently the rate may be less than 60 beats per minute.

Sinus arrhythmia is produced by variations in vagal tone during the respiratory cycle. If the sinus rate slows to an extent that causes it to be equal to or less than the intrinsic rate of the AV junction, the junctional pacemaker may assume control of the ventri-

cles, resulting in AV dissociation. Sinus arrhythmia needs to be distinguished from sinus arrest; SA block; AV block, particularly 1° AV block; atrial premature complexes; and atrial flutter or fibrillation with a high degree of AV block.

Healthy children, young adults, and elderly individuals commonly exhibit respiratory sinus arrhythmia. Sinus arrhythmia may be observed in patients with increased intracranial pressure from a variety of causes. Digitalis, morphine, and factors that increase parasympathetic tone may also exaggerate sinus arrhythmia.

No treatment for respiratory sinus arrhythmia is indicated unless the rhythm is particularly slow and producing symptoms. Atropine may be given under these circumstances to increase the heart rate.

Wandering Atrial Pacemaker. A variant of sinus arrhythmia in which the pacemaker shifts from site to site within the sinus node or nearby atrial cells is known as *wandering atrial pacemaker*. This rhythm rarely exists in the absence of an associated sinus arrhythmia and can be recognized on the ECG when the P wave varies in configuration from beat to beat, the PR interval is within normal limits and relatively constant, and the PP cycle is slightly irregular. The rate is usually between 45 and 100 beats per minute. It is important to note that the configuration of the P wave may vary slightly or markedly but remains positive in lead II and inverted in aVR. It generally varies in shape when wandering sinus pacemaker coexists with sinus arrhythmia.

Wandering atrial pacemaker may be found in healthy individuals, especially when sinus arrhythmia and sinus bradycardia exist simultaneously. The rhythm may be induced by digitalis. If wandering sinus pacemaker occurs spontaneously and persists, it may be an early indication of sick sinus syndrome.

Sinus Arrest. When impulse formation within the sinus node fails entirely, the node is said to *arrest* (Figure 10-23). The electrocardiographic consequence is the absence of the usual initiating P wave, QRS complex, and T wave. Since it produces a pause in the rhythm, sinus arrest is also known as *sinus*

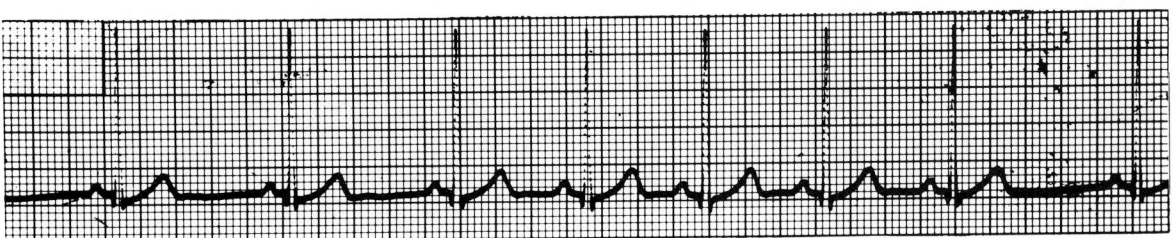

Figure 10-22 Sinus arrhythmia. The rhythm is irregular, but all other criteria are normal for a sinus rhythm. A longer strip would demonstrate the cyclic nature of the irregular rhythm. The strip was recorded from lead II.

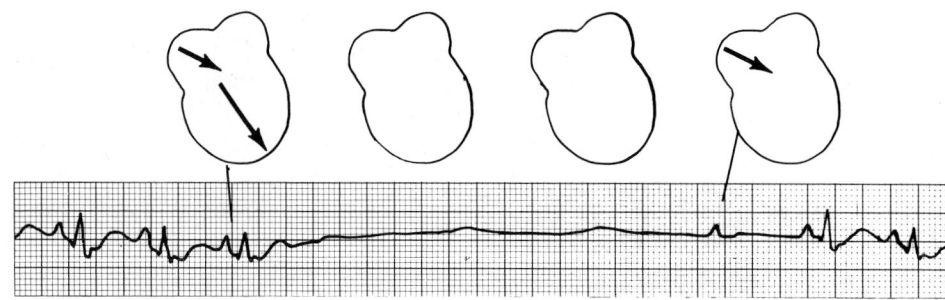

Figure 10-23 Sinus arrest, or sinus pause. During the long pause without sinus P waves, there is also an absence of a junctional escape beat.
From Conover, M. B. (1992). *Understanding electrocardiography* (6th ed.). St. Louis: Mosby—Year Book.

pause or *sinus standstill* when prolonged pauses occur without an escape mechanism.

When sinus arrest occurs, the subsidiary pacemaker sites within the AV junction or ventricles may initiate ventricular electrical activity. Commonly, an AV junctional escape rhythm appears because of its faster inherent rate of automaticity, but occasionally an idioventricular escape rhythm must assume control. Obviously, if both alternate pacemaker sites fail to take over the pacing responsibility during a prolonged sinus arrest, cardiac standstill will result.

Sinus arrest is differentiated from sinoatrial block when the pause is *not* an exact multiple of the basic cycle length. With sinus arrest the PP cycle length of the pause bears no relationship to the normal PP cycle; however, in sinoatrial block the PP cycle length for the pause is an exact multiple of the basic PP cycle or exhibits a regular irregularity. Sinus arrest must also be distinguished from marked sinus arrhythmia, second- or third-degree AV block, and nonconducted premature atrial complexes.

Normal individuals with increased vagal tone or a hypersensitive carotid sinus may experience sinus arrest. Generally the rhythm is associated with a marked sinus arrhythmia, but it may also occur without sinus arrhythmia as a result of quinidine or digitalis overdose or on a reflex basis. Other causes of sinus arrest include acute myocarditis, acute myocardial infarction with sinus node involvement, and administration of parasympathetic agents or potassium. Carotid sinus stimulation of the patient with digitalis intoxication also may result in sinus arrest. Frequent occurrence of sinus arrest with long duration is commonly caused by advanced sick sinus syndrome.

The underlying cause and cardiac status greatly influence the treatment of sinus arrest. The rhythm may be treated successfully by removing the etiological factor. If the patient is asymptomatic and the heart rate is greater than 45 beats per minute, therapy may not be warranted. However, if the patient is symptomatic, atropine bolus, isoproterenol infusion,

an artificial pacemaker, cardiopulmonary resuscitation, or some combination of these measures may be required.

Sinoatrial (SA) Block. Interference with sinus impulse conduction at the sinoatrial junction is generally thought to be the mechanism resulting in SA block. Some authors refer to SA block in three degrees, similarly to those of AV block. However, most clinicians agree that the surface ECG only permits differentiation between second-degree block (Mobitz type I and Mobitz type II) since the ECG does not record sinus node activity. Consequently, actual sinoatrial conduction time is not known. *Second-degree SA block* can be classified as *Mobitz type I* or *Mobitz type II*.

SA block should be distinguished from true SA arrest, in which there is no mathematical predictability to the recovery of sinus node activity, and sinus arrhythmia, in which the respiration causes a recognized variation in the PP interval. Mobitz type II SA block (Figure 10-24) is recognized on the ECG when there is an occasional absence of one or more complete electrical cycles (including P, QRS, and T waves) and when the PP cycle of the SA block is exactly or almost exactly a multiple of the basic PP cycle. In other words, the PP interval including the SA block is frequently three or four times the basic PP interval. If a 2:1 SA block occurs consecutively, it may be misdiagnosed as slow sinus bradycardia. If it occurs repeatedly for three, four, or more impulses, it is likely to be labeled sinus arrest even though the problem was not in SA node initiation but in transmission through the SA junction. Note that cardiac standstill results for that period of time unless a subsidiary pacemaker activates the atria and ventricles.

In Mobitz type I SA block (Figure 10-25), the long PP interval of the block is *not* a multiple of the basic PP cycle. This rhythm can be diagnosed only when the Wenckebach pattern of the block can be identifed. In this instance the PP intervals prior to the long pause become progressively shorter until an entire cycle is dropped. As with Mobitz type II SA block, the AV

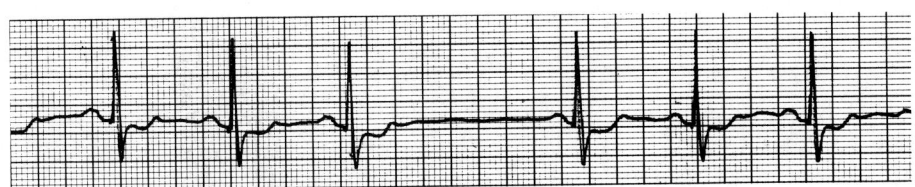

Figure 10-24   Type II SA block. The PP interval spanning the pause is twice that of the sinus cycle.

From Conover, M. B. (1992). *Understanding electrocardiography* (6th ed.). St. Louis: Mosby–Year Book.

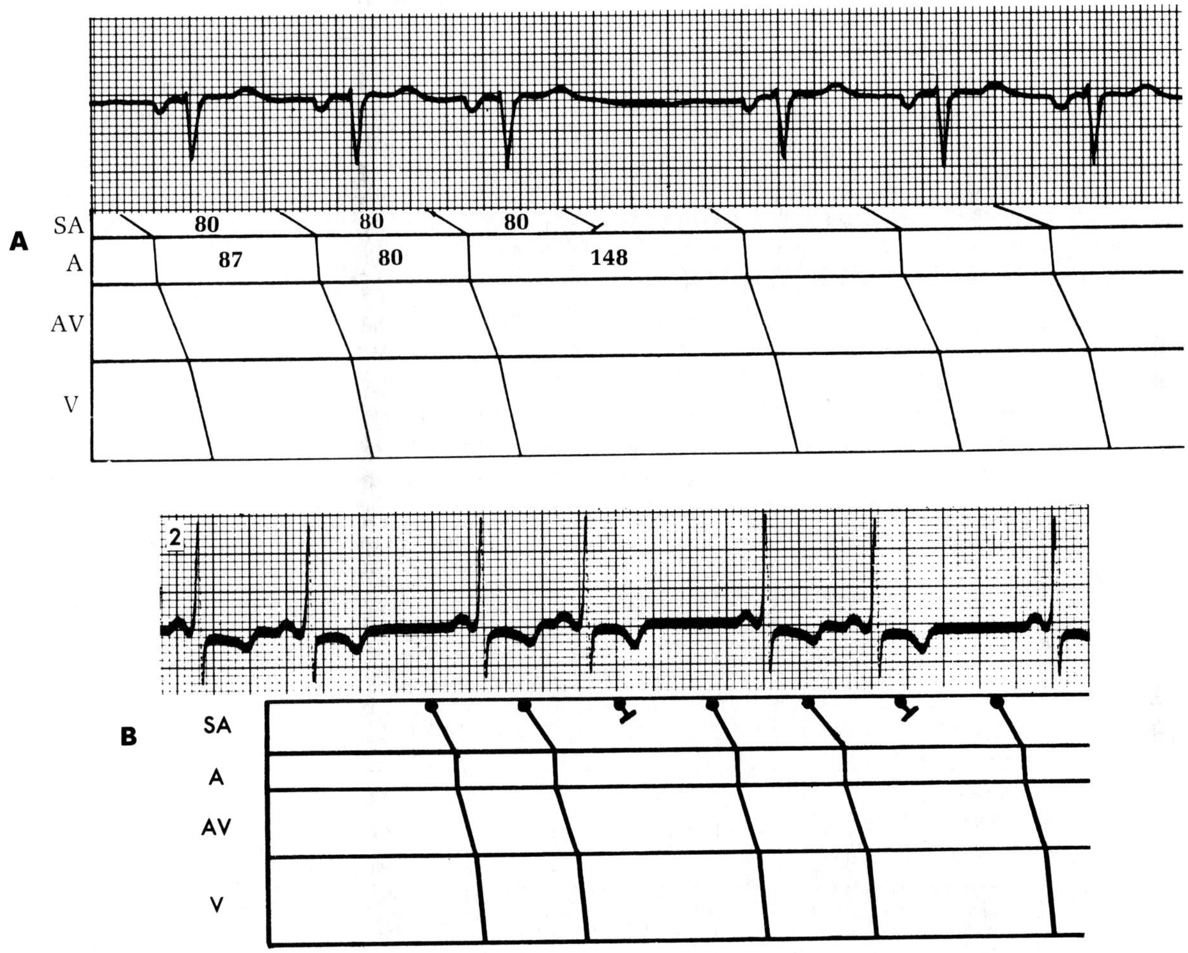

Figure 10-25   *A,* Type I SA block (or SA Wenckebach) with 4:3 group beating, dropped P waves, and shortening PP intervals prior to the pause. *B,* Type I SA block with 2:1 conduction; note the group beating and dropped P waves.

From Conover, M. B. (1992). *Understanding electrocardiography* (6th ed.). St. Louis: Mosby–Year Book.

junction may escape for one or more impulses to control the ventricles.

SA block is usually a transient rhythm but may continue for a long time. Like sinus arrest, it may be found in healthy individuals with increased vagal tone or a hypersensitive carotid sinus, as well as in individuals experiencing myocarditis or acute inferior wall myocardial infarction. Quinidine or digitalis toxicity and hyperkalemia may induce SA block. If the rhythm is not drug induced and if it occurs frequently,

sick sinus syndrome may be implicated.

Generally a transient SA block produces no symptoms and requires no treatment. However, when the block persists and no subsidiary pacemaker escapes to control the ventricles, or if an escape rhythm produces a particularly slow ventricular rhythm, the patient may experience dizziness or perhaps fainting episodes. Therapy in these instances depends on the underlying cause and the underlying cardiac status. Therapeutic methods are those used for sinus arrest.

Sick Sinus Syndrome. Sick sinus syndrome is manifested by a variety of disturbances in sinus impulse formation and conduction. The ECG of sick sinus syndrome may exhibit marked sinus bradycardia, sinus arrest, and SA block. Episodes of atrial tachyarrhythmias may alternate with episodes of bradyarrhythmias resulting in a brady–tachyarrhythmia syndrome, a common manifestation of sick sinus syndrome. These ECG findings are *not* drug induced.

Clinical significance and treatment of sick sinus syndrome depend on the severity of the sinus node dysfunction. Unless the sinus node dysfunction is a temporary phenomenon, permanent pacemaker therapy (along with antiarrhythmic drug therapy if needed) is usually required.

Atrial Dysrhythmias

Rhythm disturbances of atrial origin may be initiated from any site within the atria other than the SA node. Atrial dysrhythmias are almost always produced by active impulse formation and, therefore, almost always appear as some form of an atrial tachyarrhythmia. The rhythm disturbances of atrial premature complex, atrial tachycardia, multifocal atrial tachycardia, atrial flutter, and atrial fibrillation is discussed in this section.

Atrial Premature Complex. Premature impulse formation from within the atria but outside the SA node results in what is known as *atrial premature complex (APC)*. The most obvious feature is the premature occurrence of the complex (Figure 10-26). Other ECG findings include: (1) a P wave configuration unique to the site of origin which differs from the P wave of the sinus complexes; (2) PR intervals of variable duration but frequently within the normal range; however, they may be abnormally short or abnormally long; (3) a postectopic pause which is usually not fully compensatory (the interval between the normal complex preceding the premature complex and the normal complex after the APC is not two times the normal PP cycle); and (4) the interval

from the ectopic P to the preceding P wave of the basic rhythm (coupling interval) is usually constant. The QRS following the premature P wave is somewhat dependent on the degree of prematurity of the extrasystole and may be normal in shape because of normal ventricular conduction, abnormal in shape because of aberrant ventricular conduction, or absent (termed *nonconducted APC)* owing to the refractory state of the ventricular myocardium (Figure 10-27). APCs may occur as a single event or they may occur more frequently. If they alternate with the basic cycle the rhythm is identifed as *atrial bigeminy.* They also may occur every third complex *(atrial trigeminy)* or every fourth complex *(atrial quadrageminy).* If six or more occur consecutively the rhythm disturbance is labeled *atrial tachycardia.*

The arrhythmogenic mechanism of atrial premature complexes is likely to be either reentrant or enhanced focal excitability. This rhythm disturbance is often observed in healthy individuals without organic heart disease. In these people it may be related to emotional stress, physical or mental fatigue, excessive smoking, or ingestion of coffee or alcohol. Atrial premature complexes are more frequent, however, in people with heart disease, particularly those with atrial disease or atrial enlargement due to mitral stenosis or cor pulmonale. They often lead to atrial flutter or fibrillation.

Infrequent APCs are generally clinically insignificant. However, when they are more frequent, occurring every sixth complex or more often, they may cause the individual to experience palpitations and require treatment. Quinidine may be the drug of choice; however, other oral antiarrhythmic agents may be prescribed.

Atrial Tachycardia. Atrial tachycardia (AT) is generally defined as six or more consecutive atrial extrasystoles (Figure 10-28); however, some may consider atrial tachycardia to be present when as few as three consecutive APCs occur. As with other atrial dysrhythmias, this rhythm disturbance originates

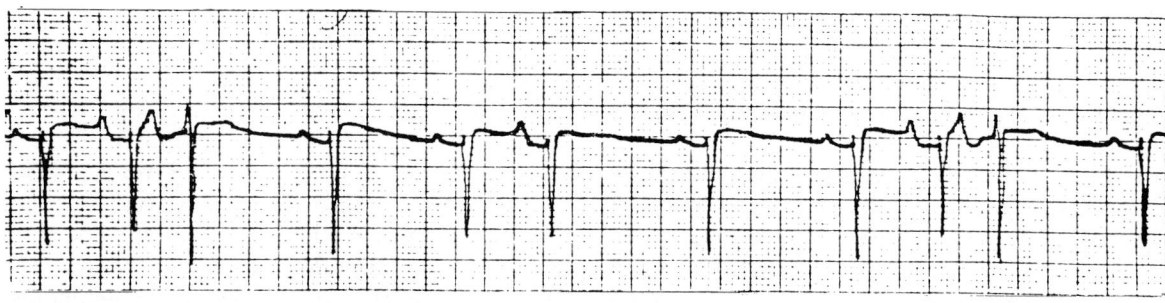

Figure 10-26   Atrial premature complexes. The second, third, sixth, ninth, and tenth P waves are premature. The third and tenth QRS complexes are slightly aberrant.

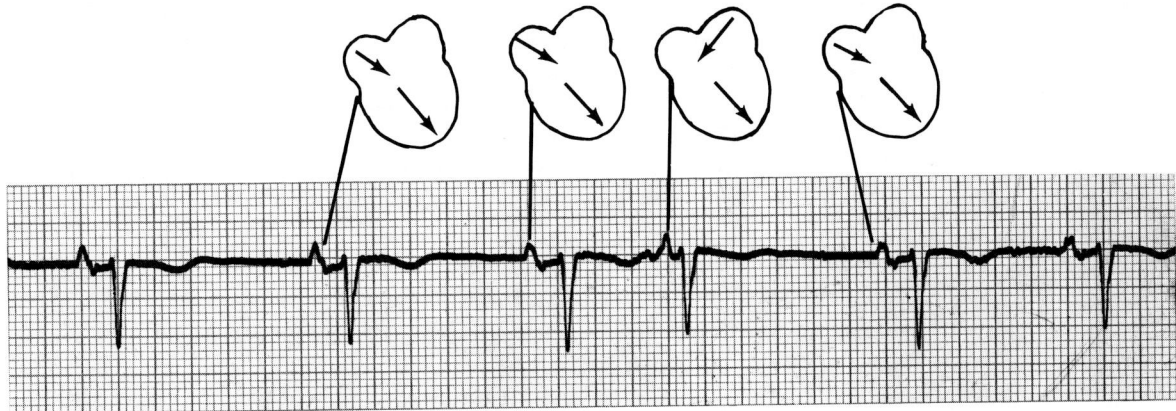

Figure 10-27   The fourth P wave initiates a premature atrial complex, conducted normally in the ventricles.
From Conover, M. B. (1992). *Understanding electrocardiography* (6th ed.). St. Louis: Mosby–Year Book.

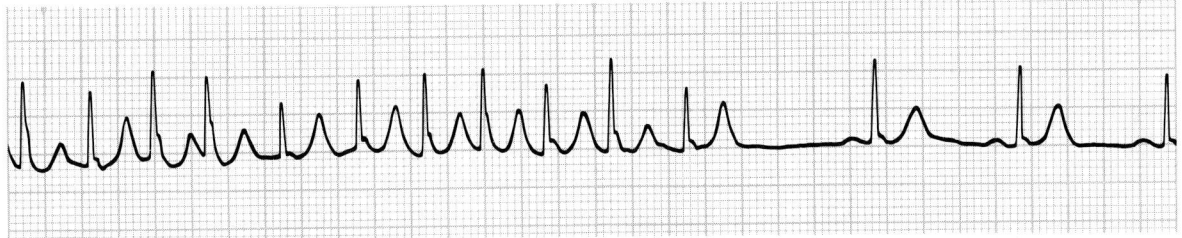

Figure 10-28   Paroxysmal atrial tachycardia at 187 per minute.
From Huszar, R. J. (1988). *Basic dysrhythmias.* St. Louis: Mosby–Year Book.

within the atria but outside the SA node. The entire atria, including the SA node, are activated by the ectopic rhythm. Consequently, the pacemaker ability of the SA node is suppressed for the duration of the rhythm. When the episode of atrial tachycardia terminates, it is often followed by a pause until sinus node function is restored.

The configuration of the ectopic P waves varies according to the site of origin, but ectopic P waves have a common morphology and are generally upright in lead II and inverted in aVR. The P waves may be hard to see but are probably superimposed on the preceding QRS complex, ST segment, T wave, or U wave. The atrial rate is usually between 160 and 250 beats per minute but may be as low as 120 beats per minute. The ventricular rate is usually equal to the atrial rate when the atrial rate is less than 200 beats per minute. However, the faster the atrial rate is, the more likely the AV junction will be physiologically refractory, allowing some of the impulses to conduct to the ventricles. With 2:1 conduction the ventricular rate will be half the atrial rate. Although the PR interval is usually within normal limits in uncomplicated atrial tachycardia, it is not commonly measured in clinical practice.

In the paroxysmal form, atrial tachycardia is usually initiated by a single APC and ends abruptly. As noted previously, when the tachycardia ends it is followed by a pause longer than the basic PP cycle, as the pacing function resumes in the sinus node. This rhythm often becomes chronic in diseased hearts.

Precisely regular PP and RR cycles are common during atrial tachycardia, but these cycles may be irregular. The configuration of the QRS complex, as with APCs, may be wide and bizarre due to abnormal conduction. This is particularly true in very rapid rates due to the partially refractory state of the ventricular conduction system. In these instances, and particularly when the P wave cannot be seen, atrial tachycardia may resemble ventricular tachycardia. Care in the diagnosis of this rhythm is therefore very important. (See Aberrant Ventricular Conduction versus Ventricular Ectopy on p. 253.)

The arrhythmogenic mechanisms of atrial tachycardia include afterdepolarizations causing triggered activity, altered automaticity or reentry. The rhythm can occur in healthy individuals and in those with heart disease. Rheumatic and coronary heart disease, particularly acute myocardial infarction, are often associated with atrial tachycardia. This rhythm disturbance may also be the result of digitalis intoxication.

Symptoms during atrial tachycardia are dependent on the disease state of the individual and the ventricular rate of the rhythm. Healthy people can tolerate paroxysmal atrial tachycardia for long periods if the rate is no greater than 180 beats per minute. In diseased hearts, though, even slow ventricular rates may cause or aggravate congestive heart failure or angina pectoris. Symptoms produced by atrial tachycardia include palpitations, chest pain, weakness, dizziness, anxiety, apprehension, and feelings of impending doom.

Medical management of atrial tachycardia may include withdrawal of the etiological factor when possible; Class IA, II, III, or IV antidysrhythmic agents (see Appendix); digitalis, if it is not the cause of the rhythm disturbance; carotid sinus stimulation; overdrive pacing; or direct current (DC) shock. Sedation in conjunction with other therapeutic measures may be beneficial.

Multifocal Atrial Tachycardia. Atrial tachycardia with variable P wave morphology and irregular ectopic PP cycles, a rate between 100 and 250 beats per minute, and varying PR intervals is identified as *multifocal atrial tachycardia (MAT)* (Figure 10-29). Other terms used to describe this electrocardiographic pattern are *chaotic atrial tachycardia, repetitive multifocal paroxysmal atrial tachycardia,* and *wandering atrial pacemaker.*

Multifocal atrial tachycardia differs from unifocal atrial tachycardia in that it does not usually appear in paroxysmal form and frequently produces a slower atrial and ventricular rate. The ventricular rate may

be as slow as 50 to 60 beats per minute but usually exceeds 100 beats per minute. This rhythm disorder may be mistaken for sinus arrhythmia, wandering atrial pacemaker, atrial flutter, or atrial fibrillation. When the multifocal P waves conduct through the ventricles in an aberrant fashion, the rhythm may be misidentified as ventricular tachycardia or ventricular fibrillation.

This rhythm disturbance is usually seen in seriously ill elderly patients with acute and chronic lung disease. It is also seen frequently in patients who have hypertensive or valvular heart disease. Digitalis intoxication may or may not be associated with MAT but probably is not a cause of the dysrhythmia. Infrequently, MAT may be identified in individuals with electrolyte imbalance, particularly hypokalemia. The mechanism of this rhythm disturbance is probably enhanced automaticity.

Antidysrhythmic drug therapy is not generally useful in treating MAT. It is usually more beneficial to treat the dysrhythmia by treating the underlying disease process.

Atrial Flutter. Rapid regular atrial deflections (F waves) that characteristically have a sawtooth appearance are the electrocardiographic hallmark of *atrial flutter* (Figure 10-30). Other features are (1) an atrial rate that is usually between 250 and 350 beats per minute; (2) a variable rate and rhythm of ventricular depolarization, depending on the atrial rate and the status of AV conduction; and (3) a QRS configuration that may be either normal or abnormal, depending on the conduction status of the bundle branches.

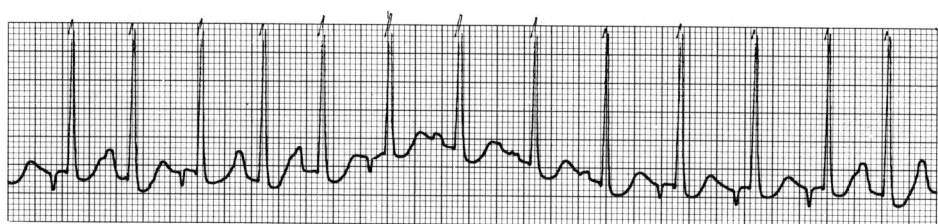

Figure 10-29   Multifocal or chaotic atrial tachycardia with at least five different P waves.
From Conover, M. B. (1992). *Understanding electrocardiography* (6th ed.). St. Louis: Mosby–Year Book.

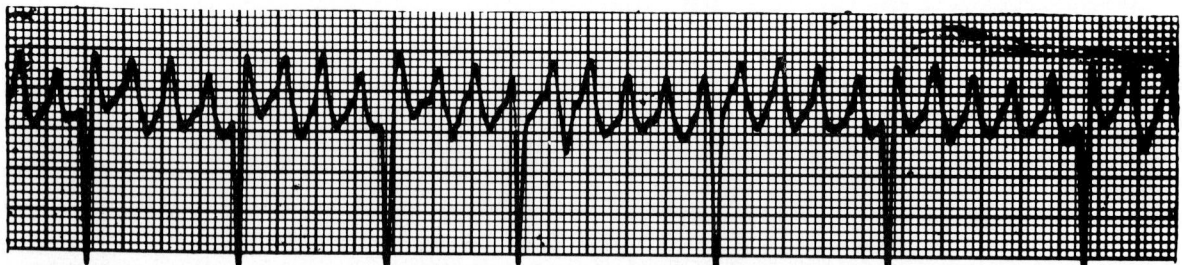

Figure 10-30   Atrial flutter. The AV conduction is variable. Note the sawtooth appearance of the "F waves."

One group of researchers[3] has identified two types of atrial flutter, which are categorized by the atrial rate. Type I has a rate of 240 to 338 beats per minute, and type II has a rate of 340 to 433 beats per minute. In the clinical setting an atrial electrogram is used to assist with the identification of these two types. The clinical significance of the two types seems to rest with their response to rapid atrial pacing. Type I can be influenced by rapid atrial pacing from the high right atrium, but type II cannot.

The arrhythmogenic mechanism of atrial flutter is unclear. However, four theories continue to be considered and tested. The theories include circus movement, multiple reentry phenomenon, unifocal impulse formation, and multifocal impulse formation. Atrial flutter may occur transiently and intermittently or it may persist in a chronic form for months and years.

This dysrhythmia is less common than atrial fibrillation and atrial tachycardia and is seen most often in elderly patients with organic heart disease. Common etiologies include coronary artery disease; rheumatic heart disease, particularly mitral stenosis; and hypertensive heart disease. Less commonly, atrial flutter is associated with thyrotoxicosis, cardiomyopathy, acute and chronic cor pulmonale, pulmonary diseases, and pericarditis. Digitalis intoxication is rarely a cause of the dysrhythmia. Infrequently, atrial flutter is identified in healthy individuals without heart disease.

Signs and symptoms of atrial flutter are dependent on a variety of factors but particularly on the nature of the underlying heart disease, the ventricular rate, and the dysrhythmia duration. With rapid ventricular rates and in elderly individuals with advanced cardiac disease, congestive heart failure (CHF) is likely to occur. Patients may experience palpitations, chest pain, and symptoms of reduced cardiac output including increased fatigability, shortness of breath, and mental confusion. Pulmonary and systemic thromboemboli secondary to atrial stasis are likely in chronic atrial flutter, especially after conversion to sinus rhythm.

Transient forms of atrial flutter generally require no treatment. Acute and chronic forms resulting in symptoms may be treated with antiarrhythmic drug therapy, rapid atrial pacing, and/or DC shock. The therapy selected depends on the clinical situation and the urgency for elimination of the rhythm.

Atrial Fibrillation. The mechanism responsible for the creation of *atrial fibrillation* is controversial but is theorized to be one of the four mechanisms mentioned in the discussion of atrial flutter. The ECG findings include atrial activity represented by fibrillatory (f) waves which replace the P wave and ventricular activity which is totally irregular (Figure 10-31). Note that in the presence of AV block, though, the ventricular rhythm may be regular. The f waves cause the baseline to oscillate randomly. The QRS configuration may be altered by (1) the superimposed f waves on a portion of the QRS complex, (2) aberrant conduction secondary to varying refractoriness of the bundle branches, or (3) ventricular preexcitation.

The atrial rate in atrial fibrillation cannot be determined. The ventricular rate is generally quite rapid, between 120 and 200 beats per minute in untreated cases of atrial fibrillation. Slower rates are possible when preceding digitalization has occurred or there is a coexisting AV conduction abnormality. Complete AV block is suggested when there is a regular junctional or ventricular escape rhythm.

Wells and associates[4] identified four types of atrial fibrillation in postoperative cardiac surgery patients. Recording of bipolar epicardial atrial electrograms (AEG) revealed atrial fibrillatory waves of varying sizes, shapes, polarities, amplitudes, and beat-to-beat intervals. Type I was characterized by discrete AEG complexes separated by an isoelectric baseline free of disturbance. Type II had discrete AEG complexes but with perturbations of the baseline between complexes. AEGs that failed to demonstrate either discrete complexes or isoelectric intervals were identified as type III. Type IV atrial fibrillation was characterized on the AEG by alternating periods of type I and type II patterns. The ability to distinguish between the

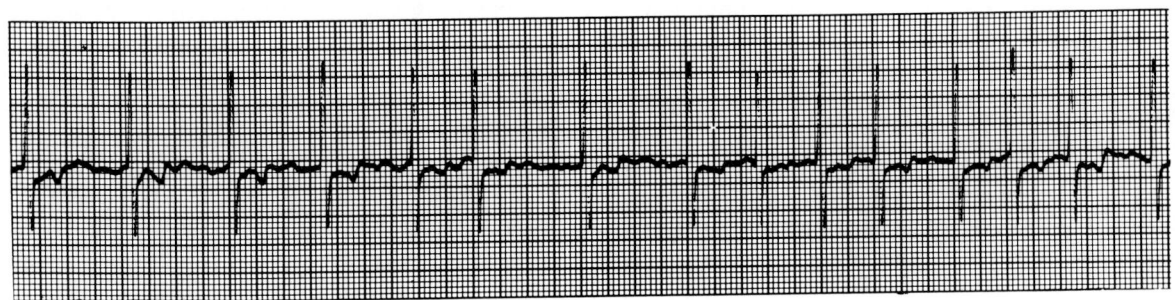

Figure 10-31 Atrial fibrillation.

types of atrial fibrillation may lead to more effective treatment of the dysrhythmia.

Atrial fibrillation is very common, occurring frequently in association with CHF and accessory pathway syndromes such as Wolff-Parkinson-White syndrome. Like atrial flutter, atrial fibrillation is often due to rheumatic, coronary, and hypertensive heart diseases or hyperthyroidism.

Less common causes of atrial fibrillation include cardiomyopathy, acute myocarditis, acute pericarditis, and chest trauma. It is rarely observed in digitalis intoxication. Healthy individuals may exhibit atrial fibrillation as a result of heavy smoking; excessive ingestion of alcohol, coffee, or tea; and sudden emotional excitement.

Symptoms resulting from atrial fibrillation vary with the presence or absence and nature of the heart disease, the presence or absence and degree of CHF, the ventricular rate, and the duration of the rhythm. Patients with transient atrial fibrillation may be symptom-free. Those with CHF may have mild symptoms of palpitations, anxiety, a fluttering or pounding feeling, and the sensation of skipped heart beats, or they may experience more severe symptoms including worsening CHF, syncope, angina, and a feeling of impending death.

Although the treatment of choice for acute onset atrial fibrillation with rapid ventricular rates, either in the presence or absence of CHF, is digitalis, it is most effective when significant CHF exists. However, intravenous diltiazem may offer more consistent control of the ventricular rate in the first several hours. Other methods for treating atrial fibrillation include antiarrhythmic agents and DC shock. Removal of precipitating factors such as alcohol or excessive thyroid is also important.

AV Junctional Dysrhythmias

Cardiac rhythms initiated in the AV junction are identified as *AV junctional dysrhythmias*. The actual site of the pacemaker is difficult to locate from the surface ECG but may be from low atrial foci, the coronary sinus ostium, the bundle of His, the node–His (N–H) region of the AV node, or possibly the atrionodal (AN) region of the AV node. Impulse formation does not originate in the nodal (N) region of the AV node. Rhythm disturbances may be initiated as an escape mechanism secondary to depressed SA node function, SA block, or AV block or occur due to enhanced automaticity of the AV junctional pacemaker. In the first case (escape mechanisms), the heart rate is often between 40 and 60 beats per minute, and in the latter (enhanced automaticity), rates are usually faster than 60 beats per minute.

The electrocardiographic features of all AV junctional dysrhythmias are similar, differing only in the time of onset in the cardiac cycle. Because the atria must be stimulated in retrograde fashion, the junctional P wave (when present) is inverted in leads II, III, and aVF, and upright in aVR. It is also upright in leads I and V_6. The P wave may occur just prior to the QRS, indicating that the atria depolarized before the ventricles; or after the QRS, indicating initial ventricular depolarization which is followed by atrial depolarization. More often the junctional P wave is superimposed on the QRS as the atria and ventricles depolarize simultaneously and, therefore, is not visible on the ECG. If the junctional pacemaker is blocked from conducting antegrade to the ventricles, the P wave will appear without a QRS complex. If it is blocked from conducting retrograde to the atria, no ectopic P waves will appear. The contour of the junctional P wave is generally abnormal.

The PR interval (or RP interval) for AV junctional complexes varies according to the location of the ectopic focus within the junction and the speed of antegrade and retrograde conduction. Generally the PR interval is equal to or less than 0.12 second and the RP intervals are between 0.10 and 0.20 second. The QRS configuration of AV junctional complexes, either escape beats or extrasystoles, is often normal but it may be wide and bizarre due to either aberrant or preexisting ventricular conduction abnormalities.

AV Junctional Escape Beats (Rhythm). An *AV junctional beat* or *rhythm* occurs as a physiologically passive escape mechanism when the SA node fails to function or is blocked from stimulating the AV junction or ventricles. The junction may escape for a single beat or for a series of consecutive beats, often a transitory event. Six or more consecutive junctional escape beats constitute an AV junctional rhythm (Figure 10-32).

The rate of impulse formation for AV junctional escape rhythm ranges commonly from 40 to 60 beats per minute but may be lower. The RR intervals are almost always regular and seldom vary by more than 0.04 second. The P wave configuration varies, depending on the activation site for the atria. If the sinus node activates the atria, the P wave will be normal in appearance but will not be associated with ventricular activation (AV dissociation). If both the sinus node and the AV junction activate the atria, atrial fusion beats result and the P configuration varies with the degree of fusion between the two impulses. When the atria are activated by retrograde conduction from the AV junction, the P wave is inverted in leads II, III, and aVF, and upright in lead aVR.

The appearance of an occasional AV junctional beat or rhythm is clinically insignificant in healthy individuals or those with diseased hearts if the beat

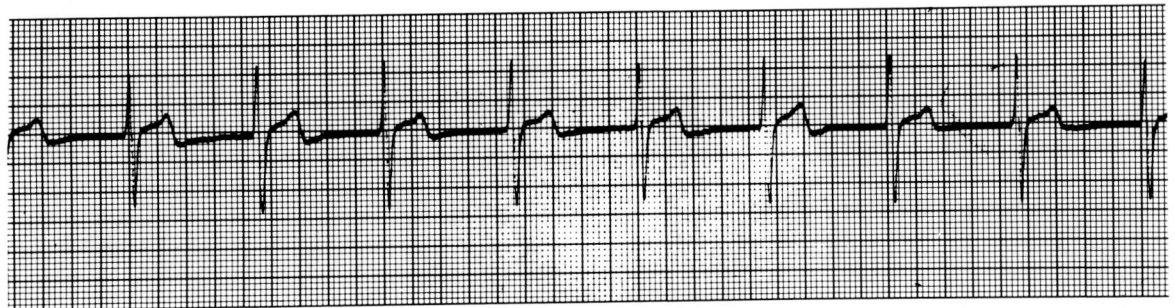

Figure 10-32   AV junctional rhythm. No P waves are evident, indicating that the atria and ventricles are activated simultaneously or that retrograde conduction to the atria is blocked.

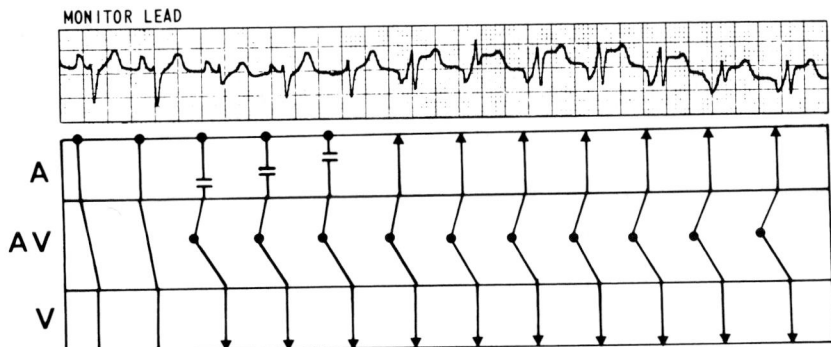

Figure 10-33   Accelerated AV junctional rhythm. After two sinus beats, an AV junctional tachycardia at a rate of 107 beats per minute takes over control of the heart. The third, fourth, and fifth P waves are atrial fusion beats.
From Friedman, H. H. (1985). *Diagnostic electrocardiography and vectorcardiography*. New York: McGraw-Hill.

or rhythm follows a postectopic pause, sinus bradycardia, sinus arrest, or SA block of short duration. An individual is often symptomatic, however, when the escape beat or rhythm occurs secondary to complete AV block, sinus arrest, or SA block of long duration, especially in the presence of serious heart disease or drug intoxication. Symptoms are generally dependent on the ventricular rate. If it is particularly slow, the patient will likely experience dizziness, mental confusion, and Adams-Stokes syndrome due to reduced cerebral blood flow and may experience angina pectoris due to reduced coronary blood flow. Congestive heart failure may develop in patients whose AV junctional rhythm is secondary to complete AV block.

Treatment of AV junctional beats or rhythm is usually unnecessary unless it occurs secondary to complete AV block or is not fast enough to maintain hemodynamics. In these cases a permanent artificial pacemaker may be required.

Accelerated AV Junctional Rhythm.   A junctional rhythm with a rate within the range of sinus rhythm and sinus tachycardia (65 to 130 beats per minute) is identified as *accelerated AV junctional rhythm*. The ECG characteristics of this dysrhythmia are generally those of an escape junctional rhythm except for the more rapid rates (Figure 10-33). As in atrial tachycardia, the QRS complex may be wide and bizarre if there is aberrant ventricular conduction, but aberrancy in this rhythm rarely occurs. It is usually the result of mildly enhanced automaticity of the AV junction. Consequently, the rhythm is not initiated by a premature complex and is without the sudden onset and termination of paroxysmal tachycardia.

Digitalis intoxication, acute myocardial infarction, intracardiac surgery, or myocarditis are the most common causes of accelerated AV junctional rhythm. It is more often associated with inferior than anterior myocardial infarction and is considered a poor prognostic sign when observed in the latter. The underlying rhythm is often chronic atrial fibrillation when the rhythm disturbance is the result of digitalis intoxication.

The key to treatment is to remove the cause when possible. Drugs used to eliminate accelerated AV junctional rhythm include quinidine and propranolol as well as other agents known for their antiarrhythmic effect on supraventricular tachyarrhythmias.

AV Junctional Premature Complex.   The electrocardiographic features of an *AV junctional premature*

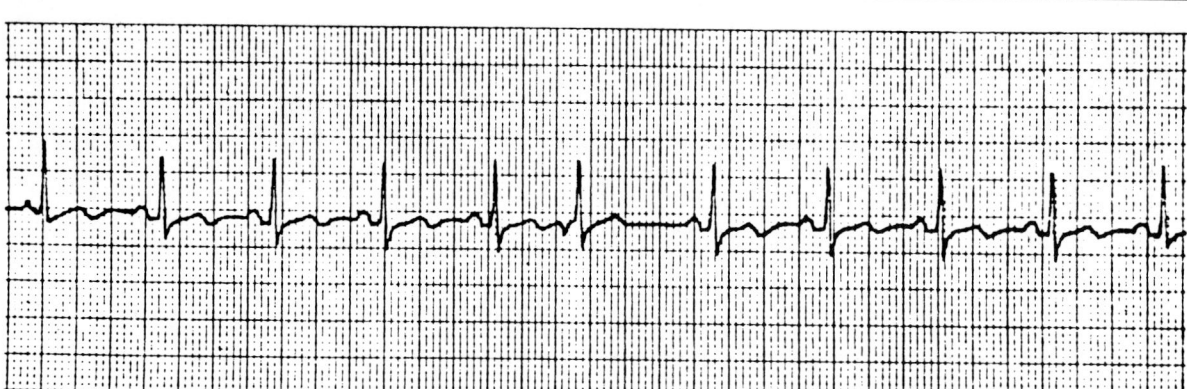

Figure 10-34   Junctional premature complex.

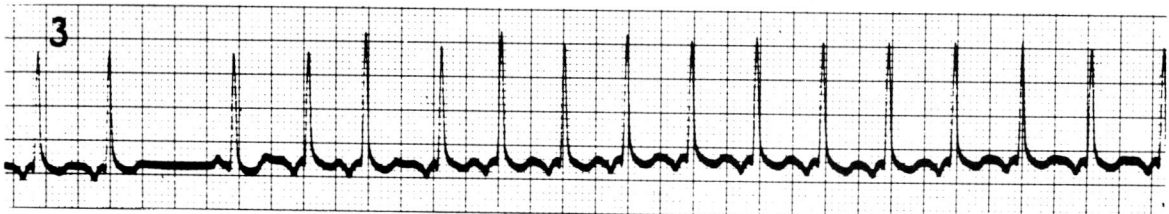

Figure 10-35   Paroxysmal AV junctional tachycardia with initial retrograde atrial activation.
From Lindsay, A. E., & Budkin, A. (1975). *The cardiac arrhythmias* (2nd ed.). Chicago: Year Book.

complex (Figure 10-34) are: (1) a premature complex in relation to the basic cycle, (2) a P wave configuration characteristic of an AV junctional beat, (3) a coupling interval that is usually constant, and (4) a postectopic pause which is usually not fully compensatory. Like atrial premature complexes, junctional premature complexes (JPC) may occur in pairs, or in bigeminal, trigeminal, or quadrageminal frequencies. A JPC must be differentiated on the ECG from APCs and ventricular premature complexes (VPC).

As with other premature complexes, the mechanism responsible for generating a JPC is likely to be either reentry or enhanced focal excitability. Although JPCs are less frequent than atrial and ventricular premature complexes, they may be observed on the ECG of a healthy individual or an individual with heart disease, and they may be induced by digitalis therapy.

Occasional JPCs generally require no treatment. Frequent JPCs or groups of JPCs may necessitate therapy to prevent an AV junctional tachycardia. When JPCs occur secondary to CHF, the use of digitalis may eliminate the dysrhythmia. Obviously, if digitalis is the suspected cause of the rhythm disturbance the drug may need to be discontinued. Other therapies include quinidine, propranolol, and other antiarrhythmic agents used for supraventricular tachyarrhythmias.

Paroxysmal AV Junctional Tachycardia. AV junctional rates ranging from 140 to 250 beats per minute characterize *paroxysmal AV junctional tachycardia* (PJT) (Figure 10-35). This rhythm is usually initiated by a premature complex and has an abrupt onset and termination. There may be a brief, irregular initial "warm-up" period if the mechanism is enhanced automaticity; otherwise the initiating beat and all subsequent RR cycles are regular and morphologically the same. The last complex of the paroxysm is followed by a brief pause until the original rhythm is reestablished. The configuration of the P wave varies, depending on the activation site for the atria, and the appearance is that described earlier in this chapter for AV junctional beats. The QRS may be normal or aberrant depending on the status of the ventricular conduction system.

The mechanism responsible for initiating PJT is either AV nodal reentry or enhanced focal excitability or automaticity. Reentry is the most common mechanism of action. Like PAT, PJT may occur in healthy individuals as well as in those with coronary artery disease, hypertension, rheumatic heart disease, or hyperthyroidism. It may also be associated with digitalis intoxication. Patients may complain of a variety of symptoms including palpitations, chest tightness or pain, weakness, dizziness, anxiety, apprehension, or perhaps a feeling of impending death.

If the rhythm can be terminated by vagal stimulation, the mechanism is most likely a reentrant one. When the mechanism is enhanced excitability or automaticity, vagal stimulation may slow the rate temporarily but the rhythm resumes its previous rate after termination of the stimulation. Treatment regimens for PJT are those used for other supraventricular tachycardias.

Paroxysmal Supraventricular Tachycardia. *Paroxysmal supraventricular tachycardia* (PSVT) is a term used to describe paroxysmal dysrhythmias of atrial and AV junctional origin. In the past, the term has been used in a generic sense to describe narrow QRS tachycardias in which atrial events have not been identifiable by surface ECGs. The mechanism recognized as being responsible for the genesis of PSVT is reentry in association with critically timed ectopic beats or sinus beats. The rhythm may be the result of reentry involving the sinus node, intraatrial cells, the AV node, an accessory pathway, a concealed AV bypass tract, or from enhanced automaticity of an atrial AV junctional focus.[5] Electrophysiology studies (EPS) are often necessary to correctly identify the site of origin of PSVT. Treatment depends on the specific cause, but generally PSVT secondary to sinus and AV nodal reentry can be effectively terminated with vagal stimulation, whereas the other forms cannot.

Ventricular Dysrhythmias

Rhythm disorders involving a pacemaker site in the ventricles are termed *ventricular dysrhythmias*. The mechanism of action generating ventricular rhythm disturbances may be either enhanced automaticity, reentry, or a combination of both. If a higher pacemaker site, the sinus node or AV junction, fails to produce a stimulus, a ventricular escape beat or an idioventricular rhythm must assume the role of pacemaker to prevent cardiac standstill. In contrast, ventricular extrasystoles may occur due to enhanced automaticity or reentry. The ventricular focus may produce a ventricular premature complex, ventricular tachycardia, ventricular flutter, or ventricular fibrillation.

Regardless of the mechanism, ventricular dysrhythmias may originate from any location within the ventricles. If the ectopic focus is in the septum near the His bundle, the QRS may be almost normal and resemble a sinus-initiated complex. However, the lower the pacemaker site within the septum, the wider and more bizarre the complex becomes. Impulses originating from the fascicles of the left bundle branch generally produce a narrow QRS complex with a right bundle branch block (RBBB) pattern (see Ventricular Conduction Abnormalities in this chapter). Sites from the left ventricle produce positive QRS complexes in the right precordial leads and negative complexes in the left precordial leads. The converse is true if the ectopic site is right ventricular; the right precordial leads exhibit generally negative QRS complexes and the left precordial leads exhibit predominantly positive QRS complexes. The QRS duration may be fairly normal but is generally wide, being 0.12 second or more. This reflects the additional time required to depolarize the ventricles through an abnormal conduction pathway.

Idioventricular Escape Beats and Rhythm. If a faster pacemaker site fails to stimulate the ventricles or if the stimulus from those sites is for some reason slower than the inherent rate of a ventricular pacemaker, the ventricles passively assume the role of pacemaker. This control by the ventricular focus may occur for a single *idioventricular beat* or consecutively in groups of beats. When six or more consecutive idioventricular escape beats appear, an *idioventricular escape rhythm* (IVR) exists (Figure 10-36).

The ECG features of either idioventricular escape

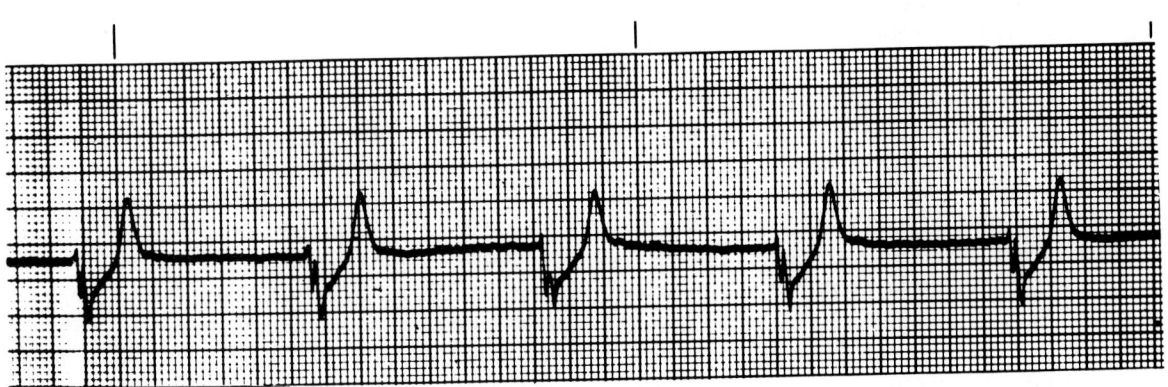

Figure 10-36   Accelerated idioventricular rhythm.
From Conover, M. B. (1992). *Understanding electrocardiography* (6th ed.). St. Louis: Mosby–Year Book.

beats or IVR are a QRS configuration and duration which vary according to the site of the ventricular origin; an irregular RR cycle, although less commonly it may be regular; a slow ventricular rate (usually between 30 and 45 beats per minute or lower); and independent atrial and ventricular activation. In the dying heart atrial activity may be nonexistent (atrial standstill).

The most common underlying rhythm disturbance that allows the ventricular pacemaker to escape is complete AV block. Occasionally, though, this escape mechanism may appear secondary to sinus arrest or SA block when the junctional pacemaker fails to respond.

Therapeutic measures for treating patients with an idioventricular rhythm are often dependent on the nature of the underlying heart disease and the severity of the problem. Frequently, a permanent artificial cardiac pacemaker is necessary to prevent excessive bradycardia.

Ventricular Standstill. When both the junction and ventricle fail to produce a QRS complex for several seconds, the heart is said to be in *ventricular standstill* or *arrest* (Figure 10-37). Ventricular standstill may occur in the presence or absence of atrial activity. It almost always is the consequence of another cardiac dysrhythmia, for example sinus arrest, SA or AV block, ventricular tachycardia, or ventricular fibrillation. It may occur during carotid sinus stimulation when supraventricular tachyarrhythmias are being evaluated. It results from depressed automaticity of the subsidiary pacemaker sites.

The significance of this rhythm disorder rests with its duration and the nature and severity of the underlying cardiac rhythm and heart disease. If the pause is brief such as after an ectopic tachycardia, the standstill is probably insignificant. However, longer pauses can be terminal if an effective cardiac rhythm is not established by cardiopulmonary resuscitation (CPR) and artificial cardiac pacing. Ventricular standstill is most commonly observed in patients with acute myocardial infarction and in those with digitalis intoxication.

Ventricular Premature Complex. The most commonly occurring dysrhythmia is the *ventricular premature complex*. This rhythm disturbance is characterized often by a wide (equal to or greater than 0.12 second) and bizarre QRS complex which is premature. It is rarely preceded by a premature P wave and is almost always followed by a full compensatory pause (Figure 10-38). The premature QRS complex is accompanied by secondary ST and T wave changes; that is, the direction of the ST segment and T wave are opposite to those of the QRS. The VPC may be

followed by a retrograde P wave if the ectopic impulse is able to conduct to the atria. The configuration of the QRS may be uniform (see Figure 10-38) or multiform (Figure 10-39). Multiform VPCs may be initiated from a single focus taking different pathways through the ventricles or from multiple foci within the ventricles. The coupling interval for unifocal VPCs is usually constant but varies when there are VPCs arising from multiple foci. When the coupling interval is very short, the QRS morphology is often more bizarre. If the coupling interval is quite long (termed a late diastolic VPC), a ventricular fusion beat may result. This is due to the fusion of the ventricular premature impulse with the sinus impulse somewhere in the ventricles.

The frequency of VPCs may be described as bigeminal, trigeminal, quadrageminal, or consecutive in pairs or triplets. Varying definitions of VT exist,[5,6,7] but it is defined here as six or more consecutive VPCs. Consecutive VPCs in groups of three, four, or five complexes are termed ventricular *salvos*. Occasionally, a single VPC may occur between two sequential normal beats without disturbing the underlying rhythm. This is identified as an *interpolated* VPC and happens when the sinus rate is slow and the VPC is particularly early.

The mechanism responsible for generating VPCs is generally thought to be either reentry or enhanced focal excitability. Ventricular premature complexes probably occur in all healthy individuals at some time or other. The incidence of VPCs increases with age. Predisposing factors include excessive ingestion of beverages containing caffeine, heavy smoking, and emotional stress. Ventricular premature complexes also occur in the presence of organic heart disease and drug intoxication. Digitalis intoxication should be suspected when ventricular bigeminy occurs during digitalis therapy and most especially when the bigeminy is in the presence of atrial fibrillation with AV junctional escape rhythm or sustained junctional tachycardia. Ventricular premature complexes are also common in patients with mitral valve prolapse syndrome. Frequent VPCs, particularly those early in the cardiac cycle, are common during the first 48 to 72 hours after an acute myocardial infarction. Ventricular premature complexes that are superimposed on the preceding T wave (R on T phenomenon) and group beats may initiate ventricular tachycardia or fibrillation (Figure 10-40). Consequently, the occurrence of VPCs under these circumstances is considered to be potentially lethal and, therefore, warrants early definitive treatment.

Therapy for VPCs is dependent on the cause and severity of the dysrhythmia. The occasional VPC in

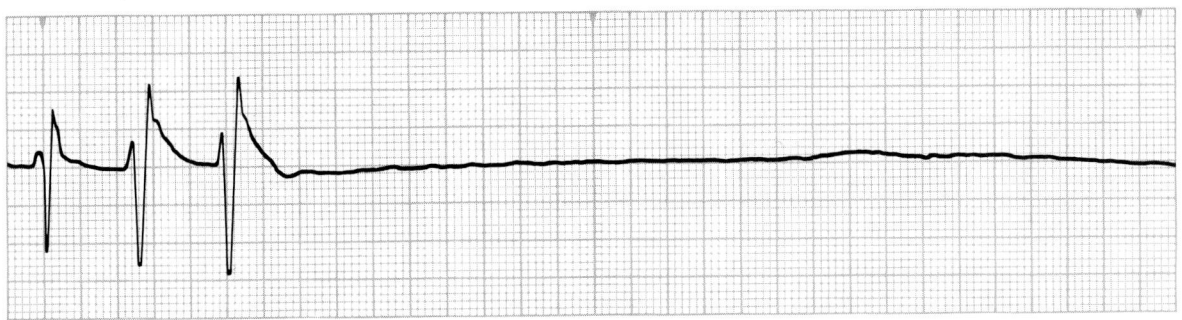

Figure 10-37   Ventricular standstill preceded by three QRS complexes at a rate of 116 per minute.
From Huszar, R. J. (1988). *Basic dysrhythmias.* St Louis: Mosby–Year Book.

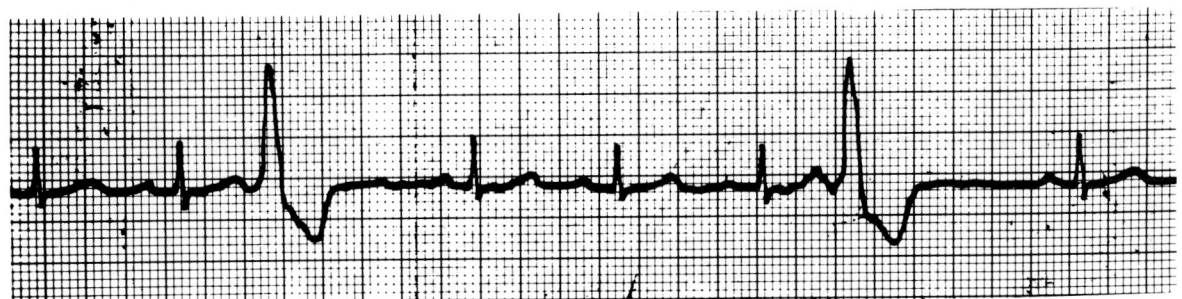

Figure 10-38   Ventricular premature complexes. Note the full compensatory pause after the first PVC.

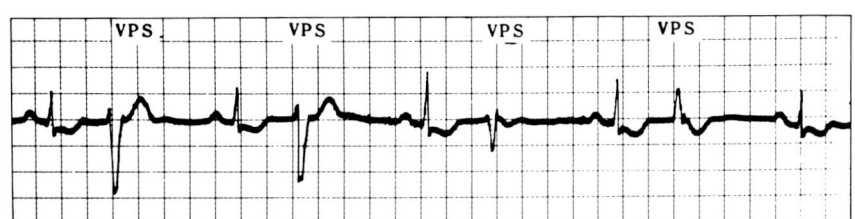

Figure 10-39   Multiform ventricular complexes with bigeminy due to digitalis intoxication.
From Friedman, H. H. (1985). *Diagnostic electrocardiography and vectorcardiography.* New York: McGraw-Hill.

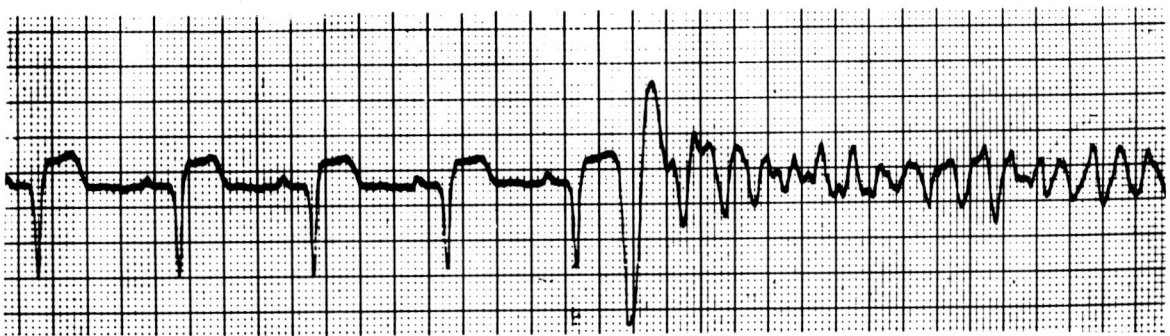

Figure 10-40   Ventricular premature complex on a T wave (R on T) initiating ventricular fibrillation in a patient with an anterior wall myocardial infarction. The rhythm was recorded from lead MCL₁.

the healthy individual is generally not treated. However, the precipitating cause (such as caffeine) should be eliminated if the incidence is frequent. Class IA, B, or C antiarrhythmic agents may be prescribed if the dysrhythmia persists. Frequent (more than six VPCs per minute), multiform, repetitive VPCs or those occurring on or near the preceding T wave in the patient with an acute myocardial infarction should be treated with an intravenous injection of lidocaine followed by a slow continuous infusion of the drug. Digitalis should be withheld immediately if it is suspected to be the cause of the dysrhythmia. Phenytoin and potassium may also be useful in treating digitalis-induced VPCs. A beta-blocker such as propranolol is the therapeutic agent for catecholamine-induced VPCs and in those associated with mitral valve prolapse syndrome.

Accelerated Idioventricular Rhythm (AIVR) (Figure 10-41). One form of ventricular rhythm is known as *accelerated idioventricular rhythm* or *slow ventricular tachycardia.* Using the strict definition for tachycardia in the adult (that is, a heart rate faster than 100 beats per minute), the latter label is a misnomer because the ventricular rate of this rhythm disturbance is between 60 and 100 beats per minute. Since this rate is faster than the usual rate of an idioventricular pacemaker cell, the preferred and less confusing term, is accelerated idioventricular rhythm.

In addition to the rate being in the range for normal sinus rhythm, other ECG criteria for an AIVR include (1) wide and bizarre QRS complexes and T waves occurring in regular rhythm; (2) brief, transient episodes of the rhythm that last only a few seconds or minutes; (3) initiating beats that occur late in diastole and are fused with a sinus conducted beat; and (4) frequent ventricular capture and fusion beats. Frequently, independent atrial rhythm is observed resulting in AV dissociation. Accelerated idioventricular rhythm is often replaced by a sinus rhythm when the sinus rate increases to a speed fast enough to suppress the ventricular pacemaker.

Accelerated idioventricular rhythm must be differentiated from accelerated AV junctional rhythm. These two rhythms may be very similar in appearance if the latter occurs in the presence of a preexisting intraventricular conduction defect. The ventricular capture and fusion beats during AIVR may serve as useful clues in the differentiation process.

An AIVR may occur in patients experiencing either acute inferior or anterior myocardial infarctions. It may also occur after reperfusion of the coronary arteries through the use of thrombolytic agents. Hypertensive, rheumatic, and congenital heart disease may also be associated with this dysrhythmia. Occasionally the rhythm may be caused by digitalis. In all instances, the mechanism of action is likely to be enhanced automaticity or focal excitability of the ventricular pacemaker, which allows that pacemaker to

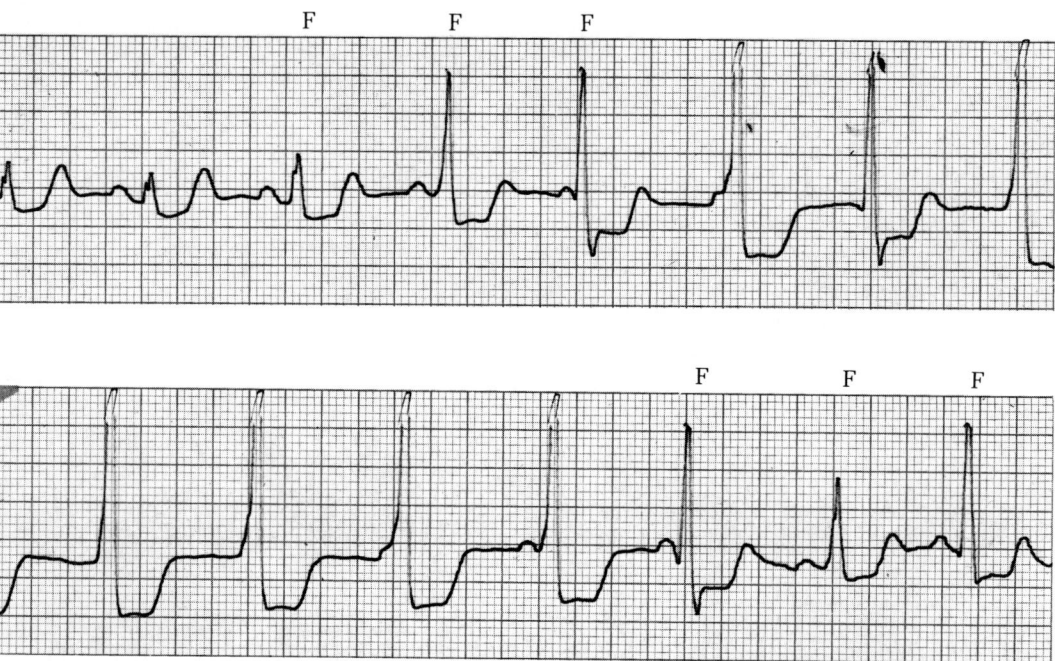

Figure 10-41   Accelerated idioventricular rhythm. Note the fusion (F) beats at the outset of the tachycardia and at the end of the tracing.

From Conover, M. B. (1992). *Understanding electrocardiography* (6th ed.). St. Louis: Mosby–Year Book.

suppress or override the slower sinus pacemaker. Often this occurs in the setting of sinus bradycardia.

Patients with AVIR generally experience no symptoms or negative effects because the rate of the rhythm is relatively normal. If treatment is necessary, therapeutic measures are directed at increasing the rate of impulse formation of the sinus node. Pharmacological agents generally used for bona fide ventricular tachycardia are usually not warranted and in fact may do more harm than good if they suppress the ventricular pacemaker when there is no other pacemaker.

Ventricular Tachycardia. *Ventricular tachycardia* (VT) exists when six or more ventricular ectopic beats occur in rapid succession (Figure 10-42). This rhythm is said to be sustained if it lasts longer than 30 seconds or nonsustained if the duration of the paroxysm is less than 30 seconds. The ventricular rate is usually between 140 and 200 beats per minute but may be slightly slower or faster. A ventricular premature complex initiates the paroxysm, and the abrupt termination of the tachycardia is followed by a postectopic pause. Frequently the initiating complex falls on the T wave of the preceding complex (R on T phenomenon), but late diastolic VPCs may also initiate the rhythm. The QRS complex of ventricular tachycardia is usually wide, often 0.12 second or more, and differently shaped than the normal supraventricular QRS. The T wave is also abnormal and has a vector opposite to that of the QRS. The rhythm is generally regular but might appear slightly irregular with variations of the RR cycle of up to 0.03 second. When dissociated sinus P waves are seen, it is usually diagnostic of VT; more frequently any P waves are "lost" in the ventricular complexes. In approximately 50% of the cases of paroxysmal ventricular tachycardia, the ventricular impulse conducts retrograde to the atria. In these cases the associated P wave follows the QRS and is usually inverted in leads II, III, and aVF, and upright in aVR. Ventricular capture and ventricular fusion beats (Dressler beats) may occur when the rate of the ventricular rhythm is less

than 150 beats per minute, but these occurrences are rare.

The same mechanisms that are responsible for ventricular premature complexes are also thought to be responsible for VT. The setting for the mechanisms of reentry and enhanced excitability is almost always advanced organic heart disease. The most common disease process causing the rhythm is ischemic heart disease resulting in acute myocardial infarction. Digitalis intoxication is also a common cause of ventricular tachycardia. Less frequently, the rhythm disturbance is seen in patients with hypertensive or rheumatic heart disease, cardiomyopathy, and mitral valve prolapse. Only rarely does ventricular tachycardia occur in individuals without evidence of heart disease.

When ventricular tachycardia occurs in patients with CHF, the failure can be aggravated by the dysrhythmia. In addition, CHF is a prime situation for the induction of ventricular tachycardia. The failure causes additional cardiac ischemia, thus changing the cell environment and promoting ventricular extrasystoles. The tachycardia then promotes further failure and decreased coronary perfusion by shortening the diastolic filling time. The resulting reduction in cardiac output may lead to syncopal episodes.

Patients who experience ventricular tachycardia may experience a wide range of signs and symptoms. Depending on the underlying heart disease and the rate of the ventricular tachycardia, the patient may be relatively free of symptoms or may be severely symptomatic and near death.

A variety of therapeutic interventions are available to prevent paroxysmal or sustained VT. The therapy of choice will depend upon the specific cause of the dysrhythmia as well as the severity of symptoms. Lidocaine IV bolus followed by a continuous infusion of the drug is the preferred therapeutic intervention when brief episodes of VT are associated with acute myocardial infarction. However, if the patient has hemodynamic instability, a sternal blow or DC shock may be necessary. For digitalis-induced VT, intrave-

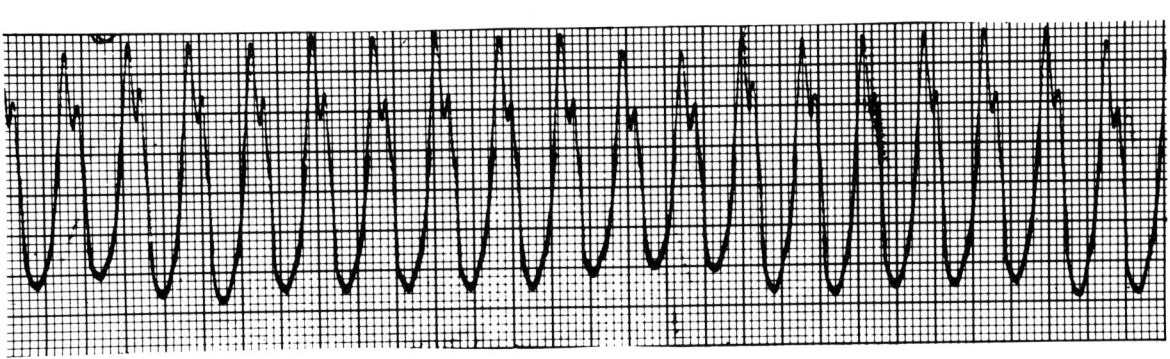

Figure 10-42 Paroxysmal ventricular tachycardia.

TABLE 10-3 **Differentiating the Origin of a Wide QRS Tachycardia**

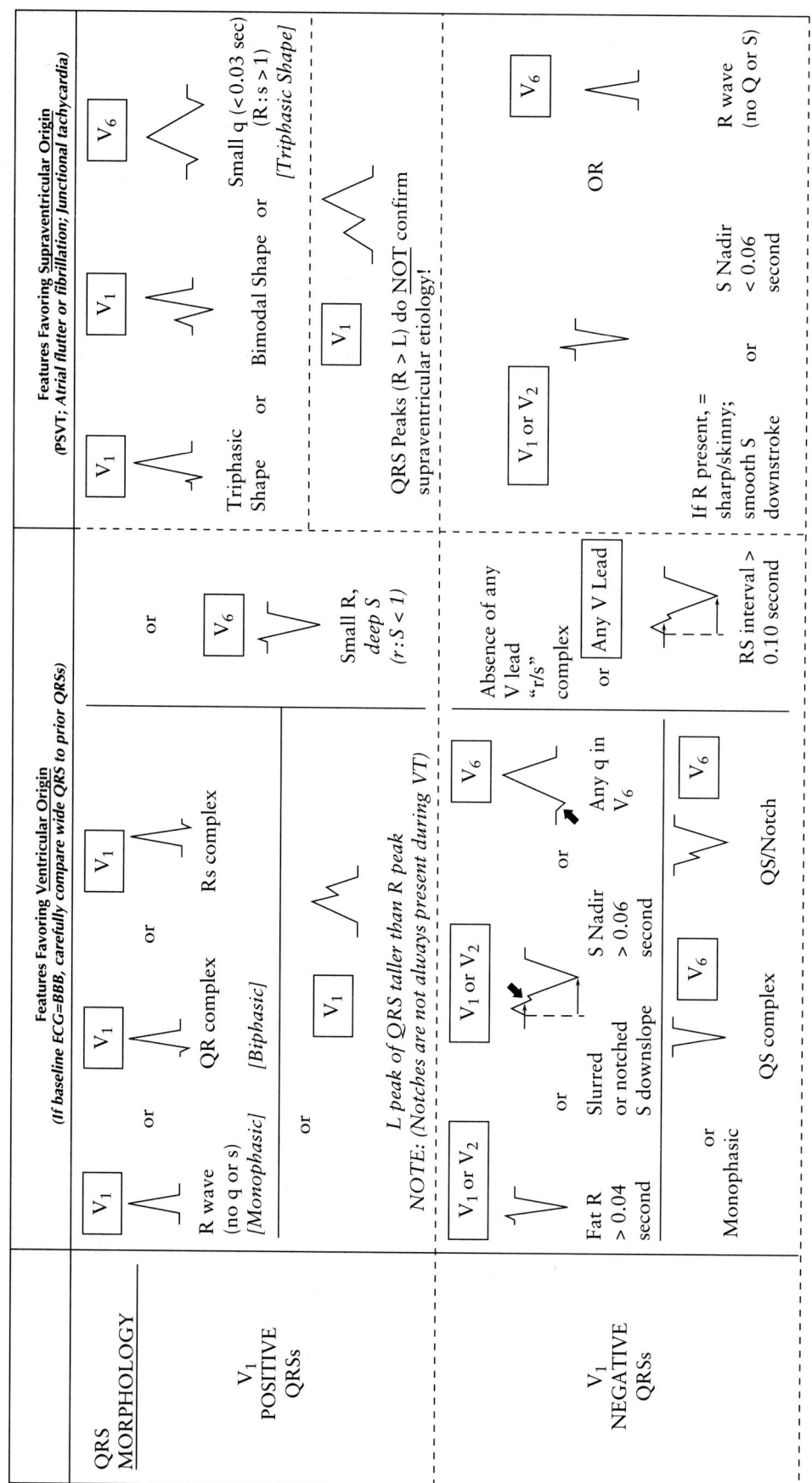

From Peck, S. A. (1990). Crush syndrome: Pathophysiology and management. *Orthopaedic Nursing, 9*(3), 38.

arrive so late that the cells are no longer refractory and the impulse conducts normally. The fourth condition determining aberrant ventricular conduction is the state of recovery of the excitability in the specialized ventricular conduction system. If there is unequal refractoriness of the bundle branches, conduction of the premature supraventricular impulse is likely to be abnormal.

The degree of aberrant conduction is dependent on the degree of refractoriness in the ventricles at the time of arrival of the supraventricular impulse. Aberrantly conducted QRSs often take the form of a right bundle branch block pattern (see Ventricular Conduction Abnormalities in this chapter) because the right bundle has a longer action potential and refractory period and is therefore more susceptible than the left bundle to conduction failure (see Figure 10-27). Less often, a left bundle branch block pattern may characterize the aberrant complex. The QRS interval may occasionally exceed 0.12 second in individuals with the right bundle branch block pattern and 0.14 second in individuals with left bundle branch block pattern.

QRS morphological clues to differentiate supraventricular dysrhythmias with aberrant ventricular conduction from ventricular ectopic impulses are listed in Table 10-3.[6]

Other distinguishing factors relate to the P:QRS relationship and tachycardia axis. When AV dissociation is confirmed during a wide QRS tachycardia by sinus Ps at an independent rate, the diagnosis of VT is very likely. If P waves are observed at consistent points before, during, or after wide QRSs, supraventricular origin is the favored diagnosis although VT does occur with retrograde atrial conduction. The axis of a wide QRS tachycardia may be abnormal in dysrhythmias of supraventricular or ventricular origin. However, indeterminate axis ($\pm 180°$ to $-90°$) is usually diagnostic of VT.

Even with these helpful hints, differentiation is sometimes difficult. Intracardiac electrograms may be needed to diagnose the problem.

AV Conduction Abnormalities

When conduction through the AV node is delayed or blocked by a prolonged refractory period in the AV junctional tissue, His bundle, or the His-Purkinje network, AV block is said to exist. The prolonged AV conduction is pathological rather than functional or physiological. AV blocks are classified as *incomplete* and *complete*, and the conduction disturbance may be described by degrees. Incomplete AV block includes first-degree, second-degree, and advanced or high-degree AV block. Complete AV block is also known as third-degree AV block. Any of these forms of AV block may be transient, intermittent, or persistent. Also, the degree of block may periodically change from one to another in the same individual.

First-degree AV Block. Prolongation of the PR interval beyond 0.20 second characterizes *first-degree AV block* (Figure 10-46). It should be noted that in this form of incomplete AV block each atrial impulse is eventually conducted to the ventricles. The PR interval is usually constant unless there is a change in the heart rate, between 0.21 to 0.40 second, but intervals as long as 0.80 second may appear.

Prolongation of the refractory period of the AV junction is the usual cause of first-degree AV block. Impaired conduction through the His bundle may also cause PR prolongation, especially with PR intervals of more than 0.28 second. This prolongation of the AV refractory period or His bundle conduction time may occur in healthy individuals but is much more common in individuals with heart disease. When first-degree AV block appears abruptly, the cause is likely to be digitalis intoxication, acute inferior myocardial infarction, or acute myocarditis. Less commonly it may be related to hyperkalemia, or to beta-blockers,

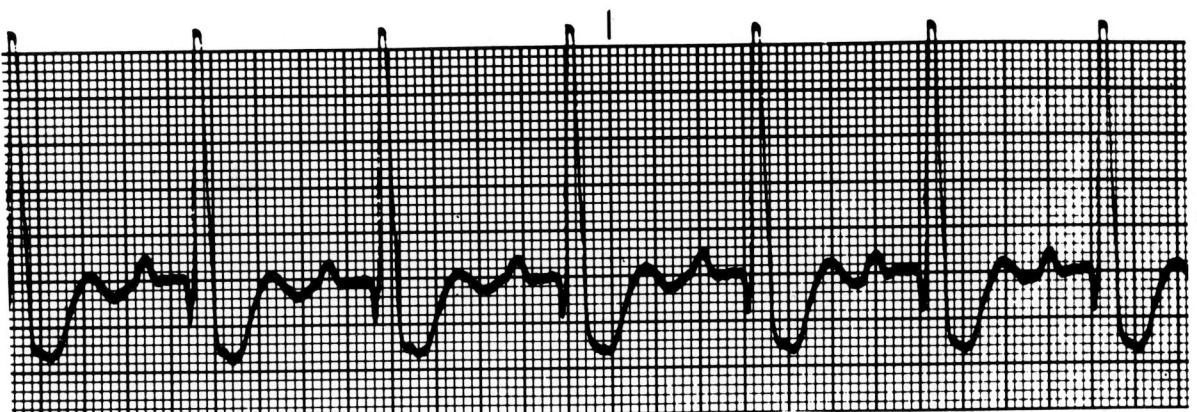

Figure 10-46 First-degree AV block. The PR interval is approximately 0.24 second.

quinidine, or procainamide therapy. First-degree AV block may occur in elderly people without established heart disease, in which case the cause may be chronic degeneration of the AV conduction system.

Therapy for first-degree AV block is generally not necessary but the cause should be investigated and corrected when possible. Individuals with first-degree AV block of recent onset should be closely monitored for a higher degree of AV block.

Second-degree AV Block: Mobitz Type I (Wenckebach AV Block). Second-degree AV block can be divided into two types identified as Mobitz type I and Mobitz type II AV block. Type I is more common than type II. Second-degree AV block: Mobitz type I is also known as *Wenckebach AV block*. This type of second-degree AV block is discussed first.

Mobitz type I AV block (Figure 10-47) is characterized on the ECG by the progressive prolongation of the PR intervals until a single P wave is not followed by a QRS. The PR interval after the blocked P will be the shortest and may be within the normal range or greater than 0.20 second. The RR intervals become progressively shorter until the P wave is blocked, thus producing the longest RR interval. This long RR interval is shorter than two PP intervals.

The AV conduction ratio is commonly 3:2 or 4:3 but may be greater (5:4 or 6:5). If the AV conduction ratio is constant, the ventricular rhythm is regularly irregular. However, the AV conduction ratio may change from time to time, that is, change from a 3:2 to a 4:3 ratio or vice versa, thereby causing the ventricular rhythm to be quite irregular.

The period from one blocked P wave to the next is the *Wenckebach period*. It is important to note that the typical Wenckebach period is not always seen in Mobitz type I AV block (such as in 2:1 AV conduction). Frequently the PR prolongation and the RR shortening are not progressive. This variation in the PP interval may be due to an underlying sinus arrhythmia or to a varying vagal tone. If the Wencke-

bach period is quite long, several successive PR intervals may show no measurable change.[5,6]

If the QRS complex is narrow in the presence of Mobitz type I AV block, the location of the block is usually in the AV node, or intranodal. This is true in 75% of cases. In the other 25%, the location of the block is the His bundle and, therefore, is infranodal. Noting the response of the rhythm to atropine or carotid sinus massage may offer a clue to the location. If the AV conduction ratio improves with carotid sinus massage and worsens after atropine administration, the block is infranodal. The opposite responses occur when the block is intranodal.[5] Occasionally a second-degree AV block: Mobitz type I is associated with an existing bundle branch block, in which case the QRS width is prolonged.[7]

The arrhythmogenic mechanism of type I AV block is thought to be prolongation of both the absolute and relative refractory periods of the AV node. This type of AV block is often transient and may be caused by mild digitalis intoxication, acute infection, uremia, electrolyte imbalance, or propranolol toxicity. In these instances the treatment for the dysrhythmia is directed at alleviating the cause. Mobitz type I AV block is often associated with acute inferior myocardial infarction. The block is generally transient due to swelling or transient ischemia of the AV node and consequently does not usually require therapy. Only rarely does Mobitz type I AV block appear in otherwise healthy individuals. Generally the block is of little clinical significance in these cases and is thought to be related to hyperactive vagal tone.

Second-degree AV Block: Mobitz Type II. When P waves are periodically blocked from conducting to the ventricles without a progressive prolongation of the PR interval or a progressive shortening of the RR interval, the conduction defect is identified as *second-degree AV block: Mobitz type II AV block* (Figure 10-48). There may be one or more dropped beats but in this conduction disturbance the PR intervals of all

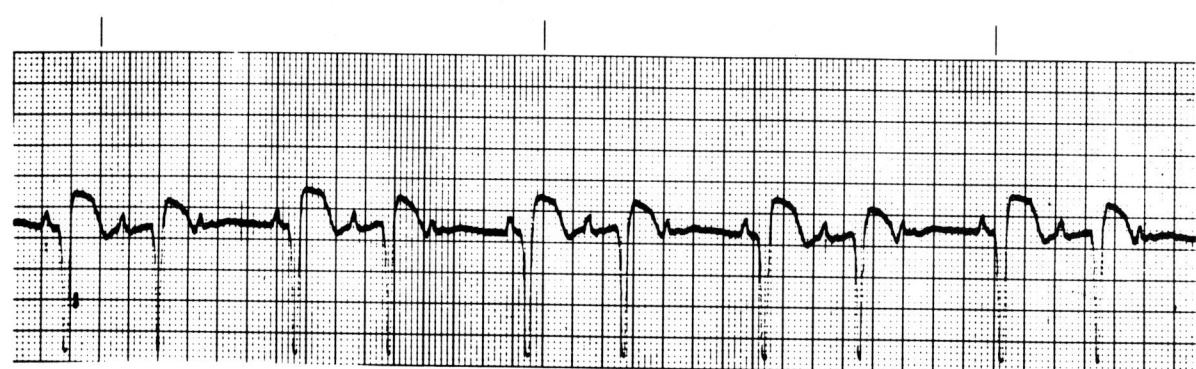

Figure 10-47   Second-degree AV block: Mobitz type I (Wenckebach AV block) with 3:2 conduction.

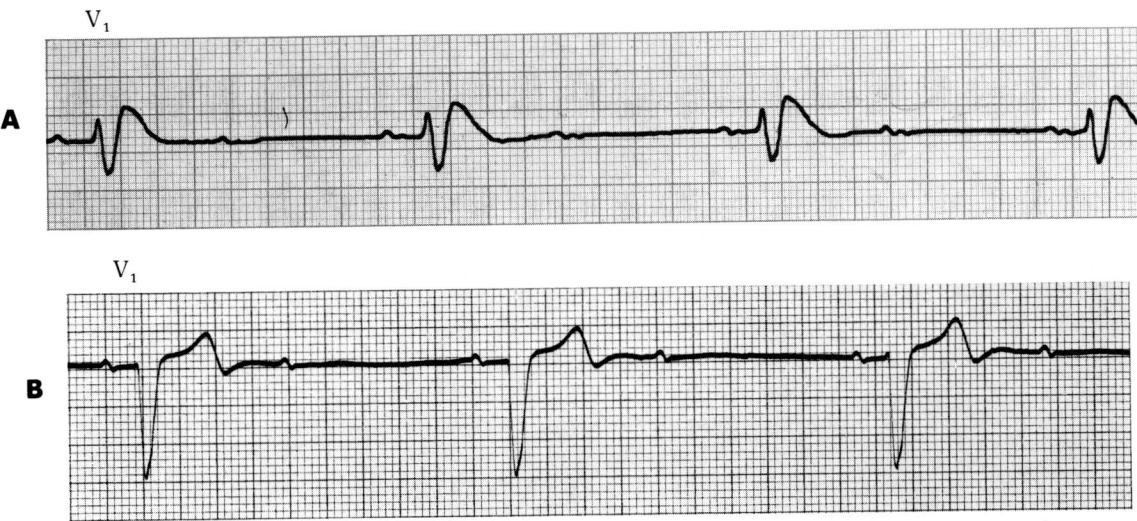

Figure 10-48   *A* and *B,* Second-degree AV block: Mobitz type II with 2:1 conduction.
From Conover, M. B. (1992). *Understanding electrocardiography* (6th ed.). St. Louis: Mosby–Year Book.

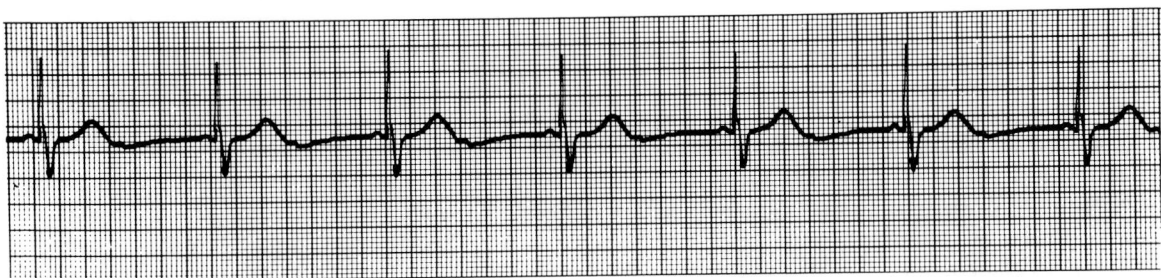

Figure 10-49   Second-degree AV block: Mobitz type II. The 2:1 AV conduction ratio is a variation of the Mobitz type II AV block. In this strip, the low-voltage, nonconducted P waves appear immediately after the T wave. The QRS complexes show slight notching in the terminal phase, which is common in this conduction abnormality.

the conducted beats are constant and usually within normal range. The QRS complex almost always exhibits a hemiblock, right or left bundle branch block, or bifascicular block pattern (see Ventricular Conduction Abnormalities in this chapter). The RR interval including the blocked P wave is a multiple of the normal PP interval.

When a 2:1 AV conduction ratio (Figure 10-49) exists, one must look at the PR interval of the conducted beats and the width of the QRS to determine whether the conduction abnormality is a type I or type II second-degree AV block. A long, continuous recording of the rhythm may show an episode of changing conduction ratios and the behavior of the PR interval and thus assist in the determination of the type of block. If the AV block decreases when the atrial rate is increased by exercise or atropine administration, the block is likely to be a type I second-degree block. When the AV block increases with an increased atrial rate secondary to these maneuvers,

the block is a Mobitz type II.[5] If recent infarction has occurred, it is helpful to note that type I is more common with inferior infarction and type II with anterior infarction.

The location of the conduction abnormality in second-degree, type II AV block is almost always in the His-Purkinje system or infranodal. The exact location may be either within the His bundle itself (intra-His) or in the bundle branches. This explains why the QRS complex in Mobitz type II block has the appearance of a ventricular conduction abnormality. The block is in actuality a form of incomplete bilateral bundle branch block in the majority of cases.

Chronic Mobitz type II AV block is probably due to a degenerative sclerotic change in the His-Purkinje system. Acute Mobitz type II AV block is almost always caused by an acute anteroseptal myocardial infarction. Symptoms may include those associated with CHF and those of lightheadedness, dizziness, fatigue and syncope, that is, Adams-Stokes attacks.

Second-degree AV block: Mobitz type II is a common precursor of complete AV block with ventricular standstill due to simultaneous bilateral bundle branch block. Since type II AV block is often irreversible, a permanent artificial pacemaker is usually indicated, irrespective of the presence or absence of symptoms.

Advanced AV Block.   Advanced or high-degree AV block is recognized on the ECG when the AV conduction ratio is equal to or greater than 3:1 (Figure 10-50). Usually the conduction ratios are even-numbered (such as 4:1, 6:1, or 8:1), with odd-numbered ratios being relatively uncommon. It is common to observe AV junctional escape complexes (less commonly ventricular escape complexes) when the conduction ratio is 4:1 or greater. When conduction ratios are very high, the conducted beats, or ventricular capture beats are relatively rare. Consequently, under these circumstances the rhythm resembles complete AV block except for the occasional conducted beat, and there is incomplete AV dissociation.

The PR intervals of the conducted beats may be normal or prolonged. They are generally constant; however, they may be variable if the Wenckebach phenomenon or concealed conduction occurs. The PP intervals are usually regular but may be irregular if there is an abnormality in sinus impulse formation or conduction. The RR intervals are almost always irregular. The QRS configuration is dependent on the site of the AV block and the origin of the QRS complex. The QRS complex of conducted beats is usually normal but may have a right or left bundle branch block configuration if there is an associated ventric-

ular conduction abnormality. If the escape mechanism arises from the AV junction, those QRS complexes are normal in configuration unless there is a coexisting bundle branch block. The QRS configuration of ventricular escape beats is differently shaped than the normal QRS, often wide and bizarre. Ventricular fusion beats have varying QRS configurations.

Advanced AV block may be caused by several mechanisms including those responsible for Mobitz type I and Mobitz type II second-degree AV block. The site of the conduction abnormality may be intranodal, in which case AV junctional escape beats can control the ventricles; or infranodal, with the escape pacemaker being from within the ventricles. As with other forms of incomplete AV block, high-degree block may be caused by drug intoxication (such as digitalis, propranolol, or guanethidine), electrolyte imbalances, acute infections, acute inferior myocardial infarction, and acute anterior myocardial infarction. The clinical significance depends on the site of the block, the ventricular rate, the presence or absence of hemodynamic instability, and the underlying etiology, but is in general very similar to that of third-degree AV block. A temporary artificial cardiac pacemaker may be necessary initially, and if the AV block is found to be infranodal and permanent, a permanent artificial pacemaker is indicated.

Third-degree AV Block.   As noted earlier, third-degree AV block is also known as *complete AV block*. This conduction abnormality is characterized on the ECG by separate and independent atrial and ventric-

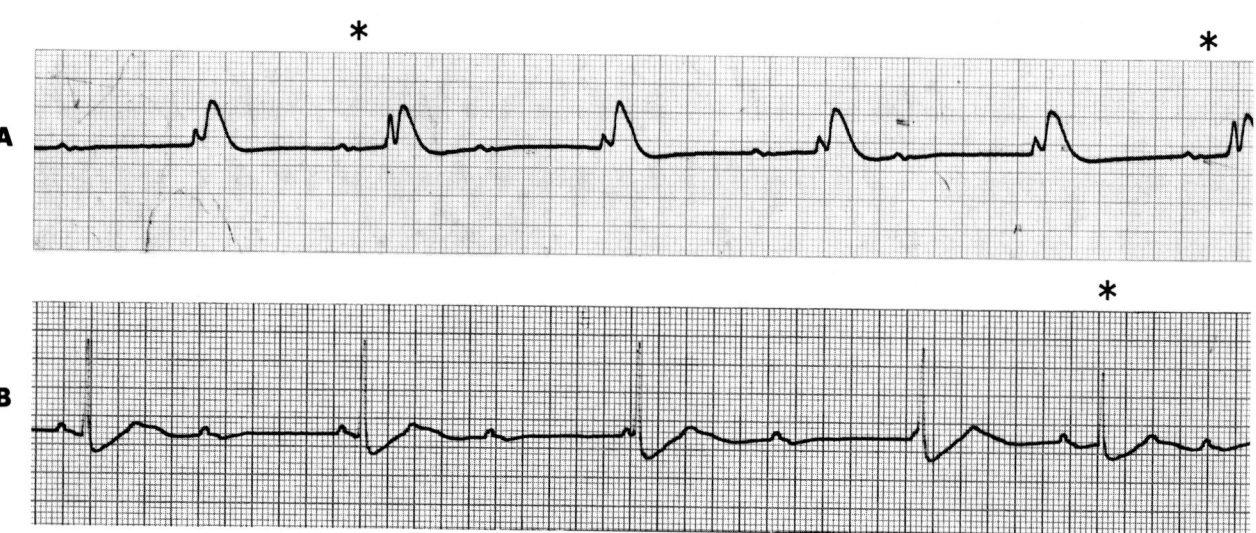

Figure 10-50   High-grade, second-degree (advanced) AV block. In tracing A, there are only 2 sinus-conducted beats (asterisks), in spite of a sinus rate of 58 beats per minute and plenty of opportunity to conduct. In tracing B, conduction occurs (asterisks) when the RP interval is at least 0.64.

From Conover, M. B. (1992). *Understanding electrocardiography* (6th ed.). St. Louis: Mosby–Year Book.

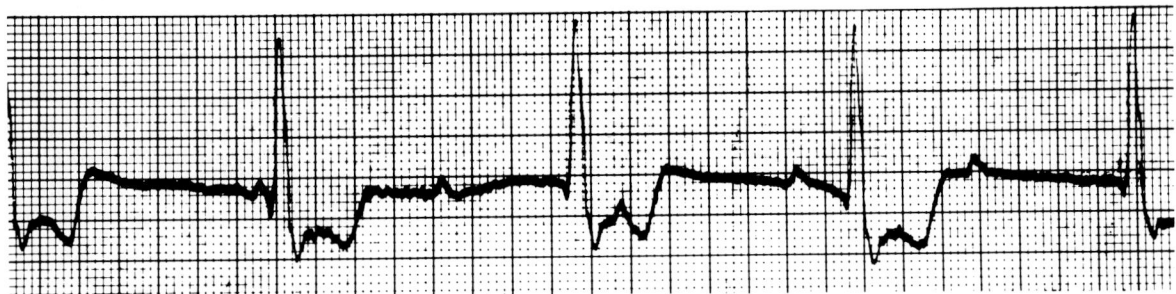

Figure 10-51   Third-degree AV block. Note the lack of association between the atria and the ventricles as indicated by the totally variable PR intervals and nonconducted P waves, some of which are in the ST segments and T waves.

ular activity (Figure 10-51). The atria are controlled by either sinus or ectopic atrial pacemakers which almost always generate impulses at a rate faster than the pacemaker cell that controls the ventricles. The ventricles are controlled by a pacemaker that is distal to the AV block. If the site of the block is intranodal, the AV junction may initiate activity at a rate of 40 to 60 beats per minute; however, if the block is in the His bundle or the bundle branches, the pacemaker cell is below that site in either the His bundle or the His-Purkinje system, often initiating signals at a rate of 20 to 40 beats per minute.

The PP interval is often regular when the sinus node acts as the atrial pacemaker but may be irregular if a sinus arrhythmia or intermittent SA block is present. The RR intervals produced by the junctional or ventricular escape complexes are usually regular; however, they too may be irregular if there are multiple pacemaker sites, irregular discharges of the pacemaker, or exit blocks of varying degrees.[7] The PR interval is totally inconsistent because of the complete dissociation of the atria and ventricles. The configuration of the QRS is dependent on the site of the subsidiary pacemaker. Normal QRS complexes result when the AV junction paces the ventricles. However, if the pacemaker site is below the bifurcation of the His bundle, the QRS is usually wide and bizarre in most leads.

Some of the causes of third-degree AV block include digitalis intoxication, acute inferior myocardial infarction, or acute myocarditis. In these instances the block is usually transient and intranodal. When an acute anterior myocardial infarction causes the complete AV block, the block is usually infranodal and permanent. Complete AV block may also be caused by congenital malformation of the AV node and by chronic degenerative changes of the His-Purkinje network in the elderly. Both these conditions produce permanent blocks. Occasionally AV block is caused by open heart surgery, particularly with aortic and/or mitral valve replacement, or by trauma.

A variety of signs and symptoms may be associated with third-degree AV block. If underlying heart disease or congestive heart failure is present, signs and symptoms secondary to those problems may be observed. Complete AV block secondary to congenital malformation may produce failure to thrive phenomena or be asymptomatic. Symptoms associated with acquired complete AV block are dependent on the severity of the underlying heart disease and the rate of the ventricular pacemaker. Slower ventricular rates may produce severe symptoms due to the resulting reduction in cardiac output.

Treatment for acute complete AV block almost always involves the use of a temporary artificial cardiac pacemaker, particularly when the site of the block is infranodal, the ventricular rate is very slow, and the individual is severely symptomatic. Emergency measures such as administration of epinephrine, isoproterenol, atropine, or a combination of these agents may be tried, and cardiopulmonary resuscitation may be necessary until a pacemaker can be placed. If the block proves to be permanent, a permanent artificial pacemaker will be necessary. Individuals with congenital complete AV block may go for years without symptoms or need of therapy; however, most will eventually require implantation of a permanent artificial cardiac pacemaker when they reach middle age and begin to develop symptoms.[7]

AV Dissociation

Mention of AV dissociation has been made on several occasions when describing rhythm disturbances such as accelerated AV junctional rhythm, accelerated idioventricular rhythm, and third-degree AV block. It is important to note that AV dissociation is never a primary rhythm disturbance but is always secondary to a cardiac dysrhythmia. By definition, AV dissociation implies that the atria and ventricles beat independently. Consequently, the P waves, atrial flutter waves, or waves of atrial fibrillation bear no relationship to the QRS complex.

Three primary rhythm disturbances produce AV dissociation. The first is slowed or impaired sinus impulse formation or SA conduction. Specific dysrhythmias of this type include sinus bradycardia, sinus arrest, and SA block. The P wave, if there is one, will originate in the sinus node and the QRS will be generated by a faster AV junctional or ventricular escape pacemaker. The second most common rhythm disturbance producing AV dissociation is acceleration of the impulse formation in an AV junctional or ventricular pacemaker. The atrial pacemaker under these circumstances may be the sinus node or an ectopic atrial pacemaker. The ventricles are controlled by an AV junctional or ventricular pacemaker that discharges faster than the pacemaker controlling the atria. These signals may be described as "accelerated" or "tachycardia" depending on the actual rate. The last cause of AV dissociation is AV conduction disturbance. Rhythm disorders of this variety are advanced AV block and complete AV block. In addition, AV dissociation results when the ventricles are stimulated by an artificial cardiac pacemaker independently of the atrial mechanism.

AV dissociation may be incomplete or complete. Incomplete AV dissociation occurs when there is an intermittent or occasional relationship between the atria and ventricles. When no capture beats exist and the atria and ventricles consistently beat independently, complete AV dissociation is said to be present.

The clinical significance of AV dissociation rests with the underlying causative rhythm disorder and the presence or absence of organic heart disease. The dissociation itself is not treated directly; rather, therapeutic measures are directed toward the basic rhythm disturbance and the underlying heart disease or drug toxicity.

Ventricular Conduction Abnormalities

The ventricular conduction system is composed of the distal portion of the His bundle, the bundle branches, and the Purkinje network (Figure 10-52). The bundle of His is a thin conductive pathway connecting the AV node with the bundle branches. At its distal end, the His bundle bifurcates into the left and right bundles. The left bundle branch arises almost perpendicularly from the common bundle, whereas

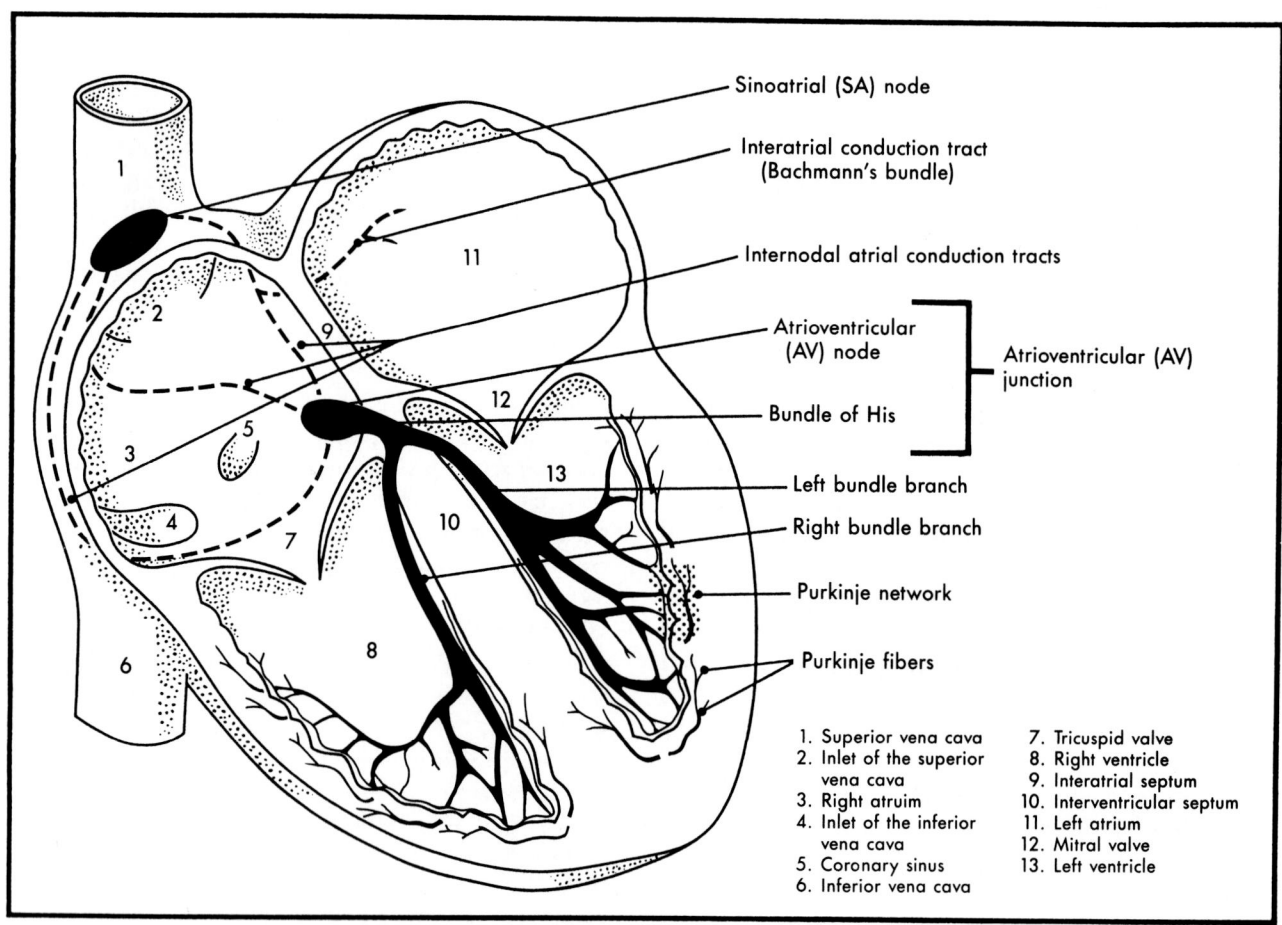

Sinoatrial (SA) node

Interatrial conduction tract (Bachmann's bundle)

Internodal atrial conduction tracts

Atrioventricular (AV) node

Bundle of His

Atrioventricular (AV) junction

Left bundle branch

Right bundle branch

Purkinje network

Purkinje fibers

1. Superior vena cava
2. Inlet of the superior vena cava
3. Right atrium
4. Inlet of the inferior vena cava
5. Coronary sinus
6. Inferior vena cava
7. Tricuspid valve
8. Right ventricle
9. Interatrial septum
10. Interventricular septum
11. Left atrium
12. Mitral valve
13. Left ventricle

Figure 10-52 Electrical conduction system.
From Huszar, R. J. (1988). *Basic dysrhythmias.* St Louis: Mosby—Year Book.

the right bundle is a more direct extension of the His bundle. The right bundle branch extends along the right side of the interventricular septum until its subdivisions merge with the Purkinje network.

Anatomists disagree about the structure of the left bundle branch. Many believe that it almost immediately subdivides into the left posterior and the left anterior fascicles. The posterior fascicle extends inferiorly and the anterior fascicle spreads superiorly beneath the left ventricular endocardium. Many individuals may also have a third subdivision, which has been identified as the septal fascicle of the left bundle branch (see Figure 10-52).[6] For the purposes of this discussion it is assumed that there are fascicular divisions of the left bundles even though some investigators dispute this concept.

The subdivisions of the bundle branch system blend into the Purkinje network. This network is widely distributed throughout both ventricles, making it possible for impulses to conduct rapidly to all sections of the ventricular muscle.

Figure 10-9 illustrates the sequence of normal ventricular activation that was described earlier in this chapter. When this activation sequence is disturbed by conduction abnormalities within the ventricles, distortions in the QRS complex result. Ventricular conduction abnormalities may occur in either of the bundle branches, the divisions of the left bundle, or a combination of sites. The most common forms of intraventricular conduction abnormalities are *right bundle branch block (RBBB)* and *left bundle branch block (LBBB)*, with the incidence being about equal. When these conduction disturbances occur, the bundle that is not blocked conducts normally, depolarizing its respective ventricle. The bundle that is blocked is unable to conduct the impulse to the ventricular fibers, so the associated ventricle will be depolarized abnormally and late. Under normal conditions both ventricles are activated simultaneously.

Left bundle branch block is generally associated with a QRS width of 0.12 second or greater in the frontal plane leads. Left bundle branch block frequently prolongs the QRS more than does RBBB. If the QRS duration is between 0.10 and 0.12 second, the bundle branch block is considered to be incomplete. It is described as a complete block only when the QRS interval is equal to or greater than 0.12 second.

Block in either the right or left bundle branch is usually caused by the same diseases responsible for AV block. However, bundle branch block is more often associated with coronary artery disease, aortic valve disease, and hypertension. These blocks are rarely idiopathic. They are generally chronic and permanent but may appear intermittently.

Fascicular blocks, or *hemiblocks*, alter the activation sequence of the left ventricle and, in so doing, alter the vector of the QRS complexes. Consequently, left anterior and posterior hemiblocks result in left and right axis deviation, respectively. They do not, however, significantly alter the QRS width.

Hemiblocks may occur alone or in association with blocks at other sites. An RBBB may coexist with either a left anterior hemiblock (LAH) or a left posterior hemiblock (LPH), creating what is sometimes described as a *bifascicular block*. Block of the right bundle and both fascicles results in a *trifascicular block* which is an expression of a *bilateral bundle branch block*.

In this chapter the ventricular conduction abnormalities of right bundle branch block, left bundle branch block, left anterior hemiblock, and left posterior hemiblock are discussed and their ECG findings described. Further discussion of the more complex ventricular conduction abnormalities of bifascicular and trifascicular block is reserved for electrocardiographic textbooks.

Right Bundle Branch Block. When conduction through the right bundle is blocked, the right ventricle is depolarized later than the left ventricle. The QRS duration may be prolonged to account for the additional time required for the right ventricle to be activated. A characteristic change in the QRS results from the abnormal ventricular activation sequence. Figure 10-53 illustrates the pattern of activation when RBBB is present. Note that the septum depolarizes in its normal left-to-right direction, producing a small r wave in V_1 and a small q wave in V_6. The left ventricle is the next area to be depolarized and results in the inscription of an S wave in V_1 and an R wave in V_6. The last area to be depolarized is the right ventricle. An R wave at the end of the QRS (often a second R wave [R'] as in this example) in V_1 and a deep and slurred S wave in V_6 represent the terminal electrical forces.

When the ventricles depolarize abnormally, they also repolarize abnormally, resulting in a T wave change. This T wave alteration is said to be *secondary* to the QRS alteration. In the case of RBBB, the secondary T wave change results in a T axis that is approximately 180° from the QRS axis. For example, in leads V_{1-3} the QRS complex of RBBB is predominantly upright; the T wave is inverted and asymmetric with the downward slope being more gradual and the upward stroke being more rapid. When combined with the ST segment it takes on the appearance of a backward check mark.

The ECG criteria for complete RBBB can be summarized as:
1. A QRS interval ≥0.12 second in V_{1-3}

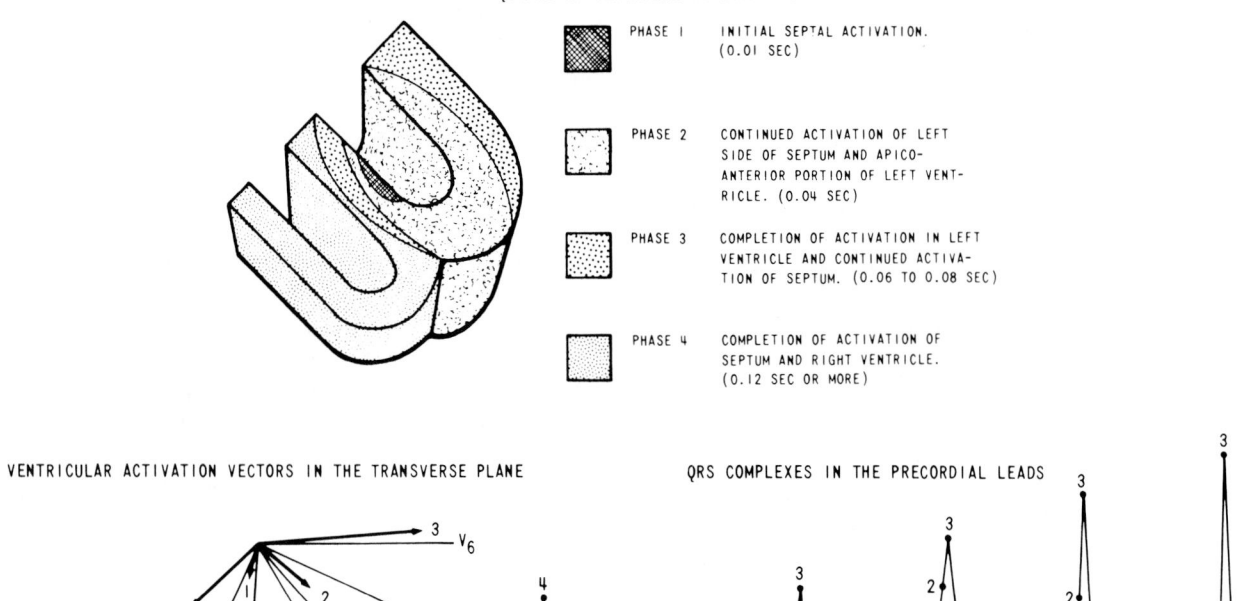

Figure 10-53 Schematic representation of ventricular depolarization in right bundle branch block. See text for description.

From Friedman, H. H. (1985). *Diagnostic electrocardiography and vectorcardiography.* New York: McGraw-Hill.

2. A triphasic QRS in V_1 (rSR') and V_6 (qRS)
3. Small q and broad S waves in the left leads (I, aVL, V_6)
4. Secondary ST, T wave changes in the right precordial leads (V_{1-3})
5. Delayed intrinsicoid deflection in V_1/normal in V_6

Figure 10-54 is an ECG from a patient with RBBB. Note the presence of each of the diagnostic criteria.

Incomplete RBBB has an abnormal R wave at the end of the QRS or rSR' morphology but often does not show secondary ST segment or T wave changes in the right precordium. The QRS width may be less than 0.12 second as well.

Other clinical conditions may produce an rSR' in V_1 and should be differentiated from RBBB. A key factor in the differential diagnosis is the QRS width, which is less than 0.12 second except when RBBB is present. Normal variants, right ventricular enlargement (especially diastolic overload), straight back syndrome, true posterior myocardial infarction, and some types of accessory pathway conduction may mimic some of the ECG changes of an RBBB.

Right bundle branch block may appear in apparently healthy individuals and those with organic heart disease. It may be identified in people with coronary artery disease, systemic hypertension, cardiac tumors, cardiomyopathy, rheumatic heart disease, and congenital heart disease. Atrial septal defects are often associated with RBBB. Acute pulmonary embolism or infarction should be suspected when RBBB of sudden onset appears. Acute CHF, acute myocardial infarction, and acute pericarditis may produce intermittent RBBB.

Left Bundle Branch Block. Block of the left bundle alters the normal activation of the ventricles beginning with septal depolarization (Figure 10-55). Rather than the usual left-to-right depolarization, the septum must depolarize in a right-to-left direction. This change in the initial vector of the QRS produces the loss of the initial r wave in V_1 and the septal q wave in V_6. Occasionally, though, the septal vector is overpowered by the right ventricular electrical ac-

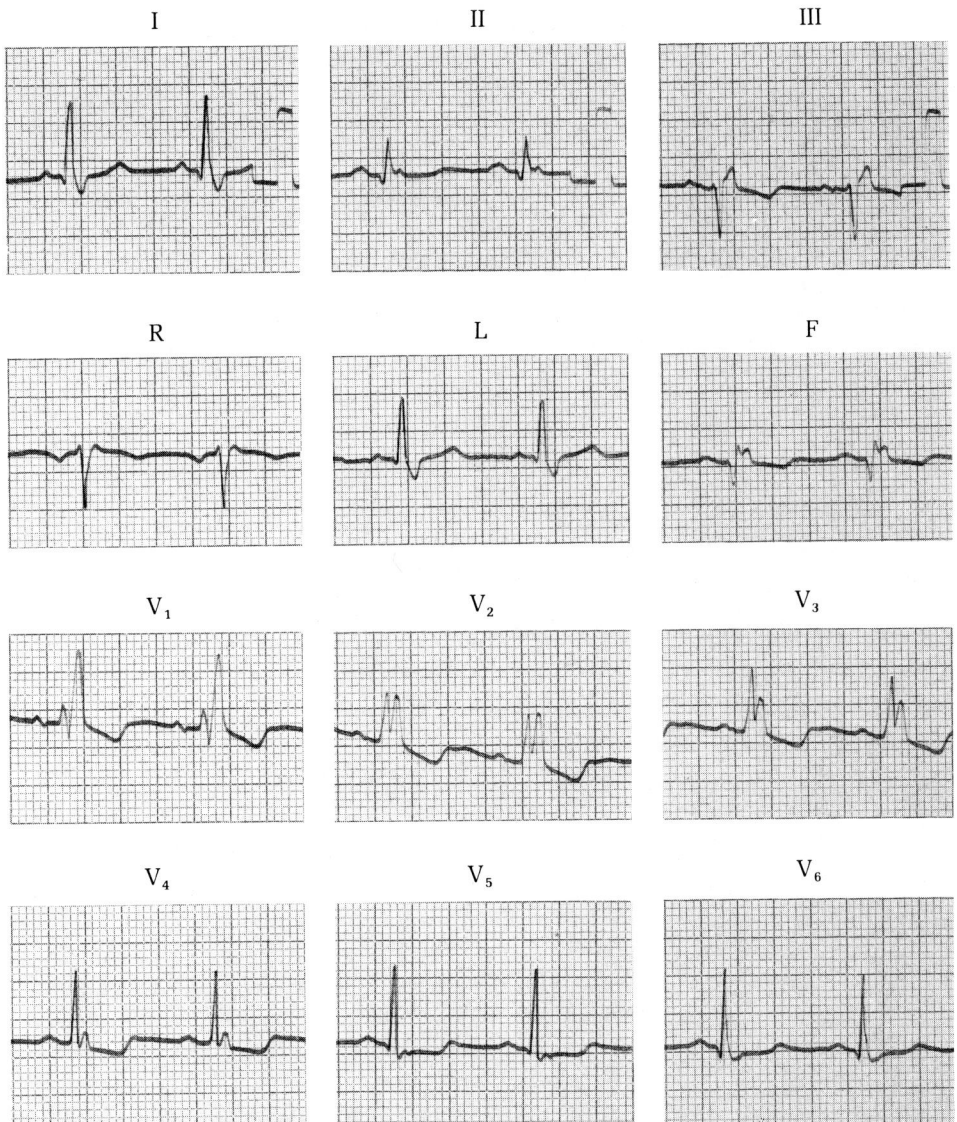

Figure 10-54   RBBB. Note the classical rSR' pattern in V_1 and the normal septal q waves and abnormal S waves in leads I, aVL, and V_6.

From Conover, M. B. (1992). *Understanding electrocardiography* (6th ed.). St. Louis: Mosby–Year Book.

tivity, in which case a small r wave may be inscribed in V_1. Following septal and right ventricular depolarization is left ventricular depolarization. Because conduction is abnormal and outside the Purkinje network, the activation time for the left ventricle is prolonged. This results in a prolonged QRS width, a broad, slurred S wave in V_1, and an R' wave in V_6. The QRS axis may be normal but more often is deviated to the left. Secondary ST, T wave changes will be present in the left lateral leads. It should be noted that if primary T wave changes (see Myocardial Infarction in this chapter) replace the secondary ST, T

wave changes in the presence of a bundle branch block, myocardial ischemia should be suspected.

The diagnostic ECG criteria for LBBB are summarized as:

1. A QRS interval ≥0.12 second
2. Absence of septal q waves in the left leads (I, aVL, V_6)
3. Mainly negative complex (QS or rS) in V_1 and always totally positive in V_6
4. Intrinsicoid deflection delayed in V_6
5. Secondary ST, T wave changes in the left lateral leads (I, aVL, V_{4-6})

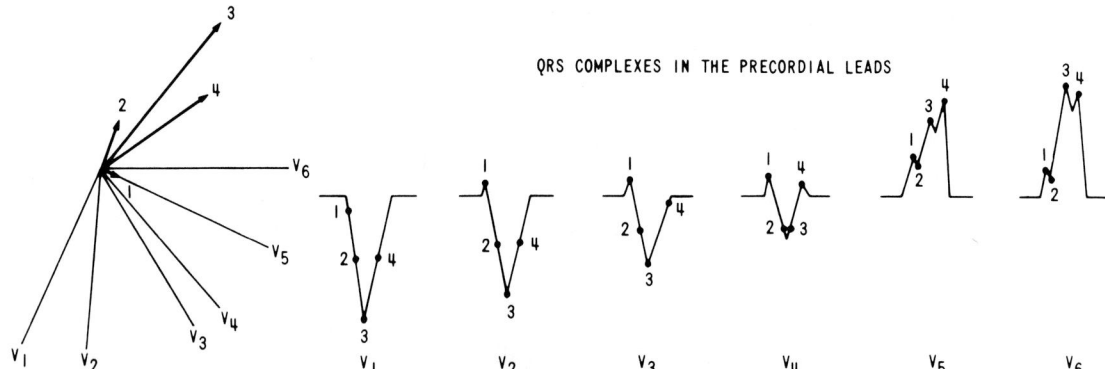

VENTRICULAR DEPOLARIZATION IN LEFT BUNDLE BRANCH BLOCK

SEQUENCE OF VENTRICULAR ACTIVATION

PHASE 1   ACTIVATION OF RIGHT SIDE OF SEPTUM AND APICO-ANTERIOR PORTION OF RIGHT VENTRICLE. (0.02 SEC)

PHASE 2   COMPLETION OF RIGHT VENTRICULAR AND RIGHT-TO-LEFT SEPTAL ACTIVATION. (0.06 SEC)

PHASE 3   ACTIVATION OF POSTEROBASAL REGION OF LEFT VENTRICLE. (0.08-0.10 SEC)

PHASE 4   ACTIVATION OF ANTEROLATERAL REGION OF LEFT VENTRICLE. (0.12 SEC OR MORE)

VENTRICULAR ACTIVATION VECTORS IN THE TRANSVERSE PLANE

QRS COMPLEXES IN THE PRECORDIAL LEADS

Figure 10-55   Schematic representation of ventricular depolarization in left bundle branch block. See text for description.

From Friedman, H. H. (1985). *Diagnostic electrocardiography and vectorcardiography* (p. 192). New York: McGraw-Hill. Reprinted by permission.

These criteria are apparent in Figure 10-56.

Left bundle branch block must be differentiated from some types of accessory pathway conduction, anteroseptal myocardial infarction, intraventricular conduction defects, idioventricular rhythm, and an artificial cardiac pacemaker–induced ventricular rhythm.[7] The QRS width and clinical history may provide clues to the correct diagnosis.

The most common cause of LBBB is hypertensive heart disease. Less often it may be associated with aortic stenosis, cardiomyopathy, and congenital heart disease. It is very rare for LBBB to exist in an individual without evidence of cardiac disease. The elderly are much more likely to have LBBB than RBBB. If an individual develops LBBB in the presence of an anteroseptal myocardial infarction or vice versa, the patient's prognosis is serious.

Left Anterior Hemiblock. Impulses usually conduct through the left anterior and left posterior fascicles simultaneously (Figure 10-57A). The left anterior fascicle normally conducts impulses to the Pur-
kinje fibers of the anterior and lateral walls of the left ventricle. However, when conduction through the anterior fascicle is blocked, the anterior and lateral walls must be activated by retrograde conduction from the posterior fascicle. The retrograde activation, which is directed left and superior (Figure 10-57B), occurs late and is essentially unopposed by other electrical activity. Consequently, the left and superior forces cause the mean vector of the QRS to shift leftward and superiorly, creating left axis deviation on the ECG (Figure 10-58). Initial forces are directed rightward and inferiorly, thus producing an initial q wave in leads I and aVL and an initial r wave in the inferior leads (II, III, and aVF).

The major ECG criterion for left anterior hemiblock is marked left axis deviation. There are conflicting opinions in the literature regarding what constitutes marked LAD. Two authors[2,5] consider axis deviation of −30° to −90° as suitable criteria for marked LAD, and others[6,7] state that −45° to −90° are the suitable limits. In this chapter, −45° is con-

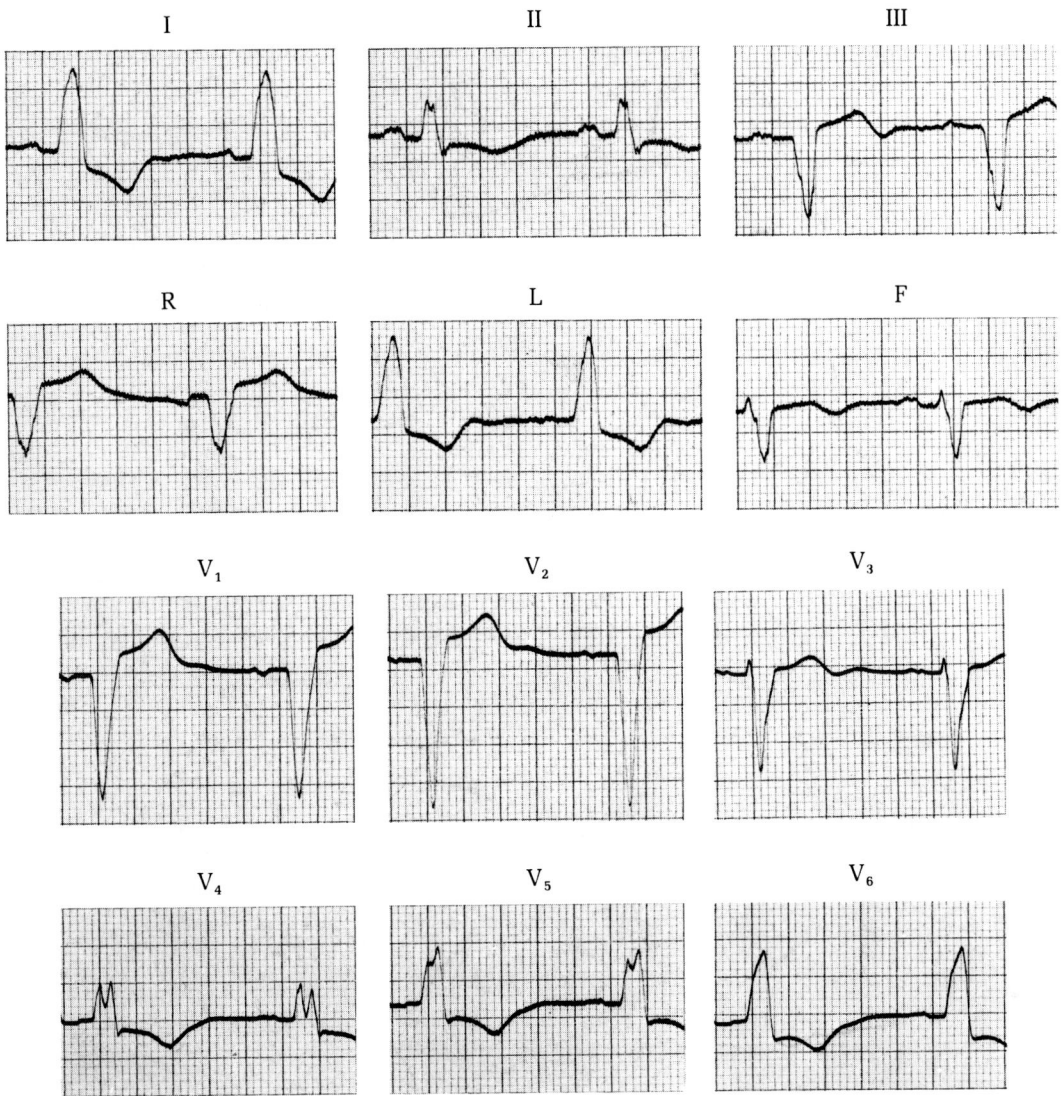

Figure 10-56 Left bundle branch block. The QRS measures 0.12 to 14 seconds. A broad biphasic R wave with a delayed intrinsicoid deflection is present in leads V₅ and V₆ and also in lead I. Significant, too, is the absence of Q waves in leads I and aVL and the left precordial leads.

From Conover, M. B. (1992). *Understanding electrocardiography* (6th ed.). St. Louis: Mosby–Year Book.

sidered to be the lower limit for marked LAD and the minimum criterion for LAH.

The electrocardiographic criteria for the diagnosis of left anterior hemiblock may be summarized as:

1. Marked left axis deviation ($-45°$ to $-90°$)
2. qR complex in leads I and aVL may be seen
3. An rS complex in leads II and III
4. A QRS width <0.12 second

It is important to note, however, that other clinical conditions (such as emphysema, ventricular preexcitation, hyperkalemia, acute pulmonary embolism, and inferior myocardial infarction) may cause marked LAD and otherwise mimic the ECG findings of left anterior hemiblock. These conditions must be ruled out before true left anterior hemiblock can be diagnosed.

Left Posterior Hemiblock. The left posterior fascicle conducts impulses to the inferior and posterior walls of the left ventricle. When this fascicle is blocked, impulses must be conducted to these areas via the anterior fascicle. The activation of the inferior and posterior left ventricular walls is late, and the impulses are directed inferiorly and rightward (see Figure 10-57C). These late forces are essentially unopposed and produce right axis deviation of the mean QRS vector. The initial QRS forces, though, are directed superiorly and to the left causing an initial r wave in lead I and an initial q wave in leads II, III,

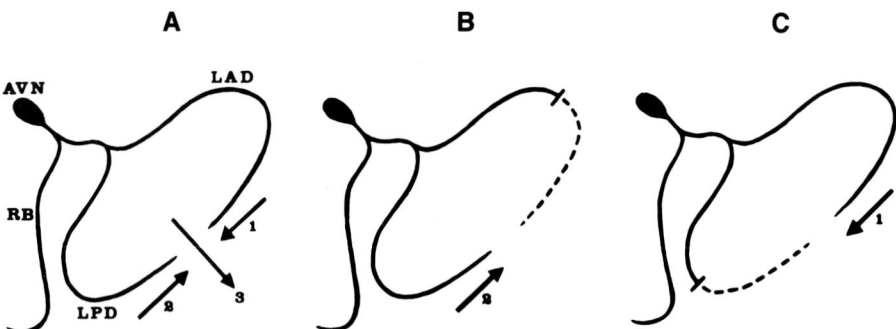

Figure 10-57 Hemiblocks. When both the anterior and posterior divisions of the left bundle branch system are intact *(A)*, the left ventricle is activated through both divisions (vectors 1 and 2) so that the resultant forces of vectors 1 and 2 will produce vector 3. However, when one of the two divisions of the left bundle branch system is blocked, the impulses must travel through the intact division only. That is, in anterior hemiblock *(B)* vector 1 is no longer present, and as a result, the left ventricle is activated through the intact posterior division (vector 2). In this case the electrical axis shifts to the left and superiorly (marked left axis deviation). For the same reason, posterior hemiblock *(C)* produces right axis deviation because the left ventricle is activated through the intact anterior division (vector 1). RB = Right bundle branch. AVN = AV node. LAD = Left anterior division. LPD = Left posterior division.

From Chung, E. K. (1985). *Electrocardiography: Practical application with vectorial principles.* Norwalk, CT: Appleton-Century-Crofts.

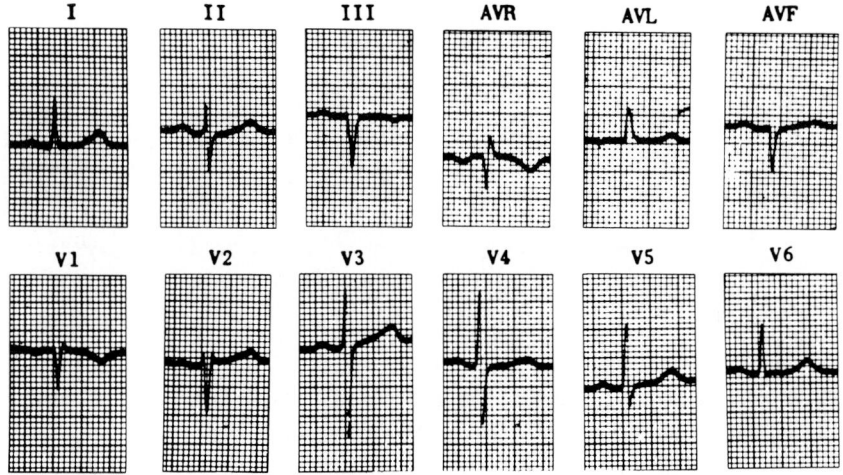

Figure 10-58 Abnormal left axis deviation (−45°) due to left anterior hemiblock in a patient with chronic coronary artery disease. The electrocardiogram is otherwise normal. There is an R' wave in leads V₁ and V₂, which indicates that the terminal QRS vector, in addition to being directed leftward and superiorly, also points anteriorly.

From Friedman, H. H. (1985). *Diagnostic electrocardiography and vectorcardiography.* New York: McGraw-Hill.

and aVF. Even though the terminal forces of the QRS occur late, the QRS width is usually less than 0.12 second.

Figure 10-59 depicts the ECG changes associated with a left posterior hemiblock. These changes can be summarized as follows:

1. Marked right axis deviation ($+105°$ to $+180°$)
2. A small r wave (rS complex) in lead I and aVL and a small q wave (qR complex) in leads III, and aVF

3. A QRS width <0.12 second

As with left anterior hemiblock, left posterior hemiblock can only be diagnosed with certainty when all other factors that might cause RAD have been ruled out. These factors include a vertical heart, chronic obstructive lung disease, right ventricular enlargement, and lateral wall myocardial infarction.

Left posterior hemiblock rarely occurs as an isolated lesion. More often it coexists with RBBB (bifascicular block), inferior wall myocardial infarction,

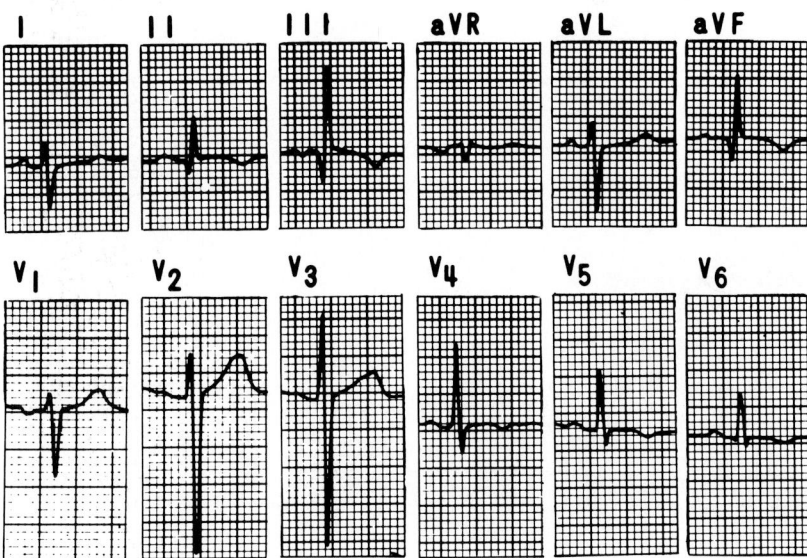

Figure 10-59 Left posterior hemiblock in a patient with recent inferior myocardial infarction. There is abnormal right axis deviation (about +120°) with an rS pattern in leads I and aVL, and qR patterns with relatively tall R waves in leads II, III, and aVF. The abnormal Q waves and inverted T waves in the inferior leads indicate a recent inferior myocardial infarction. The patient had diffuse, severe, occlusive disease of all major coronary vessels demonstrable on arteriography.

From Friedman, H. H. (1985). *Diagnostic electrocardiography and vectorcardiography.* New York: McGraw-Hill.

or both. This block may also be found, though less commonly, in individuals with cardiomyopathy, calcific aortic stenosis, and hyperkalemia.[7]

Wolff-Parkinson-White Syndrome

Wolff-Parkinson-White (WPW) syndrome is a form of ventricular preexcitation that was first described in 1930. The syndrome, characterized by a short PR interval and an abnormal configuration of the QRS complex, was formerly known as the bundle of Kent syndrome or the anomalous atrioventricular excitation syndrome. The rhythm disturbance occurs when an anomalous atrioventricular conductive pathway allows the atrial impulse to bypass the AV node and excite the ventricles sooner than would be normally expected. These pathways may be located between the free walls of the atria and ventricles or between the atrial and ventricular septa (Figure 10-60).

When the atrial impulse is able to bypass the normal AV conductive pathway in the AV node and His bundle, the normal AV conduction delay does not occur. Consequently, the PR interval is less than normal, usually between 0.08 and 0.12 second (Figure 10-61). If, however, there is a preexisting AV conduction defect, the PR interval may be prolonged and appear normal in the presence of WPW syndrome. The P wave is normal unless there is a coexisting cardiac disease.

The QRS complex in WPW syndrome is almost always prolonged (0.10 second or more). Occasionally it may be less than 0.10 second with the range being 0.08 to 0.16 second. The duration of the QRS is frequently inversely proportional to the PR interval (see Figure 10-61) and is dependent on the degree of preexcitation. The sum of the PR interval and the QRS width (PS interval) (see Figure 10-61) usually is within the normal range.

The characteristic finding in WPW syndrome is the presence of the *delta wave,* the initial slurring of the QRS complex (see Figure 10-61). This slurred initial component of the QRS complex should be present in all leads but may be more visible in some leads than in others (Figure 10-62).

The abnormal sequence of ventricular activation often leads to abnormal repolarization; consequently, secondary S and T wave changes are present (see Figure 10-61). Usually the displacement of the ST segment and the polarity of the T wave are opposite to the direction of the delta wave and the major QRS deflection.

The former delineation of Wolff-Parkinson-White syndrome into two types, A and B, is outdated. Electrophysiology studies are recommended to delineate whether the anomalous pathway involves the left free wall, the right free wall, or the anterior or posterior septum (Figure 10-63). However, the axis of the P wave during the circus movement tachycardia, the

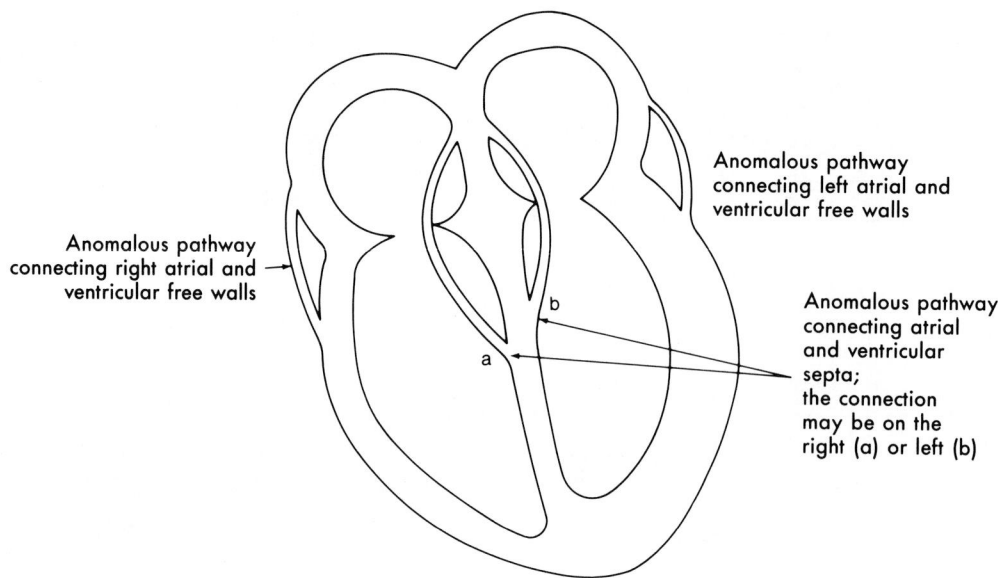

Figure 10-60   Diagrammatic representation of the four anomalous pathways of Wolff-Parkinson-White (WPW) syndrome. See text for discussion.

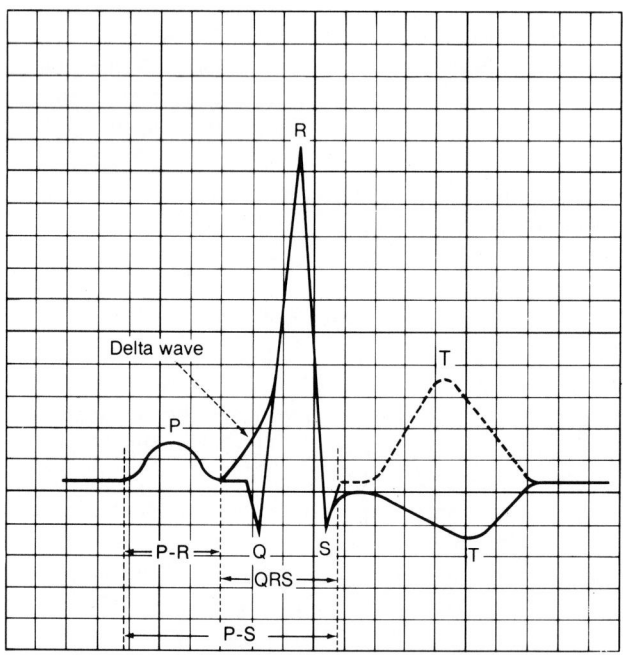

Figure 10-61   The uninterrupted line indicates anomalous conduction in WPW syndrome, whereas the broken line indicates normal conduction. Note the short PR interval, the delta wave, and the secondary T wave change. The PS interval is within the normal range. See text for further discussion.

axis of the delta wave during sinus rhythm, or both, have been used with some success in determining which type of pathway is involved. The conduction is described as *antidromic* when the supraventricular signals enter the ventricles via the accessory pathway in either free wall and conduct retrograde via the AV junction to the atria. In contrast, *orthodromic* conduction refers to the reverse: initiation via the AV junction and retrograde circus movement conduction via the accessory pathway. The term *circus movement tachycardia* (CMT) has been used to describe reentrant mechanisms involving an atrioventricular loop (usually via an accessory pathway) as opposed to reentrant AV nodal dysrhythmias.

Additional data about WPW pathways is available in advanced dysrhythmia and/or electrophysiology textbooks.

The most important clinical manifestations of WPW syndrome are paroxysmal tachydysrhythmias. They have been reported in 13% to 80% of the cases with the incidence being closely related to the population sampled: 13% in routine ECGs from clinically healthy individuals and 40% to 80% in hospitalized or cardiac clinic patients known to have the syndrome.[5,6] Paroxysmal supraventricular tachycardia is the most common form of tachydysrhythmia seen in patients with the syndrome. The tachycardia is a reciprocating or reentrant rhythm often initiated by a single premature atrial or ventricular extrasystole. When the impulse of excitation proceeds antegrade through the AV conduction system and returns to the

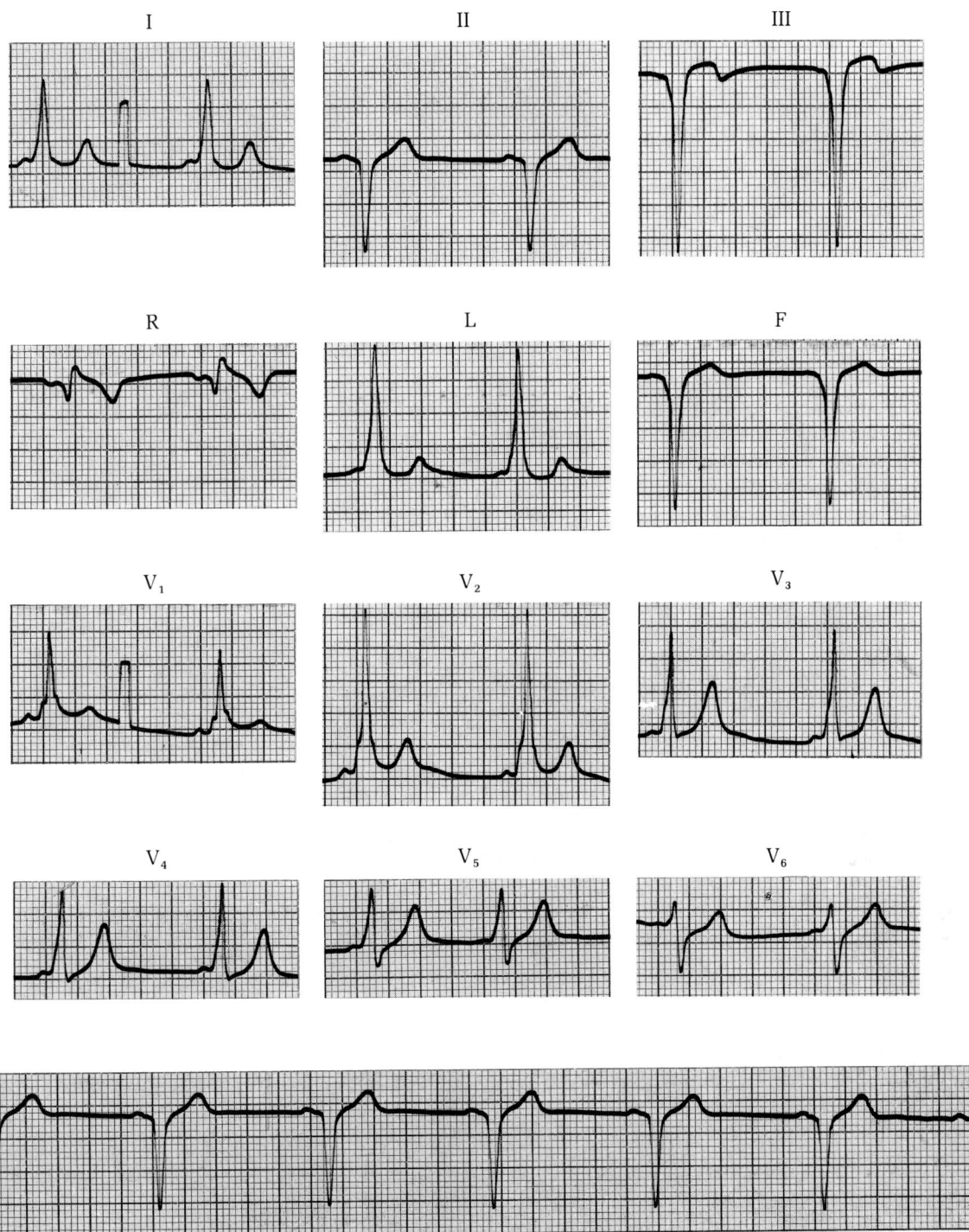

Figure 10-62 Maximal preexcitation from a posterior septal or posterior left ventricular accessory pathway. Note that the delta force actually interrupts the p wave in many leads. Note the QS waves in the inferior leads. These are the result of the orientation of the delta force toward the negative electrode of these leads.

From Conover, M. B. (1992). *Understanding electrocardiography* (6th ed.). St. Louis: Mosby–Year Book.

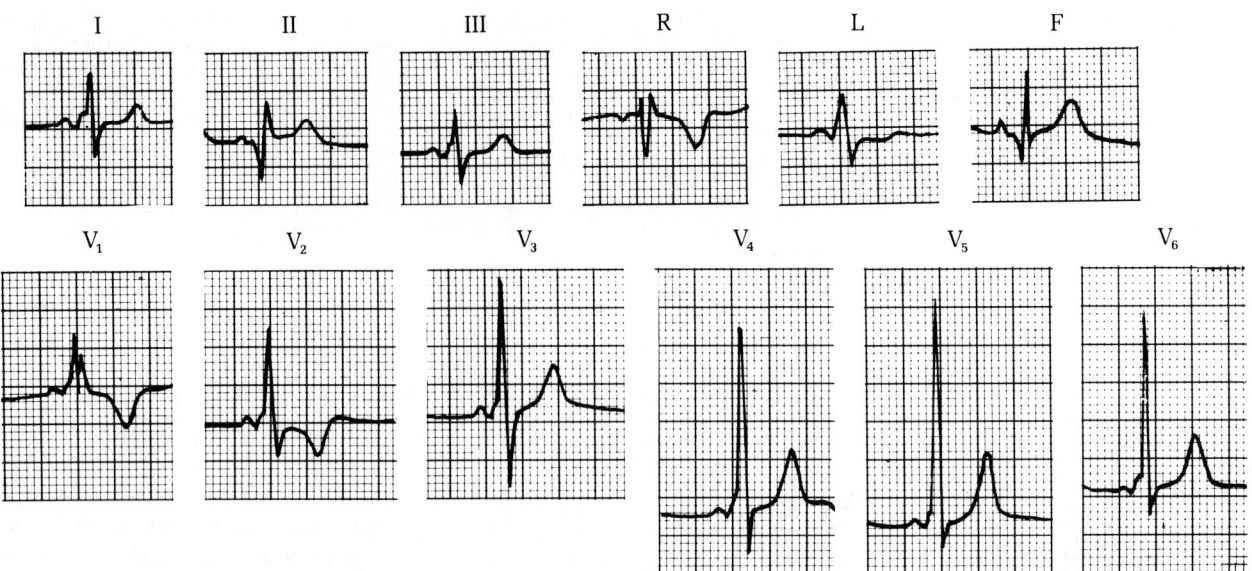

Figure 10-63 WPW syndrome, the result of a lateral left ventricular accessory pathway. Note that the ventricular complex is a fusion beat and that negative delta waves have produced Q waves in leads II and aVF.
From Conover, M. B. (1992). *Understanding electrocardiography* (6th ed.). St. Louis: Mosby–Year Book.

atrium via the bypass tract in a retrograde fashion, the delta wave is not observed, the QRS is normal, and the rate ranges between 140 and 250 beats per minute. Atrial flutter and fibrillation are less common than PSVT in WPW syndrome, but when they are present, the atrial impulses may be conducted to the ventricles via the accessory pathway and result in wide, unusually shaped QRS complexes. The ventricular rate may range from 220 to 360 beats per minute.

Wolff-Parkinson-White syndrome must be differentiated from a number of other ECG abnormalities, including bundle branch block, right ventricular hypertrophy, and myocardial infarction. WPW syndrome and atrial flutter may be mistaken for paroxysmal ventricular tachycardia or ventricular flutter.

Therapy for WPW is not warranted if no tachyarrhythmias are associated with the syndrome. Prevention of and treatment for tachycardias secondary to WPW syndrome, however, are often necessary. Vagal maneuvers may be useful in treating paroxysmal reentrant tachyrhythms, although many patients require antiarrhythmic drug therapy, either acutely or for long-term maintenance. In crisis situations of extremely rapid ventricular response to atrial fibrillation or flutter, direct current shock may be needed. When the dysrhythmias are refractory to conventional therapy, radiofrequency ablation, artificial pacemaker or surgical therapy may be needed.

The most appropriate drug for treating WPW-associated dysrhythmias is dependent on the specific electrophysiological properties of the drug and on the

TABLE 10-4 Effect of Drugs on the Refractory Periods of the Normal AV and Anomalous Pathways

	Effective Refractory Period	
Drugs	**AV Node**	**Accessory Pathway**
Propranolol	Lengthened	No change
Digitalis	Lengthened	Shortened
Lidocaine	No change	Lengthened
Quinidine	Shortened	Lengthened
Procainamide	No change	Lengthened
Phenytoin	Shortened	Variable
Amiodarone	Lengthened	Lengthened
Verapamil	Lengthened	Variable

Adapted from Chung, E. K. (1985). *Electrocardiography: Practical applications with vectorial principles* (p. 331). Norwalk, CT: Appleton-Century-Crofts.

site of the reentry mechanism (that is, the AV nodal conductive pathway or the accessory pathway). The goal of drug therapy is to change the conduction times in the pathways so that reentry is impossible. Table 10-4 lists the effect of antidysrhythmic drugs on the refractory period of the normal and anomalous pathways. Propranolol is frequently the drug of choice for normal QRS width tachycardias associated with WPW syndrome, whereas quinidine and procainamide are used for long-term treatment of reentrant rhythms that are transmitted via antegrade conduction through the accessory pathway (antidromic conduction). Digitalis may be useful in treating rhythms conducted antegrade through the AV node conduction system and retrograde through the bypass tract. However, this drug may enhance the antegrade conduction through the accessory pathway and should be used with caution in conjunction with other antiarrhythmic agents in patients with WPW syndrome and atrial fibrillation or atrial flutter. Amiodarone and verapamil have been found to be useful in treating dysrhythmias in WPW syndrome.

Nursing Management of Patients with Cardiac Dysrhythmias

The relationship between the electrical and mechanical cardiac events as well as their combined effects on cardiac output have been described earlier. It is this relationship that causes patients who are known to have or who are susceptible to developing rhythm disturbances to require close monitoring by the critical care nurse. The nurse must recognize those patients who are at risk for cardiac dysrhythmias, the potentially lethal dysrhythmias, the hemodynamic consequences of rhythm disorders, and the usual or probable therapeutic interventions for each dysrhythmia.

From the sections describing specific rhythm disorders it is clear that organic heart disease places patients in jeopardy for developing cardiac dysrhythmias. However, critically ill individuals suffering from a variety of other body system disorders or trauma are also susceptible to cardiac rhythm disturbances. Neurological trauma may result in abnormalities in the cardiac centers of the brain. Abnormal pulmonary function may cause hypoxia which affects the heart's ability to extract the amount of oxygen necessary for cellular metabolism. Altered renal function may cause electrolyte imbalances which create an abnormal ionic environment for cardiac cells. Consequently, continuous monitoring of the cardiac rhythm is recommended for all critically ill patients, and for certain patients in the acute and ambulatory care settings.

Given the right circumstances, any dysrhythmia may have potentially lethal consequences. However, certain rhythm disorders are known to produce almost immediate life-threatening hemodynamic alterations. In general, any rhythm disturbance that produces a very slow or a rapid ventricular rate is suspect. In addition, dysrhythmias that are known to lead to impending serious rhythm disturbances should be closely monitored. Vigilance on the part of the nurse is critical if the life-threatening consequences of cardiac rhythm disturbances are to be prevented or treated.

Prevention of and treatment for cardiac dysrhythmias is becoming increasingly complex. New anti-arrhythmic agents are being tested and marketed with increasing frequency. Advanced technology is creating more complex and physiologically comparable cardiac pacemakers and internal cardiac defibrillators. These advances require that the critical care nurse know about a vast array of possible therapeutic interventions. Often it is the nurse who is expected to anticipate appropriate antidysrhythmic interventions, to ensure ready availability in the critical care environment, or to administer such measures directly or indirectly.

In addition to recognizing and treating cardiac dysrhythmias, critical care nurses must be able to recognize abnormal ECG consequences associated with electrical device therapy such as artificial cardiac pacemakers and internal cardioverter defibrillators. They must be aware of other cardiac and noncardiac abnormalities that include chamber enlargement, myocardial infarction, and electrolyte imbalance. Also, the critical care nurse must be familiar with the effects of drug therapy on the ECG. A discussion of these topics follows.

ECG Effects of Device Therapy

The mechanical devices available to ensure adequate heart rhythm or to electrically terminate dysrhythmias include temporary and permanent artificial cardiac pacemakers and internal cardioverter-defibrillators (ICDs).

Artificial Cardiac Pacemakers

The electrical signals from the pulse generator of an artificial cardiac pacemaker are transmitted along either (1) transvenous leads to the endocardium of the right atrium and/or ventricle or (2) leads attached to the epicardial surface or screwed into the myocardium. A unipolar system sends the electrical stimulus directly to the lead tip (anode). After the stimulus leaves the lead (and hopefully initiates myocardial depolarization), it passes back through the chest muscles to complete the electrical circuit on the metal can of the pulse generator (cathode). The primary advantage of a unipolar pacing system relates to increased ease of ECG troubleshooting due to the large pacing artifacts.

Bipolar pacemakers also deliver the electrical signal to the anode at the lead tip. However, the cathode completing the electrical circuit is a point of electrical contact a few centimeters back from the lead tip. This smaller circle of electricity in a bipolar pacemaker minimizes the chance that external electrical signals will be transmitted to the pulse generator and interfere with pacemaker function. However, the bipolar pacing artifact is often smaller and more difficult to locate on the surface ECG. Some pacemaker systems

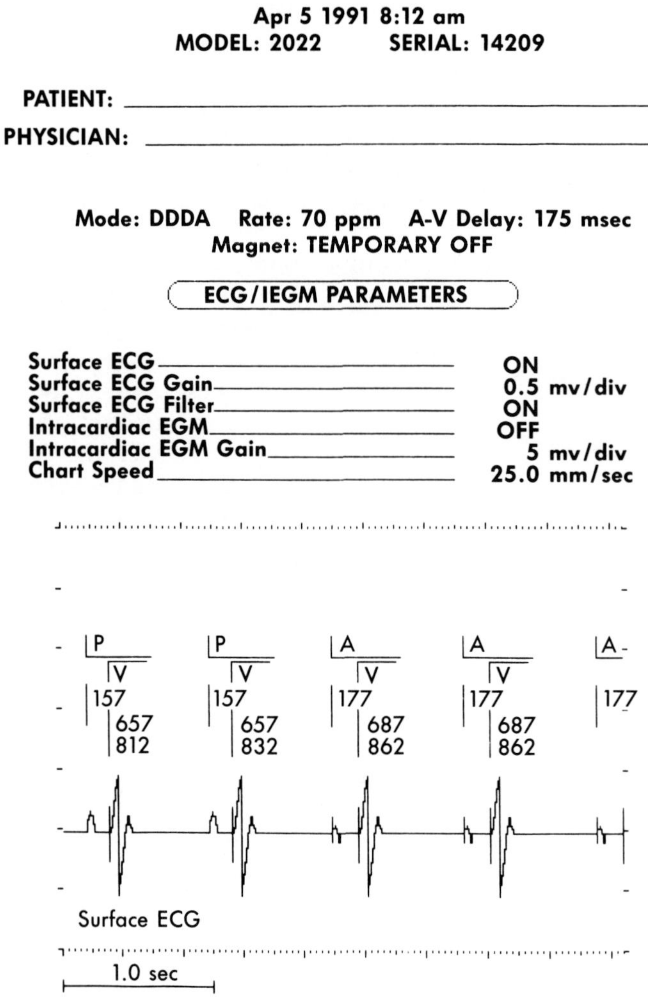

Apr 5 1991 8:12 am
MODEL: 2022   SERIAL: 14209

PATIENT: _____

PHYSICIAN: _____

Mode: DDDA   Rate: 70 ppm   A-V Delay: 175 msec
Magnet: TEMPORARY OFF

(**ECG/IEGM PARAMETERS**)

Surface ECG	ON
Surface ECG Gain	0.5 mv/div
Surface ECG Filter	ON
Intracardiac EGM	OFF
Intracardiac EGM Gain	5 mv/div
Chart Speed	25.0 mm/sec

Surface ECG

1.0 sec

Figure 10-64   Recorded strip of surface ECG from Pacesetter Programmer showing intrinsic and paced electrical events during function of Synchrony II. P = atrial event sensed by pulse generator. V = ventricular pacing. A = atrial pacing. "Live" strip from simulator on programmer.
Courtesy of Pacesetter Systems, Inc.

can be converted from bipolar to unipolar by reprogramming the pulse generator. Troubleshooting pacemaker ECGs has been enhanced by programs that provide enhanced visualization of the heart's electrical events. After ECG leads are attached to the patient, many programmers graphically display the ECG, identify the site of pulse generator firing, and sense other electrical events as well (Figure 10-64).

Since depolarization begins at the point where the electricity first reaches the myocardial cells, the ECG waveform produced by pacing on either or both heart chambers is unique. For example, the P waves initiated by atrial pacing have a different contour than the sinus-initiated P waves. In most cases, a visible pacing artifact precedes the paced atrial event. Likewise, the QRS produced by ventricular pacing has a unique contour, often wide and distorted. Once the pacemaker-initiated waveform is identified, the same

shape is expected with each pacing artifact unless the pacing lead shifts to a new position.

Pacemaker programmers are used to regulate the circuitry of a permanent pulse generator, thereby determining if there will be any interface with the heart's electrical events as well as the type of response. The asynchronous mode is a fixed-rate pacing, useful in rare instances to overdrive certain tachydysrhythmias and in routine checks of the pulse generator. Synchronous modes are demand pacemaker functions. Some pulse generators not only interface with internal heart signals but are programmed to detect and increase their rate with other events such as upper body movement, core body temperature, and respiration rate or depth. Communication among health professionals regarding the variety of pacing modes is facilitated by a code (Figure 10-65).

Normal function of a single-chamber ventricular

Position	I	II	III	IV	V
Category	Chamber(s) paced	Chamber(s) sensed	Response to sensing	Programmability, rate modulation	Antitachyarrhythmia function(s)
	0 = None	0 = None	0 = None	0 = None	0 = None
	A = Atrium	A = Atrium	T = Triggered	P = Simple Programmable	P = Pacing (antitachyarrhythmia)
	V = Ventricle	V = Ventricle	I = Inhibited	M = Multiprogrammable	S = Shock
	D = Dual (A + V)	D = Dual (A + V)	D = Dual (T + I)	C = Communicating	D = Dual (P + S)
				R = Rate modulation	
Manufacturers' designation only	S = single (A or V)	S = single (A or V)			

Note: Positons I through III are used exclusively for antibradyarrhythmia function.

Figure 10-65 NBG (North American Society of Pacing and Electrophysiology/British Pacing Electrophysiology Group) pacemaker code.

From Bernstein, A. D., et al. (1987). The NASPE/BPEG Generic Pacemaker Code for antibradyarrhythmia and adaptive-rate pacing and antiachyarrhythmia devices. *PACE, 10,* 794.

pacemaker (programmed to VVI function) is depicted in Figure 10-66. During this mode of programming, the pulse generator can pace the ventricle at a back-up rate as needed, sense intrinsic QRSs (normal or ectopic), and respond to any sensed QRSs by inhibiting the next pacing artifact.

More recently rate-responsive or rate-modulated ventricular pacing has become popular. Note in Figure 10-67 the normal function of a single-chamber ventricular pacemaker (programmed to VVI^r). This pulse generator paces the ventricle at the low rate when needed, sensing and inhibiting for any intrinsic QRSs at a faster rate. It also adjusts its rate in response to the rate and depth of respiration (Telectronics Meta-MV). Other VVI^r pacemakers use a different sensor to adjust the speed of the pacing signals to episodes of increased demand for cardiac output such as the rate of respiration, body motion, or changes in body temperature.

Figure 10-68 shows normal function of a dual-chamber pacemaker (programmed to DDD function). This pulse generator is capable of pacing the atria and ventricles at the low rate when needed. It can also sense intrinsic P waves or QRSs (normal or ectopic) up to the maximum rate setting. It is expected to trigger (fire) a companion QRS for any intrinsic Ps that do not conduct to the ventricle within the programmed AV delay. Similarly it inhibits for any QRSs

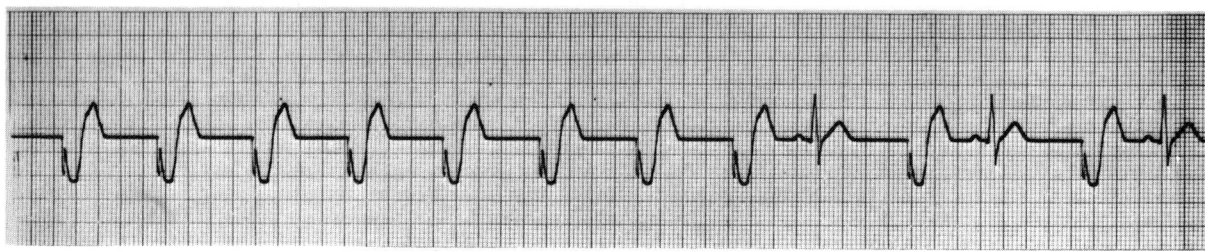

Figure 10-66 1:1 ventricular pacing with three episodes of sinus beats causing inhibition of pulse generator.

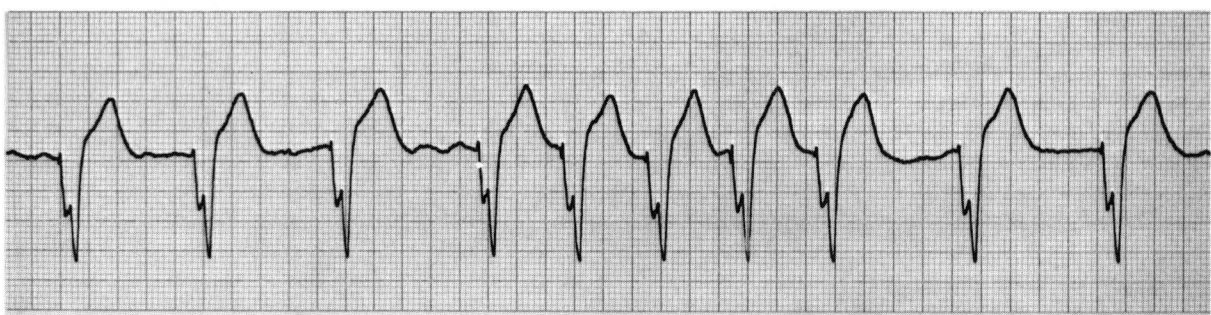

Figure 10-67 VVI^r pacing responding to normal breathing. Sensitivity adjusted so pacer rate would respond less aggressively to such signals.

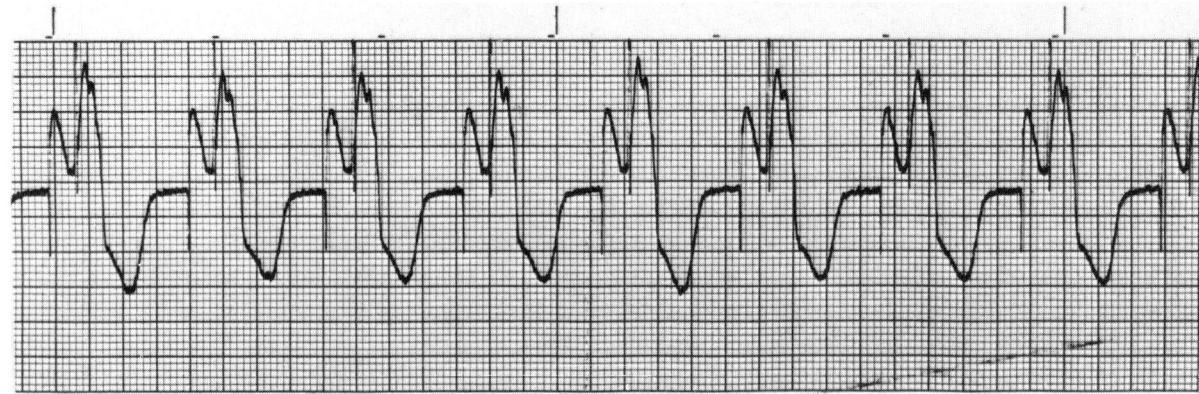

Figure 10-68 Dual chamber pacing at 72 per minute.

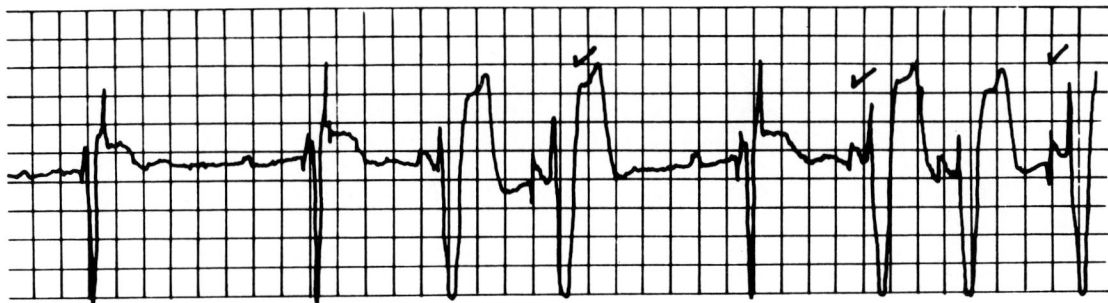

Figure 10-69 Electromagnetic interference (EMI) producing unexplained pauses in DDD pacer operation due to skeletal muscle activity near pulse generator. Simulates failure to fire and/or capture (DDD pacemaker; see usual paced beats).
From Purcell, J. A., & Burrows, S. G. (1985). CE: A pacemaker primer. *American Journal of Nursing, 5,* 56.

that come prior to its time of discharge or for QRSs that are the result of atrial events conducting through the ventricles prior to the end of the AV delay.

Some dual chamber pacemakers also have rate-responsive capability, that is, a DDD^r mode of pacing. Not only does this pacemaker respond to intrinsic atrial and ventricular events, but it can also adjust the pacing rate when signals are detected by a sensor, that is, with respiration, activity, body temperature (or with other events used to sense increased body metabolism).

More recently, antitachycardia pacing has been available for interruption of tachydysrhythmias. Once temporary pacing is proven in the electrophysiology laboratory to terminate a tachydysrhythmia, a permanent pacemaker can be selected with this feature. However, this use has been limited largely to individuals with recurrent atrial tachycardia or flutter. When antitachycardia ventricular pacing has been needed, an internal cardioverter-defibrillator is implanted at the same time to provide back-up defibrillation should the pacing attempts cause tachycardia acceleration or initiate ventricular fibrillation.

As the circuitry for pulse generators becomes increasingly sophisticated, interpreting the electrical consequences on the ECG is more difficult. A complete review of ECG pacemaker troubleshooting intervention is beyond the scope of this text. However, most pacemaker ECG abnormalities fall into one of the following categories:

Failure to emit ("fire") an electrical signal as expected
Failure of pacing artifact to depolarize the intended heart chamber (noncapture or nonconduction)
Failure to sense expected electrical or external events
Inappropriate pacing rates

Failure to Fire (Includes Oversensing). Although failure to fire can be due to a fault in the pacemaker system, one should first rule out oversensing of intrinsic or external electrical events. After it has been determined that pacing artifacts are *not* present as expected, one should investigate for oversensing of intrinsic electrical signals (such as sensing of the T wave as a QRS by a ventricular lead). Another example of oversensing is "crosstalk," where intrinsic electrical events are sensed by a lead in a different heart chamber.

Oversensing can also be due to external electrical signals (electromagnetic interference [EMI]). Often upper body skeletal muscle activity is detected as an "ECG" event, causing the oversensing (Figure 10-69). At other times failure to fire can be due to (1) a break in the pacemaker electrical circuit, such as loose lead–pulse generator connections, (2) fractured lead wire with intact insulation, or (3) depletion of the power source in the pulse generator. Rarely, failure to fire is associated with a feature of normal pacemaker programming: the use of hysteresis, a one-time longer escape interval after sensed electrical events.

Failure to Depolarize Intended Chamber. When the electrical signal does not depolarize the myocardial chamber as expected, one should rule out each of the following: (1) increased resistance to conduction in the myocardial tissues at the lead tip due to bruising or fibrosis, infarction, electrolyte disturbances, or excessive effects of antiarrhythmic medications; (2) lead dislodgement; or (3) simultaneous depolarization of the intended chamber by an intrinsic heart signal. Failure to capture is depicted in Figure 10-70.

Failure of Sensing (Undersensing). When the pulse generator fails to sense intrinsic electrical events, the sensitivity setting on the pulse generator should be evaluated. Adjusting it to the maximum sensitivity may solve the problem. More often the pacing lead is not in good position to detect the electrical signal. In other cases fibrosis may be present at the end of the lead tip or a lead fracture or an insulation or adapter defect may exist. Rarely, nonsensing is due

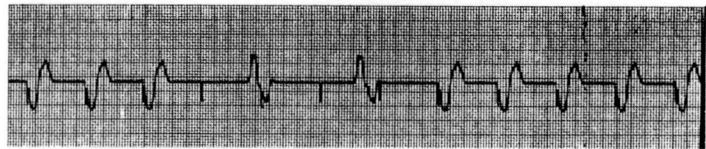

Figure 10-70 VVI pacemaker pacing at 65 per minute × 4 with loss of capture × 4 with 2 non-sensed escape beats during loss of capture.

From Purcell, J. A., Kloosterman, N. D., & Miller, L. K. (1986). Dreifus' pacemaker therapy: An interprofessional approach. In B. Riegel, & J. A. Purcell (Eds.), *Care of the hospitalized patient undergoing pacemaker therapy*. Philadelphia: Davis.

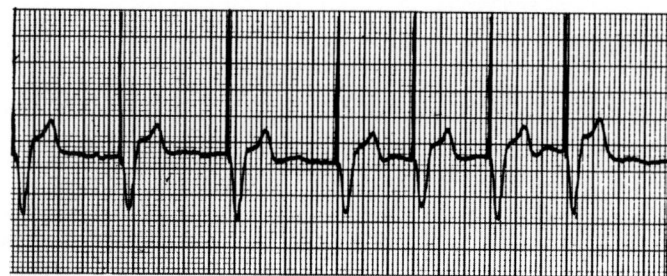

Figure 10-71 Ventricular pacing at 72 per minute for first QRS followed by 4 paced beats at rate of 100. Irregular firing induced by magnet application.

From Purcell, J. A., Kloosterman, N. D., & Miller, L. K. (1986). Dreifus' pacemaker therapy: An interprofessional approach. In B. Reigel, & J. A. Purcell (Eds.), *Care of the hospitalized patient undergoing pacemaker therapy*. Philadelphia: Davis.

to a magnetic field in close proximity to the pulse generator. This may include the presence of a pacemaker magnet over the pulse generator or close contact of the pulse generator with a large running motor (as a boat or car motor), or a "stuck" reed switch which prohibits demand pacemaker function.

Inappropriate Pacing Rates. Component failure is rare in current pulse generators but when it occurs, it allows "runaway" pacemaker rates. Although end-of-life is usually seen as a drop in the programmed or magnetic pacemaker rates, a rate increase could also be a sign of pulse generator failure. However, faster pacemaker rates are expected when there is (1) increased sensor activity to a normally functioning rate-responsive pulse generator unit, (2) application of a pacemaker magnet to the pulse generator for routine checks, or (3) inadvertent or unrecorded changes in pacemaker programming (Figure 10-71).

Internal Cardioverter-defibrillators

Since their approval by the FDA in 1987, internal cardioverter-defibrillators (ICDs) have been implanted in over 50,000 individuals. An ICD includes (1) one or more transvenous leads into the right ventricle, (2) shocking electrodes, and (3) a pulse generator implanted in the lower abdomen. Today's transvenous lead transmits the intrinsic ventricular electrical events to the pulse generator which tracks the ventricular rate. Once commercial ICD pulse generators have pacing options, this same lead will be

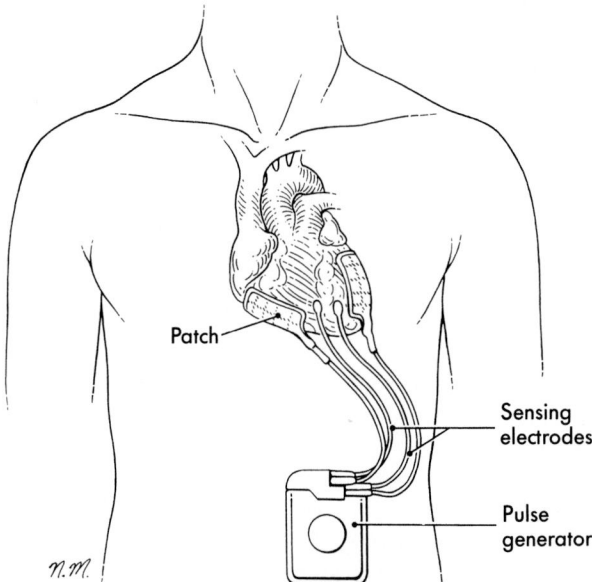

Figure 10-72 Internal Cardioverter-defibrillator. Called Automatic Implantable Cardioverter Defibrillator (AICD) by Cardiac Pacemaker, Incorporated.

Courtesy of Nancy Matthews, Department of Medical Illustrations, Emory University, Atlanta, Georgia.

able to pace the myocardium. (At present, pacing is available only in ICDs under clinical investigation.)

There are several systems for implanting commercially available shock electrodes. Common approaches include two epicardial patches (Figure 10-72) or a superior vena cava (SVC) lead in combination with one epicardial patch. The pulse generators in ICDs now undergoing clinical investigation also have back-up and antitachycardia pacing (ATP or "burst" pacing) along with increasingly sophisticated detection circuitry. At present, ICDs require major chest surgery (subcostal, sternotomy, or left lateral thoracotomy incisions) to implant the shock-delivering electrodes, and an abdominal incision for the pulse generator. However, less invasive surgery is on the horizon. Research suggests that ICD dysrhythmia conversion will be possible in the majority of patients with a patch placed subcutaneously on the left lateral chest along with a transvenous endocardial lead—shocking electrode.

Currently available ICDs provide cardioversion for tachydysrhythmias above the cutoff rate. In some cases additional screening of the QRS morphology (probability density function) is required before the unit discharges so that discharges for supraventricular tachyarrhythmias can be avoided. Although lower energy settings are available in some models, one or more shocks are commonly given at 25 to 30 joules until a new, slower rhythm results or the ICD reaches its shocks-per-episode limit. Once 35 or more seconds of a slower heart rhythm occur, the ICD is expected to reset in readiness for another episode. Up to five defibrillation attempts are provided by currently available ICDs (CPI model 1550/1600) for a continuous dysrhythmia meeting the detection criteria.

Figure 10-73 illustrates conversion of ventricular tachycardia by an ICD to sinus rhythm. Patients with ICDs require close follow-up. CPI models 1550/1600 require re-forming of the capacitors every 2 months for the anticipated 4- to 5-year battery life of the ICD.

Since the shocks are often painful and disruptive to the patient, adjustments must be made from time to time in antidysrhythmic medication to decrease the number of dysrhythmia episodes.

The long-term follow-up of an ICD should include observation for all of the following:
Failure of the ICD to detect and shock a tachydysrhythmia
Failure of the shocks to revert the rhythm to normal
Inappropriate shocks due to oversensing of internal or external electrical events
Appropriate but unnecessary shocks (occurring after short bursts of tachyarrhythmia meet detection criteria but terminate prior to delivery of the shock)
Each of these is briefly described below.

Failure to Detect or Shock. The most common reason an ICD fails to discharge during a tachyarrhythmia relates to the tachycardia cutoff rate. The nurse should always compare the heart rate during the tachycardia to the dysrhythmia cutoff rate of the ICD. It is not uncommon for the patient's tachycardia to have a new rate since the last electrophysiology test. The nurse should also check to see if the ICD is off owing to inadvertent ICD misprogramming or direct contact with a large electromagnetic field. This phenomenon has also occurred when the battery in the ICD pulse generator nears end-of-life. Checking the integrity and position of the sensing leads is also recommended. A device has been made for one type of ICD to simultaneously record the ECG and the signals being sensed by the ICD.

Failure to Revert the Rhythm. When the ICD is

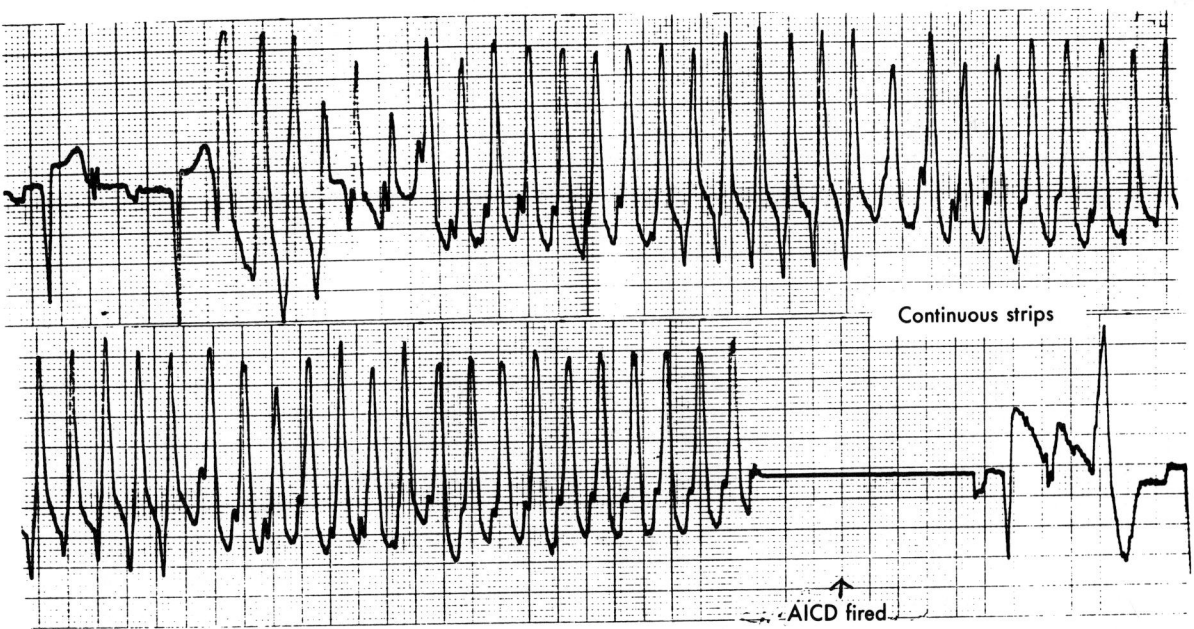

Figure 10-73 Sinus rhythm with 1st-degree AV block with rapid ventricular tachycardia (or flutter) leading to firing of internal cardioverter defibrillator and successful conversion to sinus rhythm followed by 1 PVC.

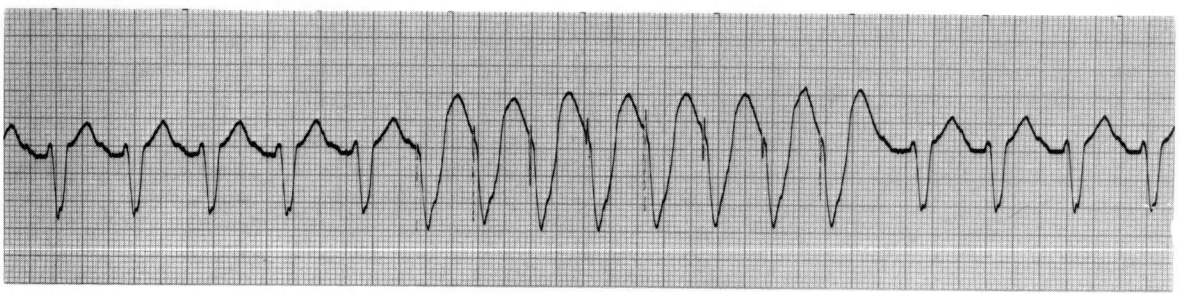

Figure 10-74   Sinus tachycardia, 1st-degree AV block and left bundle branch block with 8 cycles of 1:1 ventricular burst pacing from a Telectronics Guardian ICD followed by a continuation of sinus tachycardia.

programmed to detect only heart rate, it cannot distinguish between sinus tachycardia and supraventricular and ventricular tachyarrhythmias. Unless the body demands decrease, sinus tachycardia is likely to continue despite one or more shocks from an ICD. However, supraventricular tachycardias rarely respond to the 25 to 30 joules of an ICD and multiple ineffective shocks are likely until the rhythm reverts. When ventricular dysrhythmias are not converted by the ICD, one should evaluate for myocardial ischemia, infarction, or fibrosis at the patch–myocardial interface as well as obtain a chest x-ray to evaluate the possibility of migration of the SVC lead (if such a lead is in place). In addition, certain antiarrhythmic medications can increase the defibrillation threshold, requiring more energy than available in an ICD for conversion of the dysrhythmia. In some cases even though the ICD appears to have an adequate battery, a reduced energy source can be detected by a failure to convert the rhythm.

Inappropriate Shocks due to Oversensing. When an ICD is placed along with a separate permanent pacemaker, a bipolar system is advisable to minimize the potential for the ICD to oversense the pacing artifact. Otherwise, the ICD is likely to detect both the QRS and the pacing spike, counting the double heart rate. In some cases, ICDs have sensed large T waves or electromagnetic interference (EMI) in addition to the basic heart rate and shocked inappropriately.

Short Runs of Dysrhythmia / "Appropriate" Shocks. Occasionally patients will experience short runs of a tachydysrhythmia that are long enough to be detected by the ICD but not long enough to continue until the ICD is charged and the shock delivered. Often the ICD will be turned off during hospitalization while IV medications are given to decrease the number of ectopic events. Some ICDs can be reprogrammed to lengthen the sensing requirements.

Failure to Revert the Rhythm. The newer ICDs (under clinical investigation) offer ventricular burst pacing, allowing one or more bursts of fixed-rate rapid pacing artifact during the tachycardia in an attempt to terminate the episode. Although some patients notice minor symptoms at the outset of the dysrhythmia, burst pacing usually offers no discomfort to the patient. These ICDs cannot differentiate between supraventricular and ventricular tachycardia and will attempt burst pacing for any heart rate above the ICD cutoff rate; the device will therefore attempt dysrhythmia conversion with burst pacing (Figure 10-74).

Antitachycardia pacing is more likely to terminate monomorphic ventricular tachycardia at rates lower than 170 per minute rather than polymorphic ventricular tachycardia. If the morphology of the tachycardia has changed since EP testing, discontinuation of some antiarrhythmic agents or the addition of others may be needed to return the rate and type of ventricular tachycardia to a monomorphic variety.

Chamber Enlargement

Characteristics of cardiac *hypertrophy*, an increase in the size of the cardiac muscle fibers secondary to increased pressure loads, and cardiac *dilatation*, an increase in a chamber's diameter secondary to increased volume loads, are virtually indistinguishable on the ECG. Consequently, the term *chamber enlargement* has been adopted by many to refer to either hypertrophy or dilatation of a cardiac muscle mass or chamber. Diagnostic ECG criteria for atrial and ventricular enlargement are presented in this section.

Atrial Abnormality, Enlargement, or Hypertrophy

The normal configuration for the P wave has already been described (see Waves, Complexes, and Intervals in this chapter). An abnormality in the voltage, duration, morphology, or direction of the P wave usually indicates either the enlargement of one or both of the atrial chambers or an intra- or interatrial conduction defect. The specific diagnosis for the P wave alteration cannot be made with certainty by electrocardiography; therefore, the term *atrial abnormality* more correctly describes alterations in P wave morphology and is being used more frequently for this

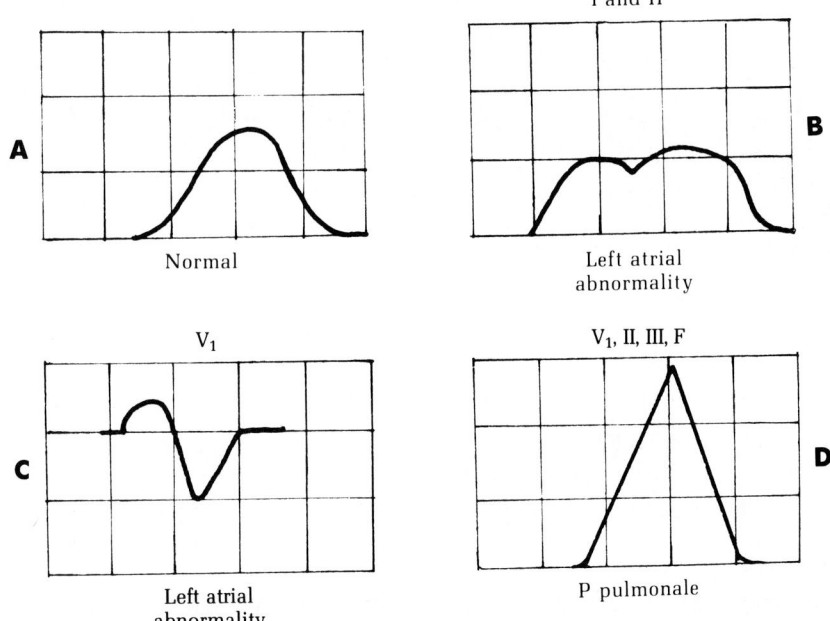

Figure 10-75   The normal P wave *(A)* compared with the P wave in left atrial abnormality *(B, C)* and P pulmonale *(D)*. From Conover, M. B. (1992). *Understanding electrocardiography* (6th ed.). St. Louis: Mosby–Year Book.

purpose. The term *atrial enlargement* is used in this chapter only because it is the term commonly used in clinical practice.

Left Atrial Enlargement.   Depolarization of the left atrium is represented on the ECG by the mid- and late portions of the P wave. Therefore, if activation of the left atrium is abnormal, the ECG reflects the abnormality via changes in the mid- and terminal components of the P wave. Diagnostic criteria for left atrial enlargement (LAE) are:

1. P-terminal force in leads V_{1-2} equal to or greater than 1 mm in both width and depth (Figure 10-75)
2. P wave duration prolonged at 0.12 second or more
3. Notched and slurred P wave with a peak-to-peak interval of 0.04 second in leads I, II, and aVL (see Figure 10-75)

Other authors require that the ratio of the duration of the P wave to the PR segment be greater than 1.60[5] and that the P axis be between 0 and +45° in the frontal plane.

Figure 10-76 is an ECG from a patient with mitral stenosis. Note the ECG characteristics of LAE.

Left atrial enlargement is commonly the result of mitral valve disease, particularly mitral stenosis. For this reason, the term *P mitrale* is often used when referring to the P wave of LAE. A useful clue for remembering the ECG criteria of LAE is to associate this term with the "M-shaped" (for mitral) or wide, notched P wave characteristic of *left* atrial enlargement due to mitral valve disease.

Other conditions in which the ECG characteristics

of left atrial enlargement may be found include aortic valve disease, coronary artery disease, acute myocardial infarction, acute pulmonary edema, constrictive pericarditis, hypertrophic obstructive cardiomyopathy (HOCM), dilated cardiomyopathy, coarctation of the aorta, endocardial cushion defects, and other conditions causing diastolic overloading of the left ventricle. Patients with systemic hypertension also frequently demonstrate characteristics of LAE on their ECGs.

Right Atrial Enlargement.   The initial component of the normal P wave reflects depolarization of the right atrium. Hence, when the right atrium is enlarged, the initial component of the P wave is altered. Diagnostic criteria for right atrial enlargement (RAE) are:

1. Tall, peaked (or tent-shaped) P waves with a height of 2.5 mm[5,6] or more in leads II, III, and aVF
2. Normal P wave duration
3. P axis of 75° or greater in the frontal plane
4. A positive deflection of the P wave in leads V_{1-2} with a height of 1.5 mm[5,6] or more

Figure 10-77 illustrates the ECG changes found in a patient with RAE. The patient in this example had cor pulmonale, which is a common cause of RAE. The term *P pulmonale* is used to describe the tall, thin, peaked P wave of RAE secondary to chronic lung disease, coronary artery disease, acute left ventricular failure, or hypoxemia.[6] It should be noted, however, that actual right atrial enlargement is demonstrable in only about one half of the patients

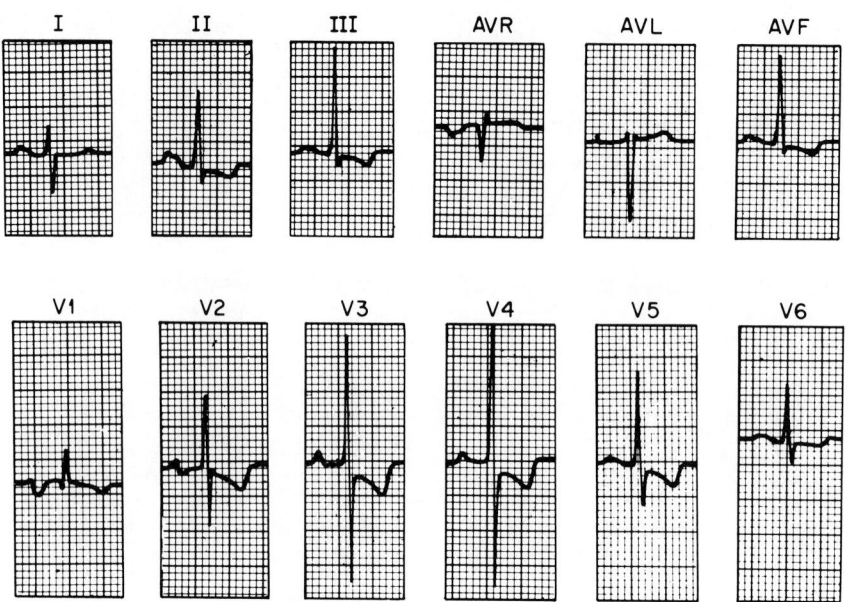

Figure 10-76   Left atrial and right ventricular enlargement and right ventricular strain in a patient with mitral stenosis. The P waves are broad and notched. There is a qR pattern with an inverted T wave in lead V₁. The ST segments are depressed and the T waves inverted in the precordial leads.

From Friedman, H. H. (1985). *Diagnostic electrocardiography and vectorcardiography*. New York: McGraw-Hill.

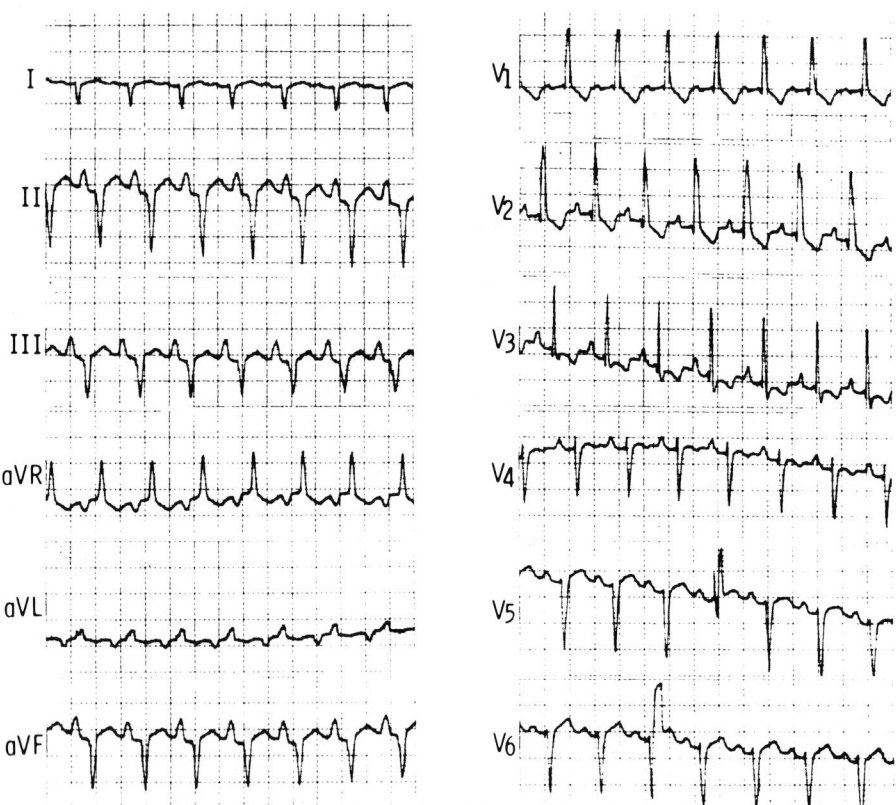

Figure 10-77   Right atrial and ventricular enlargement and right ventricular strain in a patient with advanced chronic cor pulmonale. The P waves are tall and peaked. The QRS axis is +250°. There are tall R waves in leads V₁ through V₃ with secondary T wave changes.

From Chung, E. K., & Chung, D. K. (1972). *ECG diagnosis: Self assessment*. New York: Harper & Row.

displaying the P pulmonale pattern. Occasionally, the P pulmonale pattern represents left atrial enlargement or another condition. The finding of P pulmonale in association with the finding of an abnormal P terminal force in lead V_1 and in the presence of left ventricular enlargement (LVE) favors LAE as the cause of the P pulmonale pattern. The converse of this, P pulmonale without the P terminal force in lead V_1 and LVE, but with ECG changes consistent with right ventricular enlargement (RVE) or pulmonary disease, favors RAE.

Biatrial Enlargement. When both atrial chambers are enlarged the characteristics of both right and left atrial enlargement coexist on the ECG. The diagnostic criteria for biatrial enlargement are:

1. Tall (2.5 mm or more) and wide (3 mm or more) P waves in the limb leads
2. Large diphasic P waves in the right precordial leads (V_{1-2}) with the initial component greater than 1.5 mm and the terminal component deeper and wider than 1 mm
3. Tall, peaked P waves (greater than 1.5 mm) in V_{1-2} and wide, notched P waves in the limb leads or left precordial leads (V_{5-6})[5,7]

It is important to note that the electrocardiographic findings for biatrial enlargement are largely dependent on the degree of atrial abnormality. Biatrial enlargement is found clinically in people with certain congenital heart diseases, cardiomyopathy, and rheumatic heart disease.

Ventricular Hypertrophy or Enlargement

Before considering the electrocardiographic findings associated with ventricular enlargement, it is use-ful to review the characteristics of the normal ECG (see Table 10-2), paying particular attention to the amplitude, R wave progression, intrinsicoid deflection, and axis of the QRS; the configuration of the ST segment; and the direction and shape of the T wave. This review is important because ventricular enlargement alters these elements of the ECG.

Echocardiography is far superior to electrocardiography in the diagnoses of left, right, and biventricular enlargement. However, some of the more commonly used ECG criteria for chamber enlargement are presented here.

Left Ventricular Enlargement. Left ventricular enlargement (LVE) may be secondary to either systolic overload or diastolic overload. Systolic overload of the left ventricle occurs when there is resistance to left ventricular ejection. Common causes of LVE secondary to systolic overload are systemic hypertension, aortic stenosis, and coarctation of the aorta. Diastolic overload of the left ventricle occurs when there is increased diastolic volume and pressure. The common causes of this type of overload include aortic insufficiency, mitral insufficiency, patent ductus arteriosus, and ventricular septal defect.

The most notable electrocardiographic change in LVE secondary to either systolic or diastolic overload is increased voltage of the QRS (Figure 10-78). Frequently the duration of the QRS is prolonged slightly, but it is not greater than 0.12 second. The QRS axis may be deviated to the left. Occasionally the onset of the intrinsicoid deflection is delayed in V_6. The direction of the ST and T vectors in the left limb and precordial leads is altered so that they point in a direction opposite to that of the QRS. This ST, T wave

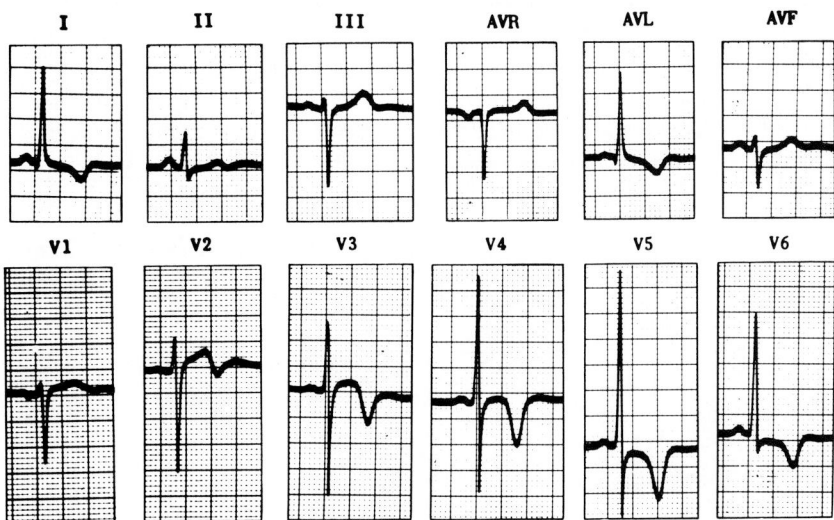

Figure 10-78 Left ventricular enlargement and strain. There is high voltage in leads aVL and V_5. The R in V_5 exceeds 30 mm. The QRS axis is +15°. The ST segments and T waves show changes characteristic of the strain pattern. This is an example of systolic overloading of the left ventricle in a patient with hypertensive heart disease.

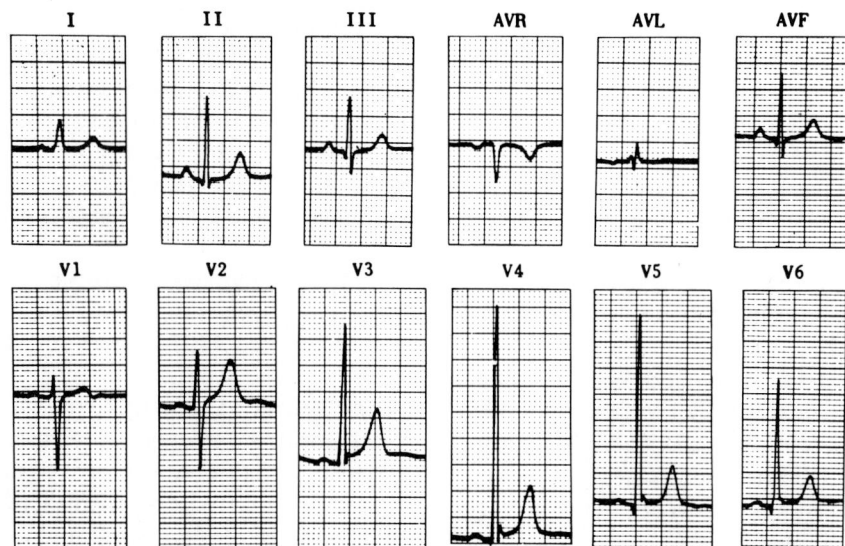

Figure 10-79 Left ventricular enlargement in an adult with aortic insufficiency. There is no deviation of the electrical axis. There is high voltage of the R waves in lead V_4 and V_5. The sum of the maximum R wave (lead V_4) and the maximum S wave (lead V_1) in the precordial leads exceeds 45 mm. The ST segments and the T waves are normal. This is an example of diastolic overloading of the left ventricle.

From Friedman, H. H. (1985). *Diagnostic electrocardiography and vectorcardiography.* New York: McGraw-Hill.

change is known as the *left ventricular strain pattern* and resembles a backward check mark (↘). The ST segment slopes gradually downward into the initial component of the T wave and the terminal component of the T wave slopes upward more rapidly. The strain pattern is generally associated with LVE secondary to systolic overload and is found more often in long-standing LVE. The pattern is intensified when dilatation and failure set in. It is important to note that the typical strain pattern found in systolic overload of the left ventricle is absent in diastolic overload of the chamber (Figure 10-79). Rather, the T waves are tall and upright in the left precordial leads of patients with diastolic overload of the left ventricle. In addition, the depth of the Q wave and the height of the R wave in leads V_{5-6} is greater in diastolic than in systolic overload LVE.

Romhilt and Estes[9] developed a point-score system for the diagnosis of LVE. This is considered to be one of the better methods for diagnosing LVE and is reproduced in Table 10-5. Other criteria also may be used to diagnose LVE (Table 10-6).[2,5,6,7] The electrocardiographic diagnosis of LVE is made when one or more of these criteria are identified and the QRS is less than 0.12 second.

It must be pointed out that a diagnosis of LVE based only on voltage criteria may be false-positive because the ECGs of some normal individuals show increased voltage in the absence of LVE. These individuals may be elderly and emaciated or may be adolescents or young adults. False-positive diagnoses may also be made when LVE is diagnosed in the

TABLE 10-5 Romhilt and Estes Point-Score System for the ECG Diagnosis of Left Ventricular Hypertrophy[9]

Characteristics			Points
1. QRS amplitude:			3
(R or S in limb lead	20 mm or more, or		
S in V_1 or V_2	30 mm or more, or		
R in V_5 or V_6	30 mm or more)		
2. ST segment (ST segment deviation in a direction opposite to that of the main deflection of the QRS):			
Without digitalis			3
(With digitalis)			(1)
3. Left atrial involvement (P terminal forces in V_1 is ≥1 mm in depth and ≥0.04 sec in duration)			3
4. Left axis deviation ≥ −30°			2
5. QRS duration ≥0.09 sec			1
6. Intrinsicoid deflection in V_5 or V_6 ≥0.05.			1
		Maximum total	13

Five points are read as LVH.
Four points are read as probable LVH.

TABLE 10-6 Diagnostic Criteria for Left Ventricular Enlargement[2,5,6,7]

Voltage of the QRS*	
Limb leads:	
R in I + S in III	More than 25 mm, or
R in I	More than 13 mm, or
S in aVR	More than 14 mm, or
R in aVL	More than 11 mm, or
R in aVF	More than 20 mm
Chest leads:	
S in V_1 or V_2 + R in V_5 or V_6	
In adults >30 years old	More than 35 mm
In adults 20-30 years old	More than 40 mm
In adults 16-20 years old	More than 60 mm, or
R in V_5	More than 26 mm, or
R in V_6	More than 20 mm, or
R + S in any V lead	More than 45 mm
Intrinsicoid Deflection (optional for diagnosis)*	
V_1 and V_2	Normal
V_5 and V_6	≥ 0.045 sec
ST segment and T wave changes*	
Left ventricular strain pattern in V_4 to V_6; in I, II, and aVL when mean QRS axis is horizontal; and in II, III, and aVF when the mean QRS axis is vertical.	

* These criteria are applicable only if the duration of the QRS is <0.12 second.

Diagnostic Criteria for Right Ventricular Enlargement[5,6,7]

1. Right axis deviation
2. r/S ratio in V_1 >1.0 and in V_{5-6} ≤ 1.0
3. Tall (or relatively tall) R wave in V_1
4. RR′ pattern in V_1
5. Deep S waves in I, aVL, and V_{4-6}

Diagnostic Criteria for Biventricular Enlargement[7]

1. Left ventricular enlargement pattern in the precordial leads and right axis deviation
2. Right ventricular enlargement pattern in the precordial leads and left axis deviation
3. Tall (or relatively tall) R waves in all precordial leads
4. Equiphasic QRS (RS pattern) complexes in the midleft precordial leads (Katz-Wachtel phenomenon)

---

presence of complete or incomplete LBBB. Accurate diagnosis of LVE may be made only when the LBBB is intermittent.[7] False-negative interpretations may be made in some individuals whose ECGs fail to record voltages exceeding maximum normal values.[6] Consequently, when making an electrocardiographic diagnosis of LVE, it is wise to evaluate carefully other factors such as body build, thickness of chest wall, and the underlying disease process.

Right Ventricular Enlargement. Like LVE, right ventricular enlargement (RVE) may be secondary to either systolic or diastolic overload. Pulmonary stenosis, pulmonary hypertension, tetralogy of Fallot, mitral stenosis, and chronic cor pulmonale are potential causes of systolic overload of the right ventricle. Diastolic overload may be caused by atrial septal defect or tricuspid insufficiency. If the resultant hypertrophy of either type of overload is mild, the ECG may not be sensitive enough to detect changes. Consequently, only marked RVE can be diagnosed with certainty on ECG (Figure 10-76).

Early ECG changes consistent with RVE are right axis deviation of the QRS and alteration of the r/S ratio in lead V_1. These changes result from the electrocardiographic dominance of the right ventricular muscle mass. The diagnostic criteria for RVE are summarized in the upper box on this page. Note that these criteria do not include a prolongation of the QRS width. This is because activation of even a mark-

edly enlarged right ventricle requires no more time than does the activation of the normal left ventricle.

The electrocardiographic findings associated with RVE may resemble those of other cardiac abnormalities. Specifically, RVE must be differentiated from a normal vertical heart, RBBB, posterior wall myocardial infarction, some types of accessory pathway conduction, left posterior hemiblock, and pseudo–right axis deviation because of a high lateral wall myocardial infarction. The QRS duration may serve as a clue when distinguishing between RVE and RBBB. The presence of a delta wave will assist with the differentiation of RVE and WPW. Distinguishing between primary and secondary ST, T wave changes will aid in the correct diagnosis of RVE versus myocardial infarction.

Biventricular Enlargement. Electrocardiographic diagnosis of biventricular enlargement is extremely difficult, especially in adults. The electrical potentials generated from the increased muscle mass of both ventricles may cancel each other so that no ECG changes indicative of ventricular enlargement are present. If one ventricle is more hypertrophied than the other, evidence of enlargement of the dominant ventricle appears. Only rarely are the signs of both left and right ventricular enlargement present on the ECG.

The diagnostic criteria of biventricular enlargement are summarized in the lower box above.[7] These findings may be present in ECGs from individuals with certain congenital lesions, cardiomyopathy, and multivalvular lesions.

Myocardial Infarction

An extended loss of blood supply to the myocardium that results in tissue death or necrosis is termed *myocardial infarction (MI)*. During an acute infarct, the necrotic tissue is surrounded by an area of injured myocardium and an area of ischemic myocardium (Figure 10-80). Each of these areas of abnormality—infarction, injury, and ischemia—produces characteristic changes in the ECG which make it possible to diagnose the specific tissue abnormality.

Characteristic ECG Changes

Necrotic myocardial tissue cannot depolarize or repolarize. Leads in which the positive electrode faces the infarcted tissue, described as *indicative*, or *direct leads*, "look through" the infarcted tissue and record the electrical activity from the opposite side of the heart (Figure 10-80). The indicative leads "see" the electrical potential move from the endocardial to the epicardial surface on the opposite myocardial wall. Because the wave of depolarization is moving away from the positive electrode, a negative deflection or Q wave is recorded on the ECG. *Reciprocal leads*, those in which the positive electrode faces the portion of the heart opposite to the infarct, record the normal endocardial to epicardial depolarization of the unaffected tissue. Because this wave of electrical potential is directed toward a positive electrode, a positive deflection or R wave is produced (see Figure 10-80). The R wave is frequently larger than normal because there are no opposing forces at the site of the infarct.

As noted earlier, Q waves produced by septal depolarization are normal in certain leads (see Table 10-2). Q waves caused by myocardial infarction may be distinguished from normal Q waves because they are larger and last longer. Pathological Q waves, those resulting from myocardial infarction, are equal to or greater than 0.04 second in duration and/or are equal to or larger than 25% of the following R wave.

The injured tissue surrounding the necrotic myocardium depolarizes incompletely and, therefore, remains electrically more positive than uninjured tissue at the end of depolarization. The relative positive electrical potential produces ST segment elevation in the indicative leads and ST segment depression in the reciprocal leads (see Figure 10-80). The elevated ST segment is typically convex upward, may be associated with larger T waves of the usual polarity (hyperacute Ts), and eventually terminates into an inverted T wave. The inverted T wave may or may not

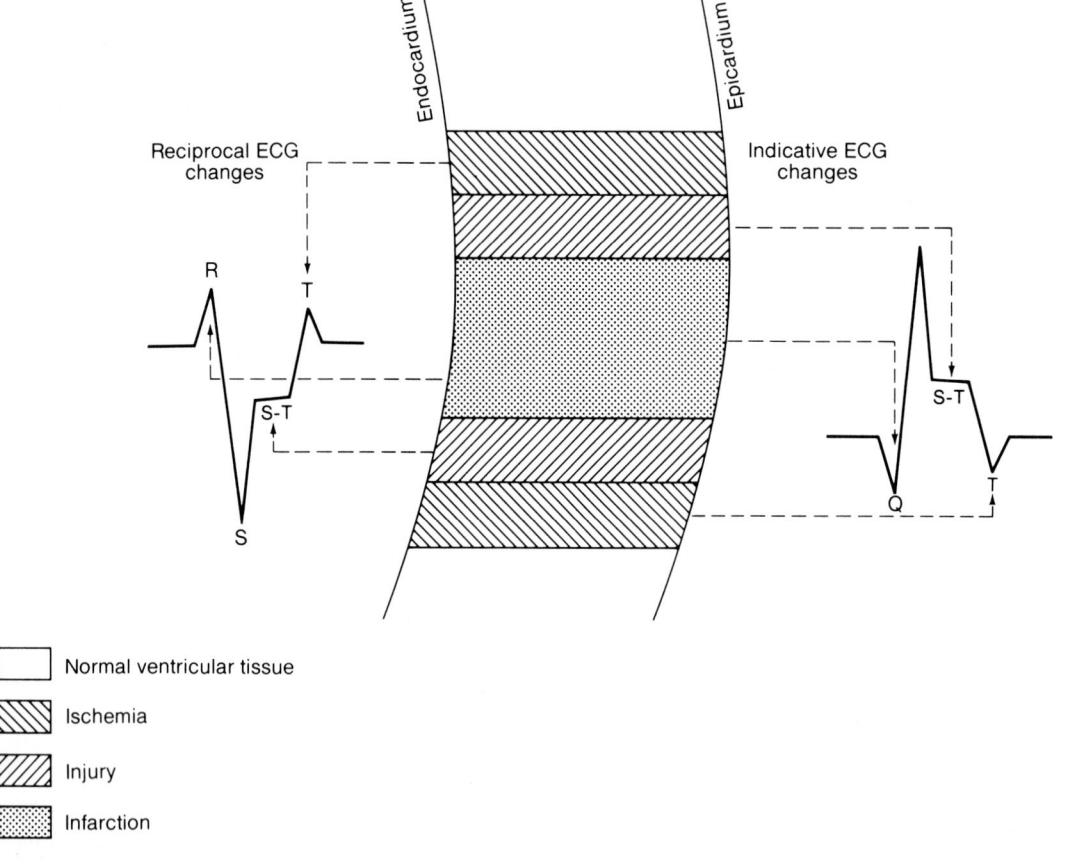

Figure 10-80 Transmural myocardial ischemia, injury, and infarction. During the acute myocardial infarction, the electrocardiogram discloses all three states. Indicative lead changes are shown on the right. Reciprocal lead changes are on the left.

be evident, depending on the age of the infarct.

Myocardial ischemia associated with an MI manifests itself on the ECG as primary inversion of the T wave in the indicative leads. These T waves are symmetrically inverted as opposed to the asymmetrically inverted T waves associated with ventricular strain and bundle branch block. Primary inversion of the T wave is thought to be due to the delay in the repolarization process which causes the ischemic zone to be electrically more negative than the unaffected area. The positive electrode facing the ischemic zone records an inverted T wave because it "sees" this increased negativity. Reciprocal leads record tall, peaked T waves (see Figure 10-80).

The ECG changes associated with myocardial infarction can be summarized as follows:
Indicative lead changes:
1. Q waves equal to or greater than 0.04 second in duration and/or equal to or larger than 25% of the associated R wave
2. ST segment elevation (positive hyperacute T waves in some cases)
3. T wave inversion
Reciprocal lead changes (when present):
1. Tall or relatively tall R waves with the initial vector greater than 0.04 second in duration
2. ST segment depression
3. Tall, peaked T waves
Although myocardial infarction can occur without any changes in the QRS complex, ST segment, or T wave, visualizing the classic ECG signs of infarct can confirm clinical impressions or enzyme alterations and avert further diagnostic testing to determine the cause of the symptoms.

Transmural versus Subendocardial Infarction

As discussed in Chapter 22, myocardial infarction may be classified into two types: *transmural* and *non-transmural*. The previously described ECG changes generally apply to transmural infarcts. Subepicardial and intramural infarcts result in ECG changes very similar to those of transmural infarcts. Subendocardial infarcts are more difficult to diagnose with certainty.

The term subendocardial infarction is generally applied to infarction involving less than the inner half of the total thickness of the ventricular wall. The ECG findings most consistently associated with acute subendocardial infarction are ST segment depression and elevation of the terminal component of the upright T waves in the leads facing the epicardial surface overlying the infarcted subendocardium. QRS changes are more variable. Typically, there is no appreciable change in the QRS complex, and the event is known as a non–Q wave infarct. However, some patients with subendocardial infarcts do demonstrate abnormal Q waves. Because of the variability of the ECG changes associated with subendocardial infarction, it is probably best that the diagnosis of this infarct type not be made from the ECG alone.

Localization of Infarcts to Anatomic Site

The anatomical site of an infarct can be located by identifying the ECG leads in which diagnostic signs of myocardial infarction appear in the QRS. Leads in which only ST segment and T wave changes are recorded are not usually helpful in localizing the infarct, but they may provide information regarding the extent of the injured and ischemic zones.

The four major infarct sites include the anterior, lateral, inferior, and posterior walls of the left ventricle (Figure 10-81). Anterior wall infarction is frequently more specifically described as anteroseptal, anteroapical, anterolateral, or extensive anterior wall infarction. A lateral infarct is occasionally described as high lateral or superior lateral infarction. Inferior wall infarction is sometimes identified as diaphragmatic wall infarction. Historically, the term *posterior* was used to describe what we now know to be inferior infarcts, so it is not uncommon to find posterior infarcts referred to as "true" posterior infarcts to distinguish between the old and new terms.

Infarcts localized in the anterior, lateral, and inferior walls produce indicative ECG changes because positive electrodes for specific leads face the infarcted site. Posterior wall infarction, however, is diagnosed when reciprocal ECG changes occur in the anterior leads. Because there are no positive electrodes facing the infarcted posterior wall, the reciprocal leads must be relied upon for diagnostic information. Following is a list of myocardial infarction sites and the associated ECG criteria.

Anteroseptal MI: Q or QS waves in leads V_{1-3} and sometimes V_4 (Figure 10-82)

Anteroapical (midanterior or localized anterior) MI: Q or QS waves in leads V_{2-4} with normal rS waves in lead V_1 and Q waves in leads I, aVL, and V_6 or decreased amplitude of the initial R waves in V_{1-4} (Figure 10-83)

Anterolateral MI: Q or QS waves in leads I, aVL, and V_{4-6} (Figure 10-84)

Extensive anterior MI: Q or QS waves in leads I, aVL, and V_{1-6} (Figure 10-85)

Lateral (superior or high lateral) MI: Q or QS waves in leads I and aVL (Figure 10-86)

Inferior (diaphragmatic) MI: Q or QS waves in two of the three inferior leads—II, III, and aVF (Figure 10-87)

Posterior ("true" posterior) MI: Tall or relatively tall R waves in leads V_{1-3} with the initial R wave duration equal to or greater than 0.04 second and the R/S ratio equal to or greater than 1 (Figure 10-88)

Text continued on p. 290.

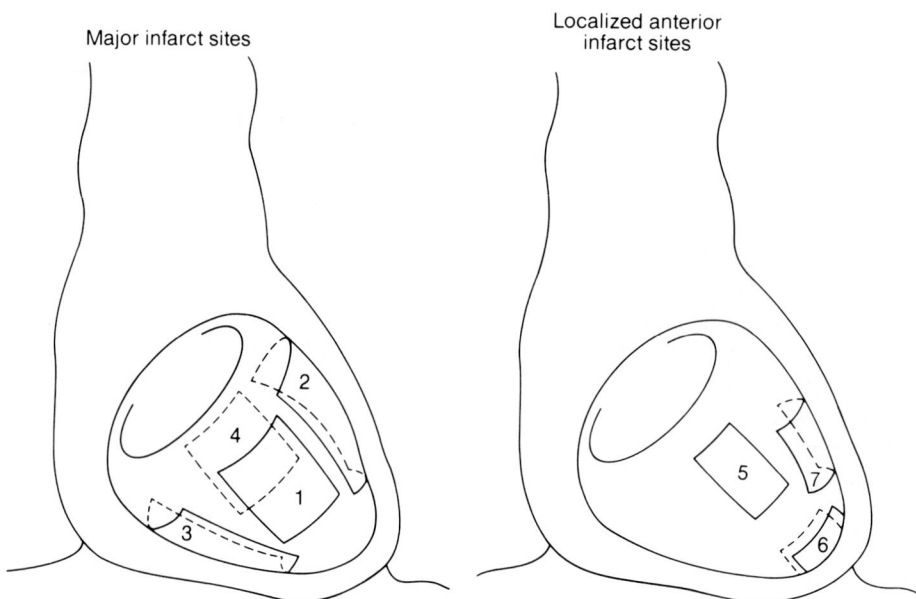

Figure 10-81   Major sites of myocardial infarction in the left ventricle. (1) Anterior wall, (2) lateral wall, (3) inferior wall, and (4) posterior wall. Anterior infarcts can be further localized to the (5) anteroseptal, (6) anteroapical, (7) antero-lateral, and extensive anterior walls.

Adapted from Friedman, H. H. (1985). *Diagnostic electrocardiography and vectorcardiography.* New York: McGraw-Hill.

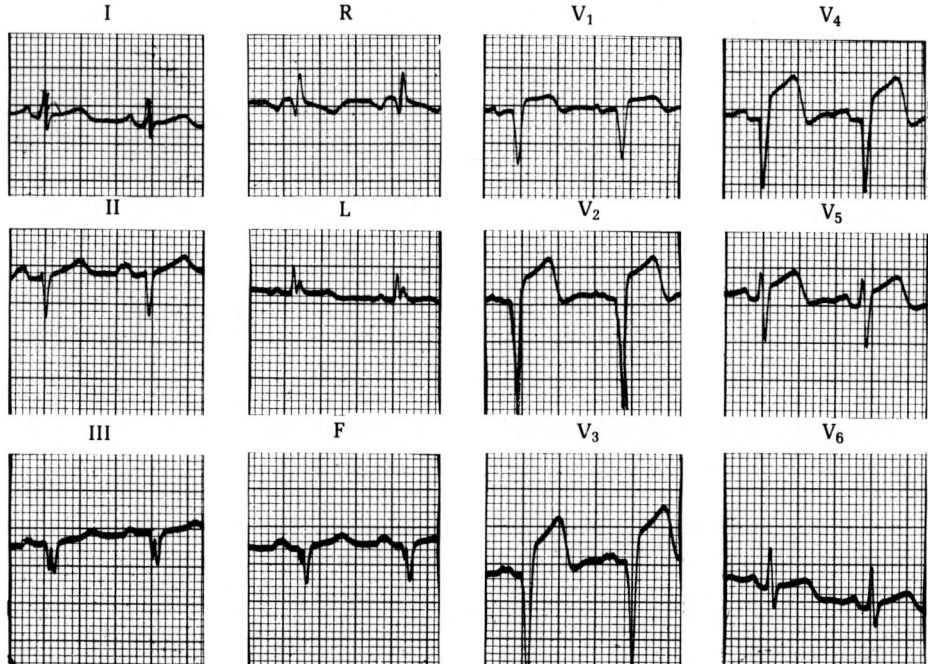

Figure 10-82   Anteroseptal MI (Q waves in V_{1-3}).

From Conover, M. B. (1992). *Understanding electrocardiography* (6th ed.). St. Louis: Mosby–Year Book.

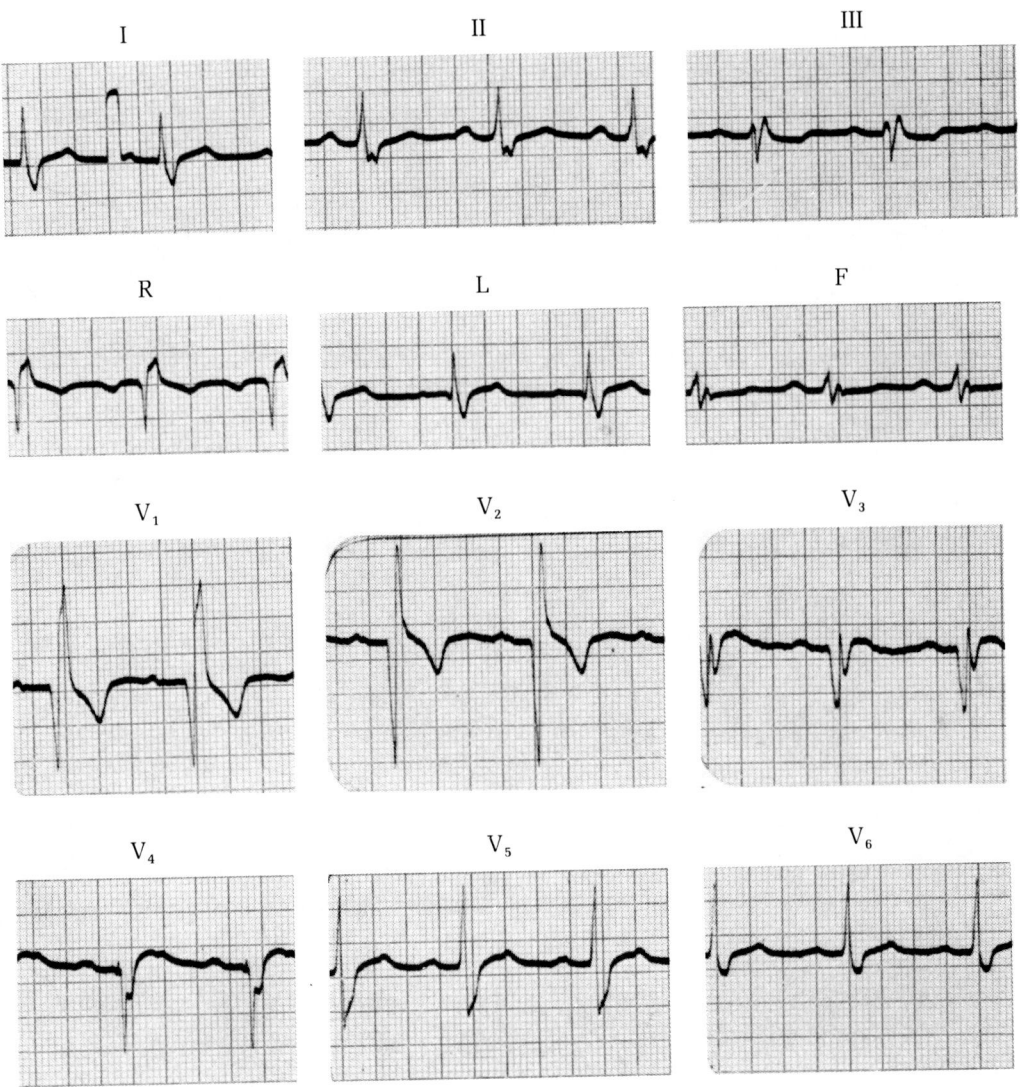

Figure 10-83   12-lead ECG showing anteroseptal myocardial infarction plus right bundle branch block. (Note terminal R wave in V₁.)

From Conover, M. B. (1992). *Understanding electrocardiography* (6th ed.). St. Louis: Mosby–Year Book.

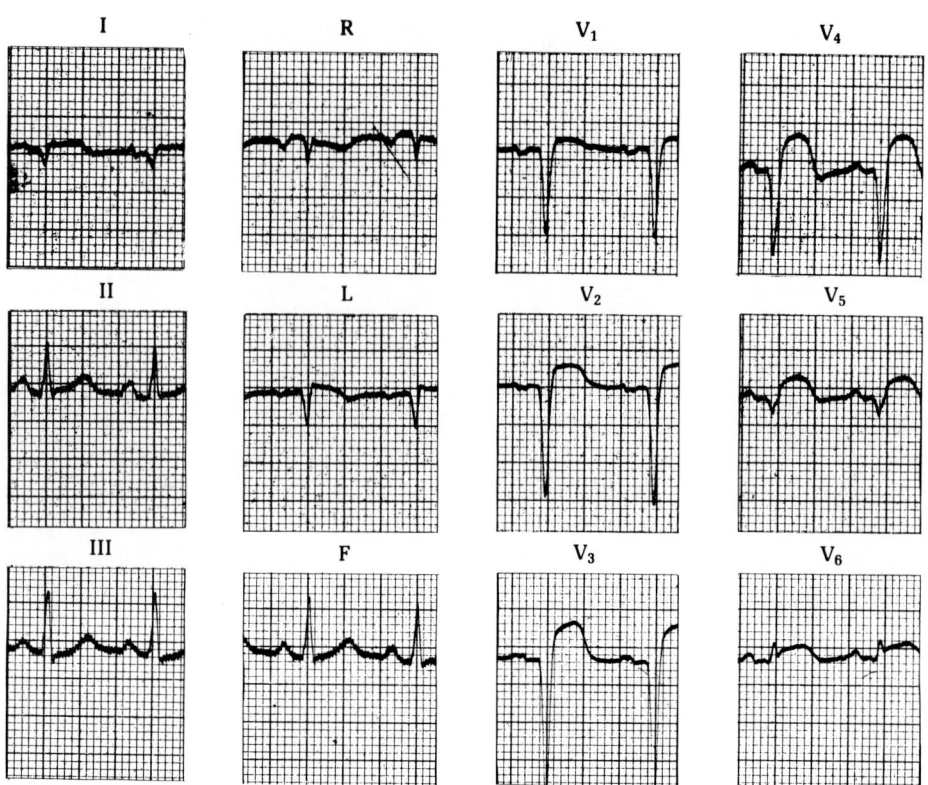

Figure 10-84   12-lead ECG showing anterolateral wall myocardial infarction (Q waves in V_2-V_6 and leads I and aVL).

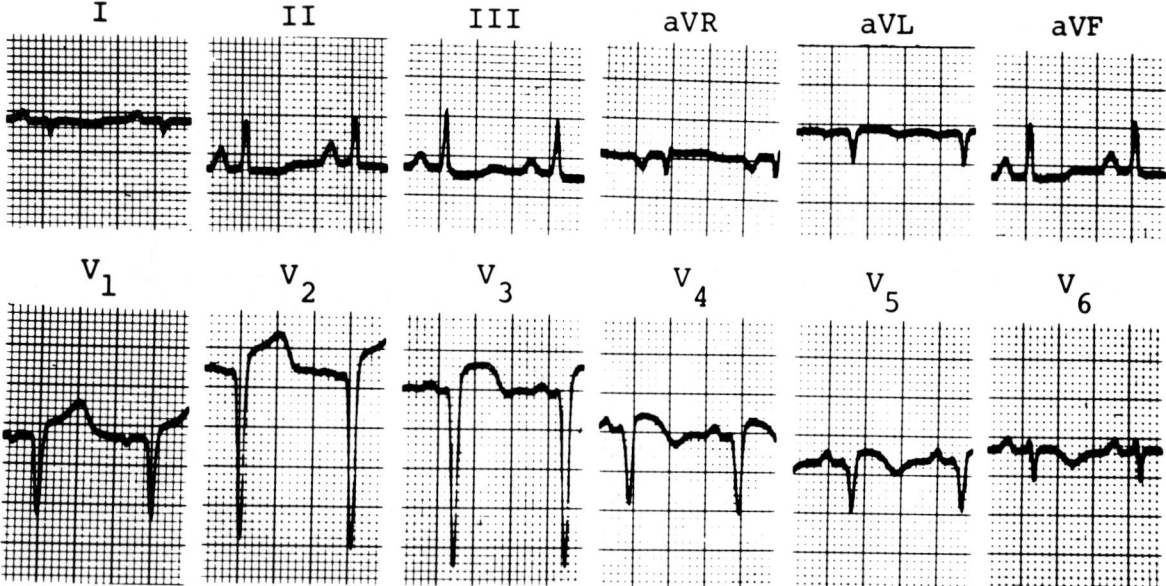

Figure 10-85   Acute extensive anterior myocardial infarction proven by autopsy. The ECG shows the loss of anterior QRS forces throughout all precordial leads with ST segment elevation and T wave inversion. QS deflections are also present in leads I and aVL. This tracing was recorded 1 week after the onset of chest pain. The patient died of cardiogenic shock. At autopsy it was estimated that about 50% of the left ventricle was infarcted.

From Chou, T. (1986). *Electrocardiography in clinical practice.* Orlando, FL: Grune & Stratton.

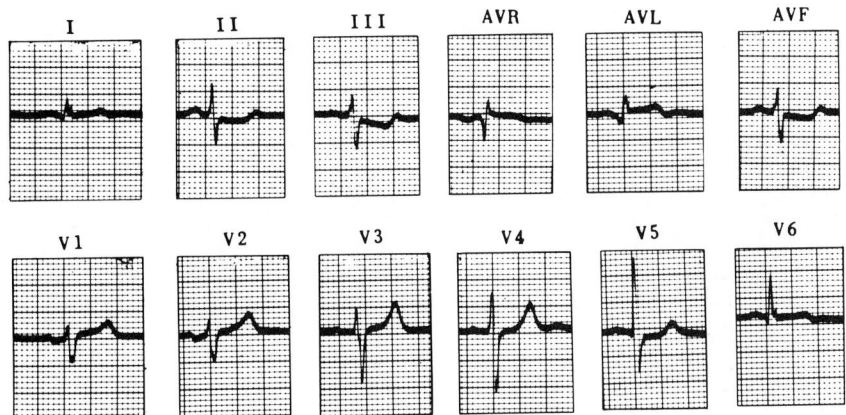

Figure 10-86   Acute superior or high lateral myocardial infarction. There are wide Q waves in leads I and aVL and broad R waves in leads III and aVF. The ST segments are elevated in leads I and aVL, with reciprocal depression in leads II, III, and aVF. The initial QRS vector points inferiorly and rightward, the ST vector superiorly.

From Friedman, H. H. (1985). *Diagnostic electrocardiography and vectorcardiography.* New York: McGraw-Hill.

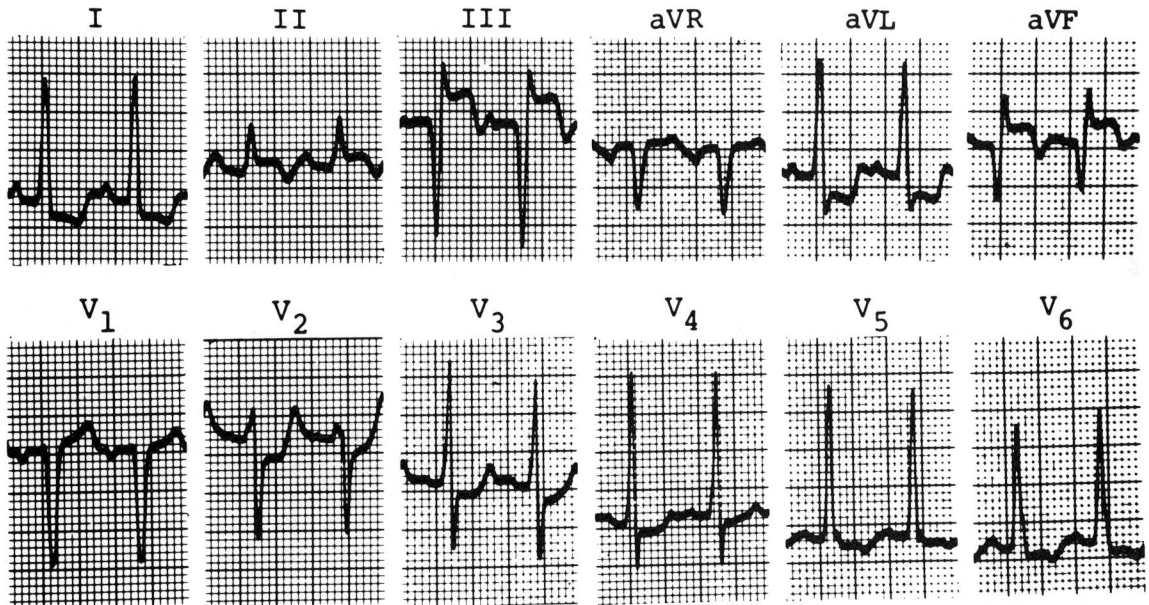

Figure 10-87   Acute inferior myocardial infarction proven by autopsy. In the ECG, the P wave in lead V_1 suggests left atrial enlargement. The abnormal Q waves in leads III and aVF with ST segment elevation and T wave inversion in leads II, III, and aVF are consistent with acute inferior myocardial infarction. There is reciprocal ST segment depression in leads I and aVL and the precordial leads, especially leads V_2 to V_4. The high voltage of the R wave in lead aVL strongly suggests left ventricular enlargement.

From Chou, T. (1986). *Electrocardiography in clinical practice.* Orlando, FL: Grune & Stratton.

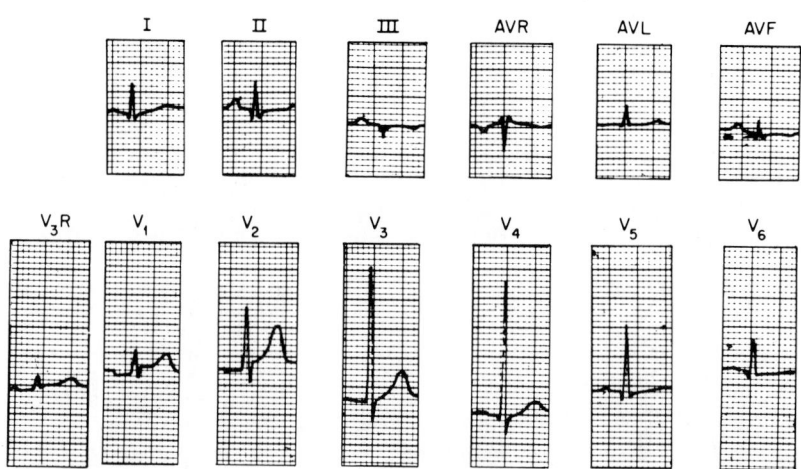

Figure 10-88   True posterior myocardial infarction. There are tall, broad R waves and tall symmetrical T waves in V_{3R}, V_1, and V_2. The patient had a typical clinical picture of myocardial infarction at the time the ECG was taken.
From Friedman, H. H. (1985). *Diagnostic electrocardiography and vectorcardiography.* New York: McGraw-Hill.

Myocardial infarction to more than one area may occur simultaneously or separately. Common infarct combinations are inferior and lateral and inferior, posterior, and lateral. Less common are simultaneous anterior and inferior infarction. On occasion the right ventricle is included in inferior or posterior myocardial infarction. This can be confirmed by clinical observations of right ventricular dysfunction in the face of normal to low left-sided filling pressures as well as early findings of ST segment elevation in right chest leads V_1, V_{3R}, and/or V_{4R} (Figure 10-89).

Evolutionary Changes of Acute Transmural Myocardial Infarction

Myocardial infarction is often described in stages: hyperacute, acute, recent, and old. The *hyperacute* stage is the initial stage occurring within minutes to hours after the onset of pain. Because it is a very transient stage, it is often missed or observed only in the ECG obtained at the outset of the experience. The ECG findings are rising ST segments with tall, peaked T waves and generally normal QRS complexes. The advent of continuous bedside ST segment monitoring will improve recognition of transient ST changes and will time the return of the ST segment to baseline, the usual hallmark of reperfusion. Recognizing alterations in the ST segment allows the nurse to treat silent ischemia, observe for life-threatening dysrhythmias at the time of reperfusion, or alert the physician immediately upon coronary spasm or acute coronary closure.

An *acute* infarct produces the usual ST segment elevation and Q wave development in the direct leads and in some cases ST segment depression and R waves in the reciprocal leads. This stage occurs within 7 to 12 hours after the onset of pain and may continue for several days. As the ST segment moves toward the baseline, the inverted T wave begins to appear and the Q wave reaches its full size. The ST segment should return to normal within the first 2 weeks after the initiation of symptoms. If ST segment elevation persists, one should consider the possibility of a ventricular aneurysm.

Recent infarcts are recognized by the typical Q and T wave inversion in the indicative leads. This stage occurs within weeks after the onset of pain and lasts for a few months or even years. *Old* infarcts are those in which the T wave has returned to normal and only the typical QRS abnormalities remain on the ECG. Occasionally the Q waves of an old infarct disappear after several years. Because of the variability in the length of the recent stage, it may be useful to define an infarct as "old" when these changes have existed for at least 2 months.[5]

It should be noted that none of the foregoing stages can be precisely described or dated. It is therefore desirable to obtain serial ECGs and to rely on the clinical history and pertinent laboratory data of the patient for a more accurate description of the age of the infarct.

Differential Diagnosis of Infarct Patterns

The ECG changes characteristic of myocardial infarction may resemble changes associated with other cardiac and noncardiac abnormalities. Therefore, a false diagnosis of myocardial infarction may be made. Following is a list of abnormalities and the infarct pattern(s) that they may mimic.[7]

Left ventricular hypertrophy and left bundle branch block: anteroseptal, anteroapical, or inferior MIs

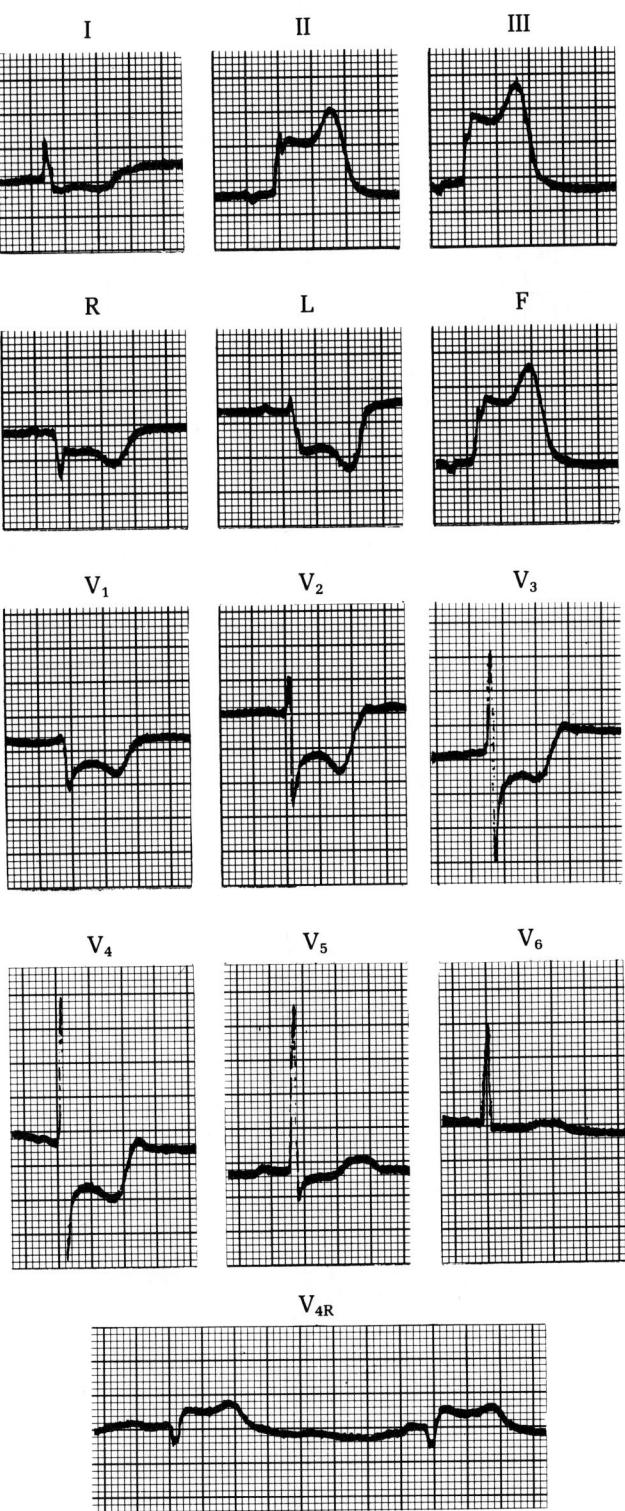

I   II   III

R   L   F

V₁   V₂   V₃

V₄   V₅   V₆

V₄R

Figure 10-89 12-lead ECG showing acute inferior wall myocardial infarction with right ventricular involvement (see V₄R). Also note the ST depression in V₁₋₄ and in leads I and aVL.

From Conover, M. B. (1992). *Understanding electrocardiography* (6th ed.). St. Louis: Mosby–Year Book.

Chronic obstructive pulmonary disease and right ventricular hypertrophy: inferior, posterior, anteroseptal, or anteroapical MIs

Left anterior hemiblock and left axis deviation: inferior or anteroapical MIs

Cardiomyopathy: any MI pattern

Hypertrophic obstructive cardiomyopathy (HOCM): inferior, posterior, or inferoposterolateral MIs

Wolff-Parkinson-White syndrome: inferior, anteroseptal, or posterior MIs

Chest deformity: inferior, anteroseptal, anteroapical, or anterolateral MIs

Ventricular aneurysm, pericarditis, cerebrovascular disease, pulmonary embolism, and hyperkalemia also may create ECG changes that mimic infarcts. Careful observation of the ECG and its recorded findings as well as close attention to the clinical history and physical examination help to prevent an incorrect diagnosis.

Effects of Electrolyte Imbalance

Recalling how the movement of electrically charged ions causes the action potential to occur, it is easy to accept that abnormalities in electrolyte concentrations can have an effect on the ECG. Two electrolytes in particular, calcium and potassium, can seriously alter the electrical function of the heart. Consequently, it is important for the critical care nurse to recognize the effects of hypocalcemia, hypercalcemia, hypokalemia, and hyperkalemia on the ECG.

Hypocalcemia

Calcium enters the cell during phase 2 of the action potential. This phase is associated with the QT interval on the surface ECG (see Figure 10-4). If the concentration of calcium is low, the movement of calcium into the cell will be prolonged. Consequently, a prolonged QT_c interval is recorded on the ECG (Figure 10-90). The degree of prolongation is inversely proportional to the calcium concentration. The QT_c prolongation is due to ST segment prolongation rather than to an increase in the duration of the T wave. Morphological changes of the T wave are common, however, and are manifested as either peaked, flattened, or sharply inverted T waves. The T wave changes may be most pronounced in the right precordial leads. Changes in the P, PR, QRS, and U are not generally seen.

Hypercalcemia

Elevated concentrations of calcium produce shortening of the ST segment on the ECG and therefore cause a decrease in the QT_c duration (Figure 10-91). Occasionally, the ST segment is so short it cannot be identified on the ECG. As the calcium concentration

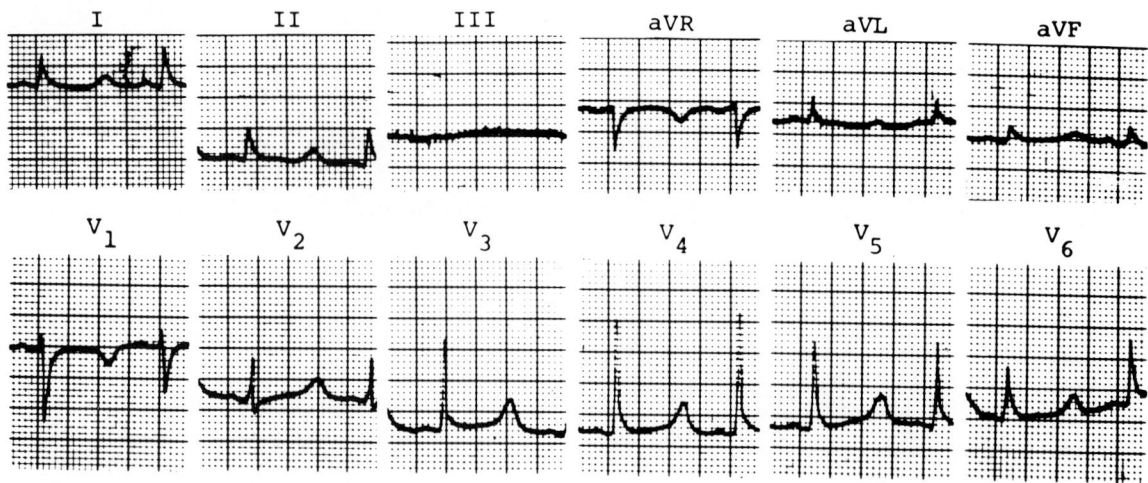

Figure 10-90 Hypocalcemia. The patient is a 69-year-old patient with uremia. The serum calcium level was 5.6 mg/100 ml. In the ECG, there is a prolongation of the QT interval, mainly because of lengthening of the ST segment.
From Chou, T. (1986). *Electrocardiography in clinical practice.* Orlando, FL: Grune & Stratton.

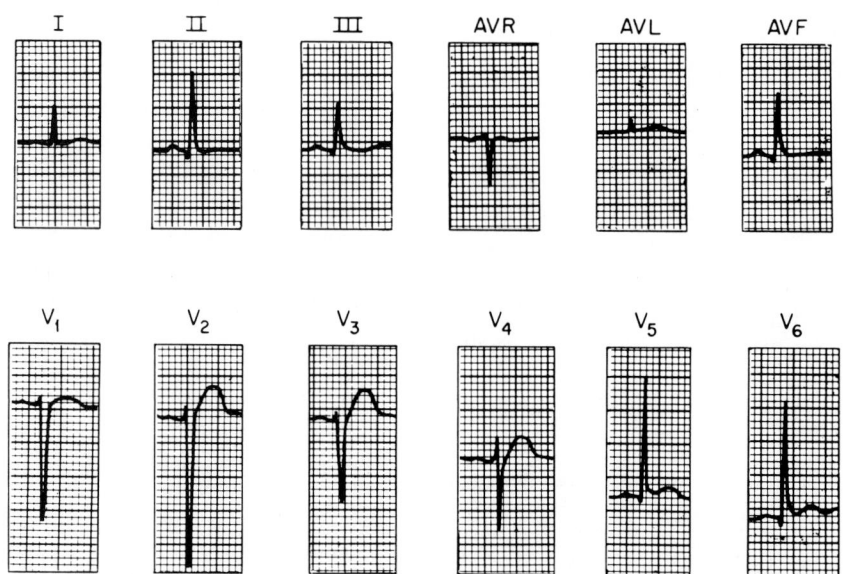

Figure 10-91 Hypercalcemia. There is a shortening of the QT_c interval and virtual absence of the segment from the beginning of the Q to the onset of the T wave ($Q-_oT$). The serum calcium was 18.7 mg/100 ml.
From Friedman, H. H. (1985). *Diagnostic electrocardiography and vectorcardiography.* New York: McGraw-Hill.

reaches and exceeds 16 mg/100 ml, the duration of the T wave may increase, causing the QT_c to appear normal. The morphology of the T wave generally does not change, however. The P wave and the QRS complex are generally not affected by hypercalcemia, but the U wave may increase in amplitude.

Hypokalemia

The electrocardiographic changes resulting from hypokalemia are due to an alteration of the ventricular action potential, particularly phase 3. Probably the first hint of a low potassium concentration ap-

pears when a prominent U wave is identified (Figure 10-92). The U wave is considered to be prominent when its amplitude is greater than 1 mm or is taller than the T wave in a given lead. The cause of the change in the U wave is not well understood. Associated with the prominent U wave are ST segment depression and decreased T wave amplitude. The changes become apparent when the serum potassium falls below 3.0 mEq/L. Very low concentrations of serum potassium may cause prolongation of the QRS complex and an increase in the amplitude and duration of the P wave; however, both of these changes

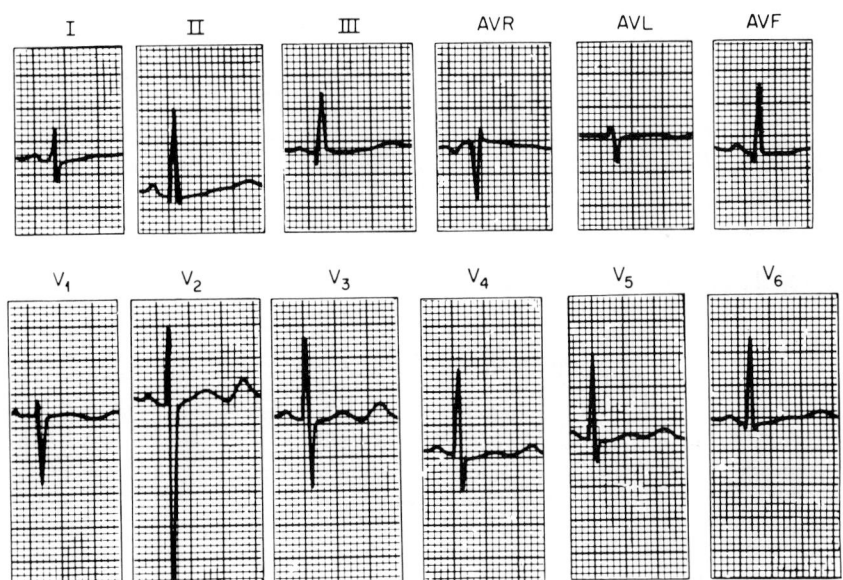

Figure 10-92   Hypokalemia. The U waves are large and the T waves flattened. The T/U ratio is less than 1.0 in leads II and V$_3$. The U wave in V$_3$ exceeds 2 mm. The ST segments have a shallow, troughlike appearance in the limb leads. The serum potassium was 2.2 mg/L.

From Friedman, H. H. (1985). *Diagnostic electrocardiography and vectorcardiography.* New York: McGraw-Hill.

are uncommon. All the ECG changes of hypokalemia are usually best seen in the midprecordial leads.

It is important to note that hypokalemia generally does not prolong the QT$_c$. Apparent prolongation of the QT$_c$ is usually the result of an inaccurate QT measurement. This occurs because the U wave is superimposed on the end of the T wave or the U is mistaken for the T wave. Great care must be taken so that a QU interval is not interpreted as a QT interval.

Hypokalemia is known to cause a variety of cardiac dysrhythmias. Patients are more susceptible to dysrhythmia when they are receiving digitalis and are hypokalemic. Supplementation with magnesium to maintain a level ≥2.0 mEq/L has been helpful in stabilizing malignant ventricular dysrhythmias presumed due to hypokalemia in patients with dilated cardiomyopathy awaiting heart transplantation. Supraventricular dysrhythmias that may be caused by hypokalemia include paroxysmal supraventricular tachycardia with block, first-degree AV block, and second-degree AV block: Mobitz type I. Ventricular dysrhythmias include premature ventricular complexes, ventricular tachycardia, and ventricular fibrillation.

Hyperkalemia

A high serum potassium is manifested on the ECG in a variety of ways. Figure 10-93 shows the progressive changes produced by hyperkalemia. The first

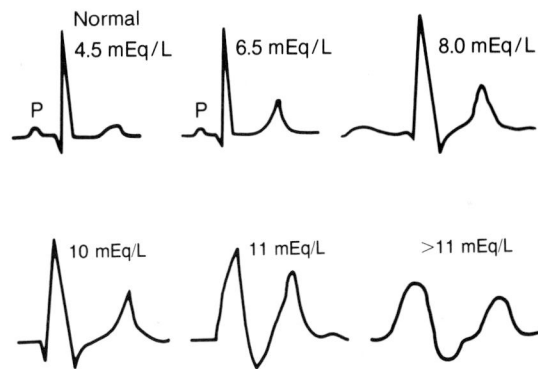

Figure 10-93   Effects of hyperkalemia on the ECG. The initial change with hyperkalemia is peaking of the T wave. With progressive elevations in serum potassium, there is loss of P waves, alteration of the ST segment, lengthening of the QRS duration, and finally ventricular fibrillation. These changes do not necessarily occur with a specific serum potassium level. See text for further discussion.

and probably most common ECG change is that of narrow, tall, peaked, tent-shaped T waves. This change, which may be seen in all leads, occurs when the serum potassium level is from 5.5 to 6.5 mEq/L (Figure 10-94). As the levels rise from 6.5 to 7.5 mEq/L, the morphology of the P, ST, and QRS begins to change; the P wave amplitude decreases, the ST segment is either depressed or elevated, and the QRS widens slightly. At advanced levels of hyperkalemia, 7.5 to 8.5 mEq/L, the P wave flattens and becomes

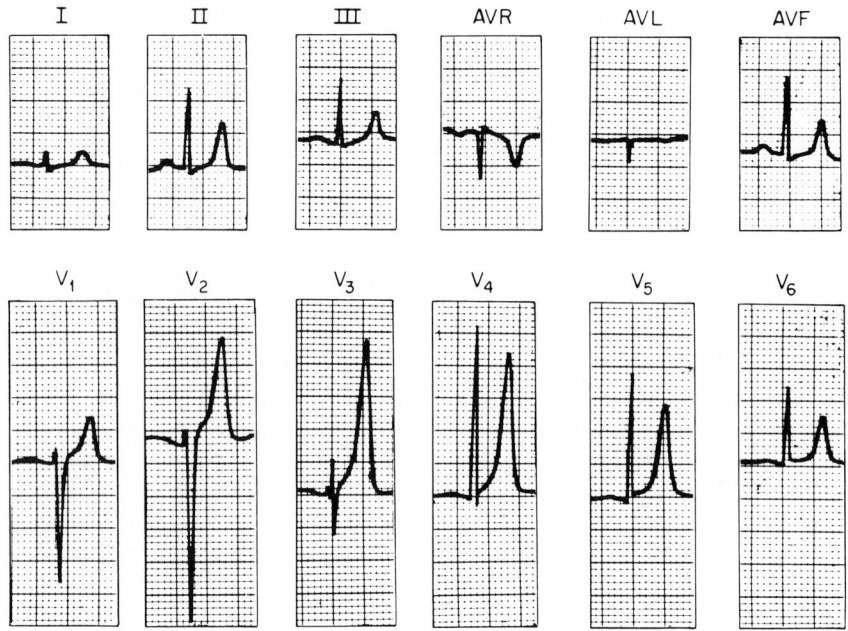

Figure 10-94   Hyperkalemia. The T waves are typically narrow, symmetrical, tall, and peaked. The serum potassium was 6.2 mEq/L.

From Friedman, H. H. (1985). *Diagnostic electrocardiography and vectorcardiography* (p. 339). New York: McGraw-Hill. Reprinted by permission.

broader, the QRS widens markedly, and various forms of AV nodal and bundle branch block appear. When the serum potassium exceeds 8.5 mEq/L, the P wave disappears; the QRS continues to broaden, resulting in various forms of intraventricular conduction blocks; and ventricular dysrhythmia, namely ventricular tachycardia, flutter, and fibrillation. Idioventricular rhythm followed by ventricular standstill may appear.

As is evident from the previous discussion, electrolyte imbalance can seriously affect the electrical function of the heart and, if not diagnosed and treated effectively, can lead to death. The critical care nurse should be constantly alert for electrolyte abnormality and should monitor the ECG for any associated changes.

Effects of Drug Therapy

The administration of cardiac and noncardiac drugs can result in direct changes in the cardiac action potential and, consequently, in the ECG. Many of the ECG drug effects are positive or therapeutic. Unfortunately, though, some can mimic pathological changes from cardiac disease processes, thus leading to incorrect diagnoses. Some may cause serious impulse formation or conduction abnormalities that if not recognized and treated can lead to the death of the patient. The critical care nurse should know which drugs are most likely to alter the ECG and should monitor the patient for the associated changes.

Digitalis

Digitalis, through either direct or indirect effects on the heart, can alter in varying degrees the automaticity, excitability, and conductivity of cardiac cells. These effects are the result of the drug's ability to inhibit the active transport of sodium and potassium across the cell membrane (direct effect), increase vagal tone (indirect effect), or both.[5] Some of these effects occur with therapeutic doses and others occur with toxic doses.

Therapeutic doses of digitalis decrease automaticity of pacemaker cells in the SA node and the atria and increase automaticity in the AV junction and the His-Purkinje system. Digitalis-induced junctional and ventricular tachyarrhythmias are the result of the latter action. The drug in usual dosages decreases excitability in atrial and His-Purkinje cells but increases ventricular excitability. Conductivity of atrial and AV junctional cells is depressed by therapeutic doses of the drug. Digitalis speeds repolarization in the ventricular myocardium, resulting in ST segment depression and flattened T waves in epicardial leads with upright QRS complexes. Therapeutic digitalis effects on the normal ECG (Figure 10-95) can be summarized as:

1. Depression of the ST segment
2. Depressed T wave amplitude, which may result in diphasic or negative T waves
3. Shortening of the QT_c interval
4. Slightly increased U wave amplitude

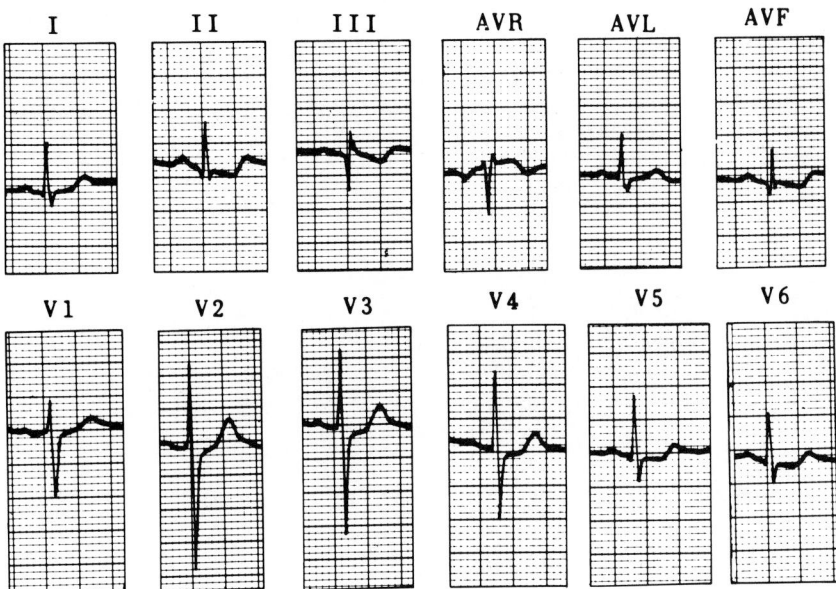

Figure 10-95   Digitalis effect. The ST segments are depressed and concave upward. The T waves are of decreased amplitude. The QT interval is shortened.

From Friedman, H. H. (1985). *Diagnostic electrocardiography and vectorcardiography*. New York: McGraw-Hill.

The ECG changes produced by digitalis are usually best observed in leads II, III, aVF, and the left precordial leads.

In abnormal ECGs, digitalis may produce prolongation of the PR interval as well as the other changes noted for normal ECGs. Digitalis may slow the ventricular rate in atrial fibrillation or terminate the dysrhythmia. However, it is important to note that the drug may cause other atrial dysrhythmias to stop, continue, or accelerate. In other words, atrial tachycardia may change to flutter, to fibrillation, and then to sinus rhythm.

Toxic levels of digitalis can increase automaticity in the SA node and atrial pacemaker cells. Sinoatrial conductibility is impaired by high drug levels and the ventricular refractory period is often shortened. Toxic effects of the drug may produce a great number and variety of dysrhythmias, including NJT, VPCs, sinus bradycardia, Mobitz type I AV block, AT with varying block, APCs, JPCs, SA block, SA arrest, MAT, atrial flutter or fibrillation, VT, VF or flutter, and VS. Therapeutic measures for these dysrhythmias are discussed in the section of this chapter that pertains to the specific rhythm disorders.

Quinidine

Quinidine is a Class I antiarrhythmic agent that has a depressant effect on the heart. Its primary electrophysiological effects are: (1) little or no change in automaticity of the SA node; (2) depressed atrial automaticity, excitability, and conductivity and pro-longed atrial refractoriness; (3) little or no effect on AV conduction; (4) depressed automaticity, slowed conduction velocity, and prolonged refractoriness of the His-Purkinje system; and (5) depressed ventricular conductivity and excitability. Its therapeutic effects on the ECG (Figure 10-96) can be summarized as:

1. Notched, flat, or inverted T waves, usually associated with prolonged T wave duration and increased U wave amplitude
2. Prolonged QT_c intervals
3. Absent ST segment elevation or depression
4. Slightly widened and notched P waves
5. Slightly prolonged PR intervals

Quinidine can also produce toxic effects that may or may not be related to dosage. Ventricular arrhythmias secondary to quinidine, for example, are not dose dependent and are probably caused by reentry. Other ECG disturbances produced by the toxic effects of quinidine are: varying degrees of AV block, intraatrial block and/or atrial standstill, marked QT prolongation, widening of the QRS complex, and ventricular tachyarrhythmias, particularly torsades de pointes.

Other Drugs

Other antirhythmic agents and drugs that act on the autonomic nervous system can produce changes in the ECG. The Appendix describes the antidysrhythmic drugs and their effects on the electrophysiological properties of the heart. Sympathomimetic drugs enhance automaticity, excitability, and con-

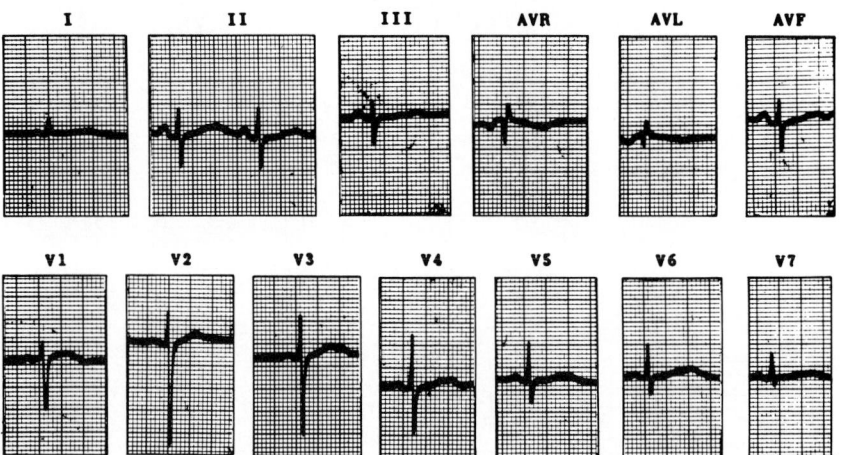

Figure 10-96   Quinidine effect. The QT interval is prolonged, the T waves are flattened, and the U waves are prominent.
From Friedman, H. H. (1985). *Diagnostic electrocardiography and vectorcardiography*. New York: McGraw-Hill.

ductivity, whereas sympathetic blocking agents have the opposite effect.

Phenothiazines and antidepressant drugs such as amitriptyline and imipramine depress intracardiac conduction. With high doses, the ST segment may become depressed and the T wave flattens or is inverted. QT_c prolongation, increased U wave amplitude, AV and ventricular conduction defects, and cardiac arrhythmias may also be produced.

REFERENCES

1. Guyton, A. C. (1991). *Textbook of medical physiology* (8th ed.). Philadelphia: Saunders.
2. Marriott, H. J. L. (1988). *Practical electrocardiography*. Baltimore: Williams & Wilkins.
3. Wells, J. L., MacLean, W. A. H., James, T. N., et al. (1979). Characterization of atrial flutter; studies in man after open heart surgery used fixed atrial electrodes. *Circulation, 60*, 665-673.
4. Wells, J. L., Karp, R. B., Kouchoukos, N. T., et al. (1978). Characterization of atrial fibrillation in man: studies following open heart surgery. *PACE, 1*, 422-437.
5. Chou, T. C. (1991). *Electrocardiography in clinical practice*. Orlando, FL: Grune & Stratton.
6. Friedman, H. H. (1985). *Diagnostic electrocardiography and vectorcardiography*. New York: McGraw-Hill.
7. Chung, E. K. (1985). *Electrocardiography: Practical applications with vectorial principles*. Norwalk, CT: Appleton-Century-Crofts.
8. Dessertenne, F. (1966). La tachycardie ventriculaire a deux foyers opposes variable. *Archives Mal Coeur, 59*, 263-272.
9. Romhilt, D. W., & Estes, E. H. (1968). A point score system for the ECG diagnosis of left ventricular hypertrophy. *American Heart Journal, 75*, 752-758.

11

Nutrition

Carolyn D. Viall

In 1974, Butterworth described the negative effects of malnutrition on hospitalized patients.[1] Following this historic article, several additional studies documented the extent of malnutrition then existing in medical and surgical patient populations. The dire consequences of malnutrition in critically ill patients, including pneumonia, wound dehiscence, increased rate of sepsis, failure to wean from ventilators, and, ultimately, increased mortality have been chronicled in the medical literature.

Over the past two decades, nutritional support has become an accepted part of medical care, as special techniques have been developed for delivery of nutrients. Recognition of malnutrition as a co-morbidity factor under the Prospective Payment System for Medicare beneficiaries has also heightened awareness of the necessity to provide nutritional support to patients. Many hospitals have interdisciplinary nutrition support teams to address the nutritional care of patients, but even without such a formal structure, nutritional care of patients can be accomplished by integrating principles of nutrition support into daily care of patients.

This chapter provides information about normal nutritional requirements and their alterations in disease and critical illness. Nutritional status assessment techniques and risk factors are defined. Specialized methods for supplying nutrients are described. This knowledge should enhance the ability of the nurse to address nutritional needs of the critically ill patient.

NORMAL NUTRITIONAL REQUIREMENTS

The intricate biochemistry of nutrition approaches the metaphysical. However, there are some constants that facilitate understanding and are useful in daily practice.

Energy

Every organism has an obligate, minimum need for energy. This energy requirement is the amount of calories or kilocalories necessary to carry on minimal, necessary body processes.* *Basal energy expenditure (BEE)* is defined as the energy required to maintain life-sustaining mechanical, transport, and synthetic processes while the body is completely at rest, at standard room temperature, and in a postabsorptive state. Basal energy expenditure can be measured by indirect calorimetry. Metabolic measurement carts that indicate a patient's oxygen consumption and expression of carbon dioxide are a means of quantifying BEE by indirect calorimetry. Use of metabolic carts to measure BEE is increasing in research and intensive care units, but in most clinical settings, BEE is still usually estimated through the use of the Harris-Benedict formula (see box below).[2] This formula provides an estimate of BEE that takes into account the effects of age, sex, and body size. Basal energy expenditure is the basis on which total energy requirements are estimated. In the clinical setting, *resting energy expenditure (REE)* is calculated; this takes into account energy requirements for minimal activity and metabolism of nutrients. Resting energy expenditure is expressed as BEE + 10% to 15%.

Basal energy expenditure is elevated by disease and critical illness. There is considerable controversy regarding the energy requirements of the critically ill patient. Different studies have demonstrated needs of 30% to 100% of BEE for patients with trauma, sepsis,

---

*A kilocalorie is the amount of heat required to raise the temperature of 1 kg of water 1° C.

> ### The Harris-Benedict Formula for Calculating Basal Energy Expenditure
>
> BEE for males = 66 + (13.7 × W) + (5 × H) — (6.8 × A)
> BEE for females = 665 + (9.6 × W) + (1.8 × H) — (4.7 × A)
> W = body weight in kg
> H = body height in cm
> A = age in years

or burns, whereas others have demonstrated much lower requirements. Regardless of these variances, the energy needs of the critically ill patient are primary and, in the face of deficit calorie input, will be met by catabolism of organ and muscle protein and adipose tissue. Use of lean body mass as an energy source represents a potentially fatal cost to the critically ill patient, since every body protein has a function. As body protein is catabolized to meet energy requirements, body function is lost.

Protein

Protein has many functions in the body. It is a vital structural component of muscle and organ tissue, erythrocytes, white blood cells, hormones, and antibodies. Proteins play a role in metabolism, as enzymes and coenzymes. Serum proteins regulate fluid and acid–base balance by maintaining osmotic pressure and serving in buffer systems.

The most important function of dietary protein is to provide amino acid precursors for synthesis of these vital body proteins. There are 20 to 25 naturally occurring amino acids. Eight of these amino acids are termed *essential* because they are necessary to prevent deficiency disease symptoms. Essential amino acids cannot be made by the body but must be consumed from the diet. Nonessential amino acids are as necessary for synthesis of new body proteins as are essential amino acids. However, nonessential amino acids can be made in the body from ingested substrates.

The synthesis of new proteins is dependent upon the presence of substrate amino acids in the body. It is essential that the patient receive an adequate amount of nonprotein calories, that is, carbohydrates and fats, to be used as an energy source so that protein can be used for synthesis of new proteins instead of being used for energy.

The recommended daily allowance (RDA) for protein intake in adults is 0.8 g protein per kilogram of body weight. Protein requirements for the critically ill patient are usually greater than the RDA requirement levels (Table 11-1). A number of factors contribute to the elevated protein needs in critically ill patients, including depletion of body protein through tissue losses from injury, surgery, and/or starvation; and drainage of serous protein through fistulas, open wounds, and/or abscesses. Catabolism of body protein is enhanced during illness or trauma because of the accompanying increase of BEE and the presence of stress-related catabolic hormones. Certain therapies, including corticosteroid administration and chemotherapy, other drug therapies, and radiation, also increase the loss of body proteins.

TABLE 11-1   **Protein Requirements during Selected Critical Illnesses**

Condition	Protein Requirements
Burns	1-4 g/kg IBW*
Cardiac cachexia	1.5-2 g/kg IBW*
Major surgery or trauma	1.5-3.5 g/kg IBW* (acute)
	1.5 g/kg IBW* (stable)
	14% to 22% of total kcal needs
Head injury	
Renal failure	
Peritoneal dialysis	1 g/kg dry body weight
Continuous ambulatory peritoneal dialysis	1.2-1.5 g/kg dry body weight
Hemodialysis	1.5 g/kg dry body weight
Cancer	1-1.5 g/kg IBW*
Chronic obstructive pulmonary disease	1.5 g/kg IBW*

*IBW = ideal body weight.

Frequently, patients with additional protein losses (e.g., draining wounds, dialysis) do not receive adequate nonprotein calories. These conditions increase their protein requirements because protein is used as an energy source as well as for synthesis of new proteins.

Carbohydrate

The major function of dietary carbohydrate is as a protein-sparing energy source. Dietary carbohydrate provides 4 kcal per gram. Carbohydrate in the form of glucose is the only energy source that can be used by the central nervous system, red and white blood cells, neutrophils, and fibroblasts. These cells are termed *obligate glycolyzers*. This has special significance for the critically ill patient since obligate glycolyzer cells are found at the frontiers of wounds and in granulating tissue. If insufficient carbohydrate is available to meet glucose demands of glycolyzer cells, protein will be catabolized (via gluconeogenesis) to supply glucose.

No RDA for carbohydrate has been established. However, it has been recommended that a minimum of 50 to 100 g of digestible carbohydrate be consumed daily to prevent ketosis. If inadequate glucose is available for energy requirements, the liver synthesizes ketone bodies as an alternate fuel source. Because glucose is the fuel of choice for many cells that are important for recovery of the critically ill patient, these patients may require much more than the minimal amount of carbohydrate.

Fat

Dietary fat is a concentrated source of energy. Fats provide 9 kcal per gram. Fats are also important as sources of fat-soluble vitamins and the essential fatty acids, linolenic and linoleic acids. Linolenic and linoleic acids must be provided from the diet or other exogenous sources, because they cannot be manufactured by the body. Although it is unusual for adults to develop symptoms of essential fatty acid deficiency, patients maintained on fat-free parenteral nutritional solutions or tube feeding formulas having very low fat content are at risk of developing symptoms of essential fatty acid deficiency.

There is no specific dietary recommendation for fat. However, adequate amounts must be consumed so that requirements for essential fatty acids are met, primarily linoleic acid. These requirements can be met if 1% to 2% of total dietary calories are provided by fat. Overall oral fat consumption should be no more than 30% of dietary calories. Although fat provides more than twice the energy per gram of carbohydrate, fat is not a source of glucose. This has special significance for the critically ill patient who requires glucose to fuel glycolyzer cells. Additionally, the ability of the critically ill patient to metabolize and use large amounts of fat may be impaired by alterations in the circulating levels of certain hormones and enzymes.

Vitamins

Vitamins do not supply energy or nitrogen to the body but are important in metabolic reactions and are required for growth and maintenance of tissue. Vitamins are classified as *fat-soluble* (vitamins A, D, E, and K) or *water-soluble* (vitamins C, B_{12}, niacin, riboflavin, thiamine, B_6, and folacin). Most vitamins cannot be synthesized by the body and must be provided by the diet or other exogenous sources. Exceptions to this are vitamins K, thiamine, folacin, and B_{12}, which can be synthesized in varying amounts by microorganisms present in the human gut; and niacin and vitamin A, which can be formed in the body if their precursors are present. Vitamins are essential to prevention of a variety of vitamin deficiency diseases. These diseases are not common among the general American population, but symptoms may occur in hospitalized patients who have greater than normal needs for vitamins or who are supported by nutritional solutions that do not meet requirements.

The RDAs for vitamins are expected to reflect average requirements for most healthy adults. Specific requirements for each vitamin required by critically ill patients are unknown. It *is* known that requirements for intravenously administered vitamins are different from the RDA for orally administered vitamins, and standards for IV dosages of vitamins have been established.[3] This has special significance for critically ill patients, since often their nutritional requirements are met by parenteral feeding.

Minerals and Trace Elements

Twenty-one minerals are known to be essential to human nutriture. Minerals that are required in very small amounts are referred to as *trace elements*. Minerals function in the body as constituents of enzymes and hormones, and as structural components. They have important roles in regulating metabolism, acid–base, and fluid balance. Minerals cannot be synthesized by the body and must be provided by the diet. Recommended daily allowances are established for calcium, phosphorus, magnesium, iron, zinc, and iodine, but because there is less information regarding requirements for other minerals, no RDAs have been established for them.

Because minerals play an integral role in regulating body processes, it is probable that the critically ill patient may require amounts that vary from the RDAs or suggested dietary intakes. It is wise to monitor a patient's serum levels of minerals and supplement closely as necessary.

NUTRITIONAL RISK FACTORS

Patients often enter the hospital in a marginal nutritional status. In addition, disease, injury, and surgery cause metabolic stress that elevates protein and calorie needs of patients. Studies show that up to 50% of patients develop malnutrition during their hospital stay.[4,5,6] Malnutrition has catastrophic effects on the ability of the critically ill patient to tolerate and recover from illness or injury. This is because the body cannibalizes its own tissues to provide energy needed to meet elevated demands for REE. When autocannibalism occurs, new body proteins are not synthesized; plasma proteins are depleted, impairing immunocompetence, so the patient is at risk for infection; and structural proteins are not produced, so wounds do not heal.

The most common types of malnutrition occurring in the critically ill population are marasmus and kwashiorkor. *Marasmus,* or severe cachexia, is a chronic condition characterized by wasting of body fat and muscle tissue and resulting from deficient intake of both calories and protein. Marasmus is easily diagnosed by clinical examination. The marasmic patient does require nutritional repletion but is likely to withstand short periods of metabolic stress because immunocompetence and wound healing ability are relatively intact. If nutritional insults are prolonged, the marasmic patient is at a particular disadvantage because he or she does not have significant reserves of endogenous nutritional substrates on which to draw.

Kwashiorkor is the result of acute protein deficiency and can develop in as short a period as 2 weeks. Typically, patients who develop kwashiorkor are those undergoing acute metabolic stress and being supported on protein-free intravenous dextrose solutions. Development of kwashiorkor is a grim prognostic indicator for the critically ill patient because of associated incompetence of the immune system. Impairment of the immune system is reflected by depressed values for total lymphocytes and lack of reactivity to skin test antigens. Immunoincompetence creates the potential for development of postoperative sepsis. Kwashiorkor is more lethal to the critically ill patient than marasmus and is more difficult to diagnose. The patient appears well nourished because muscle and fat stores remain intact. Diagnosis depends on evaluation of laboratory data. Kwashiorkor can be diagnosed when total lymphocyte count is less than $1,500/mm^3$, and serum albumin is less than 2.8 g/dl. The levels of circulating plasma proteins (such as lymphocytes, albumin, and transferrin) are rapidly depleted because of their short half-life. Because exogenous protein is not available for synthesis of replacement proteins, circulating levels rapidly fall. Nutritional support of the patient with kwashiorkor is vital to recovery. Without adequate nutritional input, the patient is at increased risk of sepsis, development of complications, and, ultimately, death.

Because the presence of malnutrition may increase the incidence of morbidity and mortality for patients experiencing metabolic stress, especially when imposed on poor nutritional status, it behooves health care professionals to identify patients who are at risk of developing nutritional deficiencies in order to prevent malnutrition-related complications. Many risk factors can be identified during nursing assessment. Inquiries regarding the ability of the patient to ingest an adequate oral diet; history of and/or impending drug treatments, radiation, and/or surgery; presence of conditions of nutrient loss or increased nutrient need; and over- or underweight or unexplained changes in weight (see box on p. 301) can be useful in identifying patients who may develop complications after surgery, illness, or injury that are secondary to malnutrition. Patients who exhibit a number of nutritional risk factors are candidates for more extensive assessment of nutritional status.

NUTRITIONAL ASSESSMENT

Nutritional assessment is the thorough evaluation of major body compartments to assess protein and energy status. This evaluation is accomplished through the use of anthropometric measurements, laboratory data, and clinical examination (Figure 11-1).

Lean Body Mass

Height, weight, midarm circumference, and calculation of midarm muscle circumference are anthropometric measurements used to evaluate lean body mass. It is accepted practice to compare the patient's values to standard values. However, these standards do not allow for individual differences and may be a source of error. It is more valuable to use the usual status of the patient as the reference for initial and serial anthropometric measurements.

A 24-hour urine collection for analysis of creatinine and 3-methylhistidine, metabolites of muscle catabolism excreted in the urine, provides biochemical data useful in assessing muscle protein turnover. A predictable amount of these metabolites is excreted daily. Total urinary excretion falls, in relation to declining lean body mass, during malnutrition. Creatinine-to-height ratio (*creatinine height index*) is calculated by dividing the amount of creatinine actually excreted during a 24-hour period by the predicted value. A creatinine height index of less than 80% indicates depletion of lean body mass.

The nurse must assure that a complete 24-hour urine collection is made. If the collection is incomplete, a false high turnover rate for muscle protein may be assumed. Since excretion of creatinine and 3-methylhistidine depends on renal function, a potential for error exists in cases of impaired renal function.

Energy Stores

Estimation of the adequacy of fat or energy stores is accomplished by evaluation of body weight and skinfold measurements. Body weight should be expressed as a percentage of usual weight so as to avoid an error that may arise from comparing a patient's weight values to standard weight values. Rapidity of weight loss is particularly important to assess, since nutritional status of the critically ill patient is extremely labile. It is important, whenever possible, to weigh the patient on admission and at routine intervals, at the same time of day and using the same scales, so that changes in weight are recognized and monitored.

Measurement of skinfold thickness is another index of body energy stores. Skinfold measurements are taken using calipers. Consistent and meticulous technique is required for reliable measurements. The patient's values for skinfold thickness should be interpreted in relation to other anthropometric measurements.

Nutritional Risk Factors

Presence of the following conditions or observations indicates the potential for malnutrition in a patient.

General

Are conditions that cause nutrient loss (e.g., malabsorption syndromes, draining abscesses or wounds, protracted diarrhea, etc.) present?

Are conditions in which there is an increased need for nutrients (such as fever, thermal injury, trauma, surgery, sepsis, chemo- or radiation therapy, etc.) present?

Has the patient been NPO for 10 days or more?

Does the patient describe food allergies, lactose intolerance, or limited food preferences? Is the patient more than 120% or less than 80% of ideal body weight, or has the patient had recent unexplained weight change?

Is the patient on a modified diet such as clear or full liquid, or one restricted in sodium, calories, protein, and/or carbohydrate?

Is the patient receiving tube feeding or parenteral nutritional solutions?

Gastrointestinal (GI)

Does the patient complain of nausea, indigestion, vomiting, diarrhea, or constipation?

Does the patient have glossitis, stomatitis, or esophagitis?

Does the patient have mechanical difficulties with chewing or swallowing?

Does the patient have any fistulas?

Does the patient have a partial or total GI obstruction?

What is the patient's dental status (edentulous? state of repair?)

Cardiovascular

Does the patient have ascites or edema?

Is the patient able to perform activities of daily living?

Genitourinary

Does input approximately equal output?

Does the patient have an ostomy?

Is the patient on hemo- or peritoneal dialysis?

Respiratory

Is the patient receiving mechanical ventilatory support?

Is the patient receiving oxygen via nasal prongs?

Integumentary

Does the patient have pressure areas on sacrum, hips, ankles, etc.?

Does the patient have rashes or dermatitis?

Are mucous membranes dry or pale?

Extremities

Does the patient have pedal edema?

Is the patient cachexic (evidenced by decreased skin turgor, reduced buccal fat pads, or general marasmic appearance)?

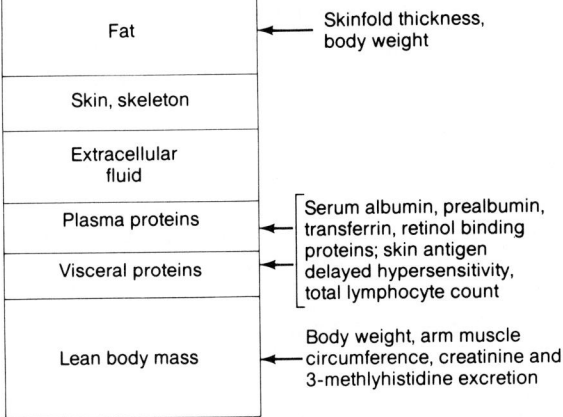

Figure 11-1 Parameters important in assessment of nutritional status.

Visceral Protein

Visceral protein status is assessed by evaluating serum concentrations of certain transport proteins. Serum albumin, transferrin, prealbumin, and retinol-binding protein have been used to assess visceral protein status because of their short half-life. These plasma proteins reflect protein malnutrition because their serum concentrations fall rapidly when protein deficiency is present. Serum albumin and transferrin levels are most commonly used in the clinical setting because they are more easily obtained and their half-life is sufficient to reflect protein depletion while being less affected by medications, therapies, and the general clinical condition of the patient. Serum albumin and transferrin concentrations of less than 3.0 g/dl and 200 mg/dl, respectively, indicate visceral protein depletion. However, these values must be interpreted with caution because dehydration or administration of blood products may falsely produce a high concentration of albumin and transferrin. Liver disease can cause a decrease in circulating levels of all transport proteins that is unrelated to nutritional status.

Nitrogen Balance

Nitrogen (N) balance is usually elevated during nutritional assessment. It is not a measure of somatic or visceral protein status but is used to estimate adequacy of protein input. A 24-hour urine collection is made and assayed for total urinary urea nitrogen (UUN) content. Frequently, the collections may be ordered for three consecutive days and an average taken of the results. Nitrogen content is reported in milligrams per deciliter. This value is used to calculate N balance using the formula:

$$N \text{ balance} = \left(\frac{24\text{-hour protein intake}}{6.25}\right) - (UUN + 4 \text{ g N})$$

The 4 grams of nitrogen are added to account for nitrogen lost in stool and other drainage. Positive nitrogen balance, or nitrogen homeostasis, is desired. Negative nitrogen balance indicates a catabolic state and necessitates an increase in protein input.

Immunocompetence

Protein malnutrition negatively affects immunocompetence by depressing neutrophil chemotaxis, total lymphocyte count (TLC), and skin reactivity to common antigens. Immunosuppression renders the critically ill, malnourished patient particularly vulnerable to infection. The immune system is assessed by determining the TLC and delayed cutaneous hypersensitivity to antigens. The total lymphocyte count is derived from a complete blood cell count with differential count. The total lymphocyte count is calculated by multiplying the percentage of lymphocytes by the white blood cell count (WBC):

$$TLC = \frac{\% \text{ lymphocytes} \times WBC}{100}$$

A TLC of less than $1,500/mm^3$ is indicative of an impaired immune system.

Skin testing with common antigens (such as mumps, streptokinase-streptodornase, *Candida albicans, Tricophytin,* tuberculin) for delayed hypersensitivity assesses immune function at the cellular level. A *positive skin test* is defined as an induration of 5 mm or more at the site of antigen injection within 24 to 72 hours. *Anergy* is defined as no response to the antigen. Anergy to skin testing indicates immuno-suppression, which may be related to malnutrition. The immune system can also be depressed by steroids, radiation, and chemotherapy. Therefore, evidence of immunosuppression in patients receiving these therapies does not necessarily indicate poor nutritional status.

Nutritional assessment consists of data collected by a variety of methods. Evaluation of nutritional status should be dynamic, and not based on data from a single source. The currently available parameters which provide nonspecific data regarding nutritional status must be reviewed as a whole to accurately evaluate and monitor the nutritional state of a patient. In addition, a thorough knowledge of the health history and biopsychological status of the patient is necessary for accurate interpretation of nutritional status assessment data, because factors other than nutritionally relevant ones can influence test results. The most important use of nutritional status assessment in the care of the critically ill is identifying patients who have the potential for developing malnutrition, preventing its occurrence, monitoring nutritional therapy, and treating existing cases of malnutrition.

NUTRITIONAL SUPPORT METHODS

Enteral feeding by tube has been used for centuries, whereas parenteral nutrition has been commonly used only since the early 1970s. Both are important techniques for providing nutritional support to the patient who cannot meet nutritional needs through an oral diet. Continuing improvements in techniques, equipment, and formulas are increasing the use of tube feeding and parenteral nutrition for hospitalized patients and outpatients.

Enteral Feeding by Tube

Nonvolitional enteral feeding was first used in 1598 when a stiff, hollow tube was used to deliver nutritional solutions into the esophagus. The practice of enteral feeding continued to develop, and by the late 1800s, stomach pumps were in common use in insane asylums for forced feeding of recalcitrant residents. Despite advances in technique, enteral nutrition by tube was not well tolerated; the assistance of four strong men was required to restrain the patient during administration of mixtures of beef broth, sugar, egg, and milk. In 1910, use of a rubber tube having a small lumen and a distal metal weight was advocated because it enhanced patient comfort and tolerance to nasoenteric feeding. By the 1970s, small-diameter, weighted feeding tubes made from biocompatible materials were commercially available. At that time, tube feeding formulas were handmade in the hospital kitchen from baby foods or blenderized house diets. Commercial availability of prepared formulas was spurred by development of special liquid diets that were first consumed by astronauts during early space flights. In the ensuing years, a plethora of commercial formulas has been introduced.

Indications

There are two major criteria which qualify patients for oral supplementation or enteral feeding by tube. Enteral nutritional support is indicated for patients who have a totally or partially functioning gastrointestinal (GI) tract and are unable or unwilling to ingest sufficient nutrients via an oral diet. Candidates include patients who are hypermetabolic because of disease, sepsis, or trauma; those who are unable to eat because of mechanical dysfunction such as esophageal or pharyngeal stricture or obstruction, maxillofacial surgery, or swallowing impairment due to cerebrovascular accident or other neurological disorder; and those who are unwilling to eat because of nausea, vomiting, or anorexia.

Patients who are able to eat an oral diet but unable to ingest enough to meet their nutritional requirements may benefit from supplementation of the diet with flavored tube feeding formulas. Oral supplements may be consumed directly from the container, or they may be incorporated into foods to increase nutritional value of the meal.

Formulas

Formulas for tube feeding or oral supplementation are available which are especially suited to the disease state, GI function, nutritional needs, and absorptive capacity of the patient. However, it is difficult to select an appropriate formula from the bewildering array of the more than 70 that are commercially available. Selection can be simplified by grouping formulas into generic categories. Type and quantity of nutrients in formulas are important criteria in assuring patient absorption and tolerance of tube feeding. Enteral formulas can be categorized as polymeric or monomeric, to indicate the form in which the nutrients are provided in a given formula.

Nutrients in *polymeric* formulas are in complex form and require digestion. Polymeric formulas range from those made from blenderized foods to those compounded from protein isolates (e.g., caseinate and soy), vegetable oils, and carbohydrates. Lactose has been eliminated as a carbohydrate source from most compounded formulas because patients with primary lactase deficiency do not tolerate it. Since secondary lactase deficiency may result from critical illness, the critically ill patient is also unlikely to tolerate lactose.

The caloric density of most of these formulas is 1 kcal per milliliter, although some provide 1.5 or 2 kcal per milliliter. The higher-calorie formulas are useful in meeting elevated energy requirements of the critically ill patient.

Most commercially prepared enteral formulas provide 14% to 17% of calories as protein. Patients whose protein needs are elevated due to trauma, sepsis, or thermal injuries may require formulas with higher protein concentrations. Polymeric formulas with a caloric density of 1 kcal per milliliter are intermediate in osmolality (300 to 450 mosm/kg water) and are tolerable, at full strength, to the nonstressed patient. Polymeric formulas with a caloric density of 1.5 to 2.0 kcal per milliliter are more hypertonic (600 to 710 mosm/kg water). More care must be given in administering a polymeric formula to the critically ill patient. The critically ill patient may require slow initiation of an isotonic formula, or dilution of a hypertonic formula, to enhance tolerance. Nurses should observe the patient for tolerance of the formula as evidenced by absence of abdominal distention, nausea, vomiting, or diarrhea. Polymeric formulas are useful as tube feedings for patients who have digestive and absorptive capacity. Many of these formulas are flavored or have a tolerable, bland taste, making them useful as oral dietary supplements.

Monomeric formulas provide nutrients in simple or "predigested" form, and very little digestion is required before nutrients can be absorbed. Monomeric formulas are compounded from nutrient sources ranging from simple crystalline amino acids and glucose molecules, to slightly more complex sources such as di- and tripeptides and modified corn starch or glucose oligosaccharides. These formulas are very low in fat. Most monomeric formulas are powdered and require reconstitution. Caloric density depends upon final dilution, but at full strength they provide 1 kcal per milliliter.

Monomeric formulas are particularly hypertonic (550 mosm/kg of water or more) because their short-chain nutrient sources contribute many osmotically active particles to the solution. Tube feeding using hypertonic formulas is often initiated with a dilute concentration to allow for gut adaptation to the osmolar load. Monomeric formulas are extremely unpalatable due to the short-chain nutrient sources. They are generally not used for oral supplementation.

A number of specialty formulas are available for use in cases of trauma, renal failure, ventilator dependence, or hepatic encephalopathy. These formulas are often used for nutritional support of the critically ill patient. The actual benefit derived from use of specialty formulas in reducing morbidity or mortality in the clinical setting remains to be proven. Moreover, the high cost of these formulas precludes routine use.

Modular nutritional components are sources of single nutrients. Carbohydrate, fat, and protein modules are commercially available and are used to supplement individual nutrients of prepared formulas, to produce formulas specifically designed to meet nutritional requirements of individual patients. Single-nutrient modules are especially useful in enteral nutritional support of the critically ill patient because the modules provide the flexibility often needed to meet special nutritional requirements.

Equipment and Supplies

Tubes specifically designed for enteral feeding are available in sizes ranging from a no. 5 French (1.7 mm) to a no. 16 French (4.3 mm); the size most frequently used is a no. 8 French (2.6 mm). The small lumen of feeding tubes greatly enhances a patient's comfort and reduces risk of aspiration.

Nasoenteric feeding tubes are constructed of silicone, polyurethane, or polyvinylchloride. Silicone and polyurethane are biocompatible materials that do not react with gastric juices. Tubes made from polyvinylchloride or other plastics, such as NG suction tubes, react with gastric juices and must be replaced more frequently than silicone or polyurethane tubes. Therefore, they are not ideal for use as feeding tubes.

Because silicone and polyurethane tubes are softer than plastic tubes, they are more comfortable but require an aid for insertion. Feeding tubes that use rigid outer guide tubes as insertion aids are available; however, the large diameter of the guide tube is a source of discomfort to the patient during intubation. Stylets are more frequently used to facilitate insertion of feeding tubes. Most tubes have been redesigned so that the outlet ports are at the distal tip of the tube. This design eliminates the possibility of mucosal damage because the stylet cannot exit through an outlet port.

Tubes tend to "sleeve up" over the stylet during removal. Some manufacturers have alleviated this problem by applying a lubricious coating to the interior of the tube. When the tube is in place, the stylet can be easily removed after the lubricant is activated by injection of about 10 ml of water into the tube. There have been some reports that, because tubes tend to collapse under negative pressure, it is difficult to check gastric residual by aspiration from feeding tubes. This is thought to be due to the softness and small lumen size of feeding tubes. Silicone tubes collapse more easily than those made from polyurethane because silicone tubes do not have very great tensile strength. Silicone tubes also have a greater tendency to rupture and stretch. Polyurethane is a superior material for feeding tubes because it has greater tensile strength.

Feeding tubes are available with and without weighted boluses. Weights are thought to help maintain tube placement, although there is some question regarding their efficacy. Most weights are made of tungsten or stainless steel, eliminating problems related to disposal of mercury.

Enterostomies are frequently used for long-term tube feeding. Gastrostomies and jejunostomies are most common, but esophagostomies are also used. Large-bore Levin-type tubes, Foley catheters, or rubber tubing are commonly used as surgically placed feeding tubes. These tubes are uncomfortable and esthetically unappealing, and they are relatively easy to dislodge or displace. Since they are not made from biocompatible materials, they require frequent replacement. Moreover, overinflation of the balloon on Foley catheters may cause intestinal obstruction or rupture.

A number of enterostomy tubes have been specifically designed to alleviate or prevent these problems. Needle catheter jejunostomy tubes are very small caliber, polyethylene tubes that can be introduced into the jejunum via a large-bore needle or trocar. These tubes are placed in the jejunum during abdominal surgery, and feeding can begin shortly after surgery. Their major disadvantage is that the very small lumen will not permit delivery of viscous formulas, necessitating exclusive use of monomeric formulas.

The majority of gastrostomy tubes require surgical placement. Percutaneous endoscopic gastrostomy (PEG) tubes can be placed via a gastroscope under local anesthesia, obviating the need for a surgical procedure.

Prior to the early 1970s enteral feeding pumps were not widely used in hospitals. Tube feeding was delivered by bolus administration or continuous gravity drip. As use of hyperosmolar feeding solutions increased, it was found that patients tolerated them better if feedings were delivered by slow, continuous infusion. Use of small-caliber feeding tubes also stimulated use of infusion pumps to assure controlled delivery of the more viscous formulas, because such formulas would not flow freely by gravity drip through small feeding tubes. Pump-assisted enteral feeding assures accurate and reliable delivery of large volumes of formula. Use of a pump assures that the patient receives formula by a slow, continuous drip, which reduces gastric pooling, thereby decreasing the potential for aspiration.

Intravenous (IV) infusion pumps have been used to deliver enteral feedings. However, in most hospitals, use of IV pumps to deliver enteral feeding is limited because pump-assisted infusion of IV solutions is of higher priority than delivery of pump-controlled enteral feeding. The use of IV pumps for delivery of enteral formulas may not result in accurate delivery because these pumps were not designed to deliver highly viscous solutions such as enteral formulas. The most recent generation of enteral feeding infusion pumps employs microprocessors which assure accuracy rates of ±5%. The newest pump models provide flexibility in range of flow rate settings because the rate can be advanced in 1-ml increments; older models offer a variety of rate settings ranging from increments of 5 ml to 50 ml. Most enteral pumps operate on both direct current and battery power. The option for battery-powered operation is an important consideration as more patients are discharged to continue tube feeding as outpatients. Feeding pumps are generally lightweight and easy to operate, making their use even more feasible in the outpatient setting. Enteral feeding pumps feature audible and visual alarms to indicate malfunction, battery status, and inadvertent change of flow rate.

The tubing and other disposable supplies used with a specific pump are not compatible between different makes of pumps. This feature may increase cost of supplies, but it assures accuracy and safety because tubing is specifically calibrated to the pump for which it is made. Also, the potential for accidental connection of enteral feeding solutions to IV lines is reduced.

Administration

Formula is delivered via the tube into either the stomach or the small intestine. Choice of a feeding site depends on the condition of the patient. Feeding into the stomach is the method of choice for the alert patient who has an intact gag reflex and an adequate rate of gastric emptying. Feeding into the stomach is advantageous because, unlike the small intestine, the stomach can tolerate high osmotic loads with less incidence of GI side effects. Most formulas are well tolerated by patients receiving gastric feeding. Bolus feedings are tolerable for the stable patient who has a gastric feeding tube; however, the critically ill patient would benefit from continuous feedings because of the complexity of care required. The relatively large volume of the stomach allows it to tolerate boluses of 200 to 250 ml.

Critically ill patients often have a depressed level of consciousness, artificial airways, depressed gag reflex, extreme debilitation, or decreased intestinal motility. Patients having these conditions are not candidates for nasogastric tube feeding because they are at a higher risk for aspiration of gastric contents. Although insertion of nasoduodenal or nasojejunal tubes is more difficult than passage of nasogastric tubes, transpyloric tube placement decreases the risk of regurgitation and aspiration of gastric contents. In addition, use of the small bowel makes early postoperative feedings possible because the small intestine is unaffected by gastric ileus. Tube migration out of the duodenum or jejunum and into the stomach is a frequent problem with nasally placed tubes, necessitating a surgically placed jejunostomy tube for longterm feeding.

Procedures used for insertion of nasoenteric feeding tubes have been well described elsewhere. Placement of the tube into the stomach is accomplished by gently advancing the feeding tube through the most patent nostril until an appropriate, premeasured length is inserted. If small bowel placement is desired, an additional 50 cm is inserted. The tube should pass into the duodenum by normal peristaltic action within 24 to 48 hours. Passage can be enhanced by having the patient lie on his or her right side. An oral or intravenous dose of metaclopramide to stimulate gastric emptying may also facilitate passage of the tube into the duodenum. Concurrent fluoroscopy during tube insertion ensures appropriate placement.

Despite the presence of weighted boluses, it is possible for feeding tubes to migrate or bcome dislodged, and it is necessary to secure the tube to the patient. Paper tape does not adhere well to silicone or polyurethane feeding tubes. Adherence may be improved by wiping the portion of the tube to be taped first with alcohol then with benzoin before placing the tape on it. Use of a transparent, moisture-vapor permeable dressing is an alternative to using paper tape (Figure 11-2).

Formula may be administered by a variety of methods. Bolus feeding is best tolerated by the patient who

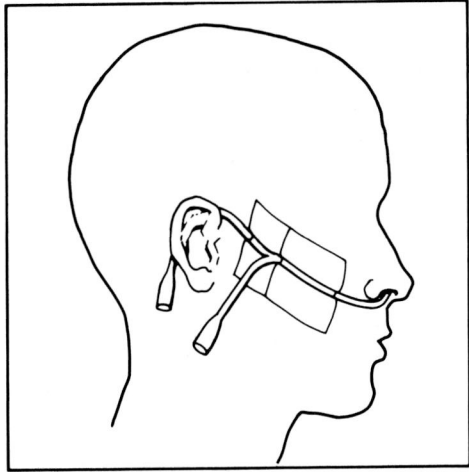

Figure 11-2 Use of a transparent moistureproof dressing to anchor feeding tubes.

Reprinted, with permission, from Gray, D. P., & Smith, P. D. (1984). *Nutritional Support Services, 4*(7), 37-38.

has a gastric feeding tube. Bolus feeding is advocated by some because it is similar to normal meal patterns and gastric distention resulting from boluses of formula may stimulate digestion. This method is more time-consuming than pump-assisted feeding because to avoid GI complications, formula should not be administered faster than 30 ml per minute. Moreover, because of decreased absorptive function of the GI tract and delayed gastric emptying time, rapid delivery of boluses may lead to gastric pooling. This can increase the potential for reflux and pulmonary aspiration of gastric contents.

The critically ill patient, and those receiving feeding into the small intestine, benefit from continuous delivery of formula. Continuous drip feeding may be accomplished by gravity or by the use of a pump. When feeding a hypertonic solution, continuous drip administration is preferred; it is associated with fewer GI complications than bolus administration because pump-assisted tube feeding assures accurate, constant delivery of formulas. Gravity flow is harder to regulate.

Regardless of the method of delivery, feeding should be initiated in small volumes and advanced slowly. It is still common practice to begin tube feeding with diluted formula, advancing to full strength over the course of 2 to 3 days. This practice is usually unnecessary for patients who have adequate GI function. Such "starter regimens" have been found to reduce nutrient intake while not significantly improving tolerance to feeding.[7] Generally, tolerance is assured if full-strength isotonic formulas are begun at flow rates of 30 to 50 ml per hour, advancing in increments of 30 to 50 ml per day, until the desired volume is reached. Feeding can be advanced from isotonic to hypertonic formulas after gut adaptation has occurred.

Enteral feeding by tube is associated with some of the complications that occur with parenteral feeding. Careful nursing care and monitoring of the patient's progress can help avoid the development of these problems. Use of routine procedures (Table 11-2) can assist in providing comprehensive care of the patient receiving tube feeding.

Complications

Side effects that may occur during tube feeding can be classified as GI, mechanical, or metabolic. Most can be alleviated through proper monitoring and management.

Gastrointestinal complications, including nausea, vomiting, diarrhea, gastric retention, and malabsorption are often considered unavoidable consequences of tube feeding. However, most complications can be relieved or prevented.

Diarrhea is the most commonly reported GI side effect of tube feeding. Numerous etiological factors may simultaneously contribute to diarrhea, each of which may require therapy before diarrhea can be resolved. Stool frequency may be due to rapid infusion of hyperosmolar enteral solutions but also may occur because of bacterial contamination of formula or malabsorption of specific components of formulas. Protein-calorie malnutrition, resulting in hypoalbuminemia and atrophy of intestinal absorptive surfaces, may cause diarrhea by decreasing absorption of nutrients from the GI tract. Frequent stools induced by antibiotic therapy may be mistakenly attributed to tube feeding. Bolus feeding is often associated with diarrhea and other GI symptoms because there is a propensity to overwhelm the absorptive capacity of the gut.

Most GI symptoms can be relieved or prevented by beginning feeding with an isotonic formula and slowly advancing the infusion rate. Use of a feeding pump to control the rate of infusion is also helpful in decreasing the incidence of GI side effects. It may be necessary in the case of malabsorption to change formulas to eliminate the offending component. The critically ill patient is frequently intolerant of lactose due to lactase deficiency. Almost all commercial formulas are lactose-free, but lactose intolerance may still be an etiological factor in development of GI complications if milk products are added to formulas. This may have greater significance as more patients are discharged from the hospital to continue tube feeding at home using homemade formulas that include lactose-containing foods. Homemade formulas do not necessarily meet the vitamin and mineral requirements for the patient.

Fat is frequently malabsorbed by patients receiving commercial formulas. This problem may be addressed by changing to a formula with a different fat source or one with a lower overall fat content.

Tube feeding formulas are rich media for bacterial growth. Administration of bacterially contaminated formulas has been associated with diarrhea; therefore scrupulous care must be taken to avoid contaminating the formula and administration system. Moreover, formula should not hang longer than 8 hours, and feeding containers and tubing should be changed every 24 hours. Some authors have suggested that the best way to minimize risk of bacterial contamination is by the use of sterile formula packaged in a closed administration system.[8]

Mechanical complications may be decreased through choice of an appropriate feeding tube, proper monitoring of tube placement, and adequate care of the tube. Mechanical side effects frequently arise from use of large-bore tubes. These tubes are extremely

TABLE 11-2   Routine Procedures for Care of the Tube-fed Patient

Procedure	Frequency	Rationale
Confirm tube placement and patency.	Prior to bolus feeding or every 4-6 hours	To prevent aspiration and avoid delivery of formula to sites other than GI tract
Check gastric residuals (use a 30-ml syringe or larger).	Prior to bolus feeding or every 4-6 hours	To assess tolerance and prevent aspiration
Hold feedings and notify physician if residual is >150 ml or patient exhibits signs of intolerance.	As necessary	To prevent aspiration and alleviate symptoms
Elevate head of bed 45° for patients who have depressed gag reflex. (This may be unnecessary for alert patients.)	During feeding and 30 min following feeding	To prevent aspiration
Hang feeding for 8 hours or less.		To decrease chance of patient intolerance due to bacterial overgrowth
Monitor gravity drip flow rates.	Every hour	To enhance tolerance by maintaining even flow rate of formulas
Irrigate feeding tube with 30-50 ml water.	After each bolus and following medications	To maintain patency of feeding tube and supplement fluid intake
Provide oral and nasal hygiene.	Daily and as necessary	To enhance comfort
Replace feeding conatiner and tubing.	Every 24 hours	To maintain sanitation of system and decrease chances of patient intolerance due to bacterial contamination
Evaluate and document:		To monitor patient tolerance and progress and avoid complications
Urine glucose and acetone	Every 4-6 hours initially, 3 times/day when stable	
Intake and output	Daily	
Stool frequency and consistency	Daily	
Body weight	Daily initially, 3 times/week when stable	
Plasma electrolytes	2-3 times/week initially, 1 time/week when stable	
Blood glucose	2-3 times/week initially, 1 time/week when stable	
Blood urea nitrogen and creatinine	2-3 times/week initially, 1 time/week when stable	
Clinical observations	Every 8 hours	To assess for change in patient status

uncomfortable for the patient and are associated with pulmonary aspiration of gastric contents. Meticulous attention to monitoring tube placement and gastric residual is also important in decreasing potential for aspiration by assuring that feeding is administered only to the GI tract, and that gastric pooling does not occur. Taping the tube helps maintain tube position. Care must be taken in taping nasoenteric tubes to avoid pressure on the nostril. Ostomy sites must be carefully dressed to avoid tissue irritation.

Feeding tubes must be carefully and frequently irrigated to maintain patency, which is particularly important if these tubes are used to deliver medications.

Feeding tubes should be flushed with 30 ml to 50 ml water before and after medications are administered. Whenever possible, liquid medications should be ordered. When this is not possible, medications should be thoroughly crushed and dissolved in water before administering. It is advisable to check with a pharmacist when medications must be delivered via a feeding tube. Crushing or dissolving drugs may alter their absorption or action. There may also be potential for drug–nutrient interactions with the tube feeding formula.

In the event of occlusion, a stylet should not be used to clear the tube because of the possibility of rupturing the tube and damaging the intestinal mucosa. Before an occluded tube is removed, an attempt can be made to clear the tube by instilling 10 ml of a carbonated beverage or warm water and clamping the tube for 1 hour. The tube is then flushed with warm water after 1 hour. A solution of ¼ tsp meat tenderizer in 60 ml of water, followed with clear water 1 hour later, has been advocated. Caution is required because frequent use of meat tenderizer will cause esophageal and gastric erosions. Use of meat tenderizer in individuals who are allergic to papain, or to MSG, is contraindicated. If these maneuvers are unsuccessful, a physician may insert an endoscopy brush or a stylet designed for clogged tubes to clear the blockage. If all of these measures fail, replacement may be needed.

Metabolic complications of tube feeding occur relatively frequently but can be prevented by proper management. Hypertonic dehydration is commonly called *tube feeding syndrome*. Tube feeding syndrome can occur when hypertonic, high-protein formulas are delivered without sufficient free water. Patients who are unable to communicate their feelings of thirst are particularly susceptible. Fluid intake of tube-fed patients must be supplemented, even though most isotonic formulas contain approximately 75% to 80% free water. Usually, 1 ml of water is required for each calorie provided by tube feeding formula.

Overhydration, or *refeeding syndrome*, can occur when feeding is reintroduced to severely malnourished patients. Patients with cardiac, renal, or hepatic insufficiency are also candidates for development of this syndrome. Refeeding syndrome is treated by decreasing the rate of feeding, then gradually advancing the rate when the fluid status of the patient normalizes. A formula providing 1.5 to 2 kcal per ml assists in providing adequate nutrition while restricting fluid volume.

Hyperglycemia occurs frequently in tube-fed patients. It is treated by decreasing the infusion rate and administering insulin to maintain the blood glucose at 200 mg/dl. Changing the formula to one with fiber or a greater percentage of calories from fat instead of carbohydrate may also assist in controlling hyperglycemia. Since hyperglycemia is an early sign of sepsis, a potential source of infection should also be investigated.

Electrolyte abnormalities occurring as a consequence of tube feeding are relatively uncommon. Such abnormalities usually arise from the underlying disease state rather than from enteral nutritional support. Hypophosphatemia may occur with rapid refeeding or secondary to insulin therapy. It can be avoided by initiating feeding slowly, and monitoring the patient's serum phosphorus levels. Specific electrolytes can be influenced by the choice of formula. The serum potassium, particularly in patients with renal failure, may be better controlled by using a formula with a lower potassium content.

Parenteral Nutrition

Patients received the benefit of intravenous glucose solutions as early as 1896. In 1952, a method for central venous access by percutaneous infraclavicular catheterization was developed by Aubaniac, which Dudrick in the late 1960s adapted to deliver hypertonic, IV nutritional solutions. The demonstration in 1967 that this technique could support weight gain and growth of human beings heralded the beginning of the modern history of parenteral nutritional support.[9]

Indications

Parenteral nutrition (PN) has been used in cases of anorexia nervosa, prolonged ileus, inflammatory bowel disease, pancreatitis, neoplastic disease, and other conditions. Metabolic support by the parenteral route was conceived as an "artificial gut." Because of expense and the potential for life-threatening complications, it should ideally be used only in situations in which the GI tract cannot or should not work, or when the patient can tolerate some enteral alimentation but not enough to meet metabolic requirements. Parenteral nutrition is often used in the critical care setting because disease or trauma frequently renders the GI tract partially or totally nonfunctional. Critical illness may increase nutritional requirements so that it is not possible for the gut to tolerate the volume or caloric density of formulas which may be required to meet the nutritional needs imposed by some hypermetabolic states.

Routes of Access

Percutaneous placement of a polyethylene or polyvinylchloride catheter into the superior vena cava via the subclavian or internal jugular vein is the most frequently used method for delivery of parenteral nutritional solutions. The catheter can be inserted at the bedside under local anesthesia, but there is a potential for technical complications including arterial puncture, pneumothorax, or hemothorax, since the catheter is inserted blindly without benefit of fluoroscopy. Another problem is that polyethylene or polyvinylchloride catheters are suitable only for short-term PN because the material of the catheter may cause thrombophlebitis, and the catheter can serve as a site for infection. Because of the potential for infection, the catheter should be used only for infusion of PN solutions.

It is common for the critically ill patient to require

several venous accesses. This need can be met by inserting bilateral subclavian catheters, but this is not ideal because it doubles the chances of catheter-related complications and increases the care required to maintain critical IV lines. A multilumen polyurethane catheter is commonly used in critical care to meet the need for multiple lines. This catheter contains three separate lumens and can be placed through a single insertion site. The multiple lumens can be used to administer blood products, medications, chemotherapy, or PN, and to withdraw blood samples. Each distinct lumen exits from the catheter at a different level, but potential incompatibilities between fluids needs to be considered. Several authors have demonstrated precipitate formation from incompatible drugs infused via separate lumens. Strict aseptic technique should be used during insertion, including sterile gown and mask and a drape large enough to accommodate the length of the guidewire.

Silastic catheters, commonly called Hickman or Broviac catheters (Figure 11-3), are used when long-term central venous access is required. Long-term silastic catheters have a number of desirable features that make them usable for months to years. The silicone material of the catheter is flexible, durable, and less thrombogenic than polyvinylchloride or polyurethane. The proximal Dacron cuff is a physical barrier to entry of bacteria to the systemic circulation via the catheter tract. The cuff also facilitates engraftment of tissue to it within 2 to 4 weeks after insertion, which helps anchor the catheter. The catheter is insered through a subcutaneous tunnel, usually around the nipple line of the chest wall, before it enters the systemic circulation. The tip of the catheter is placed in the superior vena cava, at the junction of the right

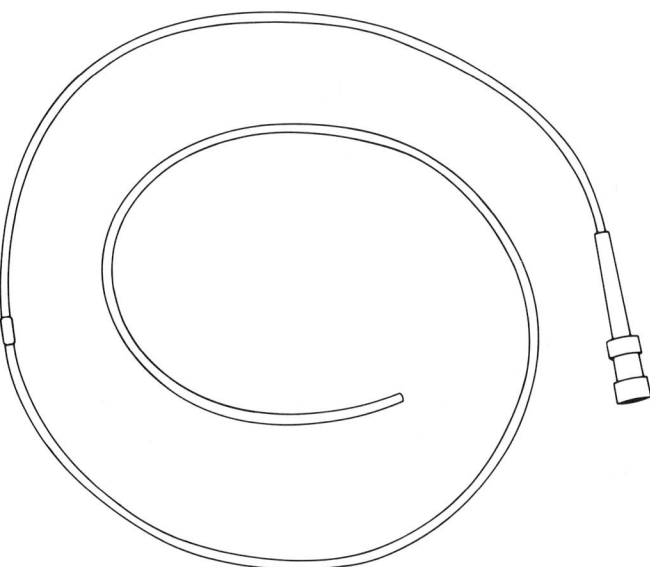

Figure 11-3 Hickman catheter.

atrium. Placement in the right atrium may cause cardiac tamponade. Because there is less potential for infection with use of this catheter, it is possible to administer multiple infusions sequentially, and to withdraw blood samples through long-term Silastic catheters.

It is not possible, however, to infuse incompatible solutions simultaneously through a single-lumen silastic catheter. Double- and triple-lumen catheters were developed to provide additional lumens for central venous access. The first lumen is used exclusively for delivery of PN solutions, and the additional lumens are used to administer other IV solutions or blood products, and to withdraw blood samples.

Long-term silastic catheters are inserted in the operating room under continuous fluoroscopy, which reduces the incidence of technical complications that can occur from blind insertion of central venous lines. Use of the operating room and the need for a surgeon's expertise to place these catheters increases the cost of using them and may discourage some physicians from prescribing long-term silastic catheters solely for the purpose of PN.

Peripherally inserted central catheters (PICC) provide some of the same benefits as long-term silastic catheters, and they can be inserted at the patient's bedside. These PICCs are made of silicone and are placed in the superior vena cava, via a percutaneous route, with the aid of an introducing device.

The development of IV lipid emulsions as a calorie source has made peripheral delivery of PN a possibility. Before IV lipids were available, peripheral parenteral nutritional support was limited to *protein-sparing* therapy (the infusion of amino acids and dextrose) because small-diameter peripheral veins cannot tolerate the hypertonic glucose solutions required to accomplish weight gain and nitrogen retention. The goal of protein-sparing therapy was to provide enough amino acids and calories in a tolerable concentration and volume to reduce catabolism of body protein by gluconeogenesis. It is obvious that this therapy cannot provide adequate calories for anabolism because 1 L of 10% dextrose in water provides approximately 354 calories.

Lipid emulsions provide 1.1 to 2 kcal per ml, and one 500-ml bottle of 20% lipid emulsion provides up to 1,000 kcal. Lipid emulsions are isotonic, and can be administered via a peripheral vein. Provision of a nutritionally complete PN solution is possible using a two-bottle system in which a lipid emulsion and an amino acid–dextrose solution are infused simultaneously through a Y connector into a peripheral IV catheter. For peripheral PN to be successful, there must be adequate venous access because, as with any peripheral IV line, sites must be changed frequently to avoid phlebitis. In addition, some patients, especially the critically ill, may not tolerate large doses of IV lipid emulsions. The use of three-in-one PN improves patient tolerance because the lipids reduce the osmolality of the dextrose and amino acids.

Solutions

Parenteral nutritional support is often called *total parenteral nutrition*, or *TPN*, because it is possible to provide all three major substrates—protein, carbohydrate, and fat—along with vitamins, minerals, trace elements and water, parenterally. Protein is provided in the form of crystalline amino acids that are commercially available in concentrations of 3.5% to 10%. A 15% amino acid solution is also available for patients needing large amounts of protein (e.g., burns, trauma), or where fluid volume is a concern. The 15% solution is costly, however, and should be reserved for use in those patients who would most benefit from it. The calories provided by protein usually are not included when calculating the amount of energy provided by PN solutions. This is because the ideal end point of amino acids is incorporation into somatic and plasma proteins. For this to occur, it is necessary to provide adequate amounts of nonprotein calories so that protein is not used as an energy source. The glucose concentrations most frequently used to supply nonprotein calories are 20%, 50%, or 70% glucose in sterile water. Intravenously administered carbohydrate provides 3.4 calories per gram, as compared to the 4 calories per gram provided by enterally administered carbohydrate.

Total reliance on glucose for energy is not ideal since its metabolism increases the cardiac output, respiratory quotient, and serum levels of catecholamines and insulin. Although glucose calories support nitrogen retention, associated weight gain may be due to increases in fat tissue and body water rather than muscle mass. Fatty deposits may develop in the liver when glucose is the only source of nonprotein calories. The critically ill patient is frequently insulin-resistant, and significant hyperglycemia may result when glucose is the sole energy source. Moreover, because glucose is not a source of essential fatty acids, the patient is at risk of developing essential fatty acid deficiency if a source is not provided. However, at least 100 g of glucose are required to meet the need for glucose by obligate glycolyzer cells and to prevent glyconeogenesis. Provision of 20% of total calories as glucose will meet these minimum requirements.

Intravenous lipid emulsions are another source of calories and are ideally used with glucose to provide calories in PN solutions. Intravenous lipid emulsions are useful in preventing essential fatty acid deficiency and side effects associated with the sole use of glucose to provide nonprotein calories. It is usual to infuse a 500-ml dose of IV lipid twice a week to preclude essential fatty acid deficiency. More frequent use of lipid emulsions may be necessary to provide calories, particularly when the use of glucose needs to be limited because of patient intolerance. Dosages for adults in excess of 2.5 g per kilogram of body weight per day should be avoided to prevent fat overload because critically ill patients are unable to eliminate excessive amounts of lipid from the bloodstream.

Requirements for parenterally administered vitamins, trace elements, and electrolytes vary from enteral requirements because the gut is bypassed. However, it is necessary to supply adequate amounts of trace elements to the patient receiving PN. Maintenance levels of IV trace elements are at least 2 mg zinc, 0.5 mg copper, 10 g chromium, and 0.15 mg manganese, but the critically ill patient, especially one with intestinal losses, requires more than these maintenance amounts.

Water needs can be met with the TPN solution. Careful calculation of fluid balance, with attention to excessive losses, should be communicated to the physician. Sterile water added to the TPN may also obviate the need for other IV fluids to be concurrently administered. Several routine medications, especially H_2 antagonists, may be added to the TPN, eliminating the need to infuse them separately.

The critically ill patient may require electrolytes in amounts different from maintenance amounts. Patients receiving antibiotics such as carbenicillin, ticarcillin, and tobramycin may require increased amounts of potassium, since these antibiotics can cause significant urinary losses of potassium. Diuretics and amphotericin also may precipitate hypokalemia through renal losses. Potassium can also be lost through the GI tract via diarrhea and small bowel drainage. Significant losses of bicarbonate may occur in the patient who has large gastric output.

Many IV fluids and certain antibiotics, such as carbenicillin and ticarcillin, contain considerable amounts of sodium. It may be necessary to reduce sodium intake by reducing or deleting sodium from PN solutions for patients receiving sodium-containing antibiotics and fluids.

Phosphorus requirements may be elevated for patients receiving phosphate-binding antacids. Corticosteroid therapy can cause renal losses of phosphate. Phosphate requirements may be increased by parenteral feeding itself because phosphate is required to metabolize glucose.

Patients receiving PN often develop hypomagnesemia simply because magnesium is overlooked when writing orders for PN solutions. Patients receiving cisplatin, amphotericin, corticosteroids, or diuretics may require increased amounts of magnesium.

Complications

Complications associated with PN can be categorized as technical, septic, or metabolic. *Technical complications* are those that occur during or in relation to catheter insertion. The most common technical complications are pneumothorax, hemothorax, air embolism, catheter embolism, arterial puncture, and subclavian vein thrombosis. These complications are more frequently associated with blind percutaneous placement of subclavian catheters. The frequency with which technical complications occur is inversely related to the experience of the physician inserting the catheter. Technical complications occur less frequently when catheters are inserted under continuous fluoroscopy. There is great potential for catheter-related sepsis; therefore, the nurse should adhere to strict aseptic technique when hanging PN solutions and caring for the catheter and tubing. Strict protocols for care and monitoring of a patient with a central venous catheter and receiving TPN should be in place and enforced.

The most common *metabolic complication* of PN is glucose intolerance. Most patients tolerate glucose infusions of 400 to 500 g delivered over a 24-hour period. Patients who are stressed, diabetic, severely malnourished or debilitated, or undergoing corticosteroid therapy, may, however, exhibit hyperglycemia and glucosuria. Blood glucose levels in excess of 200 mg/dl accompanied by urinary spillage of 2 g glucose per dl urine may lead to development of hyperglycemic, hyperosmolar, nonketotic coma. As with enteral nutrition, the sudden onset of hyperglycemia may be an early indicator of sepsis. The central venous catheter should be considered an infectious source until ruled out by blood culture and clinical observation.

Conversely, hypoglycemia may occur with sudden cessation of hypertonic glucose solutions. When discontinuing PN solutions, the infusion rate should be tapered. Usually, decreasing the rate by half for 1 to 2 hours is sufficient. If the TPN is interrupted unexpectedly, infusing $D_{10}W$ at the same rate as the TPN infused will prevent hypoglycemia.

Electrolyte abnormalities may occur rapidly with PN, especially in the critically ill patient. Aberrations in serum levels of potassium, phosphorus, and magnesium are common. Electrolytes should be monitored daily for at least the first 3 days, then three times a week in the critically ill patient.

When lipid emulsions are used, the nurse should report abnormalities in a patient's values for liver function tests, serum cholesterol, and triglycerides.

Administration

During initiation of PN, 1 to 2 L of the solution are infused during the first 24-hour period. The severely stressed or critically ill patient may require significant amounts of insulin to maintain acceptable blood glucose levels during the initial period. The insulin may be added to the TPN in subsequent days after initiation, when the patient's tolerance is determined. After 24 hours, the infusion rate can be increased in increments of 500 to 1,000 ml per day, until the volume necessary to meet nutritional requirements is attained.

Occasionally, PN solutions are "cycled" to provide a period each day during which no nutritional solutions are administered. Cycling PN solutions is thought to induce a "postabsorptive state" similar to that following oral ingestion of a meal. Cycling is claimed to prevent or resolve fatty liver deposits that can occur with continuous PN. Cycled PN is also useful when the number of IV lines is limited and silastic catheters are used to deliver medications, chemotherapy, blood products, and other IV fluids, as well as PN.

Parenteral nutrition is cycled by beginning the infusion at a lower infusion rate than the final desired rate and increasing the rate over 2 hours, or by beginning at the desired rate. The infusion is cycled over 12 to 14 hours, depending upon the patient's tolerance. When the cycle is complete, the infusion rate is tapered off by cutting the rate in half over 1 to 2 hours. Checking a blood glucose 1 hour after completion of the cycle will determine whether the patient is hypoglycemic. A bedside glucose monitor is an efficient method for performing this test.

It is not necessary to hang 10% glucose following cycles of PN administration because the infusion is tapered slowly to prevent rebound hypoglycemia.

The use of lipid emulsions in cyclic PN makes it possible to provide adequate calories in a volume that can be administered over a 12- to 14-hour period. Fat emulsions may be delivered by gravity drip or with the use of a pump. They may be delivered through a separate IV line or simultaneously with amino acid–glucose solutions through a Y connector into the central line. Lipids should be connected to the extension tubing as closely as possible to the hub of the catheter and may not go through a 0.22 μg filter. A 1.2 μg filter may be used with a three-in-one TPN solution. The lipid container should be hung lower than the PN container to prevent backflow of the lipid emulsion. The use of three-in-one PN solutions allows more convenience since all the components are infused concurrently.

When the patient is able to resume an oral diet, he or she should be weaned from PN, especially if the patient has been without oral intake for a long time, because the gut may atrophy during periods of disuse. The patient may experience symptoms of malabsorption due to decreased absorptive surface of the gut and reduced production of the digestive enzymes maltase, sucrase, and lactase. Concentrated sugars, milk products, and fats should be reintroduced slowly to the diet because these foods are frequently malabsorbed by the patient who has been NPO. Transition to an oral diet should be adjusted to the tolerance of the individual patient. Generally, following the traditional dietary progression from clear liquid to full liquid to low residue and finally to a regular diet will assure patient tolerance.

The patient should continue to receive PN until he or she is able to ingest approximately 75% of the nutritional requirements via an oral diet. Commercial nutritional supplements can be used to reach this goal, but care must be taken that they do not contribute to malabsorption. Several widely used nutritional supplements provide more than 50% of calories as carbohydrate, the majority of which is sucrose. The high fat content of most nutritional supplements also may be a factor that contributes to intolerance in patients who are being weaned from PN.

Nursing Management

Nursing interventions are aimed at preventing complications and enhancing a patient's tolerance and progress with PN. These responsibilities can be met by preparing the patient for and assisting the physician with insertion of the central venous catheter, preventing sepsis by proper maintenance of the nutritional delivery system and catheter, and evaluating patient response to the therapy. Most institutions have comprehensive policies and procedures for accomplishing these goals.

Technical complications that may occur during insertion of the central venous catheter can be reduced if the patient understands the procedure. Discussion of the need for the patient's cooperation in performing the Valsalva maneuver, patient positioning, draping, and possible sensations felt during catheter insertion are helpful in reducing anxiety and improving compliance during insertion.

When the PN catheter is inserted at the bedside, the patient is placed in the Trendelenburg position, with his or her head turned away from the insertion site and a rolled towel placed beneath the scapulae for a subclavian vein insertion. The skin is prepared by cleansing the skin with one or more antiseptic solutions (e.g., alcohol, povidone-iodine, chlorhexidine). The patient is asked to perform the Valsalva maneuver at the time of catheter insertion to prevent air embolism, and is monitored during the procedure

for evidence of complications such as pneumo- or hemothorax, or cardiac irritability.

Since PN is administered directly into the systemic circulation, meticulous care must be given to the solution, line, and insertion site to prevent infection. The IV administration set should be changed every 24 hours. Care should be taken to avoid contaminating the tubing spike when inserting it into the PN container. The catheter is clamped when the IV administration set is changed to prevent air embolism. Maintenance of a sterile occlusive dressing over the site is vital for prevention of infection. A gauze and tape dressing may be changed either daily or every other day in critical care. Transparent dressings, if used, need to be changed at least every 72 hours.

Procedures used with central venous accesses must be varied when the patient has a long-term silastic catheter. Since the catheter can be "heparin-locked" when not in use, patency should be assessed before beginning an infusion by aspiration, followed by flushing with 3 ml of saline. After the infusion is complete, the catheter must be flushed with 3 ml of 100 U per ml heparin-saline solution to prevent occlusion. Groshong long-term Silastic catheters need to be flushed with 20 ml of saline only at the end of an infusion.

It is important to use padded clamps and to change the location of clamp sites to prevent wear on the catheter. Silastic catheters of recent manufacture have a reinforced section for clamping. These measures reduce the risk of tearing or puncturing the catheter.

Other nursing responsibilities include monitoring the patient's progress and tolerance to PN. Progress should be evaluated by daily measurement of body weight to evaluate weight gain. The nurse is responsible for assuring that a complete 24-hour collection of urine, which is used for estimation of nitrogen balance, is obtained. Other nursing interventions include accurate measurement and recording of the patient's temperature and fluid input and output, and checking urine for presence of sugar and acetone, or measuring blood glucose with a bedside glucose monitor. Abnormal serum electrolyte values should be indicated to the physician as soon as possible. The catheter insertion site should be inspected for redness, tenderness, or drainage during each dressing change and signs of infection should be reported to the physician.

CASE STUDY

Mr. W. was admitted with a diagnosis of acute myelogenous leukemia. His weight was 70 kg and his serum albumin was 2.8 g/dl. His initial daily nutritional requirements were calculated to be approximately 1,700 kcal and 56 g of protein. A single-lumen silastic catheter was inserted and chemotherapy was begun.

Mr. W. lost 5 kg due to nausea, vomiting, and anorexia secondary to induction therapy. His nutritional status was compromised further when he developed an opportunistic *Candida* infection throughout his GI tract that further impaired his ability to ingest and absorb an adequate oral diet.

Mr. W. received sequential infusions of blood products, amphotericin, other medications, and IV fluids through the silastic catheter, so continuous infusion of PN was not possible. Cyclic PN was administered between 6:00 P.M. and 8:00 A.M. each day. Other necessary IV solutions were delivered through the catheter during the intervals when no PN solutions were infused.

Nutritional requirements were provided by three-in-one TPN solution. During each cycle, 1,500 ml of a solution consisting of 4.25% amino acids and 25% glucose provided 1,175 kcal and approximately 64 g of protein. An additional 500 kcal were provided by 500 ml of 10% lipid emulsion added to the amino acid–glucose solution by the pharmacy.

Ten U of insulin were added to the TPN solution during each cycle to prevent hyperglycemia. An in-line filter was not used because it was feared that insulin might adsorb to it, thus causing erratic delivery of insulin to the patient.

Serum electrolytes were evaluated each morning. Daily PN orders were written by the physician, based on the patient's electrolyte values. Electrolyte replacement was accomplished as much as possible by the nutritional solutions to obviate the need for peripheral IV lines for electrolyte replacement.

One week after cyclic PN began, evaluation of nitrogen balance showed that Mr. W. had a negative nitrogen balance of 10 g of protein. The amount of protein in the PN solution was increased by changing the 4.25% amino acid concentration to 5%. The reformulated PN solutions provided 1,675 nonprotein kcal and 75 g of protein.

Mr. W. received cyclic PN for 3 weeks. During that period, he evidenced elevated liver function values. Although elevations in liver function values can occur due to hepatitis (which may develop in patients receiving multiple blood infusions), the lipid emulsions were reduced to two times a week because it was possible that this was the reason for the elevated values. By this time, Mr. W. had begun to ingest an oral diet. His complaints of nausea and vomiting had decreased although he was still anorexic. He was encouraged to increase his daily intake of sipping, over the period of several hours, one can (250 ml) of a 2-kcal-per-milliliter, commercially prepared formula. This augmented his dietary intake by 500 kcal per day.

At the end of 4 weeks, Mr. W. was discharged, having achieved remission of his leukemia during a fairly uneventful hospital course. He had regained 4 kg of body weight and his serum albumin was 3.0 g/dl. He was encouraged to continue supplementing his diet with the commercial preparation and was given recipes that incorporated the formula in dishes he had enjoyed before his hospitalization.

SPECIAL CONDITIONS

Burns

Thermal injury is devastating since it causes impressive pain, metabolic aberrations, and nutritional costs. Recovery requires long hospitalization and comprehensive nursing care. Involvement of the entire health care team is required because input from all disciplines is necessary to facilitate healing and discharge of the patient.

Effects on Metabolism

There are two distinct metabolic phases following thermal injury. The *ebb phase* is the period immediately following injury. Shock, hypovolemia, and decreased metabolic rate and oxygen consumption are the major metabolic events of this period.

The second, or *flow phase*, begins 2 to 3 days after an injury. This period is marked by hypermetabolism, hyperventilation, elevated skin temperature, and increased evaporative water loss. Hormonal response during this period includes increased secretion of glucocorticoids and mineralocorticoids. These hormones are responsible for mounting the "survival response" which includes mobilization of necessary energy substrates. Amino acids are transferred from skeletal muscle for conversion to glucose, via gluconeogenesis by the liver. Urinary loss of nitrogen occurs as lean body mass is catabolized to produce energy. Negative nitrogen balance is enhanced by elevated serum levels of glucagon and catecholamines. These hormones are antagonistic to insulin; therefore, presence of increased serum levels of glucagon and catecholamines contributes to hyperglycemia and continued release of amino acids from the periphery.

The etiology of hypermetabolism following thermal injury is multifactorial and not completely understood. It is thought to be a result of readjustment of preburn metabolic activity to a higher level. Catecholamines are implicated as the primary mediators in this "reset" of metabolic rate. Elevated skin temperature and evaporative water loss contribute to hypermetabolism. These are also the result of adrenergic activity, which is directly proportional to the extent of the open wound and continues to influence metabolic rate until wounds are healed or grafted.

The critically ill patient undergoing disease, surgery, or injury experiences metabolic stress similar to the burned patient; therefore, the pattern of metabolic response activated by thermal injury can serve as a model of the response of the body to any major stress.

Nutritional Requirements

Basal energy expenditure of the burned patient is increased tremendously. One study[10] indicates that nutritional needs are related to the extent of the open wound and not necessarily to burn size. Age and physical condition of the patient, prior nutritional status, and the presence of chronic diseases also affect nutritional requirements.

Body weight and percentage of total body surface area burned (TBSAB) are necessary data for estimation of fluid and calorie requirements. The *rule of nines* is a rapid method for assessing burn size (see Chapter 53). This method is limited because it can be inaccurate, and it underestimates the body surface area of infants and children. Moreover, the rule of nines assesses burn size, not open wound size.

Because calorie and protein needs decrease as wound size diminishes through grafting and healing, nutritional requirements decline throughout convalescence. Therefore, the patient's nutritional needs should be routinely reevaluated to assure appropriate nutritional input.

Adequate provision of micronutrients is necessary for anabolism to occur. Although exact requirements are unknown, it is usual to supplement the diet of the burned patient with multivitamins, vitamin C, and zinc to aid in wound healing.

Nutritional Care

At one time malnutrition was considered an inevitable consequence of thermal injury. Malnutrition of the burned patient is associated with increased susceptibility to sepsis and increased morbidity and mortality in general. Loss of more than 20% of preburn body weight is common in patients with a large TBSAB. Weight loss of about 10% may be tolerated by the patient, but loss of 40% to 50% of the preburn weight is usually fatal, because this reflects corresponding loss of body function. The extreme weight loss that was once characteristic of large burns can be alleviated by use of xenografts, early wound closure, and use of nutritional support techniques.

During the ebb phase, wound care, fluid resuscitation, and major organ support are priorities. Nutritional support can begin when the patient is stable and has entered the flow phase, usually 48 to 72 hours following injury.

Consumption of an oral intake may not be possible during the first 5 to 10 days following a burn injury because of nausea, vomiting, anorexia, gastric ileus, and decreased peristalsis. Following this period, the burned patient may experience loss of appetite due to pain and, ironically, because analgesic medications may depress appetite or cause nausea. Depression, pain, and physical inability to self-feed due to scarring of the hands and mouth are powerful deterrents to attaining adequate oral intake. Frequent wound debridement and dressing changes, physical therapy, and surgical procedures are necessary, but timing of

procedures may cause pain and a decrease in appetite which reduce intake further. Moreover, it is unlikely that the patient who has large burns or chronic disease, complications from injuries, or is in poor nutritional or physical condition prior to the injury, will be able to consume amounts of food necessary to meet nutritional requirements so vastly elevated because of the injury.

Frequently, the burned patient needs "hyperalimentation." Hyperalimentation is a misnomer often applied to special modalities of nutrition support. This term is misleading since it implies that provision of more nutrients than calculated requirements is desirable. Overnutrition may, in fact, be deleterious since there is a potential for toxic effects. Input of excessive amounts of parenteral carbohydrate has been implicated in development of fatty deposits in the liver and in liver dysfunction. Moreover, excess carbohydrate may impair pulmonary function. Although these effects may be tempered when nutrients are delivered enterally, input of superfluous amounts of any nutrient may elevate BEE.

Parenteral nutrition is the route of choice when paralytic ileus persists, or GI function is impaired following a burn. Often PN is used, even though the GI tract is functioning, simply because the patient cannot tolerate the necessary volume of enterally supplied nutrients.

When the gut is functioning but the patient is unable to ingest an adequate oral diet, tube feeding should be employed. Continuous drip administration into the small bowel is the preferable method for enteral support of burned patients.

Tube feeding formulas that provide 1.5 or 2 kcal per ml are especially useful since they supply the amount of calories required in a tolerable volume. To meet specific requirements of individual patients, it may be necessary to alter the nutritional composition of a prepared formula by adding one or more modular nutritional components.

The nutritional needs of the burned patient with less than 20% TBSAB can usually be met through consumption of a high-calorie, high-protein diet supplemented with multivitamins. To avoid overwhelming the patient with the sheer volume of food, intake should be divided into several meals and nutritionally dense snacks. Commercial formulas may be used as between-meal nourishments, but it is difficult for the patient to consume large volumes. Patients complain that prepared formulas used for oral supplementation rapidly become unpalatable because the consistency may be unpleasant, and the flavor may become tiresome. In addition, the satiety value of formulas may depress the patient's appetite for meals. Nutritional modules are useful for enhancing nutrient levels of

TABLE 11-3 **Examples of Use of Modular Nutritional Components to Enhance Nutrient Density of Common Food Items**

Food Item	Calories	Protein (g)
6 oz coffee	0	0.0
6 oz coffee + 10 g Polycose*	38	0.0
4 oz chocolate pudding	160	5.0
4 oz chocolate pudding + 10 g Propac†	200	12.6
6 oz cream of tomato soup	160	5.0
6 oz cream of tomato soup + 10 ml Microlipid‡	205	5.0

* Carbohydrate module: Ross Laboratories, Columbus, OH.
† Protein module: Sherwood Medical, St. Louis, MO.
‡ Fat module: Sherwood Medical, St. Louis, MO.

the oral diet without altering the flavor of food. Carbohydrate, fat, and protein components can be added to food items (Table 11-3) to increase nutritional content.

When calorie requirements exceed 3,500 per day, it may be necessary to use both enteral and parenteral routes to deliver nutrients. An oral diet, or enteral support by tube feeding, can be augmented by peripheral or central PN. At times, an oral diet, tube feeding, and PN may be used concurrently to attain adequate nutritional input.

Regardless of the modality of nutrition support that is used, it is imperative to monitor the patient's nutritional care and status, to assure tolerance and progress toward an obtainable goal. Nutritional assessment should be dynamic so that changes in metabolic status and tolerance to nutritional therapy are noted and acted upon (see specific variables for monitoring in Methods for Providing Nutritional Support in this chapter). Care must be taken to consider the effects that burns and their treatment have on indices of nutritional status. Fluid shifts, dehydration, and transfusional therapy may affect serum concentrations of albumin, transferrin, and prealbumin. Measurements of body weight and anthropometrics are difficult to obtain and may be skewed by the presence of edema and dressings. Immunocompetence may be difficult to assess since total lymphocyte count is affected by tissue necrosis, infection, stress, and medications. Skin testing does have some utility for evaluating the immune system of burned patients; however, clinicians may not be willing to jeopardize potential skin donor sites.

Despite these limitations, nutritional assessment remains the most effective method of appraising nutritional therapy. Use of clinical judgment in evaluating results further increases effectiveness of nutritional assessment in guiding metabolic support.

Cardiac Disorders

Heart disease in America is of epidemic proportions. In coronary and intensive-care units one sees the results of cardiac disease that was years in the making. Diet is a major etiological factor in the development of cardiac disease, and one of the few over which the patient is able to have direct influence. Nutritional therapy is an integral part of overall treatment of the patient with heart disease, and it should become part of the total plan of care of the patient.

Nutritional Prevention of Cardiac Disease

Health and the opportunity for prevention of disease through dietary manipulation have been assuming increasing importance to the American population. This interest was reflected in the development of dietary goals by the U.S. Senate Select Committee on Nutrition and Human Needs in 1977. These goals were the subject of significant controversy and have been revised. A summary of the 1991 *Dietary Guidelines for Americans* includes the following:

1. Maintain or attain ideal body weight through a balance of energy expenditure and intake.
2. Increase consumption of complex carbohydrates (starches), and naturally occurring sugars while reducing consumption of refined and processed sugars.
3. Decrease total dietary fat, especially saturated fat and cholesterol.
4. Reduce sodium consumption.
5. Moderate consumption of alcohol.

Coronary artherosclerotic heart disease is the most common underlying cause of cardiac-related morbidity and mortality. Research has implicated almost every blood lipid factor in the genesis of atherosclerotic heart disease. It is believed that dietary factors influence blood lipid concentrations. Thus, the "Prudent Diet," espoused by the American Heart Association, was developed to aid Americans in reducing their risk of heart disease through dietary modification. The "Prudent Diet" provides specific recommendations that aid Americans in incorporating the U.S. Senate Dietary Guidelines into their daily dietary patterns.

The food industry has responded to the increasing interest in preventive nutrition on the part of the American public. Information regarding sodium, cholesterol, and fat content appears on food labels. A greater variety of palatable "dietetic" foods, including low-sodium, low-fat, and sugar-free items, is available. These developments are encouraging because these items are useful in enhancing adherence to restricted diets. Compliance with dietary restriction can be facilitated by assuring that the patient thoroughly understands principles of the diet before discharge from the hospital. A consultation from a registered dietitian is invaluable in teaching the patient to translate these modifications into a diet that can be maintained for life.

Coronary Artery Disease

Coronary artery disease (CAD) is the most common manifestation of cardiovascular dysfunction. Because evaluation of low-density plasma lipoproteins is considered to potentiate development of atherosclerosis, some clinicians believe dietary modification aimed toward lowering circulating levels of the offending lipoprotein(s) is helpful. An exhaustive description of the dietary regimen for each type of hyperlipidemia is beyond the scope of this chapter, but a summary of each diet is given in Table 11-4.

Another school of thought supports the use of the principles of the "Prudent Diet" for patients who have atherosclerosis, or the potential for developing it, or for patients after coronary artery bypass surgery.

Coronary Artery Bypass Grafting

The patient recovering from coronary artery bypass grafting (CABG) has elevated protein and energy needs as a consequence of major surgery. Meeting the increased nutritional requirements of patients following surgical revascularization of the myocardium is complicated by the need to severely restrict sodium during the postoperative period. Prophylactic sodium restriction is helpful in reducing the potential for thrombosis of the graft which is associated with fluid retention. When dietary sodium is restricted to 1 g or less per day, intake of milk, bread, cereals, and some vegetables is limited. All salted, cured, and many commercially prepared foods must be eliminated from the diet. Because fruit, fruit juices, and carbonated beverages contain only trace amounts of naturally occurring sodium, these foods may be consumed as the patient desires. Unfortunately, foods containing very low amounts of sodium are poor sources of protein. Low-sodium diets must be carefully planned by dietitians to be nutritionally adequate for the patient after CABG. Patients may be unable to consume an adequate diet after cardiac surgery because of unpalatability of the low-sodium diet, general weakness and fatigue, or medication-induced anorexia and gastric irritation. The nurse should encourage the patient to achieve adequate oral intake, in spite of the lack of salted foods, by teaching the patient that nutrients are vital for healing. If the patient continues to consume suboptimal amounts for more than 48 hours, the physician should be apprised and the dietitian consulted. It may be necessary to allow a familiar dish that may be relatively high is sodium content in lieu of other foods, to pique the patient's appetite. Lemon juice, vinegar, and sodium-free spices and seasonings can be used to add flavor to the otherwise bland diet.

If these measures are not successful, it may be nec-

TABLE 11-4 **Summary of Dietary Modifications for Hyperlipoproteinemia**

Dietary Modifications	Type I	Type IIa	Type IIb	Type III	Type IV	Type V
Limit kilocalories (kcal)	No	No	Yes*	Yes*	Yes*	Yes*
Limit protein	No	No	20% total kcal	20% total kcal	15% to 25% total kcal	15% to 25% total kcal
Limit carbohydrates	No	No	40% total kcal	40% total kcal	45% total kcal	50% total kcal
			← (Restrict concentrated carbohydrates) →			
Limit fat	12% to 20% total kcal	No	40% total kcal	40% total kcal	20% to 35% total kcal	12% to 30% total kcal
Emphasize PUFA†	No	Yes	Yes	Yes	Yes	Yes
Limit cholesterol	No	100-300 mg/day	100-300 mg/day	100-300 mg/day	300-500 mg/day	300-500 mg/day
Limit alcohol	Yes	Yes	0-2 oz/day	0-2 oz/day	0-2 oz/day‡	Yes

*Restrict calories to the level necessary to obtain or maintain ideal body weight.
†PUFA = polyunsaturated fatty acids (found in vegetable sources).
‡Moderate consumption of alcohol may be beneficial in some types of hyperlipidemia as it has been found to elevate serum levels of HDL.

essary to add commercially prepared supplements to the diet. Low-sodium protein modules are useful to increase protein content of menu items. When nutritional supplements are used, communication between the nurse, dietitian, and patient is vital so that attainable dietary goals can be planned which are compatible with the dietary prescription.

The patient's instruction regarding a diet reduced in calories (if the patient is above ideal body weight), fat, and sodium should be initiated as soon as possible. The nurse can enhance willingness of the patient to learn by teaching the relationship of diet to the disease process, and the potential benefits to be derived from dietary modification. Consistent, individualized instruction from a dietitian, coupled with group diet classes, is effective in teaching patients the principles of the modified diet. The patient's compliance can be facilitated if the nurse reinforces the formal diet instruction. Mealtimes can be ideal times for the nurse to review dietary principles such as sodium restriction and decreased fat intake, using the patient's menu and meal tray as visual aids. A number of patient-oriented publications, such as those prepared by the American Heart Association, contain recipes and guidelines for practical application of the diet in everyday life.

An important factor that the nurse can contribute to the diet instruction process is a positive attitude. By emphasizing the salubrious effects of the diet, the nurse can enhance the willingness of the patient to comply with necessary dietary modifications which are vital to health.

Myocardial Ischemia and Infarction

Nutritional therapy for myocardial ischemia is aimed at reducing symptoms and preventing further damage to weakened myocardial tissue. Calorie restriction may be necessary to attain ideal body weight for height. Another goal of dietary therapy is to modify fat intake in order to alter blood lipid levels. A diet low in saturated fat, cholesterol, total fat, and concentrated carbohydrates is useful in lowering calorie density of the diet and may be useful in reducing serum lipid concentrations. Since consumption of large meals may cause pain due to displacement of the diaphragm, the patient should be counseled to eat small, frequent meals. Those patients who continue to experience pain following eating usually are instructed by their physician to take nitroglycerin before meals.

If myocardial infarction occurs, the patient usually receives the traditional dietary progression from nothing by mouth during the acute phase, progressing to liquids, and finally to a soft diet. Usually, some additional modifications are imposed on this traditional dietary regimen to protect the weakened heart from further stress. Calories may be limited to preclude elevation of cardiac output. However, it must be remembered that depending upon the amount of tissue damage caused by the infarction, an adrenergic response may be evoked. This event is accompanied by an elevation in calorie and protein requirements. The clinical status of the patient must be monitored carefully so that caloric restriction that is imposed to decrease stress to the heart does not lead to nutritional depletion. Stimulants such as caffeine and extremes in food temperatures should be avoided. A moderate sodium restriction may be indicated, based on the clinical condition of the patient. Cholesterol and fat content of the diet should be limited. When the patient is able to resume consumption of solid foods, the calorie level of the diet can be increased to the amount necessary to reach or sustain ideal body weight. Dietary instruction should begin during hospitalization so that the patient understands and is able to make the necessary modifications in the diet prior to discharge.

Congestive Heart Failure

Malnutrition, and *cardiac cachexia* associated with congestive heart failure (CHF), has been recognized for centuries. Classic cardiac cachexia develops over time in the patient who has chronic CHF. Several factors are responsible. One theory purports that diminished oral intake is a voluntary compensatory mechanism that prevents stress on the failing heart by reducing cardiac output. Anorexia may occur simply because the patient is too weak to ingest adequate amounts of food. Often medications such as digitalis, opiates, and diuretics are responsible for depressed appetite. The patient with CHF frequently describes vague GI discomfort and early satiety due to the presence of pulmonary edema, which further decrease oral intake.

Conditions of nutrient loss are common due to malabsorption and failure to transport nutrients as a result of splenic, hepatic, and pancreatic hypoxia. Excessive urinary nitrogen losses occur via a nephrotic-like syndrome that is secondary to poor cardiac perfusion.

The patient with CHF is hypermetabolic due to elevated temperature and thyroid activity and the increased energy requirements of specific tissues. Energy needs are elevated because of the effects of cellular hypoxia. Poor oxygen perfusion at the cellular level necessitates energy production via less efficient anaerobic processes.

Malnutrition has serious consequences for the patient with CHF. Malnutrition can cause reduced cardiac output, decreased left ventricular mass, and low radiographic total heart volume. Successful treatment of CHF should include treatment of underlying malnutrition. Nutritional therapy must be undertaken with care to avoid overloading the impaired cardiovascular system. Provision of superfluous nutrients is not desirable since this can overtax the heart by increasing metabolic rate, cardiac output, and oxygen consumption. It is important for the nurse to measure and record fluid intake and output accurately to facilitate accurate calculation of water requirements. Fluid intake is usually limited to 1,000 to 1,500 ml per day.

Sodium replacement is titrated to maintain serum sodium at approximately 140 mEq/dl. It is usual for sodium input to be restricted to 0.5 to 2.0 g (22 to 65 mEq) per day. The nurse should monitor serum sodium levels and report abnormal values to the physician.

Parenteral nutrition is used when GI symptoms preclude enteral feeding. Use of IV lipid emulsions in combination with parenteral amino acids and glucose is advantageous because lipids are calorically dense and contribute only 500 ml to total daily fluid allowance. To further reduce volume of the TPN solution and to provide adequate protein, a 15% amino acid solution may be used.

Tube feeding with a 1.5-to-2-kcal-per-milliliter enteral formula is a means of providing concentrated nutrients in a limited volume via the enteral route. The nurse should assess the patient's hydration status to assure that he or she does not become dehydrated while receiving a high-calorie tube feeding formula.

When the patient can tolerate an oral diet, frequent, small, soft, low-sodium feedings are appropriate. Modular nutritional components and prepared formulas are vital in supplementing an oral diet because the patient with CHF is quickly fatigued by the exertion of eating. Commercial nutritional products may be added to liquids and food items to enhance nutritional value.

Nutritional support of the patient with CHF must be undertaken with caution because both over- and underfeeding have negative consequences. Strict attention to serum electrolytes, input and output records, and nursing assessment of edema and heart and lung sounds are vital to avoid worsening heart failure as a consequence of nutritional therapy.

Hypertension

An association between sodium intake and the incidence of essential hypertension has been shown by epidemiological studies.[11] Other studies have revealed that individuals who have a propensity for developing hypertension are sensitive to dietary sodium at levels of 125 to 200 mEq per day.[12] The "average" sodium content of the American diet is high, between 100 to 200 mEq per day.

The action of medications used to manage hypertension is enhanced by decreasing the amount of sodium in the diet. Generally, a diet containing 2 to 4 g of sodium per day is prescribed. This level of restriction can be met if the patient is counseled to avoid canned, processed, and cured meats, and convenience foods, unless these items are labeled as low-sodium. Use of fresh or frozen vegetables in lieu of the canned variety further decreases dietary sodium. The patient should be specifically enjoined against consumption of salted snack foods since these are a significant source of sodium and low-nutrient calories.

If the patient is obese, weight reduction may be effective in lowering blood pressure. However, it is important not to impose too many dietary modifications at one time, because one runs the risk of overwhelming the patient with lifestyle changes.

Antihypertensive medications are also associated with loss of potassium. Simply encouraging the patient to increase consumption of potassium-containing foods is not sufficient to replace potassium losses. In cases when antihypertensive medications are used, the nurse should remind the physician that oral or IV potassium replacement may be necessary.

Cardiomyopathy

Unfortunately, few articles in the literature address nutritional support of the patient with cardiomyopathy. It may be assumed that the patient is at nutritional risk for the same reasons as the patient with CHF. The poor functioning heart muscle is less efficient, requiring more energy to accomplish less work than the normal heart. Oxygen starvation of tissues interferes with absorption, transport, and metabolism of nutritional substrates. The patient may be unable to consume adequate nutrients because of weakness and fatigue, early satiety, or anorexia due to medications. The patient with severe cardiomyopathy may suffer from cardiac cachexia because of these conditions.

Nutritional therapy should be directed toward maintaining or improving the nutritional status and avoiding additional strain to the heart. The same guidelines which govern nutritional support of the patient with CHF may be applied to care of the patient with cardiomyopathy.

Valvular Disease

The most common causes of valvular disease in adults are rheumatic fever and calcification of the valve structures noted in older patients. During acute episodes of rheumatic fever, the goal of nutritional therapy is to support elevated requirements for energy and protein due to the hypermetabolism which results from fever and infection. Following recovery, prophylactic dietary modifications may include adherence to a mild sodium restriction (2 to 4 g per day), and a calorie level appropriate to obtain or maintain ideal body weight, because obesity adds to the strain on the heart.

Surgery and Trauma

The metabolic events following major surgery or multiple trauma are dictated by the changing hormonal milieu following injury. The body responds to significant trauma and surgery in the ebb and flow reactions described previously (see Burns in this section). Lesser injuries or elective surgeries do not significantly alter metabolism of body fuels or protein, although they do stimulate conservation of water and salt.

During the early flow phase, the healing wound has priority over other tissues for nutrients. The wound is in positive nitrogen balance because other tissues provide nutritional substrates through adrenergically stimulated autocannibalism. In the case of relatively minor surgery or trauma, input of large amounts of exogenous substrates is unnecessary, because metabolic requirements are not greatly increased and the patient is soon able to consume an adequate oral diet. If there is significant hypermetabolism, if nutritional input is absent or inadequate, or if sepsis and other complications occur, wound healing may suffer unless nutritional needs are met.

Frequently, surgical candidates are in poor nutritional status as a result of disease. Cancer, regional enteritis, and colitis are examples of conditions that often cause significant weight loss and impose nutritional costs in addition to those resulting from major surgery. Because patients with these conditions are already at nutritional risk, they may benefit from a period of nutritional repletion prior to surgery.

The goals for metabolic support following injury or trauma are prioritized as follows:

1. Provide fluid resuscitation and support organ function. Restoration of cardiovascular homeostasis in itself is useful in reducing catecholamine levels, thereby decreasing the period of hypermetabolism that follows major tissue damage.
2. Repair wounds and damaged tissue. The degree of adrenergic response is related to the extent of the open wound. The hypermetabolic response evoked by catecholamines is abated when wounds are closed, fractures immobilized, and septic and contaminated areas drained.
3. Provide nutritional substrates when the patient is stable and capable of using them for anabolism. This period usually does not begin until 24 to 48 hours following injury.

Nutritional Requirements

Nutritional requirements vary according to the degree of injury and resulting hypermetabolism. The patient undergoing minor elective procedures experiences limited, short-term alterations in nutritional requirements. Major surgery and trauma, on the other hand, elevate the patient's protein requirements because of the increased rates of protein synthesis and catabolism associated with these events. The elevation in protein synthetic rate accounts for some of the increase in energy expenditure experienced by patients recovering from surgery or trauma.

Because the response to injury includes obligate catabolism of amino acids, protein requirements during the acute stage may be high but level off as the patient recovers. Protein input should be monitored closely by nitrogen balance studies because these patients may quickly become intolerant of nitrogen secondary to acute renal or hepatic insufficiency. During acute stress, protein appears to be most efficiently used when approximately 15 nonprotein calories are provided with every gram of protein. As the acute phase resolves, the optimal protein/nonprotein calorie ratio increases to 1:25. Vitamin and mineral supplementation is often given although there is little agreement regarding dosages of vitamins and minerals required by trauma and surgery patients.

Nutritional Care

Choice of the feeding route depends on GI functional capability, the degree of stress and hypermetabolism present, the extent of preexisting malnutrition, and the risk of complications. Feeding by tube is the optimal route when there is adequate GI function and the patient can tolerate the volume necessary to meet nutritional requirements. Use of the GI tract precludes development of mucosal atrophy which can occur when the patient is sustained on PN over a long period. Moreover, enteral feeding is associated with fewer complications, especially less hemorrhage of the upper GI tract, than is intravenous nutritional support. Nevertheless, parenteral nutritional support is extensively used, particularly in cases of abdominal surgery, because it is thought that postoperative paralytic ileus precludes early use of the GI tract. Abdominal surgery or postoperative ileus does not necessarily contraindicate enteral feeding. Although gastric and colonic ileus may persist for 24 to 48 hours after surgery, motility of the small intestine recovers within hours. Therefore, it is possible to begin feeding into the small intestine via jejunostomy shortly after surgery. Traditionally, monomeric enteral formulas have been exclusively used for jejunostomy feeding, but polymeric formulas administered jejunally have been found to be well tolerated[7] and, unlike monomeric formulas, can be initiated in full strength because many polymeric formulas are relatively isotonic.

Protein-sparing IV solutions can be used in cases in which a relatively well-nourished patient may begin eating within 5 to 7 days of surgery. Patients who have large nutritional requirements and are not candidates for enteral feeding may require PN.

The patient undergoing metabolic stress may have a limited capacity to metabolize nutritional substrates. Intravenous infusions of about 2 to 3 mg of dextrose per kilogram per minute are generally tolerated. The energy needs of extremely hypermetabolic patients may be best met by a combination of glucose and lipid calories. Input of lipid emulsions should be limited to approximately 35% of total calorie requirements initially to assure the patient's tolerance of IV fat emulsions.

Nutritional care should be continually assessed and evaluated by the health care team. Because the metabolic consequences of surgery and trauma influence several major nutritional assessment parameters, identification of these effects is essential for accurate diagnosis of nutritional status. The fluid resuscitation that occurs following surgery or trauma affects several body compartments and may produce erroneous values when these body compartments are evaluated to assess the nutritional status of the patient. Fluid input may cause false elevation in body weight and other anthropometric measurements. Fluid retention may cause a false low value in serum protein concentrations because of dilution and extravasation from intravascular to interstitial spaces. Surgery and trauma are events that may affect common indices of a patient's nutritional status. Anergy may result from circulating immunosuppressive factor and increased suppressor T cell activity, which is associated with surgery and trauma rather than nutritional factors.

All of these changes are a result of metabolic stress, but they are usually short-lived, and are not true indicators of a nutritional deficit. Even though indicators of nutritional status may not be useful in the initial period following injury, they do provide a guide for monitoring nutritional progress. Serial assessments are necessary to follow the dynamic metabolic course following surgery and injury.

Special Considerations

The adrenergic response to *neurosurgery* is similar to that mounted as a result of major injury. However, additional factors must be considered when providing nutritional support to patients following neurosurgery or head injury. Increased energy requirements resulting from hyperventilation, increased cardiac output, fever, posturing, seizures, and general rest-lessness are superimposed on those energy requirements resulting from the effects of stress-related catecholamines. Corticosteroid therapy further increases catabolic activity and nitrogen losses. On the other hand, paralysis, ventilatory support, and barbiturate coma decrease energy expenditure.

Factors that further complicate nutritional care of the neurosurgery patient include prevention of further brain damage which can occur secondary to cerebral swelling. This necessitates fluid restriction and diuresis with mannitol and furosemide. Fluid and electrolyte status can fluctuate dramatically as a result and must be followed closely when providing nutritional support.

The obtunded patient is at risk of aspiration due to an inability to protect the airway, although the presence of an endotracheal tube or tracheostomy provides some protection. In addition, these patients are prone to vomiting because of nausea, nasogastric secretions, and changes in intracranial pressure. The presence of nausea, secretions, and changes in intracranial pressure do not preclude enteral feeding if appropriate precautions are taken (see Enteral Feeding by Tube in this chapter). Commercial formulas that provide 1.5 to 2 kcal per milliliter are especially useful because it is possible to provide adequate protein and calories in a tolerable volume. Modular nutritional components can be used to further augment nutrient density of enteral formulas. Parenteral nutrition may be necessary if the patient is unable to tolerate the volume of enteral formula necessary to meet nutritional requirements, or if the risk of aspiration is too great.

Special nutritional care is required following *surgery of the GI tract*. Surgical intervention for complications of peptic ulcer disease includes drainage, vagotomy, pyloroplasty, and partial or total removal of the stomach and/or part of the small intestine. The postgastrectomy patient is prone to develop the *dumping syndrome*. Dumping occurs when the hyperosmolar food mass rapidly enters the small intestine without first undergoing normal digestion and mixing in the stomach. Symptoms arise from 5 to 15 minutes after a meal. Symptoms include bloating, pain, nausea, diarrhea, pallor, weakness, palpitations, sweating, and increased pulse rate. One method of dietary treatment for dumping includes providing foods in numerous small meals rather than three large ones. The diet should be relatively high in protein and fat without concentrated carbohydrates. The carbohydrates used should be complex, since these are less osmotically active than simple sugars. Fluid with meals should be restricted to 4 oz because liquid enhances formation of osmolar solutes that can precipitate the dumping reaction. These dietary modifications are not necessary, however, in all patients following gastrectomy. Those patients who do suffer from dumping usually experience cessation of symptoms over time.

Following surgery of the small intestine, digestive and absorptive capability remains intact if the distal ileum, ileocecal valve, and the duodenum are not excised. If more than 50% to 75% of the small intestine is resected, malabsorption and accompanying malnutrition may occur.

Short bowel syndrome occurs after a large amount of the small intestine is removed. Malabsorption problems vary depending on the extent of excision of the small intestine, the part of small intestine resected, and the degree to which diseased tissue is excised. Nutritional therapy must be tailored to the individual needs of the patient. Fat and lactose are the nutrients most frequently malabsorbed. The consistency of the diet may require modification to omit roughage, depending on the patient's tolerance. In cases of extreme malabsorption, the patient may require tube feeding with a monomeric, low-fat formula. If very little absorptive surface of the GI tract remains, PN must be instituted.

Gastrointestinal Disorders

Diseases affecting the GI tract have the greatest potential for influencing the nutritional status of the patient because the GI tract is the site of ingestion, digestion, and absorption of nutrients. The category of GI disease includes a variety of malabsorption syndromes, inflammatory disorders, and other entities which may cause significant malabsorption and depleted nutritional status. Each condition requires specific treatment, and nutritional care is individualized according to the patient's needs and tolerance.

Nutritional Requirements

Energy needs of the patient with GI disease are based on the current clinical status, presence of preexisting malnutrition, and function of the gut. The patient with chronic disease is frequently protein-depleted due to poor intake, dyspepsia, malabsorption, and increased losses. Special attention should be given to vitamin, mineral, and trace element nutriture. The GI patient is at risk for vitamin deficiency and mineral and trace element depletion because of increased losses and failure to absorb these micronutrients.

Nutritional Care

Peptic ulcer is the lesion of the GI tract most frequently seen. Peptic ulcers may occur in the lower end of the esophagus or in the stomach or duodenum. Acute cases are treated with antacids and by elimi-

nating stimulants from the diet. Caffeine, alcohol, and spices are eliminated from the diet to decrease the production of acid. Small meals should be provided at regular intervals. Late-night snacking should be avoided since this is implicated in nocturnal production of acid. The traditional *Sippy diet,* which espouses very small, frequent feedings of milk and cream, has been proven to be noneffective and is rarely part of the modern treatment plans. The buffering capacity of milk is quite weak, and its protein content can actually increase acid production. Furthermore, the high cholesterol and saturated fat content of whole milk precludes its use in patients who have or are prone to develop atherosclerosis.[13] The patient who suffers recurrent or intractable ulcers generally requires surgical intervention to prevent erosion into adjacent structures or development of obstructions.

Malabsorption syndromes arise from three etiological factors: (1) dyspepsia due to lack of bile salts, digestive enzymes, or normal peristalsis; (2) inadequate absorption of nutrients because of a deficiency of enzymes or dysfunction of the intestinal mucosa; or (3) failure in assimilation of nutrients secondary to obstruction of the lymphatic system or portal veins or to a lack of transport mechanisms. Common malabsorption syndromes include celiac disease and inflammatory bowel disease. The patient with malabsorption syndrome is at nutritional risk because of ongoing failure to digest, absorb, and/or assimilate nutrients. Moreover, a diagnostic workup for malabsorption syndromes requires that the patient be NPO for several days prior to and during tests. Frequently this additional nutritional deprivation is superimposed on preexisting malnutrition.

Inflammatory bowel disease includes two distinct entities: Crohn's disease and ulcerative colitis. *Crohn's disease* is a progressive inflammatory process that usually affects the terminal ileum, although it may affect any part of the GI tract. Healthy bowel tissue is interposed with diseased areas, and therefore, some normal absorption may occur. Acute and chronic inflammation of the GI tract may lead to significant weight loss. Lesions of the GI tract include all layers of the mucosa and submucosa, and development of fistulas is common. Fistulas represent an additional nutritional cost because they may divert nutrients outside the GI tract.

Ulcerative colitis affects mainly the large bowel and sometimes the terminal ileum. It causes a diffuse inflammation of the mucosa but does not affect the submucosa. Eventually the absorptive surface of the GI tract is destroyed as scar tissue fills the ulcerated areas. The patient experiences significant nutritional losses due to diarrhea which occurs secondary to malabsorption of nutrients. Water and electrolytes normally reabsorbed by the large bowel are also lost.

Treatment of acute ulcerative colitis includes a period of bowel rest. Although the well-nourished patient can tolerate 3 to 5 days of being NPO, generally the patient with GI disease does not have nutritional reserves on which to call. Consequently, parenteral nutrition is an important adjunct therapy to prevent further nutritional decline in these patients. The administration of peripheral parenteral nutrition during this period is appropriate. Following the acute stage of ulcerative colitis, the patient may be advanced to an oral diet that restricts lactose and fat. The degree of dietary restriction should vary according to the patient's tolerance of foods containing fat and lactose.

Bowel rest is required by the patient with Crohn's disease when it is in the active phase. Parenteral nutrition is used frequently, but tube feeding using a monomeric formula is possible when the patient is not critically ill and when the GI tract is free of fistulas or obstructions. When remission occurs, the diet can be progressed slowly, restricting fat and lactose.

Management of fistulas that have a variety of etiologies includes keeping the patient NPO to control complications from fistula leakage. Several studies have demonstrated that with adequate PN, fistulas may close spontaneously, obviating the need for surgical intervention.[14,15]

The patient suffering from acute pancreatitis also benefits from gut rest (to decrease output of pancreatic secretions), nasogastric suction, and supportive care. Resolution of pancreatitis usually occurs within 5 to 7 days. The patient who develops complications including prolonged ileus or pseudocyst requires nutritional intervention with PN. Administration of IV amino acids has been shown to stimulate some pancreatic activity, but much less than an oral diet or tube feeding using a polymeric formula.

Follow-up of a patient's nutritional progress by serial assessments of nutritional status is especially beneficial to the GI patient. Hydration status and effects of some medications must be taken into consideration when evaluating nutritional assessment parameters, but interpretation of most measurements is fairly straightforward.

Renal Failure

Nutritional Requirements

A major goal of nutritional therapy for the patient with renal failure is to minimize uremic symptoms which occur when metabolites of protein cannot be excreted by the kidneys. Protein metabolites are generated from dietary protein and from catabolism of body proteins. Therefore, a tenet of nutritional ther-

TABLE 11-5 Recommended Protein Intake in Undialyzed Chronic Renal Failure Patients

Glomerular Filtration Rate	Recommended Protein Intake
20-25 ml/min	Up to 90 g/day
15-20 ml/min	Up to 70 g/day
10-15 ml/min	Up to 50 g/day

apy is to provide tolerable amounts of protein, accompanied by adequate amounts of nonprotein calories to prevent breakdown of muscle mass.

Input of protein that has *high biological value (HBV)* is emphasized when planning nutritional care of patients in acute renal failure (ARF) and chronic renal failure (CRF). High biological value protein sources (eggs, milk, meat, and fish) are those that contain a full complement of essential amino acids. Input of nonessential amino acids is limited so that endogenous urea is used by the body to synthesize nonessential amino acids. Provision of 70% of dietary protein as HBV protein facilitates reduction of serum urea levels because urea may be "recycled" to produce nonessential amino acids.

The type of dialysis used is a factor to consider when estimating protein needs. Continuous peritoneal dialysis (CAPD) solutions contain as much as 4.25% glucose per liter and are significant calorie sources. However, CAPD is associated with the greatest loss of protein, while lesser amounts are lost with intermittent peritoneal dialysis and hemodialysis.

Prior to initiation of dialysis, the amount of protein that can be tolerated by the patient with CRF is estimated based on the glomerular filtration rate (GFR). As the GFR declines, the amount of protein input must also be reduced (Table 11-5).

Protein requirements for patients with ARF are more difficult to estimate. Acute renal failure is frequently accompanied by conditions that may evoke overwhelming catabolism and protein losses. However, enthusiasm for providing protein must be tempered by the knowledge of the inability of the kidneys to excrete the resulting metabolites.

The failure of the malfunctioning kidney to perform its normal regulatory and endocrine functions necessitates other nutritional modifications, including attention to electrolyte, vitamin, mineral, and fluid input. Water-soluble vitamins are usually supplemented since dialysis causes loss of these nutrients. Vitamin A is generally not supplemented because serum levels are frequently elevated in patients with renal failure. Vitamin D and calcium may be supplemented but require close monitoring. Trace elements, zinc, and iron are usually supplemented.

Sodium and fluid input must be titrated to the tolerance of the individual patient. Hyperkalemia, hyperphosphatemia, and hypermagnesemia are common in renal failure because of the inability of the kidneys to excrete potassium, phosphorus, and magnesium. The potassium content of the diet is restricted to about 40 mEq/L per day. Serum levels of phosphorus are controlled through use of phosphate binders. Intake of magnesium-containing compounds is restricted and serum magnesium levels should be monitored frequently.

Nutritional Care

The patient with renal failure frequently becomes malnourished as renal failure progresses. Uremia is associated with anorexia, nausea, and vomiting. Drugs used in CRF may cause GI upset, constipation, diarrhea, and anorexia. Moreover, the sheer volume of medications the patient is required to consume daily may contribute to the inability to consume adequate amounts of food. Poor oral intake is exacerbated by a necessarily limited diet. Every opportunity should be taken to increase the calorie content of the diet while remaining within the dietary prescription for protein, sodium, potassium, and fluid. This may be accomplished through the addition of fat, oil, and sugar during food preparation. Consumption of protein-free food items, such as hard candies, jam and jelly, syrups, and breads and cookies prepared from low-protein flour, can be encouraged. Addition of commercial fat or carbohydrate modules to menu items is useful because the modules are fairly neutral in taste, provide a fair number of calories, and contribute only small amounts of volume. If nutritional intake is not adequate or continues to decline, commercial nutritional supplements may be added to the oral diet.

Frequently the critically ill patient with renal failure requires aggressive nutritional support. It is important to prevent the breakdown of tissues that results from inadequate intake, because metabolites of catabolism of body protein contribute to uremia. At least two commercial tube feeding formulas are specially formulated for use with renal failure patients. These special formulas are relatively low in protein and electrolytes and high in calories. Protein is provided as essential amino acids. These formulas are not suitable for long-term use because they are nutritionally incomplete. Moreover, they are hyperosmolar, and therefore, a period of gut adaptation is required before they are tolerated at full strength. They are extremely unpalatable because of the pres-

ence of free amino acids, and therefore, they should not be used for supplementation of the oral diet. Due to these limitations, specialty formulas should be used only in cases of short-term protein restriction, when dialysis is not an option. It is possible to use a standard polymeric formula for enteral support of the patient with renal failure. Formulas that provide 1.5 to 2 kcal per milliliter are useful for tube feeding patients with renal failure in whom volume restriction is necessary. These formulas are usually lower in potassium content than 1.0-kilocalorie-per-milliliter formulas, which facilitates management of the patient's potassium intake.

Another alternative for successful enteral support of patients with renal failure is use of modular components. Modular nutrient components can be added to standard formulas to provide for modifications of major nutrients and electrolytes required by individual patients.

Parenteral nutritional support may be necessary if the gut is nonfunctioning. Essential amino acid solutions are commercially available, but there is controversy regarding whether their use is more efficacious than use of lower concentrations of solutions containing mixed amino acids.

Patients with renal failure have alterations in glucose metabolism, so that use of hypertonic glucose concentrations must be carefully monitored to prevent complications. Intravenous lipid emulsions are especially useful for the patient who is intolerant of large glucose loads. Moreover, IV lipids are beneficial when calorie requirements are high and fluid input must be limited. When lipid emulsions are used, serum triglyceride levels should be closely monitored to assure patient tolerance to IV lipid emulsions.

Nutritional assessment is useful in following the progress of patients with renal failure. Anthropometric measurements are used to evaluate somatic protein and energy stores in the patient with CRF. These measurements are less useful in the patient with ARF since fluid status is extremely dynamic. Dramatic shifts in fluid balance can also affect the reliability of circulating proteins as markers of nutritional status in the patient with ARF. Visceral protein levels are more useful in CRF, especially when used in conjunction with parameters of somatic proteins.

Skin testing provides unreliable data regarding immune function in these patients. Estimation of nitrogen balance and creatinine height index is unreliable, if not impossible, in conditions of impaired renal excretion of nitrogenous waste products. Urea kinetics is a method for determining the rate of protein catabolism from the rate of urea generation. This method estimates protein intake by calculating the protein catabolic rate which determines the urea production, the primary product of urea catabolism.[16]

Cancer

Cachexia is the most widely recognized manifestation of cancer. The etiology of weight loss in the cancer patient is poorly understood, but a number of factors contribute to the development of malnutrition that frequently accompanies oncologic disease. Development of cancer cachexia occurs in three stages. Anorexia is the primary manifestation in the first phase, but its development is not well understood. One theory is that the tumor itself secretes "anorexigenic peptides," but isolation of these substances has yet to be accomplished. Nonetheless, early stages of cancer are typified by increasing anorexia accompanied by weight loss.

Energy requirements of cancer patients may be increased by the existence of "futile metabolic cycles," which use more energy than they produce. It has been shown that there is an increase in Cori cycle activity in some cancer patients. This Cori cycle activity produces energy via less efficient anaerobic processes.

Other factors that may contribute to cancer cachexia in the first stage are possible alterations in taste perception, development of food aversions, early satiety resulting from secretion of anorexigenic substances or mechanical effects of the tumor burden, or inability to digest or assimilate nutrients.[17]

The second stage is characterized by initiation of antineoplastic therapies and imposition of mechanical effects of the tumor (such as obstruction of the GI tract). Resection of neoplastic masses has immediate and long-term effects. Any major surgical procedure evokes the typical adrenergic response which initiates a hypermetabolic reaction (see Surgery in this chapter). Long-term effects vary according to the area and the extent of resection. Excision of tumors in the GI tract may produce difficulties in chewing, swallowing, digesting, and absorbing nutrients. Resection of the lip and tongue may interfere with the ability of the patient to retain food and saliva, to chew, and to manipulate food to the back of the mouth for swallowing. A partial laryngectomy makes swallowing difficult, and a total laryngectomy renders the patient dysphagic for some time after surgery. In addition, the protective mechanism of the epiglottis is lost, placing the patient at risk for aspiration until the skill of swallowing is relearned. Surgical treatment of cancer involving the esophagus may be accompanied by early satiety, diarrhea, and steatorrhea. Weight loss is frequently a consequence of partial gastrectomy and always occurs with total gastrectomy; either may be accompanied by the dumping syndrome. Dyspepsia may occur as a consequence of resection of the pancreas, biliary system, or small intestine. Resection of the large intestine may be associated with temporary alterations in the ability to conserve water and electrolytes. However, these aberrations are short-lived because adaptation occurs fairly rapidly.

The effects of radiation therapy are dependent on dose, site, volume of tissue treated, and time over which the dose is given. The major nutritional effects of radiation occur when the GI tract is irradiated. Acute effects include mucositis, stomatitis, esophagitis, nausea, vomiting, diarrhea, and loss of taste sensation, also known as *mouth blindness*. Later effects include malabsorption, dental caries, and radiation enteritis.

Chemotherapy is designed to destroy rapidly growing and dividing cancer cells, but normal cells that also experience rapid turnover are affected by chemotherapeutic agents. Because cells of the GI tract are rapidly growing, chemotherapy damages the GI tract, causing nausea, vomiting, diarrhea, malabsorption, and painful lesions. Moreover, nutritional status may be compromised because of possible hepatic, renal, and pancreatic toxicity of antineoplastic agents.

Patients in the third phase of cancer cachexia are extremely marasmic. The third phase of cancer cachexia is characterized by catabolism of somatic muscle and energy stores, depletion of circulating proteins, anergy, and asthenia.

It is estimated that 45% of hospitalized cancer patients lose 10% of their body weight and that an additional 25% of patients lose 20% of their body weight. Weight loss is correlated with longer length of hospital stay, a significantly higher incidence of complications, and increased mortality. Depleted serum albumin levels are also associated with higher rates of postoperative infection.

The issue of nutritional support of the cancer patient is a controversial one. Opponents cite the failure of nutritional support to positively affect prognosis. Animal studies that show acceleration of tumor growth when provided with nutritional substrate may also deter clinicians from instituting metabolic support.

It is recognized that nutritional therapy is not primary or curative cancer treatment, but nutritional therapy does have the potential for decreasing the incidence of malnutrition-associated side effects. Proponents argue that nutritional support is important adjunct therapy for the cancer patient because there are few associated complications; the possibility for prevention or alleviation of weight loss and malnutrition exists, and provision of nutritional needs contributes to a general feeling of well-being on the part of the patient. Moreover, there is no evidence of inappropriate increases in tumor growth in humans as a consequence of nutrition support. Discrepancies between tumor growth rate in animals versus humans can be explained by the fact that tumors implanted in animals grow rapidly and quickly achieve weights equal to 30% of the total weight of the animal. This is in contrast to tumors in human beings, which are slow growing and reach no more than 5% of total body weight.

Nutritional Requirements

Increased energy requirements as a result of the primary disease are not universal among cancer patients. However, it should be noted that the cancer patient does not respond to long-term inadequate nutritional intake by decreasing basal energy requirements as do normal individuals. Antineoplastic therapies may elevate energy requirements. Negative nitrogen balance and low levels of circulating proteins may persist in spite of adequate protein input, until the tumor burden is reduced and/or antineoplastic therapy is completed. Negative nitrogen balance is thought to be related to an increased rate of protein catabolism accompanied by a decreased synthesis of body proteins.

Vitamin and mineral supplementation should be provided so that the RDA for these nutrients is met and to replete diminished stores. To date, data are inconclusive regarding optimal levels of supplementation of vitamins and minerals. Particular attention should be paid to maintaining serum levels of potassium, phosphorus, and magnesium, since these electrolytes are vital for anabolism and retention of nitrogen. Potassium may be lost by the cancer patient as a result of treatments including gastric suctioning and potassium-losing diuretic and antibiotic therapies. Copious diarrhea and small-bowel drainage may also represent significant losses of potassium. Hypophosphatemia may occur during refeeding when an adequate amount of phosphorus is not supplied. Use of corticosteroids and phosphate-binding antacids is also associated with low serum phosphorus levels. Hypomagnesemia may arise from malabsorption, diarrhea, and small-bowel drainage. Hypermagnesemia may result from bone metastases and leukemias.

Nutritional Care

Dietary manipulations to deal with the sequelae of antineoplastic therapy have received wide attention in the literature. A summary is provided in Table 11-6. Dietary modifications must be adjusted to the individual patient's preferences, tolerance, and condition. Education about the importance of adequate nutritional intake and provision of encouragement and support of the cancer patient during mealtimes

TABLE 11-6 Symptom-specific Dietary Modifications

Symptom	Dietary Modification(s)
Anorexia	Small, frequent feedings.
	Emphasize high-calorie protein foods.
	Offer support and encouragement at mealtimes.
	Keep snacks available so patient can eat when appetite allows.
Dysgeusia	Serve foods at room temperature.
	Offer cold plates.
	Avoid specific foods patient cannot tolerate such as coffee or hot entrees.
Mouth dryness	Add sauces, gravies, au jus, margarine.
	Suggest pureed or liquid foods.
	Offer "slushes," popsicles, and juicy fruits.
Esophagitis	Offer soft or pureed foods.
	Avoid irritating seasonings, spices, and acidic foods such as citrus or tomatoes.
	Avoid extremes in temperature.
Stomatitis, mucositis	Avoid salty, acidic, highly seasoned foods, and carbonated beverages.
	Avoid extremes in temperature.
Early satiety	See dietary modifications for anorexia.
	Limit liquids with or just preceding meals.
Nausea, vomiting	Assure appropriate delivery of antiemetics.
	Avoid excessively sweet, strongly flavored, or greasy foods.
	Delay eating until acute nausea subsides.
	Individualize diet to patient tolerance.
	Use carbonated beverages or salty foods to relieve nausea.

are most effective in encouraging intake. Flexibility in mealtimes is useful in enabling the patient to eat whenever and whatever he or she can. If it is impossible to adjust meal service times, intake may be maximized by keeping high-protein, high-calorie food items at the bedside or in the unit refrigerator so that the patient can take advantage of times when he or she feels able to eat. Appropriate and timely delivery of antiemetic medications is invaluable in assisting the cancer patient to overcome nausea in order to eat when meals are delivered. If the patient is acutely nauseated and vomiting at mealtimes, he or she should not be encouraged to eat solid foods but should be given antiemetic medications and encouraged to sip cool liquids until the nausea subsides.

Tube feeding may be required if the patient is unable to ingest adequate nutrients by mouth because of anorexia, nausea, or mechanical obstruction. Because antineoplastic therapy or preexisting malnutrition may cause immunosuppression in the cancer patient, care must be given to maintain the sanitary condition of the tube feeding formula and system (see Enteral Feeding by Tube in this chapter). Dilution of the formula may be unwise because increased handling is required and may result in contamination of the feeding. Use of an isotonic, polymeric feeding, initiated at a slow rate, is the best way to assure tolerance and prevent infection. A monomeric, low-fat formula may be necessary, however, if the patient exhibits symptoms of malabsorption.

Parenteral nutritional support may be necessary if the patient suffers from significant malabsorption, intractable nausea and vomiting, or if the GI tract is nonfunctioning. Meticulous attention must be given to care of the catheter insertion site and delivery of PN solutions to avoid septic complications (see Parenteral Nutrition in this chapter). Long-term Silastic catheters or implanted venous access ports are frequently inserted prior to the beginning of chemotherapy to provide for deliver of chemotherapy, blood products, other medications, and PN solutions. It is possible to cycle PN solutions during hours in which the catheter is not being used for other infusions. Although it is necessary to plan delivery of all IV solutions so that none are omitted, cyclic delivery of PN formulas is helpful to assure that adequate nutritional input is attained.

The validity of traditional nutritional assessment techniques in the cancer patient has been widely debated. Most parameters of nutritional status are significantly affected by the disease and by antineoplastic therapies. Oncology patients frequently experience alterations in fluid status. Alterations in hydration status may affect the reliability of any biochemical data that are expressed as concentration per volume (such as serum albumin, transferrin, and total lymphocyte count), as well as measurements of body weight and other anthropometrics. Corticosteroids and chemotherapy cause immunosuppression which is not necessarily related to malnutrition. These therapies invalidate evaluation of the immune system as a means of evaluating nutritional status. Moreover, some chemotherapeutic agents may cause hepatic and renal dysfunction. Liver or kidney insufficiency may alter serum levels of circulating proteins and the outcome of urine tests for creatinine excretion and nitrogen

balance. Traditional nutritional assessment indices are useful in evaluating the nutritional status of the newly diagnosed cancer patient before therapy is instituted. Serial assessments must be used in combination with sound clinical judgment to assure that nutritional status is being evaluated and not simply the effects of therapy.

Pulmonary Disorders

The role that maintenance of adequate nutrition status plays in management of the patient with pulmonary disease has not been emphasized until recently. It has been reported that as many as 40% of patients suffering from chronic obstructive pulmonary disease (COPD) lose approximately 10% or more of body weight. Weight loss in COPD patients is associated with cor pulmonale, declining pulmonary function, and death. Many factors contribute to the etiology of chronic weight loss in the COPD patient. Intake is often curtailed because the patient experiences fatigue and shortness of breath caused by the exertion of eating, and lack of appetite may develop as a result of chronic sputum production. Medications frequently prescribed for the patient with pulmonary disease include bronchodilators and corticosteroids, known gastric irritants which may cause anorexia. Additional weight loss may be related to the increased energy required for the work of breathing. Malnutrition manifested by the COPD patient is generally of the marasmic type. Marasmus is recognizable on physical examination by general cachexia. The COPD patient usually has compensated for this chronically undernourished state as evidenced by relatively normal levels of circulating proteins. However, this patient is at significant nutritional risk should acute illness, infection, or trauma develop, because there are no nutritional reserves on which he or she can rely during periods of hypermetabolism.

The acutely ill patient on ventilator support is also at risk of developing malnutrition. Kwashiorkor-type malnutrition can develop rapidly if nutritional support is absent or inadequate because associated hypermetabolism causes rapid catabolism of somatic and visceral protein and energy stores, accompanied by a corresponding loss of body function.

Malnutrition has several deleterious effects that have particular significance for the patient with pulmonary disease. Lean body protein, including respiratory muscles, is catabolized during periods of hypermetabolism accompanied by inadequate nutritional input. Autocannibalism results in loss of respiratory function. Ventilatory drive is reduced as respiratory muscle mass is reduced and endurance of the remaining muscle tissue is impaired. Malnutrition is also associated with incompetence of the immune system, and thus the pulmonary patient who is unable to clear secretions has an increased risk of developing infection. Protein-calorie malnutrition causes a depletion of serum albumin level that decreases oncotic pressure, and may result in pulmonary edema. All these malnutrition-related factors contribute to decreased inspiratory force, decreased vital capacity and functional residual capacity of the lungs, impaired oxygenation, and increased minute ventilation. Presence of these effects impairs weaning from ventilator-assisted respiration.

Nutritional Requirements

Provision of overabundant amounts of nutrients to the pulmonary patient is as undesirable as is undernutrition. Input of excess calories, especially in the form of carbohydrate, is associated with an increased respiratory quotient (RQ). The RQ is the ratio of carbon dioxide produced to the oxygen consumed. It varies with the type of nutritional substrate being oxidized. Oxidation of fat results in an RQ of 0.7. When enough glucose is provided to meet basal requirements, RQ increases to 1.0. When more calories than necessary are provided, RQ rises above 1.0. An RQ above 1.0 is undesirable because this reflects production of carbon dioxide in excess of oxygen consumed, and it is associated with increased ventilatory workload. This is especially detrimental to the patient who is being weaned from ventilator support and the patient with chronic obstructive pulmonary disease. Therefore, it is beneficial to these patients to avoid provision of excess calories. Initially about 50% of energy requirements should be provided in the form of fat. The proportion may be increased to 60% to 70%.

Provision of protein in excess of requirements should be avoided in patients with pulmonary disease. Oxidation of amino acids increases minute ventilation which may result in dyspnea.

Adequate vitamin and mineral nutriture is important for nutritional support of the patient with pulmonary disease. Maintenance of normal serum phosphate levels is particularly important because hypophosphatemia has been related to respiratory failure. Hypophosphatemia may occur because of increased requirements for phosphate during hypermetabolism, movement of phosphate into the cells during metabolism of glucose, or infusion of phosphate-free PN solutions. Maintenance levels of vitamins, minerals, and trace elements should be provided and serum levels monitored to provide for increased requirements.

Nutritional Care

It is vital to provide nutritional care to patients with pulmonary disease as early as possible to forestall the development of chronic malnutrition. A high-protein, high-calorie diet accompanied by oral vitamin and mineral supplementation is the nutritional therapy of choice for the patient with chronic pulmonary disease. Since distention of the stomach can interfere with movement of the diaphragm, the patient should be encouraged to "graze," consuming numerous small snacks throughout the day, rather than concentrating nutrients into three meals. Ingestion of liquids and semisolid foods seems to provoke less shortness of breath than consumption of solids. These foods should not provide empty calories but should be nutritionally dense so that the patient benefits from the greatest nutritional input in the smallest volume possible. Addition of fats and carbohydrates to menu items is helpful to add calories. Imaginative use of eggs, milk, and cheese can boost protein content as well. Nutritional modular components and commercial supplements can increase nutrient density of the diet as well, although patients may object to their flavor and consistency.

If a patient is consuming an oral diet but is not able to meet total nutritional needs, tube feeding is necessary. It may be beneficial to cycle tube feeding. The tube feeding may be held during daytime hours so that the patient is able to eat small meals, and can be delivered by continuous drip at night. Continuous drip delivery of formula is especially beneficial to the patient on a ventilator because this decreases the risk of aspiration. Presence of the airway cuff, particularly a soft cuff, should not be construed as total protection against aspiration because it does not provide a total seal. Routine procedures designed to minimize the risk of aspiration, including proper patient position, determination of the presence of residual, adequate tube placement, and determination of tolerance of the tube feeding should be followed.

Tube feeding formulas that derive most of their energy content from carbohydrate are unsatisfactory for use in pulmonary disease. At least 20% to 50% of calories should be provided by fat. Most commercial formulas meet this requirement. The ratio of fat-to-carbohydrate calorie content of formulas can be enhanced through the addition of commercial fat modules. A high-fat formula specifically designed for use with patients with respiratory disease is available. Its clinical efficacy has not yet been widely tested.

Parenteral nutritional support may be necessary in the extremely malnourished patient whose gut has atrophied to the extent that enterally supplied nutrients are malabsorbed, or if the gut is not functioning. A mixed parenteral diet that provides approximately 50% of calories as carbohydrate and 50% as fat is ideal. The patient in sepsis and the severely catabolic patient are the exceptions to this rule. Such a patient may not be able to metabolize significant amounts of lipid calories.

The critically ill, ventilator-dependent patient should be monitored closely to ascertain the effects of nutritional support on respiratory status. Such monitoring should include measurement of minute ventilation, breathing frequency, oxygen consumption, carbon dioxide production, and arterial blood gases.

Serial nutritional assessments should be performed to facilitate evaluation of nutritional therapy, but data should be interpreted with caution. Hydration status is variable in the patient with pulmonary edema or in one receiving corticosteroid therapy. The presence of fluid overload may cause false low values in serum albumin and other serum proteins and contribute to falsely high measurements of body weight.

REFERENCES

1. Butterworth, C. E. (1974). The skeleton in the hospital closet. *Nutrition Today, 9,* 4-8.
2. Campbell, S. M. (Ed.). (1984). *Practical guide to nutritional care for dietitians and other health care professionals.* Birmingham: University of Alabama in Birmingham.
3. Shils, M. D., Baker, H., & Frank, O. (1985). Blood vitamin levels of long-term adult home total parenteral nutrition patients: The efficacy of the AMA-ADA parenteral multivitamin formulation. *Journal of Parenteral and Enteral Nutrition, 9,* 179-188.
4. Bistrian, B. R., Blackburn, G. L., Vitale, J., et al. (1976). Prevalence of malnutrition in general medical patients. *Journal of the American Medical Association, 235,* 1567-1570.
5. Reilly, J. J., Hull, S. F., Albert, N., et al. (1988). Economic impact of malnutrition: A model system for hospitalized patients. *Journal of Parenteral and Enteral Nutrition, 12,* 371-376.
6. Jeejeebhoy, K. N. (1988). Nutrient metabolism. In J. M. Kinney, K. N. Jeejeebhoy, G. L. Hill, et al. (Eds.), *Nutrition and metabolism in patient care* (pp. 60-88). Philadelphia: Saunders.
7. Moe, G. (1991). Enteral feeding and infection in the immunocompromised patient. *Nutrition in Clinical Practice, 6,* 55-61.
8. Guenter, P. A., Settle, G., Perlmutter, S., et al. (1991). Tube feeding–related diarrhea in acutely ill patients. *Journal of Parenteral and Enteral Nutrition, 15,* 277-280.
9. Rhoads, J. E., Dudrick, S. J., & Vars, H. M. (1986). History of intravenous nutrition. In J. L. Rombeau, & M. D. Caldwell (Eds.), *Parenteral nutrition* (pp. 1-8). Philadelphia: Saunders.
10. Bessy, P. Q., & Wilmore, D. W. (1988). The burned patient. In J. M. Kinney, K. N. Jeejeebhoy, G. L. Hill, et al. (Eds.), *Nutrition and metabolism in patient care* (pp. 672-700). Philadelphia: Saunders.
11. McCauley, K., & Weaver, T. E. (1983). Cardiac and pulmonary diseases: nutritional implications. *Nursing Clinics of North America, 18,* 81-96.
12. Tobian, L. V. (1979). Dietary salt (sodium) and hypertension. *American Journal of Clinical Nutrition, 31,* 2659-2662.
13. Taylor, K. B. (1977). Gastroenterology. In H. A. Schneider, C. E. Anderson, & D. B. Coursin (Eds.), *Nutritional support of medical practice* (pp. 332-340). New York: Harper & Row.
14. Ryan, J. A., Adyl, B. A., & Weinstein, A. J. (1986). Enteric fistulas. In J. L. Rombeau, & M. D. Caldwell (Eds.), *Parenteral nutrition* (pp. 419-436). Philadelphia: Saunders.
15. Soeters, P. B., Ebeid, A. M., & Fischer, J. E. (1979). Review of 404 patients with gastrointestinal fistulas. *Annals of Surgery, 190,* 189-202.
16. Bernard, M. A., Jacobs, D. O., & Rombeau, J. L. (Eds.). (1986). Renal failure. In *Nutrition and metabolic support of hospitalized patients* (pp. 226-245). Philadelphia: Saunders.
17. Kelly, K. (1986). An overview of how to nourish the cancer patient by mouth. *Cancer, 58,* 1897-1901.

12

Pain

Kathleen A. Puntillo

Pain is a sensory experience like sight, hearing, and touch. Unlike the other senses, however, pain is almost always associated with tissue injury, feelings of unpleasantness, and other negative emotions. Pain is very complex and a challenge to diagnose and treat. If left untreated, pain causes suffering. Nurses diagnose and treat this human response to prevent and limit tissue injury and its sequelae, to enhance patient comfort, and to relieve suffering.

Pain is a common response to illness and treatment conditions in critically ill patients. Many critically ill patients have undergone major surgeries, traumatic injuries, or ischemic episodes, all of which are associated with pain. In addition to the initial event being potentially painful, critical care patients are subjected to painful and stress-provoking diagnostic and treatment procedures.[1,2] The need for these often life-saving interventions must be balanced by the recognition and management of their associated pain.

Most pain in critically ill patients is acute with an identifiable cause and a time-predictable resolution. In contrast, chronic pain is longer lasting, is often difficult to treat, and is caused by physiological mechanisms that are less well understood and seem to differ from those related to acute pain.[3,4] Yet, while the time course and mechanisms of acute pain are clearer, the effects of its inadequate relief may be profound, especially in physiologically and psychologically vulnerable critically ill patients. Because of the prevalence and potential consequences of pain, critical care nurses need a thorough understanding of its physiology, assessment, and management.

THE MANY DIMENSIONS OF PAIN

Pain has many dimensions.[5,6] *Sensory* dimensions are particular characteristics of pain that are reported by individuals, including location and qualities such as burning, sharp, and dull. The ability of an individual to discriminate among these dimensions requires intricate sensory neuronal processing. Pain also has a *physiological* response dimension because of neuronal connections between fibers of the pain system and fibers of autonomic and motor pathways and hormonal systems. *Affective* pain dimensions entail emotions associated with pain—fear, anxiety, depression—through engagement of the limbic system and other emotion centers in the brain. *Behavioral* dimensions of pain are responsive actions—both voluntary and involuntary— that are due to a pain stimulus. These behaviors may consist of vocalizations, such as crying out; of movements to avoid or protect against pain; or of seeking relief, such as asking for pain medicaion. *Cognitive* dimensions of pain are the higher order processing activities that ensue when the adversive sensory stimuli are recognized. These activities include judging, deriving meaning, evaluating, and placing the pain within past and present contexts.

Completely isolating these pain dimensions is difficult, if not impossible. They are intricately interrelated. Together, they comprise the experience of pain. Knowledge of physiological pain mechanisms helps in understanding the complexity of pain and provides a supportive foundation for diagnostic and treatment activities.

THE PHYSIOLOGY OF PAIN

Peripheral Mechanisms

Sensations are derived from initial stimulation of nerve receptors in tissues and organs. *Nociceptors* are nerve ending receptors that transmit stimuli from tissues that are injured or at risk for injury.[7] The sensation will eventually be identified as pain at higher brain levels. Until that time, however, it is categorized as a noxious sensation, that is, one capable of producing injury.

Several forms of stimuli can activate nociceptors on tissue cells, causing the cells to depolarize. Depolarization is a change in the electrical voltage of a cell membrane whereby the movement of positively charged sodium (Na^+) ions into the cell increases, causing the cell interior to be less negatively charged.

TABLE 12-1 **Biochemical Substances Involved in Nociception**

Substance	Source	Effect on Primary Afferent
Potassium	Damaged cells	Activate (NT)
Serotonin	Platelets	Activate (NT)
Bradykinin	Plasma kinino-gen	Activate (NT)
Histamine	Mast cells	Activate (NT)
Prostaglandins	Arachidonic acid	Sensitize (NM)
Leukotrienes	Arachidonic acid	Sensitize (NM)
Substance P	Primary afferent	Sensitize (NM)

NT = neurotransmitter.
NM = neuromodulator.
Modified from Fields, H. L. (1987). *Pain.* New York: McGraw-Hill.

If the stimulus is strong enough, cell depolarization will result in an action potential which is transmitted as an impulse along the length of the nerve. The initiating stimulus can be mechanical, such as pressure exerted on the tissue; it may be thermal, in the form of heat; or it may be biochemical, that is, caused by substances produced by or released from cells. Table 12-1 lists substances that either alone or in combination stimulate or sensitize nociceptors by acting as neurotransmitters or neuromodulators.[8]

Neurotransmitters are chemicals that, upon attachment to cell receptors, cause a change in the polarization of the cell membrane. An excitatory neurotransmitter leads to cell firing by supporting the influx of Na^+ ions and, thus, depolarization. An inhibitory neurotransmitter hyperpolarizes a cell, making the cell interior more negative and unable to fire. Increased negativity may be due to K^+ exit from the cell or inward movement of Cl^- ions.

As can be seen in Table 12-1, other biochemical substances serve as *neuromodulators*. They may not alone cause cell firing, but they sensitize cells to make them easier to fire. Neuromodulator chemical substances such as bradykinins and histamine are also responsible for the inflammatory process associated with tissue injury in which there is swelling and redness in addition to pain.

Two types of nerve fibers transmit noxious information from peripheral receptor endings to the central nervous system (CNS), A-delta and C fibers. These nerve fibers are categorized according to their size, the presence or absence of a myelin sheath, and the specific type of stimulus that activates them. A-delta fibers, the larger of the two types, are myelinated (insulated) and transmit impulses rapidly. They are primarily activated by mechanical and thermal stimuli.[9] C fibers are small, unmyelinated, and polymodal, responding to many forms of stimuli: mechanical, thermal and biochemical substances. When A-delta fibers have been experimentally isolated and stimulated, individuals have reported feeling immediate, well localized, sharp pain. Preferential stimulation of C fibers leads to pain described as delayed, dull, and diffuse.[10] It is important for the critical care nurse to know the different characteristics of pain derived from various fiber types. This knowledge helps in understanding patient reports of the sensory dimensions of their pain and in treatment effectiveness.

Peripheral noxious nerve fibers have many origins.[11] First, there are cutaneous fibers activated by skin surface stimuli. Second, there are two types of somatic fibers: *superficial* somatic fibers innervate tissues just below the skin; *deep* somatic fibers originate in muscles, joints, and ligaments. Third, there are visceral fibers that transmit noxious impulses from internal tissues and organs. They are predominantly C fibers. Evidently there are fewer visceral fibers than cutaneous and somatic fibers.[12,13]

Visceral pain is often associated with strong motor reflexes and autonomic nervous system (ANS) activation and is described as dull, achy, and difficult to localize.[14] This difficulty in localization is believed to be due to spinal cord convergence of fibers originating from different areas. That is, there is evidence that visceral fibers converge on the same secondary nerve cells in the spinal cord as do fibers from somatic structures. A patient may report pain to be in a particular somatic structure when the origin of the stimulus may be in a distant, even visceral, tissue. This evidence helps to explain the concept of referred pain, where pain from one organ or structure is referred to another in the same dermatome, a body segment with specific sensory innervation.[8] For example, the heart and arms are believed to be in the same dermatome, and individuals often identify myocardial ischemic pain as arm muscle pain.

Spinal Cord Actions

Different nerve fibers communicate with one another at multiple synapses in the spinal cord dorsal horn. Neurotransmitters released from one fiber either depolarize (causing transmission) or hyperpolarize (blocking transmission) the second fiber. Figure 12-1 depicts several types of spinal cord dorsal horn synapses that comprise the nociception and pain processing system. First, the synapsing of primary and secondary ascending nociceptive fibers leads to impulse transmission to higher brain centers. Second, primary fibers can synapse on motor fibers whose impulses cause reflex activities such as the knee jerk

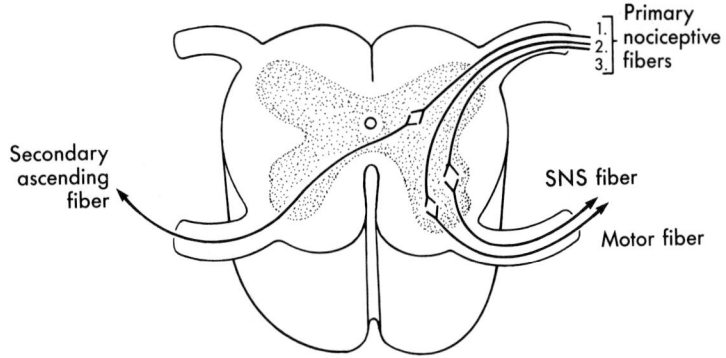

Figure 12-1 Multiple synapses of primary nociceptive fibers in spinal cord. *1,* Primary nociceptive fiber synapses with secondary ascending nociceptive fiber. *2,* Primary nociceptive fiber synapses with motor fiber. *3,* Primary nociceptive fiber synapses with fiber of the sympathetic nervous system.

response. Third, synapsing of primary nociceptive fibers with ANS cells in the spinal cord gray matter leads to autonomic responses. Also, within the spinal cord dorsal horn primary nociceptive fibers relate with other larger, myelinated sensory fibers categorized as A-alpha or A-beta. These fibers transmit nonnoxious sensory information such as touch, pressure, and vibration from the periphery to the dorsal horn. The relationship between nociceptive fibers and other non-nociceptive sensory fibers can be explained by the gate control theory.[15]

Gate Control Theory (Figure 12-2)

The gate control theory hypothesizes that both nociceptive and non-nociceptive sensory fibers synapse on the same cells that transmit pain sensations to the brain. Inhibitory interneurons in the spinal cord influence these central transmission cells by interrupting the balance between smaller (pain) fibers and large (nonpain) fibers. When larger, nonpain fibers are less active, compared to pain fibers, pain transmission cells are stimulated. When larger, nonpain fibers are stimulated, inhibitory interneurons block pain transmission to higher centers.

Higher CNS central control processes can influence the spinal cord gate by delivering descending inhibitory messages to the spinal cord. Thus, critical care nurses can use distraction, relaxation techniques, and other similar types of interventions that may activate descending inhibitory fibers and close the gate to pain.

Descending Inhibitory Fibers

Neural spinal cord activity can be interrupted by inhibitory fibers that descend directly or through a series of synapses from different brain centers. These fibers contain either endorphins or certain biogenic amines that act as inhibitory neurotransmitters in the spinal cord.

Endorphins, endogenous opioid substances such as

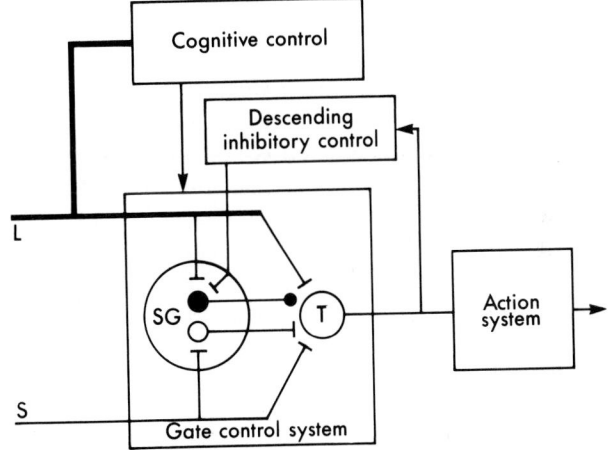

Figure 12-2 The gate control theory. Excitatory (white circle) and inhibitory (black circle) links from the substantia gelatinosa (SG) to the transmission (T) cells as well as descending inhibitory control for brainstem systems. L = large, nonpain fibers; S = small, pain fibers. See text for further description.

From Melzack, P., & Wall, P. (1983). *The challenge of pain.* New York: Basic Books.

enkephalins, are contained in fiber systems that originate in the midbrain periaqueductal gray matter (PAG) and several nuclei in the medulla. Nerve impulses descending along these fibers containing endorphins will cause their release in the dorsal horn. When endorphins occupy opioid receptors on primary or secondary nociceptive neurons, they prevent neural excitation. Cell firing is inhibited and ascending transmission of nociceptive impulses ceases.

Biogenic amines, specifically serotonin and norepinephrine, appear to have similar inhibitory actions. Pons neurons containing norepinephrine and medullary neurons containing serotonin have their ending in the dorsal horn where they synapse with ascending nociceptive fibers. Release and action of these biogenic amines lead to inhibition of ascending nociceptive transmission.[8]

These inhibitory mechanisms provide the theoretical explanations for effects of pain inhibition by various events, processes, or interventions through stimulation of descending pain inhibitory pathways. For example, stress associated with the use of restraints, fear, and hypoglycemia are proposed to induce analgesia through activation of these inhibitory systems.[16] Experimental stimulation of brain sites that contain endogenous opioids has also caused analgesia in animals[17] and in humans with chronic pain.[18] Therapeutic interventions for pain that are believed to activate pain inhibitory systems are discussed in the section on pain management.

Brain Integration

The multidimensional nature of pain is mainly due to neuronal involvement of many areas of the brain. Secondary fiber tracts originating in the spinal cord ascend to the thalamus, reticular formation, hypothalamus, midbrain, and limbic system. Tertiary fiber tracts then transmit nociceptive information from these brain structures to areas of the cortex where the sensations are identified as pain, and cognitive processing of this information occurs. The involvement of so many areas and the integration of neuronal activity helps to explain the complexity of pain in critically ill patients.

Physiological Effects of Pain

Physiological responses to pain can involve many systems because of synaptic connections between pain fibers and fibers innervating cardiovascular, musculoskeletal, and respiratory systems. The box to the right depicts the potential systemic effects of pain and potential complications that may ensue if pain is unrelieved. Sympathetic nervous system (SNS) activation increases heart rate and contractility,[19,20] with subsequent increases in myocardial oxygen consumption. Sympathetic peripheral vasoconstriction increases afterload, whereas coronary artery vasoconstriction decreases myocardial oxygen supply. Respiratory mechanics may be altered when splinting of respiratory muscles from pain alters the patient's respiratory pattern and effort. Low lung volumes and airflow lead to ineffective airway clearance and increased retention of secretions. Thus, patients may develop pneumonia, atelectasis, and ventilation/perfusion abnormalities.

Pain also has a negative effect on the musculoskeletal system, leading to contraction of skeletal muscles, muscle spasms, and rigidity. Patients will both voluntarily and involuntarily restrict mobilization, coughing, and deep breathing when it is too painful for them to perform these activities.[21] These maneuvers and activities are essential to the improvement of functional status of critically ill patients.

Potential Consequences of Pain

POTENTIAL CARDIOVASCULAR CONSEQUENCES OF PAIN

Increased heart rate, contractility $\rightarrow \uparrow$ MVo_2
Peripheral vasoconstriction $\rightarrow \uparrow$ afterload
Coronary artery vasoconstriction $\rightarrow \uparrow$ myocardial ischemia

POTENTIAL ALTERATION OF RESPIRATORY MECHANICS

Pain $\rightarrow$
  Splinting
  Altered respiratory pattern and effort
  Decreased lung volumes and flow ($\downarrow$ V_T, VC, FRC, PEFR, FEV_1)

POTENTIAL RESPIRATORY CONSEQUENCES

Ineffective airway clearance
Increased retention of secretions
Pneumonia
Atelectasis
Ventilation/perfusion abnormalities

POTENTIAL MUSCULOSKELETAL CONSEQUENCES

Pain $\rightarrow$
  Reflex motor activity
  Contraction of skeletal muscles
  Muscle rigidity
  Impaired mobilization, coughing, deep breathing

V_T = tidal volume. VC = vital capacity. FRC = functional residual capacity. PEFR = peak expiratory flow rate. FEV_1 = forced expiratory volume, 1 second.

Anxiety and Stress Responses to Pain

Anxiety is the psychological variable that is most closely related to acute pain. It has been defined as "an active organization of defense mechanisms, a reaction to an internal or external danger, and a threat to the integrity of the personality, consisting of mind and body."[22] There appears to be a close neural connection between the frontal lobe, one of the brain's cognitive centers, and the limbic system, a center for emotions.[23] These anatomical relationships help to explain the following vicious cycle: increased pain perception $\rightarrow$ increased emotional responses $\rightarrow$ increased ANS arousal $\rightarrow$ increased muscle tension, which increases pain.[23] The effect of anxiety on pain may be partially explained by the gate control theory's central control mechanisms. The central control cognitive-evaluative and motivational-affective responses at higher brain levels affect spinal cord pain input[24] by opening pain gates to transmission. Interventions that relieve anxiety by activating central inhibitory pathways may reduce pain by decreasing its spinal cord ascending transmission.

Pain has been identified as a psychological stressor in numerous critical care studies that have investigated sources of patient stressors.[1,25,26,27] The stress response to pain also has physiological effects such as initiation of hyperglycemia and increased catecholamine, cortisol, and antidiuretic hormone (ADH) secretions.[28] It is important to interrupt the mechanisms whereby pain leads to stress not only for humane reasons but for physiological well-being.

DATA ACQUISITION

Critical care nurses develop sophisticated skills in assessment of body systems. Since pain is not limited to a particular body system and is multidimensional, it should be assessed separately, as a unique human response. Nurses can use observational skills, questioning, and changes in physiological parameters to formulate an assessment of patient pain status.

Observations

People respond to pain through both reflexive and intentional behaviors. Protective defensive behaviors include guarding, withdrawal, and avoidance of movement. Palliative behaviors are attempts by the patient to seek relief such as rubbing a painful area, asking for pain medications, or moving into a more comfortable position. Affective behaviors are emotional responses to pain such as crying, moaning, screaming, or exhibiting hostility. Intubated, restrained patients are not able to express many of these pain behaviors.

The face is often a better source of pain information than the body. In fact, a particular facial pain expression has been shown to be a reliable indicator of acute pain: "brow lowering with skin drawn in tightly around closed eyes, accompanied by a horizontally stretched open mouth, sometimes with deepening of the nasolabial furrow."[29] This facial pain expression is difficult to observe in a critically ill intubated patient.

Posttransfer patients have described the behaviors they used to communicate their pain to nurses when they were in critical care units. These included use of eyes, facial expressions, or hand and leg movements when they were unable to vocalize their pain.[2] The validity of certain behaviors as indicators of pain needs to be explored further through nursing research.

Questioning

Since pain is a subjective experience, the most valid source of information about a patient's pain is that patient. In fact, pain has even been defined according to this premise as being "whatever the experiencing person says it is, existing whenever he says it does."[30] Information about the dimensions or characteristics of pain can be sought with the aid of pain description and rating instruments. Word scales, numerical rating scales (NRS), or both can be used to measure pain intensity (Figure 12-3A). Patients are asked to choose the word or number that best fits the amount or severity of their pain at that time or over a certain period. A *visual analog scale* (VAS) is a vertical or horizontal line with word anchors at both ends of the line depicting the extreme of pain intensity (Figure 12-3B). No numbers are along this line; patients are asked to make a mark along the line at the point that best depicts the pain intensity. The nurse can then measure the line length for documentation.

An evaluation of pain associated with certain activities can be made through the use of the Prince Henry Pain Scale[31] (Table 12-2). Patients' answers to the questions on this scale may indicate their ability to perform maneuvers important to their recovery

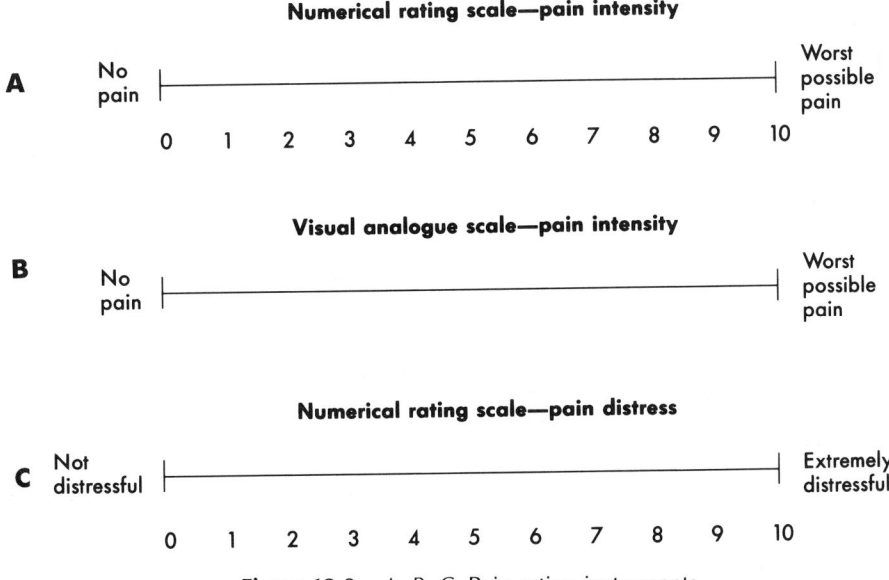

Figure 12-3 A, B, C, Pain rating instruments.

TABLE 12-2 **Prince Henry Pain Scale**

Definition	Score
No pain on coughing	0
Pain on coughing but not on deep breathing	1
Pain on deep breathing but not at rest	2
Pain at rest, slight	3
Pain at rest, severe	4

Reprinted, with permission, from Torda, T. A., & Pybus, D. A. (1984). Extradural administration of morphine and bupivicaine: A controlled comparison. *British Journal of Anaesthesia, 54,* 141-146.

such as coughing and moving. In addition, knowledge gained through use of this scale can guide patient teaching or the choice of pain management interventions. For example, if a patient relates having pain only with coughing, the critical care nurse can help with bracing techniques and teach them to the patient.

In addition to pain intensity, the emotional, or affective, component of pain can be assessed by employing an NRS that uses emotion-focused words such as "distressful" or "bothersome" (Figure 12-3C). Research subjects have been able to differentiate between pain affective words and pain intensity words,[32,33] providing support for the usefulness of both measures. Much can be gained from knowing the relationship between a patient's pain intensity and the distress associated with it. If patients report low pain intensity but high pain distress during a procedure, more information about the specific sensations they may feel during the procedure may relieve their distress.

The qualitative nature of pain can also be assessed by offering patients choices of words that describe their pain such as burning, sharp, or throbbing. This information may help in the diagnosis of pain etiology as well as in choosing appropriate interventions. For example, sharp pain may not be effectively treated by epidural opioid administration because the A-delta fibers that transmit sharp pain do not synapse near opioid receptors in the spinal cord.[34] Hence, another type or mode of analgesic may be more effective for sharp pain.

The McGill Pain Questionnaire—Short Form (MPQ-SF)[35] is an instrument that is used to select and quantify the intensity of 15 pain quality words (Figure 12-4). The first 11 of these words rate pain intensity, and the last 4 rate pain affect. This instrument also has a VAS intensity scale and a 0 to 5 present pain intensity word scale, providing the nurse one instrument with which to gain considerable information

about the patient's pain. Pictures can also be used to help patients communicate pain location. Patients can point to or make a mark on a body diagram where they are feeling pain. With use of a picture, they can more easily identify areas that they cannot reach. This information will help clinicians to avoid overlooking areas of pain.

Many instruments can assess pain in critically ill patients, even those who are unable to verbalize their answers. Both intubated and nonintubated cardiac and abdominal vascular surgery patients were able to use a VAS, NRS, body outline diagram, and MPQ-SF to communicate their postoperative and procedure-related pain.[36]

Physiological Indicators

Critical care nurses constantly monitor and assess changes in heart rate, blood pressure, and many other physiological variables that indicate ANS responsivity. As discussed earlier, SNS activation frequently accompanies an acute, painful event. This activation may be evidenced by increases in heart rate and blood pressure, pupillary dilation, and diaphoresis. There is debate as to whether these ANS responses are to the perception of the sensation of pain or to the affective and cognitive dimensions of pain. Research findings have suggested that increases in heart rate from experimental pain may be reflective of all of these pain dimensions.[37] An initial increase (first 3 seconds) in heart rate may be due to perception of the sensation. After about 6 seconds, ANS response may be due to affective or cognitive responses.

In a critical care unit, it is extremely difficult to determine whether ANS changes are due to pain or to something else, such as physiological or psychological stress. Unfortunately, there is little research to support ANS changes as indicators of pain in critically ill patients. However, a few studies have shown decreases in blood pressure and heart rate when music therapy decreased pain.[38,39] Pain, as well as blood pressure, heart rate, and respiratory rate, decreased when relaxation techniques were used with postoperative cardiac patients.[40] Still, clinicians must cautiously interpret changes in their patients' vital signs as indicators of pain, especially since so many medications given to critically ill patients influence ANS activity. However, changes in ANS parameters can be used in conjunction with patient self-reports of pain and pain behaviors to more extensively assess patient pain.

Special Challenges in the Critical Care Environment

Objective, accurate interpretation of the critically ill patient's subjective pain experience is always a

	None	Mild	Moderate	Severe
Throbbing	0) ____	1) ____	2) ____	3) ____
Shooting	0) ____	1) ____	2) ____	3) ____
Stabbing	0) ____	1) ____	2) ____	3) ____
Sharp	0) ____	1) ____	2) ____	3) ____
Cramping	0) ____	1) ____	2) ____	3) ____
Gnawing	0) ____	1) ____	2) ____	3) ____
Hot-burning	0) ____	1) ____	2) ____	3) ____
Aching	0) ____	1) ____	2) ____	3) ____
Heavy	0) ____	1) ____	2) ____	3) ____
Tender	0) ____	1) ____	2) ____	3) ____
Splitting	0) ____	1) ____	2) ____	3) ____
Tiring-exhausting	0) ____	1) ____	2) ____	3) ____
Sickening	0) ____	1) ____	2) ____	3) ____
Fearful	0) ____	1) ____	2) ____	3) ____
Punishing-cruel	0) ____	1) ____	2) ____	3) ____

Figure 12-4 Word list from McGill Pain Questionnaire—Short Form.
From Melzack, R. (1987). The short-form McGill Pain Questionnaire. *Pain, 30,* 193.

challenge, for a number of reasons. First, many critically ill patients are unable to verbalize their pain because intubation or other motor impairments such as cerebral vascular accidents (CVAs) interfere with vocalization. In these cases nurses should maximize the abilities of these patients to communicate their pain through use of pictures, word charts, and attention to nonverbal pain indicators.

Second, cultural and language differences can also affect the communication of pain. Expectations, attitudes, and meanings related to pain are learned from the family within cultural contexts.[41] In addition, languages differ in the types and numbers of words used to express pain. Hebrew, Chinese, and Japanese have very few pain expressions, whereas the English language has 16 categories of pain with 64 words.[42] When differences in language and culture exist between patients and their nurse caregivers, pain assessment and management can be significantly affected.[43] Nurses must recognize and respect these differences as they collect information about their patients' pain. The box to the right presents questions that may be helpful to nurses as they assess pain in patients who come from different cultures or speak different languages.

A third factor that makes communication and assessment of pain difficult is mobility impairment. Patients may be too weak to move or to talk. Absence of these behaviors may sometimes be erroneously construed as an absence of pain. To prevent this error, nurses can work with the patient to devise an easy method for communicating pain through simple eye or finger movements.

Nurse's Self-assessment: Culture and Pain

Do I consciously consider my patient's cultural affiliation and its potential effect on pain expression?
What is my cultural background and belief about pain and pain expression?
Do I stereotype? Or do I recognize interethnic, intraethnic variability?
What are my unit's/hospital's resources for assistance to various cultural groups? Do I make adequate use of them? Am I willing to assist in their development?
Do I use the patient's family in pain assessment and treatment activities?
What pain management practices have I found effective for people of different cultures?

Iatrogenic mobility impairments include the use of physical and chemical restraints. Wrist restraints are often used as a protective measure to avoid, for example, patient self-extubation. These restraints, however, also prevent patients from engaging in defensive and palliative behaviors, such as turning to a comfortable position or rubbing a painful area.

Sometimes critically ill patients are chemically immobilized by neuromuscular blocking agents (NMBAs). These agents interrupt motor neurons; they have no effect on sensory neurons that transmit pain. Thus, patients paralyzed with agents such as pancuronium or vecuronium are completely capable of feeling pain but are unable to report it. Unfortunately, knowledge of NMBA actions is not widespread among critical care professionals: up to 25% of approximately 258 nurses were not aware that neuromuscular blocking agents had no analgesic properties.[44] It is important for nurses to understand the mechanisms of neuromuscular blocking agents—that they are neither sedatives nor analgesics[45]—and how they interfere with the usual methods of assessing pain. To administer NMBAs without concurrent use of analgesics or sedatives is negligent nursing care that is suggestive of malpractice.

A fourth factor that makes patient pain assessment challenging is the patient's alteration in levels of consciousness (LOC). In spite of our increasing knowledge about the physiological processing of pain, it is often difficult to know at what level of consciousness pain is perceived. A reflexive response to noxious sensations occurs at spinal cord levels. This knowledge allows us to understand how a person who is comatose may withdraw from a stimulus but may not be perceiving pain. As yet, however, clinical measures do not exist to help us determine if pain perception does occur in these situations. Nurses can assume pain perception may be occurring in patients with altered LOC under circumstances in which normally painful procedures are performed and painful conditions exist.

Special Techniques for Pain Assessment

Pain assessment involves all steps of the nursing process whereby both subjective and objective data are collected. These data serve as a basis for management interventions. Through this process the nurse uses clinical judgment skills. Two techniques may assist critical care nurses in their assessment of patient pain: imagining sources of pain and using family and friends.

Assessing for Possible Sources of Pain

When patients are unable to communicate their pain, the nurse may turn to imagination and assess the patient for possible sources of pain. The box to the right presents a list of questions that can serve as a guide. These potential sources of pain may be impossible to validate. However, this type of assessment might promote prophylactic nursing care by identifying possible sources of pain.

Use of Family and Friends

The patient's family members and friends may be very valuable resources during pain assessments. They can provide information about a patient's pain history. Does the patient have chronic sources of pain such as back pain, arthritic pain, or frequent headaches? It is important, also, to know the patient's analgesic history since long-term use of opioids in-

---

Questions to Determine Sources of Pain

CUTANEOUS PAIN

Are there incisions, open wounds, abrasions, chemical or thermal injuries involving skin?

Have tubes or needles broken skin integrity?

Are there dressings, ties, restraints that are constricting or pinching the skin or pulling body hair?

Is a skin area resting on a surface (e.g., wrinkled or rough linen) that may be irritating to it?

SOMATIC PAIN

Are there immobilized joints or muscle groups?

Are there muscle groups being compressed or stretched or in positions that would increase muscle tension?

Has one position been maintained for a long time?

Has the integrity of a muscle, ligament, or joint been interrupted by a surgical incision or traumatic injury?

Is the underlying condition known to cause muscle pain or cramping?

Are medications being administered that are known to cause muscle aching or cramping?

Have tubes or needles been routed through muscles?

VISCERAL PAIN

Is the underlying condition known to originate from a visceral source?

Might there be stretching or bulging of a visceral organ, e.g., from gas in the small intestine?

Are there tubes or catheters terminating in areas with visceral fibers, e.g., parietal pleura?

Are medications being administered that are known to cause headaches?

Are there repetitive environmental noises that may be causing headaches?

---

creases susceptibility to drug tolerance. The drug-tolerant patient may not be obtaining relief from the "usual" doses of opiates.

Family members and friends can provide information about the patient's usual response to pain. Does it promote anxiety? Is pain tolerance high or low? Is the patient usually reluctant or willing to report pain. Use of family and friends may be particularly helpful when there are language barriers or cultural differences between the patient and health care providers.

Assessing Pain Relief

Patients anticipate pain relief from treatment interventions. Therefore, to evaluate a person's total pain experience adequately, assessment of pain relief needs consideration. Evaluating presence and sources of pain relief is essential to appropriate clinical management. Some interventions may even exacerbate pain.[46] Therefore, without an evaluation of pain relief, pain may increase.

Assessment of pain relief may reflect the philosophy of health care team members about medicating practices and pain relief goals. In one study, only 20% of physicians and nurses caring for surgical patients aimed for complete pain relief for their patients.[47] Even when physicians stated that their goal for pain relief was 100%, their actual analgesic practices were quite contradictory.[48] Less than one third of a sample of nurses assessed patient pain relief, believing that patients would tell them if their pain continued.[49] Telling their nurses may prove to be a problem for patients who have difficulty communicating and who may be uncertain about when and how they were last treated for pain.

It is the nurse's responsibility to follow up on pain relief. Simple pain relief instruments, like a 0 to 10 numerical rating scale for pain relief, can be used. Use of a simple word scale, such as "no pain relief," "moderate pain relief," or "complete pain relief" is another option. Results must be recorded to communicate analgesic effects to other members of the critical care team.

The Importance of Documentation

Priority needs to be given to establishing systematic documentation of pain and pain relief. This information is as important to a patient's well-being as other data collected, considering the patient's physiological and psychological vulnerability.

Research has shown that nurses' documentation of pain is incomplete.[50] Inadequate documentation can impair communication among critical care team members about a patient's pain status and diminish the ability to evaluate effectiveness of interventions. There are also legal implications, considering that lack of documentation implies that a particular nursing responsibility was left unmet.

A number of computer systems are available for nurse documentation of pain information. Alternatively, an area on the critical care flowsheet could be devoted to pain information, or a separate form devised for documentation.[51] Nurses are encouraged to assume leadership in instituting appropriate pain documentation practices.

MANAGEMENT OF PAIN

The physiological framework presented earlier provides a model for proposing interventions for pain. That is, there are many areas in the systems for pain transmission, modulation, perception, and inhibition that can be targeted with pain relief measures. Figure 12-5 illustrates target sites and examples of interventions appropriate for each site. Interventions will be

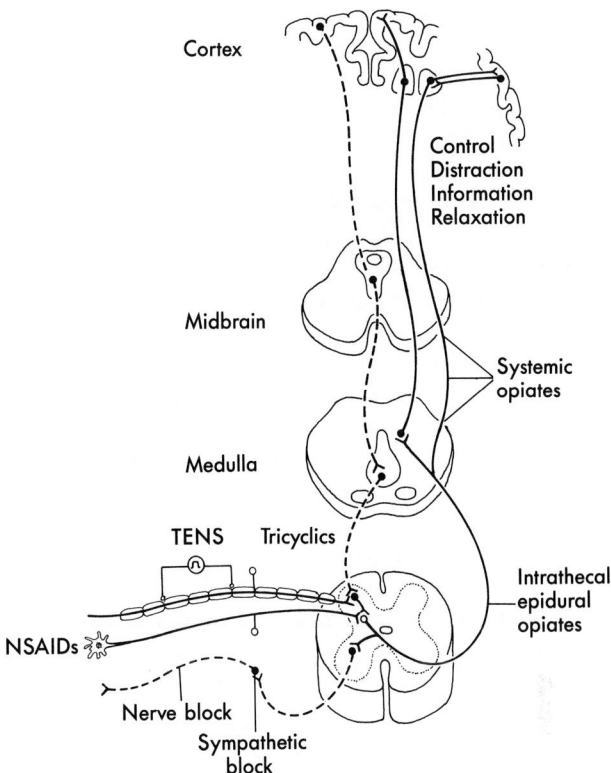

Figure 12-5 Pain therapies and their proposed action sites.

Modified from Fields, H. L., & Levine, J. D. (1984). Pain: Mechanisms and management. *Western Journal of Medicine, 141*(3), 347.

described using the pain transmission and inhibition framework.

Pain Interventions Acting in the Periphery

Nonsteroidal Antiinflammatory Agents

The actions of biochemical substances that mediate pain in the periphery can be blocked by nonsteroidal antiinflammatory agents (NSAIDs). These agents, as well as aspirin, inhibit the synthesis of prostaglandins that sensitize nerve endings. NSAIDs also inhibit the inflammatory response to tissue injury. The potential side effects of NSAIDs may preclude their use in some critically ill patients. That is, they may promote bleeding because of antiplatelet properties. They may also promote renal insufficiency because they inhibit synthesis of prostaglandins, which dilate renal arteries.[52] NSAIDs also often cause gastrointestinal (GI) irritability and upset.

Until recently, all NSAIDs available in the United States were oral agents, so their use in critically ill patients was restricted. However, ketorolac tromethamine (Toradol) is now available for intramuscular administration and is reported to have a single-dose effectiveness similar to or greater than morphine for treatment of moderate to severe postoperative pain.[53]

Caution is advised in the use of Toradol in elderly or renally impaired patients because of slower clearance rates in these individuals.[54] Nevertheless, Toradol may serve as a valuable new analgesic modality alone or in combination with opioids[52] for critically ill patients. Research on its effectiveness in this patient population is warranted.

Regional Nerve Blocks

Local anesthetic agents such as lidocaine and bupivacaine are widely used to block the transmission of pain along afferent peripheral fibers. These agents prevent nerve cell depolarization by binding to intracellular receptors and preventing Na^+ ion influx. In so doing, analgesia can be complete, and the adverse effects of systemic medications such as opioids are avoided.[55]

Although the intent in using local anesthetic agents for pain relief is to block sensory fibers, SNS and motor fibers can be blocked also, depending on the concentration and amount of drug injected.[56] When both afferent pain fiber and SNS fiber transmission are blocked, the physiological stress response to an injury and pain may be inhibited. Blockage of this response is protective in nature since stress can further tax the system.[55]

Use of local anesthetics is not without its risks, however. Vasodilation associated with SNS block may have adverse hemodynamic effects, especially in volume-depleted patients. Although allergic reactions are rare, toxic responses to local anesthetics can involve CNS and cardiovascular systems. CNS manifestations include tinnitus, numbness, tremulousness, and even convulsions. Local anesthetics may also act as myocardial depressants.[55]

Local anesthetics have been used to promote blockade of many types of peripheral nerves. Intercostal and interpleural blocks are two types often used to promote analgesia in critically ill patients. Direct injection of intercostal nerves or insertion of an epidural catheter near an intercostal nerve for local anesthetic infusion has been used to manage pain associated with trauma or surgery.[57] The mechanism of pain relief from interpleural local anesthetic administration is not entirely clear. There is a general consensus that anesthetics injected into the pleural space diffuse across the parietal pleura to the intercostal space and cause an intercostal blockade.[31,58,59]

Nurses do not yet insert interpleural catheters or inject local anesthetic agents into the interpleural space, but they assist with the procedure and are responsible for assessing effects and detecting complications.[60] Nurses are also in the position to recommend local anesthetic use as a means to interrupt peripheral pain transmission when appropriate conditions exist to support their use.

Use of Cold or Heat

Although little clinical research has been done on the effects of cold and heat on pain suppression, these treatments have often been used with success. It is suggested that vasoconstriction produced by cutaneous cold application can reduce bleeding, edema, inflammation, and sensitivity of nerve fibers and receptors.[61] Heat dilates local blood vessels, thereby increasing regional blood flow. Increased flow may support the resolution of inflammation,[61] perhaps by removing pain-producing substances from the area. Heat, however, may cause local swelling by increasing blood flow and thereby create more pressure at the area of injury. Critical care nurses are encouraged to consider the judicious use of either heat or cold for pain management since these techniques are inexpensive and easy to apply.

Massage

Massage is often one of the first nursing therapeutic measures addressed in nursing education. Unfortunately, it may be one of the first nursing activities to be deleted from a plan of care because of nursing time pressures. The physiological basis of its effectiveness for pain relief is unclear. However, the theoretical explanation may lie in the gate control theory. That is, large nonpain fibers—those that transmit pressure sensation—may be preferentially stimulated by massage so that they block pain transmission. Massage also may activate acupuncture points and release endorphins. It assists in increasing venous and lymphatic flow, consequently ridding an area of toxic substances.[62] Massage may alleviate pain mainly because of its relaxing, soothing, or distracting effects. Most people enjoy massages. However, there are times when they are an inappropriate intervention. Massage should be avoided any time there are open lesions, if the patient declines, or if it causes—instead of relieving—pain. Donovan et al.[63] questioned 158 medical-surgical patients about the effects of massage on their pain. Forty-nine percent stated that it decreased pain, 12% had an increase in pain, and 39% felt no effect on pain from the massage.[63]

Transcutaneous Electrical Nerve Stimulation (TENS)

TENS is a method by which electrical impulses are transmitted through a battery-operated device via electrodes applied to a particular area. TENS is believed to work by stimulating endogenous opioid activity[64] or by blocking afferent nociceptive impulses at the spinal cord or brainstem levels.[57] Advantages in using TENS are its few side effects and easy application. Disadvantages to its use, particularly with critically ill patients, is the need to adjust the amplitude and frequency to desired effect, as felt by the patient. The communication and mobility limitations of many of these patients may limit its applicability here. However, research and clinical experience may increase its use in critical care areas.

Interventions Acting at Spinal Cord Level

Spinal Opioids

Opioid analgesic therapy is the mainstay pharmacological treatment modality for pain in critically ill patients. Opioids mimic the actions of endogenous opioids by attaching to endogenous opioid receptors. These receptors have been located in areas of the limbic system, the periaqueductal gray matter and thalamus, the spinal cord gray matter, and the gut. Spinal cord opiate receptors are found in the substantia gelatinosa layer of the dorsal horn, the hypothesized site of gate control. Here, opiates bind to receptors on the cell body and terminals of primary afferents and inhibit the release of noxious transmitter substances such as substance P. They interfere with ascending transmission through secondary neurons, which also contain opioid receptors.[65]

Opioid actions depend on the type of receptor to which they attach. Many different types of receptors have been discovered. Most opiates currently used clinically have an affinity for mu receptors. Mu receptors are of two subtypes, mu-1 and mu-2. Mu-1 receptors are located in many supraspinal sites and mediate the analgesia effects of opiates. Mu-2 receptors may mediate respiratory depressant and GI effects of opiates such as constipation.[66]

Exogenous opiates such as morphine interact with these opioid receptors and act like endogenous opioids; that is, they are agonists. An opioid antagonist such as naloxone prevents the binding of an agonist and renders the opiate ineffective. Some opioids such as Butorphanol are mixed agonist-antagonists since they have agonist effects at one receptor type and antagonist effects at another.[67]

Certain properties of specific opiates used influence the onset, spread, and duration of analgesia obtained. Drugs like fentanyl, sufentanil, and alfentanil are very lipid-soluble and thus have a more rapid onset of action than morphine, which is one of the least lipid-soluble opiates. Duration of action is influenced by the dosage and spread of the drug, the particular pain stimulus, and the individuality of the patient.

Knowledge developed about spinal cord receptor sites has led to the administration of opioids either intrathecally (that is, into the subarachnoid space) or epidurally. Since the drug is administered close to receptor sites, less drug is needed and duration of effect is longer than with intravenous administration. Delivery modes for spinal analgesics include bolus or continuous infusion through catheters placed in subarachnoid or epidural spaces.

Epidural Opioids. The clinical use of epidural opioids has increased dramatically and has been the subject of a substantial number of research studies. Epidural opioid therapy can provide profound analgesia while minimizing adverse systemic effects from opioids.

Effects of epidural opioids have been compared to effects of IV opioid administration as needed in several kinds of postoperative critically ill patients. Patients given epidural opioids had better pain control and lower stress hormone levels,[34] better pulmonary function status,[68] increased ambulation,[69] fewer postoperative complications, lower mortality, shorter intubation time, and lower hospital and physician costs.[70] These findings support the use of epidural analgesics in certain patients.

Epidural catheters are placed at a spinal cord segment whose dermatomal distribution involves the painful area but as low as possible in the spinal cord to minimize respiratory and sedative effects due to rostral spread of the drug.[57] Epidural opioids diffuse across the dura layers and attach to dorsal horn opioid receptors. Time to onset of action depends on the lipophilicity of the opioid. The actions of lipophilic fentanyl are seen sooner than those from the less lipophilic morphine. Duration of effect is shorter with lipophilic drugs, also. Table 12-3 presents information regarding dosage, onset, and duration of effects from the most frequently used epidural opioids for postthoracotomy pain.

Critical care nurses play a very important role in epidural opioid therapy. They assist in catheter insertion, offering instruction and support to the patient. Depending on institutional policy, they may administer intermittent epidural bolus injections after the initial dose, using established protocols. Care is taken to assure proper epidural catheter placement and to inspect the injection site area for evidence of infection or leakage. Before the opioid is injected, the catheter should be aspirated. Blood return may indicate catheter migration into an epidural blood vessel; clear fluid aspirate may be cerebrospinal fluid. In either case, the analgesic injection should be postponed and a physician notified.[71] Meticulous aseptic technique should be used at all times. Only preservative-free opioids are administered, since preservatives may be neurotoxic.

Critical care nurses also play an essential role in monitoring analgesic effectiveness and indications of adverse effects. Respiratory depression can occur 1 to 2 hours after injection if the opioid has CSF or vascular access. Late respiratory depression, occurring up to 12 hours after injection, occurs from rostral spread of the opioid to brainstem areas.[72] Respiratory depression, one of the most serious consequences, is estimated to occur less than 0.5% of the time.[73]

TABLE 12-3   **Intraspinal Opioids for Postthoracotomy Pain**

Drug	Single Dose*	Infusion†	Onset, min	Duration, hr‡
EPIDURAL				
Morphine	1-6 mg	0.1-1.0 mg/hr	30	6-24
Meperidine	20-150 mg	2-20 mg/hr	5	6-8
Fentanyl	25-150 μg	25-100 μg/hr	5	3-6
Sufentanil	10-60 μg	10-50 μg/hr	5	2-4
SUBARACHNOID				
Morphine	0.1-0.3 mg	. . .	15	8-24
Fentanyl	5-25 μg	. . .	5	3-6

* Doses must be carefully adjusted for patient age and catheter position.
† When using epidural infusion, adjust concentration to allow infused volume to be approximately 10 ml/hr for accuracy and convenience of administration. For infusion with bupivacaine, use 0.0625% bupivacaine solution.
‡ Duration of analgesia is variable; it tends to increase with dose and patient age.
From Stevens, D. S., & Edwards, W. T. (1990). Management of pain in the critically ill. *Journal of Intensive Care Medicine, 5,* 271.

Other side effects of epidural opioids include pruritus, urinary retention, nausea, vomiting, and headache.[71,72] Many of these side effects can be treated with pharmacological and nursing comfort measures. The opioid antagonist naloxone is administered as an IV bolus to reverse respiratory depression effects. A continuous IV naloxone infusion can be used concurrently with epidural opioid infusions to reverse many of the other side effects while analgesia is maintained. It is suggested that naloxone acts at brainstem opioid receptor sites to counteract side effects while opioid analgesia is maintained at the spinal cord level.[73] Figure 12-6 presents an algorithm to assist critical care nurses in assessment and decision making associated with use of epidural opioids for their patients. Leib and Hurtig[74] provide detailed guidelines for epidural analgesia nursing assessment and intervention.

Intrathecal Opioids. Opioids administered into the intrathecal (subarachnoid) space will rapidly bathe dorsal horn opioid receptors. Therefore, intrathecal doses needed to achieve effective analgesia are much lower than epidural doses.

Intrathecal morphine infusions were used to manage pain effectively in 8 critically ill patients with primarily traumatic or surgical injuries when IV analgesics had proved ineffective.[75] In this group of patients, analgesia was inferred by decreases in pulse and better coordination with ventilators. Pain was not directly assessed.

Intrathecal opioids are used with caution because of the concern about repeated invasion of the spinal canal and the seriousness of side effects, including a more marked respiratory depression than seen with epidural opioids as well as CNS infections.[73] Significant overdoses can occur if a larger, epidural dose of opioids is given intrathecally due to frank error or because an epidural catheter migrates into the subarachnoid space.

Combined Spinal Opioids and Local Anesthetics

Spinal opioids and local anesthetics are often used in combination to obtain the beneficial effects of each. Each has a different action site, type of effect on neurons, and type of neural response inhibited. That is, spinal opioids act at receptors, interfere with neuron excitability, and inhibit nociception. Local anesthetics block conduction across the membrane of spinal nerves; inhibit impulse transmission; and may block SNS, other sensory fibers, and motor fibers as well as pain fibers.[72] Actions of local anesthetics are dose and concentration dependent; smaller fibers are affected first.[56] Block of pain and SNS fibers occur first because these sensations are transmitted along smaller fibers. As dosage and concentration are increased, fibers transmitting other sensations such as touch, pressure, and vibration are affected. Large motor fibers are the last to be affected by a block.

When continuous, combined infusions of spinal opioids and local anesthetics are used for pain control, patients may become hypotensive from SNS blockade. It may be possible to control the hypotension with IV fluids, thus negating the need to terminate the analgesic infusion. Patients receiving local anesthetic infusions over time may experience tachyphylaxis, a tolerance (nonresponsiveness) to the drug's effect, requiring the use of increasingly higher local anesthetic doses. A motor blockade could interfere with mobilization or, more important, respiration if the block involved respiratory muscles. Altered respiration is less of a concern for patients receiving controlled mechanical ventilation.

Spinal local anesthetics have been used successfully to treat myocardial infarction pain[76] and postopera-

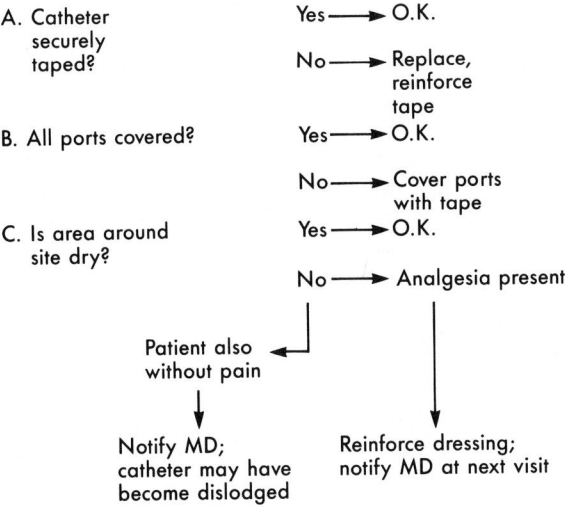

I. Is the system intact?

A. Catheter securely taped? Yes → O.K.

No → Replace, reinforce tape

B. All ports covered? Yes → O.K.

No → Cover ports with tape

C. Is area around site dry? Yes → O.K.

No → Analgesia present

Patient also without pain

Notify MD; catheter may have become dislodged

Reinforce dressing; notify MD at next visit

D. Are all the parts of the infusion system clearly identified as epidural system?

Yes → No

O.K.   Apply I.D. tapes

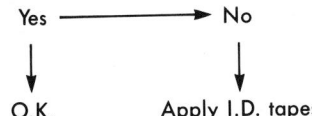

II. Is there effective analgesia?

Yes   No

Maintain infusion; anticipate potential complications

Is the system intact?

Yes   No

→ Notify MD

(1) Assess; Is there preexisting tolerance to opioids?

(2) Administer supplemental narcotics as needed

(3) Use nursing measures to assist with pain relief

No   Yes

O.K.   May have increased narcotic need

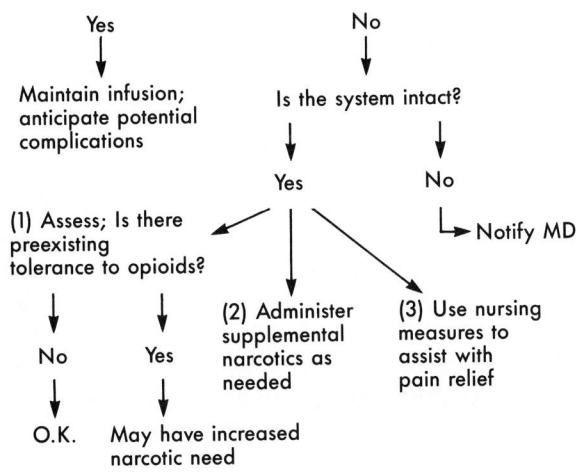

III. Are side effects present?

A. Is there ↓ respiratory rate?   ↓ respiratory volume?
↑ pCO_2?   ↓ LOC?

Yes

Consider presence of respiratory depression

Early, due to systemic/epidural vein uptake

Late, due to CSF distribution; involvement of respiratory

Prepare to:
- Notify MD
- Administer Narcan as prescribed (may need to readminister)
- Use ventilatory support measures if necessary

B. Is there nausea/vomiting?
C. Is there urinary retention?
D. Is there pruritus?
E. Are there allergic reactions?
F. Is there evidence of infection?

1. Administer medications as prescribed
2. Notify MD if necessary
3. Use nursing comfort measures

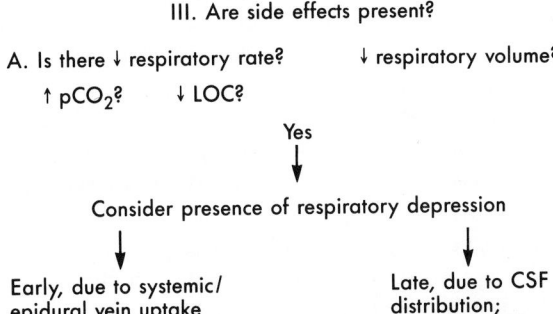

Figure 12-6 Epidural opiate administration—assessment and troubleshooting.

tive (abdominal and thoracic) pain.[77] Those who received a combination of spinal morphine and bupivacaine had less pain and used less supplemental narcotics than did those who received IV opioids, epidural morphine, or epidural bupivacaine alone.

Alpha-2 Adrenergic Agonists

Alpha-2 adrenergic agonists such as clonidine show promise as a new category of drugs for pain. Critical care nurses may be more familiar with clonidine's antihypertensive actions; it is currently not approved by the Food and Drug Administration for analgesic use. Clonidine appears to activate descending nonopioid biogenic amine pain inhibitory pathways discussed earlier. The actions of clonidine are similar to the bioamine norepinephrine contained in pons-to-spinal-cord neurons. When clonidine is applied to the spinal cord area that contains alpha-2 receptors, pain transmission is inhibited.[8] In fact, animal studies have shown that a combined treatment of intrathecal clonidine and subcutaneous morphine provided better analgesia than each drug administered alone.[78] Research on the effects of spinally administered clonidine on pain relief has been encouraging.[79] Its critical care use may be forthcoming.

Interventions Acting at the Midbrain/Brainstem Level

Tricyclic Antidepressants

Tricyclic antidepressants (TCAs) are drugs that potentiate the actions of the biogenic amine system discussed earlier. Neurons containing serotonin and norepinephrine originate in brainstem areas and project to the spinal cord. TCAs inhibit the inactivation of these neurotransmitters, thus prolonging their effect. The analgesic effect from TCAs appears to be separate from their antidepressant effect and requires lower doses.[8]

TCAs have not yet been used to any great extent for pain management in critically ill patients. They could be considered, however, especially for those who are depressed and have long stays in the critical care unit.

Systemic Opioids

Intermittent Opioid Injections. The traditional method of providing analgesics to critically ill patients is through the use of IV injections as needed (that is, PRN). Systemically administered opioids travel through the circulatory system to the limbic system, midbrain, thalamus, and spinal cord, all of which contain high concentrations of opioid receptors.[73] Onset of action after IV injection is rapid, and duration of effect is short.[80] Advantages of the use of IV opioids are their familiarity to critical care professionals; their effectiveness for short-term, time-limited pain; their absence of accumulation; and rapid reversal of adverse effects.[81] Many of these advantages, however, can be disadvantages due to the unpredictable pharmacokinetic actions of opioids, especially in critically ill patients.[82] Specifically, with intermittent dosing, it is difficult to maintain a therapeutic range of effect over time and avoid side effects. Also, patients become uncomfortable, anxious, and stressed during times of decreased analgesia.[80]

Continuous Opioid Infusions. Continuous opioid infusions allow for titration of the drug to a level of analgesic effectiveness and maintenance of steady plasma levels within a therapeutic range. This method can help minimize respiratory depression and oversedation.[64] A goal in the use of continuous opioid infusions is to achieve a minimum effective analgesic concentration (MEAC). With MEAC, an opioid plasma level that provides adequate pain relief for a particular individual is achieved and maintained.[82] Given interpatient variability, there is no single specific MEAC.

The first step in achieving MEAC is to frontload opioids through IV injections until patient analgesia is reached.[57] Table 12-4 provides guidelines that can be used for frontloading. After frontloading achieves analgesia, this analgesia can be maintained by continuous opioid infusions. Stevens and Edwards[57] provide a method of determining the continuous infusion rate: (1) approximately one half the amount of opioid needed for frontloading will be needed to maintain analgesia *during each half-life of the drug;* (2) most of the frequently used opioids have a half-life of approximately 3 hours. Thus, if 12 mg of morphine is needed for frontloading, 6 mg (half the dose) is divided by 3 half-life hours. Therefore, the continuous IV infusion rate would be estimated at 2 mg per hour.

It is important for patient safety to consider the individual's specific hepatic, renal, and general physiological status rather than to use these guidelines as "hard and fast" rules. It is also important to frontload again and recalculate the continuous infusion rate if the patient's pain status changes, such as might occur after a painful procedure is performed.

Continuous opioid infusions provide distinct advantages over intermittent injections. A steady comfort level can be maintained, and anxiety associated with peaks and valleys of pain can be avoided. Patients may even sleep more comfortably knowing they will not awaken in pain.[81]

Transdermal Opioid Administration. A relatively new method of opioid administration is through the transdermal route. Fentanyl patches of various sizes are applied to nonhairy skin areas from which the drug is absorbed.[57] Onset of action is delayed for

TABLE 12-4   **Guidelines for Frontloading Intravenous Analgesics**

Drug	Total Frontload Dose, mg/kg	Increments	Side Effects/Cautions
Morphine	0.08-0.12	0.03 mg/kg every 10 min	Histamine effects, nausea, biliary colic; reduce dose for elderly.
Meperidine	1.0-1.5	0.30 mg/kg every 10 min	Reduce dose or change drug for impaired renal function.
Codeine	0.5-1.0	One third of total every 15 min	Nausea.
Methadone	0.08-0.12	0.03 mg/kg every 15 min	Do not administer maintenance dose after analgesia achieved; accumulation; sedation.
Levorphanol	0.02	50-75 µg/kg every 15 min	Similar to methadone.
Hydromorphone	0.02	25-50 µg/kg every 10 min	Similar to morphine.
Pentazocine	0.5-1.0	One half of total every 15 min	Psychomimetic effects; may cause withdrawal in narcotic-dependent patients.
Nalbuphine	0.08-0.15	0.03 mg/kg every 10 min	Less psychomimetic effect than pentazocine; sedation.
Butorphanol	0.02-0.04	0.01 mg/kg every 10 min	Sedation; psychomimetic effects like nalbuphine.
Buprenorphine	Up to 0.2	One quarter of total every 10 min	Long-acting like methadone and levorphanol; may precipitate withdrawal in narcotic-dependent patients; unlike methadone can be given subcutaneously for maintenance after analgesia.

From Stevens, D. S., & Edwards, W. T. (1990). Management of pain in the critically ill. *Journal of Intensive Care Medicine, 5,* 277.

approximately 12 hours, and steady state is reached in 36 to 48 hours. MEAC has been maintained for approximately 16 hours after the patch was removed.[83]

The effectiveness of transdermal fentanyl patches for postoperative pain has been investigated. No differences in pain intensity were noted between abdominal surgery patients who received either transdermal fentanyl or a placebo patch. However, the placebo group of patients received significantly more PRN opioids in the 12- to 48-hour period after patch application.[83] The effectiveness of and indications for transdermal opioid administration for critically ill patients have yet to be investigated.

Nonpharmacological Relaxation Techniques

Emotional—motivational dimensions of pain are due to neuroanatomical involvement of the reticular formation and limbic systems of the brain.[84] Distressful emotions such as anxiety along with increased muscle tension can exacerbate pain.

According to the gate control theory, descending inhibitory tracts, which may arise from those brain areas associated with the negative emotions, may prevent the transmission of pain from spinal cord levels. Certain interventions, such as relaxation techniques, may activate these descending inhibitory systems.

Relaxation is a method of behavioral control in which a person performs techniques that will reduce or eliminate pain.[84] Several forms of relaxation techniques have been suggested for use such as deep breathing exercises, muscle relaxation, hypnosis, and visual imagery.[85] All of these techniques require some degree of training which may preclude their widespread use with critically ill patients. However, the nurse can work with patients to decrease their pain by using a simple relaxation script such as that proposed by Faucett.[85] (The box on p. 344 depicts a deep breathing technique.)

There is limited research supporting the effectiveness of relaxation on decreasing pain in critically ill patients. Results from relaxation taught to cardiac surgical patients have been variable. Progressive relaxation had no significant effect on one sample,[86] but systemic relaxation helped to decrease distress associated with ambulation pain in another sample.[87]

A Technique for Guiding Deep Breathing

Guiding begins as the chest starts to fall with exhalation. The nurse says:

"I want you to take a couple of *deep* breaths *in* now."

Vocal tone and emphasis draw attention to the nurse's voice and engage the patient in following directions. The word "deep" is timed to occur right before the end of the falling motion of the chest and the word "in" right at the beginning of the rise of the chest. The word "in," by coinciding with the actual physiological sensation of air intake, reinforces the association of the nurse's voice and words with changes in breathing.

As the chest continues to rise, full expansion is encouraged by repeating the words:

"Deep . . . deep . . . deep"

"And   then   let   your   breath   out slowly . . . slowly . . . slowly."

As the breath turns again to inhaling, the nurse retains control over the breathing rate and depth by saying:

"Take another *deep* breath *in* now."

Usually two or three breaths in this manner are enough to divert attention and to promote relaxation without hyperventilation.

From Faucett, J. (1991). Care of the critically ill patient in pain: The importance of nursing. In K. A. Puntillo (Ed.), *Pain in the critically ill: Assessment and management.* Gaithersburg, MD: Aspen.

More recently, Miller and Perry[40] found that a slow, deep breathing relaxation technique decreased pain, heart rate, blood pressure, and respiratory rate in cardiac surgical patients. All patients who had the relaxation training in this study were pleased with the intervention.

Interventions Acting at the Cortical Level

Distraction

The attention given to pain is part of cognitive processing and thus of the cognitive dimension of pain. Attention is directed away from pain through use of active or passive distractors.[88] The process may be active when the patient performs a task that competes with the painful stimulus, such as counting backwards or reciting phrases. Or the process may be passive distraction by means of auditory or visual stimuli, such as focusing on viewing pictures or figures or listening to music.[88]

The relationship between pain and an auditory stimulus can be partially explained by the fact that both systems interact at reticular-formation and thalamic levels. Thus, auditory input may be able to override pain input.[89]

Music has been shown to decrease procedural (abdominal wound packing) pain[90] as well as postoperative surgical pain.[91] Music has been studied as an intervention for pain in critically ill patients, also. In one study, music selected by 22 ICU patients or their family members decreased both self-reported pain and anxiety.[38]

Use of music is a highly feasible distraction intervention as well as a method of relaxation for pain management of many critically ill patients. It requires very little staff time, energy, or technology. In fact, music listened to through earphones may block annoying ICU noises and may promote sleep as well as decrease pain.

Keeping the Patient Informed

Providing certain individuals with information about what they can expect to experience from a procedure or an event helps to decrease the sensory or distress components of pain. Information about the sensations a person might experience from a procedure seems to be more important in relieving pain distress than does information about the procedure itself.[33] Information may best help people who are anxious, vigilant, or need to control a situation.[24] It may be less effective for those who cope with a stressful situation by ignoring it or having anxious feelings.[85]

Critically ill patients undergo many pain-producing procedures such as dressing changes, endotracheal suctioning, or chest tube removal. Therefore, providing information about the sensations accompanying these procedures may help relieve pain. Information can be combined with other treatments to optimize effect.

Clinicians should also consider providing information to patients about what they may experience from *interventions* for pain. This information may include the potential numbing, tingling effects of anesthetic agents; dysphoria from ketamine; or itching and other sensations associated with epidural opioids. Providing information may encourage patients to report these experiences and may improve patient tolerance of pain management interventions.

Patient-controlled Analgesia

With patient-controlled analgesia (PCA), patients are able to self-administer their analgesic medications. PCA is now widely and successfully used for many patients who are not critically ill. Patients can self-administer the analgesics at the onset of pain perception. Thus, cognitive processes are employed. The individual makes a judgment about pain and sedation levels and can choose a balance between them. If patients feel "in control" of their pain management, anxiety and distress associated with pain can be minimized.[82]

Many computerized PCA pumps have been manufactured. The relative advantages of each can be determined by an individual institution, using research findings and cost–benefit analyses. With PCA systems, patients receive intermittent boluses of a certain amount of analgesic over a certain time period, both of which are predetermined. Most PCA systems allow for the delivery of continuous, background infusions of a preset analgesic amount to maintain MEAC.

Although numerous research studies have established the effectiveness of PCA (see Stanik[92] for a review), little research has been conducted of PCA use in critically ill patients. Patients must be able to activate the PCA device and have a clear enough sensorium to determine need. Yet, this treatment modality may be applicable to a number of patients, and nurses are encouraged to consider its use. PCA offers some degree of control to critically ill patients who find themselves in an environment over which they otherwise have little control.

Opioid Tolerance, Dependence, and Addiction

Understanding opioid tolerance, dependence, and addiction is an extremely important part of patient care. There are significant differences among these three phenomena. *Tolerance* is a physiological state in which increasingly greater amounts of opiates are needed to achieve a similar analgesic effect.[93] *Physical dependence* on opioids is present if a withdrawal syndrome occurs when opioids are withheld. It, too, is a physiological process that may be due to rebound CNS noradrenergic activity that is depressed by chronic opioid use.[94] *Addiction* is a psychological dependence on opioids evidenced by compulsive drug-seeking behavior. Addiction is often associated with physiological dependence. It is essential to the provision of appropriate care that health professionals recognize these differences.

When opioids are used to treat patients in pain, addiction is extremely rare (<1%).[95] Yet over 20% of 2,459 RNs believed addiction occurs in at least a quarter of patients receiving opioids for pain.[96] Certainly, more education about opioid effects is warranted.

Dissociative Anesthetics

Ketamine is a dissociative anesthetic that has been used for general anesthesia as well as for postoperative or treatment-related analgesia. Dissociative anesthetics cause an individual to feel separated from the surrounding environment.[97] They induce sedation, amnesia, and analgesia in doses lower than those needed to produce anesthesia.[98]

Ketamine can be administered intramuscularly or IV; its effects do not seem to be opioid mediated since they are not blocked by naloxone.[98] Unlike opioids, ketamine activates the SNS. Thus, arterial blood pressure, cardiac output, and heart rate are increased. Ketamine also decreases airway resistance and may reverse bronchospasm.[97] These actions may be advantageous in certain compromised, critically ill patients. A ketamine infusion reportedly produced sedation, inotropy, and bronchodilation in a ventilated ICU patient.[99]

Ketamine is structurally similar to phencyclidine (PCP), as they both interact with sigma receptors. This relationship helps to account for the unpleasant effects that may accompany its use, such as visual disturbances, delerium, or excitement.[97] Concurrently administered benzodiazepine helps counteract dysphoric effects and induce amnesia.[99]

Nurses are encouraged to consider advocating the use of ketamine when appropriate patient conditions arise. These conditions can include a patient's inability to tolerate opioid side effects, states of inadequate analgesia, or episodic procedural pain such as that felt during burn or wound dressing changes.

Pharmacological Adjuvants: The Benzodiazepines

Benzodiazepines (BNZs) have sedative, amnesic, and anxiolytic effects and are often used in conjunction with analgesics for pain management. Since BNZs do not themselves have analgesic properties,[57,100] they should not be used as a substitute for analgesics. They may contribute to pain management by diminishing anxiety associated with pain, reducing levels of consciousness to decrease perception of pain, and blocking recall of painful procedures or other experiences.

Benzodiazepines reduce anxiety by a facilitory action of gammaaminobutyric acid (GABA) receptors. When GABA receptors are activated, there is increased conductance of Cl^- ions across the neural cell membrane. Hyperpolarization and thus cell inhibition ensue. Because BNZs facilitate this GABA action, they also inhibit cells. The anxiolytic effect may be due to actions on cells that comprise pathways in the limbic system; the sedation effect may result from decreased alertness associated with anxiety; and the amnesic effect may be due to GABA involvement in memory functions.[101] Because BNZs are also muscle relaxants,[102] they may contribute to relief of pain associated with muscle rigidity and spasms.

Benzodiazepines, most particularly midazolam, diazepam, and lorazepam, are frequently used in critical care units[100] for combination analgesia–sedation therapy. The challenge is to assess the effects of these drug combinations on pain, on anxiety, and on level of sedation, and to know which of these prevailing problems—if any—are being effectively managed.

Nurses are also responsible for monitoring the presence of potential side effects of the BNZs. (Readers are referred to Doherty[103] for an extensive review of BNZ actions, administration techniques, and adverse effects.) When BNZs are used in conjunction with opiates, adverse opiate effects of decreased mean arterial pressure, decreased systemic vascular resistance, and respiratory depression may be potentiated.[64]

An associated risk of BNZ use has been, until recently, the inability to reverse its effects pharmacologically. Recently, however, flumazenil has been introduced as a BNZ antagonist. Acting at BNZ receptors, it reverses all CNS effects of BNZs.[104] Flumazenil could be used to reverse long-term or short-term (such as procedure-related) sedation, to reverse BNZ overdosages, or to facilitate weaning from mechanical ventilation.[104] The use and effects of flumazenil in critical care have not been investigated.[100]

EVALUATING THE EFFECTIVENESS OF INTERVENTIONS

Numerous pharmacological and nonpharmacological interventions have to be considered in treating pain in critically ill patients. It is important that health care professionals chose interventions according to each individual's situation. It is equally important that the effectiveness of these interventions be evaluated. This evaluation can entail subjective patient responses that their pain has been alleviated, or at least minimized to the extent possible. Evaluation of effectiveness can also include observations that physiological responses to pain have subsided and psychological consequences of pain have been resolved.

COLLABORATION FOR PAIN MANAGEMENT

Pain management is a multidisciplinary process. Pharmacologists, psychologists, physicians, and critical care nurses all play extremely important roles by contributing their specific knowledge and expertise. Assessing and managing pain in critically ill patients are challenging and often difficult responsibilities that must be shared. Collaboration among health professionals for the purpose of providing pain relief maximizes successful patient outcomes and prevents needless patient suffering.

REFERENCES

1. Paiement, B., Boulanger, M., Jones, C. W., et al. (1979). Intubation and other experiences in cardiac surgery: The consumer's views. *Canadian Anaesthetists' Society Journal, 26,* 173-180.

2. Puntillo, K. A. (1990). The pain experiences of intensive care unit patients. *Heart Lung, 19,* 526-533.

3. Bonica, J. J. (Ed.). (1990). Postoperative pain. In *The management of pain* (2nd ed.) (pp. 461-480). Philadelphia: Lea & Febiger.

4. Portenoy, R. K. (1989). Mechanisms of clinical pain: Observations and speculations. *Neurologic Clinics, 7,* 205-230.

5. Melzack, R., & Casey, K. K. (1968). Sensory, motivational, and central control determinants of pain. In D. R. Kenshalo (Ed.), *The skin senses* (pp. 423-443). Springfield, IL: Thomas.

6. Price, D. D. (1988). *Psychological and neural mechanisms of pain.* New York: Raven.

7. International Association for the Study of Pain: Subcommittee on Taxonomy. (1986). Classification of chronic pain: Descriptions of chronic pain syndromes and definitions of pain terms. *Pain, S216-S221.*

8. Fields, H. L. (1987). *Pain.* New York: McGraw-Hill.

9. Meyer, R. A., Campbell, J. N., & Raja, S. N. (1985). Peripheral neural mechanisms of cutaneous hyperalgesia. In H. L. Fields, R. Dubner, & F. Cervero (Eds.), *Advances in pain research and therapy* (pp. 53-71). New York: Raven.

10. Torebjork, E. (1985). Nociceptor activation and pain. In A. Iggo, L. L. Iverson, & F. Cervero (Eds.), *Nociception and pain* (pp. 227-234). London: The Royal Society.

11. Janig, W. (1987). Neuronal mechanisms of pain with special emphasis on visceral and deep somatic pain. *Acta Neurochirurgica, 38*(Suppl.), 16-32.

12. Cervero, F. (1985). Visceral nociception: Peripheral and central aspects of visceral nociceptive systems. In A. Iggo, L. L. Iverson, & F. Cervero (Eds.), *Nociception and pain* (pp. 325-337). London: The Royal Society.

13. Cervero, F. (1988). Visceral pain. In R. Dubner, G. F. Gebhart, & M. R. Bond (Eds.), *Proceedings of the Vth World Congress on Pain* (pp. 216-226). Amsterdam: Elsevier.

14. Ness, T. J., & Gebhart, G. F. (1990). Visceral pain: A review of experimental studies. *Pain, 41,* 167-234.

15. Melzack, R., & Wall, P. (1965). Pain mechanisms: A new theory. *Science, 150,* 971-978.

16. Basbaum, A. I., & Fields, H. L. (1984). Endogenous pain control systems: Brainstem spinal pathways and endorphin circuitry. *Annual Review of Neurosciences, 7,* 309-338.

17. Reynolds, D. V. (1969). Surgery in the rat during electrical analgesia induced by focal brain stimulation. *Science, 164,* 444-445.

18. Hosobuchi, Y. (1980). The current status of analgesic brain stimulation. *Acta Neurochirurgica,* (Suppl. 30), 219-227.

19. Bouckoms, A. J. (1988). Pain relief in the intensive care unit. *Journal of Intensive Care Medicine, 3*(1), 32-51.

20. O'Gara, P. T. (1988). The hemodynamic consequences of pain and its management. *Journal of Intensive Care Medicine, 3,* 3-5.

21. Bonica, J. J., & Benedetti, C. (1980). Postoperative pain. In R. E. Condon, & J. J. DeCosse (Eds.), *Surgical care: A physiologic approach to clinical management* (pp. 394-414). Philadelphia: Lea & Febiger.

22. Cazzullo, C. L., & Gala, C. (1987). Cognitive and emotional aspects of pain. In M. Tiengo, A. Cuello, J. Eccles, et al. (Eds.), *Advances in pain research, Vol. 10* (pp. 255-263). New York: Raven.

23. Mindus, P. (1987). Anxiety, pain and sedation: Some psychiatric aspects. *Acta Anaesthesiologica Scandinavica, 32,* S7-S12.

24. Schalling, D. (1985). Anxiety, pain, and coping. *Issues in Mental Health Nursing, 7*(1-4), 437-460.

25. Ballard, K. (1981). Identification of environmental stressors for patients in a surgical intensive care unit. *Issues in Mental Health Nursing, 3,* 89-108.

26. Jones, J., Hoggart, B., Withey, J., et al. (1979). What the patients say: A study of reactions to an intensive care unit. *Intensive Care Medicine, 5*(2), 89-92.

27. Wilson, V. S. (1987). Identification of stressors related to patients' psychologic responses to the surgical intensive care unit. *Heart Lung, 16,* 267-273.

28. Kehlet, H. (1986). Pain relief and modification of the stress response. In M. J. Cousins, & G. D. Phillips (Eds.), *Acute pain management* (pp. 49-75). New York: Churchill Livingstone.

29. LeResche, L., & Dworkin, S. F. (1984). Facial expression accompanying pain. *Social Science Medicine, 19,* 1325-1330.

30. McCaffery, M. (1979). *Nursing management of the patient with pain.* Philadelphia: Lippincott.

31. Stromskag, K. E., Reiestad, F., Holmqvist, E. L., et al. (1988). Intrapleural administration of 0.25%, 0.375%, 0.5% of bupivacaine with epinephrine after cholecystectomy. *Anesthesia and Analgesia, 68,* 430-434.

32. Jamner, L. D., & Tursky, B. (1987). Discrimination between intensity and affective pain descriptors: A psychophysiological evaluation. *Pain, 30,* 271-283.

33. Johnson, J. E. (1973). Effects of accurate expectations about sensations on the sensory and distress components of pain. *Journal of Personality and Social Psychology, 27,* 261-275.

34. El-Baz, N., & Goldin, M. (1987). Continuous epidural infusion of morphine for pain relief after cardiac operations. *The Journal of Thoracic and Cardiovascular Surgery, 93,* 878-883.

35. Melzack, R. (1987). The short-form McGill Pain Questionnaire. *Pain, 30,* 191-197.

36. Puntillo, K. A. (1991). Dimensions and predictors of pain in critically ill thoracoabdominal surgical patients. DNSc disseration. University of California, San Francisco.

37. Moltner, A., Holzl, R., & Strian, F. (1990). Heart rate changes as an autonomic component of the pain response. *Pain, 43,* 81-89.

38. Stone, S. K., Rusk, F., Chambers, A., et al. (1989). The effects of music therapy on critically ill patients in the intensive care setting. *Proceedings of the 16th Annual National Teaching Institute of the American Association of Critical-Care Nurses* (p. 624). Atlanta, GA, May 15-18, 1989.

39. Updike, P. (1990). Music therapy results for ICU patients. *Dimensions of Critical Care Nursing, 9*(1), 39-45.

40. Miller, K. M., & Perry, P. A. (1990). Relaxation technique and postoperative pain in patients undergoing cardiac surgery. *Heart Lung, 19,* 136-146.

41. Bates, M. S. (1987). Ethnicity and pain: A biocultural model. *Social Science Medicine, 24*(1), 47-50.

42. Bagchi, A. K. (1987). Pain and language. *Acta Neurochirurgica, 38,* S182-S184.

43. Douglas, M. K. (1989). Physiologic and behavioral responses to acute myocardial ischemic pain in Mexican male patients. DNSc dissertation. University of California, San Francisco.

44. Loper, K. A., Butler, S., Nessly, M., et al. (1989). Paralyzed with pain: The need for education. *Pain, 37,* 315-316.

45. Wild, L. R. (1991). Neuromuscular blocking agents in the critically ill patient: Neither sedating nor pain relieving. *AACN Clinical Issues in Critical Care Nursing, 2*(4), 778-787.

46. Donovan, M. I., & Dillon, P. (1987). Incidence and characteristics of pain in a sample of hospitalized cancer patients. *Cancer Nursing, 10*(2), 85-92.

47. Weis, O. F., Sriwatanakul, K., Alloza, J. L., et al. (1983). Attitudes of patients, housestaff, and nurses toward postoperative analgesic care. *Anesthesia and Analgesia, 62,* 70-74.

48. Marks, R. M., & Sachar, E. J. (1973). Undertreatment of medical inpatients with narcotic analgesics. *Annals of Internal Medicine, 78,* 173-181.

49. Graffam, S. (1981). Congruence of nurse-patient expectations regarding nursing intervention in pain. *Nursing Leadership, 4*(2), 12-15.

50. Camp, L. D., & O'Sullivan, P. S. (1987). Comparison of medical, surgical and oncology patients' descriptions of pain and nurses' documentation of pain assessments. *Journal of Advanced Nursing, 12,* 593-598.

51. Leisifer, D. (1990). Monitoring pain control and charting. *Critical Care Clinics, 6,* 283-294.

52. Amodio, M., & Koo, P. J. (1988). Nonsteroidal anti-inflammatory and adjuvant analgesics. *Highlights on Antineoplastic Drugs, 6,* 31-39.

53. Buckley, M. M., & Brogden, R. N. (1990). Ketorolac: A review of its pharmacodynamic and pharmacokinetic properties and therapeutic potential. *Drugs, 39*(1), 86-109.

54. Arzeno, S. (1990). *Toradol.* Palo Alto, CA: Syntex Laboratories.

55. Rung, G. W., & Marshall, W. K. (1990). Nerve blocks in the critical care environemnt. *Critical Care Clinics, 6,* 343-367.

56. Covino, B. G., & Scott, D. B. (1985). Handbook of epidural anaesthesia and analgesia. Orlando, FL: Grune & Stratton.

57. Stevens, D. S., & Edwards, W. T. (1990). Management of pain in the critically ill. *Journal of Intensive Care Medicine, 5,* 258-291.

58. Covino, B. G. (1988). Interpleural regional analgesia. *Anesthesia and Analgesia, 67,* 427-429.

59. Kvalheim, L., & Reiestad, F. (1984). Interpleural catheter in the management of postoperative pain. *Anesthesiology, 61,* A231.

60. Bragg, C. L. (1991). Interpleural analgesia. *Heart Lung, 20,* 30-38.

61. McCaffery, M., & Beebe, A. (1989). Pain: Clinical manual for nursing practice. St. Louis: Mosby.

62. Tappan, F. (1984). Massage. In P. D. Wall, & R. Melzack (Eds.), *Textbook of pain* (pp. 735-740). Edinburgh: Churchill Livingstone.

63. Donovan, M., Dillon, P., & McGuire, L. (1987). Incidence and characteristics of pain in a sample of medical-surgical inpatients. *Pain, 30*(1), 69-78.

64. Hamill, R. J. (1991). Pain management in the intensive care unit. In J. W. Hoyt, A. S. Tonnesen, & S. J. Allen (Eds.), *Critical care practice* (pp. 496-511). Philadelphia: Saunders.

65. Sabbe, M. B., & Yaksh, T. L. (1990). Pharmacology of spinal opioids. *Journal of Pain and Symptom Management, 5*(3), 191-203.

66. Pasternak, G. W. (1988). Multiple morphine and enkephalin receptors and the relief of pain. *Journal of the American Medical Association, 259,* 1362-1367.

67. Inturrisi, C. E. (1989). Clinical pharmacology of opioid analgesics. *Anesthesiology Clinics of North America, 7*(1), 33-49.

68. Welchew, E. A., & Thornton, J. A. (1982). Continuous thoracic epidural fentanyl. *Anaesthesia, 37,* 309-316.

69. Rawal, N., Sjostrand, U., Christofferson, E., et al. (1984). Comparison of intramuscular and epidural morphine for postoperative analgesia in the grossly obese: Influence on postoperative ambulation and pulmonary function. *Anesthesia and Analgesia, 63,* 583-592.

70. Yeager, M. P., Glass, D. D., Neff, R. K., et al. (1987). Epidural anesthesia and analgesia in high-risk surgical patients. *Anesthesiology, 66,* 729-736.

71. Olsson, G. L., Leddo, C. C., & Wild, L. (1989). Nursing management of patients receiving epidural narcotics. *Heart Lung, 18,* 130-138.

72. Dyble, K. M. (1991). Epidural and intrathecal methods of analgesia in the critically ill. In K. A. Puntillo (Ed.), *Pain in the critically ill: Assessment and management* (pp. 95-113). Gaithersburg, MD: Aspen.

73. Benedetti, C. (1987). Intraspinal analgesia: An historical overview. *Acta Anaesthesiologica Scandinavica, 31*(Suppl. 85), 17-24.

74. Leib, R. A., & Hurtig, J. B. (1985). Epidural and intrathecal narcotics for pain management. *Heart Lung, 14,* 164-174.

75. Rawal, N., & Tandon, B. (1985). Epidural and intrathecal morphine in intensive care units. *Intensive Care Medicine, 11,* 129-133.

76. Toft, P., & Jorgensen, A. (1987). Continuous thoracic epidural analgesia for the control of pain in myocardial infarction. *Intensive Care Medicine, 13,* 388-389.

77. Slack, J. F., & Faut-Callahan, M. (1991). Comparing the efficacy of epidural analgesia and local anesthesia for pain management of critically ill patients. *AACN Clinical Issues in Critical Care Nursing, 2*(4), 729-740.

78. Drasner, K., & Fields, H. L. (1988). Synergy between the antinociceptive effects of intrathecal clonidine and systemic morphine in the rat. *Pain, 32,* 309-312.

79. Maze, M., & Tranquilli, W. (1991). Alpha-2 adrenoceptor agonists: Defining the role in clinical anesthesia. *Anesthesiology, 74,* 581-605.

80. Teeple, E. (1990). Pharmacology and physiology of narcotics. *Critical Care Clinics, 6,* 255-282.

81. Wild, L. (1991). Intravenous methods of analgesia for pain in the critically ill. In K. A. Puntillo (Ed.), *Pain in the critically ill: Assessment and management* (pp. 79-93). Gaithersburg, MD: Aspen.

82. Veselis, R. A. (1990). Intravenous narcotics in the ICU. *Critical Care Clinics, 6,* 295-313.

83. Gourlay, G. K., Kowalski, J. L., Plummer, D. A., et al. (1990). The efficacy of transdermal fentanyl in the treatment of postoperative pain: A double-blind comparison of fentanyl and placebo systems. *Pain, 40,* 21-28.

84. Chapman, C. R. (1985). Psychological factors in postoperative pain. In G. Smith, & B. G. Covino (Eds.), *Acute pain* (pp. 22-41). London: Butterworths.

85. Faucett, J. (1991). Care of the critically ill patient in pain: The importance of nursing. In K. A. Puntillo (Ed.), *Pain in the critically ill: Assessment and management* (pp. 115-136). Gaithersburg, MD: Aspen.

86. Bafford, D. C. (1977). Progressive relaxation as a nursing intervention: A method of controlling pain for open-heart surgery patients. In M. Batey (Ed.), *Communicating nursing research: Vol. 8. Nursing research priorities: Choice or chance* (pp. 284-290). Boulder, CO: Western Interstate Commission for Higher Education.

87. Horowitz, B. F., Fitzpatrick, J. J., & Flaherty, G. G. (1984). Relaxation techniques for pain relief after open heart surgery. *Dimensions of Critical Care Nursing, 3,* 364-371.

88. Fernandez, E. (1986). A classification system of cognitive coping strategies for pain. *Pain, 26,* 141-151.

89. Gardner, W. J. (1960). Suppression of pain by sound. *Science, 132*(3418), 32-33.

90. Angus, J. E., & Faux, S. (1989). The effect of music on adult postoperative patients' pain during a nursing procedure. In S. G. Funk, E. M. Tornquist, M. T. Champagne, et al. (Eds.), *Key aspects of comfort: Management of pain, fatigue, and nausea* (pp. 166-172). New York: Springer.

91. Locsin, R. (1981). The effect of music on the pain of selected post-operative patients. *Journal of Advanced Nursing, 6*(1), 19-25.

92. Stanik, J. A. (1991). Patient-controlled analgesia with critically ill patients: A risk/benefit analysis. *AACN Clinical Issues in Critical Care Nursing, 2*(4), 741-747.

93. American Pain Society. (1989). *Principles of analgesic use in the treatment of acute pain and chronic cancer pain* (2nd ed.). Skokie, IL: Author.

94. Gossop, M. (1988). Clonidine and the treatment of the opiate withdrawal syndrome. *Drug and Alcohol Dependence, 21,* 253-259.

95. Porter, J., & Jick, H. (1980). Addiction rare in patients treated with narcotics. *New England Journal of Medicine, 302,* 123.

96. McCaffery, M., Ferrell, B., O'Neil-Page, E., et al. Nurses' knowledge of opioid analgesic drugs and psychological dependence. *Cancer Nursing, 13,* 21-27.

97. Marshall, B. E., & Wollman, H. (1980). Intravenous anesthetics. In A. G. Gilman, L. S. Goodman, & A. Gilman (Eds.), *The pharmacological basis of therapeutics* (6th ed.) (pp. 296-297). New York: Macmillan.

98. Maurset, A., Skoglund, L. A., Hustveit, D., et al. (1989). Comparison of ketamine and pethidine in experimental and postoperative pain. *Pain, 36,* 37-41.

99. Park, G. R., Manara, A. R., Mendel, L., et al. (1987). Ketamine infusion. *Anaesthesia, 42,* 980-983.

100. Aitkenhead, A. R. (1989). Analgesia and sedation in intensive care. *British Journal of Anaesthesia, 63,* 196-206.

101. Oreland, L. (1987). The benzodiazepines: A pharmacological overview. *Acta Anaesthesiologica Scandinavica, 32,* S13-S16.

102. Crippen, D. W. (1990). The role of sedation in the ICU patient with pain and agitation. *Critical Care Clinics, 6,* 369-392.

103. Doherty, M. H. (1991). Benzodiazepine sedation in the critically ill patient. *AACN Clinical Issues in Critical Care Nursing, 2*(4), 748-761.

104. Amrein, R., Hetzel, W., Bonetti, E. P., et al. (1988). Clinical pharmacology of dormicum (midazolam) and anexate (flumazenil). *Resuscitation, 16,* S5-S27.

13

Sleep and the Critically Ill Patient

Dorrie K. Fontaine

Sleep is one of the most basic and natural processes in which all humans engage. As an activity, it occupies roughly one third of our lives, yet it is often taken for granted. Most commonly, the vital and controversial role that sleep plays in the maintenance of high-level wellness is only appreciated when sleep has been lost or disrupted. Fortunately, otherwise healthy individuals usually need only to adjust their activities or environment and to sleep normally to completely reverse the impact of previous sleep compromise, a process typically accomplished within several days.

In contrast, individuals admitted to critical care units are at risk for life-threatening physiological vulnerability. Continuous monitoring, intensive treatment, and aggressive interventions are the rule. As a result, the critically ill patient is subjected to further compromise in both the quality and quantity of sleep. Compounding the problem is the patient's inability to adjust the environment to promote normal sleep. Thus, sleep disruption tends to have potentially significant and cumulative effects.

Sleeplessness remains a major stressor reported by patients in critical care settings.[1] In the 1990s, nurses will encounter critically ill patients with accompanying sleep disorders such as sleep apnea. Recognizing the importance of sleep and the need for intensified research, the U.S. Congress has created a multidisciplinary National Institutes of Health Commission on Sleep.[2] Critical care nurses have an important role in promoting effective sleep patterns in the critically ill patient. Sleep is an important topic for nursing because of its importance to patients and the opportunity for independent nursing therapies. The positive outcomes of effective sleep may enhance recovery and quality of life for the critically ill patient.

This chapter discusses information about the nature and physiological correlates of normal sleep, considers the nature and impact of disruptive influences inherent in the critical care setting, and presents wide-ranging strategies to promote sleep.

NORMAL SLEEP

Scientific research involving simultaneous monitoring of the electroencephalogram (EEG), electrooculogram (EOG), and electromyogram (EMG) has shown that sleep is composed of two very distinct types of activity: REM, or rapid eye movement, and non-REM (NREM) sleep. Far from the traditional view of sleep as a quiescent state, REM sleep involves intense physiological activation with an associated muscle atonia. NREM sleep, on the other hand, is associated with progressive relaxation. It is divided into stages 1 to 4, with stages 3 and 4 collectively referred to as slow-wave sleep (SWS).[3]

Sleep Stages

The pattern of NREM sleep occurs characteristically as an individual progresses from alert wakefulness to the sleep stages 1 through 4. Stage 1 sleep, a transition phase, is described as subjectively light sleep with a low arousal threshold and a slower EEG frequency than the alpha rhythm of wakefulness.[3] Hallmarks of stage 2 sleep include sleep spindles and K complexes, considered the brain's unique signature of sleep. A sleep spindle is a burst of rhythmic waveforms at 14 to 16 hertz (cycles per second) interspersed with occasional high amplitude slow waves.[4] Sleep researchers debate whether the onset of "true sleep" occurs with NREM stage 1 or stage 2.[3]

Stages 3 and 4 NREM sleep are associated with high voltage, slow-frequency waves in the EEG, and thus are referred to as SWS. The primary criterion to differentiate stage 3 and 4 is the percentage of these slow waves on EEG. Stage 3 sleep, occurring when at least 20% of the sleep record consists of slow waves, is transitional to stage 4, which accounts for slow waves on greater than 50% of the sleep record.[3] Throughout NREM sleep, the EOG reflects gradual slowing or cessation of eye movements, and the EMG waveform progressively declines in association with the profound muscle relaxation characteristic of NREM sleep.

REM sleep was named for the characteristic sporadic bursts of extremely rapid conjugate eye movements seen on the EOG. These movements may be visible to an observer through closed eyelids. The EMG during REM sleep is essentially flat and reflects hyperpolarization of motor neurons in the brainstem and spinal cord. This hyperpolarization prevents distal impulse transmission and results in functional paralysis of large postural and skeletal muscles. In contrast, cerebral cortical metabolic activity greatly increases during REM sleep, and, not suprisingly the EEG resembles the waking state.[4] REM sleep has been defined as a highly activated brain in a paralyzed body.[3] REM sleep is associated with dreaming. In sleep studies where subjects are awakened during REM sleep they report dreams 80% of the time.[3]

Sleep Architecture

Sleep most commonly occurs rhythmically in a continuous bulk period once a day, typically during the dark portion of the daily cycle of light and dark. A specific repeating pattern of NREM and REM sleep makes up the sleep cycle. The term *sleep architecture* refers to the structure and timing of sleep cycles and the quantitative relationship of each sleep stage to the total sleep period.[5]

Sleep architecture is often plotted as a sleep histogram, as depicted in Figure 13-1 with accompanying EEG waveforms. The typical sleep cycle demonstrates a 90-minute pattern whereby sleep is entered through NREM stage 1 with a descent through stage 4, a more abrupt ascent back through stage 2, and entry into REM sleep[4] (Figure 13-2). The length of time within each cycle that is occupied by a particular sleep stage is determined by the cycle's temporal relationship to the total sleep period. A night's sleep typically consists of five to six sleep cycles. Early in the sleep period, NREM stages dominate the cycle and REM sleep periods are very brief. As the sleep period progresses, the proportions reverse somewhat, and cycles near the end of the sleep period tend to be dominated by REM periods of successively longer duration. Thus, most NREM sleep occurs during the early sleep period, while the majority of REM sleep is obtained later in the bulk sleep period.[5]

Normative sleep data suggest approximate sleep stage percentages and awakenings for a typical night. For example, young adults spend approximately 1% of the sleep period awake, 5% in stage 1 sleep, 46% in stage 2 sleep, 6% in stage 3 sleep, 14% in stage 4 sleep, and 28% in stage REM sleep.[5] Awakenings are few in healthy individuals.

Daytime naps taken in the late afternoon are characterized by cycles relatively dominated by NREM sleep, as if the total sleep period had begun early.[6] Afternoon naps can reduce NREM stages 3 and 4 during the subsequent total sleep period. Morning naps, on the other hand, are characterized by cycles dominated by REM, as if reflecting continuation of the preceding sleep period.[6]

Normal sleep architecture is grossly disrupted for patients in critical care settings. Studies measuring

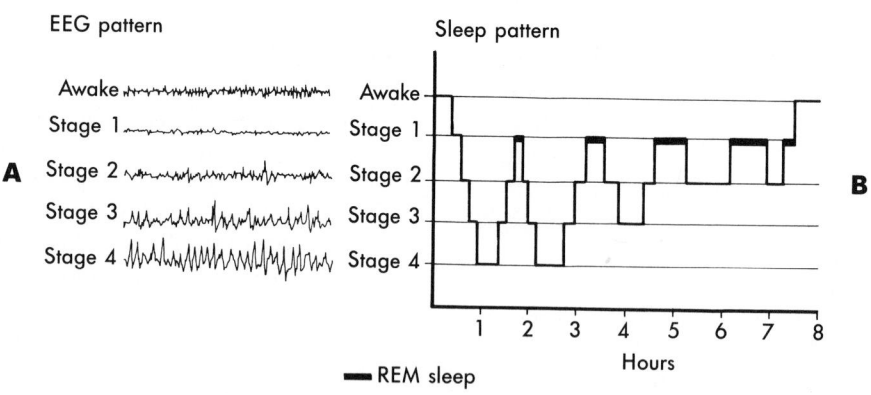

Figure 13-1 *A,* Examples of the EEG pattern during the various stages of sleep; each trace represents about 30 seconds of recording. *B,* A typical night's sleep pattern in an adult. REM sleep is indicated by black bars.

Adapted from Institute of Medicine. (1990). *Basic sleep research.* Washington, DC: National Academy Press.

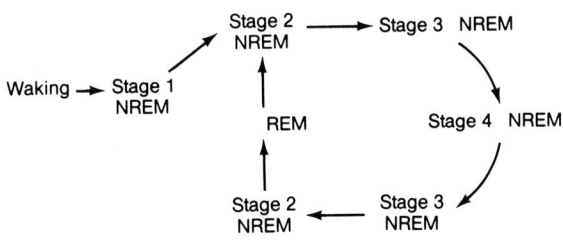

Figure 13-2 The sleep cycle. The average time between two REM sleep periods equals approximately 90 minutes.

sleep stages of critically ill patients consistently document increased wake time and stage 1 sleep with diminished or absent slow wave and REM sleep, and a severely increased number of awakenings.[7-12] Chronic nocturnal sleep restriction can lead to altered sleep architecture in the critically ill patient.[3] Patients with cardiopulmonary illnesses such as congestive heart failure[13] and obstructive sleep apnea also experience abnormal sleep structure.[14]

Circadian Influences on Sleep

Most physiological processes have a circadian rhythm, a predictable rise and fall approximately every 24 hours. Temperature is one example of a rhythm with consistent peaks and troughs. Others include hormone secretion such as growth hormone, metabolic parameters, and emotional functioning.[15] Knowledge of circadian rhythms and the basic sleep cycle can assist the critical care nurse to encourage sleep at times most in tune with the individual's unique biologic rhythms.

Sleep regulation is associated with a complex circadian organization.[15] The majority of total sleep time within a 24-hour period occurs in one uninterrupted or monophasic period. Sleep onset occurs best on the falling limb of the temperature cycle, and sleep is most efficient during the lowest point of the temperature cycle.[3] This indicates that individuals attempting to sleep out of phase with the internal circadian pacemaker will experience poor quality or disrupted sleep.

Light is a powerful *zeitgeber,* an environmental synchronizer that assists in entraining sleep by promoting the circadian cycle of sleep and wakefulness. In fact, the light–dark cycle may be the most powerful zeitgeber. Many critical care settings could benefit from more natural lighting and lights that are lowered during typical sleep times.

Alertness and body temperature are believed to peak in early to midevening and are minimal in the early morning hours.[6] The relative inability to sleep in the early evening may thus be associated with an increased body temperature. Critical care nurses can use this information to encourage morning naps to provide potentially needed REM sleep or afternoon naps to add SWS.

Age-related Changes

The single most significant determinant of sleep architecture is age.[16] Sleep patterns change dramatically across the life span. It is well documented that newborns may spend 50% of their total sleep in REM sleep, adolescents have the largest amount of SWS, and older adults typically have no stage 4 sleep.[4] Studies of healthy older adults report an increased number of awakenings, more time in bed but less time asleep, and a decreased auditory arousal threshold.[16]

Changes in sleep with aging are believed due in part to a loss of effective circadian regulation[17] or a decrease in the number of catecholaminergic neurons in the locus coeruleus, a group of neurons in the brainstem.[18] Elderly individuals may awaken earlier in the morning because the circadian temperature cycle has shifted. The elderly frequently exhibit an advanced sleep phase syndrome which is a pattern of falling asleep earlier. Nearly one third of older adults complain of waking too early.[17] However, the elderly make up for lost nighttime sleep with naps during the day, refuting the myth that the elderly require less sleep.

The most critical finding for sleep in the elderly is the increase in interindividual variability.[3] Gender differences suggest an increased amount of lighter sleep and more respiratory disturbances in older men, with more frequent awakenings for older women.[19,20] Two areas of concern for sleep in the older adult are the increased incidence of sleep-disordered breathing and the widespread use of sedative-hypnotics.[17]

Theories of Sleep Function

Sleep theorists have embraced restoration and energy conservation as potential functions for sleep. It is suggested that SWS is needed for body repair, whereas REM sleep is useful for mind repair.[21] One controversial sleep theorist believes sleep to be essential for the brain but optional for the body.[22] Others have hypothesized that sleep promotes protein synthesis, information processing and memory storage, cognitive function, and enforcement of rest.[4] Major controversy exists over the precise function for sleep with the suggestion that sleep may serve an instinctive, protective, or adaptive purpose, or only to prevent sleepiness.

The importance of sleep for the quality of daytime wakefulness and functioning is often ignored.[6] This concept is vital to the critically ill patient during recovery who may be expected to turn, deep breathe, wean from the ventilator, and even get out of bed

tial implications for the critical care patient who may spend days to weeks with a monotonous view.

Noise

Excessive noise is a frequent complaint of critical care patients. Researchers have identified that sound levels in critical care units are often between 60 and 80 decibels,[62,63] while sleep occurs best at levels lower than 35 decibels.[64] Many noises may be unfamiliar or frightening to the patient. Communication between caregivers may be loud and not particularly therapeutic to the patient who is attempting to sleep.[65] Critical care nurses can easily become desensitized to the level of noise in their unit and block it out, whereas patients have no way to escape. It thus becomes a cruel environmental feature that inhibits sleep.

Frequent Caregiver Disruptions

Although it is widely noted that critical care nursing is life-saving for patients, many stressors described by patients originate from the perception of too-frequent interventions and interruptions by their caregivers. Sleep disruption clearly follows many caregiver interruptions. Monitoring techniques have increased the sophistication of assessment to the degree that hands-on manipulation of the sleeping or napping patient should not need to occur. Juggling the competing priorities of chest physiotherapy, wound care, and other treatments does not always give sleep the priority the patient believes it deserves. The 5 A.M. patient bath, too common in critical care settings, needs to be evaluated in terms of the knowledge that important REM sleep could be occurring during this time.

Situational Disruptions

Isolation and Loneliness

Patients admitted to critical care units are completely removed from many things familiar to them. Family and significant others are usually allowed to visit only infrequently, although there is a trend toward renewed interest in the family and policies of flexible visiting. Communication with family members may be strained and promote a sense of loneliness and isolation.

Discomfort and Pain

Patients in critical care settings often complain of inadequate pain relief,[66] and this may be a major reason for sleep disruption in the critically ill (see Chapter 12). Pharmacological agents, especially narcotics, are frequently used, but pain relief is not achieved. The use of an additional drug, an alternative drug, or an administration route such as patient controlled analgesia needs to be considered. Nonpharmacolog-

ical methods to achieve pain relief and perhaps sleep are underutilized. These methods could include distraction, relaxation, massage, imagery, and music. In a recent study, only a minority of subjects reported any use of factors other than medications to relieve their pain.[66]

Patients experience discomfort while being mechanically ventilated and this may make it difficult to sleep or rest. In one study, 35% of 158 ventilated patients complained of difficulty sleeping.[67] Forced immobilization with tubes and monitoring devices prolongs the discomfort of the critically ill and may make getting in a comfortable position to sleep impossible.

Relief of pain is probably the major area where critical care nursing can have the most significant impact on sleep. Patients would sleep more effectively if nurses put into practice what is already scientifically known about pain relief.

Pharmacological Agents

Caregivers order and administer analgesic, sedative, and hypnotic agents in recognition of the prevalence of pain, anxiety, and fear in the critically ill patient. However, many of these commonly used agents disrupt sleep.

Narcotics, benzodiazepine hypnotics, and other pharmacological agents cause havoc with normal sleep architecture. While it is essential to provide patients with the benefits of these medications, a knowledge of the drugs' effects on sleep patterns is necessary. A consulting pharmacologist is often a crucial health team member to evaluate a patient's potential for the polypharmacy of critical care. The goal is to provide the least drug to achieve a therapeutic goal with the minimum amount of side effects. Many drugs surprisingly affect the sleep cycle. Table 13-1 identifies significant sleep effects with medications commonly used in critical care.

Although it is not clear that patients benefit from long-term use of hypnotics, 0.3% of all adults use them and may be abruptly weaned when entering a critical care unit.[68] The elderly are especially likely to be chronic users of hypnotics, and this needs to be assessed on admission. Of significance is the recent recommendation against using the often advocated L-tryptophan as a sleep aid. Reports of associated eosinophilia, myalgia, and other symptoms suggest it should not be recommended until further evidence assures its safety.[68]

Sleep Fragmentation and Deprivation

In contrast to the normal practice of obtaining essentially all the 24-hour quota of sleep in one uninterrupted period of repeating sleep stage cycles, patients in critical care units are likely to experience

TABLE 13-1 **Drugs That Affect Sleep**

Drug		Effects on Sleep	Comments
Barbiturates	Acute:	↑ TST ↓ WASO ↓ REM ↑ Stage 2, ↑ spindles ↑ or ↓ SWS	Rapid development of tolerance Withdrawal insomnia Daytime sedation
	Withdrawal:	↓ TST	
Benzodiaze-pines	Acute:	↓ SL (most agents) ↑ TST ↓ WASO ↓ REM ↑ Stage 2, ↑ spindles ↓ SWS (most agents; some ↑ SWS)	Agents vary in onset and duration of action Daytime sedation (with long-acting agents) Tolerance develops (with short-acting agents) Withdrawal insomnia (with short-acting agents)
	Withdrawal:	↓ TST	
Chloral hydrate		↑ TST → REM → Stage 2 → SWS	Little information regarding tolerance or withdrawal
Alcohol	Acute:	↑ TST (1st half of night; ↓ 2nd half) ↓ WASO (1st half of night; ↑ 2nd half) ↓ REM (1st half of night) ↑ SWS	Acute effects variable
	Chronic:	→ TST → REM ↓ SWS	
	Withdrawal:	↓ TST ↑ WASO ↑ REM ↓ SWS	Degree of REM rebound may correlate with likelihood of withdrawal delirium
Narcotics	Acute:	↑ WASO ↓ REM ↓ SWS (total)	Effects vary with specific agents
	Chronic:	→ WASO → SWS	Hypersomnolence may occur during with- drawal
	Withdrawal:	↓ WASO	
Miscellaneous stimulants (nicotine, co- caine)		↑ SL ↓ TST ↓ REM	
Antidepressants (tricyclic and monoamine oxidase in- hibitors)	Acute:	↓ WASO ↓ REM ↑ Stage 2 ↑ SWS	Sleep effects vary with sedative potential of specific agent; MAOIs may cause ↑ WASO
	Withdrawal:	↑ WASO ↑ REM	
Lithium		↓ REM ↑ SWS	
Phenothiazines		↑ TST ↑ SWS	Effects mild and variable, according to spe- cific agent; REM effects inconsistent

Abbreviations: SL = sleep latency. WASO = wakefulness after sleep onset. REM = rapid eye movement sleep. TST = total sleep time. SWS = slow-wave sleep.
Modified from Buysse, D. J., & Reynolds, C. F. (1990). Insomnia. In M. J. Thorpy (Ed.), *Handbook of sleep disorders* (pp. 394-397). New York: Marcel Dekker.

Continued.

TABLE 13-1 **Drugs That Affect Sleep—cont'd**

Drug	Effects on Sleep	Comments
Reserpine	↑ WASO ↑ REM ↑ SWS	Can cause insomnia, nightmares
Diuretics	↑ WASO	Probably acts via nocturia, hemodynamic effects
Cimetidine	↑ SWS	Can cause daytime sedation
Baclofen	↑ TST	
L-Dopa	→ TST → or ↑ REM → SWS	In toxic doses, causes insomnia, delirium
Steroids	↑ WASO	

frequently interrupted and sporadically occurring cycles.[69] Patients in a respiratory intensive care unit who were physiologically monitored for EEG, EOG, and EMG were found to have limited sleep with frequent awakenings.[11] Surprisingly, 50% of their sleep was obtained during the day. This suggests how truly sleep deprived these individuals were who took every available opportunity to sleep.

Numerous studies document the severe sleep fragmentation that typically is a hallmark of critical care.[7-12,43,44,69] This sleep disruption leads to acute sleep deprivation which is endemic to the critical care setting. Polygraphic studies of medical intensive care patients and multiple trauma patients have identified consistent disruptions in sleep architecture including increased wake time, increased number of awakenings, decreased SWS, and decreased REM sleep.[10,11,12] The use of sedatives and necessary analgesics may contribute to this loss of SWS and REM.

An important consideration in sleep stage disruption is that each time the patient is interrupted after falling asleep, the sleep cycle must begin anew rather than returning to the stage from which arousal occurred. Repeated failure to complete full 90-minute cycles therefore leads to relative dominance of NREM sleep stages 1 and 2. This fragmented, light sleep is best exemplified in studies where critical care patients had an average of 30 to 50 awakenings per night based on EEG data.[10,12] Not all awakenings are due to caregiver disruptions; pain, discomfort, anxiety, noise, and other factors certainly play a role.

Loss of REM and SWS leads to the development of debtlike phenomena. After selective deprivation of these stages, rebounds—consistent quantitative increases in the "debted" types of sleep—occur in subsequent bulk sleep periods. Specifically, the stage for which the debt has been developed is entered both more often and from stages that normally do not precede the deficient stage.

Only about one third of lost sleep may be made up in an acute situation. This recovery sleep typically contains most of the missing stage 4 NREM sleep but only about one half of the missing REM sleep. It is therefore concluded that NREM stage 4 sleep is preferentially rebounded.

NURSING MANAGEMENT

Normal sleep in the critical care setting is essentially impossible. Environmental and situational disruptions to customary sleep patterns are inherent, rampant, and likely self-perpetuating without aggressive nursing therapy. Perhaps one of the major challenges to critical care nurses is to integrate interventions designed to limit sleep disruption into the complex, ever-changing plan of care required for critically ill patients. An important first step is a thorough sleep assessment, taking into account sleep patterns at home as well as an understanding of the detrimental effect of the critical care environment on the quantity and quality of sleep.

Data Acquisition

The ubiquitous "patient slept well" found in nurses' notes throughout the world belies the real problem that patients state they experience with hospital sleep in general and critical care sleep in particular. Nurses' observation and recording of sleep pattern and patient's subjective report of quality sleep is typically absent in many hospital records.[70] This makes decision making regarding the diagnosis of sleep pattern disturbance impossible and creates missed diagnoses a majority of the time. Lack of assessment of sleep leads to underrecognition of the problem. Initially, assessment of sleep patterns of critical care patients begins with the admission database.

Often referred to as sleep hygiene, the sleep routine that a patient follows at home not only needs to be recorded but should guide nursing care wherever possible. Areas to include are time of going to bed and rising, number of awakenings, room temperature, number of pillows, type of bed, and position of bed and patient, use of hypnotics, and any other bedtime rituals. Naps should be noted, especially in the elderly, and a history of snoring, a risk factor for OSA, may be important to note. Other areas to consider are normal work hours; patterns of smoking, alcohol, and caffeine use; and exercise routine.[71] This assessment is useful and needs to be consistently reviewed. Research demonstrates that patient sleep preferences, even when documented, may not be taken into account.[70]

Patient sleep times need to be recorded, especially in patients at high risk for experiencing prolonged stays in critical care settings. Measurement of patient sleep in critical care settings is much like assessing pain, in that the subjective component is the most important. With large individual variability in sleep, the absolute hours or minutes a patient spends asleep are not as critical as how rested that patient feels or how he or she subjectively rates the quality of sleep in the critical care setting.

Because the gold standard of sleep measurement, recording EEG, EOG, and EMG is not practical, nurses must rely on observational skill and patient self-report to assess sleep. Patients typically report the quality of their sleep by relying on perceptions of how quickly they fell asleep (sleep latency), how frequently they awakened, and finally, how much of the night they spent awake (wake after sleep onset). Nurses should therefore monitor these very same sleep variables carefully and question the patient when possible about sleep latency, awakenings, and wake after sleep onset. Research has demonstrated that while nurses' observation and patients' subjective assessment of sleep do not always correlate,[7] nurses can reliably ascertain wake after sleep onset based on good correlation with recorded sleep data.[10] This can occur if careful monitoring of patient sleep state includes watching for potential signs of sleep: closed eyes; not moving; decreased or variable heart rate, blood pressure, and respiration; and decreased awareness of surroundings. Obviously this will not be effective in patients receiving neuromuscular blocking agents or patients with anxiety and pain who may choose to lie still with eyes closed.

Nurses erroneously believe that just because they provide an opportunity to sleep, patients will quickly sleep; unfortunately this is not the case. Subjective patient assessment to validate nursing observation of sleep is truly the key, with careful communication strategies initiated such as a word board or magic slate for the intubated patient. Documentation on a flow sheet is the final step in patient assessment.

All patients in critical care settings are at risk for sleep pattern disturbance and need to have the nursing care plan reflect this. However, for patients with prolonged physiological instability who require a lengthy critical care stay, sleep-promoting interventions have a higher priority than for patients who will recover more quickly and return home. Unfortunately, this is the very group of patients for whom life-sustaining care and sleep promotion seem at odds, and justifiably a novice nurse chooses the former. This is unfortunate since creative nursing care can move sleep up on the priority "to do" list and share equally with life-saving care. Positive patient outcomes of faster recovery may ensue due to the beneficial, although incompletely known, effects of sleep on healing. Today's sophisticated monitoring techniques allow nursing activities such as monitoring hourly hemodynamic parameters to occur without disrupting patient sleep. Turning patients should be based on sound physiological rationale, not a 2-hour checklist.

The following information is a summary of patient outcome criteria and the recommended strategies critical care nurses should use to promote and maintain sleep in the critically ill.[15,30,40,58,60,62,63,71,72] However, these prescriptive interventions have not been investigated to any degree, and many have been recommended in the nursing sleep literature for nearly 20 years, some since Florence Nightingale's writings. Isolated studies rather than programs of research in sleep have contributed to intuitive, non-research based interventions in this area. A study of the positive effects of white noise on the sleep of postoperative cardiac surgery patients is an example of an isolated investigation where more work would suggest stronger utilization of the findings.[73]

■ NURSING DIAGNOSIS

Sleep pattern disturbance, related to environmental and/or situational disruptions, sleep fragmentation, and/or sleep deprivation.

OUTCOME STANDARD AND CRITERIA

The desired outcome for the critically ill patient from nursing therapies designed to promote sleep is a subjectively well-rested patient able to engage in recovery activities such as turning, getting out of bed, or even weaning from the ventilator without subjective evidence of excessive tiredness or sleepiness.[41,74] An additional outcome is that the patient will report factors that prevent or inhibit sleep and identify personal techniques to induce sleep.[59]

According to the AACN's *Outcome Standards for Nursing Care of the Critically Ill,* sleep deprivation is an etiology-related factor for the nursing diagnosis Altered Sensory Perception. Sleep pattern disturbance was not addressed separately. Although no outcome is therefore specific to sleep, the outcome standard for altered sensory perception states: Response to sensory-perceptual stimuli is appropriate. The outcome criteria are (1) oriented to person, place, time and (2) accurate description of the environment. These patient outcomes could also be used to evaluate interventions to promote sleep.[75]

NURSING INTERVENTIONS

Recommended nursing therapies to deal with sleep pattern disturbance can be categorized as surveillance activities, shielding, and modification of the patient-environment interface. *Surveillance activities* are per-

---

Nursing Strategies for Sleep Pattern Disturbance

SURVEILLANCE

Obtain and use sleep history to plan care.

Assess quality and quantity of sleep using appropriate methods.

Document sleep/wake time for all high-risk patients.

Monitor patient for psychophysiological signs of sleep deprivation.

Determine if sleep occurs during the limited opportunity provided.

SHIELDING

Increase nurses' sensitivity to sounds and lights in the ICU.

Prevent excessive lights and noise from alarms and limit staff conversation.

Evaluate the need for nursing care interruptions.

Use a nursing care plan to individualize and block sleep times.

Allow an opportunity for uninterrupted sleep time during day and night.

Promote comfortable positioning of the patient for sleep.

Explain environmental sounds and provide other information to lower patient anxiety.

MODIFICATION

Provide adequate pain relief and evaluate continuous analgesia or epidural anesthesia for promoting effective sleep.

Include backrubs and patient's own presleep routine.

Use relaxation techniques and imagery or music therapy.

Administer hypnotics according to patient protocol and evaluate their effectiveness.

Maximize patient privacy through the use of curtains and doors.

Post sign at designated sleep times—**Patient Sleeping.**

Provide large clocks and natural lighting.

Evaluate bed for comfort and sleep quality.

Ease visitor restrictions if this encourages patient to sleep.

From Fontaine, D. K. (1987). Sleep deprivation in the critical care unit. *Critical Care Nursing Currents, 5*(4), 22. Reprinted, with permission, from Ross Laboratories.

formed to initially assess and then monitor the patient in an ongoing manner for sleep pattern disturbance. *Shielding* refers to nursing therapies designed to protect the patient from the damaging environmental effects of critical care. Noise abatement strategies ranging from new unit design to closing of patient doors and limiting loud, nontherapeutic conversation that serves to raise patient anxiety levels are examples here. *Modification strategies* include those that will chemically alter a patient's internal environment to promote sleep, such as intravenous narcotic with patient-controlled analgesia or, external modification, with the use of light restriction and most especially, relaxing rigid visiting hours. The box to the left details nursing recommendations in these three categories.

Nursing research is needed to suggest which interventions work best with different patient populations such as the elderly, cardiac surgery patients, or those with multisystem trauma. As Giblin stated:[60]

> Further research is needed to evaluate the effectiveness of the nursing interventions and therapies used to support or improve sleep. Systematic documentation of the factors related to sleep disturbance, its defining characteristics, the interventions and therapies used to facilitate normal sleep in the clinical setting, together with documentation of patient outcomes, can provide a basis for testing the diagnosis of sleep pattern disturbance and validating the positive influence of sleep on recovery.

REFERENCES

1. Simpson, T. F., Armstrong, S., & Mitchell, P. (1989). American Association of Critical-Care Nurses Demonstration Project: Patients' recollections of critical care. *Heart Lung, 18,* 325-332.

2. Sassin, J. F. (1990). Prologue: The development of sleep disorders medicine. In M. J. Thorpy (Ed.), *Handbook of sleep disorders* (pp. 1-9). New York: Marcel Dekker.

3. Carskadon, M. A., & Dement, W. C. (1989). Normal human sleep: An overview. In M. H. Kryger, T. Roth, & W. C. Dement (Eds.), *Principles and practice of sleep medicine* (pp. 3-13). Philadelphia: Saunders.

4. Institute of Medicine. (1990). *Basic sleep research.* Washington, DC: National Academy Press.

5. Williams, R. L., Karacan, I., & Hursch, C. J. (1974). *Electroencephalography (EEG) of human sleep: Clinical applications.* New York: Wiley.

6. Dinges, D. F., & Broughton, R. J. (1989). *Sleep and alertness: Chronobiological, behavioral, and medical aspects of napping.* New York: Raven.

7. Aurell, J., & Elmqvist, D. (1985). Sleep in the surgical intensive care unit: Continuous polygraphic recording of sleep in nine patients receiving postoperative care. *British Medical Journal, 290*(6474), 1029-1032.

8. Broughton, R., & Baron, R. (1978). Sleep patterns in the intensive care unit and on the ward after myocardial infarction. *Electroencephalography and Clinical Neurophysiology, 45,* 348-360.

9. Dohno, S., Paskewicz, D. A., Lynch, J. J., et al. (1979). Some aspects of sleep disturbance in coronary patients. *Perceptual and Motor Skills, 49,* 199-205.

10. Fontaine, D. K. (1989). Measurement of nocturnal sleep patterns in trauma patients. *Heart Lung, 18,* 402-410.

11. Hilton, B. A. (1976). Quantity and quality of patients' sleep and sleep-disturbing factors in a respiratory intensive care unit. *Journal of Advanced Nursing, 1,* 453-468.

12. Richards, K. C., & Bairnsfather, L. (1988). A description of night sleep patterns in the critical care unit. *Heart Lung, 17,* 35-42.

13. Hanly, P. J., Millar, T. W., Steljes, D. G., et al. (1989). Respiration and abnormal sleep in patients with congestive heart failure. *Chest, 96,* 480-488.

14. Kimoff, R. J., Cosio, M. G., & McGregor, M. (1991). Clinical features and treatment of obstructive sleep apnea. *Canadian Medical Association Journal, 144,* 689-695.

15. Dinges, D. F. (1989). The influence of the human circadian timekeeping system on sleep. In M. H. Kryger, T. Roth, & W. C. Dement (Eds.), *Principles and practice of sleep medicine* (pp. 153-162). Philadelphia: Saunders.

16. Prinz, P. N., Vitello, M. V., Raskind, M. A., et al. (1990). Geriatrics: Sleep disorders and aging. *New England Journal of Medicine, 323,* 520-526.

17. Treatment of sleep disorders of older people. (1990). *NIH Consensus Development Conference Consensus Statement, 8*(3).

18. Brody, H. (1978). Cell counts in cerebral cortex and brainstem. In R. Katzman, R. D. Terry, & K. L. Bick (Eds.), *Alzheimer's disease: Senile dementia and related disorders: Vol. 7. Aging* (pp. 345-351). New York: Raven.

19. Rediehs, M. H., Reis, J. S., & Creason, N. S. (1990). Sleep in old age: Focus on gender differences. *Sleep, 13,* 410-424.

20. Hoch, C. C., Reynolds, C. F., & Monk, T. H. (1990). Comparison of sleep-disordered breathing among healthy elderly in the seventh, eight, and ninth decades of life. *Sleep, 13,* 502-511.

21. Naitoh, P., Kelly, T. L., & Englund, C. (1990). Health effects of sleep deprivation. *Occupational Medicine, 5,* 209-237.

22. Horne, J. (1988). *Why we sleep: The functions of sleep in humans and other mammals.* Oxford: Oxford University Press.

23. Rechtschaffen, A., Bergmann, B. M., Everson, C. A., et al. (1989). Sleep deprivation in the rat: Part 10. Integration and discussion of the findings. *Sleep, 12,* 68-87.

24. Karnofsky, M. L. (1986). Progress in sleep. *New England Journal of Medicine, 315,* 1026-1028.

25. Gaillard, J. M. (1990). Neurotransmitters and sleep pharmacology. In M. J. Thorpy (Ed.), *Handbook of sleep disorders* (pp. 55-76). New York: Marcel Dekker.

26. Remmers, J. E. (1990). Sleeping and breathing. *Chest, 97*(Suppl. 3), 77S-80S.

27. Douglas, N. J., White, D. P., Weil, J. V., et al. (1982). Hypoxic ventilatory response decreases during sleep in normal men. *American Review of Respiratory Disease, 125,* 286-289.

28. Hara, K. S., & Shepard, J. W. (1990). Sleep and critical care medicine. In R. J. Martin (Ed.), *Cardiorespiratory disorders during sleep* (2nd ed.) (pp. 323-363). Mount Kisco, NY: Futura.

29. Landis, C. A. (1988). Arrhythmias and sleep pattern disturbances in cardiac patients. *Progress in Cardiovascular Nursing, 3,* 72-80.

30. Shaver, J., & Giblin, E. C. (1989). Sleep. *Annual Review of Nursing Research. 8,* 71-93.

31. Flenley, D. C. (1989). Chronic obstructive pulmonary disease. In M. H. Kryger, T. Roth, & W. C. Dement (Eds.), *Principles and practice of sleep medicine* (pp. 601-610). Philadelphia: Saunders.

32. Erickson, R. S. (1989). Physiologic adaptations during sleep. In S. L. Underhill, S. L. Woods, & E. S. Sivarajan Froehlicher (Eds.), *Cardiac nursing* (2nd ed.) (pp. 158-164). Philadelphia: Lippincott.

33. Verrier, R. L. (1991). Stress, sleep, and vulnerability to ventricular fibrillation. In M. R. Brown, G. F. Koob, & C. Rivier (Eds.), *Stress: neurobiology and neuroendocrinology* (pp. 437-461). New York: Marcel Dekker.

34. Wooten, V. (1989). Medical causes of insomnia. In M. H. Kryger, T. Roth, & W. C. Dement (Eds.), *Principles and practice of sleep medicine* (pp. 456-475). Philadelphia: Saunders.

35. Parsons, L. C., & Ver Beek, D. (1982). Sleep-wake patterns following cerebral concussion. *Nursing Research, 31,* 260-264.

36. Thorpy, M. J. (Ed.). (1990). Classification and nomenclature of the sleep disorders. In *Handbook of sleep disorders* (pp. 155-178). New York: Marcel Dekker.

37. Reite, M. L., Nagel, K. E., & Ruddy, J. R. (1990). *Concise guide to the evaluation and management of sleep disorders.* Washington, DC: American Psychiatric Press.

38. Williams, R. L. (1988). Sleep disturbances in various medical and surgical conditions. In R. L. Williams, I. Karacan, & C. A. Moore (Eds.), *Sleep disorders: Diagnosis and treatment* (2nd ed.) (pp. 265-291). New York: Wiley.

39. Fletcher, E. C. (1990). Respiration during sleep and cardiopulmonary hemodynamics in patients with chronic lung disease. In R. J. Martin (Ed.), *Cardiorespiratory disorders during sleep* (2nd ed.) (pp. 215-249). Mount Kisco, NY: Futura.

40. Phillips, B. A., Cooper, K. R., & Burke, T. V. (1987). The effect of sleep loss on breathing in COPD. *Chest, 91,* 29-32.

41. Erickson, R. S. (1989). Sleep in patients with cardiovascular disease. In S. L. Underhill, S. L. Woods, E. S. Sivarajan Froehlicher, et al. (Eds.), *Cardiac nursing* (2nd ed.) (pp. 1052-1061). Philadelphia: Lippincott.

42. Kutz, I., Garb, R., & David, D. (1988). Posttraumatic stress disorder following myocardial infarction. *General Hospital Psychiatry, 10,* 169-176.

43. McFadden, E. H., & Giblin, E. C. (1971). Sleep deprivation in patients having open-heart surgery. *Nursing Research, 20,* 249-254.

44. Woods, N. F. (1972). Patterns of sleep in postcardiotomy patients. *Nursing Research, 21,* 347-352.

45. Walker, B. B. (1972). The postsurgery heart patient: Amount of uninterrupted time for sleep and rest during the first, second, and third postoperative days in a teaching hospital. *Nursing Research, 21,* 164-169.

46. Orr, W. C., & Stahl, M. L. (1977). Sleep disturbances after open heart surgery. *American Journal of Cardiology, 39,* 196-201.

47. Westbrook, P. R. (1990). Sleep disorders and upper airway obstruction in adults. *Otolaryngologic Clinics of North America, 23,* 727-743.

48. Guilleminault, C., & Dement, W. C. (1988). Sleep apnea syndromes and related sleep disorders. In R. L. Williams, I. Karacan, & C. A. Moore (Eds.), *Sleep disorders: Diagnosis and treatment* (2nd ed.) (pp. 47-71). New York: Wiley.

49. Findley, L. J., Unverzagt, M. E., & Suratt, P. M. (1988). Automobile accidents involving patients with obstructive sleep apnea. *American Review of Respiratory Disease, 138,* 337-340.

50. Sher, A. E. (1990). Obstructive sleep apnea syndrome: A complex disorder of the upper airway. *Otolaryngologic Clinics of North America, 23,* 593-608.

51. Levinson, P. D., & Millman, R. P. (1991). Causes and consequences of blood pressure alterations in obstructive sleep apnea. *Archives of Internal Medicine, 151,* 455-462.

52. Martin, R. J. (1990). The sleep-related worsening of lower airways obstruction: Understanding and intervention. *Medical Clinics of North America, 74,* 701-714.

53. Sher, A. E. (1990). The upper airway in obstructive sleep apnea syndrome: Pathology and surgical management. In M. J. Thorpy (Ed.), *Handbook of sleep disorders* (pp. 311-335). New York: Marcel Dekker.

54. Sher, A. E. (1990). Surgery for obstructive sleep apnea. In F. G. Issa, P. M. Suratt, & J. E. Remmers (1990). *Sleep and respiration* (pp. 407-415). New York: Wiley-Liss.

55. Esclamado, R. M., Glenn, M. G., McCulloch, T. M., et al. (1989). Perioperative complications and risk factors in the surgical treatment of obstructive sleep apnea syndrome. *Laryngoscope, 99,* 1125-1129.

56. Koopman, C. F., & Moran, W. B. (1990). Surgical management of obstructive sleep apnea. *Otolaryngologic Clinics of North America, 23,* 787-808.

57. Sanders, M. H., Johnson, J. T., Keller, F. A., et al. (1988). The acute effects of uvulopalatopharyngoplasty on breathing during sleep in sleep apnea patients. *Sleep, 11,* 75-89.

58. Dracup, K. A. (1988). Are critical care units hazardous to health? *Applied Nursing Research, 1,* 14-21.

59. Carpenito, L. J. (1989). *Nursing diagnosis application to clinical practice* (3rd ed.). Philadelphia: Lippincott.

60. Giblin, E. (1990). Rest and sleep: Current bases for practice. In S. G. Funk, E. M. Tornquist, M. T. Champagne, et al. (Eds.), *Key aspects of recovery: Improving nutrition, rest, and mobility* (pp. 46-54). New York: Springer.

61. Ulrich, R. S. (1984). View through a window may influence recovery from surgery. *Science, 224,* 420-421.

62. Baker, C. (1984). Sensory overload and noise in the ICU: Sources of environmental stress. *Critical Care Quarterly, 6*(4), 66-80.

63. Hilton, B. A. (1985). Noise in acute patient care areas. *Research in Nursing and Health, 8,* 283-291.

64. World Health Organization. (1980). *Environmental health criteria 12: Noise.* Geneva: Author.

65. Noble, M. A. (1979). Communication in the ICU: Therapeutic or disturbing? *Nursing Outlook, 27,* 195-198.

66. Puntillo, K. A. (1990). Pain experiences of intensive care unit patients. *Heart Lung, 19,* 526-533.

67. Bergbom-Engberg, I., & Haljamae, H. (1989). Assessment of patients' experience of discomforts during respirator therapy. *Critical Care Medicine, 17,* 1068-1072.

68. Gillin, J. C., & Byerly, W. F. (1990). The diagnosis and management of insomnia. *New England Journal of Medicine, 322,* 239-248.

69. Helton, M. C., Gordon, S. H., & Nunnery, S. L. (1980). The correlation between sleep deprivation and the intensive care unit syndrome. *Heart Lung, 9,* 464-468.

70. Closs, S. J. (1990). Factors affecting the sleep of patients on surgical wards in Scotland. In S. G. Funk, E. M. Tornquist, M. T. Champagne, et al. (Eds.), *Key aspects of recovery: Improving nutrition, rest, and mobility* (pp. 223-231). New York: Springer.

71. Goodmote, E. (1991). Alterations in rest and sleep patterns. In M. E. Shekleton, & K. Litwack (Eds.), *Critical care nursing of the surgical patient* (pp. 240-257). Philadelphia: Saunders.

72. Sanford, S. (1983). Sleep and the cardiac patient. *Cardiovascular Nursing, 19*(5), 19-24.

73. Williamson, J. (1992). The effects of ocean sounds on sleep after coronary artery bypass graft surgery. *American Journal of Critical Care, 1,* 91-97.

74. Swearingen, P. L., & Keen, J. H. (1991). *Manual of critical care: Applying nursing diagnoses to adult critical illness* (2nd ed.). St. Louis: Mosby-Year Book.

75. American Association of Critical-Care Nurses. (1990). *Outcome standards for nursing care of the critically ill.* Laguna Niguel, CA: Author.

14

Thermal Balance

Barbara J. Holtzclaw

Variations in body temperature serve as important clinical indicators of patient progress and recovery. Historically, fever was of primary concern, because it provided a reliable index of the patient's ability to respond to and combat infection. Today's critical care nurse confronts alterations in thermal balance that often result from factors external to the patient. Advances in medical science and technology have created complex conditions that intensify thermoregulatory problems caused by disease or injury:

Patients who would have succumbed to critical illnesses in the past can survive with compromised thermoregulatory ability.

New physical and pharmacological therapies deliberately or inadvertently alter body temperature.

New devices measure temperature from several body sites and require greater judgment by caregivers for interpretation.

These factors are common to every critical care unit where environmental, therapeutic, and pathological factors often combine to alter thermal balance. Not only do new therapies change the complexity of thermal alterations, but scientific advances markedly enhance their recognition and management. New discoveries challenge age-old traditions related to measurement, assessment, and maintenance of thermal balance in the critically ill.

Because alterations in thermal balance are essentially disorders of heat loss or heat gain, assessment and intervention require a clear understanding of the dynamics of heat exchange and thermoregulation. Early recognition and appropriate nursing action are of particular importance in averting more serious complications.

THERMOREGULATION: A DELICATE BALANCE

Thermal balance is a dynamic state: a delicate equilibrium in which the heat generated by the body is equivalent to the heat lost to the environment. Healthy humans maintain internal, or "core" body temperature within a relatively narrow range (about 36.4° to 37.5° C) even when exposed to extremely high or low external temperatures. In health, heat-regulating mechanisms are inconspicuously efficient and noticeable only in extremes of environmental temperature or physical activity. During illness, exaggerated or inefficient thermoregulatory responses may provide clues to underlying pathology.

As a homeotherm, the human's marvelous capability to maintain a constant internal temperature lies in the ability to effectively control heat. Heat is produced as a by-product of the body's never-ceasing expenditure of energy. Metabolic reactions within cells, friction created by circulating blood and contracting muscles, and virtually all types of energy expenditure within the body continually generate heat. Heat is always in motion, passing from warmer molecules to cooler ones, and inevitably to the environment. Through a complex system of physiological and behavioral controls, the body actively generates, conserves, and redistributes heat to achieve a fairly stable internal temperature. Thermal balance is tipped in the direction of heat generation during fever, when shivering and rising metabolic activity occur in response to infection or pyrogenic substances. If thermoregulatory processes are severely impaired by drugs or injury, central control mechanisms become ineffective. This thermal instability makes the person extremely vulnerable to changing environmental temperature and much like the poikilothermic, "cold-blooded," amphibians or reptiles.

Body Heat Generation

Metabolic and Chemical Heat Production

A major source of heat is derived from the combustion of foodstuff. Nearly 75% of the energy of ingested food becomes heat during processing and transfer to cells. The remaining 25% is used for cellular function, which includes the formation of peptide linkages for protein synthesis from adenosine triphosphate (ATP). Even these cellular stores of energy are ultimately released as heat during the eventual breakdown and turnover of body proteins.[1]

The rates at which cellular metabolic processes produce heat are regulated by adrenal and thyroid hormones. When the sympathetic nervous system is stimulated, norepinephrine and epinephrine increase cellular metabolic activity. In neonates, this is the primary mechanism for heat production. Sympathetic stimulation caused by the infant's falling body temperature leads to oxidization of a specialized type of mitochondria-rich brown fat to liberate heat. This chemical, or nonshivering, thermogenesis consumes large amounts of oxygen in the process. This mechanism presents a significant problem to the low-birth-weight infant, whose respiratory function is often underdeveloped and whose brown fat stores are minimal.[2] Failure to provide warmth by external means may quickly compromise oxygenation. Beyond the first year of life, brown fat declines and nonshivering thermogenesis is relatively insignificant. By adulthood, it probably accounts for no more than 10% to 15% of heat production.[1]

The influence of thyroid hormone is less immediate, with related changes in metabolic rate and heat production being more gradual. Thyroxine speeds up the activity rates of most body cells by increasing the number and function of cell mitochondria that produce ATP from adenosine diphosphate (ADP) by oxidative phosphorylation. Excessive thyroxine production can raise metabolic rate 100% above normal, while absence of the hormone can decrease this value to nearly half the normal rate.[1] The effects of the thyroid on heat production are directly related to its ability to increase the rates of chemical reactions within all body cells.

Temperatures are lower during sleep and generally peak in late afteroon. Corticosteroids are thought to influence these normal fluctuations of 0.2° to 0.3° C that vary with circadian changes. Monthly temperature variations follow ovulatory cycles in women and are also hormone related.[3]

Kinetic Heat Production

Sudden exposure to the cold usually provokes an increase in musculoskeletal activity that can generate a dramatic increase in body heat production. Contraction of muscle fibers creates friction that raises heat production significantly for short periods. Some cold-induced muscle activity is voluntary, and some is reflexive. Persons going outdoors on a cold day commonly tense their muscles, "hug" themselves, and walk more briskly than usual. However, the primary source of heat production in adults comes from an involuntary increase in skeletal muscle activity in the form of shivering. Phasic contractions of skeletal muscle during vigorous shivering raise metabolic rate three to five times the resting value. Unfortunately, large amounts of body heat are lost during shivering. As muscles generate heat, it is carried by circulation to cooler regions nearer the skin. The movement of shaking extremities further dissipates heat to the environment. In all, the body can conserve only about 11% of the heat generated by shivering to replace heat loss.[4] This makes shivering a metabolically expensive and relatively ineffective process for maintaining thermal balance.

The influence of musculoskeletal activity in heat production depends on functional musculature and the availability of metabolic fuel for energy. In the critical care setting, muscle activity is often impaired in persons with neurological disease or injury, or suppressed by neuromuscular blocking agents. These individuals are unable to summon their primary source of immediate heat production when environmental temperatures fall. Consequently, they require greater vigilance in care to protect them from inadvertent heat loss.

Heat Exchange Dynamics

Heat is a form of energy that is familiar to nurses, both in terms of its measurement (temperature) and its relationship to food (calories). Principles of thermodynamics govern the nature of heat, whether in a living body or an inanimate object. The transfer of heat is further influenced in living animals by physiological mechanisms. Knowledge of these properties is essential to understanding the measurement, assessment, prevention, and management of alterations of thermal balance.

Physical Properties

Heat changes the character of many things, causing molecules to move more rapidly and substances to expand. Substances differ in the specific speed and temperature at which these changes take place, and in the character they assume when heated. The character of water, for example, is reversible at rising and falling temperatures. When water changes from liquid to vapor as it heats beyond the boiling point (100° C), it then returns to liquid again as temperatures fall. Protein substances, on the other hand, are irreversibly denatured by heat and become insoluble. Awareness of this characteristic is crucial to caring for patients with fever or hyperthermia, whatever the cause. Proteins within the central nervous system are particularly vulnerable to damage from high temperatures. As core temperatures rise above 41° C, meningeal irritation and convulsions are common. Above 44° C, irreversible denaturation of proteins and enzymes leads quickly to death.[1]

Substances have specific characteristics that influence the gain and loss of heat. These characteristics help to explain why the amount of heat delivered to one object is not always the same as the heat lost from an adjacent object. They also explain why heat is not transferred uniformly between different objects or to different types of patients in the same way.[5] First of all, not every substance has the same "heating effect" as water. It takes 20 g of mercury, for example, to raise or lower the temperature to the same extent 1 g of water would. Using water as a reference point, *specific heat* is expressed as a ratio. When 1 g of another substance loses 1° C when mixed with 1 g of water, the specific heat is determined by measuring the heat gained by the water. In the body, the movement of heat from solid tissue through cellular and vascular fluids will reflect this ratio and in turn determine heat capacity. *Heat capacity* is the quantity of heat (calories per gram) required to raise temperature in the substance a given amount (1° C). Because heat capacity is the product of specific heat and mass, the larger the object or animal, the greater the heat capacity. Animals are composed of both liquid and solid matter, each with different heat capacities. Total heat capacity of the human body is thus derived from a sum of heat capacities. Calculation of specific heat and heat capacities enhances (1) prediction of the amount of heat and caloric expenditure necessary to rewarm hypothermic patients and (2) concern about thin adults or low-birth-weight infants who lose or gain heat easily to gradients with cooler or warmer objects in clinical settings.

Physical mechanisms influencing the transfer of heat are: radiation, conduction, convection, and evaporation. In *radiation,* heat passes as radiant energy through air or space from warm to cool objects. It is not necessary for the source of radiant heat to glow or to change the ambient temperature for heat to be radiated.[5] Radiant waves, such as infrared and ultraviolet, may even be invisible to the eye. Because heat always moves from warmer to cooler regions, exposed skin radiates heat from the body surface to the cooler environment. Patients sitting next to a closed window can radiate heat through the glass to the cooler environment outside. By contrast, radiant heat from lamps and sunlight, even through a closed window, can warm exposed skin despite cool surroundings.

Transfer of heat by *conduction* is influenced in part by the nature of the substance involved. Substances differ in their ability to conduct heat, with metals tending to be more rapid conductors than other substances. Poor conductors such as wool fabric and goose down serve as insulators that tend to trap heat when worn as clothing.

Convection transfers heat by movement of air or liquid over an object. Air conditioner vents, drafts, breezes, and wound irrigations are common sources of heat loss for patients. Heat gain by convection is achieved through convective air warming blankets, hot showers, and forced air heaters.

Moisture loss from wet skin or exposed mucous membranes constitutes a major source of *evaporative heat loss* for hospitalized patients during bathing, dressing changes, and surgical procedures. Low humidity, high environmental temperature, and the presence of air currents all facilitate evaporative heat loss.[1]

Distribution, Conservation, and Loss of Body Heat

Physiological Factors

The human body, as a homeotherm, does not respond passively to the physical mechanisms affecting heat transfer. Instead, physiological processes actively distribute or conserve body heat. Circulating blood is a primary factor in heat distribution: heat loss to the environment is enhanced by vasodilation and diminished by vasoconstriction. Movement of heat through the body is further facilitated by conduction and countercurrent exchange from circulating blood. Body tissues differ in their composition and propensity to conduct, transfer, or retain heat. A layer of subcutaneous body fat provides exceptional heat-conserving insulation, similar to that of a layer of clothing. Fat is insulative because its rate of heat conduction is only about one third the rate of other tissues.[1] Thin or emaciated patients may require added clothing or covering in a cool room or during transport because they lack this insulation. Vasomotor control is able to either decrease or increase the insulative factor of superficial tissues by regulating the perfusion of skin and subcutaneous layers. Vasoconstriction of superficial vascular beds creates a thick insulative "shell" of poorly perfused tissue. Conversely, vasodilation perfuses superficial capillary beds with warm blood near the surface of the skin where it is easily lost to the environment by conduction and convection. Vasodilation produced by neurological disorder or vasoactive drugs, such as nitroglycerine or sodium nitroprusside may inadvertently promote heat loss. These effects are often seen when vasodilatory drugs are given during postoperative recovery, where anesthetic agents suppress other warming mechanisms.

Behavioral Factors

When healthy individuals sense significant temperature changes, they respond behaviorally to influence heat loss or gain. They may move from outdoors to inside, open or shut a window, turn on a fan or eliminate drafts, adjust the heat or air conditioning, add or subtract clothing, or simply seek more comfortable surroundings. These actions seem simple and instinctive to healthy persons, but they serve a significant adaptive function in thermoregulation. When patients are seriously ill or debilitated, such activities are difficult or impossible. Some patients may also lack the physical or cognitive abilities to communicate discomfort or needs related to temperature.

The Hypothalamic "Thermostat"

"Set Point" Range

Thermal balance is regulated by a complex feedback system that is coordinated by the *hypothalamic control center*. The system includes: (1) sensory inputs from central and peripheral thermoreceptors, (2) hypothalamic integration and comparison, and (3) output effector mechanisms. Core temperature is maintained within an optimal range specific for the individual. This range varies widely among people, but limits generally range from 36.2° to 37.8° C. This temperature range constitutes a thermostatic threshold known as the hypothalamic "set point." When core temperatures rise above or fall below this range, compensatory cooling or warming responses occur to regain the optimum temperature.

Central and Peripheral Feedback System. Sensory information about heat loss and gain is transmitted to the preoptic-anterior area of the hypothalamus from central and peripheral thermoreceptors. Central thermoreceptors are found in the brain and spinal cord. Peripheral sensors for heat have been found in the abdominal viscera, but the predominant source of peripheral thermal stimuli is the skin. Although hypothalamic thermoreceptors are acutely sensitive to the central stimulus of blood temperature, afferent impulses from skin often elicit more immediate responses. This warning system is protective to the body, in that compensatory mechanisms such as vasoconstriction and shivering can avoid heat loss long before central temperatures drop. Cutaneous receptors are functionally different for sensing heat and cold. There are nearly ten times the number of cold receptors as there are heat receptors, and neither are uniformly distributed over the skin. There are heavier concentrations of heat-loss sensors in the hands, feet, and face than in other body areas. Thus, cold feet and hands may bring on chills without temperature changes occurring in the trunk or other areas. Heat-sensitive impulses from skin are transmitted over type C nerve fibers, while cold sensitive impulses travel by small myelinated A fibers and nonmyelinated C fibers. Sensations of heat loss are transmitted over ten times as quickly as those transmitting warmth. Sensory fibers enter dorsal roots of the spinal cord, cross to the opposite side, then traverse the lateral spinothalamic tract to the thalamus, rostral reticular system, and hypothalamus.[6]

Thermal Signals Integration. Thermosensory impulses from the periphery are transmitted via the spinal tracts to the preoptic anterior hypothalamus where they are integrated or summed with central inputs. Thermosensitive structures in skin appear to dominate as input, with rate of temperature change serving as an important stimulus. Gradual cooling, for example, allows a person to experience a drop of several degrees in environmental temperature without shivering. However, sudden exposure of warm skin, even with a less drastic drop in temperature, will cause shivering.

Comparator Function of the Preoptic Regions. Integrated signals from the periphery, the reticular formation, and local sensors in the central nervous system are received in the preoptic regions of the brain, ventral to the anterior commissure, near the walls of the third ventricle. Compression or injury in this area of the brain can cause abnormal thermoregulation because this region functionally acts as the thermostatic comparator. It compares sensory input information to the optimum set point range and relays the stimulus to efferent control centers. Gradients or discrepancies between set point and integrated temperature stimulate efferent responses.[1]

Effector Systems Maintaining Thermal Balance

Effector systems are stimulated by the hypothalamic control center to activate compensatory warming and cooling mechanisms. During heat loss, signals are sent to the primary shivering center and the sympathetic nervous system is stimulated. During heat gain, signals cause inhibition of sympathetic centers governing shivering, vasoconstriction, and chemical thermogenesis, while stimulating cholinergic fibers to induce sweating. Each of these effects enhances the physical properties of heat transfer: to generate, conserve, or redistribute heat in a way to preserve optimum core temperature.[1]

Neuroendocrine Thermoregulatory Effects

Hypothalamic stimulation of the sympathetic nervous system brings about temperature changes by influencing vascular and skeletal muscle tone, sweating, and metabolic rate. Because catecholamines play such an important role in inhibiting or stimulating thermoregulatory responses, sympathetic stimulation caused by alarm or emotional stimuli can influence body temperature. An example is seen in the perceptible feelings of being "hot under the collar" in an anxiety-provoking situation. The same situation may also induce peripheral vasoconstriction, making the hands cold and clammy. Sympathomimetic drugs often stimulate thermoregulatory responses whereas catecholamine antagonists inhibit them.

Vasomotor Control of Blood Flow

Sympathetic control of the vasculature is both direct, by neural impulses, and indirect, a result of circulating catecholamines. By perfusing either deep or superficial vascular beds, heat is conserved, redistributed, or lost to the environment.

Sudomotor Systems Affecting Evaporative Heat Loss

Sweat glands have either a cholinergic or adrenergic nerve supply, although both types are affected by circulating catecholamines. Cholinergic sweating is of primary importance to thermoregulation as it supplies large portions of the skin with moisture for evaporative heat loss. Adrenergic sweating is less important to temperature control, because of the smaller localized areas involved. Also, because adrenergic sweat has less water than cholinergic sweat, it evaporates less readily.[1]

Gamma Efferent Control of Shivering

Shivering that results from heat loss is not an autonomic function. The *primary shivering center*, located in the dorsomedial portion of the posterior hypothalamus, mediates shivering via the extrapyramidal gamma efferent motor system. Motor impulses reach skeletal muscles through descending pathways that pass through the midbrain just lateral to the red nucleus, into the lateral reticular formation of midbrain, pons, and medulla oblongata and finally through the lateral funiculus of the spinal cord.[1] Pathways continue in the spinal cord via anterior motoneurons which give rise to nerve fibers that leave the cord by anterior roots. Nerve fibers innervate skeletal muscle fibers by two primary structures: large type A alpha fibers, which operate the muscle motor unit, and smaller type A gamma fibers, which activate the muscle spindle fusimotor system. The tremor of cold-induced shivering is created by tension of the muscle spindle which sets up a feedback oscillation of phasic contractions.[6]

Behavioral Responses as Effector Systems

Central thermoregulatory controls influence behaviors that affect heat loss or gain. Changes in temperature elicit reflexive postural changes, even in sleep, where heat loss causes people to "curl up" in bed and warmth makes them "spread out" their limbs. Uncomfortably cool or warm conditions are difficult to ignore, and even healthy individuals usually cannot relax under these conditions. Thus, when sensed deviations in temperature stimulate purposeful activities to change the thermal environment, this, too, becomes a behavioral effector mechanism.

DATA ACQUISITION

Temperature Measurement

Body Sites

Several factors must be considered when measuring body temperature. Perhaps one of the most important is "which body temperature?" Every body region has its own normal temperature range, and the suitability of one measurement site over another depends largely on the thermal stability of the patient. "Central temperatures" might ideally be measured from the brain, if that were possible. However, they are most easily accessible from regions close to the brain, such as the oral cavity, tympanic membrane, or auditory canal. The terms "central temperature" and "core temperature" are often used as synonyms, although there are imprecisions in the use of both terms. *Core temperature* is considered in much of the literature as that of the deep tissues of the body (the visceral regions). However, the same term is used to refer to the regions regulated by the hypothalamic set point. In that case, core temperature refers to the integrated input sensed by the hypothalamic "thermostat." To avoid confusion in terms when discussing measurement, the specific temperature sites (oral, tympanic membrane, pulmonary artery, bladder, or skin) should be stated. Temperature reflecting the deep tissues of the body are best measured from regions closest to the warmest organ, the liver. In euthermia, measurements from the rectum or the pulmonary artery might reflect these temperatures equally well.[7]

Selecting a temperature site that reflects central or core temperature is more difficult when rectal, pulmonary artery, and bladder temperatures become widely divergent. This divergence often occurs in conditions in which there is significant sympathetic stimulation, profound heat loss, or circulatory shunting. This is the case during rewarming after hypothermic bypass or during circulatory shock. In critical care settings, pulmonary artery (PA) temperatures can often be obtained from patients already being monitored by hemodynamic monitoring systems. In euthermic humans, PA temperatures closely parallel those of the brain and are usually higher than those routinely measured from other sites. Some investigators consider PA values the best indicator or "gold standard" for core temperature measurement.[8] However, the use of such an invasive device for temperature measurements alone is not warranted.

Tympanic membrane (TM) thermometers have been found to correlate closely with PA temperatures in euthermic, hypothermic, and febrile states.[9,10] They are purported to provide central temperature measurement because the tympanic membrane receives abundant arterial blood supply from the external carotid artery. Thermistor-tipped esophageal probes are often used to monitor temperature during surgery. Esophageal temperature readings have been found to closely track TM values, yet the proximity of the esophagus to respiratory passages may make it unreliable when inspired gases are warmed during anesthesia. The indwelling probe may be undesirable and uncomfortable for some patients. Nasopharyngeal temperatures are poor indicators of central temperature, correlated poorly with PA temperatures, are highly influenced by the heat of warmed inspired gases, and are uncomfortable to the conscious patient.

Rectal measurements, a traditional method used in infants and in unconscious adults or those unable to cooperate, have been shown to be no more valid or reliable than more aesthetically acceptable methods. Rectal temperatures normally run about 0.5° C higher than oral temperatures, except during hypothermic rewarming, where rectal values lag behind other sites. Cold blood, returning from the lower extremities, tends to retard the return to normal temperatures. Risk of rectal perforation and inconvenience have led to a decline in use.

Oral temperatures are more convenient and when obtained correctly are highly correlated with pulmonary artery and rectal measurements. Oral temperatures unfortunately tend to be influenced by inspired air, differences in location within the mouth, chewing gum, drinking cool or hot fluids, and talking.

Axillary temperature measurement is, in effect, skin or surface temperature. In euthermia it generally measures 0.5° C lower than oral temperature. Its validity as a reflection of core temperature depends on vascular supply. During the defervescence phase of fever, superficial vessels are dilated and skin temperature is more closely correlated with that of the brain. During chilling or vasoconstriction, skin temperatures correlate poorly with central measures. Urinary bladder temperatures and those from freshly voided urine have been found to correlate well with PA temperatures in euthermic states. The difficulty in collecting fresh urine of sufficient quantity makes the measurement of urine temperature impractical for monitoring critically ill patients.

Measurement Instruments

The ideal instrument for measuring body temperature is accurate, safe, comfortable and convenient. Standard mercury-in-glass thermometers, used for so many years in clinical settings, fall short in several of these criteria. Although many nurses believe that glass thermometers are more accurate than electronic models, studies show otherwise.[11] Significant differences in accuracy and reliability are found among glass thermometers purchased in quantity from the same manufacturer. Some brands are shown to have a "shelf life" and become inaccurate when left unused. Most glass thermometers are inadequate for monitoring hypothermic patients because they do not measure below 34.4° C (94° F). Mercury-in-glass thermometers take from 6 to 10 minutes to register, with larger and feverish patients requiring less time than children and afebrile persons. These thermometers also have the disadvantage of not providing continuous measurement; they must be shaken down anew with each measurement. Glass breakage is common, making these thermometers dangerous for use with children and uncooperative patients. Mercury, the temperature-sensitive liquid sealed in the thermometer, is highly toxic. Ingestion or aspiration of mercury from a thermometer compounds the danger of broken glass.

Electronic thermometers offer a wider range of temperature measurements. They register more quickly, and digital readings pose less ambiguity in interpretation. As with glass thermometers, reliability and accuracy are major concerns. All electronic thermometers require regular checks and calibration against a scientific standard. Electronic thermometer probes have the advantage of continuous measurement over time but the disadvantage of requiring an indwelling line or means of attachment to the body. Electronic temperature probes are used on skin, in vascular lines, and in nasopharyngeal, gastrointestinal, urinary bladder, and tympanic membrane sites. A common problem with indwelling temperature probes is malposition or displacement. With tympanic membrane probes, perforation is possible. Faulty probes on indwelling vascular lines or urinary catheters are problematic in that malfunction often requires replacement with a new sterile system.

A hand-held thermometer recently introduced into clinical use measures temperature by infrared light reflectance. The thermometer is used primarily for tympanic membrane readings, although one model is capable of scanning for skin surface readings. The light reflectance thermometer is safe, requiring no deep insertion of probes and produces reading in less than 10 seconds.[9] Proper technique is needed, however, to assure consistent measurements over time. The instrument is directed into the ear canal, much like an otoscope, and variations in reading occur if the angle directs the probe toward the wall of the ear canal.

Body Temperature as a Vital Sign

Body Temperature in Context of Other Findings

No single measurement of body temperature is meaningful without consideration of the site and context of the patient's condition. Temperature is indeed a vital sign, and as such must be observed over time, compared with baseline readings, and correlated with physiological, psychological, and environmental events occurring at the same time. Age, body size, fat distribution, hydration, physical exertion, immunocompetency, and neuroendocrine status are among the constitutional factors that directly affect body temperature.

Temperature Variations in the Critically Ill

Tissue damage from surgery, trauma, radiation, and ischemia create responses reflected in body temperatures. Body temperature varies with exposure to pyrogens and extremes in environmental temperature. Finally, in the care of critically ill patients, the loss of body temperature control reflects a serious decline in vital functions. Vigilant nursing action is required to maintain the patient's optimum temperatures necessary to preserve cellular function.

Patients at Increased Risk

While assessment of thermal balance should include all patients, certain critically ill patients are at particular risk.

Newborn and Low-birth-weight Infants

The nurse caring for low-birth-weight infants should continuously monitor body temperature. Because of the thin skin and scanty subcutaneous tissue, skin temperatures are usually well correlated with core measures. Visual cues, such as mottled skin, are less an indicator of temperature than they are of oxygenation. The two factors are closely linked, however. The normal neonate's primary defense against cold is the burning of brown fat, stimulated by sympathetic stimulus. When the infant is chilled, catecholamines rise, increasing metabolic rate and the need for more oxygen. Immature infants are deficient in brown fat and become hypoxic quickly as oxygen demand increases. Much heat is lost during the birth process and transport to the nursery. Still more is lost during examination and surgical procedures or when the infant must be moved outside the protection of the isolette. Heat is easily lost from low-birth-weight infants by (1) conduction, particularly to good conductors such as metallic surfaces; (2) convection to drafts caused by open isolette doors or movement of the caregiver; (3) evaporation of body moisture through extremely thin skin; and (4) radiation from exposed skin, even through the window of the iso-

lette. Heat must be actively restored to the immature infant's body by warming lights, heating units, or in some cases by skin-to-skin contact with the mother.

Frail Elderly Patients

The frail elderly are at risk for alterations in thermal balance if exposed to extremes in environmental temperature. Metabolic and vasomotor function declines to a moderate extent during the mid-sixties, but by age 80 there is significant reduction in the ability to generate and conserve heat.[12] Elderly patients tend to lose heat more quickly because they have decreased muscle mass and are unable to conserve heat by vasoconstriction as well as younger persons do. The ability to shiver or promote heat by muscular activity may be impaired if neurological or musculoskeletal function has declined. Assessment should include frequent objective measurement, because the elderly are not always aware of their thermal status. Fever in the elderly is a serious sign and should never be taken lightly. Sometimes fever is caused by dehydration, a factor that can induce fever in all ages. In addition, fever may quickly lead to dehydration in the elderly because cell hydration tends to decline with advancing age. The metabolic cost of fever may use calories the older patient can ill afford to spare.

Neurologically Impaired Patients

Patients who are neurologically impaired cannot respond physiologically and behaviorally to changes in temperature. Unconscious or neurologically impaired patients may lack sensation or awareness of temperature changes. Those with motor deficits may be unable to change positions or adjust clothing to conserve or dissipate heat. Drugs and anesthesia may interrupt both the sensory and motor functions necessary to conserve or generate heat. Awareness of environmental changes and protection from heat loss are anticipatory actions that may prevent loss of thermal balance. Objective measurements of body temperature are crucial in this population to assess thermal status.

Surgical Patients

Patients who undergo surgery are particularly vulnerable to intraoperative heat loss. Normal compensatory warming mechanisms are inactivated by anesthetics, neuromuscular blocking agents, and other drugs. The operative theater is kept cool, primarily for comfort of staff who must work under heavy gowns. Heat is lost by conduction to metal instruments, radiation from the exposed wound or viscera, convection from the laminar flow of air filtering systems, and evaporation from moist skin and mucous membranes. Hypothermic patients may require active rewarming if the heat deficit is great or the patient is neurologically or metabolically compromised. The elderly patient, in particular, has difficulty regaining this heat.

Burn Patients

Patients with burns or other thermal injuries often must deal with temperature problems at both ends of the continuum. First, the injury itself has caused tissue damage by denaturation of cell proteins. Underlying muscle damage may ultimately interfere with behavioral and kinetic activities for heat conservation. Skin loss from the initial burn, or through debridement of the eschar, leaves the patient vulnerable to evaporative heat loss from the moist denuded area. Hypothermia is a threat when large areas of skin are lost. Fever frequently complicates the course of the patient's care because of the inflammatory response to the burn and the patient's vulnerability to infection. Shivering further raises caloric and oxygen expenditure exerted by fever. Continuous temperature measurement and assessment of hydration are essential with the severely burned patient. Dehydration, or shifting of fluid out of the vascular space, may further derange the thermostatic set point. If the patient's thermoregulatory control is severely impaired, temperature may drift either to hypothermic or febrile levels in a poikilothermic state.

Patients with Acute Traumatic Injury

Accident victims, whatever the cause, persons found unconscious, or casualties of environmental disasters should be assessed immediately on admission for alterations in thermal balance. Some of this population suffer hyperthermia from exposure to high temperatures, but by far the most common alteration is hypothermia. Persons who have been found ill or injured outside in the snow or cold are certainly candidates for hypothermia. Less obvious, but no less common, are those who have lain unattended and uncovered on the cold surface of the street or ground while waiting for assistance. Neurological injury, shock, pain, and blood loss contribute to the person's inability to generate or conserve heat. The age and physical condition of the person also add risk factors to the possibility of inadvertent heat loss seen in these situations. The elderly, for example, may suffer significant heat loss if they lie unattended for several hours after a fall, even if it occurs indoors in temperate weather.

ALTERATIONS IN THERMAL BALANCE

Abnormal body temperatures are often, but not always, the first indication of alterations in thermal balance. Temperature measurement alone, taken out of the context of other assessment data, may lead to inappropriate nursing decisions. For example, interventions aimed at cooling a febrile patient may instead promote shivering and further heat production. The choice of intervention in most circumstances depends on the mechanisms leading to the alteration. On the other hand, temperatures above 40° C denature the protein of the brain cells, causing irreversible damage; therefore, action must be aimed at reducing body heat, regardless of the cause.

To avoid confusion, the term *thermal balance* should be used to refer to the status of equilibrium between heat loss and gain. *Alteration in thermal balance* implies no causation (just as alteration in fluid balance does not). As such, the term can be used to describe nearly all patient care problems related to heat loss and gain, whether or not they involve altered thermoregulation. There are a number of situations in which thermoregulatory mechanisms and responses are intact, but cool or warm environmental conditions overcome a weak or debilitated patient's physiological reserves. In fever, body temperature is closely regulated, but at a higher than normal level.[1] Thermoregulatory mechanisms remain intact and actually play a part in driving the body temperature higher.

The term *altered thermoregulation* implies incapability of homeothermic mechanisms to respond to heat gain and loss rather than the actual level of the body temperature. Disorders may affect any part of the delicate balance of sensory input, central integration, and effector systems to regulate body heat. Thermal balance becomes precarious when there is neurological impairment. Cells in the brain and spinal cord are easily damaged by compression, oxygen and glucose deprivation, toxins, and high temperatures. Therefore, loss of hypothalamic control and central regulation may be sequelae of traumatic injury, systemic shock, tumors, ischemia, chemical toxins, or exposure to excessive heat.

Fever: A New Thermostatic Range

Fever, also called *hyperpyrexia*, occurs in response to certain substances called pyrogens. When the pyrogen enters the body, a chain of reactions take place called the *febrile response*. Pyrogens include infectious organisms, toxic drugs, chemical compounds, blood products, neoplastic cells, and foreign bodies. Whatever the offending agent, antigenic properties cause the body to release endogenous fever-inducing factors called cytokines. Cytokines act as intercellular messengers that recruit host defenses.

Altered Set Point

During fever, the thermostatic range of acceptable core temperatures, or set point, is reset at a higher level. As the regulating reference point rises, existing body temperatures are sensed as too cool, and warming mechanisms are activated.

The Febrile Response and Thermoregulatory Function

Compensatory vasoconstriction shifts the warm blood away from the skin to conserve heat, but in doing so causes the skin to feel cool. Shivering generates body heat so that core temperature rises. This phenomenon is known as the *chill phase* of fever, which seems so paradoxical: the shivering patient complains of "freezing to death" as temperatures soar to febrile levels. Core temperature is driven up to the new set point range causing warming mechanisms to subside; the *plateau phase* follows (Figure 14-1). Heat continues to accumulate within the body, eventually exceeding the set point range, so compensatory cooling mechanisms are activated. This *defervescence phase* of fever is often dramatic: the patient throws back bed covers and complains of "burning up," as diaphoresis and vasodilation ensue to allow heat to dissipate to the environment.

Neurochemical Mediators

Much of what is known about the neurochemical basis of fever has been elucidated within the past three decades.[13] The idea that organisms might produce substances that were pyrogenic emerged early in the twentieth century. As early as 1960, these exogenous pyrogens were assumed to have an indirect fever-inducing effect, which triggered release of "true" endogenous mediators of fever derived from the animal's own tissues. Prostaglandins and cyclic nucleotides were implicated as naturally occurring fever mediators in the early 1970s, but the search for the precise mechanisms of fever and the identification of the true definitive endogenous pyrogen still continues.[13]

Potential Benefits

Recent research indicates there may be numerous endogenous pyrogens capable of inducing fever as well as endogenous cryogens which attenuate or limit the extent of fever. Interleukin-1, or a closely related substance, has been identified as a probable endogenous pyrogen. This discovery renews the age-old debate over the beneficial aspects of fever as an immunostimulant. Interleukin-1 is known to stimulate antibody formation and to mobilize lymphocytes in response to antigen or mitogen. Prostaglandins and related cytokines are still thought to be major factors in fever production. Prostaglandin antagonist drugs, such as aspirin, remain mainstays of fever therapy.

Patterns

Fever is a dynamic process, with the unstable set point often rising higher, renewing the cycle of chills, plateau, and defervescence. The tendency for fevers

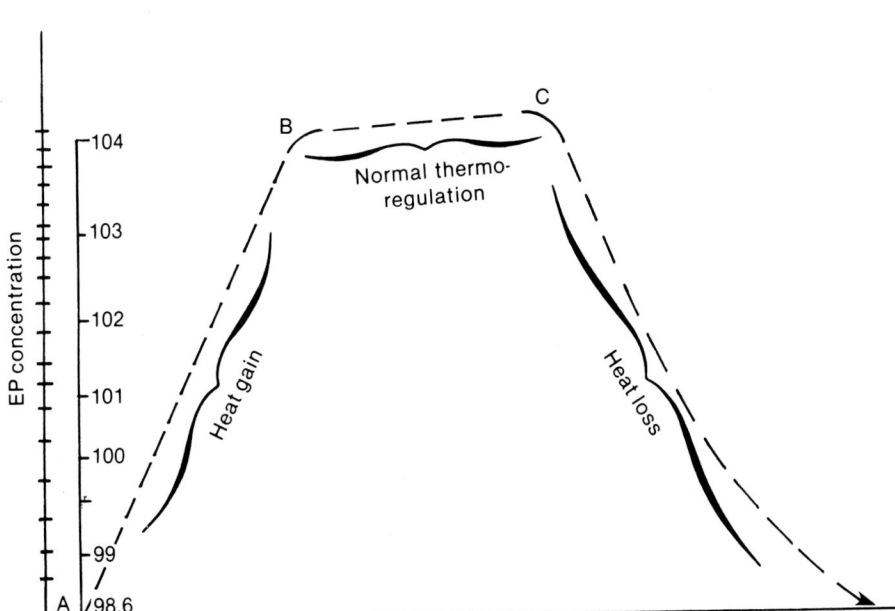

Figure 14-1   Phases of the febrile episode related to endogenous pyrogen (EP) activity on hypothalamic set point. Dotted line from *A* to *B* indicates chill phase during which warming mechanisms are activated to lessen discrepancy between body temperature and set point; from *B* to *C*, the plateau phase during which discrepancy is alleviated; and from *C* to *D*, the defervescence phase during which falling EP or accumulated heat mandates heat loss.

From Groer, M. W., & Shekleton, M. E. (1990). *Basic pathophysiology: A holistic approach* (3rd ed.). St. Louis: Mosby–Year Book.

to "spike" and fall at different times of the day has long provided diagnostic clues. In cases of noninfectious pyrogens, the onset of fever may help to isolate the causative agent. With known pyrogens, the intensity of the febrile response reflects both the potency of the antigen and the sensitivity of the host response. In cases of septicemia or bacteremia, core temperature rises early as organisms release substances into the systemic circulation that trigger the febrile response. Collection of specimens for blood culture are typically aimed at the onset or peak of such a temperature spike, when organisms are most prevalent. Watching patterns in the febrile course assists in evaluating therapy. Fever patterns show effects of antibiotic therapy and help differentiate between and among infectious and noninfectious processes. Naproxen, a nonsteroidal antiinflammatory drug, has been used to rule out neoplastic fever in patients with cancer. Because the drug is ineffective in reducing infectious fevers but is antipyretic in neoplastic fever, it provides a method of differential diagnosis.[14]

Hazards and Complications

Although fever may provide some immunostimulant effects, the response is usually accompanied by a feeling of lassitude. Headache and facial flushing are among the most common subjective symptoms. Shivering contributes to generating higher body heat during the chill phase of fever. The muscular exertion leads to fatigue and is often distressful. Violent febrile shivering, called *rigors,* accompanies therapy with some blood products and drugs. Amphotericin B infusions, for example, induce shivering in 50% to 78% of patients receiving initial treatments. Nursing studies indicate that the incidence and severity of amphotericin B—induced shivering can be reduced by protecting the dominant skin sensors of the hands and feet with insulative wraps.[15] Intravenously administered meperidine and acetaminophen are also used to treat febrile shivering.

Fever increases metabolic rate approximately 13% for each degree Celsius of temperature elevation, with the primary source of heat generation coming from febrile shivering. Vigorous shivering can increase energy expenditure up to 400% above resting levels in healthy subjects. This increase constitutes a major metabolic cost for patients with severe preexisting depletion of body protein stores.

Many infectious fevers appear to be self-limiting, but occasionally central temperatures will exceed 40° C and continue rising. Because neural cells are among the most sensitive to heat, the thermoregulatory centers in the brain become deranged. Therapeutic cooling measures must be instituted before irreversible cellular damage occurs.

Hyperthermia: Impaired Heat Loss Mechanisms

Hyperpyrexia versus Hyperthermia

In fever, thermoregulatory mechanisms function well, but at a higher level. This is not true of *hyperthermia,* which occurs when there is dysfunction of thermoregulatory ability. Hyperthermia occurs when there is injury to the hypothalamus or when a person's heat loss mechanisms are overwhelmed by high environmental heat. With malfunction of the body's control centers, compensatory cooling mechanisms no longer help to eliminate the heat. Central temperatures can rise above 42° C where cellular damage becomes inevitable.

Heat Stroke

One type of hyperthermia is *heat stroke,* which occurs when a person becomes so overheated that the heat-regulating ability of the hypothalamus fails to function.[16] A leading cause of death in athletes, it is also seen in hot humid weather when elderly and debilitated persons have no fans or air conditioning. This type of hyperthermia causes body temperature to rise above 40.6° C and sets in motion a cascade of cellular events that will lead to death if the patient is not treated. Action to cool the patient must be aggressive and may include infusions of cool intravenous fluids, use of cooling blankets, and ice-water immersion. Antipyretic drugs are usually of little value when the patient is hyperthermic. As the hyperthermic person is subjected to cooling treatments, shivering is a common complication that may require treatment with meperidine. Wrapping the hands and feet in insulative wraps prior to placement on a cooling blanket may diminish the severity of shivering during the cooling process.[17]

Malignant Hyperthermia

Malignant hyperthermia (MH) is a hereditary disorder leading to uncontrolled heat generation when affected persons are given potent inhalation anesthetics and most skeletal muscle relaxants. Halothane and methoxyflurane are potent inducers of MH crises, whereas cyclopropane and enflurane are less often involved. It is fortunately rare, occurring in about 1 in 15,000 courses of anesthesia, with males under age 50 or infants of less than 1 year of age most often affected. During an MH crises, the muscle cell membrane becomes unstable. Myoplasmic calcium levels rise, and skeletal muscles develop rigid contractures. While calcium levels remain relatively low in the myoplasm, patients may manifest only fever and acid—base disorders. However, as calcium levels rise, severe muscle rigidity develops. These violent muscle contractions generate heat, which may raise temperatures to 44° C. Irreversible neurological damage and death are inevitable without medical intervention. Death may be related to acute pulmonary edema, impaired coagulopathy, and acidosis.

It is important to recognize that fever may not be the earliest sign.[18] More often, tachycardia or ventricular arrhythmias appear before the onset of muscle rigidity and fever. Respiratory distress and unstable blood pressure are also early signs. Rigidity usually begins in the extremities, jaws, or chest. Management includes restoration of electrolyte and acid–base balance, ventilatory support, and cooling measures. Sympathomimetic drugs further aggravate the myopathy and tissue hypoxia, so they cannot be used to manage the hypotension. Intravenous dantrolene should be given to treat the MH crisis as soon as it is recognized in a patient. Dantrolene acts directly on excitation–contraction coupling and blocks contraction of skeletal muscle. Initially, 1 mg per kg is administered, then repeated as necessary until a total of 10 mg per kg is received.

Acute MH episodes should be suspected if a previously asymptomatic patient develops a dysrhythmia, pulmonary distress, and hypotension after receiving an anesthetic. Persons with possible hereditary links to the disease should be tested before receiving anesthesia. Susceptible persons with the disorder should carry medical identification with them to warn caregivers should the need for emergency surgery arise.

Induced Hyperthermia

Induced hyperthermia for cancer treatment is an emerging modality, although the idea is not new. High temperatures were known to have an inhibitory effect on some infectious organisms. Patients were sometimes inoculated with fever-producing organisms to cause temperature elevations before the advent of effective antimicrobial drugs. "Fever boxes" were used to combat the spirochete that causes syphilis. By raising body temperature to levels incompatible with cell metabolism, the newer modalities are aimed at metastatic and nonmetastatic tumors. Microwaves are used for either regional or whole-body hyperthermia, and the treatment is often combined with other ionizing radiation and pH-altering drugs. The patient is supported during the treatment to avoid injury to vital body cells, but long-term consequences following induced hyperthermia need further exploration.

Hypothermia: Profound Heat Loss

Stages and Correlates

The term *hypothermia* is used to describe a range of conditions from mild to profound (Table 14-1). When profound heat loss occurs for a prolonged pe-

TABLE 14-1   **Levels of Hypothermia and Corresponding Clinical Changes**

Level	Core Temperature
Mild	32° to 37° C
Moderate	28° to 32° C
Deep	17° to 28° C
Profound	<17° C

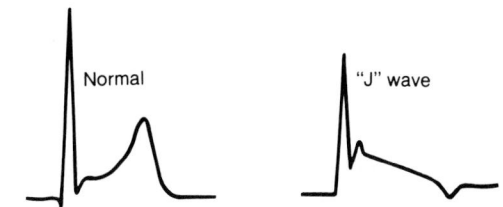

Figure 14-2   The Osborn, or "J" wave, is pathognomonic of hypothermia. It is seen in lead V_4 at junction of QRS complex and ST segment.

riod, vasoconstriction and shivering eventually become ineffective in generating or recovering sufficient heat to regain that being lost. This is why a cooling blanket will eventually reduce the febrile patient's core temperature, despite compensatory shivering and vasoconstriction. At brain temperatures below 20° C, thermoregulatory ability is suppressed, and the person becomes poikilothermic. Lacking thermoregulatory ability, body temperature is governed by environmental conditions. Initially, the heart rate, cardiac output, and mean arterial pressure rise, while the amplitude of ECG signals fall. Shivering begins, with a compensatory rise in respiratory rate and oxygen consumption. Urine flow increases, and cold diuresis continues into moderate hypothermia.

As cooling progresses, the patient becomes hemodynamically unstable. When the patient reaches a core temperature of about 31° C, neurological signs include confusion and stupor, exaggerated tendon reflex, and hyperactivity. Heart rate declines and ECG abnormalities increase, hastened by poor oxygenation. Premature ventricular beats are common throughout cooling. The humplike Osborn wave, also called the *J wave*, is seen in lead V_4 at the junction of the QRS complex and ST segment and is pathognomonic of hypothermia (Figure 14-2). Because the J wave is detected in only about a third of hypothermic patients,[19] its absence should not rule out the diagnosis. Below 28° C, atrial fibrillation and other dysrhythmias are common. The patient is unconscious and apneic with an absence of neurological reflexes. At about 10° C, the QRS disappears, and only the P wave persists. Blood viscosity increases as temperature falls and with cold-induced diuresis contributes to the sludging and coagulopathy during hypothermia. Acid—base changes are often dynamic, reflecting initial alkalosis from overventilation and diuresis and progressive acidosis from pooled circulation and shivering-induced lactic acid.

Situations Leading to Hypothermia

Inadvertent or accidental *hypothermia* occurs frequently when people suffer exposure in mountainous, cold, or snowy climates. It is seen increasingly in emergency rooms during winter among the elderly or debilitated, homeless persons without shelter, persons found unconscious from alcohol intoxication, and accident victims. Although remarkable recoveries of hypothermic patients have been reported in healthy persons, survival is less likely when hypothermia accompanies severe trauma.[19] If core temperature falls below 32° C, survival of the trauma patient may be impossible. In hospitals, neonates and patients undergoing surgery are at risk for inadvertent hypothermia. Immature thermoregulatory systems or the effects of neuromuscular blocking drugs and anesthesia combine with environmental conditions that promote heat loss. Thin fatty insulation, weak musculature, and reduced metabolic rate also predispose patients to hypothermia.

Preventive measures are aimed at conserving heat during patient transport and surgical procedures. During surgery, heated blankets, warming vests, caps, leggings and plastic hoods, reflective drapes, and heated humidified inspired gases are among the measures used to conserve heat. Conductive and convective warming blankets, radiant lights, and warmed humidified gases are employed in the postoperative recovery area to restore lost heat.

Induced hypothermia is a treatment modality used to reduce elevated temperatures in fever and hyperthermia, or to reduce body temperature to subnormal levels during operative procedures. During cardiac surgery and neurosurgical procedures, deep and profound hypothermia is induced to reduce cell metabolism and oxygen demand. Heat is removed as the patient's blood is circulated through the heat exchanger in the cardiopulmonary bypass pump. Close supervision and drug management allow the anesthetized patient to tolerate deep hypothermia surprisingly well during the surgical procedure. At the end of the surgical procedure, the patient is rewarmed by the bypass pump heat exchanger, but owing to the differences in regional heat capacities throughout the body, heat is poorly distributed. By the time many patients are returned to the recovery unit, they are hypothermic. This is a period of great hemodynamic instability made more difficult by compensatory warming mechanisms. As effects of anesthetic drugs and muscle relaxants diminish, shivering and vasoconstriction increase metabolic rate and oxygen consumption. Cardiac output, heart rate, and blood pressure increase in response to the sympathetic activity and increased muscle activity. Lactic acid accumulates from shivering muscles. Return of pooled blood from cold unperfused regions brings fixed acids and metabolites that contribute to acidosis.

Shivering

Intravenously administered meperidine is used to suppress shivering in the rewarming cardiac surgery patient, although tremors often persist until euthermic temperatures return.[20] Neuromuscular blocking agents may be used to maintain the paralyzed state until the patient is euthermic in some cases.

Thermal Instability

During induction and recovery from hypothermia, thermal instability is common. Nurses should be alert to several conditions that complicate this period. *Drift* may result when skin temperatures are cooled or warmed rapidly by artificial or environmental means. Drift refers to the tendency for core temperatures to follow skin temperatures rapidly when thermoregulatory reflexes are compromised and in patients with poor muscle and vascular tone. Changes may exceed 1° C in 15 minutes.[17] *Afterfall,* or the tendency for core temperature to continue falling after cooling procedures are discontinued, poses a serious threat to the hypothermic patient. When thermoregulatory activity is suppressed, heat continues to flow from the body's deep regions to the cooler periphery. If afterfall is undetected and untreated, temperatures may fall below 30° C. *Overshoot* is a problem that occurs during rewarming when regulatory mechanisms rebound or overcompensate. Vigorous shivering and profound vasoconstriction may cause core temperatures to rise to febrile levels.

NURSING MANAGEMENT

■ NURSING DIAGNOSIS

Nursing assessment and diagnosis of alterations in thermal balance must include considerations of the patient's physiological status, psychological responses, and medical regimen. Goals of appropriate nursing actions are determined in the context of underlying physiological dynamics and the plan of medical and pharmacological treatment. In each situation, the origin of the alteration should be defined by answering the following questions:

Is the alteration induced to achieve a therapeutic goal, as in hypothermia or hyperthermia?

Is the alteration pathological and secondary to other predisposing conditions?

If the alteration is pathological, what are the therapeutic goals?

What nursing actions will support therapeutic goals while minimizing adverse effects to the patient?

The physiological processes and dynamics of heat transfer, described earlier, provide a basis for understanding the changing condition of the patient. They also help explain why and how specific interventions can assist a patient in gaining or losing heat. Important points related to the origin of the physiological alteration and the goals of nursing and medical management for the conditions of fever, hyperthermia, and hypothermia are outlined in Table 14-2.

The critical care nurse plays a vital role in assisting patients to maintain thermal balance that exceeds vigilant monitoring and execution of medical measures.

TABLE 14-2 **Relationships between Physiological Alterations and Therapeutic Goals**

	Fever	Hyperthermia	Hypothermia
Physiological Alteration	"Set point" elevated by pyrogen. Thermoregulatory ability intact. Thermoregulation may become impaired if temperature rises above 40° C. Shivering, vasoconstriction, and hypermetabolic activity warm body to febrile level. Diaphoresis phase cools the body.	Hypothalamic injury or high environmental temperature overwhelms ability to lose heat. Impaired thermoregulation.	Low environmental temperature overwhelms ability to conserve and generate heat. Eventually impairs thermoregulation. Can occur in temperate climate if thermoregulation impaired by hypothalamic injury, drugs, or alcohol.
Therapeutic Goals and Medical Management	Stabilize set point through hydration and prostaglandin-inhibiting drugs. Maintain central temperature below 40° C. Antimicrobial therapy, if indicated.	Actively lower body temperature by surface cooling or central heat exchange. Restore central temperature to below 40° C. Sometimes iced IV fluids and immersion in ice water are used. Antipyretic drugs usually ineffective.	Slowly restore body heat. Have cardiac support ready. At 27° to 30° C, danger of dysrhythmias from cardiac irritability. CPR can intensify it so is avoided except in apnea, ventricular fibrillation, or cardiac arrest. More aggressive rewarming is possible in special care units with cardiac care support, where central heat exchanger, microwave-warmed fluids, and warm humidified airway rewarming are used.
Nursing Care	Adapt coverings and environmental temperature to phase of the febrile episode: wraps when chilling; light, dry clothing during diaphoresis. Avoid drafts, sudden changes in room temperature. Avoid cool baths and fans that may lead to shivering unless rising temperature impairs thermoregulation.	Wrap hands and feet with insulative material prior to placement on hypothermia cooling blanket to diminish shivering stimulus as temperature falls. Watch for temperature drift or afterfall. Shivering also significantly increases oxygen consumption, so watch for adequate oxygenation during cooling.	Shivering will occur during rewarming. Radiant heat to reduce skin stimulus for shivering. Slower rewarming makes skin-to-core gradients less abrupt and creates less shivering stimulus. Observe closely for temperature drift until euthermia is restored. As thermoregulatory mechanisms return, watch for temperature overshoot to febrile levels.

First, the nurse must remain abreast of new advances and therapies related to thermoregulation through constant inquiry and reappraisal of knowledge. With supportive environmental and protective measures, the nurse helps those at risk avoid the physiological burden of thermal changes. Effective nursing assessment is based on understanding the dynamic nature of thermal balance with surveillance for potential as well as actual alterations. Reasoned judgment is essential in interpreting thermal events early in their course, so intervention can forestall or alleviate more serious sequelae. Finally, the nurse in critical care can be an active participant in the quest for new knowledge about thermal balance. As investigators, consultants, and participants in research studies, nurses continue to find new information and test interventions that address this important dimension of care.

REFERENCES

1. Guyton, A. C. (Ed.). (1991). Body temperature, temperature regulation and fever. In *Textbook of Medical Physiology* (8th ed.) (pp. 797-808). Philadelphia: Saunders.
2. Darnall, R. A. (1987). The thermophysiology of the newborn infant. *Medical Instrumentation, 21*(1), 16-22.
3. Reinberg, A., Smolensky, M. (1990). Chronobiology and thermoregulation. In E. Schonbaum, & P. Lomax (Eds.), *Thermoregulation: Physiology and biochemistry* (pp. 61-94). New York: Pergamon.
4. Hemingway, A. (1963). Shivering. *Physiological Reviews, 43*, 397-422.
5. Black, W. Z., & Hartley, J. G. (1985). Thermodynamics (pp. 1-21). New York: Harper & Row.
6. Kleinebeckel, D., & Klussmann, F. W. (1990). Shivering. In E. Schonbaum, & P. Lomax (Eds.), *Thermoregulation: Physiology and biochemistry* (pp. 235-253). New York: Pergamon.
7. Earp, J. K., & Finlayson, D. C. (1991). Relationships between urinary bladder and pulmonary artery temperatures: A preliminary study. *Heart Lung, 20*(3), 265-270.
8. Erickson, R. S., & Yount, S. T. (1991). Comparison of tympanic and oral temperatures in surgical patients. *Nursing Research, 40*(2), 90-93.
9. Shinozaki, T., Deane, R., & Perkins, F. M. (1988). Infrared tympanic thermometer: Evaluation of a new clinical thermometer. *Critical Care Medicine, 16*, 148-150.
10. Terndrup, T. E., Allegra, J. R., & Kealy, J. A. (1989). A comparison of oral, rectal, and tympanic membrane-derived temperature changes after ingestion of liquids and smoking. *American Journal of Emergency Medicine, 7*, 150-154.
11. Abbey, J. C., Anderson, A. S., Close, E. L., et al. (1978). How long is that thermometer accurate? *American Journal of Nursing, 78*(8), 1375-1376.
12. Morrison, R. C. (1988). Hypothermia in the elderly. *International Anesthesiology Clinics, 26*, 124-133.
13. Kluger, M. J. (1991). Fever: Role of pyrogens and cryogens. *Physiological Reviews, 71*(1), 93-127.
14. Chang, J. C. (1987). How to differentiate neoplastic fever from infectious fever in patients with cancer: Usefulness of the naproxen test. *Heart Lung, 16*(2), 122-127.
15. Holtzclaw, B. J. (1990). Effects of extremity wraps to control drug induced shivering: A pilot study. *Nursing Research, 39*(5), 280-283.
16. Groer, M. W., & Shekleton, M. E. (1990). *Basic pathophysiology: A holistic approach* (3rd ed.). St. Louis: Mosby.
17. Abbey, J. C., Andrews, C., Avigliano, K., et al. (1973). A pilot study: The control of shivering during hypothermia by a clinical nursing measure. *Journal of Neurosurgical Nursing, 5*(2), 78-88.
18. Britt, B. A. (1984). Malignant hyperthermia: A pharmacogenetic disease of skeletal and cardiac muscle [Editorial]. *New England Journal of Medicine, 290*, 1140.
19. Jurkovich, G. J. (1989). Hypothermia in the trauma patient. *Advances in Trauma, 4*, 111-140.
20. Holtzclaw, B. J., & Geer, R. T. (1986). Shivering after heart surgery: Assessment of metabolic effects. *Anesthesiology, 85*(3A), A18.

15

Communication

Catherine Nuss Kotecki

Sensitive and individualized verbal and nonverbal communication with the critically ill patient is a major method for bringing the art of healing into the highly scientific intensive care setting.[1]

The art of nursing is founded, in part, on excellent communication between nurse and patient. Virginia Henderson described the art of nursing as being able to get into the patient's skin and to know and feel what he does, in order to better care for him.[2] The art of nursing includes caring about a patient, recognizing the patient's individuality and humanity, and assisting the patient to derive meaning from disease and illness. In critical care nursing, especially, the art of nursing is realized in the processes and skills of communication.

Many juxtapositions occur in critical care nursing today. The need for family and significant other involvement in care is contrasted with legal–ethical issues and patients' rights. As the influence of technology increases, so does its dehumanizing effect. Ethical dilemmas arise because technology has taken patients where they may not have intended to go. The communication process is a key to making informed care decisions, exploring human and moral decision making, and increasing human interaction in the critical care unit.

Communication is not just talking to the patient. It includes listening and responding to patients' cues, permitting them to lead the conversation, and directing them through areas of informational conversation. The goal of communication is the formulation of a plan of care for the patient that will improve the individual's outcomes. Effective communication in the critical care unit assists the person to place a potentially life-changing event in perspective. Effective communication also assists patients in making their needs known. In the face of physical disability, the nurse directs the patient to alternative channels of communication so that self-expression is not lost.

It has been shown that nurses and patients have a physical reaction to each other, as well as a psycho-logical reaction. Researchers from the University of Maryland have looked at patient–staff interactions with respect to a variety of physiological responses. One study reviewed patients' cardiac responses to interviews in a coronary care unit.[3] Patient reaction to being interviewed by the nurse varied, but the heart rate always changed in response to the interview. In 12 of the 19 patients, the heart rate increased significantly from preinterview levels. The postinterview heart rate was lower in 6 of the 19 patients. Moreover, the patient's heart rate decreased when the nurse spoke and increased when the patient spoke.

This study supported earlier findings that the mere act of speaking influences a patient's heart rate and blood pressure. The authors concluded, "In a series of studies, we have shown that a subject's verbal activity, the content of communication, status of the interviewer, and the content of the immediate social environment can all interact to produce rapid and highly significant shifts in blood pressure and heart rate in both normotensive and hypertensive subjects."[3]

Nurses and patients make an impression on each other. Communication is encouraged by positive nonverbal cues, by asking appropriate questions, encouraging patients to continue, mirroring what is said, and observing and following a patient's cues. In a study of nurse–patient interaction on a general nursing unit, nurses were found to block attempts at communication more than they encouraged it. They did so by asking closed or leading questions; missing or recognizing, but responding negatively to direct or indirect cues; use of cliché; maintaining superficiality; changing the subject; and avoidance.[4]

ACHIEVING EFFECTIVE COMMUNICATION

Effective communication in the critical care unit can be realized in three kinds of outcomes: (1) improved patient outcomes, (2) improved family–staff relationships, and (3) more satisfying staff–staff relationships. Research has demonstrated the relationship between positive communication strategies and improved patient outcomes in a variety of clinical areas. For example, Owens and Hutelmeyer[5] tested the hypothesis that patients who are educated pre-operatively about the possibility of unusual sensory or cognitive experiences will either not have such ex-periences or will feel more comfortable, or more in control of the experiences, if they do occur. The au-thors concluded that, when patients are supplied with information about what to expect and how to deal with it, they are better able to cope. The authors further stress that nurses need communication skills to elicit responses from patients.

The reduction of anxiety when a patient is trans-ferred out of the coronary care unit can also be linked to nursing interventions that have communication as a consideration. Schwartz and Brenner[6] examined the effectiveness of specific nursing interventions in re-ducing stress associated with coronary care unit trans-fer. They found that either communication with the nurse from the step-down unit, or the patient's family involvement in the transfer period, was a factor in reducing transfer stress. Overall, the patients in the experimental group who received information about their transfer—either from the nurse or from family members—scored lower in stress as reported by pa-tient, family, and nurse, and had fewer cardiovascular complications after transfer.

Positive outcomes of communication in the critical care unit are also related to the nurse's ability to influence a patient's care through family involvement. The family of the critically ill patient was initially identified as a source of stress for intensive care nurses.[7,8] Later, both positive and negative factors were identified regarding family involvement in the critical care unit. One positive factor, a source of satisfaction for the critical care nurse, was the devel-opment of a relationship between the nurse and the patient's family. Knowing more about the patient made it more rewarding to provide care.[8]

Other researchers[9] found that patients' interactions with family or friends were no more stressful than patients' interactions with the staff. Nursing staff members further discovered that they were able to direct the families' perception of the CCU experience to a more positive light through the use of interven-tion that alleviated anxiety related to a lack of infor-mation.[10,11,12]

Research has also been directed toward determin-ing the needs of families of critically ill patients. The thought is that, once the families' needs are met, they will be better able to help their loved ones cope with their illnesses.[13,14,15] Communicating with patients' families is now considered an important and positive part of the critical care nurse's role. Chapter 17 dis-cusses the role of families in critical care.

Discord in interpersonal relationships among staff members and between nursing staff, physicians, and administration is frequently cited as the greatest source of job-related stress in critical care.[16,17] One study cited patient care as the most stressful factor, followed by the environment, the patient's family, administration, and interaction with other critical care nurses.[18] The use of good interpersonal relation-ships and communication skills among the staff can ease some of the stress and tension that arise from working in a critical care unit.

COMMUNICATION CHALLENGES IN CRITICAL CARE

The special nature of the environment of the crit-ical care unit and the relationships among people in that environment lead to three assumptions about communications:

1. Time pressure means that interactions between nurse and patient must occur in a compressed framework.
2. Critical illness caused by physiological compro-mise alters, interferes with, or destroys the pa-tient's usual pathway of communication.
3. The nursing interview, the traditional starting point of the nurse–patient relationship, is not a practical vehicle for communication in the critical care setting.

Time is a governing factor in the critical care nurse's day. The nurse has a tremendous responsi-bility for communicating with patients because no extended, gradual time to develop the nurse–patient relationship is available. Very often, important in-formation is gathered between tests or treatments. This may also be the only time available to talk with the patient and give comfort or support. A frequent nursing dilemma is how to conduct an interview with a patient who wants to discuss concerns, with time limiting what can be discussed.

Making the most of every patient interaction is crucial. The need for sensitive care that realizes the patient's needs and yet incorporates the nurse's need for information makes communication in critical care especially challenging. Skilled communication tech-niques that elicit the patient's feelings and assist the acceptance of feelings and discussion of concerns en-compass and transcend the traditional nursing inter-view. The nurse who can compress these skills into the fast, demanding pace of the critical care unit is justified in saying that the art of critical care nursing is being practiced.

The physiological status of critically ill patients frequently prohibits communication along usual pathways. Patients who are intubated or neurologi-cally compromised are frequently unable to speak. This situation, coupled with time pressure, presents a challenge for communication. The nurse who has alternative methods of communication ready to use greatly assists the patient in making needs known.

COMMUNICATION MODELS

Communication is the imparting or sharing of information, messages, feelings, and experience through signs, speech, gestures, touch, or writing. The sharing of ourselves with one another on levels ranging from the cursory to the intimate may well be unique to humans. A framework of communication in critical care nursing that reflects the diversity of nurses and their patients can be derived from different sources.

Systems Model

A systems model is a generic way of looking at communication between individuals.[19] This model utilizes general systems terminology. The sender, receiver, and message are ultimately influenced by the channel, which includes the environment and distractions in the environment, and results in feedback.[20] The following is an example of how a critical care nurse could use a communication model that is based on a systems framework. When the nurse meets a patient for the first time, he or she waits to see what the patient will say and do, then evaluates the verbal and nonverbal messages and decides how to interact with the patient. Depending on the content and context of the message, as well as nonverbal cues, the nurse formulates a response to the patient, sends his or her own message, and thereby completes the interaction.

In this example, the nurse is the recipient of the message and the stimulus for the message to occur. The patient is the sender of the message. The channel is the way in which the message is sent: orally, in writing, or in nonverbal anger. Communication is influenced by environmental factors such as noise, other people, and lack of privacy in the critical care unit. Characteristics of successful communication, based on a systems model approach, are presented in the box to the right.

Nursing Theory

Nurse theorists recognize that the process of communicating is central to the human experience. They focus on the specific communication of the nurse and patient. Peplau[2] saw the nurse–patient interaction as the key element of nursing. Within the nurse–patient relationship is a mutuality that legitimizes growth in the nurse as well as the patient. Through the process of mutuality, the patient and nurse establish care goals and move together to meet those goals. Personal interactions are seen as "educative." The nurse–patient relationship is viewed as a therapeutic relationship with elements that distinguish it from a social

> ### Characteristics of Successful Communication in a Systems Model[25]
>
> - The sender and receiver have the physical, intellectual, and perceptual ability to receive, analyze, and send messages.
> - The relationship between the sender and receiver affects the communication process.
> - The receiver attends to the message that the sender initiates.
> - Both verbal and nonverbal communication is used.
> - Nonverbal behavior is consistent with verbal communication.
> - The sender and receiver have similar meanings for words.
> - The message sent is appropriate to the context of the communication and is complete.
> - The timing of the message is appropriate to the content and the context.
> - Feedback is relevant to the persons and context, clearly stated, and appropriately timed.
> - The sender has the opportunity and is able to correct the information/message.
> - Both the sender and receiver are affirmed and gratified by the communication.

relationship. This relationship is also described as unique.

Much like Peplau, King describes a process of interaction that leads to goal setting between the nurse and the patient. Assumptions of King's Goal Attainment Theory include the recognition of the humanity and worth of the individual and the importance of patient involvement in the care process. Both Peplau's and King's models require that a patient be able to participate fully in the care regimen.[2] Therefore, the patient must be aware and alert. The participation of every critical care patient is difficult to achieve. The person who has experienced neurological trauma, shock, or cardiovascular collapse cannot collaborate in mutual goal setting. However, patients who have experienced myocardial infarction, coronary artery bypass surgery, or angioplasty are likely to benefit from use of the Peplau or King model of communication.

Martha Rogers' unique Science of Unitary Man may be useful for patients in the critical care unit who are not conscious or aware of their surroundings. In Rogers' model, communication occurs through the nurse and patient's intermingling energy fields: dynamic wave patterns that change frequency and can operate in physical, social, psychological or biological domains.[21] Therapeutic touch is a communication strategy that can be explained by a transference in energy fields. As described by MacRae, communication through the transference of energy in the process of therapeutic touch can promote a feeling of well-being and facilitate healing.[22]

Technological Caring

Caring is proposed as the essence of nursing and a framework in which all nurse–patient interactions must operate. Watson defines caring as the "moral ideal of nursing, whereby the end is protection, enhancement, and preservation of human dignity."[23] Caring is a concept that can be applied to all nurse–patient situations. Caring is imperative in the critical care setting to override the influence of and dependence on technology that dehumanizes individuals.

Technological caring is a model of care proposed by Ray.[24] It emphasizes the integral part of communication in the caring process and encompasses the concerns of today's critical care nurse. Ray used a phenomenological research approach and asked nurses to answer the question, "What is the meaning of human care and the experience of caring for me as a nurse and for my patient?" Five themes of human care experiences were raised by the eight nurses interviewed:

1. The experience of caring in the critical care unit is a process of growth.
2. Technical achievement is one of the meanings of being a critical care nurse.
3. Giving and receiving is the bonding process in nursing.
4. Being with the patient and family and one another is communication and community.
5. The experience of conflict is in ethical decisions that must be made.[24]

These themes of caring include communication in practice, through technology, and in ethical decision making as a part of the critical care nurse's role.

The importance of communication with the critically ill patient is found in many models and theories of nursing. Each critical care nurse has a personal view of communication with patients that must be explored, developed, and refined in order to communicate effectively with the critically ill patient.

CASE STUDY

Mr. V. is a 70-year-old white male with recurrent ventricular tachycardia. Most recently, he has been in the CCU with congestive heart failure and ventricular tachycardia. He had been home only 48 hours when he was admitted to the cardiovascular step-down unit with angina. After stabilization of pain and vital signs, his demeanor was one of alertness, apprehension, and vigilance. The vigilant look was noticed by the primary nurse. When asked how he was feeling, Mr. V. responded that he felt fine: no chest pain, palpitations, or shortness of breath. The nurse responded by telling Mr. V. that the expression on his face showed anxiety. Was

something upsetting Mr. V. that he wished to talk about? Mr. V. expressed concern that he was in the "step-down" unit. He explained that this meant to him he was "going down hill," "down for the count," and he would soon be "down and out." After Mr. V. explained his perception of what the step-down unit meant to him, the astute nurse was able to explain what it means to be in the step-down unit. The nurse also reviewed Mr. V.'s therapies, treatment goals, and progress and was able to offer encouragement and support.

In this example, the nurse is alerted to a miscommunication by the incongruities of the patient's facial expression and verbal message. When the patient states he is fine, the nurse determines that he is not fine, but in fact is extremely upset. From the perspective of a systems model, the nurse realizes that verbal and nonverbal messages must be congruent if effective communication is to take place, and that the sender and the receiver must have the same meaning of words. The nurse interacts with the patient until Mr. V. realizes the true meaning of the step-down unit, what his course of treatment is, and what his outcomes are projected to be.

COMMUNICATION IN THE CRITICAL CARE SETTING
Personal Communication

In the previous section, broad models of communication were presented. The pivotal point in the process of communication is the individual nurse–patient interaction. Much of what comes out of this interaction is directly influenced by the nurse. Research in different clinical settings strongly suggests that it is the nurse who initiates, directs, and controls the communication process.[4,25,26,27,28] If the nurse approaches the encounter with a jocular and humorous approach, it is likely that the patient will respond in kind. Likewise, if the nurse is businesslike, the patient will also be businesslike.

Skilled communication is required in each of the many roles of the critical care nurse: advocate, patient educator, clinician, and coordinator of care. In the critical care environment, the nurse also serves as an interpreter to patients, family, and even hospital staff.

Lubbers and Ray[29] identify the essential skills in interpersonal communication as listening, instructing, interviewing, motivating, advising, and giving feedback. Communication activities given first priority by health care personnel include listening, routine information exchange, management of conflict, small group work, and instructing.[29] Listening is an important skill, since research shows nurses to be in control of the communication process. The listening ability of the nurse is crucial to the ability of the patient to communicate needs, yet time to listen to the patient is frequently not available in the fast-paced critical care environment. Therefore, the critical care nurse must be very attentive, making time to explore the meaning of what the patient is expressing.

The communication skills of nurses may be influenced by personality type. The work of Carl Jung[30] suggests this relationship. Personality includes a characteristic orientation to people in general, and this orientation directs communication. Interactions between people of complementary personality types may be more satisfying than interactions between people whose personality differs.

Psychologist Karen Horney developed three classifications of people based on their interpersonal response traits: (1) moving toward others, (2) moving against others, and (3) moving away from others. According to Horney's system, the person who moves toward others seeks approval and affection from others. This person has a strong need to be loved and accepted. One significant person is the focus of the person's attention and trust. Persons who engage in behavior that is described as going against others have a hostile or aggressive communication style and need to exert control over their surroundings. Such a person will look at situations from the point of benefits to self. The person whose orientation is moving away from others is emotionally detached and removed from people. This person is self-sufficient and has a great need for privacy. Three questions exemplify these three interpersonal styles. The person who moves toward others asks, "Will they like me?" The person who goes against others asks, "How can I use others?" The person who moves away from others asks, "Will I be bothered?"[31]

The communicating strategy of the critical care nurse must consider personal communication skills and styles of self, patients, and family. The nurse should ask family and patients open-ended questions that reflect concerns related to the current situation. The nurse must follow up on patient responses with more than reflective technique. Finally, critical care nurses have the responsibility to evaluate their own personal style of communication and to improve and expand their effectiveness. Critical care nurses can strengthen their communication ability by asking themselves questions such as: "Have I made time during my shift to talk with my patients about their needs, feelings, and concerns?", "Did I allow patients and family members time to finish their statements before responding?", and "Did I use open-ended questions and follow with appropriate probing?"

Communication Barriers

Two barriers to communication in the critical care setting are identified by critical care nurses: language and culture. The diversity of ethnic groups within the hospital necessitate an awareness of cultural diversity and a plan to overcome language barriers.

Language

Language is the channel in which messages are sent and received. Language may be made unintelligible by a physiological barrier such as aphasia or a cultural barrier such as language differences. When this happens, communication does not occur, or occurs at a severely limited level. The cultural barrier of different languages may be frustrating and time-consuming at the least and life-threatening at worst. Most patients appreciate any attempt on the nurse's part to understand or speak the language. If the nurse does not have a working knowledge of the patient's language and it is a common one in the area, the hospital system should be providing interpreters. Perhaps the single major factor that should be considered in caring for patients who do not speak English is that more time will be needed to provide nursing care.

Interpreters working in the critical care area should be specifically trained to translate for patients and their families. Interpreters should know basic policy information about the unit, such as visiting hours and the availability of other patient and family services. Translating is more than interpreting what a person has said. When translators are used, the nurse still directs the conversation along therapeutic lines. Factors that are important to consider when patient interpretation occurs are: tone of voice, the use of jargon, semantics, or polishing of phrases that may alter or change the patient's meaning; and the importance of anecdotal information in relation to the patient's health problem. A final factor to consider is that a person who speaks English as a second language may lose that ability when stressed by a critical illness.[32]

A patient's privacy and confidentiality are difficult to maintain when visitors, housekeeping, or dietary aides are pressed into service as translators. Family members are usually not trained in medical language or translating techniques and, although convenient, they may not be appropriate interpreters in certain situations. The nurse also must be sensitive to cultural variations regarding who is privileged to be spokesperson for the family. Although a younger daughter may have a good command of English, if the oldest brother is spokesperson, the nurse should make every attempt to communicate with him or at least obtain his consent to talk with others of lesser stature in the family. This is particularly true in Asian cultures where age is accorded a high measure of respect.

Language barriers can be largely overcome through the use of skilled interpreters and an understanding of how language is translated. When translators are not available, or a patient speaks a little-known language, the nurse may press others into service to obtain information about the patient's language and culture. Sources of information about language include the hospital medical library, social services, and community-based organizations. Written material with basic information about the critical care unit may assist some patients and families in determining what is occurring. Audiotapes in the person's language will also be helpful.[33] Without written or spoken language communication, gestures and facial expressions may be the only available means to communicate with the patient. Demonstration is helpful in teaching respiratory techniques. Small-scale models of hospital equipment may help the patient relate hygiene needs to the nurse with minimal effort. Ingenuity and resourcefulness on the part of the nurse will facilitate communication and provide access to important patient information.

The scientific language that health care professionals use within the hospital setting constitutes a foreign language—complete with symbols and abbreviations. Many common or basic medical terms are misunderstood, misconstrued, or misinterpreted by the general public. In a study of public understanding of medical terms, lack of understanding of the following terms was found to exist: virus, strep throat, herpes, tumor, Pap smear, and uterus.[34] Patients who were elderly, uneducated, or lacking in medical background were identified as being less able to define terms correctly. Women had as much difficulty as men in their understanding of the terms "uterus" and "Pap smear." The educational level of the person proved to be the strongest indication of knowledge. Multiple misconceptions and interpretations of phrases commonly used in the hospital were found to exist. Interpretation of the phrase, "It will only hurt a little," varied from a "quick pinch" to "will hurt a lot." One way to bridge misconceptions is to use the person's own language and terminology when possible, and to repeat information in different ways.

Culture

Culture is the reference point or orientation that shapes and guides our beliefs, actions, and reactions to others and the environment around us. "Communication is the medium by which our cultural heritage is maintained, conveyed, and translated as time passes. From this point of view, culture should invite, arouse, and excite the curious individual to seek out and discover the ways in which his own culture is expressed."[19] When two people from different cultures communicate, the understanding that there is no "right" or "wrong" culture facilitates the communication process. Ethnocentric behavior or attitudes prevail when one believes the only "correct" culture is one's own. Ethnocentric health care professionals look down their noses at health care practices

and ideas that are not in line with modern western medical thinking. When this message is conveyed to patients and their families, the communication barrier widens. Patients or families may withhold information important to optimum health because they fear ridicule or embarrassment.

Cultural relativism is an attempt to understand each cultural trait in relation to a whole culture without being critical of the trait or culture. The nurse who practices cultural relativism does not pass judgments on cultural health care practices but instead tries to create a bridge between the patient's cultural system and modern medicine to ensure optimal health for the patient.[35]

Additionally, a patient may combine the practices of different cultures. For example, an Asian patient may be hospitalized and submit to western medical practices, such as medications, diagnostic testing, and oxygen therapy, while still using herbal medicine, acupuncture, and hot and cold foods to supplement the medical regimen. The blending of healing practices from the old and new cultures to treat critical illness requires skill and discernment on the part of the nurse.[36]

The elements of a culture having the greatest significance for nursing may include (1) family organization; (2) care during birth, sickness, and death; (3) age- and sex-related values; (4) language; (5) time orientation; (6) sleep and hygiene habits; (7) modesty; (8) communication of satisfaction and dissatisfaction; (9) value of personal accomplishment; (10) food habits; and (11) religious orientation. In complex societies such as our own, people do not share a common culture, even if we share a common language. The term "cultural scene" may be helpful in determining cultural variations within a large, complex society.[37] Thus, certain of the previously mentioned cultural elements may characterize one cultural scene, while other elements may predominate in another.

Emotional reactions to critical illness and their expression may be based on cultural variables such as ethnic origins, religious orientation, socioeconomic status, or geographic location. Coping mechanisms used during past crisis situations or what the patient feels are expected emotions at a particular time also influence how emotion is displayed in critical care. Stereotyping of a patient's emotions based on ethnic origin is not accurate since a person's emotions are based on many variables. The nurse who does not "expect" patients or families to emote in a certain way can do much to facilitate communication as each set of emotions is viewed in light of the circumstance or context in which it occurs. When inappropriate emotion is perceived, the nurse may well explore why the emotion is occurring, the feeling behind it, and the person's perception of the occurrence before "labeling" it as inappropriate.

Cultural biases begin to emerge as territory and personal space are chosen and defined. Because of the status accorded to health care workers, nurses are offered frequent and easy access to a person's intimate space. *Intimate distance* of space occurs within 18 inches of two people. Touch, the feel of one's breath, and body odors are exchanged within this distance. Personal space is the extension of ourselves to the point where we feel comfortable interacting with others. The extent of personal space may depend on how one feels about the person with whom one is communicating. Additionally, personal space and intimate distances are culturally influenced with people from some cultures feeling very comfortable interacting in close proximity and others preferring increased distance.

Critical care nurses working in a person's intimate space have the responsibility to provide the patient with sensory preparation on certain procedures. Draping and covering a patient to ensure modesty are essential. When asked by the patient to stop a certain procedure, the nurse should stop, even just for a moment, and reassess what is occurring. Would there be another way, or a different person or equipment that would ease the patient's discomfort? Respect, understanding, and compromise are needed in critical care to preserve a patient's autonomy.

Personal distance is between 1½ feet and 4 feet in distance. Nurses are more comfortable working in this range, as there is an increased flexibility in caring for the patient through touch and close contact but with the ability to move away from the patient. Conversation can range from serious talk to light banter. It is easier to change the subject in this distance, or avoid topics that may be disturbing to the patient or nurse. The foot of the bed is a comfortable personal distance to assume for many health care professionals. Awareness of the patient's desires regarding distance and comfort zone when discussing topics of concern can help the communication process.

Social distance, 4 to 12 feet, is characterized by activity. The symbol of social distance is the nurses' station, where activity is directed. The nurses' station may be off limits to anyone but nurses and physicians, or it may allow more contact with families, technicians, and students. Within the social distance setting, a person can choose to join certain groups or persons, or ignore them by bustling through the unit and avoiding eye contact. By maintaining social distance within the unit, the nurse may be able to step away from the patient for a moment or two and regain his or her thoughts, away from the demands that intimate personal distance contact places on an individual.[19]

NURSING MANAGEMENT

■ NURSING DIAGNOSIS

Impaired communication, related to foreign language and cultural barriers.

OUTCOME STANDARD

Communication is effective.

OUTCOME CRITERIA

- The patient is able to communicate needs satisfactorily
- The patient is able to communicate feelings of being accepted and understood by caregivers

NURSING INTERVENTIONS

- Determine which of the following interventions would be appropriate for the non-English-speaking patient:

  Use of interpreters, language guides, tapes, picture books or flash cards to communicate patient needs and information.

  Identify alternative sources of information if the preceding are not available, such as support services, library services, and community support groups with specific cultural emphasis.

  Allow additional time for teaching sessions, or patient care conferences.

  Use gestures, signs, models, or pictures when language is not understood. Tone of voice and eye contact are important.

  Touch is culturally determined; determine cultural reference to touch and plan accordingly.

  When possible, use trained interpreters.

- Monitor use of medical terminology

  Offer explanations of medical terms used by others.

  Rephrase directions or explanations to the simplest terms.

  Use the patient as the point of reference.

- Identify nonverbal cues from the patient and establish respect for the patient's intimate space

  Personal space is culturally determined.

  Some patients may need to have their family present at all times; attempt to be flexible with visiting.

  Maintain patient dignity when performing procedures.

  Elicit patient's desires with respect to care needs, for example, when is the preferred time for personal care? Who should be involved?

- Assist patient in expression of emotions and provide privacy for patient and/or significant others as desired

THE NEUROLOGICALLY IMPAIRED PATIENT

Communicating with the person who has experienced neurotrauma and is experiencing the loss of control over self and future is particularly challenging. The nurse may also encounter communication problems in patients experiencing neurological impairment as a result of metabolic and respiratory alterations.

Assessment of Communication Ability

The assessment of an individual's communication ability has to go beyond the standard neurological or Glasgow Coma Scale evaluation. The baseline assessment is important because the person with a neurological trauma is likely to have a long hospitalization, and there may be few changes from baseline over time. The communication assessment presented is meant to build upon the standard neurological assessment performed by the critical care nurse. There are seven parameters in the communication assessment: environmental response, emotional condition, cognitive functioning, speech output, comprehension, verbal behavior, and writing ability. Table 15-1 presents assessment parameters and guidelines for evaluating communication ability.

Aphasia

Aphasia is the loss of the ability to process, understand, or express words as thoughts, symbols, or ideas in a manner that communicates the intent of the sender to the receiver. Three main types of aphasia are generally identified: *receptive, expressive,* and *global.* The critical care nurse may encounter aphasia as part of a patient's primary problem, such as a brain abscess, or as a secondary problem, as in the case of a patient who needs care for a duodenal ulcer and who has also had a cerebrovascular accident. Rehabilitation of the patient who experiences aphasia takes time and occurs over several months. Full rehabilitative potential is not usually reached until the patient has been discharged from the hospital.[38,39]

In light of this, the critical care nurse works with the aphasic patient who is not ready for speech therapy, who may be physiologically unstable, and whose neurological sequelae are still evolving, thereby presenting a changing pattern of communicative abilities. Time and patience are needed to help patients become aware of how the disability affects their relationship to the environment and others. The anatomic approach to understanding aphasia correlates lesions in the cerebral cortex with causes of aphasia. It is the approach most frequently taken and will be used in this discussion. Table 15-2 lists characteristics of the different types of aphasia.

The left hemisphere is considered dominant for speech in most people, although connection and transmission of impulses occur in both hemispheres through the thalamus and mesencephalic areas. It is generally accepted that 90% of right-handed people have language dominance in the left hemisphere and 50% to 60% of left-handed people have language dominance in the left hemisphere. Some people have a right hemisphere dominance for language or mixed language function divided between the two hemispheres. The tendency for hemisphere dominance is thought to be hereditary. Through learning and use, the hemisphere's dominance develops further. This is illustrated by the case of young children with lesions in their dominant hemisphere. Usually, speech function is not totally lost but is taken over by the non-injured hemisphere. The nondominant hemisphere's role in speech and language can be further developed if the dominant hemisphere's lesion is slow growing.

In *sensory aphasia* the basic deficit occurs when the area of auditory comprehension, located at the superior part of the superior temporal convolution, is destroyed. The person is able to hear sounds and words but is unable to comprehend them. This is also reflected in the patient's inability to "hear" oneself speak. Resulting speech is lacking in content, although it is correct in grammar, rhythm, and articulation.[39] *Literal paraphasia* is said to exist if incorrect sounds are substituted such as "bat" for "cat." In *verbal paraphasia,* one word is substituted for another, such as "fork" for "spoon." The communication barrier that exists in the patient with sensory aphasia makes it difficult to determine the patient's meaning in a sea of words. Quite often, the patient is initially unaware that communication is ineffective, although in time the realization occurs that something is amiss. The patient is then likely to become angry with others at their lack of communicative ability.

Expressive aphasia results when there is a lesion in the area of the inferior frontal gyrus of the frontal lobe, anterior to the facial and lingual areas of the motor cortex.[40,41] The ability to formulate a sentence originates in Broca's area. It is transmitted to the motor cortex where transmission of impulses to motor speech areas produces speech. The motor cortex is responsible for control of movement of the lips, jaw, tongue, soft palate, and vocal cords. Patients become frustrated by the inability to articulate the thought that has formed in their minds. "Because Broca's area is so near the left motor area, disease often affects the ability to speak of those with right-sided paralysis, whereas left-sided paralysis almost never results in speech disturbances."[42] The converse is also true, that melodic areas for singing and automatic speech located on the right side of the brain enable those with expressive aphasia to hum, sing, or curse with fluency.

The person with expressive aphasia is very aware of the inability to communicate. Feelings of anger, hostility, hopelessness, depression, and withdrawal may further widen the communication barrier. When conversing with the patient, the nurse should allow more time than usual and stick to one main topic per short conversation time. Nurses need to be aware of

TABLE 15-1 Assessment of Communication Ability

Parameter	Assessment Guidelines
ENVIRONMENTAL RESPONSE	
Awareness	Document patient's position in bed.
	Observe response to cues and events in the environment.
	Note patient's attention capacity.
	Observe patient's response to introduction of self.
	Observe nonverbal behavior.
EMOTIONAL CONDITION	
Anxiety	Note signs of apprehension, restlessness, inability to concentrate, hold conversation, or focus on task or situation.
Denial	Note if patient avoids discussion of illness when introduced into the conversation, or changes the topic.
	Note whether plans for the future are realistic.
	Observe for inappropriate laughter or boasting.
Anger	Observe whether the patient exhibits rage or uncontrolled anger.
Withdrawal	Note if the patient is withdrawn from self, others, and the environment.
COGNITIVE FUNCTIONING	
Short-term memory	Determine patient's ability to remember by asking questions related to events prior to interview time, within a 24-hour span.
Long-term memory	Determine patient's ability to remember past events by asking him or her to recite medical history.
	Validate responses to recent and remote occurrences.
Ability to learn	Document ongoing efforts of patient teaching and response.
	Discuss with patient new information, reinforce throughout the day, document patient's response.
	Discuss how new information will be applied to current lifestyle.
SPEECH	Engage patient in conversation in order to assess ability to speak and content of speech patterns assessing specifically for word choice, syntax, and grammar.
	Evaluate fluency of speech: What is articulation ability?
	How much effort is needed to form words, and is the person successful?
	Evaluate rate of speaking: Normal rate is 100-125 words/min. Does patient use correct intonation, pitch, and stress of words?
COMPREHENSION	Determine patient's ability to understand the meaning of spoken words, ability to follow simple and complex commands, repeat back what is said and respond correctly in a conversation.
VERBAL BEHAVIOR	Evaluate output and effort to produce speech.
	Evaluate nonverbal speech and ability to correct speech errors.
	Observe emotional tone to speech. Is the patient upset or frustrated by speech efforts?
WRITING ABILITY	Can the patient write clearly with the dominant hand?

their own verbal style to prevent overburdening the expressive aphasic patient with excessive words and questions.

Anomic and *conduction aphasia* refer to two types of lesions that occur in the association between Broca's and Wernicke's area. *Anomic aphasia* occurs when there is a lesion in the angular gyrus. The speech of the anomic individual is fluent and rhythmic, but there is difficulty naming objects or places. The patient engages in circumlocutory speech in an attempt to make meanings known.

Conduction aphasia exists when there is a lesion in the arcuate fasciculus that prevents transmission of neuronal impulses from Wernicke's area to Broca's area. Comprehension is intact, but the speech is characterized by literal paraphasias. The affected person

TABLE 15-2 **Characteristics of Aphasia by Type**

Type	Alternate Names	Anatomical Area of Involvement	Speech Characteristics	Language Comprehension
Expressive aphasia	Broca's aphasia, nonfluent aphasia, motor aphasia, anterior aphasia, apraxia of speech	Lateral Inferior portion of frontal lobe of dominant hemisphere	Slow, labored speech. "Telescoping" the omission of small words or ends of nouns and verbs. Poor naming ability. Ability to repeat more than one word is poor. Writing is similar to speech pattern. Reading comprehension good. May be fluent at swearing or humming.	Good.
Receptive aphasia	Wernicke's aphasia, fluent aphasia, sensory aphasia	Superior temporal convolution of dominant hemisphere	Fluent speech, normal rate, rhythm, good grammar. Content of speech is lacking. Content of writing similar to speech. Poor reading comprehension. Repetition is poor. Object naming poor.	Poor. Lacks auditory comprehension.
Anomic aphasia	General agnosia	Angular gyrus, near Wernicke's area	Speech fluent or rhythmic. Difficulty in naming objects or places. Circumlocutory speech.	Good.
Conduction		Arcuate fasciculus, between frontal and temporal lobes sphere	Difficulty in repeating words, substitutes incorrect sounds (literal paraphasia). Substitutes incorrect words (verbal paraphasia).	Good.
Global		Several areas in dominant hemisphere	Combination of characteristics, depending on area of involvement.	Poor to good, depending on area of involvement.

will have trouble repeating words spoken by another.[41]

Global aphasia exists if there is damage to multiple areas in the left cerebral cortex and the person is left with few language skills. Poor comprehension and inability to name objects and repeat words, coupled with nonfluent speech, make communication difficult with this patient. Perhaps the best hope for communication lies in recognition of sign language, gestures, pantomime, or cues.

The proportion of the cerebral cortex related to receptive and expressive aphasia is small. The remaining areas are called *association areas,* which coordinate incoming sensory data and may influence motor function in response to sensory data.

The aphasic patient presents the critical care nurse with a special challenge in the communication process. The nurse must alter existing patterns of communication to fit the physiological deficits of the patient. In turn, the nurse helps the patient use alternate means of communicating when speech is incomprehensible. The nurse's awareness of the relationship between the area of cerebral damage and clinical signs will help the nurse formulate effective communication strategies.

Neurological Trauma

Hearing is generally thought to be the last sense to be lost in severe sensory compromise or limitation. Therefore, auditory stimulation is frequently a part of the care plan for patients with neurological trauma. For head-injured and comatose patients, the playing of radios, TVs, and tapes is considered a means of interacting. Staff and family are encouraged to talk to the patient. Although the belief is widely held that auditory stimuli are perceived by comatose patients, little research data are available to support these measures.

Sisson[43] used EEG tracings, coma score, and behavioral observation to evaluate the response of comatose, head-injured patients to auditory stimuli. Five subjects were evaluated on their response to a tape of popular music during one week. Specific behavioral and EEG changes led the author to conclude that persons in coma do perceive and respond to auditory stimuli.[43]

Music may be considered to be a neutral auditory stimulus, whereas conversation is not. Johnson, Omery, and Nikas[44] evaluated the effects of neutral and emotionally referenced conversation on the intracranial pressure of comatose, head-injured patients. The emotionally referenced conversation was in the form of a change of shift report. Neutral conversation referred to child care and carpooling arrangements. The conversations were held "over" the patient. No statistically significant difference was found between the effects of the two conversation types on the intracranial pressure (ICP) of patients as a group. No significant increase in the ICP occurred during emotionally referenced conversation, but the ICP decreased significantly during the conversation that was not related to the patient. Further, the investigators noted wide individual differences in response to the conversations; these differences were not reflected in overall group measures. The authors concluded that the findings are "important to nursing practice because they indicate that patient response to conversation may need to be considered on an individual basis."[44] As with the Sisson[43] study, the depth of the coma seemed

to be a contributing factor in the response of the individual. Individuals with a Glasgow Coma Scale score of 5 or less may not be able to interpret language and, therefore, have no response to it.

Persons who have had spinal cord injuries also have difficulty in communicating with their environment, but from a different perspective. Such individuals experience a loss of control over self, future, and environment, which may lead to a sense of powerlessness (see Chapter 6).[28,45] The powerless individual is unable to interact with others in ways meaningful for the future. By enhancing communication ability, the critical care nurse can help reverse feelings of powerlessness.

THE PATIENT RECEIVING MECHANICAL VENTILATION

Critical care nurses are experts in anticipating and meeting the physical needs of the patient who has a tracheostomy or who is intubated for purposes of mechanical ventilation. Meeting the patient's communication needs may be a different matter: frequently overlooked but no less important. Patients who are responsive and aware of their surroundings yet unable to communicate present a tremendous challenge to the critical care nurse. Since the AACN Delphi study of research priorities was published in 1983, interest in identifying and meeting the patient's need for communication has increased.[46] A climate of care and a desire to communicate effectively with ventilator patients now exist.

The communication needs of a patient receiving mechanical ventilation may be physiological, physical, psychological or emotional, or situational. The patient with an impaired airway may have alterations in oxygenation that alter the level of consciousness. The patient with PCO_2 narcosis cannot communicate adequately until PCO_2 levels are brought down. Thus, there may be a physiological basis for the inability to communicate in addition to the physical impairment created by intubation.

Psychological factors related to the intubation or tracheostomy may alter the patient's perception of self and the surroundings, thereby inhibiting communication. Roberts[47] postulates that critically ill patients revert to earlier developmental stages and perceive the ventilator as an extension of themselves. Smith[48] expounds on this idea and says that "until the individual reestablishes his body boundaries, he may be unable to assimilate other information in a meaningful way." The patient confined by a ventilator has a limited view of the environment and consequently an altered sense of proprioception. Energy expended in continually orienting oneself to person and place prevents interaction with the environment and the people in it.

Assessment and Strategies

In contrast to their physically relaxed appearance, mechanically ventilated patients may be emotionally detached from their environment. In a review of communication strategies, Connolly[26] presents a theme of impaired communication as described by individuals who were intubated. Perceptions of communication difficulties were identified in five areas: (1) an inability to communicate, (2) insufficient explanations of events and occurrences, (3) inadequate understanding of what was occurring, (4) a fear of danger related to not being able to speak, and (5) difficulty in finding alternative communication methods.

Situational factors such as time and patience are crucial in communicating with the intubated patient. To communicate, the patient requires more energy and time than usual. The nurse bears the responsibility of assisting patients in making their needs known. Communication of needs to the nurse may be critical: Viner[49] related an experience of being attached to a ventilator that was not plugged in. A mistake by the janitor had left him airless.

How can the communication process be facilitated when intubation or tracheostomy leaves the patient unable to speak? The communication board is the most common type of adjunctive agent for nurse–patient communication. Yet one study found that patients in the intensive care unit often do not have their eyeglasses available, and therefore they cannot see the communication board.[50] This situation highlights a common occurrence: a multitude of methods for communicating with patients but no continuity or consistency in applying them.

The initial step to take when a patient cannot communicate verbally is a complete communication assessment as described in detail in Table 15-1, encompassing determination of verbal ability, comprehension of spoken word and contextual cues, nonverbal expression, and interface with the environment. The nurse then uses the communication assessment to plan nursing care that will meet the ventilated patient's need both to express and to receive information. The communication plan should be feasible for the nurse and patients and appropriate to the environment. A variety of communication needs must be addressed by appropriate methods.[26]

The first area is one of immediate need. Can the patient respond to a yes/no question by a nod of the head, a blink of the eye, or by raising a hand. This can cover emergency questions: Are you in pain? Can you breathe? Are you getting enough air? Immediate communication can employ verbal or nonverbal strat-

egies. The nurse must be prepared to move through several strategies in rapid succession to ascertain the patient's needs.

Frequently the intubated patient tries to mouth words. It is difficult to read lips when a patient is orally intubated. Tape and the presence of an naso-gastric tube also make it difficult to read lips and facial expressions. If the nurse cannot read lips, another strategy must be employed, such as writing out letters on the nurse's hand. If that is not effective, letters may be written in the air or a marker and paper can be employed. Whatever the method, it must be mutually agreed upon by the nurse and the patient. It is also important that patients be able to initiate communication of their needs. If the nurse is only going to ask questions and have the patient respond to them, the patient has lost freedom of expression.

A study of nurse–patient interactions involving intubated patients[51] showed that communication was usually nurse initiated. Of 217 observed interactions between nurses and patients, only 34 were patient initiated. Of the 34, 4 were expressions of anger or hostility, with the rest being classified as positive. One third of the positive patient-initiated actions received a negative response from the nurse, such as silence during care or expression of disapproval. Praise or encouragement, explanations, or directions from the nurse were classified as positive.

This study found that the most common nursing action or reaction to patients was silence, with patients responding to that silence by remaining silent themselves. The researchers concluded that critical care nurses in their study "may have been unable to recognize and/or deal with their patient's responses to illness and hospitalization, or they may have been unable to deal with their own reaction to the patient or situation."[51] This study strongly suggests that intubated patients may wait for the nurse to initiate communication and, when nothing is forthcoming, remain silent. The responsibility of the critical care nurse is clear. Any attempt on the part of the intubated patient to communicate must be fostered and encouraged.

After the immediate communication needs of the patient have been identified and met, an intermediate strategy for communication needs to be developed if the patient will remain mechanically ventilated for several days. Stovsky[50] identifies assist devices that can be used for the patient who has a short-term ventilator experience. The strategies include the use of marker and paper, the "magic slate," magnetic letter board, alphabet board, and picture board. When these methods are used, it is crucial that patients be positioned in such a way that their hands are free to write, that the materials be within the patient's visual field, that the patient wear any needed vision aids, and that the patient have the physical strength and ability to handle the items.

The appropriateness of the communication device for the patient's physical defects must be completely assessed, especially for the long-term ventilator-depedent patient. Computer technology has the potential to assist the long-term communication. Several computer programs that use word processing and project a voice are available. The patient must be willing to learn the computer software and typing skills to use these techniques effectively. The use of word-processing methods necessitates reading and writing skills, physical strength, manual dexterity, and knowledge of the keyboard. These requirements tend to limit the successful use of the bedside computer, perhaps only to stable long-term ventilator-dependent patients.[52]

NURSING MANAGEMENT

The nursing diagnosis "Impaired Verbal Communication" describes a state in which "an individual experiences a decreased or absent ability to use or understand language in human interaction."[53] Etiological and contributing factors include laryngeal edema; tracheostomy; laryngectomy; intubation; or surgery of the head, face, neck, or mouth.[54] Other related factors include age, physical or psychosocial stress, anger or depression, neurological or cerebral impairments, respiratory impairment, pain, fatigue, speech impediments, and language barriers.[53] Defining characteristics of impaired verbal communication are presented in the box below.

■ NURSING DIAGNOSIS

Impaired verbal communication, related to inability to articulate words.

OUTCOME STANDARD

Communication is effective.

OUTCOME CRITERIA

- The patient is able to communicate needs satisfactorily using alternatives to language
- Patient expresses satisfaction with method of communication

NURSING INTERVENTIONS

- Assist the patient in determining an alternative means to communicate for immediate and long-term purposes
- Experiment with different methods of communication until an acceptable method is found
- Provide time and a quiet environment during communication; watch for nonverbal cues that indicate the patient may have a need
- Guide and direct patient's efforts at communication so others may understand them
- Do not waste time on methods that do not work; encourage patient to express feelings nonverbally
- Reassure patient that speech will return after tracheostomy or endotracheal tube is removed (if this is true)
- If tracheostomy will be permanent, plan for alter-

Defining Characteristics of the Nursing Diagnosis Impaired Verbal Communication[25,55,56]

SIGNIFICANT CHARACTERISTICS
Inability to speak (cannot speak, does not wish to, or cannot speak dominate language)
Inappropriate speech

SECONDARY CHARACTERISTICS
Stuttering or slurred speech
Word finding difficulty
Weak or absent voice
Decreased auditory comprehension
Deafness or inattention to voice or sound
Confusion

RELATED CHARACTERISTICS
Dyspnea
Inability to modulate speech, find words, name or identify objects, or speak in sentences
Difficulty in phonation
Disorientation
Too little or too much attention to stimuli
Speech impediments
Physical condition

Disregard for speaker
Reliance on nonverbal communication
Inability to organize words
Use of unfamiliar words
Inconsistent nonverbal messages
Message inappropriate to context
Excessive or insufficient verbiage
Ill-timed message
Inadequate listening skills
Disparity of punctuation
Absent or inappropriate feedback
Discordant information
Disconfirmation
Absence of gratification
Inability or reluctance to express feelings
Withdrawal from interaction
Unrestrained or inappropriate emotional expression
Imaginary or false perceptions
Incongruent communication styles
Lack of assertive skills

native methods of communication to facilitate discharge planning; involve patient and family in this process
- Assess patient's satisfaction and desire to change communication strategies

COMMUNICATING BY TOUCH

Touch can be used to balance technology in the critical care unit. Human contact through touch provides comfort, offers assurance, directs attention and promotes healing. Critical care nurses may take touch for granted, because it is so much a part of the nursing routine. Increased attention to the kinds of touch and their use as part of the nurse–patient interaction may help patients cope with their critical care experience and offer the nurse a feeling of fulfillment.

An abundance of literature on the use of touch as a nursing strategy has become available. One research area concerns the use of therapeutic touch as a modality of healing. The second major domain of touch is caring touch, which includes affective, expressive, comforting, and nonprocedural touch. A final domain is that of procedural touch or touch that is task related or intervention specific. The type of touch employed as a strategy can be influenced by many patient- and nurse-related factors.

Therapeutic Touch

The concept of therapeutic touch is a contemporary interpretation of several ancient healing practices. It is based on the concept of *prana*, a Sanskrit word that represents the idea that a healthy person has an abundance of vitality that can be transferred to any person who is ill. The illness is believed to be caused by a lack of vitality. Therapeutic touch is defined as the art of interpersonal energy transfer for the purpose of healing.

Therapeutic touch was pioneered in nursing by Dr. Delores Krieger in the early 1970s.[57] Dr. Krieger was influenced by eastern culture, religion, and biological experimentation using healers to promote change and growth in animals and plants. She was particularly influenced by the work of Canadian biochemist Bernard Grad and healer Oskar Estebany in healing mice and causing plants to grow. Dora Kuntz, an observer of paranormal healing, taught Dr. Krieger the technique of therapeutic touch. Dr. Krieger translated the work of Grad and Estebany into a series of experiments on human subjects.

Working in New York hospitals, Dr. Krieger tested a hypothesis that therapeutic touch would change the hemoglobin levels of patients. In a pilot test, hemoglobin levels were shown to increase significantly from pretest measurements in 28 patients after they were treated with therapeutic touch. In a second study, 16 registered nurses administered therapeutic touch to 32 patients. A control group of a like number of patients and nurses in which therapeutic touch was not used was also included in the study. Once again, hemoglobin values were found to significantly increase in the group of patients who received therapeutic touch. These studies represent the beginning of interest in therapeutic touch for the nursing community.

As a process, therapeutic touch involves the transference of energy from one human energy field to another. Healers first center themselves and become aware of the intention to help the patient. Healers have an awareness of the self as an open system. Next, healers assess the patient by placing their hands approximately 4 to 6 inches over the patient's body, moving from head to toe. As part of the healing process, the healer then redirects areas of tension, which represent illness, to other areas of the body. At all times the healer concentrates on the energy field of the patient and the interaction of the energy fields between self and the patient.[22]

Krieger found that therapeutic touch (1) initiated a powerful relaxation response, sometimes within 2 to 4 minutes after the treatment has been initiated; (2) reduced pain and promoted a sense of well-being, and (3) initiated or accelerated the healing process. An important assumption of therapeutic touch is that the healer has a belief system that is compatible with the beliefs of therapeutic touch and its effectiveness. Another key for the effectiveness of therapeutic touch is the belief that humans are capable of transformation and transcendence.[58]

Therapeutic touch has been used in a variety of settings with different types of patients. An early study by Heidt[59] examined the effect of therapeutic touch on anxiety in hospitalized patients in a cardiovascular unit. Patients were randomly assigned to one of three groups, and each received a 5-minute intervention of therapeutic touch, no touch, or casual touch. As measured on the Spielberger State Anxiety Measure, patients in the therapeutic touch group had significantly less anxiety after intervention.[58] Some authors criticize this study for its design, which included only one dependent variable to measure anxiety, and for the inappropriate statistical analysis.[60]

Therapeutic touch may be useful in promoting relationships, reducing anxiety, and promoting healing in the critically ill patient. Limited research has been done using therapeutic touch in a population of critically ill patients. A major drawback to the use of therapeutic touch in critical care is the training and belief system that it requires to be effective. If a trained healer is present on the staff, and the patient desires the use of therapeutic touch, it could be employed as a nursing strategy.

Caring Touch

Caring touch is a domain of touch as identified by Estabrooks.[61] It includes affectional, protective, expressive, nonprocedural, comforting, and encouraging touch. As a strategy for nursing care, encouraging touch requires no special training but requires an emotional intent to care for the patient. As with therapeutic touch, the nurse must possess sufficient emotional and physical energy to care.[61] Components of caring touch and their descriptors are presented in the box below.

Under the domain of caring touch is affectional touch as described by Schoenhofer.[62] *Affectional touch* is defined as tactile communication from one person to another that has as its primary purpose the transmission and receipt of recognition, acceptance, protection, and caring concern. Schoenhofer described the use of affectional touch in the intensive care unit in a study of 30 patients. Interactions of patient–nurse dyads were observed for 1-hour periods between 7:30 A.M. and 10:20 P.M. The number of instances of affectional touch were recorded, along with other variables such as place touched and quality of touch. A total of 30 hours of observation were recorded. During this time there were 84 instances of touch, a frequency of 2.8 times per hour. In 6 of the 1-hour periods, no touch event occurred. In 181 instances, avoidance of affectional touch was recorded.

Components and Descriptors of Caring Touch

AFFECTIONAL TOUCH
Recognition
Acceptance
Protection
Concern

COMFORTING TOUCH
Loving
Warm
Being there
Compassion
Sad
Soothing/calming
Supportive

ENCOURAGING TOUCH
Supportive
Reassuring
Spirit raising

Procedural or task touch was not recorded in this study. The author points out that the interraters had some difficulty in classifying affectional touch, because it so often seemed to coincide with procedural touch. Also important was the observation that there were more instances of the avoidance of affectional touch than actual events of touch.[62]

Weiss[63] studied nervous system arousal in patients hospitalized with cardiac disease as measured by cardiovascular response and state anxiety. Areas of high neural arousal were the hands, feet, head, and face. Body locations either conducive or not conducive to arousal were given comfort touch, procedural touch, and no touch in association with stressful and nonstressful stimuli and the results compared by physiological and psychological measures of anxiety. Touch had no apparent adverse effect. Heart rate, diastolic blood pressure, and anxiety score decreased with touch. No age or gender differences in physiological measures were found, but a significant reduction in anxiety scores occurred in men.[63]

Glick[64] found a similar result using the Speilberger State Anxiety Measure on 33 patients with myocardial infarction after transfer to a stepdown unit. Caring touch lowered state anxiety scores for male patients under age 60. Caring touch applied to the hands, feet, face, and/or head was found to have no deleterious effect on neural arousal and may be an instrument in decreasing anxiety, especially for men.[62] Research suggests that caring touch is not used as much as it could be in the intensive care unit setting.[61,64]

If caring touch is to be used effectively, the quality and duration of touch and the gender of the patient need to be considered. Touch may be most effective when used on an area of the body that is highly innervated, such as the face. Additionally, women appear to be more receptive to touch than men are, and thus may require less frequent touch or one that is lighter in pressure. Pressure must be applied for touch to be recognized by the patient. Location of touch, the pressure with which touch is applied, and the intent of the touch are the major factors determining the significance of the touch interaction in helping the patient.[61,62,63,64]

Procedural Touch

Task-related, or *procedural, touch* may be the most important kind of touch the critical care nurse uses. Inherent in procedural touch is the touch that makes up the everyday care that the patient receives from the nurse. It is frequently dismissed as not important or even as harmful to the patient, but it warrants attention because it is so crucial to the nurse–patient relationship. As identified by Estabrooks,[60] procedural touch is dispassionate and is necessary to provide care for the patient. It differs from therapeutic touch and caring touch because it is not an optional strategy that the nurse may employ. However, caring touch may be incorporated into procedural touch.[61] Schoenhofer[62] found it difficult to separate procedural touch from caring touch because one frequently proceeded the other. It was not unusual for Schoenhofer to observe a nurse holding the patient's hand and requesting permission to perform a procedure before doing so. Similarly, at the end of a procedure, hand holding or stroking would serve to comfort the patient.

Procedural touch can be performed in a manner that distances the nurse from the patient. For example, if a nurse is performing cardioversion, distancing from the patient is necessitated by the risk to the nurse from the procedure. However, nurses may also use distancing to protect themselves emotionally in situations that are ethically or morally difficult. Distancing should not be employed on a regular basis.

Additional attributes of touch include its intensity, its meaning for the patient, and its frequency and location. As already mentioned, Weiss[63] demonstrated that the areas which are neurally sensitive to touch and which evoke a patient response when touched are the feet, face, hands, and head. In planning procedures or the initiation of caring touch, the nurse must take this information into consideration. Patterns of touch may be related to variables that are influenced by the nurse, the patient, or the environment. Communication in the critical care environment can be significantly enhanced by an awareness of touch as a healing tool.

CASE STUDY

Mr. M., age 35, was admitted with an anterior wall myocardial infarction at a community hospital and then transferred to a major university teaching center. After cardiac catheterization, he was transferred to the coronary care unit. Results of the catherization revealed a 50% occlusive lesion high on the right coronary artery, and a 90% occlusion of the left anterior descending artery. After catheterization, Mr. M. received a standard nitroglycerin drip and supplemental oxygen at 2 L per minute. His vital signs were stable, and he was free of chest pain. Upon hearing the extent of his cardiac disease and that an angioplasty or surgery would be likely, Mr. M. became upset and verbally abusive to nursing staff and his family; he threatened to leave the hospital. Although antianxiety medication had been administered, Mr. M. was clearly in a state of crisis.

The nurse wanted to communicate caring and concern to the patient and also to protect him from harm caused by his high anxiety state. The patient was receptive to procedural touch, so the nurse used that mechanism first. By skillfully and carefully checking Mr. M.'s blood pressure, assessing his catheterization site, and checking peripheral pulses, the nurse established contact with him and communicated competence. After procedural touch had been applied, the nurse used caring touch to elicit the patient's concerns and communicate concern. The nurse sat on the edge of the bed, face to face with the patient, and held the patient's hand firmly. The nurse encouraged the patient to express his concerns, which he began to do. After discussing concerns for a while, the nurse moved to the patient's feet and began to massage them while encouraging the patient to take deep breaths and relax. The nurse spent approximately 20 minutes with the patient applying caring touch. After this time the patient was much calmer and able to verbalize his fears. He gave up on the idea of leaving the hospital. During this time his heart rate had decreased from 98 beats per minute to 88 beats per minute. No ectopic beats were observed at any time during the episode.

This case illustrates how procedural touch can be used with caring touch as an intervention that will benefit the patient who is experiencing an anxiety crisis.

REFERENCES

1. Obier, K., & Haywood, L. J. (1973). Enhancing therapeutic communication with acutely ill patients. *Heart Lung, 2,* 49-53.
2. Meleis, A. (1985). *Theoretical nursing: Development and progress.* Philadelphia: Lippincott.
3. Thomas, S. A., Friedman, E., Noctor, N., et al. (1982). Patients' cardiac response to nursing interviews in a CCU. *Dimensions of Critical Care Nursing, 1,* 198-205.
4. Clark, J. M. (1981). Communication in nursing. *Nursing Times, 77,* 12-18.
5. Owens, J. F., & Hutelmeyer, C. M. (1982). The effect of preoperative intervention on delirium in cardiac surgical patients. *Nursing Research, 31,* 60-62.
6. Schwartz, L. P., & Brenner, Z. R. (1979). Critical care unit transfer: Reducing patient stress through nursing interventions. *Heart Lung, 8,* 540-546.
7. Eisendrath, S., & Dunkel, J. (1979). Psychological issues in intensive care unit staff. *Heart Lung, 8,* 751-758.
8. Dunkel, J., & Eisendrath, S. (1983). Families in the intensive care unit: Their effect on staff. *Heart Lung, 12,* 258-560.
9. Fuller, B. F., & Foster, G. M. (1982). The effect of family/friend visits vs. staff interaction on stress arousal of surgical intensive care patients. *Heart Lung, 11,* 457-463.
10. Gardner, D., & Stewart, N. (1978). Staff involvement with families of patients in critical care units. *Heart Lung, 9,* 105-110.
11. Chatham, M. A. (1978). The effect of family involvement on patients' manifestations of postcardiotomy psychosis. *Heart Lung, 7,* 995-999.

12. Doerr, B. C., & Jones, J. W. (1979). Effect of family preparation on the state anxiety level of the CCU patient. *Nursing Research, 28,* 315-316.

13. Molter, N. E. (1979). Needs of relatives of critically ill patients: A descriptive study. *Heart Lung, 8,* 332-339.

14. Rasie, S. M. (1980). Meeting families' needs helps you meet ICU patients' needs. *Nursing 80, 10,* 32-35.

15. Rodgers, C. D. (1981). Needs of relatives of cardiac surgery patients during the critical care phase. *Focus on Critical Care, 10,* 50-55.

16. Friedman, E. H. (1982). Stress and intensive care nursing: A ten year reappraisal. *Heart Lung, 11,* 26-28.

17. Gardner, D., Parzen, Z. D., & Stewart, N. (1980). The nurses' dilemma: Mediating stress in critical care units. *Heart Lung, 9,* 103-106.

18. Oskins, S. L. (1979). Identification of situational stressors and coping methods by ICU nurses. *Heart Lung, 8,* 953-960.

19. Hein, E. C. (1980). *Communication in nursing practice* (2nd ed.). Boston: Little, Brown.

20. Wiedenbach, E., & Falls, C. E. (1978). *Communication: Key to effective nursing.* New York: Teresias.

21. Rogers, M. E. (1970). *An introduction to the theoretical basis of nursing.* Philadelphia: Davis.

22. MacRae, J. (1990). *Therapeutic touch: A practical guide.* New York: Knopf.

23. Watson, J. (1988). *Nursing: Human science and human care: A theory of nursing.* New York: National League for Nursing.

24. Ray, M. A. (1987). Technological caring: A new model in critical care. *Dimensions in Critical Care Nursing, 6,* 166-173.

25. McFarland, G. K., & Naschinski, C. E. (1985). Impaired communication: A descriptive study. *Nursing Clinics of North America, 20,* 775-786.

26. Connolly, M. A., & Shekleton, M. E. (1991). Communication with ventilator dependent patients. *Dimensions in Critical Care Nursing, 10,* 115-121.

27. Johnson, M. M., & Sexton, D. L. (1990). Distress during mechanical ventilation: Patients' perceptions. *Critical Care Nurse, 10,* 48-57.

28. Sullivan, J. (1990). Individual and family responses to acute spinal cord injury. *Critical Care Nursing Clinics of North America, 2,* 407-414.

29. Lubbers, C. A., & Roy, S. J. (1990). Communication skills for continuing education in nursing. *Journal of Continuing Education in Nursing, 21,* 109-112.

30. Heinrich, K. T. (1988). What's my type? Teaching interviewing skills. *Nurse Educator, 13,* 34-38.

31. Duldt, B. W., Giffin, K., & Patton, B. R. (1988). *Interpersonal communication in nursing.* Philadelphia: Davis.

32. Diaz-Duque, O. F. (1982). Overcoming the language barrier: Advice from an interpreter. *American Journal of Nursing, 82,* 1380-1382.

33. Kubricht, D. W., & Clark, J. A. (1982). Foreign patients: A system for providing care. *Nursing Outlook, 30,* 55-57.

34. Spiro, D., & Heidrich, F. (1983). Lay understanding of medical terminology. *Journal of Family Practice, 17,* 227-229.

35. Leininger, M. (1984). Transcultural nursing: An essential knowledge and practice field for today. *The Canadian Nurse, 80,* 41-45.

36. Yep, J. (1991). A family member responds: Please understand us. *Journal of Christian Nursing, 8,* 6-8.

37. Spradley, J. P., & McCurdy, D. W. (1972). *The cultural experience, ethnography in complex society.* Kingsport, TN: Kingsport.

38. Pickersgill, M. J., & Lincoln, N. B. (1983). Prognostic indicators and the pattern of recovery in aphasic stroke patients. *Journal of Neurology, Neurosurgery and Psychiatry, 46,* 130-139.

39. Piotrowski, M. M. (1978). Aphasia: Providing better nursing care. *Nursing Clinics of North America, 13,* 543-554.

40. Marshall, R. C., & Phillips, D. S. (1983). Prognosis for improved verbal communication in aphasic stroke patients. *Archives of Physical Medicine and Rehabilitation, 64,* 597-600.

41. Louis, M. C., & Povse, S. M. (1980). Aphasia and endurance: Considerations in the assessment and care of the stroke patient. *Nursing Clinics of North America, 15,* 265-282.

42. Blanco, K. M. (1982). The aphasic patient. *Journal of Neurosurgical Nursing, 14,* 34-37.

43. Sisson, R. (1990). Effects of auditory stimuli on comatose patients with head injury. *Heart Lung, 19,* 373-378.

44. Johnson, S. M., Omery, A., & Nikas, D. (1989). Effects of conversation on intracranial pressure in comatose patients. *Heart Lung, 18,* 56-63.

45. Richmond, T. S. (1990). Spinal cord injury. *Nursing Clinics of North America, 25,* 57-69.

46. Lewandowski, L. A., & Kositsky, A. M. (1983). Research priorities for critical care nursing: A study by the American Association of Critical-Care Nurses. *Heart Lung, 12,* 35-44.

47. Roberts, S. L. (1980). Piaget's theory reapplied to the critically ill. *Advances in Nursing Science, 2,* 61-78.

48. Smith, S. A. (1989). Extended body image in the ventilated patient. *Intensive Care Nursing, 5,* 31-38.

49. Viner, E. D. (1985). Life at the other end of the endotracheal tube: A physician's personal view of critical illness. *Progress in Critical Care Medicine, 2,* 3-13.

50. Stovsky, B., Ruby, E., & Dragonette, P. (1988). Comparison of two types of communication methods used after cardiac surgery with patients with endotracheal tubes. *Heart Lung, 17,* 281-289.

51. Salyer, J., & Stuart, B. J. (1985). Nurse-patient interaction in the intensive care unit. *Heart Lung, 14,* 20-24.

52. Cronin, L. R., & Carrezosa, A. A. (1984). The computer as a communication device for ventilator and tracheostomy patients in the ICU. *Critical Care Nurse, 4,* 72-76.

53. McLane, A. (Ed.). (1987). *Classification of nursing diagnosis: Proceedings of the Seventh Conference.* St. Louis: Mosby.

54. Sawyer, D. L., & Bruya, M. A. (1990). Care of the patient having radical neck surgery or permanent laryngostomy: A nursing diagnosis approach. *Focus on Critical Care, 17,* 166-173.

55. Carpenito, L. J. (1990). *Nursing diagnosis: Application to clinical practice.* Philadelphia: Lippincott.

56. Kim, M. J., McFarland, G. K., & McLane, A. M. (1987). *Pocket guide to nursing diagnosis* (2nd ed.). St. Louis: Mosby.

57. Krieger, D. (1975). Therapeutic touch: The imprimatur of nursing. *American Journal of Nursing, 75,* 784-787.

58. Krieger, D. (1990). Therapeutic touch: Two decades of research, teaching and clinical practice. *Imprint, 37,* 83, 86-88.

59. Heidt, P. (1981). Effect of therapeutic touch on anxiety level of hospitalized patients. *Nursing Research, 30,* 32-37.

60. Clark, P. E., & Clark, M. J. (1984). Therapeutic touch: Is there a scientific basis for the practice? *Nursing Research, 33,* 37-41.

61. Estabrooks, C. A. (1989). Touch: A nursing strategy in the intensive care unit. *Heart Lung, 18,* 392-400.

62. Schoenhofer, S. O. (1989). Affectional touch in critical care nursing: A descriptive study. *Heart Lung, 18,* 146-153.

63. Weiss, S. J. (1990). Effects of differential touch on nervous system arousal of patients recovering from cardiac disease. *Heart Lung, 19,* 474-480.

64. Glick, M. S. (1986). Caring touch and anxiety in myocardial infarction patients in the intermediate cardiac care unit. *Intensive Care Nursing, 2,* 61-66.

16

Teaching and Learning

Anne E. Belcher

At no previous time in the evolution of critical care nursing have patient education and staff development assumed the positions of importance they now enjoy. The major reason for the increased emphasis on these essential nursing functions is the impact of the prospective payment system on health care. By limiting hospitals' reimbursement for services rendered, the government and increasing numbers of other third-party payers make each day of patients' stay a critical one—not just for the provision of care but also for comprehensive instruction and discharge planning.

For many patients, the intensive care unit may be the only care setting where they are hospitalized. In addition, increasing numbers of these patients are being discharged to home or to another facility in a stable but critically ill condition. Because of these changes in the delivery of critical care, nurses should be addressing such educational issues as:

- How should patient education be provided to the critically ill patient?
- How can discharge planning be provided in a timely and effective way?
- How should staff development be provided to nurses in the critical care setting?
- What techniques are most effective in meeting the educational needs of critically ill patients and the nurses caring for them?

DEFINING PATIENT EDUCATION

Patient education, viewed as part of the nursing process, is a planned, organized activity that takes into consideration the patient's individual right and need to know about health maintenance and promotion, prevention of illness, treatment, and rehabilitation. It is not only a patient's right but also a nursing responsibility.

Narrow[1] defines patient teaching as a process of helping patients to learn those things that will enable them to live a longer and/or fuller life and helping them learn how to reach their optimal level of physical and mental health. The emphasis on process is an important one. The American Hospital Association[2] describes planned patient education as a process that includes the conduct of a needs assessment; the setting of objectives; the development of an action plan; and the implementation, documentation, and evaluation of that plan.

The target population for patient education consists of those individuals and their families who have entered the health care delivery system for diagnosis, treatment, and rehabilitation. The services developed in response to patient and family educational needs should include information about ways to use various health care services, preparation for medical and nursing procedures, assistance in managing disease during hospitalization and after discharge, and behavior modification for health promotion and disease prevention.

Current Status and Future Directions

The goals of patient education are (1) to inform individuals about health, illness, and disability, and the ways in which they can improve and protect their own health, including more efficient use of the health care delivery system; (2) to motivate people to want to change to more healthful practices; (3) to help persons learn the skills needed to adopt and maintain healthful practices and lifestyles; and (4) to advocate changes in the environment that facilitate healthful conditions and behavior.

Patient education has assumed what has been called "a degree of motherhood status"; everyone agrees that it is an essential service and every health profession wants to be involved in it. The issues on which critics now focus are those of:

- Access: for whom should services be provided?
- Patient privilege: what should be taught?
- Professional privilege: who should teach it?

• The nature of evaluation: process or outcome?

Among several reasons for the increased interest in patient education are its income-producing potential and its efficiency-enhancing effect on health services. Burke[3] notes that educated patients are more likely to comply with prescribed therapy; experience lessened stress and anxiety; and sustain shorter hospital stays, fewer emergency room admissions, and reduced mortality. Miller[4] also notes that patients who have had preoperative instruction spend less time in the hospital, have fewer postoperative complications, experience less pain, and resume normal activities sooner.

The self-care perspective on patient education[5] has as its goal the anticipation of risk, derived from patients' perceived needs and preferences. The patient-learner determines alone or in collaboration with the nurse the content, teaching and learning methods, and criteria for evaluation. This approach lessens patient dependency on the nurse and other health care providers.

The focus of self-care education is on increased awareness of the hazards of health care, the "how-tos" of reducing the risk of iatrogenic illness, and methods for changing the health care system to conform to patients' needs and preferences. This approach relies on the knowledge and skills the patient already has, such as traditional family health practices or home remedies, or autonomous self-healing. The nurse's key strategy is to encourage circumstances wherein problem-posing skills of the patient are acknowledged and supported.

Given the current climate of forced shorter hospitalization, increasing demands on available time, and the need to give acutely ill patients highly technical information as quickly as possible, nurses must learn to teach patients and families more effectively in less time. Harrell and Frauman[6] suggest the following cost-containment strategies for patient education: (1) teach patients in groups with printed or audiovisual materials; (2) train other, less costly personnel such as volunteers to do some aspects of patient education; and (3) focus on assessing individual patient needs and directing learning activities.

A philosophical issue that affects the process of patient education in a variety of ways is that of beliefs about learning. Although most learning theorists define learning as an enduring change in behavior,[7] some educational program planners prefer to focus on learning as gaining new knowledge or skills. One's perspective on learning thus guides the selection of teaching strategies and, more important, the criteria used for learner evaluation. It is certainly less time- and resource-consuming to view learning as primarily the attainment of information and abilities, but the long-range goal of self-care cannot be assured without a focus on resultant changes in patient and family behavior.

Factors That Affect Teaching and Learning

Factors frequently identified by nurses as hindering patient teaching are low patient motivation; poor availability and quality of teaching aids; noise; lack of sufficient time; patients' impaired sensory perception, that is, poor eyesight or poor hearing; poor reading ability; and lack of family involvement. Other nurse-related factors include the *lack* of (1) patient teaching as a priority, (2) knowledge regarding the content, (3) teaching skills, (4) communication among members of the health care team, and (5) resultant *lack* of continuity of instruction and evaluation.

The enhancement of patient motivation, a complex challenge, is discussed in a separate section, as is the availability and quality of teaching aids. Nurses can learn to control noise in a variety of ways such as putting a sign on the patient/classroom door, prearranging quiet time, using settings distant from noise sources, and selecting teaching times when there is decreased activity in the area. Nurses can also more effectively manage their time by using "routine" patient contacts for teaching, for example, during the bath or meals, by supplementing one-to-one or classroom instruction with self-instructional audiovisual materials, and by sharing teaching activities with colleagues. Patients' impaired sensory perception may require assistive devices such as corrective lenses, a magnifying glass, a hearing aid, posters, and other enlarged image or print media. Patients with poor reading ability will also benefit from visual aids such as photographs, diagrams, movies, and video tapes. In some instances it is necessary to involve the family or significant others in patient teaching sessions so that they can assist the patient with self-care. Teaching these persons may also heighten their involvement in and commitment to the patient's self-sufficiency.

Dealing with nurse factors requires a variety of strategies. Corkadel and McGlashan[8] describe a series of classes designed for staff nurses that addressed the areas of role clarification and resource utilization, nurse–patient rapport, content review, learning needs assessment, assessment of readiness to learn, teaching strategies, and documentation. Hinthorne[9] developed a Patient Teaching Flow Sheet to help nurses perform and document patient teaching (see boxes on p. 399). Whitehouse[10] also designed a patient teaching record. It includes general topics as well as specific information presented, documentation of time and

Hinthorne's Directions for the Use of the Patient Teaching Flow Sheet

1. As the patient is admitted and you are interviewing him for the patient profile you have an excellent opportunity to assess the patient's learning needs. Enter these in the column "Teaching Needs" in terms of patient behavior. See box below.

2. At this time you can decide the teaching methods that would be most appropriate for this patient. Enter these in the column "Teaching Approach." See example.

3. As the staff initiates these approaches, the date is entered. This communicates to all members of the health team just exactly what the teaching plan is. Thus anyone on the staff can initiate an approach at the time most conducive for patient learning.

4. When the patient demonstrates that he has achieved the objective, note the date and sign it.

5. If the patient is unable to learn (confused, forgetful) please note this across the top of the Teaching Sheet.

6. If you are able to teach the family or significant others, please note this across top of sheet, i.e., "Daughter Taught."

7. In these cases use the sheet as you would for the patient. Family should be included in all teaching situations when possible.

From Hinthorne, R. (1983). Teaching nurses how to teach patients. *Nursing Management, 14*(9), 30-33.

teacher, comments shared by the nurse and patient, and an evaluation section. Planned conferences using real patient situations can serve as both a learning experience for the staff and an instructional planning session for the patient. Whatever methods are used to overcome nurses' real or perceived barriers to patient teaching, nursing administration should evidence its support by providing time, money, and recognition to the nursing staff.

DEFINING STAFF DEVELOPMENT

The term *staff development* describes a process that involves both formal and informal learning opportunities to assist individuals to perform competently in fulfillment of role expectations within a specific setting. Both internal and external resources may be used to facilitate this process. The primary goal of nursing staff development is to provide opportunities for employed nursing personnel to acquire further knowledge, skills, and attitudes needed to perform their assigned functions safely and effectively in the provision of nursing care to patients and their families.

Current Status and Future Directions

Nursing staff development has traditionally focused on orientation and inservice education, but there is now an increasing emphasis on continuing education with experientially and educationally prepared teachers, a wide variety of teaching strategies, and systematic evaluation of learners and programs. The shortage of professional nurses combined with the high patient acuity in the critical care setting chal-

Problem-oriented Flow Sheet for General Patient Teaching

MEDICAL RECORD	PROBLEM-ORIENTED FLOW SHEET—GENERAL Problem Numbers and Titles (Do Not Abbreviate)				
Patient Teaching Teaching Needs	Teaching Approach	Date	Verbalizes and/or demon. know.	Signature
Identify action dosage, side effects of Digoxin Lasix	1. Write out for patient	5/1		
	2. Explain as you give medicine × 3 day	5/1		
	3. Question patient	5/4	5/4	D. Miller
Select proper food: 2 GmNa, Hi K	1. Dietitian consult	5/2		
	2. Hand out list	5/2		
	3. Discuss		5/6	D. Miller
Explain A & P of heart	1. Video "I Am Joe's Heart"	5/4		
	2. Discuss			
Recognize symptoms which require medical attention	1. Hand out list	5/6		
	2. Discuss			

From Hinthorne, R. (1983). Teaching nurses how to teach patients. *Nursing Management, 14*(9), 30-33.

lenges the staff development educator to provide clinically relevant education in a timely and cost-effective manner. This is the present state of affairs and seems likely to continue in the foreseeable future.

Factors That Affect Teaching and Learning

Because nurses are working longer shifts and caring for patients with greater acuity, staff development must be timely, clinically relevant, and presented in a convenient a comfortable environment. As nurses participate in increasing numbers in shared governance, they will be more involved in the determination of staff development foci and in program planning. In some models of shared governance, the staff development educator is unit based, thus a part of the "team" and in touch with the needs of the nurses on that unit for educational experiences. This individual, because of physical proximity to the nurses in the clinical setting and because of expertise in the specialty (e.g., critical care nursing) can provide (1) applicable staff development programs tailored to the needs of the nurses in the setting; (2) ongoing, unit-based leadership for educational activities; and (3) peer support to nurses wishing to develop their own teaching skills. As summarized by Robinson,[11] unit-based staff development nurses provide opportunities for the professional development of staff nurses while offering the necessary leadership and peer support needed to foster commitment.

LEARNING NEEDS ASSESSMENT

Assessment of the individual's learning needs is conducted to anticipate or recognize needed behavior change, to establish mutually identified educational goals, to determine the preexisting knowledge base, and to correct misinformation. Assessment can be accomplished through individual and family interviews, written questionnaires, chart audit, review of the research literature, evaluation of relevant health care and illness statistics, and conferences with family and with nurse colleagues and other members of the health care team. Much can be learned by listening with a third ear—that is, hearing what the individual does *not* say as well as what is said. Facilitative responding, listening carefully and reflecting back to the learner the feelings and content of statements, may help both learner and teacher to identify general and specific learning needs.

"Therapeutic seeding," described by Corkadel and McGlashan,[12] is a technique used to "plant ideas" via suggestion in the learner's mind. Given time to think about the idea, the learner can then identify personal learning needs. An example of this technique is "Many of our cardiac patients have questions about their postdischarge diet. Perhaps you have some, too."

Factors That Affect Learning Needs

Each person's learning needs are affected by such factors as knowledge, past experience, values, priorities, and willingness to change. Determining the individual's preexisting knowledge, skills and attitudes provides a point of reference for identifying learning needs. The person may reveal incorrect or inaccurate knowledge or skills that need to be corrected as soon as possible so that learning can proceed from a sound base. The adult's experience in life and as a learner can either help or hinder learning. Positive feelings about oneself as a person and as a learner can heighten the individual's desire to learn and willingness to change, whereas failures in life and in learning may cause fears and anxiety that prevent learning. In addition, past experiences that conflict with what the individual is asked to learn may lead to resistance to change.

Adults value information and skills that help them to live their lives more happily and more productively—both to avoid and solve problems, and to be self-directed and independent. The adult's priorities for learning relate to these goals. Some may be indirectly health related, such as living on a restricted diet, maintaining or regaining sexual function, or resuming the role as family wage earner. The nurse should encourage the person to share these priorities so that mutually satisfying goals can be set.

Age can be a useful indicator of a person's priorities, according to Taylor.[13] For example, teenaged to young adult patients consider appearance the highest priority. Learning about bowel, bladder, or sexual function is also a high priority; other teaching is secondary until these needs are addressed. Middle-aged persons also consider appearance an important priority; they want to understand problems with bowel, bladder, or sexual function but are uncomfortable discussing them and worry most about family acceptance of changes in body image. Elderly persons tend to consider function a higher priority than appearance, are uncomfortable discussing bodily functions, and often accept the inevitability of loss affecting body image, especially if it prolongs life or brings comfort.

Learning from Patients about Their Needs

Barrett and Schwartz,[14] interested in what and how much patients want or need to know, administered a questionnaire to 15 hospitalized patients. Patients' knowledge level varied with regard to causes, effects, and prognosis of the illness, treatments, and tests, but most said they wanted to know (1) the name of the illness, (2) how the illness affected their body, (3) what to expect about recovery, (4) what to expect from medical tests, and (5) how the condition would affect their life.

Although most patients want at least some information about their illness and treatment, some would rather "let the doctor decide" or have a family member receive the information. Such a patient's "need not to know" should be periodically reassessed and questions answered as the patient poses them.

Patients also have much to teach nurses, which in turn makes patient teaching more individual and effective. Taylor[15] offers several tips for learning from patients about their needs:

- Discover what the patient already knows.
- Ask the patient about his or her treatment; for example, "How have you been doing this procedure?" or "Which way is best for you?"
- Reinforce book learning with real-life examples.
- Do not be defensive about a patient's criticism.
- Learn from the things the patient doesn't say, including nonverbal behavior such as strained facial expression, nail biting, excessive eating, or smoking.

Learning from Nurses about Their Needs

Monette[16] believed that needs assessment "ought to involve the testing of felt needs so as to uncover the real needs," because a felt need may be symptomatic of a real need and only the learners can "decide to learn and to act upon their learnings." The staff development educator may facilitate this process by providing standards or criteria against which "learners can make comparisons and determine the nature and magnitude of their need."[17]

Specific strategies for assessing learning needs have been described in the literature. For example, MacDonald and Grogin[17] asked nurses to relate their personal accounts of both satisfying and unsatisfying nursing experiences. These were analyzed and categorized according to Maslow's theory of basic human needs to determine whether a gap existed (and the nature of that gap) between what the nurses knew and what they needed to know in order to have a sense of accomplishment. Sullivan and others[18] designed questionnaires with a list of generic topics as well as those specific to the specialty. Items were placed in the sequence of knowledge (Likert-type scale), skills (prioritizing), and demographic information (forced choice and fill-in-the-blank questions). The results were illustrated in the Johari window (Figure 16-1). The Arena space contained learning needs ranked as priority by nurse managers and staff. The

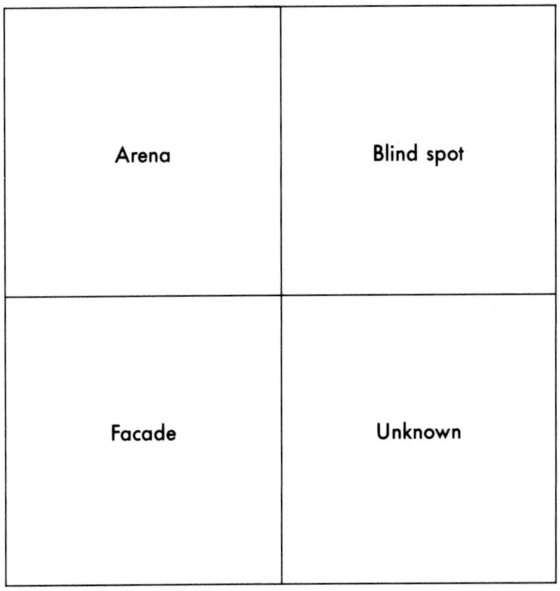

Figure 16-1   Johari window.

From Sullivan, P., Saver, C., Moyer, D., et al. (1991). Needs assessment: Process and application. *Journal of Nursing Staff Development* 7(1), 33.

Blind Spot consisted of topics identified only by staff nurses as priority learning needs. The Facade contained topics identified by the nurse managers as priority for the staff nurses, while the Unknown contained all the topics that neither nurse managers nor staff nurses selected as priority learning needs.

This use of the Johari window is helpful to the nurse educator in organizing learning needs as they are identified by staff nurses and nurse managers. Selection of priorities for staff development would ideally come from Arena first, with Blind Spot or Facade topics chosen on the basis of such factors as available resources (e.g., expert teachers, time, and space), "mandatory" areas dictated by accrediting agencies or institutional policy, and problems highlighted by quality assurance activities.

The Johari window strategy is also useful to the educator in identifying appropriate motivational strategies. For example, if it is deemed necessary to offer a program to staff nurses from the Facade, the educator will need to persuade the learners of its benefit to them over and above the nurse manager's decision that they need the information or skill. If the educator chooses a topic from the Blind Spot, the nurse managers must be provided with data supporting the selection, such as changing clinical practice, specialty certification requirements, or the timeliness of focusing on the staff nurses' requests when they perceive that the nurse manager always has the final vote.

Needs assessment models include individual self-fulfillment, discrepancy, competency, and demographic. *Self-fulfillment data* are usually collected via individuals' completion of a questionnaire, telephone interview, or suggestion boxes. The problem with these methods is that they often assess learners' interests or wants rather than needs. *Discrepancy* approaches are used to diagnose the gap between what is and what ought to be in order to solve or eliminate the problem. *Competency* models assess individuals' learning needs in relation to a standard of performance. For example, nurses can be rated by selves, managers, or peers. *Democratic* models involve the learners or a representative sample in learning need identification using such techniques as Nominal Group Process and the Delphi Technique.[19] Learning needs may also be derived from organizational needs through such methods as quality assurance and risk management. Society is another source of learning needs, such as those reflected in regulatory requirements and changing societal conditions such as child, spouse, and elder abuse.[20]

NEED AND READINESS TO LEARN: POTENTIAL OBSTACLES

Individualizing a learner's instruction requires an in-depth assessment of the learner's current knowledge, skills, and attitudes; previous health and educational experiences; preferred learning modes; and cultural, social, and economic factors. Stanton[21] developed a diagrammatic representation of the factors that she believes govern both needs and readiness to learn (Figure 16-2). These include intellectual capac-

ity, developmental stage, personal characteristics, prior experiences, sociocultural group, religious group, prevalent life needs, and stage of illness. Any number of these factors may also be obstacles to learning. For example, Caron and Roth,[22] in studying the effectiveness of a program that taught a peptic ulcer regimen, identified three specific sets of obstacles: the patient's lack of understanding of certain key concepts, such as acid neutralization; erroneous concepts previously learned, for example, the ineffectiveness of antacid therapy; and fears and concerns present at the time of illness, including fear of loss of job or spouse.

Murray and Zentner[23] described these and other prohibitors to teaching and learning that need to be acknowledged and considered in planning for learning:

- Language or reading response: individuals decode instructional messages in relation to background situations, prejudices, and moods, which affect belief and comprehension.
- Culture: new ideas and practices are judged in relation to existing customs and beliefs.
- Myths and unconscious resistance.
- Personal prejudices related to such characteristics as race, personality, status, or sex.

To overcome language as a prohibitor, a variety of audiovisual aids should be used as adjuncts to verbal explanations, such as motion pictures, videotapes, slides, and photographs. In response to culture as a prohibitor, there are a variety of useful strategies: (1) Consult important persons whose prestige can lend influence to the recommended change in behavior, and then refer to that person in teaching sessions; (2) develop a feeling for the culture's beliefs, attitudes, knowledge, and behavior; (3) be aware of subcultural variations; (4) identify family and/or community decision makers; (5) appeal to the group's desire for health; and (6) help the individual and family to maintain a realistic perspective on effects of changed behavior.

Myths need to be identified and refuted with facts and figures whenever possible; they may be the basis for both conscious and unconscious resistance. Personal prejudices may inhibit the effectiveness of both teacher and learner. Recognition of these feelings as well as open discussion and negotiations regarding their resolution are essential if this barrier is to be overcome.

The stage of the patient's illness affects readiness to learn, which is described as a state of being both willing and able to make use of instruction. Lee[24] refers to these stages of illness as impact, regression, acknowledgment, and reconstruction. These are briefly described as follows:

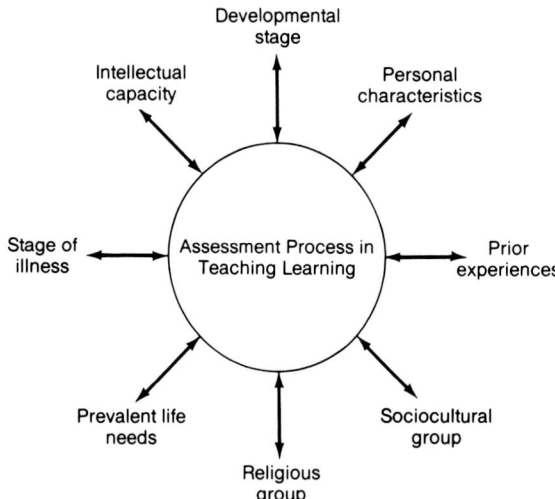

Figure 16-2 Stanton's diagrammatic representation of factors that govern need and readiness to learn.

From Stanton, M. (1985). Teaching patients: Some basic lessons for nurse educators. *Nursing Management, 16,* 59.

1. *Impact*: the patient's initial emotional reaction to a trauma or illness. Feelings of anxiety, fear of dying, loss of control, despair, and discouragement are evident.
2. *Regression*: sets in with physiological stability; denial is the defense mechanism usually used by the patient in flight from reality. This stage gives the patient time to prepare for dealing with the crisis. Some patients express their fear of the loss of belonging and love through anger, others joke about the illness or make unrealistic plans for postdischarge activities.
3. *Acknowledgment*: also called the *mourning period*, when the patient's self-esteem and self-confidence are at an all-time low. The patient reviews precrisis events to identify and prevent the recurrence of its causes; the patient may also acknowledge his or her change in body image.
4. *Reconstruction*: brings hope for the future with the patient's renewed sense of self-worth and potential.

No teaching should begin in the impact stage, although the patient's and family's questions should be answered and nursing actions explained. In the regression stage, teaching should be realistic, presented in a nonthreatening manner, and with reality given in small doses. Effective teaching can best begin in the acknowledgment stage, when the patient accepts and often asks for explanations and educational materials. Reconstruction may be enhanced by a focus on rehabilitation training, with instruction offered in a positive, nonblaming manner.

Factors that strongly influence readiness to learn are comfort, energy, motivation, and capability. Comfort is both physical and psychological and should be provided during each session. Physical discomfort may be due to pain, nausea, fatigue, hunger, thirst, weakness, or dizziness. Emotional discomfort includes fear, anxiety, worry, depression, and anger. The learner's energy level is related to the physical status before illness as well as to the current stage of illness, psychological status, and stress level.

Motivation to Learn

Motivation is an important variable that must be considered, both in assessing learner readiness and in selecting teaching strategies. In its truest sense motivation is concerned with what gains individuals' attention, what directs their actions, and what keeps them learning (changing their behavior). Both intrinsic and extrinsic factors have been identified as contributing to motivation. The most frequently cited variables are:
- A positive orientation toward learning, as evidenced by such behaviors as persistence, a high need for

achievement, a high level of aspiration, a positive self-concept, and positive feelings about past learning experiences
- Curiosity about things, events, people, and relationships
- A need for social recognition
- Desire for conformity
- The desire to avoid failure

According to many nurse-teachers, learners are motivated if they want to do the things the teacher thinks they should want to do, such as quit smoking, eat "right," exercise regularly, or stop worrying. In reality, persons are motivated to learn and do those things that help them to solve problems and avoid distress.

Some principles of motivation to use in working with individuals are:
- A sense of satisfaction has the most positive effect on future motivation.
- Learners, in general, progress only as far as they need to in order to achieve their objectives or goals.
- Genuine participation, not pretended sharing, enhances learner motivation at each step of the learning process.
- To the extent possible, there must be freedom from discouragement or threats.
- Feedback must be closely connected to learners' efforts when they are evaluating their own performance.
- Both positive reinforcement, such as praise and attention, and negative reinforcement, including removal of discomfort and lessening of fears, should be used to increase the likelihood of a response recurring.
- Always help the person to see the applicability of the desired knowledge, skills, and attitudes to the solution of personally identified problems.

Capacity to Learn

The capacity to learn is composed of the following factors:
- Aptitude; the amount of time required by the learner to actually learn the behavior or information. Aptitude is affected by the learner's individual differences and experiences
- The ability to understand instructions
- The opportunity or time allowed for learning
- The learner's perseverance, which is affected by motivation, physical stamina or endurance, ability to cope with frustration, and number of external distractions[25]

Often the learner's ability to understand instructions reflects knowledge of hospital vocabulary. Byrne and Edeani,[26] in a follow-up to earlier studies, found a significant difference between nurses' perceptions of patients' knowledge and patients' actual understanding of medical terminology. Although knowledge of medical terms had increased significantly over the two decades prior to the study, many black adults (44%), Hispanic adults (33%), and white adults were reported as functionally or marginally illiterate.[27] Apse and Stetle[28] found that the better educated the patient, the better the understanding of medical terms, and the older the patient, the fewer clinical terms known. Investigators suggest that not only should nurses make themselves and their colleagues more aware of this issue but also that (1) fewer technical terms be used in patient education materials, (2) patients be oriented to hospital terminology, and (3) a handbook of commonly used medical terms be compiled and distributed to patients. The patient's and family's feedback should be elicited to determine whether they comprehend the instruction given.

Instructions should also be specific and simple, such as "take the tablet three times a day with food," rather than "take the tablet after every meal." Repeat instructions both orally and in printed materials whenever time and resources permit.

Cognitive Dissonance

A factor called *cognitive dissonance* can greatly influence learning. The basic premise of this concept is that one's knowledge, beliefs, and attitudes are generally consistent with one another. If given information that is not consistent, one experiences discomfort that may motivate one to change or, alternatively, may reinforce the "correctness" of present knowledge, beliefs, and attitudes.[29] For example, persons who smoke, when taught that smoking causes cancer, believe this to be true. They may subsequently quit, rationalize that they are not susceptible and continue to smoke, or accept the risk and continue to smoke. Observing that a learner is denying susceptibility or accepting risk, the teacher may discuss the inconsistency between knowledge and behavior with him or her. A learner may then do one of the following to modify the inconsistency:

- Revise the initial decision to fit more closely the nurse's belief in the dangers of smoking
- Diminish the importance of the teacher's perceptions by such actions as questioning the available statistics
- Look for other aspects of the problem on which to agree, for example, some types of cigarettes are more dangerous than are others
- Change the perception of certain aspects of the situation by scheduling a chest film or implementing an exercise plan

Other strategies that a person might use to cope with the dissonance are denial, projection (criticize the teacher), or suppression, to name a few.

The teacher can help the learner resolve the dissonance in a manner that leads to abstinence from smoking by focusing on the underlying issues such as stress, peer pressure, or weak self-image; by helping to plan step-by-step alterations, for example, changing to a brand of cigarettes lower in tar, or smoking only a certain number of cigarettes each day; or by referral to a credible smoking cessation program and support group.

SPECIFICATION OF OBJECTIVES

The formulation of objectives should be accomplished by the teacher in collaboration with the learner. As Stanton[30] notes, specifying learner behaviors is helpful for the following reasons:

- It makes clear to teacher and learner what the expected outcome(s) is (are).
- It guides the teacher in selecting appropriate content, learning activities, and/or media.
- It directs the teacher toward valid methods of evaluating learner outcomes.

It is important to differentiate among the domains of learning—cognitive (thinking), psychomotor (doing), and affective (feeling)—in order to teach and evaluate in a valid and fair manner. Simple words and phrases should be used so that both teacher and learner are clear regarding the expected outcomes. For example, objectives relating to dietary modification might be:

- Cognitive: Name five foods high in sodium.
- Psychomotor: Prepare a green, leafy vegetable using low-sodium seasoning.
- Affective: Report the daily substitution of fresh fruits for salt snacks within 1 week.

TEACHING TECHNIQUES

Although some teaching techniques are more effective than are others with certain persons and in certain situations, there are no specific rules to apply in their selection. It is important that the technique correlate with the learning objectives, that it be familiar and nonthreatening to the learner, and that the teacher have experience with and/or comfort in its use. Murray and Zentner[31] organized teaching techniques according to desired behavioral outcomes:

1. Acquiring generalizations about experiences: lectures, symposiums, reading, audiovisual materials, and discussion based on printed materials.
2. Applying information to experience: problem-solving discussions, laboratory experiments, case studies, group activities such as role playing and simulation.

3. Skill development: role playing, coaching, demonstration, and return demonstration.
4. Creating new attitudes: reverse role playing, simulation games, and experience-sharing discussion.
5. Changing values: biographical or autobiographical reading, drama, experienced speakers, support groups, and values clarification activities.

Varied Teaching Strategies

As an educator, the nurse needs a varied repertoire of strategies from which to choose. Many of those to be described are traditional but still useful; others are relatively new and worthy of consideration.

Lecture is useful for providing information efficiently to large numbers of persons. The teacher retains control of the content, the time, and the amount and nature of interaction. Lecture is most appropriate when memory and logical organization of information are required.

The drawbacks of lecture include (1) poor retention, with approximately 40% of content forgotten in 20 minutes; (2) the tendency of the learners to remember the quality of the presentation rather than the content; and (3) the difficulty learners have in requesting clarification of specific points. Useful techniques for enhancing a lecture include adding a question and answer period, using meaningful examples for the learners, providing a content outline for note taking, and using slides or other media to stress important points.[32]

A *panel presentation* uses the expertise of four to eight persons in a planned conversation on a specific topic. A moderator, who has prepared questions in advance, initiates and sustains the discussion. This technique, as well as debate, is useful for presenting conflicting points of view. In both instances, the learner is passive, so that the moderator may wish to elicit questions from the audience.

Demonstration is appropriate for instruction in psychomotor skills. The teacher serves as a model of attainable skill and can provide immediate feedback to the learner when a return demonstration is requested. Anatomical models and equipment enable the learner to see and touch as well as listen, all of which enhance learning skills.

Class size should be limited so that all learners can see the demonstration; videotaped demonstrations can increase visibility. Return demonstration enables learners to practice the skill, with immediate feedback after the learner completes the procedure. Sufficient equipment, time and space are needed, as well as a low teacher/learner ratio.

The use of *discussion* actively involves the learner by encouraging his or her input and questions, with an opportunity for feedback and reinforcement. The peer group can provide another, perhaps more influential level of pressure for change to which the learner may be more responsive.

Group discussions are often used as a follow-up to a lecture, film, or other large group presentation. Forming small groups for discussions enables learners to analyze the content in greater detail and to apply it to individual situations. This technique is also useful when dealing with individual or group attitudes, values, and beliefs. The teacher must keep the group on target, make sure each learner has a chance to participate, and avoid anyone's dominating the discussion.

Adom and Wright[33] found in their study of hospitalized adults that two thirds preferred *group teaching*, perhaps because they felt less alone in a group in which their fears and questions were voiced by others as well as themselves. In addition, the patients in this study gained reassurance from shared feelings in the group setting, perceived that sufficient time and attention had been given to them as individuals, and felt well prepared for surgery. Nurses, however, indicated a greater preference for individual teaching, perhaps because they were more familiar and comfortable with this method. Nevertheless, nurses perceived that group teaching was more time-effective and, therefore, of increasing value with shortened length of stay and decreased staff.

Case studies and critical incidents enable learners to apply previously learned information to situations derived from real life. *Case studies,* accounts of problem situations, help learners develop problem-solving skills by requiring them to decide what to do next or what was done correctly (or incorrectly) in the situation. A *critical incident* presents the learner with only the most important or dramatic aspect of the situation. The learners need to ask the appropriate questions to elicit the needed data from the teacher.

Simulation games and *role playing* are effective in actively involving persons in learning. They are particularly useful for providing a relatively safe environment in which to test new or modified attitudes, values, and beliefs.

Simulation provides the learner with a situation that duplicates, as nearly as possible, the actual environment, for example, mass casualty exercise or patient emergency. Learners, under the pressure of the experience, must make decisions and use skills that would be needed in such situations. An effective simulation requires much advance planning and is often expensive; the more realistic it is, the more effective it will be.

Instructional games, while expensive, difficult to

develop, and time-consuming, involve learners in mastering the learning objectives. A "debriefing" session is needed at the end of the game to reinforce the objectives and review the outcomes.

In *role play* each learner is given information about the situation and the individual characters, as well as about other characters involved. After the participants act out the scenario, the learners as a group critique the behaviors/interactions. Videotaping the session enables participants to critique their own performance as well. The teacher needs to be skilled in group dynamics and sensitive to learner tolerance of this technique.

Independent study is especially beneficial to those who enjoy learning on their own, with the teacher serving as guide, facilitator, and evaluator. The variety of audiovisual and printed materials available provides the flexibility and individual approach that many learners prefer.

Charts, graphs, diagrams, posters, and photographs can be used to supplement verbal or written descriptions and to provide added detail or relationships. These are particularly useful when the learner needs to see the object, activity, or concept being discussed.

Audiotapes are difficult to use for learning because of the concentration required and the dependence on only the sense of hearing. If supplemented with printed materials or slides, they are more effective. Audiotapes are most appropriate when the person needs to learn to differentiate between or among sounds such as heart sounds or those of a dialysis machine or volumetric infusion pump.

The 16-millimeter movies are useful for group instruction, especially if the objectives specify movement or interaction, both verbal and nonverbal. Elderly patients and the learning disadvantaged are particularly responsive to this medium. Slides, transparencies, and filmstrips can be integrated with other media (audiotapes) and methods (lecture) and can be presented at variable rates, which is particularly helpful to middle-aged and elderly learners who may need more time to study the pictures or print.

Videotapes provide visualization and action, are a familiar medium to most, and can be stopped at intervals for a patient's questions if a teacher is present. Some learners cannot keep up with the fast-paced format; others dislike the "talking heads" with whom they cannot interact. Many hospitals and other health care institutions are developing centralized education channels on television. If this format is used, the teacher should be available to answer learners' questions and to evaluate their learning.

Relatively new to the catalogue of education media is the computer, which offers an active learning en-vironment. Computer-assisted instruction offers patients the advantages of self-paced learning, frequent testing for comprehension with immediate feedback, individualized questions and information, and simulation of real-life situations.

Selecting and Evaluating Media

Many nurses and patients contract a condition known as "media-itis," which is caused by an overdose and/or prolonged exposure to inappropriate visual and auditory stimuli. This condition is a direct result of the belief that each instructional session should contain audiovisual materials and that everyone learns more effectively when they are utilized.

In determining the appropriateness of using these materials for education, nurses need to consider the objective(s) to be attained by the learner, the size of the group, the availability of equipment, the teacher's skill in using equipment, and the location of the program. Questions to be considered when evaluating audiovisual materials are listed in the box on p. 407.

Use of Printed Materials

In developing printed teaching materials, application of a number of principles should make these materials more effective and useful:

- Use a title that describes clearly the purpose and contents of the material, such as "Sexual Function after Myocardial Infarction."
- Use purpose stagements—e.g., when the information should be used (as prescribed, as needed), and what materials are needed (quiet room, comfortable clothing).
- Present information clearly and concisely (number items, organize from simple to complex, provide rationale for actions).
- Highlight possible errors or precautions ("It is important to . . ." "Caution . . ." "Be sure to . . .").
- Select visuals to meet the objectives and facilitate learning, then use them correctly (label figures, diagrams, charts), use clear photographs, eliminate distractions.
- Use easy-to-read type and other visual devices such as different type styles and sizes, color, arrows, boxes, while avoiding clutter and distracting variety.
- Test the material for readability using such tools as the Smog Readability Formula. Do not assume that learners read at the level of their completed education. Glazer-Waldman, Hall, and Weiner[34] found in a sample of 81 literate patients that only 40% could read at the sixth-grade level.

Morton[35] describes a staff development activity using printed materials that is called "The 10-Minute Learning Break." Each clinical unit must have a stan-

Evaluating Audiovisual Materials

- Do the visuals (slides, photos, posters) portray scenes, people, and items familiar to the learner?
- Do the visuals contain material that may be offensive to cultural background (clothing, lifestyle, or character)?
- Are the verbal cues appropriate to the learner's level of literacy? Are terms defined? Is medical terminology kept to a minimum when appropriate?
- If the objective is to teach a skill, is there an opportunity to practice?
- If the objective is to modify attitudes, beliefs, or values, does the program ask for a commitment to action?
- Are correct responses provided to the learner?
- Is the informational content accurate and up to date? Is it presented at the appropriate developmental and literacy levels? Has it been approved by recognized and respected health care associations?
- Does each picture or sequence of pictures represent a single concept?
- Is the graphic information legible?
- Are the visuals properly lighted so that details are easily seen?
- Are the voices clear? Is music appropriate to mood?
- Does the program have an identifiable introduction, body, and conclusion?
- Does the introduction gain and maintain the learner's interest? Identify the objective of the presentation? State the reasons (if applicable) for the learner's participation? Show the need for change? Demonstrate workable action? Is there enough repetition?
- Does the program appeal to and maintain learner interest?

dard location, such as a bulletin board or communication book in which the nurse educator can post a one- or two-page flyer. The flyer is prepared by the educator weekly or monthly and contains content that can be read in 10 minutes or less. "Theme" flyers such as "Leadership Break," "Self-Esteem," "Stress Management," "Five-Minute Facts" (clinical content), and "Did you Know . . ." can be used to reinforce concepts and skills or pique staff interest in upcoming programs.

Focus on Sensory Information

Preparing patients for diagnostic or therapeutic procedures has traditionally focused on specific information such as the equipment to be used and the steps in the procedure. McHugh, Christman, and Johnson[36] found that sensory information was also helpful to patients in coping. These authors defined sensory information as "information about our environment that is acquired by way of our sensory modalities—sight, hearing, touch, taste, and smell." Their proposition was that giving patients information about typical experiences they could anticipate during a procedure would help them form realistic mental images (schemata), which would lead them to expect certain things to occur. A series of studies indicated that (1) patients told about sensations created by pumping a blood pressure cuff on the arm to the level of 250 mmHg reported less distress than those not informed, (2) patients given sensory information coped more effectively with gastroendoscopic examinations, and (3) preparatory information decreased the length of the postoperative hospital stay for patients undergoing cholecystectomy. Patients in these studies were given sensory information describing both objective and subjective features of the event, including length of the procedure, nature and location of objects in the environment, and physical sensation.

Guidelines for giving patients preparatory information were provided:
- Describe but do not evaluate physical sensations ("It will ache or burn" but not "You'll really feel awful").
- Tell patients the cause of the sensations.
- Focus on commonly occurring aspects of the experience.

General indicators of the effect of a diagnostic or therapeutic procedure on a patient include the amount of sedation needed, verbal and facial expressions, degree of cooperation, and subsequent length of hospitalization.

DISCHARGE PLANNING

Each patient preparing for a transition in care setting needs to learn something, whether it be knowledge, skills, or attitudes. Because patients in increasing numbers are being discharged directly from the critical care setting, both they and their families need to learn how to perform procedures, how to organize resources, and how to recognize and respond to signs and symptoms of complications or exacerbation of problems. Patients who are discharged to an extended care facility need to know what their options are, how their care needs will be met, and how to handle the financial aspects of the transfer. Patients transferring from the critical care area to another unit within the acute care facility also need to know who will be caring for them and what care to expect.

Postponing discharge instruction until shortly before the patient leaves the critical care setting is ineffective for two important reasons: (1) the patient's attention span and ability to concentrate are limited by anxiety about the planned transition in care and (2) teaching done with the pressure of a deadline is usually less well presented and may confuse rather than enlighten the learner.

The decision about whether to include family or significant others in discharge planning is based on three criteria: (1) the individual or group will be affected by the patient's change in behavior (learning); (2) the individual or group can lend support to a change; or (3) the individual or group has responsibility with the patient for a behavior change.[37]

EVALUATION OF TEACHING AND LEARNING

Evaluation usually receives the least attention in education, perhaps because it is viewed as too time-consuming and difficult to implement. One way to facilitate evaluation is to develop measurable learner objectives and outcomes that guide the selection of measurement procedures and the judgment of learner attainment.

The use of written tests may be useful, although one must be concerned with validity (does the test measure what it is supposed to measure?), reliability (generalizability), readability, practicality (ease of administration and grading), and resources needed (paper, pencil, desk).

Observation is another useful tool, particularly if a checklist or rating scale is developed that includes the desired outcomes in measurable terms. Psychomotor skills are best evaluated with a performance rating scale or checklist completed during a learner demonstration.

Antecdotal notes are useful for noting behaviors in all domains—cognitive, psychomotor, and affective. Both objective and subjective data can be included from which a judgment can be made.

Interviews serve dual purposes: (1) to measure changes in knowledge and attitudes, and (2) to elicit the learner's opinions about the teaching program and instruction. It is useful to record compliments and complaints as a basis for improving the effectiveness of the teaching. Family members and significant others should also be asked for opinions on the effectiveness of the teaching session or program.

Documentation of instruction and learner outcomes is essential. It serves as an indispensable form of communication among health care professionals to ensure continuity and as a legal record of a learner's attainment. The patient's record should also reflect the patient's and family's response to teaching, including doubts, fears, satisfaction, and confidence.

Communication should also occur via such avenues as nursing care plans, planning conferences, and nursing rounds. All methods of communication pro-

---

Suggestions for Effective Teaching[39]

- Be consistent in your approach to the learner.
- Show enthusiasm for the content and its value.
- Present yourself as a role model (neat, erect, alert, calm).
- Know your content and present it in an organized manner so that the learner has confidence in what you are saying.
- Continually evaluate the effectiveness of your teaching, seeking input from peers and learners.
- Use available teaching methods, resources, and referral systems as appropriate.
- Communicate orally and in writing with other nurse-teachers about the learner's level of understanding and attainment of objectives.
- Respect the learner as an individual with wants and needs that may differ from those of the health care system.
- Give the learner the rationale for any guidelines or prescriptions.
- Do not equate ability to learn with educational level.
- Distinguish between learning ability and misunderstandings caused by cultural, ethnic, religious, or developmental differences.
- Learn about the learner in order to identify teachable moments.
- Stimulate the person's desire to learn rather than using such external motivators as threats or bribes.
- Give frequent feedback and reinforcement.

---

vide an opportunity to evaluate the effectiveness of instructional programs.

Broader foci for evaluation in education have been suggested by Price and Cordell.[38] Their premise is that scientific methods must be applied to the teaching and learning process in order to validate the process. Some of the more frequent areas of investigation, which can serve as the basis for replication as well as new ideas, include changes in learners as a result of educational experiences; surveys of techniques, materials, evaluation methods, and so on; effects of "teaching style" on educational outcomes; and comparison of group and individual instruction.

HELPFUL HINTS

Murray and Zentner[39] list suggestions for effective teaching which have a common-sense appeal, enhancing their value to the nurse teacher in the box above.

Some of the most rewarding aspects of nursing are derived from education. As Woldum et al.[40] point out so clearly in their philosophical perspective on the nurse as teacher:

- Believe in yourself as a teacher and in the value of this role in your practice.
- See yourself as an extension of the learner.
- Seek peer support for your teaching activities.
- See yourself as an important advocate for the learner without encouraging dependence.
- Risk questioning your beliefs about education in order to be open to new perspectives.
- Let the learner teach you whenever possible.
- View every communication with the patient as a form of instruction.
- Be aware of, acknowledge, and collaborate with other health care providers in providing teaching.
- Accept responsibility and accountability for documenting education.
- Experiment with innovative and creative teaching and evaluation techniques.

In this era of prospective payment, high technology, and growing consumer awareness, the nurse faces the challenge of educating a more complex and knowledgeable patient and nurse population. Use of the teaching–learning process, which includes the assessment of learner needs, specification of objectives, selection of teaching techniques, and evaluation of teaching and learning enables the critical care nurse to provide cost-effective education while maintaining quality patient care.

REFERENCES

1. Narrow, B. (1979). *Patient teaching in nursing practice*. New York: Wiley.
2. American Hospital Association. (1982). *Policy and statement. The hospital's responsibility for patient education services*. Chicago: Author.
3. Burke, C. (1985). Patient education and cost containment. *Computers in Healthcare, 6*, 38-42.
4. Miller, A. (1985). When is the time ripe for teaching? *American Journal of Nursing, 85*(7), 801-804.
5. Levin, L. (1978). Patient education and self-care: How do they differ? *Nursing Outlook, 26*, 170-175.
6. Harrell, J., & Frauman, A. (1985). Prospective payment calls for boosting productivity. *Nursing and Health Care, 6*(10), 535-537.
7. Bigge, M. (1976). *Learning theories for teachers*. New York: Harper & Row.
8. Corkadel, L., & McGlashan, R. (1983). A practical approach to patient teaching. *The Journal of Continuing Education in Nursing, 14*, 9-15.
9. Hinthorne, R. (1983). Teaching nurses how to teach patients. *Nuring Management, 14*(9), 30-33.
10. Whitehouse, R. (1979). Forms that facilitate patient teaching. *American Journal of Nursing, 79*(7), 1227-1229.
11. Robinson, J. (1991). Focus. Patient education: Opportunity and necessity. *Journal of Nursing Staff Development, 7*(1), 97-98.
12. Corkadel, L., & McGlashan, R. (1983). A practical approach to patient teaching. *The Journal of Continuing Education in Nursing, 14*, 9-15.
13. Taylor, P. (1982). Patient teaching: Keys to more success more often. *Nursing Life, 2*, 25-32.
14. Barrett, N., & Schwartz, N. (1981). What patients really want to know. *American Journal of Nursing, 81*(9), 1642.
15. Taylor J. (1984). Are you missing what your patients can teach you? *RN, 47*, 63-69.
16. Monette, M. (1977). The concept of educational need: An analysis of selected literature. *Adult Education, 27*(2), 116-127.
17. MacDonald, R., & Grogin, E. (1991). Personal accounts of satisfying and unsatisfying nursing experiences as a needs assessment strategy. *Journal of Continuing Education in Nursing, 22*(1), 11-15.
18. Sullivan, P., Saver, C., Moyer, D., et al. (1991). Needs assessment. Process and application. *Journal of Nursing Staff Development, 7*(1), 31-35.
19. Delbecq, A., Van de Ven, A., & Gustafson, D. (1975). *Group techniques for program planning: A guide to nominal group and delphi processes*. Glenview, IL: Scott, Foresman.
20. Jazwiec, R. (Ed.). (1991). Learning needs assessment. Part 1: Concepts and process. *Journal of Nursing Staff Development, 7*(2), 91-94.
21. Stanton, M. (1985). Teaching patients: Some basic lessons for nurse educators. *Nursing Management, 16*, 59-62.
22. Caron, H., & Roth, H. (1978). An evaluation of a program for teaching clinic patients the rationale of their peptic ulcer regimen. *Nursing Digest, 6*, 56-57.
23. Murray, R., & Zentner, J. (1976). Guidelines for more effective health teaching. *Nursing 76, 6*, 44-53.
24. Lee, J. (1970). Emotional reactions to trauma. *Nursing Clinics of North America, 5*, 577-587.
25. Wolf, V., & Quiring, J. (1971). Carroll's model applied to nursing education. *Nursing Outlook, 19*(3), 176-179.
26. Byrne, F., & Edeani, D. (1984). Knowledge of medical terminology among hospital patients. *Nursing Research, 33*(3), 178-181.
27. Kozol, J. (1985). *Illiterate America*. Garden City, NJ: Doubleday.
28. Apse, A., & Stetler, C. (1985). Avoiding terms of bewilderment. *Nursing 85, 15*, 42-43.
29. Miller, J. (1974). Cognitive dissonance in modifying families' perceptions. *American Journal of Nursing, 74*(8), 1468-1470.
30. Stanton, M. (1985). Teaching patients: Some basic lessons for nurse educators. *Nursing Management, 16*, 59-62.
31. Murray, R., & Zentner, J. (1976). Guidelines for more effective health teaching. *Nursing 76, 6*, 44-53.
32. Holmes, S. (1991). Getting started. *Journal of Nursing Staff Development, 7*(1), 42.
33. Adom, D., & Wright, A. (1982). Dissonance in nurse and patient evaluations of the effectiveness of a patient-teaching program. *Nursing Outlook, 30*, 132-136.

34. Glazer-Waldman, H., Hall, K., & Weiner, M. (1985). Patient education in a public hospital. *Nursing Research, 34*(3), 184-185.

35. Morton, P. (1991). The 10-minute learning break. *Journal of Continuing Education in Nursing, 22*(1), 39-40.

36. McHugh, N., Christman, N., & Johnson, J. (1982). Preparatory information: What helps and why. *American Journal of Nursing, 82*(5), 780-782.

37. Rorden, J., & Taft, E. (1990). *Discharge planning guide for nurses.* Philadelphia: Saunders.

38. Pirce, J., & Cordell, B. (1984). Patient education evaluation: Beyond intuition. *Nursing Forum, 21*(3), 117-122.

39. Murray, R., & Zentner, J. (1976). Guidelines for more effective health teaching. *Nursing 76, 6,* 44-53.

40. Woldum, K., Ryan-Morrell, V., Towson, M., et al. (1985). *Patient education. Foundation of practice.* Rockville, MD: Aspen.

17

Family Care

Sandra B. Dunbar

Rhonda M. McLain

The admission of a family member or loved one to a critical care unit often creates as much of a crisis for the family system as it does for the individual who is critically ill. Concerns about the patient's survival, anxiety about short-term and long-term quality of life, and the overall response to the highly technological environment of the critical care unit create special needs for family members and significant others. Changes in roles and responsibilities within the family, as well as new illness-related demands, add to the family's stress. Many complex and unfamiliar medical, ethical, economic, and legal issues can increase the sense of helplessness and loss of control for the family. Although it is appropriate that the nurse focus primarily on the critically ill patient, incorporating family care into critical care nursing practice is of great importance to the health of both the patient and family.

The family serves as a critical link between society and the individual, and the incorporation of family care into critical care nursing practice is essential to foster patient recovery and to minimize disruption to the family system. The goal of family care in the critical care setting is to support the family system and to preserve family resources during crises so that the family system will be able to cope with the long-term implications of the life-threatening illness. When returning the patient to the family is not feasible or realistic because of the nature of the illness or injury, then supportive nursing interventions are aimed at reducing the impact of the crisis and the changes forced on the family.

Direction for the critical care nurse's role with families is found in the Scope of Practice statement developed by the American Association of Critical-Care Nurses (AACN), which defines critical care nursing as the interaction of the critically ill patient, the critical care nurse, and the critical care environment.[1] The critically ill patient is viewed as having not only life-threatening physiological needs but also needs pertaining to the maintenance of psychological, emotional, and social integrity. The familiarity, comfort, and support provided by social relationships can enhance effective coping. Therefore, the concept of the critically ill patient incorporates the patient's family, significant other(s), or both. AACN's *Outcome Standards for Nursing Care of the Critically Ill*[2] underscores the importance of fostering family coping in the provision of appropriate and high quality patient care. In addition, the growing nursing research literature addressing family needs and interventions is uncovering important family perspectives about effective and ineffective nursing actions. The role of the critical care nurse with the family in crisis has evolved over two decades and will continue to evolve as both experiential and research data provide direction for practice.

ASSUMPTIONS ABOUT FAMILIES

Before family needs and interventions are discussed, several assumptions about family care should be articulated. These assumptions provide a context for what follows. The first assumption relates to what is meant by "family." The family has traditionally been defined as a system of individuals related to one another by strong reciprocal affection and loyalty; members enter through birth, adoption, or marriage and leave through death. This definition is no longer adequate because modern families are often small, have flexible structures, and contain members who may be distant from one another. Members of contemporary families must often rely on others not bound by marriage, birth, or adoption for support for roles traditionally filled by family members. Thus, a nurse often focuses on those individuals deemed most significant to the patient. One implication of this assumption is that nurses may encounter families with values and roles quite different from their own.

An introspective analysis of one's assumptions and attitudes about family constellations, family functioning, and family roles is an important step toward accepting the family diversity encountered in critical care nursing practice.

The second assumption is that critical care nurses are not family therapists. Families bring to the critical care setting their history and lifetime of relationships, some of which may have been dysfunctional for years. Critical care nurses do not have the time or skills to serve as a family therapist in these situations. A life-threatening illness of a family member may either augment family problems or may actually serve as a trigger for family growth and beginning resolution of problems. An astute critical care nurse must recognize when additional family therapy or counseling may be beneficial and make the appropriate referrals.

The third assumption is that critical care nurses do not have to meet all family needs by themselves. Overall responsibility for family care remains with the nurse, but the implementation may be partially delegated to other members of the health care team such as a chaplain or social worker when appropriate. The primary responsibilities of the nurse are to assess family needs and devise a plan of care that informs and supports families as they in turn provide support to the critically ill patient.

FAMILY RESPONSES TO CRITICAL ILLNESS
Families in Crisis

Crisis has been defined as "a struggle for adjustment and adaptation in the face of problems that are for a time insolvable."[3] Adjustment and adaptation to a problem are determined, in part, by the perceived significance of the situation and the resources available to cope with the problem. An imbalance between the perceived significance of the problem and resources for coping leads to a crisis.

Admission of a family member to the ICU is an acute situation that upsets the emotional equilibrium of the family group. The family's response to this situational crisis depends on the ability of those involved to draw on coping skills learned from life experiences. When people are confronted with a problem that cannot be resolved in the usual way, increased stress occurs from the threat that physical, psychosocial, or sociocultural needs will not be met.[3] The frustration accompanying unmet needs upsets the emotional equilibrium, and subjective feelings such as anxiety, fear, guilt, and helplessness are experienced.

Family responses to the critical illness of a loved one and the critical care environment present many challenges to the nurse. Fear and anxiety are common reactions. Critical illness may occur suddenly and unexpectedly as with trauma or acute myocardial infarction. Even when the patient has been ill for some time before requiring critical care, family members may express feelings of shock and disbelief that the situation could have accelerated to the point of critical illness.

Not only may family members be fearful of losing the patient as a result of the illness, they may also fear touching the patient out of concern that they might disrupt the medical support being provided. Yet touch between a patient and members of the family may be the only link the patient has with a normal and "human" view of self.

Helplessness is another common reaction of the family to the critical care environment. The machinery, lines, and devices can be extremely intimidating to anyone who does not work with them regularly. Serious illness itself places family members who desperately want to help in a very helpless position. As they stand by and witness all that is being done, perhaps even causing considerable suffering for the patient, they struggle with feelings of inadequacy.

What determines whether an imbalance will occur between coping resources and perceived significance of the situation? Moos[4] suggests that the cognitive appraisal of the situation leads to identification of basic adaptive tasks needed to cope with the crisis of physical illness. Background and personal characteristics, illness-related factors, and physical or social environmental factors can affect the perceptions of the crisis situation.

Family members are confronted with the basic adaptive tasks of: (1) dealing with pain and incapacitation, (2) dealing with the hospital environment and special treatment procedures, (3) developing adequate relationships with professional staff, (4) preserving a satisfactory self-image, (5) preserving a reasonable emotional balance, and (6) preserving relationships with family and friends.[4] Preparing for an uncertain future completes the list of adaptive tasks identified by Moos.[4] The importance of the task and the coping skills used to accomplish the tasks will vary among individuals. Despite these common tasks required for coping with the crises of physical illness, the outcome of a crisis varies among individuals. Once again, this difference is accounted for by personal characteristics, the nature of the illness, and physical and social environmental factors.

Age, intellect, emotional and cognitive development, religious beliefs, and previous coping experiences are among the personal characteristics that influence the outcome of a crisis. Perception of the situation, identification of adaptive tasks, and the use of coping skills are also affected by these personal characteristics.[3,4]

The nature of the injury or illness as well as associated symptoms and prognosis influence the family adaptive process. Additional concerns about pain and suffering and anticipation of disability or disfigurement further influence adjustment. The physical and social environment can provide additional stressors or can be a resource for coping. The unknown environment of the hospital and the unfamiliar sights of the intensive care unit can certainly create further stress.

Patient relationships with families and staff, interactions between staff and families, and social support from the community are part of the human environment that affects crisis outcome. Sociocultural norms and expectations are also part of the environment that can influence coping skills used.

Not only do these determinants of outcome influence cognitive appraisal, adaptive tasks, and coping skills, these factors are interdependent. Background and personal characteristics such as age, emotional development, and previous coping experiences can determine whether factors in the physical and social environment are stressors or resources.[4]

To facilitate a healthy outcome from the potential crisis situation, critical care nurses need to identify those factors that may add to family stress. Once family needs are identified, nursing interventions can facilitate adaptation to the crisis.

Family Needs

Consideration of the stated needs of families, as well as their responses to the critical care environment, is an important aspect of planning comprehensive care. Nursing research has revealed the most significant needs of family members of critically ill patients. Identified by family members themselves, the needs of family members change somewhat from the time of admission to the time when the immediate crisis has passed.

The most frequently reported needs of family members are listed in the box above to the right. Informational needs are frequently identified as most important. Family members want to know as much as possible about the patient's diagnosis and condition, the plan of treatment, and the prognosis. Knowing what is being done for the patient, the purpose of the equipment, and what they as family can do for the patient are high-priority information needs.[5]

The need for assurance also is very important at this time of crisis. Family members want to feel that their questions are being answered honestly and in terms they can understand. Reassurance that they will be called at home for any change in condition helps to establish a small sense of control.

The need for hope has repeatedly been identified

Family Needs
To have questions answered honestly
To know the prognosis
To have hope
To be called at home about changes
To talk to the physician every day
To know specific facts about the progress of the patient
To have understandable explanations
To feel that hospital personnel care about the patient
To be assured that the best possible care is being given to the patient
To know why things were done for the patient

---

as a highly rated need. Family members want to know that the staff is competent and that they care about patients in a personal way. Seeing staff who exhibit a knowledgeable and caring attitude toward the patient fosters hope.

Personal comfort and welfare are generally ranked as less important to family members in the early phase of critical illness than rankings of this need obtained at later time points. The importance of access to a telephone, of feeling accepted by hospital personnel, or of having a waiting room nearby is reported differently in the different studies.

Many factors can affect family needs. The duration of intensive care and the type of illness or injury appear to influence needs identified by family members as important. To know the prognosis, to see the patient frequently, and to receive information once a day are a few of the needs that change in priority over time.[6] As family members are reassured about the care the patient is receiving and become more comfortable in the hospital environment, their concerns about being involved in the care of the patient, about visitation, and about their own comfort increase.

The type of injury or illness seems to influence the importance of needs for family members. Mathis[7] found that the need to know the prognosis was not included in the top ten needs listed by family members of patients with acute brain injury, possibly because of the uncertainty of the condition. Other populations studied include the families of coronary and trauma patients. Because there is some discrepancy among the needs identified as important, more research is needed to learn about needs of families of different patient populations.

Assessing and reassessing family needs is important. Nurses' perceptions of what family members need are not always accurate.[8,9] For example, nurses have underrated the importance to family members of the need to know the prognosis, to feel accepted by hospital staff, to be called at home about changes in condition, and to feel the best possible care is being given to the patient.

At the time of admission and during the first several days, the two greatest needs identified by family members are to feel that the highest quality care is being delivered to the patient and to feel there is hope.[6] Families have identified as immediate concerns the need for information, estimation of probable outcome, honesty, and to feel confident that they would be contacted if there were any changes in the patient's condition.

Another interesting finding, singled out in the study by Bouman,[6] is that families find talking with the same nurse every day particularly reassuring. Continuity of care is clearly considered an advantage by family members. Perhaps such continuity supports the development of a trusting relationship or is related to inability to tolerate frequent changes of any kind when stressed. Interestingly, families have related a willingness to forego frequent visitation and efforts to provide for their personal comfort as long as their priority needs are met.

Once the initial crisis is past, the needs of family members change. The opportunity to visit frequently becomes more important. In addition, families may welcome the opportunity to participate in the patient's care. Availability of a telephone and a comfortable place to wait near the patient become more important. As their worry about the patient stabilizes, family members become more aware of their own personal needs. The need to talk about their feelings and fears may also become more important once the initial scare has dissipated. Such talk may center on the events preceding or precipitating the critical illness, the extent of the therapies being administered to the patient, or the possibility of the patient's death. On the other hand, some family members have described the need to have a place within the hospital where they can be alone.

Regardless of the timing, families require several essential aspects of care. A caring attitude from the staff is always perceived as a need; initially it is considered a priority for the patient, but families eventually look for caring behaviors to include them as well. Honesty, frequent updates about the status and progress of the patient, and hope are additional ongoing needs for families. Regardless of the probable outcome for the patient, family members express a strong need for even a small measure of hope at all times.

Staff Responses to Families

Despite increasing awareness of the importance of families to patients in the critical care setting and a growing knowledge of the needs of family members, the establishment of nurse–family relationships continues to be an issue. Factors reported to affect staff responses to family include lack of time, a stressful environment, limited knowledge about dealing with families, and a lack of confidence in the nurse's own skill.[10]

Nurses may feel threatened by having family members watch them provide care or perform procedures, fearing questions or even criticism of the care they are providing. Limited education about emotional issues and limited experience in dealing with them contributes to nurses' hesitancy to establish a relationship with families. Nurses may feel it is easier to deal with the patient's physical problems than with the family's psychosocial needs.

Perhaps the most important factor is the stressful environment in which critical care nurses work. Supporting families creates additional demands on time and energy. Strategies to overcome some of these barriers are discussed in subsequent sections. Despite the drawbacks, nurses who continue their involvement with families often find this relationship to be a very rewarding part of their work.

NURSING CARE OF FAMILIES

The nursing process is an excellent approach for providing care for families of critically ill patients. Although all phases of the nursing process—assessment and diagnosis, setting goals, interventions, and evaluation—can be used with families, these phases are nonlinear and frequently merge very quickly. For example, identification of a knowledge deficit within a family may yield an educational intervention that creates additional stress or produces changes in coping behaviors. Thus, the critical care nurse must use an ongoing system of family care that results in planned and documented assessment of family needs, mutually agreed upon goals, interventions, and evaluation with consistent communication to others involved in the care of the patient and family.

Family Assessment

Initial Assessment

A systematic and planned approach facilitates obtaining information about the critically ill patient as a family member and about specific needs of an individual family. The initial assessment has two major components and requires data about the patient and family members (see box on p. 415).

When critically ill patients are able to participate in an initial family assessment, parameters related to their role as a family member include their perceptions of the role they usually assume in the family, anticipated changes in the family due to the critical illness, and immediate worries or concerns. Deliberate early discovery of this information leads to an enhanced nurse–patient relationship by improving understanding of who the patient is and identification of patient concerns that might not be readily disclosed. Initial assessment data obtained from the patient should also include his or her desire for family participation in care and visitation, who should be involved in both care and decision making, and support usually received from family. Patients should be asked what they think their family can do for them while in the unit. This is particularly important for a patient with a chronic illness whose family may be significantly involved in the care provided at home. Assessment of the patient's perspective regarding family roles and involvement in care is usually quite informative. When the patient cannot participate in this initial assessment because of the severity of illness or injury, impaired cognitive state, or impaired communication ability, then obtaining the family's perspective on these issues can be helpful.

The initial patient and family assessment data should be incorporated into the nursing care plan. Such an assessment enables the nurse to meet family needs effectively and efficiently. An initial preliminary assessment provides baseline information and allows early identification of problems that may require ongoing monitoring or referral. This information can usually be obtained by the primary nurse, clinical nurse specialist, or case manager without conflict with patient care, and subsequently can be shared with other members of the health care team. Participation in structured and informal family assessments provides an important opportunity for initiation and development of the nurse–family relationship.

The critical elements of the initial family assessment relate to the immediate needs of the family (see box to the left). Determining the structure of the family as well as location and availability of the family to the patient and to each other is useful in planning supportive and information-sharing measures. Knowledge of the family's perspective of the role the patient assumes in the family as well as the anticipated changes in roles can help the nurse to appreciate the degree of dependence or independence usually displayed by the patient. Identification of the usual and current decision-maker in the family as well as a spokesperson will direct the flow of information between the nurse and family members. Determining a single family spokesperson who will have open privileges to call the unit for information and then serve as the source of information for the rest of the family may facilitate meeting a family's need for information without placing an inordinate burden on the nurse to interact with many family members. Cultural influences may dictate or determine who should be the family spokesperson.[11]

Initial assessment of the family's understanding of the patient situation involves determining their perception of the need for critical care, their understanding of the patient's condition and the plans for care, their previous experiences with critical care, and their expectations related to care and outcome. These data are more easily obtained when the critical care nurse uses a warm, caring manner to assess family knowledge and expectations and to provide important information, answer questions, and clarify misconceptions.

The initial assessment should also note past coping strategies employed by the family and their perceptions of the effectiveness or ineffectiveness of these strategies to resolve family crises. This kind of discussion typically leads to nurse-guided identification of coping strategies that might be helpful in the current situation. A history of dysfunctional patterns of coping, such as alcohol or substance abuse, may emerge from this discussion and lead to subsequent referral.

Assessment of logistical needs such as for transportation, special services, lodging, parking, and use of a telephone leads to identification of significant effects imposed on the family by the critical illness. This information can be used to devise a visitation schedule that will meet the family's logistical needs and facilitate involvement in patient care if desired. Again, early referral to social services may result from this assessment.

Ongoing Assessment

The initial assessment can provide important information upon which to base an initial family care plan, but ongoing assessment is critical to evaluate care and monitor family needs in response to changes in the patient, whose health status may be improving, not improving, or actually deteriorating. Ongoing family assessment incorporates some of the same parameters as the initial or preliminary assessment (family coping, family roles) and adds the dimensions of family health, family support, and family decision-making (see box below).

Continued assessment of family coping examines family members' response to new information and to changes in the patient's condition. As the patient's situation unfolds and changes are made in the plan of care, assessing the family's continued interpretation and processing of information yields important

data about their anxiety, fears, and expectations. Identification of other stressors or changes in the family is also important to appreciate the total family response. For example, the birth of a child, a graduation, career advancement or loss of employment, a wedding, or an illness or death of another family member may occur during the critical illness. The impact and meaning of these family events as well as who is most affected by these events should be assessed.[12] The nurse is often asked whether the news of significant distressing family events should be imparted or withheld from the patient. Anticipating the patient's response and mobilizing support is critical and can be done only if the nurse is familiar with the family situation. Additionally, the nurse can encourage and promote celebration of joyous family events to improve the patient's mood when appropriate.

Social support is assessed by determining how the family is actually supporting its members as well as by identifying significant individuals or groups who have the potential to support the family. Cultural variations in family structure and roles may lead to unique differences in perceptions of the sick role and intradependence of families[12] and subsequently to family members' response to critical illness. For example, family obligations in some cultures result in large numbers of people coming to the hospital to be with the patient and immediate family.[13] Assessment of social support should include more than just the number of family members present in the waiting room. Observation of family behaviors and interactions in the family waiting area provide an ideal method for obtaining family support information. The stress of waiting in a situation fraught with uncertainty and in which families have little control can readily manifest in strained family interactions.[14] Since this type of observation is rarely feasible for the critical care nurse, assessment of family support is more efficiently accomplished by interacting with the family spokesperson and determining if particular problems are occurring. Anticipating family needs and guiding family members toward information and supportive interactions are helpful strategies.

As the patient's status changes, assessment of family perceptions about anticipated role changes and resources required to adapt to these changes is important. For example, changes in employment status for the patient or family member may be anticipated and require additional referral or further consideration. Guided anticipation of role change may uncover family members' feelings of resentment regarding new demands and responsibilities to be assumed or the potential for overprotectiveness of the patient after discharge. Misconceptions about the impact of the illness and potential for family conflict can be addressed early to reduce family stress.

Ongoing Family Assessment

FAMILY COPING

Family responses to new information
Family responses to changes in patient condition
Concurrent family stress
Expression of feelings, emotions
Perceptions of helpful nursing behaviors
Actual and potential social support

FAMILY DECISION MAKING

Response of family members during decision making

FAMILY SUPPORT/INVOLVEMENT WITH PATIENT

Ability to support critically ill family member
Ability to support each other

FAMILY ROLES

Changes in responsibilities at home
Anticipated changes in roles

FAMILY HEALTH BEHAVIORS

Sleep/rest
Nutrition
Personal health

ECONOMIC ISSUES

FAMILY SATISFACTION

Opportunity for visitation
Involvement in care
Information

FAMILY KNOWLEDGE

Patient care and rationale
Understanding of illness
Required lifestyle changes
    Rationale
    Skills to implement changes

Attention to the health needs of individual family members is essential for the family to preserve its resources and maintain its integrity. Ensuring that family members are eating, sleeping, participating in usual exercise activities, and taking their own medications when necessary helps them to maintain their personal health and enhances their coping. In addition, identification of potential health risks that may be present in either the patient or family leads to family-focused health education that has a greater impact on behavior than does isolated individual patient teaching.

Economic issues for families of critically ill patients can be enormous. Anxiety about the costs of hospitalization creates stress compounded by the short-term and long-term impact of critical illness on family finances. In the immediate situation, family members may need to take a leave of absence from employment, travel great distances to be with loved ones, and accrue expenses related to lodging and eating outside the home. Families may also be involved in making decisions about insurance coverage, investigating Social Security benefits, changing bank accounts, replacing damaged motor vehicles, and selling real estate,[15] none of which are simple events under normal circumstances. Assessment of family coping with these problems can lead to early referral to social services and alternative means of support.

Assessing family satisfaction with visiting procedures, communication, their involvement in the patient's care, and receipt of information is part of the ongoing assessment plan. Interest in the family's level of satisfaction imparts a caring concern to the family and helps build trust in the nurse–family relationship. When possible, the family's sources of dissatisfaction should lead to modification of the plan of care or explanations about why such change is not feasible at present.

As stated earlier, families of critically ill patients have consistently ranked the need for information as a very high priority. Ongoing nursing assessment of the family's need for information can be conducted by determining the family's knowledge about the patient's progress, planned care, and the rationale for selected procedures or nursing activities. When lifestyle modifications (such as diet changes, smoking cessation, risk factor reduction) are anticipated, the family's understanding and role in such changes are assessed as a prerequisite to initiating educational strategies.

Assessment of Special Populations

The assessment parameters outlined in the previous section should be modified as dictated by special family circumstances. For example, families of patients who are scheduled to undergo cardiac surgery may have received extensive preparatory information and guidance prior to hospitalization. On the other hand, families of patients who have suffered spinal cord injuries or unplanned admissions to a critical care unit need additional assessment and interventions to plan for unexpected major life changes. Parents of critically ill infants and children pose special concerns beyond the scope of this chapter.[16] When family members have been primary caretakers for a chronically ill patient in the home, the period of hospitalization may be an important time of respite from the day-to-day demands. Thus, these family members may have different needs for involvement in care, or they may prefer to be more actively involved in care than others. McLain[17] found that families of patients with multiple trauma focused more on concerns about prognosis and needed reassurance that the best care possible was being provided. Mathis[7] found conflicting results in that the "need to know the prognosis" was not of the greatest importance for families of patients with acute brain injury. Thus, nursing assessment should focus on specifically identified needs in these groups.

■ NURSING DIAGNOSIS

Impaired coping by family members of critically ill patients can be diagnosed when "the family member or significant other is unable to provide support, comfort or assistance that is needed by the patient."[2] Recognition of impaired coping emerges from a systematic assessment as outlined earlier and the presence of indicators such as inappropriate support behaviors; withdrawal from the patient; denial; inappropriate repetitive questions and information seeking; inability to make family decisions; inability to mobilize resources; and inadequate self-care behaviors related to sleeping, eating, and hygiene.[3] Family members may also verbalize their inability to cope with the many stressors of the situation. The label of impaired coping should be used cautiously since many behaviors such as expressions of anger, distrust, or frequent complaints are attempts by the family to cope and may be long-held patterns or cues to related needs. The diagnosis of "impaired family coping" in critical care settings should be made by focusing on the family's behavior and on their ability to support the critically ill patient.

OUTCOME STANDARD

Family coping is effective as evidenced by available and supportive family, intrafamily cooperation with decision making, and expressions of ability to cope.[2]

Further indicators include the ability to process and internalize information, and seek/utilize appropriate resources for their own support.

NURSING INTERVENTIONS

Interventions to promote effective coping include providing information as discussed below. Additional strategies that may be used by critical care nurses include:

1. *Problem-solving alternatives:* Guide the family thinking through alternative ways of addressing the immediate demands of the situation to reduce the stress.
2. *Social support:* Encourage the family to contact their social network of kin and friends who can be supportive; encourage a healthy dependence on others for emotional support and routine assistance as needed.
3. *Relaxation techniques:* Provide families with information about use of different relaxation exercises and benefits of distractive therapy during long periods of waiting.
4. *Specify support role:* Clarify how the family can be supportive to the patient through the use of touch, emotional expression, and encouragement. Provide specific ways the family can be involved with care (e.g., feeding, massaging the patient's back, obtaining x-rays or records from other facilities, bringing in personal items, as dictated by the situation).
5. *Encourage expression:* Allow time on a routine basis for the family to express their concerns and feelings. Initiate family discussions and patient status reports rather than waiting for questions.[17,18]
6. *Self-care activities:* Encourage adequate sleep, nutrition, and usual exercise for family members; refer to social services for lodging assistance as needed. Reassure families they will be called or notified immediately if the patient's status changes while they are away from the unit.

These interventions are general and can be adapted to the individual family situation as needed. Two additional approaches to improving family coping may be family support groups and strategies to foster hope.

Family Support Groups. Family support groups have been reported to meet a range of family needs and to enhance family coping in selected situations.[19] Such groups provide an opportunity to share information and to compare experiences with critical illness. Support groups may also be organized around an education theme so that families with similar needs for teaching can receive and discuss information. Not all family members benefit from family support groups.[19,20] A group of family members with similar needs or of patients with similar severity of illness may be most effective. For example, an education support group of spouses of cardiac patients or liver transplant patients can be more focused than a group of families with patient diagnoses as diverse as spinal cord injury, thoracic surgery, and diabetic metabolic acidosis. Halm[20] provides a detailed discussion of strategies used in successful family support groups, including how to define the purpose and membership of the group, planning group logistics, using group process and effective group leadership, and evaluating the support group.

Fostering Hope. Strategies for developing and maintaining hope for families in crisis are integrally related to improving coping. Hope is frequently referred to as an effective coping strategy. In addition, hope expressed by family members to their critically ill loved one has the potential to foster patient hope. Hopelessness can be diagnosed in families when they exhibit helplessness and a sense of despair; a sense of "giving up"; powerlessness and lack of autonomy; and immobilization in terms of solving problems, setting realistic goals, and taking action.[21] Factors contributing to hopelessness in critical care include lack of control, depersonalization, pessimistic staff attitudes, perceptions of poor regard for the family, and physical setbacks of the patient.[22] Critical care nurses must remain cognizant of family needs to prevent this extreme of the hope–hopelessness spectrum from occurring.

Specific sources of hope for families of critically ill patients include being physically present with their loved one, reassurance that competent care is being provided, and knowing what to expect.[22] A study of family-identified hope-inspiring strategies revealed that the three most frequently used strategies by family members were prayer and faith; relationships with competent, caring caregivers; and family support and bonds.[23] These findings were similar to strategies to promote hope identified by critically ill patients.[24]

Specific hope-inspiring strategies for families and specific outcomes are presented in Figure 17-1. In addition to the previously discussed coping strategies, these hope-inspiring strategies include:

• Promoting a caring relationship
• Eliminating distortions or misconceptions that threaten hope
• Providing visitation and opportunities to be with the critically ill family member
• Decreasing uncertainty
• Providing expert, competent care
• Encouraging the expression of hope so that its contagion to the patient is maximized
• Promoting spiritual well-being and the use of spiritual resources
• Controlling the environment to protect privacy
• Exploring the meaning of the crisis and potential for positive family growth or change
• Using humor as appropriate

A concerned, caring approach with families has been advocated throughout this chapter and the related nursing literature as a strategy to promote hope.

Critical care nurses can employ a great deal of creativity and in return receive great satisfaction from developing unique strategies for families. These strategies might include displaying family photographs to promote the staff's ability to view the critically ill patient as a member of the family system, examining ways to establish privacy for large families, and supporting family rituals related to religious or cultural beliefs. When families perceive that staff care for them, hope is fostered.

Critical care nurses often encounter a dilemma when the family's hope is contrary to realistic patient outcomes or survival. Before pressing the hard realities, a gentle investigation of the family's understanding of the probable outcome may often reveal that they do not lack understanding but choose to hope for a "miracle." So long as their hope does not interfere with patient care or the need to make important decisions, the family should be allowed this coping choice. Such acceptance is not viewed as allowing or encouraging false hope; rather, it represents a willingness to meet the individual needs of both

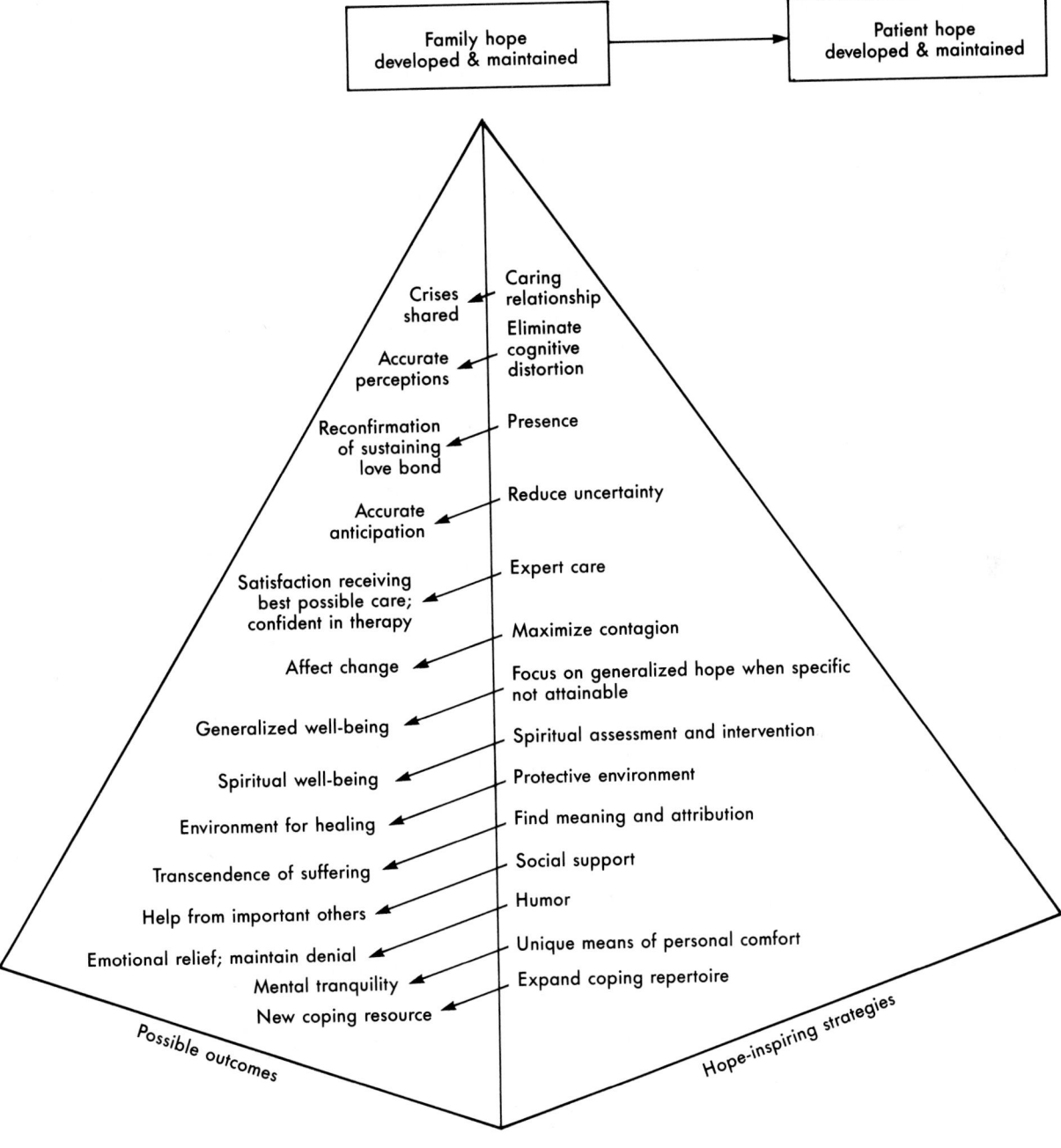

Figure 17-1   Hope-inspiring strategies for families with potential outcomes.
From Miller, J. (1991). Developing and maintaining hope in the families of the critically ill. *AACN Clinical Issues in Critical Care Nursing, 2,* 309.

patient and family. Of all the nursing interventions to assist families in coping with the critical care environment, the concern and caring demonstrated by allowing even a small measure of hope is perhaps the most significant and compassionate of all. When the critical care nurse is not able to foster specific hope for a particular outcome such as recovery, families can be redirected with shorter-term expectations and refocused on hope for alternatives such as reduced pain, spiritual peace, or a peaceful and dignified death.[22,25]

■ NURSING DIAGNOSIS

Knowledge deficit is defined as an individual's lack of cognitive knowledge or psychomotor skills that may alter health status.[26] The recurring importance of the need for information in research supports nursing assessment and interventions related to the diagnosis of knowledge deficit for family members of the critically ill.

Contributing factors for knowledge deficit in families are varied. The occurrence of a medical or surgical condition that requires critical care nursing is the major factor leading to exposure to an unfamiliar environment, previously unknown individuals upon whom a loved one is totally dependent, equipment that is often intimidating, and procedures that, though necessary, can cause discomfort for the patient.

Questions eliciting information about family members' knowledge and experience with critical illness can assist in making an appropriate diagnosis of knowledge deficit. Determining the knowledge level of family members regarding the severity and prognosis of the illness and the treatment plan can assist the nurse in meeting their informational needs. Assessing the coping strategies and support systems available to family members as early as possible can increase the nurse's ability to identify appropriate interventions.

OUTCOME STANDARD

The primary outcome standard is that family members will have an increased feeling of control over the situation and ultimately be able to express appropriate understanding and information regarding the situation.[26]

NURSING INTERVENTIONS

Interventions to assist in meeting the identified outcomes can be simple or complex. Because the degree of knowledge deficit varies, the first step is to assess the family members' current knowledge level. The nurse should focus on their understanding of the condition of the patient, the plan of care, and the prognosis. Understanding the psychological responses of the family members is also important to facilitate

meeting this need. A high anxiety state will limit the information that family members are able to understand.

General information about the environment of the hospital and the critical care unit should be provided to all family members. As soon as possible, family members need to be oriented to the unit, the waiting room, and the hospital. Identification of hospital resources such as pastoral services or the business office can be provided in a written format. Simple things like posting cafeteria hours in the waiting room can assist the family in taking care of their own needs. Orientation to the waiting area, such as the availability of a phone and restroom, or any regulations, can increase the comfort of the family while their anxiety and fear are high.

During the first visit to the critical care unit, careful information should be given regarding any equipment and specific instructions about what family members can do. Knowing that they can touch their family member or that the alarms are being monitored can help reduce the anxiety that the family members often experience. Information about the hospital and unit environment can be provided informally or more formally through structured family groups. Many alternatives are available depending upon existing hospital and unit resources.

Information about the patient should be provided as honestly and consistently as possible. Information regarding the condition and status of the patient should be based on assessment of current family knowledge. Questions need to be answered as honestly as possible. To reduce confusion, identification of one family member to act as liaison to other family members can be helpful. When several health care workers are providing information, consistent information must be given. Promoting physician–family interaction can facilitate this goal. Several studies have identified the need to talk to the physician once a day as very important, yet frequently this need is unmet.[5]

■ NURSING DIAGNOSIS

Family members have identified the need to see the patient frequently as a priority concern.[5] The nature of a critical care unit with its high acuity, aggressive diagnostics and therapies, and unstable patient conditions often makes it difficult to meet these needs. Separation of family members can lead to feelings of frustration and helplessness.

Just as the diagnosis of *social isolation* can affect critically ill patients, problems related to family separation can affect family members of the critically ill. *Family separation* can be defined as a condition of separation of members of a family or support system who usually have access to each other.

The defining characteristics, like those for social isolation, are subjective. Expressions of unhappiness or discomfort with the separation, a desire to see the family member, and feelings of helplessness or uselessness are some of the characteristics that lead to this diagnosis. Because the diagnosis is subjective, the defining characteristics will vary according to the family system and individual coping strategies.

OUTCOME STANDARD

The desired outcome is expression of satisfaction with familial relationships and with the social opportunities provided by family members of the hospitalized person.

NURSING INTERVENTIONS

Visiting time plays a significant role as an intervention for achieving the desired outcome. Visiting time is important both for family members and the critically ill patient. Research concerning family members of critically ill patients provides evidence that family members can influence the physiological and psychological states of the patient. Doerr and Jones[27] found that educating family members prior to their visit in the ICU decreased not only the anxiety of the family members but of the patient as well. Henrickson[28] identified a positive relationship between family presence and intracranial pressure of patients with head injuries.

Although visitation is generally considered to have a positive effect on patients, adverse effects have also been identified. Visits by family members have been identified as a stressor for selected patients, causing an increase in stress as exhibited by elevations in heart rate and blood pressure.[29,30]

The effect of visitation on patients must be considered when evaluating visitation as an intervention in meeting family needs. Visiting policies vary greatly as to the number of visits allowed, the length of time of visits, and the number of age of visitors.[10,31] Visiting hours may be highly structured or may be very flexible. Patient and family satisfaction appears to be higher with liberal policies. On the other hand, nurses are as likely to be satisfied with a liberal policy as a conservative one.[31]

The optimal visiting policy remains unclear. Consideration should be given to the preference of the patient as well as the family members. The physical condition of the patient is another factor that affects the determination of the best visiting policy to meet family and patient needs. The literature suggests that other personal characteristics, such as age and socioeconomic status, affect patient and family satisfaction with visiting.[30,31]

Contracting of visiting hours is one method that may benefit both patients and family. As part of the admission assessment and family orientation to the critical care unit, a determination of family and patient needs regarding visitation can assist the nurse in meeting those needs. Visitation can be agreed upon by all individuals involved. In this way, when the patient's condition or unit's demands do not allow for liberal or "open" visiting, family members have some control over when they see their loved one. Consideration of the many variables that can affect satisfaction with visitation can help alleviate the feelings of frustration and helplessness associated with family separation.

■ NURSING DIAGNOSIS

Anticipatory grieving is a condition in which an individual grieves before an actual loss occurs. It may be related to factors such as potential loss of a significant person, loss of physiological processes, loss of role, or loss of personal possessions.[26,32] Families of critically ill patients may experience anticipatory grieving related to one or more of these factors. Persons who experience or anticipate a significant loss manifest several common emotions and needs. Spouses of critically ill patients in a coronary unit have been found to express the same needs as those of spouses of terminally ill patients.[33,34]

Anticipatory grieving can be identified in specific patient and family situations when family assessment data reveal expressions of distress regarding potential loss, denial of obvious impending loss, guilt, anger, choked feelings, or sorrow.[32] Changes in eating, sleeping, and activity patterns and altered communication patterns are minor defining characteristics of anticipatory grieving.

OUTCOME STANDARD

The outcome standard is that the family will participate in constructive anticipatory grief work as evidenced by discussion of thoughts and feelings related to the anticipated loss; identification of appropriate resources; participation in own self care activities related to nutrition, rest and activity; and maintenance of constructive interpersonal relationships.[32]

NURSING INTERVENTIONS

Many of the nursing interventions aimed at fostering coping are also useful in facilitating anticipatory grieving. More specifically, family members should be encouraged to express their perceptions about the potential loss and encouraged to verbalize their fears and concerns about the impact of such a loss on the family system. When the potential loss is related to a family role or disruption in current lifestyle (e.g., ability to drive), the family can be guided through constructive problem solving and short-term goal setting. The family can be encouraged to identify specific sources of support such as friends, extended family, and church. Families should be reassured that it is normal to experience intense and chaotic feelings during this time. If the situation allows, the critical care nurse may also facilitate the ability of the family and critically ill patient to share concerns, emotions, or fears as well as plans and hopes. Once again, encouraging the family to maintain their own health and stamina is critical.

Another important consideration in assisting a family undergoing anticipatory grieving is to avoid reinforcing denial. Although nurses usually allow the use of denial and disbelief in initial stages of coping with a loss or anticipated loss, continued reinforcement of denial is inappropriate. The Patient Self-Determination Act of 1991 encourages a greater use of living wills and durable power of attorney for health care, giving family members an increased role in making decisions about a critically ill family member's care, initiations of heroic medicine, and termination of life support. In situations where recovery is unlikely, critical care nurses are increasingly initiating discussions about resuscitation and guiding families who must make extremely difficult decisions.

Serving as an advocate for the critically ill patient and family is an important role assumed by critical care nurses. The process of advocacy can be influenced and complicated by the nurse's attitudes and beliefs as well as by factors within the institution. Critical care nurses often find themselves interpreting for families what other health professional have said as well as interpreting the family's ideas to other health professionals. Gadow[35] offers a holistic approach to patient advocacy. When applied to the family member, this approach may be useful because it involves values clarification through significant engagement of the nurse and person (family member). In addition to having the legitimate authority and appropriate information to make patient decisions, the essential components of Gadow's advocacy approach include the nurse–person relationship and disclosure of the nurse's values about the situation or decision. The nurse's self-disclosure helps affirm the importance of articulating values and beliefs. The approach also stresses articulation of the kind of life the patient desires or deems acceptable and the use of these values in making decisions.

Self disclosure is a critical factor in this model of advocacy. Critical care nurses therefore need to be aware of their attitudes about death and the many ethical and legal situations encountered by family members. Likewise, critical care nurses must be able to communicate their opinions to families. Nursing education has traditionally encouraged nurses to keep their opinions to themselves and to avoid biasing patient or family decisions. Gadow[35] emphasizes that holistic advocacy can occur *only* when nurse and family share and validate feelings. In a study of critical care nurses' interactions with families of potential organ donors, Vernale[36] found that nurses frequently expressed their own positive feelings about organ donation. Families who are confronted with significant decisions about initiating or terminating life support, donating organs, or withholding treatment, can be supported through the anticipatory grieving process by nurses who know the importance of values clarification and self-disclosure.

Evaluation of Family Care

Quality can be defined as a continuous improvement in services to meet the needs and expectations of those receiving the services. Taking this definition one step farther, the Joint Commission on Accreditation of Healthcare Organizations (JCAHO) defines quality in relation to expected or desired outcomes.[37] Quality care means that desired patient outcomes are achieved. Monitoring is necessary to determine the effectiveness of the nursing interventions described previously.

Several approaches are possible when incorporating family care into the quality improvement program of a critical care unit. One such approach uses the ten-step model described by JCAHO. These ten steps facilitate the monitoring and evaluation of care. Each step can be applied to the care of family members.[38]

Assignment of responsibility and *delineation of the scope of care* are the first steps in the process. Family care is the responsibility of all staff in the critical care unit. Identifying the scope of care is necessary so that an understanding of the roles of staff with family members is achieved. As described in the AACN *Standards of Practice*, critical care nurses include the care of family in their scope of practice.[39] The inclusion of family in critical care should be defined through the structure standards of the unit or other unit policies. A written unit philosophy concerning families facilitates the delineation of this scope of practice.

Once the scope of care is determined, *identification of the important aspects of care* is the next step. Important aspects of care are those activities that are considered high volume, high risk, or problem prone. Family members of patients with specific conditions, such as transplant patients, may have support identified as an important aspect of care. Other aspects of care concerning families may include orientation to the unit, education, and emotional support.[38] The aspects of care are based upon the delineated scope of care.

Indicators are then developed to monitor those important aspects of care. An indicator may be developed to assess family knowledge after orientation to the critical care unit has been provided. This indicator can be monitored by identifying specific criteria for what family members should know after the orientation. Another potential indicator may be based upon the desired outcomes. To ensure validity of the indicator, it must be objective, measurable, and well defined.

The next step is to *determine thresholds for evaluation*. The threshold identifies the acceptable level of performance and acts as a signal for identifying quality-of-care issues. At this point, *data can be collected, organized, and evaluated*. Data collection for outcome monitoring requires direct feedback from family members. Interviews and questionnaires are two methods that can be used to obtain feedback. Evaluation of data allows for identification of opportunities to improve care.

On the basis of the evaluation of data, *an action plan can be developed and implemented*. For example, the data may identify a need for a more comprehensive orientation of family members to the ICU. An action plan is then developed to delineate strategies to meet this need. A videotape or information booklet could be developed for family members to address frequently asked questions. Once the action plan is implemented, an *evaluation of the action plan* is conducted to assess its effectiveness and whether or not the problem has been resolved.

The final step requires *communication* to the hospital-wide quality improvement committee. The initial findings, actions taken, and final outcome need to be shared to complete the assigned responsibility.

An alternative approach for evaluating family care is to develop a program based on the standards of the unit, incorporating structure, process, and outcome as described by Marker.[40] Structure standards describe the mechanisms that facilitate the operation of a system. For a nursing unit, the structure standards describe the operation of the unit and include all policies that govern the unit. An example is the unit visitation policy. Outcome monitoring can be accomplished by means of this standard. Family and patient satisfaction are the desired outcomes.

Process standards guide the implementation of care by staff. An example of a process standard is a unit protocol that describes the implementation of family orientation, who does it, and what is told to all family members. An outcome monitor can be developed that assesses family members' knowledge of the critical care environment. Standards of care are an additional type of process standard for which outcome monitoring can be accomplished.

Desired family outcomes can be developed for related structure and process standards. Outcome standards for family members will focus primarily on education or coping responses with the goal generally focused on some kind of behavioral change. Evaluation of care and continual monitoring of the effectiveness of the care is important for families. Just as patient care is guided by the nursing process, so should this process guide the care of family members.

ORGANIZATIONAL STRATEGIES

Overcoming barriers to successful family care involves a thorough evaluation of (1) existing family policies and strategies in a particular unit, (2) institutional factors and resources, and (3) critical care nurses' knowledge and confidence in working with families. Adopting a family-centered approach to critical care involves a conscientious effort by nurses, physicians, administrators, and other members of the health care team. Critical care nurses can assume an important leadership role in removing institutional and philosophical barriers to family care by serving as role models, bringing family issues to the forefront of discussion with other health care providers, and facilitating the acquisition of resources needed to implement family care.

One frequently noted barrier to family care is lack of time and competing priorities. The high patient acuity seen in critical care units creates a paradoxical situation in that nurses find themselves prioritizing what can and cannot be done at the time when the need for family care is at its peak, and family care is frequently placed last. The use of patient classification systems to determine staffing may actually compound this situation if the classification system does not accommodate appropriate family care needs. Many acuity systems account for only the educational needs of families rather than taking into account comprehensive care needs. Clearly, developing nurse–family relationships requires time as well as a planned, systematic approach.[41]

Focusing on the positive benefits to both staff and patients strengthens adoption of a family-centered approach. Developing strong nurse–family relationships increases the opportunity for critical care nurses to receive positive feedback and feel satisfied with their care; it opens avenues for the nurse to develop a richer understanding of the patient's needs.[14,42] Helping families through the grieving process also enhances the nurse's response to dying patients and provides an opportunity for resolving the family's personal grief.[42]

In a survey of over 200 critical care nurses, Hickey and Lewandowski[10] found that nurses were more likely to become involved with families if they were aware of what had been communicated by physicians. This finding is not surprising: critical care nurses often find themselves translating what has been misheard or misperceived by anxious family members. This study underscores the need for an interdisciplinary approach to family care. Critical care nurses can take the lead in planning and leading family conferences that incorporate other members of the health care team in improving consistency of communication, problem solving, and family decision making. When conferences are not possible, critical care nurses can initiate other interdisciplinary strategies to help families get the information or support they need. One example is a family communication system by which family members can write their questions or express their concerns to nurses or physicians when they are unable to be present for face-to-face interactions. Another approach is for the nurse to serve as a family advocate to enhance communication of the family's concerns or decisions.

Developing the knowledge and skills to provide family care requires as much education as does learning the techniques involved in obtaining and interpreting hemodynamic data. Yet family needs and interventions are frequently omitted from critical care educational and orientation programs. Lack of confidence and overall discomfort with family issues can be very real barriers to family care. Assuming individual responsibility for learning more about families in crisis and initiating discussion among staff during rounds, during report, and in specially developed sessions are some of the mechanisms that can be used to create not only individual change but change within the larger critical care unit.

Finally, a thorough investigation of existing and required resources needed to accomplish family care should be conducted. Family waiting rooms are frequently small, crowded, and impersonal. Soliciting the assistance of volunteer workers and the support of administration could lead to a new environment that facilitates family-oriented care. The wealth of nursing research on family needs can direct this and many other aspects of moving toward family-focused care.

REFERENCES

1. American Association of Critical-Care Nurses. (1985). *Scope of practice statement.* Newport Beach, CA: Author.
2. American Association of Critical-Care Nurses. (1990). *Outcome standards for nursing care of the critically ill.* Laguna Niguel, CA: Author.
3. Caplan, G. (1964). *Principles of preventive psychiatry.* New York: Basic Books.
4. Moos, R. (1977). *Coping with physical illness.* New York: Plenum.
5. Hickey, M. (1990). What are the needs of families of critically ill patients? A review of the literature since 1976. *Heart Lung, 19,* 401-415.
6. Bouman, C. C. (1984). Identifying priority concerns of families with relatives in the intensive care setting. *Dimensions of Critical Care Nursing, 3,* 313-319.
7. Mathis, M. (1984). Personal needs of family members of critically ill patients with and without acute brain injury. *Journal of Neuroscience Nursing, 16,* 36-44.
8. Norris, L., & Grove, S. (1986). Investigation of selected psychological needs of family members of critically ill adult patients. *Heart Lung, 15,* 194-199.
9. Irwin, B., & Meier, J. (1973). Supportive measures for relatives of the fatally ill. In M. V. Batey (Ed.), *Communicating Nursing Research,* Vol. 5 (pp. 119-128). Boulder, CO: Western Interstate Council for Higher Education, Western Council on Higher Education for Nursing, and Western Society for Research in Nursing.
10. Hickey, M., & Lewandowski, L. (1988). Critical care nurses' roles with families: A descriptive study. *Heart Lung, 17,* 670-676.
11. Janosik, E. H. (1988). Variations in ethnic families. In J. R. Miller, & E. H. Janosik. *Family-focused care.* New York: McGraw-Hill.
12. Lynn-McHale, D., & Smith, A. (1991). Comprehensive assessment of families of the critically ill. *AACN Clinical Issues in Critical Care Nursing, 2,* 195-209.
13. Boyle, J., & Andrews, M. (1988). *Transcultural concepts in nursing care.* Glenview, IL: Scott, Foresman/Little, Brown.
14. Rodgers, B. (1990). The intensity of waiting: Life outside the intensive care unit. *Focus on Critical Care, 17*(4), 325-329.
15. Mirr, M. (1991). Decisions made by family members of patients with severe head injury. *AACN Clinical Issues in Critical Care Nursing, 2*(2), 242-251.
16. Miles, M. S. (1989). Parents of critically ill premature infants: Sources of stress. *Critical Care Quarterly, 12,* 69-74.
17. McLain, R. (1987). Needs of families of trauma patients. Unpublished master's thesis. Atlanta, GA: Emory University.
18. Loos, F., & Bell, M. F. (1990). A family interviewing strategy. *Dimensions of Critical Care Nursing, 9,* 46-53.
19. Halm, M. (1991). Strategies for developing a family support group. *Focus on Critical Care, 18,* 444-459.
20. Sabo, K., Kraay, D., Rudy, E., et al. (1989). ICU family support group sessions: Family members perceived benefits. *Applied Nursing Research, 2,* 82-89.
21. Miller, J. (1992). *Overcoming powerlessness.* Philadelphia: Davis.
22. Miller, J. (1991). Developing and maintaining hope in families of the critically ill. *AACN Clinical Issues in Critical Care Nursing, 2,* 307-315.
23. Edwards, S. (1990). Hope-inspiring strategies of critically ill family members. Unpublished master's thesis. Atlanta, GA: Emory University.
24. Miller, J. (1989). Hope-inspiring strategies of critically-ill patients. *Applied Nursing Research, 2,* 23-29.
25. Leske, J. (1991). Overview of family needs after critical illness: From assessment to intervention. *AACN Clinical Issues in Critical Care Nursing, 2,* 220-226.

26. Carpenito, L. (1992). *Nursing diagnosis application to clinical practice.* Philadelphia: Lippincott.

27. Doerr, B., & Jones, J. (1979). Effect of family preparation on the state of anxiety level of the CCU patient. *Nursing Research, 28,* 315-316.

28. Henrickson, S. L. (1987). Intracranial pressure changes and family presence. *Journal of Neuroscience Nursing, 19,* 14-17.

29. Brown, A. (1976). Effect of family visits on the blood pressure and heart rate of patients in the coronary care unit. *Heart Lung, 5,* 291-296.

30. Simpson, T. (1991). Critical care patients' perceptions of visits. *Heart Lung, 20,* 681-688.

31. Stockdale, L., & Hughes, J. (1988). Critical care unit visiting policies: A survey. *Focus on Critical Care, 15,* 45-48.

32. Kim, M., McFarland, G., & McLane, A. (1991). *Guide to nursing diagnoses.* St. Louis: Mosby.

33. Breu, C., & Dracup, K. (1976). Implementing nursing research in a critical care setting. *Journal of Nursing Administration, 6,* 14-17.

34. Hampe, S. (1975). The needs of the grieving spouse in a hospital setting. *Nursing Research, 24,* 113-120.

35. Gadow, S. (1990). Existential advocacy: Philosophical foundations of nursing. In T. Pence, & J. Lantrall (Eds.), *Ethics in nursing: An anthology* (NLN Public No. 20-2294). New York: National League for Nursing.

36. Vernale, C. (1991). Critical care nurses' interactions with families of potential organ donors. *Focus on Critical Care, 18,* 335-339.

37. Joint Commission on Accreditation of Healthcare Organizations. (1991). *Accreditation manual for hospitals.* Chicago: Author.

38. Krumberger, J. (1991). Linking critical care family research to quality assurance. *AACN Clinical Issues in Critical Care Nursing, 2(2),* 321-328.

39. American Association of Critical-Care Nurses. (1989). *Standards for nursing care of the critically ill* (2nd ed.). Norwalk, CT: Appleton & Lange.

40. Smith-Marker, C. (1988). *Setting standards for professional nursing: The Marker Model.* Baltimore: Resource Applications.

41. Artinian, N. (1991). Strengthening nurse–family relationships in critical care. *AACN Clinical Issues in Critical Care Nursing, 2,* 269-275.

42. Dunkel, J., & Eisendrath, S. (1983). Families in the intensive care unit: Their effect on staff. *Heart Lung, 12,* 258-261.

Decreased Adaptive Capacity

Pamela H. Mitchell

The movement to define nursing care largely in terms of nursing diagnoses has posed a particular problem for critical care nursing. This problem stems from the fact that nursing, medicine, and other disciplines such as respiratory therapy collaboratively manage multiple dynamic pathophysiological states in critically ill patients and are therefore mutually accountable for patient outcomes. In contrast to nursing practice with less acutely ill persons, the collaborative management of the critically ill patient comprises a large part of critical care nursing practice. The North American Nursing Diagnosis Association (NANDA) defines nursing diagnosis as "a clinical judgment about individual, family, or community responses to actual or potential health problems/life processes. Nursing diagnoses provide the basis for selection of nursing interventions to achieve outcomes for which the nurse is accountable."[1] If one accepts the premise of this definition that diagnosis must direct interventions for which nursing has primary accountability, it is possible to define areas of clinical judgment even in the highly multidisciplinary critical care arena where nursing interventions are directly relevant to immediate outcomes.

Some have addressed the problem by renaming pathophysiological states (for example cardiogenic shock becomes decreased cardiac output; increased intracranial pressure becomes altered tissue perfusion, cerebral). However this semantic ploy does not solve the problem, because independently prescribed nursing measures do not directly treat decreased cardiac output any more than they directly treat cardiogenic shock, for example. Even when nurses are exercising considerable latitude in independent judgment within protocols in managing cardiogenic shock (or decreased cardiac output), they are still treating the pathophysiological state in collaboration with physicians—which is not considered nursing in the strictest interpretation of the definition of nursing diagnosis.

Carpenito[2] terms these situations collaborative problems and by implication would contend that the bulk of critical care nursing practice consists of managing collaborative problems. Within these collaborative problems, however, is a subset of true nursing diagnoses, managed independently (although largely unconsciously) by nurses. This subset of diagnoses are diminished capacities of the several physiological systems to adapt to the demand of external or internal stimuli. Nurses manage these states of decreased adaptive capacity by (1) decreasing the demand on the system or (2) increasing the capacity to adapt. This chapter presents the concept of decreased adaptive capacities and illustrates the concept and associated nursing management with examples from selected physiological systems.

ADAPTIVE CAPACITY

Adaptive capacity is the capability of any dynamic system to maintain or restore stability in the face of internal or external challenge to that stability. A *dynamic* system is one that is not constant at any one state but rather has continual oscillation or movement around a given point. For example, while we speak of mean arterial blood pressure as if it were a fixed point, we know that the values of the systolic and diastolic pressures change with each heartbeat.

Stability in a physiological system is best understood as a homeokinesis, or dynamic oscillating equilibrium, rather than as a homeostasis, or steady state equilibrium. In stable homeokinetic systems, perturbations (stimuli that act to alter the system) produce relatively little change in the regular oscillation. An unstable system shows a large response to the same magnitude of stimulus.[3,4,5] *Adaptation,* then, is the decrement or diminution in response to a given stimulus.

For example, if a person stands up rapidly, blood pressure drops markedly secondary to hydrostatic effects. Standing up is a perturbation to the cardiovascular system; the initial large drop in blood pressure is a response. However, if the pressure-sensing and neural inputs to the cardiovascular system are functioning normally the drop in pressure will last only one to two heartbeats; "normal" blood pressure is rapidly restored and is at a level sufficient to maintain cerebral blood flow. This all occurs so rapidly in normal persons that we are ordinarily unaware of the dynamic changes occurring.

Adaptive capacity therefore is the range in which physiological regulatory mechanisms operate to promote a small or brief response to input of various magnitudes. The greater the capacity, the more stability is maintained. The less the capacity the greater the magnitude and duration of response to small amounts of input.

In critically ill persons, one or more dynamic physiological systems are unstable, or at high risk for becoming unstable. Therefore, overall critical care therapy aims to restore stability to that system. In the meantime, nursing therapy aims at decreasing unnecessary stimuli to the system, or at increasing responsive capacity when external challenges are necessary. For example, adaptive demands on the person with cardiovascular instability are decreased by minimizing the physical demands of bathing, rapid position change, upper extremity activity, and the psychophysiological demands of fear or anxiety. Nurses judge the readiness of the person's cardiovascular system to respond to the challenge of activity by monitoring heart rate, blood pressure, color, and speed of return of parameters to baseline after increased activity. Nurses also monitor patient response to family visits in terms of potential physiological demand of these visits, balanced against the capability of family to assist in decreasing adaptive demand by decreasing patient anxiety. This monitoring is not delegated by another discipline but is an integral part of nursing therapy.

This assessment and monitoring of adaptive capacity is further illustrated by the fact that in more enlightened coronary care units, judgments about progressing patients' activity is entirely a nursing judgment. In less enlightened units, physicians prescribe increases in activity, often based on number of days since the cardiac event rather than on the individual patients' response to graded activity.

DECREASED ADAPTIVE CAPACITY, INTRACRANIAL

The diagnostic category *decreased adaptive capacity, intracranial* is not an official NANDA diagnosis but is used in practice and is the most extensively developed of the possible adaptive capacity categories.[6,7,8] It is used here to illustrate how it is different from the pathophysiological state intracranial hypertension (or increased intracranial pressure) and how

the nursing therapy for the decreased adaptive capacity interdigitates with medical therapy for the pathophysiological state.

Decreased intracranial adaptive capacity is defined as a clinical state in which intracranial fluid dynamic mechanisms that normally compensate for increased intracranial volume are compromised, resulting in *repeated disproportionate increases* in intracranial pressure (ICP) in response to a variety of noxious and nonnoxious stimuli. Therefore the single measurable characteristic that allows us to make the diagnosis is: repeated increases in ICP of greater than 10 mmHg over baseline for more than 5 minutes following any or a variety of external stimuli (such as nursing care maneuvers or environmental noise). In a single small study, all patients with this diagnosis had five or more episodes of disproportionate increase in 24 hours.[8]

The diagnosis may occur in patients with a variety of brain injuries or disorders that raise intracranial pressure. However, the presence of elevated ICP alone (≥ 15 mmHg) does not establish the diagnosis. Thus this is not a state that is simply equivalent to increased ICP (alternatively called intracranial hypertension). Not all patients with increased ICP exhibit disproportionate increase in ICP above baseline in response to noxious and nonnoxious stimuli. Those who do are at particular risk for further damage to brain tissue by virtue of decreased cerebral tissue perfusion or mechanical compression of brain tissue. The diagnosis *decreased adaptive capacity, intracranial* allows the nurse to identify this subset of critically ill patients for whom nurse-prescribed interventions such as positioning or managing the frequency and magnitude of environmental stimuli can be applied to reduce adaptive demand or increase the adaptive capacity of the intracranial system. Making the diagnosis is dependent upon the availability of electronic monitoring of intracranial pressure and preferably systemic blood pressure. The nurse's use of data from the monitoring system to make the diagnosis and to intervene as described is totally within the scope and accountability of nursing practice.

Physiologically, intracranial adaptive capacity reflects the relationship among the three components of the intracranial system: blood, brain, and cerebrospinal fluid (CSF). When the volume of each of the three components is within a normal physiological range, activities that challenge the system such as coughing, straining, or turning over in bed neither produce any change in ICP nor result in a sharp, steep change with rapid return to normal values. Movement of cerebrospinal fluid from the cranium into the spinal dural sac is the primary regulatory mechanism that underlies the adaptive capacity of the intracranial system. When this mechanism and the minor mechanisms of increased CSF absorption, decreased CSF production, and brain shift are exhausted, ICP increases rapidly in response to formerly innocuous stimuli. This change from little or no response to large response to the same stimulus is shown in Figure 18-1. If we were able to see this same mechanism in individual patients, we could say that those who were on the steep and rounded part of the ICP curve have decreased adaptive capacity, while those who remain on the flat portion have adequate adaptive capacity.

The term *elastance* ($\Delta P/\Delta V$) or its inverse compliance ($\Delta V/\Delta P$) is commonly used in clinical physiology to describe this same nonlinear relationship between changes in pressure and volume in body cavities such as the lungs or cranial cavity. Although the concept of decreased elastance expresses the same idea as decreased adaptive capacity for certain systems, such as intracranial dynamics, it does not capture altered capacities or reserves in other body systems.

Unfortunately, we cannot deduce an individual's position on the pressure–volume curve from clinical signs; therefore this diagnosis can be made only if the patient is undergoing intracranial pressure monitoring and manifests repeated disproportionate increases in ICP. However, certain characteristics identified in the clinical research literature help identify patients with increased ICP who are at high risk for the diagnosis.

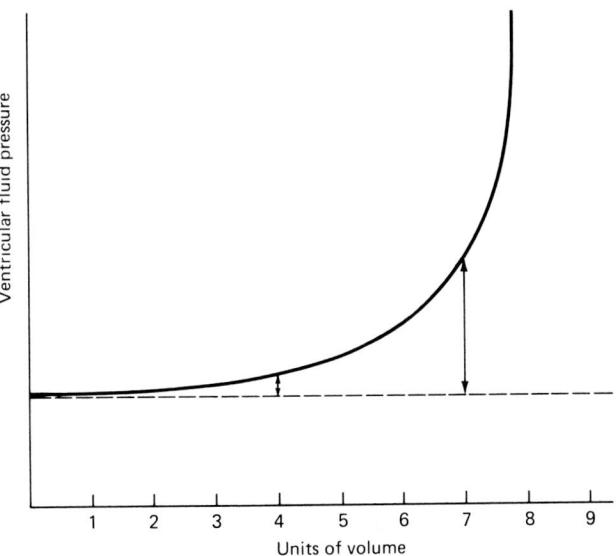

Figure 18-1   Intracranial volume–pressure curve. Note that for the addition of any given unit of volume (abscissa) a markedly different rise in pressure occurs, depending on location (flat or steep portion) on the curve. Thus, adding one unit of volume at the second arrow results in nearly four times the increase in pressure from the same volume at the first arrow.

The following characteristics should be considered as predictors of patients who are at high risk to manifest repeated disproportionate increases in ICP in response to stimuli:

1. Disproportionate increase in ICP following a single environmental or nursing maneuver stimulus: In patients with communicating hydrocephalus, increases in ICP with the first instance of passive turning to a particular position were predictive of similar increase on the subsequent turns to the same position.[9]
2. Volume pressure response tests: Volume/pressure ratio (VPR) greater than 2 or pressure–volume index (PVI) less than 10. These diagnostic procedures are highly predictive of disproportionate increases in ICP but are not currently performed independently by critical care nurses.[10,11]
3. Elevated P_2 waveform:[12,13] An elevated P_2 waveform correctly identified 100% of patients with disproportionate increase but had a false-positive rate of 50%, for an overall positive predictive value of 75% and an error rate of 20% in 15 patients with a variety of pathological conditions.[8]
4. Baseline ICP equal to or greater than 10 mmHg in head-injured patients: Willis[8] found this factor to have a higher positive predictive value (100%) than did the elevation of the P_2 wave because there were no false positives. However, the presence of false negatives (those with baseline $\geq$10 mmHg but who did not manifest disproportionate increases) decreased the sensitivity (prediction of true positives) to 77%. The overall error rate was 13%.
5. Wide amplitude waveform: Rauch, Mitchell, and Tyler[7] reported that a wide-amplitude tracing was 100% sensitive for disproportionate increase (i.e., all patients with disproportionate increase also had wide tracing) but had a 65% rate of false negatives to some stimuli, for example suctioning.

This diagnosis might be used in the following way for a patient with severe closed head injury whose baseline ICP remains 15 to 20 mmHg and who has 10 to 15 mmHg increases in ICP whenever the nurses attempt to turn the patient from supine to lateral positions. The formal *diagnostic statement* might be: Decreased intracranial adaptive capacity related to exhaustion of intracranial compensatory mechanisms as evidenced by more than five episodes in 24 hours of disproportionate increase in ICP (>10 mmHg for > 5 minutes) in response to any of a variety of nursing activities (for example suctioning, turning, hygiene). The *outcome criterion* (for stimulus: passive turning in bed) might be: No more than three episodes of ICP increase > 10 mmHg for 5 or more minutes immediately following passive turning. The *intervention* would be: *reduce adaptive demand* by using kinetic bed to continuously change patient positions. The rationale: Research has shown that the slow turning of this bed does not increase overall ICP.[14,15]

Alternatively, if the patient shows a few but not so consistently disproportionate increases in ICP, one might consider the following intervention plan: *Increase adaptive capacity* by doing the following whenever the patient is turned manually:

1. Locate head elevation position for this patient that optimizes cerebral perfusion pressure (may be flat or slight head elevation).[16]
2. Maintain head in 90° alignment throughout the turning process.
3. Use turning sheet to minimize interrupted tactile sensation to patient.

All of these interventions are totally within the scope of independent nursing practice and are prescribed within the context of medical interventions to maintain baseline ICP below 20 mmHg and to maintain cerebral perfusion above 60 mmHg. A variety of pharmacological and mechanical measures are used for these purposes, all of which are available to the nurse to use as needed for increasing adaptive capacity if it is believed that a particular activity, for example suctioning, may exceed the patient's available capacity.

THE CONCEPT IN OTHER PHYSIOLOGICAL SYSTEMS

The idea of adaptive capacities has conceptual appeal for considering diagnoses that guide nursing intervention in patients with other kinds of disorders. For the diagnosis *decreased intracranial adaptive capacity* the defining characteristics and high-risk predictive factors are expressed in terms of volume and pressure, whereas adaptive capacities of a system such as the immune system might be measured in terms of cellular reactivity, for example anergic response. If we think of adaptive capacities as system-specific reserve capability the concept would have applicability to a wide range of physiological responses in maintaining or promoting physiological stability in critically ill patients. The challenge to clinicians and clinical nurse researchers is to specify the measurable defining characteristics and indicators of adaptive capacity and response in a variety of human subsystems.

REFERENCES

1. North American Nursing Diagnosis Association. (1990). *Definition of nursing diagnosis. Adopted at the 9th Conference.* St. Louis: Author.
2. Carpenito, L. J. (1989). *Nursing diagnosis: Applications to clinical practice* (3rd ed.). Philadelphia: Lippincott.
3. Iberall, A. S., & Cardon, S. Z. (1964). Control in biologic systems: A physical review. *Annals of the New York Academy of Science, 117,* 445-518.
4. Garfinkel, A. (1983). Introduction to special issue on dynamic models for physiology. *American Journal of Physiology (Regulatory Integrative Comparative Physiology), 14,* R453-R454.
5. Yates, F. E. (1982). Outline of a physical theory of physiologic systems. *Canadian Journal of Physiology and Pharmacology, 60,* 217-248.
6. Mitchell, P. H. (1986). Decreased adaptive capacity, intracranial: A proposal for a new nursing diagnosis. *Journal of Neuroscience Nursing, 18,* 170-175.
7. Rauch, M. E., Mitchell, P. H., & Tyler, M. L. (1990). Validation of risk factors for the nursing diagnosis of decreased intracranial adaptive capacity. *Journal of Neuroscience Nursing, 22,* 173-178.
8. Willis, M. L. (1991). Interpretation of intracranial pressure waveforms: The predictive value of P_2 elevation in the diagnosis of decreased intracranial adaptive capacity. Unpublished master's thesis. Seattle: University of Washington.
9. Mitchell, P. H., Ozuna, J., & Lipe, H. P. (1981). Moving the patient in bed: Effects of turning and range of motion on intracranial pressure. *Nursing Research, 30,* 212-218.
10. Miller, J. D., & Leech, P. (1975). Effects of mannitol and steroid therapy on intracranial volume-pressure relationships in patients. *Journal of Neurosurgery, 42,* 274-281.
11. Marmarou, A., Shulman, K., & Rosende, R. (1978). A non-linear analysis of the cerebrospinal fluid system and intracranial pressure dynamics. *Journal of Neurosurgery, 48,* 332-334.
12. Germon, K. (1988). Interpretation of ICP pulse waves to determine intracranial compliance. *Journal of Neuroscience Nursing, 20,* 334-349.
13. Cardoso, E. R., Rowan, J. O., & Galbraith, S. (1983). Analysis of cerebrospinal fluid pulse wave in intracranial pressure. *Journal of Neurosurgery, 59,* 817-821.
14. Gonzalez-Arias, S. M., Goldberg, M. L., Baumgartner, R., et al. (1983). Analysis of the effect of kinetic therapy on intracranial pressure in comatose neurosurgical patients. *Neurosurgery, 13,* 654-656.
15. Clemmer, T. P., Green S., Ziegler, B., et al. (1990). Effectiveness of the kinetic treatment table for preventing and treating pulmonary complications in severely head-injured patients. *Critical Care Medicine, 18,* 614-617.
16. March, K., Mitchell, P. H., Grady, S., et al. (1990). Effects of backrest position on ICP and CPP. *Journal of Neuroscience Nursing, 22,* 375-381.

19

Elder Responses in Critical Care

Suzanne S. Prevost

The elderly population is the fastest growing segment of U.S. society. In 1900, 3.1 million people, or 4% of the nation's population, were over the age of 65. By 1985, the elderly cohort had increased to 28.5 million, or 12% of the population. By the year 2020, over 50 million Americans, nearly 20% of the total population, will fall into the elderly category.[1]

As the demographics of society are changing, the population of critically ill patients is changing as well. In 1987, 70% of acute care beds and 30% to 40% of critical care beds were occupied by elderly patients.[2] Elderly patients are now filling up to 70% of the beds in some critical care units, depending on the type of facility and unit, and the demographics of the surrounding community.

During the 1980s, critical care nurses developed subspecialties in neonatology and pediatrics to address the needs of patients in these age groups. On the opposite end of the aging continuum, elderly patients comprise another unique population with age-specific needs and responses to critical illness. Throughout the 1990s, this new subspecialty of gerontologic critical care must expand to promote optimal outcomes for this rapidly growing population.

AGEISM

One factor that may have considerable impact on the outcomes of elderly patients is the attitudes of care providers. A very prevalent negative attitude in American society is known as ageism. *Ageism* is:

> a process of systematic stereotyping of and discrimination against people because they are old. . . . Ageism allows the younger generations to see older people as different from themselves; thus they subtly cease to identify with their elders as human beings.[3]

Elders are victims of negative stereotyping more frequently than any other age group. Negative attitudes toward elders, lack of knowledge related to aging, and a reluctance to participate in the care of elderly patients have been documented by researchers in a variety of health care settings. A potential linkage between negative attitudes and negative behaviors has been hypothesized but has not been consistently supported. Educational programs and increased knowledge on aging have been shown to be effective in promoting more positive attitudes.[4,5] The addition of gerontologic content to basic critical care courses and continuing education programs should enhance care.

ETHICAL DILEMMAS

Negative attitudes or responses are often elicited by the preponderance of ethical dilemmas associated with the care of elderly patients in the critical care unit. Nurses struggle with whether the care they are providing is ethically the right thing to do for individual patients. Dilemmas commonly encountered with this group involve the ethical principles of autonomy, nonmaleficence, and distributive justice.

Autonomy

Autonomy, or the right to self-determination, is a fundamental principle underlying health care delivery in the United States. There is a common belief that people have the right to make decisions about the care they will receive. This principle is frequently violated in caring for elderly patients. Often, health care providers make hasty decisions regarding the elder's lack of intellectual competence based on slight symptoms of confusion or disorientation.

Communication barriers related to the critical care environment, the nature of critical illness, and the deficits of aging make the process of informed decision making very difficult. Frequently, it is easier and more expedient to turn to the spouse or adult children of the patient to obtain consent. Family members are often eager to take on the decision-making role and determine what they feel is best for the patient. It is the critical care nurse's responsibility to see that communication, particularly when it involves treatment decisions, is directed first and foremost to the patient, then to the family.

Nonmaleficence

Nonmaleficence is the ethical duty to do no harm. This principle arises when the use of highly intrusive procedures or devices is considered in caring for critically ill elderly patients. Care providers must carefully evaluate whether the action has the potential to produce more harm, or suffering, than good for the patient. In these circumstances, calculation of the risk/benefit ratio differs greatly from calculations for patients in other age groups. Whenever possible, treatment decisions should be based on the individual's informed preferences.

Distributive Justice

The concept of distributive justice deals with the fair allocation of scarce resources. Two resources whose availability frequently create dilemmas in critical care are critical care beds and critical care nurses. The criteria used in making decisions about distribution of scarce resources are often biased against elderly patients.

For example, suppose two patients, an 80-year-old and a 6-year-old, both injured in a motor vehicle accident, require critical care admission, but only one bed is available. Who would receive the bed? Similarly, if staffing in the critical care unit will permit a one-to-one nurse/patient ratio for only one of these two patients, the child or the elder, who would receive the extra nursing care?

Two factors that are considered in such cases are societal contribution and potential quality of life of the patient. If critical care is provided and the patient survives the present illness, will he or she be able to make a valuable contribution to society? Will the remaining life be one of quality? The concepts of societal contribution and quality of life are generally applied by health care providers to young adults or middle adults. The meaning of these concepts to the elderly population may be very different. Does an individual who is no longer capable of employment still have the capacity to make a valuable contribution to society? If a person can no longer provide for self-care, does the person continue to have quality of life? Both sides of these questions can be supported depending on who is defining the concepts and where their interests lie.

DATA COLLECTION

A multidimensional approach is essential in the assessment of elderly patients. These patients tend to present with an acute illness compounded by the presence of one or more chronic illnesses. An episode of critical illness can have a dramatic and sometimes irreversible impact on functional and cognitive abilities, as well as physiological processes. A comprehensive assessment should include the components listed in the box below. It is important to evaluate any sudden changes in these areas that may have occurred in the days or weeks preceding illness or hospitalization.

The general approach to assessment of the elderly patient is somewhat different than the approach to patients in other age groups. For many critically ill patients, the primary focus of assessment and related interventions is the physical examination, followed by diagnostic testing. With elderly patients the history component of assessment must be emphasized. An

---

Components of Elder Assessment

1. Chief Complaint
   Symptoms
   Impact on physiology, function, and cognition
   Relationship to previously known illnesses
2. Health History
   Illnesses
   Hospitalizations
   Health-seeking behaviors
3. Medications
   Prescribed
   Over-the-counter
   Patterns of adherence
   Impact on function or lifestyle
4. Functional Status
   Mobility
   Activity
   Assistance required

   Typical daily patterns
5. Cognitive Ability
   Orientation
   Memory
   Intellectual function
6. Support Systems
   Significant others
   Spirituality
   Housing arrangements
   Recent lifestyle changes
7. Physical Examination
   Inspection, palpation, percussion, auscultation
   Differentiation between age-related changes and pathological conditions
8. Laboratory Tests
   Altered values related to current acute illness, previous illnesses, medications, or age-related changes

accurate and comprehensive history is essential to the planning of appropriate goals and interventions. For example, if two 80-year-old patients are being treated in a critical care unit for pneumonia, the long-term goals are likely to be very different if the histories revealed that one of the patients had been comatose in a long-term care facility, whereas the other had been living independently.

Interviewing Techniques

The history should be taken in a well-lit room since elderly people require more light than younger adults to see clearly. Glare from windows or examination lights should be controlled because the elderly are often very sensitive to glare. Visual or auditory distractions, such as beeping infusion pumps, should be reduced or eliminated if possible.

More than 30% of elderly patients have hearing impairments,[6] even though many do not realize or admit it. The following modifications can enhance the effectiveness of communication to the hearing impaired:

Face the client so that lips and gestures are clearly visible.

Speak toward the good ear.

Speak slowly and distinctly in short phrases.

Speak loudly without shouting.

Use expressions, gestures, and body language.

Communication should be directed to the patient, rather than the family, if at all possible. If the patient's orientation level or memory is questionable, information should be validated with the family. Use of the patient's proper title (Mr., Mrs., Miss, or Ms.) and last name will help establish an air of respect and dignity.

Perhaps the most difficult aspect of obtaining an accurate history is the time required. The elderly patient's history encompasses many more years and experiences than that of a younger person. Elderly people process thoughts more slowly, are slower in providing verbal responses, and are easily distracted. Patience is difficult to display within the urgency of the critical care environment, yet it is essential for effective communication with elderly individuals.

Functional Status

Assessment of functional status is the evaluation of the patient's ability to perform activities of daily living (ADLs).[7] This component of assessment is often overlooked because full independence is assumed for the majority of patients younger than 65 years. Even though only 5% of Americans over 65 are living in institutions,[8] 45% require some degree of assistance in performing ADLs.[9] Accurate assessment of functional status is essential to initiating appropriate discharge planning. Since most elderly patients have al-

ready experienced some degree of functional loss, appropriate goals are to return to the preillness functional level and to prevent further functional loss, rather than anticipating full recovery. According to the Katz Index of ADLs,[10] the critical parameters of function include bathing, dressing, toileting, transferring, continence, and feeding.

Cognitive Ability

Although assessment of orientation is the most common cognitive evaluation used in critical care, it is the least sensitive indicator of mental function.[11] Two of the most widely accepted instruments for cognitive assessment of elderly persons are Folstein's Mini-Mental State Exam (MMSE)[12] and Pfeiffer's Short Portable Mental Status Questionnaire (SPMSQ).[13]

The MMSE evaluates orientation, registration, attention, calculation, recall, language, and ability to follow a three-part command (e.g., "Take a paper in your hand, fold it in half, and put it on the floor."[12]) The SPMSQ is a 10-item instrument designed to test current events, remote memory, and mathematical ability. Two of the questions are "What is your telephone number?" and "What was your mother's maiden name?"[13]

Physical Examination

One of the greatest challenges in caring for the elderly patient is differentiating between changes due to age and those due to pathological conditions.[14] Table 19-1 illustrates some of the most common age-related physical changes. Additional age-related findings are included in the following paragraphs. As was noted with history taking, the approach to physical examination must be tailored to the individual needs of the elderly patient.

Vital Signs

Patients should be allowed to rest for 5 to 10 minutes before assessment of vital signs to avoid falsely high pulse and respiratory rates related to exertion. A baseline pulse should be assessed at the apical site for a full minute because dysrhythmias occur frequently with advanced age. Blood pressure should be assessed in both lying and sitting positions, if possible, to assess for orthostatic changes. Temperatures tend to be 1° to 2° F lower in the elderly. Temperature is an unreliable indicator of infection because thermoregulatory capacity is altered in the elderly.

Skin

Two commonly occurring skin abnormalities are pruritus and pressure sores. Some of the most common disorders associated with pruritus include renal failure, hepatitis, diabetes mellitus, and drug toxicity.

TABLE 19-1   **Age-related Physical Changes**

Physical Change	Associated Alterations
CARDIOVASCULAR	
Thickening and ↑ rigidity of cardiac valves	Systolic ejection murmurs
↓ Response to beta-adrenergic stimulation	↓ Tachycardic response to stress or exercise
↓ Elasticity in arterial walls	↑ Systolic and diastolic blood pressure
	↑ Pulse pressure
	↑ Peripheral vascular resistance
↓ Number of pacemaker cells in sinoatrial node	↑ PR and QT intervals
	Atrial dysrhythmias
↓ Baroreceptor response	Orthostatic hypotension
↑ Amount of lipofuscin (yellow-brown lipid pigment) in myocardium	↓ Cardiac output
PULMONARY	
↑ Anteroposterior diameter of chest	Barrel-shaped chest
	↓ Breath sounds
↓ Number and elasticity of alveoli	↓ PaO$_2$ levels
	↑ Incidence of pneumothorax with coughing
↑ Rigidity of rib cage and intercostal cartilage; atrophy of intercostal muscles	↓ Compliance
	↑ Residual volume
	↓ Vital capacity
	↑ Incidence of fractured ribs
Epithelial atrophy of cilia	Pooling of secretions
	Depressed cough reflex
NEUROLOGICAL	
Degeneration of cerebral and spinal vasculature	↓ Cerebral blood flow: ↑ sensitivity and ↓ recovery from hypoxic states
↓ Secretion of neurotransmitters: ↓ nerve conduction velocity	↓ Reflexes and reaction time
↓ REM sleep periods	Wakeful periods at night, need for naps
↓ Number of neurons in the brain	↓ Short-term memory
Lipofuscin accumulation in neurons	Altered proprioception, increased tendency to fall
GASTROINTESTINAL	
↓ Salivary flow	Xerostomia
	Altered starch metabolism
↓ Esophageal peristalsis	Dysphagia, heartburn
Atrophy of skeletal muscle in pharynx	↓ Gag reflex
	↑ Potential for aspiration
Atrophy of gastric mucosa, shrinking of gastric lumen	Delayed gastric emptying
	↓ Hydrochloric acid secretion
↓ Basal metabolic rate	↓ Caloric needs
↓ Blood flow to intestines, slowed peristalsis	↓ Bowel sounds
	↑ Tendency for constipation
↓ Number of hepatic cells	Altered drug metabolism
↓ Hepatic blood flow and fat soluble vitamins	↓ Absorption of fats
↓ Rectal muscle tone	↑ Potential for impaction or incontinence
GENITOURINARY	
↓ Thirst sensation	↑ Tendency for dehydration
↓ Number of nephrons, renal blood flow, and GFR	↑ BUN and creatinine
	↓ Drug excretion
↓ Smooth muscle tone and sphincter tone in bladder	↓ Bladder capacity, frequency, urgency, potential incontinence

TABLE 19-1   **Age-related Physical Changes—cont'd**

Physical Change	Associated Alterations
MUSCULOSKELETAL	
Demineralization of spine	↓ Height
Thinning of intervertebral disks	Kyphosis, altered balance
General muscular atrophy	↓ Lean muscle mass: weight loss, ↓ strength and endurance
	↓ Drug tolerance
	↓ Range of motion
Stiffening of ligaments, tendons, and synovial membranes	↑ Tendency for fractures
Osteoporosis and ↓ bone density	
INTEGUMENTARY	
Epidermal atrophy, collagen changes of dermis	Wrinkled skin, ↓ turgor
Dermal atrophy	Paper-thin skin, ↑ tendency for skin tears and sheering
Atrophy of sweat glands	Heat intolerance
↓ Sebaceous gland secretion	Dry skin
↑ Capillary fragility	↑ Susceptibility to bruising
IMMUNE	
Degeneration of the thymus, ↓ T helper cell activity	↓ Response to antigenic stimuli
	↓ Immunological competence
Altered thermoregulatory response	Delayed or absent pyrexia with infection
SENSES	
Vision	
Lacrimal gland atrophy	↓ Tear production
Yellowing, opacity of lens	↓ Accommodation
	↓ Color discrimination
Iris becomes rigid	↓ Pupillary response
	↑ Sensitivity to glare
↓ Blood supply to retina	↓ Visual acuity
	↓ Peripheral vision
Lipid deposition on cornea	White circular discoloration (arcus senilis)
Hearing	
↑ Thickness of cerumen	Cerumen impaction may decrease hearing
Thickening of tympanic membrane	Difficulty understanding fast speech
Loss of cells in the organ of Corti	Sensorineural hearing loss
↓ Efficiency of the cochlea	Poor discrimination of high-pitched sounds (F, G, S, T, Z)
Hardening of the stapes	Conductive hearing loss, usually unilateral
Smell	
Loss of olfactory fibers	↓ Sense of smell
	↓ Appetite
Atrophy of mucous membranes	↑ Susceptibility to mucosal irritation from nasogastric tubes, etc.
Taste	
↓ Number of taste buds, especially for sweet and salty tastes	↓ Sense of taste
	↓ Appetite
	Food tastes sour or bitter
↓ Sensation in oral mucosa	↑ Susceptibility to alterations of mucosa
↓ Blood supply to the mouth	Pale gums
	Delayed healing
Touch	
↓ Number and sensitivity of pain receptors	↓ Pain medication required

Pruritus is often associated with disorientation or confusion related to these disorders.

The presence of and potential for pressure sores should be included in the assessment. The risk assessment scale developed by Bergstrom et al.[15] identifies sensory perception, moisture, activity, mobility, nutrition, friction, and shear as the primary indicators of pressure sore risk. Additional approaches may be used according to individual patient needs and physician preferences.

Head

Hair color, texture, and distribution provide an indirect reflection of the patient's nutritional status. Hair loss due to balding usually ends during the mid-sixties. A large quantity of hair loss beyond age 65 is usually related to a nutritional deficit. Pupillary response is generally sluggish and may be difficult to evaluate due to cataracts. The presence of glaucoma and use of glaucoma medications is very common among elderly patients. The mouth should be carefully inspected for mucous membrane alterations which may be related to nutritional problems and/or diminished sensation.

Thorax

Breath sounds and heart sounds are often difficult to evaluate because of increased anteroposterior diameter. Third and fourth heart sounds are frequently heard in elders, and systolic ejection murmurs are heard in 60% to 80% of the population.[8] Premature atrial contractions, premature ventricular contractions, and atrial fibrillation are the most common dysrhythmias in the elderly.[16]

Abdomen

Some of the most significant age-related gastrointestinal changes are diminished perfusion, peristalsis, and absorption. Therefore, the potential for constipation, fecal impaction, and bowel obstruction should be carefully evaluated.

Musculoskeletal System

Both height and weight decrease with age. Tendon reflexes diminish and may disappear totally in old age. Other common findings include swollen, tender inflamed joints; decreasing range of motion; muscular atrophy; and kyphosis.

ILLNESS PRESENTATION IN ELDERLY PATIENTS

The signs and symptoms of specific illness processes often differ in the elderly population from those seen in younger adults. Many illnesses tend to present with a generalized bad feeling, rather than specific symptoms such as localized pain or fever. For example, elderly patients experiencing a myocardial infarction often present with shortness of breath and confusion. The first symptom of a urinary tract infection is often incontinence rather than dysuria. One of the most interesting phenomena commonly seen in elders is the presentation of hyperthyroidism, which often produces lethargy, weakness, and depression. Changes in the elderly patient's cognition, functional status, appetite, energy level, and mood should all be evaluated as potential symptoms of underlying pathology.

The diagnostic process is further complicated by several factors. Both patients and health care providers tend to regard these generalized symptoms as a normal response to aging. Therefore, diagnosis and treatment are often delayed. Most patients have some degree of multiple-organ pathology. Symptoms of one illness may mask those of another illness. Many patients also consume a complex regimen of prescription and over-the-counter drugs. When multiple drugs are combined with age-related and pathological processes and a declining ability to metabolize and excrete these substances, the incidences of drug interactions and toxicity become very high.

This phenomenon is particularly problematic in critical care units where patients are treated with multiple, highly potent, interactive medications. In many cases, normal dosage ranges and anticipated responses are not well established in the elderly population. New medications should be initiated at the lowest possible dose for elderly patients, with close observation for potential side effects and interactions.

NURSING MANAGEMENT

Several nursing care problems can be anticipated among elderly patients in critical care areas. A listing of some of the most common nursing diagnoses is included in the box on p. 437.

Psychosocial alterations such as anxiety, fear, hopelessness, powerlessness, and spiritual distress are typical responses of the elderly patient admitted to the critical care unit. Anxiety has been described as "a direful terror of imminent catastrophe."[17] This is a normal response to critical illness, and particularly so for the elderly patient. Often, these patients have had first-hand experience with friends or family members who were admitted to critical care units and were not discharged alive, or were discharged with a lower level of functioning. Often, the fears of discomfort and dependency are greater than the fears of death. Some of the most valuable interventions that the nurse can provide are to assure that the patient is sufficiently informed of the prognosis and treatment options, and to act as an advocate in supporting the patient's autonomous decisions.

Altered sleep patterns are a common concern

Common Nursing Diagnoses for Critically Ill Elderly Patients

Anxiety	Knowledge deficit
High risk for aspiration	Altered nutrition: less than body requirements
Altered bowel elimination: constipation	Oral mucous membrane alterations
Altered bowel elimination: incontinence	Powerlessness
Decreased cardiac output	Self-care deficit
Ineffective coping	Sensory–perceptual alterations
Fatigue	High risk for impaired skin integrity
Fear	Sleep pattern disturbance
High risk for fluid volume deficit	Social isolation
High risk for fluid volume excess	Spiritual distress
Hopelessness	Ineffective thermoregulation
Impaired communication	Altered tissue perfusion
High risk for infection	Altered urinary elimination: incontinence

---

among well elders. This problem is aggravated by the critical care environment and can rapidly lead to disorientation and confusion. The nurse is responsible for controlling environmental stimulation as much as possible, reorienting the patient whenever necessary, and attempting to maintain a normal circadian pattern.

Support of family members and significant others is also an extremely important nursing responsibility in caring for critically ill elderly patients. Elders are often dependent upon family members both before and after a critical care experience. It is essential to maintain these relationships and draw upon the support they can provide to optimize hope for the patient. The nurse should explain to the family that some degree of functional and/or cognitive setback is likely to occur during critical illness, although it may be temporary.

Many physiological responses of the elderly to critical illness are associated with age-related physiological changes (Table 19-2). Nursing measures to anticipate and prevent negative responses are the best defense. For example, the potential for aspiration is related to several factors including diminished gag reflex, decreased esophageal peristalsis, and delayed gastric emptying. In light of this knowledge, preventive measures can be instituted. The presence of the gag reflex should be assessed before oral feeding is begun. The patient should be placed in an upright position during feeding and for 30 minutes afterward. Patients should be permitted and encouraged to eat slowly and should be observed closely during the first few meals. Nursing management of three of the most frequently cited problems for this population follows.

■ NURSING DIAGNOSIS

Anxiety, related to fear of the unknown.

OUTCOME STANDARD AND CRITERIA

Anxiety is reduced or absent as evidenced by:
- Patient verbalization of concerns

- Reduction or absence of anxiety symptoms

NURSING INTERVENTIONS

- Encourage patient to express concerns about ICU admission and care because verbalization decreases anxiety and offers opportunities to clarify misconceptions
- Orient patient to critical care environment and explain all procedures to reduce fear of the unknown
- Assess family and significant others' needs regarding critical illness to reduce fears and promote support
- Encourage participation of significant others to promote utilization of familiar support systems and provide distraction
- Encourage use of familiar personal articles (e.g., Bible, rosary, pillows from home) to promote comfort with the critical care environment
- Face the patient; speak slowly and calmly to enhance communication despite sensory deficits
- Remove excess stimulation (e.g., dim lights during rest periods, control distracting noises) because of high tendency for sensory overload in ICU
- Provide honest and complete information about diagnosis, treatments, and prognosis to promote patient autonomy and informed consent
- Consistently touch the patient in a caring and reassuring manner because elderly persons have an increased need for touch to reduce feelings of isolation

■ NURSING DIAGNOSIS

Potential impairment of skin integrity, related to altered mobility.

OUTCOME STANDARD AND CRITERIA

- Skin remains intact
- Skin color, texture, and moisture are normal for the patient
- Erythema, blisters, ulcers, and abrasions are absent

NURSING INTERVENTIONS

- Turn and reposition patient at least every 2 hours,

TABLE 19-2 Commonly Used Pressure Sore Products and Equipment Prevention

	Prevention — Risk			Treatment — Stage			
	Low	Moderate	High	I	II	III	IV
PRESSURE REDUCTION/RELIEF							
Mattresses/overlays							
Foam*	X	X		X			
Air		X	X	X	X		
Water		X	X	X	X		
Gel		X	X	X	X		
Flotation		X	X	X	X	X	X
Air or fluidized			X			X	X
FRICTION/SHEAR CONTROL							
Turning sheets	X	X	X	X	X	X	X
Trapeze		X	X	X	X	X	X
MOISTURE CONTROL							
Cornstarch/powder	X	X	X	X			
Aeration devices		X	X	X	X	X	X
Moisture barrier Creams		X	X	X	X		
TOPICAL THERAPY†							
Saline				X	X	X	X
Wound gels					X	X	X
Nonirritating cleansers (e.g., Cara-Klenz)				X	X	X	X
Sharp debridement						X	X
Enzymatic agents						X	X
WOUND COVERINGS‡							
Plasticized coatings			X	X			
Transparent dressings			X	X	X	X	
Hydrocolloid dressings			X	X	X	X	
Absorptive dressings					X	X	X
Gauze					X	X	X

*Foam overlays should be at least 4 inches thick to provide pressure reduction.
†Hydrogen peroxide, povidone-iodine, Dakin's Solution, and acetic acid—all destroy fibroblasts in granulating wounds.
‡Wet-to-dry dressings provide nonselective debriding which can remove healthy granulating tissue along with necrotic tissue.
Modified from Prevost, S. (in press). Management of pressure sores. In R. Boggs, & M. King (Eds.), *AACN procedure manual for critical care* (3rd ed.). Philadelphia: Saunders.

with minor position changes between (ROM, weight shifts) because pressure-induced ischemia can begin to develop within 30 minutes

- Use utilization pressure-reducing devices such as 4-inch block foam to promote comfort and augment pressure reduction achieved by positioning
- Use pressure-relieving devices for severely compromised patients (e.g., air-fluidized beds) because these devices reduce tissue interface pressure below the capillary closing pressure of 25 to 32 mmHg. Because of expense, these are recommended only for patients who cannot be turned or who have breakdown on more than one surface

- Keep head of bed at 30° or lower, if tolerable, to reduce potential for friction and shear from sliding down in bed
- Use assistive devices for positioning (drawsheets, trapeze, and lifts) to facilitate bed mobility and reduce friction
- Contain urinary or fecal incontinence by anticipating and providing for elimination needs. Pad the bed with natural fiber sheets or blankets and provide perineal care as needed to protect skin from maceration and bacterial contamination. Vinyl or plastic-coated pads increase maceration potential by containing moisture close to the skin

- Contain diaphoresis with bathing as needed and bed padding to decrease potential for maceration over bony prominences and in skin folds
- Protect bony prominences by covering (heel and elbow protectors, polyurethane or hydrocolloid dressings) to protect areas from friction
- Support nutrition and hydration status by monitoring daily intake and output and weight gains or losses, and by encouraging oral intake; offer fluids frequently in small quantities (50-100 ml) rather than just at meals. Rationale: NPO status for more than 3 days, unintentional weight loss, serum albumin <3.5 gm/dl, and serum transferrin <150 mg/dl are all associated with increased pressure sore development

Additional detail on interventions for the prevention and treatment of pressure sores is listed in Table 19-2 on p. 438.

■ NURSING DIAGNOSIS

Altered thought processes, related to confusion, sleep deprivation, drug interactions, or toxicity.

OUTCOME STANDARD AND CRITERIA

- Patient verbalizes orientation to person, time, and place
- Confusion, disorientation, and hallucinations are absent
- Patient demonstrates ability to control own behavior and participate in or cooperate with care

NURSING INTERVENTIONS

- Obtain information on patient's usual level of cognitive function prior to illness/hospitalization from significant others to establish baseline and develop reasonable goals
- Assess current cognitive ability: orientation, thought processes, arithmetic skills, memory, problem solving, and mood so increased confusion can be recognized if it develops. Rationale: Elderly client can no longer compensate for overwhelming internal and external stressors
- Evaluate potential stressors that may produce thought process alterations: drug interactions, excessive doses and toxicity, infection and fever, hypoxia, dehydration, hyper- or hypoglycemia, electrolyte imbalances, sensory–perceptual deficits, sensory overload or deprivation, or sleep deprivation, all known causes of confusion and disorientation in the elderly patient
- Speak clearly and slowly and allow patient considerable time to respond because reaction time and response time are slower in the elderly patient. Patients can adapt to some cognitive deficits by taking more time to process thoughts
- Provide consistent caregivers to place fewer memory demands on the patient
- Encourage frequent visitation and participation by

significant others to provide familiar support system and possibly reduce need for restraints
- Evaluate need for sensory aids and provide them (glasses, hearing aid, adequate lighting) because sensory impairment or deprivation will increase confusion

REFERENCES

1. Pegels, C. (1988). *Health care and the older citizen: Economics, demographics, and financial aspects.* Rockville, MD: Aspen.
2. Bellamy, P., & Oye, R. (1987). Admitting elderly patients to the ICU: Dilemmas and solutions. *Geriatrics, 42*(3), 61-68.
3. Butler, R. (1975). *Why survive? Being old in America.* New York: McGraw-Hill.
4. Robb, S. (1979). Attitudes and intentions of baccalaureate nursing students toward the elderly. *Nursing Research, 28,* 43-50.
5. Wilson, J., & Hafferty, F. (1983). Long-term effects of a seminar on aging and health for first-year medical students. *Gerontologists, 23*(3), 319-324.
6. Christ, M., & Hohlock, F. (1988). *Gerontologic nursing.* Springhouse, PA: Springhouse.
7. Lueckenotte, A. (1990). *Pocket guide to gerontologic assessment.* St. Louis: Mosby.
8. Matteson, M., & McConnell, E. (1988). *Gerontological nursing: Concepts and practice.* Philadelphia: Saunders.
9. Newman, D., & Smith, D. (1991). *Geriatric care plans,* Springhouse, PA: Springhouse.
10. Katz, S., Ford, A., Moskowitz, R., et al. (1963) Studies of illness in the aged. The Index of ADL: A standardized measure of biological and psychosocial function. *Journal of the American Medical Association, 185,* 94-98.
11. Giduz, B., Snow, T., Sanchez, C., et al. (1986). *Geriatric first aid kit.* Chapel Hill: University of North Carolina, Program on Aging.
12. Folstein, M., & Folstein, S. (1975). Mini-mental state: A practical method for grading cognitive state of patients for the clinician. *Journal of Psychiatric Research, 12,* 189-198.
13. Pfeiffer, E. (1975). A short portable mental status questionnaire for the assessment of organic brain deficit in elderly patients. *Journal of the American Geriatric Society, 23,* 433-441.
14. Carnevalli, D., & Patrick, M. (1986). *Nursing management for the elderly* (2nd ed.). Philadelphia: Lippincott.
15. Bergstrom, N., Braden, B., Laguzza, A., et al. (1987). The Braden scale for predicting pressure sore risk. *Nursing Research, 36*(4), 205-210.
16. Moser, M. (1982). The management of cardiovascular disease in the elderly. *Journal of the American Geriatric Society, 30,* S20-S29.
17. Matteson, M., & McConnell, E. (1988). *Gerontological nursing: Concepts and practice* (p. 530). Philadelphia: Saunders.

PART FOUR

Cardiovascular Patient Care Problems

20

Anatomy and Physiology of the Cardiovascular System

Joan Vitello-Cicciu

When considering the anatomy and physiology of the cardiovascular system, it is helpful to begin with a sense of awe and admiration for the heart as a remarkably simplistic organ in which motion is continuous during a lifetime. The appreciation for the importance of the living heart perhaps was considered by William Harvey in the 17th century when he looked into the chest of an animal and noted "that there is a time when it moves, and a time when it is motionless."[1]

As knowledge about this remarkable organ expanded, it was noted that the heart has two fundamental tasks: (1) to pump blood without interruption to supply oxygen and nutrients to the billions of cells within the body, and (2) to be able to adjust its pumping action to supply more or less blood to the tissues upon demand.

A thorough knowledge of cardiovascular anatomy and physiology provides the foundation on which treatment for cardiovascular disorders can be directed. John Morgan[2] substantiates this perspective by commenting, "As every disease we labour under is a disorder of the vital animal or natural functions; a thorough acquaintance with these in their sound state is implied before we can pretend to understand their morbid affections, or how to remedy them."

CARDIAC ANATOMY

External Appearance

The heart is a cone-shaped muscle situated in the middle of the mediastinum where it is overlapped by the two pleural sacs. It occupies most of the space between the posterior surface of the sternum and the anterior surface of the vertebrae. The heart is projected approximately two thirds to the left of the midsternal line in what is known as the *levocardiac position*.

The normal heart size in the average adult is approximately 12 cm long and 9 cm wide. The weight varies in individuals depending on such factors as age and sex. The upper part of the heart is called the base and is formed by the right and left atria. The great vessels are suspended from the base. The lower part of the heart, called the apex, rests on the upper surface of the diaphragm.

The anterior surface of the heart consists mostly of the right ventricle (Figure 20-1). The pulmonary trunk arises upward from the right ventricle and bifurcates into the left and right pulmonary artery under the arch of the aorta. The right atrium is situated above the right ventricle. The groove known as the *atrioventricular (coronary) sulcus* separates these two chambers. The curved shape of the right atrium forms the right lateral border of the heart in the frontal plane. The superior vena cava forms the upper right margin. It can be visualized entering the right atrium from above through the pericardium.

The left lateral border or apex of the heart consists of the left ventricle (LV). The groove known as the *anterior interventricular sulcus* demarcates the right ventricle from the left. The remaining portion of the left border of the heart is formed by the left atrial appendage and the pulmonary trunk. The aorta arises behind the pulmonary trunk from the LV. The space between the aortic arch and pulmonary trunk is called the *aortic window*. The ligamentum arteriosum and the left recurrent laryngeal nerve reside in this space.

Cardiac Tissue

Pericardium

The heart and roots of the great vessels are contained in a relatively fixed position by the pericardium, a fibroserous sac. This sac contains two surfaces known as the *fibrous* and *serous pericardium*.

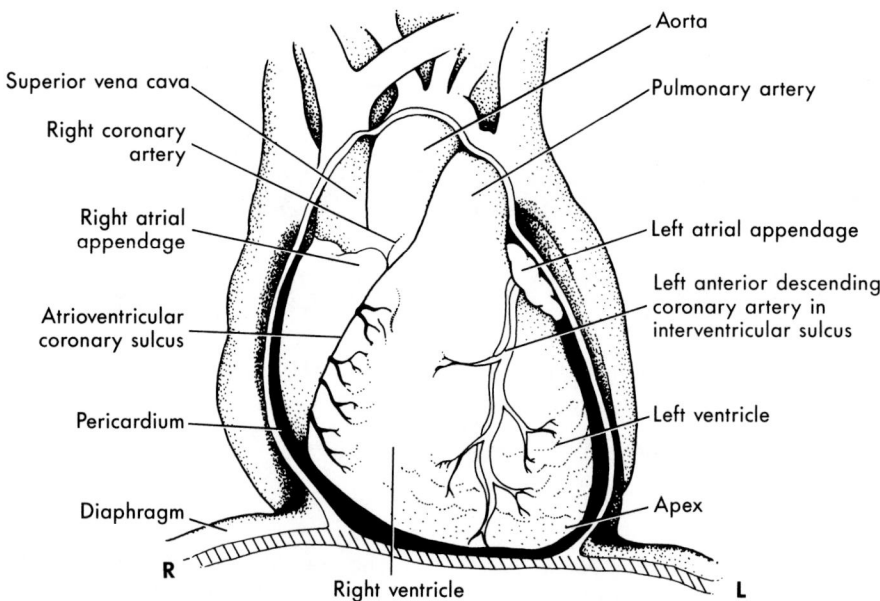

Figure 20-1   Schematic drawing showing the normal relations of the pericardium, great vessels, ventricles, and atria as viewed in the frontal position. R = right; L = left.

The *fibrous pericardium* is the outer surface which consists of white, glistening fibrous tissue giving the pericardium its shape and appearance. The *serous pericardium* consists of two linings known as the *visceral* and *parietal layers*.

The *visceral pericardium* or *epicardium* lines the surface of the heart. It also covers a small portion of the venae cavae, aorta, coronary blood vessels, and nerves. The *parietal layer* is continuous with the visceral layer and intimately adheres to the fibrous pericardium. This layer is attached by ligaments to the manubrium, the xiphoid process, vertebral column, and diaphragm. The visceral and parietal layers are separated by the pleural cavity or space which contains about 10 to 20 ml of thin, clear pericardial fluid that lubricates the contracting surfaces of the visceral and parietal layers.

The compliance of the pericardium is limited, containing the heart in a stationary position, as previously mentioned. Since it resists stretching, it also prevents acute cardiac overdistenion. In addition, the pericardium serves as a barrier to infection and neoplastic invasion.

Myocardium

The myocardium is the cardiac muscle tissue that composes the largest portion of the heart wall. It consists of three major types: (1) the specialized conduction fibers, (2) the atrial muscle fibers, and (3) fibers of the ventricles. Each type is discussed later in this chapter.

Endocardium

The endocardium is the innermost tissue layer of the cardiac wall. It contains connective tissue, elastic fibers, and endothelial cells which line the heart chambers and valves. The endocardium is in continuation with the tunica intima layer of the great vessels. These endothelial cells form a smooth surface for blood contact to deter clot formation.

Cardiac Chambers

Atria

The right and left atria serve as volume reservoirs and conduits for blood that is being sent into the ventricles. The atria are divided by the interatrial septum which contains the fossa ovalis. The right atrium (RA) is a thin-walled structure approximately 2 mm thick. The inflow tracts, specifically the superior and inferior venae cavae, which deliver unoxygenated blood, enter through the posterior wall of the atrium, known as the *sinus venarum*. The opening to the coronary sinus that drains venous blood from the coronary circulation is located between the inferior vena cava and the tricuspid valve.

The left atrium (LA) is not usually seen in the anterior view. It lies posterior and to the right of the left ventricle. The wall thickness is approximately 3 mm, which is slightly thicker than the RA. Four pulmonary veins serve as inflow tracts bringing oxygenated blood from the lungs through the posterolateral wall of the LA. The posterior wall of the LA forms

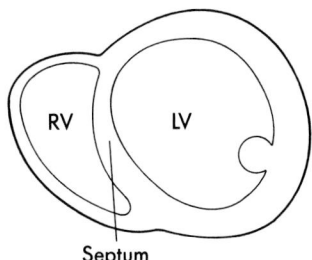

Figure 20-2 The striking structural difference between the left and right ventricular chambers. The interventricular septum protrudes into the right ventricle, causing a crescent shape, which is in marked contrast to the circular left ventricle.

Adapted from Hurst, J. W. (Ed.). (1974). *The heart, arteries, and veins* (4th ed.). New York: McGraw-Hill.

most of the posterior surface of the heart and is anterior to the esophagus and thoracic aorta.

Ventricles

The right and left ventricles function as the pumping chambers of the heart (Figure 20-2). The right ventricle (RV) is an anterior crescent-shaped structure that lies underneath the sternum. It contains trabeculations, or fibromuscular bands, from which the papillary muscles originate. These trabeculations serve as stabilizers for pacing catheters. The RV is approximately 3 to 5 mm thick and can be divided into an inflow and an outflow tract. The inflow tract consists of the trabecular muscles and the tricuspid valve which directs incoming blood from the RA toward the smooth-walled infundibulum or outflow tract. The infundibulum forms the superior aspect of the chamber. It is divided from the inflow tract by a band of muscle, the *crista supraventricularis,* which joins other constrictor muscles from the outflow tract to direct blood superiorly and posteriorly out through the pulmonic valve. During ventricular systole, this chamber contracts like a bellows to eject venous blood through the pulmonary artery into the pulmonic circulation.

The LV is an egg-shaped structure. It is three to five times thicker than the RV with a wall thickness of 13 to 15 mm. This wall thickness reflects the degree of high-pressure work that is required of the LV. The LV free wall is the portion of the LV exclusive of the septum. A small portion of the LV and the interventricular septum form a blunt tip referred to as the *cardiac apex.* Because of the forward tilt of the heart, the movement of this apical portion during ventricular contraction is referred to as the *point of maximal impulse (PMI)* or *apical impulse,* which can be located on physical examination at the fourth to fifth inter-

costal space at the midclavicular line. The funnel-shaped inflow tract, consisting of the mitral annulus, both mitral leaflets, and their chordae tendineae, directs blood in from the LA. Blood flows in an anterior leftward motion and is ejected from the LV through the outflow tract in a superior rightward direction at a 90° angle to the inflow tract. The LV pumps like a corkscrew when ejecting blood out to the aorta.

Cardiac Valves

Three functional properties of the cardiac valves are (1) preventing regurgitation of blood from one chamber to another, (2) permitting rapid antegrade flow without imposing resistance on that flow, and (3) withstanding high-pressure loads. Valves open and close in response to pressure gradients; that is, valves open when pressure in the preceding chamber is higher and close when the gradient reverses.

The AV valves are structurally the more complex of the two sets of valves (Figure 20-3). Situated between the atria and ventricles, the tricuspid valve on the right and mitral valve on the left are functionally very similar. Each has a fibrous supporting ring, the annulus, and has two large primary cusps (leaflets). The cusps are opposite one another and connected via chordae tendineae, which descend as if from an inverted parachute to the papillary muscles. Note that the chordae tendineae arise from the large anterior and posterior cusps of the mitral valve and individually insert into two sets of papillary muscles. The tricuspid has a third intermediate cusp (septal) which inserts with the anterior and posterior cusps into a total of three sets of papillary muscles.

During ventricular filling, the valves serve as a conduit that transfers blood from the atria to the ventricles (Figure 20-3). With ventricular contraction, the papillary muscles exert tension on the chordae; this tension tends to allow the valve leaflets to balloon upward and draw together. Should the chordae tendineae rupture or the papillary muscle suffer acute ischemia, the result can be severe valvular regurgitation or insufficiency.

The semilunar valves of the heart each consist of three cuplike cusps which are similar in shape. Structurally, they are very dissimilar to the AV valves; since a much greater pressure load is imposed on them, their design is much simpler. After termination of ventricular systole, the high pressure within the pulmonary artery and aorta drops, causing retrograde flow of blood toward the ventricles, thus filling the aortic and pulmonary cusps with blood and snapping them shut. The event can be seen on the normal arterial waveform and is known as the *dicrotic notch.*

The *sinuses of Valsalva* are two outpouchings im-

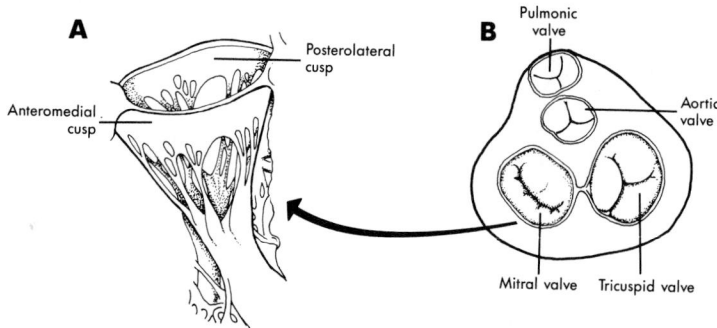

Figure 20-3   Anatomical structure of atrioventricular valves. *(A)* The funnel-shaped mitral valve is schematically demonstrated on the left, with the two cusps attaching via chordae tendineae to individual sets of papillary muscles. *(B)* Schematic representation of the closed mitral and tricuspid valves. Though very similar structurally, the tricuspid has a larger intermediate cusp, which attaches to a third set of papillary muscles.
Adapted from Spalteholz, W. (1933). *Hand atlas of human anatomy.* Philadelphia: Lippincott.

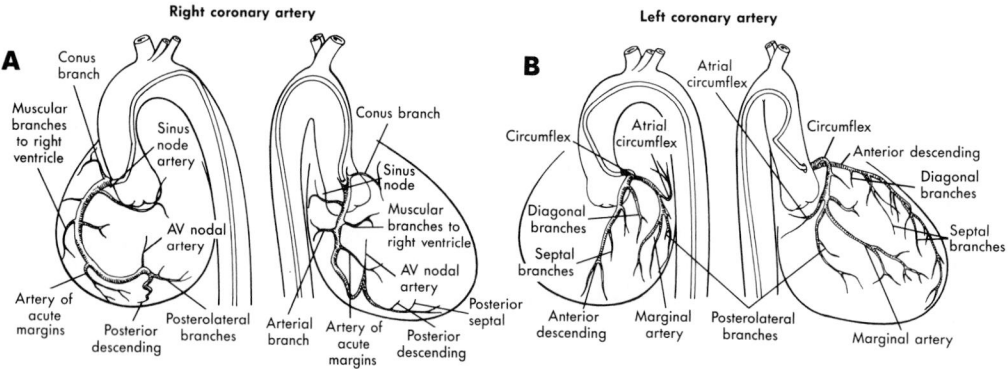

Figure 20-4   Normal coronary anatomy from right and left posterior oblique positions. *A,* Right artery: (1) conus branch, (2) sinus node artery, (3) muscular branches to right ventricle, (4) artery of acute margins, (5) AV nodal artery, (6) posterior descending, (7) posterior septal, (8) posterolateral branches, (9) arterial branch. *B,* Left coronary artery: (1) anterior descending, (2) circumflex, (3) diagonal branches, (4) septal branches, (5) atrial circumflex, (6) marginal artery, (7) posterolateral branches.
Adapted from Ayres, S., & Gianelli, V. (1971). *Cardiology: A clinicophysiologic approach.* New York: Appleton-Century-Crofts.

mediately behind the semilunar cusps. In the aorta, they prevent obstruction of the coronary ostia by the valve cusps.

Coronary Artery

The right and left coronary arteries arise from the coronary ostia in the aortic root (Figure 20-4). In almost all individuals, the left coronary artery emerges from a single ostium in the coronary sinus of the aorta, while the right coronary sinus sometimes gives rise to two ostia, the smaller of which becomes the conus artery.

The left main coronary artery is of variable length but divides, usually within 2 to 10 cm, into the left anterior descending (LAD) and left circumflex arteries. The branches of the main vessel take a diagonal route over the left ventricular free wall and are fre-

quently referred to as the *diagonal left ventricular branches.* They are generally situated between the anterior descending and circumflex arteries. The LAD supplies the LV ventricular free wall, the septum, and portions of the right ventricle. In addition, it usually supplies the anterior as well as portions of the posterior and inferior apex. The circumflex artery usually emerges at a 90° angle from the main left coronary artery and courses toward the lateral left ventricle and apex. Branches from the circumflex artery supply the posterior and lateral walls of the left ventricle. In about 10% of persons, the circumflex artery gives rise to the AV nodal artery; in such cases the left coronary and its branches supply the entire left ventricle and septum.

The right coronary artery arises from the right aortic sinus and courses down the right atrioventricular sulcus. In 85% to 95% of hearts, it makes a 90° turn and crosses the crux of the heart and becomes the posterior descending artery.

If the conus artery does not originate directly from the aorta, it is the first branch off the right coronary artery (RCA). The sinus node artery emerges from the RCA in approximately 50% of persons; in the remainder it emerges from the circumflex artery. In the majority of cases, the RCA supplies the RA and RV and gives rise to branches supplying the inferior surface of the LV. The determination of right or left coronary artery dominance is made by evaluating whether the right coronary artery or the left circumflex artery crosses the crux (the point at which the interventricular sulcus and coronary sulcus meet on the posterior wall) to become the posterior descending artery (PDA). The heart is said to have right coronary dominance if the right coronary artery becomes the PDA. The AV nodal artery arises from the right coronary in right-sided dominance and supplies the AV node and bundle of His.

Interarterial vessels connect, or anastomose, with each other. These vessels foster collateral circulation and can be found through the full thickness of the myocardium. The greatest amount of collaterals is located near the endocardial surface. The number of these collaterals can increase in response to demand imposed by atherosclerotic heart disease, chronic anemia, or hypoxemia.

Coronary venous drainage is accomplished via three drainage routes referred to as the coronary sinus, anterior RV cardiac veins, and the thesbian veins. The coronary sinus located in the posterior atrioventricular groove near the crux of the heart, receives chiefly LV blood from the great, middle, and small cardiac veins. The coronary sinus then empties this compilation of venous return into the right atrium. Anterior RV cardiac veins drain venous blood from the RV and empty directly into the RA. The thesbian veins empty primarily into the RA and RV, but some may empty into the LV constituting a physiological shunt of unoxygenated blood into the systemic circulation.

Lymphatic System

The lymphatic vessels are the principal routes by which protein and other large particulate matter can be removed from the interstitium; it is fundamentally a drainage system facilitated by cardiac contraction. The distribution of the lymphatics parallels that of the venous system in that they both have extensive superficial and deep collecting systems. Only cartilage, epithelium, and tissues of the central nervous system lack lymph supply. In addition to returning fluid and protein to the circulation, the lymphatic system removes debris such as bacteria, toxins, and degenerating tissues.

Cardiac Nerves

The heart is innervated by cholinergic fibers from the vagus nerve and by adrenergic fibers from the upper thoracic spinal cord through the cardiac plexus via superior, middle, and inferior cervical ganglia.

Vagal fibers are predominantly found in the SA node, AV node, and atrial muscle fibers. The right vagus nerve fibers supply the SA node and control the heart rate and force of atrial contraction, whereas the left vagus nerve supplies chiefly the AV node.

Sympathetic nerve fibers extend to the atria and ventricles. Most of these fibers influence ventricular contraction. Vagal fibers also extend to both ventricles but do not seem to affect ventricular contraction as do the sympathetic fibers.

Sensory fibers also transmit impulses through the cardiac nerves up to the central nervous sytem. These sensory fibers are located in the pericardium, ventricular walls, and coronary blood vessels.

Systemic Circulation

The walls of the aorta and large arteries are extremely thick and tough. Functionally, they transport blood under high pressure to the tissues through their role as a pressure reservoir. With left ventricular ejection, the walls within the aortic arch distend as the arterial pressure rises, thereby transmitting a pressure pulse down the aorta and on into the arteries. When the ventricular contraction ceases, the arterial pressure gradually falls, but sufficient tension remains within the walls to drive blood through the capillaries to the tissues and overcome peripheral resistance. By so doing, the systemic arterial pressure of approximately 90 mmHg maintains forward flow, as demonstrated in Figure 20-5. The elasticity of the aorta allows it to act as a compression chamber and reservoir during LV ejection which converts pulsatile to continuous flow in diastole. This process is called the *windkessel effect*.

Between the arteries and veins lie the capillaries, whose walls are composed only of endothelial cells. The thin capillary walls are essential in permitting rapid diffusion of substances between the blood and tissue. Because of their very small caliber they can support pressures of up to 100 mmHg in the lower extremities during standing. At heart level, the capillary pressure is normally between 20 and 30 mmHg.

The veins are very thin-walled and normally are under very low pressure. They accommodate large volumes of blood with very little fluctuation in pressure. Contrasted with the arterial circulation, in which even small increases in volume can induce large

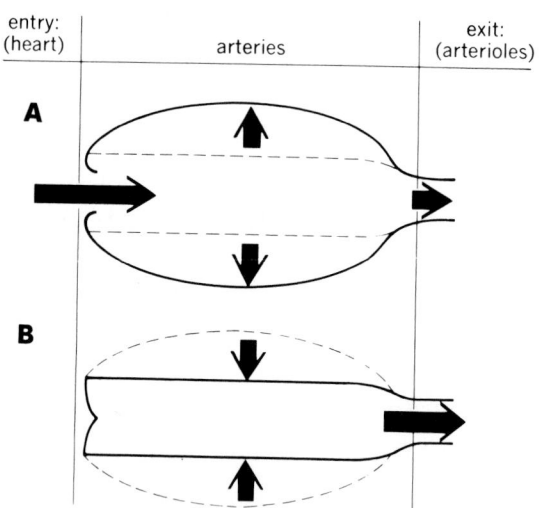

Figure 20-5   *A,* During systole, much of the blood is stored in the elastic arteries, although some forward flow does occur. *B,* In diastole, the stored tension within the walls (elastic recoil) is instrumental in modifying pulsatile flow into constant flow throughout the cardiac cycle.

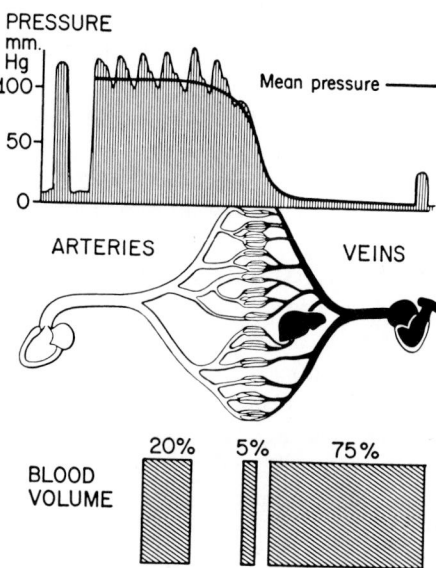

Figure 20-6   The volume of blood stored in the distensible venous circulation is between 60% and 75% and can change dramatically. Arterial volume, however, remains at about 20% of total blood volume and does not vary significantly.
From Rushmer, R. (1976). *Cardiovascular dynamics* (4th ed.). Philadelphia: Saunders.

pressure fluctuations, the principal function of the venous sytem as a low-pressure, variable-volume reservoir becomes apparent. In fact, almost three quarters of the systemic circulation is stored within the venous circulation in the large capacitance veins (Figure 20-6). Note the very small amount of blood within the capillaries, where the most important function of the cardiovascular system occurs.

Conduction System

The cardiac cells involved in conducting an electric current are known as the *pacemaker* or *automatic cells.* They are discussed in greater detail in Chapter 10. Located at the junction of the superior vena cava and the right atrium lies the normal pacemaker of the heart, the *sinoatrial node* (SA node). An electric impulse is initiated at this node and travels through the internodal pathways to the *atrioventricular (AV) node,* located in the right atrium, directly above the tricuspid valve and anterior to the coronary sinus. Once the impulse travels through the AV node, it courses along the common *bundle of His,* which divides almost immediately into the right and left bundles. The left bundle further divides to form two direct pathways to the anterior and posterior papillary muscle. The impulse then travels and permeates through the many small fibers of the *Purkinje network,* beginning at the endocardium, and finally terminates within the ventricular myocardium.

CARDIAC PHYSIOLOGY
Myocardial Structure

The cells that compose the cardiac muscle are the specialized electrical conduction cells known as pace-

maker cells (previously discussed) and the *working myocardial cells.* These working myocardial cells consist of atrial and ventricular fibers which are involved in the contractile force of the heart. The pacemaker cells are somewhat smaller than the ventricular fibers.

The cardiac muscle as a whole is often compared to skeletal muscle because of its striated appearance and color as well as some of its functional characteristics. It should be noted, however, that myocardial muscle shares many similarities with certain types of visceral smooth muscle such as the ureter, uterus, and gastrointestinal tract. These muscles appear to have inherent rhythmicity and to be able to conduct a wave of excitation in a manner similar to that of the myocardium.

Microscopically, an individual myocardial cell is approximately 40 to 100 μm in length and 10 to 20 μm in diameter.[3] The long end of each cell is connected by a thickened portion of the sarcolemma known as an *intercalated disk.* These disks may vary in type, but they serve functionally as a barrier between cells. Although these disks separate the cells, these cells as a whole still function as a syncytium—that is, as a single cell—because these disks offer little electrical resistance, allowing the electric current to spread simultaneously throughout the fibers.

Surrounding each cell is the surface membrane known as the sarcolemma. It is composed of the plasmalemma, which is a semipermeable membrane layer, and the glycocalyx. In the center of each cell is the nucleus. Lysosomes are located near the nucleus. These vesicles contain hydrolytic enzymes which have the potential of lysing cellular membranes and other cellular components.

Myofibrils are long rodlike structures that give the heart muscle its striated appearance. These structures run the length of a cell and are composed of repeating units called the sarcomeres. The *sarcomeres* are the contractile unit within the myofibrils arranged in parallel rows along the long axis (Figure 20-7). The average length of a sarcomere is 1.6 to 2.2 μm. Multiple sarcomeres are found in any given cell and are joined end to end at Z bands to form myofibrils. Extending from each Z band toward the middle of the sarcomere can be seen a thin filament that is predominantly composed of the protein actin. The thick filaments of myosin are found in the middle of the sarcomere, the A band where they overlap with the thin actin filaments. The central light area or H zone is occupied only by the thicker filaments, while the I band contains only the actin filament.

It is postulated that cross bridges protrude from the myosin filaments at regular intervals, and it is these cross bridges that, during contraction, cause lateral movement of the actin and myosin filaments so that they slide past one another, bringing about the development of tension and shortening within the muscle. During contraction, it appears that the widths of the I band and H band shrink as the actin is drawn past the myosin and the Z bands draw closer together, while the A bands remain of one length during both stretching and contraction of the fiber. The physiology of mechanical contraction is discussed in further detail in the next section, Excitation–Contraction Coupling.

In close proximity to the sarcomeres are the *mitochondria*, which are vitally important in cardiac metabolism. These bodies are the source of high-energy compounds such as ATP (adenosine triphosphate) needed for production of chemical energy for myocardial contraction as well as for synthesis of nutrients. The prodigious oxygen demands of the heart can be appreciated by noting that between 30% and 50% of the myocardium is occupied by mito-

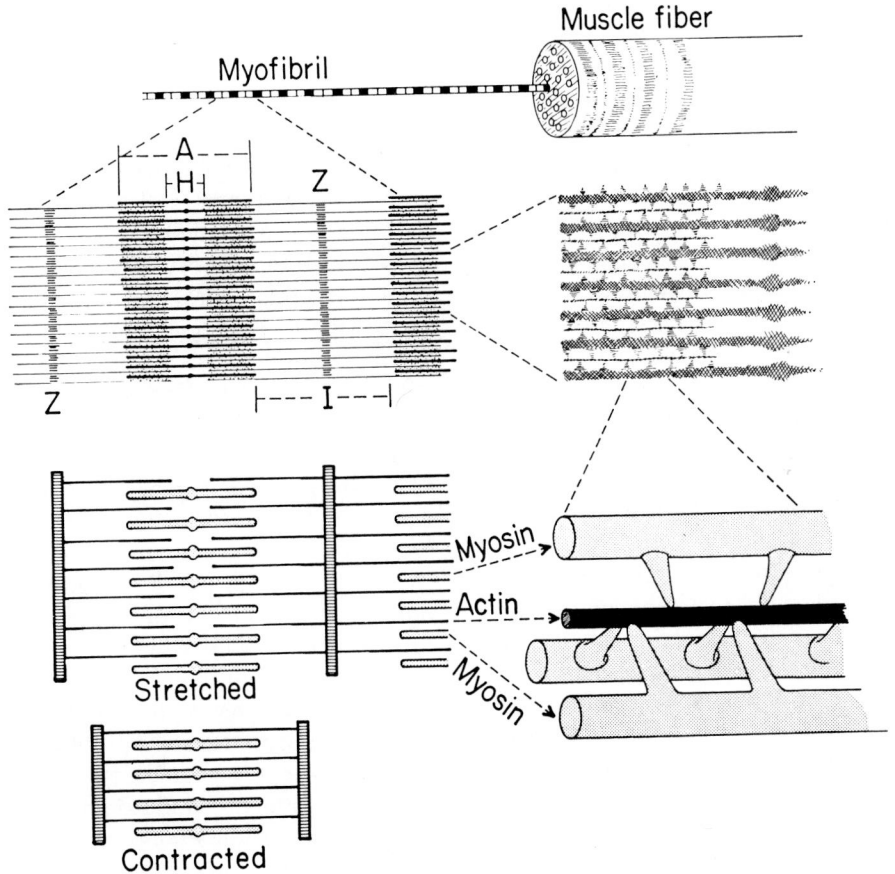

Figure 20-7 Structural components of myocardial muscle fiber. The myofibrils are composed of thick myosin and thin actin filaments. Many cross bridges may be seen periodically between the two filaments, which are activated during contraction so that the myosin filaments are able to draw the actin filaments, resulting in much greater interdigitation of actin and myosin.

From Rushmer, R. (1970). *Cardiovascular dynamics* (3rd ed.). Philadelphia: Saunders.

chondria. When ischemia exists within the heart, the balance between energy supply and demand can become most precarious. There is some suggestion that a deficiency of ATP may be an important factor in influencing infarct size and in the development of cardiac failure.[3]

Additional intracellular components consist of the *transverse tubular system* and the *sarcoplasmic reticulum*. The *transverse tubular system* is considered to be the place at which the electrical action potential permeates through the cell to trigger muscle contraction and acts as an intracellular transport system for calcium. The *sarcoplasmic reticulum* is a tubular network surrounding each myofibril. This network stores calcium internally and is thought to release this intracellular calcium once an action potential has been generated. Once calcium is released, it migrates to the myofibrils where it is involved in binding of the actin and myosin molecule. A more detailed discussion of the role of calcium in myocardial contraction follows.

Excitation–Contraction Coupling

To comprehend cardiac physiology, it is essential that the electrical and mechanical events be understood. The electrical events were discussed in Chapter 10. This section discusses the mechanical events that are preceded by electrical events. The method by which the electrical wave of depolarization at the cell membrane produces the mechanical contraction is known as *excitation–contraction coupling*. The major pathological alterations in myocardial contractility have their basis in the degeneration of this very complex and intricate mechanism.

Calcium seems to have a dual role in cardiac contraction: as a trigger for initiation of contraction and as a regulating factor for the contractile process. The method for release of calcium from its storage place in the sarcoplasmic reticulum appears to result from the Ca^{2+} ions which enter the cell during the plateau of the action potential. These Ca^{2+} ions are thought to release large quantities of Ca^{2+} from the sarcoplasmic reticulum, allowing activation of the contractile process.[3] Thus, depolarization of the cell membrane initiates the release of the internal store of Ca^{2+} into the cytoplasm. When the wave of depolarization stimulates the release of Ca^{2+}, the ion activates myosin to interdigitate with actin.

Interdigitation of the actin and myosin filaments depends upon two more proteins that are present within the thin filaments: *troponin* and *tropomyosin*. During relaxation these two proteins appear to inhibit activation of the myosin cross bridges. When calcium is released during excitation, however, the inhibition is reversed and calcium is bound to troponin so that the myosin cross bridge is activated to draw the thin

filament toward itself. It appears that the amount of calcium available to bind with troponin has a direct bearing on the strength of the cardiac contraction.

During repolarization of the muscle, relaxation occurs as Ca^{2+} is pumped back into the reticulum until its concentration is insufficient to utilize ATP and cross bridges can no longer be formed. Complete recovery of the cell coincides with the return of Ca^{2+} to its storage sites.

Other potential influences on cardiac contractility are those caused by abnormal extracellular concentrations of electrolytes, specifically Ca^{2+} and potassium (K^+). Increased concentrations of potassium can cause hyperpolarization of the resting membrane and result in cardiac arrest. Hypercalcemia may cause serious spastic contraction of the heart and induce systolic arrest while a decrease in ionized Ca^{2+} can decrease the force of contraction.

The Frank-Starling Phenomenon

Much like that of the skeletal muscle fiber, the force of myocardial contraction is a function of the initial muscle length. The classic studies by Frank in 1895 demonstrated that the myocardial fiber responds with a more forceful contraction when it is stretched. Also referred to as the *length–tension relationship*, the results of Frank's work further demonstrated that there are physiological limits to the relationship; excessive stretch of the muscle fiber results in development of less tension, resulting in a decrease in contractility.

Maximal force is developed at a length of 2.2 μm. At that length the actin and myosin filaments are able to provide the greatest number of cross bridges, or force-generating sites. When stretch exceeds a length of 2.4 μm, less interdigitation of thick and thin filaments occurs, and fewer contractile sites are activated. Wiggers, and later Starling, continued Frank's work by studying the heart in an isolated heart–lung preparation and demonstrated that the length–tension relationship for the sarcomere can be applied graphically within the heart by substitution of ventricular filling pressure for tension and end-diastolic volume for fiber length. Clinically, this means that the heart can contract more forcefully during systole when it is filled to a greater degree during diastole provided the filling is within certain physiological limits. This principle whereby an increase in ventricular filling (preload) produces significant increases in stroke volume is known as the *Frank-Starling law of the heart*.

The normal ventricle is very compliant. Initially the ventricle can accept large increases in volume without a significant increase in pressure. This concept can be illustrated in the Frank-Starling curve (Figure 20-8). Physiological limits operate here as well. However, should increases in ventricular end-

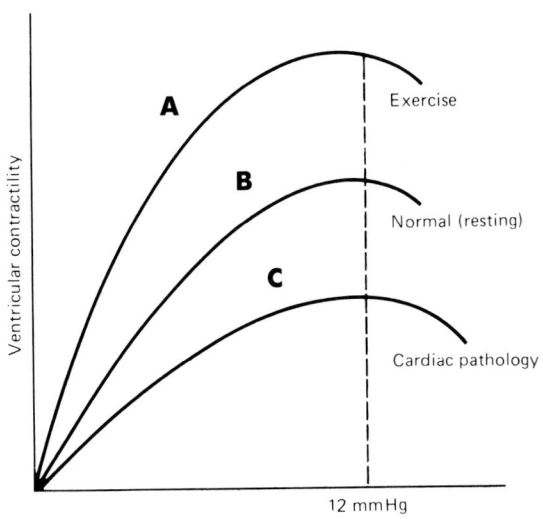

Left ventricular end-diastolic filling pressure (LVEDP)

Figure 20-8   Schematic drawing of the Frank-Starling law of the heart. *A,* Stretching of the myocardial fiber will within physiological limits produces an augmentation of ventricular contraction. Since myocardial fiber length cannot be measured, left ventricular end-diastolic filling pressure (LVEDP) is utilized to assess ventricular ejection. Peak ventricular ejection generally occurs at a ventricular filling pressure of 12 mmHg, represented by the dashed line. *B,* Sympathetic effects can shift the curve to the left, resulting in more rapid increase of ventricular ejection. *C,* Pathology can shift the curve to the right, causing greater filling pressures for the same or lesser ventricular ejection volume. Thus, filling pressures greater than 12 mmHg are generally required in the diseased heart for optimal performance.

diastolic volume cause an elevated filling pressure within the ventricle, further increases in diastolic filling result in a decrease in ventricular performance, the so-called descending limb of the Starling curve (Figure 20-8*A*). In the normal heart, optimal tension is achieved at a filling pressure of about 10 to 12 mmHg, which corresponds to a fiber length of 2.2 μm. Usually end-diastolic pressure is approximately 0 to 7 mmHg and myocardial length about 2 μm, resulting in normal ventricular performance on the ascending limb of the curve.

The Cardiac Cycle

To comprehend cardiac physiology, it is essential that the sequential relationships between the electrical and mechanical events be understood. Figure 20-9 demonstrates the interrelation of those events along with the resulting pressure and volume changes within the cardiac chambers.

Correlation of Electrical and Mechanical Activity

With generation of an action potential within the sinus node and corresponding movement of Ca^{2+} into the cells, atrial depolarization occurs and a P wave is

recorded on the electrocardiogram. Atrial pressure rises immediately thereafter, and atrial contraction occurs, adding an additional third to the volume of blood which becomes the ventricular diastolic filling volume. Within 0.2 second following atrial depolarization, the wave of excitation activates the ventricles, resulting in the ventricular action potential and the inscription of the QRS complex, and generating ventricular contraction and the resulting rapid rise in ventricular pressure. The QRS complex, then, precedes ventricular systole very slightly. During either right or left atrial pressure monitoring, pulsations that occur in either of the atria can be depicted as waveforms (pressure peaks) (see Figure 20-9). The *a* wave is produced by atrial contraction. The *c* wave occurs at the onset of ventricular systole and results from an initial bulging of the AV valves. This wave is often not seen in hemodynamic monitoring. The *v* wave, which corresponds to the TP interval on the ECG, results from atrial filling behind closed AV valves, causing an increase in atrial pressure.

The T wave signals the beginning of ventricular repolarization. Atrial repolarization cannot be measured because it occurs simultaneously with ventricular systole and the resulting ventricular relaxation. Hence, ventricular diastole follows the T wave.

Ventricular Systole

The initial portion (phase 1) of ventricular contraction raises pressure within the chamber. As described previously, the sharp rise in pressure is caused by contraction of the papillary muscles which exerts pressure on the chordae tendineae so that the leaflets of the AV valves are drawn closer together. The resulting pressure increase closes them tightly. Thus, phase 1 of ventricular contraction is called *isovolumic* or *isovolumetric*. Since all four valves are closed, the contracting muscles elevate ventricular pressure without a change in volume. This period includes lengthening of some as well as shortening of other ventricular muscle fibers and is termed isovolumetric, meaning "maintenance of a constant volume."

During phase 2 of ventricular systole, known as the rapid ventricular ejection phase, intraventricular pressure exceeds the diastolic pressure within the outflow tract, approximately 80 mmHg in the aorta (Figure 20-9) and 8 mmHg in the pulmonary artery; the semilunar valves are opened, and ejection begins. In the initial portion of ventricular ejection, left ventricular pressure rises above that of the aorta, producing a very rapid flow. In phase 3, known as the reduced ejection phase, ventricular pressure drops below aortic pressure, and the velocity of outflow diminishes. The amount of blood ejected from each ventricle under resting conditions, the *stroke volume,* is about 70 to 80 ml.

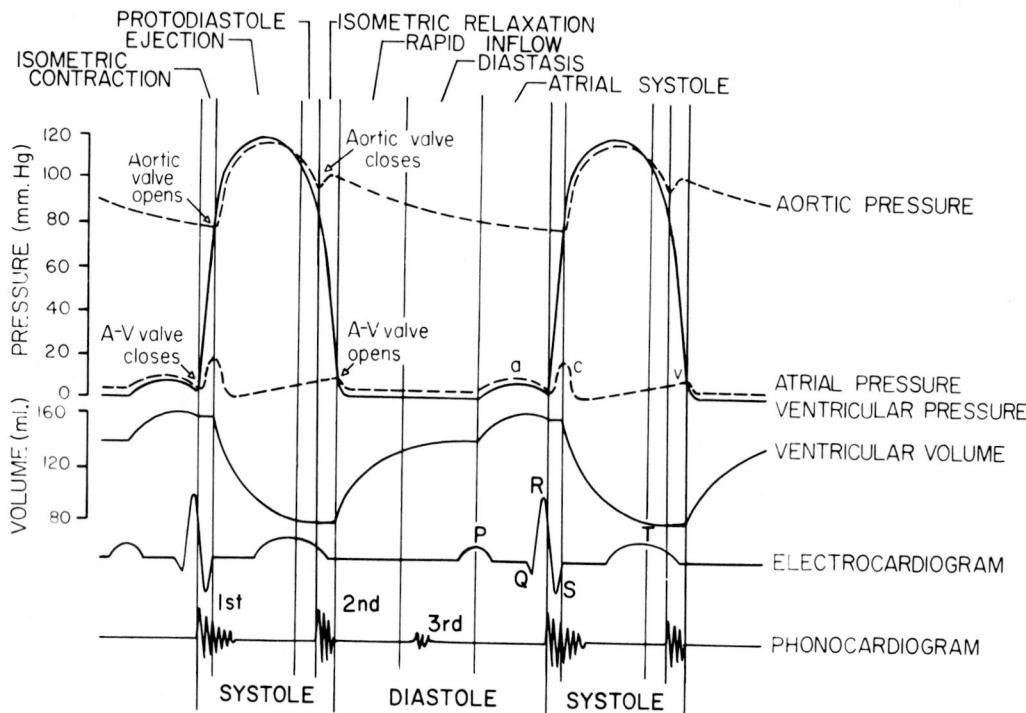

Figure 20-9 Interrelationship of the electrical and mechanical events in the cardiac cycle. Also depicted are the heart sounds (phonocardiogram) and intraventricular volume.
From Guyton, A. C. (1991). *Textbook of medical physiology* (8th ed.). Philadelphia: Saunders.

With cessation of ventricular contraction and the ensuing pressure drop within the arteries, the semilunar valves close and systolic ejection ceases. Under resting conditions, the ejected stroke volume equals 50% to 60% of ventricular diastolic volume. The residual volume is influenced by many factors; among them are preload, afterload, contractility, and heart rate.

Right Ventricular Ejection. The geometric differences between the two ventricles were mentioned earlier (see Figure 20-2). Right ventricular ejection performance resembles that of a bellows, since the surface area of the two walls is large in relation to the area contained between them, and very slight movement from the free wall toward the septum is quite effective in accomplishing systolic ejection. The right ventricular muscle shortens, but this is less effective than the bellows action.

It is apparent that the right ventricular structure is suited to perform as a high-volume, low-resistance pump; severely deleterious effects can occur from an acute pressure load on the right ventricle, such as a massive pulmonary embolism. The effect of right ventricular ischemia and infarct on cardiac performance is being investigated.

Left Ventricular Ejection. The power of LV contraction and its efficiency are largely determined by reduction of circumference. In contrast to the RV, the left chamber has a small surface area in relation to its volume. The *law of Laplace (P = T/R)* states that the muscle tension *(T)* necessary to maintain a level of pressure *(P)* is reduced as the radius *(R)* is decreased. A chronically dilated, hypertrophied ventricular chamber requires greater muscle tension and, therefore, a greater energy supply, to sustain a given ventricular pressure. Because the LV with each ejection must overcome a pressure gradient of over 90 mmHg, it is structurally designed as a high-pressure pump. When subjected to excessive volume loads, however, the resulting ventricular dilatation may severely compromise left ventricular efficiency.

Ventricular Diastole

Phase 1 of ventricular diastole is called the *isovolumic* or *isovolumetric relaxation*. A precipitous drop in ventricular pressure occurs without a change in volume. As blood accumulates within the atrial chambers during ventricular systole, atrial pressures rise significantly. When diastolic pressures fall below levels less than those within the atria, the AV valves open and the rapid filling phase (phase 2) begins. Phenomena such as diastolic recoil or diastolic suction significantly affect the rapid filling phase, during which ventricular volume apparently increases without a significant elevation of filling pressure. Rushmer[4] believes that diastolic recoil largely explains the more complete systolic ejection that occurs in tachycardia. He postulates that some of the contractile tension occurring during systole is stored within the walls of the left ventricle; with sudden diastolic relaxation, the ventricular walls appear to spring outward during early ventricular filling. This diastolic recoil causes a drop in diastolic filling pressure, thus greatly augmenting filling. During tachycardia, when filling time is very brief, this phenomenon becomes even more important in contributing to a rise in cardiac output.

After the period of early ventricular filling, blood flow diminishes and effectively ceases. This phase 3, the middle third of diastole, is known as the *period of diastasis* and occurs only if the ventricular diastolic period is sufficiently long. Since there is no blood flow and the AV valves are open, the pressures within the atria and ventricles are equal during the period of diastasis. During phase 4, atrial contraction occurs following atrial depolarization. The amount of blood entering the ventricle during atrial contraction is variable and is influenced by the following: (1) duration of the PR interval, (2) heart rate, and (3) chamber filling pressures. Blood flow resulting from atrial contraction will follow the path of least resistance, forward into the LV or retrograde into the great veins.

The atrial contraction is not essential for adequate cardiac performance at normal activity levels. During exercise or any increase in metabolic demand resulting in tachycardia, however, the atrial contribution can be significant, particularly if the heart rate becomes so rapid that it affects the rapid filling phase.

Heart Sounds

The exact cause of the heart sounds remains controversial, but they are caused at least in part by the sudden acceleration and deceleration of blood within the ventricular chamber at the time of valvular closure and muscular contraction. Heart sounds reflect the mechanical events of the heart. Refer to Chapter 21 for more detailed discussion of heart sounds.

Components of Arterial Pressure

Systolic Pressure

The normal LV ejects the majority of its stroke volume (SV) during the early period of ventricular systole, the rapid ejection phase. As already described, the left ventricular pressure momentarily exceeds aortic pressure (Figure 20-9). Following the rapid ejection phase, the peak systolic pressure is reached, which is determined by the mass of ventricular volume, the rate of ejection, and the compliance of the arterial vessels. A relatively small stroke volume injected into a distensible aorta will raise aortic pressure slightly, while a very rapid ventricular ejection into a rigid arteriosclerotic vessel significantly elevates arterial pressure.

Diastolic Pressure

During ventricular diastole, arterial pressure falls to a low level just prior to the next contraction. The rate of pressure drop is influenced by many factors; among them are the systolic pressure, the rate of flow through the periphery (peripheral runoff), and the length of diastole. End-diastolic pressure is determined mainly by total peripheral resistance and heart rate.

Mean Arterial Pressure

The average pressure throughout the phasic cardiac cycle is known as the *mean arterial pressure*. It can be measured by recording the area under the curve of an arterial pressure tracing and dividing the area by the concurrent time period. Normally, the mean is slightly less than the average of the systolic and diastolic pressures and it can be grossly approximated by adding one third of the pulse pressure (difference between the systolic and diastolic pressures) to the diastolic pressure. The average adult with a systolic pressure of 120 mmHg and a diastolic pressure of 80 mmHg has a mean arterial pressure of 93 mmHg.

The mean pressure varies directly with systolic and diastolic fluctuations. In the newborn it is normally about 70 mmHg, but it is approximately 100 to 110 mmHg in the adult. With arteriosclerosis the arterial mean pressure can rise to 140 mmHg. Because the mean arterial pressure is the average pressure responsible for the arterial to venous pressure gradient, it has a very important influence on tissue perfusion.

Pulse Pressure

Pulse pressure is defined as the difference between the systolic and diastolic pressures. Thus, it can be affected by factors that determine systolic or diastolic pressure, particularly arterial capacitance or stroke volume.

The pulse pressure, according to Berne and Levy,[5] can be used to assess both arterial capacitance and stroke volume. Normally the pulse pressure is approximately 40 mmHg. If arterial compliance is reduced, as in arteriosclerosis, pulse pressure will be higher than if the arterial wall were normally distensible. The elevated pressure increases left ventricular work and energy requirements. Increases in total peripheral resistance resulting from conditions such as hypertension will obviously increase arterial pressure if the same volume is to be maintained.

Heart rate, then, will change the pulse pressure

according to the degree by which stroke volume and compliance of the arterial tree are changed. If a tachycardia and the resulting normal increase in arterial pressure are accompanied by a drop in arterial compliance, pulse pressure will be increased, assuming stroke volume is constant. Conversely, if the volume of blood ejected from the left ventricle is reduced without a change in arterial compliance, the pulse pressure will usually decrease. In summary, factors that tend to increase systolic pressure and/or cause a drop in diastolic pressure will tend to augment the pulse pressure.

Transmission of the Arterial Pulse Wave

Since the left ventricular stroke volume is ejected with such force and velocity, it tends to accumulate in the aortic root (the first portion of the aorta), causing stretching and increased tension within the aortic wall. The transmission of the stretching and development of tension into each adjacent section of the aorta and arterial vasculature results in a measurable pressure waveform and palpable pulse within the peripheral arterial circulation. The rate at which the pressure waveform is transmitted depends upon arterial compliance.

The shape of the arterial waveform changes as the pressure pulse reaches the more peripheral segments of the arterial tree; the systolic peak becomes significantly higher, as much as 20 to 40 mmHg higher within the brachial and femoral arteries than in the central aorta due to an increase in the pulse pressure; and the dicrotic notch (point of closure of the aortic valve) becomes increasingly more distorted and eventually disappears. In addition, a peak is often seen on the diastolic portion of the peripheral arterial waveform. The changes in morphology of the transmitted aortic waveform decrease with age, and in older individuals with severe arteriosclerosis there may be relatively little difference between central and peripheral waveforms.

Control of Cardiac Output

Cardiac output is defined as the amount of blood that is pumped from the left ventricle into the aorta per minute. Although the right ventricle ejects an equivalent amount of blood into the pulmonary artery, it is not included in measurement of total cardiac output. *Venous return* is considered as the amount of blood that is returned to the right atrium. Venous return may differ from the cardiac output for short periods because blood can be stored in some areas of the circulation; the cardiac output and venous return are eventually equivalent amounts and are inextricably related to one another.

The normal volume of cardiac output in the average adult, is about 5,000 ml/min or 5.0 L. Because the cardiac output varies considerably in accordance with body size, the cardiac index is used to achieve an accurate estimate of blood flow in proportion to body surface area. The average 70-kg male has an estimated standard cardiac index of approximately 3 L/min.

Cardiac output is calculated as the product of the heart rate multiplied by the amount of blood ejected from the left ventricle with each contraction, which is the stroke volume. Clinical alterations in cardiac output means that the heart must adjust either frequency of beating or the stroke volume. Alteration of heart rate is chiefly controlled through the autonomic nervous system, while alteration of the stroke volume involves a much more complex group of control mechanisms (Figure 20-10). With sympathetic stimulation, the cardiac output can more than double by utilizing the systolic and diastolic reserve capacities. The normal resting cardiac output is achieved through the product of a resting stroke volume of 80 ml and a resting heart rate of 70 beats per minute. The heart rate can increase to an effective rate of 180 beats per minute while the ventricles respond to the inotropic sympathetic effects. If only the rate of the SA node is increased by electrical stimulation or specific localized sympathetic excitation upon the SA node, without generalized peripheral effects, cardiac output will probably not increase.

The *stroke volume* is calculated as the difference between the end-diastolic volume within the left ventricle and the residual volume of blood within the ventricle following systole. The major factors that influence stroke volume are diastolic filling (preload), afterload, and contractility.

Diastolic filling (preload) is defined as the volume or pressure of blood in the ventricle at the end of diastole (EDV or EDP).[6] It is dependent upon total blood volume and peripheral circulatory regulation. Atrial contraction can augment diastolic filling by as much as 35%. Increase in stroke volume is effected by the length–tension relationship of the Frank-Starling mechanism within physiological limits. The effects are augmented through the inotropic effects of the sympathetic nervous system.

Afterload, or wall tension, is the pressure in the artery leading from the ventricle that the ventricle must overcome to eject its stroke volume.[6] Afterload is determined primarily by aortic end-diastolic pressure but is influenced by other factors influencing resistance as well: aortic distensibility, peripheral vascular resistance, and characteristics of the blood itself, namely, the mass of the column of blood in the aorta

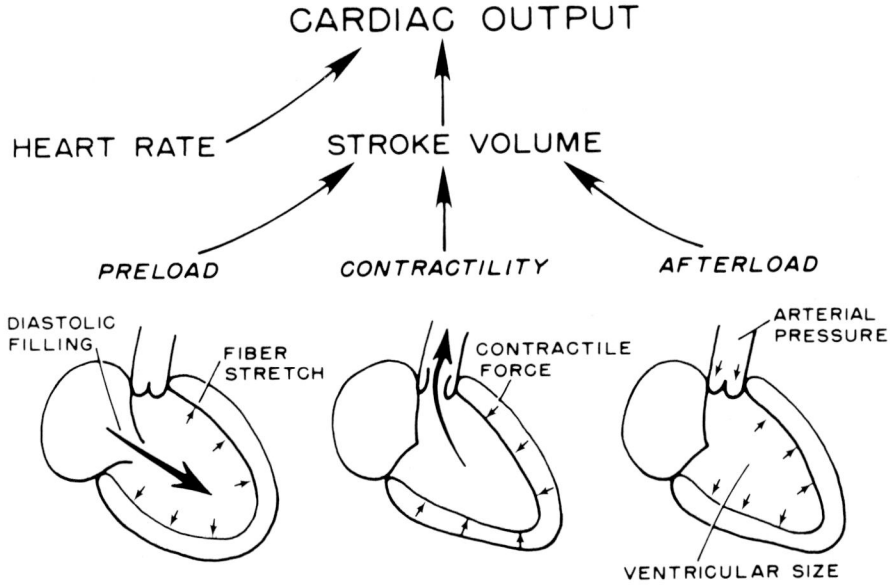

Figure 20-10   Factors influencing cardiac output. Among the complex variables that affect cardiac output are changes in heart rate and four factors which influence stroke volume: (1) diastolic filling pressure, (2) ventricular distensibility, (3) arterial pressure, and (4) myocardial contractility.
From Price, S., & Wilson, L. (1992). *Pathophysiology* (4th ed.). St. Louis: Mosby–Year Book.

and the viscosity of the blood. The effect of afterload on the normal ventricle is possibly augmentation of contractility insofar as a smaller afterload will enable the heart to contract more rapidly. This relationship is often referred to as the *force–velocity relationship*. Within the diseased heart, however, severely deleterious effects may result from the resistance imposed by normal aortic impedance (afterload).

Ventricular contractility is defined as the intrinsic ability of the myocardium to contract. The contractile state can be either increased or decreased by inotropic agents, hypercalcemia, hypoxia, hypercapnia, or disease states.

Cardiac output, then, is dependent on the interrelationships developed between (1) heart rate, (2) stroke volume, (3) venous return or diastolic filling pressure, (4) aortic end-diastolic pressure, and (5) myocardial contracility.

Venous Return

Cardiac output and venous return are, in the broad sense, inseparable. The heart can obviously pump no more blood than it receives from the peripheral circulation; therefore, venous return and cardiac output must eventually be equal, although temporary differences can exist.

Guyton[6] describes the role of the heart as permissive in its regulation of cardiac output. Up to a physiological limit of 13 to 15 L/min, the heart will pump the amount of blood that returns to the right atrium. If venous return exceeds that amount, sympathetic stimulation is required. The normal resting venous return is approximately 5 L/min; therefore, the normal cardiac output is also 5 L/min.

Control of Heart Rate

The normal adult heart beats at a frequency of between 60 and 100 beats per minute. This frequency occurs because of spontaneous electrical pacemaker activity (automaticity) of cells in the SA node (see Chapter 10). The heart will beat intrinsically at a rate approximately 100 beats per minute irrespective of any extrinsic influences. In the clinical setting, alterations in heart rate frequently occur in normal human subjects in response to changes in cardiac output. In fact, heart rate appears to play more of a role in normalizing the cardiac output than does stroke volume.

The principal regulators of cardiac rate are nerves of the autonomic nervous system: sympathetic and parasympathetic fibers. Another regulator is the sympathetic secretion of epinephrine and norepinephrine from the adrenal medulla. These aforementioned controls may either increase or decrease the heart rate from its intrinsic rate. In addition, these regulators influence the conduction velocity through the AV node. For example, the sympathetic fibers increase the conduction through the AV node, thereby shortening the PR interval on the ECG, whereas the parasympathetic fibers will do the reverse.

Other factors can also vary the heart rate. These include ions, circulating hormones, physical factors such as temperature, and atrial wall stretch.

Autonomic Control

The divisions of the automatic nervous system exhibit tonic influence on the heart rate. Increased parasympathetic stimulation along with reciprocal decrease in sympathetic activity results in a drop in rate. Acceleration of the heart rate is produced by the opposite action of the two divisions of the nervous system.

The parasympathetic cardiac fibers originate in the cerebral medulla and have their innervation primarily in nodal tissue and the atria. Animal experimentation has revealed that the right vagus nerve affects the sinoatrial node predominantly, and that the left vagus has its greatest effect on atrioventricular (AV) conduction tissue.[5] Some ventricular innervation occurs at the base of the ventricles near the conduction tissue. However, ventricular muscle is relatively unresponsive to acetylcholine, and thus, the parasympathetic effect on the ventricles is presumed to be insignificant.

The effect of vagal stimuli is transient since the acetylcholine is rapidly dissipated by the enzyme cholinesterase, of which the SA and AV nodes have abundant stores.

The sympathetic nerve fibers arise from the thoracic spinal cord and penetrate the myocardium in a manner similar to the parasympathetic nerve fibers; that is, left and right fibers appear to be functionally specific. Under experimental conditions, the left sympathetic fibers appear to augment cardiac contractility more than they accelerate the heart rate. The right sympathetic fibers electively increase heart rate with relatively little effect on contractility. In addition, fibers from the right primarily innervate the SA node and atria, while those from the left have their predominant influence within the ventricles.

In contrast to acetylcholine, norepinephrine remains active following release from the nerve endings; relatively little undergoes degradation within the tissues. Most of the remaining norepinephrine is taken up again by the nerve terminals. Norepinephrine acts on the beta receptors within the myocardium (most of the adrenergic receptors within the nodal regions and myocardium are beta receptors) and on the alpha receptors within the coronary arteries.

The antagonistic interaction between acetylcholine and the catecholamines is very complex and poorly understood. Normally, in the resting heart, the parasympathetic system predominates in controlling the SA node. In addition to these neurotransmitters, the heart rate is also controlled by the higher centers in the brain and by baroreceptors.

Control by Higher Neural Centers

Impulses from the cerebral cortex can substantially affect the heart rate; fear, excitement, and anger can all induce significant acceleration in rate. Areas within the hypothalamus can also effect changes in the heart rate, especially in response to variations in environmental temperature. The cerebral medulla also appears to play a pivotal role in the reflex regulation of the cardiovascular system. The ventrolateral medulla is referred to as either the *medullary cardiovascular center*[7] or the *cardiovascular control area*.[8] This center or area is further divided into the pressor (lateral area of medulla) and depressor (medial and caudal area of medulla) regions. Stimulation of the pressor region will increase heart rate and contractility, whereas stimulation of the depressor region will have the reverse effect.

Baroreceptor Reflex

An elevation in right atrial pressure sufficient to cause distention causes a reflex acceleration of heart rate. In 1915, Bainbridge hypothesized that tachycardia resulted from a vagal reflex. The effect of the Bainbridge reflex is somewhat controversial and is probably offset by the effect of the baroreceptors in the carotid sinus and aortic arch. Thus, the Bainbridge reflex is regarded as having minor effect on heart rate.[8]

Stretch receptors of the ventricles have been identified within the epicardium and deep within the myocardium. A potent stimulus can induce bradycardia, hypotension, and a drop in the respiratory rate.

The reciprocal relationship between arterial pressure and heart rate has been called *Marey's law of the heart*. The stretch receptors within the carotid sinus and aortic arch respond to an increase in arterial pressure with a reflex bradycardia. The well-known carotid sinus reflex, similar to occipital pressure, can produce a bradycardia and can frequently convert a tachydysrhythmia to normal sinus rhythm.

The carotid sinus reflex is so sensitive in some individuals that tight collars or sudden movement of the head can cause syncope by inducing bradycardia and hypotension. Such syncopal reactions can be produced by many other types of stimuli. Called a *vasovagal response*, the reaction can be elicited by stimulation of the upper respiratory tract during endotracheal suctioning and during intubation of the trachea and the esophagus.

Since the gastrointestinal tract has afferent fibers leading to the medulla, nausea and vomiting in addition to rectal stimulation can be associated with a reflex bradycardia. Generally, stimulation of visceral pain fibers can cause a marked bradycardia. Pressure on the eyeball, as well as painful stimulation of skeletal muscle, may elicit a significant reduction of heart rate. Conversely, somatic pain in the skin frequently produces tachycardia.

The phenomenon of phasic acceleration and deceleration in heart rate simultaneous with inspiration and expiration, known as *sinus arrhythmia,* is common. Since intrathoracic pressure drops during inspiration, increasing venous return, sinus arrhythmia has been attributed to stimulation of the Bainbridge reflex causing increased heart rate. With the corresponding increase in left ventricular output and resulting rise in arterial pressure, a decrease in heart rate occurs through excitation of the aortic baroreceptors.

Control of Stroke Volume

The fundamental control mechanism for the stroke volume is the Frank-Starling law of the heart. Though the experiments done by Starling were in isolated hearts on heart-lung machines and many complex variables exist within the intact animal and human heart, the basic qualitative relationships regarding ventricular performance can be extrapolated and applied to ventricular function.

When the Starling mechanism was mentioned earlier in this chapter, it was referred to as an intrinsic method for autoregulation of cardiac performance. Its most basic effect is to guarantee equal stroke volumes from the right and left ventricles, should there be a momentary increase in diastolic volume; thus the term *autoregulation.* The mechanism through which the heart can automatically respond is one it shares with all striated muscle: the length–tension relationship. Increasing the length of the ventricular fiber (preload) in practice, measured as filling pressure (Figure 19-8B), shifts the curve to the left, augmenting ventricular contractility.

The normal left ventricle is extremely distensible and accepts increases in diastolic volume, or preload, without significant increase in ventricular filling pressure (end-diastolic pressure). Generally, peak contractility occurs at a fiber length of 2.2 μm or a filling pressure of 12 mmHg. Further increases in filling pressure beyond the physiological limits of the length–tension relationship lead to a reduction in ventricular effectiveness. Once fiber length reaches 4 to 4.5 μm corresponding to a filling pressure of 14 or 15 mmHg, ventricular end-diastolic pressure rises very rapidly.

In the noncompliant, stiff ventricle, the situation is very different. A higher filling pressure occurs with a given fiber length; the performance curve shifts to the right, as shown in Figure 20-8C. The end result,

then, is a reduction in ventricular performance combined with higher filling pressures.

There is evidence that other types of cardiac autoregulation exist, unrelated to increases in preload or ventricular fiber length. Afterload may lead to ventricular adaptation by augmenting ventricular contractility (Anrep effect); however, this is theorized to be only a temporary measure. Other examples of the augmentation of ventricular contractility can be seen in tachycardia and with premature beats. Berne and Levy theorize that the increased contractility seen with elevation of heart rate is based on increases in intracellular calcium (*Treppe,* or staircase, phenomenon).[5] Similarly, the phenomenon known as *postextrasystolic accentuation* may be caused by elevated intracellular calcium. It is well known that a premature beat generally produces a feeble contraction, which probably relates to low concentrations of calcium. The fact that the beat following the premature (extrasystolic) beat is usually much stronger relates not only to the increased time for diastolic filling during the long pause following the premature beat, but, according to Berne and Levy, may be potentiated by increased concentrations of intracellular calcium as well.[5]

Myocardial Contractility

Myocardial contractility, as previously stated, is the intrinsic ability of the heart to contract or to generate power in order to propel blood. It is important to distinguish myocardial contractility from cardiac performance. *Cardiac performance* refers to such measurements as stroke volume and cardiac output. These are certainly affected by contractility, but cardiac performance is also modulated by mechanical and other factors.[8] The strength of contraction may be affected by two means: (1) intrinsic regulation, which is the basic contractile property of the heart itself; and (2) extrinsic regulation, which is the effect that is modified by certain outside (extrinsic) conditions.

There are three primary intrinsic regulators of myocardial contractility.[8] The first involves the Frank-Starling law of the heart (previously discussed) whereby an increase in diastolic filling or stretch within physiological limits will increase the force of contraction. This characteristic of the myocardium to contract more forcefully when stretched is referred to as *heterometric autoregulation.* The second regulator of myocardial contractility is the myocardial response to an increased load imposed during contraction (force–velocity relationship) whereby an increase in aortic diastolic pressure usually results in a decrease in strength, velocity, and duration of contraction due to the afterload burden. The third regulator of myocardial contractility is heart rate. Recall the previously mentioned staircase phenomenon, or *Treppe* effect, whereby an increase in heart rate allows more Ca^{2+} to enter the cell each minute. This in turn causes intracellular Ca^{2+} to be released from the sarcoplasmic reticulum in greater quantities for each action potential. Thus, a sudden increase in heart rate modulates an increase in the strength of contraction.

Three general types of external factors may alter myocardial contractility: (1) neurohormonal effects, (2) chemical and pharmacological effects, and (3) pathological effects.[8]

Neurohormonal

The neurohormonal effect is primarily caused by the autonomic nervous system or by catecholamines secreted by the adrenal medulla. Sympathetic innervation has already been reviewed with respect to control of the heart rate. The atria are liberally supplied with both parasympathetic and sympathetic nerves, while the ventricles are mainly supplied by sympathetic nerves. Generally, the sympathetic nerves augment contractility; the parasympathetic nerves diminish the strength of ventricular contraction.

The amount of sympathetic activity can be estimated by comparing the quantity of norepinephrine within the atria, in the SA and AV nodes, and within the ventricles; ventricular concentration of norephinephrine is triple that in the atria and nodes.

Sympathetic stimulation within the heart is inotropic; within the atria, stimulation can cause a 20% to 30% increase in atrial contractility. The effect of sympathetic activity within the ventricle is more complicated and is dependent upon the relationship of the factors listed earlier which influence contractility in addition to affecting heart rate. The stroke volume may or may not increase; the primary benefit from the inotropic effect of sympathetic activity is thought by some investigators to be the increased rate and velocity of pressure change, ventricular outflow, and change in ventricular dimensions. The net result is ejection of the same or slightly higher stroke volume in a much shorter period of time, and more frequently per minute, thereby increasing cardiac output. The results of sympathetic effects on cardiac function are summarized in Figure 20-11.

The vagal inhibitory effect on the nodes and other conduction tissue within the atria and AV junction is

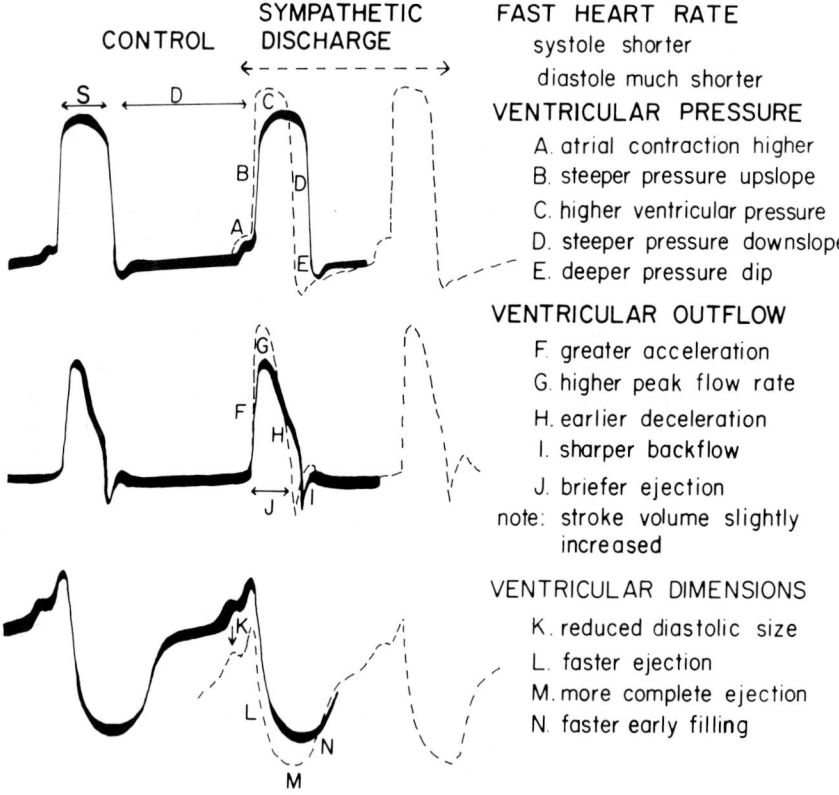

Figure 20-11 Summary of sympathetic effect on cardiac performance. The major results of sympathetic discharge are in increasing the following: (1) ventricular functioning, (2) heart rate, (3) pressure rise and fall within ventricles, (4) ejection velocity, (5) change in velocity (acceleration), (6) deceleration, and (7) change in ventricular dimensions.

From Rushmer, R. (1976). *Cardiovascular dynamics* (4th ed.). Philadelphia: Saunders.

very potent. The existence of parasympathetic influence within the ventricle has now been demonstrated. Its effect is the reverse of sympathetic: Left ventricular pressure falls, as does the maximum rate of pressure development.

Chemical

Chemical effects on contractility may be produced by potassium (hyperkalemia), calcium (hypocalcemia and hypercalcemia), carbon dioxide (hypercapnia), and pH (acidosis). Hyperkalemia, hypocalcemia, hypercapnia, and acidosis will bring about a decrease in contractility (negative inotropic effect) whereas hypercalcemia may increase the force of contraction resulting in tetany. Clinically this is rarely seen, since tetany would more likely cause respiratory arrest before significant cardiac effects of hypercalcemia would be seen.

Pharmacological

Pharmacological effects on contractility include those of digitalis, sympathomimetic drugs, or calcium, which would all increase the force of contraction. Contractility also is increased in varying degrees by corticosteroids, serotonin, angiotensin, and aldactone. Negative inotropic agents include most beta blockers, some calcium channel blockers, barbiturates, quinidine, procainamide, lidocaine, and disopyramide.

Pathological

Pathological effects for the most part depress myocardial contractility. These conditions would include anoxia, ischemia, heart failure, myocarditis, and metabolic acidosis.

Measurement

Contractility cannot be directly measured in patients. Indirect measurements such as left ventricular stroke work or cardiac work, dP/dT, and systolic time intervals can be employed to assess contractility.

Coronary Blood Flow

In the resting state, coronary flow is about 5% of the cardiac output (100 to 150 ml/min). As metabolic demands increase, blood flow can increase to more than four to five times the resting value. The myocardial oxygen extraction remains fixed at 65% to 70% of stroke volume, regardless of physiological conditions, which provides arterial PO_2 of 18 to 20 mmHg and a venous oxygen saturation of about 30%. That is the lowest value for venous oxygen saturation in the body. The heart functions exclusively on aerobic metabolism and cannot sustain an oxygen debt as can skeletal muscle. The most basic

regulator, then, of coronary flow is the degree of oxygen need. Since oxygen extraction is maximal, the sole mechanism for meeting increased oxygen demand is an increase in coronary flow.

Coronary blood flow is intermittent; it is dependent on phasic aortic pressure and faces significant resistance within the myocardium. External compression during systole severely reduces flow within the left ventricle. Although the right ventricle is subjected to the same factors, the lower right ventricular pressures result in relatively mild changes in coronary flow. The left ventricular coronary flow, however, occurs almost exclusively during ventricular diastole. In addition, the thickness of the left ventricular wall causes some variance in flow from endocardium to epicardium. Normally, however, the endocardium is compensated during diastole for the increased systolic epicardial flow. With pathological conditions such as severe atherosclerosis, severe reduction of flow can occur within the endocardium.

Since the major regulator of coronary flow is oxygen deficiency, it is believed that hypoxia causes coronary arteriolar dilation, but whether this occurs directly or from the release of neurotransmitters is unclear. The primary method appears to be automatic regulation of flow through arteriolar constriction and dilation. Influence of the sympathetic nervous system or of catecholamines (norepinephrine and epinephrine) is complex; coronary blood flow increases either through dilation or from increased heart rate and perfusion pressure.

Collateral coronary circulation within the vasculature is apparently present from infancy in the form of arterial anastomoses and is particularly plentiful within the ventricular septum, apex, right ventricular anterior surface, and in the atria. Epicardial anastomoses exist between all three major coronary vessels of the left ventricle. The crucial determinant for success of the anastomoses is the rapidity with which occlusion occurs, because the anastomotic connections become functional only when there is a longstanding need for increased flow. Other determining factors in the development of adequate collateral circulation are the location of the anastomosis to the occluded artery and the amount of disease in adjacent vessels.

Myocardial Oxygen Consumption (MVO_2)

The oxygen demands of the myocardial tissue may exceed the ability of coronary blood flow to deliver enough oxygen (supply) to the heart muscle. This potential imbalance between supply and demand often leads to myocardial ischemia if the increase in myocardial demand is not met by an increase in coronary blood flow. Therefore, the clinician needs to know what factors increase the MVO_2 consumption rate in order to reduce the oxygen demand. These include: (1) increased heart rate, (2) rise in arterial pressure, (3) increased contractility, and (4) increased wall tension. The last of these, myocardial wall tension, plays an extremely important role in determining oxygen consumption, particularly in the event of cardiac decompensation.

Myocardial oxygen consumption is the amount of oxygen (in the form of chemical energy, ATP) expended during each contraction. It is determined chiefly by the amount of tension developed by the myofibrils (ventricular wall tension) and by the inotropic state. The resulting O_2 consumption of the heart is approximately 8 ml/100 g every minute. Basal metabolism accounts for about one fourth of MVO_2 consumption in a resting state while the remaining three fourths are expended for muscle contraction. Moreover, the chemical energy expended during phase 1 of ventricular systole, known as the isovolumetric contraction phase of the cardiac cycle, accounts for over 50% of total MVO_2 consumption.[7] To clinically estimate the MVO_2 rate, the *rate–pressure product* is considered to be the simplest index of energy demands of the heart. It is obtained by multiplying peak systolic pressure by heart rate.

Vascular Circulation

Blood Flow Determinants

An important determinant of blood flow is viscosity. Several factors influence the viscosity of blood; principal among them are the hematocrit and the internal diameter of the vessel. An increase in the percentage of cells within the blood, the hematocrit, from the normal of 40 to 70 or 80, can triple the viscosity and seriously impair blood flow.

Within the small vessels, blood flow decreases markedly. Because of the slower velocity, blood viscosity can increase tenfold. When an artery or vein divides (bifurcates), the cross-sectional area of the branches taken together exceeds that of the vessel of origin. Since the volumes of blood moving through each segment of the circulation are equal, changes in a cross-sectional area necessarily influence the velocity of blood flow. In the aorta, blood travels very rapidly. It slows significantly within the capillaries (large cross-sectional area), and accelerates in the veins, where the cross-sectional area once again is smaller. The relatively slow capillary blood flow provides sufficient time for exchange of oxygen and nutrients through the capillary walls.

Blood flow is directly proportional to the pressure difference between two ends of a vessel and inversely proportional to the resistance imposed by character-

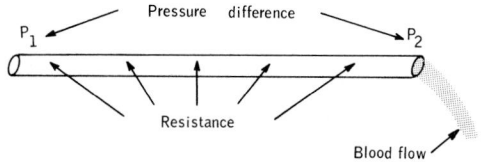

Figure 20-12 Factors influencing blood flow: pressure resistance and pressure gradient (P_1 and P_2).
From Guyton, A. C. (1991). *Textbook of medical physiology* (8th ed.). Philadelphia: Saunders.

istics within the vessel. The relationship is expressed in Figure 20-12, for which any vessel within the circulation is depicted. Were there no pressure difference or gradient between P_1 and P_2, there could be no blood flow. The resistance, which includes any factor that serves to impede flow, can be calculated from measurements of blood flow and pressure gradients within the vessel.

In a resting individual, blood flow within the circulation occurs at a rate of approximately 100 ml/sec. The normal arterial to venous pressure gradient within the total circulation is around 100 mmHg. The resistance within the circulation (total peripheral resistance), then, is 100 ml/sec to 100 mmHg, or one peripheral resistance unit (PRU). Another type of measurement of total peripheral resistance is obtained by relating the cardiac output and arterial pressure. An individual with a cardiac output of 5,000 ml/min and arterial pressure of 100 mmHg would have a calculated peripheral resistance of 0.02 PRU. The systemic resistance will vary considerably when vasoconstriction or vasodilation occur, increasing with the former and dropping as vascular capacity is increased through vessel dilatation.

The effect of vessel diameter on blood flow is graphically demonstrated in Figure 20-13. In Figure 20-13*A*, increasing the vessel diameter by fourfold increases blood flow by 256-fold with no change in pressure gradient. The basis behind such marked changes in flow with relatively small changes in vessel diameter is explained in Figure 20-13*B*. Blood flows within a vessel in layers; the layers closest to the vessel wall experience the greatest "drag" and move very slowly, while the layers farther away from the vessel wall move with increasing velocity. The phenomenon is known as *streamlining*, or *laminar flow*. The greater the internal diameter of the vessel, the greater the number of layers that can form, thereby increasing flow.

The major factors influencing blood flow are often expressed through *Poiseuille's law*,[5] which states that the flow ($\dot{Q}$) of fluid through a tube is directly proportional to the pressure gradient ($P_1 - P_2$) across the tube, to the fourth power of the radius of the tube

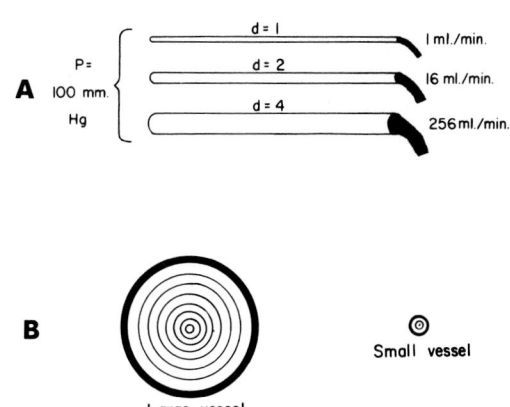

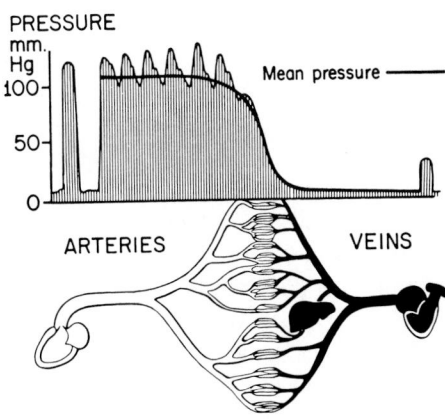

Figure 20-13   Effect of increasing vessel diameter on (A) blood flow increasing velocity of (B) concentric rings of blood flowing at varying velocity; the farther away from the vessel wall, the more rapid the flow.
From Guyton, A. C. (1991). *Textbook of medical physiology* (8th ed.). Philadelphia: Saunders.

Figure 20-14   Resistance and resulting loss of pressure within the circulation. Arterial pressure diminishes very rapidly in the small resistance vessels of the circulation. In the venous vessels, the pressure gradient is very low.
From Rushmer, R. (1976). *Cardiovascular dynamics* (4th ed.). Philadelphia: Saunders.

(r^4), and inversely proportional to the length of the tube (L) and the viscosity (n) of the fluid:

$$\dot{Q} = \pi(P_1 - P_2)r^4 \div 8Ln$$

with $\pi/8$ serving as a geometric proportional value. Resistance, then, increases in direct proportion to the viscosity and length of the vessel but decreases in direct proportion to the vessel diameter (the fourth power of the radius of the vessel) and pressure gradient.

Although the relationships of Poiseuille's law are helpful in isolating the dynamics of blood flow, several factors hinder a qualitative application. The formula is based on a system of rigid tubes which, unlike distensible blood vessels, cannot increase in length or diameter; in addition, there are other factors unique to the fluid characteristics of blood which are not considered in the Poiseuille relationship.

The caliber of blood vessels is unquestionably significant in determining pressure gradients and flow through different segments of the circulation. Approximately 80% of the pressure drop occurs in the terminal arteries and arterioles (Figure 20-14). The resistance imposed by the arteriolar circulation must, in addition, be related to the cross-sectional area. Since the different types of vessels lie in a series arrangement with one another and the various vascular beds are parallel, it is apparent that the total flow is a sum of the individual flows through each vascular bed (Figure 20-14). Since resistance is increased both by an increase in cross-sectional area and by a reduction in vessel diameter, it follows that the resistance of each individual resistance bed exceeds the

total systemic resistance. The resistance of the renal circulation, for instance, will exceed that of the total peripheral circulation, since far greater volumes of blood will flow through the total circulation than through the renal vasculature.

Law of Laplace

The law of Laplace, which was used earlier to explain the relationship between cardiac dilation and resulting increase in oxygen consumption also operates within the vascular system. The relationship as applied to blood vessels states that the tension sustained by the wall of a cylinder is directly proportional to the product of the pressure within the cylinder and its radius. In other words, the smaller a blood vessel, the less tension is required to maintain a given pressure. At normal aortic and capillary pressures, the tension necessary to support the pressure exerted on the wall of the aorta is over 10,000 times as great as that in the capillary.

Vascular Smooth Muscle

Vascular smooth muscle shares some characteristics of cardiac and skeletal muscle. The contractile process operates in a similar manner, since it is contingent on the action of the proteins actin, myosin, and troponin-tropomyosin. In addition, the ability of certain of the smooth muscles to exhibit automaticity has already been reviewed. Since it is very difficult to separate the structural components of smooth muscle, no consistent pattern of myofibril organization has been observed. The actual mechanism that causes vascular smooth muscle shortening is unknown, since the relationship of the actin and myosin filaments during contraction and the mechanism for calcium release can only be inferred. The relationship between stimulation and contraction seems to vary, although the contractile time of smooth muscle is generally much more prolonged than that of cardiac and skeletal muscle. Neural and hormonal stimuli (epinephrine, angiotensin) usually elicit a contractile response.

The sympathetic nervous system innervates a majority of the arterial and venous circulation. Arterioles apparently have a relatively greater concentration of neuromuscular connections, which is in keeping with their role as resistance vessels. It is this property of relative contraction or relaxation that determines the tone of vascular smooth muscle. Although sympathetic control is very important, it is crucial to understand that the routine control of the peripheral circulation is independent of extrinsic mechanisms.

Arterial Circulation

The essential feature of the arterial circulation is its function as a pressure reservoir in order to convert its intermittent ventricular ejection into relatively constant flow i.e., the windkessel effect. The intrinsic properties of normal arteries that permit such a function have been reviewed. The fact that the arteries are capable of storing a portion of energy received from the heart during systolic contraction within their elastic walls is critically important in maintaining flow to the tissues in a pulsatile circulation. The greater the distensibility or compliance of the arterial circulation, the more constant is blood flow during diastole and systole. In addition, the arterial circulation has an important influence on the workload imposed on the heart. Since the phasic pumping of the heart requires much more energy expenditure from the heat than would be demanded for steady flow, the capability for the normal arterial circulation to transmit

pressure throughout the diastolic phase of the heart results in a decrease in cardiac workload. On the other hand, loss of the property of elastic recoil within the arterial circulation can profoundly increase cardiac work.

It is known that the major resistance within the peripheral circulation is exerted by the extremely muscular arterioles and their precapillary sphincters. The distention properties of the venae cavae and of the aorta are exemplified by a comparison of the relative diameter, wall thickness, and proportion of elastic tissue with those of the arteriole and sphincter (Figure 20-15). It is through constriction and dilation of these resistance vessels, thereby changing internal diameters, that blood flow is distributed to the tissues. Note that the capillary walls contain only endothelial tissue, a structural composition that is highly appropriate for rapid diffusion. Although much of the arterial pressure head is dissipated prior to reaching the capillary bed, the capillaries must be able to withstand significant pressure to effect a sufficient pressure gradient for maintenance of blood flow.

Capillary Dynamics

Normally the regulation of blood through the vast capillary network is controlled very precisely. An exact amount of blood is provided to the tissue in accordance with its metabolic demands. Blood flows continuously through the arterioles and then into metarterioles through the precapillary sphincter and on into the capillary. Two types of capillaries can be seen in Figure 20-16: thoroughfare channels (TC), which serve as direct channels from the arteriole to the venule, and the true capillaries (C). By reviewing Figure 20-16, it will be recalled that the capillaries are not invested with muscle, while the thoroughfare channels are supplied with smooth muscle which is more pronounced at the arterial end.

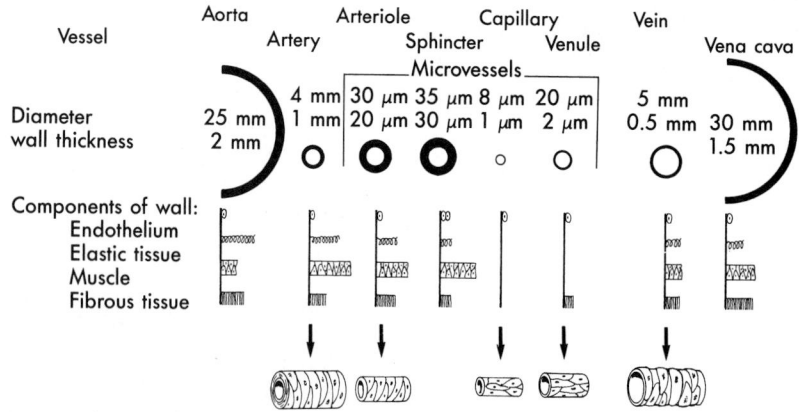

Figure 20-15 Schematic representation of anatomy of circulatory vasculature. Comparison of internal diameters, musculature, wall thickness, and vascular components.

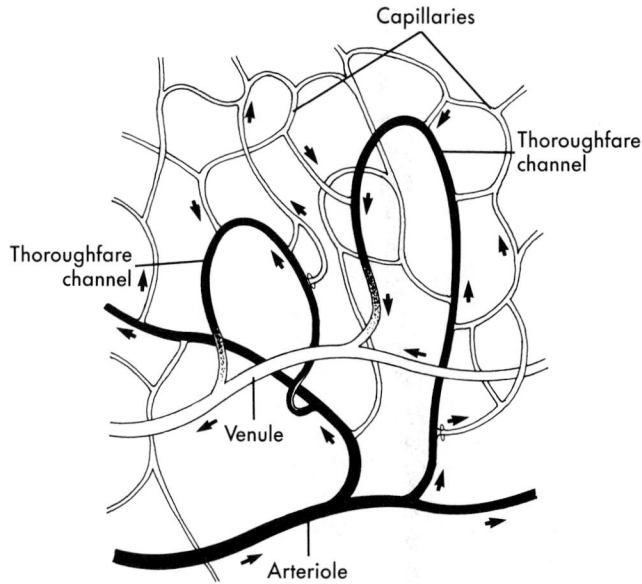

Figure 20-16 Schematic representation of the microcirculation. The arrows indicate blood flow direction. Circular structures on arteriole and venule indicate smooth muscle fibers, and branching solid lines are indicative of sympathetic nervous innervation.

Adapted from Vander, A. H., Sherman, J. H., & Luciano, D. S. (1975). *Human physiology* (2nd ed.). New York: McGraw-Hill. Adapted from Zweifach, B. W. (1965). *Fed. Proc. 24*, 1074.

Through dilation and constriction of the precapillary sphincters, thoroughfare channels, and arterioles, blood flow is controlled according to the specific needs of a group of cells. Since the process involves rhythmic movement of the vessels, it is also called *vasomotion*. With dilation of these vessels, a steeper pressure gradient occurs and, therefore, an increase in blood flow. With constriction, the arterial pressure gradient is decreased, resulting in either reduction or cessation of blood flow.

The most important method for exchange of substances through the capillary wall is diffusion. Though there are many factors which affect the rate at which a substance diffuses across the capillary wall, the chief influence is derived from the concentration gradient between the two sides of the membrane. The greater the difference between the concentrations of any substance, the more rapidly will it diffuse across the cell membrane. Tiny passageways connect the interior of the capillary with the exterior. Substances that are insoluble in the lipid capillary membrane can diffuse only through these capillary "pores."

Starling Equilibrium

Maintenance of fluid within the vascular system is the very basis of capillary dynamics. According to the *Starling equilibrium*, or law of the capillaries, filtration or reabsorption of fluid across the capillary wall depends on the interrelation of four forces. Figure 20-17 depicts the four major factors involved in fluid transfer: (1) capillary pressure, which tends to filter fluid out of the capillary membrane to the tissues; (2)

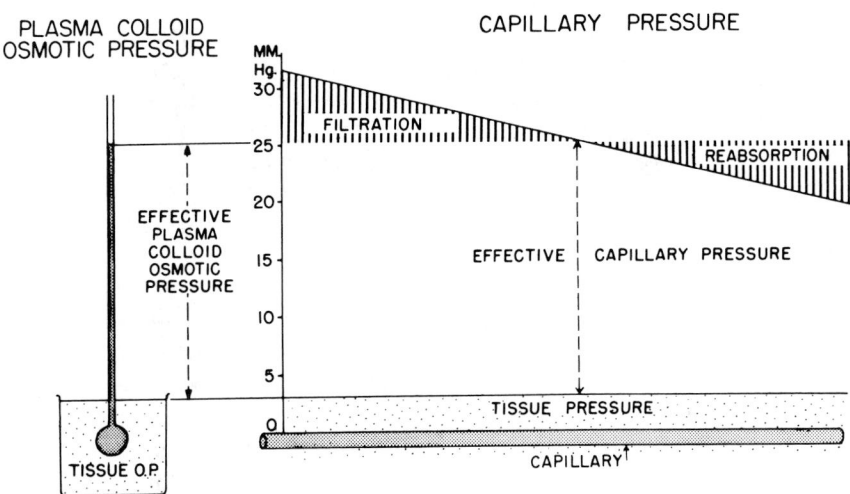

Figure 20-17 Capillary fluid exchange. Factors favoring filtration occur at the arterial end of the capillary and reabsorption at the venous end. The determination is the result of a balance between four pressures: (1) arterial and venous capillary mean pressures, (2) plasma colloidal pressure, (3) tissue colloidal osmotic pressure, and (4) interstitial fluid pressure. The lymphatic system is involved in maintenance of normal capillary dynamics. See text for further explanation.

From Rushmer, R. (1976). *Cardiovascular dynamics* (4th ed.). Philadelphia: Saunders.

interstitial fluid pressure, which maintains a negative value, tending to draw fluid back into the interstitium; (3) plasma colloid osmotic pressure (oncotic pressure), which promotes absorption of fluid through osmotic attraction back into the capillary; and (4) interstitial fluid colloid osmotic pressure, which osmotically attracts fluid into the interstitium (tissue space).

Tables 20-1 and 20-2 depict the forces that tend to move fluid (filtration) out of the arterial end of the capillary (outward forces) and the forces that tend to favor reabsorption at the venule end of the capillary (inward force). The net outward force of 13 mmHg tends to move fluids out of the arterial end where a net inward force of 7 mmHg favor reabsorption of fluids at the venule end of the capillary.

TABLE 20-1 Analysis of the Forces Causing Filtration

FORCES TENDING TO MOVE FLUID OUTWARD
Capillary pressure	30 mmHg
Negative interstitial free fluid pressure	3 mmHg
Interstitial fluid colloid osmotic pressure	8 mmHg
Total outward forces	41 mmHg

FORCES TENDING TO MOVE FLUID INWARD
Plasma colloid osmotic pressure	28 mmHg
Total inward force	28 mmHg

SUMMATION OF FORCES
Outward	41 mmHg
Inward	28 mmHg
Net outward forces	13 mmHg

From Guyton, A. C. (1991). *Textbook of medical physiology* (8th ed.). Philadelphia: Saunders.

TABLE 20-2 Analysis of the Factors Favoring Reabsorption

FORCES TENDING TO MOVE FLUID INWARD
Plasma colloid osmotic pressure	28
Total inward force	28

FORCES TENDING TO MOVE FLUID OUTWARD
Capillary pressure	10
Negative interstitial free fluid pressure	3
Interstitial fluid colloid osmotic pressure	8
Total outward forces	21

SUMMATION OF FORCES
Inward	28
Outward	21
Net inward force	7

From Guyton, A. C. (1991). *Textbook of medical physiology* (8th ed.). Philadelphia: Saunders.

Strategic factors in preventing fluid loss from the capillaries are the plasma proteins. The major determinant in the maintenance of the colloidal osmotic pressure is the protein albumin. Since the protein molecule is so large, it cannot diffuse readily into the tissue space, but the few molecules that do diffuse into the interstitium are removed by the lymph system. In addition, a phenomenon known as *Gibbs-Donnan equilibrium* enhances the osmotic attraction of proteins. Since proteins are anions, they attract an equal number of cations, predominantly sodium, to achieve electrical balance. This increases the osmotic attraction of proteins by about 50%. In addition, the Donnan effect increases in proportion to increasing concentrations of proteins. In other words, additional grams of protein over the first few have much greater oncotic attraction than do the original few grams, a fact that makes hypoalbuminemia increasingly significant. The plasma oncotic pressure is estimated to be about 28 mmHg. Within the interstitium, the oncotic pressure is approximately 8 mmHg.

The pressures, when combined, favor filtration, or movement outward, at the arterial end of the capillary. The low hydrostatic pressure at the venous end of the capillary reverses the balance. There the oncotic pressure exceeds the filtration (outward) force, and reabsorption into the venule occurs. The Starling equilibrium states that in a steady state, the positive filtration forces favoring diffusion outward at the arterial end of the capillary are equal to the forces favoring reabsorption at the venous end. The total amount of fluid leaving the circulation is almost equal to the amount of fluid being reabsorbed in the venous end. The small amount of excess fluid and protein that accumulates within the interstitial space is removed by the lymphatic drainage system.

Edema Formation

It is immediately evident that a significant increase in capillary pressure, which causes an imbalance of filtration and reabsorptive forces, can produce an accumulation of fluid within the tissues. Similarly, edema can result from a reduction of oncotic pressure; from an increase in the permeability of the capillary such that excessive protein is lost from the plasma, causing reduction of oncotic pressure within the plasma; and from an increase in colloid osmotic pressure within the tissue spaces.

Exchange across Capillary Membrane

The permeability of the capillaries is not consistent in all tissues. Lymph flow can be used to determine capillary permeability, and the lymph flow from the heart, lungs, intestines, and kidneys reveals a higher concentration of protein than does that from the skin and connective tissues. The liver capillary system is far more permeable than the others, so that protein concentration within the lymph flow almost equal to that of plasma.

Other factors affecting the rate of exchange of substances across the capillary are: (1) the area of capillary available for filtration, (2) thickness of the capillary wall, (3) viscosity of the filtrate, and (4) the sum of hydrostatic and osmotic pressures, as discussed earlier.

Although filtration and absorption are critically important in the maintenance of normal capillary dynamics, they play a relatively minor role in the normal exchange of substances. Diffusion is the governing factor in the exchange of water, gases, waste products, and substrates across the capillary membranes. Since the principal limiting factors of diffusion are concentration gradient, molecular size, and lipid solubility, small molecules like water and glucose diffuse with little restriction.

The major factor that determines the rate of lymph flow is the interstitial fluid pressure. A rise in tissue pressure, which can result from a rise in capillary pressure, reduction in oncotic pressure, increase in capillary permeability, or increase in tissue oncotic pressure, will accelerate lymph flow.

As in the veins, lymphatic vessels are liberally supplied with one-way valves that prevent backflow and contribute to the lymphatic pump. Contraction of the muscles, passive movements of parts of the body such as respiration or abdominal movement, arterial pulsations, and external compression of the tissues all stimulate the lymphatic pump. In addition, there is evidence that certain lymphatics possess independent contractility which performs similarly to a type of peristalsis. About 120 ml of lymph per hour flows through the thoracic system of a resting adult. Although it is a very small volume in comparison to total capillary exchange, were protein not removed by the lymph vessels, it would significantly increase tissue oncotic pressure and cause severe edema.

Venous Circulation

The veins function not only as conduits for blood flow but as a variable-volume reservoir, thereby helping to regulate cardiac output. Marked changes in venous capacity can occur without a significant effect on venous pressure. Thus, the veins are a capacitance system. *Capacitance,* as defined by Berne and Levy, is the increment of volume accommodated per unit change of pressure.[5] Assuming normal arterial and venous pressures, a 1-mmHg increase in venous pressure would accommodate 20 times more blood within the venous system than within the arterial system for the same pressure change.

Since the pressure at the point of outflow from a series of tubes to a large extent determines the pressure gradient, an understanding of the right atrial pressure and its role as reflecting the central venous pressure (CVP) is important. Three factors contribute to the regulation of right atrial pressure or the CVP: (1) capacitance of the venous sytem (C), (2) total blood volume (V), and (3) the pumping ability of the heart (P). Normally the mean right atrial pressure, or CVP, is about equal to the atmospheric pressure around the body, which is zero. With hypervolemia or ventricular failure resulting from a reduction in contractility or pumping ability, the CVP may rise to very high levels. The effect within the peripheral veins is a backing up of blood, resulting in distention. Usually, many of the large veins which lie adjacent to the ribs and abdominal organs are almost totally collapsed, therefore offering considerable resistance to venous flow. Normally the pressure gradient between peripheral venous pressure and right atrial pressure is approximately 6 to 10 mmHg. As right atrial pressure climbs above its norm, blood begins to distend the large veins, correspondingly decreasing resistance; elevated peripheral venous pressure is, therefore, not seen until the later stages of failure, or until all the collapsed veins have opened, which is usually seen when right atrial pressure exceeds 4 to 6 mmHg.

Effects of Hydrostatic Pressure

The pressure resulting from the weight of fluid within a chamber is called *hydrostatic pressure;* at the surface of the fluid, the pressure equals atmospheric, but for each 13.6-mm distance under the surface, pressure increases 1 mmHg. In a standing, immobile person with a normal right atrial pressure (zero), venous pressure within the feet will be 90 mmHg. The same relationship exists within the arterial system.

Were the arterial pressure within the same individual equal to 100 mmHg, arterial pressure at the feet would approximate 190 mmHg. It is only at the phlebostatic axis, which is at the level of the tricuspid valve, that venous pressures are not significantly affected by hydrostatic influence. Regardless of the position of the body, the pressure will not vary more than about 1 mmHg.

The venous pump and the valves enable the standing individual to overcome hydrostatic pressure as long as muscle compression occurs. As in the lymphatic vessels, the veins are supplied with unidirectional valves so that muscle compression causes blood to flow back toward the heart. In the quietly standing individual, of course, the venous pump cannot function, and extravasation of fluid from the capillaries into the tissues can occur fairly rapidly, causing edema and possibly significant loss of volume from the vascular space.

Although the resistance imposed by the veins and venules does not approach that of the arterioles, it is important to note that constriction and dilation of the postcapillary venous vessels can cause marked changes in blood volume. Constriction of the venules will produce an increase in capillary pressure and result in enhanced filtration of fluid from the capillary. Dilation, along the precapillary constriction, can result in expansion of blood volume and dehydration of the tissues.

Control of Arterial Pressure

Everyday control of variations in arterial pressure is exercised mainly by the circulatory reflexes. Were it not for this vital integrative role, arterial pressure and, thereby, vital cerebral and cardiac perfusion could be dangerously compromised by changes in position, or by extreme localized demand for increased flow. When simply assuming the erect position from the supine, the tendency is for cerebral arterial pressure to drop precipitously; however, by excitation of the circulatory reflexes, increased sympathetic tone through vasoconstriction maintains cerebral flow.

Circulatory Reflexes

The most important of the cardiovascular reflexes are the baroreceptors, or stretch receptors. Although baroreceptors are situated within the walls of most large thoracic and neck arteries, the highest concentrations are within the carotid sinus, which is located in the internal carotid artery slightly above the bifurcation of the external and internal carotid arteries. With a rise in arterial pressure, the baroreceptors respond extremely rapidly through inhibition of the vasomotor center in the medulla and stimulation of the vagal center (Figure 20-18). The vagal center functions primarily as a countercheck on the heart in that excitation produces bradycardia, while inhibition results in tachycardia. The overall effects of the baroreceptors are vasodilation due to suppression of the vasomotor center, and reduction of heart rate and contractility (previously discussed), which results in a decrease in arterial pressure. Conversely, arterial pressure is augmented through opposite effects of the baroreceptors—should there be a drop in arterial pressure. Because these neural receptors mitigate increases and decreases in arterial pressure, they are called *buffer nerves,* and the baroreceptors are a buffer system.

The baroreceptor response can be obviated if the hypertension or hypotension persists for a protracted length of time. The major effect of the circulatory reflexes exists in acute changes. However, over a

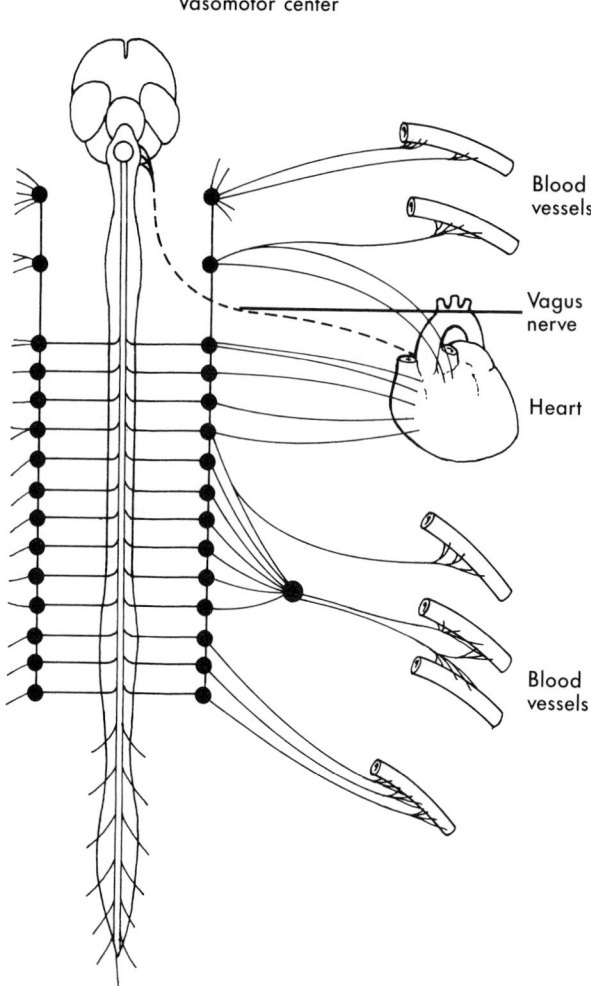

Vasomotor center

Blood vessels

Vagus nerve

Heart

Blood vessels

Figure 20-18   Neural control (vasomotor center) of the circulatory system through sympathetic and vagal nervous innervation.

Adapted from Guyton, A. C. (1990). *Textbook of medical physiology* (7th ed.). Philadelphia: Saunders.

longer period, the baroreceptors simply adapt by decreasing their rate of excitation to normal, although the blood pressure remains very high or very low.

Other Types of Cardiovascular Reflexes

Chemoreceptors located at the bifurcation of the internal and external carotid arteries and within the aortic arch are sensitive to hypoxia and hypercapnia, which causes stimulation of the vasomotor center and results in elevation of arterial blood pressure.

The *atrial baroreceptors,* called *low-pressure receptors,* include two types of receptors. The A receptors are synchronous with the *a* wave of atrial contraction, while the B receptors are stimulated by the *v* wave occurring during atrial filling. Experimentally, these receptors, when stretched, have demonstrated a slight reflex vasodilation of peripheral arterioles, which in turn may decrease arterial pressure.[6] These receptors are stretched in response to an increase in blood volume within the atria. It is thought that stimulation can also cause an increase in urinary flow, either a decrease or increase in heart rate, and reduction of arterial pressure, at least experimentally.

Spinal cord receptors become evident following cervical spinal cord transection. Initially following the trauma, arterial pressure drops but can eventually return to near-normal levels, probably through local sympathetic vasoconstriction.

Other potential reflexes occur within the pulmonary vasculature. Distention of the pulmonary vessels can cause reduction in both heart rate and arterial pressure. Distention of the abdominal viscera may elicit a depressor response. Lastly, pain can cause either vasoconstriction or vasodilation; usually, however, pain elicits a sympathetic response.

The cardiac and respiratory reflexes are very closely related. It can be safely surmised that anything affecting the respiratory center will also stimulate the vasomotor center. Elevations of PCO_2 and reduction of pH produce vaosconstriction. Conversely, vasodilatation results from a drop in PCO_2 or rise in pH.

Intrinsic Control

Through variations in capillary pressure which are a direct result of changes in arterial pressure, changes in vascular volume via capillary-to-tissue fluid shifts can effectively participate in arterial pressure control. Although capillary fluid shift takes longer than the cardiovascular reflexes to become fully effective (about 1 hour), this system can be twice as effective as the baroreceptors in restoring normal ranges of arterial pressure. Refer to the previous discussion on capillary dynamics for a review of normal fluid balance.

Long-term Regulation

The crucial role of the kidneys in long-term regulation of arterial pressure cannot be overemphasized. It is estimated that an increase in arterial pressure from 100 mmHg to 200 mmHg can increase water and sodium excretion approximately sixfold. Hypotension, of course, has the opposite effect of increasing reabsorption of water and salt, thus augmenting blood volume and, therefore, pressure.

The kidneys can begin to respond to an acute situation within a few hours; for complete effect, though, several days are necessary.

Variables Affecting Circulation

The actual method by which each local tissue is able to regulate its blood flow is unknown, but several theories have been proposed. Since a decrease in the available oxygen supply or an increase in the metabolic activity of tissue causes an immediate increase in blood flow, it is postulated that hypoxia is a stimulant for the phasic opening and closing of the precapillary sphincters. Another possibility is that an unknown vasodilator substance accumulates within the tissue as a result of increased metabolic activity. Proposed vasodilator substances are carbon dioxide, adenosine, and hydrogen.

Autoregulation

A phenomenon that has received considerable attention is the ability of the vessels to maintain blood flow in the face of marked changes in arterial pressure. Changing arterial pressure from a low of 80 mmHg to 175 mmHg has remarkably little effect. The mechanisms previously discussed are able to obviate the effects of acute changes in pressure.

Another example of a type of autoregulation is known as *reactive hyperemia*. If arterial flow to a specific organ or vascular bed is occluded, flow to the affected area quadruples after the occlusion is removed. This phenomenon may be observed in an extremity following occlusion via a tourniquet—for example, the arm may be seen to redden considerably, and dilation of blood vessels is observed.

If the change in arterial pressure persists for an indefinite period or if the metabolic demands of a tissue increase chronically, a system of long-term autoregulation develops over days and weeks. An example of this type of chronic local autoregulation probably occurs with coarctation of the aorta. Coarctation is a congenital condition in which an area of partial occlusion occurs within the aorta and causes an extremely high pressure above the occlusion and a lower than normal pressure below it. Despite the enormous pressure gradient, blood flow to the upper and lower body appears to be equal within several weeks.

Earlier in this section, an almost linear correlation was made between the vascularity of the tissue and its metabolic demands: the higher the activity, the more vascular the tissue. It appears that this increase in vascularity may develop on demand. For an example, consider coarctation once more. Should the arterial pressure below the coarctation drop to 80 mmHg, the number of vessels probably increases so that blood flow is not compromised. In the upper extremities, however, where the arterial pressure may be 220 mmHg, the reverse situation occurs; the vessels decrease both in number and in size. The rate at which the tissue can adjust its vasculature undoubtedly relates to many factors, not the least of which is age.

Collateral circulation can be considered as a mechanism of long-term autoregulation. In the discussion relating to the coronary circulation, the observation was made that the anastomotic connections were assumed to be present from early life but that their use as channels for blood flow only occurred following occlusion or insufficiency within a vessel. The same pattern for utilization of collateral vessels appears to exist in most vascular systems.

Fluid Balance

A review of the intrinsic control mechanisms within the circulation would be incomplete without at least brief attention to the integral role of the blood and extracellular fluid volumes on circulatory control, and of the key role of the kidneys in maintaining fluid balance. Proper function of the intrinsic vascular mechanisms in maintenance of adequate tissue perfusion is dependent on sufficient blood volume and an adequate pressure gradient (arterial pressure) to move blood through the circulatory system.

Simplistically, extracellular fluid volume is maintained through daily ingestion of fluid and sodium. With increases in the extracellular fluid volume, proportionate amounts will remain in the plasma as increased blood volume until the point at which capillary balance is lost and fluid extravasates into the tissues, resulting in edema.

As blood volume increases, venous return to the heart is increased, raising both cardiac output and arterial pressure. With an increase in arterial pressure, the rate of urine production correspondingly increases to restore plasma and extracellular fluid volumes to their normal levels. For example, at a normal arterial pressure of 100 mmHg, the kidneys form glomerular filtrate at a rate of approximately 1 ml/min. Elevating the arterial pressure to 150 mmHg will increase the rate of filtrate production to about 4 ml/min.

Neural Control of Circulation

Located within the cerebral medulla and a portion of the pons is the vasomotor center, depicted in Figure 20-18. From the vasoconstrictor portion of the vasomotor center, sympathetic fibers descend to synapse in the thoracolumbar region of the spinal cord and to innervate all major blood vessels except the capillaries. Through this massive innervation of the entire vasculature, sympathetic stimulation alters arterial and venous resistance.

The vasomotor center is able to maintain sympathetic vasoconstrictor tone through continual transmission of impulses, the frequency of which is increased or decreased in relation to stimulation received from the cardiovascular reflexes and hormones. This continual activity of the vasomotor center causes release of the sympathetic hormone nor-

epinephrine from the nerve endings, and elicits through its alpha-adrenergic effect on the blood vessels a partial state of contraction, or tone.

Within the vasomotor center, near the vasoconstrictor center, lies a depressor or inhibitory portion. Its function is, at intervals, to inhibit impulse transmission from the vasoconstrictor center, thus permitting vasodilation.

The major effect of neural control is demonstrated within the microcirculation. Though innervation exists in all major vessels, localized reduction in blood flow is effected through constriction of the resistance vessels, whereas circulating blood volume is increased through constriction of the venous, or capacitance, vessels. In response to any increase in metabolic demand, whether exercise or shock, circulating blood volume is increased and cardiac contractility enhanced through an elevation in venous return to the right side of the heart. Arterial pressure, in addition, is augmented by arterial and venous vasoconstriction.

Control of the vasomotor center can be exercised by other higher nervous centers. Areas within the diencephalon, mesencephalon, and pons can have either a stimulative or a suppressive effect. The hypothalamus as well can have a powerful influence on neural control of the vasculature. Many coordinative responses that involve the circulatory system are known to center within the hypothalamus: temperature control, osmotic regulation of circulating plasma through water balance, and cardiovascular responses to exercise. Experimental excitation of the hypothalamus is known to produce vast alterations in arterial pressure, heart rate, and cardiac contractility. Lastly, vasomotor control can be affected to some extent by the cerebral cortex, as investigation of areas such as biofeedback and relaxation therapy has demonstrated.

Hormonal Influences on Circulation

Humoral or hormonal regulation means control of the circulation by substances such as hormones, ions, or both secreted into or absorbed by the bloodstream. The most important of the humoral or hormonal substances is aldosterone. Secreted by the cortex of the adrenal gland, aldosterone is important in regulation of blood volume through its control over sodium and water concentrations within the extracellular fluid. Stimulated by a decrease in cardiac output, total body volume, or reduction in sodium concentration, aldosterone promotes increased renal tubular reabsorption of sodium and, indirectly, chloride and water. The end result is an increase in plasma and extracellular fluid volume.

Epinephrine, norepinephrine, and acetylcholine exert their major influence when released at sympathetic and parasympathetic nerve endings. Stimulation of sympathetic nerves also prompts the adrenal medulla to secrete epinephrine and norepinephrine as circulating catecholamines. Large quantities of epinephrine (80%) and smaller quantities of norepinephrine (20%) circulate in the bloodstream and are transported to all the tissues of the body.[6] The effect of these circulating catecholamines is similar in nature to the direct effect of neural sympathetic stimulation; however, these adrenal hormones have a much longer effect (5 to 10 times greater) due to the slow removal from the bloodstream.[6] Norepinephrine produces profound vasoconstriction of virtually all the blood vessels of the body. This vasoconstrictive effect (alpha-adrenergic) greatly increases total peripheral vascular resistance and, therefore, causes significant elevation of the arterial pressure. Epinephrine exerts its influence primarily on the beta receptors in the heart, thereby augmenting cardiac output more significantly than the blood pressure.

Vasodilator substances known as *kinins* can be identified within the blood following obstruction of flow or decrease in oxygen. Little is known about kinins other than their very potent vasodilator effect. *Bradykinin* and *kallidin* are two kinins that can be activated with relative ease and function throughout the circulation to cause significant arteriolar dilation and also increased capillary permeability.

Angiotensin is formed through the release of renin from the kidney. When renin acts on another substance to produce angiotensin I, an activating enzyme converts angiotensin I to angiotensin II. The mechanism for renin release is uncertain, but it is believed to be governed by variations in arterial pressure because increased renin secretion follows hypotension. Renal vascular constriction and low serum sodium also influence the rate of renin production. Angiotensin has very powerful vasoconstrictive effects on the arterioles, but there is apparently little or no significant influence on the venous system. The renin mechanism has, in addition, an important role in raising aldosterone secretion in response to hypotension and reducing it in response to elevations in arterial pressure.

Similar to angiotensin, antidiuretic hormone (ADH), also known as vasopressin, is a potent vasoconstrictor that acts primarily on the arterioles. It is produced in the neurohypophysis and is secreted by the posterior pituitary gland. In the past, most physiologists regarded ADH as having inconsequential effects on vascular control; however, recent experiments in hemorrhage have demonstrated an increased concentration of ADH—enough to increase the arterial pressure by as much as 60 mmHg.[6] In addition, ADH is important in regulating water reabsorption in the renal tubules and thereby controlling fluid volume.

Serotonin is concentrated predominantly in the intestinal and other abdominal tissue as well as within platelets. It can have very powerful vasodilator as well as vasoconstrictor effects. The role of serotonin in controlling the peripheral circulation is being investigated.

Histamine is probably not involved in normal circulatory control. Almost every tissue within the body releases histamine in response to injury. The result is local vasoconstriction, surrounding vasodilation, and edema. Histamine causes intense dilation of the arterioles and constriction within the venous system, a combination that produces edema. The hormone is involved with allergic responses and tissue injury such as burns in addition to trauma.

Prostaglandins and Atrial Natriuretic Peptide or Factor

The prostaglandins are a group of chemically related substances contained or synthesized in almost all tissues of the body. Certain prostaglandins can have either potent vasodilator or vasoconstrictor effects on vascular tone. Some prostaglandins may be involved in the vascular response to injury and during immune reaction.[7] These substances are presently under heightened research inquiry.

Atrial natriuretic peptide (ANP) or factor is contained within the atrial tissue of the heart and is secreted through the coronary sinus.[9] Two peptides have been discovered, atriopeptin I and atriopeptin II.[10] Atriopeptin I appears to discriminately relax intestinal smooth muscle, whereas atriopeptin II relaxes both vascular and intestinal smooth muscle. Both possess natriuretic and diuretic properties.

The ANP is thought to be released continuously at low levels and to have a short half-life. It is released into the bloodstream in response to atrial distention or sodium-volume loading. The main effect that ANP has demonstrated in clinical studies is to decrease the workload of the heart by causing dilating both arterioles and veins, thereby reducing preload and afterload.[9,11,12] The ANP also participates in opposing the renin-angiotensin-aldosterone system by suppressing renin and aldosterone secretion, thereby increasing the glomerular filtration rate and facilitating renal excretion of sodium.[12] This mechanism of ANP may be very important for patients in acute or chronic congestive heart failure. Clinical studies of patients with acute CHF who have received ANP infusion have demonstrated improved LV function.[9] However, additional clinical studies are warranted to determine clinical efficacy before widespread administration of ANP is advocated.

REFERENCES

1. Harvey, W. (1941). An anatomical disquisition on the motion of the heart and blood in animals. In F. A. Willius, & T. E. Keys (Eds.), *Cardiac classics*. St. Louis: Mosby.

2. Morgan, J. (1968). A discourse upon the institution of medical schools in America. In M. B. Strauss (Ed.), *Familiar medical quotations*. Boston: Little, Brown.

3. Braunwald, E., Sonnenblick, E. H., & Ross, J. (1992). Mechanisms of cardiac contraction and relaxation. In E. Braunwald (Ed.), *Heart disease* (4th ed.). Philadelphia: Saunders.

4. Rushmer, R. F. (1981). *Cardiovascular dynamics*. Philadelphia: Saunders.

5. Berne, R. M., & Levy, M. N. (1992). *Cardiovascular physiology* (6th ed.). St. Louis: Mosby.

6. Guyton, A. C. (1991). *Textbook of medical physiology* (8th ed.). Philadelphia: Saunders.

7. Mohrman, D. E., & Heller, J. E. (1991). *Cardiovascular physiology*. New York: McGraw-Hill.

8. Smith, J. J., & Kampine, J. P. (1990). *Circulatory physiology* (3rd ed.). Baltimore: Williams & Wilkins.

9. Saito, Y., Nakao, K., Nishimura, K., et al. (1987). Clinical application of atrial natriuretic peptide in patients with congestive heart failure: Beneficial effects on left ventricular function. *Circulation, 76,* 115-130.

10. Currie, M. G., Geller, D. M., Cole, B.R., et al. (1984). Purification and sequence analysis of bioactive atrial peptides (atriopeptins). *Science, 223,* 67-90.

11. Birney, M. H., & Penney, D. G. (1990). Atrial natriuretic peptide: A hormone with implications for clinical practice. *Heart Lung, 19*(2), 174-185.

12. Epsiner, E. A., & Richards, A. M. (1989). Atrial natriuretic peptide, an important factor in sodium and blood pressure regulation. *Lancet, 1*(8640), 707-710.

21

Data Acquisition from the Cardiovascular System

Joan Vitello-Cicciu

Janet S. Eagan

NURSING HISTORY

The clinical evaluation of any cardiovascular (CV) patient admitted to a critical care unit consists of a nursing history, physical assessment, and data from diagnostic procedures. When a seriously ill patient is admitted to a unit, he or she may be incapable of providing a history. In this instance, any available data should be obtained from significant others, emergency technicians or paramedics, helicopter personnel, or previous records. When no history can be gathered, the critical care nurse must rely on subsequent data obtained from the physical assessment and diagnostic procedures.

Ideally, the nursing history should be obtained from the patient on arrival in a unit, but life-threatening medical problems that need immediate assessment and intervention must take precedence. One of several frameworks for obtaining a nursing history has been proposed by Gordon.[1] Before discussing this framework, an understanding of Gordon's views of the scope of nursing is a prerequisite.

Gordon[1] divides the scope of nursing into two focuses. The first deals with the patient's medical problems. These are viewed as "collaborative problems" between medicine and nursing and are most frequently encountered in the critical care setting. The other focus deals with purely "nursing problems," referred to as "nursing diagnosis." Gordon[1] defines these diagnoses as "actual or potential problems which nurses by virtue of their education and experience are capable and licensed to treat."

Nursing diagnoses are formulated on the basis of the data obtained from the nursing history. To facilitate the collection of admission history information, Gordon[1] has suggested 11 assessment categories.

These categories are referred to as *functional health patterns.* Gordon's model encompasses a biopsychosocial perspective of the patient. This holistic view is important in understanding that a problem in one pattern area may affect function in other areas.

A detailed explanation concerning each pattern is beyond the scope of this chapter. However, a list and description of each 11 functional health patterns can be found in Table 21-1. Specific questions related to each pattern that can facilitate the collection of information are also found in Table 21-1. Moreover, salient aspects of the nursing history should include data regarding the patient and family's history of hypertension, diabetes, lipid abnormalities, and rheumatic fever or other types of heart disease. In addition detailed information should be obtained regarding smoking history, alcohol intake, industrial exposure, travel history, viral infections, medications, dietary patterns, stressful events, and exercise capacity.

Once the nursing history is completed and the nursing diagnoses have been identified, a plan of care should be formulated that is aimed at resolving the patient's problems. This plan of care is based on the steps of the nursing process. Thus, interventions and outcomes will be the elements contained in a standard nursing care plan developed to treat these problems. In addition, to facilitate psychological as well as physiological recovery, the plan of care should include the patient's significant others.

PHYSICAL ASSESSMENT

The next step in the clinical evaluation of a cardiovascular patient is performance of a physical assessment. Included in this process are inspection, palpation, percussion, and auscultation. The cardinal

TABLE 21-1   **Gordon's 11 Functional Health Patterns**

Functional Health Patterns	Description	Questions Relating to Patterns
1. Health perception and health management pattern	Describes client's perceived pattern of health and well-being and how health is managed	What brought you here to the hospital? How has your health been before this incident? Are you taking any medications or following any special regimens to maintain your health? What do you feel has caused this illness?
2. Nutritional and metabolic pattern	Describes pattern of food and fluid consumption relative to metabolic need and pattern indicators of local nutrient supply	Any recent weight loss or gain? Could you describe your daily food intake? Do you follow any dietary restrictions? Any problems with healing, dentures, or digestion?
3. Elimination pattern	Describes patterns of excretory function (bowel, bladder, skin)	Any problem moving your bowels? How often? Any problem urinating? How frequently do you have to urinate? Do you wake up at night to urinate?
4. Activity and exercise pattern	Describes pattern of exercise, activity, leisure, and recreation	Describe the type, amount, and frequency of exercise you do on a regular basis. Does your occupation require exercise? Do you have sufficient energy for all your activities?
5. Cognitive and perceptual pattern	Describes sensory, perceptual, and cognitive pattern	Describe your vision and hearing. Any changes? Any trouble feeling hot or cold? Describe your memory. Any changes? What's the easiest way for you to learn something?
6. Sleep and rest pattern	Describes patterns of sleep, rest, and relaxation	How many hours do you sleep each night? Do you have trouble falling asleep or with early awakening? Do you take anything or follow a nightly ritual to induce sleep?
7. Self-perception and self-concept pattern	Describes self-concept pattern, perceptions of self (e.g., body comfort, body image, feeling state)	How would you describe yourself to another? What are your strengths and weaknesses? What do you feel about your life? Future goals?
8. Role and relationship pattern	Describes pattern of role engagements and relationships	What are your primary responsibilities? Who makes decisions? Any major changes recently? Who are the most significant persons available to you?
9. Sexuality and reproductive pattern	Describes client's pattern of satisfaction and dissatisfaction with sexuality pattern; describes reproductive patterns	Any changes or problems with your sexual relations? For female question, self-breast exam. For males, testicular exam.
10. Coping, stress, and tolerance pattern	Describes general coping pattern and effectiveness of the pattern in terms of stress tolerance	What are the major stressors in your life? How do you feel you handle stress? How have you handled a past crisis? Any significant losses or changes in your life?
11. Value and belief pattern	Describes pattern of values, beliefs (including spiritual), or goals that guide decisions or choices	Is religion important to you? List three things you value most in life. Would you like to see a member of the clergy?

Adapted from Gordon, M. (1991). *Manual of nursing diagnosis, 1991-1992*. St. Louis: Mosby–Year Book.

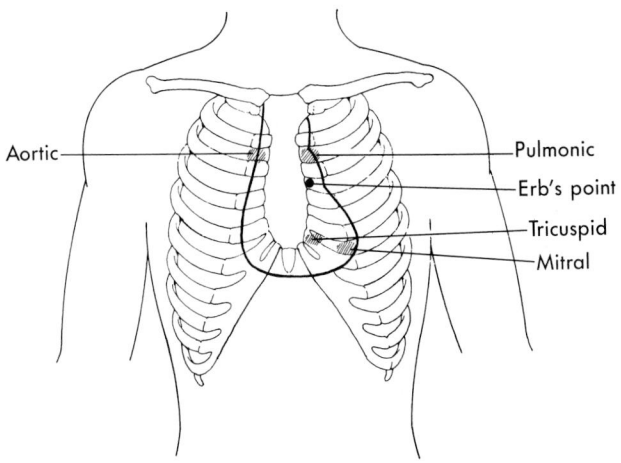

Figure 21-1   Cardinal areas for inspection, palpation, and auscultation.

Adapted from Hochstein, E., & Rubin, A. L. (1964). *Physical diagnosis.* New York: McGraw-Hill.

areas for inspection, palpation, percussion, and auscultation are illustrated in Figure 21-1.

Inspection

The observations noted on inspection should include level of consciousness, posture, facial expressions, and mobility. In regard to the skin, the critical care nurse should look for cyanosis, pallor (anemia), ruddiness (polycythemia), glossy or shiny skin surface (Raynaud's disease), the presence of ulcers (vascular insufficiency), loss of hair, petechiae, jaundice (liver congestion due to right-sided heart failure), and peripheral edema. Inspection should also reveal any bounding pulses occurring in the upper extremities. Corrigan's pulse is an example of a bounding arterial pulsation that can be present in severe aortic regurgitation.

The eyes can reveal underlying cardiovascular disorders. Exophthalmus, or protrusion of the eyeball, can occur in advanced congestive heart failure in the presence of severe pulmonary hypertension and significant weight loss.[2] The presence of corneal arcus, a circumferential light ring around the iris, is frequently associated with hypercholesterolemia and premature atherosclerosis. Roth's spots, which are white spots in the center of hemorrhages, can occur in infective endocarditis. Yellow plaques called xanthelasmas may be found in patients with atherosclerosis.[3]

The ear lobes may reveal diagonal creases, called McCathy's sign. These creases may be an indicator of coronary artery disease (CAD). They have also been noted in patients who present with acute myocardial infarction.[4]

The nails may evidence clubbing in the setting of hypoxemia or infective endocarditis. There may also be splinter hemorrhage in the nail beds and Osler's nodes, which are painful, tender red nodules associated with emboli in infective endocarditis.

The chest may reveal pectus excavatum, a depressed sternum often associated with aortic aneurysms. The abdomen may be enlarged and tender from venous congestion as a sequela of right ventricular failure. The lower extremities should be inspected for edema, clubbing, petechiae, and absence of hair.

Venous Pulsations

The internal and external jugular veins should be inspected for abnormal pulsations and elevated pressure. The normal venous pulse includes two outward pulsations known as the *a* and *v* waves. A third positive, the *c* wave, which is graphically recorded using instrumentation, can rarely be detected clinically and thus has no significance in the assessment of the venous pulse.[5] The *a* wave corresponds to right atrial contraction and is seen just prior to the first heart sound. It occurs after the *p* wave on an ECG. The *v* wave is produced during diastole as a result of atrial filling and corresponds in time to ventricular contraction. It follows the second heart sound and can be seen after the QRS complex. In order to visualize these pulsations, the head of the bed should be elevated 15° to 45° with a pillow placed directly under the patient's head and shoulders so as not to cause neck flexion. In inspecting the venous pulse, the nurse should observe a "double flicker," with both *a* and *v* waves being of equal prominence.[5] Giant *a* waves, for example, are seen in any condition that impedes emptying from the right atrium into the right ventricle. Thus, large *a* waves can be seen in tricuspid stenosis and with such dysrhythmias as junctional rhythms, complete heart block, premature ventricular contractions, and ventricular tachycardia. Conversely, the *a* wave is absent in atrial fibrillation.

The *v* wave is affected when any condition increases or decreases the right atrial (RA) pressure during diastole. For example, tricuspid insufficiency can produce amplified *v* waves because of the retrograde flow of blood into the right atrium.

Ideally, the internal jugular vein should be used when measuring jugular venous pressure (JVP). This vein courses under the sternocleidomastoid muscle, in parallel with the carotid artery. When the internal jugular cannot be visualized, the external jugular vein may be used. The angle of Louis is used as a zero reference point. Also known as the sternal angle, it is a bony protrusion on the sternum found at the second intercostal space, and is located 5 to 7 cm above the right atrium (Figure 21-2).

Measurement of the JVP is begun by drawing an imaginary horizontal line from the sternal angle away from the body. The patient should be positioned in

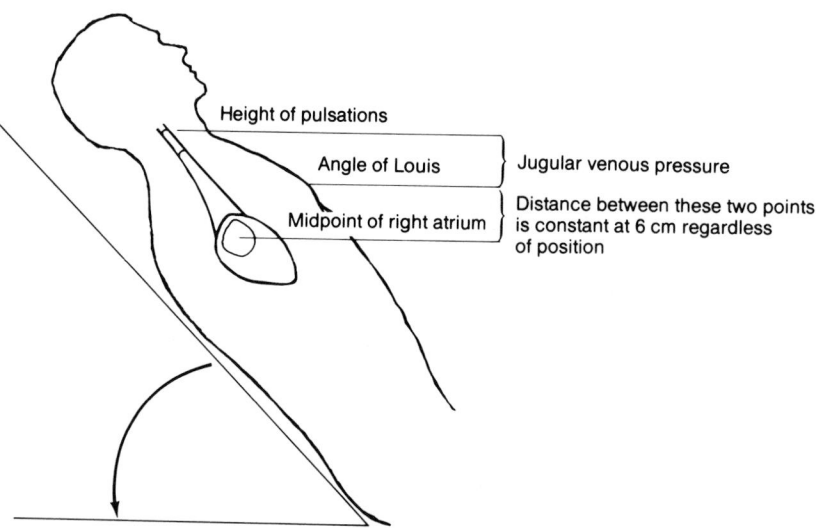

Figure 21-2   Measurement of JVP: Calculated by measuring the distance between angle of Louis and height of column of blood visible in the internal jugular vein.

bed at 30° to 45° of truncal elevation to locate the highest point of jugular pulsations. Another horizontal imaginary line is drawn from this point. The vertical distance from this horizontal line at the height of the column of blood to the other horizontal line at the sternal angle is the measurement made in centimeters. Documentation of this pressure may be written as follows: The internal jugular pulse is 3 to 5 cm above the sternal angle at 45° of truncal elevation.

Another method used to calculate the jugular pressure is to add the vertical distance in centimeters to the 5- to 7-cm distance known to exist from the sternal angle to the right atrium. As an example, if the vertical distance is 5 cm, the central venous pressure can be estimated to be 10 to 12 cm. Elevation of the JVP can occur with congestive heart failure, right ventricular infarcts, tricuspid valvular defects, constrictive pericarditis, hypervolemia, and obstruction of the superior vena cava.

Carotid Arterial Pulsations

The critical care nurse should inspect the carotid artery for bounding or weak pulsations. Abnormal large bounding pulses may be associated with hypertension, complete heart block, hypoxia, anemia, or anxiety states. A weak pulse may be related to left ventricular failure, aortic stenosis, or any other condition that causes diminished stroke volume.

Anterior Chest Pulsations

Pulsations should also be observed on the anterior chest. Table 21-2 lists the abnormalities of the heart detected by inspection and palpation. Possible etiologies are also listed.

Respiratory Movement

In concluding the inspection, the nurse should observe for the adequacy of chest expansion; breathing patterns, especially the use of accessory muscles to breathe (may be an indication of respiratory distress); and the quality and quantity of the respiratory rate.

Palpation

Precordial palpation is done to confirm and qualify visible findings and detect the presence of other normal and abnormal pulsations or vibrations. The nurse should be positioned on the right side of the patient. Palpation begins by placing the palmar surface of the fingers and hand over visible areas of pulsation and then moving over the entire precordium, palpating systematically. When areas of pulsation or vibration are felt, the fingertips are used to denote the rate, rhythm, and intensity of the pulsation.

Beginning at the base of the heart, the nurse then palpates for pulsations, thrills, and heaves or vibrations in the aortic area at the second or third intercostal space (ICS) to the right of the sternum. A thrill in this area may signify aortic stenosis and abnormal pulsations may be suggestive of an aortic aneurysm. Palpation of this area is enhanced when the patient is sitting up or leaning forward.

In the pulmonic area (second or third ICS to the left of the sternum), a slow, sustained, forceful pulsation may be associated with pulmonary hypertension or mitral stenosis. Erb's point, located in the third intercostal space on the left sternal border (LSB) should be palpated, since murmurs of aortic and pulmonic origin may be referred to this area. Gradually, palpation is continued over the parasternal area until

TABLE 21-2　Heart Abnormalities Detected by Inspection and Palpation

Precordium	Abnormality	Examples of Possible Cause
Aortic area 　2nd and 3rd interspaces to 　　right of sternum	Forceful pulsation	Rheumatic heart disease Systemic hypertension Ascending thoracic aortic aneurysm
	Thrill	Aortic stenosis
Pulmonary area 　2nd and 3rd interspaces to 　　left of sternum	Forceful pulsation	Essential pulmonary hypertension Left-to-right intracardiac shunt Mitral stenosis, pulmonary embolism, diffuse 　　pneumonia
	Thrill	Obstruction of right ventricular outflow tract
Right ventricular area 　Lower sternal border to the 　　immediate right and left of 　　sternum	Thrill Lift or heave	Ventricular septal defect Obstructions of right ventricular outflow tract Mitral stenosis Left-to-right intracardiac shunts Skeletal deformities
Left ventricular area 　4th to 6th interspaces 　Left midclavicular line or be- 　　yond	Strong apical impulse or 　abnormally large PMI Dyskinetic apical impulse Thrill Gallop	Left ventricular hypertrophy Aortic valve diseases Left ventricular aneurysm Mitral valve disease Myocardial dysfunction, mitral or aortic valve 　disease, HCVD
Epigastric area	Strong pulsation of ab- 　dominal aorta Pulsation of liver	Abdominal aortic aneurysm Congestive heart failure

the right ventricular area is reached. An abnormal pulsation of the right ventricular area may be indicative of right ventricular (RV) enlargement. A substantial heave may suggest pulmonic stenosis, mitral stenosis, or left ventricular (LV) failure. The epigastric region is then palpated to detect the presence of pulsations. The apical area is palpated next to determine the strength of the point of maximal impulse (PMI). The PMI is about the size of a quarter and is normally felt in about half the population. The apical area is most easily palpated with the patient either in the left lateral decubitus position or seated and leaning forward. Thrills in this area may be associated with mitral stenosis or regurgitation. A displaced PMI occurs with LV hypertrophy. In addition, a systolic bulge suggestive of an LV aneurysm may be present in the apical area. Location of areas of palpation and abnormalities that may be detected by such inspection may be found in Table 21-2.

Abnormal arterial pulsations may occur as a manifestation of diminished left ventricular function, increased cardiac output, or may be secondary to dysrhythmias. Configurations of normal and abnormal arterial pulse waves are illustrated in Figure 21-3.

Lastly, during palpation the critical care nurse should ascertain skin temperature, diaphoresis, and skin texture.

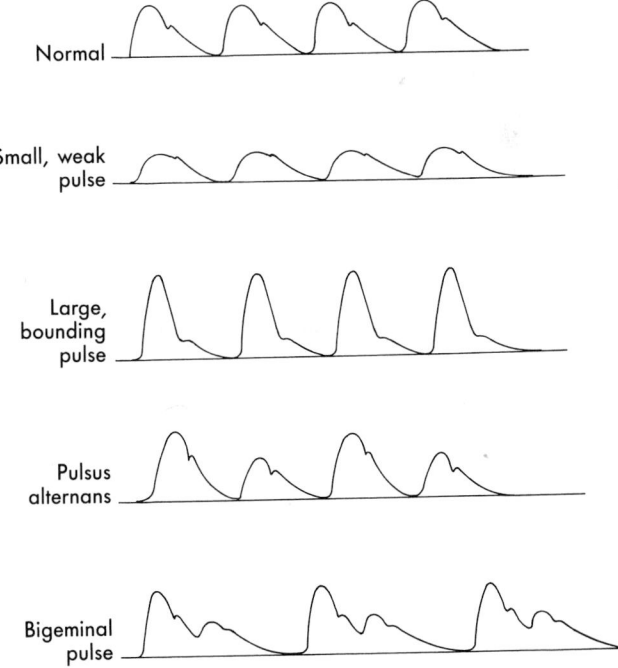

Figure 21-3　Arterial pulse waves.

Percussion

Percussion is no longer routinely used in the cardiovascular assessment because imaging techniques have supplanted it. When percussion is used, it is performed to outline the left and right borders of cardiac dullness, although the findings may not be as reliable as palpation. This technique may often be omitted from a routine physical assessment.

Auscultation

Auscultation of the heart includes listening to the rate and rhythm of the heartbeat, auscultating blood pressure, evaluating normal heart sounds, and determining the presence or absence of extra heart sounds, murmurs, and pericardial friction rubs. These sounds may be evaluated with either a stethoscope or Doppler probe.

Examining the heart by auscultation ideally begins with a warm, well-lighted, and particularly quiet space. The patient is placed in the same positions for auscultation as palpation: lying, left lateral, sitting, and leaning forward. Both the diaphragm and the bell of the stethoscope are used.

The entire precordium, including areas of radiation (axilla and carotid arteries), is auscultated; however, particular attention should be paid to the areas in which valve closure sounds are best heard. These areas include the aortic area at the second right intercostal space adjacent to the sternal border, the pulmonic area in the second left intercostal space, the tricuspid area situated at the fifth left intercostal space near the sternal edge, and the mitral or apical area located at the fifth left intercostal space medial to the midclavicular line.

The examiner may begin with the diaphragm of the stethoscope at the aortic area, at which the second heart sound (S_2) is loudest, move to the pulmonic area, and inch the stethoscope down the left sternal border to the mitral or apical area. Another approach is to begin at the apical area, at which the first sound (S_1) is loudest, and move upward to the left sternal border and across the sternum to the aortic area. Beginning at the aortic or the apical area first, the examiner listens to and assesses the rate and rhythm of the heart to establish a baseline for comparison in each area examined. The course of auscultation is then reversed using the bell of the stethoscope.

In each area auscultated, the following components of the cardiac cycle are assessed:

1. The characteristics of S_1 (intensity, splitting, effects of respiration)
2. The characteristics of S_2 (intensity, splitting, effects of respiration)
3. The presence or absence of extra sounds in systole and diastole
4. The presence or absence of murmurs in systole and diastole
5. The presence or absence of pericardial friction rubs

Heart Rate and Rhythm

The normal rate and rhythm of the heart are determined by the conduction system. In the normal heart, the small bundle of fibers comprising the sinoatrial (SA) node initiates the cardiac impulse. Known as the *cardiac pacemaker*, the SA node is located in the wall of the right atrium at the entrance of the venae cavae. The SA node automatically discharges an electrical impulse which is then conducted throughout the atria to the atrioventricular (AV) node, another small bundle of cardiac fibers located in the posterior lower right atrium near the septum. After a slight delay, allowing for completion of atrial systole, the impulse is conducted through a bundle of electrically specialized conducting tissue, the *His bundle*. The bundle divides into right and left branches, each passing down the corresponding side of the interventricular septum, and then spreads into a fine network of Purkinje fibers. These fibers infiltrate into all portions of the ventricular myocardium. The impulse reaches the ventricles almost simultaneously and excites the muscles, causing ventricular contraction.

Variations in the rate and rhythm of the heart are classified as dysrhythmias and are caused by (1) variation in the rate of discharge of the SA node, (2) ectopic impulses which compete with the SA node, or (3) abnormal conduction of impulses from the SA node through the heart. (See Chapter 10 for further discussion of cardiac electrical activity.)

Blood Pressure

In a critical care unit, blood pressure (BP) should ideally be obtained on both arms. Using a properly sized cuff, the nurse should slowly inflate the cuff approximately 30 mmHg above the disappearance of the radial pulse. The pressure difference between arms should be less than 10 mmHg.[6] A greater difference may suggest obstructive lesions of the aorta or the innominate, or subclavian artery; supravalvular aortic stenosis; subclavian steal syndrome; aortic dissection; aortic arch syndrome; or patent ductus arteriosus.

Abnormal blood pressure findings such as pulsus paradoxus (decrease in systolic BP during inspiration) may be present in such conditions as constrictive pericarditis, cardiac tamponade, or restrictive cardiomyopathy. Pulsus alternans (alternation of the sound intensity of each beat) may be indicative of LV failure. Orthostatic changes (changes in response to position changes) may reflect hypovolemia or alterations in vascular resistance. Differences in pulse pressure (the difference between systolic and diastolic blood pressure) may also be indicative of cardiac abnormalities. For example, a widened pulse pressure may be present in aortic insufficiency (regurgitation) or in certain congenital abnormalities. A narrowed pulse pressure is usually present in severe aortic stenosis, hypovolemia, or states that are associated with increased outpouring of catecholamines.

Normal Heart Sounds

Normal heart sounds are vibrations produced, at least in part, by the closure of valves and by the flow of blood through the heart. The first heart sound (S_1) is high-pitched but is slightly lower in frequency and longer in duration than the second heart sound (S_2).

An S_1 is louder than an S_2 at the apex. If any difficulty arises in differentiating between S_1 and S_2, the timing of S_1 correlates with that of the carotid pulse and it is usually heard as one sound. The S_1 sound occurs as a result of closure of the atrioventricular (mitral [M_1] and tricuspid [T_1]) valves and can be heard over the entire precordium but is heard best at the apex.

Since the pressure gradients are greater on the left side of the heart than on the right side, sometimes there will be a minimal difference in closure of the mitral and tricuspid valve. This interval between M_1 and T_1 is referred to as a split of the first heart sound which produces an audible separation between these two components of S_1.

The second heart sound is high-pitched and slightly shorter in duration than S_1. The S_2 sound occurs upon closure of the semilunar (aortic and pulmonic) valves and may be heard most audibly at the base of the heart. It may vary in character when related to loudness as does S_1; however, particular attention should be given to the "splitting" phenomenon of S_2 which explains why two sounds are heard when listening. Other variations of S_2 will be presented following this discussion.

Splitting of S_2 may be physiological or pathological. Physiological splitting is audible on inspiration at the pulmonic or aortic area when the aortic valve (A_2) closes before the pulmonic valve (P_2) as in the normal heart. This accentuated asynchronous closure of A_2 and P_2 on inspiration is due to an increased venous return to the right ventricle during inspiration. The prolongation of right ventricular systole delays closure of the pulmonic valve, increasing the time interval between closure of A_2 and P_2.

Pathological splitting of S_2 indicates the presence of disease. When the split does not vary with inspiration or expiration, it is referred to as *fixed splitting* and occurs in such conditions as pulmonic stenosis and atrial septal defect. *Wide splitting* refers to an increase in the normal splitting time of S_2 on inspiration along with an S_1 split. This occurs in right bundle branch block in which prolonged electrical conduction delays right ventricular contraction and pulmonic valve closure. *Paradoxical splitting* refers to a reverse phenomenon in which splitting of S_2 occurs on expiration rather than inspiration. In left bundle branch block, a delay in left ventricular contraction may cause the aortic valve to close after the pulmonic valve, producing a single sound on inspiration and a split sound on expiration.

In further assessing S_2, attention should be given to the intensity of the aortic and pulmonic components of S_2. An accentuated aortic component of S_2, as heard in arterial hypertension and aortic regurgitation, results from an increase in arterial pressure which forces the aortic valve to close. A diminished aortic component of S_2 occurs when the arterial pressure is low, as in shock, and aortic valve closure is soft. Aortic stenosis also produces a diminished second sound because the valve leaflets are relatively immobile.

An accentuated pulmonic component of S_2 occurs when back pressure in the pulmonary artery increases and forces the pulmonary valve to close, as in pulmonary hypertension. Other conditions in which an accentuated P_2 is heard are mitral stenosis, left ventricular failure, and atrial septal defect. A diminished pulmonic component of the second heart sound is also heard in pulmonic stenosis when the pressure against the pulmonic valve is less than normal.

Extra Heart Sounds

Extra heart sounds can basically be classified in relation to location in the cardiac cycle and are named and described accordingly. The sounds are heard in either systole or diastole, except for pericardial friction rubs, which are heard in both.

Ejection clicks may be heard in the early, middle, or late phase of cardiac systole. These clicks are thought to be related to prolapse of either the mitral or tricuspid valve. Early systolic ejection clicks are either aortic or pulmonic in origin and occur immediately after S_1. Aortic ejection clicks are heard at the base and apex of the heart and occur in diseases of the aortic valve and in aortic aneurysms. The click does not change with respiration.

Pulmonic ejection clicks are heard in the pulmonic area, diminish with inspiration, and occur in pulmonic stenosis and pulmonic hypertension. Middle and late systolic clicks are not as well defined as early systolic clicks but are frequently associated with systolic murmurs of mitral regurgitation.

The opening snap (OS) of mitral stenosis is a high-pitched, short, snappy sound heard in the early phase of diastole. An OS is best heard along the LSB medial to the apex; however, it does radiate widely and can be differentiated from a third heart sound (S_3) because it occurs earlier in the cardiac cycle.

The third heart sound (S_3) can be physiological or pathological. It is a common and usually normal finding in children and young adults. In the middle-aged and older person, however, it is considered abnormal and usually indicative of LV failure. In fact, the presence of an S_3 sound should be sought in any patient with a cardiac condition. It is a low-pitched sound that occurs early in diastole during rapid ventricular filling, causing vibrations in the left ventricle. An S_3 sound can be heard best at the apex with the bell of the stethoscope.

The fourth heart sound (S_4) may also be physiological or pathological. It may be occasionally heard normally in young children, but not as often as is an S_3. It is usually an abnormal sound that is believed to be a late ventricular filling sound caused by the accelerated flow of blood into the ventricles produced by atrial contraction. It is a low-pitched sound that occurs late in diastole just before the first heart sound. It is heard best at the apex with the bell of the stethoscope. A pathological S_4 is usually associated with hypertensive cardiovascular (CV) disease, coronary artery disease, or aortic stenosis. It may be the first evidence of CV disease and can be an important contribution to the data regarding the CV system of a patient.

A pericardial friction rub is usually described as a transient scratching, grating, or squeaking high-pitched sound indicative of pericarditis. It is heard best with the diaphragm of the stethoscope in the region between the apex and left sternal border. The timing of the pericardial friction rub is associated with cardiac movement and consists of three short components: atrial systole, ventricular systole, and ventricular diastole. Often, two components are heard; however, all three components are diagnostic and help to differentiate a pericardial rub from a pleural friction rub, which has two components.

Gallop Rhythm

Gallop rhythm is a term used to describe the rhythm of the heart when an S_3, S_4, or both sounds are perceived by auscultation and possibly palpation. The presence of an S_3 sound is referred to as a *protodiastolic gallop*. The term *summation gallop* is used when presystolic (S_4) and protodiastolic (S_3) gallops combine to form a single, loud, evenly spaced sound in diastole. Gallop rhythms are heard best with the bell of the stethoscope.

Murmurs

Murmurs are audible vibrations that originate within the heart and great vessels. These sounds represent turbulence of blood flow caused by (1) an increased rate of blood flow through normal structures (such as is caused by exercise), (2) the forward flow of blood across a partially obstructed or narrowed valve (such as in valvular stenosis), (3) blood flow into a dilated chamber, or (4) the backward flow of blood across an incompetent valve or defect (such as in valvular insufficiency).

Murmurs are usually classified as *systolic*, *diastolic*, or *continuous* because of the location in the cardiac cycle. To determine the significance of a murmur, certain factors must be identified and described in the process of cardiac assessment. These factors include:
1. The timing of the murmur within the cardiac cycle which may be in early, or late systole, or in diastole, or it may be considered holosystolic
2. Characteristics
   a. Intensity (graded on a scale from 1 to 6)
      (1) Difficult to hear; barely audible, very faint
      (2) Very soft, but can be heard without straining
      (3) Moderately loud
      (4) Loud
      (5) Very loud, but requires stethoscope chestpiece to be placed on chest
      (6) Extremely loud; heard with chestpiece off chest
   b. Pattern (crescendo, decrescendo, or diamond-shaped)
   c. Pitch (high, medium, low)
   d. Quality (harsh, musical, blowing, or rumbling)
3. Location on the precordium (location of greatest intensity, that is, the apex, tricuspid, aortic, or pulmonic area)
4. Radiation (areas in which the murmur is less audible but still perceptible)
5. Posture and exercise (the body position or activity under which murmur is heard)
6. Stethoscope chestpiece used to hear the murmur (bell or diaphragm)

Systolic Murmurs

Systolic murmurs may be physiological or pathological and occur between S_1 and S_2 sounds. They may be further described as *early systolic* or *midsystolic* because of their relationship or proximity to S_1 and S_2 sounds.

There are basically two types of systolic murmurs: ejection and regurgitant. *Systolic ejection murmurs* occur when ventricular contraction forces blood, under high pressure, forward through the aortic valve, pulmonic valve, or septal defect into normal or dilated vessels which are at lower pressures. Systolic ejection murmurs occur with such conditions as aortic and pulmonic stenoses. Aortic and pulmonic stenoses produce midsystolic murmurs that are diamond-shaped, medium-pitched, and harsh, and heard with either the bell or diaphragm chestpiece.

Regurgitant murmurs occur in systole when the mitral or tricuspid valves do not close sufficiently to prevent the backflow of blood into the atria during ventricular contraction as seen in mitral and tricuspid insufficiency or mitral valve prolapse. These murmurs are holosystolic and heard over their respective valvular areas. They are both high-pitched and blowing, with the intensity remaining relatively the same. Mitral and tricuspid regurgitant murmurs differ characteristically in the effect of respiration and manner of radiation. The intensity of the murmur of tricuspid regurgitation increases with inspiration and may radiate only to the left midclavicular line. The murmur of mitral regurgitation does not change with inspiration and radiates into the left axilla. They are best heard with the diaphragm chestpiece.

Diastolic Murmurs

Diastolic murmurs occur after S_2 and before S_1 and are also further classified as early, mid-, late, or holosystolic. Diastolic murmurs are usually pathological and may be ejection, filling, or regurgitant in nature.

The *ejection* or *filling* murmur of mitral stenosis may range from a very faint to a loud rumble with a crescendo or descrescendo pattern. It is low-pitched, heard best with the bell chestpiece, and usually localized at the apex in a very small area.

Regurgitant murmurs, as in aortic insufficiency, occur when blood flows back into the ventricle at the beginning of diastole, continuing throughout the diastolic phase in a descrescendo pattern. The intensity varies from very faint to loud, depending on the degree of valvular insufficiency. It is a very high-pitched,

blowing murmur that is heard best with the diaphragm chestpiece at the aortic area. (See Chapter 24 for further discussion of valvular murmurs.)

Continuous murmurs are less common and represent the presence of both systolic and diastolic murmurs. These are evident in conditions in which arteriovenous communication exists, such as patent ductus arteriosus.

DIAGNOSTIC PROCEDURES

The third and final component in the clinical evaluation of a patient involves the interpretation of data obtained from diagnostic procedures. This section focuses on those procedures that enable the critical care team to assess a patient with cardiovascular disease.

Atrial Electrograms

The recording of atrial electrograms (AEGs) can significantly facilitate the bedside diagnosis of complex rhythm and conduction disturbances. The surface ECG will generally permit an accurate identification of the QRS width and an assessment of the ventricular activation sequence. The recognition of the low-amplitude P wave, however, can be unreliable, especially in patients with ECG baseline artifacts, tachydysrhythmias, and conduction disturbances. The atrial electrogram overcomes this problem by recording the atrial activity as a large amplitude A wave that can be readily identified. Atrial electrograms can be recorded as either unipolar or bipolar signals (Figure 21-4). The unipolar atrial electrogram is a recording of the electrical difference between the atrial electrode and the skin electrode and has the appearance of a conventional ECG with amplification of the P wave. A standard electrocardiographic amplifier can be used to record a unipolar atrial electrogram by connecting the left arm lead to an atrial electrode and the right arm lead to a skin electrode with the lead selector in the I position. Most electrocardiographic amplifiers also require an additional

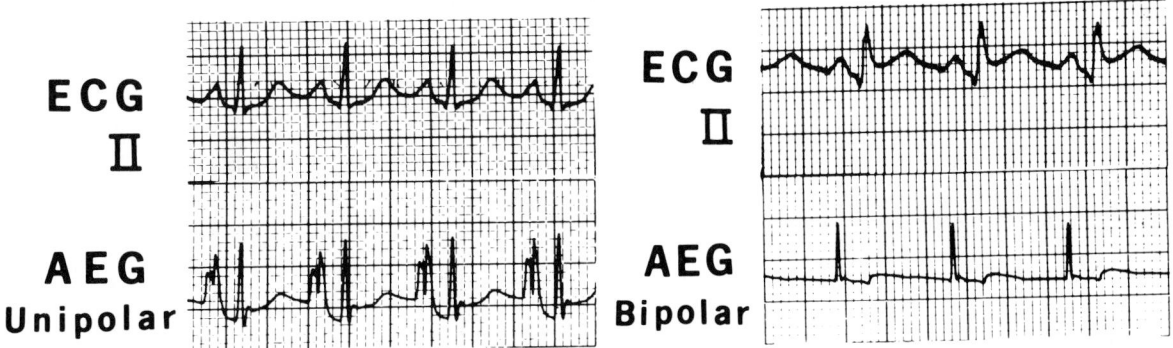

Figure 21-4 Simultaneous recording of lead II electrocardiogram and unipolar atrial electrogram (AEG) or bipolar atrial electrogram. See text for definition and recording techniques.

skin electrode as an indifferent reference lead (generally the right leg). Recording the atrial electrogram as a unipolar signal has the advantages of requiring only a single atrial electrode and of providing information about both the atrial and ventricular rhythm on a single data channel. The disadvantages include baseline noise introduced via the skin electrode and superimposition of the atrial and ventricular signals. The bipolar atrial electrogram is a recording of the atrial electric impulses recorded from two atrial electrodes and consists of isolated A waves.

A standard electrocardiographic amplifier can be used to record a bipolar electrogram by connecting one atrial electrode to each arm lead and recording with the lead selector in the I position (Figure 21-5). With computerized ECG machines, it is possible to obtain both a bipolar and a unipolar tracing by attaching both arm leads to two atrial wires with alligator clamps and attaching the conventional limb leads to each leg. By changing the format and using the manual mode, one can obtain a simultaneous lead I, II, and III. Lead I is the bipolar lead and leads II and III are the unipolar leads. Since the bipolar atrial electrogram records only information about the atrial rhythm, a simultaneous ECG is required to evaluate the relationship between the atrial and ventricular rhythms. The advantages of recording the atrial electrogram as a bipolar signal include a high signal/noise ratio and isolated atrial signal without interference from ventricular activity. The disadvantages are the requirement for two atrial electrodes and the need for a second data channel to display the simultaneous ECG. The polarity of the atrial electrogram can be reversed by interchanging the lead connections.

Atrial electrograms can be recorded from epicardial electrode wires, permanent pacemakers, and esophageal electrodes. Patients undergoing cardiac surgery can have electrode wires sutured to the atrial epicardium and brought out through the chest wall for temporary postoperative atrial electrogram recording and pacing.[7] The routine placement of two epicardial atrial wires and one or two ventricular wires has proved to be extremely valuable in the management of these patients. Prior to discharge, the wires are pulled free and removed.

Atrial electrograms can also be recorded by passing an electrode catheter down the esophagus and positioning the electrodes at the level of the atrium. This approach has the advantage of being noninvasive but cannot be used for atrial pacing. An esophageal "pill electrode" with fine connecting wires can be more easily swallowed and left comfortably indwelling for many hours for electrogram monitoring even while eating. Since the pill electrode is well tolerated by patients and can provide a high-quality atrial electrogram, this noninvasive technique makes the use of atrial electrograms practical for a much larger patient population with complex dysrhythmias.

Independent of the technique used for recording the atrial electrogram, great care must be exercised to protect the patient from microshock. All recording equipment must be electrically isolated from current leakage of less than 10 μA. Precautions must be used to avoid additional sources of current leakage from electric beds, televisions, radios, razors, or hair dryers. To prevent accidental contact with potential sources of current, the electrode terminal connectors should never be left uncovered. Frequent periodic checks of

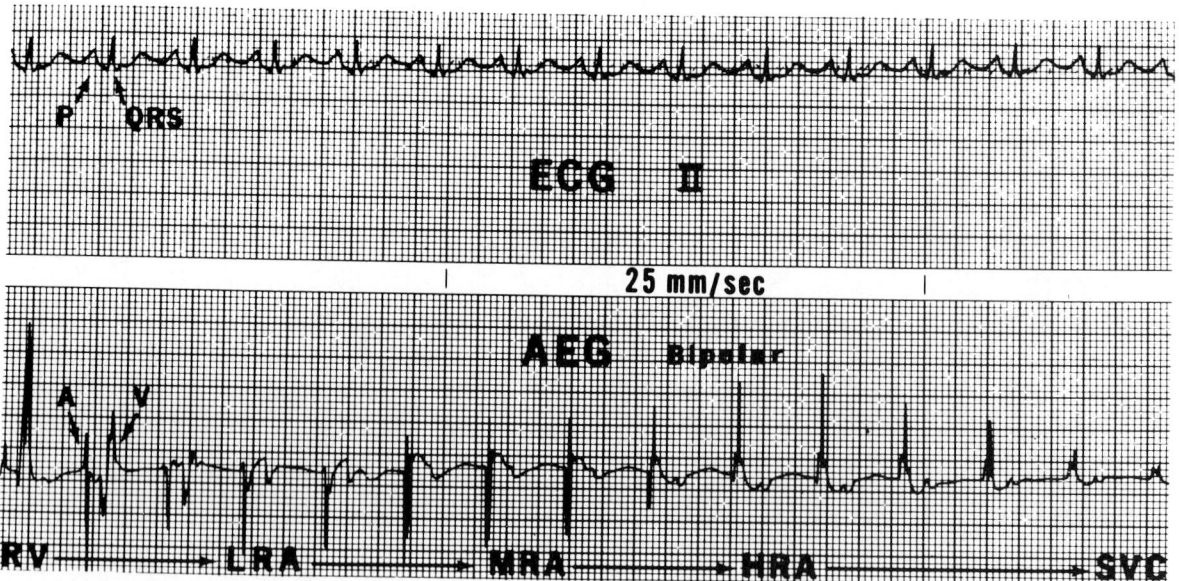

Figure 21-5   Simultaneous recording of a lead II electrocardiogram and an atrial electrocardiogram.

the recording equipment for ground faults and current leakage are mandatory.

Atrial electrograms are useful in the evaluation of patients with tachydysrhythmias, atrioventricular dissociation, heart block, and premature beats. Specific examples in which an atrial electrogram may be necessary to establish correct diagnoses include the differentiation of ventricular tachycardia versus supraventricular tachycardia with bundle branch block, atrial tachycardia (or flutter) with 2 to 1 conduction versus sinus tachycardia, and premature ventricular contractions (PVCs) versus aberrantly conducted premature atrial contractions (PACs). The ability to identify both the atrial and ventricular complexes accurately simplifies these electrocardiographic dilemmas into a straightforward rhythm analysis and diagnosis.

Blood Tests

To determine whether a patient has sustained a myocardial infarction (MI), a clinician evaluates the patient's pain history, associated electrocardiographic changes, and elevations of serum enzyme levels. The enzymes frequently assessed are creatine phosphokinase (CK) and lactate dehydrogenase (LDH). In the past, a third enzyme, serum glutamic oxaloacetic transaminase (SGOT), was also assessed when making this diagnosis. However, owing to its lack of specificity, clinicians today use mainly the CK and LDH total enzymes and isoenzymes when diagnosing an MI. These enzymes are released from myocardial cells that have undergone necrosis. Roberts[8] estimates that 30 to 60 minutes of prolonged ischemia can result in cellular membrane damage and resultant enzyme leakage.

LDH can be isolated in serum within 8 to 12 hours after infarction, peaks in 3 days, and returns to baseline within 10 to 14 days. An elevated LDH value is not specific for myocardial infarction because this enzyme is also found in liver, kidney, and red blood cells. Therefore, an elevation of LDH may be recorded in liver and kidney abnormalities as well as in hemolyzed blood samples.

To increase the specificity of LDH in confirming the diagnosis of MI, one needs to examine the five isoenzymes of LDH, which are LDH_1, LDH_2, LDH_3, LDH_4, and LDH_5. Cardiac muscle contains a predominance of the LDH_1 isoenzyme. Under normal circumstances, the serum level of LDH_1 is less than LDH_2. After infarction, the heart releases LDH that includes LDH_1. This elevates the total LDH level and raises the level of LDH_1 above that of LDH_2. Galen[9] reports that this "flipped" pattern in LDH isoenzymes is present within 48 hours in 80% of acute infarctions.

The cardiac enzyme creatine phosphokinase (CK) is more sensitive in diagnosing MI than LDH or SGOT. CK is mainly contained in heart and skeletal tissue and to a lesser extent in the gastrointestinal tract and brain. CK can be detected in the serum approximately 4 hours after an MI, peaks in 12 to 24 hours, and returns to baseline in 72 to 96 hours. Although the most sensitive of the three enzymes, total CK may be elevated in conditions other than MI. Elevated CK levels are seen with repeated intramuscular injections or postoperatively. Evaluation of the isoenzymes of CK, especially the MB isoenzyme, is necessary to increase the specificity of the test.

The CK-MB isoenzyme is found predominantly in cardiac muscle tissue. It is released into the serum after infarction and necrosis of cardiac tissue occurs. At present, it is the most specific laboratory enzymatic test indicative of an MI.

Serial sampling of cardiac enzymes is recommended after a suspected MI or if chest pain occurs with concomitant EKG changes. Sampling intervals will vary depending on the timing of the suspected MI. For example, if the MI is in the evolutionary stages of development, it is recommended that serial CK and CK-MB levels be obtained and assayed on admission and about 12 or 24 hours later.[10] However, if the MI occurred up to 24 hours prior to admission, a total LDH level should be obtained. If the LDH is elevated then LDH isoenzymes should be sampled.[10]

Cardiac Catheterization

From a historical perspective, cardiac catheterization has evolved over the last 60 years since the first attempt by Werner Forssman in 1929 to pass a catheter into his own right heart. The 1930s saw the perfection of right heart catheterization by such investigators as Klein, Padillo, Cournand, and Richards.[11] The technique of left heart catheterization was first introduced by Zimmerman and Lason in the 1950s. Seldinger created the percutaneous technique, which is the currently accepted procedure for both left and right heart catheterization, in 1953. In 1959, Sones developed selective coronary arteriography, which has become the "gold standard" in the cadre of diagnostic procedures for coronary artery disease.

Cardiac catheterization is an invasive hemodynamic and angiographic procedure performed for several diagnostic purposes. It may also be used as a baseline technique before and after such procedures as balloon angioplasty, valvuloplasty, atherectomy, laser angioplasty, and stent insertions.[12] Moreover, future research will use the cardiac catheter to focus on coronary vasoreactivity and atherosclerotic changes.[12] As a hemodynamic procedure, the data which can be obtained include chamber and vessel pressures, volumes, waveforms, and calculations of cardiac outputs.

Angiography, which is the injection of contrast material into the ventricle (ventriculography) or coronary artery (arteriography), is employed when visualization of the chamber or artery is necessary. Filming methods such as cineangiography or angiocardiography provide visualization of ventricular motion. This is especially helpful in looking for wall motion abnormalities, ventricular function, valvular defects, septal defects, and aneurysms.

Right Heart Catheterization

With right heart catheterization, a catheter is inserted through either the basilic or femoral vein. It is sequentially introduced through the right heart chambers into the pulmonary artery. Through this catheter, pressures, volumes, and tracings of the right atrium, right ventricle, pulmonary artery, and pulmonary artery wedge position may be obtained for evaluation.

Right-sided Valvular Function. Tricuspid and pulmonic valvular function can be assessed for the purpose of determining the presence and/or severity of stenosis or regurgitation. In evaluating stenosis, for example, the physician can determine the presence of a pressure gradient (normally, there should be none) and calculation of the valve orifice size. If valvular stenosis is present, ventriculography can be employed to indicate mobility and calcification of the valve leaflets. Tricuspid regurgitation is evaluated on the basis of waveform tracings and the degree of regurgitation seen angiographically. The grading of regurgitation ranges from 1+ to 4+, whereby 4+ is the most severe gradation. The evaluation of pulmonic regurgitation is accomplished by looking for a widened pulmonary arterial pressure, an increase in right ventricular end-diastolic pressure, and demonstration of regurgitation via ventriculography.[11]

Shunts. In addition to valvular assessment, left-to-right shunts can be detected during the angiography procedure. This is accomplished by drawing blood samples sequentially from the pulmonary artery, right ventricle, right atrium, superior vena cava (SVC), and inferior vena cava (IVC). A significant finding for the presence of a shunt is a "step up" in blood oxygen saturation found during this retrograde sampling. The visualization and localization of a shunt are further elucidated via angiography.

Cardiac Outputs. Cardiac outputs (CO) can be obtained in the catheterization laboratory via four different methods: quantitative angiography, the Fick method, the indicator dilution method, and the thermodilution method. The thermodilution technique is discussed in the section, Hemodynamic Monitoring.

Quantitative angiography involves obtaining ventricular end-systolic (ESV) and end-diastolic volumes (EDV) from the ventriculogram. Once these volumes have been obtained, stroke volume (SV) can be determined by subtracting the end-systolic volume from the end-diastolic volume (SV = ESV − EDV). Total CO is then calculated. It should be noted that this cardiac output differs from that obtained by the Fick method. The Fick cardiac output is the forward cardiac output. From a clinical standpoint, this would have significance in valvular regurgitation in which some of the total cardiac output flows in a retrograde pattern. Thus, the regurgitant volume could be easily obtained by simply subtracting the forward CO from the total CO (regurgitant volume = total CO − forward CO).

The Fick method is based on the principle proposed by Fick in 1870. This principle states "that in a steady state, the flow of blood through an organ (such as the lungs) is equal to the amount of a substance (oxygen) absorbed by the blood flowing through the organ (consumption), divided by the difference in oxygen concentration between the blood entering and leaving the organ (arteriovenous O_2 difference).[11] This formula can then be computed as follows:

$$\text{Cardiac output} = \frac{\text{Oxygen consumption (ml/min)}}{\text{Arteriovenous } O_2 \text{ difference (ml/100 ml blood)}}$$

Normal oxygen consumption is approximately 250 ml/min. The arteriovenous O_2 difference is about 50 ml. Thus, the cardiac output is normally about 5 L/min. If this cardiac output is adjusted to the body surface area, the value is referred to as the *cardiac index*.

The indicator-dilution method for determining CO involves the injection of green dye (indocyanine green) into the right atrium; the concentration of the indicator is sampled at a peripheral site downstream, after the indicator has adequately mixed with the blood. A blood sample is continually withdrawn through a photoelectric instrument called a *densitometer*. A curve is recorded from the densitometer whereby the CO is calculated through computers from the known amount of the indicator that was injected and the area of the time concentration curve.

Left Heart Catheterization

Left heart catheterization is performed either through a retrograde approach from the femoral artery to the aorta and then through the aortic valve, or through a transseptal approach across the right atrium through the foramen ovale into the left atrium. Hemodynamically, left-sided pressures and volumes are assessed. Elevations of left-sided pressure can result from such CV disorders as myocardial infarction, cardiomyopathy, hypertension, cardiogenic shock, and valvular disease.

Left-sided Valvular Function. Pressure gradients across the valve orifice are determined to assess for either mitral or aortic stenosis. The valve orifice is visualized during angiography for mobility and calcification. The aortic valve is evaluated at this time for the presence of bicuspid or unicuspid defects.

Heightened v waves on the left atrial tracing are diagnostic of mitral regurgitation. Severe regurgitation is determined when the v waves are greater than twice the mean left atrial pressure.[13] In advanced mitral regurgitation, it is also common for the patient to have a reduced cardiac output. During the catheterization procedure, the regurgitant fraction will also be calculated. The formula is as follows:

Regurgitant stroke volume = total left ventricular
stroke volume − forward stroke volume

Elevated a waves and a significant systolic pressure difference between the LV and aorta are the findings on catheterization that indicate aortic stenosis. Angiographically, the stenotic orifice can be visualized during systole along with the mobility of the cusps. Aortic regurgitation is determined by a widened aortic pulse pressure and elevated end-systolic volume. The amount of blood regurgitated can be as great as 60% or more of the forward stroke volume and occurs mainly in early diastole.

Left Ventriculography. Left ventriculography is also useful in providing the following information: (1) anatomy and function of the ventricle, (2) presence and location of ventricular aneurysms, (3) abnormalities in wall motion, (4) presence of ventricular septal defects, (5) calculation of LV wall thickness and mass, and (6) LV ejection fraction.

Abnormalities of wall motion are commonly seen in patients with prior myocardial infarcts. The critical care nurse should become familiar with such abnormalities. These abnormalities will be further discussed in Chapter 22 regarding myocardial infarction.

Coronary Arteriography

Coronary arteriography, developed by Sones in 1959, is usually performed to assess the coronary arterial circulation. This procedure defines the presence and extent of coronary arterial lesions. It also assists physicians to quantify the degree of stenosis as well as to assess collateral circulation. These findings are then used to determine the feasibility of performing percutaneous transluminal coronary angioplasty (PTCA), other procedures, or coronary artery bypass surgery (CABG). In addition, the presence of vasospasm can be determined by coronary arteriography.

Complications

The mortality associated with cardiac catheterization is relatively low. Morbidity noted with left heart catheterization is significantly greater than that noted with a right-sided procedure. One of the more serious complications associated with left heart catheterization via the femoral approach is the formation of a thrombus which can occlude the femoral artery. Careful vascular checks need to be performed. Dissection of a coronary artery also may occur with arteriography. Hemorrhage at the insertion site is another complication that necessitates applied pressure at the site of insertion upon withdrawal of the catheter.

Chest X-ray

The chest x-ray is a convenient, noninvasive method for assessing the cardiac silhouette, its chambers and great vessels, and the pulmonary system. Cardiac enlargement, valvular calcification, aortic dilatation, thoracic tumors, pulmonary infiltrate, pleural effusion, hemothorax, and pneumothorax are abnormalities commonly recognized with the standard posterior-anterior and lateral views. The radiographic findings of pulmonary edema, pulmonary hypertension, left-to-right cardiac shunts, and various types of congenital heart disease are also reasonably specific.

Portable chest films taken in the anterior-posterior (AP) view in the critical care setting are different from those posteroanterior (PA) films taken in the x-ray department. These AP films are taken in such a way that the x-ray beam passes from front to back instead of posteriorly to anteriorly, which places the heart farther from the x-ray film than in the PA projection and thus casts a larger shadow on the x-ray film. The result is that the AP film provides poor visualization of the cardiac silhouette, which limits its diagnostic value. Moreover, heart size cannot be compared accurately between AP and PA projections but can be compared with similar sequential AP or PA projections.[13]

The assessment of left ventricular function and pulmonary venous pressures from a chest x-ray lacks both sensitivity and specificity. A cardio-thoracic ratio (a technique used to measure overall cardiac size comparing the maximal cardiac diameter against the maximal thoracic diameter measured to the inner border of the ribs) of greater than 1:2 is a late sign of left ventricular failure and may also occur from right ventricular dilatation and pericardial effusions.[14] The estimation of pulmonary vein engorgement is subjective in light of the fact that an x-ray pattern of pulmonary edema may be present when the pulmonary venous pressure is normal. Fluid that leaks into the alveolar space may be noted on x-ray for up to 24 hours after pulmonary venous hypertension has been reversed, and noncardiac causes of pulmonary edema produce an x-ray picture of pulmonary edema with normal pulmonary venous pressure.[13]

Other extraneous findings that may be noted on chest x-ray include valvular prostheses, epicardial pacing wires, sternal closure wires after cardiac surgery, mediastinal or pleural chest tubes, endotracheal tubes, electrocardiogram leads, and pacemakers.

In the critical care setting, the patient should be positioned in an erect position if possible. The portable chest x-ray should be taken during deep inspiration because this is a factor that affects the size and contour of the heart.

Fast Computed Tomography

Fast computed tomography (CT) is a radiological diagnostic technique with a new application in the diagnosis of cardiovascular pathophysiology. Since cross-sectional views or slices of a targeted area can be obtained within 50 ms, the indication for this technology in assessing cardiac disorders has emerged.[15]

Other developments in this technology are the ability to obtain multiple gated views of the heart in accordance with the electrocardiogram (cine CT) and the advantage of using a contrast material to refine tomographic images. Cine CT provides data abstracted from multiple views of the heart obtained simultaneously and displays it in a "closed-loop cine format."[16] This technique has many applications in measuring cardiac volumes. Contrast-enhanced CT scans demonstrate a clear outline of the internal and external cardiac wall margins, thereby providing information regarding specific cardiac regions, chamber mass, and wall thickening.[15] Information about wall thickening is important when assessing myocardial function.

Indications for fast CT are as follows: (1) to identify ventricular aneurysms, intracardiac thrombus, wall dimension changes with systole and diastole, intracardiac masses, certain pericardial diseases; (2) to assess ventricular function; (3) to measure myocardial mass; (4) to determine graft patency after coronary artery bypass surgery; and (5) to document thoracic aortic disease.[16] Current research is examining the future applicability of this technology in assessing additional dimensions of cardiac disease such as myocardial perfusion.[17]

Echocardiography

Echocardiography is a noninvasive technique that uses high-frequency ultrasonic waves to yield information about cardiac structures and function. This technique employs a transducer capable of both sending and receiving sound waves. This transducer contains a piezoelectric substance which, when stimulated by an electric current, expands and contracts to produce mechanical energy which produces waves that are sent outward. Conversely, when a sound wave is reflected back toward the transducer, it converts this mechanical energy back into electric energy which can be recorded.

Feigenbaum[18] cites the advantages of using ultrasonic waves as being that (1) they are reflected by very small objects, (2) they can be directed, and (3) they obey the laws of reflection and refraction. The disadvantages are that they are poorly transmitted in a gaseous medium; therefore, good transducer-to-skin contact is imperative.

During an echocardiogram, the patient is placed in a supine position, and the transducer is placed on the chest wall. An ultrasonic coupling gel is used to facilitate sound wave transmission. The technician directs ultrasonic sound waves toward the heart and records the echos of these waves as they reflect back from various cardiac structures. This procedure is usually quick and painless for the patient.

Several types or modes of echocardiography are currently available: unidimensional, two-dimensional, Doppler, color Doppler flow mapping and transesophageal.

Unidimensional Echocardiograms

Three modes of unidimensional echocardiograms are available: A mode, B mode, and M mode. The A mode monitors the amplitude of returning signals or sound waves and converts them to spikes that can be visualized and recorded on an oscilloscope. The stronger the wave, the taller the height of the spike. The B mode transforms the returning sound waves to dots that are displayed on the oscilloscope, in which the stronger waves evidence brighter dots. Lastly, the M mode, which is the most common, records both amplitude and motion. The M-mode echocardiogram has the advantage of enabling the physician to study cardiac structures in motion as they function at various points in the cardiac cycle.

The M-mode echocardiogram uses a single beam of ultrasonic waves and measures the distance of structures from the transducer in a vertical axis with time on a horizontal axis. Therefore, although called unidimensional, M-mode echocardiography actually is composed of two dimensions, distance and time. The major disadvantage of this type of echocardiography is that it lacks spatial orientation. Figures 21-6 and 21-7 are examples of M-mode echocardiograms.

Two-dimensional Echocardiograms (2-D)

The two-dimensional or 2-D echocardiogram records returning sound waves on a planar image, thus allowing a spatial orientation for viewing cardiac structures. This is accomplished with a more advanced transducer that emits a planar beam of sound waves, not a single beam. The disadvantage of a 2-D echocardiogram is that it cannot record a complete heart chamber or valve as a whole. Composite views must be examined to avoid missing important data.

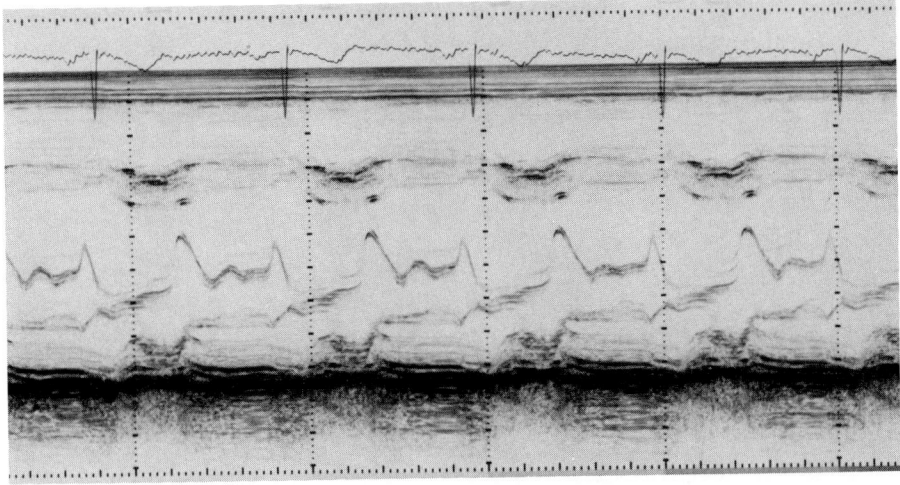

Figure 21-6   Normal mitral valve (M-mode echocardiogram).

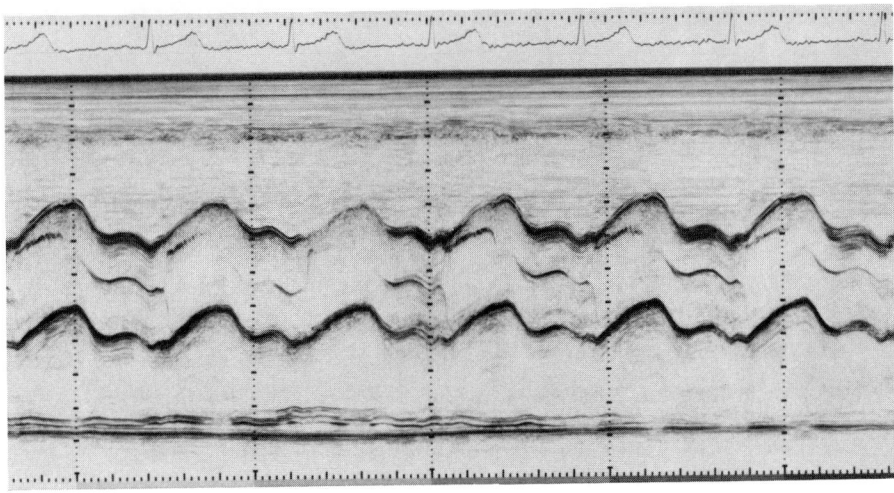

Figure 21-7   Normal aorta/aortic valve/left atrium (M-mode echo).

An example of this type of echocardiogram is found in Figure 21-8.

Doppler Echocardiograms

Unlike unidimensional and two-dimensional echocardiograms which record returning sound waves, Doppler echocardiograms record the velocity of moving objects by measuring the frequency of change of emitted and reflected ultrasonic waves. The clinical applicability of this technique is in assessing the circulation in peripheral arteries and veins, examining blood flow in the heart and great vessels, and in assessing regurgitant valvular disorders. The disadvantages of this technique are the following: (1) it cannot record a high velocity, (2) it cannot record velocities that lie within structures greater than 13 cm from the transducer, (3) it cannot be recorded on a graphic display, and (4) much variability exists with the dif-

ferent angles at which the transducer is held.

A new development in this field has been the introduction of pulsed Doppler echocardiography. When combined with the previously described continuous Doppler technique, pulsed Doppler echocardiography has the advantage of recording views of the heart while also examining Doppler signals.

Color Doppler Flow Mapping

Color Doppler flow mapping is an advance in technology used in ultrasonography. Its major advantage is that it provides a spatial display of low velocities in relation to surrounding structural detail. This combination of structure and flow allows a more precise study of the patterns of intracardiac flow.[19] Clinical applications of this technique are the assessment of valvular disorders and septal defects.

This technique employs a pulsed mode. Pulses are

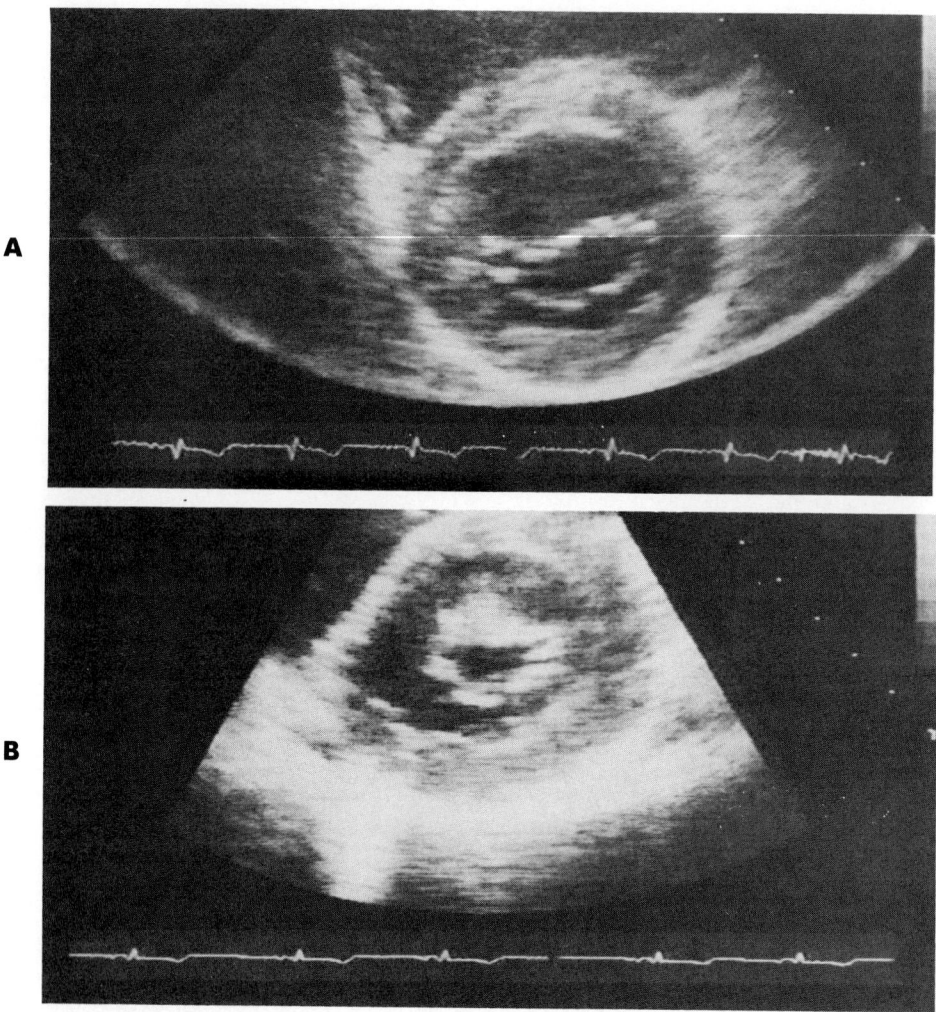

Figure 21-8   *A,* Normal mitral valve parasternal short axis (2-D echocardiogram). *B,* Mitral stenosis (2-D echocardiogram).

delivered sequentially. Spatial information is gained first, and the remainder of the pulses reveal data on hemodynamic flow.

Flow velocities are color-coded in two ways. The first color codes blood flow in relation to the transducer. One color is assigned to blood flowing toward the transducer and a second to blood flowing away from the transducer. The second manner by which color is coded is in accordance with velocity variance. This technology color-codes flow according to the variance within the flow itself. Flow that is irregular and turbulent has a high degree of variance. Different colors are assigned to the differing rates of flow variance. Both types of data are useful when studying valvular lesions.

Flow velocities are further evaluated by digital computer analysis. This technology examines the color-coded flow velocities in two ways. Each color may be illustrated separately or the intensities of the differing flow velocities may be quantified. This information aids data interpretation.

Transesophageal Echocardiography

Transesophageal echocardiography (TEE) is a new application of echocardiography in the diagnosis of cardiac conditions. This invasive technique employs the antegrade passage of a flexible echoscope, similar to a gastroscope but equipped with an ultrasound transducer at its tip. Once it is positioned, echocardiographic views of the left ventricle may be gained. Upon withdrawal of the scope, both ventricles and atria, the mitral, aortic, and tricuspid valves, and the thoracic aorta can be visualized.[20] The procedure requires local oropharyngeal anesthesia. Although it is generally associated with only minor complications such as hoarseness or atrial dysrhythmias, vocal paralysis has been reported.[20]

The indications for TEE are evolving with the technology. Current indications are as follows: intracardiac vegetations; prosthetic cardiac valve function; intraatrial thrombus or mass; congenital heart defects, especially atrial septal defects and partial anomalous pulmonary venous return; dissection of the thoracic aorta; inconclusive transthoracic echocardiography; and valve anatomy before and after valvuloplasty.[20] In addition, intraoperative TEE has been employed to diagnose prosthetic valve failure[21] and perioperative myocardial infarction.[22,23] Some data suggest that TEE is superior to transthoracic echocardiography in some patients.[20,24,25,26] Last, TEE can employ color flow Doppler technology to reveal data about valvular incompetence and septal integrity.[27]

Clinical Applications

Echocardiography can be used for noninvasive study of cardiac function, valvular disorders, complications resulting from a myocardial infarction, the functional effects of ischemia, cardiomyopathy, pericardial effusions, endocarditis, and congenital heart defects.

Cardiac Function Assessment. Information regarding left ventricular performance can be calculated with the aid of echocardiography. A shortening fraction which reflects performance, similar to an ejection fraction, can be estimated from measurements of the left ventricular end-systolic (DES) and end-diastolic dimensions (DED) gained from an echocardiogram.

Mitral Stenosis. Both the M-mode and 2-D echo are useful in evaluating mitral stenosis (MS). Evidence of fibrosis or calcification of the valve leaflets which commonly is found in MS exists when there is an increased number of reflected echos. Thickening of the leaflets, minimal leaflet separation during diastole, and abnormal valve motions are other M-mode findings of MS. Two-D echocardiography can also quantify the size of the valve orifice.

Other echocardiographic data to support the existence of MS are the effect of MS on other cardiac structures. Left atrial dilatation and occasional pulmonary hypertension as a result of the outflow obstruction caused by MS may be documented. Figures 21-8A and 21-8B illustrate normal and stenotic mitral valves.

Finally, Feigenbaum[28] reports that the echocardiogram is useful to evaluate whether a mitral valve replacement (MVR) or a commissurotomy is required for MS. Likewise, information gained by echocardiography is useful in determining the feasibility of valvuloplasty. Both commissurotomy and valvuloplasty require a noncalcified, nonregurgitant valvular apparatus. An in-depth discussion regarding this valvular defect is found in Chapter 24.

Mitral Regurgitation. Regurgitant lesions are better evaluated by Doppler echocardiography than by other modes of echocardiography because this method detects turbulent blood flow indicative of these lesions. Two-dimensional and unidimensional echocardiography can provide data to support the diagnosis of mitral regurgitation (MR) by assessing left atrial dilatation. This occurs as the left atrium expands to compensate for the regurgitant volume. An increased left ventricular stroke volume is recorded as blood exits the left ventricle through two outflow tracts, normally via the aortic valve and abnormally through the incompetent mitral valve. Lastly, an increased left ventricular end-diastolic dimension is noted due to the increased volume in the left ventricle. Refer to Chapter 24 for more information regarding MR.

Mitral Valve Prolapse. Because of changes in the mitral valve structure, the mitral valve balloons or protrudes backward into the left atrium during ventricular systole in mitral valve prolapse (MVP). Both 2-D and M-mode echocardiograms are helpful in documenting the abnormal backward motion of the mitral valve in MVP. More information on MVP is located in Chapter 24.

Aortic Stenosis. The diagnosis of aortic stenosis (AS) via echocardiographic data is supported by the findings of thickened and/or calcified leaflets, decreased separation of the leaflets during systole, and doming of the valve on the 2-D echocardiogram. Absence of these characteristics does not completely exclude the diagnosis, however. Figures 21-9A and 21-9B contrast a normal and a stenotic aortic valve.

Pulsed Doppler echocardiography may be helpful in the diagnosis of AS by documenting turbulent blood flow in the aorta. Lastly, the presence of left ventricular hypertrophy, secondary to this outflow tract obstruction, can often be calculated with echocardiography. More information on AS may be found in Chapter 24.

Aortic Insufficiency. As in mitral regurgitation, Doppler echocardiography is useful in assessing the turbulent blood flow that results from the regurgitant lesion of aortic insufficiency (AI). Direct evaluation of AI by echocardiography is not a useful technique; therefore, indirect assessment of the secondary effects of AI on the left ventricle and mitral valve serves as supportive data for this disorder. Dilatation of the left ventricle due to volume overload as well as heightened septal motion reflect AI. Lastly, fluttering of the mitral valve from the regurgitant diastolic flow through an incompetent aortic valve is diagnostic of AI.

The usefulness of echocardiography in determining the optimum time for an aortic valve replacement is documented by Feigenbaum[28] and Fernandez.[29] Aortic insufficiency is further discussed in Chapter 24.

Tricuspid and Pulmonic Valvular Disorders. Tricuspid stenosis exhibits motion abnormality on an echocardiogram similar to that of mitral stenosis. Evidence of tricuspid regurgitation can be found by calculating the degree of secondary right ventricular di-

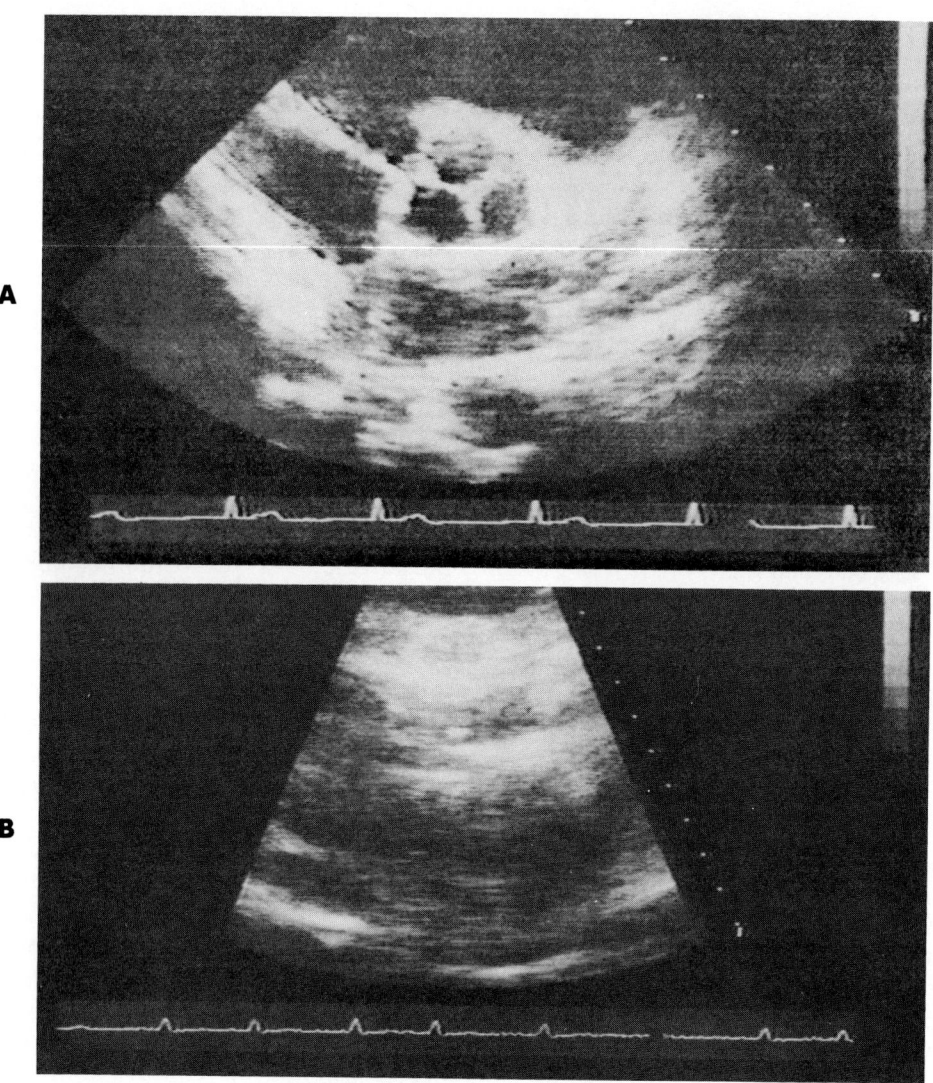

Figure 21-9 *A,* Normal aortic valve (2-D echo) contrasted with *B,* aortic stenosis.

latation from volume overload and the degree of turbulent regurgitant blood flow by Doppler echocardiography. The pulsed Doppler echocardiogram also aids in the diagnosis of pulmonic valvular regurgitation.

Septal Defects. Wenger and Hellerstein[30] report that ventricular septal defects occur in about 1% of patients who sustain an acute transmural MI. Echocardiography is very useful in isolating the defect and documenting the amount of shunted blood. Two-D echocardiography is useful in identifying both ventricular and atrial septal defects by direct visualization. The M-mode echocardiogram provides data to support this diagnosis by evaluating the hemodynamic consequences of enlargement in chambers affected by the shunt. Doppler echocardiography is also useful in evaluating turbulent bloodflow that results

from shunting of blood through a septal defect.

Lastly, a technique called *contrast echocardiography* is helpful in evaluating shunts. In this technique, agitated normal saline solution is injected via a brachial vein. The path of the bubbled normal saline solution is followed on an echocardiogram. Shunts are detected if bubbles traverse the septum and do not follow the normal pathway.

Papillary Muscle Rupture. Necrosis of the left ventricular papillary muscles is common with an acute MI and exceeds a 50% incidence in patients with a fatal MI, but papillary muscle rupture occurs in less than 1% of patients who sustain a fatal MI[30] Echocardiographic evidence of papillary muscle rupture consists of prolapsing of a part of a mitral valve leaflet during systole.

Aneurysm. The incidence of a ventricular aneurysm secondary to a transmural MI is approximately 20% as supported by Wenger and Hellerstein.[30] Echocardiography is useful in estimating the size of an aneurysm as well as myocardial function. Feigenbaum[28] states that 2-D echocardiography is superior to M-mode echocardiography in detecting these abnormalities and in assessing residual ventricular function. An aneurysm is suspected if there is dilatation, thinning, and dyskinesis of a part of the ventricular wall. For more information regarding complications of an MI, refer to Chapter 22.

Evaluating Thrombi. Thrombi can be clearly visualized by use of echocardiography as their densities reflect echoes. Because 15% to 20% of patients with an acute myocardial infarction develop thrombi,[29] the echocardiogram may be useful in documenting thrombosis and guiding management.

Evaluating Ischemia. During systole, the left ventricular wall normally thickens. Ischemic tissue does not thicken during systole and can therefore be identified and quantified by echocardiography.

Cardiomyopathy. Two types of cardiomyopathies can be evaluated with the aid of echocardiography, *dilated* (congestive) and *hypertrophic*. In dilated cardiomyopathy, echocardiographic findings reveal a dilated and poorly functioning left ventricle with possible involvement of other cardiac chambers as well as the mitral valve. While 2-D and M-mode echocardiography evaluate chamber changes, pulsed Doppler echocardiography is useful in assessing coexisting mitral regurgitation.

Echocardiographic findings in patients with hypertrophic cardiomyopathy illustrate left ventricular hypertrophy. In contrast to the findings noted in dilated cardiomyopathy, there is no cardiac enlargement, and a hypercontractile state exists.

The echocardiogram is the "gold standard" for diagnosing one form of hypertrophic cardiomyopathy, idiopathic hypertrophic subaortic stenosis (IHSS). Two classic features of IHSS are abnormal septal hypertrophy, causing an outflow obstruction of the left ventricle, and an abnormal systolic anterior motion (SAM) of the mitral valve secondary to this obstruction. Early midsystolic closure of the aortic valve may also be present secondary to the outflow obstruction. For additional information on cardiomyopathies, refer to Chapter 23.

Pericardial Effusions. Pericardial effusions can be visualized on both M-mode and 2-D echocardiograms. Two-D echocardiograms, however, allow for the most accurate quantification of pericardial effusions, especially if the fluid is loculated. Since fluid is less dense than tissue, a pericardial effusion appears on an echocardiogram as an echo-free space between the pericardium and the epicardium. Feigenbaum[18]

states that the echo helps differentiate cardiac tamponade from an effusion, which is noted as compression of the right ventricle.

Endocarditis. Vegetations associated with valvular endocarditis can often be recorded by echocardiography. If present, the vegetations usually affect one valve leaflet to a greater degree than others and appear asymmetrical. When valvular function is impaired, secondary changes in cardiac chambers may be recorded on the echocardiogram. Absence of these findings, however, does not entirely rule out the possibility of endocarditis.

Electrocardiography

Electrocardiography depicts important information regarding the electrical forces produced by the heart during the cardiac cycle. The electrocardiogram (ECG) is a simple, noninvasive recording taken from the body surface in contrast to atrial electrograms or His bundle recordings, which are taken within the tissue. Refer to Chapter 10 for a more in-depth discussion regarding electrocardiography.

The ECG is useful as a clinical tool in depicting abnormalities associated with certain cardiac pathology. For example, atrial enlargement and ventricular or biventricular hypertrophy can be detected on an ECG. These chamber enlargements may be related to a valvular defect, systemic or pulmonary hypertension, heart failure, or a cardiomyopathy. Specific ECG changes relating to coronary artery disease, valvular defects, hypertension, and cardiomyopathy are discussed in the relevant chapters.

In addition to being used as a diagnostic tool, the ECG is also affected by drugs and electrolytes. Drugs such as digoxin and quinidine alter the normal appearance of an ECG. Digoxin, for example, produces a scooping effect in the ST segment, and quinidine prolongs the QT interval. Electrolytes such as potassium and calcium also affect the ECG. Variations in potassium levels produce changes in T wave morphology (hyperkalemia) or the appearance of U waves (hypokalemia). Calcium levels either shorten (hypercalcemia) or lengthen (hypocalcemia) the QT interval.

Caution needs to be exercised in relying on the ECG. Although the 12 leads provide 12 different views of the heart in assessing for abnormalities, the ECG alone should not be used to make a clinical diagnosis.

Electrophysiological Studies

Cardiac electrophysiology is a recently developed discipline in cardiology and cardiovascular nursing. Simply defined, it is "the direct study and manipulation of the electrical activity of the heart utilizing electrodes placed inside the cardiac chambers."[31] This technique provides information regarding sinus node function, atrioventricular conduction, and tachyarrhythmias. Cardiac electrophysiology guides medical therapy by yielding data regarding the effectiveness of different antiarrhythmic drugs on tachyarrhythmias and determines which type of pacemaker is most effective in terminating sustained tachydyserhythmias. Lastly, through the technique of cardiac mapping, cardiac electrophysiology assists in locating the origin of dangerous, repetitive dysrhythmias and in directing surgical interventions.

A cardiac electrophysiological study is performed in a controlled environment. It requires the use of catheters with multiple electrodes at their distal ends capable of stimulating the heart and of recording its response. Figure 21-10 illustrates common placement sites for these catheters. Michelson, Spielman, and Greenspan[32] point out that the catheter may be placed within the outflow tract of the right ventricle as well as the left ventricle, but the more common sites are high in the right atrium, across the tricuspid valve, in the apex of the right ventricle, and in the coronary sinus.

The catheter electrodes are then connected to a switchbox. The switchbox designates the electrode used for monitoring and stimulating. It is connected to a console that records and displays electrical activity on an oscilloscope.

Passive Applications of Cardiac Electrophysiology

Vacek, Smith, and Phillips[31] classifed the uses of cardiac electrophysiology into three categories: passive, active, and interventional (refer to the box below for a complete list). The *passive* applications of cardiac electrophysiology are merely observational. The catheter electrodes record the electrical activity in different cardiac structures. If an abnormal pathway exists such as in heart block or conduction via an ac-

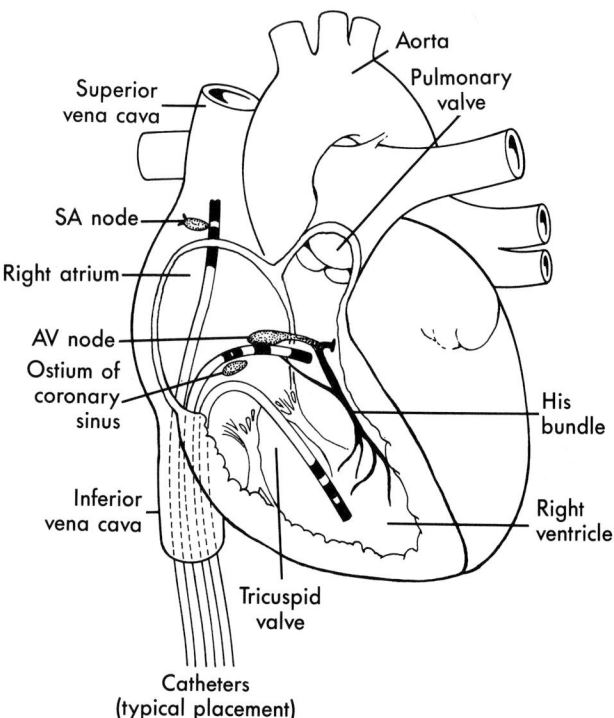

Figure 21-10   Common placement sites for catheters used in electrophysiological studies.

Adapted from Vacek, J., Smith, W., & Phillips, J. (1984). Cardiac electrophysiology: An overview. *Practical Cardiology, 10*(13), 83-97.

Applications of Cardiac Electrophysiology

PASSIVE

Intrinsic pacemaker site and activity

Sequence of atrial, conducting-system, and ventricular activation

Characteristics of AV node and His bundle

Observation of spontaneous phenomena
Heart block
Intraatrial or intraventricular conduction abnormalities
Tachydysrhythmias

Overt bypass-tract presence and position

ACTIVE

SA-node function and conduction of impulses through peri-SA-node tissues (sinus-node recovery time, SA conduction time, response to carotid-sinus massage or drugs) (direct measurement of SA-node activity still experimental)

AV-node and His bundle properties in response to pacing or premature stimuli (or both) (internal changes and assessment of dual AV-node pathways)

Tachycardia initiation and termination

Concealed bypass-tract presence and position; response of both overt and concealed bypass tracts to pacing or premature stimuli (or both)

Mapping of endocardium for sites of tachycardia initiation and wavefront propagation characteristics

INTERVENTIONAL

Trials of the effects of drugs on induced tachyarrhythmias or on conduction properties of various portions of the cardiac electrical system

Consideration of efficacy and practicality of implantable pacemakers and defibrillators

Cold ablation (cryoablation) or electrical (direct-current shock) ablation of AV node or bypass tracts when part of a reentrant tachycardiac circuit is unresponsive to pharmacological manipulation

From Vacek, J., Smith, W., & Phillips, J. (1984). Cardiac electrophysiology: An overview. *Practical Cardiology, 10*(13), 83-97.

cessory pathway, it is recorded. Since such events may be transient, they often go undetected when only passive cardiac electrophysiology is employed.

Active Applications of Cardiac Electrophysiology

During cardiac electrophysiological testing, the heart can be stimulated and its response assessed, which is helpful in provoking transient dysrhythmias. Sinus node disorders, atrioventricular conduction disturbances, supraventricular tachycardias (SVT), and ventricular tachycardias (VT) can be evaluated with this technique.

Ventricular Tachycardia. For patients with a history of malignant ventricular tachycardias, provoking the dysrhythmia and studying its cause and the location of origin yield valuable information to guide therapy. A number of protocols for programmed premature stimulation exist, all of which require a basic rhythm that is either sinus or paced. A ventricular or atrial premature beat is then stimulated to occur in late diastole. This beat is then programmed to occur earlier and closer to the T wave of the previous beat until the effective refractory beat is reached or the desired rhythm provoked. The effective refractory period is the longest distance between the patient's baseline rhythm and a programmed extra systole that does not produce a ventricular response. If one extra systole fails to produce a ventricular response, the procedure is repeated with a second or third programmed beat.

The desired end point when evaluating patients with a history of malignant ectopy is usually to elicit VT. Podrid and Lambert[33] report that, if well tolerated, this rhythm can be terminated in 88% of patients with a programmed extra systole. To decrease the risk of provoking sustained VT, some authorities use nonsustained VT as an end point.

In addition to studying factors affecting VT, cardiac electrophysiology employs mapping to locate the origin of the VT reentrant dysrhythmia. Two types of mapping techniques exist: endocardial and epicardial.

In *endocardial mapping*, several percutaneous electrodes are implanted on the heart, approximately 15 to 20 sites on the left ventricle, 3 on the right, and 3 sites over any aneurysm. Recordings are taken with the patient in sinus rhythm and again during VT. The location of the earliest activation time correlates to the location of the reentry circuit. During the mapping, which is a surgical procedure, the location is verified with a finger probe which measures the activation time in the endocardium.

Epicardial mapping is also performed during surgery and involves applying electrodes directly to the epicardium. Again, the earliest activation time is sought. Since mapping is performed while the patient is on bypass, bypass time is lengthened. A prolonged bypass time exposes the patient to a number of potential complications. Podrid and Lambert[33] also report that in 10% to 15% of these patients, VT cannot be replicated; therefore, the origin cannot be identified.

Supraventricular Tachycardia. Cardiac electrophysiological studies are used to define the mechanism of supraventricular tachycardia (SVT) and, therefore, are helpful in treating patients with symptomatic medical refractory SVT. AV nodal reentry (Chapter 10) is the most common cause of SVT as supported by Denes and Ezri,[34] and Kienzle et al.[35] This reentry circuit can be located in the AV node or accessory pathways between the atria and ventricles. These pathways are endowed with different properties of conduction. Once the mechanism responsible for the SVT is isolated, drug therapy aimed at the specific site of the problem can be instituted.

Drugs affecting the AV node are employed if the node is the site of reentry. Digoxin, verapamil, and beta-blocking medications prolong the conduction time and refractory period of the AV node and may be helpful. If the problem is the retrograde accessory pathways, drugs such as procainamide, quinidine, and disopramide, which alter the conduction properties of the retrograde pathway, may be used.[35]

Cardiac electrophysiological studies are useful in guiding therapy in patients with a preexcitation syndrome. These patients experience dysrhythmias secondary to accessory pathways. Ezri[36] states that the major benefit of studying this group of patients is to avoid using drugs that may exacerbate the dysrhythmia.

Atrioventricular Conduction Disturbances. Cardiac electrophysiological studies are useful to examine transient conduction disturbances, to locate the site of the disturbance, and to discern the need for permanent pacemaker implantation. This technique is helpful in evoking transient His-Purkinje disease for which a permanent pacemaker may be indicated. It is also useful in evaluating symptomatic patients with bifascicular block to determine the need for permanent pacing. Lastly, this technique is beneficial in assessing asymptomatic patients with chronic heart block.

Sinus Node Disorders. The usefulness of cardiac electrophysiological testing for sinus node dysfunction or sick sinus syndrome is controversial because this dysrhythmia is often identified by less invasive techniques. Denes and Ezri[34] and Ezri[36] believe the decision regarding pacemaker use in these patients should be based on clinical symptomatology at the time of occurrence of bradydysrhythmias.

Cardiac electrophysiological testing is useful in patients with undocumented cardiac syncope. It provides objective data regarding sinus node function.

Applications of Cardiac Electrophysiology

Assessing the Effectiveness of Antiarrhythmic Therapies. Cardiac electrophysiological studies provide objective data regarding the effectiveness of antiarrhythmic medications. Data from certain investigators have shown that antiarrhythmic therapy may potentiate dysrhythmias.[37] Although work by Naccarelli et al.[38] alludes to the benefits of basing antidysrhythmic treatment on the data obtained from electrophysiological study, the effectiveness of this approach remains controversial.[39]

Determining the Mode of Implantable Pacemakers/Defibrillators. Pacemakers can terminate dysrhythmias by a number of mechanisms: overdrive pacing, underdrive pacing, or direct countershock. Cardiac electrophysiological testing helps determine which pacemaker mode is most effective in terminating a patient's dysrhythmia and, thus, guides therapy.

Cold or Electrical Ablation. Electrophysiological testing is used in extreme circumstances to isolate and destroy accessory pathways of the arrhythmogenic area by cryoablation or direct electric shock. Careful studies of the patient's coronary circulation need to be conducted prior to the procedure. This procedure is contraindicated if the area is located near a major artery due to the threat of a significant myocardial infarction.

Complications

At present, there are insufficient data regarding the risk of cardiac electrophysiological testing. Kaufman and Schwartz[40] report a 1% to 2% morbidity rate. Potential complications secondary to cardiac electrophysiological testing are the following: excessive bleeding, hematoma formation at the catheter insertion site, catheter-induced vascular dissection, phlebitis, thrombophlebitis, pneumothorax, and pulmonary emboli. The risk of cardiac perforation and infection is small. The need for cardioversion from sustained VT or fibrillation is approximately 20%, as cited by Podrid and Lambert.[33]

Hemodynamic Monitoring

Invasive hemodynamic monitoring in the critical care setting has become a safe, convenient bedside technique used to monitor pressures and waveforms in critically ill patients. On-line continuous monitoring is invaluable when caring for the critically ill in whom hemodynamics may change rapidly. Through the use of various catheters, the critical care team is provided with valuable information concerning pressures, waveforms, oxygen saturation, cardiac outputs, and venous or arterial blood gas parameters.

Therapy in the critically ill patient is often directed at maintaining an adequate cardiac output. Variables that directly regulate cardiac output include stroke volume, preload, afterload, contractility, and heart rate (Chapter 20). Heart rate is controlled by both the parasympathetic and sympathetic nervous systems. Changes in rate brought on by neural control directly affect cardiac output by altering ventricular filling time. For example, in the setting of bradycardia (parasympathetic influence) the ventricular filling time is prolonged, whereas a tachycardia (sympathetic influence) reduces it. Alterations in ventricular filling time will in turn affect stroke volume and subsequently cardiac output. In the setting of diminished cardiac output, both direct and indirect, or derived, parameters are useful in assessing preload, afterload, and contractility which determine appropriate therapy.

Right ventricular preload is usually assessed in the critical care setting using such parameters as central venous pressure (CVP) or right atrial pressure (RAP). However, the recent advent of a new pulmonary artery catheter will enable clinicians to assess right ventricular end-diastolic volume, right ventricular stroke volume, and ejection fraction of the right heart.[41] Parameters used to assess left ventricular preload include pulmonary artery end-diastolic pressure (PAEDP), pulmonary artery wedge pressure (PAWP), and left atrial pressure (LAP). The parameters that are used to reflect right or left ventricular afterload, respectively, are pulmonary arterial pressure, pulmonary vascular resistance, aortic end-diastolic pressure, and systemic vascular resistance. Lastly, right and left ventricular stroke work and cardiac work indices are the derived parameters used to indirectly assess contractility in the critical care setting. Another derived parameter that can be obtained via hemodynamic monitoring is the rate–pressure product (RPP), which is used as an indirect determinant of myocardial O_2 consumption (Chapter 20).

Arterial Line (A-line) Catheter

Use of an indwelling arterial catheter (A-line) is common in many critical care units. These catheters permit constant monitoring of peripheral arterial pressures and frequent blood sampling. Indwelling arterial catheters can be placed in the radial, ulnar, brachial, femoral, or pedal artery, either percutaneously or via a surgical cutdown procedure. The radial artery is the site most frequently cannulated. Prior to radial insertion, the Allen's test should be performed to assess circulation to the distal extremity.

In addition to these intraarterial catheters, the central aorta can be cannulated with an intraaortic balloon (IAB) catheter. This catheter has two lumens: one that transports gas to and from the balloon, and a second one which serves as a central aortic A-line.

The data that can be obtained from an A-line are

systolic, diastolic, and mean pressures. These pressures are discussed in more detail later in this section.

The most frequent complication of arterial line use results from accidental disconnection of the catheter from the transducer. This complication can be minimized if careful attention is paid to maintenance of intact connections. Other complications of A-line use are thrombus, local obstruction with resultant distal ischemia, embolization, and infection.

Right Atrial or Central Venous Pressure Catheters

Right atrial pressure (RAP) catheters or central venous pressure (CVP) catheters are used to measure the mean pressure of the right atrium. The RAP or CVP measurement is obtained by either a water manometer or a transducer. If a water manometer is used, the reading is recorded in cmH_2O. If, however, the transducer is employed, the reading will be recorded in mmHg. Due to the different molecular weights of substances (water or mercury) used to obtain the measurement, the readings are not interchangeable. Because mercury is 1.34 times heavier than water, conversion from a mercury reading to a water reading requires multiplying the pressure by 1.34.

Example: 7 mmHg × 1.34 = 9.38 cmH_2O

As with arterial catheters, RAP catheters can be inserted in a variety of sites. The subclavian vein is the optimum site for RAP catheter insertion, although cannulation of the internal jugular, cephalic, antecubital, basilic, saphenous, and femoral veins are alternatives. The approach taken can be either by percutaneous or surgical cutdown procedure. Once inserted, a confirmatory chest x-ray is required to verify the position of the catheter. Some complications associated with RAP catheter insertion and position include pneumothorax, hemothorax, pulmonary embolism, perforation of the right atrium or ventricle, air embolism, and cardiac tamponade.

Pulmonary Artery Catheter

A pulmonary artery (PA) catheter is a flow-directed, balloon-tipped catheter. This catheter measures the pressure in the right side of the heart and in the pulmonary vasculature. Newer generations of these catheters include (1) the thermodilution pulmonary artery pacing catheter, which permits ventricular pacing; (2) a fiberoptic catheter that allows continuous monitoring of mixed venous oxygen saturation ($S\bar{v}O_2$); (3) a catheter with additional lumen ports for fluid resuscitation; and (4) a catheter that calculates right ventricular stroke volume, right ventricular end-diastolic volume and pressure, and right ventricular ejection fraction.[41]

Before any type of PA catheter is inserted, the patient must be assessed for underlying complete left bundle branch block (LBBB), because there is a small risk of developing a right bundle branch block (RBBB) during insertion, and complete heart block might result. Hurst[42] advocates the prophylactic insertion of a temporary pacemaker or a pacing thermodilution PA catheter in patients with a preexisting LBBB. An alternative in patients with an LBBB is to have an external transthoracic pacemaker on standby during the insertion.

A pulmonary artery catheter may be inserted via a brachial, subclavian, or femoral vein and is advanced into the right atrium, through the tricuspid valve into the right ventricle, and finally out the pulmonic valve into the pulmonary artery. When the catheter is traversing the right ventricle, the small balloon at its distal end is inflated to allow the normal cardiac circulation to direct the catheter into the pulmonary artery, and to minimize the potential of catheter-induced ventricular irritability. Pressure readings from the RV are obtained only on insertion of the catheter.

Once the catheter is in the pulmonary artery, systolic, diastolic, mean, and wedge pressures can be obtained. The pulmonary artery wedge pressure (PAWP) can be obtained by inflating the balloon at the distal tip of the catheter with air, permitting the pulmonary artery catheter to advance until it occludes a pulmonary arterial branch. When the balloon is inflated, blood flow in this branch is impeded from the right side of the heart toward the lungs. The distal part of the catheter records the pressure that is reflected backward through the capillary bed from the left atrium. During diastole, the mitral valve opens, allowing the pressure in the left ventricle to be transmitted through the left atrium backward against the tip of the pulmonary artery catheter. This reflected left ventricular pressure is captured by the catheter when the balloon is inflated and is referred to as the pulmonary artery wedge pressure (PAWP). Once the catheter has been inserted, a confirmatory chest x-ray is necessary for validation of placement if fluoroscopy has not been used.

Special attention should be paid to the potential problems associated with the use of these catheters, which include (1) catheter-induced ventricular irritability, which may warrant that lidocaine be kept at the bedside during insertion; (2) catheter whip artifact caused by acceleration forces induced by ventricular systole, which may require high-frequency filters; (3) balloon rupture, which requires careful attention to prevention of overinflation; and (4) catheter migration to other areas, which requires repositioning of catheters and documentation of proper placement by chest x-ray. Complications associated with PA catheter use include infection, pulmonary infarction, pulmonary artery rupture, pulmonary embolism, and air embolism.

Left Atrial Catheter

The left atrial (LA) catheter may be inserted in some patients following cardiac surgery. While the distal end of the LA catheter lies in the left atrial appendage, it exits through a small incision to the right of the mediastinal incision near the epigastric area and permits recording of left atrial pressures (LAP).

Because the LA line enters the left heart circulation, the presence of any foreign material such as air or debris poses the risk of embolization to the brain or coronary arteries, and therefore the LA line should be inspected frequently. Gentle aspiration of foreign material is imperative. In addition, the administration of any drugs through this catheter is usually not permitted. Complications associated with use of the LA catheter include emboli, infection, bleeding associated with withdrawal, and cardiac tamponade.

Special Considerations Regarding Monitoring Systems

In assembling the equipment for hemodynamic monitoring, sterile technique needs to be maintained. Before hemodynamic monitoring is initiated, each transducer must be leveled, balanced, and calibrated. Leveling is performed so that the transducer will be positioned at the height of the right atrium. The most accurate method to accomplish this is to position the air–fluid interface of the transducer stopcock at the fourth intercostal space in the midaxillary line. This location is often referred to as the phlebostatic axis. Balancing refers to a zero reference (usually atmospheric pressure). This is attained by positioning the transducer stopcock so that the transducer is opened to air. The transducer is then calibrated to a known pressure. The procedure varies with each monitor; moreover, some newer monitors have internal calibration factors. It is recommended that specific guidelines by each manufacturer be followed.

Once these tasks have been accomplished, the system must be kept patent by a constant flow of solution (may or may not contain heparin) via an intraflow device. This device allows for a constant flow of 3 to 4 ml per hour. This flush solution also needs to be pressurized by some means to prevent backup of blood into the catheter.

Certain considerations need to be addressed to ensure accuracy of pressure readings. These include (1) catheter and tubing length, (2) type of tubing used, (3) catheter diameter, (4) secure connections, and (5) air bubbles and blood clots. The catheter and tubing length should be kept to a minimum. Tubing that is too long may result in an overshoot of the systolic

pressures and lowering of diastolic pressures. Therefore, the recommended length of tubing is 3 to 4 feet. The tubing must also be stiff and noncompliant because soft, compliant tubing may cause distortion by absorbing transmitted pressure. This in turn will create falsely low pressure readings. The diamter of the catheter is probably of least importance than others. In the clinical setting, there is a trade-off between using a large-size catheter which ensures an adequate signal transmission, or a smaller catheter which reduces the risk of thrombosis. Catheter size is thus largely dependent on physician preference and the size of the patient's vessels.

Air bubbles and blood clots pose an additional problem in that both are compressible and produce a decrease in the amplitude of the wave. Thus, the critical care nurse needs to eliminate each.

In addition to these considerations, the critical care nurse needs to take special precautions regarding electrical hazards. There is an inherent risk for developing microshock in patients with catheters placed directly in the heart.

Hemodynamic Parameters

In the critical care unit, it is important for nurses to be able to identify, monitor, and interpret hemodynamic parameters. This section focuses on only those parameters that assess cardiac output, stroke volume, preload, afterload, contractility, and myocardial oxygen consumption. A summary of these parameters is found in Table 21-3 along with normal values and formulas.

Cardiac Output. The cardiac output is obtained via the pulmonary artery catheter using the thermodilution method, which involves injecting a solution of known temperature into the blood and measuring the resultant change downstream. Iced or room temperature solution is injected via the proximal port of the PA catheter, producing a temperature change in the blood that is detected by a thermistor located at the distal end of the catheter. A computer records the thermodilution curve and calculates a digital value from the area under this curve.[43] It is recommended that the injectate be injected in less than 4 seconds to prevent distortion of the temperature concentration curve. It has been suggested that CO be measured during end-expiration. Riedinger and Shellock[44] dispute the necessity of taking CO at end-expiration because most current CO computers correct for the potential problem of respiratory-associated baseline drift by electronically averaging the blood temperature over a shortened time period prior to the injection of indicator solution. This averaging offers a stable baseline during the period of cardiac output measurement, eliminating the need for proper timing of the injection.

TABLE 21-3 **Summary of Hemodynamic Parameters**

	Normal Values	Calculations	Definition
CO	4-8 L/min	SV × HR	Blood ejected from the heart into systemic circulation per minute
CI	2.5-4.0 L/min	$\dfrac{CO}{BSA}$	Cardiac output adjusted for body size
SV	60-135 ml per beat	$\dfrac{CO \times 1000}{HR}$	Volume of blood ejected from the ventricle per beat
SVI	45-85 ml/m² per beat	$\dfrac{SV}{BSA}$	Stroke volume adjusted for body size
CVP	2-6 mmHg 2.7-12 cmH₂O	1 mmHg = 13.6 mmH₂O or 1.36 cmH₂O	Reflects filling pressure of RV and mean pressure of systemic veins (i.e., venous return)
PAEDP	8-10 mmHg		Reflects filling pressure to LV (usually 1 to 5 mmHg higher than PAWP)
PAWP	5-15 mmHg		Reflects filling pressure of LV if no obstruction exists between catheter balloon tip and LV (i.e., mitral stenosis)
PVR	155-255 dyn/sec/cm⁻⁵	$\dfrac{(PAM - PAWP) \times 80.0}{CO}$	Resistance to RV ejection offered by pulmonary pressure
SVR	950-1,300 dyn/sec/cm⁻⁵	$\dfrac{(MAP - CVP) \times 80.0}{CO}$	Resistance to LV ejection offered by aortic pressure
RVSWI	8.5-12 g-m/m²	$\dfrac{RVSW}{BSA}$	Work performed by RV to generate pressure per beat, adjusted for body size
RCWI	0.54-0.66 kg-m/m²	$\dfrac{CO \times PAP_m \times 0.0136}{BSA}$	Work performed by RV to generate pressure per minute adjusted for body size
LVSWI	35-85 g-m/m²	$\dfrac{LVSW}{BSA}$	Work performed by LV to generate pressure per beat, adjusted for body size
LCWI	3.4-4.2 kg-m/m²	$\dfrac{CO \times MAP \times 0.0136}{BSA}$	Work performed by LV to generate pressure per minute adjusted for body size
RPP	<12,000	SYS. BP × HR	Indirect determinant of MVo₂ consumption
EF	60% to 75%	$\dfrac{\genfrac{}{}{0pt}{}{(LVEDV)}{RVEDV}}{SV} \times 100$	Percentage of the total (LVEDV) or RVEDV that has been ejected per beat

The thermodilution method provides a quick, accurate assessment (±20%) of the CO. A major disadvantage, however, is the potential for inaccuracy when thermodilution is used in low output states, intracardiac shunts, or pulmonary/tricuspid regurgitation, dysrhythmias, or mechanical ventilation. Thus, clinicians should also inspect the thermodilution curve itself and not accept the digital display of cardiac output alone. Moreover, if the reliability of the CO is questionable, the critical care nurse should assess CO by measuring the arteriovenous oxygen content difference.[45] This can be obtained by the following formula:

Arteriovenous O₂ content difference = (% oxygen saturation of arterial blood − % O₂ saturation of mixed venous blood) × hemoglobin (g/dl) × 1.36 ml of O₂ per gram of hemoglobin

The normal arteriovenous O₂ content is 3.0 to 5.0 ml/dl. In conditions that decrease CO, the peripheral tissues extract more oxygen from hemoglobin causing an increase in the arteriovenous oxygen difference. Conversely, the oxygen content difference decreases with an increase in CO.[45]

Many conditions may result in a decreased CO. Tachycardia is one example that may precipitate a low CO because of a decrease in ventricular filling time and a reduction in stroke volume. Additional conditions that lower CO are factors that reduce preload such as massive vasodilation, diuresis, dehydration, third space shifting of fluids, dysrhythmias, and increased intrathoracic pressure. Factors such as ischemia, myocardial infarction, and negative inotropic drugs also yield a lower CO by decreasing contractility. Lastly, any factor that increases afterload or the vascular resistance such as hypothermia, increased sympathetic stimulation, or hypertension may limit CO. Conversely, variables that cause an increase in CO include exercise, anxiety, certain atrioventricular shunts, and sepsis in the early stage.

Cardiac Index. The cardiac index (CI) is more precise than CO in reflecting LV output because it takes into account the individual patient's body size. The CI represents a patient's CO in relation to his or her body surface area. Any factors which decrease or increase CO will directly affect the cardiac index (Chapter 20).

Stroke Volume (SV). The SV is obtained by dividing the cardiac output by the heart rate. Factors that affect preload, afterload, and contractility directly affect SV.

Stroke Volume Index (SVI). The SVI is a sensitive measurement of stroke volume because it reflects the body surface area of an individual. The normal SVI value and formula are in Table 21-3.

Preload Parameters. The CVP or RAP is a determinant of the right ventricular end-diastolic pressure or preload and is recorded as a mean pressure. This mean pressure corresponds to RV end-diastolic pressure because during diastole when the tricuspid valve is open, there is communication between the right atrium and ventricle. In the past, these pressures were considered to be a reliable measure of left ventricular preload, but with the advent of pulmonary arterial catheters, these pressures were found not to accurately reflect LV preload.

The RAP and CVP reflect venous return to the right atrium; thus, any condition that reduces venous return results in a decrease in these pressures. Some of these conditions include hemorrhage, shock, third space shifting, burns, diuresis, vomiting, venous pooling, and increased intrathoracic pressure. Interventions used in some of these circumstances are aimed at augmenting venous return such as with the administration of crystalloid or colloid therapy. Conversely, interventions used to decrease these pressures

include diuretics and venodilators. The positioning of patients is another variable that may alter venous return. For example, patients in the semierect position may experience a decrease in venous return and those who are recumbent may have an increase in venous return.

The waveform of a right atrial tracing characteristically has three positive pressures (a, c, v) and two negative descents (x, y) (Figure 21-11). An explanation of each waveform and correlation to the ECG are found in Table 21-4.

Left ventricular preload parameters such as the pulmonary artery end-diastolic pressure (PAEDP) are obtained via the PA catheter. The PAEDP is obtained during diastole. It will approximate the PAWP with the exception of such conditions as mechanical ventilation, elevated pulmonary vascular resistance, heart rates that exceed 125 beats per minute, chronic obstructive lung disease, and pulmonary embolism. The PAEDP is usually 1 to 4 mmHg higher than the PAWP.

The PAWP is a damped, time-delayed version of a left atrial pressure tracing. It reflects left ventricular filling pressure and is extremely useful in managing cardiac patients. Readings should be obtained at the end of expiration. Studies have indicated that both PA and PAW pressures can be accurately measured with the backrest of the bed elevated from 0° to 45°.[46] Conditions in which the PAWP cannot be used as a reflection of left ventricular preload include mitral stenosis, mitral regurgitation, left atrial tumors, and pulmonary venous obstructions. Elevations in the PAWP occur with left ventricular failure.

The advantages of obtaining a PAWP in reflecting left ventricular performance are obvious. The disad-

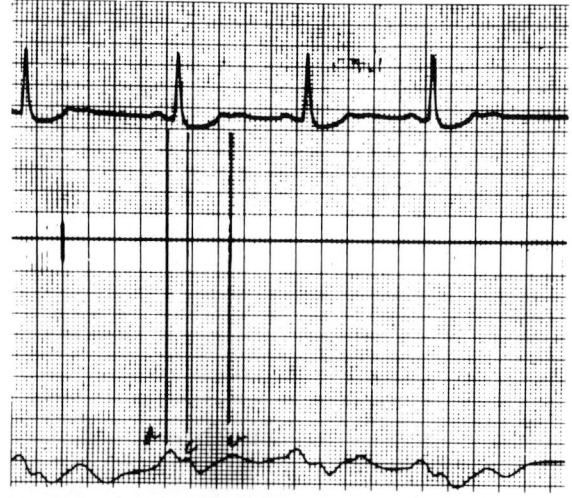

Figure 21-11 Normal right atrial pressure waveform showing a, c, and v waves, and x and y descents.
Courtesy of Hewlett-Packard, Waltham Division.

TABLE 21-4   **Summary of Right Atrial, Pulmonary Artery Wedge, and Left Atrial Waveforms**

Waveforms	Normal Right Atrial	Correlation to ECG	Pulmonary Artery Wedge Pressure or Left Atrial	Correlation to ECG
a	Produced by atrial contraction; precedes arterial pulsation	Corresponds in time to PR interval of ECG	Produced by left atrial systole	Follows P wave of ECG
x	Negative descent caused by a reduction in pressure after atrial contraction		Decline in pressure related to a decrease in LA volume	
c	Depicts movement of the tricuspid valve toward the atrium	Corresponds to RST junction on ECG	Produced by closure of mitral valve—may not be seen	
v	Occurs at end of ventricular systole	Corresponds to TP interval	Results from filling of LA and bulging back of mitral valve during ventricular contractions	Follows T wave complex on ECG
y	Reflects a decrease in RA volume during filling of RV		Reflects decrease in LA during filling of LV	

Adapted from Daily, E., & Shroeder, J. (1989). *Techniques of bedside hemodynamic monitoring* (4th ed.). St. Louis: Mosby.

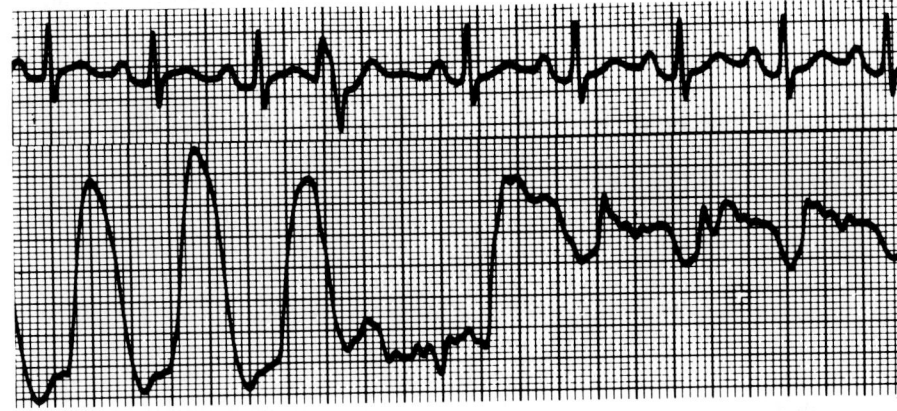

Figure 21-12   Normal PA and PAW pressure waveforms showing *a* and *v* waves and *x* and *y* descents.
Courtesy of Hewlett-Packard, Waltham Division.

vantages are (1) threat of balloon-induced pulmonary artery rupture and hemorrhage as a result of repeated balloon inflation and (2) migration of the catheter to a distal artery yielding a permanent wedge tracing and potential pulmonary infarct if not repositioned. The risk of pulmonary artery rupture or infarct can be minimized with careful adherence to the procedures for balloon inflation (1.5 ml maximum). Frequent balloon inflations may not be necessary when the PAEDP approximates the PAWP.

The normal PA wedge tracing has a characteristic atrial pattern described in the CVP parameter section. A more detailed explanation of this waveform along with correlation to the ECG is found in Table 21-4 and Figure 21-12.

An abnormal PA wedge tracing is found in mitral regurgitation. An elevated *v* wave tracing is considered to be the hallmark of this type of valvular defect. In mitral regurgitation the PAWP does not accurately reflect LVEDP and displays a falsely high value.

The left atrial pressure (LAP) is the third parameter used to assess LV preload. The major limitation of LAP monitoring is that the catheter can be placed only during cardiac surgical procedures and thus is not a commonly obtained pressure in critical care units. However, the LAP is the most accurate esti-

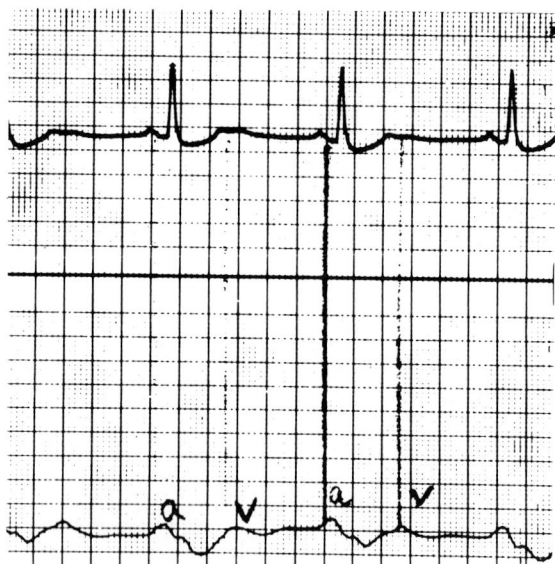

Figure 21-13   LA pressure waveform demonstrating similarity to PAW waveform. This pressure is normal.
Courtesy of Hewlett-Packard, Waltham Division.

mation of LVEDP in the absence of mitral valve disease. The waveform is the exact tracing as found in Figure 21-13. A detailed description of the positive and negative descents of LAP will also be found in Table 21-4.

Afterload Parameters. Right ventricular afterload can be evaluated using the pulmonary vascular resistance whereby the systemic vascular resistance and aortic end-diastolic pressure may be used as a reflection of left ventricular afterload. The formulas to calculate these derived parameters are found in Table 21-3.

Pulmonary vascular resistance (PVR) is a measure of impedance or resistance by the pulmonic arterial circulation to RV ejection. It can be calculated with a programmed calculator or by using the formula found in Table 21-3. Certain conditions elevate the PVR and may cause a subsequent reduction in cardiac output. These include hypoxia or hypercapnia, which induces vasoconstriction; acute respiratory distress syndrome; positive end-expiratory pressure; pulmonary embolism; pulmonary interstitial edema; chronic obstructive lung disease; inflammatory states; and mitral stenosis. The critical care nurse needs to be aware of conditions that may increase the PVR and report them to the physician.

Systemic vascular resistance (SVR) is a measure of resistance by the systemic arterial circulation to LV ejection. Certain states or conditions elevate the SVR and reduce CO. Vasoconstriction, inotropic agents, polycythemia vera, and hypovolemic/cardiogenic shock all cause increased sympathetic stimulation. Af-

terload reducers such as nitroprusside or nitroglycerin are frequently employed in these conditions. Decreases in SVR occur with vasodilatation, moderate hypoxemia, vasodilator agents, and anemic states.

Two other parameters can be used as a reflection of afterload: the mean arterial pressure and the aortic end-diastolic pressure. The mean arterial pressure is defined as the average pressure during the cardiac cycle. This pressure correlates to the pressure that the left ventricle must overcome to open the aortic valve during the phase of isovolumetric contraction and can be easily obtained from an arterial catheter. Conditions that elevate or decrease the SVR produce similar changes in aortic end-diastolic pressure.

Contractility Parameters. There are no direct methods of measuring contractility, but an indirect value may be obtained by calculating the amount of work that the right or left ventricle does during systolic ejection. These indirect measures of contractility are referred to as *right ventricular stroke work* (RVSW), *right ventricular cardiac work* (RVCW), *left ventricular stroke work* (LVSW), and *left ventricular cardiac work* (LVCW).

The RVSW parameter measures the amount of work the right ventricle generates per beat when ejecting blood and is based on the calculation for work: Work = pressure generated × volume of blood pumped. It is a product of the mean arterial blood pressure and stroke volume. The conversion factor of 0.0136 converts pressure to work. It can be calculated either by a programmed calculator or using the formula cited in Table 21-3. A decrease in RVSW is suggestive of a right ventricular infarct, which can depress contractility. The right ventricular stroke work index (RVSWI) is a more precise determinant of RV stroke work in that it reflects the body surface area of a patient. The right ventricular cardiac work (RVCW) closely resembles the RVSW insofar as it measures the amount of work the right ventricle does each *minute* when ejecting blood. The right ventricular cardiac work index (RVCWI) reflects the body surface area and can be calculated as cited in Table 21-3. A decrease in either RVCW or RVCWI is also indicative of depressed RV contractility.

The LVSW is a measurement of the amount of work the left ventricle generates per beat during ventricular ejection. It is similar to RVSW in that it is based on the calculation of work. The LVSW is a product of the MAP and the SV. In the presence of depressed contractility and decreased LVSW, inotropic agents are needed to strengthen cardiac contraction. An increase in LVSW may be related to conditions in which there is an increase in MVo_2. This increase can be detrimental in patients with coronary artery disease, who by virtue of their disease have diminished blood supply and may develop further ischemia because they are unable to satisfy the demand for O_2. The LVSWI is also a more exact measurement of SW in that it is indexed to the patient's body surface area. The left ventricular cardiac work parameter measures the amount of work the left ventricle does each minute during systole. The indexed value (LVCWI) is also calculated similarly to the RVCWI in Table 21-3. A decrease in either LVCW or LVCWI is also indicative of depressed LV contractility.

Rate–Pressure Product. The rate–pressure product (RPP) is an indirect assessment of myocardial oxygen consumption and is calculated as the product of systolic blood pressure and heart rate. If the RPP is greater than 12,000 it indicates an increase in MVo_2, which is an important consideration in patients who have ischemic heart disease and are vulnerable to further damage when demand exceeds supply.

Mixed Venous Oxygen Saturation Monitoring

Mixed venous oxygen saturation ($S\bar{v}o_2$) monitoring is a relatively new concept in the assessment of critically ill patients. $S\bar{v}o_2$ monitoring provides data relative to the body's oxygen supply and demand. It is a useful parameter to monitor the cardiac and pulmonary systems as well as the effect of stressors and clinical interventions upon tissue oxygen consumption.

This technology employs reflection spectrophotometry. Light waves sent via a fiberoptic fiber are reflected by the red blood cells, transmitted by a second fiberoptic fiber, and analyzed and transformed into a digital display. The color of the blood determines the amount of reflected light and in turn the color is determined by the amount of oxygenated and deoxygenated hemoglobin and the density of red blood cells.[47]

The system components consist of an optical module, which produces light waves, and two fiberoptic fibers, the first to transmit the light waves and the second to conduct the reflected light waves. These components are housed within the pulmonary artery catheter. Another important component is the microprocessor which analyzes the reflected light and transforms it into a continuous digital display for clinical use.

The digital display represents the oxygen saturation of the hemoglobin within the pulmonary artery. Since this location is the terminal endpoint for the venous return from all parts of the body, this venous blood is said to be "mixed" and globally reflective of the whole body.

The normal $S\bar{v}o_2$ is 60% to 80%. Refer to Table 21-5 for a more detailed interpretation of $S\bar{v}o_2$ levels.

TABLE 21-5 Interpretation of $S\bar{v}o_2$

Range of $S\bar{v}o_2$	Physiological Condition	Clinical Examples
Normal $S\bar{v}o_2$ (60% to 80%)	Oxygen supply is balanced with oxygen demand	Tissue perfusion is adequate
Low $S\bar{v}o_2$ (<60%)	Oxygen demand exceeds oxygen supply	Shivering, hyperthermia, seizures, pain
	Alteration of components of oxygen delivery system:	
	Decreased CO	Hypotension, hypovolemia, shock failure, dysrhythmias
	Insufficient/abnormal Hb	Anemia, hemorrhage, carbon monoxide poisoning
	Reduced arterial oxygen saturation, related to:	
	Alveolar hypoventilation, shunt (generalized/localized)	Drug overdose Adult/neonatal respiratory distress syndrome, pneumonia, atelectasis
	Ventilation/perfusion mismatching	Asthma, chronic obstructive pulmonary disease
High $S\bar{v}o_2$ (>80%)	Oxygen supply exceeds oxygen demand	Septic shock, hypothermia, cyanide poisoning, excess inotropic therapy, cirrhosis, pharmacological paralysis
	Technical problems that interfere with $S\bar{v}o_2$ reading	Wedged pulmonary artery catheter, clot formation, noncalibrated monitor
	Alteration in one of the components of the oxygen delivery system:	
	Increased oxygen delivery	Hyperoxia, increased Fio_2

Source: Gardner, P. E., & Laurent-Bopp, D. (1987). Continuous $S\bar{v}o_2$ monitoring. *Progress in Cardiovascular Nursing, 2,* 13.

Significant changes in the $S\bar{v}O_2$ level, defined as +5% to 10% for more than 5 minutes necessitate investigation into the possible etiologies.[47]

The $S\bar{v}O_2$ is affected by four major variables: the cardiac output, hemoglobin levels, arterial oxygen saturation, and tissue oxygen consumption. Whereas tissue oxygen consumption reflects the body's demand, the cardiac output, hemoglobin level, and arterial oxygen saturation represent oxygen supply. The cardiac output is the circulatory drive transmitting the oxygen-laden hemoglobin. Any decrease in the cardiac output reduces tissue oxygen supply reflected in a low $S\bar{v}O_2$. Conversely, any increase in cardiac output increases tissue oxygen supply and raises the $S\bar{v}O_2$. An increased cardiac output is the body's first compensatory mechanism in response to a fall in oxygen delivery or a rise in oxygen demand.

The second compensatory mechanism is increased cellular oxygen extraction. In a critically ill patient, cardiac compromise may prohibit any augmentation of cardiac output in response to changes in delivery or demand. Thus, increased oxygen extraction becomes the major compensatory mechanism and results in a reduced $S\bar{v}O_2$ level.

Similarly, hemoglobin levels directly relate to the $S\bar{v}O_2$ because hemoglobin circulates approximately 98% of the oxygen contained within the blood. Any decrease in hemoglobin, such as with anemia or hemorrhage, lowers the $S\bar{v}O_2$, whereas conditions that raise hemoglobin levels, such as blood transfusions, raise the $S\bar{v}O_2$.

Additional variables affecting oxygen affinity to hemoglobin will further affect tissue oxygen supply. These are blood temperature, hydrogen ion and carbon dioxide concentration, and 2,3,DPG.

The last major variable directly affecting oxygen supply is arterial oxygen saturation ($S\bar{v}O_2$). This is the percentage of oxygenated hemoglobin within 100 ml of blood. Normally the $S\bar{v}O_2$ is 98% to 99%. In pulmonary disease, infections, or any other conditions resulting in shunting of blood, less oxygen-laden arterial hemoglobin is available to the cells so that the returning $S\bar{v}O_2$ level is further reduced.

Oxygen demand is represented by tissue oxygen consumption or the amount of oxygen the tissues require. It is inversely related to $S\bar{v}O_2$. Normal oxygen demand is approximately 250 ml per minute. Some conditions increasing oxygen demand are fever, shivering, or pain. If a compensatory increase in cardiac output is insufficient, greater oxygen extraction occurs, lowering the $S\bar{v}O_2$. Conversely, hypothermia and paralyzing agents reduce oxygen demand and increase $S\bar{v}O_2$ levels. Patients in septic shock initially may present with an elevation in $S\bar{v}O_2$ secondary to venodi-

lation that manifests an attempt to shunt blood to major organ systems.

The indications for $S\bar{v}O_2$ monitoring of the critically ill cardiac patient are clear. This technology is also helpful in the postoperative care of cardiac surgical patients. These patients frequently experience postoperative low cardiac output states, hypovolemia, anemia, and hypoxemia, which directly affect oxygen supply. They often exhibit fever, dysrhythmias, and pain, which increase oxygen demand in a compromised cardiovascular state. The critically ill patient in cardiogenic shock, with the propensity for multisystem failure, is another indication for $S\bar{v}O_2$ monitoring. Lastly, this technology is useful in assessing the effectiveness of therapeutic interventions such as pharmacological agents like inotropes, vasodilators, or paralytic agents as well as nursing interventions such as positioning or suctioning.

Magnetic Resonance Imaging (MRI)

Magnetic resonance imaging (MRI) is a relatively new noninvasive diagnostic technique. At present, three types of MRI techniques are being applied clinically to provide data on tissue structure, function, or metabolism. This technique can provide detailed anatomical images of cardiac structure. Cine-MRI and MR velocity imaging both yield data on cardiac function. Lastly, information gained from magnetic resonance spectroscopy (MRS) affords insight into cellular metabolism for the study of cardiac ischemia, injury, and reperfusion.

MRI is concerned with the nucleons (protons and neutrons) of the atomic nucleus. Atoms with an odd number of nucleons or atomic mass have both a charge and an inherent spin around their axes. Since any moving charge creates a magnetic force, these spinning atomic nuclei have their own magnetic fields, or moments. A substance is composed of many nuclei whose magnetic moments occur randomly. When subjected to an external magnetic field, random magnetic moments align themselves in either a parallel or antiparallel relation to the external field.

If these nucleons are further subjected to a second force, or radiofrequency, they are pulled from their equilibrium with the first external magnetic field. When the radiofrequency is discontinued, the nucleons return to their prior position of alignment with the first external magnetic field and release a signal known as *free induction decay*. This signal is one type of data analyzed in MRI. A second type of data obtained by MRI is the *relaxation time*, or the time it takes for a nucleon to return to its original position after exposure to a radiofrequency force.[48] The relaxation time of nucleons differs depending on the tissue type, presence of disease, and differences in tissue water content.

Magnetic Resonance Imaging Study

In MRI, the free induction decay signal and relaxation time are used to construct a three-dimensional image. Protons are the nucleons studied in MRI because they are abundant in humans and sensitive to MRI. Hydrogen (H^+) is the proton of choice.

A moving object such as the heart poses a threat to image clarity. To minimize image distortion, the delivery of the radiofrequency force is gated, that is, timed to coincide with a consistent period in the cardiac cycle. Gating to the ECG has been found to minimize image distortion and improve imaging.[45,50]

One advantage of MRI over x-ray is its superiority in differentiating tissues: MRI detects changes in tissue chemistry. A second is that bone is not visible with MRI. Therefore, MRI is not limited to specific windows around bony structures to view the heart as in echocardiography.

The applicability of MRI in evaluating the cardiovascular system is varied. It permits viewing the heart on many planes and yields visualization of the cardiac chambers, ventricular wall, aorta, pulmonary artery, and septum during systole as well as diastole. Early detection of lipid deposits on coronary artery intima is possible. Myocardial wall dimensions are more clearly outlined with MRI than by other cardiac imaging techniques.[51] The clinical utility of these data is in the extent of myocardial thinning secondary to infarction and septal integrity.

Clinical cardiovascular indications for MRI are the following: thrombosis; tumors; cardiomyopathy; congenital and ischemic heart disease; disease of the aortic arch, pericardium, and pulmonary artery; septal defects; ventricular aneurysms[16]; and coronary artery bypass graft patency.[52] Figures 21-14 and 21-15 depict cross-sectional views of the heart taken with MRI.

Cine Magnetic Resonance Imaging (Cine-MRI)

Anatomical and functional data regarding the cardiovascular system are provided by cine-MRI. This technique takes multiple views of the heart during the cardiac cycle and displays them in a cinematic format to study myocardial wall motion, valve abnormalities, and blood flow.[52] Clinical applications of cine-MRI are to study left and right ventricular function and dimensions, regurgitant valvular pathophysiology, certain congenital abnormalities, and abnormal blood flow patterns as in septal defects.[16,52]

Magnetic Resonance (MR) Velocity Imaging

The MR velocity imaging technique provides functional data on the cardiovascular system by isolating

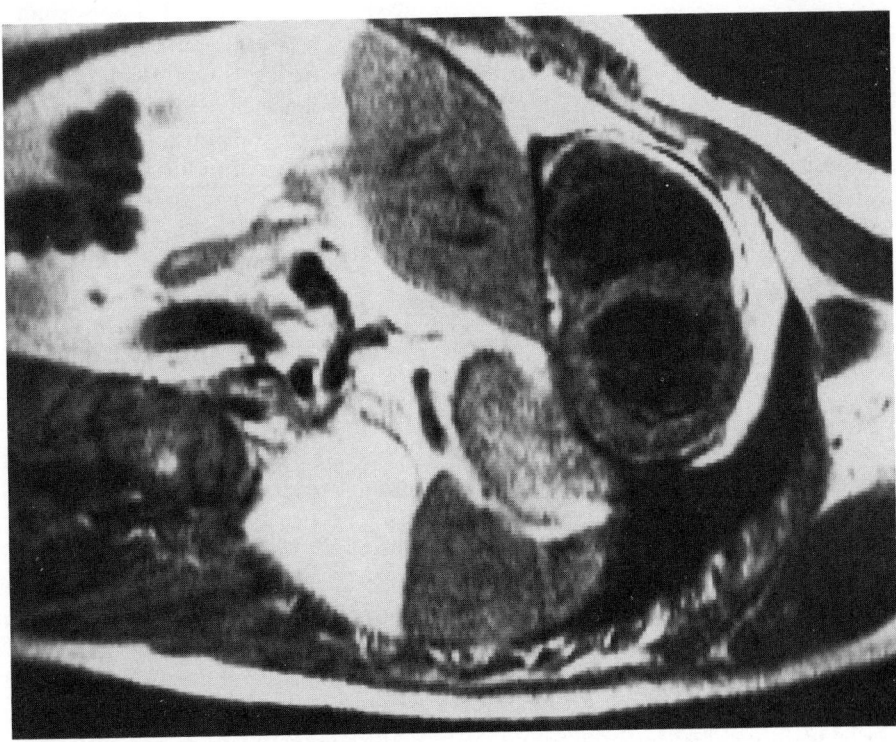

Figure 21-14   Cross-sectional view of heart taken by MRI.

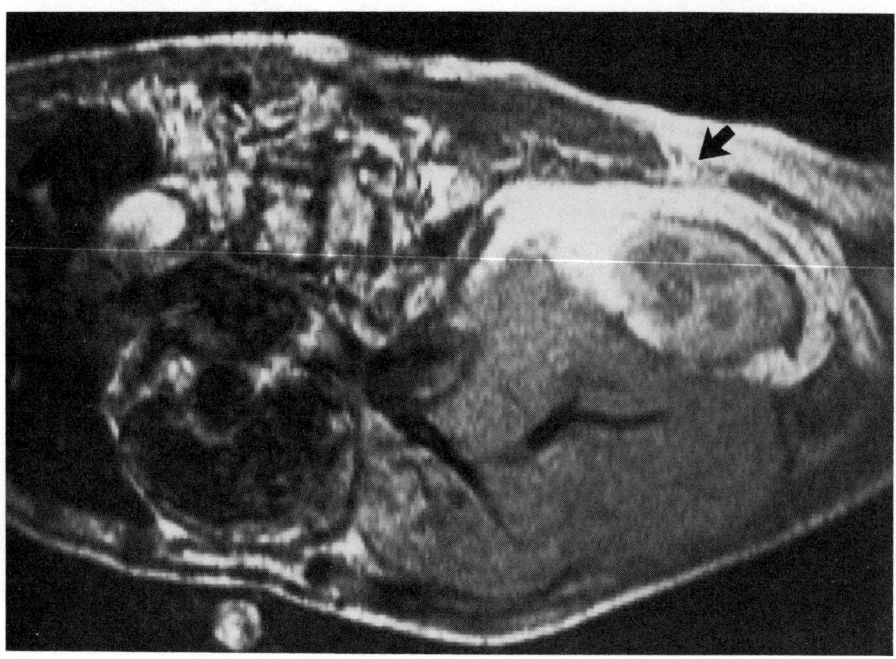

Figure 21-15   Cross-sectional view of heart taken by MRI.

data on blood velocity. Magnetic pulses are delivered and targeted to moving spinning nuclei as in blood while signals from stationary nuclei are minimized.[16] These data may be useful in calculating cardiac output and assessing a variety of cardiovascular disorders.

Magnetic Resonance Spectroscopy (MRS)

Spectroscopic MRI provides data regarding cellular metabolism by transforming the free induction decay signal into a frequency spectrum and revealing the chemical composition of nuclei. Hydrogen-1, carbon-13, sodium-23, fluorine-19, and phosphorus-31 are elements possessing nuclei that are sensitive to MRS. Upon stimulation by an outside magnetic force, these nuclei characteristically release their own unique frequency. This frequency will differ if the environment of the nuclei is altered. Therefore, the frequency emitted will be altered if it is located in ischemic, injured, or reperfused myocardium. This then becomes the basis for the clinical application of MRS in ischemic cardiac disease.[16]

Currently, research is concentrating on MRS of phosphorus-31 (^{31}P). This element can be easily studied and is critical to cellular metabolism, tissue pH, and membrane integrity. Three types of phosphorus are detected by MRS: adenosine triphosphate (ATP), phosphocreatine (PCr), and inorganic phosphorus (Pi). In ischemia, reduced ATP and PCr levels and increased Pi can be identified and quantified.[53]

The applicability of this information to clinical practice is discussed in the literature. ^{31}P spectroscopy has been used to examine the effectiveness of therapeutic interventions in reducing ischemic arrest–induced acidosis[54] and one case of metabolic familial cardiomyopathy.[53] Others have used ^{31}P spectroscopy to document the effect of potassium cardioplegia and hypothermia on high-energy phosphates and cellular pH during ischemia.[55] This technology requires further development before it becomes applicable to clinical practice. Technical challenges that remain include the reduction of motion-induced artifact, the risk of misinterpreting signals emitted from other structures, and the poor ability to localize areas of ischemia or infarction.

Contraindications

MRI is contraindicated in patients with neurostimulating devices or pacemakers. A pacemaker may be reprogrammed to an asynchronous mode. Patients with aneurysm clips should not undergo this technique because of the danger of dislodging the clips.

Safety

To date, there are no reports of ill effects associated with MRI. The only potential ill effect from the magnetic radiofrequency fields is tissue heating, but Morganroth et al.[48] state that this has not been actualized even when higher magnetic fields were employed. Finally, unlike x-ray or radionuclide techniques, MRI does not use ionizing radiation.

Radionuclide Testing

Radionuclide tests, or nuclear scans, use radionuclide substances to study cardiac function, perfusion, myocardial viability, and extent of infarction or ischemia. When stable radionuclide substances are converted to an unstable form, energy is emitted in the form of gamma rays. These gamma rays, the radioactive decay of the radionuclide substance, are monitored by a device known as a gamma scintillation camera.

Myocardial Infarct Imaging Techniques

Myocardial infarct imaging is a radionuclide technique that identifies the size and location of a myocardial infarction. For certain subsets of patients, this technique is necessary to confirm the diagnosis of an MI. In patients who experienced a MI days before admission, have muscle disease, and have electrocardiographic (ECG) findings of a left bundle branch block, previous MIs, paced rhythm, or subendocardial changes, enzymatic and ECG evidence of an MI may be inconclusive, and diagnosis may depend on a myocardial infarct imaging study.

Technetium pyrophosphate (^{99m}Tc), the radionuclide used in myocardial infarct imaging, was previously used for bone scanning. In myocardial scanning, ^{99m}Tc accumulates in infarcted tissue and is detected as an area of increased concentration or a "hot spot" by the gamma scintillation camera (Figure 21-16).

Although the exact mechanism by which the ^{99m}Tc is deposited in necrotic myocardium is disputed, some theories have been postulated. One such theory is the binding of the radionuclide with damaged mitochondria; a second theory alludes to the role of calcium crystals present in necrotic tissue as postulated by Wacker.[56]

Myocardial infarct imaging can identify an MI within 10 to 12 hours of infarction. The imaging reaches a diagnostic peak within 72 hours and is negative after 4 to 5 days. Identification of an MI that has occurred 7 to 10 days earlier is not feasible.

Myocardial infarct imaging relies on myocardial blood flow, calcification, and size of infarction for adequate uptake of ^{99m}Tc. Technetium pyrophosphate uptake is more concentrated in areas surrounding an infarction than in the center. In a large anterior MI, for instance, the damaged myocardium may appear as a doughnutlike area of increased uptake, corresponding to the zone of injury, surrounding a center area of decreased uptake which corresponds to the necrotic or infarcted tissue. Areas of calcification are also associated with increased uptake. Lastly, 3 g or more of infarcted myocardium must be present for imaging to be diagnostic. Gerson[57] and Willerson[58] have identified new three-dimensional techniques that permit the imaging of smaller infarcts.

Although very specific in identifying an MI, ^{99m}Tc scanning is a useful diagnostic tool for a variety of cardiac conditions. Viral myocarditis, trauma, left ventricular aneurysms, unstable angina, tumor, calcification of valves, and amyloidosis are examples. Willerson[58] identified other conditions, excluding MI, that result in positive findings such as decreased myocardial perfusion secondary to hypotension, delayed clearance secondary to renal insufficiency, or excessive injection of the radionuclide. It has been found that persistently abnormal results are associated with more severe disease, congestive heart failure, and persistent angina.[59]

Myocardial Perfusion Imaging Techniques

There are currently two types of myocardial perfusion imaging techniques, single photon emission computed tomography (SPECT) and positron emission tomography (PET). Since PET studies may also provide data on myocardial metabolism, they are discussed in detail in the following section.

The SPECT radionuclide studies commonly employ either thallium-201 (^{201}Tl) or technetium-99m sestamibi (Tc-99m sestamibi). Both radionuclides are circulated via the coronary circulation and, therefore, have a rapid uptake in perfused mycardium. Areas of decreased uptake, or "cold spots," correlate with ischemic or infarcted tissue.

Researchers are currently comparing the effectiveness of these two agents. Both agents can be detected

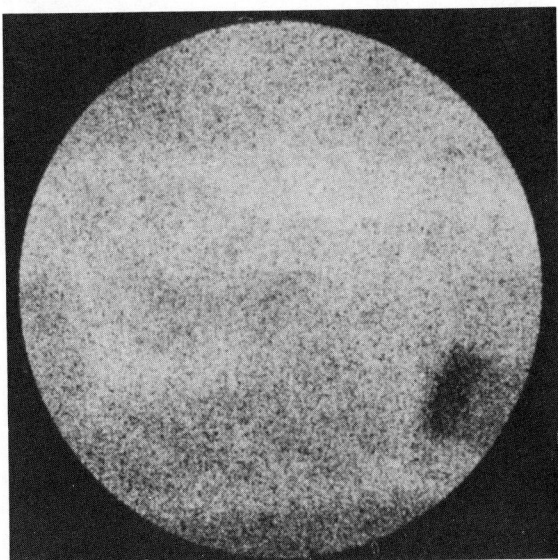

Figure 21-16 Pyrophosphate scan depicting area of increased uptake.

by gamma cameras. The first radionuclide used in SPECT studies was [201]Tl. It has a more rapid uptake in the myocardium than Tc-99m sestamibi but has the disadvantage of a longer half-life and a more rapid redistribution rate. Because of the longer half-life, a smaller quantity of the radionuclide can be administered. Therefore, first-pass studies of ventricular function that follow a bolus injection of the radionuclide through the heart and provide data about myocardial function and structure cannot be obtained. The long half-life also tends to reduce image quality because of lower nuclear counts, especially in women with large breasts or obese patients. The rapid distribution rate of ^{201}Tl requires that studies be conducted immediately after injection of the radionuclide tracer. If this is not feasible and ^{201}Tl is allowed to diffuse into hypoperfused areas, segments of ischemic myocardium may be masked.

Tc-99m sestamibi possesses a shorter half-life. Consequently, a larger dose can be administered and data from first-pass studies can be obtained. Its slow rate of redistribution permits perfusion studies to be performed hours after injection—a clear advantage in the patient with unstable angina. If Tc-99m sestamibi is introduced during the anginal episode, areas of decreased perfusion secondary to ischemia remain evident despite the time required for patient stabilization.

SPECT studies differ from planar scintigraphy in that the planar technique provides only three different views of the heart. The SPECT studies provide a three-dimensional re-creation of a cardiac image compiled from 32 frames taken at six angle intervals across a 180-degree arch.[60]

SPECT studies may be combined with exercise testing to increase sensitivity and specificity and to quantify transient perfusion defects associated with ischemia. In a thallium exercise scintigraphy study, the patient exercises in a cardiovascular laboratory. Once the patient's peak exercise capacity is attained, ^{201}Tl is introduced. Areas of decreased tracer uptake ("cold spots") identify areas of decreased myocardial perfusion (Figure 21-17).

To differentiate between ischemia and infarction, a repeat scan is performed approximately 4 hours after the ^{201}Tl injection. Ischemia is identified if reperfusion manifests in the previously documented cold spots, although cold spots may require more time for reperfusion to occur. The existence of ischemia is supported by the documented clinical improvement in such areas after revascularization. Studies are examining the effectiveness of a second dose of ^{201}Tl at follow-up to detect ischemic areas.[61,62,63]

Like ^{201}Tl, Tc-99m sestamibi may be used with exercise testing. Its slow rate of redistribution makes

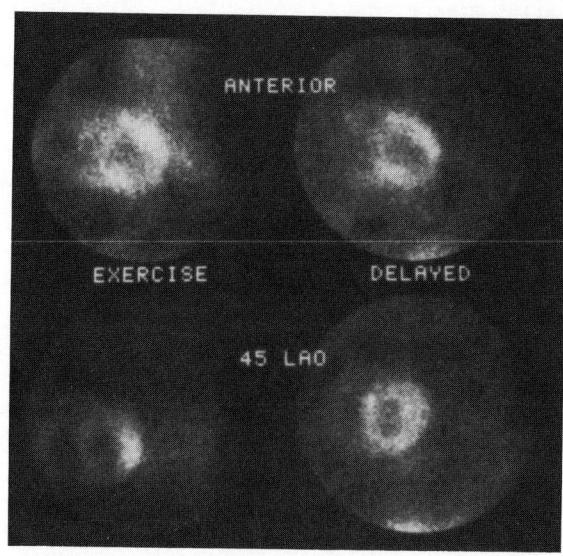

Figure 21-17   Exercise thallium scan with reperfusion indicating septal and inferoapical ischemia.

it unsuitable for delayed follow-up scans. Two injections are required. The first quantifies perfusion at rest. The second is given at peak exercise to quantify areas of decreased perfusion or myocardium at risk. Current research is examining the optimal timing of these two injections.[64]

Indications for SPECT include the following: (1) to identify high-risk patients, (2) to evaluate the effectiveness of therapeutic interventions, and (3) to quantify perfusion defects.[60]

Myocardial Perfusion and Metabolic Studies

Positron emission tomography (PET) is the only study currently available that can assess myocardial perfusion and cellular metabolism. This test uses radioisotopes that decay and emit a positive electron. When the emitted positive electron collides with a negative electron, it emits two gamma photons. The simultaneous emissions of these two gamma photons are monitored, recorded, and used to create tomographic images of the heart.[65]

Positron emission tomography can document myocardial perfusion with a high degree of specificity and sensitivity. The radioisotopes used for these perfusion studies are ^{13}N ammonia and rubidium-82 ([82]Rb). A second capability unique to the PET scan is the ability to monitor cellular metabolism by means of its substrates. For example, ^{18}F deoxyglucose is used to monitor glucose utilization and ^{11}C palmitate to track free fatty acid metabolism.[16] Clinically, these techniques may be used to demonstrate areas of viable myocardium existing in segments of absent or inadequate perfusion. Studies that verify the accuracy of the technique suggest a future therapeutic use.[66,67]

PET scans may also be used to quantify areas of myocardial ischemia and infarction and to assess collateral circulation to the myocardium.[68]

Myocardial Function Imaging Techniques

Two radionuclide techniques allow for evaluation of ventricular function. Both require the injection of a radionuclide tracer.

One technique, the *first-pass technique,* was discussed earlier. The major advantage of this technique is the ability to obtain data regarding ventricular size and function quickly.[69] The disadvantage is that incorrect patient positioning and variable injection techniques may alter the results.

Equilibrium scans assess ventricular function. The technique differs from the first-pass method in that a delay of several minutes after injection and before scanning allows the tracer to be mixed homogeneously in the blood. The scintigraphic camera is synchronized with the cardiac cycle and divides the RR interval into multiple intervals or gates. The counts emitted by the radionuclide tracer in each gate are recorded, and an image is made of the heart and its function throughout the cardiac cycle. The advantage of the equilibrium technique is in assessing regional wall motion and ventricular shape.[69]

These radionuclide tests may be combined with exercise stress testing to yield a variety of information. A higher sensitivity has been reported when combined exercise radionuclide angiocardiography was employed as opposed to conventional exercise testing.[70] The ability to assess the effectiveness of therapies as a second benefit of this procedure has also been noted.[71]

The effect of inadequate exercise levels on the sensitivity of the test must be considered when utilizing this technique and interpreting the results.[72]

REFERENCES

1. Gordon, M. (1991). *Manual of nursing diagnosis* (2nd ed.). St. Louis: Mosby–Year Book.
2. Braunwald, E. (1988). The physical examination. In E. Braunwald (Ed.), *Heart disease: A textbook of cardiovascular medicine* (3rd ed.). Philadelphia: Saunders.
3. Silverman, M. E., & Hurst, J. W. (1990). Inspection of the patient. In J. W. Hurst, R. B. Logue, R. C. Schlant, et al. (Eds.), *The heart* (7th ed.). New York: McGraw-Hill.
4. Lichstein, E. (1974). Diagonal ear lobe crease: Prevalence and implications as a coronary risk factor. *New England Journal of Medicine, 290,* 615-616.
5. Thompson, D. A. (1981). *Cardiovascular assessment.* St. Louis: Mosby.
6. Gould, B. A. (1985). Is the blood pressure the same in both arms? *Clinical Cardiology, 8,* 423-426.
7. Sulzbach, L. M. (1985). The use of temporary atrial wire electrodes in patients who had cardiac surgery. *Heart Lung, 14,* 540-548.
8. Roberts, R. (1981). Diagnostic assessment of myocardial infarction based on lactic dehydrogenase and creatine kinase isoenzyme. *Heart Lung, 10*(3), 486-504.
9. Galen, R. S. (1977). Myocardial infarction: A clinician's guide to the isoenzymes. *Resident and Staff Physician, 23,* 67-75.
10. Lee, T., & Goldman, L. (1986). Serum enzyme assays in the diagnosis of acute myocardial infarction. Recommendations based on a quantitative analysis. *Annals of Internal Medicine, 102,* 221-233.
11. Grossman, W., & Barry, W. H. (1988). Cardiac catheterization. In E. Braunwald (Ed.), *Heart disease: A textbook of cardiovascular medicine* (3rd ed.). Philadelphia: Saunders.
12. Rackley, C. E., & Satler, L. F. (1989). The cardiac catheter: Past, present & future. *American Journal of Cardiology, 64,* 1034-1036.
13. Sanderson, R. G. (1983). Diagnostic techniques. In R. G. Sanderson, & C. L. Kurth (Eds.), *The cardiac patient.* Philadelphia: Saunders.
14. Canobbio, M. (1984). Chest x-ray interpretation. *Focus on Critical Care, 11*(2), 18-24.
15. Lipton, M. J., Higgins, C. B., Farmer, D., et al. (1984). Cardiac imaging with a high speed cine CT scanner: Preliminary results. *Radiology, 152,* 579-582.
16. Caputo, G. R., & Higgins, C. B. (1990). Advances in cardiac imaging modalities: Fast computed tomography, magnetic resonance imaging, and positron emission tomography. *Investigative Radiology, 25,* 838-854.
17. Gould, R. G., Lipton, M. J., McNamara, M. T., et al. (1988). Measurement of regional myocardial blood flow in dogs using ultrafast CT. *Investigative Radiology, 23,* 348-353.
18. Feigenbaum, H. (1981). *Echocardiography* (3rd ed.). Philadelphia: Lea & Febiger.
19. Simpson, I. A. (1990). Color doppler flow mapping: Providing insight into cardiac hydrodynamics. *Journal of Medical Engineering and Technology, 14*(4), 133-142.
20. Paulides, G. S., Hauser, A. M., Stewart, J. R., et al. (1990). Contribution of transesophageal echocardiography to patient diagnosis and treatment: A prospective analysis. *American Heart Journal, 120*(4), 910-914.
21. Tanaka, M., Abe, T., Takeuchi, E., et al. (1991). Intraoperative echocardiography of a dislodged Bjork-Shiley mitral valve disc. *Annals of Thoracic Surgery, 51*(2), 315-316.
22. Shintani, H., Nakano, S., Matsuda, H., et al. (1990). Efficacy of transesophageal echocardiography as a perioperative monitor in patients undergoing cardiovascular surgery. *Journal of Cardiovascular Surgery, 31,* 564-570.
23. Chung, H., Seyone, C., & Rakowski, H. (1991). Transesophageal echocardiogram may fail to diagnose perioperative myocardial infarction. *Canadian Journal of Anesthesia, 38*(1), 98-101.

24. Galvin, I. F., Black, I. W., Lee, C. L., et al. (1991). Transesophageal echocardiography in acute aortic transection. *Annals of Thoracic Surgery, 51*(2), 310-311.

25. Kranzan, I., Tunick, P. A., Freedberg, R. S., et al. (1991). Transesophageal is superior to transthoracic echocardiography in the diagnosis of sinus venosus atrial septal defect. *Journal of the American College of Cardiology, 17*(2), 537-542.

26. Burstow, D. J., McEniery, P. T., & Stafford, E. G. (1990). Fenestrated atrial septal aneurysm: Diagnosis by transesophageal echocardiography. *Journal of the American Society of Echocardiography, 3*(6), 499-501.

27. Konstadt, S. N., Louie, E. K., Black, K. S., et al. (1991). Intraoperative detection of patent foramen ovale by transesophageal echocardiography. *Anesthesiology, 74*(2), 212-216.

28. Feigenbaum, H. (1988). Echocardiography. In E. Braunwald (Ed.), *Heart disease: A textbook of cardiovascular medicine* (3rd ed.) (pp. 400-408). Philadelphia: Saunders.

29. Fernandez, G. (1983). Echocardiography for the general internist. *Comprehensive Medicine, 9*(10), 46-56.

30. Wenger, N., & Hellerstein, H. (1984). *Rehabilitation of the coronary patient.* New York: Wiley.

31. Vacek, J., Smith, W., & Phillips, J. (1984). Cardiac electrophysiology: An overview. *Practical Cardiology, 10*(13), 83-97.

32. Michelson, E., Spielman, S. R., Greenspan, A. M., et al. (1979). Electrophysiologic study of the left ventricle. Indication and safety. *Chest, 75,* 592-596.

33. Podrid, P., & Lambert, S. (1983). Electrophysiologic approach to ventricular arrhythmias: A review. *Cardiovascular Review and Reports, 2*(4), 231-237.

34. Denes, P., & Ezri, M. D. (1983). Clinical electrophysiology—a decade of progress. *Journal of the American College of Cardiology, 1,* 292-305.

35. Kienzle, M., Doherty, J., Marcus, N., et al. (1984). When do electrophysiologic studies benefit arrhythmia patients? *Journal of Cardiovascular Medicine,* January, 41-55.

36. Ezri, M. D. (1983). Electrophysiologic testing in the diagnosis and management of cardiac arrhythmias. *Chest, 84,* 481-491.

37. Velebit, V., Podrid, P., Lown, B., et al. (1982). Aggravation and provocation of ventricular arrhythmias by antiarrhythmic drugs. *Circulation, 65,* 886-894.

38. Naccarelli, G. V., Prystewsky, E. N., Jackmen, W. N., et al. (1982). Role of electrophysiologic testing in managing patients who have ventricular tachycardia unrelated to coronary artery disease. *American Journal of Cardiology, 50,* 165-171.

39. Michelson, E. L., & Medina, R. P. (1985). Introduction to clinical electrophysiologic studies. *Cardiovascular Clinics, 16*(1), 1-36.

40. Kaufman, L, & Schwartz, J. (1984). Diagnostic endocardial electrical recording and stimulation. *Annals of Internal Medicine, 100*(3), 452-454.

41. Spinale, F. G. (1990). Thermodilution right ventricular ejection fraction: Catheter positioning effects. *Chest, 98*(5), 1259-1265.

42. Hurst, J. M. (1984). Invasive hemodynamic monitoring: An overview. *Journal of Emergency Nursing, 10*(1), 11-22.

43. Sedlock, S. (1981). Cardiac output: Physiologic variables and therapeutic interventions. *Critical Care Nurse, 2*(1), 14-22.

44. Riedinger, M. S., & Shellock, F. G. (1984). Technical aspects of the thermodilution method for measuring cardiac output. *Heart Lung, 13*(3), 215-222.

45. Sharkey, S. W. (1987). Beyond the wedge: Clinical physiology and the Swan-Ganz catheter. *American Journal of Medicine, 83,* 111-121.

46. Chulay, M., & Miller, T. (1984). The effect of bedrest elevation on pulmonary artery and pulmonary capillary wedge pressures in patients after cardiac surgery. *Heart Lung, 13*(2), 138-140.

47. Hardy, G. R. (1988). S$\bar{\text{v}}$O$_2$ continuous monitoring technique. *Dimensions of Critical Care Nursing, 7*(1), 8-17.

48. Morganroth, J., Parisi, A., & Pohost, G. (1983). *Noninvasive cardiac imaging.* Chicago: Year Book.

49. Ratner, A. V., & Pohost, G. M. (1988). Nuclear magnetic resonance imaging of the heart. In E. Braunwald (Ed.), *Heart disease: A textbook of cardiovascular medicine* (3rd ed.) (pp. 400-407). Philadelphia: Saunders.

50. Viamonte, M. (1985). New images of imaging. *Emergency Medicine, 17*(8), 52-67.

51. Henkelman, R. M. (1990). Technologic advances in magnetic resonance imaging and spectroscopy for cardiovascular applications. *Current Opinions in Radiology, 2,* 542-546.

52. deRoos, A., & van Voorthursen, A. E. (1989). Magnetic resonance imaging of the heart—morphology and function. *Current Opinions in Radiology, 1,* 166-173.

53. Aisen, A. M., & Chenevert, T. L. (1989). MR spectroscopy: Clinical perspective. *Radiology, 173*(3), 593-599.

54. Pieper, G. M., Todd, G. L., Wu, S. T., et al. (1980). Attenuation of myocardial acidosis by propanolol during ischemic arrest and reperfusion. *Cardiovascular Research, 14,* 646-653.

55. Flaherty, J. T., Weisfeldt, M. L., Bulkley, B. H., et al. (1982). Mechanism of ischemic myocardial cell damage assessed by phosphorus-31 nuclear magnetic resonance. *Circulation, 65,* 561-570.

56. Wacker, F. J. (1980). Current status of radionuclide imaging in the management and evaluation of patients with cardiovascular disease. *Advances in Cardiology, 27,* 40-50.

57. Gerson, M. C. (1983). Myocardial imaging in myocardial infarction: Technetium vs. thallium. *Cardiovascular Clinics, 13*(3), 223-242.

58. Willerson, J. T. (1983). How reliable is myocardial imaging in the diagnosis of myocardial infarctions? *Cardiovascular Clinics, 13,* 33-50.

59. Olson, H. G. (1977). Follow up technetium-99m stannous pyrophosphate myocardial scintigrams after acute myocardial infarctions. *Circulation, 56,* 181-187.

60. Mahmarian, J. J., & Verani, M. S. (1991). Exercise thallium[201] perfusion scintigraphy in the assessment of coronary artery disease. *American Journal of Cardiology, 67*, 2D-11D.

61. Rocco, T., Dilsizian, V., McKusick, K., et al. (1989). Redistribution after thallium reinjection: Relationship to coronary anatomy and regional wall motion. *Journal of Nuclear Medicine, 30*, 740.

62. Dilsizian, V., Rocco, T., Freedman, N., et al. (1990). Enhanced detection of ischemic but viable myocardium by the injection of thallium after stress-redistribution imgaging. *New England Journal of Medicine, 323*, 141-146.

63. Ohtani, H., Tamaki, N., Yoshiharo, Y., et al. (1990). Value of thallium-201 reinjection after delayed SPECT imaging for predicting reversible ischemia after coronary artery bypass grafting. *American Journal of Cardiology, 66*, 396-399.

64. Tailefer, R. (1990). Technetium-99m sestamibi myocardial imaging: Same day rest-stress studies and dipyridamole. *American Journal of Cardiology, 66*, 80E-84E.

65. Phelps, M. E., Hoffman, E. J., Mulani, N. A., et al. (1975). Application of annihilation coincidence detection into transaxial reconstruction tomography. *Journal of Nuclear Medicine, 16*, 210-224.

66. Tillisch, J., Marshall, R., Schelbert, H., et al. (1986). Reversibility of wall motion abnormalities: Preoperative determination using positron tomography ^{18}F deoxyglucose and ^{13}N ammonia. *New England Journal of Medicine, 314*, 884-888.

67. Ludbrook, P. A., Geltman, E. M., Tiefenbrann, A. J., et al. (1983). Restoration of regional myocardial metabolism by coronary thrombolysis in patients. *Circulation, (Abstract Vol. 68, No. 325.)*

68. Gould, K. L. (1990). Positron emission tomography and interventional cardiology. *American Journal of Cardiology, 66*, 51F-58F.

69. Burrow, R. D. (1977). Analysis of left ventricular function from multiple gated acquisition cardiac blood pool imaging. Comparison to contrast angiography. *Circulation, 56*, 1024-1028.

70. Jones, R. I. (1981). Accuracy of diagnosis of coronary artery disease by radionuclide measurements of left ventricular function during rest and exercise. *Circulation, 64*, 586-601.

71. Bodenheimer, M. M., & Helfant, R. H. (1983). Exercise radionuclide angiography: Role in diagnosis and management of cardiovascular disease. *Cardiovascular Clinics, 13*, 243-251.

72. Brady, T. J., Thrall, J. H., & Pitt, B. (1980). The importance of adequate exercise in the detection of coronary heart disease by radionuclide ventriculography. *Journal of Nuclear Medicine, 21*, 1125-1130.

22

Coronary Artery Disease

Joan Vitello-Cicciu

Anne M. Morrissey

Despite a recent decline in mortality, coronary artery disease (CAD) is a predominant health problem in our nation today. Each year over 500,000 people die of its complications.[1] This disease process is characterized by progressive narrowing of the lumen of coronary arteries, referred to as *atherosclerosis*.

Coronary artery disease affects all ethnic groups, all areas of the world, and all socioeconomic classes. Its ramifications are not limited to its impact on morbidity or mortality. Complications of CAD such as angina pectoris, myocardial infarction (MI), congestive heart failure (CHF), and cardiogenic shock create physical, psychosocial, and economic hardships. Moreover, individuals who manifest these complications often require costly critical care interventions.[1]

Many advances have been made in the treatment of coronary artery disease and its complications. Medical and nursing research have provided many options to patients as well as to the members of the health care interdisciplinary team. Developments such as coronary artery bypass graft (CABG) surgery, intraaortic balloon counterpulsation, percutaneous transluminal coronary angioplasty, laser angioplasty, thrombolytic therapy, and cardiac rehabilitation programs have opened new doors for acutely ill cardiovascular patients and for the quality of life they may experience. Drug therapies such as beta-adrenergic blocking agents, calcium channel antagonists, and longer-acting nitrates have improved care.

With all these advances, critical care nurses need to expand their skill and knowledge base to maintain expertise in patient assessment and early intervention to prevent complications.

ATHEROSCLEROSIS

Atherosclerosis leads to the development of thick, hard atherosclerotic plaques referred to as *atheromas* or *lesions* that obstruct the lumen in coronary arteries as well as in other medium-sized or large arteries. In the coronary arteries, plaque formation predominates within the first few centimeters.[2] Atherosclerosis manifests itself in varying forms, depending upon the organ it affects.

The clinical effects of these plaques are related to their space-occupying characteristics, which usually result in stenosis of the vessel, or to the propensity for thrombi to develop over a plaque, which may totally occlude the vessel. For example, deposition of atherosclerotic plaques in the coronary arteries leads to ischemic heart disease which can provoke angina or an acute myocardial infarction (MI). Lesions found in the coronary vessels may also be a source for emboli which can occlude distal vessels or the collateral circulation. In the kidneys, these lesions may cause renal failure, renovascular hypertension, or both. Atherosclerotic plaques in the cerebral arteries can induce organic brain syndrome and stroke. Atherosclerotic plaques may also account for the development of peripheral vascular disease in the lower extremities and aneurysms (because of weakening of the wall) in the lower abdominal aorta.

Lesions

The lesions of atherosclerosis include the fatty streak, the fibrous plaque, and the advanced or complicated lesion. These lesions are located primarily within the intima (innermost layer which contains endothelial cells) of the coronary artery; however, with more advanced lesions, involvement of the medial layer (contains smooth muscle cells) has also been noted.[3] Each intimal lesion is thought to contain three elements: (1) smooth muscle cells; (2) large amounts of connective tissue matrix consisting of collagen, elastic fibers, and proteoglycans; and (3) intracellular and extracellular lipid. In addition to these components, platelets and monocytes/macrophages are thought to contribute to the atherosclerotic process.[3] The genesis of the lesions remains controversial.

However, there is consensus that these lesions progress over a period of years and that plaque formation is not only a preventable process but also a reversible one.

Fatty Streak

The fatty streak, found in infants and children, is considered by some to be the earliest lesion of atherosclerosis.[3] These clinically insignificant lesions are thought to be the precursor of the more complex fibrous plaque. Fatty streaks in the young are often found at the same anatomical sites as the fibrous plaque at older ages, supporting the concept of a precursor–product relation between these two types of lesions.[4]

The fatty streak is a yellowish, grossly flat, lipid-rich lesion consisting of monocytes, macrophages, and some smooth muscle cells. The lipid found in these smooth muscle cells is chiefly composed of cholesterol and cholesterol esters. These lipid-rich cells are commonly referred to as *foam cells*. These lesions may balloon out and protrude slightly into the lumen of the artery but are usually not obstructive to blood flow. Fatty streaks have been found in the coronary arteries in children and continue to accumulate in these vessels in young adults.

Fibrous Plaque

Fibrous plaques, or atheromas, are white, pearly, fibrous elevations of the intima which may protrude into the lumen of the artery, causing occlusion of the vessel.[3] Controversy exists regarding whether fibrous plaques are derived from fatty streaks. These lesions are thought to develop around the age of 25.[3] During the development of the fibrous plaque, the principal change that takes place within the intima of the artery is the proliferation of smooth muscle cells, which in turn forms a fibrous cap. Smooth muscle cells are not usually found in the intima. They are contained chiefly in the medial layer of the artery. It is thought that the proliferation of smooth muscle cells is derived from the cells in the medial layer, although the exact mechanism of this needs to be further elucidated.[4]

One hypothesis of smooth muscle cell proliferation comes from the work of Ross in the 1970s.[4] They observed that when the arterial intima was damaged platelets would stick or disintegrate on the damaged site, liberating a platelet factor known as the *platelet-derived growth factor (PDGF)*. This PDGF, in turn, promoted proliferation of smooth muscle cells.[4]

More recent studies by the same investigators found that PDGF promotes smooth muscle migration from the media to the intima and also binds to receptor sites on smooth muscle cells.[4] Once these smooth muscle cells proliferate in the intima, they combine with accumulated lipids to form a fibrous

cap of connective tissue that protrudes into the arterial lumen.

The accumulation of lipids is chiefly cholesterol in the form of low-density lipoproteins (LDL) or β-lipoprotein. These lipoproteins are discussed in further detail in the section Risk Factors.

The deep central core of the fibrous plaque also contains lipid and cell debris that is thought to result from necrosis related to inadequate blood supply to the central core.[3] This necrotic core appears on gross examination as having a soft, porridgelike consistency. The proportions of all the components of a fibrous plaque vary from plaque to plaque. These proportions also may differ during the evolution or regression of a certain plaque.

Advanced or Complicated Lesion

The advanced or complicated lesion is a degenerative fibrous plaque (Figure 22-1). The lipid-rich necrotic central core is thought to enlarge and become calcified.[4] As this lesion degenerates, the fibrous cap may rupture, hemorrhaging into the plaque and possibly leading to thrombus formation.[4] If thrombosis occurs, the clot increases the thickness of the plaque, reducing the diameter of the lumen. Myocardial infarction or sudden death may ensue. As the medial layer atrophies, the intimal lesion progresses, and the number of medial smooth muscle cells declines, an aneurysm may form.[4]

Pathogenesis

Investigations have disclosed that the pathogenesis of atherosclerosis involves several cell types such as the arterial smooth muscle cells of the medial layer, endothelial intimal cells, and macrophages.[3] In addition, there are two major processes; namely, smooth muscle cell proliferation and lipid accumulation (previously discussed), which contribute to progressive atherosclerosis having clinical significance. Theories regarding the pathogenesis of atherosclerosis include the lipogenic or lipid insudation theory, the response to injury theory, and the monoclonal theory.

Lipogenic Hypothesis

According to the lipogenic hypothesis, markedly elevated levels of plasma low-density lipoprotein (LDL) in some individuals are associated with the development and progression of a fibrous plaque. The elevated levels of LDL may be a result of heredity, hypothyroidism, or ingestion of a high-fat or a high-cholesterol diet. According to Ross,[3] some studies in hyperlipidemic animals suggest that factors in LDL promote proliferation of smooth muscle cells and their formation of a connective-tissue matrix. In addition, it is thought high concentrations of LDL act as an irritant or chemical agent that weakens the en-

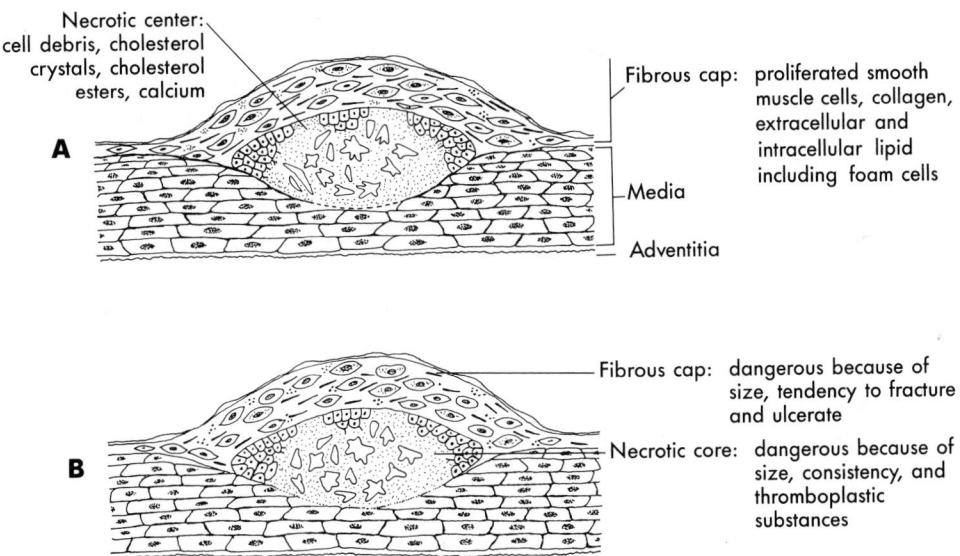

Figure 22-1 *A,* Major components of the advanced or complicated (clinically important) atherosclerotic plaque. *B,* Diagram depicting relationship of plaque components to clinical effects.

dothelial barrier of the intima. Once injury has occurred to the vessel wall, LDL fractions seem to permeate the intima and initiate proliferation of smooth muscle cells, although the exact mechanism is not known. Further research in this area is warranted to extrapolate the exact mechanisms by which LDL is transported across the endothelial cells of the intima. This information could then be used to develop preventive measures.

Response to Injury Hypothesis

According to the response to injury hypothesis, endothelial cells that normally act as a protective barrier for the intimal layer are injured by mechanical or chemical means.[4] This injury leads to structural and/or functional changes in the endothelial cells, such as platelet adhesion, platelet aggregation, and proliferation of smooth muscle cells into the intima. The theory suggests that an abnormal response to injury may be precipitated by such risk factors as cigarette smoking, hypertension, and hyperlipidemia. In a revision of the response to injury theory, Ross[4] proposes that at least two pathways may lead to formation of intimal smooth muscle proliferative lesions (Figure 22-2). In experimentally induced hypercholesterolemia, for example, injury to the endothelium may induce a growth factor secretion and also attachment of monocytes to the endothelium. The attached monocytes may continue to secrete growth factors. Once the subendothelial migration of the monocytes occurs (referred to as *macrophages* once they are inside the cell), fatty streak formation appears to develop, along with the release of other growth factors such as PDGF. The fatty streaks are

thought to be directly converted to fibrous plaques through release of these growth factors. Platelet adherence is promoted in certain cases when the macrophages lose their endothelial cover. The platelets also release PDGF which in turn can induce both smooth muscle migration and proliferation.[3,4]

Other investigators have found that the monocytes which adhere to the endothelium are transformed into macrophages once the monocytes migrate into the intima.[5,6] These macrophages have been found to be scavengers of plasma lipoproteins and cholesterol, promoting lipid accumulation in the intima. Additionally, the macrophages may become the foci for platelet aggregation and development of mural thrombi.[5,6]

The second proposed pathway suggests that there is a release of growth factor by the cells of the intact but injured epithelium. This release of a growth factor is thought to stimulate migration of smooth muscle cells from the media into the intima, where they proliferate and incite fibrous plaque formation and further lesion progression. Ross[4] suggests that this second pathway may be related to risk factors such as hypertension, cigarette smoking, or diabetes mellitus, which injure the endothelium.

Monoclonal Therapy

The monoclonal theory of atherosclerotic pathogenesis proposes that each atherosclerotic lesion begins with a single smooth muscle cell and the remaining proliferative cells within the lesion are descendants or clones of that single cell. This hypothesis was first proposed by Benditt and Benditt.[7] These investigators liken the monotypic lesion to a benign

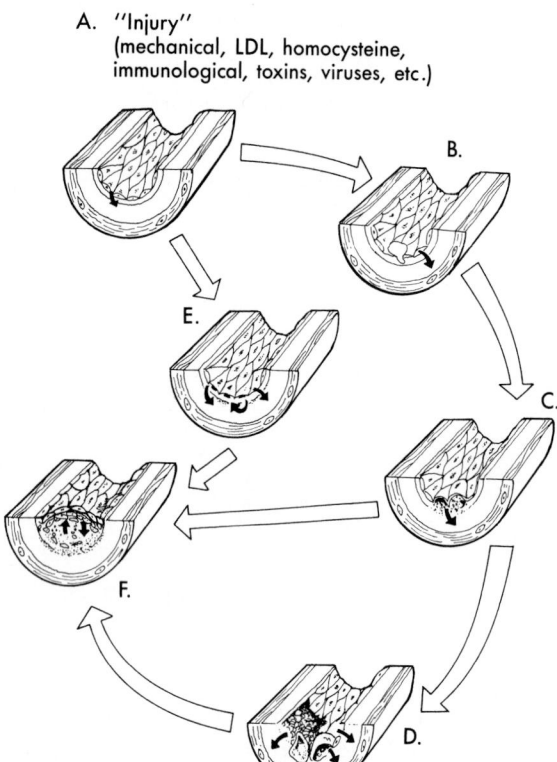

A. "Injury"
(mechanical, LDL, homocysteine,
immunological, toxins, viruses, etc.)

Figure 22-2 Advanced intimal proliferative lesions of atherosclerosis may occur by at least two pathways. The pathway demonstrated by the clockwise (long) arrows to the right has been observed in experimentally induced hypercholesterolemia. Injury to the endothelium (A) may induce growth secretion (short arrow). Monocytes attach to endothelium (B), which may continue to secrete growth factors (short arrow). Subendothelial migration of monocytes (C) may lead to fatty-streak formation and release of growth factors such as PDGF (short arrow). Fatty streaks may become directly converted to fibrous plaques (long arrow from C to F) through release of growth factors from macrophages or endothelial cells or both. Macrophages may also stimulate or injure the overlying endothelium. In some cases, macrophages may lose their endothelial cover and platelet attachment may occur (D), providing three possible sources of growth factors—platelets, macrophages, and endothelium (short arrows). Some of the smooth muscle cells in the proliferative lesion itself (F) may form and secrete growth factors such as PDGF (short arrows). An alternative pathway for development of advanced lesions of atherosclerosis is shown by the arrows from A to E to F. In this case, the endothelium may be injured but remain intact. Increased endothelial turnover may result in growth-factor formation by endothelial cells (A). This may stimulate migration of smooth muscle cells from the media into the intima, accompanied by endogenous production of PDGF by smooth muscle as well as growth-factor secretion from the "injured" endothelial cells (E). These interactions could then lead to fibrous plaque formation and further lesion progression (F).

neoplasm that arise through transformation of cells by mutagenic agents such as toxins, viruses, or chemical agents. Other studies conflict with this hypothesis, and additional research is needed.[3]

A great deal of new information about the genesis of atherosclerosis at the cellular and molecular levels is continually emerging. Many of these investigations employ animal studies; however, experimentally-induced atherosclerotic plaque in animals has been found to develop differently from the human atherosclerotic lesion. Furthermore, successful attempts to induce regression of animal plaques require additional confirmation by controlled, randomized studies in humans beyond the limited investigations conducted thus far. Moreover, substantial inquiry into the role of certain risk factors in the pathogenesis of atherosclerosis is also necessary.

RISK FACTORS

Recognition of risk factors associated with the development of CAD has been attained chiefly through epidemiological studies. The Framingham Heart Study[8] was one of the first to discern such risk factors as age, sex, familial tendency, hyperlipidemia, hypertension, obesity, cigarette smoking, diabetes, and personality traits.[1,8,9,10]

In grouping all these risk factors, two categories emerge: (1) those risk factors regarded as unavoidable or unalterable—age, sex, heredity, and geography, and (2) those considered avoidable or alterable, including hypertension, hyperlipidemia, cigarette smoking, hyperglycemia, obesity, physical inactivity, personality traits, and oral contraceptive use. Moreover, all these risk factors (unavoidable and avoidable) tend to have a multiplicative or synergistic effect on each other. That is, an individual in whom several risk factors are present appears to be at greater risk than the sum of individual risks would suggest. Risk factors for developing heart disease are listed in the box on p. 513.

Risk factors may be addressed by either primary or secondary measures. *Primary prevention* involves risk factor modification before clinical manifestations of coronary artery disease occur. *Secondary prevention* of risk factors refers to those measures begun to minimize the progression of CAD or to prevent recurrences of catastrophic events such as MI in patients with documented CAD.

Nonalterable Risk Factors

Age, Sex, Familial History

Fifty percent of all myocardial infarctions reportedly occur in patients 65 years or older.[1] Moreover, of those who succumb, approximately 80% are more than 65 years old.[1] Thus, a direct relationship is ev-

Coronary Heart Disease (CHD) Risk Factors

Male gender
Family history of CHD before 55 years of age (parent or sibling)
Cigarette smoking
Hypertension
Diabetes mellitus
Definite cerebrovascular or peripheral vascular disease
Obesity (≥30% overweight)
Known low HDL-C (≤35 mg/dl)

From Department of Health and Human Services, Public Health Service, National Institutes of Health. (1989). *Report of the expert panel on the detection, evaluation, and treatment of high blood cholesterol in adults.* (Publication No. 89-2925). Bethesda, MD: National Institutes of Health.

ident between advancing age, CAD, and mortality.

A decline in the incidence of CAD has been noted in both sexes. A greater incidence is seen in men than women by age 50 to 55 years, but women close this gap after menopause. In fact, the incidence of CAD is greater in women than in men after age 75.[11] Furthermore, myocardial infarction has become a "silent epidemic" among women; it is the *number one killer* of U.S. women over the age of 40.[11] This alarming mortality is higher for black females (22% higher) than white females.[1,9,11] Moreover, one of three women over the age of 65 has developed some form of cardiovascular disease.[11] Risk factors for women are the same as for men with the additional concerns for the use of oral contraceptives in premenopausal women and hormone replacement in postmenopausal women.[12] Refer to reference 12 for an excellent review of CAD in women.

There is increasing evidence of a familial risk associated with the development of atherosclerosis. Investigations in molecular biology have shed some light on the interrelationship of genes, lipids, and atherosclerosis.[13] This information centers on *apoproteins*, protein moieties that facilitate the transport of lipids in the blood. The predominant apoprotein of low-density lipoprotein (LDL) is APO B and of high-density lipoprotein (HDL) is APO A-1.[14,15] These apoproteins have been localized on specific chromosomes. Several studies have implicated these apoproteins as significant risk factors for CAD.[14,15] In fact these apoproteins may be more precise indices of CAD than LDL or HDL.[13] Future blood screening tests may include these apoproteins.

A family history of MI continues to be a risk factor. In one prospective study, a parental (maternal or paternal) history of MI was implicated as a risk factor

among healthy men in health professions.[16] The younger the parent had been at the time of MI, the higher the risk.[16]

Alterable Risk Factors

Several major and minor risk factors are considered avoidable or alterable. The major alterable risk factors include hypertension, hyperlipidemia, cigarette smoking, and hyperglycemia.

Hypertension

Over 60 million Americans have hypertension.[1] This disease is more common in blacks, obese persons, and women taking oral contraceptives. Women over the age of 65 have a greater propensity to develop hypertension than their male counterparts.[11] In fact, more than half of all women over age 55 currently suffer from hypertension.[11]

Hypertension is associated with an increased risk of developing CAD. Moreover, this risk greatly increases with the coexistence of hypertension and hypercholesterolemia.[17] It is often referred to as the "silent killer" because an individual may have the disease for up to 10 to 20 years or longer without being aware of its existence. By the time hypertension is discovered, vital organs may have been damaged. It is thought that the mechanism by which hypertension is related to CAD is that the chronic, persistent tension in the arterial walls that hypertension exerts, leads to injury and/or structural changes in the intimal layer of the coronary vessels.[3] These changes accelerate the development of atherosclerosis which may in turn lead to angina and myocardial infarction.

Systolic blood pressure elevation has been found to be a better predictor of mortality associated with CAD than diastolic blood pressure, especially in the elderly and in men over 50.[18]

A sequela of hypertension, left ventricular hypertrophy (LVH), is also strongly associated with the risk of a coronary event. This finding comes from the Framingham study whereby it was documented that 44% of deaths related to CAD were heralded by electrographic evidence of LVH.[10] This ventricular enlargement develops to compensate for the increase in wall tension exerted to overcome high aortic pressure gradients. Thus, left ventricular hypertrophy develops when there is continued impedance to left ventricular ejection. Left ventriculalr hypertrophy is depicted on the ECG by increased voltage of the QRS complexes and the typical "R wave plus S wave" voltage that is greater than 35 mm in certain precordial leads.

Another noteworthy development involves the metabolic abnormalities of hyperinsulinemia and insulin resistance prevalent among hypertensive individuals.[19] In individuals with these coexistent metabolic abnormalities, alterations in lipids have been noted including an increase in LDL and VLDL levels and a decrease in HDL.[19] Thus, the additive effect of hypertension and insulin resistance may accelerate the development of CAD.

Identification and early treatment of hypertension is imperative in preventing the complications associated with prolonged, elevated blood pressure. Discussion of the treatment of hypertension is beyond the scope of this chapter. The reader is referred to references 9 and 18 for more information.

Hyperlipidemia or Hyperlipoproteinemia

Among the numerous risk factors for the development of atherosclerosis, one of the best documented is the association between blood lipids and CAD. No population with a severely reduced dietary intake of cholesterol has been found to develop atherosclerotic heart disease. Atherosclerosis apparently does not occur until a certain threshold amount of cholesterol-rich lipoproteins has been reached in the body. This threshold tends to be quite variable and is dependent on the individual as well as the presence of other risk factors. The etiology of sustained levels of serum cholesterol (hypercholesterolemia) in atherosclerotic heart disease may be genetically induced; secondary to a metabolic disorder such as hypothyroidism; or caused by the elevated intake of a high-fat, high-cholesterol diet.

The term *hyperlipidemia* is used in reference to an elevation of one or more of the commonly known lipids referred to as cholesterol, triglycerides, and phospholipids. These lipids are insoluble in plasma and do not freely circulate in the blood. They are bound to apoproteins. Together they are transported in the serum in the form of lipoprotein complexes. Prospective studies have shown inconclusive results in implicating serum triglycerides as a coronary risk factor. In contrast, results from several prospective studies have unequivocally indicated that the risk of CAD in an otherwise healthy person is directly related to the concentration of plasma cholesterol.[20] Also, the National Cholesterol Education Program (NCEP) recommends that lipoproteins be measured after an initial total cholesterol greater than 200 mg/dl.[21]

Lipoproteins are produced in the gut and liver, and each has distinct functions in transporting exogenous and endogenous lipids. An elevation of lipoproteins is referred to as *hyperlipoproteinemia*. Lipoproteins are broken down into the following subgroups or fractions, based on their density and chemical breakdown: chylomicrons, very-low-density lipoproteins (VLDL), intermediate-low-density lipoproteins (ILDL), low-density lipoproteins (LDL), and high-density lipoproteins (HDL).

Chylomicrons are derived from exogenous dietary fat. They are metabolized in the small intestine. Chylomicrons are composed mainly of triglycerides and small amounts of cholesterol. When released into the systemic circulation, they are hydrolyzed rapidly by the enzyme lipoprotein lipase. After chylomicrons undergo hydrolysis in the circulation, the remnants are transported to the liver for the removal of cholesterol. After 12 to 14 hours of fasting, chylomicrons are usually absent in plasma, and their presence in fasting plasma is considered to be an abnormal finding.[9] Elevations of chylomicrons have not been linked with premature CAD, although the remnant particles of chylomicrons could lead to atherosclerosis.[9]

Another type of lipoprotein, very-low-density lipoproteins (VLDL), are produced by the liver and contain APO B100. The main functions of VLDLs are to transport triglycerides from the liver to peripheral tissue and to serve as a precursor for LDL. Increases in triglyceride levels are associated with high dietary intake of carbohydrates. An excess of VLDL is associated with hypertriglyceridemia and premature atherosclerosis.[9]

Intermediate-low-density lipoproteins (ILDL) are an intermediate form in the metabolism of VLDL to LDL. In certain types of hyperlipoproteinemia ILDL-like particles have been associated with premature coronary artery disease.[9]

Low-density lipoproteins (LDL) are obtained from the breakdown of VLDL. They serve primarily to transport large amounts (50% to 75%) of cholesterol from the liver to peripheral tissues. Apo-B is the apoprotein present in LDL. This lipoprotein has been most directly linked with CAD because patients with elevated levels of LDL tend to have CAD more often than those with normal levels of LDL. It has been found that patients with this type of hyperlipoproteinemia have concomitant hypercholesterolemia.

High-density lipoproteins (HDL) are produced in the hepatocyte and secreted from the liver. These lipoproteins appear to have a protective effect against atherosclerosis.[9,18] The cause and effect of this inverse relationship remain to be elucidated. It is also thought that the ratio of HDL to LDL may be a *better* predictor of coronary risk than either value alone.[9] High concentrations of HDL are noteworthy in such groups as children and premenopausal women, who tend as groups to have low coronary risk. It has also been found that exercise, reduction in obesity, cessation of cigarette smoking, and, lastly, consumption of alcoholic beverages, may elevate HDL levels.[9] Subfractions of HDL have been identified through in vitro studies.[9] HDL_2 and HDL_3 are the two subfractions most extensively studied. HDL_2 may be the protective fraction against atherosclerosis.[9]

TABLE 22-1   Classification of Hyperlipidemias

Type	Lipoprotein Abnormality
I	Markedly ↑ chylomicrons Normal cholesterol, ↑ triglycerides
IIA	↑ LDL, ↑ cholesterol, normal triglycerides
IIB	↑ LDL and VLDL, ↑ cholesterol, ↑ triglycerides
III	Floating beta lipoproteins, ↑ cholesterol and triglycerides
IV	↑ VLDL, normal cholesterol, ↑ triglycerides
V	↑ Chylomicrons and VLDL, cholesterol greatly ↑, triglycerides present, ↓ LDL

Adapted from Gotto, A. M. (1984). Practical approach to phenotyping hyperlipoproteinemia. In P. D. Kligfield (Ed.), *Cardiology reference book*. New York: Co-Medica.

Hyperlipidemias are classified into five types based on evaluation of laboratory data. Table 22-1 lists these categories and illustrates the lipoprotein abnormality found in each type. Lastly, a major thrust to educate health care professionals and the general public regarding cholesterol has been the establishment of the National Cholesterol Education Program (NCEP) by the National Heart, Lung and Blood Institute in 1985 regarding the detection, evaluation, and treatment of high blood cholesterol.[21] The critical care nurse should become familiar with these recommendations in reference 21.

Cigarette Smoking

Cigarette smoking has been considered one of the major health hazards in the United States. It has been associated with even more deaths from CAD than from cancer. According to the Framingham study, cigarette smokers had a risk of CAD two to four times greater than the risk for nonsmokers.[22] The risk is also multiplicative or synergistic in that moderate cigarette smoking doubles or triples the susceptibility to CAD when associated with other risk factors.[18] Other factors associated with an increased risk of developing CAD include the age one started smoking, the number of years one smoked, the number of cigarettes smoked per day, and how deeply one inhales the smoke.[9,18] Furthermore, the risk of infarction has also been shown to correlate with the number of cigarettes (>15 per day) smoked for both women and men.[9,18] In addition, women who take oral contraceptives and smoke have a significantly increased vulnerability to myocardial infarctions.

Some mechanisms by which cigarette smoking may induce coronary artery disease include the following:
The inhalation of cigarette smoke may expose arterial cells to mutagens that alter the smooth muscle cells and cause them to proliferate.[3]

Higher levels of LDL, cholesterol, and triglycerides as well as lower levels of HDL have been found in men and women who smoked more than 15 cigarettes daily as compared to nonsmokers.[9,18]
Cigarette smoking was found to increase the adhesiveness of platelets, perhaps leading to thrombus formation.[9]
Carboxyhemoglobin, a substance which is increased in cigarette smokers, competes with oxygen to bind with hemoglobin and, thus, reduces the oxygen carrying capacity in blood. It has been found to interfere with coronary oxygen supply.[9]
Increased myocardial demand for oxygen secondary to nicotine inhalation has been noted.[9]
Nicotine causes release of catecholamines, thereby increasing heart rate and myocardial oxygen consumption (MVO_2).
Further research is necessary, however, to identify the specific cellular mechanisms that are altered by cigarette smoking.

It has been suggested that cessation of cigarette smoking decreases the risk of atherosclerosis and may induce regression of lesions. The risk decreases about 50% within the first year following cessation and approaches the same risk as that of nonsmokers in about 2 to 10 years. Also, the level of HDL has been found to increase while levels of LDL decrease once cigarette smoking has been discontinued.[18]

Hyperglycemia

The Framingham study clearly identified a relationship between CAD and hyperglycemia which was as strong for men as it was for women.[8] It has been found that the type of diabetes was also significant. For example, type 1 (adult-onset, non-insulin-dependent) diabetes was associated with more deaths from CAD than type 2 (juvenile-onset, insulin-dependent).[8] More deaths from renal disease occurred in type 1 disease. Both male and female type 2 diabetics have a 50% greater incidence of developing CAD than type 1 diabetics.[8]

Several complex interrelationships between hyperglycemia and CAD have been proposed. The first involves the effect of insulin and glucose on the arterial wall. High serum insulin levels may incite proliferation of smooth muscle cells and synthesis of cholesterol and triglyceride.[23] Second, hyperglycemia may increase the adhesiveness of platelets and may cause other abnormalities of coagulation, setting the stage for thrombus development.[23] Last, some studies suggest that diabetics tend to have decreased levels of high-density lipoproteins, increasing their vulnerability to CAD.[9,18]

Control of hyperglycemia alone has not been shown to eliminate the risk of CAD. It appears that concomitant reduction of other risk factors such as obesity, hypertension, and hypercholesterolemia may be necessary.[18]

Minor Risk Factors

Minor risk factors have been associated with an increased incidence of CAD; among these are obesity, physical inactivity, personality traits, and oral contraceptive use.

Obesity

Obesity is considered to contribute significantly to the severity of such major risk factors as hypertension, hyperglycemia, and hyperlipidemia. Patients who are obese also tend to have higher levels of LDL linked to premature atherosclerosis and lower levels of HDL. Hypertriglyceridemia is the most common abnormality among obese persons. The epidemiological significance of all these lipid abnormalities and obesity needs further clarification.[9]

Physical Inactivity

Recognition of exercise as a factor associated with decreased coronary risk is relatively recent. Several studies have shown that HDL levels are below normal in sedentary people compared to elevated HDL levels noted after both short- and long-term exercise.[18] According to Wenger and Schlant,[18] the following favorable effects are achieved through exercise: (1) decreased weight, (2) increased cardiovascular functional capacity, (3) reduced myocardial oxygen demand, (4) decreased platelet adhesiveness and improved fibrinolysis, and (5) electrical stability of the myocardium. These effects suggest that regular exercise is a positive influence for decreasing the risk of CAD, although additional research is necessary to confirm exercise as a direct factor in the prevention of coronary artery disease.

Personality Traits

The psychosocial factors most consistently related to coronary artery disease are personality and behavioral traits. The Western Collaborative Study showed that men with type A personality traits developed coronary artery disease at two times the rate of individuals with a type B personality.[24] The Framingham study also supported this finding.[9]

Individuals with type A personality are characterized by a chronic struggle to obtain an unlimited number of items from the environment in the shortest time, despite environmental constraints. These individuals characteristically behave in a hostile, impatient, aggressive, and highly competitive manner. In contrast, the type B personality tends to be more patient, less aggressive, and less concerned with either deadlines or any habitual sense of time urgency.

To date, the exact mechanism whereby personality traits contribute to the pathogenesis of CAD is unknown. However, people with type A personalities tend to have increased circulating catecholamines. These endogenous amines may cause hypertension and abnormal platelet function, contributing indirectly to the development of atherosclerotic heart disease.[18,25]

Oral Contraceptives

A history of oral contraceptive use seems to be associated with an increased incidence of CAD in postmenopausal women. An increased risk of myocardial infarction is also associated with those premenopausal women who have concomitant hypertension and diabetes. Another significantly high risk group for the development of an MI are women who take oral contraceptives and who smoke cigarettes.

Oral contraceptives have also been found to raise blood pressure and alter serum levels of lipoproteins. These contraceptives create disturbances in the clotting cascade and favor thrombus formation. In addition, the use of these agents may cause an increase in body weight, an elevated triglyceride concentration, and a decrease HDL levels.[18] However, all of these mechanisms need further investigation to clarify the role of oral contraceptives in the promotion of atherosclerosis.

Research

Data from both epidemiological and clinical studies indicate that coronary artery disease in humans may be due to multiple risk factors and not only to hypercholesterolemia. Reduction of risk factors through primary prevention is thought to have the most beneficial effect if done before clinical findings of CAD become evident. Data indicating the ability to hinder or reverse CAD in humans by modification of risk factors is mounting. A landmark study known as the Lipid Research Clinics Coronary Primary Prevention trial demonstrated for the first time a direct cause-and-effect relationship between plasma lipoproteins and cholesterol levels with morbidity and mortality from CAD.[26] This trial was a randomized double-blind study that tested the efficacy of lowering cholesterol levels in reducing the risk of CAD over a period of 7.4 years. The sample population consisted of 3,806 middle-aged men with type 2 hyperlipoproteinemia (elevated LDL levels). The treatment group (1,906 subjects) received the bile acid cholestyramine. The control group (1,900 subjects) received a placebo. Both groups were also placed on a moderate cholesterol-lowering diet. The investigators monitored LDL levels as well as the occurrence of coronary artery disease, death, or definite nonfatal myocardial infarction. The treatment group was found to have lower levels of LDL in comparison to the placebo group. The treatment group also had a significantly decreased incidence of CAD in comparison to the placebo group. This trial provided a strong cause-and-effect relationship between LDL and the pathogenesis of coronary heart disease.[22]

The importance of each risk factor may also be influenced by the genetic composition of each individual. Approaches to the prevention, treatment, or progression of CAD continue to be developed as researchers discover how each of these risk factors is related to the specific cellular structural and/or functional interactions that lead to atherosclerosis.

ANGINA PECTORIS

In the majority of cases, angina pectoris is associated with an atherosclerotic lesion causing greater than 75% occlusion of the lumen of a specific coronary artery. Angina pectoris is a symptom of myocardial ischemia which literally means "choking of the chest," from the Greek word *anchein*, meaning "to choke." It is a manifestation of the disparity between myocardial oxygen demand and supply. The ability of the heart to increase blood flow when oxygen demand increases is limited by the intraluminal obstruction of the atherosclerotic lesion. This fixed arterial obstruction in turn leads to an insufficient arterial oxygen supply in the coronary vasculature and results in ischemia and chest pain, especially when the demand exceeds the supply. This type of angina is often referred to as *classic, effort,* or *exertional angina,* because the fixed coronary artery lesion impedes myocardial blood flow, leading to ischemia at a certain level of exertion.

A different type of angina presents itself typically at rest, suggesting that a discrepancy in supply suddenly exists as the demand remains relatively constant. This finding led investigators, notably Prinzmetal and coworkers in the 1950s, to probe for functional changes in the lumen of the coronary vessel.[27] They were able to document the presence of coronary vasoconstriction or coronary vasospasm in patients who experienced pain spontaneously at rest, and in whom ST segment elevation was depicted on the ECG during pain. Prinzmetal referred to this rest pain as *coronary spasm, variant angina,* or *spontaneous angina,* but the condition is often called Prinzmetal's angina to acknowledge his investigations. Prinzmetal-type angina can occur in two subsets of patients: those with atherosclerotic lesions and those with normal or near-normal coronary arteries.

Some clinicians use the term mixed angina to describe a combination of pure exertional angina and coronary vasospasm.[28] Typically, these patients have a fixed obstruction with concomitant vasoconstriction (spasm). These lesions precipitate ischemia, with or without increased oxygen demand.

Other causes of angina include systemic hypertension, aortic stenosis or regurgitation, cardiac dysrhythmias, anemia, and hyperthyroidism.

Clinical Manifestations

The chest pain of classic angina pectoris is typically described as substernal chest discomfort or pain with a sensation of pressure or heaviness that occurs with activity and is relieved by rest. The pressure may be associated with a burning or itching in the chest. This chest discomfort gradually increases in intensity and is followed by a gradual fading away. Occasionally, some diabetic patients may not complain of chest pain, only dyspnea, because they have developed peripheral neuropathy that prevents chest pain from being experienced.

The sensation of angina may appear in many locations but the most common is the middle or lower sternum, or over the left precordium, which may be confused with indigestion. Patients may complain of left shoulder pain or upper arm pain that may be mistaken for arthritis. When pain extends down the arm, usually the fourth and fifth fingers are involved. Rarely, patients may complain of jaw pain, and occasional patients describe pain in the posterior thorax or intrascapular area. If a careful assessment is not made, the pain may be attributed to back ailments. When describing angina, patients commonly use their fist to describe the location of discomfort rather than pointing with their finger (*Levine's sign*).

Patients may also develop associated symptoms during an anginal attack. These symptoms include nausea, vomiting, diaphoresis, dyspnea, and exhaustion. They may appear pale or dusky with signs of labored breathing. Their skin may be clammy and cool. Certain cardiac dysrhythmias may occur with angina related to transient ischemia of a small area of heart tissue. In addition, patients may experience an increase in heart rate and blood pressure. Usually these signs and symptoms subside with resolution of the anginal attack.

Stimuli that may provoke an anginal episode include physical activity, exposure to cold or heat, heavy eating, sexual intercourse, emotional stress factors, cigarette smoking, and rapid eye movement (REM) sleep. Physical activity commonly provokes an anginal attack because it increases myocardial oxygen demand. The discomfort usually occurs during the attack, rather than after the activity. The "second wind" phenomenon refers to a small group of patients who characteristically develop symptoms during the activity but whose discomfort disappears while the activity is continued.

Exposure to hot or cold weather places an increased workload on the heart, thereby increasing myocardial oxygen demand. Heavy eating may precipitate an anginal attack because there is an increase in gastrointestinal oxygen demand which, in turn, increases cardiac output to the gut, thereby placing more demand on the heart. Sexual intercourse also increases the workload on the heart and therefore increases oxygen demand. Emotional stress factors such as anger, fear, and enthusiasm are known precursors of angina in that they increase circulating catecholamines which increase heart rate and contractility, thereby increasing myocardial oxygen demand. Another trigger for angina includes mental activities associated with cognitive tasks such as mental arithmetic. Angina is believed to be precipitated by cigarette smoking because the nicotine is thought to stimulate the release of epinephrine, which increases the work of the heart. Angina is also thought to occur during rapid eye movement (REM) sleep because of stimulation of the sympathetic nervous system which, in turn, increases myocardial oxygen demand by increasing heart rate, blood pressure, and contractility.[29]

A recent premise is that ischemia occurs in a circadian pattern. Several investigations have documented that overt as well as silent ischemic episodes tend to manifest in the early morning hours, peak at about noon, and subside during the afternoon and evening.[30,31,32] This same diurnal pattern has been noted in patients with an acute MI, sudden cardiac death, and postinfarction ventricular activity.[31] It tends to support the concept that the stenotic lesion leads to a dynamic rather than a fixed obstruction. The dynamic nature of the obstruction means that blood flow through the area of stenosis is variable.[30] This variability can be attributed to changes in smooth muscle tone, platelet aggregability, and other factors that may alter lumen size (Figure 22-3) during a day.

The duration of angina pectoris precipitated by effort is usually 1 to 5 minutes, once the patient discontinues the activity. Angina provoked by emotional stress typically lasts longer than effort angina because emotional factors are less easily controlled than is physical activity.[33]

The chest pain of coronary vasospasm or variant angina (Prinzmetal) is typically similar to classic or effort angina but differs in that the pain occurs at rest. This rest pain often presents in a cyclic or predictive pattern, occurring around the same time every day in a particular individual. Notably, rest pain tends to occur in the early morning hours. It has been suggested that the etiology of this occurrence may be related to increased levels of endogenous circulating catecholamines present in the body in the early morning or perhaps due to the decrease or absence of endothelium-derived relaxing factor (a substance produced by normal epithelium).[34] Associated symptoms include syncope, dyspnea, and palpitations.

Precipitating factors of variant angina have also been identified. For example, cigarette smoking, alcohol, and cocaine have been implicated in inciting variant angina.[34,35,36] This type of angina has also been

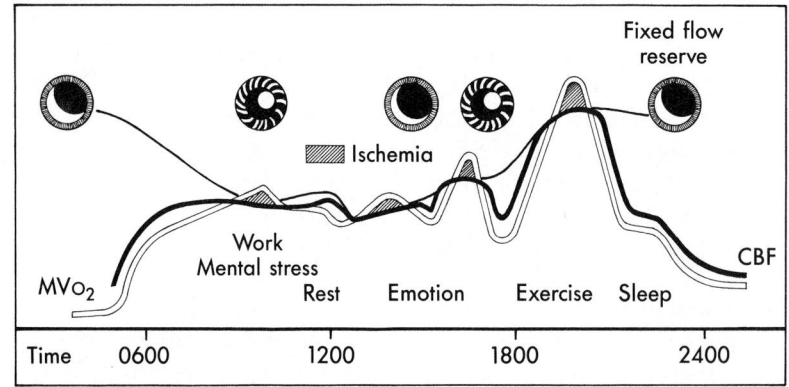

Figure 22-3 Revised concept of myocardial ischemia suggests that the coronary artery stenosis must be considered as a dynamic rather than a fixed obstruction. Changes in smooth muscle tone, in platelet aggregability, and other factors alter lumen size so that flow reserve is variable. When sympathetic nervous system activation takes place in the early morning, increases in myocardial oxygen demand may or may not be met by appropriate increases in coronary flow. Cognitive and emotional activities seem to increase myocardial oxygen demand above the level that can be met by coronary flow. Hence, this revised concept explains how ischemia may occur many times throughout the day and tends to be most frequent in the hours after waking and is infrequent in the late evening and early morning hours. Here, ischemia is most often silent.

reported in non-bypassed coronary arteries following surgical revascularization.[34,37]

Categories of Angina

Stable Angina

Stable angina is also referred to as *classic angina*, and is usually triggered by physical exertion or emotional stress as previously discussed. This type of pain tends to remain unchanged over several months. The pain typically lasts 1 to 5 minutes and is relieved by rest. Thus, each attack of stable angina is similar to the previous episode and is relieved by the same mode of therapy.

Unstable Angina

Unstable angina, preinfarction angina, or crescendo angina are terms used to describe the first episode of angina, pre- or postinfarction angina, or stable angina in which there has been a change in the timing, frequency, intensity, duration, and quality. Unstable angina is easily provoked with lower exercise workloads than stable angina. Pain is greater than that of stable angina, typically lasting longer (10 minutes), despite rest and the use of sublingual nitroglycerin. Moreover, unstable angina is harder to control with pharmacological therapy and may mimic the symptoms of a myocardial infarction. The patient with unstable angina may also be in jeopardy for myocardial infarction and sudden death.

Variant Angina

Variant angina (Prinzmetal-type) is precipitated by constriction (transient and abrupt) of a coronary artery. As previously noted, variant angina is usually associated with a reduction in the diameter of the coronary artery resulting in myocardial ischemia in the absence of an increase in myocardial oxygen demand. However, this pain may manifest not only at rest but during and after exertion. It may be intense, prolonged, and not quickly relieved by sublingual nitroglycerin. Ergonovine maleate and dopamine have been found to induce coronary artery spasm. The ECG in variant angina typically depicts transient ST elevations. These elevations are often mistaken for the acute injury pattern associated with MI. Moreover, these elevations are transient and return to normal once the spasm is relieved. Treatment for variant angina includes nitrates and calcium channel blockers.

Silent Ischemia

The term *silent ischemia* (asymptomatic myocardial ischemia) has been defined as the presence of objective evidence of ischemia (as shown by electrocardiographic, exercise test, or radionuclide findings) in asymptomatic patients with or without documented coronary artery disease.[31,32,33] This definition is in contrast to *unrecognized* myocardial ischemia in which symptoms have been misinterpreted by health care professionals or the patient does not report the symptoms, thus delaying medical treatment.[38] Three subsets or categories of silent ischemia have been suggested.[39] Type 1 are those patients who have no accompanying symptoms of angina but show ST segment shifts on exercise testing or ambulatory ECG monitoring. Type 2 are those patients asymptomatic postinfarction who demonstrate ST segment changes on exercise testing or ambulatory monitoring. Type 3 includes those with angina pectoris who have multiple episodes of silent ischemia as documented by 24-hour Holter (ambulatory) monitoring. According to Pratt,[40] it is postulated that patients with silent ischemic episodes may have higher pain thresholds than others. This syndrome is probably related to a reduction in myocardial oxygen supply secondary to vasospasm in contrast to an increase in myocardial oxygen demand as noted in classic angina. However, the pathophysiology of silent ischemia is under investigation.

Therapy for silent ischemia is similar to treatment for symptomatic ischemia including nitrates, beta-adrenergic blockers, calcium channel blockers, coronary angioplasty, and surgery. Refer to reference 38 for discussion of this topic.

Syndrome X

A subset of patients with angina-type chest pain who present with angiographically normal coronary arteries and no evidence of vasospasm has recently been identified. These patients also may have a positive exercise stress test. There is some evidence that the myocardial ischemia in these patients may be at the microvascular level described as syndrome X.[41] This syndrome is currently under intensive investigation.

Data Collection

Electrocardiogram

The electrocardiogram (ECG) at rest is of limited importance in the diagnosis of angina pectoris related to atherosclerotic heart disease, except in diagnosing an old myocardial infarction. Normal resting ECGs have been noted in approximately 70% of patients with stable angina pectoris.[33] Transient ST depression of 1 mm or greater has been recorded in some patients during an episode of angina pectoris and has also been observed in patients experiencing silent ischemia but no pain.[33] This ST segment depression is characteristic of myocardial ischemia.

In variant angina, the ECG may be diagnostic. As

previously mentioned the ECG will display transient ST segment elevations in the leads relative to the ischemic areas. Interestingly, there have also been reports of ST segment depression in such patients.[42] Evaluations of ST segments are considered by many as pathognomonic for coronary spasm, but they in no way rule out the presence of an atherosclerotic lesion at the site of the spasm.[34] Concomitant with this typical finding of variant angina may be a multitude of dysrhythmias. Ventricular dysrhythmias such as premature beats, ventricular tachycardia, or ventricular fibrillation may be present. Atrioventricular block such as second- and third-degree heart block may also occur during chest pain indicative of spasm of the right coronary artery.[34]

Holter (ambulatory) monitoring is useful in the evaluation of patients believed to have atherosclerotic heart disease, silent ischemia, or coronary spasm. It enables clinicians to document ischemic changes such as ST segment depression during activities and over an extended period.

The exercise electrocardiogram is another worthwhile tool used to reveal ECG changes during and after exercise in contrast to the resting ECG in patients with stable angina pectoris. It is usually contraindicated in patients displaying unstable angina pectoris. Exercise stress testing can be accomplished using a bicycle ergometer, treadmill, or the master two-step test. The patient is exercised under controlled ECG monitoring conditions until certain findings are noted or until the patient reaches a predetermined heart rate. Patients believed to have multivessel CAD or left main vessel disease may have any or all of the following:[33]

Onset of ST segment depression within the first 3 minutes of exercise

Persistent ST segment depression 8 minutes after exercise

Downward sloping or 2-mm ST depression for at least 0.8 second

Low maximum heart rate/blood pressure product

Interest in the exercise test has shifted from diagnostic to prognostic uses.[33] For example, patients who demonstrate ischemic ST segment changes during stage 1 or stage 2 have been noted to have a poorer prognosis.[33] The exercise stress test has limited diagnostic capabilities, especially in asymptomatic patients. There is a high incidence of false positives noted in this group.[33] Other factors that may cause false positives include hypokalemia, anemia, Wolff-Parkinson-White syndrome, and ventricular hypertrophy. False positives have also been noted in young women. In contrast, patients with triple vessel disease have a 20% chance of a false positive test.[33]

The exercise stress test is also of limited value in patients with coronary vasospasm because spasm rarely occurs during exercise. However, a recent normal exercise test in a patient who then presents with a pain history similar to unstable angina should alert clinicians to the likelihood of coronary spasm. The exercise stress test is also useful in diagnosing silent ischemia in asymptomatic patients after a positive stress test.

Radionuclide Imaging

Radionuclide imaging with thallium-201 or isonitrile compounds and radionuclide angiography with technetium can evaluate patients with suspected CAD or determine the extent and severity of the disease during exercise stress testing. Patients with stable angina are candidates for either test. The patient with unstable or variant angina usually is not a candidate for such testing.

In the thallium exercise stress test, thallium is injected once the patient becomes physically exhausted or develops angina. Following injection, myocardial scintigraphic images are obtained to reveal regions of underperfusion that develop with exercise. The amount of thallium present in each region is determined by two factors: (1) the amount of coronary blood flow to that region, and (2) the degree of viable myocardium. Ischemic or infarcted myocardial regions receiving little or no blood flow accumulate minimal or no amounts of the injected thallium. Such regions are referred to as "cold spots" and are suggestive of the presence of coronary artery disease.

Nuclear imaging with technetium bound to human serum albumin or red blood cells allows evaluation of global and segmental ventricular performance. This test is more useful in diagnosing myocardial infarction and is further described in that section. Newer cardiac imaging techniques such as position emission tomography (PET) scan and magnetic resonance imaging are emerging as more useful modalities in distinguishing ischemic from infarcted tissues. Refer to Chapter 21 for more detailed information.

Cardiac Catheterization and Coronary Arteriography

The data from cardiac catheterization and coronary arteriography are used to assess the hemodynamic status of the heart, left ventricular performance, and the presence, severity, and/or distribution of coronary artery disease. These invasive tools are also used to ascertain whether a particular patient may be a suitable candidate for either medical or surgical interventions. Pacing-induced ischemia is also used in conjunction with cardiac catheterization to assess LV performance and lactate metabolism.

Left heart catheterization is performed to obtain

left ventricular (LV) and aortic pressures as well as volumes. There appears to be a correlation between abnormal elevations of left ventricular end-diastolic pressures or decreased cardiac output and the number of vessels with more than 75% occlusion of the lumen. The severity of vessel disease does not, however, solely have a reciprocal relationship with hemodynamic abnormalities. The left ventricular end-diastolic pressure may also be elevated as a reflection of decreased left ventricular compliance or LV failure or both. Decreased compliance or failure may be a sequela of acute ischemia or scar formation from a previous MI.

Left ventricular angiography permits visualization of LV wall motion and determination of the ejection fraction. During diastole, the normal configuration of the outline of the LV cavity is that of an ellipsoid (Figure 22-4). During systole, the ventricular walls are squeezed inward, especially the anterior and posterior walls. At the peak of systolic ejection, the normal appearance of the LV cavity is thought to resemble a pear core or an ice cream cone in the right anterior oblique (RAO) projection. Abnormalities (asynergy) are noted whenever the LV outline either enlarges in one area or loses its normal characteristics (see Figure 22-4). In patients with angina, asynergy has been noted during anginal attacks that cause ischemia but is reversible once the ischemic episode resolves.

Ejection fractions are calculated from the ventriculogram and are a reflection of the systolic performance of the left ventricle. The normal ejection fraction is approximately 60% to 75% of the total left ventricular end-diastolic volume. A decrease in ejection fraction of less than 40% to 50% is indicative of impaired left ventricular function in patients with angina.

Coronary arteriography permits assessment of the presence of CAD and grading of severity of lesions. A lesion in the left main coronary artery is considered significant when the obstruction is 50% or greater. In arteries other than the left main a reduction of 50% or more in diameter or 75% or more in cross-sectional area is considered a severe risk for myocardial ischemia.[43]

The indication for cardiac catheterization and coronary arteriography in patients with stable angina is not as urgent as in patients with unstable angina who require more immediate interventions. Those stable patients are often referred for an elective cardiac catheterization when symptoms are causing limitations in lifestyle and the need for surgery may become an issue. These patients may also require catheterization to confirm the presence of CAD. Unstable patients, on the other hand, are believed to be candidates for immediate catheterization. When possible, these patients are medically stabilized prior to catheterization. Patients with unstable angina are often found to have severe obstruction and multivessel disease.

Coronary arteriography also permits definitive di-

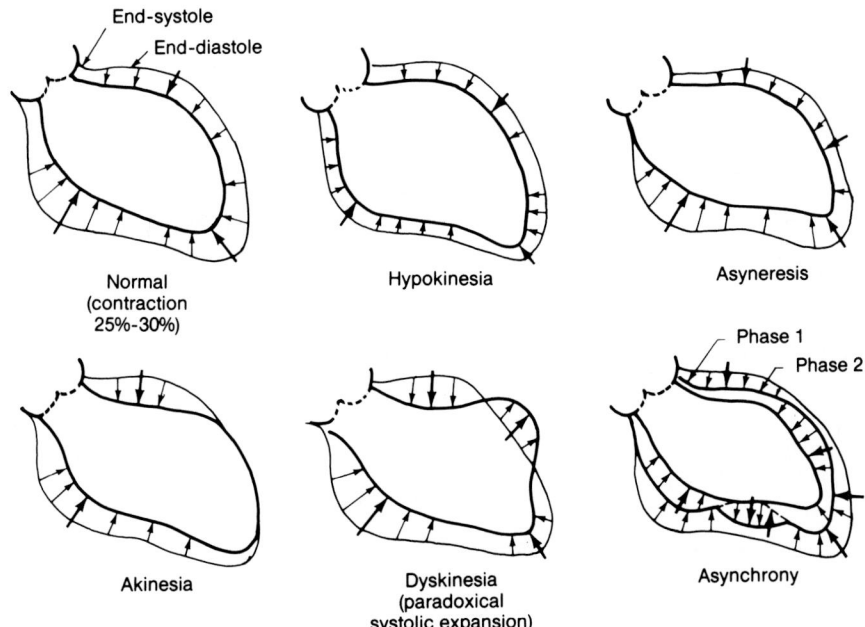

Figure 22-4 Figures which depict normal and abnormal cardiac contraction. Arrows represent motion from end-diastole to end-systole.

From Herman, M. V., & Gorlin, R. (1969). Implications of left ventricular asynergy. *American Journal of Cardiology, 23,* 588.

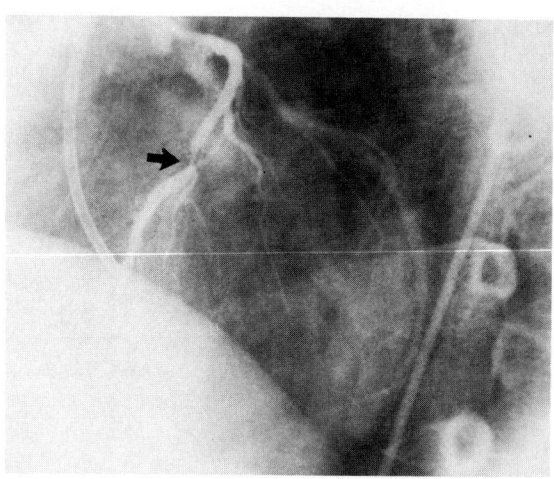

Figure 22-5 Arteriography of a patient who develops spasm (arrow) in the artery during the catheterization procedure.

agnosis of the presence of coronary artery spasm (Figure 22-5). This is often accomplished with the intravenous injection of ergonovine maleate, an agent found to induce uterine smooth muscle contraction in obstetric patients. The usual response to ergonovine in a patient with variant angina is near or total occlusion of an artery. This test also helps to differentiate pure coronary artery vasospasm from spasm superimposed on a fixed lesion. Therapeutic interventions are directed differently once this distinction is made. The safety of the ergonovine test has, however, been questioned. It is recommended that this test be performed only in settings whereby the immediate injection of intravenous nitroglycerin or calcium channel antagonists can be administered to prevent irreversible spasm which may lead to an MI.

Angioscopy

As the field of invasive and interventional cardiology expands, methods for determining what is occurring on the inner surface of the coronary arteries are developing. One such method is *angioscopy*, visualization of the inner surfaces of the cardiac blood vessels of the heart by means of a fiberoptic balloon-tipped catheter.

The use of instruments to view intracardiac structures and large vessels intraoperatively was introduced as early as 1913. The use of a balloon to displace blood for better visualization was introduced in the mid-1940s.[46] However, early coronary angioscopes were too large to be used percutaneously and had no means of guidance.[47] Only relatively recently has the development of smaller, more flexible catheters; extremely thin, high-quality fiberoptics; and miniature lenses permitted therapeutic and diagnostic catheterization of the coronary arteries.[48]

Although coronary angiography remains the standard means for diagnosing coronary artery stenosis and viewing the coronary anatomy, it cannot determine intraluminal changes such as plaque rupture and thrombosis. Investigators using angioscopy have detected free floating clots, membranelike obstructions, and atherosclerotic debris undetected by angiography.[47]

The limitations of angioscopy include increased procedure time and loss of resolution when the videotaped image is converted to a photographic print. Pathological changes that lie beyond the view of the angioscope are not detected.[46] The potential adverse effects of angioscopy include perforation of the vessel wall, dissection, dislodgement of atherosclerotic plaque, thrombus formation, and spasm.[48]

Angioscopy is currently being evaluated in protocols for unstable angina, plaque morphology, and suboptimal results of percutaneous transluminal balloon angioplasty. Researchers in Japan are working with the angioscope in determining the pathological changes that occur in patients with dilated cardiomyopathy.[49]

The patient is prepared for angioscopy as for a PTCA. The percutaneous coronary angioscope is designed similarly to the coronary balloon angioplasty catheter[46] (Figures 22-6 and 22-7). It is thin, flexible, and steerable. The imaging system is composed of a fiberoptic imaging bundle, a television camera, a videomonitor, and a videotape recorder.[44]

Using standard angioplasty technique, the lesion is crossed with the angioscopic guide wire. The angioscope is then advanced over the guide wire. The angioscopic balloon is inflated with 1 to 2 atm of pressure to occlude blood flow. Two to ten ml of warmed lactated Ringer's solution is flushed through to create a blood-free field, and the images are recorded on videotape[46] (Figure 22-8). The angioscopy balloon is deflated and removed, and a standard angioplasty is then performed.

After the angioplasty, repeat angioscopic and angiographic views are taken. The lesion appearance is characterized by the presence or absence of plaque, thrombus, and dissection.[46] Based on this information, the need for further treatment (i.e., atherectomy, systemic anticoagulation, or thrombolytic therapy) is determined.

The nursing care for these patients is basically the same as is described in the section discussing PTCA. Pressures, cardiac rhythm, ST segment changes and patient comfort are monitored. White and associates found that all of their patients experienced transient ST and T wave changes and mild chest pain while the angioscopic balloon was inflated,[44] but the discomfort and ischemic changes resolved with balloon deflation. They also found that patients tolerated an-

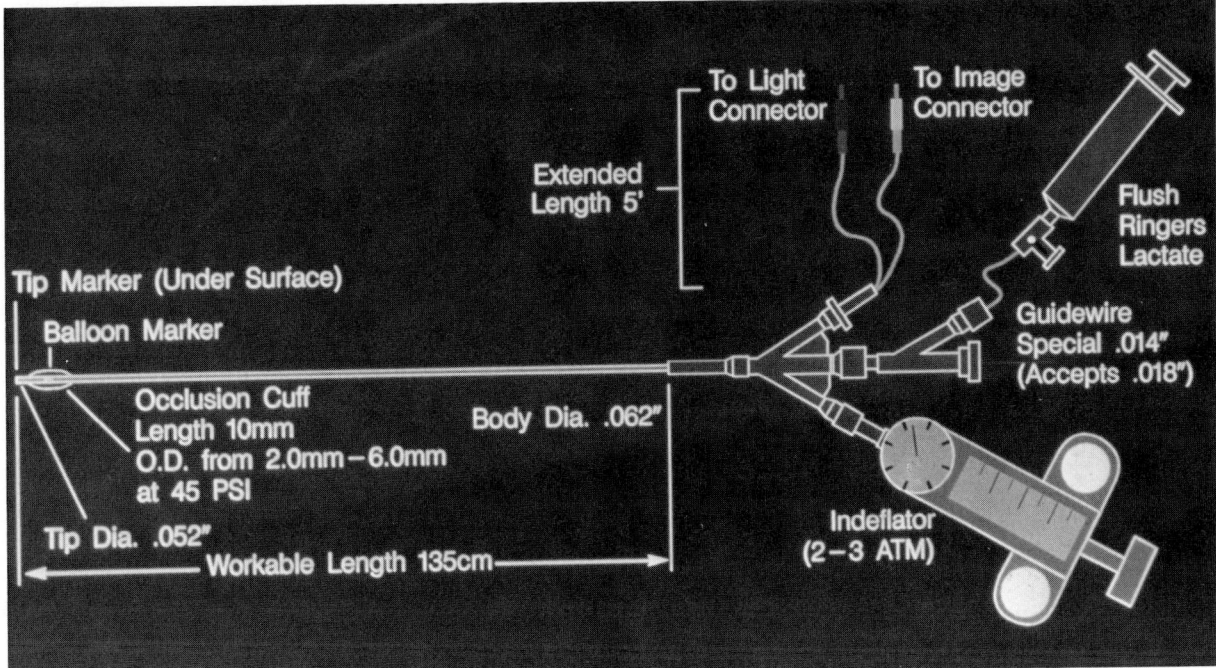

Figure 22-6   Diagram of angioscope catheter.

gioscopic imaging for longer periods (up to 45 seconds) following the PTCA. After the procedure, these patients are treated in the manner described for PTCA.

The morphological appearance of coronary lesions, described according to angiographic parameters, has become extremely important in determining the diagnosis, prognosis, and treatment of patients with CAD. Some investigators believe that angioscopy employing current technology provides superior imaging of coronary lesions.[44] Research continues in the use of this new diagnostic tool. (See Chapter 21.)

Medical Management

Admission to a critical care or coronary care unit is usually reserved for patients who (1) present with the first episode of angina, (2) have suspected variant angina requiring confirmation, or (3) have unstable angina. Patients are often admitted to rule out myocardial infarction. The goal of treatment for these patients is either to increase the coronary blood supply or decrease the myocardial oxygen demand or both. This goal may be accomplished through medical or surgical interventions. Certain patients with CAD may also be offered alternatives such as percutaneous transluminal coronary angioplasty (PTCA) laser angioplasty, or other interventional procedures that are discussed later in this section.

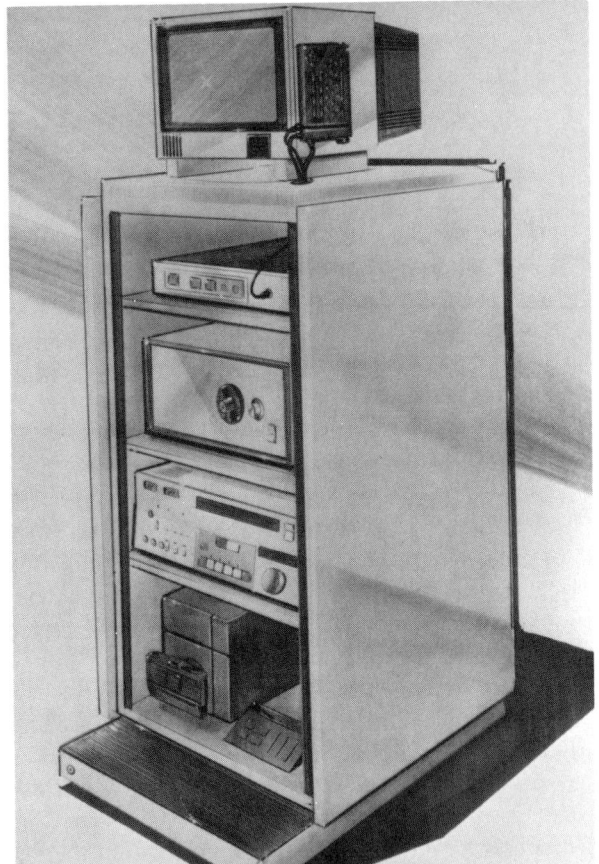

Figure 22-7   Imaging equipment. Top to bottom: Monitor to view artery, calibration and focus equipment, light source, video cassette recorder, and hardcopy printer.

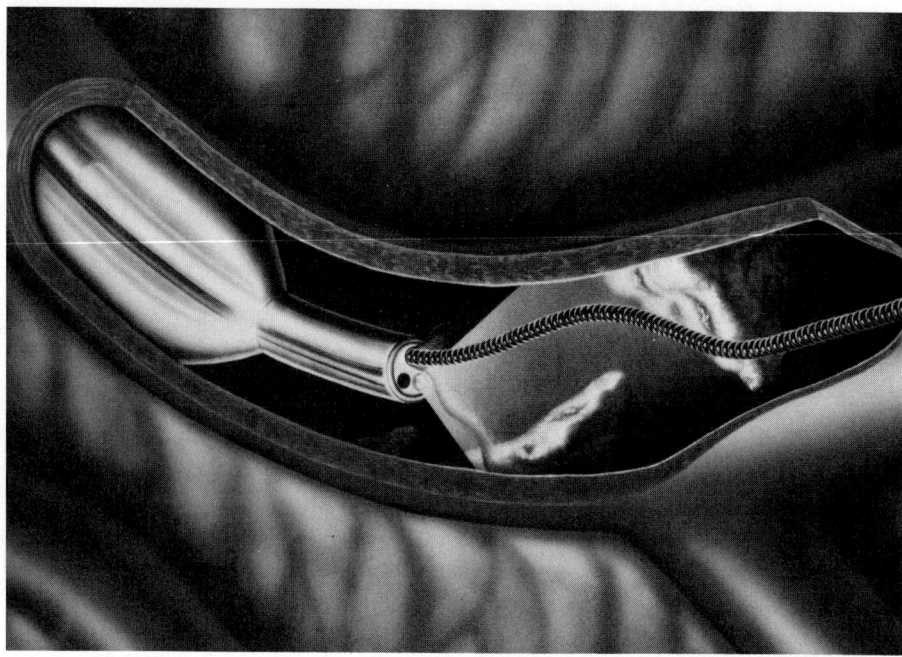

Figure 22-8 View of the coronary occlusion with angioscope catheter. Guidewire across lesion with catheter proximal to the lesion.

Medical interventions for patients with CAD include pharmacological therapy, dietary modifications, reduction of other risk factors, activity modification, and counterpulsation. Patients with vasospasm are treated medically with pharmacological agents unless a mixed lesion is documented.

Pharmacological Management

Three classes of agents are currently used for patients with CAD or spasm: nitrates, beta-adrenergic blocking agents (beta blockers) and calcium channel antagonists.

Nitrates are the first-line agents employed for both angina and coronary spasm. Nitrates act by dilating vascular and selected smooth muscle throughout the body, primarily causing venous dilation and, to a lesser degree, arterial dilation. The venous dilation decreases venous return to the right side of the heart (preload). The reduced preload, in turn, reduces wall tension which decreases the oxygen requirements or demand. The minimal arterial dilatory effect causes a slight decrease in blood pressure. Nitrates are also thought to exert an effect on the coronary arteries specifically to increase coronary blood flow in some patients with coronary obstruction and to increase collateral blood flow to ischemic myocardium.[50] Nitrates are administered in sublingual, oral, intravenous, and topical forms.

Nitrates are classified as short-acting and longer-acting. Nitroglycerin, a shorter-acting nitrate, is often used sublingually to alleviate an acute anginal attack or episode of coronary spasm because of its rapid onset of action. It may also be used as prophylaxis prior to an activity that is known to precipitate attacks.

Intravenous or intracoronary nitroglycerin is often employed after provoking spasm with ergonovine maleate for therapeutic purposes. Continuous intravenous infusion of nitroglycerin may be used to control angina. The longer-acting nitrates such as isosorbide dinitrate and isosorbide 5-mononitrate are used to increase exercise tolerance and prevent further anginal episodes or spasm attacks. Table 22-2 summarizes the effects of the commonly used nitrates.

Beta-adrenergic blocking agents are used alone or in combination with nitrates or calcium channel blockers for treating stable and unstable angina. Investigations suggest that combined therapy may be more effective in treating stable angina than either nitrates or beta blockers alone.[51] The mechanism of action of the beta blockers is to inhibit the binding of catecholamines at receptor sites. These drugs compete at binding sites to block the effects of catecholamines. Such blockade selectivity inhibits both inotropic and chronotropic actions produced by beta-adrenergic stimulation. The clinical effect of these drugs, therefore, is a reduction in the resting and exercising heart rate, a reduction in myocardial contractility, and a reduction in myocardial oxygen consumption. Most of the beta blockers have been found

TABLE 22-2 **Summary of Commonly Used Nitrates**

Drug	Route of Administration	Dosage	Onset of Effect	Duration of Effect
Nitroglycerin (Nitrostat; Susadrin)	Sublingual	0.3-0.6 mg	30 sec	15-30 min
Nitroglycerin (Nitrostat SR; Nitro-Bid)	Oral	2.5-19.5 mg	1 hr	2-4 hr
Nitroglycerin (Nitro-Bid; Nitrodisc; Nitro-Dur; Nitrol ointment; Transderm)	Transdermal	1-2 in (ointment) 10-60 cm² (patches)	1 hr	6-24 hr
Nitroglycerin (Tridil)	Intravenous	10-200 µg/min	Immediate	—
Isosorbide dinitrate (Isordil; Sorbitrate; Dilatrate)	Sublingual	2.5-10 mg	5 min	1-2 hr
Isosorbide dinitrate (Isordil; Sorbitrate; Dilatrate)	Oral	10-60 mg	30 min	4-6 hr
Isosorbide 5-mononitrate (ISMO)	Oral	10-40 mg	30 min	8-21 hr

Modified from Cohn, J. (1990). Drugs used to control vascular resistance and capacitance. In J. W. Hurst, R. C. Schlant, C. E. Rackley, et al. (Eds.), *The heart* (7th ed.). New York: McGraw-Hill.

to increase exercise capacity in coronary artery disease and to increase diastolic filling time, thereby extending coronary perfusion time.

The use of beta blockers in coronary spasm is controversial. The benefit of these agents in spasm is as yet undetermined.[39] Some clinicians believe that beta blockers control the symptoms of variant angina by blocking the adrenergic effect which may induce coronary spasm.[52] Others believe that beta blockers may be ineffective because some of these agents only reduce myocardial oxygen consumption. Others caution that beta blockers may be ineffective for spasm because of their failure to exert vasodilatory effects on coronary blood flow.[53] Despite the drawbacks of beta blockers, they have been used alone or concomitantly with other agents in treating vasospasm.

The role of beta blockers in treating silent ischemia is evolving. Beta blockers have been found to be efficacious in reducing the incidence of silent ischemic attacks as evidenced by ambulatory ECG.[54]

Propranolol (Inderal) is the most widely used beta blocker for control of angina as well as for dysrhythmias and hypertension in CAD. It is usually contraindicated in second- or third-degree heart block, bronchial asthma, cardiogenic shock, congestive heart failure, and with concurrent use of any adrenergic-stimulating psychotropic agent. Propranolol is also known to have a quinidine-like effect which depresses cardiac function. Therefore, the patient should be monitored for manifestations of congestive heart failure.

Metropolol (Lopressor) is a beta blocker that is more cardioselective in that it has more effect on the B_1 receptors of the heart than B_2 receptors. It is used for angina and hypertension and can be used judiciously with bronchospastic disease. Both propranolol and metropolol have short half-lives requiring frequent dosages. Nadolol (Corgard) and atenolol have longer-half-lives, permitting less frequent dosages (one dose a day) for patients who have difficulty complying with drug regimens.

Calcium channel antagonists are widely used for angina. The primary mechanism of action of these agents is inhibition of the movement of calcium ions across myocardial and vascular smooth muscle, which produces (1) vasodilatation of the coronary arteries and collateral vessels; (2) a decrease in myocardial contractility, which leads to a decrease in myocardial oxygen demand; (3) vasodilatation of the peripheral arteries, resulting in a decrease in systemic blood pressure; and (4) a decrease in cardiac conduction.[55] Because of the coronary vasodilator effect, these drugs are useful in angina and spasm. Compared to the nitrates, the onset of action of calcium channel antagonists is somewhat slower, but they are much longer-acting.[55]

The three most widely used calcium channel antagonists are verapamil (Isoptin, Calan), diltiazem (Cardizem), and nifedipine (Procardia). All of these have been found effective in stable angina, reducing anginal attacks and improving exercise capacity. Each drug works differently on the heart to produce clinical effects.

Verapamil and diltiazem decrease the heart rate by depressing the rate of sinus node discharge and attenuating the conduction velocity through the atrioventricular (AV) node. This negative chronotropic effect is useful in controlling tachydysrhythmias associated with CAD. Nifedipine is not useful in tachydysrhythmias because of the reflex tachycardia associated with its use. All three agents have been found to depress cardiac contractility; therefore, each has a negative inotropic effect. In addition, nifedipine exerts the greatest vasodilatory effects of these agents.[55]

Several clinical trials have supported the use of all

three calcium channel antagonists for coronary spasm and rest pain associated with unstable angina.[52,55] These drugs have been able to block spontaneous and drug-induced spasm.

Patients with unstable angina in which medical management is difficult may require a combination of long-acting nitrates, a beta-adrenergic blocker, and calcium channel antagonists. In a randomized double-blind trial, combined therapy of nifedipine, nitrates, and propranolol reduced the number of unstable anginal attacks and reduced the number of patients requiring surgery for relief of chest pain.[56] The hemodynamic effects of each of these different types of drugs may be efficacious. However, adverse reactions such as heart block, severe bradycardia, and congestive heart failure mandate careful patient selection and surveillance.[55]

Activity Modifications

Patients with stable angina are encouraged to engage in activities that do not precipitate an anginal attack. Walking is often one of the recommended exercises. Those patients who wish to engage in more vigorous activity should participate in a supervised structural exercise program to gradually increase their exercise capacity so as not to precipitate anginal attacks. Prior to engaging in any activity that may precipitate angina, the use of prophylactic nitroglycerin is encouraged.

The type of exercise is also an important variable in the patient with CAD. Dynamic (isotonic) exercise involving the large muscle groups is favored over static (isometric) exercises, which may actually increase myocardial oxygen demand. Patients should also be instructed not to engage in dynamic exercises immediately after a large meal because of the shunting of blood flow to the gastrointestinal tract.

Activity restrictions are frequently employed for the patient with unstable angina. Because of the seriousness of this type of angina, patients are often hospitalized, placed on bed rest, and given combined pharmacological agents. If their condition improves, gradual ambulation is encouraged. However, if despite medical therapy the condition worsens, these patients will require standard interventions such as counterpulsation, percutaneous transluminal coronary angioplasty, or coronary artery bypass surgery before progressive activity is undertaken. In addition, some patients may be candidates for several interventions still under investigation in many tertiary centers.

Nutritional Management

The study that provided evidence that dietary modifications and drug therapy (antilipids) was effective in lowering blood cholesterol and LDL levels was the Lipid Research Clinics Coronary Primary Prevention Trial.[26] This study has been discussed in the section Risk Factors. A consensus development conference was convened in 1984 by the National Institutes of Health for the twofold purpose of reviewing the scientific evidence from this study and making specific recommendations on blood cholesterol reduction. The panel concluded that the scientific evidence "established beyond a reasonable doubt that lowering definitely elevated blood cholesterol (specifically blood levels of low density lipoprotein cholesterol) reduces the risk of heart attacks due to coronary heart disease."[57] Recent recommendations have been made regarding which people should be referred to physicians based on their cholesterol level (Table 22-3). In addition to reducing the plasma cholesterol level, special attention is paid to LDL levels and HDL levels obtained from a lipid analysis. Plasma LDL levels are often compared to HDL levels as a ratio such as LDL/HDL when the LDL level ranges between 100 to 200 mg/dl. Patients with an LDL/HDL ratio of 5:1 should be considered for drug therapy. However, if a patient has an LDL level that exceeds 200 mg/dl, aggressive drug therapy concomitant with diet restrictions is warranted regardless of the HDL level.[57]

Dietary modifications that lower cholesterol levels include restricting total fat, saturated fat, and cholesterol. In addition, weight reduction is an important component of a dietary plan. Foods such as poultry, fish, shellfish, lean red meats, and low-fat dairy products should be encouraged. Amounts of fruits, vegetables, breads, grains, and legumes also should be increased. Those foods to be avoided include fried foods and foods that are high in saturated fat such as palm and coconut oil (found in nondairy creamers).

The consumption of fish has received much attention, primarily because of the eicosapentaenoic acid (EPA) contained in fish oil. Kromhout, Bosschieter, and Coulander[58] observed a group of men in the town of Zutphen, the Netherlands, for 20 years. In the 20-year study, an inverse relationship was observed between fish consumption and death from coronary artery disease. Fish contains EPA, which has been shown in vitro to be the precursor of platelet thromboxane A_3 and of prostaglandin I_3. Thromboxane A_3, unlike thromboxane A_2, has demonstrated no platelet-aggregating power. In addition, prostaglandin I_3 has been shown to be an effective antiaggregating substance. The high levels of EPA are, therefore, theorized to lead to an antithrombotic state because of reduced platelet aggregation. In vivo, EPA has also been shown to reduce the plasma concentrations of triglycerides and VLDL.[9] Thus, patients with type IIB and IV hyperlipidemia may benefit from EPA.

TABLE 22-3 **Classification of People for Referral on the Basis of Cholesterol Level**

Blood Total Cholesterol Level	Recommended Action
Desirable blood cholesterol <200 mg/dl	1. Repeat cholesterol measurement within 5 years or with physical examination. 2. Provide dietary and risk factor education.
Borderline high cholesterol 200-239 mg/dl	1. Refer to physician for follow-up* if history of CAD or if 2 or more other CAD risk factors are present. If no reported history of CAD or less than 2 other risk factors, refer to physician within 1 year for repeat cholesterol management. 2. Reinforce dietary education.
High blood cholesterol ≥240 mg/dl	1. Refer to physician for follow-up.*

*Individuals should be referred to physician within 2 months.
Source: National Cholesterol Education Program, Department of Health and Human Services, Public Health Services, National Institutes of Health. (1990). *Report of the expert panel on population strategies for blood cholesterol reduction.* (Publication No. 90-3046). Bethesda, MD: DHHS.

Platelet aggregation, which has been discussed in the section Pathogenesis of Atherosclerosis, may promote smooth muscle cell proliferation leading to atherosclerotic lesions. Thus, the effects of EPA may influence the pathogenesis of atherosclerosis by this mechanism as well as by other means.[59]

Lastly, Kromhout, Bosschieter, and Coulander concluded from their study that one or two fish dishes per week may have some preventive value against the development of atherosclerosis.[58] Many questions remain regarding the therapeutic effect of EPA. Additional studies are required to substantiate the benefits and provide more insight into the correlation between consumption of fish and coronary heart disease before widespread use is advocated.

Risk Factor Reduction

Patients with CAD should be motivated to adopt healthier lifestyles and to minimize their risk factors. As was previously mentioned, the number of risk factors can have an additive or synergistic effect on the development and progression of CAD, and therefore these factors need to be controlled individually as well as collectively.

Patients with documented or suspected CAD should be encouraged to stop smoking cigarettes, filtered or nonfiltered. They should also be instructed to adhere to pharmacological regimens to reduce high blood pressure when present.

Stress reduction is important for the patient who is under a great deal of stress. Critical care nurses need to encourage the verbalization of feelings and explore ways of reducing stress associated with the patient's present illness. Often, such patients and significant others require follow-up counseling.

Obesity is another risk factor requiring careful consideration. The overweight patient should be encouraged to change his or her eating habits to lose weight and maintain optimal body weight. Furthermore, results from the Framingham study suggest that weight reduction may decrease the risk of CAD and increase the functional exercise capacity in patients with CAD.[60]

Patients with systemic hypertension require careful management. Pharmacological agents such as beta blockers and diuretics are recommended for the control of hypertension, especially for patients with systolic pressures over 160 mmHg or diastolic blood pressures over 95 mmHg. In certain patients with mild hypertension, the initial intervention may be to alter concomitant risk factors such as obesity, sedentary lifestyle, excessive alcohol intake, and use of oral contraceptives.[18]

It appears that management of hyperglycemia alone does not prevent atherosclerotic development, but multifactorial risk reduction in association with control of hyperglycemia is important.[18] In patients with clinical manifestations of atherosclerosis, dietary restrictions as well as drug therapy may be employed.

Dietary restrictions include decreased saturated fats, complex carbohydrates, and sodium intake, especially for patients who are hypertensive or who have congestive heart failure. Drug therapy may include oral hypoglycemic agents or exogenous insulin preparations. The critical care nurse should also be aware that diabetic patients on nonselective beta blockade therapy may not manifest the sympathetic response during hypoglycemic reactions; thus, careful consideration must be given to avoiding hypoglycemia in patients receiving beta blockade therapy.

Intraaortic Balloon Counterpulsation

For unstable angina patients, intraaortic balloon pump (IABP) counterpulsation is considered may reverse ischemia and protect the myocardium if all conventional modes of therapy have failed, including bed rest, intravenous calcium channel antagonists, beta blockers, and nitrates. Ischemia must be documented according to clinical, hemodynamic, and electrocardiographic criteria. Persistent refractory ischemia is considered an indication for balloon pumping in certain institutions. There are many other indications for the IABP. However, the intent of this section is to relate the IABP to the patient with unstable angina or medically refractory myocardial ischemia.

The intraaortic balloon pump has demonstrated efficacy in the reversal of myocardial ischemia for unstable angina patients. During balloon pumping, a favorable balance between myocardial oxygen supply and demand can be restored by the simultaneous increase in coronary perfusion pressure and the reduction in cardiac work achieved with this intervention.

Instrumentation and Technique. The IABP, a counterpulsation device, was first introduced into the critical care setting in 1969 and it is now the more widely used of the ventricular assist devices. Many systems are commercially available, and the specific vendor's operating guidelines should be consulted.

The intraaortic balloon catheter (available in several sizes with one or more lumens) is introduced either percutaneously (usual method) or by surgical cutdown into the femoral artery. The catheter is then advanced in a retrograde fashion to lie in the descending thoracic aorta 1 or 2 cm distal to the origin of the left subclavian artery. Once in position, the catheter is connected to a console, and the balloon is inflated with helium or CO_2 according to user preference. Most of the IABP catheters currently marketed have a sheath. Under investigation is a new sheathless catheter that may be less damaging to the vascular status of a patient.

The device operates by synchronized displacement of blood in the aorta by inflation and deflation of the balloon (Figure 22-9). The inflation–deflation cycle is precisely set (timed) by the clinician in synchrony with the mechanical events of the cardiac cycle. Because the timing of balloon inflation and deflation is opposite that of ventricular systole, balloon activation is referred to as *counterpulsation.*

Inflation is timed to occur at the beginning of diastole. The arterial waveform is used for accurate timing. The dicrotic notch, which depicts aortic valve closure (beginning of phase I in diastole), must be identified on the arterial trace, and the balloon is then inflated. Minor corrections in accordance with specific manufacturers' instructions are recommended to adjust the timing from a radial or femoral arterial line to account for slight delays in waveform transmission from the aorta to these distal recording sites. If a central aortic root line is used, then precise inflation at the dicrotic notch is suggested. The inflated balloon displaces a volume of blood equal to its own volume size, resulting in a pressure elevation in the aorta referred to as the *diastolic augmented pressure.*

Deflation of the balloon is set to occur just prior to the next aortic valve opening, specifically during isovolumetric contraction of the left ventricle (phase 1 systole). As gas is removed from the balloon, the intraaortic volume is decreased and, therefore, aortic end-diastolic pressure is reduced. This reduction in aortic pressure lowers the pressure the left ventricle must overcome to eject its stroke volume during the next systole. The balloon deflation, therefore, facilitates systolic unloading and emptying. The waveform achieved during balloon deflation should depict a 10- to 15-mmHg lowering of the balloon aortic end-diastolic pressure in contrast to the patient's unaugmented aortic end-diastolic pressure.[61]

Mechanism and Outcome. The physiological effects of balloon inflation and deflation are significant. During balloon inflation, elevation of the diastolic pressure (diastolic augmentation) has important ef-

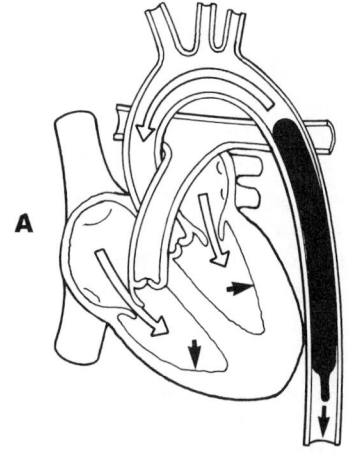 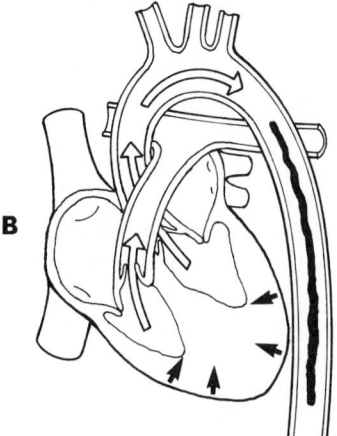

Figure 22-9   Mechanical events of IAB *(A)* inflation (diastole) and *(B)* deflation (systole).

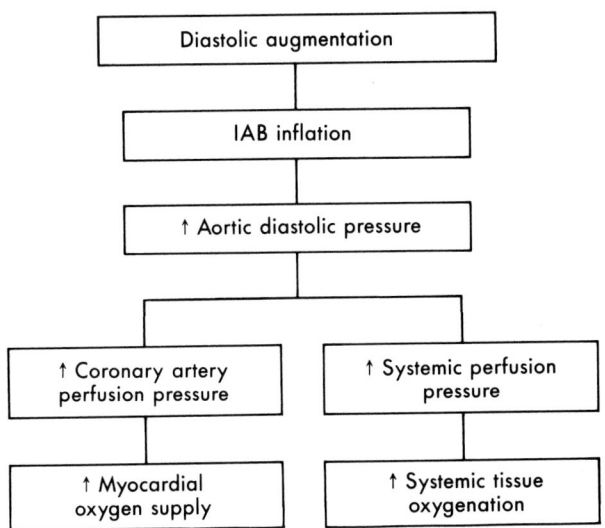

Figure 22-10   Diastolic augmentation.

From Eagan, J. S., Stewart, S. L., & Vitello-Cicciu, J. M. (1991). Quick reference to cardiac critical care nursing. In J. M. Vitello-Cicciu (Ed.), *Quick reference to critical care nursing series.* Gaithersburg, MD: Aspen.

fects in terms of coronary flow and tissue perfusion (Figure 22-10). Coronary flow is phasic because the branches of the coronary arteries are deeply embedded in the myocardium. During systole these intramyocardial branches are compressed, increasing the resistance to flow. During diastole, however, the coronary vascular resistance is minimal; therefore, coronary filling occurs primarily during diastole. The timing of pressure augmentation during balloon pumping is, therefore, optimal. Elevating diastolic pressure increases coronary perfusion pressure and potentially increases coronary blood flow and oxygen supply. In addition, the augmented diastolic pressure increases the systemic perfusion pressure, in turn increasing systemic tissue oxygenation.

Even though coronary perfusion pressure is elevated by balloon pumping, variable effects on total coronary blood flow may occur. In some instances, total coronary blood flow is elevated by diastolic augmentation; in others it is unchanged or even reduced. This variability results because the dominant mechanism controlling coronary blood flow is autoregulation within the coronary bed—not coronary perfusion pressure. Autoregulation is an intrinsic mechanism altering coronary blood flow in response to tissue need for oxygen. The process of autoregulation maintains a precise balance between myocardial oxygen supply and demand. Local tissue hypoxia or oxygen lack is the most potent stimulus for increasing coronary blood flow and oxygen supply through coronary vasodilatation. Conversely, a reduction in oxygen demand induces a corresponding reduction in coronary blood flow through vasoconstriction. Because

counterpulsation reduces myocardial work and oxygen demand, overall coronary blood flow may be reduced during balloon pumping via autoregulated vasoconstriction, despite the elevation of aortic diastolic pressure.

Typically, absolute increases in total coronary blood flow are noted when the myocardium has been underperfused because of hypotension prior to initiation of balloon pumping. In this instance, the myocardium is flow-deprived by the low-pressure state and is maximally dilated by the resultant tissue hypoxia. Consequently, elevation of pressure elevates flow. However, in the absence of hypotension, the balloon essentially supplements the autoregulatory process, offering a reserve in coronary perfusion pressure and oxygen supply.

In contrast to the variable effects on total coronary blood flow, favorable localized effects on flow do occur with diastolic augmentation. Flow to myocardium threatened by significant obstructive lesions is pressure-dependent. The normal autoregulatory ability is impaired by disease. Therefore, flow to these potentially ischemic regions may improve with elevation of diastolic pressure. In addition, the balloon may increase coronary collateral development. In summary, diastolic augmentation increases the available myocardial oxygen supply, may improve the distribution of coronary blood flow to potentially ischemic regions of the myocardium, and improves peripheral tissue perfusion.

Balloon deflation has significant effects because it facilitates systolic emptying of the ventricle and, therefore, afterload reduction (Figure 22-11). Afterload reduction produces a number of physiological alterations. Because the resistance to ventricular ejection is reduced, the systolic pressure the left ventricle must generate to open the aortic valve and eject blood is correspondingly lower. As a result, the ventricle does not have to generate as much pressure during systole, and cardiac work is reduced. Finally, a reduction in cardiac work lowers myocardial oxygen demand and oxygen consumption. In essence, afterload reduction improves myocardial efficiency and reduces cardiac work and oxygen demand. Clinically, the effect of balloon deflation is, therefore, manifested by an increase in cardiac output and a reduction in left ventricular end diastolic pressure, left atrial pressure, and pulmonary wedge pressure.

In summary, the physiological effects of intraaortic balloon counterpulsation is the alteration of diastolic pressure to enhance the key components of cardiac work such as an elevation of diastolic pressure and a lowering of systolic work while maintaining tissue perfusion. Myocardial oxygenation is improved with a reduction in oxygen demand and an increment in

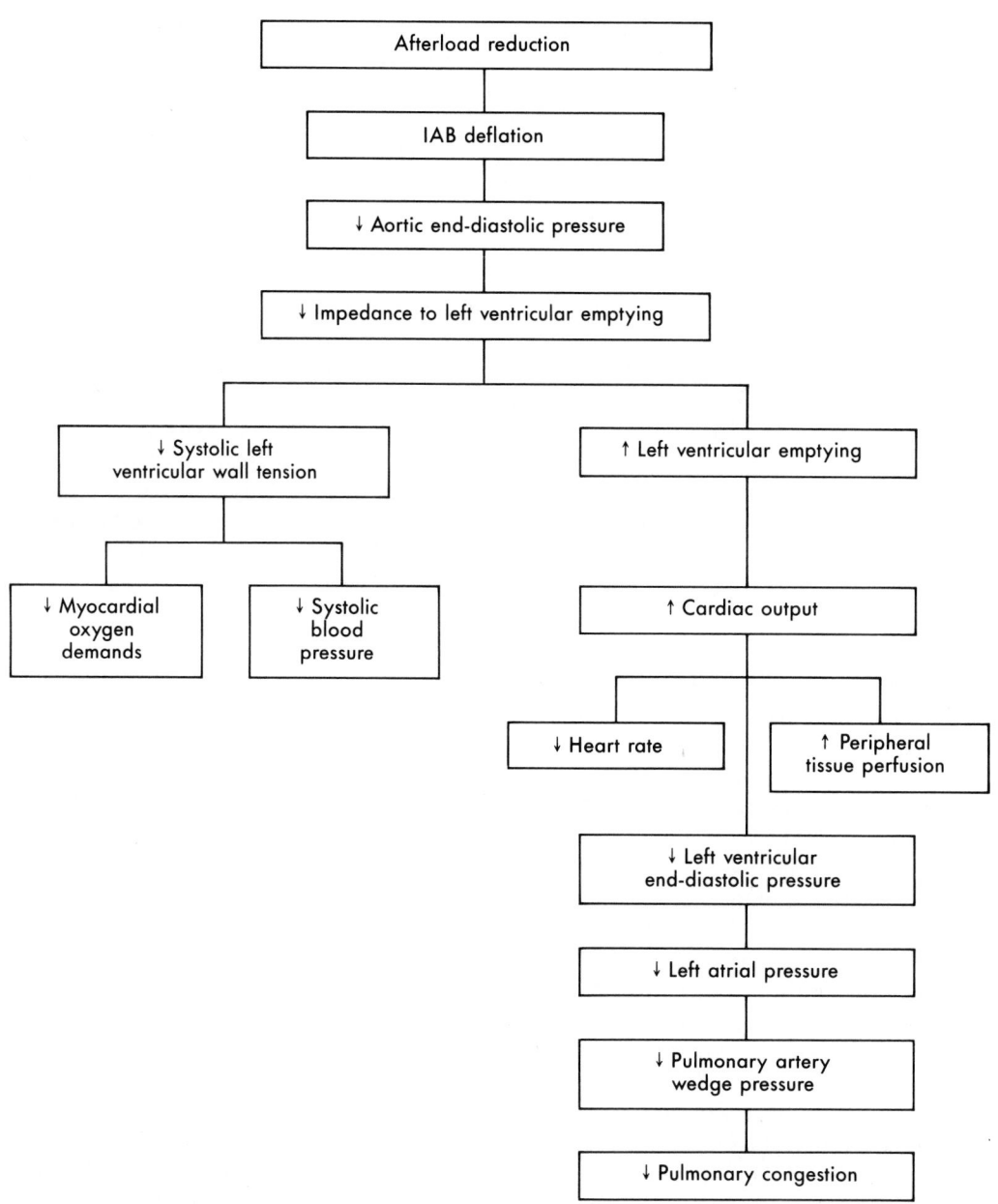

Figure 22-11   Afterload reduction.

From Eagan, J. S., Stewart, S. L., & Vitello-Cicciu, J. M. (1991). Quick reference to cardiac critical care nursing. In J. M. Vitello-Cicciu (Ed.), *Quick reference to critical care nursing series.* Gaithersburg, MD: Aspen.

oxygen supply. All of these effects are especially desirable for unstable angina patients with persistent ischemia who are at high risk for infarction.

Contraindications. The absolute contraindications to intraaortic balloon pumping are anatomical considerations. For the most part, the relative contraindications involve ethical issues that must be decided at the discretion of the patient, family, and physician.

Absolute contraindications to IABP therapy are the following: (1) aortic aneurysm, (2) aortic dissection, and (3) moderate to severe aortic valve insufficiency.

Severe aortoiliac disease may also be a contraindication because it may preclude insertion of the IABP catheter. Aortic wall damage also precludes insertion because of the hazard of progressive damage with potential aortic rupture secondary to the mechanical stress of pumping. Balloon inflation in the setting of aortic valve insufficiency increases the retrograde flow into the left ventricle during diastole, worsening the underlying dysfunction. Severe aortoiliac disease significantly increases the incidence of arterial trauma and peripheral embolization. Extensive atherosclerosis in the peripheral arterial vessels may prevent passage of the balloon catheter through the femoral artery. If balloon pumping is required urgently, consideration may be given to an alternative approach intraoperatively through the aortoiliac system or retrograde via the ascending aorta into the descending aorta.

Nursing Responsibilities. Nursing care of the patient undergoing balloon pumping does not differ significantly from the care of any critically ill patient. It is assumed that nurses caring for these patients possess a sound knowledge of hemodynamic monitoring, cardiac pacing, cardiac rhythm analysis, and patient assessment. Expertise in these areas is essential to provide safe and effective patient care during balloon pumping.

An initial clinical assessment must be completed prior to insertion. The following information is critical to the anticipated insertion procedure: Status of peripheral pulses must be determined. Pulses must be checked and the quality recorded. Significant peripheral vascular disease may prevent the passage of the balloon catheter through the iliofemoral system and increase the risk of arterial trauma during insertion. Also, postinsertion assessment of pulses is meaningless without accurate baseline data for comparison. A history of bleeding tendencies or medication sensitivity must be noted. Anticoagulants and antibiotics are routinely administered during the insertion procedure. The patient's expectations and preparation for the procedure must be assessed to guide subsequent teaching and support efforts. Depending on time constraints and the presenting problem, additional information elicited should be tailored accordingly.

Once the admission procedure has been completed, the first priority is to establish quality electrocardiographic and hemodynamic monitoring signals. The ECG is of primary importance during balloon pumping because it provides the triggering signal for balloon action. To coordinate balloon and cardiac action effectively, the balloon console must sense the R wave of the electrocardiogram. To ensure that the console senses only the R wave and not other ECG waves, a lead should be selected that demonstrates maximal R wave amplitude and minimal amplitude of all other ECG components, including pacing artifacts. This is most easily accomplished by recording a 12-lead ECG, reviewing all leads, and identifying the lead with the required ECG configuration. The electrodes can then be placed on the patient's chest to duplicate the desired lead. If none of the standard 12 leads is adequate, the electrodes can be systematically moved over the precordium until the ideal electrode placement is identified.

Insertion of the arterial line is the next priority when a double-lumen catheter is not inserted. An arterial line is necessary to time balloon action accurately. The arterial tracing represents the mechanical activity of the heart, whereas the ECG reflects the electrical activity. Because the intraaortic balloon is a mechanical assist device, accurate synchronization can only be obtained by means of the arterial tracing. On certain consoles, the ECG trace is used as a guide for "initial" timing adjustments prior to initiation of pumping. This is possible because a rough relationship exists between the electrical and mechanical cycles. Ventricular contraction begins approximately at the R wave and continues through the peak of the T wave; consequently, a deflation marker can be placed in the PR interval with the inflation marker superimposed on the peak of the T wave. Once pumping begins, precision timing is possible only by observing the arterial tracing for waveform alterations indicative of effective balloon pumping.

The percutaneous route is the most commonly used method for patients with unstable angina. Once the catheter has been placed, the balloon catheter is unwrapped and sutured to the leg prior to connection to the pump console. Then counterpulsation may be initiated. Balloon location must be confirmed immediately after insertion either by fluoroscopy or a chest film. Proper timing is then adjusted from the arterial tracing (Figure 22-12). Timing must be set by trained personnel because inappropriate timing can increase cardiac work and compromise myocardial function.

During the insertion procedure the nurse should assess for any patient's complaint of acute or sudden back pain. This could be a clue to acute aortic dissection of the catheter and requires life-saving measures. The hemodynamic and clinical response to balloon pumping should be evaluated every 15 to 60 minutes as the patient's condition dictates.

Patients requiring counterpulsation for refractory myocardial ischemia usually experience either complete relief from pain or a reduction in the frequency of ischemic episodes. Recurrent angina should immediately be brought to the attention of the responsible physician, since more aggressive therapy might be required to control the ischemia.

Evaluation of perfusion to the involved extremity should be performed hourly because ischemia of the extremity distal to the IABP may occur. This may manifest as limb-threatening vascular problem if not continually assessed. Another observed vascular emergency is balloon entrapment whereby a leak in the catheter causes blood to form within the catheter itself.[62] A hard blood clot develops within the catheter which prevents the catheter from being withdrawn and occludes arterial flow at the level of entrapment.

Peripheral pulses and skin temperature and color should be checked relative to preinsertion status. It

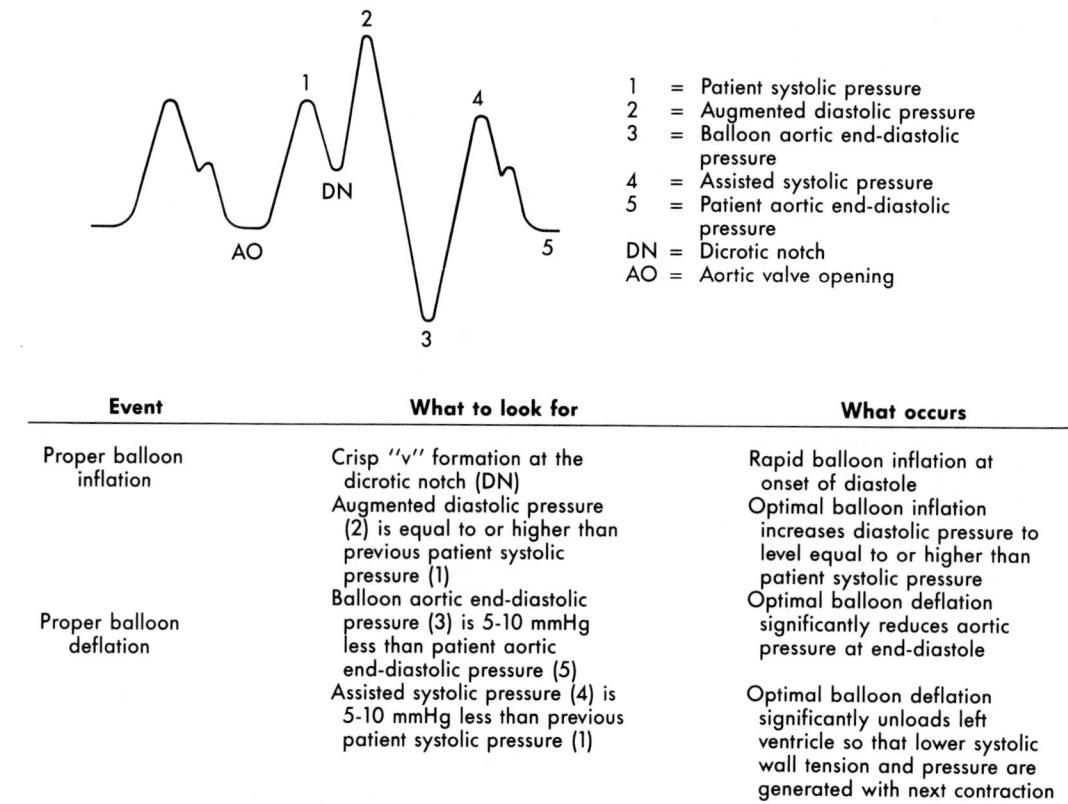

1	= Patient systolic pressure
2	= Augmented diastolic pressure
3	= Balloon aortic end-diastolic pressure
4	= Assisted systolic pressure
5	= Patient aortic end-diastolic pressure
DN	= Dicrotic notch
AO	= Aortic valve opening

Event	What to look for	What occurs
Proper balloon inflation	Crisp "v" formation at the dicrotic notch (DN)	Rapid balloon inflation at onset of diastole
	Augmented diastolic pressure (2) is equal to or higher than previous patient systolic pressure (1)	Optimal balloon inflation increases diastolic pressure to level equal to or higher than patient systolic pressure
Proper balloon deflation	Balloon aortic end-diastolic pressure (3) is 5-10 mmHg less than patient aortic end-diastolic pressure (5)	Optimal balloon deflation significantly reduces aortic pressure at end-diastole
	Assisted systolic pressure (4) is 5-10 mmHg less than previous patient systolic pressure (1)	Optimal balloon deflation significantly unloads left ventricle so that lower systolic wall tension and pressure are generated with next contraction

Figure 22-12   Optimal timing of intraaortic balloon counterpulsation.

From Eagan, J. S., Stewart, S. L., & Vitello-Cicciu, J. M. (1991). Quick reference to cardiac critical care nursing. In J. M. Vitello-Cicciu (Ed.), *Quick reference to critical care nursing series*. Gaithersburg, MD: Aspen.

is essential that the quality of posterior tibial and dorsalis pedis pulses be assessed and recorded. The Doppler flow technique can be used to locate difficult-to-palpate pulses. When evaluating pulses, the opposite leg can be used for comparison, but it must be remembered that either leg can be the site of embolization from the aortoiliac tree. Peripheral pulses, when located initially, should be marked to facilitate subsequent localization. See Chapter 25 for further discussion.

Timing must be evaluated and adjusted as needed. Even if timing adjustments are not a nursing responsibility, nurses must be able to distinguish between normal and abnormal arterial waveform configurations. Quality hemodynamic signals must be preserved to ensure the accuracy of timing adjustments and to permit valid interpretation of hemodynamic status.

Hematologic studies must be evaluated closely to detect abnormalities. Platelet counts may fall because platelet integrity is interrupted by the balloon surface and the mechanical trauma. Infusion of rheomacrodex at 10 to 20 ml/hr minimizes this fall in platelets. Rarely is the administration of platelets required unless active bleeding with thrombocytopenia is noted. Hematocrits may also fall secondary to the inevitable blood loss during insertion and subsequent blood sampling. Anticoagulation status should be monitored closely with anticoagulation precautions in effect.

Respiratory considerations during balloon pumping are straightforward. The balloon should not interfere with respiratory care or chest physical therapy. The only procedural modifications are positional. The head of the bed should not be elevated over 45°, nor should the involved leg be flexed at the hip. Either one of these maneuvers could kink and crack the balloon catheter at the site of insertion in the groin, or could displace the catheter proximally into the aortic arch, potentially traumatizing the intima. The patient can be turned from side to side with only mild angulation of the affected extremity. The leg to which the catheter is attached should be restrained if the patient's cooperation cannot be achieved. During chest physical therapy, inducing artifact in the electrocardiogram should be avoided, because it is the ECG that provides the triggering stimulus to the balloon.

Renal parameters are significant because renal perfusion is a sensitive index of cardiac output. Persistent oliguria in patients receiving IABP therapy may be secondary to an inadequate cardiac output. However, unexplained oliguria should prompt assessment of balloon-related causes. The position of the balloon should be reevaluated on x-ray. Poor perfusion of the kidneys could also indicate renal embolization during insertion.

Similarly, neurological or psychological signs and symptoms can have multiple origins. Disturbances of mentation can be secondary to low cardiac output, embolization, hypoxia, or psychosis. Careful evaluation and documentation is therefore required. Psychological stress needs to be addressed. Patacky and coworkers[63] found that patients who were placed on the IABP perceived more stress than patients who were not on the IABP. Additional major stressors reported by patients receiving IABP therapy were (1) admission to CCU, (2) being unable to move about freely in bed because of equipment, (3) frequent sleep interruptions, (4) noise, and (5) the lack of knowledge and understanding of their illness and treatment. The implications for nursing based on this study indicate that stress can be minimized by clear explanations regarding the CCU environment, routines, and equipment components of patient care to patients and their families; providing emotional support by listening to patients and families; and establishing an atmosphere to promote communication. Efforts to reduce sensory overstimulation and sleep deprivation are essential.

The number of indwelling catheters and the high frequency of invasive procedures predisposes these patients to infection. If surgery is necessary, preoperative infection increases the likelihood of postoperative endocarditis and other septic complications. Therefore, strict sterile technique must be maintained during line management and dressing changes. Antibiotic coverage may be used 24 to 48 hours after insertion. Signs and symptoms of infection must be monitored closely.

Ideally, the indication for weaning is evidence of potential hemodynamic independence. On occasion, however, the balloon must be removed because of ischemia to the involved extremity. The contribution of the balloon pump to circulatory support can be progressively reduced over a period of hours. The weaning process can be accomplished either by gradual reduction in the frequency of balloon support or in the volume of balloon inflation. Reduction in frequency is preferred. Most units have a weaning control to reduce the ratio of inflation cycles. Typically, patients are weaned from 1:1 to 1:8 over a period of hours. The duration of weaning depends on the patient's condition and the physician's preference. The primary nursing responsibility is to evaluate the patient's tolerance of the weaning process. Specific or-

ders should be obtained prior to initiation of weaning to guide the weaning process. The criteria for resumption of balloon pumping at a higher frequency should be predetermined. Indications for substituting pharmacological means of support, such as vasopressors or volume, should be established. Weaning intolerance is evidenced by rising pulmonary wedge pressure, falling mean arterial pressure, falling cardiac output, oliguria, cardiac dysrhythmias, or chest pain.

It must be remembered that despite the fact that the patient's stability is the usual indication for balloon removal, the procedure should be approached with the same care as balloon insertion. The patient must be prepared psychologically and physically for the procedure. Antibiotics may be reinstituted one half hour before removal begins. The patient is draped and the balloon is removed. Firm pressure must be applied over the insertion site for 30 minutes to 1 hour. Pulses should be evaluated during removal and immediately thereafter. Balloon removal represents the final stage of the weaning process, and patients should be observed closely for tolerance.

Percutaneous Transluminal Coronary Angioplasty

Percutaneous transluminal coronary angioplasty (PTCA) is used to dilate occluded coronary arteries. In 1964, Dotter and Judkins first introduced this procedure in the treatment of peripheral vascular disease to improve vascular patency.[64] They used a catheter and a guide wire to dilate arterial narrowings of the femoral and iliac arteries. It was not until 1977 when Dr. Andreas Gruentzig developed a double-lumen catheter small enough to be used in the coronary circulation that PTCA became an alternative treatment for CAD.[65]

Little is understood of the mechanism by which the technique improves vascular patency. Originally, Dotter and Judkins postulated that the luminal diameter of the occluded vessel is increased by compression of the atheromatous intima.[64] Today the exact mechanism by which balloon angioplasty increases vessel patency remains unsettled. Several theories have been presented. Waller[66] reported plaque fracture, intimal atherosclerotic flaps, and localized medial dissection as the major mechanism of balloon angioplasty in human coronary arteries. Another method of coronary artery expansion by balloon angioplasty seems to be the "stretching" of the plaque-free wall segments. The angioplasty balloon is inflated across the eccentric plaque lesion, inducing some stretching of the normal wall segment and little or no damage to the remaining portions of the arterial wall. The combination of vessel stretching and mild plaque compression is another possible mechanism of action of balloon angioplasty. This theory involves the use of an oversized angioplasty balloon to stretch the entire coronary segment that is stenosed by plaque.[66]

The patient who may undergo PTCA must also be a suitable candidate for surgery in the event of complications. Thus, this patient must fulfill the criteria for surgery and indicate a willingness to have the PTCA procedure. This procedure is traditionally used for lesions in any of the three coronary vessels except the left main coronary artery, but the ideal candidate usually has one or two proximal or midvessel stenoses. Patients chosen for PTCA usually have stable angina that has caused lifestyle changes or unstable angina of short duration (less than 6 months) despite optimal medical therapy. The patient may also have multivessel disease and still be considered a candidate for PTCA.

Because of improvements in balloon technology and clinician expertise the indications for PTCA have now expanded to include patients with multivessel lesions, bifurcation lesions, and prior bypass surgery.[67] The approach used in multivessel lesions is to dilate the most severe lesion first to ascertain the probability of successful angioplasty. If the more severe lesion cannot be dilated, the patient will need surgery.

Until recently, bifurcation lesions were not considered appropriate for PTCA. However, when a small side branch supplies a sizeable area of viable myocardium, this branch can be protected by using specialized angioplasty techniques. These consist of using two balloons that are inflated simultaneously or a double-wire technique in which the balloon in the main artery is dilated first followed by inflation of the balloon in the side branch.[67]

Approximately 50% of patients undergoing bypass surgery present with recurrent angina in 5 to 10 years due to progressive disease in the native or graft vessel. It has been noted that vein graft lesions seem to have a higher rate of restenosis than native vessels.[67] Balloon angioplasty has thus been a successful alternative for these patients as well.

It is generally agreed that left main artery stenosis should not be dilated because of the danger of total vessel occlusion and the extent of myocardium at risk.[68] In addition, lesions at the coronary ostia are typically resistant to dilation and are also associated with a high rate of restenosis. Finally, patients with severely reduced ventricular function may also not be suitable candidates for PTCA.

The procedure for PTCA is very similar to the procedure for cardiac catheterization. Informed consent is obtained prior to the procedure and the patient is kept NPO the day of the procedure in the event that surgery becomes necessary. Patients at our institution are started on aspirin and persantine, and some are given a calcium channel blocker before the procedure. A guiding catheter is inserted via a femoral or branchial artery and advanced retrograde into the ascending aorta. Some physicians may perform a right heart catheterization for measurement of baseline filling pressures and to insert a transvenous pacing lead to permit emergency cardiac pacing. The guiding catheter is positioned in the coronary ostium. Angiography is performed to identify the lesion. A dilatation catheter with the balloon attached is advanced through the guiding catheter into the stenotic area of the artery. When the catheter has been strategically placed over the area of occlusion, the balloon is inflated in a stepwise fashion until it reaches 4 to 10 atm of pressure. The balloon is inflated for approximately 15 to 90 seconds (if patient can tolerate it) and then deflated. Balloon inflations are repeated until angiographic appearance is satisfactory (Figure 22-13). Once favorable results have been achieved, the angioplasty balloon is removed and repeat angiography is performed to visualize the distal flow. At the completion of the procedure, the sheath is left in place, and the patient is then transferred to a nursing unit.

According to individual hospital protocols, some patients may be started on IV nitroglycerin prior to the procedure and remain on it during the procedure. In addition, some patients receive sublingual nifedipine and intracoronary nitroglycerin if coronary artery spasm is suspected or demonstrated. During the procedure, patients usually receive heparin to prevent thrombus formation, which is stopped when the procedure is finished. The femoral sheath is removed 4 to 6 hours after the heparin is stopped to allow for metabolism of the heparin and to prevent bleeding. Some patients need calcium channel antagonists after the procedure. After successful PTCA, patients receive antiplatelet drugs or coumadin.

A registry of patients who have undergone PTCA has been maintained by the National Heart, Lung, and Blood Institute (NHLBI).[69] This registry compiles data on the results of this procedure. According to the NHLBI an estimated 300,000 PTCAs were performed in 1990. The success rate of angioplasty was 92%. Nonfatal MIs occurred as a complication in 3.4% of these patients. Another 2.9% of these patients underwent emergency bypass surgery. The mortality for PTCA was 0.8%. These numbers are representative of most of the centers in the United States.[70] Failure of angioplasty was most commonly due to an inability to achieve reduction of the stenosis rather than an inability to cross the lesion.[70]

Despite advances, PTCA continues to have some limitations. Abrupt closure of the vessel shortly after balloon removal requires immediate interventions to restore coronary blood flow.[67] These patients are

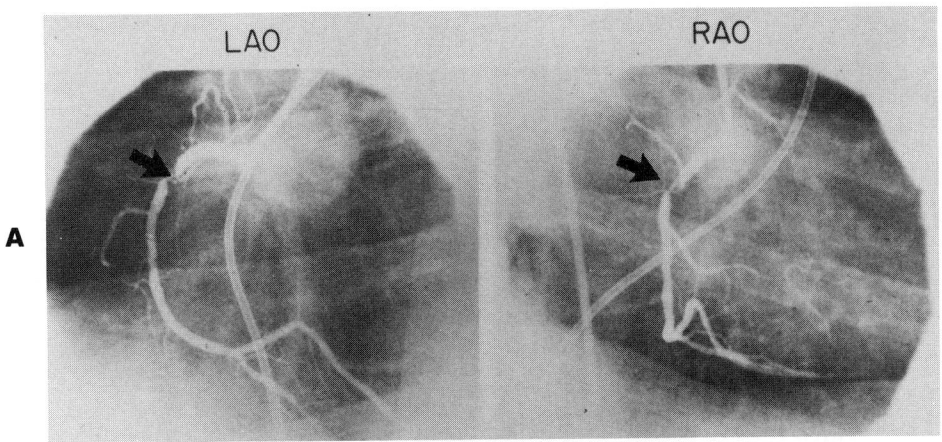

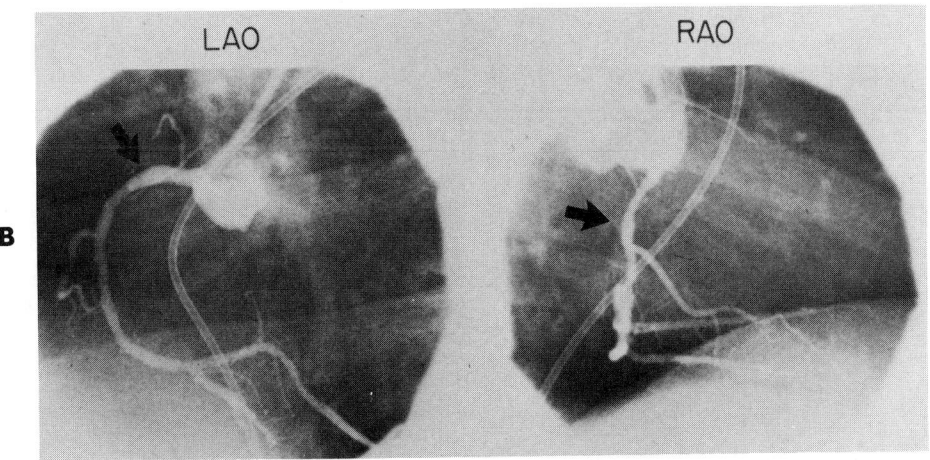

Figure 22-13   *A,* Arteriography of a patient in the LAO and RAO projections, which depict a proximal RCA lesion (95%) stenosis amenable to angioplasty. *B,* After PTCA, in the same patient, flow has been established through the vessel as depicted by the arrows.

treated with repeat balloon angioplasty or some of the newer technologies such as lasers, stents, or atherectomy. If all interventions attempted are unsuccessful, the patient may be sent for cardiac surgery. Abrupt closure occurs is about 7% of patients undergoing angioplasty. Restenosis, the narrowing of a previously dilated artery, continues to occur at a rate of 30% within the first 6 months of the PTCA procedure.[67,70] So far, according to the statistics from the NHLBI registry, restenosis does not present with a life-threatening problem (MI) or death. It is also interesting to note that repeat angioplasty yields a low complication rate. The majority of patients do not develop restenosis and report no further complaints of angina.

Researchers are attempting to identify factors such as platelet aggregation or new thrombus formation that may predispose patients for restenosis. Pharmacological trials have been attempted in an effort to reduce restenosis. Warfarin, calcium channel antagonists, prolonged intravenous heparin, prostacycline infusion, and fish oil supplements have all been reported ineffective.[67] At this time no therapy has been found as beneficial as aspirin and persantine.[67]

At present, cardiologists choose a balloon catheter smaller than the calculated adjacent artery for use in a PTCA. Some authorities propose that successful results can be achieved with optimal selection of the balloon/artery ratio and balloon pressure application. Furthermore, it has been suggested that anatomical or procedural factors may be responsible for restenosis.[71] Research is needed in relation to anatomical or procedural factors which could be responsible for restenosis. Further inquiry into the role of antiplatelet drugs and calcium channel blockers in preventing restenosis must also be addressed.

The patient's condition at the conclusion of the PTCA procedure dictates the intensity of care. Most patients receive cardiac monitoring for at least 4 to 6 hours to detect signs of myocardial ischemia. Isoenzymes are drawn on return from the catheterization laboratory. After the femoral sheath is removed, adequate assessment of the site for bleeding or hematoma formation is completed. The patient may ambulate several hours later.

If the patient should develop chest pain soon after the procedure, standard acute coronary care procedure is followed. This includes a 12-lead ECG to document ischemia, vasodilator or drug therapy to relieve pain, and serial CK and isoenzyme assays (CK and LDH) to document the presence or absence of significant myocardial damage. If the pain persists, indicating an abrupt reduction in blood flow due to reocclusion of the dilated artery, the patient may be returned to the catheterization laboratory for repeat angiography and, perhaps, angioplasty.

Laser Angioplasty

Percutaneous transluminal coronary angioplasty (PTCA) remains the standard for the nonsurgical treatment of coronary artery disease. In the 1980s the number of PTCAs performed annually increased from 10,000 to 250,000; it is expected to reach 450,000 by 1993.[72] Acute vessel closure and chronic restenosis are problems associated with balloon angioplasty. Standard balloon angioplasty fractures the plaque. To address the problems of abrupt closure and restenosis, clinical investigations are exploring methods of removing rather than fracturing the plaque, for example, laser technology. The goal of laser therapy is to remove the atherosclerotic lesion with minimal damage to normal adjacent tissue.[73]

The term *laser* is an acronym derived from *light amplification by stimulated emission of radiation*. Lasers artificially excite or stimulate atoms, forcing the release of energy in the form of light.[74] Sakallaris described laser light as being composed of photons (excess energy released from an atom) and holding three unique properties:

1. Laser light is coherent (photons are in phase in time and space).
2. Photons are collumated (the waves are parallel and do not diverge from each other as they travel outward).
3. Photons are monochromic (have identical wavelength).[75]

The theory of stimulated emission, the basis of the creation of a laser beam, was first articulated by Albert Einstein. As a charged atom is struck by a photon, the atom is stimulated to release energy in the form of photons that have equal wavelengths and that leave the atom together in the same direction and in phase with each other. This process produces a laser beam (stimulated emission). Four components are required

to produce a laser beam: (1) a constantly charged atom, (2) stimulation of the charged atom with a photon, (3) amplification of light generated by the process of stimulated emission, and (4) a mirror to reflect the photons released from the charged atoms so that the photons will reverse course, travel back through the charged atoms, and generate release of more photons. The photons bouncing back and forth between the mirrors in the laser apparatus produce a fine laser beam.[75] The laser beam may be generated in an uninterrupted wave (continuous wave laser) or delivered in short bursts or pulses (pulsed laser).[74]

The clinical purpose of laser energy is to destroy targeted tissue. This occurs through three mechanisms: photothermal, photochemical, and photoablative interactions. The *photothermal* mechanism employs energy in the form of heat to vaporize tissue. The *photochemical* interaction involves the use of photosensitized dyes, which selectively concentrate in the target tissue, undergo a series of reactions upon exposure to laser light, and cause cellular death. In *photoablative* interaction cellular molecular bonds are disrupted by entering photons.[74]

The degree of tissue destruction and the damage to the surrounding normal tissue are influenced by the intensity and the duration of exposure to the laser beam, the wavelength of the laser beam, the type of laser, and the type of medium in which the energy is delivered.[74] Halfman-Franey and Coburn state that continuous wave lasers have been shown to cause three zones of tissue injury.[73] The central zone is crater formation due to tissue vaporization. The second zone, surrounding the crater, is burned tissue. The outermost zone is a region of shock injury. Pulsed lasers emit a single pulse or a train of discrete light pulses alternating with relaxation periods. Theoretically, the relaxation time allows the target tissue to conduct heat away from the lased area, thereby avoiding thermal injury. Pulsed lasers cause less thermal damage to adjacent cells than the continuous wave type.[73]

Several types of lasers are in use. The argon, carbon dioxide, and Nd:YAG are most commonly used in cardiovascular intervention. The excimer laser and SMART laser are also under investigation.[73]

Argon laser: The blue-green light of the argon laser is transmitted through clear tissue and is readily absorbed by pigmented tissue, particularly red or orange. Argon lasers produce a predictable level of plaque penetration without perforation.[73]

Carbon dioxide laser: The beam from the CO_2 laser is absorbed by water; it brings intercellular water to a boiling point so that the cells vaporize. It is possible to direct this laser beam for precise tissue ablation.[73]

Nd:YAG laser: The Nd:YAG (neodynium-yttrium-garnet) laser welds together disrupted tissue elements thermally and thereby decreases the incidence of abrupt reclosure and restenosis associated with PTCA.[73]

Excimer laser: This recently developed pulsed laser is still experimental but has several advantages over other types. The energy from the excimer laser is (1) intensely absorbed by the atherosclerotic plaque, (2) can precisely ablate plaque without causing thermal injury, and (3) can effectively ablate calcified plaque.[73] Litvack et al.[72] have used the excimer laser to recanalize aortocoronary saphenous vein grafts.

SMART laser: This low-density laser is also currently under investigation. The system uses computerized plaque detection and targeting to prevent vessel perforation. It is designed to provide precise plaque removal without thermal damage and to remove plaque at low energy levels which will not harm normal tissue.[73]

The major complication resulting from laser therapy is vessel perforation. Other complications include aneurysm, abrupt closure, dissection, and spasm. Reperfusion dysrhythmias, embolization, bleeding at the insertion site, and impaired circulation to the involved extremity have also been noted.[73,74]

There are several techniques used in the cardiac catheterization laboratory with laser therapy. One method is to use laser energy alone to remove the plaque from the coronary artery (laser angioplasty). A second type of angioplasty involves using laser energy to create an opening in the plaque, followed by balloon angioplasty (laser-assisted balloon angioplasty). A third type, thermal welding balloon angioplasty, involves the absorption of laser energy from the interior of the inflated balloon resulting in the creation of a smooth lumen that is the size and shape of the angioplasty balloon being used.[73]

The Laserprobe, which is under investigation, has a metallic tip at the end of a fiberoptic catheter that converts laser energy to heat (Figure 22-14). When the heated tip reaches the obstruction, it tends to predilate the plaque, creating a groove for the rest of the probe to follow and leaving behind a thin layer of carbonized plaque.[73]

The patient is prepared for laser angioplasty as for a standard PTCA. Because this is an investigational procedure, the patient needs a thorough explanation, and a consent must be signed. In the cardiac catheterization laboratory the patient is prepared, and monitoring instrumentation is set up as for a standard PTCA. The one added feature is that the patient and the staff must wear protective eyewear appropriate to the wavelength being used. The patient's neurological, respiratory, hemodynamic, and cardiac status are monitored throughout the procedure. As stated

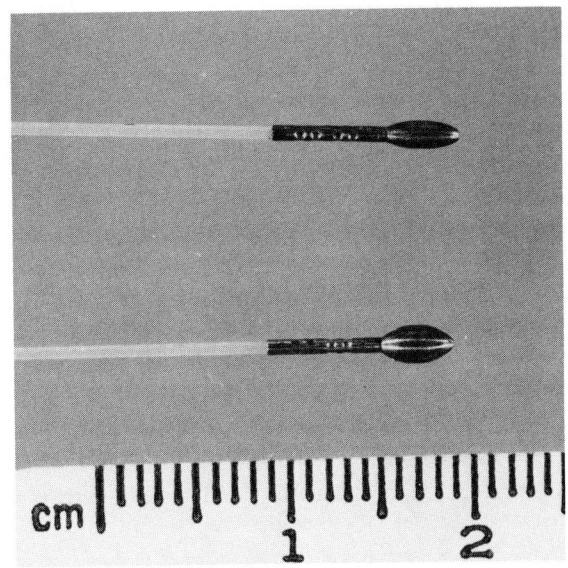

Figure 22-14 Illustration of the laser probe delivery system used to vaporize atheromatous lesions.

by Sakallaris, transient reperfusion dysrhythmias are usually seen during the procedure.[75] After the procedure, the patient is returned to the unit and cared for as a routine PTCA. If there are no problems, the patient is discharged on the third day. Aspirin and a calcium channel blocker are prescribed.

Laser angioplasty can remove atherosclerotic plaque from coronary arteries and can be used in conjunction with balloon PTCA. Preliminary data reveal a restenosis rate of 30% to 40% in elective procedures.[76] More research is needed on techniques like angioscopy, laser pulsing modes, and alternative laser catheter designs to improve tissue abatement and decrease injury to the surrounding normal tissue.[74]

Atherectomy

An approach being used to overcome the problems of abrupt closure and restenosis with PTCA is the atherectomy. *Atherectomy* involves a percutaneous approach to removal of plaque from a coronary artery instead of the fracturing of plaque accomplished by conventional PTCA. Atherectomy removes the obstructive material and leaves a smoother surface to diminish the probability of restenosis.[77] Several theories exist regarding the potential mechanisms of how atherectomy may reduce the restenosis rate:[78]

1. Removal of atheroma may provide a wider lumen that is able to accommodate subsequent cellular hyperplasia without appreciable obstruction to blood flow.
2. The radical stretch injury that is caused by high-pressure balloon inflation may be reduced with atherectomy.
3. Removal of smooth muscle cells from within or

beneath the atheroma or neointima may reduce the number of cells available for replication and thereby reduce the substrate for restenosis.[78]

Halfman-Franey and Coburn[73] state that this device may be more applicable than balloon angioplasty in occluded arteries and in stenotic vessels that are calcific, eccentric, or ulcerated. Kaufman and associates[79] believe that atherectomy is a safe procedure in stenosed vein grafts. Muller, Ellis, and Topol[80] are using atherectomy of the left main coronary artery in patients being treated by percutaneous cardiopulmonary bypass.

Complications associated with atherectomy include abrupt closure (possibly necessitating emergent coronary bypass surgery), dissection, distal embolization, side branch occlusion and transient thrombosis.

Several types of atherectomy devices are available. The directional coronary atherectomy (DCA) is a double-lumen catheter (known as the Simpson Atherocath) that cuts and retrieves the atherosclerotic lesion. The Auth atherectomy catheter is a single-lumen device with a rotating abrasive tip consisting of a diamond-coated brass burr. The high speed rotary burr grinds occluding atheroma into fine particles that pass harmlessly through the capillary circulation.[73] The transluminal extraction catheter fragments the plaque via the steel cutting head and then suctions it out of the body by means of a vacuum. The DCA is discussed here.

Patient preparation is similar to that for a PTCA. In the cardiac catheterization laboratory a no. 10 or 11 French sheath (vs. a no. 8 French for PTCA) is inserted in the femoral artery. A guiding catheter is then positioned at the opening of the stenosed coronary artery. A guide wire is then passed through the catheter and positioned across the lesion. The Simpson Atherocath is advanced over the wire to the lesion. Once the distal end of the Atherocath is positioned across the stenosis, the balloon is inflated, and the cutter is slowly advanced until it travels the length of the housing opening. Atheroma protruding into the opening is shaved off the vessel wall and captured in the end of the catheter. The balloon is deflated to allow for repositioning of the cutter or removal of the catheter.[73] The procedure is repeated until a satisfactory angiographic result is achieved. The tissue specimens are then retrieved and can be sent for analysis (Figure 22-15).

The nursing care of the patient during an ather-

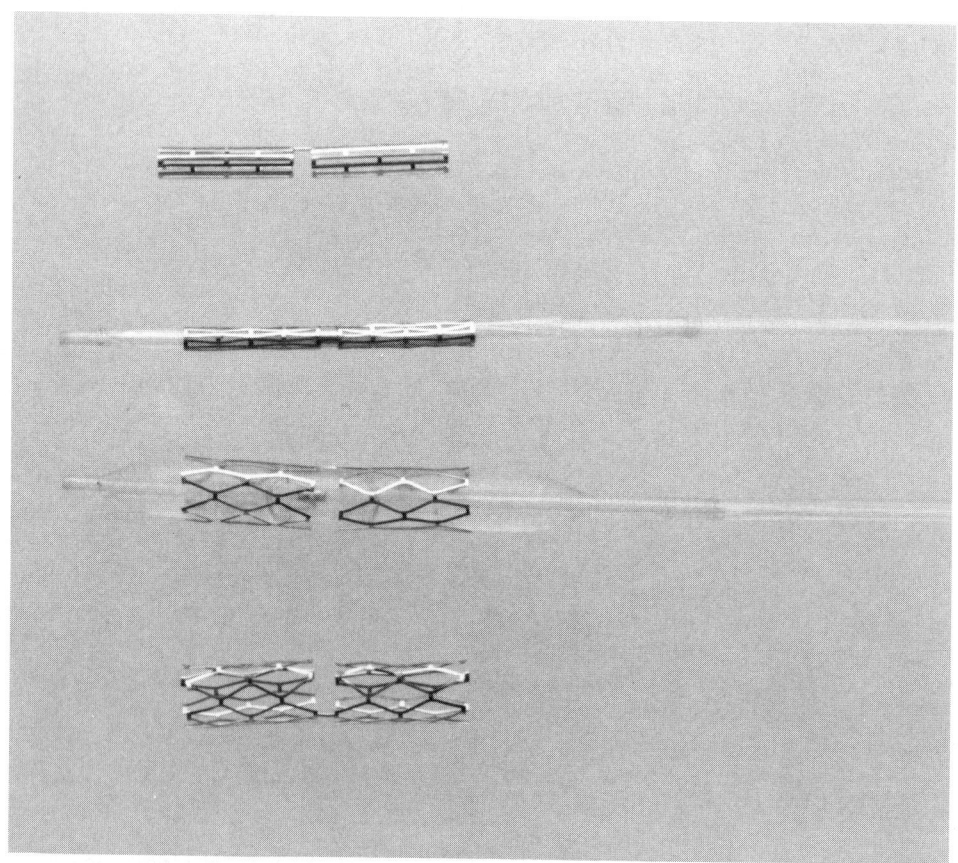

Figure 22-15 Palmaz-Schatz stent.
Courtesy of Johnson and Johnson Interventional Systems Co.

ectomy is similar to that given during PTCA. Neurological, respiratory, hemodynamic, and cardiac status are monitored. Most patients do not experience any chest discomfort. Some patients are disturbed by the noise of the cutter and require the reassurance that only the stenotic lesion is being removed.

After the procedure these patients are monitored closely, as they are after a PTCA. In our institution they are brought to the coronary care unit because of the size of the sheath. As part of any atherectomy procedure, the groin site and pedal pulses must be monitored attentively because of the high risk for vascular compromise. The sheaths are pulled 4 hours after the procedure, and a sandbag is placed on the site. If there are no complications, the patient is discharged 48 hours after the procedure. Aspirin and a calcium channel blocker are prescribed.

It has been proposed that atherectomy may decrease restenosis rates by creating a smooth luminal surface and optimal flow conditions with minimal injury to the vessel wall;[79] however, the reported restenosis rate for atherectomy is roughly 30%.[76] A study done by Garratt et al.[78] demonstrated that intimal hyperplasia occurs after atherectomy in a manner similar to that seen after PTCA. They suggested that careful patient selection and modification of atherectomy instrumentation and technique to provide better control of the depth of tissue resection may improve long-term results after coronary artery and vein graft atherectomy.

Stents

Despite improvements in operator technique and angioplasty equipment, patients undergoing PTCA are still faced with the 5% possibility of abrupt closure or the 30% chance of restenosis.[81] Abrupt closure occurring after PTCA is usually related to a combination of thrombosis, dissection, and spasm, as previously described.[82] Late restenosis is attributed to areas of abnormal flow separation and stasis that contribute to platelet-thrombus formation and later smooth muscle cell proliferation.[73] Intracoronary stents provide a nonsurgical method for keeping vessels open after balloon dilatation.[83] The method is currently being investigated in the United States and Europe.

The first use of stents began with Charles Dotter in 1969.[84] He placed stainless steel coils into the peripheral arteries of dogs with favorable results. There was little interest in Dotter's work until the early 1980s, when several researchers developed stent designs. Most of these designs failed because of stent thrombogenicity and unreliable placement characteristics.[73] In 1986, Sigwart placed the first stent in human coronary circulation.[85] At present, three stents are being investigated.[73]

The Wallstent is a self-expanding mesh of stainless steel filaments that fits over the end of a delivery catheter. The stent is contained by a sleeve, and a catheter delivers it to the desired location. After the stent is positioned in the artery, the sleeve is withdrawn, and the stent expands. Complications such as migration and thrombosis can occur with the underexpansion of the stent, whereas overexpansion can cause thrombosis and excessive intimal proliferation.

The Palmaz-Schatz stent is a balloon-expandable composed of two shorter segments of slotted tubes connected by a small (1-mm) bridging strut. Collapsed, this stent rests on a standard balloon delivery system. At the target site, the stent is expanded by balloon inflation. When the balloon is deflated and removed, the stent remains embedded in the vessel wall.

The third type of stent being examined has thermal memory. Stents fabricated of alloys of nickel and titanium (nitinol) assume a coil configuration when they come into contact with warm blood or saline.[73] Nitinol stents are shaped at high temperatures into a coil configuration and are then straightened at room temperature to pass through a catheter as a straight wire.[86] They are deployed at the site of the stenosis. These coils may change shape because of temperature changes in the catheter lumen or during deployment. They cannot be dilated at a later date if the stent lumen restenoses.

Of the three basic types, the balloon-expandable has the fewest complications at this time.[86]

Stents are used to treat acute vessel occlusion, vessel wall dissection, restenosis despite repeated attempts at balloon dilatation, and after PTCA to prevent restenosis of totally occluded coronary arteries. The use of stents in treating saphenous vein bypass graft stenosis is under investigation.[87]

Stent therapy is contraindicated in patients who are unable to take long-term anticoagulation which is necessary because of the risk of stent-related thrombosis.[87] Patients are selected for stent placement on the basis of the lesion. Short segmental blockages in a relatively straight artery are associated with the most promising results because of the design, length, and thickness of the expandable stent.[82]

Once the patient has given consent for the stent procedure, care is similar to that for a PTCA. A dextran drip (100 ml/hr) is added to the regimen of heparin, aspirin, dipyridamole, and calcium channel blocker 2 hours before the procedure. The patient is prepared as for a PTCA. Insertion of the modified Palmaz-Schatz stent (Figure 22-15) is discussed here.

A standard balloon dilatation is performed, the PTCA balloon is withdrawn, and a stent-loaded balloon catheter is passed over a guide wire. At the target site, the stent is expanded by a single balloon inflation of 6 to 10 atm for 5 to 10 seconds.[88] The patient is given 10,000 units of heparin intravenously in the catheterization laboratory followed by 2,500 units per hour during the procedure to keep the activated clotting time (ACT) 2 to 2.5 times greater than normal. After the stent is placed, the patency of the artery is evaluated by angiography. At the completion of the procedure the arterial and venous sheaths are sutured in place.

Postprocedure, the patient is monitored closely for thrombosis, spasm and the potential for hemorrhage. According to the protocol outlined by Halfman-Franey and associates,[82] the dextran is infused at a rate of 150 ml/hr, and low-dose nitroglycerin is continued until the following morning.

The predominant acute complication of metallic stents is closure from thrombosis.[81] Halfman-Franey and associates state that the success of any vascular stent depends on rapid endothelialization (because endothelium provides an ideal flow surface) and endothelium cannot grow on bare metal. It can, however, grow on a thin layer of fibrin and thrombus.[82] Thrombosis is essential for healing, but it must be controlled, and close attention must be paid to anticoagulation. When the ACT is less than 175 seconds, it is considered safe to remove the sheaths.[82] One to 2 hours after sheath removal, the heparin drip can be restarted. The PTT and ACT are measured every 4 hours. The PTT should be maintained at 50 to 80 seconds. Aspirin and dipyridamole are continued, and warfarin is added after the sheath is pulled.[82] Because of the risk of bacterial seeding, subbacterial endocarditis (SBE) prophylaxis should be administered during the first 8 weeks following stenting.[76]

Aggressive anticoagulation extends the patient stay to 5 days.[76] Patients are discharged home on a regimen of aspirin, dipyridamole, calcium channel blockers, and warfarin. Calcium channel blockers and dipyridamole are continued for 3 months. Coumadin therapy is continued for 1 to 3 months, but aspirin is continued indefinitely. Patients are scheduled for follow-up visits at 1 and 2 weeks and at 1, 2, 3, 6, and 12 months. A repeat cardiac catheterization is scheduled for 6 and 12 months.

Research continues to determine the best design for intracoronary stents. The ideal stent would be biocompatible to allow for controlled thrombosis, flexible so it can be guided through tortuous vessels, visible by fluoroscopy, retrievable to eliminate the need for surgery in the event of a problem, and would have the ability to deliver medication to inhibit restenosis.

Ultrasonic Angioplasty

Studies using high-energy ultrasound to disrupt thrombi and plaque show that ultrasound angioplasty can induce selective injury to thrombi and plaque only.[89] Rosenschein and coworkers selected patients undergoing bypass surgery for totally occluded femoral-popliteal arteries. They performed ultrasonic angioplasty using a device composed of a flexible aluminum ultrasound transmission wire attached at its proximal end to a transducer that converts electrical energy to ultrasonic energy. The ultrasound energy is transferred via the wire to the lesion.

As this procedure was to be performed during surgery, a routine surgical incision of the femoral artery was made. Once the artery had been incised, an ultrasound wire was inserted into the artery and advanced under fluoroscopy to the stenotic area. Angioplasty was begun at low energy levels that were gradually increased. When the lesion was opened at a certain energy level, that level was maintained as the ultrasound wire was passed back and forth through the stenotic area two to four times. At the completion of the surgical procedure peripheral angiograms were performed and analyzed.

The investigators found that ultrasound angioplasty substantially improved flow with minimal damage to the arterial wall.[89] Minimal injury to the affected arteries may indicate that recanalization before the media and adventitia had been damaged. Injury to the media is believed to stimulate the smooth muscle cell proliferation associated with restenosis after angioplasty. If this hypothesis is correct, the ability of ultrasound angioplasty to cause selective injury may lower the rate of restenosis postprocedure.

This study was the first clinical trial of ultrasonic angioplasty in peripheral vascular disease. The investigators believe that the results of this study indicate that ultrasound angioplasty can be used successfully in the treatment of total occlusions.[89] More research needs to be done in this area. The potential exists for ultrasound to become a useful treatment for totally occluded coronary arteries.

Percutaneous Cardiopulmonary Bypass

One method of circulatory support in the event of circulatory collapse is percutaneous cardiopulmonary bypass support (PCBS).[90] A PCBS system is a preassembled cardiopulmonary bypass circuit composed of a blood pump, heat exchanger, oxygenators, and interconnecting tubing. This system can be set up and primed in 5 minutes, an advantage in life-threatening circumstances.[91] It can rapidly infuse large volumes, thereby maintaining a normal cardiac output. A major advantage of PCBS is that the system is able to provide adequate perfusion even when no intrinsic cardiac rhythm exists.

Because PCBS can be readily initiated, the indications for its use are expanding. Some centers initiate PCBS preprocedure in high-risk angioplasty patients to maintain hemodynamic stability. This is called *supported PTCA*. A high-risk angioplasty may be defined as one in which the patient has poor left ventricular function (ejection fraction less than 25%) or the vessel or vessels to be dilated supply more than one half of the remaining viable myocardium.[90] Other hospitals use the PCBS system for patients in whom an abrupt closure (closure of the treated artery during PTCA or shortly after completion) causes hemodynamic instability or cardiac arrest. This is termed *rescue PTCA*. The system can also be used for patients at high risk during an aortic valvuloplasty. During a valvuloplasty, as the balloon is inflated across the aortic valve there is substantial reduction in cardiac output potentially causing hypotension and ventricular dysrhythmias.[92]

Patients with left main lesions are usually not candidates for balloon angioplasty because they are at high risk for abrupt closure and hemodynamic collapse. Some studies suggest that in patients with left main lesions PCBS should be instituted and an atherectomy performed.[93] Patients experiencing cardiogenic shock from an acute MI can be hemodynamically stabilized by PCBS and then undergo a PTCA.[94] Patients experiencing refractory ventricular fibrillation can be hemodynamically stabilized by PCBS even if the dysrhythmia still exists.[94]

Some studies have examined initiating PCBS in patients who were hypothermic and in refractory ventricular fibrillation. These patients were rewarmed by PCBS for 2 hours and were successfully defibrillated; however, they did not survive. Studies indicate that PCBS is most effective for patients whose arrest was related to cardiac causes; the survival rates were poor in patients with trauma or septic shock.[95]

Institutional criteria are usually established to determine whether patients are appropriate candidates for emergent PCBS. At our institution, patients are excluded for emergent PCBS if CPR has been continuing for more than 30 minutes without signs of neurological response; if the patient has a known aortic aneurysm or significant aortic insufficiency; or if severe peripheral vascular disease would preclude the insertion and placement of the femoral cannulas. The box to the right lists the criteria for emergent PCBS.

Two major advantages of PCBS are that it can be initiated emergently at the bedside without the need for fluoroscopic equipment and that it can be initiated during CPR. However, the system has several disadvantages. First, there is incomplete left ventricular unloading after a prolonged cardiac arrest; thus, the PCBS system should not be used for more than 6 hours.[90] Second, the large size of the cannulas contraindicates use of the systems in patients with significant iliofemoral disease.

Initiation of Therapy. Once the decision is made

to initiate PCBS, an arterial and venous access to the femoral system is obtained by a physician. As access is being gained, the PCBS is being primed by the perfusionists. The patient is usually given 300 units of heparin per kg of body weight to ensure an activated clotting time (ACT) of ≥400 seconds. No. 18 to 20 French cannulas are used for percutaneous insertion. The venous cannula is placed just proximal to the junction of the inferior vena cava and the right atrium. The arterial cannula rests just distal to the aortic bifurcation (Figure 22-16). After placement of the cannulas the system is checked for air bubbles. Once the lines are free of air, blood is actively aspirated out of the right atrium via the venous cannula using a vortex

---

Clinical Inclusion Criteria for Emergency PCBS

PATIENTS MUST:

1. Be surgical candidates prior to their PTCA/valvuloplasty procedure and remain an appropriate candidate in the view of the surgeon.
2. Have shock or refractory dysrhythmias unresponsive to initial medical therapy with evidence of adequate neurological function.
3. Have massive myocardial infarction despite initial trials of alternative reperfusion therapy.

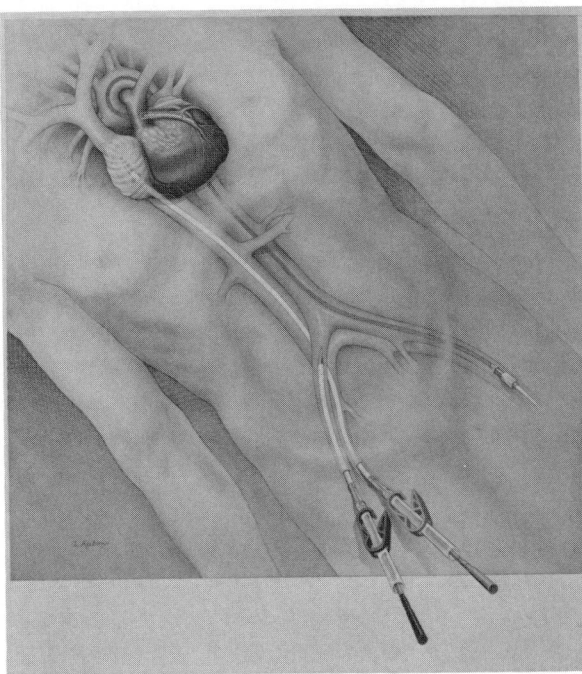

Figure 22-16 Placement of percutaneous bypass catheters. The arterial catheter is placed in the femoral artery. The venous catheter is at the junction of the inferior vena cava and the right atrium.

Courtesy of Bard Cardiopulmonary Division of C. R. Bard, Inc.

pump. Blood circulates through the bypass system where it is oxygenated, heated, and returned to the body via the arterial cannula. After the PCBS has been instituted (Figure 22-17), baseline hemodynamic pressures are obtained: arterial pressure, right atrial pressure, pulmonary artery pressures, and pulmonary wedge pressure. Cardiopulmonary bypass is initiated at a flow rate of 2 L/min and can be increased by increments of 0.5 to 5 L. Patients undergoing a supported PTCA usually require a flow rate of 2 to 3 L. For patients with poor left ventricular function, or

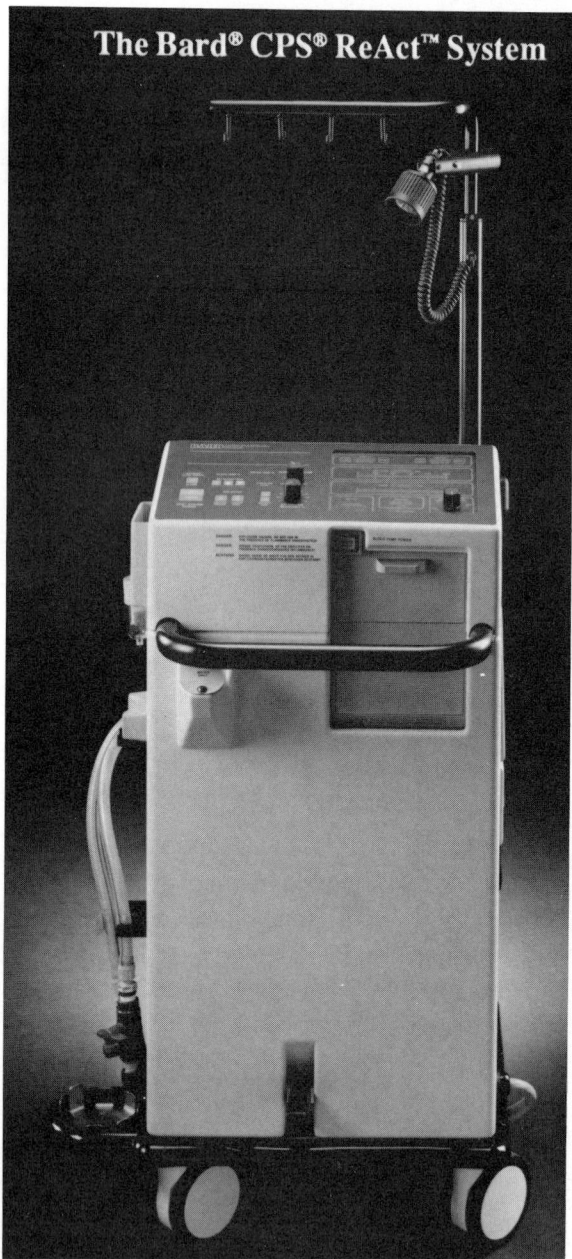

Figure 22-17   Percutaneous cardiopulmonary bypass system.

Courtesy of Bard Cardiopulmonary Division of C. R. Bard, Inc.

those having an angioplasty of the only remaining patent vessel, higher flow rates may be required. The best physiological assessment of blood flow adequacy is venous blood oxygen saturation.[90] Angioplasty or valvuloplasty begins at this point for patients undergoing a supported procedure. Patients who were undergoing a rescue PTCA would be transported to the operating room.

Initiating PCBS requires a large team: a cardiologist, cardiothoracic surgeon, anesthesiologist, perfusionist, and cardiac catheterization laboratory nurses and technicians. The operating room is usually on standby to accept the patient.

PCBS-supported PTCA or Valvuloplasty. During a supported PTCA or valvuloplasty, patients have received some sedation but are awake during the procedure. The nursing care in the cardiac catheterization laboratory includes assessing the patient's neurological, respiratory, cardiac and volume status; monitoring medications; and providing emotional support to the patient. The ACT is measured every 15 minutes. Heparin boluses are given and the heparin drip adjusted. A dextran drip also is administered.

As the cannulas and catheters are inserted the patient feels little discomfort because of the local anesthetic. There is also no discomfort as the catheters are moved into the coronary artery. As the angioplasty wire and balloon are advanced inside the stenosed coronary artery, the patient may experience some discomfort (angina) due to the decreased blood flow. Increasing the flow rate from the bypass system can eliminate this discomfort. Patients need to be encouraged to report all symptoms.

At the completion of the supported PTCA or valvuloplasty, cardiopulmonary support is gradually withdrawn over 5 minutes by reducing the flow rate. Fluid infusions are given to keep the pulmonary wedge pressure in the range of 8 to 10 mm or to the prebypass level.[90] The femoral arterial and venous cannulas are sutured into place, and the patient is transferred to the critical care unit. The patient must remain flat with the head of the bed elevated only 15°.

The femoral arterial and venous cannulas are removed 5 to 7 hours after the last dose of heparin or when the ACT is less than 240 seconds.[90] After the cannulas are removed, manual compression is applied for at least 15 minutes, and a compression clamp is applied. The pressure is adjusted so that pedal pulses remain either palpable or confirmed by Doppler ultrasound. After 90 minutes, the clamp is very gradually released if there is no evidence of bleeding. When the PTT decreases to under 60 seconds, a heparin infusion (600 to 800 units/hr) is started. The pulmonary artery catheter is removed the next day.[90]

The nursing care of patients following supported

PTCA/valvuloplasty is similar to that given after routine procedures. The one exception is that special attention must be paid to the femoral area through which the bypass system was passed. The groin site should be checked frequently for any sign of bleeding or hematoma. Pedal pulses should also be checked for any change. The following day a CBC should be obtained and the creatinine level assessed.

Patients whose coronary arteries close abruptly or who have a large dissection during their PTCA may be given PCBS prior to their emergent CABG. (The box on p. 541 lists the clinical inclusion criteria.) If these complications occur, the patient requires nursing care as previously described. If the patient is conscious, the physician will explain to the patient that an emergent CABG will take place. As PCBS is initiated, the patient is sedated and intubated. Patients need reassurance and need to be told that their families will be notified. Often these patients are being resuscitated before PCBS is initiated, and there is no opportunity for any teaching.

In patients undergoing an emergency CABG, PCBS is terminated after conventional bypass is underway. At the completion of the surgery, the femoral cannulas are removed, and the artery and vein are sutured.

The most common complications seen are those involving the bypass cannula insertion sites such as pseudoaneurysm of the femoral artery and enlarging hematoma. Sometimes these complications require surgical repair. Blood transfusions are sometimes required, but this need is decreasing because the cannulas are now being removed at 6 to 7 hours postinsertion.

Patients undergoing a supported PTCA are usually hospitalized for 3 to 5 days. Two to four weeks after discharge, these patients undergo noninvasive flow studies on the PCBS site to determine if a pseudoaneurysm or arteriovenous fistula has developed.

Percutaneous cardiopulmonary bypass support initiated in the cardiac catheterization laboratory makes PTCA feasible in patients who were not previously candidates.[90] PCBS is also believed to allow prolonged balloon inflations, thereby reducing restenosis and improving the angiographic results. For those who experience an abrupt closure during PTCA, PCBS provides a means of attaining hemodynamic stability prior to an emergency CABG. Circulatory support systems such as this will allow patients with more complex coronary artery disease to be treated in the cardiac catheterization laboratory.

Surgery

Coronary artery bypass grafting (CABG) is the predominant surgical intervention for CAD. Some centers are also doing coronary endarterectomies for coronary artery disease. These interventions are discussed in greater detail in Chapter 26.

NURSING MANAGEMENT

Patients admitted to a coronary care unit or a critical care unit are usually those patients who manifest symptoms of unstable angina requiring further evaluation. Patients with unstable angina may present at the time of admission with chest discomfort. Immediate attention must be given to providing relief of the discomfort; the drug of choice is usually nitroglycerin. The degree and intensity of the discomfort or pain determine the route of administration. Most often, if pain resolution cannot be obtained with oral or sublingual nitrates, which is likely with unstable angina, intravenous therapy is required. A second priority on admission is the application of electrodes for continuous ECG monitoring to observe for ischemic changes. It is also necessary during an anginal attack to obtain a 12-lead ECG to document the presence of ischemic changes in leads viewing the area of ischemia. After these priorities have been addressed, the critical care nurse should obtain a nursing history, including patient assessment, and identify the patient's problems based on the data obtained. Early interventions aimed at resolving these problems as well as minimizing or preventing potential problems are then implemented. In addition to the nursing history, the physical assessment and data from diagnostic procedures are incorporated in the database.

Gordon's functional health patterns, as described in Chapter 21, provide a framework upon which a biopsychosocial nursing history may be obtained.[96] Refer to that chapter for a more detailed explanation of these health patterns. As part of the nursing history, specific information regarding cardiac risk factors, family history of heart disease, and pain history, especially activities that precipitate discomfort or pain, is elicited. Previous medical history, medication history, occupation (may be a source of stress), and anticipated changes in lifestyle secondary to coronary artery disease should also be obtained.

The physical assessment of the patient with unstable angina provides minimal information because the examination usually depicts normal data. Specific signs and symptoms during an anginal attack have been previously described. Auscultation of heart sounds during an anginal attack may reveal a paradoxical splitting of the second heart sound (S_2), pulsus alternans, or the presence of a transient S_3 or a fourth heart sound (S_4). In addition, there may also be a transient systolic murmur of mitral regurgitation secondary to papillary muscle ischemia. Most of these findings are considered nonspecific findings in unstable angina patients because they are often associated with stable angina or acute MI.[97]

Laboratory data may reveal elevated serum cholesterol levels and specific lipoproteins. Cardiac enzymes should not be elevated unless necrosis is present.

Once the database is completed, both actual and potential problems may be identified. These problems are classified into high-risk diagnoses or nursing diagnoses which can be treated independently by the nurse. A nursing care plan aimed at minimizing or preventing either type of problem may be formulated from the database. Nursing interventions and outcomes will be discussed for these diagnoses.

■ NURSING DIAGNOSIS

Pain (angina), related to an imbalance between myocardial oxygen supply and demand.

OUTCOME STANDARD AND CRITERIA

Pain is absent or controlled as evidenced by:
- A decreased use of pharmacological agents
- A decrease in nonverbal cues
- A decrease in incidence of pain
- A decrease in duration and intensity of pain
- Ability to verbalize factors that precipitate or aggravate pain and describe preventive actions

NURSING INTERVENTIONS

- Instruct patient to notify nursing staff immediately of pain or chest discomfort
- Observe for nonverbal cues such as facial grimaces, restlessness, and posturing suggestive of pain or discomfort
- Monitor and document pain characteristics such as intensity, duration, localization, and radiation; and associated and alleviating factors so as to discern angina from other etiologies
- Administer medications such as nitrates, beta blockers, and calcium channel antagonists to relieve or prevent chest discomfort or pain
- Assess the patient's response to prescribed medications to determine the degree of relief obtained
- Explore with patient what factors precipitate or aggravate pain and then discuss possible changes in daily activities or lifestyle that may be necessary to prevent angina attacks
- Decrease physical activity during anginal attack
- Remove or reduce stress-provoking stimuli from a patient's environment, such as bright lights, loud, sudden noises, and frequent interruptions
- Provide for long, uninterrupted restful periods by organizing plan of care with other health care disciplines
- Obtain a 12-lead ECG during chest discomfort and report ischemic changes
- Employ energy conservation measures

■ NURSING DIAGNOSIS

Anxiety, related to unfamiliar ICU environment, unknown future, or lack of knowledge regarding disease process.

OUTCOME STANDARD AND CRITERIA

Anxiety is reduced or absent as evidenced by:
- Verbalization of an increase in psychological comfort and support
- Absence or diminution of restlessness or irritability
- Verbalization of disease process and realistic expectations regarding future
- Vital signs within normal ranges
- Verbalization of effective techniques to reduce anxiety

NURSING INTERVENTIONS

- Assess level of anxiety in patient and significant others and validate
- Observe for signs of increasing anxiety through verbal or nonverbal cues
- Encourage patient and family communication regarding concerns or lack of knowledge
- Inform patient and significant others of proposed treatment options as previously discussed with physician
- Discuss the disease process
- Discuss risk factors that contribute to the development of CAD and identify which of those risk factors are present and can be modified
- Instruct patient regarding signs and symptoms of angina that may occur as well as signs and symptoms of progression to an MI
- Assist with identification of appropriate resources that patient or family may use to help patient reduce anxiety associated with the disease process
- If patient's anxiety increases, encourage relaxation techniques such as slow deep breathing and imagery exercises
- Begin instruction regarding medications—specifically their actions, side effects, and prophylactic use of antianginal drugs. Stress importance of adhering to precribed medications
- Begin to explore necessary lifestyle changes related to disease process
- Reduce sensory overload if contributing to anxiety

HIGH-RISK NURSING DIAGNOSES

High-risk nursing diagnoses for the patient with unstable angina include:
- High risk for decreased activity tolerance, related to deconditioning or fear of repeated angina attacks
- High risk for sleep pattern disturbances, related to ICU environment and treatment regimens
- High risk for disturbance in self-concept, related to patient/family response to changes in lifestyle
- High risk for injury, related to failure to follow prescribed regimen

Along with these nursing interventions, critical care nurses need to be aware of the physician's plan of therapy. Most patients with unstable angina stabilize or progress into such coronary events as MI or congestive heart failure. If progression occurs, the patient may also require counterpulsation or surgery. The critical care nurse needs to prepare the patient and significant others for these interventions and also to provide teaching about diagnostic procedures such as cardiac catheterization or gated blood pool scans.

The prognosis of unstable angina has improved. This improvement can be attributed to advances in drug therapy, modification of risk factors, and more aggressive treatment modalities such as counterpulsation and PTCA. As additional information regarding the pathogenesis of atherosclerosis in CAD is elucidated, secondary prevention measures may also improve this prognosis.

MYOCARDIAL INFARCTION

As a serious complication of coronary artery disease, myocardial infarction (MI) remains the leading cause of death in the United States. The development of an MI is a manifestation of a serious interruption in blood supply to a segment of myocardium over time. As previously discussed, the supply is often fixed because atherosclerotic plaques partially occlude the lumen. It appears that an acute disruptive incident within an atherosclerotic coronary segment leads to sudden cessation of blood supply. This abrupt cessation of blood flow results in diminished or absence of oxygen supply to the heart resulting in ischemia, injury, and necrosis to the area of the myocardium supplied by that particular artery. The time course for damage to occur seems to be an interval ranging from minutes to 4 to 6 hours.[98,99]

Etiology

Myocardial infarction may be associated with any condition that produces prolonged, unrelieved ischemic episodes which cause irreversible damage and necrosis to myocardial cells. Unlike ischemic precordial chest pain (angina), which is caused by an imbalance between myocardial blood supply and demand, an MI is caused by total obstruction in blood supply to a region of myocardium and is largely unrelated to myocardial demand.[99] The majority of MI patients have underlying atherosclerosis; however, these lesions are not thought to be solely responsible for occluding the coronary vessel. Thrombosis has been implicated as the major precipitator of the abrupt interruption in blood supply. Coronary spasm and platelet aggregation have also been suggested as causative factors in the precipitation of an MI.

Thrombosis

It is evident from the recent literature that thrombus formation is a major factor in the etiology of an MI.[3,30,99,100] A thrombus that has been found to form over a previously narrowed atheroma (75% to 80% occluded) is usually the acute disruptive event that leads to total cessation of blood to the area of myocardium supplied by that atherosclerotic coronary artery. The precipitating events that incite thrombus formation appear to be plaque rupture, hemorrhage into the plaque, or erosion of the intima over the fibrous cap.[99] According to Factor and Kirk,[98] a number of studies have correlated coronary thrombosis with rupture or cracks of the thin fibrous cap and release of the plaque constituents into the coronary lumen. Plaque rupture may incite thrombus formation through one or a combination of mechanisms: (1) contact of platelets with denuded collagen, leading to thrombocyte adherence and the accumulation of a platelet plug; (2) release of tissue thromboplastin from the plaque contents, inciting the initiation of the clotting cascade; and (3) mechanical obstruction of the vascular lumen by the plaque components. Other sequelae associated with an arterial thrombus besides total occlusion of the lumen include distal embolization of microthrombi, promotion of growth of an atherosclerotic plaque, or complete endogenous lysis or dissolution of the clot. Obviously spontaneous lysis of the clot is the most desirable outcome.[101]

The incidence of thrombosis is thought to be 60% or greater as noted in postmortem investigations of subjects who had sudden cardiac death.[102] Because thrombus formation plays a major role in the evolution of an infarct, interventions have been aimed at dissolving clots. Such discoveries as thrombolytic agents are helping to unravel the mysteries regarding the etiology of MI.

Coronary Artery Spasm

Spasm of the coronary artery has been implicated as a cause of acute MI in patients with or without atherosclerosis. One speculation regarding vasospasm is that it may stimulate thrombus formation by damaging the coronary endothelium and inciting platelet aggregation and leukocyte infiltration.[103,104] In patients with underlying atherosclerosis, vasospasm has been documented following treatment of acute MI with streptokinase[105] and following PTCA.[106] Spasm following PTCA was noted at and distal to the site of balloon dilatation.[106]

Several mechanisms for vasospasm have been proposed. First, platelet aggregation appears to be associated with the release of certain vasoconstrictor substances such as thromboxane A and serotonin which in turn may cause vasospasm.[107] Second, atherosclerotic arteries have been found to have an abnormal vasodilator function perhaps attributable to a deficiency in the production or release of an endothelium-derived relaxing factor.[108] As an example, patients with early or advanced atherosclerosis receiving the vasodilator acetylcholine (intracoronary route) demonstrated vasoconstriction of the coronary arteries.[109] Because of these possible mechanisms, attention is being paid to developing pharmacological agents that can either inhibit the release of thromboxane A and serotonin or induce more production of the relaxing factor.

Platelet Aggregation

Blood flow turbulence at the site of a stenotic area creates a favorable milieu for platelet adhesion and aggregation. Platelet aggregation follows myocardial tissue injury because platelets migrate to the site of injury and envelop the damaged surface. Moreover, these platelets are thought to release serotonin, adenosine diphosphate (ADP), catecholamines, and PDGF into the plasma. In turn, additional platelets adhere and aggregate at the site of vessel injury. The platelet aggregation can further impede blood flow at the area of stenosis, resulting in prolonged ischemic episodes and tissue necrosis.

Pathophysiology

Myocardial infarction usually develops distal to a totally occluded coronary artery. The amount of cells that become necrotic is determined by the amount of blood that is able to flow into the ischemic zone after the abrupt occlusion and by the time it takes for flow to be resumed, if at all. Flow can be reestablished into the affected region, either retrograde via collateral vessels from distant coronary beds, or antegrade through clot lysis, or by retraction of a wall that has been in spasm.[99]

There is a sequential transmural pattern by which the jeopardized myocardium undergoes a wavefront of necrosis. This wavefront theory of necrosis highlights two facts.[110,111] First, myocardial damage is progressive, and second, it is time dependent. Progression occurs in such a way that necrosis begins in the subendocardium and extends toward the epicardium. If blood flow ceases for more than 30 to 40 minutes, there is a strong probability that the myocardium may be irreversibly injured.[30] In the epicardial layers, tissue salvage is relative to the restoration of blood flow to this region or the presence of sufficient collateral circulation to this area to prevent tissue necrosis.[98]

The time for prolonged, unrelieved ischemic episodes to cause cellular death is thought to range from 25 minutes to several hours (3 to 6 hours).[3,30,98,100] Cellular death is also dependent on the following factors: (1) the rate of development of the obstruction; (2) the coronary artery that is occluded; (3) the quantity of myocardium supplied by that artery; (4) the quantity of collateral flow available to the ischemic cells; and (5) the presence site, and severity of any coronary artery spasm.[99,100]

Three types of irreversible cell injury can be identified histologically. These include coagulation necrosis, contraction band necrosis, and myocytolysis.[99] *Coagulation necrosis* occurs when the blood supply to that region is permanently impeded. The cells in this region are rendered functionally and electrically silent. The tissue becomes pale or white because the area is devoid of blood. Within 6 to 12 hours, the necrotic cells thin and stretch out. Over the course of several weeks, the necrotic cells are replaced by newly formed granulation tissue, and within a year the affected area becomes a dense collagen scar.

Contraction band necrosis results from a period of prolonged ischemia followed by reperfusion of the area.[99] Thus, this type of necrosis occurs when myocardial blood flow is temporarily interrupted. The tissue typically appears as a red infarct which depicts the restoration of blood to the necrotic region. This reperfusion may cause some frank hemorrhage into the extracellular spaces. Patients in whom contraction band necrosis has been noted are those with spasm, those with nontransmural MIs, those who have died after cardiac surgery, or those who have had cardiopulmonary bypass which temporarily interrupted flow to the heart. Moreover, this type of necrosis may become the most prevalent form seen in acute MI patients given the current emphasis on reperfusion.

The third type of necrosis is *myocytolysis*, which is predominantly found on the border of infarcts or in the subendocardium.[99] Subcellular damage occurs with this type of ischemic cell injury along with a balloonlike degenerative appearance of these cells. Some of these cells have been found to survive for a time, although the ultimate fate of these damaged cells needs to be elucidated. When any of these cells die, they are replaced by scar tissue.

Intracellular Alterations

Myocardial cells normally utilize glucose (postprandial state) and free fatty acids (unfed state) as an energy source to form adenosine triphosphate (ATP) during aerobic metabolism. With ischemia, there is a decrease in oxygenated blood supply to these cells, and they revert to anaerobic metabolism. Through the process of glycolysis (which requires a supply of glycogen) glucose becomes the main fuel source in anaerobic metabolism. The formation of ATP is severely reduced by anaerobic metabolism: anaerobic metabolism supplies less than half the energy requirements of the cell.[100] In addition, lactic acid is produced by anaerobic metabolism, causing the intracellular pH to lower, resulting in acidosis. Acidosis, in turn, can inhibit the phosphorylation of glycogen to glucose, further reducing the production of ATP as well as depression contractility.[100]

As a result of anaerobic metabolism, ischemic tissue is able to meet a significantly smaller proportion of its energy requirements. Therefore, when the demand exceeds the supply, the limited high-energy phosphate stores of ATP are depleted rapidly, and irreversible injury develops in the ischemic tissue. The injured cell membranes lose their functional integrity and leak their cytoplasmic contents into the circulation, releasing enzymes such as lactic dehydrogenase (LDH), creatine kinase (CK), and serum glutamic oxaloacetic transaminase (SGOT), which can be clinically measured.

Classification

In the past infarcts were categorized as transmural or nontransmural according to the extent of the ventricular wall that was affected. The nontransmural category included subendocardial, subepicardial, or intramural infarcts. The presence or absence of a Q wave on the ECG was the criterion used to distinguish a transmural from a nontransmural infarct. Recent evidence has highlighted the limitation of this classification system. Postmortem examinations have revealed transmural infarcts in subjects who had had no Q waves or ECG, and nontransmural infarcts in subjects whose ECGs had displayed Q waves. Therefore, it is now advocated that MIs be classified according to what is actually depicted on the ECG, that is, as a Q-wave or non-Q-wave infarct.[30,112]

Q-wave infarcts are chiefly a result of an occlusive coronary thrombus superimposed at the site of a severe stenotic segment (plaque) of a coronary artery.[112] As previously mentioned, such occlusive thrombi are thought to be caused by endothelial injury to the atherosclerotic plaques. In comparison, many non-Q-wave infarcts are associated with multivessel stenosis and a transient reduction in coronary blood flow that is not severe and is probably unrelated to thrombus formation. The thrombus may have been spontaneously lysed. Interestingly, more patients are being diagnosed with non-Q-wave than Q-wave infarcts, perhaps because of the widespread use of creatine kinase MB fraction assays in patients with ECG changes.[30] These patients tend to have smaller infarcts and reduced in-hospital mortality compared to patients with Q-wave infarcts. However, the patients with non-Q-wave infarcts appear to be at increased risk for early reinfarction, postinfarction angina, and death owing to the high likelihood of recurrent ischemia.[30,112]

The ECG criteria for a non-Q-wave infarct are prominent T waves and/or hyperacute ST segment elevations in the leads facing the injury. These ECG changes manifest within a few minutes to hours or days, eventually evolving into a pattern of Q waves and T wave inversions. In contract, a non-Q-wave infarct depicts T wave inversions and/or ST segment depressions of varying degrees on the ECG. These changes revert to normal in the hours to days after myocardial injury.

Treatment for these different cohorts of patients differs. For example, the patients with Q-wave infarct probably should receive thrombolytic therapy if there are no contraindications. Conversely, patients with non-Q-wave infarcts are usually treated with platelet-active agents (aspirin and in some cases heparin), nitrates, and calcium channel blockers to enhance coronary blood flow.[112]

Location

The size and location of an infarct is dependent on several variables. These variables include (1) the site and degree of occlusion of the coronary artery, (2) the occurrence and intensity of coronary artery spasm near the occluded vessel, (3) the extent of the tissue supplied by that vessel, (4) development and extent of collateral blood vessels distal to the occluded vessel, and (5) O_2 requirements of the poorly perfused myocardium.[100]

To comprehend the locations of infarcts, the critical care nurse must know which coronary artery supplies each area of the myocardium. As a review, the coronary arteries are classified as (1) the left main coronary artery, which extends about 5 cm from the left coronary ostium and subdivides into the left anterior descending (LAD) and left circumflex (LCX) artery; and (2) the right coronary artery (RCA). The coronary arteries and the area each supplies are listed in Table 22-4.

Most infarcts occur in the left ventricle and interventricular septum. However, approximately one third of patients with inferior infarcts sustain some damage to the right ventricle. Right ventricular infarcts are thought to occur in the setting of a transmural infarction of either the inferior-posterior wall or the posterior wall of the septum. Atrial infarcts have also been reported. These atrial infarcts tend to be manifested more on the right than on the left side, and in atrial appendages rather than in the lateral or posterior walls.[100] Patients with atrial infarcts frequently exhibit atrial dysrhythmias due to obstruction of the sinus node artery.[100]

The majority of anterior wall infarcts are caused by occlusion of the LAD. Other areas which may be affected by occlusions in the LAD are portions of the septum, anterolateral wall, papillary muscle, and inferioapical wall of the LV. Anterior infarcts tend to be larger than inferior infarcts and generally tend to have a greater degree of LV impairment in contrast to inferior infarcts. Anterior infarcts also tend to have a worse prognosis for patients than inferior infarcts,

TABLE 22-4 **Summary of the Coronary Arteries and the Major Areas and Structures Supplied**

Coronary Artery	Major Areas and Structures Supplied
Right coronary	1. SA node (55%) 2. AV node (90%) 3. Bundle of His 4. Right atrium and right ventricle 5. Inferior/diaphragmatic surface of left ventricle 6. Posterior third of septum 7. Posterior/inferior division of left bundle
Left main	1. Massive LV area
Left anterior descending	1. Anterior wall of left ventricle 2. Anterior two thirds of septum 3. Bundle of His 4. Right bundle branch 5. Anterior/superior division of the left bundle branch 6. Posterior/inferior division of the left bundle branch 7. Apex of LV
Left circumflex	1. SA node (45%) 2. AV node (10%) 3. Inferior/diaphragmatic surface of left ventricle 4. Lateral wall of left ventricle 5. Left atrium 6. Posterior/inferior division of the left bundle branch

probably because of the greater extent of LV injury.[113]

Lateral or inferolateral wall infarcts of the LV can be attributed to occlusion in the left circumflex artery (LCX). Occlusions of the RCA can cause inferior, inferoposterior, as well as right ventricular (RV) infarcts.

True posterior infarcts usually result from occlusion in the LCX artery. These types of infarcts are somewhat more difficult to diagnose because there are no specific leads that directly face the injured area. Clinicians therefore look for reciprocal changes in leads V_1 and V_2 on the ECG. However, Bar et al.[114] noted that a Q wave in V_6 is an excellent marker for posterior asynergy and is a useful criterion for the presence of a true posterior MI when concomitant Q waves are noted in inferior leads on the ECG.

Data Acquisition

History

The majority of patients (70% to 80%) admitted after an acute myocardial infarction present with chest pain.[30] The remaining 29% to 30% of acute MIs may be silent and only detected by ECG.[30] The pain is typically more severe than angina, is prolonged (usually >15 to 20 minutes), and most often, is unrelieved by nitroglycerin. When describing the pain, some patients report radiation or localization to the neck, jaw, back, shoulder, substernal region, left arm, or near the epigastric area, which may cause patients to think that they have indigestion and to treat themselves with antacids. Patients may be clutching their chest and sitting forward and may appear diaphoretic, pale, and restless, along with being nauseated, and some may vomit. Gastrointestinal symptoms such as nausea, vomiting, and hiccoughing are often associated with a vagal reflex.

Physical Examination

On physical examination, the overall cardiovascular status is evaluated. Patients generally look acutely ill, are in severe discomfort, and display facial grimaces indicative of pain. Their skin color may be either normal or a gray, ashen appearance, and the skin may be moist, warm, or cool.

Vital signs are affected by the autonomic nervous system. Excessive sympathetic stimulation as a compensatory mechanism can be seen in 40% of patients with an acute anterior infarction and in 25% of patients with an inferior infarction.[115,116] Under these circumstances, the blood pressure is elevated and the heart rate may be rapid and irregular due to premature ventricular contractions (PVCs). Sympathetic overactivity may be attributed to either pain or anxiety or to the stimulation of cardiac chemoreceptors by substances emitted from acutely ischemic or infarcted cells.[116]

Parasympathetic overactivity, the result of activation of the vagal reflex, has been reported in 30% of patients with anterior infarcts and 65% of those experiencing an inferior infarct. This vagal reflex is often referred to as the Bezold-Javisch reflex.[116] The resultant bradycardia exhibited by these patients is often associated with concomitant hypotension. The hypotension is reversible when atropine and fluids are administered.

The respiratory rate is usually elevated immediately after an MI as a sequela of the pain and anxiety. The respiratory rate should return to normal once the pain and psychological stress are decreased, unless the patient develops ventricular failure.

An elevation in body temperature may occur 24 to 48 hours postinfarction as a result of tissue necrosis. Acute pericarditis can also cause an elevation in body temperature 2 to 3 days following an MI.

Heart sounds are often muffled because of the reduced left ventricular contractility, but they are more distinctive as healing occurs. The presence of an S_4 sound is considered to be a common sign in patients with ischemic heart disease. This sound is best heard between the left sternal border and apex.[100] A fourth heart sound may be an indication of a decrease in LV compliance and reflect elevations in LVEDP. With RV infarcts, an S_4 is best heard at the left sternal border.

Patients with extensive infarctions may also have an S_3 sound, which reflects severe LV dysfunction, decreased LV compliance, and LV dilatation. An S_3 sound is a common finding with Q-wave infarcts, in contrast with non-Q-wave infarcts. It is best heard at the apex with a patient in the left lateral decubitus position. It has been reported that mortality is higher in patients with a documented S_3 sound in the immediate postinfarct phase than in patients without this sound.[100] In the presence of papillary muscle dysfunction, there may also be systolic murmurs resulting from acute mitral regurgitation. A pericardial friction rub may also be auscultated in the setting of an acute MI in approximately 20% of patients.[100]

Breath sounds need to be auscultated for baseline purposes as soon as possible after admission to a critical care unit. Moist bibasilar crackles may be found in patients who subsequently develop left ventricular failure postinfarction.

In patients who exhibit RV infarcts, the jugular veins are distended. The jugular venous pressure is also elevated in cardiogenic shock and reduced in the presence of hypotension or hypoperfusion. Palpation of the carotid pulse indicates the status of the LV stroke volume. For example, a small, weak pulse is indicative of reduced stroke volume, while a sharp, brief upstroke is often felt in patients with mitral regurgitation, or a ruptured interventricular septum when there is a left-to-right shunt.[100]

Diagnostic Procedures

In addition to a history suggestive of MI, other data required to make the diagnosis include ECG abnormalities suggestive of ischemia, injury and necrosis, and serial enzyme assays. Discussion in this section centers on these data as well as information obtained from such procedures as echocardiography, radionuclide studies, and cardiac catheterization.

ECG. As previously discussed, infarcts are now classified as Q-wave or non-Q-wave infarctions. The pathological changes seen in the majority of patients who sustain a Q-wave infarct include development of abnormal, persistent Q waves; elevation of the ST segment; and symmetrical inversion of the T wave. Ischemia produces ST segment depression as well as T wave inversion. Injury is depicted as ST segment elevation and T wave inversion. Infarction is noted with the appearance of pathological Q waves which

either exceed 0.04 second (1 mm) wide or are 25% (one fourth), or one third the height of the R wave in leads facing the infarcted area. These changes are often referred to as indicative changes.

The sequence of events of an MI as noted on the ECG begins with the hyperacute phase in which the ST segment and T waves are elevated in those leads facing the injured area. The T waves invert after several hours or days, and pathological Q waves eventually appear. As the infarct resolves, the ST segments revert to the baseline, and eventually the T waves return to normal. The pathological Q waves persist for months to years.

Reciprocal changes or mirror images of the ECG disturbances noted in the leads facing the injured areas appear in those leads opposite to the site of injury. Notably, there are ST depressions. Many patients with inferior wall infarctions who demonstrate ST depression in V_1 to V_4 leads have been shown to have extensive global and regional wall dysfunction and are at high risk for further complications of ischemic heart diease.[115] Table 22-5 lists the sites of an MI and the leads associated with indicative and reciprocal changes.

Non-Q-wave infarcts are treated aggressively because data suggest a mortality comparable to that of Q-waves infarcts.

The ECG changes that occur with non-Q-wave infarcts may be associated initially with ST segment depression and T wave inversions. However, many etiologies (tachycardia, electrolyte disturbance, pericarditis) may demonstrate these same ECG changes. Thus, ECG changes in patients with a non-Q-wave infarct are typically nonspecific. Willerson and Buja[112] caution that the ECG cannot distinguish transmural from nontransmural damage with certainty. They

TABLE 22-5 Sites of an MI and Leads Associated with Indicative and Reciprocal Changes

Type of Infarct	Leads with Indicative Changes	Leads with Reciprocal Changes
Inferior	2, 3, aVF	I, aVL and right and midprecordial chest leads V_1-V_4
Extensive anterior	I, aVL, V_1-V_6	2, 3, aVF, aVR
Anteroseptal	V_1-V_4	
Anterolateral	I, aVL, V_3-V_6	
High anterolateral	I, aVL	
Lateral	I, aVL, V_5-V_6	2, 3, aVF
True posterior	V_6 (Bar et al.)	V_1-V_2

conclude that transmural infarct patients present with Q-wave infarcts and/or infarcts associated with greater than 50% R wave loss across the ECG leads reflecting the infarction. Conversely, nontransmural infarcts are demonstrated in patients without subsequent Q wave or R wave loss who also have ST segment depression and T wave inversions.

Cardiac Enzymes. Enzymes are released from necrotic myocardial cells and enter the circulation. The most important of these enzymes, creatine kinase (CK) and lactic dehydrogenase (LDH), are found to be elevated in an acute MI. Certain isoenzymes of CK and LDH are more specific for acute MI because these isoenzymes are located predominantly in myocardial tissue. The isoenzymes of CK specific for myocardial damage are the MB band of CK (CK-MB) which elevates 2 to 4 hours after an MI. The isoenzymes for LDH are LDH_1 and LDH_2, which are changed to a characteristic "flipped pattern."[117] Under normal circumstances, the value of LDH_2 exceeds that of LDH_1; however, in the setting of an MI, LDH_1 exceeds LDH_2.[117]

The current recommendation for sampling enzymes if an MI is suspected is to obtain a CK and its MB fraction on admission and again 12 to 24 hours later.[30] In the setting of reperfusion, sampling should be obtained at approximately 8 hours because of the "washout phenomenon" after reperfusion. Washout refers to enzymes being flushed into the circulation as blood flow is restored to the injured myocardium. A rapid rise in enzymes will occur with a peak of CK in 10 to 15 hours instead of the normal 12 to 24 hours.[118]

If the clinician suspects that an MI may have occurred 20 hours before, sampling of the LDH isoenzymes will increase the likelihood of diagnosis.[30] Refer to Chapter 21 for further discussion of enzymes.

Echocardiography. Echocardiography is often employed to estimate the extent of myocardial damage and to identify regional wall motion abnormalities associated with an MI. It can also be used to detect intracardiac thrombi following an infarct. If thrombi are discovered, anticoagulant therapy may be warranted. In addition, echocardiography is useful in detecting myocardial complications associated with an AMI.

In one study, serial 2-D echocardiograms were performed in 43 consecutive patients with documented MIs to predict the short-term clinical outcome.[119] The researchers concluded that an echocardiogram obtained on the day of admission could be used to accurately define the extent and severity of the acute MI and could be used to predict whether the short-term clinical course would be complicated.

Two-dimensional echocardiograms may also prove useful in differentiating new from old infarcts.[120] In addition, other useful data can be obtained by 2-D echocardiograms, such as the detection of small pericardial effusions in patients with postinfarction pericarditis, ventricular septal defects, and mitral regurgitation.[100]

Radionuclide Studies. Many advances in nuclear cardiology have substantially improved diagnostic capabilities to detect an acute MI. Common radionuclide tests used in detection of an MI, assessing infarct size and IV function, are the technetium-99m (^{99m}Tc) pyrophosphate (PYP) scan; thallium-201 myocardial perfusion scintigraphy; radionuclide ventriculography (RVG), also known as gated blood-pool scans; and positron emission tomography.

Thallium-201 and ^{99m}Tc PYP are both radioactive cell tracers that can be absorbed by either normal or abnormal myocardial cells. ^{99m}Tc PYP scans use hot spot imaging to detect myocardial infarction. In theory, technetium pyrophosphate binds to calcium in infarcted tissue; therefore, the accuracy of this test is dependent on the amount of calcium contained within necrotic tissue. It has been reported that the maximal sensitivity of this type of imaging is 24 to 72 hours after an MI because the calcium in necrotic tissue is eventually reabsorbed.[117] Newer isotopes that have been employed in humans include ^{99m}Tc-labeled antimyosin antibody, which has been proposed to detect regions of myocardial necrosis, and indium III, which is used to image platelets at sites of cardiac thrombosis.[121]

Thallium-201 utilizes thallous chloride, which is chemically similar to potassium, as its isotope. This type of imaging is referred to as "cold spot imaging" in that infarcted tissue does not absorb this isotope and shows up as a blank or cold spot image. Thallium scans can be used in the evaluation of acute as well as old infarcts; however, there appear to be some doubts about the accuracy of these scans. Newer techniques, such as thallium-201 tomography and rubidium-82 positron-emitted tomography, may be useful for the localization of infarcts. In addition, magnetic resonance imaging (MRI) continues to be investigated and may play an important role in cardiovascular diagnosis in the future.

Gated blood-pool scans, or RVGs, are used to assess cardiac function (ejection fraction) and to analyze wall motion abnormalities in infarcted areas by which aneurysms may be detected. Radionuclide ejection fractions tend to be lower in patients with anterior infarctions in contrast to inferior infarctions.[121] Gated blood-pool scans are not used to specifically localize infarcts.

Positron emission tomography (PET) evaluates the extent of an MI by assessing myocardial blood flow and cellular metabolism.[121] This noninvasive technique allows measurements of local myocardial tissue concentrations of certain radioactive isotope tracers. Two tracers, F-2-fluoro-2-deoxyglucose (FDG) and N-13 ammonia, have been employed to identify and differentiate between myocardial ischemia and infarction in humans.[122] The FDG tracer is a glucose compound that measures glucose uptake in ischemic tissue. Glucose utilization increased in ischemic cells because these cells are incapable of normally metabolizing free fatty acids (FFAs) when becoming ischemic and revert to anaerobic glucose metabolism. The N-13 ammonia isotope tracer measures the degree of flow (perfusion) to myocardial tissue. Thus, areas that have necrotic tissue will not depict any uptake of the N-13 ammonia tracer.

When both tracers were used, the extent of the infarct as well as the degree of ischemic tissue could be noted.[122] It was found that neither FDG nor N-13 ammonia uptake occurred in necrotic tissue. This is regarded as a match or concordance between FDG and N-13 ammonia. On the other hand, it was found that in ischemic regions, there was an increase in the uptake of FDG but virtually no uptake of N-13 ammonia. This mismatch between the two tracers shows a discordant increase in FDG activity relative to N-13 ammonia which is found to be consistent with the increased extraction of glucose in ischemic myocardium.

Positron emission tomography has considerable diagnostic potential not only for detecting infarctions but ischemic regions as well. Further evaluation will be necessary to perfect this technique. Its application to other cardiovascular disorders such as cardiomyopathy may be enormous as well. Refer to Chapter 21 for more in-depth discussion of radionuclide studies.

Cardiac Catheterization and Angiography. Data from cardiac catheterization following an acute LV infarction may reveal elevations in the LVEDP and LVEDV, as well as elevations in LVESP and LVESV. In addition, there is a reduction in the ejection fraction after an MI. Left ventriculography may reveal wall motion abnormalities, referred to as patterns of dysnergy or asynergy, as previously described. Figure 22-4 depicts these abnormalities. Under normal conditions, the LV cavity resembles an ellipsoid during diastole. During systole, the walls move inward such that at the peak of systolic ejection the LV outline resembles an ice cream cone or a pear. Hypokinesis is depicted as generalized reduction in wall motion, whereas akinesis is revealed as a segment in which there is no wall motion. Dyskinesis is the paradoxical bulging of a segment during systole. This paradoxical bulging occurs in patients soon after sustaining an MI

TABLE 22-6 Correlation between the Extent of Dyskinetic Segment and Clinical Manifestations

Dyssynergy	Clinical Manifestations
1. Abnormal segment → 11% of the left ventricle	LVEDP rises above 12 mmHg
2. Abnormal segment → 14%	Decreased ejection fraction
3. Abnormal segment → 30%	Clinical evidence of LV failure
4. Abnormal segment → 40% to 50%	Clinical evidence of cardiogenic shock

From Donat, W. E., & Weiner, B. H. (1985). Syndromes of left ventricular failure. In J. M. Rippe, R. S. Irwin, J. S. Alpert, et al. (Eds.), *Intensive care medicine.* Boston: Little, Brown.

(most often anterior infarcts) due to an initial increase in segmental LV compliance.[123] This wall motion abnormality leads to decreased stroke volume and a decrease in overall ejection fraction. Left ventricular compliance decreases in time as the infarct evolves, which, in turn, may led to less dyskinesis and improvement in the ejection fraction. Correlations between the extent of the dyskinetic segment and clinical manifestations have also been noted.[123] These are found in Table 22-6.

Data from right and left heart catheterization in right ventricular infarctions usually reveal higher pressures on the right side than on the left. An increase in right atrial pressure and right ventricular end-diastolic pressure on inspiration is common. The pulse pressures in the right ventricle and pulmonary artery also may be decreased.[124]

Medical Management

Pepine suggests classifying MI phases according to timing to facilitate appropriate therapeutic interventions.[30] This classification includes:

Evolving infarction: presentation in the initial hours of infarction up to 6 hours after the onset of symptoms; these patients have reversible and nonreversible ischemic injury.

Completed infarction: the period from approximately 6 hours after the onset of symptoms until hospital discharge when little or no reversible injury is present.

Convalescent phase: the period from after discharge until approximately 8 to 12 weeks during which the infarcted segment heals and the risk of complications subsides. During this period, the patient attempts to return to previous activities of daily living.

Objectives in Management of Acute Myocardial Infarction

Evolving Infarction Phase (onset to 6 hours)
1. Admit to CCU
2. Confirm diagnosis
3. Assess risks and benefits of thrombolytic therapy
4. Attempt to preserve ischemic myocardium

Completed Infarction Phase (>6 hours to just before discharge)
1. Prevent complications
2. Identify patients who are at early high risk
3. Initiate secondary prevention

Convalescent Infarction Phase (predischarge evaluation to 8 weeks)
1. Assess risk
2. Begin rehabilitation
3. Continue secondary prevention

Adapted from Pepine, C. J. (1989). New concepts in the pathophysiology of acute myocardial ischemia and infarction and their relevance to contemporary management. *Cardiovascular Clinics, 20,* 3-18.

The objectives of managing patients with an acute MI are summarized according to this classification in the box above.[30]

Evolving Phase

In the evolving phase of an AMI, the first objective is to admit a patient to an emergency room, then to a coronary care unit or designated critical care unit for continuous ECG monitoring. Critical care nurses in all these areas must have demonstrated competency in the immediate recognition and treatment of life-threatening dysrhythmias. Most of the deaths that occur within the first 2 hours after an AMI are related to dysrhythmias. The patient is also at significant risk for dysrhythmias after reperfusion therapy and for the following 24 hours after an AMI.

Some centers use lidocaine routinely; however, the prophylactic use of lidocaine in patients suspected of having an AMI is controversial. Several conflicting studies existed prior to the meta-analysis by McMahon et al.,[125] who pooled data from 14 randomized trials of approximately 9,000 patients. They concluded that in patients treated with lidocaine, there was a 33% decrease in the incidence of ventricular fibrillation as compared with those not receiving prophylactic lidocaine. Conti[126] suggests the use of prophylactic lidocaine only in two subsets of patients: those receiving thrombolytic therapy and those in whom early balloon angioplasty is indicated. The use of lidocaine in both of these situations is to prevent the reperfusion dysrhythmias associated with the interventions. Moreover, lidocaine use in patients re-

ceiving a beta blocker may be unnecessary because beta-adrenergic blocking agents decrease the incidence of ventricular fibrillation.[126,127]

The second objective is to confirm the diagnosis with presenting symptoms and an electrocardiogram. Blood samples for creatine kinase isoenzymes assays are collected at this time. Relief of chest pain is another priority in the evolving phase to decrease the myocardial oxygen demand associated with the pain. Small doses of morphine sulphate (4 to 8 mg) are usually given at 10-minute intervals. Patients with hypersensitivity to morphine can be treated with meperidine (25 to 50 mg) at 10-minute intervals. Persistent or recurrent chest pain unrelieved by morphine sulfate can be treated with continuous IV nitroglycerin (NTG) which allows for a constant controlled blood level. Although there is no reported optimal dosage of NTG, it is recommended that the IV rate be titrated between 10 to 20 mg/min with an endpoint of pain relief but short of causing symptomatic hypotension or headache.

During diagnosis of an AMI, health care personnel should assess the appropriateness of early reperfusion therapy, ideally in the emergency room. This decision is critical because of the window of time (4 to 6 hours) to salvage viable myocardium. Thrombolytic therapy has become the mainstay of treatment to reperfuse the infarcted area and to limit the infarct size. Thrombolytic therapy involves use of thrombolytic agents to dissolve coronary artery thrombi.

Currently used thrombolytic agents include two of the three generations listed in the box below.[128] Of the first-generation agents, streptokinase and urokinase, *streptokinase* is the more widely studied (Figure 22-18). It is a synthetic protein derived from the *Streptococcus* organism. One of its side effects is the po-

Three Generations of Thrombolytic Agents

First Generation
 Streptokinase
 Urokinase
Second Generation
 TPA
 APSAC
 Prourokinase (SCUPA)
Third Generation
 Synergistic combinations (e.g., TPA and SCUPA)
 Hybrids
 Chimerics
 Fibrin-antibody conjugated SCUPA, TPA

From Topol, E. J. (1990). Thrombolytic intervention. In E. J. Topol (Ed.), *Textbook of interventional cardiology.* Philadelphia: Saunders.

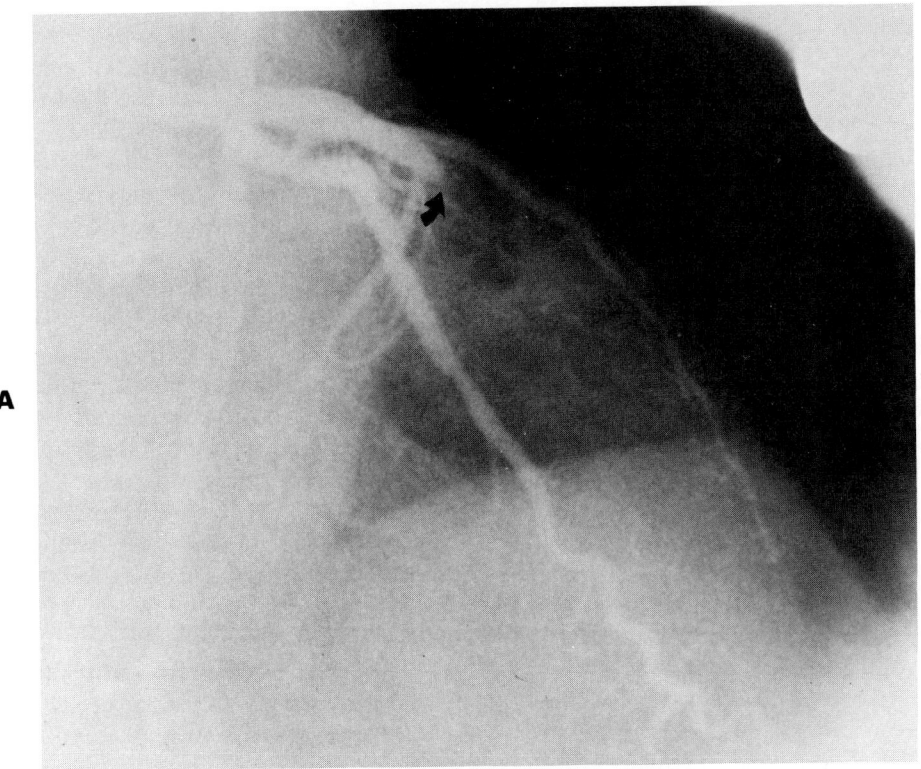

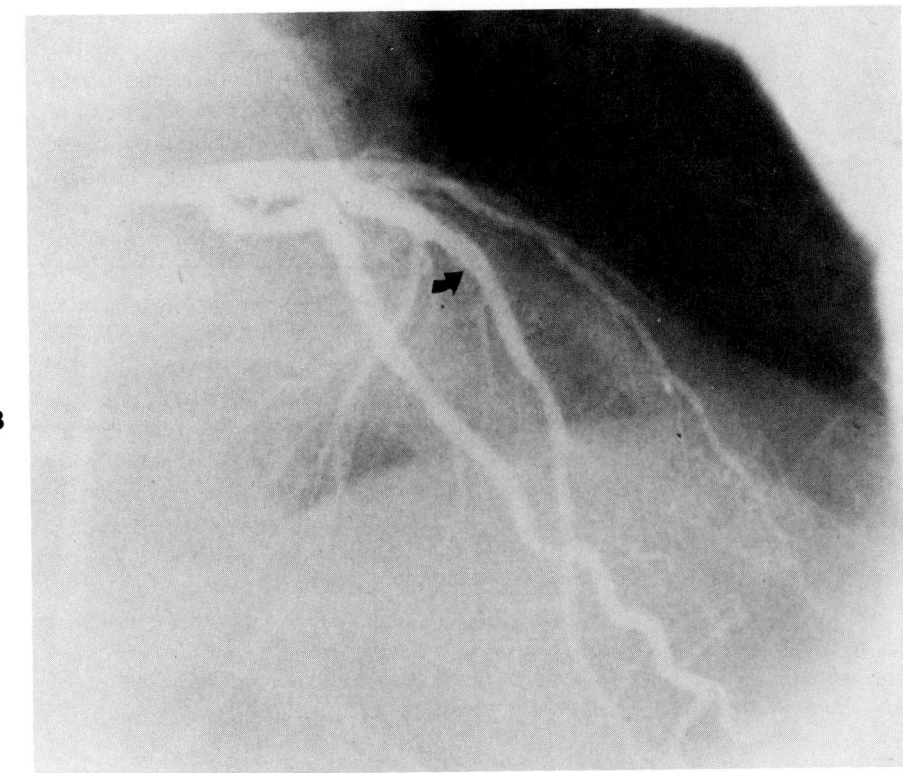

Figure 22-18   *A,* Arteriogram of a patient which depicts abrupt cessation of flow (arrow) in the LAD of a patient who presented with an anterior MI. *B,* The same patient received intracoronary streptokinase and had reestablished flow (arrow) to the affected myocardium.

tential for an allergic reaction. Although anaphylactic shock is possible, it is rare. Usual symptoms associated with administration of streptokinase are fever, flushing, and rash. Sudden hypotension, another side effect associated with streptokinase, necessitates the use of vasopressor agents. Use of streptokinase within 6 months preceding admission precludes its administration because high antibody titers have been found in patients who have received the drug.[30] Streptokinase is classified as a non-clot-specific agent, which means that this drug activates circulating non-clot-bound plasminogen to form complexes that activate plasmin formation, thus creating a systemic lytic state. This systemic lysis predisposes patients to increased bleeding complications.

Urokinase is a naturally occurring proteolytic enzyme isolated from human urine. Its mechanism of action is similar to streptokinase is that it is a non-clot-specific agent yielding a systemic lytic state. Side effects associated with its administration include fever and bleeding. It also costs 10 times as much as streptokinase for the same treatment dose.

The second generation of thrombolytic agents includes tissue plasminogen activator (TPA), anisoylated plasminogen streptokinase (APSAC), and single-chain urokinase plasminogen activator (SCUPA). Of these agents, TPA is the most extensively studied agent to date.

TPA is an endogenous enzyme produced by human vascular endothelial cells. It has a marked affinity for the plasminogen-fibrin complex. It is a clot-specific agent, which means it activates plasminogen only at the site of a clot. Therefore, TPA does not produce a systemic lytic state like streptokinase and urokinase. The advantages of TPA are its clot specificity, its short half-life of 3 to 5 minutes, and its failure to produce allergic reactions. The disadvantages of TPA is its relatively high cost in comparison to streptokinase.

APSAC is the acyl derivative of streptokinase. It is generally considered to be a non-clot-specific agent similar to streptokinase and urokinase. A major advantage is that it can be administered in bolus form.[128,129] Its much longer half-life (compared to streptokinase) provides more effective clot dissolution.[128,129]

SCUPA is a naturally occurring enzyme that is converted to urokinase in the presence of fibrin. It is thought to be (fibrin) clot-specific.[128] SCUPA has a short half-life and is metabolized by the liver.

In comparative reperfusion and patency studies, the clot-specific agents (TPA and SCUPA) have shown a faster patency rate (velocity of reperfusion 71% to 76%) with approximately 75% patency established by 90 minutes of therapy in comparison to streptokinase (50%) and urokinase (64%).[128] By 24 hours

after therapy, the two classes of agents have nearly equivalent patency rates (85%), although streptokinase patency rates decrease to 25% when the drug is given later (5 to 7 hours).[128]

Other agents currently under investigation in the United States and abroad include the third generation of agents which are synergistic combinations of TPA and SCUPA, hybrids, chimerics, and fibrin-antibody conjugated forms of SCUPA and TPA.[130] These agents alone or in combination may provide for more rapid, prolonged and efficient thrombolysis. Results from ongoing clinical studies in the future may elucidate specific indications for the use of these agents.

The regimens recommended for administration of currently available agents depend on timing of the AMI. It is currently suggested that TPA be administered to patients if 3 hours or more have passed since the onset of symptoms. To reduce cost, streptokinase is given to patients presenting earlier than 3 hours.[131] Pepine[30] suggests that thrombolytic therapy should be considered for patients with acute anterior wall MI except those with a history of recent bleeding (6 weeks), peptic ulcer disease, stroke, or surgery, or those with coexisting pathological conditions such as cancer.

Administration of thrombolytic therapy has shifted from intracoronary to intravenous techniques. Settings where thrombolytic agents are employed are also shifting, from catheterization laboratories to emergency rooms, and, in some select cases, to ambulances. The goal of thrombolytic therapy is to salvage viable myocardium and limit infarct size by prompt administration. The most dramatic reductions in mortality and preservation of LV function occur when the drug is given very early, within 2 to 4 hours of presenting symptoms; in other words, "time is muscle." Several randomized trials have clearly demonstrated that thrombolytic therapy improves survival in selected patients and may reduce mortality in patients up to 1 year after an AMI.[128]

Several controversies surround thrombolytic therapy. Its use in elderly patients has been questioned because the propensity for bleeding with lytic therapy is higher in this group. Many early clinical trials excluded patients 75 years or older. More recent studies demonstrate a significant survival benefit in patients over age 60.[129] These findings substantiate the need for individual evaluation of candidates for thrombolytic therapy; taking functional and physiological status into account.

Earlier use of thrombolytic agents was limited to patients presenting with anterior wall infarcts. Evidence now supports the use of thrombolytic therapy in inferior wall infarctions, especially those associated with ST segment depression in ECG leads V_1 to V_4.[132]

Another controversy is whether to administer thrombolytic therapy in patients who present with chest pain of more than 6 hours' duration. Two studies have shown some reduction in mortality in patients receiving thrombolytic therapy after 6 hours.[129] Several ongoing trials are addressing the issue of potential benefits of late reperfusion. For now, it seems prudent that thrombolytic therapy not be routinely administered after 6 hours.[129]

The success of thrombolytic therapy as evidenced by vessel recanalization was previously evaluated by coronary arteriography because these agents were first employed by the intracoronary route. Since arteriography is not routinely obtained with IV administration, other clinical markers have been used as outcome criteria (Table 22-7). The clinical reliability of these markers is controversial. For example, relief of chest pain may result from narcotic administration and may not reflect reperfusion to ischemic myocardium. Return of ST segment elevations to normal may indicate relief of coronary vasospasm.

Thrombolytic therapy is now a major pharmacological measure in managing AMI. However, some patients are not candidates for such therapy or present in a late phase of AMI. Conventional therapy must be used for these patients.

Completed Phase

The completed phase of an AMI begins about 6 hours after the onset of symptoms and ends with the predischarge evaluation. During the first 24 to 48 hours of this phase patients may be restricted to bed rest with commode privileges. The perils of immobility must be weighed against the need to decrease oxygen demand. Controversy also surrounds the use of supplemental oxygen. Clinicians differ regarding the benefit of oxygen therapy in all uncomplicated MIs but concur that oxygen is indicated for patients who are hypoxic. Noninvasive O_2 saturation monitoring can help determine which patients could benefit from supplemental oxygen.

During the completed phase of an AMI, patients should be stratified to identify those at high risk. Pharmacological therapy with intravenous nitroglycerin, beta blockers, and perhaps calcium channel blockers may be used. Mechanical interventions may include coronary arteriography and subsequent PTCA or CABG surgery, especially in high-risk patients. Prevention of complications is the cornerstone of treatment during this phase. If congestive heart failure is imminent, measures such as diuretics and inotropic agents should be instituted.

Nitrates, especially intravenous nitroglycerin, may be useful in AMI to (1) reduce the incidence of coronary spasm which could further impede blood sup-

TABLE 22-7   Clinical Markers of Successful Coronary Thrombolysis

Marker	Etiology
Sudden and marked relief of chest pain	Relief of ischemia
Resolution of the ST segment injury pattern on the ECG	Reperfusion of myocardium
Early peak of CK-MB isoenzymes at 10-15 hours after event onset	Washout of enzymes from infarct area after restoration of blood flow
Reperfusion dysrhythmias	Washout and changes in extracellular electrolytes
Improvement in left ventricular wall motion (seen in radionuclide imaging)	Salvage of myocardial segments by reperfusion

From Eagan, J. S., Stewart, S. L., & Vitello-Cicciu, J. M. (1991). *Quick reference to cardiac critical care nursing.* In J. M. Vitello-Cicciu (Ed.), *Quick reference to critical care nursing series.* Gaithersburg, MD: Aspen.

ply, (2) improve coronary collateral blood flow, (3) dilate coronary arteries, (4) decrease myocardial oxygen demand,[30] (5) alleviate ischemic pain, and (6) treat pulmonary edema.[126] Nitroglycerin IV should be started at a low dose of $10\mu/min$ and increased every 2 to 5 minutes in increments of $10\mu g$, usually not to exceed 200 $\mu g/min$.[126] The end-point should be cessation of pain without symptomatic hypotension or severe headache.

Beta blockers may be used in AMI to decrease myocardial oxygen demand by modulating sympathetic discharge so as to reduce heart rate, blood pressure, and contractility. In numerous clinical studies, beta blockers given orally weeks after an AMI have been shown to be effective.[53,100,126] Use of beta blockers in the evolving phase of AMI has also been recently studied.[53,100] Conflicting results in reducing infarct size have been reported, and the use of beta blockers in the acute phase remains controversial. Metopolol has been approved by the FDA for IV use in MI and is recommended by some clinicians.[100,126] The drug is given intravenously at a dosage of 5 mg every 2 to 5 minutes to a total dose of 15 mg. Oral administration begins 6 to 8 hours later at 50 mg twice daily; dosage is increased to 100 mg twice daily if tolerated. Contraindications to the use of beta blockers include bronchospasm, significant bradycardia or hypotension, heart failure, or heart block. The critical care nurse needs to be aware of situations that necessitate stopping or withholding beta blockers:[100]

- Second- or third-degree AV block or lengthening of first-degree block >0.24 second
- Increasing rales (one third of the lung filled) or wheezes on auscultation
- Heart rate <50
- Blood pressure <90 mmHg systolic
- PAWP >20 to 24 mmHg

Calcium channel blockers may be used in AMI to reduce myocardial oxygen demand by lowering blood pressure and myocardial contractility. They also dilate coronary vessels, reduce the incidence of vasospasm, and protect ischemic cells from reperfusion injury. However, some trials have demonstrated no appreciable effect on mortality or reinfarction and have indicated that the prophylatic issue of calcium channel blockers in the acute phase is not likely to be beneficial and may even be detrimental in some high-risk patients.[133]

A modality used in limited settings during AMI is direct PTCA, which is a primary intervention without the preceding use of a thrombolytic agent. Its use is limited to institutions with skilled physicians and fully equipped catheterization laboratories, and therefore, it is not generally applicable at present. This may be unfortunate because excellent patency rates of 85% with a reduced incidence of recurrent ischemia have been reported with direct PTCA.[134] So far no randomized controlled studies demonstrated an improvement in patient survival with direct PTCA.[134]

PTCA following thrombolysis has been evaluated as either an immediate (18 hours to 7 days) or a delayed intervention. In three randomized trials (TAMI, European Cooperative Study Group, and Timi-IIA), mortality, bleeding complications, and the need for emergency bypass were higher in the immediate angioplasty group than in the deferred angioplasty group.[134] Considering these discouraging results, interest in immediate angioplasty following thrombolysis has waned. Delayed (48 hours) PTCA may reasonably be indicated for patients with specific conditions such as recurrent ischemia, postinfarction angina, or hemodynamic instability.[134] Moreover, Morris, Walter, and Hurst[135] recommend that immediate PTCA without prior use of thrombolytic agents be performed for patients already hospitalized, who could undergo angioplasty as quickly as the vessel would be opened with a lytic agent. The advantages are a higher rate of reperfusion, a reduced risk of bleeding, and less residual stenosis.

Coronary artery bypass surgery has been performed to reduce infarct size in patients in the evolving phase of an AMI. This therapy can be effective only if it is instituted within 4 to 6 hours. Logistically, this is generally impossible, and thus CABG will not gain widespread acceptance in the routine treatment of an AMI. However emergent, CABG surgery for

AMI is recommended in the following situations:[131]
- In-hospital patients with evolving AMI (within 3 hours of examination) who are developing cardiogenic shock and in whom previous reperfusion therapies have failed
- Patients with postinfarction angina and coronary anatomy unsuitable for PTCA, especially multivessel disease
- Coronary occlusion during or immediately following PTCA
- Cardiogenic shock dependent on intraortic balloon counterpulsation

Convalescent Infarction Phase

The convalescent phase includes the period just before hospital discharge and 8 to 12 weeks postinfarction. Risk should be assessed using criteria that include age; history of previous MI, heart failure, or ventricular dysrhythmias; LV function; and data from noninvasive studies.[30] Data from the risk assessment determine further treatments such as PTCA or CABG surgery. Rehabilitation regimens should be instituted during this phase. Lastly, secondary preventive measures such as the use of beta blockers or aspirin should be considered.

Most patients are treated with heparin or aspirin to minimize the risk of reocclusion.[100] To date, no studies have been conducted regarding the efficacy of heparin in relation to timing and proper dosages required in AMI. However, several large randomized studies have found that overall mortality and recurrent MI are significantly reduced in patients receiving intravenous or high-dose subcutaneous heparin.[136] In fact, Pepine advocates the use of IV heparin in patients without contraindications for anticoagulation,[30] such as patients who have developed large anterior infarcts, heart failure, enlarged hearts, or atrial fibrillation. Moreover, patients who exhibit mural thrombus on echocardiogram should receive several months of warfarin therapy.[131]

In light of findings suggesting residual thrombus may persist after thrombolytic therapy, it would seem prudent to administer anticoagulant therapy during convalescence. Chesebro et al.[101] recommend that a heparin bolus of 150 U/kg be given concomitantly with lytic agents followed by an infusion of 1,000 U per hour to maintain heparin levels. The heparin infusion should be adjusted 12 hours later to maintain the APTT at two to three times the control for 3 to 5 days.

The use of aspirin has been shown to increase vessel patency, reduce the incidence of recurrent MI, provide some benefit in preventing an AMI, and reduce mortality following an AMI.[133] The Secondary International Study of Infarct Size (ISIS-2) demonstrated a 40% reduction in mortality in patients receiving a combination of aspirin and streptokinase.[137] Aspirin at 80 mg/day combined with warfarin achieves maximal persistent lysis of any residual thrombosis.[101,126,133] In patients with no evidence of severe residual stenosis, aspirin (160 mg/day) alone may be as effective.[101]

Complications

Numerous complications are associated with MI. The critical care nurse is pivotal in assessing for these complications and in intervening to prevent further deterioration. An in-depth discussion is beyond the scope of this chapter, but significant complications will be highlighted.

Reocclusion

A recently noted complication of AMI is reocclusion of the affected vessel. The benefits of opening a closed artery have been clearly delineated from the standpoint of myocardial salvage. The use of thrombolytic therapy and PTCA have achieved reperfusion rates in more than 75% of patients presenting with an AMI. However, a reported 10% of patients experience reocclusion of the affected vessel.[101,128] Reocclusion may be caused by rethrombosis, which may be related to the thrombolytic agent used, the residual diameter (cross-sectional area) of the infarct-related artery at 90 minutes after thrombolytic therapy, and the adequacy of antithrombotic measures such as antiplatelet and anticoagulation therapy.[101] Residual thrombus that remains after either thrombolytic ther-

apy or PTCA is highly thrombogenic and has a strong affinity for platelet deposition.[101] If the vessel is partially occluded, symptoms of myocardial ischemia may prevail. If total occlusion occurs, the clinical picture of an evolving MI will be manifested.

The critical care nurse should assess the patient for signs of reocclusion; these are return of ischemic pain, elevated ST segments, and worsening of the hemodynamic status. If reocclusion is strongly suspected, thrombolytic agents may be readministered. TPA can be used for a second time, but streptokinase should not be readministered because of the danger of allergic reaction.[30] The incidence of bleeding is higher with a second course of thrombolytic treatment than with the first.

Mechanical interventions such as PTCA or CABG surgery also can be employed for reocclusion depending on the nature and presenting clinical picture of reocclusion.

Reperfusion Injury

Another complication associated with restoration of blood supply to infarcted myocardium is reperfusion injury (Figure 22-19). Reoxygenation of hypoxic cells may kill or damage them.[138,139,140] This phenomenon is referred to as the *oxygen paradox*.[141] This complication may occur with thrombolytic therapy, PTCA, or CABG.

Histologically, coronary reperfusion triggers a series of events that disturb the integrity of cell membranes, leading to additional necrosis, explosive

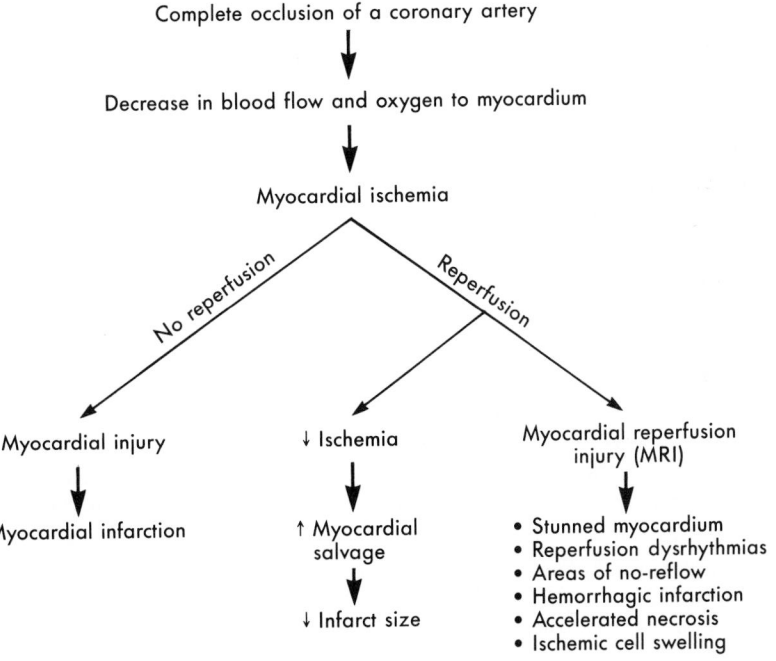

Figure 22-19   Evolution of an acute myocardial infarction.
From Misinski, M. (1990). Myocardial reperfusion injury. *Critical Care Nursing Clinics of North America,* 2(4), 652.

swelling of irreversibly injured myocytes, and ultimately to cell death.

The role of calcium in reperfusion injury is very controversial.[139,141] There is agreement that a dramatic influx of calcium into the cell occurs at the time of reperfusion, and that this seems to hasten cellular injury: the *calcium paradox*.[141] Whether this celluar calcium overload occurs as a primary or secondary event is not known.[142,143,144]

The "no-flow phenomenon" is another facet of reperfusion injury. It results from capillary shutdown produced by osmotically swollen cells. Histologically, the injured segment displays patchy blood flow[145] or none,[146] prolonging tissue ischemia thereby accelerating cell death.[145,147]

Lastly, *oxygen free radicals* (molecules that contain an odd number of electrons and are, therefore, unstable and highly reactive) appear to play a pivotal role in reperfusion injury.[138,139,140] When oxygen is reintroduced to hypoxic cells, a series of biochemical reactions occur. These reactions produce large quantities of the superoxide anion (O_2^-), which is a highly reactive oxygen metabolite that is very injurious to tissues. This superoxide anion in turn engages in chain reactions that produce more oxygen free radicals such as hydrogen peroxide (H_2O_2) and the hydroxyl radical (OH^-). Each of these metabolites can further damage cells and impair contractile function. As a defense mechanism against free radicals, cells normally contain certain protective enzymes called *oxygen free radical scavengers*. Two such enzymes are superoxide dismutase (SOD) and catalase. SOD metabolizes the superoxide anion and catalase metabolizes H_2O_2. These oxygen free radical scavengers are now being extensively investigated experimentally and clinically to determine their efficacy in decreasing reperfusion injury. Refer to references 138 to 140 for additional discussion of reperfusion injury.

Myocardial Stunning. The terms *stunned myocardium* or *postischemic ventricular dysfunction* define viable myocardium that has been reperfused yet exhibits prolonged but transient impaired contractile function, lasting hours to days.[138] The return of myocardial function is dependent on the duration and intensity of ischemia, the preexisting condition of the tissue at the onset of ischemia, and the quantity of collateral flow.[148] The exact mechanism causing stunning is not known but is thought to be multifactorial.[98,148] Inotropic agents have been used successfully in animal models to increase the force of contraction in stunned myocardium. Clinicians can assess for stunned myocardium in those patients whose LV function appears impaired. This assessment should ideally be done in the completed MI phase instead of in the immediate postinfarction period. If LV dysfunction is present, the judicious use of inotropes may improve myocardial function.[98,148] Lastly, clinicians should be aware that continued episodes of postischemic injury could prolong stunning.

Hibernating Myocardium. An ischemic myocardium (supplied by a narrow artery) in which cells remain viable but LV contraction is impaired is described as *hibernating myocardium*. The condition may persist for months to years without acute manifestations, probably because the reduction in blood flow or increase in oxygen demand is sufficiently gradual to allow for down-regulation, or a decrease of myocardial functioning ability to match oxygen supply.[149] Thus, a new equilibrium is established between myocardial oxygen supply and demand at a lower level that does not result in necrosis.[30] Clinically, hibernating myocardium can be detected by positron emission tomography.

Reperfusion Dysrhythmias. In animal models, dysrhythmias have been observed when blood flow was restored to reversibly injured tissue. Dysrhythmias associated with reperfusion include: ventricular fibrillation, ventricular tachycardia, bradydysrhythmia, and accelerated idioventricular rhythms. The exact physiological mechanism of these dysrhythmias has not been established but may be multifactorial.[138] Interestingly, the administration of oxygen free radical scavengers appears to reduce the incidence of reperfusion dysrhythmias, substantiating the theory that oxygen free radicals are implicated in causing such electrical disturbances.[150] These dysrhythmias are managed clinically as they would normally be treated.

Ventricular Irritability

The most frequent complication in the first 48 hours after an AMI is ventricular irritability. Investigators have attempted to profile the patient at risk for developing ventricular dysrhythmias. According to Wessman,[151] studies have revealed the following:

1. Older patients who experienced episodes of ventricular irritability had greater frequency and severity of episodes than younger patients.
2. Gender was not significant.
3. There was a greater likelihood of ventricular dysrhythmias following an acute MI in patients with diseases such as Parkinson's disease, peptic ulcer, diabetes, or pulmonary disorders.
4. The presence of congestive heart failure, hypertension, angina, or palpitations was associated with a greater likelihood of developing ventricular dysrhythmias.
5. Patients with transmural as opposed to subendocardial infarcts had a higher incidence of ventricular irritability.
6. Patients with anterior infarcts had an increased risk for ventricular dysrhythmias.

The critical care nurse must be able to identify MI patients at increased risk of life-threatening ventricular dysrhythmias in order to institute preventative measures. Refer to the previous discussion regarding lidocaine for additional information.

Approximately one third of patients with an MI develop sinus tachycardia.[135] The etiology of sinus tachycardia varies from patient to patient, but factors associated with its development include pain, anxiety, hypovolemia, vasoactive medications, LV failure, pericarditis and RV infarcts. Persistent sinus tachycardia may be an ominous sign of severe LV dysfunction.[135] It must be noted that sinus tachycardia increases MVO_2 consumption and also decreases diastolic filling time and coronary artery perfusion time. Thus, in the setting of an MI, sinus tachycardia should be treated directly or by removing the underlying cause.

Supraventricular dysrhythmias such as atrial flutter and fibrillation commonly occur in the post-MI patient. Atrial flutter occurs less frequently than atrial fibrillation in MIs. Atrial flutter is often associated with a 2:1 block and a rapid ventricular response. The critical care nurse needs to be aware that the rapid ventricular rate may intensify hemodynamic compromise to MI patients and that excessive rates which exceed 100 beats per minute need to be reported quickly so that therapy can be instituted promptly.[135] Drug therapy may be unsuccessful in treating the rapid ventricular rate; therefore, early cardioversion or overdrive atrial pacing is recommended for patients with atrial flutter.[135,152] Atrial fibrillation may be more amenable to treatment with such drugs as digitalis, verapamil, or quinidine.[152]

Vagotonia following an AMI may produce bradydysrhythmias. Sinus bradycardia is a frequent sequela of an inferior MI. This disturbance is usually not treated unless the patient manifests hemodynamic deterioration, in which case atropine may be administered as a vagolytic agent.

Ventricular conduction disturbances also may occur in the setting of an AMI. It is often the critical care nurse who must recognize these disturbances early to prevent deterioration to complete heart block.

Insertion of a temporary pacing wire is generally indicated after an MI for either prophylactic or therapeutic reasons. Those indications are found in the box below. Prior to insertion of a pacing wire, these patients may require pharmacological interventions such as atropine and isoproterenol for significant hemodynamic compromise.

Congestive Heart Failure. Prompt, continuous clinical assessment is necessary to the early recognition of congestive heart failure (CHF). The degree of LV failure is associated with the extent of the infarcted area as well as the degree of LV segmental contraction.[123] Clinical and hemodynamic criteria have been used to classify CHF[153] (Table 22-8). These criteria provide clinicians with a logical approach to therapy. For example, patients in subset II might require diuretic therapy, whereas patients in subset III

Indications for Temporary Pacing Following Acute Myocardial Infarction

A. Prophylactic (usually anterior MI)
   1. Transvenous pacing indicated; noninvasive transcutaneous pacer less desirable
      a. Usually anterior MI
      b. New RBBB and LAHB
      c. New RBBB and LPHB
      d. Alternating BBB
      e. Mobitz II 2° AVB
      f. Complete heart block
   2. Optional indication for transvenous pacing; noninvasive transcutaneous pacing indicated
      a. 1° AV block and old bilateral BBB
      b. 1° AVB and new BBB
B. Therapeutic (any MI)
   1. Medically refractory bradycardia with symptoms (CHF, chest pain, syncope)
   2. Heart rate <50 beats/min
   3. Atrial or AV sequential pacing for AV dissociated rhythms and hemodynamic compromise

Adapted from Love, J. C. (1991). Conduction disturbances following acute MI. In J. W. Rippe, R. S. Irwin, J. S. Alpert, et al. (Eds.), *Intensive care medicine* (2nd ed.). Boston: Little, Brown.

TABLE 22-8   **Correlative Classification of Clinical and Hemodynamic Criteria after an Acute MI**

Subset	Clinical Appearance	Hemodynamic Criteria	
I	No pulmonary congestion or peripheral hypotension	≤18 mgHg	>2.2 L/min/m²
II	Pulmonary congestion without peripheral hypotension	≥18 mmHg	>2.2 L/min/m²
III	Peripheral hypotension without pulmonary congestion	≤18 mmHg	<2.2 L/min/m²
IV	Pulmonary congestion and peripheral hypotension	≥18 mmHg	>2.2 L/min/m²

Adapted from Forrester, J. S., Diamond, G. A., & Swan, H. J. (1977). Correlative classification of clinical and hemodynamic function after acute MI. *American Journal of Cardiology, 39*, 137-145.

should benefit from additional volume. Common signs and symptoms of CHF are dyspnea, tachypnea, crackles, and an S_3 gallop. The chest x-ray usually reveals pulmonary congestion. In addition, elevations of hemodynamic parameters such as LVEDP, LAP, and PAW are often noted along with a decrease in the cardiac index. Arterial blood gases may reveal hypoxemia depending on the severity of the heart failure.

Patients with anterior MIs tend to have more severe failure in contrast with inferior infarcts because the extent of damage is usually greater with anterior lesions. In the acute setting, the goal of therapy for patients exhibiting LV failure is twofold: (1) to diminish blood volume and preload with the use of diuretics or nitroglycerin (NTG) and (2) to decrease afterload with intravenous vasodilators such as nitroprusside (Nipride). Oral vasodilators such as prazosin, captopril, and hydralazine, along with digitalis preparations, are used in the chronic phase of heart failure.

Cardiogenic Shock. The most serious form of acute congestive heart failure is cardiogenic shock (subset IV), which is the leading cause of in-hospital mortality in MI patients. Cardiogenic shock usually occurs in massive MIs in which 40% or more of the LV is damaged.[123] Hemodynamically, these patients manifest marked hypotension (systolic BP <80 mmHg), low cardiac index less that 1.8 L min/m², decreased urinary output, elevated heart rates, and concomitant high filling pressures (pulmonary artery wedge pressure that exceeds 18 mmHg). They also have pulmonary congestion and arterial hypoxemia. A vicious cycle ensues in which there is continued myocardial ischemia related to decreased cardiac output and coronary blood flow which, in turn, leads to further ischemia. Therapeutic interventions include the use of inotropic agents such as dopamine and dobutamine to increase contractility and the use of vasodilators such as Nipride or NTG to reduce impedance to LV ejection (afterload) and, thereby, to increase forward flow.

Dopamine is also used in cardiogenic shock for its ability to increase renal blood flow. However, dopamine can be deleterious because it increases MVo_2 consumption and has a tendency to induce dysrhythmias. Nipride or nitroglycerin as vasodilators reduce afterload and allow the LF to eject a larger stroke volume, thereby decreasing the LV end-diastolic pressure. These drugs also decrease MVo_2 consumption; however, Nipride, because of its arterial vasodilatory properties, may decrease coronary artery perfusion. Thus, the critical care nurse needs to be congnizant of these properties and possible complications that may result.

The intraaortic balloon pump, previously dis-

cussed on pp. 527 to 533, is also employed for MI patients. The use of the IABP in the setting of cardiogenic shock does not improve overall survival, and in fact many of these patients became "balloon dependent," with a few being successfully weaned from the device. The overall mortality from cardiogenic shock due to extensive myocardial damage remains high, in the 80% to 90% range, despite aggressive interventions. However, there are certain circumstances whereby cardiogenic shock is exacerbated, including vagally induced hypotension, intravascular volume depletion, acute RV failure, and surgically treatable entities such as ventricular septal rupture, papillary muscle rupture, chordae tendineae rupture, and left ventricular aneurysms. When cardiogenic shock is induced by the aforementioned complications, it is usually reversible. Newer modalities to treat cardiogenic shock consist of thrombolytic therapy or emergency PTCA. These interventions are of limited use in patients with cardiogenic shock because the shock usually manifests 24 to 48 hours after an MI when necrosis has occurred and successful reperfusion is unlikely to improve LV function.[100]

Right ventricular infarcts are a rare but important cause of cardiogenic shock. As previously mentioned, RV infarcts occur in the presence of inferior or inferioposterior infarcts of the LV. It has been estimated that RV infarcts occur in approximately 15% to 30% of all infarctions, but only 1% to 2% of these manifest in shock.[124] Right ventricular infarcts can be diagnosed on the basis of the hemodynamic alterations that are noted in these patients. There is a disproportionate increase in the right atrial pressures in contrast with the pulmonary wedge pressures in the setting of normal pulmonary artery pressures. Radionuclide ventriculography or echocardiography may be helpful in detecting the RV infarct as evidenced by wall motion abnormalities and a decreased RV ejection fraction. Echocardiograms may also reveal RV dilatation. The ECG may be helpful in revealing posterior RV necrosis by the presence of a Q wave or ST segment elevation in lead V_{4R}.[154] The goal of therapy for these patients is to administer fluid therapy despite the apparent elevation in right atrial pressure. Arterial vasodilators should be used when RV infarcts occur concomitantly with LV failure to facilitate systolic unloading of the LV and in turn decrease the impedance to RV outflow.[100] Inotropic agents (dopamine or dobutamine) may also be employed when volume alone is unable to correct hypotension.[122] Pacing such as atrioventricular sequential pacing is advocated for bradycardia or AV block.[123]

Acute Mitral Regurgitation

Another complication that may occur after an MI, acute mitral regurgitation, is caused by papillary muscle rupture (usually posterior medial papillary muscle) which usually occurs in inferior infarcts within the first several days after hospitalization.[100,155] Unfortunately, papillary muscles are subendocardial structures: they are supplied by terminal end-branches of the coronary arterial system, rendering them highly vulnerable to ischemia. Infarction of a papillary muscle may also be limited to a subendocardial MI.

When a papillary muscle ruptures, there is incomplete closure of the mitral valve leading to acute regurgitation of blood from the left ventricle into the left atrium. The clinical manifestations of acute mitral regurgitation are pulmonary congestion, and a new, loud pansystolic murmur with a thrill heard best at the apex. If a pulmonary artery catheter is in place, the appearance of large *v* waves is noted. These patients require mitral valve replacement on an emergency basis. The IABP and/or vasodilators have been used as temporary measures in some cases prior to surgery in the hope of decreasing the regurgitation and encouraging forward flow which is accomplished by decreasing the resistance to LV ejection.

Interventricular Septum Rupture

Another surgically correctable complication of an MI is rupture of the interventricular septum, more commonly associated with anterior or anterior-lateral MIs.[100] It tends to develop in first-time MI patients who have not developed adequate septal collateral flow.[135] Although a rare complication (1% to 2%), it requires surgical intervention because the mortality is high if left untreated. Characteristically, when there is a large septal rupture, a left-to-right shunt occurs with an abrupt and dramatic overloading of the right ventricle. These patients exhibit signs and symptoms of right-sided failure along with dyspnea and reduced LV forward output. Small ruptures may manifest only a new cardiac murmur. Right and left heart catheterization and angiography confirm the diagnosis with a "step-up" in O_2 saturation in blood sampled from the pulmonary artery and right heart chambers as well as shunting of contrast material from left to right at the ventricular level. IABP or vasodilators may be temporarily employed to reduce the resistance to LV ejection and thereby to decrease the left-to-right shunt while the patient is awaiting surgery. Timing of surgery has been controversial, but early surgical repair is now considered the preferred treatment.[156]

Left Ventricular Free Wall Rupture

Left ventricular free wall rupture accounts for up to 5% to 10% of hospital deaths after MI.[98] Complete rupture of the free wall is thought to be caused by several factors, including thinning of the apical wall, marked intensity of necrosis at the terminal end-branches of the arterial blood supply, inadequate collateral flow, and the shearing effect of muscular contraction against a stiffened necrotic area. A profile typical of a patient at high risk for developing this dreaded complication is a hypertensive elderly female who has had a left anterior or lateral transmural infarct in the terminal area of the LAD. Ruptures commonly occur 3 to 5 days after infarction, and some have been reported up to 4 weeks later.[100] A pericardial friction rub may be auscultated prior to the rupture.[135] A tear or a dissection hematoma in the necrotic area of the myocardium is the precipitating event leading to hemopericardium and sudden death from cardiac tamponade. Patients with LV free wall rupture can survive when the rupture is immediately recognized and surgically treated.

Ventricular Aneurysm

True ventricular aneurysms develop most often after an anterior or apical transmural MI in approximately 12% to 15% of MI patients.[100,135] An aneurysm is a circumscribed, akinetic outpouching of the left ventricle which develops from increased wall tension that stretches the infarcted muscle. The aneurysm is a weak, thin-walled structure that bulges (dyskinesis) with each systolic contraction, occurring most often at the apex in the anterior wall of the left ventricle. Persistent ST segment elevation after 3 weeks following an MI is a characteristic yet not sensitive ECG finding of an LV aneurysm. Two-dimensional echocardiography and radionuclide angiography are useful in diagnosing an aneurysm. Mural thrombi may adhere to the aneurysmal wall, which puts patients at risk for systemic emboli. Other complications associated with ventricular aneurysms are CHF, angina pectoris, and ventricular dysrhythmias. Medical intervention includes treatment of CHF symptoms, prophylactic anticoagulation, and antidysrhythmic agents. When the patient with an aneurysm develops any of the above complications, an aneurysmectomy is recommended.

False (pseudo) aneurysms have been reported to occur in the post-MI phase and are usually due to an initial, incomplete rupture of the LV wall. The rupture is sealed with thrombus, and a hematoma develops which prevents the sequela of hemopericardium. A false aneurysm is in direct contact with the LV cavity through a narrow opening. False aneurysms are problematic because of their tendency to rupture in contrast with true aneurysms that rarely rupture.[100]

Left Ventricular Thrombosis

Left ventricular thrombi are common findings in patients following an acute MI. They frequently occur with extensive infarcts and are located in the apex of the left ventricle.[100] These thrombi can be recognized on the echocardiogram. Prophylactic anticoagulation is used to prevent systemic emboli which may result from these thrombi.

Pericarditis

Pericarditis can manifest in two forms. Early pericarditis is a direct inflammatory response to transmural damage in approximately 15% of patients on the second to fourth days after infarction. Late pericarditis is a delayed autoimmune response often referred to as *Dressler's syndrome.*[100,157]

Early pericarditis is clinically diagnosed by a pericardial friction rub which is transient in nature. Patients may also exhibit chest pain which may be confused with postinfarction angina or pain resulting from extension of an MI. This chest pain differs from angina in that it is positional and exacerbated with inspiration. The ECG may reveal diffuse ST segment elevation during the acute phase, which may also lead to confusion regarding extension of a preexisting infarct. However, it is imperative that the critical care nurse be aware that these ST elevations are diffuse and exist in many leads (I, II AVL, AVF, V_3 to V_6) and that the patient will not develop pathological Q waves. During the evolutionary phase of early pericarditis, the ST segment returns to normal, and the T waves invert in most of the leads in which ST segment elevations existed. The T waves eventually return to the baseline configuration within days or weeks, although a few patients may be left with some degree of T wave inversion for an indefinite period.[157]

Treatments in early pericarditis include antiinflammatory agents such as aspirin, indomethacin (Indocin), and nonsteroidal antiinflammatory drugs (ibuprofen) or corticosteroids. The critical care nurse should be aware of the possibility of cardiac tamponade when patients with early pericarditis receive systemic anticoagulants.[157]

Late pericarditis or Dressler's syndrome is not often seen in the critical care unit because it usually occurs 2 to 4 weeks after the infarction.[100,155] The etiology of late pericarditis remains unknown; however, investigations suggest that it is probably an autoimmune antibody response against certain pericardial or myocardial antigens that are produced by myocardial necrosis.[157] Clinical manifestations of Dressler's syndrome are persistent fever between 101° and 102° F, leukocytosis, malaise, and dull chest pain which is positional and intensified by deep inspiration. Patients often obtain pain relief by leaning forward. Pericardial friction rubs are also noted in this type of pericarditis. Antiinflammatory agents such as aspirin or ibuprofen are also employed in the treatment of this syndrome. Patients need to be told that this syndrome is self-limiting and usually requires no further medical intervention.

NURSING MANAGEMENT

The nursing priorities for the patient with an MI must include the recognition and treatment of all the complications previously discussed along with the psychological impact of the infarction on the patient. The critical care nurse needs to obtain a complete biopsychosocial assessment of the MI patient using Gordon's[96] functional health patterns as described in Chapter 21. This tool guides the nurse, along with the information obtained from the physical examination in collecting data from which to deduce nursing problems or diagnoses that may be treated within the scope of nursing.

Specific features to be noted on physical examination pertaining to the MI patient include height, weight, presence of edema, skin color and temperature, quality of respirations, presence and location of crackles, normal and abnormal heart sounds, cardiac murmurs, thrills, heaves or rubs, arrhythmias, blood pressure, jugular venous pressure, and mental status.

Laboratory data may reveal elevated serum enzymes such as LDH and CK with elevations in their respective isoenzymes. Data may also reveal an elevated sedimentation rate, elevated serum cholesterol, and specific lipoproteins.

The psychological impact of the infarction is dependent on many factors such as the patient's age, functional status, previous coping mechanisms, and personality. Patients may experience a wide array of emotions ranging from anxiety, denial, and depression to anger. These emotions are similar to those experiencing grief or loss as described by Kubler-Ross.[158] Miller's[159] composite of assessment criteria and interventions required for these responses are found in Table 22-9.

Upon completion of the database, nursing diagnoses may be identified. A nursing care plan aimed at minimizing or preventing the patient's problems should be formulated and evaluated. Patient outcomes and nursing interventions are discussed in terms of nursing diagnosis.

The nursing diagnosis for the MI patient is similar to that of the unstable angina patient in that chest pain is a major problem. In MI, however, pain is due not to a temporary reduction in tissue perfusion secondary to an imbalance in myocardial supply and demand but to an abrupt cessation of blood supply that causes death of the myocardial tissue.

■ NURSING DIAGNOSIS

Pain (MI), related to an absence of tissue perfusion to the myocardium, resulting in tissue necrosis.

OUTCOME STANDARD AND CRITERIA

Pain is absent or controlled as evidenced by:
- Verbalization that pain is relieved or tolerable
- Rating on pain scale is reduced

TABLE 22-9   **Emotional Reactions to Perceived Losses Associated with Acute Myocardial Infarction**

Behaviors	Assessment	Interventions
ANXIETY		
Apprehensiveness: appears tense, scares easily	What is the patient's major concern? The patient's family?	Maintain close nurse–patient interaction, especially during episodes of high anxiety.
Severe insomnia	Is anxiety mild or severe?	Provide continuity of staff assignments.
Talks incessantly	Is anxiety related to a specific situation (cardiac arrest, monitoring equipment)?	Give continual orientation to CCU environment, personnel, procedures.
Weepy, trembling, jittery	How has the patient coped in the past?	Encourage verbalization, use active listening.
Tachycardia, dysrhythmia		Decrease anxiety by allowing patient to control situation.
DENIAL		
Verbally denies severity of illness	Does patient manifest complete or partial denial?	Accept denial when need is recognized.
Stoic or inappropriately cheerful	Is denial excessive or will it interfere with rehabilitation?	Do not foster denial.
Refuses to comply with medical regimen	Are other coping mechanisms available to patient?	Convey feeling of concern.
Unrealistic statements in the face of reality		Maintain specificity when the patient generalizes, avoids, or attempts to change the subject.
ANGER AND HOSTILITY		
Voices anger or resentment	What appears to be the trigger for anger?	Be calm, matter-of-fact.
Open opposition to medical regimen	What are the patient's usual aggression patterns?	Explore reasons for anger.
Sarcasm	What other coping mechanisms is the patient using?	Acknowledge angry feelings.
Inappropriate sexual behavior	What purpose is the behavior achieving?	Provide supportive environment, active listening.
Passive-aggressive behavior		Acknowledge concerns about sexuality.
DEPRESSION		
Changes in sleep pattern: early morning awakening	Was the patient depressed before the MI?	Limit number of people caring for the patient.
Loss of concentration	Is it directly related to the illness?	Provide empathy and understanding of mood.
Helplessness	What losses has the patient experienced in the past?	Give appropriate information to allay misconceptions.
Pessimism, crying	Can the patient deal with anger openly?	Encourage ventilation and catharsis.
Irritability		Let patient know this is a normal response.
Decreased self-esteem		
Decreased energy, increased fatigue		

From Miller, N. (1989). Acute myocardial infarction. In B. Riegel, & D. Ehrenreich (Eds.), *Psychological aspects of critical care nursing*. Gaithersburg, MD: Aspen.

- Vital signs return to normal after administration of narcotics

NURSING INTERVENTIONS

- Instruct patient to notify nursing staff of pain or chest discomfort
- Observe for nonverbal cues such as facial grimaces, restlessness, and posturing suggestive of pain or discomfort
- Monitor and document pain characteristics such as intensity, duration, localization, and radiation
- Administer analgesia such as morphine sulfate for pain as ordered to prevent increased intensity. Evaluate pain relief and effectiveness of interventions
- Check vital signs prior to admission of narcotics and after 30 minutes
- To promote psychological reassurance, assure patient that analgesia should relieve discomfort
- Assess the response to the analgesic agent by asking patient whether or not relief has been obtained using a scale of 1 to 10 (1 = low, 10 = high)
- Instruct patient regarding the effects of analgesia
- Decrease physical activity during chest discomfort
- Avoid excessive sympathetic stimulation such as caffeine beverages, fever, volume depletion, and anxiety
- Obtain a 12-lead ECG during chest discomfort and report any changes

■ **NURSING DIAGNOSIS**

Activity intolerance, related to: (1) decrease in myocardial workload capacity; (2) knowledge deficit regarding activity progression after infarction; (3) deconditioning effects of prolonged bed rest; and (4) potential sleep deficit secondary to care requirements.

OUTCOME STANDARD AND CRITERIA

Activity level prescribed is tolerated as evidenced by:

- Demonstration of ability to progressively increase level of activity without developing chest discomfort
- Verbalization of an increase in activity tolerance
- Verbalization of decreased shortness of breath or fatigue with minimal activity
- Appropriate heart rate, blood pressure, and respiratory rate with increased activity

NURSING INTERVENTIONS

- Assess prior activity level on admission to the critical care unit
- Assist patient to complete those activities of daily living that do not lead to excessive increases in heart rate, blood pressure, respirations, or electrical disturbances such as dysrhythmias
- Plan and implement incremental increases in activity such as bed rest to chair to ambulation so as not to abruptly increase myocardial workload
- Monitor blood pressure and heart rate prior to and immediately after activity and 3 minutes later
- Instruct patient regarding factors that increase myocardial workload, such as strenuous activity, stress, smoking, heavy meals, isometric exercises, and Valsalva maneuvers
- Instruct patient to stop an activity if the following signs of cardiac decompensation are present: increased heart rate, dyspnea, or chest pain
- Instruct patient to rest between activity periods
- Encourage passive and active ROM exercises while patient is on bed rest
- Minimize the effect of postural hypotension by allowing bed to chair activity once the patient is hemodynamically stable, and by allowing patient to dangle feet at bedside
- Have patient plantar and dorsiflex feet while in bed to prevent stasis of blood
- Encourage frequent changes in body position during bed rest
- Decrease environmental stimulation to promote sleep periods
- Assess quality and response to sleep by asking patient about his or her sleep periods
- Provide adequate rest periods for the patient between therapeutic care activities

HIGH-RISK NURSING DIAGNOSIS

High-risk nursing diagnosis identified for the MI patient include:

- High risk for fear or anxiety, related to diagnosis and prognosis of MI
- High risk for disturbance in self-concept, related to loss of healthy body image and role in family

The nursing management of an individual with an acute MI who becomes a patient in the critical care setting is challenging. The patient often may develop serious potential complications. Nursing personnel must constantly assess for these complications and institute preventive measures to minimize or prevent them. Lastly, the critical care nurse must also be aware of the many therapeutic modalities for the acute MI patient to educate and prepare both the patient and significant others for such alternatives.

REFERENCES

1. American Heart Association. (1991). *Heart facts.* Dallas: Author.
2. Guyton, A. C. (1991). *Textbook of medical physiology* (8th ed.). Philadelphia: Saunders.
3. Ross, R. (1990). Factors influencing atherogenesis. In J. W. Hurst, R. C. Schlant, C. E. Rackley, et al. (Eds.), *The heart* (7th ed.). New York: McGraw-Hill.
4. Ross, R. (1986). The pathogenesis of atherosclerosis—an update. *New England Journal of Medicine, 314,* 488-500.
5. Faggiotto, A., Ross, R., & Harker, L. (1984). Studies

of hypercholesterolemia in the non-human primate: Part 1. Changes that lead to fatty streak formation. *Atherosclerosis, 4,* 323-340.

6. Faggiotto, A., & Ross, R. (1984). Studies of hypercholesterolemia in the non-human primate: Part 2. Fatty streak conversion to fibrous plaque. *Arteriosclerosis, 4*(4), 341-356.

7. Benditt, E. P., & Benditt, J. M. (1973). Evidence for a monoclonal origin of human atherosclerotic plaques. *Proceedings from the National Academy of Science USA, 70,* 1753-1756.

8. Kannel, W. B. (1978). Recent findings of the Framingham study. *Resident and Staff Physician, 24,* 56-71.

9. Gotto, A. M., & Farmer, J. A. (1992). Risk factors for coronary artery disease. In E. Braunwald (Ed.), *Heart disease: A textbook of cardiovascular medicine* (4th ed.). Philadelphia: Saunders.

10. Kannel, W. B. (1976). Some lesions in cardiovascular epidemiology from Framingham. *American Journal of Cardiology, 37,* 269-282.

11. American Heart Association. (1989). *Silent epidemic: The truth about women and heart disease.* Dallas: Author.

12. Murdough, C. (1990). Coronary artery disease in women. *Journal of Cardiovascular Nursing, 4*(4), 35-40.

13. Taylor, W. J. (1990). Genetics and the cardiovascular system. In J. W. Hurst, R. C. Schlant, C. E. Rackley, et al. (Eds.), *The heart* (7th ed.). New York: McGraw-Hill.

14. Maciejko, J. J., Holmes, D. R., Kottke, B. A., et al. (1983). Apolipoprotein A-1 as a marker of angiographically assessed coronary artery disease. *New England Journal of Medicine, 309*(7), 385-389.

15. Freedman, D. S., Srinivasan, S. R., Shear, C. L., et al. (1986). The relationship of apolipoproteins A-1 and B in children to parental myocardial infarction. *New England Journal of Medicine, 315*(12), 721-726.

16. Colditz, G. A., Rimm, E. B., Giovannucci, E., et al. (1991). A prospective study of parental history of M.I. and coronary artery disease in men. *American Journal of Cardiology, 67*(11), 933-938.

17. Assmann, G., & Schulte, H. (1987). The prospective C.V. Munster Study: Prevalence and prognostic significance of hyperlipidemia in men with systemic hypertension. *American Journal of Cardiology, 59*(14), 9G-17G.

18. Wenger, N. K., & Schlant, R. C. (1990). Prevention of coronary atherosclerosis. In J. W. Hurst, R. C. Schlant, C. E. Rackley, et al. (Eds.), *The heart* (7th ed.). New York: McGraw-Hill.

19. Zemel, P. C., & Sowers, J. R. (1990). Relation between lipids and atherosclerosis. Epidemiologic evidence and clinical implications. *American Journal of Cardiology, 66,* 7I-12I.

20. National Institutes of Health Consensus Development Conference Statement. (1984). *Lowering blood cholesterol to prevent heart disease,* (Vol. 5, No. 7). Bethesda, MD: U.S. Department of Health and Human Services.

21. Department of Health and Human Services, Public Health Service, National Institutes of Health. (1989). *Report of the expert panel on the detection, evaluation, and treatment of high blood cholesterol in adults.* (NIH Publication No. 89-2925). Bethesda, MD: National Institutes of Health.

22. Kannel, W., & Stokes, J., III. (1985). The epidemiology of coronary artery diseae. In P. Cohn (Ed.), *Diagnosis and therapy of coronary artery disease.* Boston: Martinus Nijhoff.

23. Boucek, R., Morales, A., Romanelli, R., et al. (1984). Genetic considerations of coronary artery disease. In J. Sangston (Ed.), *Coronary artery disease: Pathologic and clinical assessment.* Baltimore: Williams & Wilkins.

24. Rosenman, R. H., Brand, R. J., Sholtz, R. I., et al. (1976). Multivariate prediction of coronary heart disease during 8.5 year follow-up in the Western Collaborative Group Study. *American Journal of Cardiology, 37,* 903-910.

25. Williams, R. B., Friedman, M., Glass, D. C., et al. (1977). Mechanisms linking behavioral and pathophysiological processes. In T. M. Dembroski, S. M. Weiss, J. L. Shields, et al. (Eds.), *Coronary-prone behavior.* New York: Springer-Verlag.

26. Lipid Research Clinics Program. (1984). The Lipid Research Clinics coronary primary prevention trial results: Part 1. Reduction in incidence of coronary heart disease. *Journal of the American Medical Association, 251,* 351-374.

27. Prinzmetal, M., Kennamer, R., Merliss, R., et al. (1959). Angina pectoris. A variant form of angina pectoris. *American Journal of Medicine, 27*(88), 375-388.

28. Maseri, A., Chierchia, S., & Kaski, C. (1985). Mixed angina pectoris. *American Journal of Cardiology, 56,* 30E-33E.

29. Friedberg, C. K. (1972). Angina pectoris. *American Heart Association Monograph No. 37.* New York: American Heart Association.

30. Pepine, C. (1989). New concepts in the pathophysiology of acute myocardial ischemia and infarction and their relevance to contemporary management. *Cardiovascular Clinics, 20,* 3-18.

31. Tofler, G. H., Brezinski, D., Schafer, A. I., et al. (1987). Concurrent morning increase in platelet aggregability and the risk of an M.I. and sudden cardiac death. *New England Journal of Medicine, 316,*(24), 1514-1518.

32. Muller, J. E., & Tofler, G. H. (1990). Introduction a symposium: Triggering and circadian variation of onset of cardiovascular disease. *American Journal of Cardiology, 66,* 1G-6G.

33. Hurst, J. W. (1990). Atherosclerotic coronary heart disease: Historical benchmarks, methods of study and clinical features, differential diagnosis and clinical spectrum. In J. W. Hurst, R. C. Schlant, C. E. Rackley, et al. (Eds.), *The heart* (7th ed.). New York: McGraw-Hill.

34. Gaca, J. M., Gore, J. M., & Kirshenbaum, H. D. (1991). Coronary spasm and variant angina. In J. M.

Rippe, R. S. Irwin, J. S. Alpert, et al. (Eds.), *Intensive care medicine* (2nd ed.). Boston: Little, Brown.

35. Sato, A., Taneichi, Y., Sekine, I., et al. (1983). Prinzmetal's variant angina induced only by alcohol ingestion. *Clinical Cardiology, 4,* 193-195.

36. Schachne, J. S., Roberts, B. H., & Thompson, B. D. (1984). Coronary artery spasm and myocardial infarction associated with cocaine use. *New England Journal of Medicine, 310,* 1665-1666.

37. Buxton, A. E., Goldberg, S., Harken, A., et al. (1981). Coronary artery spasm immediately after myocardial revascularization. Recognition and management. *New England Journal of Medicine, 304,* 1249-1253.

38. Assey, M. E. (1990). The recognition and treatment of silent myocardial ischemia. In J. W. Hurst, R. C. Schlant, C. E. Rackley, et al. (Eds.), *The heart* (7th ed.). New York: McGraw-Hill.

39. Cohn, P. F. (1985). Silent myocardial ischemia: Classification, prevalence and prognosis. *American Journal of Medicine, 79,* 2-6.

40. Pratt, C. (1986). Silent ischemia. In R. Roberts (Ed.), *Current perspectives in coronary care.* Selected proceedings of two symposia in Bermuda and San Diego, August, 1986.

41. Holdright, D. R., Rosano, G. M., Sarrel, P. M., et al. (1992). The ST segment. The herald of ischaemia, the siren of misdiagnosis or syndrome X. *International Journal of Cardiology, 35*(3), 293-301.

42. Shurbrooks, S. (1979). Variant angina: More variants of the variant. *American Journal of Cardiology, 43,* 1245-1247.

43. Franch, R. H., King, S. B., & Douglas, J. S. (1990). Techniques of cardiac catheterization including coronary arteriography. In J. W. Hurst, R. C. Schlant, C. E. Rackley, et al. (Eds.), *The heart* (7th ed.). New York: McGraw-Hill.

44. White, C. J., Ramee, S. R., & Collins, T. J. (1991). Percutaneous coronary angioscopy current status and future directions. *Current Trends in Cardiovascular Medicine,* January/February, 6-11.

45. Cortis, B. S., Harris, D. M., & Principe, J. (1986). From angiography to angioscopy: Informal discussion. *Texas Heart Institute Journal, 13*(30), 281-289.

46. Ramee, S. R., White, C. J., Collins, T. J., et al. (1991). Percutaneous angioscopy during coronary angioplasty using a steerable microangioscope. *Journal of the American College of Cardiology, 17*(1), 100-104.

47. Siegel, R. J., Jang-Seong Chan, G., & Forrester, J. S. (1990). Angiography, angioscopy, and ultrasound imaging before and after percutaneous balloon angioplasty. *American Heart Journal, 120*(5), 1086-1090.

48. Advanced Cardiovascular Systems, Inc. (1991). Angioscope catheter. *ACS angioscope system manual, 7.*

49. Uchida, Y., Nakamura, F., & Oshima, T. et al. (1990). Percutaneous angioscopy of the left ventricle in patients with dilated cardiomyopathy and acute myocarditis. *American Heart Journal, 120*(3), 677-687.

50. Cohn, J. N. (1990). Drugs used to control vascular resistance and capacitance. In J. W. Hurst, R. C.

Schlant, C. E. Rackley, et al. (Eds.), *The heart* (7th ed.). New York: McGraw-Hill.

51. Parmley, W. W. (1982). The combination of beta-adrenergic blocking agents and nitrates in the treatment of stable angina pectoris. *Cardiology Review Reports, 3,* 1425-1430.

52. Conti, C. R., Hill, J. A., Feldman, R. L., et al. (1986). Treatment of coronary artery spasm and variant angina. *Journal of Intensive Care Medicine, 1,* 66-74.

53. Rishman, W. H., & Sonnenblick, E. H. (1990). Beta-adrenergic blocking drugs. In J. W. Hurst, R. C. Schlant, C. E. Rackley, et al. (Eds.), *The heart* (7th ed.). New York: McGraw-Hill.

54. Frishman, W. H., & Teicher, M. (1987). Antianginal drug therapy for silent myocardial ischemia. *American Heart Journal, 114,* 140-144.

55. Frishman, W. H., & Sonnenblick, E. H. (1990). Calcium channel blockers. In J. W. Hurst, R. C. Schlant, C. E. Rackley, et al. (Eds.), *The heart* (7th ed.). New York: McGraw-Hill.

56. Gerstenblith, G., Ouyang, P., & Achuff, S. C. (1982). Nifedipine in unstable angina. A double blind randomized trial. *New England Journal of Medicine, 306*(15), 885-889.

57. U.S. Department of Health and Human Services Public Health Service. (1985). *Cholesterol counts—steps for lowering your patient's blood cholesterol* (NIH Publication No. 85-2699). Baltimore, MD: National Institutes of Health.

58. Kromhout, D., Bosschieter, E., & Coulander, C. (1985). The inverse relation between fish consumption and 20 year mortality from coronary heart disease. *New England Journal of Medicine, 312,* 1205-1210.

59. Glomset, J. A. (1985). Fish, fatty acids and health [Editorial]. *New England Journal of Medicine, 312,* 1253-1254.

60. Ashley, F. W., & Kannel, W. B. (1974). Relation of weight changes to changes in atherogenic traits: The Framingham study. *Journal of Chronic Disease, 27,* 103-144.

61. Craver, J. M., & Hatcher, C. R. (1990). Techniques of using the intraaortic balloon pump. In J. W. Hurst, R. C. Schlant, C. E. Rackley, et al. (Eds.), *The heart* (7th ed.). New York: McGraw-Hill.

62. Millham, F. H., Hudson, H. M., Woodson, J., et al. (1991). Intraaortic balloon pump entrapment. *Annals of Vascular Surgery, 5,* 381-384.

63. Patacky, M. G., Garvin, B. J., & Schwirian, P. M. (1985). Intra-aortic balloon pumping and stress in the coronary care unit. Patient's perceptions of psychological stress. *Heart Lung, 14,* 142-148.

64. Dotter, C. T., & Judkins, M. P. (1964). Transluminal treatment of atherosclerotic obstruction. Description of a new technique and a preliminary report of its application. *Circulation, 30,* 654-670.

65. Gruentzig, A. (1978). Transluminal dilatation of coronary artery stenosis. *Lancet, 1,* 263-265.

66. Waller, B. (1989). "Crackers, breakers, stretchers, drillers, scrapers, shavers, burners, welders, and mill-

ers." The future treatment of atherosclerotic coronary artery disease—morphological assessment. *Journal of the American College of Cardiology, 13*(5), 969-987.

67. Sipperly, M. E. (1989). Expanding role of coronary angioplasty: Current implications, limitations and nursing considerations. *Heart Lung, 18*(5), 507-513.

68. Cowley, M. J., Vetrovec, G. W., DiSciascio, G., et al. (1985). Coronary angioplasty of multiple vessels: Short term and long term results. *Circulation, 72,* 1314-1320.

69. Dorros, G., Cowley, M. J., Janke, L., et al. (1984). In-hospital mortality rate in the National Heart, Lung and Blood Institute percutaneous transluminal coronary angioplasty registry. *American Journal of Cardiology, 53,* 17C-21C.

70. Faxon, D. P. (1991, June). PTCA: Current results in single and multivessel disease. Presented at New England Cardiovascular Scientific Session on Interventional Cardiology: Present and Future, Framingham, MA.

71. Mata, L. A., Bosch, X., David, P. R., et al. (1985). Clinical and angiographic assessment six months after double vessels percutaneous coronary angioplasty. *American Journal of Cardiology, 6*(6), 1239-1244.

72. Litvack, F., Grundfest, W. S., Goldenberg, T., et al. (1990). Percutaneous excimer laser coronary angioplasty. *American Journal of Cardiology, 66*(15), 1027-1032.

73. Halfman-Franey, M., & Coburn, C. (1990). Techniques in cardiac care: Lasers, stents and atherectomy devices. *AACN Clinical Issues in Critical Care Nursing, 1*(1), 87-109.

74. Eagan, J. S. (1989). Lasers: Applications in cardiovascular atherosclerotic disease. *Critical Care Nursing Clinics of North America, 1*(2), 311-326.

75. Sakallaris, B. R. (1987). Laser therapy for cardiovascular disease. *Heart Lung, 16*(5), 465-471.

76. Baim, D. S. (1991, June). New technologies for revascularization: Atherectomy, stents, lasers and beyond. Presented at New England Cardiovascular Society Scientific Sessions on Interventional Cardiology: Present and Future, Framingham, MA.

77. Sanborn, T. A. (1990). Percutaneous peripheral atherectomy: What are its indications? *Journal of the American College of Cardiology, 15*(3), 689-690.

78. Garratt, K. N., Holmes, D. R., Bell, M. R., et al. (1990). Restenosis after directional coronary atherectomy: Differences between primary atheromatous and restenosis lesions and influence of subintimal tissue resection. *Journal of the American College of Cardiology, 16*(7), 1665-1671.

79. Kaufman, U. P., Garratt, K. N. & Vlietstra, R. E. (1990). Transluminal atherectomy of saphenous vein autocoronary bypass grafts. *American Journal of Cardiology, 65*(15), 1430-1433.

80. Muller, D. W., Ellis, S. G., & Topol, E. J. (1989). Atherectomy of the left main coronary artery with percutaneous cardiopulmonary support. *American Journal of Cardiology, 64*(16), 967-970.

81. Holmes, D. R., Vlietstra, R. E., Reiter, S. J., et al. (1990). Advances in interventional cardiology. *Mayo Clinic Proceedings, 65*(4), 565-583.

82. Halfman-Franey, M., Tukan, T., Bergstrom, D., et al. (1991). Using stents in the coronary circulation: Nursing perspectives. *Focus on Critical Care, 18*(2), 132-142.

83. Martin, S., Chesnick, P. A., & Young, J. B. (1990). Invasive cardiac procedures after myocardial infarction: Which procedure when and its relationship to thrombolysis. *Journal of Emergency Nursing, 16*(3, pt. 2), 202-207.

84. Dottler, C. T. (1969). Transluminally placed coil spring endarterial tube grafts: Long term patency in canine popliteal artery. *Investigational Radiology, 4,* 329-332.

85. Sigwart, U., Puel, J., Mirkovitch, V., et al. (1987). Intravascular stents to prevent occlusion and restenosis after transluminal angioplasty. *New England Journal of Medicine, 316,* 701-706.

86. Halfman-Franey, M., & Levine, S. (1989). Intracoronary stents. *Critical Care Nursing Clinics of North America, 1*(2), 327-337.

87. Murphy, J. G., Garratt, K. N., Schwartz, R. S., et al. (1990). Intracoronary stenting: Bailout or bypass. *Catheterization and Cardiovascular Diagnosis, 21*(4), 260-262.

88. Schatz, R. A., Baim, D. S., Leon, M., et al. (1991). Clinical experience with the Palmaz-Schatz coronary stent: Initial results of a multicenter trial. *Circulation, 83*(1), 148-161.

89. Rosenschein, U., Bernstein, J. J., DiSegni, E., et al. (1991). Ultrasonic angioplasty in totally occluded peripheral arteries: Initial clinical, histological, and angiographic results. *Circulation, 83*(6), 1976-1986.

90. Shawl, F. A. (1990). Percutaneous cardiopulmonary bypass support in the catheterization laboratory: Technique and complications. *American Heart Journal, 120*(1), 195-203.

91. O'Neill, P., Menendez, T., Host, R., et al. (1989). Prolonged ventricular fibrillation—salvage using a new percutaneous cardiopulmonary support system. *American Journal of Cardiology, 64*(8), 545.

92. Vogel, R. A. (1988). The Maryland experience: Angioplasty and valvuloplasty using percutaneous cardiopulmonary support. *American Journal of Cardiology, 62*(18), 11k-14k.

93. Muller, D. W., Ellis, S. G., & Topol, E. J. (1989). Atherectomy of the left main coronary artery with percutaneous cardiopulmonary bypass support. *American Journal of Cardiology, 64*(1), 114-116.

94. Shawl, F. A., Domanski, M. J., Hernandez, T. J., et al. (1989). Emergency percutaneous cardiopulmonary bypass support in cardiogenic shock from acute myocardial infarction. *American Journal of Cardiology, 64*(16), 967-970.

95. Phillips, S. J. (1989). Percutaneous cardiopulmonary bypass: Applications and indications for use. *Annals of Thoracic Surgery, 47*(1), 121-123.

96. Gordon, M. (1991). *Manual of nursing diagnosis* (5th ed.) St. Louis: Mosby—Year Book.

97. Rutherford, J. D., & Braunwald, E., (1992). Chronic ischemic heart disease. In E. Braunwald (Ed.), *Heart disease: A textbook of cardiovascular medicine* (4th ed.). Philadelphia: Saunders.

98. Factor, S. M., & Kirk, E. S. (1990). Pathophysiology of myocardial ischemia. In J. W. Hurst, R. C. Schlant, C. E. Rackley, et al. (Eds.), *The heart* (7th ed.). New York: McGraw-Hill.

99. Bulkley, B. H. (1990). Pathology of coronary atherosclerotic heart disease. In J. W. Hurst, R. C. Schlant, C. E. Rackley, et al. (Eds.), *The heart* (7th ed.). New York: McGraw-Hill.

100. Pasternak, R. C., Braunwald, E., & Sobel, B. E. (1992). Acute myocardial infarction. In E. Braunwald (Ed.), *Heart disease: A textbook of cardiovascular medicine* (4th ed.). Philadelphia: Saunders.

101. Chesebro, J. H., Badimon, L., & Fuster, V. (1990). New approaches to treatment to an M.I. *American Journal of Cardiology, 65,* 12C-19C.

102. Cavies, M. J., & Thomas, A. (1984). Thrombosis and acute coronary artery lesions in sudden cardiac ischemic death. *New England Journal of Medicine, 310,* 1137-1140.

103. Gertz, S. D., Merin, G., Pasternak, R. C., et al. (1981). Endothelial cell damage and thrombus formation after partial arterial constriction. *American Journal of Pathology, 63*(3), 476-486.

104. Joris, I., & Majno, G. (1981). Endothelial changes induced by arterial spasm. *American Journal of Pathology, 102*(3), 346-358.

105. Hackett, D., Davies, G., Chierchia, S., et al. (1987). Intermittent coronary occlusion in acute myocardial infarction. Value of combined thrombolytic and vasodilator therapy. *New England Journal of Medicine, 317,* 1055-1059.

106. Fischell, T. A., Derby, G., Tse, T. M., et al. (1988). Coronary artery vasoconstriction routinely occurs after percutaneous transluminal angioplasty. *Circulation, 78,* 1323-1334.

107. Willerson, J. T., Golino, P., Eidt, J., et al. (1989). Specific platelet mediators and unstable coronary artery lesions. Experimental evidence and potential clinical implications. *Circulation, 80,*198-205.

108. Griffith, T. M., Lewis, M. J., Newby, A. C., et al. (1988). Endothelium-derived relaxing factor. *Journal of the American College of Cardiology, 12,* 797-806.

109. Ludmer, P. L. (1986). Pardoxical vasoconstriction induced by acetylcholine in atherosclerotic coronary arteries. *New England Journal of Medicine, 315,* 1046-1051.

110. Reimer, K. A., Lowe, J. E., Rasmussen, M. M., et al. (1977). The wavefront phenomenon of ischemic cell death: Part 1. Myocardial infarct size vs. duration of coronary occlusion in dogs. *Circulation, 56,* 786-794.

111. Reimer, K. A., & Jennings, R. B. (1979). The "wavefront phenomenon" of myocardial ischemic cell death: Part 2. Transmural progression of necrosis within the framework of ischemic bed size (myocardium at risk) and collateral flow. *Lab Investigation, 40*(6), 633-644.

112. Willerson, J. T., & Buja, L. M. (1989). Q wave vs. non-Q wave myocardial infarction. *Cardiovascular Clinics, 20,* 183-192.

113. Hands, M. E., Lloyd, B. L., Robinson, J. S., et al. (1986). Prognostic significance of electrocardiographic site of infarction after correction for enzymatic size of infarction. *Circulation, 73*(5), 885-891.

114. Bar, F. W., Brugada, P., & Wassen, W. R. (1984). Prognostic value of Q waves, R/S ratio, loss of R wave voltage, ST-T segment abnormalities, electrical axis, low voltage and notching: Correlation of electrocardiogram and left ventriculogram. *Journal of American College of Cardiology, 4*(1), 17-27.

115. Alpert, J. S. (1991). A comparison of anterior and inferior myocardial infarction. In J. M. Rippe, R. S. Irwin, J. S. Alpert, et al. (Eds.), *Intensive care medicine* (2nd ed.). Boston: Little, Brown.

116. Hancock, E. W. (1982). Ischemic heart disease: Acute myocardial infarction. *Scientific American,* June, 1-22.

117. Vinsant, M. O., & Spence, M. I. (1989). *Commonsense approach to coronary care.* St. Louis: Mosby.

118. Gore, J. M., Roberts, R., & Ball, S. P. (1987). Peak creatinine kinase as a measure of effectiveness of thrombolytic therapy in acute myocardial infarction. *American Journal of Cardiology, 59*(15), 1234-1238.

119. Horowitz, R. S., Morganroth, J., & Parrotto, C. (1981). Prognosis in acute myocardial infarction determined by serial 2-D echocardiography. *Circulation, 64*(Suppl. II), IV-94.

120. Chandrarantna, P. A. N., Ulene, R., Reid, C. L., et al. (1983). Differentiation between new and old myocardial infarction by color encoding and time averaging two-dimensional echocardiograms. *Circulation, 68*(Suppl. III), III-3.

121. Zaret, B. L., & Berger, H. J. (1990). Techniques of nuclear cardiology. In J. W. Hurst, R. C. Schlant, C. E. Rackley, et al. (Eds.), *The heart* (7th ed.). New York: McGraw-Hill.

122. Marshall, R. C., Tillisch, J. H., Phelps, M. E., et al. (1983). Identification and differentiation of resting myocardial ischemia and infarction in man with position computed tomography, 18F-labeled fluorodexyglucose and N-13 ammonia. *Circulation, 67,* 766-778.

123. Frances, G. S., Donat, W. E., & Weiner, B. H. (1991). Syndromes of left ventricular failure. In J. M. Rippe, R. S. Irwin, J. S. Alpert, et al. (Eds.), *Intensive care medicine* (2nd ed.). Boston: Little, Brown.

124. Barnard, D., & Alpert, J. S. (1991). Right ventricular infarction. In J. M. Rippe, R. S. Irwin, J. S. Alpert, et al. (Eds.), *Intensive care medicine* (2nd ed.). Boston: Little, Brown.

125. MacMahon, S., Collins, R., Peto, R., et al. (1988). Effects of prophylactic lidocaine in suspected acute myocardial infarction: An overview of results from the randomized controlled trials. *Journal of the American Medical Association, 260*(13), 1910-1916.

126. Conti, C. (1989). Conventional drug therapy of patients with acute myocardial infarction. *Cardiovascular Clinics, 20,* 249-258.

127. Ryder, L. (1983). A double blind trial of metopolol in acute M.I. Effects on ventricular tachyarrhythmias. *New England Journal of Medicine, 308*(11), 614-618.

128. Topol, E. J., & Wilson, V. E. (1990). Pivotal role of early and sustained infarct vessel patency in patients with acute myocardial infarction. *Heart Lung, 19,* 583-595.

129. Kline, E. M. (1990). Clinical controversies surrounding thrombolytic therapy in acute M.I. *Heart Lung, 19,* 596-603.

130. Collen, C. (1988). Fibrin specific thrombolytic agents. *Annales de Biologie Clinique. 46,* 195-200.

131. Lavie, C. J., Gersh, B. J., & Chesebro, J. H. (1990). Reperfusion in acute M.I. *Mayo Clinic Proceedings, 65,* 549-564.

132. Bates, E. R. (1989). Expanding indications for thrombolytic therapy for acute myocardial infarction. *Practical Cardiology, 15,* 23-33.

133. Yusuf, S., Sleight, P., & Held, P. (1990). Routine medical management of acute myocardial infarction. Lessons from overviews of recent randomized controlled trials. *Circulation, 82*(Suppl. II), II-117-II-134.

134. Ellis, S. (1990). Interventions in acute myocardial infarctions. *Circulation,* (Suppl. IV), IV-43-IV-50.

135. Morris, D. C., Walter, P. F., & Hurst, J. W. (1990). The recognition and treatment of myocardial infarction and its complications. In J. W. Hurst, R. C. Schlant, C. E. Rackley, et al. (Eds.), *The heart* (7th ed.). New York: McGraw-Hill.

136. Lopez, L. M., & Mehta, J. L. (1987). Anticoagulation in coronary heart disease, heparin and warfarin trials. *Cardiovascular Clinics, 18*(1), 215-229.

137. ISIS-2 (Second International Study of Infarct Survival) Collaborative Group. (1988). Randomized trial of intravenous streptokinase, oral aspirin, both or neither among 17,187 cases of suspected acute myocardial infarction. *ISIS-2 Lancet, 2,* 349-360.

138. Misinski, M. (1990). Myocardial reperfusion injury. *Critical Care Nursing Clinics of North America, 2*(4), 651-662.

139. Bodwell, W. (1989). Ischemia, reperfusion and reperfusion injury: Role of oxygen free radicals and oxygen free radical scavengers. *Journal of Cardiovascular Nursing, 4*(1), 25-32.

140. Black, L., Coombs, V. J., & Townsend, S. N. (1990). Reperfusion and reperfusion injury in acute myocardial infarction. *Heart Lung, 19*(3), 274-284.

141. Hearse, D. J., Humphrey, S. M., & Bullock, G. R. (1978). The oxygen paradox and the calcium paradox. Two facets of the same problem? *Journal of Molecular Cellular Cardiology, 10,* 641-668.

142. Altschuld, R. A., Hostetler, J. R., & Brierley, G. P. (1981). Response of isolated rate heart cells to hypoxia, reoxygenation and acidosis. *Circulation Research, 49,* 307-315.

143. Ganote, C. E., & Kattenbach, J. P. (1979). Oxygen-induced enzyme release: Early events and a proposed mechanism. *Journal of Molecular Cellular Cardiology, 11,* 389-406.

144. Hess, M. L., & Manson, N. H. (1984). Molecular oxygen: Friend and foe—the role of the oxygen free radical system in the calcium paradox, the oxygen paradox and ischemia/reperfusion injury. *Journal of Molecular Cellular Cardiology, 16,* 969-985.

145. Nayler, W. G., & Elz, J. S. (1986). Reperfusion injury: Laboratory artifact or clinical dilemma? *Circulation, 74,* 215-220.

146. Jennings, R. B., Ganote, C. E., & Reimer, K. A. (1975). Ischemic tissue injury. *American Journal of Pathology, 81,* 179-191.

147. Ambrosio, G., Weisman, H. F., Mannisi, J. A., et al. (1989). Progressive impairment of regional myocardial perfusion after initial restoration of postischemic blood flow. *Circulation, 80*(6), 1846-1861.

148. Kloner, R. A., Przyklenk, K., & Patel, B. (1989). Altered myocardial states. *American Journal of Medicine, 86*(Suppl. IA), 145-225.

149. Braunwald, E., & Rutherford, J. D. (1986). Reversible ischemic left ventricular dysfunction: Evidence for the hibernating myocardium. *Journal of the American College of Cardiology, 8,* 1467-1470.

150. Nejima, J., Knight, D. R., Fallon, J. T., et al. (1989). Superoxide dismutase reduces reperfusion dysrhythmias but fails to salvage regional function or myocardium at risk in conscious dogs. *Circulation, 79*(1), 143-153.

151. Wessman, J. P. (1985). Preventing ventricular dysrhythmia following myocardial infarction. *Dimensions of Critical Care Nursing, 4*(1), 24-32.

152. Becker, R. C., & Mills, R. M. (1991). Arrhythmias following myocardial infarction. In J. M. Rippe, R. S. Irwin, J. S. Alpert, et al. (Eds.), *Intensive care medicine* (2nd ed.). Boston: Little, Brown.

153. Forrester, J. S., Diamond, G. A., & Swan, H. J. (1977). Correlative classification of clinical and hemodynamic function after acute myocardial infarction. *American Journal of Cardiology, 39,* 137-145.

154. Sendon, J. L., Coma-Canella, I., Alcasena, S., et al. (1985). Electrocardiographic findings in acute right ventricular infarction: Sensitivity and specificity of electrocardiographic alterations in right precordial leads. V4R, V3R, V1 and V3. *Journal of the American College of Cardiology, 6,* 1273-1279.

155. Aurigemma, G. P., & Waksmonski, C. A. (1991). Miscellaneous problems after myocardial infarction. In J. M. Rippe, R. S. Irwin, J. S. Alpert, et al. (Eds.), *Intensive care medicine* (2nd ed.). Boston: Little, Brown.

156. Caspi, Y., Merin, G., Safadi, T., et al. (1988). Surgical treatment of post infarction ventricular septal defect without concomitant myocardial revascularization. *Journal of Cardiovascular Surgery, 29*(4), 383-386.

157. Leon, M. B., & Cohen, L. S. (1984). Guidelines for patient management. In N. K. Wenger, & H. K. Hellerstein (Eds.), *Rehabilitation of the coronary patient.* New York: Wiley.

158. Kubler-Ross, E. (1969). *On death and dying.* New York: MacMillan.

159. Miller, N. (1989). Acute myocardial infarction. In B. Riegel, & D. Ehrenreich (Eds.), *Psychological aspects of critical care nursing.* Gaithersburg, MD: Aspen.

23

Cardiomyopathy

Joan Vitello-Cicciu

Molly Johantgen

Cardiomyopathy is a general term used to refer to a disease that affects the myocardial layer of the heart, resulting in systolic and/or diastolic dysfunction. Other general terms that are used synonymously with the term cardiomyopathy are listed in the box below.

More specifically, Goodwin, Roberts, and Wenger[1] classify cardiomyopathies into three types based on the pathophysiological abnormalities of each: (1) *dilated*, or *congestive*; (2) *hypertrophic*; and (3) *restrictive*, or *obliterative*. In the dilated congestive type, there is diffuse dilatation of all four heart chambers; thus, it is currently referred to as *dilated cardiomyopathy*. The hypertrophic form involves some degree

---

Cardiomyopathy Synonyms

Diffuse myocardial disease
Idiopathic cardiomegaly
Idiopathic myocardial disease
Myocardiopathy
Myocardosis
Primary myocardial disease

---

of obstruction to the left ventricular outflow tract, whereas the restrictive type contains rigid walls caused by the fibrosis that has occurred. This rigidity restricts ventricular filling during diastole, causing the pathophysiological alterations to those noted in constrictive pericarditis. These three types are illustrated in Figure 23-1.

Despite the pathophysiological differences of the three types of cardiomyopathies, there are strong similarities: (1) by definition, the etiology is idiopathic, or unknown; (2) the myocardium is affected in all three types, and the pathological changes may extend into the endocardial and pericardial layers; and (3) the sequelae of each form are often cardiomegaly and heart failure.

Wynne and Braunwald[2] further classify cardiomyopathies into primary and secondary forms. In the *primary form*, the heart is the only organ affected, and there is no involvement of valves or other cardiac structures. The cause of primary cardiomyopathy is not usually known (idiopathic). In *secondary cardiomyopathy*, the myocardial abnormality is related to another abnormality or condition and other organs

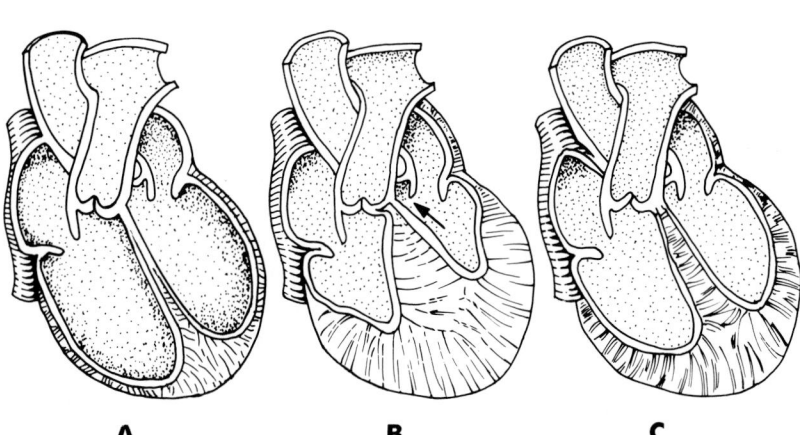

A   **B**   **C**

Figure 23-1 Types of cardiomyopathies: *A*, Dilated, congestive cardiomyopathy. *B*, Hypertrophic: Left ventricular outflow tract obstruction. *C*, Restrictive: Abnormal diastolic function: rigid, fibrotic ventricular walls which restrict ventricular filling.

TABLE 23-1 **Secondary Causes**

Dilated	Hypertrophic	Restrictive
Alcohol	Genetic (heredity)	Endomyocardial fibrosis
Hypertension	Systemic hypertension	
Pregnancy		Hemochromatosis
Coxsackie B virus	Pheochromocytoma	
Arbovirus		Amyloidosis
Cobalt	Neurofibromatosis	Sarcoidosis
Adriamycin		Glycogen storage disease
Daunorubicin	Lentigenosis	
Hyperthyroidism	Friedreich's ataxia	Lymphoma
Muscular dystrophy (Duchenne type)	Norepinephrine	Neoplastic tumor
Limb girdle dystrophy		Scleroderma
Refsum's disease		Loeffler's endocarditis
Emetine		

Adapted from Wynne, J., & Braunwald, E. (1988). The cardiomyopathies and myocarditides. In E. Braunwald (Ed.), *Heart disease: A textbook of cardiovascular medicine* (3rd ed.). Philadelphia: Saunders; and Wenger, N. K. Abelmann, W. H., & Roberts, W. C. (1990). Cardiomyopathy and specific heart muscle disease. In J. W. Hurst, R. C. Schlant, C. E. Rackley, et al. (Eds.), *The heart* (7th ed.). New York: McGraw-Hill.

are affected. Table 23-1 lists some of the secondary causes of the three types of cardiomyopathy.

DILATED CARDIOMYOPATHY

The dilated type is the most common of the cardiomyopathies. The striking characteristics of this form are cardiomegaly and impairment of systolic pump function, which leads to congestive heart failure. Cardiomegaly is a result of the dilation of all four chambers which gives the heart its globular-shaped appearance. The ventricles, however, are usually more dilated than the atria. Hypertrophy may or may not coexist with dilated cardiomyopathy, but the coronary arteries are most often free of disease.

According to Goodwin and associates,[1] a variety of noncardiac disorders or conditions may cause this form of cardiomyopathy. They include alcohol use, viruses (Coxsackie B virus, polio virus, influenza), hypertension, pregnancy (occurs in last trimester or 6 months postpartum), hyperthyroidism, and pheochromocytoma. The myocardial damage caused by these secondary disorders may sometimes lead to extensive areas of fibrosis as revealed by histological examination.

Pathophysiology

The contractile function of the ventricles is impaired as the disease progresses. The inadequacy of the systolic pump leads to an elevated end-systolic volume (ESV). Poor contractility reduces the stroke volume as well as the ejection fraction.

Cardiac ouput may initially be augmented through compensatory increases in heart rate, but because of the lack of adequate cardiac reserve, cardiac output will be inadequate during exercise or in stress situations. Over time, both the atria and ventricles become dilated because of an increase in end-systolic volume; atrial dilation is due to restricted emptying of blood into the ventricle during diastole. This progressive chamber dilation and resultant increase in fiber stretch cause eventual decreases in the rate and degree of myofibril shortening. According to the law of Laplace, dilation causes greater wall tension and increased workload. This increased workload is manifested as an increase in myocardial oxygen consumption (MVo_2).

Retention of blood in the cardiac chambers due to increased end-systolic volume encourages thrombus formation which may predispose a patient to systemic or pulmonary emboli. Postmortem examination has revealed the most common sites of intracavity thrombus formation, which are (in descending order of frequency): the left ventricle, the right ventricle, the right atrial appendage, and the left atrial appendage.[1]

Dilation of the ventricles may also alter the valvular annulus and interfere with the spatial relationship of the valvular structure. These changes may cause secondary atrioventricular valvular insufficiency (regurgitation).

In the end stage of dilated cardiomyopathy, cardiac output declines. Furthermore, the right side of the heart eventually fails as well, leading to biventricular failure accompanied by the clinical manifestations of systemic and pulmonic congestion.

Data Acquisition

History

Dilated cardiomyopathy occurs most commonly in middle age and affects men more frequently than women.[1] Symptoms of cardiomyopathy are insidious. The initial insult is to the left ventricle; end-systolic volume begins to increase as does ventricular end-diastolic pressure. Progressive pulmonary symptoms are manifested as failure progresses, involving the left atrium and the pulmonary venous circulation. Dyspnea, initially on exertion, advances to orthopnea, then to paroxysmal nocturnal dyspnea (PND), and finally to dyspnea at rest. These prominent symptoms are frequently accompanied by fatigue and weakness.

Signs and symptoms of right-sided heart failure become evident in the end stage of the disease process, and include increased jugular venous distention (JVD), hepatomegaly, splenomegaly, ascites, and peripheral edema. Patients frequently complain of abdominal pain, reflecting congestion in the liver. There is danger of embolic phenomena should there be separation of mural thrombi with migration into the pulmonic or systemic circulation. The end stage of this progressive failure process is marked by pump failure or cardiogenic shock as left ventricular function is further impaired and compensatory mechanisms fail.

Physical Assessment

The patient with dilated cardiomyopathy will appear breathless on exertion, perhaps even at rest, depending on the stage of the disease. The skin may be cool, pale, and cyanosed. Peripheral edema, ascites, jugular venous distention, and pulsatile liver engorgement may be detected by palpation. Left, and occasionally right, precordial heaves may also be present, but they will differ from those commonly felt in patients with pronounced ventricular hypertrophy, the latter being more sustained. The apical impulse is usually laterally displaced as a reflection of left ventricular dilation.

S_3 and S_4 heart sounds are often present on auscultation. These sounds may fuse with rapid heart rates and form what is known as a *summation gallop*. Blood pressure auscultation frequently reveals a reduction in pulse pressure that is related to an inadequate stroke volume. There also may be systolic murmurs, reflecting mitral and/or tricuspid valve regurgitation.

Diagnostic Procedures

The chest x-ray often reveals enlargement of both ventricles and dilation of the atria. Pleural effusions, sequelae of left ventricular failure, may also be present.

Sinus tachycardia may be exhibited on the electrocardiogram (ECG). This increase in heart rate is frequently seen in the presence of ventricular failure and is due to compensatory mechanisms aimed at augmenting cardiac ouput when stroke volume declines. Various atrioventricular conduction disturbances may also be evident, as well as left bundle branch block and supraventricular and ventricular tachyarrhythmias. Atrial fibrillation, a common supraventricular tachyarrhythmia, has been found in approximately 25% of patients with documented dilated cardiomyopathy.[1]

The appearance of pathological Q waves may indicate the presence of extensive left ventricular fibrosis as opposed to necrosis. When Q waves are seen in these patients, however, coexisting myocardial infarction should be ruled out. The patient with cardiomyopathy may evidence abnormalities of the ST segment and T waves on the ECG. Chamber enlargement and axis deviation are often noted as well. Pul-

sus alternans, a morbid sign, indicates severe left ventricular failure.

The echocardiogram may reveal an enlarged ventricular cavity with poor left ventricular free wall movement related to the progression of the disease. In addition, there may be concomitant dyssynergy of the septum and regurgitant valvular lesions caused by alterations in the valve structure. Moreover, two-dimensional echocardiography is useful in detecting thrombi in the cardiac chambers.

Left ventricular function is generally assessed by radionuclide techniques. Ventricular ejection fraction and end-systolic and end-diastolic volumes are useful in evaluating disease progression and the response to therapy.[3] Left ventricular function may also be assessed by echocardiography.

Cardiac status may be directly assessed using invasive methods commonly employed in the cardiac catheterization laboratory. Catheterization of the heart of patients in end-stage dilated cardiomyopathy reveals elevated volumes and pressures on both sides of the heart, reflecting biventricular failure. Both the left ventricular ejection fraction and cardiac output are decreased in dilated cardiomyopathy. Left ventriculography depicts enlargement of the chamber and abnormal wall motion. If thrombi are present in the ventricles, they may be visualized as a filling defect, and mitral regurgitation may also be observed.

Some investigators have employed the technique of transvenous myocardial biopsy to evaluate patients with dilated cardiomyopathy.[4] Additional use of transvenous myocardial biopsy is to determine efficacy of corticosteroids in patients with inflammatory causes of dilated cardiomyopathy.[5]

Medical Management

Medical treatment of dilated cardiomyopathy is palliative rather than curative. Treatment is aimed at alleviating the symptoms of congestive heart failure, improving stroke volume, preventing thromboembolic complications, and maintaining normal conduction. These end points become the collaborative problems that both medicine and nursing work toward achieving.

Cardiac glycosides, such as digoxin, are used for their positive inotropic effects. Corticosteroids are also used, but their value in management of this type of cardiomyopathy remains controversial. They have been found useful in treating patients with subacute myocarditis and dilated cardiomyopathy secondary to autoimmmune disorders, but reports in the literature reveal them to be of little or no value in treatment of established dilated cardiomyopathy.[6]

Diuretics are employed to decrease blood volume in patients in failure, and anticoagulation therapy is used to prevent systemic and pulmonary embolism. When tachdysrhythmias are poorly tolerated by the patient, antidysrhythmic agents are used. Lethal ventricular dysrhythmias are frequently noted in patients with dilated cardiomyopathy and are treated aggressively with antidysrhythmic agents.[7] When the ECG reveals serious atrioventricular or intraventricular conduction defects, a pacemaker may be required.

Sympathetic overstimulation has been suggested as a feature of dilated cardiomyopathy. Beta-adrenergic blocking agents have been used to: (1) reduce myocardial energy requirements; (2) improve compliance; and (3) lower arterial pressure by decreasing the force of systolic contraction. However, the reduction in contractility and increase in left ventricular volume by beta blockers in the dilated cardiomyopathy patient may decrease with efficacy.[8]

Use of vasodilator therapy, to lessen symptoms of failure and increase exercise tolerance is advocated by some authorities.[9] Vasodilators are classified according to action site. Arteriolar vasodilators, such as hydralazine and nifedipine, decrease arteriolar resistance and lessen impedance to ejection (afterload). With reduced impedance the left ventricle may empty its contents with less energy expenditure; thus, MVO_2 consumption is reduced.

Venodilators decrease filling pressure (preload) by redistributing intravascular volume from the central to the peripheral vasculature. By redistributing venous volume the signs and symptoms of pulmonary congestion may be relieved. Nitrates are the more commonly used of the venodilators.

Balanced vasodilators, such as nitroprusside, prazosin, and captopril, have both arteriolar and venule effects. Their action is to reduce both afterload and preload. Vasodilator therapy is contraindicated when systolic blood pressure levels are below 100 mmHg, and in the presence of cardiogenic shock.[1]

Diltiazem, a calcium channel blocker, administered in conjunction with conventional therapy of digoxin, diuretics, and vasodilators has demonstrated symptomatic improvement in patients with dilated cardiomyopathy. The reduction in myocellular calcium causing a vasodilatory action, and reduction in contractility and heart rate by diltiazem enhance the action of the vasodilator and digoxin.[10]

Although no clear data have demonstrated the efficacy of angiotensin converting enzyme inhibitors (ACE inhibitors) in dilated cardiomyopathy, the report of the Cooperative North Scandinavian Enalapril Survival Study (CONSENSUS) strongly supports the use of enalapril in end-stage congestive heart failure. In the CONSENSUS study, enalapril significantly improved the prognosis of patients in NYHA grade IV heart failure.[7]

Myocardial contractility may be enhanced through use of such positive inotropic agents as amrinone, dopamine, and dobutamine. Both metabolic and hemodynamic advantages, such as increases in cardiac output and coronary blood flow have resulted from infusing dobutamine or amrinone over a short period into patients with dilated cardiomyopathy.[11,12] Home dobutamine infusions may be safely administered in end-stage dilated cardiomyopathy as in end-stage congestive heart failure. This therapy provides an alternative to hospitalization in patients who cannot be weaned from the drug.[13]

Physiological dual-chamber pacing in patients whose end-stage dilated cardiomyopathy has become refractory to medical therapy has demonstrated improvement in clinical symptoms. This mode of pacing reduced preload, improved systolic and diastolic blood pressure, and normalized heart rate.[14]

The only surgical treatment for end-stage dilated cardiomyopathy is cardiac transplantation. Mitral valve replacement may be used as a palliative measure for patients with concomitant mitral regurgitation, which may provide temporary relief of congestion.

NURSING MANAGEMENT

Patients with dilated cardiomyopathy typically experience many admissions to critical care units during the course of the disease. According to Wold,[15] severe congestive heart failure, emboli, or dysrhythmias are the reasons for most admissions; these require vigorous intervention by the health care team. In addition to implementing the various treatments, the nurse is involved with guiding the patient and significant others in dealing with the human responses generated by this devastating disease.

Data from the patient's history, the nursing and medical physical examinations, laboratory evaluations, and other diagnostic tests form a database upon which a personalized nursing care plan is formulated. Data acquisition using the functional health patterns assessment described in Chapter 21 is begun as soon as possible after patient is admitted to the critical care unit. Critical data that should be retrieved during the inverview process include:

1. Description of dyspneic episodes and the measures that the patient has used to relieve the symptoms, as well as the situations that exacerbate them
2. The level of physical activity that the patient is capable of attaining
3. Dietary habits, including sodium and fluid intake
4. Medical history, especially hypertension, dysrhythmias, diabetes, and thyroid disease
5. Medications currently taken
6. Smoking habits

7. Alcohol consumption (alcohol could be the etiology of this form of cardiomyopathy)
8. Recent pregnancy, if applicable (another etiological factor of this disease)
9. Patterns of sleep
10. Recent weight gain or loss

The data obtained from physical examination by the nurse should focus on the patient's overall cardiovascular status. Specific attention should be paid to inspection of general skin color, posture, pattern and depth of breathing, presence of ascites, peripheral edema, nail-bed changes, a tendency to use accessory muscles for breathing, the presence of jugular venous distention, muscle atrophy, and poor skin turgor.

Heart sounds, breath sounds, blood pressure, and bowel sounds should be auscultated. Palpation should include the location of the apical impulse, verification of heaves, abdominal distention, and peripheral pulses.

The complete database also includes nursing assessment of the level of factual awareness possessed by the patient and significant others regarding the disease. The plan of care should include periodic evaluation of the level of comprehension to avoid unnecessary anxiety and confusion. Moreover, the nurse must frequently evaluate the psychosocial impact of the disease on the patient and significant others.

Once the data from the nursing assessment, physical examination, and diagnostic tests are obtained, the nurse has a complete biopsychosocial database from which to identify nursing diagnoses, which may be treated independently within the practice of nursing. The formulation of a plan of care aimed at minimizing or preventing these problems directs specific interventions and outcome criteria.

Nursing diagnoses for the patient with dilated cardiomyopathy are classified into actual and high-risk problems.

■ **NURSING DIAGNOSIS**

Activity intolerance, related to fatigue secondary to limited cardiac reserve and lack of knowledge regarding energy conservation measures.

OUTCOME STANDARD AND CRITERIA

Activity level prescribed is tolerated as evidenced by:
- Decreased fatigue and heart rate
- Increase in respiratory rate and blood pressure appropriate to level of activity
- Verbalization of factors that increase fatigue
- Demonstration of ability to take pulse during activity

NURSING INTERVENTIONS
- Initiate a schedule of activities that includes bed to chair for at least 20 minutes tid to prevent further deconditioning
- Help patient prioritize activities he or she values the most to achieve realistic goals
- Develop progressive activity regimen with patient and significant others including physical therapy and occupation therapy, aimed at increasing patient's functional capacity
- Consult physical therapist (PT) for exercise training after discharge
- Consult occupational therapist (OT) for energy conservation activities
- Measure the patient's heart rate, blood pressure, respiratory rate, and emotional tolerance; and assess his or her ECG pattern before and after incremental increases in activity level
- Implement active and passive range-of-motion exercises
- Plan adequate rest periods to decrease energy expenditure
- Assess patient's readiness for instruction of energy conservation measures
- Teach the patient how to assess pulse rate during activities

■ **NURSING DIAGNOSIS**

Impaired gas exchange, related to excess fluid retention.

OUTCOME STANDARD AND CRITERIA

Gas exchange will improve as evidenced by:
- Stable or improved ABGs with a decreased FiO_2 requirement
- A decrease or absence of crackles on auscultation
- Absence of an S_3
- Stable weight
- Decreased amount of tissue edema
- Equal or negative fluid balance
- Optimal cardiac output

NURSING INTERVENTIONS
- Monitor and report alterations in heart rate, blood pressure, pulmonary artery diastolic and/or wedge pressure, level of consciousness, urine output, arterial blood gases, and fluid balance
- Examine for tissue edema by palpation and note abnormalities
- Examine the jugular veins for distention and report increased distention
- Auscultate the lung fields for signs of pulmonary congestion and report increasing signs of congestion
- Assess hepatojugular reflux
- Auscultate the heart for an S_3, which is indicative of failure
- Weigh the patient daily at the same time and on the same scale to assess fluid status
- Monitor the patient's response to prescribed diuretic therapy
- Consult with dietitian for specific food and beverage restrictions

- Restrict fluids as prescribed
- Administer vasodilator therapy as prescribed, and monitor effectiveness
- Administer positive inotropic agents as prescribed and monitor effectiveness
- Assess the patient's and significant others' readiness for instruction regarding prescribed dietary and fluid restrictions

HIGH-RISK NURSING DIAGNOSES

Patients with a diagnosis of dilated cardiomyopathy are more vulnerable to develop the following nursing diagnoses:

- High risk for powerlessness, related to the patient's and significant others' response to chronic illness
- High risk for fear, related to the patient's and significant others' response to uncertain prognosis and progressive nature of condition
- High risk for sleep pattern disturbances, related to excess fluid volume, fear and depression, and the critical care environment
- High risk for injury, related to the use of numerous pharmacological agents
- High risk for ineffective individual and family coping, related to the patient's and significant others' response to the uncertainty of the chronic disease process
- High risk alteration in health maintenance, related to knowledge deficit

Management of the patient with dilated cardiomyopathy presents a particular challenge to the critical care nurse. The patient leaves the critical care unit following resolution of perhaps only one of a series of acute episodes. But the underlying disease persists. Thus, the patient and significant others are dependent on a continuity of both the physical and supportive care provided by critical care practitioners.

HYPERTROPHIC CARDIOMYOPATHY

Hypertrophic cardiomyopathy (HC) has been described by many names, primarily in relation to its pathological characteristics or clinical features. In the United States it has been known until recently as idiopathic hypertrophic subaortic stenosis (IHSS). It has also been known as hypertrophic obstructive cardiomyopathy (HOCM), asymmetrical septal hypertrophy (ASH), and muscular aortic stenosis.

The classic definition of HC is that of a disease of unknown etiology that is characterized by a hypertrophied, nondilated ventricle in the absence of a cardiac or systemic disease that could produce left ventricular hypertrophy.[16]

Pathophysiology

The primary abnormalities that characterize HC are thickening of the ventricular septum greater than the left ventricular free wall, and disorganization of the myocardial fibers within the ventricular septum. Secondary abnormalities associated with HC include: (1) a fibrous plaque on the mural endocardium of the outflow portions of the septum, (2) a decrease in ventricular cavity size or a lack of ventricular dilation related to the hypertrophy of the septum and the left ventricular free wall's (LVFW) inability to distend outward, (3) anterior and posterior mitral valve thickening in response to the small ventricular cavity, and (4) left atrial dilation in adults in response to the increased ventricular filling pressure.[1]

Varying patterns of hypertrophy occur within the ventricular septum which may include portions of the anterolateral LVFW. These patterns range from hypertrophy that affects all regions of the left ventricle except the basal anterior ventricular septum (Figure 23-2). The most common form of hypertrophy involves a substantial portion of ventricular septum and anterolateral LVFW. This form is most commonly associated with individuals who experience moderate to severe obstruction of the left ventricular outflow tract.

The etiology underlying the disorganization of the myocardial fibers of the ventricular septum is unclear. This disorganization and disarray has been noted in other diseases as well as in normal hearts, but the extent of cellular involvement is much greater in HC than in other cases. Two theories concerning the etiol-

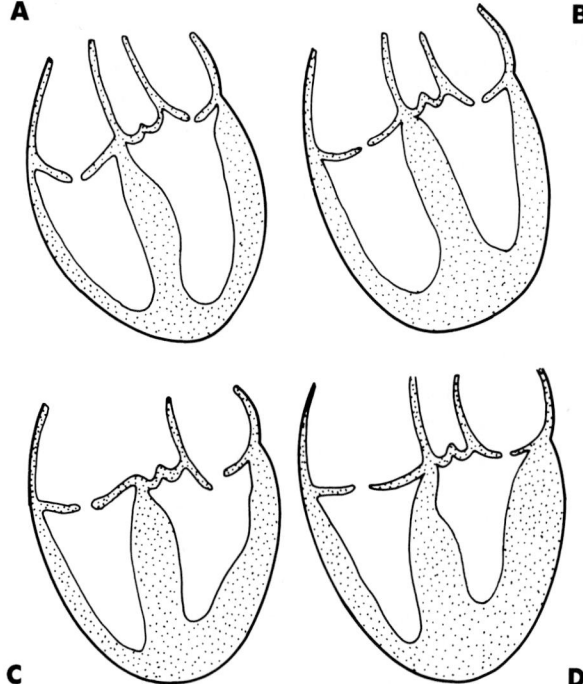

Figure 23-2 Types of hypertrophy. *A,* Type 1: Hypertrophy of anterior septum. *B,* Type 2: Hypertrophy of entire septum. *C,* Type 3: Hypertrophy of the septum and anterior-lateral LVFW. *D,* Type 4: Hypertrophy of septum and LVFW except the basal anterior septum.

ogy of the myofibril disarray have been proposed. The first is that there is a congenital aberration of catecholamine function in the embryonic heart.[1] The second theory is that a primary abnormality of collagen leads to an abnormal and disorganized fibrous skeleton that in turn leads to the cellular disarray.[2]

Both the fibrous mural plaque and thickening of the mitral valve appear to result from trauma of the anterior mitral leaflet apposing the septum during systole. This defect is generally correlated with both a dynamic increase in the left ventricular outflow gradient in obstruction[17] and systolic anterior motion of the mitral valve.[18] Systolic anterior motion (SAM) is validated by echocardiogram and is depicted as the posterior leaflet coapting with a midportion of the anterior leaflet in the left ventricle during systole. Many individuals have some degree of mitral regurgitation related to SAM or to the abnormal bending and pulling of the papillary muscles from hypertrophy, especially when occurring in the anterolateral area.

The interaction of the asymmetric hypertrophy within the left ventricle with the chaotic architecture of the myofibrils produces several hemodynamic changes in the left ventricle. Venticular compliance decreases, diastolic filling volume increases, and the pressure gradient across the outflow tract is elevated when obstruction is present. The decreased ventricular compliance produces a prolonged diastolic filling time. The isovolumetric relaxation period is prolonged due to a delay in opening of the mitral valve. Opening of the mitral valve is hindered by the slow rate of reduction of left ventricular pressure. The rapid filling period is prolonged because the end-diastolic period is shortened. Finally, the initial systolic contraction is rapid and powerful, expelling the majority of the stroke volume in the first half of systole.[1]

Data Acquisition

Individuals with HC initially seek medical attention with a history of dyspnea, angina, palpitations, dizziness, or syncope. A few individuals remain asymptomatic but experience sudden death prior to diagnosis. The event that precedes the sudden death is unknown. Studies indicate that the prevalence of sudden death is higher among individuals with HC and asymptomatic ventricular tachycardia (VT) as compared to those with HC but without VT as recorded by Holter monitoring.[19,20] In one reported case, however, a 52-year-old woman with HC was monitored during a syncopal episode and found to have lost the left ventricular outflow tract murmur. She had an unrecordable blood pressure, suggesting that a hemodynamic mechanism that reduces left ventricular volume may be the primary cause of death.[20]

Individuals with HC are often active, athletic people whose condition is diagnosed during young adulthood.[1] The presence of a pressure gradient is indicated on physical examination by three dominant signs. A systolic murmur of late onset is auscultated at the left sternal border and apex and radiates to the axilla. The murmur is increased by standing or performing a Valsalva maneuver. The systolic murmur reflects the late onset of a left ventricular outflow gradient and mitral regurgitation. The arterial pulse is abrupt and ill-sustained and has a jerky quality due to the powerful initial contraction followed by a collapse in pressure from the obstruction. Turbulent blood flow through the left ventricular outflow obstruction may also produce a thrill on palpation.

The electrocardiogram in HC reflects ventricular hypertrophy and atrial abnormality. These abnormalities are depicted as an increase in QRS voltage and the depressed T wave of left ventricular hypertrophy. Additional ECG abnormalities noted are Q waves in the inferior and left precordial leads, left anterior hemiblock, left atrial enlargement, a short PR interval, and asymptomatic ventricular dysrhythmias.[19] Atrial fibrillation is present in approximately 20% of patients.

Echocardiography, which includes the standard M-mode and the wide-angle, two-dimensional mechanism, has been used to identify the extent and regions of hypertrophy noninvasively. Findings on the echocardiogram may reveal a dilated atrium, septal hypertrophy, a narrowed LV outflow tract, and an abnormality of the anterior mitral valve leaflet. Magnetic resonance imaging may be used in concert with the echocardiogram to specify the areas of hypertrophy noninvasively.[21]

Cardiac catheterization is the definitive test used to diagnose HC and to evaluate the extent of obstruction when present. Endomyocardial biopsy of the left ventricular muscle performed during the cardiac catheterization is a further adjunct in diagnosing HC.

A gated blood-pool imaging scan may be performed to determine the functional type of cardiomyopathy and myocardial perfusion. Furthermore, the use of thallium-201 on single photon emission computed tomographic scintigraphy is helpful in identifying septal abnormalities and progression in myocardial disease.[22]

Medical Management

Treatment protocols pertinent to the patient with HC are directed toward relief of symptoms and prevention of complications. The underlying pathophysiology of the disease provides the guideline for treatment. Interventions that increase or maintain left ventricular end-diastolic volume and reduce ventricular contractility are generally employed.

The primary pharmacological therapy is beta-adrenergic blockade. Beta-adrenergic blockers (1) inhibit inotropic and chronotropic actions; (2) prolong cardiac diastole, thereby decreasing contractility; (3) decrease myocardial oxygen consumption; (4) improve the distensibility of the left ventricle; and (5) increase diastolic filling time.

Calcium channel blocking agents, specifically verapamil, nifedipine, and diltiazem, are used as an alternative to beta-adrenergic blockade in the long-term management of HC. Verapamil is the more widely studied agent in HC. It has been found to produce significant increases in left ventricular stroke volume, a decreased heart rate, and increased exercise tolerance through increased diastolic filling.[23] Unfortunately, serious side effects can cause suppression of the SA node and inhibition of the AV node, vasodilation, and a negative inotropic action. These properties may lead to hypotension and an increase in obstruction, pulmonary edema, and death.[24] Nifedipine has a greater vasodilatory effect and produces fewer conduction disturbances than verapamil. Studies describing clinical improvement using nifedipine are inconsistent.[25] Diltiazem has been shown to improve left ventricular relaxation and diastolic filling time without altering left ventricular systolic function.[26]

In those patients who exhibit frequent ventricular ectopy or ventricular tachycardia, amiodarone has been shown to decrease the frequency of atrial and ventricular tachyarrhythmias.[27] In addition, amiodarone has a weak beta-adrenergic blocking effect. Unfortunately, the drug's onset of action is 5 to 10 days, and cumulative effects may result.

Until recently atrial fibrillation was regarded as a medical emergency in patients with HC because of the loss of atrial kick and tachycardia reducing left ventricular volume. A study by Robinson and associates[28] demonstrated that patients with atrial fibrillation who were treated with conventional drug therapy on amiodarone had a mortality similar to that of patients in sinus rhythm.

In severe disease, the treatment of congestive heart failure is difficult. Digoxin and diuretics are contraindicated in the early stage because of the obstruction; however, these are used because there is little risk of provoking further obstruction. The goal of treatment, then, is to decrease the congestive failure. When medical management is ineffective, surgical interventions such as septal myotomy-myectomy or mitral valve replacement may reduce the outflow obstruction.[1] In one study, patients treated by partial septal myectomy were observed over 10 to 20 years. It was reported that in 26 of 36 surviving patients, the surgery relieved the obstruction and mitral regurgitation and concomitantly reduced symptoms.[29] Although mitral valve replacement has been advocated, the myotomy-myec-

tomy alone has become the surgical procedure of choice.[2] The myotomy-myectomy procedure appears to reduce symptoms but has not shown to improve long-term survival when compared with medical therapy.[25]

Protection from infective endocarditis with antibiotic prophylaxis is indicated in patients with HC both before and after a surgical procedure. It has been reported that approximately 50% of individuals with HC without prophylactic antibiotic therapy develop infections involving the mitral and aortic valves.[30]

Progressive depressed LV function is often refractory to medical and surgical therapies. Many patients may be considered candidates for cardiac transplantation.[25]

NURSING MANAGEMENT

The individual with HC who enters the critical care area may be categorized as: (1) newly diagnosed, having recently incurred angina or a "sudden death" episode; (2) admitted to the hospital for other medical or surgical problems for which HC is a complicating factor; or (3) having progressive disease in which congestive heart failure is being treated. Depending upon the category or stage of diagnosis, some of the nursing diagnoses may change.

Initially, a nursing history needs to be completed which focuses on: (1) the presenting symptoms, (2) time and duration of symptoms, (3) associated factors with onset of symptoms and relieving techniques of the symptoms, (4) background knowledge concerning the disease, (5) family history, (6) contributing diseases, (7) medications, (8) type of work or employment, (9) position in family, (10) hobbies, and (11) coping mechanisms. A physical examination including vital signs, pulse characteristics, ECG, and heart sounds indicates the clinical manifestations of HC.

■ NURSING DIAGNOSIS

Altered health maintenance, related to knowledge deficit regarding activity intolerance, outflow tract obstruction, medications, and energy conservation measures.

OUTCOME STANDARD AND CRITERIA

Health maintenance is normal as evidenced by:
- Verbalization of reduced chest pain, syncope, and shortness of breath during activity
- Verbalization of methods to decrease obstruction and undesirable side effects of prescribed medications
- Demonstration of methods to reduce obstruction
- Demonstration of health behaviors needed to manage condition
- Knowledge of signs and symptoms that should be reported to health care team

NURSING INTERVENTIONS
- Instruct patient on signs and symptoms of activity

intolerance, taking pulse rate during activity
- Instruct patient in methods of reducing LV outflow tract obstruction, such as avoiding dehydration, strenuous exercise, straining or Valsalva, very hot environments, and rapidly rising to a standing position
- Instruct patients regarding the potential side effects of prescribed medications
- Assess readiness for instruction in reducing exercise and physical work through energy conservation measures

■ **NURSING DIAGNOSIS**

Ineffective coping, related to fear of chronic fatal disease and sense of vulnerability.

OUTCOME STANDARD AND CRITERIA

Coping is effective as evidenced by:
- Verbalization of fears
- Demonstration of positive coping methods for stress reduction
- Identification of support system
- Identification of personal strengths and weaknesses and acceptance of emotional support from nursing staff and health care team
- Absence of ineffective coping behaviors

NURSING INTERVENTIONS
- Assess individual's present coping status as evidenced by ability to relate facts and verbalize feelings regarding disease
- Keep lines of communication open among patient, significant others, and staff
- Identify patient's positive support system
- Explore patient's and significant others' stress-reducing coping methods that have been useful in the past
- Assess the patient's and significant others' readiness for instruction in methods of stress reduction
- Assist patient in problem-solving techniques
- Provide support and reinforcement of adaptive behavior, such as problem solving, ability to make decisions
- Consult with significant others regarding desire for CPR training
- Consult and refer to appropriate professionals (e.g., chaplain, social service, psychologist, psychiatrist)
- Identify factors that hinder patient's ability to cope with disease

HIGH-RISK NURSING DIAGNOSES

Patients with a diagnosis of hypertrophic cardiomyopathy are more vulnerable to the same high-risk nursing diagnoses previously discussed under Dilated Cardiomyopathy. Two additional high-risk diagnoses pertain to the fact that, as a group, these patients tend to be active, athletic young adults, and the diagnosis of HC may necessitate changes in lifestyle. Therefore, the high-risk nursing diagnoses for such a cluster of patients include:

- High risk for noncompliance with medical therapy, related to a change in lifestyle.
- High risk for ineffective coping (significant others and/or patient), related to change in lifestyle and body image.

RESTRICTIVE CARDIOMYOPATHY

Restrictive cardiomyopathy, an infiltrative disorder of the myocardium, is not commonly seen. It resembles constrictive pericarditis in clinical presentation. The distinguishing characteristic of restrictive cardiomyopathy is an abnormal diastolic function resulting from abnormal cardiac stiffness. This abnormal diastolic filling leads to a decrease in cardiac output and eventual heart failure.

Pathophysiology

Many specific pathological processes may develop into restrictive cardiomyopathy, including myocardial fibrosis, hypertrophy, or infiltration, but the cause is often unknown (idiopathic). These processes increase rigidity of the ventricular walls and impede ventricular filling. Secondarily, restrictive cardiomyopathy may be caused by amyloidosis, hemochromatosis, glycogen deposition, endomyocardial fibrosis, fibroelastoses, neoplastic infiltration and pseudoxanthoma elasticum.[2]

The clinical and hemodynamic features of restrictive cardiomyopathy and constrictive pericarditis are similar but not the same. According to one authority, the left ventricular end-diastolic pressure in restrictive cardiomyopathy is greater than the right ventricular end-diastolic pressure, while in constrictive pericarditis both pressures are equal.[31] Restrictive cardiomyopathy does not demonstrate the extent of the deep and rapid early decline in ventricular pressure at the onset of diastole or the square root sign as in constrictive pericarditis. Finally, the left ventricular relaxation period is prolonged in restrictive cardiomyopathy but remains normal in constrictive pericarditis.[32] Table 23-2 summarizes the differentiating characteristics of restrictive cardiomyopathy from constrictive pericarditis.

Data Acquisition

Individuals with restrictive cardiomyopathy commonly present with chest pain, dyspnea on exertion, and fatigue resulting from pulmonary congestion and diminished cardiac output. Exercise tolerance is limited because of the heart's inability to increase cardiac output. In advanced cases, an elevated central venous pressure and pulmonary artery pressure are present. Atrial pressure waveforms have a prominent y descent followed by a rapid rise and plateau, and the a wave is of equal amplitude to the v wave.[33] Jugular venous distention, peripheral edema, ascites, anasarca, and

TABLE 23-2   **Characteristics Differentiating Restrictive Cardiomyopathy from Constrictive Pericarditis**

	Restrictive Cardiomyopathy	Constrictive Pericarditis
Ventricular end-diastolic volume	Left > right	Equal
Square root sign	+ + + +	+ +
Left ventricular relaxation time	Prolonged	Normal
Left ventricular mass	Increased	Normal
Biatrial size	Increased	Normal
Left ventricular filling rate	+ +	+ + + +
Diastolic thinning of posterior wall	+ + + +	+ +
Interval between minimum cavity size and mitral valve opening	Prolonged	Normal

+ = increased.

hepatomegaly may be noted. A concomitant S_3 or S_4 sound is commonly auscultated, with mitral valve and tricuspid valve regurgitation murmurs frequently noted.

The electrocardiogram frequently shows sinus tachycardia, which is a compensatory mechanism to maintain cardiac output. Atrial fibrillation occurs frequently with atrial dilation. Biventricular hypertrophy with decreased voltage is also seen. High-degree AV blocks occur with amyloid diseases.

The echocardiogram differentiates restrictive cardiomyopathy from other cardiomyopathies or constrictive pericarditis.[34] Findings from the echocardiogram may include: (1) an enlarged atrium (caused by increased LV filling pressure), (2) increased ventricular wall size, (3) pericardial effusion, and (4) decreased ventricular chamber resulting from hypertrophied walls. Embolic phenomenon and the degree of ventricular stiffness can be seen as well. Radionuclide imaging techniques differentiate the systolic and diastolic function of the ventricles, including volumes and the ejection fraction. Cardiac catheterization defines the hemodynamic features and ventricular dynamics particular to restrictive cardiomyopathy.

Endomyocardial biopsy is sometimes used to further distinguish restrictive cardiomyopathy from constrictive pericarditis.[35]

Medical Management

The medical treatment for restrictive cardiomyopathy is similar to that for congestive heart failure. Treatment is symptom limiting and focuses on fluid restriction, diuretic therapy, anticoagulation, and digitalization if atrial fibrillation is present. Paracentesis

may relieve pressure from ascites. When recurrent pericardial effusion occurs, pericardioperitoneal shunts have relieved tamponade.

Surgical treatment of restrictive cardiomyopathy is that of resection of thickened endocardial tissue. Mitral and tricuspid valve replacement is done when needed. Acute symptoms have been relieved with these surgical procedures, but long-term effectiveness is uncertain. Placement of a permanent pacemaker is done to relieve AV blocks when they occur.

Nursing Management

As with the other cardiomyopathies, a careful and complete nursing history and physical examination guide the nurse in formulating nursing diagnoses, goals, and interventions. The primary nursing diagnosis common for patients with restrictive cardiomyopathy is activity intolerance related to fatigue, but this type is secondary to restrictive diastolic filling. The high-risk diagnosis is congestive heart failure related to restrictive diastolic filling. The nursing interventions are the same as previously discussed in the dilated cardiomyopathy section.

REFERENCES

1. Wenger, N. K., Abelmann, W. H., & Roberts, W. C. (1990). Cardiomyopathy and specific heart muscle disease. In J. W. Hurst, R. C. Schlant, C. E. Rackley, et al. (Eds.), *The heart* (7th ed.). New York: McGraw-Hill.
2. Wynne, J., & Braunwald, E. (1988). The cardiomyopathies and myocarditides. In E. Braunwald (Ed.), *Heart disease: A textbook of cardiovascular medicine* (3rd ed.). Philadelphia: Saunders.
3. Goldman, M. R., & Boucher, C. A. (1980). Value of radionuclide imaging techniques in assessing cardiomyopathy. *American Journal of Cardiology, 46,* 1232-1236.
4. Parrillo, J. E., Aretz, H. T., Palacios, I., et al. (1984). The results of transvenous endomyocardial biopsy can frequently be used to diagnose myocardial diseases in patients with idiopathic heart failure. *Circulation, 69*(11), 93-101.
5. Hobbs, R. E., Pelegrin, D., Ratcliff, N. B., et al. (1989). Lymphocytic myocarditis and dilated cardiomyopathy: Treatment with immunosuppressive agents. *Cleveland Clinic Journal of Medicine, 56,* 628-635.
6. Latham, R. D., Mulrow, J. P., Virmani, R., et al. (1989). Recently diagnosed idiopathic dilated cardiomyopathy: Incidence of myocarditis and efficacy of prednisone therapy. *American Heart Journal, 117,* 876-882.
7. Caforio, A. L. P., Stewart, J. T., & McKenna, W. J. (1990). Idiopathic dilated cardiomyopathy. *British Medical Journal, 300,* 890-891.
8. Goodwin, J. F. (1988). Overview and classification of the cardiomyopathies. In J. A. Shaver (Ed.), *Cardio-*

myopathies: Clinical presentation, differential diagnosis, and management. Philadelphia: Davis.

9. Camerini, F., Mestroni, L., Neri, R., et al. (1984). Vasodilators in left ventricular failure. *Italian Cardiology, 14,* 685-693.

10. Figulla, H. R., Rechenberg, J. V., Wiegand, V., et al. (1990). Beneficial effects of long-term diltiazem treatment in dilated cardiomyopathy. *Journal of the American College of Cardiology, 13,* 653-658.

11. Marcus, R. H., Raw, K., Patel, J., et al. (1990). Comparison of intravenous amrinone and dobutamine in congestive heart failure due to idiopathic dilated cardiomyopathy. *American Journal of Cardiology, 66,* 1107-1112.

12. Unverferth, D. V., Margorien, R. D., Altshuld, R., et al. (1983). The hemodynamic and metabolic advantages gained by a three-day infusion of dobutamine in patients with congestive cardiomyopathy. *American Heart Journal, 106,* 29-34.

13. Miller, L. W., Merkle, E. J., & Herrmann, V. (1990). Outpatient dobutamine for end-stage congestive heart failure. *Critical Care Medicine, 18*(Suppl.), S-30-S-33.

14. Hochleitner, M., Hörtnagl, H., Ng, C., et al. (1990). Usefulness of physiologic dual-chamber pacing in drug-resistant idiopathic dilated cardiomyopathy. *American Journal of Cardiology, 66,* 198-202.

15. Wold, B. (1983). Dilated cardiomyopathy: Considerations for the coronary care nurse. *Heart Lung, 12,* 544-553.

16. Goodwin, J. F. (1974). Prospects and predictions for the cardiomyopathies. *Circulation, 50,* 210-219.

17. Shah, P. M., Taylor, R. D., & Wong, M. (1981). Abnormal mitral valve coaptation in hypertrophic obstructive cardiomyopathy: Proposed role in systolic anterior motion of the mitral valve. *American Journal of Cardiology, 48,* 258-262.

18. Pollick, C., Rakowski, H., & Wigle, E. D. (1984). Muscular subaortic stenosis: The quantitative relationship between systolic anterior motion and the pressure gradient. *Circulation, 69,* 43-49.

19. Maron, B. J., Savage, D. D., Wolfson, J. K., et al. (1981). Prognostic significance of 24-hour ambulatory electrocardiographic monitoring in patients with hypertrophic cardiomyopathy: A prospective study. *American Journal of Cardiology, 48,* 252-257.

20. McKenna, W., Harris, L., & Deanfield, J. (1982). Syncope in hypertrophic cardiomyopathy. *British Heart Journal, 47,* 177-179.

21. Higgins, C. B., Byrd, B. F., III, Stark, D., et al. (1985). Magnetic resonance imaging in hypertrophic cardiomyopathy. *American Journal of Cardiology, 55,* 1121-1126.

22. Fine, D. G., Clements, I. P., & Callahan, M. J. (1989). Myocardial stunning in hypertrophic cardiomyopathy: Recovery predicted by single photon emission computed tomographic thallium-201 scintigraphy. *Journal of the American College of Cardiology, 13,* 1415-1418.

23. Hanrath, P., Schluter, M., Sonntag, F., et al. (1983). Influence of verapamil therapy on left ventricular performance at rest and during exercise in hypertrophic cardiomyopathy. *American Journal of Cardiology, 52,* 544-548.

24. Epstein, S. E., & Rosing, D. R. (1981). Verapamil: Its potential for causing serious complications in patients with hypertrophic cardiomyopathy. *Circulation, 64,* 437-441.

25. Bonow, R. O., Maron, B. J., Leon, M. B., et al. (1988). Medical and surgical therapy of hypertrophic cardiomyopathy. In J. A. Shaver (Ed.), *Cardiomyopathies: Clinical presentation, differential diagnosis, and management.* Philadelphia: Davis.

26. Suwa, M., Hirota, Y., & Kawamura, K. (1984). Improvement in left ventricular diastolic function during intravenous and oral diltiazem treatment in patients with hypertrophic cardiomyopathy: An echocardiographic study. *Amerian Journal of Cardiology, 54,* 1047-1053.

27. McKenna, W. J., Harris, L., Rowland, E., et al. (1984). Amiodarone for long-term management of patients with hypertrophic cardiomyopathy. *American Journal of Cardiology, 54,* 802-810.

28. Robinson, K., Frenneaux, M. P., Stockins, B., et al. (1990). Atrial fibrillation in hypertrophic cardiomyopathy: A longitudinal study. *Journal of the American College of Cardiology, 15,* 1279-1285.

29. Beahrs, M. M., Tajik, A. J., Seward, J. B., et al. (1983). Hypertrophic obstructive cardiomyopathy: Ten to twenty-one year follow up after partial septal myectomy. *American Journal of Cardiology, 51,* 1160-1166.

30. Chagnac, A., Rudniki, C., Loebel, H., et al. (1982). Infectious endocarditis in idiopathic hypertrophic subaortic stenosis: Report of three cases and review of literature. *Chest, 81,* 346-349.

31. Hirota, Y., Kohriyama, T., Hayashi, T., et al. (1983). Idiopathic restrictive cardiomyopathy: Differences of left ventricular relaxation and diastolic waveforms from constrictive pericarditis. *American Journal of Cardiology, 52,* 421-423.

32. Francis, V. R., Paulsen, W. H. J., Sagar, K. B., et al. (1985). Improved echocardiographic differentiation of restrictive cardiomyopathy from constrictive pericarditis. *Circulation, 72*(4) (Suppl. III), III-355.

33. Benotti, J. R., Grossman, W., & Cohn, P. F. (1980). Clinical profile of restrictive cardiomyopathy. *Circulation, 61,* 1206-1212.

34. Lekakis, J., Schick, E., Falk, R., et al. (1985). Left ventricular diastolic function in differentiating constrictive pericarditis and restrictive cardiomyopathy. *Circulation, 72*(4) (Suppl. III), III-355.

35. Schoenfeld, M. H., Supple, E. W., Dec, W. W., et al. (1985). Restrictive cardiomyopathy versus constrictive pericarditis: Role of endomyocardial biopsy in avoiding unnecessary thoracotomy. *Circulation, 72*(4) (Suppl. III), III-355.

24

Valvular Heart Disease

Joan Vitello-Cicciu

Diane Panton Lapsley

ACUTE RHEUMATIC FEVER AND RHEUMATIC HEART DISEASE

Acute rheumatic fever is a systemic connective tissue disease in which damage occurs to the collagen fibrils and to the ground substance of connective tissue. This disorder is characterized by inflammatory lesions that pervade connective and endothelial tissue. It has been linked to a group A beta-hemolytic streptococcal infection. Rheumatic fever is thought to be an autoimmune response to the streptococcal organism. There is no definitive evidence as to the underlying mechanism by which damage occurs.[1] Rheumatic fever has declined, probably because hemolytic streptococcal infections are now prevented by penicillin. It develops in 1% to 3% of patients with a prior untreated streptococcal infection.[2] Those who have had previous attacks are more susceptible to recurrent episodes and should be on continuous antibiotic therapy as prophylaxis against recurrences.[3]

Rheumatic heart disease (rheumatic carditis) is defined as a cardiac disorder that occurs as a sequel to an episode of acute rheumatic fever. It is the major acquired heart disease in children and the leading cause of death in persons aged 5 to 24 years. A delayed diffuse inflammatory reaction resulting from acute rheumatic fever can affect the pericardium, myocardium, and endocardium.

Rheumatic pericarditis is characterized by thickening of the visceral and parietal layers and the formation of exudate in the pericardial space. Serosanguineous fluid may accumulate, leading to pericardial effusion. During the healing process, the cells initiate the scarring process that contributes to fibrosis and adhesions. These may lead to adherence of the pericardium onto the epicardium; however, constrictive pericarditis usually does not occur.[4,5]

Rheumatic myocarditis is characterized by the presence of Aschoff bodies, which are areas of edema, destruction of tissue, and scarring. In addition to these Aschoff bodies, an extensive cellular infiltrate is found in the interstitial tissue, this infiltrate is thought to cause ineffective contractility leading to cardiomegaly and heart failure.[4] The coronary arteries are usually not involved in this pathophysiology and remain free of disease.

Rheumatic endocarditis usually is limited to valvular involvement and does not infiltrate the mural endocardium. In descending frequency, the mitral, aortic, tricuspid, and rarely the pulmonic valves are affected. During the initial stages of valvulitis, there is inflammation and edema of the valve leaflets and formation of tiny beadlike vegetations referred to as *verrucae*. These verrucae grow along the lines of contact of the valve leaflets.

As the pathology progresses, blood, fibrin, and platelets are deposited along the coapting edges of the valves. They are also found in the commissures as well as in the chordae tendineae of the atrioventricular (AV) valves. According to McCarthy,[5] as sequelae of the above, the leaflets of the affected valves adhere to one another, and fusion of the commissures develops. There is also shortening, fibrosis, and fusion of the chordae tendineae. In the later stages, granulation tissue develops and fibrotic changes occur leading to fibrosis and thickening with eventual calcification of the valve leaflets. These pathological changes, which often take years to manifest, will produce stenosis, regurgitation, or combined stenosis and regurgitation of the involved valves. Valvular stenosis and regurgitation are detailed later in this chapter.

Although not diagnostic, certain laboratory findings are consistent with acute rheumatic fever. These consist of an elevated antistreptolysin O titer (ASOT) after the streptococcal infection, an increased erythrocyte sedimentation rate (ESR) indicative of inflammation, and the appearance of a C-reactive protein (CRP).

The clinical features of acute rheumatic fever include: (1) systemic manifestations such as fatigue, malaise, and fever; (2) a migratory polyarthritis involving inflammatory movement from one large joint to another; (3) erythema marginatum, which is a painless, nonpruritic redness of the trunk and proximal extremities that is more pronounced with local heat; (4) Sydenham's chorea (rare occurence), which is depicted as aimless, irregular movements and labile emotional state; (5) abdominal pain secondary to hepatic engorgement or inflammatory sinusitis; and (6) small, painless, subcutaneous nodules located over bony prominences which are often overlooked.

Treatment consists of bed rest, analgesics, and nonsteroidal antiinflammatory agents (NSAIDs) until the fever and acute manifestations abate. The streptococcal organism is treated with antibiotic (penicillin preferred) therapy. The acute phase of the disease usually resolves within 12 weeks.

INFECTIVE ENDOCARDITIS

Infective endocarditis affects the lining of the heart, predominantly affecting the valves. It may be caused by an inflammatory lesion found in collagen vascular diseases or rheumatic fever, or by an infectious process caused by invading microorganisms.[5] The most common microbes involved are bacteria, fungi, yeasts, and rickettsiae. Of these, the gram-positive bacteria cause the highest incidence of reported cases. Rarer organisms implicated in this disease are viruses, parasites, mycobacteria, and chlamydia.

Infective endocarditis occurs most frequently in men over the age of 60. The left valves of the heart are affected more often than the right. Predisposing factors to infective endocarditis include parenteral drug abuse, insertion of indwelling catheters, dental procedures, urinary tract infections, skin and wound infections, congenital heart disease, rheumatic fever, cardiac surgery, and various instrumentation procedures. The overall incidence of this disease appears to have declined, but this is misleading in the sense that a decreased incidence in nonaddicted persons with native heart valves is balanced by an increased incidence in drug addicts and patients with prosthetic heart valves. This discussion centers on native valves affected by endocarditis. Endocarditis in patients who have undergone valve replacement is discussed in the section concerning valvular prostheses.

Endocarditis is no longer being classified into acute and subacute forms.[6,7,8] Many clinicians have discovered that acute cases of endocarditis can be converted to a subacute status with aggressive antibiotic therapy, and, conversely, subacute cases can suddenly become life-threatening.[9] A clinical differentiation remains useful, however, because clinical manifestations of the two forms differ in duration, nature of complications, and final outcome.[9,10]

In the acute form, the causative agents are of higher virulence. They include *Staphylococcus aureus*, *Streptococcus pneumoniae*, and *Neisseria menigitidis*. The onset of acute endocarditis is rapid as compared with a more insidious progression found in the subacute type. The acute type is associated with a fulminating course resulting in rapid destruction of the valves and a greater incidence of abscesses developing in the ring of the annulus.

The two most common invading organisms found in subacute endocarditis are *Streptococcus viridans* and *Staphylococcus epidermidis*. Less valvular destruction occurs from these organisms, but they may form large vegetations that may result in systemic emboli and occlusion of major arteries.[1]

Another feature that differentiates these two forms is the types of valves affected. Acute endocarditis usually affects normal valves, whereas subacute endocarditis is often found in previously damaged valves.

Regardless of the type, the pathological process is essentially the same. One of the causative microorganisms traveling in the bloodstream attaches itself to the endocardial lining of a normal, diseased, or prosthetic valve. Once attached, these organisms become enmeshed in deposits of fibrin, bacteria, platelets, and inflammatory cells which then are referred to as *vegetations*. These vegetations, which range in size and shape, settle on the valves and invade the leaflets. The color of the vegetations may vary from pink, red, yellow, or green initially, becoming gray when healed. Fungal infections are notorious for developing very large vegetations leading to emboli that can occlude large arteries.[9]

Vegetations interfere with normal alignment of the cusps and subsequently cause incomplete closure or regurgitation, which manifest as murmurs. The absence of a cardiac murmur has been reported in some patients (10%) with subacute endocarditis and in approximately one third of patients stricken with acute endocarditis involving the left side.[9]

The clinical manifestations exhibited in patients with endocarditis are based on three underlying pathophysiological mechanisms: generalized infection, valvular destruction, and embolism. Generalized infection accounts for such symptoms as weight loss, general malaise, anorexia, night sweats, and arthralgias. Fever is found in the majority of cases but will vary depending on the type of infection. For example, the patient with acute endocarditis presents with a fever associated with shaking chills. With subacute endocarditis, the fever is usually an intermittent, low-grade type, and without shaking chills.

Regurgitant murmurs are associated with valvular destruction and correspond to the affected valve. For

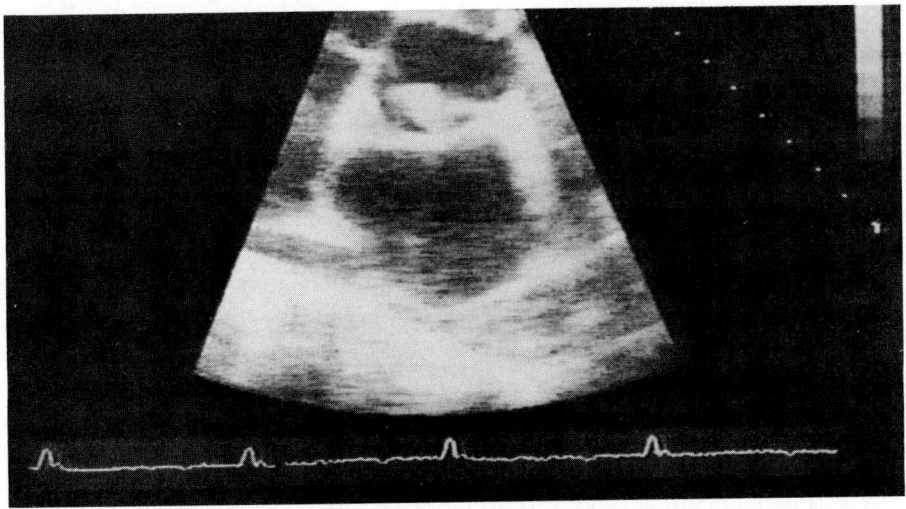

Figure 24-1   An example of a vegetation seen on an aortic valve.

example, with mitral regurgitation, a systolic murmur results; with aortic insufficiency, the murmur is audible in the early diastolic phase. The regurgitation may become severe enough to produce hemodynamic alterations leading to congestive heart failure.

Embolism may result when fragments of the vegetations break off and travel downstream. Fragments on the right side of the heart may embolize to the lungs while fragments located on the left side may cause embolization to the coronary, cerebral, and systemic circulation. Sepsis may occur at the site of embolic infarct in acute endocarditis, whereas secondary inflammatory reactions may result from emboli in subacute endocarditis. The spleen is reported to be the most common site of emboli in left-sided endocarditis along with the heart, brain, and kidneys. Thus, patients may manifest with splenomegaly, myocardial infarction, stroke, or renal infarction.

In addition, small emboli that migrate to the skin and mucous membranes cause certain classic findings such as Osler's nodes, Janeway's lesions, and Roth's spots. *Osler's nodes* are painful, tender, erythematous papules found in the pads of the fingers and toes. *Janeway's lesions* are flat, tiny, irregular, nontender red spots found on the palms of the hands and soles of the feet of some patients. *Roth's spots* are the result of retinal hemorrhages, appearing as white or yellow centers surrounded by red, irregular halos. In addition to these, patients may also exhibit splinter hemorrhages, petecchiae, and clubbing.

The diagnosis of endocarditis is established by blood cultures. The offending organism is identified, and its sensitivity to antibiotics is assessed. In addition, anemia may also be present along with an elevation in the ESR. The white blood count (WBC) may be elevated in acute endocarditis, or it may be normal or subnormal in subacute endocarditis. In about 50% of cases, the urinalysis may reveal microscopic hematuria.[11]

Fluoroscopy and two-dimensional echocardiography have been found helpful in identifying vegetations and complications such as valvular ring abscesses. Figure 24-1 depicts a vegetation found on an aortic valve during echocardiography.

Medical treatment involves use of the appropriate bactericidal agent based on sensitivities. The dose of antibiotic is routinely based on bactericidal titer levels. Duration of antibiotic therapy is generally from 4 to 6 weeks. The critical care nurse needs to be aware of the side effects of antibiotics and to assess the patient frequently for signs and symptoms of toxicity.

The use of valvular replacement surgery for acute endocarditis is increasing in many centers. Current indications for surgery include patients who develop congestive heart failure from severe regurgitant valves, evidence of valvular ring abscesses, multiple embolic events, conduction disturbances, *Brucella* infection, prosthetic valve infection, and failure to control sepsis.[9,11] The goals of surgery are to remove infective tissue and to replace a diseased valve so as to restore valvular function.

In caring for patients with infective endocarditis, the critical care nurse needs to employ strict aseptic technique and to monitor for the development of complications. A widening of the pulse pressure, for instance, should alert the nurse to the possibility of worsening aortic regurgitation. Health teaching is important for both the patient and family and should include antibiotic prophylaxis for instrumentation procedures, importance of maintaining proper oral hygiene, and discussion regarding the signs and symptoms of complications that should be immediately reported.

VALVULAR DYSFUNCTION

Valvular dysfunction may result from either congenital or acquired causes. For many years, rheumatic heart disease accounted for nearly all cases of acquired valvular heart disease.[12] The valves on the left side of the heart are more commonly affected because of constant exposure to high pressures. Any abnormality of a valve, either congenital or acquired, exposes the valve to extraordinary hemodynamic stress and can thereby accelerate the degenerative changes that cause dysfunction.[12] The degenerative changes causing a narrowing of the valve (mitral or aortic) orifice are classifed as *stenosis*. Changes leading to valvular insufficiency due to improper closing of the mitral or aortic valves are classified as *regurgitation*.

MITRAL STENOSIS

Mitral stenosis, a narrowing of the mitral orifice, is usually caused by rheumatic fever.[13] Most patients who develop rheumatic heart disease from rheumatic fever are women. The latency period from the time of rheumatic fever to the onset of clinical symptoms of mitral stenosis is about 19 years.[14]

Pathophysiology

The major long-term pathological changes in the mitral valve caused by rheumatic fever are (1) fusion of the commissures; (2) fibrosis and thickening of the leaflets; (3) shortening, fibrosis, and fusion of the chordae and/or papillary muscles; and (4) calcification of the leaflets.[15] Thickening and shortening of the mitral valve structures result in a funnel-shaped valve with the valve orifice having a "fish mouth" or "buttonhole" shape.[13]

The normal mitral valve has a cross-sectional area of 4 to 6 cm^2. Normal flow across the valve is 150 to 200 ml per second of diastole.[16] There is usually no detectable pressure gradient across the normal mitral valve even when flow is increased with exercise.

As the valve area is reduced, the gradient across the valve increases. When the valve area is reduced to 3 cm^2, the gradient is approximately 2 mmHg; at 2 cm^2, the gradient increases to 4 to 6 mmHg; and at 1 cm^2, the gradient rises to 18 to 28 mmHg at rest.[14]

Critical mitral stenosis occurs when the mitral valve opening is reduced to 1 cm^2. This leads to elevations in left atrial pressure (LAP), which in turn leads to elevated pulmonary venous and pulmonary artery wedge pressure (PAWP). Dyspnea on exertion (especially after exercise, emotional stress, infection, or with atrial fibrillation) results from the increased rate of flow across the mitral orifice causing elevations in LAP. With a further rise to 25 to 30 mmHg, the LAP will exceed plasma oncotic pressure and episodes of orthopnea and/or paryoxysmal nocturnal dyspnea

(PND) develop. Right-sided heart failure may develop after chronic elevations in pulmonary capillary pressures produce pulmonary hypertension and exert increased and constant pressure against the right ventricle.

Years of elevated LAP lead to left atrial hypertrophy and may precipitate the development of atrial fibrillation. Systemic thromboembolic episodes occur in approximately 25% of patients with atrial fibrillation.[16]

Data Acquisition

History

The principal symptom of mitral stenosis is dyspnea, which is graded according to New York Heart Association (NYHA) classifications. Dyspnea initially occurs with extreme exertion (NYHA Class II), then with moderate exertion (NYHA Class III), and finally with minimal exertion with episodes of orthopnea, PND, or pulmonary edema (NYHA Class IV). Complaints of fatigue are also common with severe mitral stenosis. If atrial fibrillation develops, patients may also complain of palpitations.

Other symptoms of mitral stenosis include hemoptyis, which may develop as frank pulmonary hemorrhage from a ruptured pulmonary vein; as frothy pink blood-tinged sputum from pulmonary edema; or as a result of pulmonary infarction.[2] Symptoms of "asthma" which develop after adolescence may also suggest mitral stenosis. Hoarseness (Ortner's syndrome) may develop from compression of the left recurrent laryngeal nerve by a dilated left atrium, enlarged tracheobronchial lymph nodes, and a dilated pulmonary artery.[13] Systemic venous hypertension with increased jugular venous distention (JVD), hepatomegaly, ascites, splenomegaly, and peripheral edema develop when severe mitral stenosis leads to pulmonary vascular resistance and right-sided heart failure.

Thromboembolism may be the presenting symptom in some patients. The rhythm of most of these patients (80%) is atrial fibrillation. Thromboemboli accounted for one fourth of all deaths in patients with mitral valve disease before the development of anticoagulation and surgical treatment. Patients who are over 35 years of age and have atrial fibrillation, a low cardiac output (CO), and dilation of the left atrial appendage are at the highest risk of emboli.[13]

Physical Assessment

Patients with severe mitral stenosis may appear with "mitral facies" (pinkish-purple patches on the cheeks). The degree of dyspnea will depend on the severity of the stenosis. Palpation reveals a point of maximum impulse (PMI), which is usually normal, and a right ventricular heave if pulmonary hypertension is present. An apical diastolic thrill may be elicited with the patient in a left lateral recumbent position.

Auscultation will usually reveal a loud S_1, a normal S_2, and an opening snap heard with the diaphragm of the stethoscope and caused by the snapping of the narrowed mitral valve during early diastole. If these heart sounds are present, the classic diastolic rumble may be heard with the bell of the stethoscope near the apex with the patient in the left lateral recumbent position. The diastolic rumble and opening snap are often reduced with inspiration and augmented during expiration.[13] As the severity of mitral stenosis increases, and valve leaflets are markedly calcified or

thickened, the S_1 sound will decrease in intensity while the diastolic rumble progresses from a mid-diastolic to presystolic to pandiastolic murmur.

Diagnostic Procedures

The electrocardiogram (ECG) demonstrates a widened P wave in lead 2 that may be notched, bifid, or with a flat top (P mitrale) due to left atrial enlargement. Evidence of P mitrale is found in 90% of patients with significant mitral stenosis who are in normal sinus rhythm.[13] If the patient is in atrial fibrillation, the *f* waves are usually coarse (Figure 24-2), although the voltage of the *f* wave is not an indication of left atrial size.[14] A right axis shift (mean QRS axis

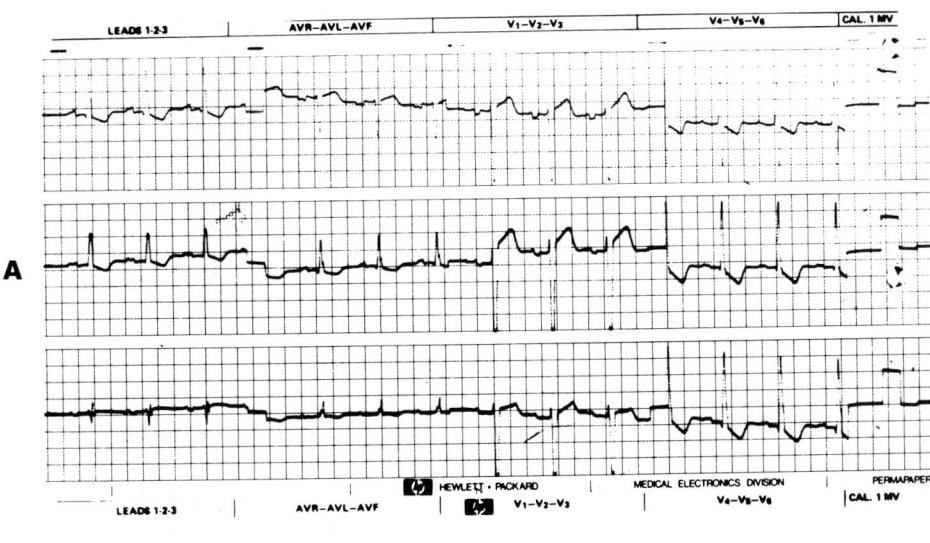

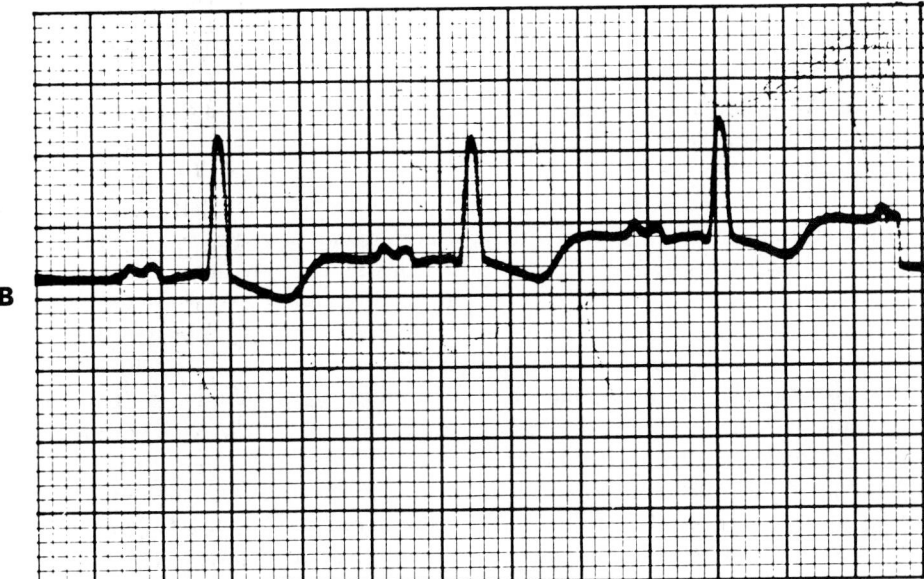

Figure 24-2   Electrocardiograms of a patient with mitral stenosis. *A,* 12-lead ECG of a patient with mitral stenosis. *B,* Lead II of same patient depicting mitral stenosis.

greater than $+90°$) usually occurs when the mitral valve orifice is less than 1.3 cm^2 and right ventricular hypertrophy has developed.

The chest x-ray may reveal a "double density" in the midportion of the cardiac silhouette, a "straight left heart border," or Kerley B lines.[16] Enlargement of the left atrium, pulmonary artery, and right ventricle, and redistribution of fluid to the upper lobes become present when severe mitral stenosis leads to elevation of pulmonary artery pressure. Exercise testing may also be employed to determine functional capacity, response to exercise, and augmentation of auscultatory findings.

Echocardiographic evidence of anterior movement of the posterior mitral valve leaflet during diastole occurs in 90% of patients with mitral stenosis.[13] The degree of calcification of the mitral valve and measurement of left atrial size are also determined with the echocardiogram. (Refer to Chapter 21 for a discussion of echocardiography.)

Cardiac catheterization may be used to assess the severity of obstruction as well as adequacy of left ventricular contractility. Impaired left ventricular function is associated with poor surgical results.[16]

Medical Management

Medical treatment of mitral stenosis is aimed at preventing complications such as systemic embolism or bacterial endocarditis, as well as treatment of atrial fibrillation. All patients with mitral stenosis receive penicillin prophylaxis for infections, surgery, or any instrumentation procedures. Anemia or infections should be promptly treated. Occupations that demand strenuous physical exertion should be avoided.

Patients who become symptomatic are initially treated with oral diuretics and restriction of sodium intake. Patients with hemoptysis from elevated pulmonary vascular resistance are treated with sedation and aggressive diuresis. They should be instructed to maintain an upright position when sitting to facilitate breathing. A decrease in PAWP and congestion after sublingual nitroglycerin has been reported.[17] The relief of pulmonary congestion has been noted with combined dobutamine and isorbide dinitrate (Isordil) therapy.[18]

Dysrhythmias, atrial fibrillation in particular, are treated with digitalis glycosides to slow the ventricular rate. For patients with mild mitral stenosis in whom atrial fibrillation has developed for the first time, cardioversion may help restore normal sinus rhythm. The patient must receive anticoagulation for 3 weeks prior to cardioversion. Successful cardioversion should be followed by treatment with quinidine sulfate and digitalis glycosides to maintain normal sinus rhythm. Repeat cardioversion is not recommended if the patient reverts to atrial fibrillation while on adequate doses of quinidine sulfate or if the left atrium is significantly enlarged.[13] The rate of successful cardioversion is low in patients who have been symptomatic for over 3 years and who have a left atrial size of over 5.2 cm as documented by echocardiography.[19]

Braunwald[13] reported systemic embolism occurring in 1% to 2% of patients with mitral stenosis after electrical or chemical cardioversion. Risk of embolization increases in patients with paroxysmal atrial fibrillation and repeated conversions to normal sinus rhythm. Anticoagulant therapy can help prevent venous thrombosis and pulmonary embolism and can reduce the frequency of systemic embolism in patients who have experienced previous embolic episodes and who have had rheumatic heart disease and heart failure and/or atrial fibrillation.

It takes approximately 5 to 10 years after the onset of symptoms for most patients with mitral stenosis to progress from mild disability to total disability.[13] Mortality of medically treated patients at 10 years was 70% in one study.[14] Surgery has been recommended for symptomatic patients, especially if thromboembolism has occurred. Patients in NYHA Class II and III are ideal surgical candidates with excellent results and low operative risk.[16] A major contraindication to surgery is active rheumatic endocarditis, which is rare.[13] An alternative to surgery in some selected cases is mitral valvuloplasty. This procedure is discussed in further detail at the end of this chapter.

Patients who are in NYHA Class IV represent a slightly greater surgical risk. These patients should remain on bed rest with intensive medical therapy prior to surgery. If blood urea nitrogen or creatine levels continue to rise despite aggressive diuresis, surgery should not be delayed because medical therapy has reached its limit.[16]

The three surgical techniques for treatment of mitral stenosis are (1) closed mitral commissurotomy, (2) open mitral commissurotomy, and (3) mitral valve replacement. Closed mitral commissurotomy (CMC), which does not require cardiopulmonary bypass, is performed with the aid of a transventricular dilator and is an effective procedure for patients who do not also have mitral regurgitation, atrial thrombosis, or serious valve calcification with shortening or fusing of chordae. Postoperative improvement has been reported in 86% of patients, with an 18-year survival rate of 89.5%.[13] Low operative mortality for this type of surgery has been reported—1.5% for the first procedure, and 6.7% for closed valvotomy.[13]

Open mitral commissurotomy (OMC) has been termed the "precise" method of mitral commissurotomy. This technique, which requires cardiopulmonary bypass, allows for more precise visualization of the commissures as well as slitting of fused chordae or papillary muscles, and removal of left atrial thrombi. Operative mortality of OMC has been reported to be between 0% to 4.4%, and 10-year survivals have been reported to be between 81% to 95%.[13,20] Most patients who were NYHA Class III preoperatively improve to NYHA Class I or II postoperatively.

Mitral valve replacement is necessary for patients with an immobile, extremely calcified rheumatic mitral valve.[16] Hospital mortality for patients with NYHA Class IV has been reported to be 32%, while those in NYHA Class III were 3%.[21] Nine-year survival after mitral valve replacement was 72%.[21] Pulmonary hypertension was reported to decrease within 24 hours of valve replacement for mitral stenosis.[22] Prosthetic heart valves are discussed at the end of this chapter.

AORTIC STENOSIS

Valvular aortic stenosis (AS) is usually congenital or degenerative rather than rheumatic in origin.[13] These congenital malformations are more common in men and usually consist of unicuspid, bicuspid, or unequal valve leaflets. Any of these malformations may cause increased turbulent flow leading to fibrosis, calcification, and eventually to stenosis.[13]

Pathophysiology

The aortic valve orifice, normally 2.6 to 3.5 cm^2, is reduced in AS. This reduction causes obstruction to the flow of blood from the left ventricle into the aorta during ventricular systole. Left ventricular pressure rises, increasing systolic wall stress and thereby ventricular wall thickening (concentric hypertrophy). A systolic pressure gradient, known as an *aortic valve gradient,* develops between the left ventricle and aorta.[2]

The left ventricle hypertrophies as a compensatory mechanism to maintain an adequate cardiac output. A large pressure gradient across the aortic valve may be sustained for many years without a reduction in cardiac output, development of left ventricular dilation, or the development of symptoms.[13] Critical obstruction to left ventricular outflow occurs when the aortic orifice is less than approximately 0.4 cm^2 per square meter of body surface area, or when there is a peak systolic pressure gradient exceeding 50 mmHg in the presence of normal cardiac output.[13] Persistent pressure overload to the left ventricle may eventually lead to left ventricular dilation, left atrial enlargement, and pulmonary and systemic vascular changes. Ultimately, the left ventricle may fail completely, leading to a critically low cardiac output.

Data Acquisition

History

Chest pain, syncope, dyspnea, and heart failure are the classic clinical manifestations of severe aortic stenosis. Exertional angina occurs in about two thirds of patients with severe aortic stenosis and may be due to coronary atherosclerosis or to the markedly increased myocardial oxygen demand.[13] Dizziness or syncope, which occurs in 15% to 30% of patients, may result from (1) the abrupt decrease in cardiac output during effort without compensatory increase in systemic vascular resistance (SVR), (2) an abrupt fall in SVR in the presence of a fixed output, (3) or an arrhythmia.[13,23] Left ventricular failure eventually occurs with symptoms of fatigue, cough, progressive dyspnea on exertion, orthopnea, and paroxysmal nocturnal dyspnea. If unrelieved, death is likely within 2 years in patients with heart failure, 3 years in those with syncope, and 5 years in those with angina.[13]

Physical Assessment

Aortic stenosis typically produces a harsh crescendo–decrescendo systolic ejection murmur which begins after the S_1 sound. This murmur is loudest at the second right sternal edge with radiation to the left lateral sternal edge and carotids. A thrill is often present. The murmur of aortic stenosis can be augmented by inhalation of amyl nitrite or by squatting or lying flat.[13] Delay in aortic valve closure often produces paradoxical splitting of the S_2 sound, except in severe stenosis, in which A_2 is inaudible.

A widened pulse pressure with a normal diastolic pressure is common in compensated aortic stenosis. Narrowing of the pulse pressure may occur with decompensation. The prolonged ejection phase noted in aortic stenosis produces a slow rise of the arterial pulse which is best felt in the carotid artery. Left ventricular hypertrophy produces a sustained thrust or heave of the apical impulse. Displacement of the apical impulse downward and to the left occurs after left ventricular failure develops. The *a* wave on a jugular venous pulse becomes prominent once right ventricular compliance decreases secondary to left ventricular failure.

Diagnostic Procedures

The ECG demonstrates normal sinus rhythm with signs of left ventricular hypertrophy occurring from high-grade stenosis. Decompensated severe aortic stenosis may produce ECG evidence of left atrial hypertrophy. In one study, only 9% of patients with aortic stenosis who died suddenly had demonstrated normal ECGs.[23] Conduction abnormalities such as first-degree atrioventricular block, bundle branch block, and intraventricular conduction disturbances are fairly common among patients with aortic stenosis resulting from infection, disease, or calcification of the conduction system.

Chest x-ray may demonstrate concentric hypertrophy of the left ventricle, poststenotic dilation of the aorta, and calcification of the valve cusps. The heart shadow may depict a change in configuration, but not in size. Cardiomegaly is visualized, however, with decompensated aortic stenosis.

The echocardiogram demonstrates a poststenotic dilation of the aorta, and left ventricular wall thickening. Dilation of the left ventricle occurs with myocardial failure. Mobility of the aortic valve can also be assessed via the echocardiogram.

Cardiac catheterization can determine the severity of obstruction and assess the functional status of the left ventricle as well as the coronary circulation. Cardiac catheterization is discussed in Chapter 19.

Medical Management

Medical therapy for the asymptomatic patient with aortic stenosis consists of antibiotic prophylaxis for the prevention of infective endocarditis. Those with high-grade lesions should be advised to avoid strenuous physical exertion. Digitalis glycosides are used when evidence of either an increased left ventricular volume or a decreased ejection fraction is noted. Diuretics should be used with caution since hypovolemia may decrease the elevated left ventricular end-diastolic pressure, decrease cardiac output, and produce orthostatic hypotension. The use of beta-blocking agents may depress myocardial function and may induce left ventricular failure.[13]

Atrial dysrhythmias occur in less than 10% of patients with aortic stenosis.[13] The appearance of atrial fibrillation necessitates treatment with cardioversion, quinidine, or procainamide, because loss of atrial contraction may further impair left ventricular function.

Systemic emboli are rare in patients with aortic stenosis. Emboli which do occur are often due to calcific flecks coming from the aortic valve rather than from thrombi.

Patients with severe aortic stenosis with left ventricular dysfunction and myocardial ischemia have responded well to cautious administration of nitroprusside. Ikram et al.[24] reported a decrease in cardiac index in patients with aortic stenosis and preserved left ventricular function when given nitroprusside. Patients with impaired left ventricular function had an increase in cardiac index when given nitroprusside.[24]

Use of the intraaortic balloon pump (IABP) has brought about marked clinical improvement in patients with decompensated aortic stenosis. The hemodynamic benefit from the IABP in these patients was reportedly derived almost entirely from augmentation of the diastolic coronary filling pressure because left ventricular systolic pressure was not decreased.[25]

Once patients with aortic stenosis become symptomatic with angina or syncope, the average survival time is 2 to 3 years. Patients with congestive heart failure demonstrate an average survival time of $1\frac{1}{2}$ years.[13] Without surgery, mortality from onset of symptoms is approximately 25% at 1 year and 50% at 2 years, with more than half the deaths occurring suddenly.[13]

Surgical therapy primarily consists of aortic valve replacement with either mechanical or tissue valves. Surgical mortality ranges from 2% to 8% for patients without left ventricular failure and from 10% to 25% for those with left ventricular failure or a depressed ejection fraction.[13] Five-year survival has been reported to be less than 50% in medically treated patients while surgically treated patients' survival was 75% to 80%.[26] Even patients over the age of 60 at the time of surgery demonstrated improved left ventricular function and a 10-year survival of 57.5% using life-table analysis after surgical treatment.[27] The V. A. Cooperative Study Group recommends surgical intervention for patients with moderate or severe aortic stenosis or insufficiency before the onset of significant left ventricular dysfunction, since the strongest predictor of postoperative left ventricular dysfunction is preoperative dysfunction.[28]

Aortic valvuloplasty or balloon dilatation of the aortic valve is a nonsurgical technique employed under very specific circumstances. This procedure is discussed in further detail at the end of this chapter.

MITRAL REGURGITATION

Mitral regurgitation (insufficiency) occurs when the mitral valve fails to close completely, allowing blood to flow back into the left atrium during ventricular systole.

Chronic rheumatic heart disease remains the most common cause of mitral regurgitation. Other causes include isolated rupture of the chordae tendineae, mitral valve prolapse, ischemic papillary muscle dysfunction, and infective endocarditis. Mitral regurgitation results from a disruption of the functional components which may include the valve leaflets, papillary muscle, mitral valve annulus, chordae tendineae, or the left ventricle itself.

Pathophysiology

The degree of mitral regurgitation gradually increases over many years. The patient with chronic mitral regurgitation may remain asymptomatic for decades. The symptoms and outcome of chronic mitral regurgitation depend on the rate of progression, onset of atrial fibrillation, development of pulmonary hypertension, and coexisting coronary artery disease.[15]

With chronic mitral regurgitation, the increased volume of blood ejected back into the left atrium will cause stretching and thinning of the atrial wall. The large, thin-walled atrium accommodates the large volume of blood ejected into it during ventricular systole. The left atrial pressure decreases to near normal during ventricular diastole. The left ventricle dilates and becomes hypertrophied in response to the increased volume from the left atrium so that a sufficient cardiac output is maintained.[2] Pulmonary hypertension is not likely to develop in a patient with mitral regurgitation that has increased over time.

In contrast, patients with acute mitral regurgitation develop a rapid increase in left atrial pressure due to the sudden volume overload of a normal left atrium secondary to myocardial infarction or to chest trauma that causes rupture of the papillary muscle or chordae. This sudden increase in left atrial pressure is reflected in the pulmonary vascular bed, producing interstitial edema that leads to pulmonary edema.[29] Pulmonary hypertension may develop from compression of the pulmonary vascular bed. The left ventricle dilates rapidly without hypertrophy, producing a decrease in the ratio of left ventricular mass to left ventricular end-diastolic volume.[13]

The volume of mitral regurgitant flow in either chronic or acute mitral regurgitation depends on the size of the regurgitant orifice and on the pressure gradient between the left ventricle and left atrium. Flow is decreased by any agent that decreases left ventricular size (i.e., cardiac glycosides, diuretics, or vasodilators). Regurgitant flow is increased by any agent that enlarges the left ventricle by increasing preload or afterload or depresses myocardial function, as do vasoconstrictors. A decrease in ejection fraction signifies severe impairment of contractility.

Data Acquisition

History

Patients with chronic mitral regurgitation initially complain of fatigue and, later, dyspnea on exertion. Palpitations may also occur. Symptoms of left ventricular failure frequently appear late in the course of chronic mitral regurgitation due to the gradual increase in volume overload. Hemoptysis is a rare finding in mitral regurgitation. A common complication of chronic mitral regurgitation is atrial fibrillation, which is related to the size of the left atrium and affects 75% of patients.[14] Other common complica-

tions include systemic emboli (usually occurring in the presence of atrial fibrillation) and bacterial endocarditis.

Those who develop acute mitral regurgitation have been in relatively good health with an abrupt onset of symptoms. The intensity of symptoms and immediate prognosis depend on the cause and the amount of sudden volume overload to the left atrium. A patient with rupture of a few chordae from subacute bacterial endocarditis or trauma usually describes easy fatigue, dyspnea, pedal edema, and occasional intermittent chest pain, while a patient with rupture of a papillary muscle from acute myocardial infarction presents with severe hypotension and florid pulmonary edema.[30] In the latter instance, 75% of patients die within the first 24 hours of rupture without surgical intervention, and 95% die within the first 2 weeks.[30]

Physical Assessment

Chronic mitral regurgitation produces a carotid pulse which tends to collapse in quality from early closure of the aortic valve. This collapsing quality is less marked as the severity of mitral regurgitation increases and left ventricular failure increases. The hyperkinetic apical pulse will be displaced leftward and downward. A parasternal lift is usually present.

Auscultation of the patient with chronic mitral regurgitation reveals a widely split S_2 sound (A_2 early) accompanied by a short, mid-diastolic flow rumble due to the increase in left atrial stroke volume flowing across the mitral valve. The hallmark of mitral regurgitation is a pansystolic, harsh, blowing murmur best heard at the apex and radiating to the axilla or back. This murmur can be increased or decreased with certain maneuvers. Maneuvers that decrease left ventricular volume by decreasing impedance to left ventricular outflow, decrease venous return, or increase myocardial contractility (such as sudden standing or inhalation of amyl nitrite) will result in a decreased murmur. Maneuvers that increase left ventricular volume by increase in venous return, decrease in myocardial contractility, bradycardia or increase in impedance to left ventricular emptying (such as squatting or administration of phenylephrine or methoxamine) will increase the murmur of mitral regurgitation.[13]

Patients with acute mitral regurgitation exhibit a rapid upstroke and fall-off of the carotid pulse. The jugular venous pressure may be elevated, indicating right ventricular failure. On palpation, the apical impulse may be prominent but is usually not displaced or sustained. A widely split S_2 sound (A_2 early) with increased P_2, as well as S_3 and S_4 sounds are present.

An apical systolic murmur with a decrescendo character which may radiate throughout the chest is also present.

Diagnostic Procedures

The ECG of a patient with chronic mitral regurgitation demonstrates normal sinus rhythm with left atrial hypertrophy in the early stage and then atrial fibrillation. As the degree of mitral regurgitation increases, evidence of left ventricular hypertrophy and associated ST and T wave changes secondary to strain may be present.

With acute mitral regurgitation, sinus tachycardia is the most obvious ECG sign. Volume overload of the left atrium may produce a large terminal negative force of the P wave in the precordial leads.

The chest x-ray of a patient with chronic mitral regurgitation initially demonstrates an increase in cardiac size due to left ventricular dilatation. As regurgitation increases, left atrial enlargement becomes evident. Pulmonary changes of upper lobe redistribution are seen when the left atrial pressure exceeds 12 to 18 mmHg. When left atrial pressure exceeds 18 to 20 mmHg, pulmonary edema is evident on the chest x-ray.

With acute mitral regurgitation, the chest x-ray shows little or no left ventricular or left atrial enlargement. Enlargement of the upper pulmonary vascular lobes as well as pulmonary edema are present on chest x-ray.

The echocardiogram assesses the severity of regurgitation by measuring left ventricular end-diastolic dimension, septal and posterior ventricular wall motion, left atrial size, and ventricular contractility. Chronic mitral regurgitation usually produces a volume overload pattern and a large left atrium. Acute mitral regurgitation usually produces evidence of normal volume and some increase in left atrial size, a fluttering of the mitral valve leaflet, and a decrease (with ruptured papillary muscle) or hyperdynamic (with ruptured chordae) ventricular wall motion.

Radionuclide ventriculography may be used to calculate the ejection fraction and left ventricular cavity size to estimate the severity of chronic mitral regurgitation. Cardiac catheterization is required prior to surgery to quantify left ventricular size and contractility, the degree of regurgitation, and intracardiac pressures and to identify concurrent lesions or coronary artery disease. Dalen and Alpert[14] recommend that exercise hemodynamics be assessed in the catheterization laboratory for any patient with compensated chronic mitral regurgitation who demonstrates normal hemodynamics at rest. Catheterization data help to classify the severity of mitral regurgitation and the status of the left ventricle.[14] A dilated, poorly contracting left ventricle may be a contraindication for surgery. Giant v waves on a PAWP tracing suggest an acute, severe regurgitation into a noncompliant left atrium.

1. Minimal to mild mitral regurgitation (1 to 2+ on a scale of 4) = normal left ventricular end-diastolic pressure (LVEDP) and PAWP (less than 12 mmHg) at rest and exercise. Ejection fraction is greater than 55%.

2. Moderate chronic mitral regurgitation (3+) = marked dilatation of left atrium and ventricle. Normal or slightly increased LVEDP and PAWP at rest. Ejection fraction may be slightly decreased. Exercise may cause slight increase in ejection fraction and decrease in LVEDP due to vasodilatation, or cause an increase in LVEDP and PAWP secondary to pulmonary hypertension and an increase in mitral regurgitation.

3. Severe chronic mitral regurgitation (4+) = gross dilatation of left atrium and ventricle with increased LVEDP and PAWP at rest. Ejection fraction is less than 50%.

Data from cardiac catheterization are also used to determine a "regurgitant fraction," which is the ratio of blood volume regurgitated into the left atrium during systole divided by the total volume of blood ejected into both the left atrium and aorta by the left ventricle during systole. A correlation exists between the calculated regurgitant fraction and the degree of mitral regurgitation. A patient with severe chronic mitral regurgitation demonstrates a regurgitant fraction of 0.6 or greater.[14]

Medical Management

Medical treatment for all patients with chronic mitral regurgitation, even those who are asymptomatic, consists of antibiotic prophylaxis for any dental or surgical procedure. If atrial fibrillation develops, digitalis glycosides are given to control ventricular rate, and anticoagulation is started to prevent systemic emboli. Patients with moderate mitral regurgitation (NYHA Class II) require the addition of a no-added-salt diet, but patients with moderately severe regurgitation (NYHA Class III) require addition of diuretics. If digitalis glycosides, a no-added-salt diet, and diuretics do not control left ventricular failure and the patient has severe regurgitation (NYHA Class IV), afterload reduction with an angiotensin inhibitor or oral hydralazine may be required.

For patients with acute mitral regurgitation, early stabilization is required to allow for identification of the responsible mechanical defect. Vasodilators are used to decrease preload and afterload because any increase in left ventricular volume may worsen mitral valve dysfunction. The PAWP should be maintained at 15 to 18 mmHg. Patients who are in shock or have severe coronary artery disease do poorly with vasodilators alone because the decrease in coronary perfusion pressure compromises left ventricular function. In this case, use of the intraaortic balloon pump should be considered to decrease afterload while maintaining perfusion pressure. Use of inotropic agents such as dopamine or dobutamine to increase arterial diastolic pressure must be monitored with caution because the increase in systemic vascular resistance may aggravate myocardial ischemia and mitral regurgitation.

Of patients with chronic mitral regurgitation who are treated medically, 60% survive 10 years after diagnosis. As previously mentioned, the occurrence of acute mitral regurgitation carries an extremely poor prognosis with medical treatment. Surgical mortality ranges from 2% to 7% in patients with pure or predominant chronic mitral regurgitation who are NYHA Class II or III.[13] Braunwald[13] recommends medical management for 4 to 6 weeks for those patients with acute mitral regurgitation prior to surgical therapy. The development of renal or pulmonary failure indicates a need for immediate surgical intervention. Five-year survival has been reported as 70% for patients with rheumatic mitral regurgitation and 30% for those with myocardial dysfunction secondary to ischemic heart disease.[13]

Surgical therapy is aimed at improving the patient's symptoms, relieving severe pulmonary hypertension, and decreasing LVEDV and mass. The V. A. Cooperative Study recommended surgery for significant mitral regurgitation or mitral stenosis/mitral regurgitation before left ventricular ejection fraction decreases below 0.50, the end-systolic volume index increases above ml/m² or pulmonary hypertension develops because left ventricular size and systolic function will likely be normal postoperatively, and survival and functional class will be enhanced.[31] Patients with marked left ventricular dysfunction may remain symptomatic after surgical treatment. Patients may show a decrease in ejection fraction and an increase in end-systolic volume immediately after surgery because abolition of mitral regurgitation may increase afterload. These patients may require vasodilator treatment in the immediate postoperative period.

Surgical techniques used to treat mitral regurgitation are valve repair/reconstruction and valve replacement. Valve repair/reconstruction, in which the disrupted functional component is repaired, has shown stable functional results, a low surgical mortality, and an acceptable rate of reoperation.[32] It has been suggested that some of the left ventricular dysfunction observed after mitral valve replacement may

be due to the excision of the native valve, whereas mitral valve repair retains the tethering effect of chordal attachments which may prevent postoperative dilatation.[33] David, et al.[34] found a significant increase in exercise ejection fraction and stroke volume postoperatively in mitral valve replacement patients in whom the chordae and papillary muscles were preserved.

MITRAL VALVE PROLAPSE

One of the most prevalent valvular abnormalities is mitral valve prolapse (MVP). It has been estimated that 5% to 10% of the population are afflicted with this condition. Typically, it is described as a displacement (prolapse) of the posterior cusp of the mitral valve in a posterior direction into the left atrium during systole. This syndrome has been given many synonyms—Barlow's syndrome, floppy mitral valve syndrome, and mitral leaflet prolapse—all of which are used interchangeably.

This syndrome is most prevalent in women aged 20 to 40 years, although it has been detected in males of all ages. A hereditary link is suggested by the tendency for MVP to occur in families; it is thought to be transmitted as an autosomal dominant trait.[13] In addition, MVP tends to be associated with such extracardiac defects as scoliosis, kyphosis, and pectus excavatum and carninatum. It has also been known to coexist with ischemic heart disease and mitral stenosis.

Pathophysiology

Mitral valve prolapse may lead to mitral regurgitation that occurs when the posterior leaflet bulges back into the left atrium during the maximal ejection phase of systole. This billowing back of the leaflet places stress on the chordae tendineae and papillary muscles, interfering with their ability to close the valve. Blood consequently flows in a retrograde fashion into the left atrium during ventricular contraction instead of flowing foward through the aortic valve.

Data Acquisition

History

Most persons with MVP are asymptomatic. When symptoms do occur, patients usually report chest discomfort, palpitations, minimal dyspnea, fatigue, and anxiety. The chest discomfort is atypical of anginal pain in that it is of longer duration, is not precipitated by exertion, and is manifested as brief attacks of severe piercing pain localized at the apex. The critical care nurse will need to differentiate this pain from angina, especially if the patient has coexisting coronary artery disease. Palpitations are usually the result of dysrhythmias that may be a manifestation of the increased adrenergic tone found in patients with MVP. This outpouring of catecholamines could also be responsible for the dyspnea and anxiety that frequently accompany the palpitations.

Physical Assessment

Most cases of MVP are diagnosed on routine physical examination. The most specific sign of this syndrome is the presence of a nonejection click on auscultation. This click is a snapping extra heart sound that tends to occur in mid- to late systole. It is generally heard best at the lower left sternal border or at the apex. Positioning of the patient into the left lateral decubitus position or in an upright position enhances the click. The straining phase of a Valsalva maneuver or the inhalation of amyl nitrite will also produce a more audible click. The presence of an apical systolic murmur varies with the degree of mitral regurgitation. This systolic murmur is a late systolic–crescendo type that can be loud and musical. Holosystolic murmurs are usually an indication of pronounced mitral valve prolapse resulting in a more severe form of mitral regurgitation.

Diagnostic Procedures

The ECG may reveal some abnormalities in patients who are symptomatic with MVP. Typically, there can be inverted T waves and nonspecific ST segment changes in the inferior and left precordial leads. These changes can be a manifestation of the ischemia to the papillary muscles due to the strain placed on these muscles by the prolapsed valve leaflets.

A multitude of dysrhythmias have been reported in association with this disorder, the most serious being ventricular tachycardia and ventricular fibrillation, which are found in patients who also manifest the aforementioned ECG changes.

Echocardiography, specifically two-dimensional, is regarded by some as the single best technique to define this disorder. Typically, the echocardiogram shows the posterior mitral valve leaflet bulging back into the left atrium during systole.[13]

Stress ECGs and thallium-201 exercise scans are employed when there is a need to differentiate MVP from coronary artery disease. This is especially important when patients with suspected MVP have chest discomfort.

Left ventricular angiography may be used to evaluate the degree of regurgitation. This invasive procedure is not, however, routinely done to confirm the diagnosis of MVP. The angiographic procedure permits visualization of valve leaflet movement during systole. The integrity of the valve leaflets can also be seen. Decreased ventricular contraction, dilatation, and even calcification of the mitral annulus have been seen on angiography in some patients with MVP.[13] As an adjunct in evaluating the severity of the mitral regurgitation, volumes and pressures are obtained to ascertain its hemodynamic consequences.

Medical Management

Most persons with MVP are asymptomatic, as previously stated. No treatment is recommended for asymptomatic patients unless ECG abnormalities are documented or signs of advanced mitral regurgitation (MR) are present. Asymptomatic patients need reassurance that their condition is benign and usually uncomplicated. They also need to be told that their prognosis for life is good.

Patients who are asymptomatic but who have a systolic murmur require more frequent follow-up. The question of prophylaxis for bacterial endocarditis, which is a well-documented complication, remains controversial. Braunwald[13] recommends antibiotic prophylaxis in patients with a midsystolic click and/or systolic murmur.

Beta blockers, especially propranolol are employed for patients with documented dysrhythmias and for the group of patients with increased adrenergic tone. Propranolol is also used to decrease the tension on the stretched chordae tendineae.

Mitral valve prolapse has been surgically treated. Mitral annuloplasty may be useful if the patient has such major symptoms as chest pain, dysrhythmias, and dyspnea.[35] A retrospective study reported relief of one or more symptoms in 60% of patients.[36] Mitral valve replacement has also been performed in patients with refractory ventricular dysrhythmias and severe atypical chest pain.[37,38]

The majority of patients with MVP are never admitted to a critical care unit. Only patients with severe MR or refractory ventricular dysrhythmias are likely to be seen in this setting. Nursing therapies for this subset of patients are the same as for patients with mitral regurgitation and are discussed in that section.

AORTIC REGURGITATION

Aortic regurgitation occurs when the aortic valve fails to close completely, allowing blood to flow back into the left ventricle during ventricular diastole. This process may be either chronic or acute. Pathological processes that affect the aortic valve, leading to chronic aortic regurgitation, are inflammation (due to rheumatic fever, syphilis, rheumatoid arthritis, etc.), structural (unicuspid, bicuspid, aneurysm), disruptive (trauma, infective endocarditis, dissection), congenital, or stress from hypertension.[39] Acute aortic regurgitation may occur from infective endocarditis, dissecting aortic aneurysm, chest compression injuries, spontaneous rupture of the valve cusps, or post-operative disruption of the valve leaflets during aortic valvuloplasty.[40]

Pathophysiology

Aortic regurgitation produces a volume overload to the left ventricle during diastole. The volume of blood regurgitated into the left ventricle determines whether the volume overload is mild, moderate, or severe. Regurgitant volume is determined by (1) the area of the regurgitant valve orifice, (2) the diastolic pressure gradient between the aorta and left ventricle, and (3) the duration of diastole.[39]

In chronic aortic regurgitation, the left ventricle compensates for the gradual increase in preload by dilation and concentric hypertrophy. In acute aortic regurgitation there is no time for this adaptation to occur. Therefore, patients with chronic aortic regurgitation develop an increased end-diastolic volume without increased end-diastolic pressure, while those with acute aortic regurgitation develop a dramatic increase in left ventricular end-diastolic pressure with only minor increases in end-diastolic volume.

Data Acquisition

History and Physical Assessment

Patients with chronic aortic regurgitation may be asymptomatic for decades. When symptoms do occur, the patient usually complains of chest discomfort and/or symptoms of congestive heart failure (especially dyspnea and fatigue). Patients with acute aortic regurgitation present with symptoms of severe left-sided failure (dyspnea at rest, orthopnea, paroxysmal nocturnal dyspnea, fatigue, exhaustion) which have occurred suddenly. Heart failure, in acute aortic regurgitation, is usually progressive and rapidly fatal unless surgical intervention is accomplished.[40] Symptoms of low foward cardiac output (fatigue and exhaustion) are overshadowed by symptoms of pulmonary congestion in patients with acute aortic regurgitation.

Hemodynamic findings of patients with acute, severe aortic regurgitation and chronic, severe, decompensated aortic regurgitation are similar except for the marked increase in left ventricular end-diastolic and end-systolic volume seen in the chronic patient. Arterial blood pressure usually demonstrates a low diastolic pressure (the Korotkoff sounds may even reach zero) in a patient with moderate or severe chronic aortic regurgitation. Because the systolic blood pressure is normal or increased, the patient with chronic aortic regurgitation usually demonstrates a widened pulse pressure, but patients with acute aortic regurgitation do not usually develop widened pulse pressures. The carotid arterial pulse will rise to a single, rapidly collapsing peak with acute aortic regurgitation. A pulsus alternans may be present in acute severe aortic regurgitation but is unusual in patients with chronic aortic regurgitation.[41]

The apical pulse may be normal with acute aortic regurgitation. A parasternal lift indicative of right ventricular dilatation may be felt after pulmonary hypertension has developed. With chronic aortic regurgitation, the apical impulse is displaced to the left and downward. Left ventricular enlargement produces a large and forceful impulse. A water-hammer pulse may be present due to the forceful ejection of blood in early systole and regurgitation during early diastole.

On auscultation, the S_1 sound may be decreased or absent if premature closure of the mitral valve occurs, which makes it difficult to separate systole from diastole in acute aortic regurgitation. The S_2 quality varies, depending on the integrity of the aortic valve leaflet—if intact, the S_2 sound is well-preserved, but if destroyed, the S_2 is absent. An S_3 sound is a common finding in the patient with aortic regurgitation. The diastolic murmur of aortic regurgitation is best heard with the diaphragm of the stethoscope with the patient sitting up or leaning forward and expiring deeply.[39] The murmur is usually brief, soft, and of medium pitch. With chronic aortic regurgitation of mild severity, the diastolic murmur occurs early with a decrescendo pattern. The Austin Flint murmur of antegrade flow across a decreasing mitral valve orifice is usually mid-diastolic with acute severe aortic regurgitation, and mid-diastolic and/or presystolic with chronic severe aortic regurgitation.[40] A systolic ejection murmur is common in both acute and chronic aortic regurgitation.

Diagnostic Procedures

The ECG will reflect left ventricular hypertrophy, especially in the precordial leads. Conduction disturbances may occur with aortic regurgitation secondary to inflammatory processes. The ECG is usually normal except for sinus tachycardia, without evidence of left ventricular hypertrophy with acute, severe aortic regurgitation.

As the severity of chronic aortic regurgitation increases, the left ventricular contour enlarges, producing a "boot-shaped" heart silhouette on chest x-ray. The aortic knob and ascending aorta become prominent in patients with moderate to severe chronic aortic regurgitation. Patients with acute aortic regurgitation do not demonstrate cardiac enlargement. These patients exhibit increased venous redistribution to the upper lobes because of pulmonary venous and capillary hypertension secondary to an increased left ventricular end-diastolic pressure and left atrial pressure.

Echocardiographic evidence of increased diastolic

chamber dimension occurs with chronic aortic regurgitation but not with acute aortic regurgitation. The increased volume of the left ventricle during diastole may also cause fluttering of the anterior mitral valve leaflet.[39]

Cardiac catheterization is used to document the severity and extent of aortic regurgitation as well as left ventricular function. Aortic regurgitation is gauged on a 1-to-4 + scale according to severity (minimal to severe). No increase in left ventricular filling pressures occurs with compensated chronic aortic regurgitation. Left ventricular filling pressures increase as volume overload increases. Hemodynamic abnormalities occur at rest in 57% of patients with NYHA Class IV and 30% of patients in NYHA Class I, and with exercise in 100% of patients in NYHA Class IV and 47% of patients in NYHA Class I.

Medical Management

Medical therapy for chronic aortic regurgitation consists of antibiotic prophylaxis for all patients. Once left ventricular failure develops, digitalis glycosides, diuretics, and vasodilators are necessary to improve left ventricular function and to reduce the aortic regurgitant fraction.

Long-term vasodilator therapy with oral hydralazine reduces the volume overload and the left ventricular end-diastolic volume in clinically stable, moderate-to-severe aortic insufficiency.[42] The medical management in acute aortic regurgitation consists of minimizing congestive heart failure. Digitalis glycosides, diuretics and nitroprusside (to maintain a PAWP between 16 to 20 mmHg), and inotropic agents (dopamine or dubotamine) to augment myocardial contractility may be necessary. Use of the intraaortic balloon pump (IABP) is contraindicated in patients with significant aortic regurgitation because the augmented diastolic pressure from the IABP is transmitted directly to the left ventricle, compounding the deleterious effects of valvular insufficiency.[43] Favorable hemodynamic effects of sublingual nifedipine, intravenous hydralazine, and oral prazosin have been reported.[13,44,45,46]

Surgery is usually not indicated for asymptomatic patients with severe chronic aortic regurgitation who have good exercise tolerance and normal left ventricular function. Surgery is advocated for symptomatic patients with severe aortic regurgitation who have impaired left ventricular function. The surgical risk of aortic valve replacement depends on the condition of the patient, the state of left ventricular junction, and the skill of the surgical team.[13]

Patients with acute aortic regurgitation due to active endocarditis had an 80% mortality after surgery while those with chronic aortic regurgitation who had

surgery within 3 years of symptoms of heart failure had a mortality rate of zero.[47] After aortic valve replacement, patients whose heart size did not decrease during the first 6 months have demonstrated a 57% mortality compared with 15% mortality for those whose hearts did decrease in size.[42] Evidence of severe left ventricular dysfunction preoperatively has been associated with poor postoperative prognosis.[48]

NURSING MANAGEMENT

The nursing management of a patient with valvular dysfunction who presents to the critical care unit is challenging. The patient is in a state of hemodynamic instability whether it is related to acute valvular dysfunction secondary to another disease process (acute myocardial infarction) or to decompensation as a result of chronic valvular dysfunction. Intensive medical and nursing management is necessary to stabilize the patient and to prepare for the possibility of valvular heart surgery.

Nursing diagnoses for the patient with valvular dysfunction are classified into actual and high-risk problems.

■ NURSING DIAGNOSIS

Activity intolerance, related to insufficient oxygen for activities of daily living as evidenced by dyspnea, shortness of breath, fatigue, vertigo, tachycardia, or other altered hemodynamic responses.

OUTCOME STANDARD AND CRITERIA

Activity level prescribed is tolerated as evidenced by:

- Verbalization of decreased shortness of breath, fatigue, and vertigo during increased activity
- Verbalization of increased activity tolerance
- Demonstration of appropriate heart rate, blood pressure, and respiratory rate with increased activity
- Demonstration of ability to monitor heart rate during activities of daily living

NURSING INTERVENTIONS

- Assess patient's classification of disease status according to NYHA classification system
- Assist patient to complete those activities of daily living that do not lead to excessive increase in heart rate, blood pressure, respiratory rate, or electrical disturbances
- Provide adequate periods of rest for the patient between therapeutic care activities (such as completion of activities of daily living, therapeutic tests)
- Plan and implement incremental increase in activity (such as passive or active range of motion while on bed rest, increase in active participation in activities of daily living)
- Instruct the patient about signs of increased fatigue or exercise intolerance (such as increased heart rate,

respiratory rate, shortness of breath)

- Encourage patient to rest and/or decrease level of activity if the signs or symptoms of exercise intolerance are present
- Help patient prioritize activities
- Develop a plan to enable patient to achieve desired activities
- Assess the patient's readiness to learn energy conservation measures
- Provide positive reinforcement to encourage increases in activity
- Encourage patients to wear proper walking shoe (slippers may not be supportive)

The following nursing interventions support the medical plan of care for the medical diagnoses of congestive heart failure related to valvular heart disease:

- Monitor and assess the patient's blood pressure, pulse, respiratory status (dyspnea, orthopnea, pulmonary edema), heart sounds (S_1, S_2 systolic and diastolic murmurs), apical pulses, jugular venous distention, hepatic enlargement, and peripheral edema. Assessment should be done based on the patient's condition (every 10 to 15 minutes during unstable periods, every 4 hours when stable)
- Monitor hemodynamic variables such as pulmonary artery pressure, pulmonary wedge pressure, and cardiac output to assess cardiac function. Measurements should be taken as prescribed by the physician based on the patient's condition
- Administer medications as prescribed: digitalis glycosides, diuretics, and vasodilators, and evaluate patient's response to therapy
- Monitor hemodynamic status of patient with intraaortic balloon pump (IABP) when applicable. Assess timing of IABP to assure maximum hemodynamic benefit to patient
- Assess degree of oxygenation by obtaining arterial blood gases and administer oxygen if necessary
- Assess the patient's fluid status (daily weight, intake and output, serum BUN, creatinine and electrolytes, urinary specific gravity)
- Assess the patient for signs of cardiogenic shock (hypotension, tachycardia, urine output less than 30 ml/hr, decreased peripheral perfusion, increased respiratory rate, mental status change)
- Assess the patient's electrical conduction system by continuous ECG monitoring and 12-lead ECG recordings for evidence of electrical disturbances (such as sinus or atrial tachycardia, atrial fibrillation, ventricular dysrhythmias, or conduction disturbances)
- Administer medications to control ventricular rate (digitalis glycosides, verapamil) and rhythm (quinidine sulfate, procainamide) as prescribed
- Assess for signs of acute mitral or aortic regurgitation (dyspnea at rest, fatigue, PND, pulmonary edema, hepatomegaly, hypotension, pedal edema). Collaborate with physician for therapeutic interventions (such as diuretics, fluid restriction)

HIGH-RISK NURSING DIAGNOSES

Patients with a diagnosis of valvular dysfunction are more vulnerable to develop the following nursing problems:

- High risk for injury, related to risk of bleeding secondary to anticoagulation therapy
- High risk for self-care deficit, related to dyspnea and fatigue
- High risk for sleep pattern disturbances, related to nocturnal dyspnea
- High risk for powerlessness, related to progressive nature of valvular condition

PROSTHETIC HEART VALVES

The ideal prosthetic heart valve does not exist. Since the implantation of the first prosthetic valve in 1952 by Hufnagel, many mechanical and biological prostheses have been introduced, and many have failed. Failure has often been attributed to poor hemodynamic performance, high incidence of thrombosis on the valve surface leading to obstruction and/or emboli, mechanical failure, cracking or fracture of valve components, excessive hemolysis, rapid degeneration, and durability of the device.[49,50] Characteristics that are considered desirable in the design of an ideal substitute valve include: (1) durability, (2) optimal hemodynamic performance, (3) absence of thrombogenicity, (4) minimal hemolysis, (5) resistance to infection, (6) quiet movement, (7) low cost, and (8) ease of insertion.[51,52]

Achieving optimal hemodynamic performance is considered one of the most important features of prosthetic heart valves. The aim in the design of an artificial valve is to permit laminar as opposed to turbulent flow. To achieve laminar flow, the direction of flow through the valve should ideally be central and smooth. If the construction of the valve is such that turbulent flow is created, then complications may develop, such as intimal proliferation, thrombosis formation leading to obstruction and/or embolization, and, finally, hemolysis. Furthermore, the transvalvular gradient which normally should be zero is increased with turbulent flow patterns. Although significant advances in the development of artificial valves have been achieved, no type of valve has yet met all these ideal characteristics.

Mechanical versus Biological (Tissue) Valves

Prosthetic heart valves are classified into two broad categories: (1) mechanical, and (2) biological (tissue) prostheses.

Mechanical Valves

Mechanical valves include the three most commonly employed types: caged-ball, tilting disk, and bileaflet. Another type, the caged-disk valve, was found to be associated with a high degree of obstruction, thrombosis, and hemolysis[52] and is rarely used.

The *caged-ball valve* has been used extensively since 1960 (Figure 24-3). Models of this type include the Starr-Edwards, Harken, Sutter Silastic (formerly called the Smeloff-Cutter), DeBakey, Magovern, and Brownwell-Cutter. The two most frequently used valves are the Starr-Edwards and the Sutter types. In the early years, some of these valves were associated with prosthetic disproportion. When placed in small annuli, the large, cumbersome valves obstructed blood flow.[53] The use of caged-ball prostheses is now recommended only in patients with aortic or mitral regurgitation who have an enlarged left ventricle or ascending aorta.[52] These valves as a group also have a tendency to promote thrombosis, a problem that plagues all mechanical prostheses. Thus, patients with these devices require ongoing anticoagulation therapy.

Caged-ball prostheses also have less than desirable hemodynamic characteristics. Blood flow through these valves is not central, leading to all the complications of turbulent flow patterns. Hemolysis is usually not clinically problematic because the bone marrow under normal conditions is able to overcome the development of anemia and thrombocytopenia[52]; however, in some patients hemolysis may be clinically significant. Another undesirable feature of these valves is that they are the most audible of all the prosthetic valves. This can be a nuisance to some patients.

The one important advantage of the caged-ball

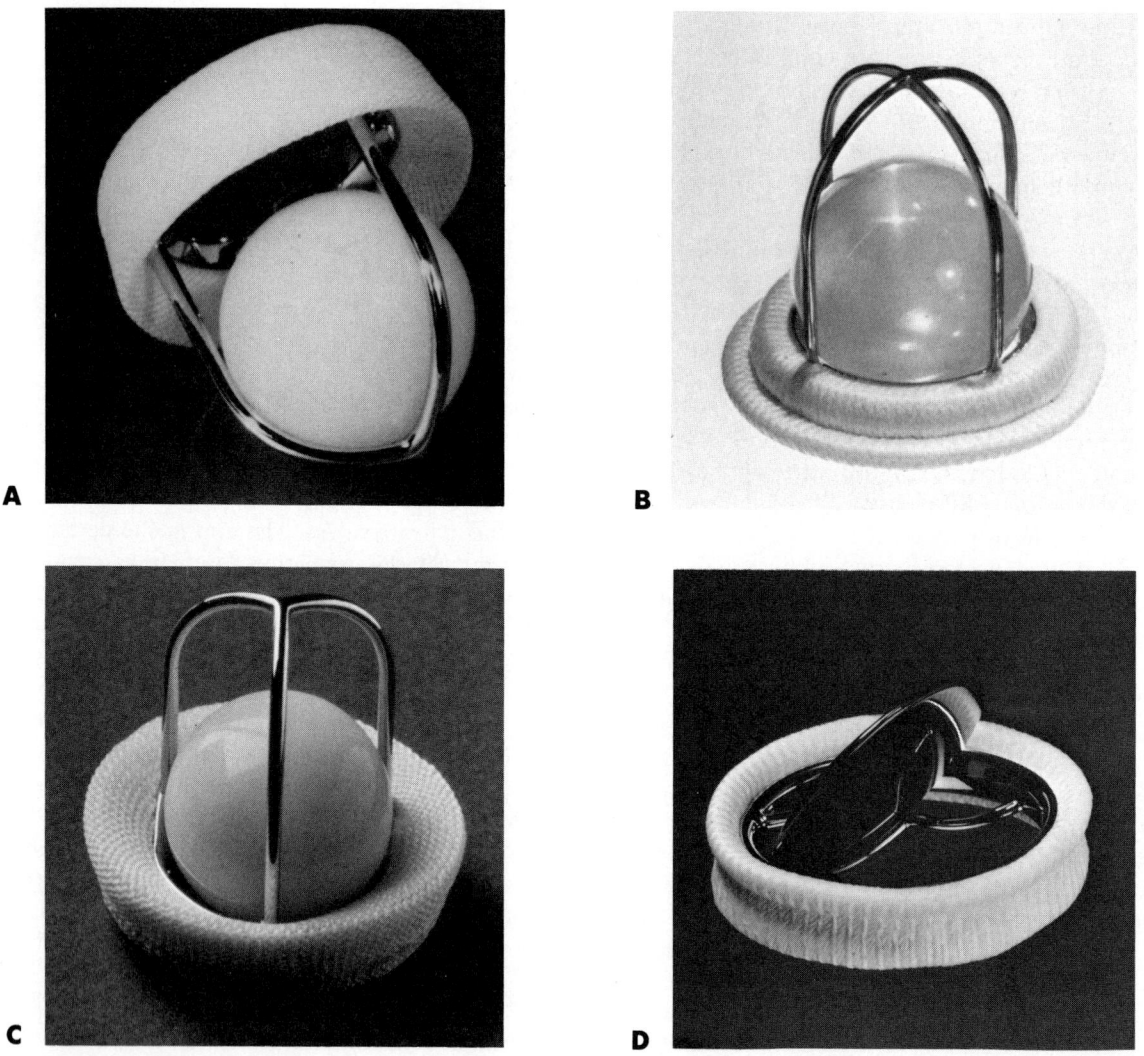

Figure 24-3 *A*, Aortic position. *B*, Model 6120. *C*, Model 1260, caged-ball. *D*, Bjork-Shiley spherical disk valve for aortic position.

A-C, Courtesy of American Edwards; D, Courtesy of Shiley, Inc.

prostheses is durability. They are not subject to rapid degeneration and wear and have an excellent record of being implanted for up to 20 years.[13]

Tilting disk valves came into use in the mid to late 1960s. Earlier models included the Wada-Cutter, Lillehei-Kaster, and Bjork-Shiley (spherical disk model; see Figure 24-3). Because the Wada-Cutter and Bjork-Shiley valves were associated with a high incidence of thrombosis and lack of durability leading to valve failure, their use was discontinued after 1976. A new generation of tilting disk valves including the Medtronic-Hall (formerly the Hall-Kaster) and the Bjork-Shiley convexo-concave models. These valves have a single disk that rests against the sewing ring when the valve is closed. When the valve opens, the disk tilts at an angle that allows a semicentral flow of blood through the orifice. These valves produce less hemodynamic obstruction and have a lower transvalvular gradient than their caged-ball valve counterparts.

Thrombosis remains a problem with the tilting disk valves, necessitating ongoing anticoagulation therapy. Durability also remains a serious problem, especially with the Bjork-Shiley convexo-concave models. These valves were withdrawn from the U.S. market by the manufacturer in 1986 because of reported problems with strut fracture and disc embolization. Over 20,000 U.S. patients have these valves, however, so health care personnel need to be cognizant of these potential problems.[54] The Lillehei-Kaster valves in contrast have had an acceptable reliability record. Only three cases of disk embolization have been reported.[55]

A great improvement in the hemodynamic performance of mechanical valves has been achieved with *bileaflet valves*, specifically the St. Jude Medical valves (see Figure 24-3). These valves (Omniscience, Omnicarbon, Duromedics) typically have a two-leaflet design. The leaflets move apart as they open to create a central orifice for blood flow. This central orifice in

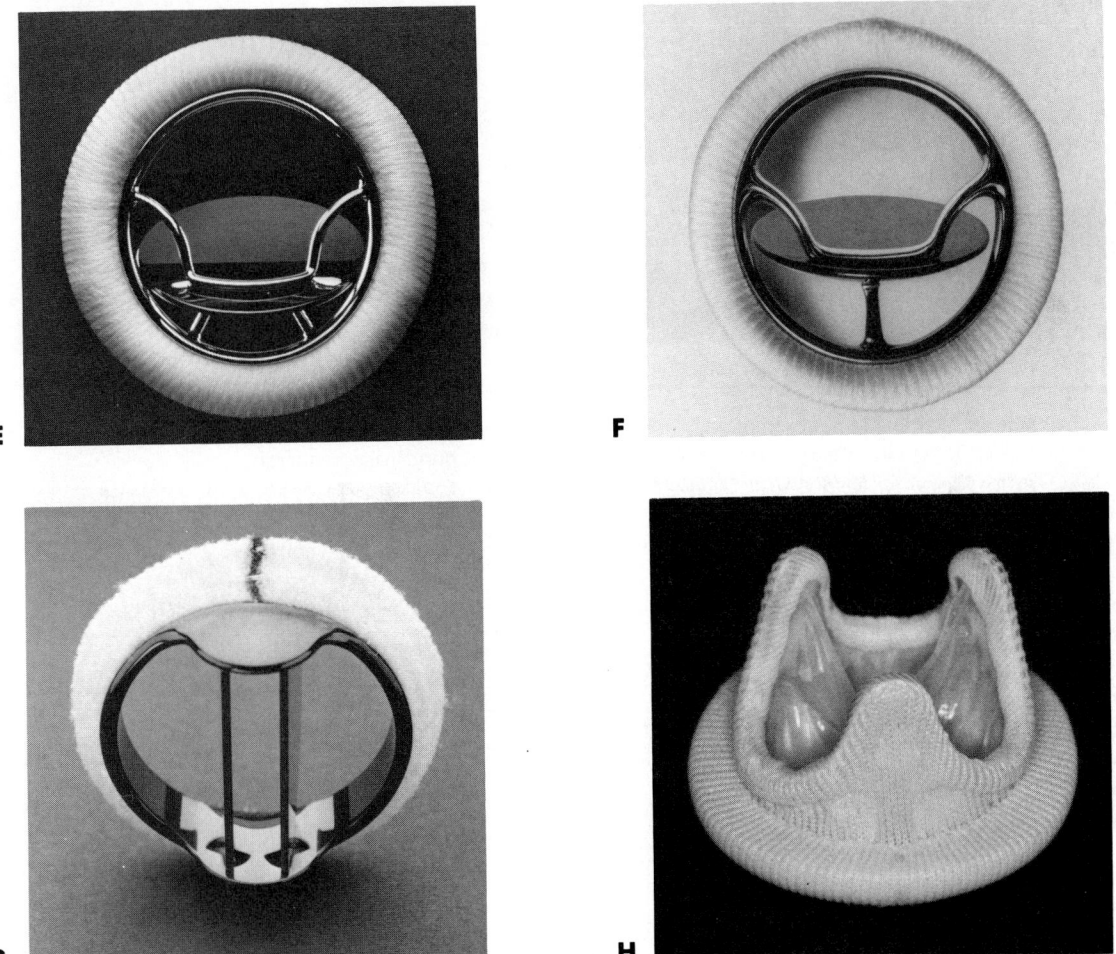

E   **F**

G   **H**

Figure 24-3, cont'd.   *E,* Bjork-Shiley spherical disk valve, mitral position. *F,* Bjork-Shiley monostruct valve. *G,* St. Jude Medical Heart Valve, aortic position. *H,* Hancock porcine mitral valve, model 342R.

E and *F, Courtesy of Shiley, Inc. G, Courtesy St. Jude Medical, Inc. H, Courtesy of Johnson & Johnson, Cardiovascular.*   *Continued.*

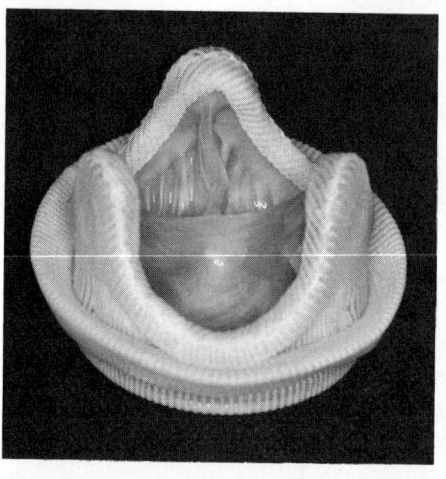
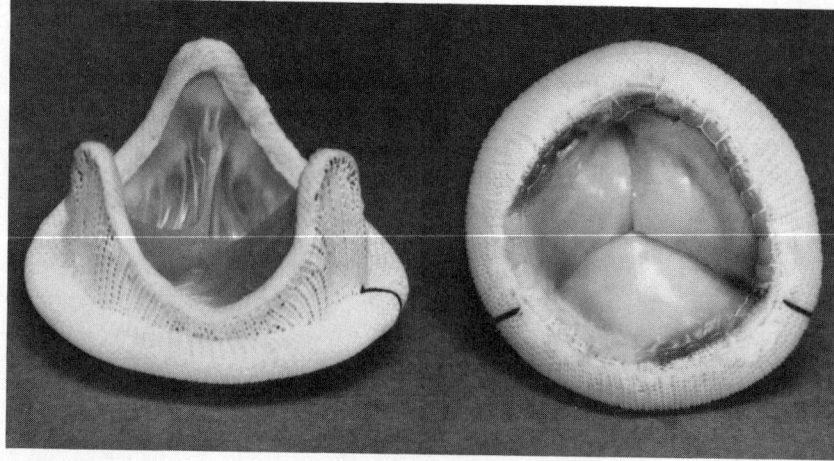

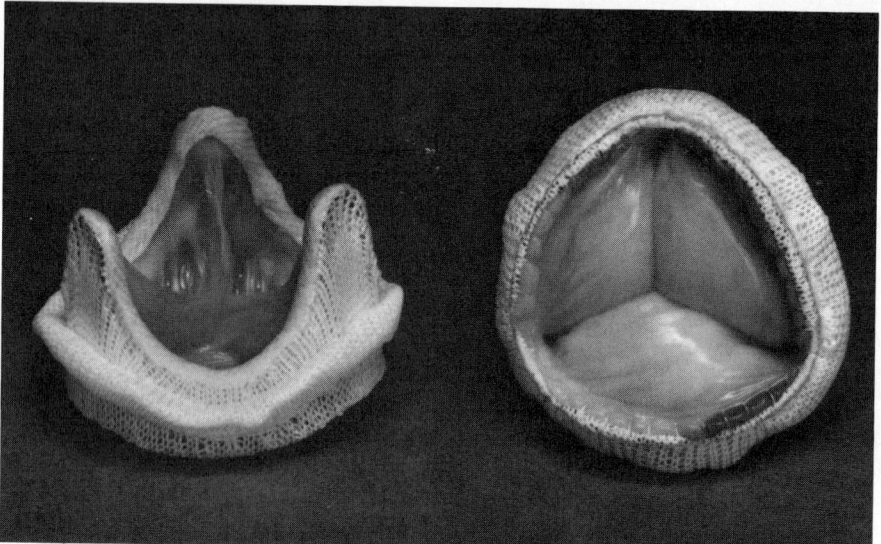
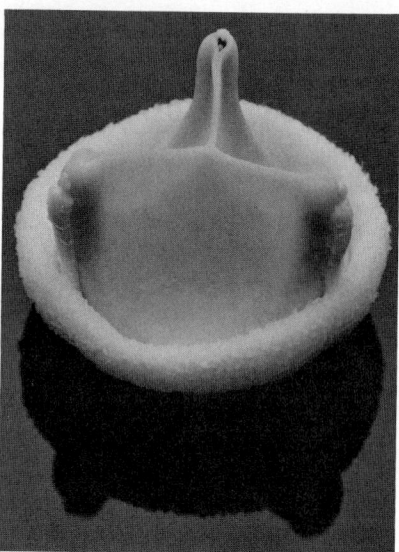

Figure 24-3, cont'd. *I,* Hancock porcine aortic valve, model 242. *J,* Carpentier-Edwards porcine valve, mitral position. *K,* Carpentier-Edwards porcine valve, aortic position. *L,* Ionescu-Shiley pericardial xenograft.

I, Courtesy of Johnson & Johnson, Cardiovascular. *J* and *K,* Courtesy of American Edwards. *L,* Courtesy of Shiley, Inc.

turn eliminates turbulence and reduces the transvalvular gradient to a minimal amount. However, these valves are vulnerable to thrombosis, necessitating long-term anticoagulation therapy. To date the St. Jude valves have an excellent clinical performance and durability record.[56] They are currently the most widely implanted valve type.

Biological Valves

The first biological tissue valve was implanted in 1962 by Heimbecker.[49] Since that time, a number of tissue types classified as isografts, allografts, and xenografts have been employed. Table 24-1 lists types of tissue valves and their biological source.

In the 1960s, isografts were initially considered to be satisfactory. The use of the native pulmonic valve

TABLE 24-1   Classification of Biological Valves

Types	Source
Allograft (isograft)	Fascia lata, pulmonic valve
Homologous (allograft)	Cadaver aortic valve, dura mater
Heterologous (xenograft)	Bovine aortic valve, porcine aortic valve, bovine pericardium

Source: Oyer, P. E., & Stinson, E. B. (1983). Biologic valves. In W. L. Glenn (Ed.), *Thoracic and cardiovascular surgery.* Norwalk, CT: Appleton-Century-Crofts.

to replace the diseased aortic valve was first reported by Ross in 1967. He then replaced the native pulmonic valve with a homograft.[49] This technique fell into disuse because it required a prolonged operation and durability could be attained with newer biological valves. Fascia lata could be fashioned to form a trileaflet aortic valve. The early results with this valve were reportedly excellent. After clinical investigation over several years, fascia lata valves were found to have a high incidence of endocarditis and rapid tissue degeneration.[49] Thus, long-term durability could not be achieved, and they were discontinued in the early 1970s.

The use of allograft tissue has been limited by availability. Too few donors have been obtained to supply all the patients requiring valve replacement. However, allograft valves are still used in England and New Zealand and are enjoying a resurgence of interest in the United States since cryopreservation of donor valves has increased the availability of these valves. For example, allograft valves are being used with increasing frequency in the Boston area.

Currently, the most extensively used biological valve is the xenograft. Xenograft valves that have been frequently implanted are the porcine (Hancock, Carpentier-Edwards; see Figure 24-3) and the bovine pericardium (Ionescu-Shiley) molded from the pericardium of 16-to-18-month-old calves. The use of bovine aortic valves had been restricted because of the inability to obtain a wide range of sizes. Recently, the Ionescu-Shiley bovine pericardial valve has been discontinued due to its limited durability record especially in the mitral position. The major advantage of the xenografts is their minimal thrombogenicity. Long-term anticoagulation therapy is generally not necessary. Isolated reports of thromboembolic events have occurred predominantly during the first 3 months with the xenograft implanted in the mitral position.[13] Therefore, anticoagulants may be ordered by some physicians for up to 6 months following mitral valve replacement. Circumstances that may require long-term anticoagulation with implanted xenograft valves are chronic atrial fibrillation and left atrial enlargement or a history of thromboembolic events.[13]

The most serious disadvantage with the porcine xenograft is its lack of clinical durability. Progressive deterioration and calcification on the valve surfaces of porcine tissue valves have occurred as early as 5 to 7 years postoperatively.[55] The issue of durability remains unclear because preservation techniques for porcine valves have changed. The next decade may reveal the answer.

Another disadvantage of the porcine xenografts is related to their initial structural design in small sizes.

Small-sized aortic porcine valves tended to have a small orifice size. This rendered the valves stenotic and as a result they had a higher transvalvular gradient than their mechanical counterparts in the same size. Moreover, when implanted into a small annulus they were obstructive to flow. However, the modified orifice Hancock bioprosthetic valve appears to have overcome the problem of obstruction.

Selection of Prosthetic Valves

Considerations in choosing a prosthetic valve include: (1) age of the patient, (2) activities of daily living, (3) medical history, (4) willingness and/or ability to follow an anticoagulation regimen, and (5) cardiac anatomy.[13,51,53] Critical care nurses should be aware of these considerations in the physician's selection of an artificial valve. This knowledge enhances the teaching of patients and significant others regarding the advantages and disadvantages of each type of device.

Age can be an important criterion from the standpoint of durability. Braunwald[13] advocates the use of a mechanical valve prosthesis in patients under 65 who have no contraindications to anticoagulation. In patients over 65, durability is less of an issue, but the risk of hemorrhage from anticoagulants or noncompliance may be greater. Thus, the use of a tissue valve would seem warranted in this subset.

Tissue valves are preferred for patients whose activities of daily living increase the risk of bleeding. The question of which type of valve to implant in women of childbearing age remains controversial. Proponents of tissue valves believe that pregnancy increases the risk of thromboembolism and that patients with mechanical valves who take anticoagulants have an increased risk of fetal hemorrhage during pregnancy.

Patients with a medical history of bleeding usually receive a tissue valve as do patients in whom willingness or the ability to follow an anticoagulation regimen is doubtful. Elderly patients often receive tissue valves because of the potential problems associated with an anticoagulation regimen.

Cardiac anatomy is another important consideration. Patients with small left ventricular cavities or tiny mitral annuli will probably benefit from the St. Jude–type valve in comparison with the bulky caged-ball devices.

Auscultation

To assess for possible malfunctioning of a prosthetic heart valve, an understanding of the normal auscultatory findings is appropriate. The opening and closing sounds associated with certain types of valves in either the mitral or aortic position are discussed.

Caged-ball Valves

Caged-ball valves are noted characteristically for their distinct, high-pitched, audible opening and closing sounds. These prostheses emit a prominent opening click in both the aortic and mitral position which is notably louder than the mitral or aortic closure sound. The second or third right intercostal space (aortic) or the apex (mitral) are the preferred landmarks to auscultate these sounds. Caged-ball valves are associated with grade II/VI to III/VI early decrescendo or systolic ejection murmurs.[57] These murmurs are accentuated in conditions which augment the stroke volume. The presence of a diastolic murmur is not considered to be a normal finding.

Tilting Disk Valves

The commonly used tilting disk valves, excluding the St. Jude model, generally are not associated with an audible opening sound in either mitral or aortic position but do produce distinct closing sounds.[57] Absence or diminution of a closing sound during sinus rhythm is considered to be an abnormal finding. Systolic murmurs are often noted in the mitral and aortic positions with tilting disk valves. A mitral prosthetic valve produces a II/VI early-to-midsystolic ejection murmur, whereas an aortic prosthetic valve produces a basal early-to-midsystolic ejection murmur.

Tissue Valves

Porcine tissue valves have crisp, high-pitched opening and closing sounds which are typically less prominent than those produced by their mechanical counterparts. In the mitral position, approximately one half of patients with implanted tissue valves have opening sounds which can be heard in the apical area. In addition, there may be apical diastolic rumbling or systolic murmurs. Prosthetic malfunction should be considered if a new diastolic murmur appears, or a change in the character or intensity of a murmur becomes apparent. Opening sounds are not generally heard in the aortic position; however, closing sounds are auscultated in many patients. A midsystolic murmur may be audible at the lower left sternal border. No diastolic murmur should be heard in the aortic position with tissue valves.

Complications

A detailed explanation of all possible complications associated with every type of valve is beyond the scope of this section. Discussion focuses on four major complications: inadequate valve seating, valvular obstruction related to thrombus formation or mechanical failure, thromboembolism, and prosthetic endocarditis.

Inadequate valve seating is usually related to suture displacement. Adherence between the valve ring and the annulus is lost and acute valvular regurgitation results. These patients generally recover poorly from surgery, and develop congestive heart failure despite medical interventions. Inadequate seating should be suspected in patients who also develop a new regurgitant murmur. Treatment for this complication is to replace the valve.

Valvular obstruction related to thrombus formation or mechanical failure can be life-threatening or fatal if total obstruction occurs. Parameters by which to assess for this complication are a sudden or persistent decline in cardiac output, or a change in intensity or timing of a valve click. Echocardiography is useful in detecting this complication. Replacement of the prosthetic valve is usually necessary, especially if a mechanical failure is the precipitating factor.

Thromboembolism is usually a result of inadequate anticoagulation therapy. For this reason, nurses need to educate patients and significant others regarding the possibility of this complication. Prothrombin times must be periodically assessed to ascertain proper blood levels. The organs to which arterial emboli migrate most often are the brain, heart, and kidneys. Therefore, careful assessment of the level of consciousness, cardiac function, and urinary output are necessary to evaluate clinically for the presence of emboli.

Prosthetic valve endocarditis (PVE) has similar clinical features to those discussed in the section related to infective endocarditis. Only the differences will be mentioned. Predisposing factors to this type of endocarditis are sternal wound infections or sternal osteomyelitis.[9] A relatively recent decline in early PVE is probably related to prophylaxis antibiotic therapy and improved surgical technique.

The most frequent causative microorganisms in both early (less than 2 months postoperatively) or late (more than 2 months postoperatively) PVE are *Staphylococcus epidermidis* or *aureus*. Streptococcal infection, when implicated, is seen in late PVE and carries a better prognosis than a staphylococcal infection.

The site of endocarditis varies with the type of tissue valve. For example, with the majority of mechanical valves the infection is beneath the site of attachment and, as a result, a ring abscess occurs. With tissue valves the infection is usually limited to the cusps and, therefore, is associated with a better prognosis. When two prosthetic valves have been replaced, the infection for the most part involves the most downstream prosthesis.[50]

Clinical findings consist of a fever (95% of cases),

leukocytosis (50% of cases), new or changing regurgitant murmur (50% of cases), and gram-positive blood cultures (85%). Two-dimensional echocardiography is a useful diagnostic test in suspected PVE.[58]

A review by Cowgill et al.[59] found the average mortality rate for PVE to be 54% for the last decade. When early surgery was performed in appropriate circumstances the mortality was reduced from 61% to 38%. Generally accepted indications for surgery include: (1) severe congestive heart failure, (2) persistent sepsis despite appropriate therapy, (3) fungal infection, (4) valve obstruction, (5) unstable prosthesis as evidenced by fluoroscopy, and (6) new onset of heart block.[60]

PERCUTANEOUS BALLOON VALVULOPLASTY

The procedure known as percutaneous valvuloplasty or balloon valvular dilatation offers a nonoperative treatment option for specific patients experiencing aortic or mitral stenosis. Balloon valvuloplasty is of limited use in patients with aortic or mitral stenosis.

Aortic Valvuloplasty

Balloon aortic valvuloplasty was first performed in children in 1983 and was later tried in adults with calcific aortic stenosis in 1986.[62] A dilating balloon catheter is inserted into the femoral or brachial artery and advanced retrograde across the aortic valve. The balloon is then inflated around the orifice of the stenotic aortic valve. The postulated mechanisms of valvular dilatation are fracture of the calcified nodules or frame of the valvular cusps, commissural separation, leaflet stretching or tearing, or annulus rupture.[61] Regardless of the mechanism, the desired outcome of valvuloplasty is to increase the valve orifice area and to decrease the existing transvalvular gradient.

Pooled results from many multicenter trials indicate that patients treated by aortic valvuloplasty have experienced serious adverse effects and complications such as ventricular perforation, acute aortic insufficiency, embolic events, vascular damage, restenosis, and death. Rates of restenosis and death are both relatively high, with a 1-year survival ranging from 50% to 80%.[62] Considering these grim results, current indications for this procedure include: (1) short-term palliation of symptoms in patients for whom surgical aortic valve replacement must be deferred because of high expected surgical risk, as in the case of pregnancy; (2) a bridge to valve replacement in patients who have poor LV function that may improve postprocedure; (3) patients with aortic stenosis who require urgent noncardiac surgery such as bowel surgery or repair of an abdominal aortic aneurysm and in whom this procedure may permit the patient to tolerate general anesthesia.[62,63,64]

Mitral Valvuloplasty

The historical perspective of this procedure parallels the sequence of aortic valvuloplasty, beginning with children and extending to adults. It differs from aortic valvuloplasty in that a balloon dilatation catheter is inserted antegrade into the right heart, advanced transseptally across the right atrium into the left atrium, then across the mitral valve to be inflated. In addition, one or two balloons may be inflated to achieve the desired outcome, as in aortic valvuloplasty.

The mechanism of this type of valvuloplasty is thought to be separation of the fused commissures similar to the mechanism of closed commissurotomy.[62] Complications associated with this procedure include cardiac perforation, massive mitral regurgitation, cardiac tamponade, the need for emergency mitral surgery, pulmonary edema, cerebrovascular accidents, and embolic events.[62] Procedural mortality rates pooled from large studies indicate a range between 0.5% and 2%.[62] Restenosis rates are more favorable with mitral valvuloplasty than with aortic valvuloplasty. The average rate of restenosis is approximately 5% per year. One-year survival is also good with an average greater than 90%.[62]

These favorable findings have led to the following current indications for mitral valvuloplasty: (1) as a first-line treatment option for patients with noncalcified mitral stenosis, especially in the young or pregnant woman; and (2) as a palliative treatment for patients with calcific disease who are not surgical candidates.[62,63]

REFERENCES

1. Caplan, C. H. (1983). Diseases of the pericardium, myocardium and endocardium. In N. Levinsky (Ed.), *Medicine essentials of clinical practice.* Boston: Little, Brown.
2. Packa, D., & Vitello, J. M. (1984). Valvular heart disease. In B. Bullock, & P. Rosendahl (Eds.), *Pathophysiology.* Boston: Little, Brown.
3. American Heart Association. (1977). Committee on rheumatic fever bacterial endocarditis: Prevention of rheumatic fever. *Circulation, 55,* 1-4.
4. Stollerman, G. H. (1992). Rheumatic and heritable connective tissue diseases of the cardiovascular system. In E. Braunwald (Ed.), *Heart disease* (4th ed.). Philadelphia: Saunders.
5. McCarthy, R. J. (1983). The medical cardiac patient. In R. G. Sanderson, & C. L. Kurth (Eds.), *The cardiac patient.* Philadelphia: Saunders.
6. Lerner, P. I., & Weinstein, L. (1966). Infective endocarditis in the antibiotic era. *New England Journal of Medicine, 274,* 199-206.

7. Come, P. C. (1982). Infective endocarditis: Current perspectives. *Comprehensive Therapy, 8*(7), 57-70.

8. Arbulu, A., & Asfau, I. (1983). Infective endocarditis. In W. Glenn (Ed.), *Thoracic and cardiovascular surgery*. Norwalk, CT: Appleton-Century-Crofts.

9. Weinstein, L. (1984). Infective endocarditis. In E. Braunwald (Ed.), *Heart disease: A textbook of cardiovascular medicine* (2nd ed.). Philadelphia: Saunders.

10. Agarwal, A. K. (1985). Infective endocarditis. *Comprehensive therapy, 11*(3), 17-25.

11. Durack, D. T. (1990). Infective and non-infective endocarditis. In J. W. Hurst, R. C. Schlant, C. E. Rackley, et al. (Eds.), *The heart* (7th ed.). New York: McGraw-Hill.

12. Pape, L. A. (1986). Pathogenesis and etiology of valvular heart disease. In J. E. Dalen, & J. S. Alpert (Eds.), *Valvular heart disease* (2nd ed.). Boston: Little, Brown.

13. Braunwald, E. (1984). Valvular heart disease. In E. Braunwald, (Ed.), *Heart disease: A textbook of cardiovascular medicine* (2nd ed.). Philadelphia: Saunders.

14. Dalen, J. E. (1986). Mitral stenosis. In J. E. Dalen, & J. S. Alpert (Eds.), *Valvular heart disease* (2nd ed.) (pp. 47-110). Boston: Little, Brown.

15. Isom, O. W., Shemin, R. J., & Whidden, L. L. (1983). Rheumatic mitral valve stenosis. In W. L. Glenn (Ed.), *Thoracic and cardiovascular surgery*. Norwalk, CT: Appleton-Century-Crofts.

16. Dalen, J. E. (1986). Mitral stenosis. In J. E. Dalen, & J. S. Alpert (Eds.), *Valvular heart disease* (2nd ed.) (pp. 47-110). Boston: Little, Brown.

17. Bornheimer, J. F., Kim, J. S., Sambasivan, V., et al. (1982). Effects of nitroglycerin on supine and upright exercise in mitral stenosis. *American Heart Journal, 104*(6), 1288-1293.

18. Kawashita, K., Kambara, H., Kadota, K., et al. (1983). Radiocardiographic assessment of dobutamine and isosorbide dinitrite therapy in patients with mitral stenosis and pulmonary congestion. *Japan Circulation Journal, 47*(3), 283-288.

19. Flugelman, M. U., Hasin, Y., Katznelson, N., et al. (1984). Restoration and maintenance of sinus rhythm after mitral valve surgery for mitral stenosis. *American Journal of Cardiology, 54*(6), 617-619.

20. Breyer, R. H., Mills, S. A., Hudspeth, A. S., et al. (1985). Open mitral commissurotomy: Long term results with echocardiographic correlation. *Journal of Cardiovascular Surgery, 26*(1), 46-52.

21. Chaffin, J. S., & Daggett, W. M. (1979). Mitral valve replacement: A nine year follow-up of risks and survivals. *Annals of Thoracic Surgery, 27*(4), 312-319.

22. Tryka, A. F., Godleski, J. J., Schoen, F. J., et al. (1985). Pulmonary vascular disease and hypertension after valve surgery for mitral stenosis. *Human Pathology, 16*(1), 65-71.

23. Levinson, G. E. (1981). Aortic stenosis. In J. E. Dalen, & J. S. Alpert (Eds.), *Valvular heart disease* (2nd ed.). Boston: Little, Brown.

24. Ikram, H., Low, C. J. S., Crozier, I. G., et al. (1992). Hemodynamic effects of nitroprusside on valvular aortic stenosis. *American Journal of Cardiology, 69*(4), 361-366.

25. Folland, E. D., Kemper, A. J., Khuri, S. F., et al. (1985). Intraaortic balloon counterpulsation as a temporary support measure in decompensated critical aortic stenosis. *Journal of the American College of Cardiology, 5*(3), 711-716.

26. McAnulty, J. H. (1984). Timing of surgical therapy for aortic valve stenosis, goals of therapy. *Herz, 9*(6), 341-345.

27. Murphy, E. S., Lawson, R. M., Starr, A., et al. (1981). Severe aortic stenosis in patients 60 years of age or older: Left ventricular function and 10 year survival after replacement. *Circulation, 64*, 184-188.

28. Hwang, M. H., Hammermeister, K. E., Oprian, C., et al. (1989). Preoperative identification of patients likely to have left ventricular dysfunction after aortic valve replacement. Participants in the Veterans Administration Cooperative Study on Valvular Heart Disease. *Circulation, 80*(3), I-65-I-76.

29. Kay, J. H., Carlish, R. A., & Dunne, E. F. (1983). Mitral insufficiency. In W. L. Glenn (Ed.), *Thoracic and cardiovascular surgery*. Norwalk, CT: Appleton-Century-Crofts.

30. Howe, J. P., & Alpert, J. S. (1986). Acute mitral regurgitation. In J. E. Dalen, & J. S. Alpert (Eds.), *Valvular heart disease* (2nd ed.). Boston: Little, Brown.

31. Crawford, M. H., Souchek, J., Oprian, C., et al. (1990). Determinants of survival and left ventricular performance after mitral valve replacement. *Circulation, 81*(4), 1173-1181.

32. Nunley, D. L., & Starr, A. (1984). The evolution of reparative techniques for the mitral valve. *Annals of Thoracic Surgery, 37*(5), 393-397.

33. Bonchek, L. I., Olinger, G. N., Siegal, R., et al. (1984). Left ventricular performance after mitral reconstruction for mitral regurgitation. *Journal of Thoracic Cardiovascular Surgery, 88*(1), 122-127.

34. David, T. E., Burns, R. J., Bacchus, C. M., et al. (1984). Mitral valve replacement for mitral valve regurgitation with and without preservation of chordae tendineae. *Journal of Thoracic Cardiovascular Surgery, 88*, 718-725.

35. Deveraux, R., Kramer-Fox, R., & Kligfield, P. (1989). Mitral valve prolapse: Causes, clinical manifestations, and management. *Annals of Internal Medicine, 111*(4), 305-317.

36. Reece, I. J., Cooley, D. A., Painvin, G. A., et al. (1985). Surgical treatment of mitral systolic click syndrome: Results in 37 patients. *Annals of Thoracic Surgery, 39*, 155-158.

37. Ross, A., DeWeese, J. A., & Yu, P. W. (1978). Refractory ventricular arrhythmias in a patient with mitral valve prolapse. Successful control with mitral valve replacement. *Journal of Electrocardiography, 11*, 289-295.

38. Malpartida, F., Arcas, R., Alegria, E., et al. (1980). Surgical treatment for chest pain in mitral valve prolapse. *Chest, 78*(1), 101-104.

39. Alpert, J. S. (1986). Chronic aortic regurgitation. In J. E. Dalen, & J. S. Alpert (Eds.), *Valvular heart disease* (2nd ed.). Boston: Little, Brown.

40. Benotti, J. R. (1986). Acute aortic insufficiency. In J. E. Dalen, & J. S. Alpert (Eds.), *Valvular heart disease* (2nd ed.). Boston: Little, Brown.

41. O'Rourke, R. A., & Walsh, R. A. (1986). Recognition and treatment of acute aortic regurgitation. *Journal of Intensive Care Medicine, 1*(1), 33-46.

42. Greenberg, B., Massie, B., Bristow, D., et al. (1988). Long term vasodilator therapy of chronic aortic insufficiency. A randomized double-blinded, placebo-controlled clinical trial. *Circulation, 78*(1), 92-103.

43. Cutler, B. S. (1986). The intraaortic balloon and counterpulsation. In J. M. Rippe, R. S. Irwin, J. S. Alpert, et al. (Eds.), *Intensive care medicine*. Boston: Little, Brown.

44. Shen, W. F., Roubin, G. S., Hirasawa, K., et al. (1984). Noninvasive assessment of acute effects of nifedipine on rest and exercise hemodynamics and cardiac function in patients with aortic regurgitation. *Journal of the American College of Cardiology, 4*(5), 902-907.

45. Shen, W. F., Roubin, G. S., Hirasawa, K., et al. (1984). Abnormal left ventricular response to isometric exercise in pure, isolated aortic regurgitation: Beneficial effects of nifedipine. *American Journal of Cardiology, 54*(6), 605-609.

46. Greenberg, B. H., & Rahimtoola, S. H. (1980). Long term vasodilator therapy in aortic insufficiency. Evidence for regression of left ventricular dilatation and hypertrophy and improvement in systolic pump function. *Annals of Internal Medicine, 93*(3), 440-442.

47. Osamura, Y., & Tasaka M. (1984). Observations on the timing of operative intervention for aortic regurgitation. *Japan Circulation Journal, 48*(10), 1162-1168.

48. Louagie, Y., Brohet, C., Lopez, E., et al. (1984). Early surgery for severe aortic regurgitation. *Journal of Cardiovascular Surgery* (Torino), 25(4), 304-312.

49. Oyer, P. E., & Stinson, E. B. (1983). Biologic valves. In W. L. Glenn (Ed.), *Thoracic and cardiovascular surgery*. Norwalk, CT: Appleton-Century-Crofts.

50. Davila, J. C. (1989). Ideal heart valve substitute. *Annals of Thoracic Surgery, 48*, 20-23.

51. Weiland, A. P. (1983). A review of cardiac valve prostheses and their selection. *Heart Lung, 12*, 498-504.

52. Geha, A. S. (1980). Mechanical valve prostheses. In W. L. Glenn (Ed.), *Thoracic and cardiovascular surgery*. Norwalk, CT: Appleton-Century-Crofts.

53. Bonchek, L. I. (1981). Current status of cardiac valve replacement: Selection of a prosthesis and indications for operation. *American Heart Journal, 101*, 96-106.

54. Shiley advises physicians on fractures of the convex-oconcave heart valves. (1990). *FDA Bulletin, 20*(2), 6.

55. Lillehei, C. W., Nakib, A., Kaster, B. E., et al. (1989). The origin and design of three new mechanical valve designs: Toroidal disc, pivoting disc, and rigid bileaflet cardiac prostheses. *Annals of Thoracic Surgery, 48*, 35-37.

56. Wang, J. H. (1989). The design simplicity and clinical elegance of the St. Jude Medical Heart Valve. *Annals of Thoracic Surgery, 48*, 55-56.

57. Smith, N. D., Raizada, V., & Abrams, J. (1981). Auscultation of the normally functioning prosthetic valve. *Annals of Internal Medicine, 95*, 594-598.

58. Cunha, C. L. P., Guiliani, E. R., Callahan, J. A., et al. (1980). Echophonocardiographic findings in patients with prosthetic heart valve malfunction. *Mayo Clinic Proceedings, 55*, 231-242.

59. Cowgill, L. O., Addonizio, V. P., Hopeman, A. R., et al. (1986). Prosthetic valve endocarditis. *Current Problems in Cardiology, 11*, 618-664.

60. Harrison, E. C., Rashtain, M. Y., Allen, D. T., et al. (1988). An emergency physician's guide to prosthetic heart valves: Valve related complications. *Annals of Emergency Medicine, 17*(7), 704-710.

61. Cribier, A., Savin, T., Berland, J., et al. (1987). Percutaneous transluminal balloon valvuloplasty of adult aortic stenosis: Report of 92 cases. *Journal of the American College of Cardiology, 9*(2), 381-386.

62. McKay, R. G. (1991). Balloon valvuloplasty is the treatment of choice for an increasing number of patients with valvular heart disease. Paper presented at the New England Cardiovascular Society's Scientific Session on Interventional Cardiology: Present and Future, Framingham, MA.

63. Cohn, L. (1991). Balloon valve dilatation is not the treatment of choice for an increasing number of patients with valvular heart disease. Paper presented at the New England Cardiovascular Society's Scientific Sessions on Interventional Cardiology: Present and Future, Framingham, MA.

64. Zaibag, M. A., & Ribeiro, P. (1990). The future of balloon valvotomy. In E. J. Topol (Ed.), *Textbook of interventional cardiology* (pp. 912-926). Philadelphia: Saunders.

25

Vascular Disease

Jeanne Doyle

Molly Johantgen

Joan Vitello-Cicciu

The arteries and veins are the roads and pathways by which the blood circulates through the body. The aorta is the largest of these conduits, delivering oxygenated blood directly from the heart. This chapter discusses abnormalities of the aorta, peripheral arteries and veins, vascular trauma, and compartment syndrome and the integral role that the critical care nurse plays in the care of patients with such abnormalities.

AORTIC DISEASE

Arterial Anatomy

The aorta is a large but thin and tough vessel that must absorb the pumping of approximately three billion heartbeats in an average lifetime. It consists of the thin inner intima, thick media, and thin outer adventitia (Figure 25-1). The aortic intima is a single endothelial layer that is easily traumatized. The media is composed of intertwining sheets of elastin arranged in a spiral design to increase strength. A small amount of smooth muscle and collagen lies between the elastic membranes, providing additional tensile strength and elasticity. The outer adventitia contains collagen and the vasa vasorum and lymphatics, which nourish the aortic wall.

The aorta is divided into (1) the ascending aorta, which arises from the base (aortic valve) of the heart

and extends to the arch; (2) the arch of the aorta, from which the brachiocephalic and carotid vessels originate; (3) the descending thoracic aorta, which continues from the arch to the diaphragm; and (4) the abdominal aorta, which continues from the thoracic aorta to the aortic bifurcation.

Aortic Aneurysm

An *aneurysm* is defined as an abnormal dilatation of an artery. Aneurysms may be classified as "true" or "false." True aneurysms involve all three layers of the arterial wall. False aneurysms are in fact not aneurysms at all but are pulsatile hematomas which develop from disruption of one or two layers of the arterial wall.

The most common underlying disease affecting the aorta is atherosclerosis. Although atherosclerosis is initially an intimal process, hemorrhage into the plaque may invade the medial layer, causing weakening and generalized dilatation of the aorta. Atherosclerotic aneurysms characteristically affect the abdominal aorta below the renal arteries most severely and the ascending aorta least frequently. Advancing age has been linked with decreased elastin content within the aorta, which also may contribute to weakness in the aortic wall.

Risk factors such as smoking, hyperlipidemia, and hypertension parallel those involved in coronary artery disease. Refer to Chapter 22 for discussion of these risk factors. It is interesting to note, however, that aneurysm formation occurs eight times more often in smokers than in nonsmokers,[1] and patients with aneurysms may have elevated levels of triglycerides and low-density lipoproteins (LDL).[2] Hypertension increases injury to the endothelium and may accelerate medial degeneration because of increased hemodynamic stress in persons with underlying molec-

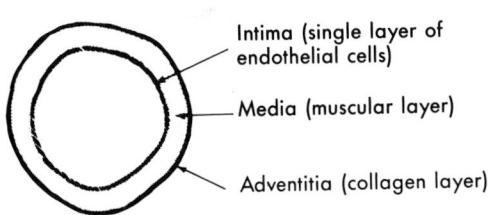

Figure 25-1 Cross-sectional representation of layers in arterial wall.

ular defects of elastin and collagen. Moreover, acute hypertension has been shown experimentally to decrease blood flow to the vasa vasorum, thereby decreasing nutrient flow into the media and causing ischemia and weakening of that layer.

Additional theories regarding aneurysm formation include: (1) a familial tendency toward the disease; (2) a sex-linked type of inheritance pattern suggested by the high incidence of aneurysm formation in males; and (3) abnormal amounts and function of certain enzymes in the aortic wall such as elastase and collagenase.[3,4,5]

Marfan's disease is a nonatherosclerotic disorder of connective tissue involving massive degeneration of elastic fibers in the aortic media, which can result in aneurysm formation. Medial degeneration is most severe at the aortic root and ascending aorta; therefore, aneurysm of the proximal aorta is the most frequent manifestation noted in Marfan's syndrome. *Marfan's syndrome* is an inherited disorder that in its most complete presentation has four clinical characteristics in addition to a family history of the disorder: skeletal abnormalities consisting of long extremities, particularly long hands and feet; a high arched palate; deformities of the thorax; and lax ligaments or sparse muscle mass. Many persons with Marfan's syndrome present with symptoms of aortic rupture prior to age 40.

Syphilis, autoimmune disease, and trauma also cause aortic wall destruction that can result in aneurysm formation. Congenital anomalies such as coarctation of the thoracic or abdominal aorta are rare but may be associated with aneurysm formation (see box below).

Underlying Causes of Aortic Disease

Hypertension	Congenital anomalies
Atherosclerosis	Trauma
Medial degeneration	Smoking
Age	Genetic link
Marfan's syndrome	Sex-linked trait
Idiopathic cystic medial	Cellular enzyme dys-
degeneration	function
Aortitis	Hyperlipidemia
Bacterial aortitis	
Mycotic aneurysm	
Syphilitic aortitis	
Nonspecific aortitis	
Takayasu's disease	
Giant cell arteritis	
Ankylosing spondylitis	
Reiter's syndrome	

Adapted from Lindsay, J., Jr., DeBakey, M. E., & Beall, A. C., Jr. (1982). Diseases of the aorta. In J. W. Hurst, R. B. Logue, C. E. Rackley, et al. (Eds.), *The heart: Arteries and veins.* New York: McGraw-Hill.

Most common kinds of aneurysms

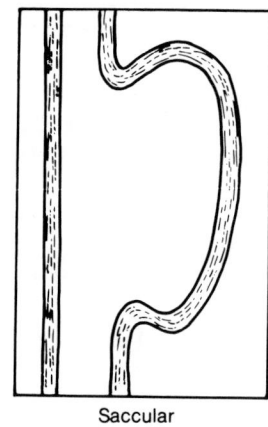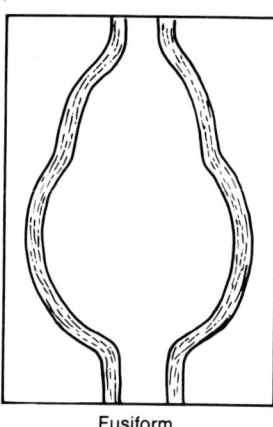

Saccular   Fusiform

Figure 25-2 Two most common types of true aortic aneurysms.

Once begun, aneurysm formation is promoted by the law of LaPlace. A vicious cycle begins with increased tension on the aortic wall, which leads to expansion of the aortic wall diameter, that further increases the tension, producing progressive dilatation of the aneurysm. The rate of expansion of an aneurysm is unpredictable, and, therefore, there is no "safe" aneurysm.

Two types of true aneurysms are seen in the aorta. *Fusiform* aneurysms result from a diffuse area of weakness producing a spindle-shaped deformity, whereas in *saccular* aneurysms a balloonlike dilatation is present. The lumen of an aneurysm usually contains layers of laminated clot, portions of which may break loose, embolizing to areas distal to the aneurysm[6] (Figure 25-2).

The primary concern with aortic aneurysms is the risk of aortic rupture. The incidence of aortic rupture is directly proportional to aneurysm size; the likelihood of rupture increases dramatically when the aneurysm is 6 cm in diameter or more. Aneurysms of smaller diameter are also at risk of rupture, but the incidence is far lower.

Rupture of an aneurysm is the extravasation of blood beyond the walls of the aneurysm. This rupture may occur anteriorly into the peritoneal cavity or posteriorly into the retroperitoneal space. The location of the rupture is related to the severity of the bleeding. Anterior rupture into the peritoneal cavity is life-threatening, with profound bleeding and exsanguination, often before resuscitative measures can be instituted. Posterior rupture into the retroperitoneal space is often tamponaded by anatomic structures such as the spinal cord. Rapid recognition of a posterior rupture often allows for successful surgical repair.

Symptoms of aneurysmal rupture include unremitting back or abdominal pain, weakness, nausea, or vomiting, or unconsciousness consistent with hypovolemia. Rupture may also precipitate myocardial ischemia, pulmonary edema, or high output failure. Lastly, severe tenderness of a mass in the abdominal aorta is suggestive of imminent aneurysmal rupture.

Data Acquisition

History and Physical Assessment. In general, patients who have an aneurysm are asymptomatic until the aneurysm reaches a size at which it impinges on other organs or begins to leak. Depending on the location of the aneurysm, the physical examination may reflect pressure on or involvement of other organs.

Persons with ascending aortic aneurysms may be asymptomatic or may have dyspnea and chest pain. Physical examination is significant for a widened pulse pressure, a bounding pulse, an aortic diastolic murmur, and/or an aortic valve regurgitation murmur.

An aortic arch aneurysm may impinge on the lungs, trachea, pulmonary artery, superior vena cava, innominate veins, or laryngeal nerve. Symptoms include dyspnea, stridor, hoarseness, hemoptysis, cough, or chest pain. Physical findings may include distended jugular and arm veins, left vocal cord paralysis, abnormal pulsations of the upper anterior chest, signs of pleural fluid such as absent breath sounds or dullness on percussion, and signs of congestive heart failure such as crackles and an S_3.

The most common symptom of an aneurysm of the descending thoracic aorta is pain. The pain is often located in the posterior thorax between the shoulders. However, some patients have pain in the lower back, abdomen, shoulders, arms, or neck. The pain is described as dull and may be intermittent or constant. Aneurysms of the descending thoracic aorta can rarely be detected by physical examination. A pulsatile mass at the base of the neck or left supraclavicular fossa may be noted if there is enlargement of the aneurysm, and hoarseness from pressure on the laryngeal nerve sometimes occurs. Leaking of the aneurysm may cause a significant increase in pain and hemoptysis.

Abdominal aneurysms generally produce no symptoms until there is pressure on the lumbar nerves, inferior vena cava, or duodenum. Back pain that is dull and constant is caused by pressure on the lumbar nerves. Abdominal pain and bloating may indicate a stretching of the duodenum over an enlarging aneurysm.

Diagnostic Procedures. The diagnosis of an aortic aneurysm is frequently an incidental finding on a chest x-ray, abdominal film, or a routine physical examination. The aneurysm is further delineated by invasive and noninvasive methods including aortography, echocardiography, ultrasound, computed tomography (CT), and digital subtraction angiography (DSA).

Doppler echocardiography of the aortic root and ultrasound studies of the descending thoracic aorta are noninvasive techniques for defining an aneurysm within the thorax. Computed tomography may also be used to determine the size, location, and extent of the aneurysm and the amount of mural thrombus that may be present. Aortography and cardiac angiography define areas of obstruction and ischemia and outline the inner wall of the aneurysm. Unfortunately, aortography may fail to delineate the actual size of the aneurysm because of intraluminal thrombus formation. In instances when ascending aneurysms have caused aortic valvular insufficiency, the electrocardiogram may indicate left ventricular hypertrophy (increase in QRS voltage) and strain (ST depression and T wave inversion).[7]

Abdominal aortic aneurysms may be defined as to size, location, and extent through the use of cross-sectional ultrasound, abdominal x-rays, aortography, computed tomography, digital subtraction angiography, or magnetic resonance imaging (MRI). Digital subtraction angiography may yield information similar to aortography but eliminates the use of an intraarterial injection.[8] Of all these procedures, ultrasound is currently considered the method of choice for assessing patients with abdominal aortic aneurysms.[8]

Medical Management

Medical management of a patient with an aortic aneurysm involves frequent monitoring of aneurysmal size (as by ultrasound every 6 months) to indicate the need for surgical repair (at a diameter of 4 to 5 cm). Control of contributory risk factors such as hypertension, hypercholesteremia, hyperlipidemia, and smoking through modifications in diet, exercise, and medications and the cessation of smoking is also important. In the presence of a large aneurysm or rupture, operative repair is the only effective therapy.

For the patient facing elective surgical repair, medical therapy involves complete evaluation of the coronary arteries, carotid arteries, and peripheral vasculature. This exam includes a comprehensive cardiovascular history, physical examination, and other studies such as an electrocardiogram, Doppler blood flow studies, and a serum lipid profile, since atherosclerosis is the most frequent underlying cause of aneurysm formation. Surgical treatment of significant coronary artery occlusions or carotid artery stenoses may precede repair of the aneurysm.

Leaking or rupture of an aneurysm is a surgical emergency. Treatment of hypovolemia, minimization of leakage with an external counterpulsation device, e.g., MAST trousers, and administration of intravenous fluids to maintain a systolic blood pressure of

80 to 100 mmHg are required with the onset of rupture.[8,9]

Surgical repair consists of replacing the section of the aorta that contains the aneurysm by a synthetic graft that is sewn into the proximal and distal aorta. Depending upon the area of aneurysm repair, the surgical procedures vary in the method of and the need for maintaining distal circulation. For aneurysms involving the ascending aorta and the aortic arch, cardiopulmonary bypass is needed, and aortic valve replacement may be required if aortic regurgitation is severe. In aneurysms below the left subclavian artery, the aorta is clamped proximally and distally while the surgical repair is done. The blood pressure is lowered and controlled by use of vasodilators such as sodium nitroprusside.

Aortic Dissection

Acute dissection of the thoracic aorta occurs more frequently than rupture of an abdominal aortic aneurysm. If not treated, it has a 90% mortality rate.[10]

A longitudinal tearing of the aortic media by a dissecting hematoma is the primary feature of aortic dissection. A sudden laceration of the aortic intima opens the way for blood propelled by the force of arterial pressure into a false lumen between the intima and the media. The underlying pathogenesis of dissection may include (1) medial degeneration as noted in Marfan's syndrome, aging, and hypertension; (2) intimal damage as in atherosclerosis, syphilis, infection, or trauma; (3) shearing stress related to the beating of the heart, especially affecting the ascending aorta and related to the hemodynamic forces of the pulse wave and (4) chemical toxins.[8,11]

The types of dissection have been classified according to the areas most frequently affected within the aorta (Figure 25-3). DeBakey types II and III arise from the ascending aorta: type II extends from the ascending aorta beyond the arch, while type III is confined to the ascending aorta. DeBakey type I begins in the descending thoracic aorta beyond the left subclavian artery and extends distally.

The prompt diagnosis and management of patients with acute aortic dissection has reduced mortality significantly.[10] Men are more frequently affected than women, and dissection most often occurs during the sixth or seventh decade of life. However, persons with Marfan's syndrome who experience acute dissection are usually in their early thirties.

Data Acquisition

History and Physical Assessment. Most patients with aortic dissection have a history of long-standing hypertension. Often, the dissection occurs as a result of a malignant hypertensive episode.

The most frequent presenting symptom of acute

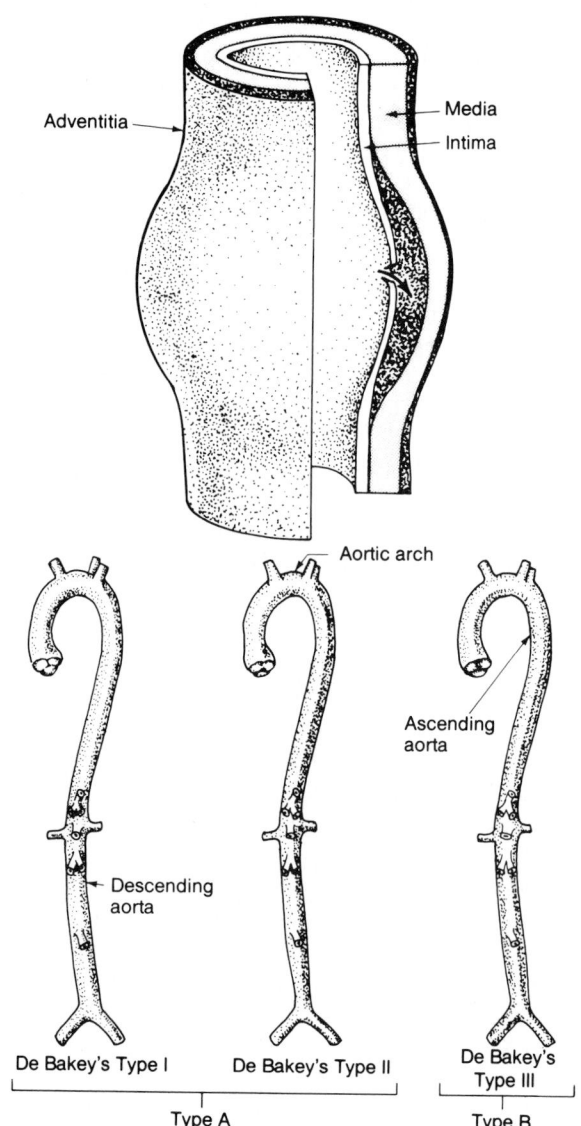

Figure 25-3   Aortic dissections classified according to DeBakey's typing.

From Urk, F., & Oakes, A. (1983). Assessing the patient with acute aortic dissection. *Focus on Critical Care, 10,* 16.

dissection is the onset of intense pain described as sharp, tearing, knifelike, or ripping, occurring in the chest and spreading toward the back and into the abdomen. The pain also has a tendency to travel along the path of the dissecting hematoma.[8] Determination of the location of the pain is useful in localizing the dissection.

The manifestations of aortic dissection are determined by the path taken by the dissecting hematoma: the circulation in major arteries originating from the aorta may be compromised, leading to myocardial infarction, cerebral insufficiency, cerebral vascular accident, paraplegia, necrosis of the bowel, or renal failure.

If the dissection has disrupted the aortic valve, precordial systolic murmurs are usually noted, and a diastolic murmur of aortic regurgitation with concomitant symptoms of pulmonary edema may be present. Strokelike symptoms of paralysis or hemiplegia may evolve from partial to complete occlusion of one or both carotid arteries. Nausea and vomiting with hematemesis or melanotic stools may indicate erosion of a thoracic dissection into the esophagus.[12] Blood pressure may differ significantly between arms, indicating compromise of blood flow into one or both subclavian arteries. Loss or decrease of femoral pulses associated with pain may indicate dissection into the aortic bifurcation, disrupting blood flow to the legs.

The patient with an acute dissection is in severe distress and presents with signs of shock (pallor, sweating, peripheral cyanosis, restlessness), yet the blood pressure is usually elevated. In some patients the systolic pressure may be greater than 200 mmHg.

Diagnostic Procedures. Initial blood studies of the patient admitted to the critical care unit are usually within normal limits unless the patient is actively bleeding, in which case there is a decrease in red blood cell count, hemoglobin, and hematocrit values. A baseline electrocardiogram assists in ruling out signs of myocardial ischemia or infarction. There may be signs of left ventricular hypertrophy as a sequela of hypertension.

The chest x-ray assists in confirming the diagnosis by detecting a widening of the mediastinum with left pleural effusion, indicating possible rupture into the pleural cavity.[10] Further confirmation may be obtained by the use of computed tomography, transesophageal echocardiography, and MRI.[8,13] Aortography provides definitive diagnosis of aortic dissection, delineating the area of intimal tearing, false channels, compression of the true aortic lumen, and aortic valve competence.

Medical Management

Once aortic dissection is suspected, immediate treatment is instituted to lower blood pressure and reduce the pulsatile force of left ventricular ejection. Medication and rest are instituted in the critical care unit to reduce blood pressure and myocardial contractility and thereby slow the progression of the dissecting force until the patient is stabilized for further diagnostic procedures or surgery. While antihypertensive drugs are administered, blood pressure, cardiac rhythm, central venous pressure, pulmonary artery pressures, and urine output must be carfully monitored to detect complications such as hypotension, cardiac dysrhythmias from the medication, and progression of dissection causing ischemia or infarction of the kidneys, mesentery, or lower extremities.

Sodium nitroprusside (Nipride) or trimethaphan camsylate (Arfonad, a ganglionic blocking agent), are frequently used to lower blood pressure. Sodium nitroprusside used alone can increase ejection force; thus concurrent use of beta-adrenergic blocking agents such as propranolol is essential to decreasing contractility. Propranolol is contraindicated if bradycardia, asthma, or congestive heart failure is present. Trimethaphan camsylate decreases blood pressure and myocardial contractility; however, tachyphylaxis, or rapid immunization to a toxic dose, is a common problem, so this drug is used less often than sodium nitroprusside. Reserpine given in doses of 1 to 2 mg every 4 to 6 hours intramuscularly also decreases blood pressure and pulsatile force. However, the side effects of drowsiness, depression, and increased gastric acid formation, as well as difficulty in controlling the administration of the drug, reduce the frequency of use in medical management of aortic dissection.

Decrease of cardiac workload with diuretics such as furosemide or other loop diuretics contributes to limiting contractility and, therefore, progression of the dissection. Pain is managed primarily through reduction of blood pressure and limited amounts of morphine sulfate.

Patients with nonprogressive isolated dissection in an area of the aorta that does not affect major arteries may be treated medically. Persons of advanced age and those with severe associated disease or severe neurological injury caused by the dissection are not candidates for surgery. Other patients may choose between continued medical therapy or surgical intervention when their condition is stable (see box).

Factors Determining Interventions in Acute Aortic Dissection

MEDICAL
Initial stabilization of patient
Uncomplicated DeBakey type III dissection
Stable, isolated arch dissection
Chronic dissection—uncomplicated dissection presenting 2 or more weeks after onset
Inoperability because of advanced age, severe concomitant medical problems, or severe neurological injuries

SURGICAL
Aortic valve regurgitation
Failure of drug therapy
Cardiac tamponade
Compromise of a major branch of the aorta
Types I and II dissection
Type III dissection complicated by compromise of vital organs, rupture, retrograde extension into the ascending aorta, or Marfan's syndrome

Adapted from Finnerty,[14] Lindsay et al.,[15] and Eagle and De-Sanctis.[18]

Immediate surgical intervention is indicated when there is acute aortic valve regurgitation, failure of drug therapy to control the progression of dissection, cardiac tamponade, or compromise of a major branch of the aorta.[14] Surgical therapy involves repair of the intimal tear and obliteration of the entry into the dissecting aortic wall. Repair of dissections involving the ascending aorta (DeBakey types II and III) requires cardiopulmonary bypass and myocardial preservation techniques such as cold cardioplegia and hypothermia. If there is aortic valve regurgitation due to dissection of the intima into the valve annulus, the valve is resuspended or replaced with a prosthetic valve. Splitting of the layers of the aortic wall in conjunction with underlying disease such as atherosclerosis may make the aorta very friable, difficult to suture, and susceptible to free bleeding. A tube graft is sutured in place, using Teflon strips to reinforce the suture line externally, within the true lumen and within the false lumen. The aortic wall is sutured around the graft for reinforcement and hemostasis (Figure 25-4).

Repair of distal or DeBakey type I dissections consists of resecting the descending thoracic aorta above the origin of dissection, closing the inner and outer layers of the false lumen by suturing, and replacing the excised aorta with a graft.[15] Reimplantation of major branches of the aorta may be necessary, depending upon the extent of the dissection.

NURSING MANAGEMENT

Nurses in the critical care setting are crucial to the survival of patients with aortic aneurysms or acute aortic dissection. Discerning observation and assessment of the patient entering the critical care environment assist in determining the diagnosis of rupture or dissection and expedite appropriate patient care.

Depending on the patient's level of consciousness and degree of discomfort, the following information can be ascertained from the patient or significant others as part of the initial nursing history:

1. A complete description of the pain, including its onset, duration, type, intensity, location, radiation, and any contributing factors that increase or decrease its severity.
2. Past medical history of hypertension, carotid artery disease, coronary artery disease, peripheral vascular disease, Marfan's syndrome, syphilis, or severe infections.
3. The presence and duration of symptoms such as hemoptysis, hematemesis, melena, hoarseness, dyspnea, changes in sensation or movement of extremities, or changes in vision.

The physical examination is a comprehensive physical assessment focusing on the factors in the box on p. 613.

All too often the patient who presents acutely because of aneurysmal rupture or aortic dissection exhibits shock. The interventions by nurses are often aimed at minimizing or treating this shocklike state. In this case, shock is the medical diagnosis. Nursing interventions support the medical plan of care for shock.[16] Most of these patients and their significant others are anxious, have a sense of impending doom, and verbalize fear because of the severity of the condition.

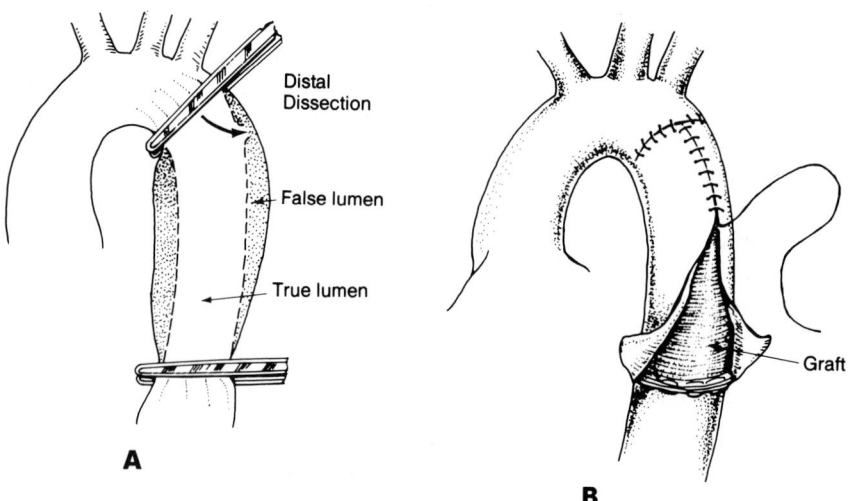

A   **B**

Figure 25-4   Surgical repair of type III aortic dissection. *A*, The clamps in place for a distal dissection. The distal clamp does not encompass the distal extent of the dissection. *B*, The graft is in place, and the adventitia is being closed.

From Little, A. G., & Anagnostopoulos, C. E. (1991). Aortic dissections. In W. W. L. Glenn (Ed.), *Thoracic and cardiovascular surgery* (4th ed.). Norwalk, CT: Appleton & Lange.

Factors of Comprehensive Physical Assessment

Blood pressure, both range and difference between extremities
Pulse pressure
Heart rate and rhythm
Pulse quality and bilateral changes in quality
Skin temperature and color
Heart sounds
Presence of palpable heaves, thrills, or bruits in the anterior chest or abdomen
Breath sounds
Respiratory rate and depth and use of accessory muscles
Distention of jugular veins or upper extremity veins
Level of consciousness
Bowel sounds
Urine output
Presence of paresthesia or decreased motor function
Pain on palpation of the abdomen
Decreased field of vision

■ **NURSING DIAGNOSIS**

Fear, related to acute hospitalization, severity of condition, and unpredictable outcome.

OUTCOME STANDARD AND CRITERIA

Fear is absent or reduced as evidenced by:
• Verbalization of decrease in fear
• Differentiation between real and imagined situations
• Identification of support system to reduce fear
• Verbalization of realistic outcomes
• Pulse and respirations within normal limits

NURSING INTERVENTIONS
• Promote communication of patient and significant others with members of health care team
• Assess level of fear
• Provide a sense of empathic understanding through quiet presence and touch
• Inquire regarding patient's knowledge about the actual condition and prognosis
• Identify patient's positive support system
• Discuss with patient and significant others coping methods previously used in fearful situations
• Provide support and reinforcement of adaptive behavior such as problem solving
• Consult with appropriate resources (clergy, social service department, psychologist) to provide additional support
• Allow for adequate rest periods if possible between procedures or required activities
• Continually monitor for increased level of fear as evidenced by increases in heart rate and respiratory rate

HIGH-RISK NURSING DIAGNOSES

High-risk nursing diagnoses that may be applicable for the patient with an aortic aneurysm or acute aortic dissection include:
• High risk for alteration in comfort (pain), related to decreased tissue perfusion
• High risk for impaired physical mobility, related to decreased tissue perfusion
• High risk for skin breakdown, related to decreased tissue perfusion

PERIPHERAL VASCULAR DISEASE

Peripheral vascular disease (PVD) is defined as any pathophysiological process that disrupts blood flow through arteries or veins of the extracranium, thorax, abdomen, or extremities, although the term is often used synonymously with lower extremity arterial insufficiency. Though rarely a cause of death in and of itself, PVD can result in profound morbidity in such forms as stroke, limb amputation, or chronic venous insufficiency. Additionally, symptomatic PVD often heralds the presence of "central" vascular disease, that is, coronary artery disease, with resultant risk of cardiac death and disability.

Because lower extremity arterial and venous diseases are the most commonly encountered clinical problems, they are the focus of this section.

Lower Extremity Arterial Disease

Pathophysiology

The leading cause of arterial insufficiency in the lower extremities is atherosclerotic occlusive disease. Other causes include acute thromboembolic problems, vasospastic disease (Raynaud's phenomenon), inflammatory processes (e.g., Buerger's disease, arteritis) and, less commonly, fibromuscular dysplasia, increased muscular compartment pressure (compartment syndrome), and congenital vascular diseases. Although a discussion of atherosclerosis forms the framework of this section, some of these other causes warrant brief mention.

Acute Arterial Occlusion. Acute disruption of arterial blood flow results from either thrombosis of a previously stenotic arterial lesion or embolism of a blood clot or atherosclerotic debris into the arterial circuit. Abrupt arterial thrombosis usually results in more insidious symptoms, since preexisting arterial narrowing has often prompted the development of collateral arteries. Arterial embolism, on the other hand, causes very dramatic signs and symptoms of acute arterial insufficiency, namely, the six P's: pain, pallor, pulselessness, paresthesia, paralysis, and poikilothermia. Emboli most often originate from mural thrombi lining the myocardium in patients with chronic dysrhythmias and/or ventricular dysfunction secondary to myocardial infarction. They can also originate from arterial aneurysms lined with thrombus (most often from the abdominal aorta or popliteal artery) or roughened intimal surfaces of stenotic arterial lesions. Depending on their size, arterial emboli can lodge anywhere from the aortic bifurcation, disrupting arterial flow to both legs, to tiny vessels in the toes.

When acute occlusion of arterial flow threatens the viability of the limb(s), immediate intervention in the form of arteriography, thrombolytic therapy, and/or surgery is indicated. These treatment options are discussed later in this section.

Vasospastic Disease. Vasospastic arterial disease is also known as *Raynaud's disease* or *phenomenon*. Raynaud's affects more women than men, and symptoms usually present from late adolescence to middle age. The hands are affected more commonly and severely than the feet. Reported causes of Raynaud's disease include ineffective basal heat production, stress, and overstimulation of the sympathetic nervous system.

Raynaud's is triphasic in nature, the first phase being characterized by marked blanching of the skin, predominantly in the hands and feet, caused by severe vasoconstriction of the cutaneous blood vessels. During the blanching phase, patients complain of a cold, numb feeling in the affected digits. The second phase manifests as cyanosis resulting from dilatation of cutaneous arterioles and venules. Because vasoconstriction is diminished in the final phase, reactive hyperemia characterized by reddish discoloration, burning, and throbbing pain are experienced.

Most mild cases of Raynaud's can be successfully managed with conservative measures such as avoiding extremes in temperature, particularly cold, and avoiding stress. Historically, drugs have proved to be of little value, although several reports describe the effectiveness of nifedipine in treating this syndrome.[17,18] With advanced Raynaud's, characterized by severe persistent vasoconstriction, full-thickness tissue necrosis may necessitate amputation of one or more digits.

Thromboangiitis Obliterans. Also known as *Buerger's disease,* thromboangiitis is an inflammatory occlusive disease involving small to medium-sized arteries and veins in the extremities. The existence of Buerger's disease as a distinct clinical entity is highly controversial among experts in peripheral vascular disease, although the current consensus is that the specific pathological condition does exist, albeit with decreasing incidence in western cultures.[19] Unlike Raynaud's disease, Buerger's disease occurs more commonly in the lower extremities and predominantly in young male cigarette smokers. Histologically, the "lesion" of Buerger's disease is characterized

by full-thickness inflammation of the vessel walls with associated thrombosis.

Signs and symptoms of Buerger's disease result from decreased arterial blood flow to tissues beyond the occlusive lesion and may parallel those of atherosclerotic arterial occlusive disease, discussed below. The diagnosis is usually determined from factors such as age of onset, associated risk factors, and the presence of venous as well as arterial involvement.

Atherosclerotic Occlusive Disease

Atherosclerosis is the leading cause of arterial occlusive disease in the extremities of patients older than 30 (see Chapter 22). Atherosclerosis, the most common form of arteriosclerosis obliterans, is histologically characterized by structural changes in the arterial wall as well as the development of intraluminal plaque, narrowing the route of blood flow through the artery.

Atherosclerosis is also characterized by accumulation of lipids and connective tissue in the arterial wall, increased intimal permeability and platelet aggregation secondary to injury, and proliferation of smooth muscle cells. The earliest precursor of atherosclerosis, the fatty streak, has been detected in autopsy specimens in the first decade of life. Although some fatty streaks are apparently reversible, others progress to fibromuscular lesions and to complex nonreversible lesions containing lipids, platelets, fibrin, and cellular debris. Mature atherosclerotic lesions may be further complicated by intimal ulceration and intraplaque hemorrhage.

Risk Factors. The pathogenesis of atherosclerosis is exceedingly complex and undoubtedly multifactorial. Several modifiable risk factors have been linked with this process, most notably cigarette smoking, hypertension, and hyperlipidemia.

Smoking. Innumerable reports implicate cigarette smoking as the single independent risk factor most closely associated with atherogenesis in both the coronary and the peripheral arteries.[20] Additionally, cigarette smoking adversely affects the course of existing arterial occlusive disease. Besides the marked vasoconstrictive effect of nicotine, inhalation of carbon monoxide in cigarette smoke increases circulating carboxyhemoglobin levels. Since carbon monoxide has a greater affinity for hemoglobin than oxygen, oxygen transport to ischemic tissues is impaired and hypoxic injury to the intimal lining of the artery results. Increased platelet aggregation and thrombus formation secondary to enhanced platelet adhesiveness have also been reported.

Hypertension. It is well documented that persons with sustained hypertension are at increased risk of atherosclerotic development. The detrimental mechanism of hypertension is perhaps best explained by the constant trauma of elevated blood pressure, causing damage to and thus increasing the permeability of the intimal endothelium. This theory is further supported by the propensity for atherosclerotic plaque to develop at points of arterial branching or narrowing, where blood flow is turbulent and blood pressure is increased.

Hyperlipidemia. As previously mentioned, incorporation of lipoproteins into the arterial wall is the hallmark of atherosclerosis. Increased serum concentrations of cholesterol (190 mg per 100 ml blood) and/or fasting triglycerides (150 mg per 100 ml blood) as well as low-density lipoproteins and very-low-density lipoproteins are noted in relation to the incidence of atherosclerotic lesions in humans. Conversely, increased serum concentration of high-density lipoproteins has been shown to exert an antiatherogenic effect.

Other commonly implicated atherosclerotic risk factors include diabetes mellitus, advanced age, male sex, unfavorable family history, obesity, and psychophysiological stress. The presence of more than one risk factor often exerts a multiplicative atherogenic risk.

Data Acquisition

A thorough history and physical assessment can provide the examiner with a nearly conclusive diagnosis of lower extremity arterial occlusive disease. In addition to a functional assessment of health patterns,[21] the nursing history should focus on (1) a detailed description of the patient's presenting complaint (emphasizing understanding), (2) a body systems review with specific questioning as to the presence of systemic atherosclerosis (e.g., history of stroke, transient ischemic attacks, angina, myocardial infarction, or renovascular hypertension), and (3) the presence of known atherosclerotic risk factors.

History. Specific questioning about the presenting complaint (usually leg pain or discomfort), focusing on precipitating factors, character and location of pain, and relief methods, will often differentiate true ischemic pain from other potential causes of leg pain, such as neurogenic or musculoskeletal syndromes.

Arterial stenosis or complete occlusion in the presence of collateral vessels can precipitate symptoms of intermittent claudication distal to an occlusive lesion. Intermittent claudication is defined as muscular leg discomfort that is precipitated by exercise, is reproducible, and is relieved by a short period of rest. Depending on the location of the arterial obstruction, intermittent claudication may involve muscles of the calf, thigh, and/or buttocks. Cessation of exercise even for a minute or two relieves the discomfort. With risk factor modification and continuance of exercise,

intermittent claudication is often self-limiting and may improve with time. The need for surgery is determined by the clinical course of the patient with intermittent claudication.

More extensive arterial occlusion often results in ischemic rest pain. As the name implies, blood flow in the limb is inadequate to meet even the basal metabolic tissue demands at rest. Pain is usually described as relentless, burning, and throbbing in the most distal portion of the limb, usually in a toe or toes and in the forefoot. Patients frequently describe the pain as being worse with leg elevation, necessitating sleeping upright in a chair so as to keep the ischemic limb dependent. Unlike intermittent claudication, ischemic rest pain is an ominous finding, heralding impending ulceration or tissue necrosis and threatening the viability of the limb unless adequate arterial circulation can be restored.

Physical Assessment. In conjunction with a thorough history and systemic physical examination, assessment of the arterial circulation can confirm or exclude a diagnosis of arterial occlusive disease. The examiner should employ the skills of inspection, palpation, and auscultation in order to thoroughly examine the arterial system. (Percussion is not applicable to examination of the arterial system.)

Inspection. Inspection of a chronically ischemic lower limb often evidences several characteristic signs. Most obvious is the presence of atrophic skin and nail changes in the toes and foot. Typically, the nails are thickened, cornified, and misshapen. The skin of the foot is often thin, shiny, and scaly in appearance, due to atrophy of subcutaneous tissue. Since distal hair follicles are inadequately nourished, absence of hair growth is evident. Additionally, the ischemic limb is often cool or cold to touch.

Severe ischemia is often associated with position-related color changes in the foot. Elevation of an ischemic limb, even at a slight angle, results in the development of cadaveric pallor of the toes and foot. Blanching occurs because the capillary perfusion pressure is inadequate to pump blood "uphill" to the distal portion of the limb. In contrast, putting an ischemic limb in a dependent position (sitting) results in the development of dependent rubor and cyanosis. The toes and forefoot become red to deep bluish purple in color, secondary to pooling of blood in maximally dilated arterioles and venules. The time it takes to develop dependent rubor following leg elevation is directly proportional to the degree of ischemia.

Ischemic tissues are very susceptible to breakdown, and alterations in skin integrity are common. The ischemic limb should be carefully inspected for evidence of arterial ulceration or tissue necrosis (gangrene). Even minor trauma can result in skin disruption and the potential for infection. Also, patients with long-standing arterial insufficiency may suffer from ischemic neuropathy, increasing their risk of traumatic injury, which is exacerbated in diabetic patients with concomitant diabetic neuropathy.

Arterial ulcers are prone to develop on the toes, in the interdigital spaces, and over bony prominences, which are most susceptible to pressure and/or friction necrosis. Gangrene may develop following such simple trauma as stubbing a toe or wearing poorly fitting shoes.

Palpation. Pulse assessment is the mainstay of a vascular examination. All peripheral pulses, including the carotid, brachial, radial, femoral, popliteal, dorsalis pedis, and posterior tibial, should be evaluated for quality and symmetry as well as presence or absence.

Weakness or absence of a pulse is indicative of stenosis or occlusion of an artery proximal to that anatomic location. For example, presence of a femoral pulse and absence of a popliteal pulse indicate obstruction of the superficial femoral artery.

Pulse assessment, like any skill, can be easily mastered with practice. If the examiner is uncertain as to whether a pulse is present, it is safest to document it as absent. Having a colleague count the patient's radial pulse aloud or checking the examiner's pulse may help differentiate the examiner's pulse projected through the fingertips from the patient's pulse. Keep in mind that one would not expect to palpate pulses in the foot of a markedly ischemic limb.

Auscultation. Auscultation of the arteries may evidence a bruit over a stenotic lesion. In the presence of stenosis, bruits are most commonly audible in the carotid arteries, the abdominal aorta and its major branches, and the femoral arteries. A completely occluded artery will *not* project a bruit.

Noninvasive Diagnostic Procedures. The Doppler ultrasound flowmeter can provide an adjunct to auscultation. This device amplifies the sound of blood flow through the vessel and often makes it possible to detect pulsatile flow through an artery in the absence of a palpable pulse.

Perhaps the most valuable noninvasive diagnostic test for lower extremity arterial disease, and certainly the most commonly employed, is segmental leg pressure measurement. Using the Doppler blood flow velocity detector and a technique identical to that of determining brachial blood pressure (see box above), the examiner can compare the *systolic* blood pressure in the leg with that in the arm. Though determinations can be made at various levels in the leg, a quick test in routine clinical practice is to compare the higher of the dorsalis pedis or posterior tibial artery systolic pressure in each limb with the brachial systolic pres-

---

Procedure for Use of Ultrasound Blood Flow Detector (Doppler) Flowmeter for Arterial Assessment of the Lower Extremity

1. Place a blood pressure cuff on the lower leg just above the ankle
2. Apply acoustic coupling gel to the Doppler probe or on the dorsum of the foot. This permits percutaneous transmission of high-frequency sound wave to underlying blood vessel. (Avoid using water-soluble lubricants or ECG transmission gel, as they are corrosive to the probe)
3. With the Doppler turned on, place the probe over the expected anatomic location of the dorsalis pedis (DP) artery. Manipulate the probe until *pulsatile** flow is audible
4. Holding the probe in place, inflate the blood pressure cuff until the pulse is obliterated. Slowly release the pressure in the cuff, recording the first audible return of pulse as the systolic artery pressure
5. Repeat procedure to determine systolic pressure in posterior tibial (PT) artery, behind medial malleolus
6. In the same manner, determine the brachial artery systolic pressure
7. Compare the ankle pressure (higher of DP or PT) to the arm pressure to calculate the ankle/brachial index (ABI)

Example:

$$ABI = \frac{\text{Ankle pressure} = 80 \text{ mmHg}}{\text{Brachial pressure} = 120 \text{ mmHg}} = 0.66\dagger$$

---

* Differentiate carefully between arterial pulsatile flow and consistent, windlike venous flow.
† May also be expressed as 66%, or 2/3 normal ABI of 1.00. The lower the index, the more severe the ischemia.

---

sure. This comparison, known as the ankle/brachial index (ABI), is determined by dividing the "ankle" pressure by the arm pressure. The result is most commonly expressed as a fraction, decimal, or percentage. With normal circulation, the ankle pressure should equal or exceed the brachial pressure (i.e., ABI ≥1.00). Patients with intermittent claudication often have an ABI in the symptomatic limb in the range of 0.4 to 0.8, and those with severe ischemic rest pain lie between 0.0 and 0.4.

Invasive Diagnostic Procedures. The "gold standard" against which all other diagnostic modalities are compared is arteriography, the roentgenography of the arteries after intraarterial injection of radiopaque contrast material which outlines the arterial circuit. A quality arteriogram will delineate the specific anatomic location of obstruction, clarify the underlying etiology (e.g., atherosclerosis vs. fibromuscular dysplasia) and depict the arteries proximal and distal to the obstructing lesion. Thus, it provides the vascular surgeon with a "road map" of the arterial circuit, clarifying the surgical treatment options. However, because a thorough health history and vascular assessment are nearly conclusively diagnostic, an arteriogram is indicated only when further intervention is planned, not solely to further strengthen the examiner's findings.

The nurse should be knowledgeable about the technique of arteriography in order to adequately prepare the patient for the procedure (see Chapter 21). The patient should be assured that throughout the procedure the heart function and vital signs will be closely monitored by the radiology staff.

Following the procedure, the patient requires careful nursing assessment. Arteriography carries with it the risk of intimal disruption at the site of catheter insertion, acute arterial occlusion, or arterial embolization, any of which may impair arterial inflow to the limb. These risks are most significant in patients with preexisting atherosclerotic disease. A significant change in circulatory status in the limb should be reported immediately to the physician.

The nurse should carefully monitor the patient's fluid balance for 72 hours following arteriography and throughout the perioperative period. The rationale for this is twofold: (1) the contrast medium is hyperosmolar and precipitates an osmotic diuresis, and (2) the contrast medium is nephrotoxic and can precipitate acute tubular necrosis (acute renal failure), particularly in the diabetic patient with preexisting nephropathy.[22,23] Documentation of intake and output minimizes the risk of dehydration and provides a useful parameter by which to monitor renal function. Additionally, the postprocedure serum creatinine and BUN can be compared with the admission baseline results as another indicator of renal function.

Bed rest, with the punctured extremity immobile, is maintained for 8 to 12 hours following the procedure to minimize the risk of disrupting the healing arteriotomy, with consequent hematoma or bleeding. Barring complications, the patient can resume sitting, ambulating, and routine daily activities following this period.

Medical Management

The majority of patients with symptomatic lower extremity arterial occlusive disease—that is, those with intermittent claudication—are treated medically. The goal is to control modifiable risk factors such as cigarette smoking, hypertension, hyperlipidemia, diabetes mellitus, obesity, and stress, in the hope of preventing disease progression. Numerous reports studying the natural history of intermittent claudication conclude that with risk factor modification, particularly cessation of smoking, and routine exercise (walking is sufficient), only a small percentage of patients develop worsening symptoms or threatened limb viability within a 5-year follow-up period.[24,25]

Historically, vasodilating drugs have proved to be of little value in the treatment of peripheral arterial occlusive disease, because no known agent selectively dilates vessels in ischemic areas or in exercising skeletal muscle.[26] In fact, vasodilators may worsen symptoms, secondary to decreases in systemic blood pressure that further compromise flow to ischemic areas. Additionally, the efficacy of these drugs is limited by the fact that atherosclerosis has resulted in increased rigidity of the vessel walls, making them structurally incapable of dilating.

A multicenter trial, however, has evidenced an exception to the general rule that drugs are ineffective in treating intermittent claudication. Favorable objective results with the agent pentoxifylline (Trental) were reported to include increase of walking distance and minimization of limb paresthesias as compared with the placebo effects.[27] Pentoxifylline acts primarily by reducing blood viscosity and thus increasing blood flow in the microcirculation by increasing red blood cell flexibility and decreasing platelet aggregation and fibrinogen.[28] Future clinical trials are needed to substantiate these findings.

As mentioned previously, exercise in the form of walking to the point of discomfort, resting a short time, then continuing to walk is also an important component of treatment for patients with intermittent claudication. Although the cause of claudication—that is, inadequate oxygenation of working muscles—is similar to that of angina pectoris, an important distinction must be made. Persons with exertional angina must cease further exertion to preclude increases in myocardial oxygen demand and the risk of infarction, whereas stimulation of exercising leg muscles to the point of pain is thought to promote the development of collateral circulation. Although collateral vessels are normally insignificant in blood transport, they become important in bypassing a localized arterial obstruction, gradually increasing in size to carry more blood and thus stabilize or improve symptoms.

Occasionally, patients with severe limb-threatening ischemia and rest pain are faced with a nonreconstructible situation (that is, diffuse disease with no bypassable lesion) or are prohibitive surgical risks because of coexisting medical problems. The goals of medical management of these patients are prevention of skin breakdown, ulceration, and infection, and treatment of gangrenous necrosis, if present. *Gangrene* is full-thickness tissue necrosis and is nonreversible even with an adequate blood flow. If the necrotic areas of the toes or foot are dry, they can be left open to air. The limb should be assessed daily for evidence of gangrenous progression. With purulent exudate, suggestive of infected necrotic tissue, wound cultures should be obtained and intravenous antibiotic therapy initiated. The draining area can be bandaged with a normal saline wet-to-dry dressing. A foot or lower leg x-ray can determine the presence of underlying osteomyelitis. If the infected necrotic limb precipitates systemic septicemia, local or limb amputation may be a lifesaving treatment.

Other nonsurgical treatment options include the use of percutaneous transluminal angioplasty and thrombolytic therapy, each being appropriate in certain clinical situations.

Percutaneous Transluminal Angioplasty. In selected patients, percutaneous transluminal angioplasty (PTA) is a safe and effective treatment option. PTA involves mechanical dilation of a narrowed or occluded artery using a specially designed balloon-tipped catheter. The technique of PTA parallels that of arteriography, and preparation of the patient is identical. The balloon catheter is directed to the desired anatomic point using fluoroscopic control, and dilation is achieved by repeated inflations of the balloon tip to a predetermined size, minimizing the risk of overdistention and vessel rupture.

The atheromatous lesions that have proved to be most successfully managed with PTA are focal narrowings in the iliac or common femoral arteries. Refinements in technique and equipment are improving the results of PTA in arteries distal to the common femoral.

PTA actually causes a "cracking" of the intimal plaque, leaving behind a rough intimal surface which results in platelet aggregation and the potential for thrombus formation.[29] Therefore, following PTA, patients are often treated with anticoagulants or antiplatelet-aggregating agents, such as aspirin and/or dipyridamole (Persantine).

In the hands of a skilled vascular radiologist, and in patients who are at high risk for complications from surgical intervention, PTA can provide a safe, effective, and well tolerated treatment option.

Laser-assisted Angioplasty. As the name of this technique implies, a laser is used to "assist" in angioplasty. The laser is used to open a totally occluded artery so that an angioplasty catheter can be passed through this total occlusion to dilate the narrowing. Thus, the use of a laser allows angioplasty to be performed on totally occluded arteries that may previously have been untreatable.

Complications associated with laser-assisted angioplasty include perforation, vasospasm, reocclusion, dissection and thrombus or hematoma formation.[30,32] Wright and associates reported discouraging results with laser-assisted angioplasty in peripheral arteries, with a significant clinical failure rate noted after 6 months.[32]

Patient preparation for this procedure is similar to that for a PTA. However, patients should be informed that pain may be felt at the treatment site during the application of the laser but will subside when the laser is turned off.[33] The reader is referred to Chapter 22 for additional information on use of lasers.

Ultrasound Angioplasty. The use of ultrasound angioplasty as a means of recanalizing totally occluded peripheral arteries is on the horizon. Rosenscheim et al.[34] have reported the successful intraoperative use of ultrasound angioplasty in seven patients with totally occluded femoral arteries. Further studies are currently underway investigating the feasibility of this method.

Thrombolytic Therapy. The thrombolytic enzymes urokinase and streptokinase were approved for clinical use in 1979. In the peripheral arterial circulation, they can be used to treat acute thromboembolic events as well as occlusion of arterial bypass grafts (Figure 25-5). Additionally, in the venous circulation they are used to treat extensive deep venous thrombosis and massive pulmonary emboli. A newer thrombolytic agent, recombinant tissue plasminogen activator (rt-PA), has been used in comparative studies with streptokinase and urokinase. This agent has been found efficacious in the treatment of acute pulmonary embolism.[35] However, rt-PA is much more costly than either of the two approved drugs, limiting its current use. Further comparative studies are needed to elucidate the efficacy and safety of these agents before widespread clinical use of any one agent can be advocated.

Streptokinase is obtained from bacterial culture (filtrates of group C beta-hemolytic streptococci), whereas urokinase is extracted from human urine or fetal kidney tissue culture. Both these thrombolytic agents work by converting plasminogen to plasmin, resulting in the degradation of fibrin clots, fibrinogen, and other plasma proteins. They can be administered either intravenously (systemically) or directly into an arterial occlusion via a localizing catheter. Their action is immediate, and lysis is halted rapidly following discontinuation. Table 25-1 provides a comparison of dosage recommendations, methods of laboratory monitoring, adverse reactions, and cost of urokinase and streptokinase, the major difference being cost. Because of its source, urokinase is nearly ten times more expensive than its bacterial counterpart.

Activation of the fibrinolytic system is confirmed

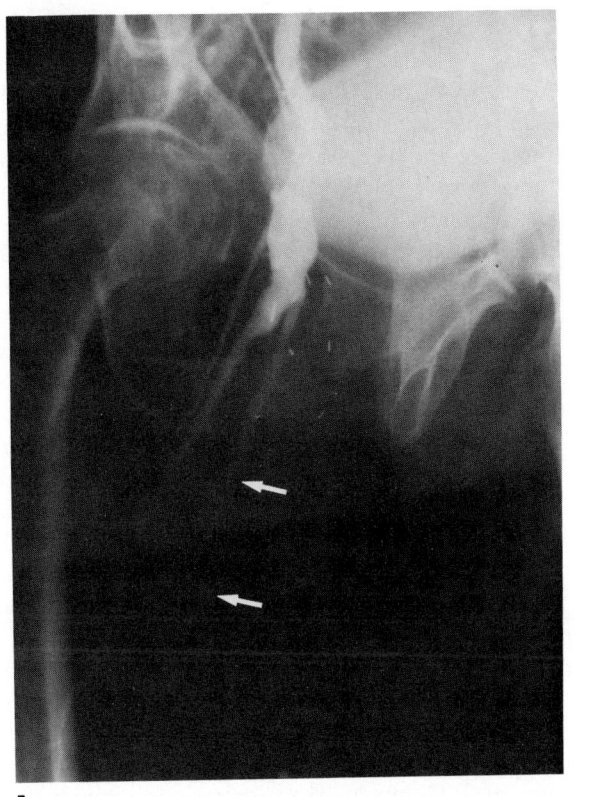
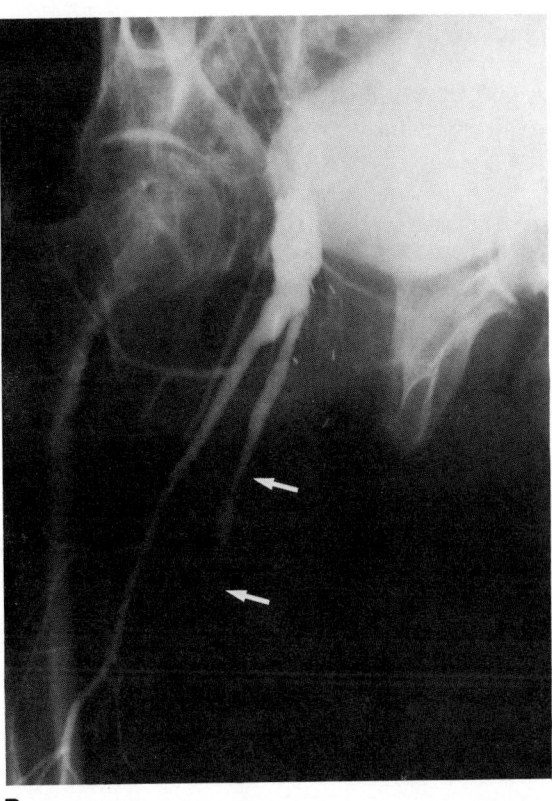

A   **B**

Figure 25-5   Arteriogram demonstrating *(A)* occlusion of right femoropopliteal bypass graft (arrows) and *(B)* partial patency of same graft following treatment with intraarterial urokinase.

TABLE 25-1   **Comparison of Urokinase and Streptokinase as Thrombolytic Agents**

	Urokinase	Streptokinase
Origin	Isolated from human urine or fetal kidney tissue	Filtrate of group C beta-hemolytic streptococci
Mechanism of action	Immediate-acting enzymatic protein that converts plasminogen to plasmin, resulting in breakdown of fibrin clot	Immediate-acting nonenzymatic protein that converts plasminogen to plasmin, resulting in breakdown of fibrin clot
Dosage/route of administration	IV: bolus of 4,400 U over 10-20 min	IV: bolus of 250,000 IU over 20-30 min
	Maintenance dose 4,400 U/hr via controlled infusion pump	Maintenance dose 100,000 U/hr, via controlled infusion pump
	Intraarterial: up to 100,000 U/hr*	Intraarterial: 5,000-100,000 U/hr*
	Available in powder form	Available in powder form
	Reconstitute with sterile saline	Reconstitute with sterile saline
Therapeutic monitoring	Thrombin time 2 to 5 times control (in seconds) assures lytic state	Thrombin time 2 to 5 times control (in seconds) assures lytic state
Adverse reactions	Pyrogenic	Pyrogenic
	Risk of hemorrhage	Risk of hemorrhage
		Allergic reaction, particularly in patients with recurrent streptococcal infection or retreatment with streptokinase
Cost	$2,000 for 12-hr treatment	$300 for 24-hr treatment

* Wide variation in recommended dosage.

by prolongation of the thrombin time to two to five times the control value. The thrombin time should be checked 4 hours after initiating treatment and every 8 to 12 hours throughout therapy.[36]

Both agents are pyrogenic, though urokinase is less so. Fever is managed with antipyretics. Additionally, streptokinase has been associated with allergic reactions in 10% to 12% of patients, because preexisting antibodies to streptococci are common. Anaphylaxis can occur in 2% to 3% of patients.[37] Symptoms of an allergic reaction are treated with antihistamines and/or corticosteroids. These agents should be on hand before initiating treatment.

The major complication associated with the use of fibrinolytic agents is hemorrhage, which reportedly occurs in about 10% of patients but is only rarely life-threatening.[37] Nonetheless, patients treated with thrombolytic agents should not be concurrently treated with anticoagulants or antiplatelet agents.

Angioscopy. Angioscopy involves the use of a fiberscope that permits direct intravascular visualization of peripheral arteries. This method has been used both percutaneously and surgically. It provides radiologists and vascular surgeons information on atherosclerotic plaque formation and composition, on the results of angioplasty and atherectomy procedures, on placement of stents, and in situ vein bypass valvulotomy procedures. Disadvantages of angioscopy include vessel spasm, which may be overcome by using smaller fiberscopes; vessel perforation; intimal disruption; air emboli; intimal trauma; and hemorrhage. According to Anderson,[38] intraoperative angioscopy may also decrease operating time (in turn reducing patient expenditures) and may reduce exposure of patients and operating room personnel to radiation from x-rays. However, the cost of the entire angioscopic system is relatively high, which limits its present use. Refer to Chapter 22 for additional discussion of this modality.

Surgical Management

Surgical intervention in management of arterial occlusive disease is indicated for patients with ischemic rest pain, with or without tissue necrosis. As mentioned previously, rest pain is premonitory of threatened limb viability without restoration of arterial inflow. In most cases, every attempt is made to preserve a limb, and amputation is limited to areas of full-thickness tissue necrosis (toe, forefoot). Unfortunately, limb amputation may be the only treatment option in cases of extremely diffuse atherosclerotic occlusion.

Arterial revascularization by means of bypass procedures is the most commonly employed surgical approach. Each patient must be considered individually when deciding on the best surgical option, taking into consideration factors such as the patient's general health, the location of the occlusive lesion along with the quality of the arteries proximally and distally, the availability of a suitable conduit with which to bypass the lesion, and the natural history of atherosclerosis.[39] Five-year survival rates are markedly lower in patients with clinically symptomatic systemic atherosclerosis than in age-matched asymptomatic patients, coronary artery disease carrying with it the most ominous prognosis.

The most commonly encountered arterial occlusive lesions are aortoiliac, superficial femoral, and tibial. Aortoiliac disease refers to arterial obstruction of blood flow into the lower extremities. It is often bilateral but may produce more severe symptoms in one leg. Symptoms range from exertional muscle pain and discomfort distal to the obstruction (as in the buttocks, thigh, and calf) to rest pain with or without tissue necrosis. Bypass approaches for aortoiliac occlusion include (1) aortobifemoral bypass (Figure 25-6); (2) unilateral aortofemoral grafting, bypassing the more severely diseased iliac artery in the symptomatic extremity (Figure 25-7); and (3) extraanatomic bypass, either axillobifemoral (Figure 25-8) or femorofemoral (Figure 25-9), restoring blood flow beyond an occlusive lesion. Extraanatomic bypass is safest in high-risk surgical patients. All these procedures are done with synthetic graft material, either Dacron velour or polytetrafluoroethylene (PTFE, Gore-tex). These synthetic materials are plagued with patency problems. In an attempt to improve patency in the long term, studies are underway to grow an endothelial cell layer within these synthetic grafts to make them more similar to native blood vessels.[40]

Occlusive disease in the superficial femoral artery occurs most commonly in the mid to distal thigh, anatomically where the artery tapers and passes through the adductor canal posteriorly, above the knee (Figure 25-10). The most common surgical approach in this situation is femoropopliteal bypass anastomosed proximal and distal to the occlusion, with the conduit of choice being an autogenous (usually saphenous) vein because of the superior patency rates of autogenous veins over synthetic material.[41]

Arterial obstruction of one or more tibial vessels is an especially common finding in the diabetic patient[42] and not unheard of in the nondiabetic smoker. As surgical techniques and instrumentation have improved, vascular surgeons have succeeded in improving patency rates to a distal tibial vessel. Depending on the quality of the vessels proximally, the bypass graft can originate at either the femoral or popliteal level. As with femoropopliteal bypass grafting, the conduit of choice is an autogenous vein, which has superior long-term patency.

Previously, use of an autogenous vein as an arterial

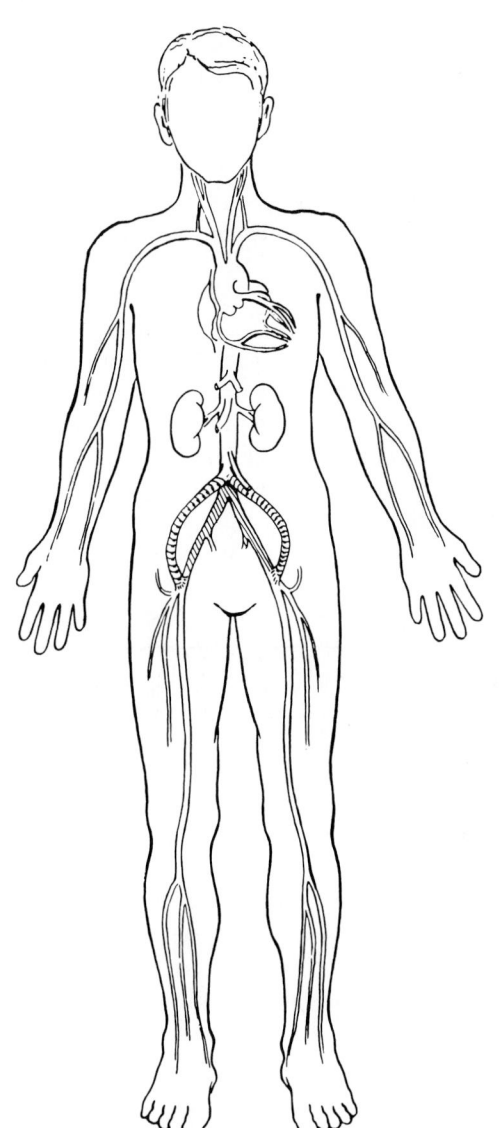

Figure 25-6 Aortoiliac occlusion and revascularization—aortobifemoral prosthetic bypass graft.

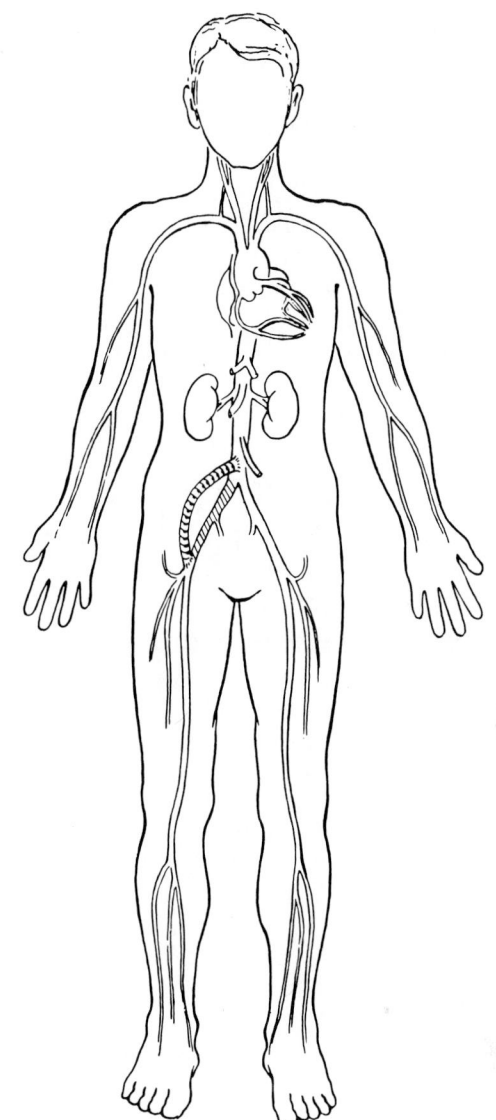

Figure 25-7 Right iliac artery occlusion and revascularization—unilateral aortofemoral prosthetic bypass graft.

bypass graft involved ligating its branches and storing it in a preservative solution until the bypass was performed. Because of the vein permitting only unidirectional flow, the vein had to be reversed before being anasatomosed to the artery proximal and distal to the occlusion. A major limitation to the reversed saphenous vein bypass is the size mismatch created because the large end of the saphenous vein is sewn in as the distal anastamosis into the smaller end of the artery. The smaller end of this vein in turn is sewn into the large end of the artery. This mismatch may cause hemodynamic problems.

In the late 1970s Leather and Karmody[43] introduced the in situ saphenous vein technique to eliminate this problem. With the in situ technique, the saphenous vein is left in place. After the vein is transected proximally and distally, a valvutome is used to cut the valve leaflets, rendering the valves incompetent and permitting antegrade flow. The vein is then sewn to the artery above and below the obstruction, and the proximal and distal veins are ligated. By eliminating the size mismatch, this procedure reduces the incidence of blood flow obstruction.[44] Postoperative nursing care is the same as that for other bypass graft techniques.

Apart from bypass procedures, surgical approaches to lower extremity arterial occlusive disease include endarterectomy and amputation. *Endarterectomy* involves opening the occluded portion of the artery and removing the obstructing plaque. Because this technique also necessitates excision of the artery's intimal lining, the denuded surface tends to be thrombogenic and prone to thrombotic occlusion. Thus, endarterectomy is usually reserved for localized le-

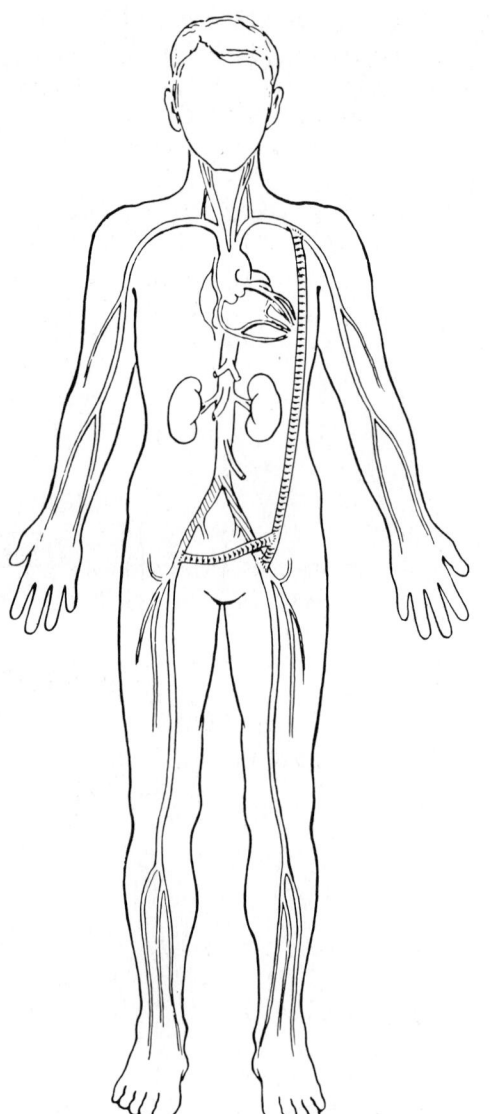

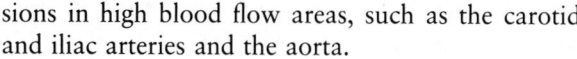

Figure 25-8   Aortoiliac occlusion and revascularization—left axillofemorofemoral prosthetic bypass graft.

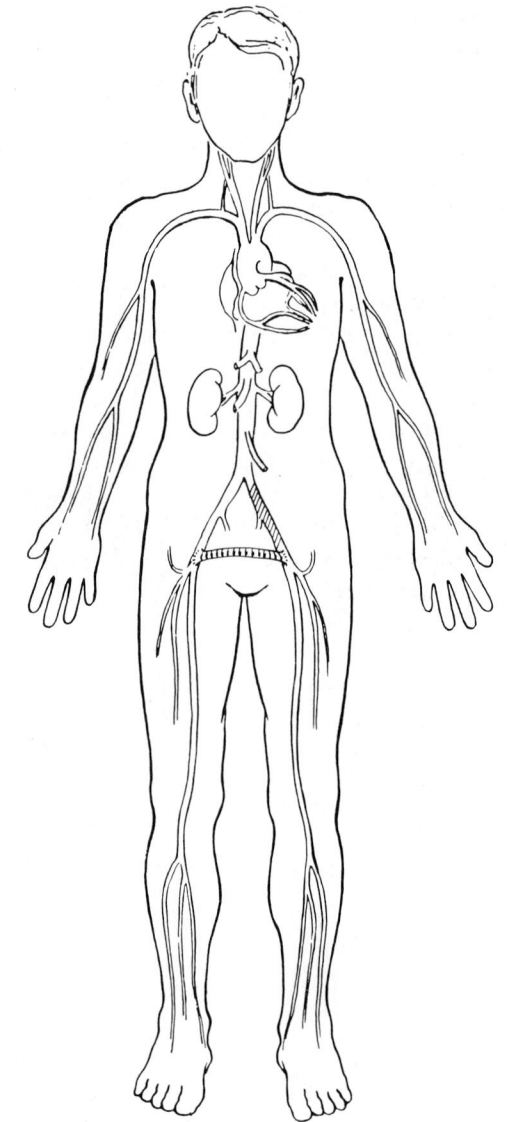

Figure 25-9   Left iliac artery occlusion and revascularization—right-to-left femorofemoral prosthetic bypass graft.

sions in high blood flow areas, such as the carotid and iliac arteries and the aorta.

Despite continually improving results with arterial revascularization, *limb amputation* may be the only treatment option to obliterate excruciating rest pain, gangrene, and/or infection. Consideration is given to preservation of as much of the limb as possible to facilitate rehabilitation. Below-knee versus above-knee amputation often means the difference between returning to ambulation with a prosthesis and total loss of independence, especially for elderly patients. Limb loss is a devastating outcome. Providing emotional support to the patient and family, as well as recognizing and coordinating rehabilitation needs, is a critical nursing role.

NURSING MANAGEMENT

Nurses in the critical care setting may encounter patients with severe lower extremity ischemia. These patients may have severe cardiopulmonary dysfunction, brittle diabetes, or end-stage renal failure with concomitant lower extremity atherosclerosis. The use of certain therapeutic modalities, such as intraaortic balloon counterpulsation or femoral artery catheters for dialysis access, may further impair already compromised arterial blood supply.

The nurse in this setting should carefully assess the adequacy of the patient's lower extremity circulation by means of a thorough history and physical examination as described previously. Prevention is the hallmark of nursing care for patients with arterial occlu-

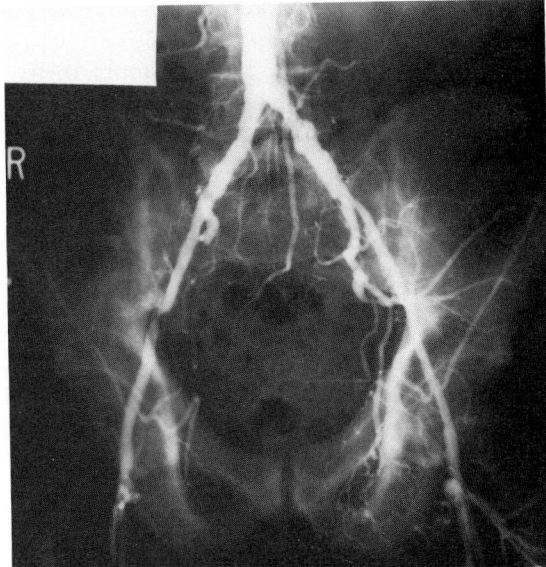

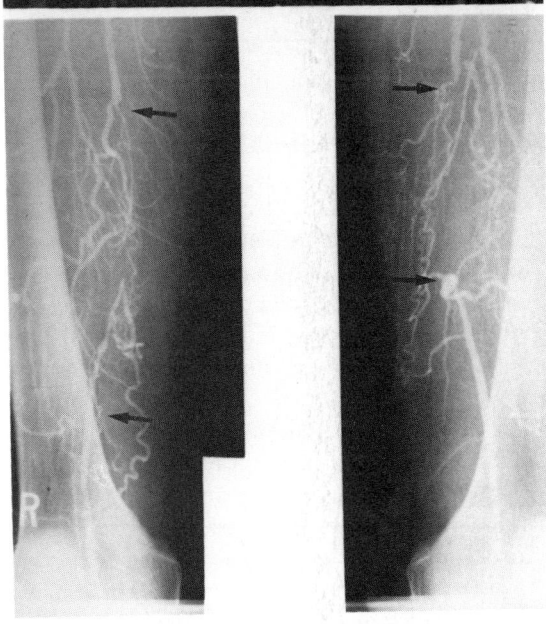

Figure 25-10 Arteriogram depicting diffuse iliac disease and complete occlusion of superficial femoral arteries, with reconstitution of popliteal arteries bilaterally (arrows).

sive disease. Because these patients are at high risk for alteration in skin integrity, especially associated with a history of diabetes, a plan of care should be devised aimed at preventative measures.

■ **NURSING DIAGNOSIS**

Impaired skin integrity of foot and leg, related to impaired blood flow.

OUTCOME STANDARD AND CRITERIA

Skin is intact, or skin integrity is improved, and risk for further impairment is reduced as evidenced by:

• No mechanical, thermal, or chemical skin break-

down of ischemic limb
• Verbalization of understanding of increased risk for skin breakdown
• Active participation in daily foot care

NURSING INTERVENTIONS

• Prevent mechanical trauma:
  Minimize pressure of mattress and bedclothes by using heel protectors, footboard, a sheepskin pad at foot of bed and static and low air loss mattress overlays and beds
  Use lambswool between toes to prevent interdigital friction necrosis
  Moisturize ischemic foot and leg with alcohol-free lubricant lotion to prevent cracking of skin
  Protect foot with shoe or slipper when patient is out of bed
  Inspect ischemic limb every 4 hours for evidence of pressure necrosis, especially at bony prominences such as phalanges, heel, and malleoli. Reposition ischemic limb every 2 hours
  Do not apply antiembolism stockings to ischemic limb
• Prevent thermal trauma:
  Avoid extremes in temperature; do *not* use heating pads in attempt to enhance vasodilatation
  Keep ischemic limb covered loosely with bedclothes. If socks are worn, remove frequently to inspect foot
• Prevent chemical trauma:
  Use only mild isotonic solutions on ischemic limb
  Avoid use of enzymatic debriding agents or hypertonic bactericidal agents such as full-strength povidone-iodine solution
  If foot soaks are prescribed, use mild soap solution and test water temperature before immersing ischemic limb
• Teach patient about necessity of meticulous foot care, reinforcing awareness of increased risk of skin breakdown arising from compromised arterial circulation
• Encourage patient to participate actively in daily foot care

■ **NURSING DIAGNOSIS**

Pain, related to impaired blood flow.

OUTCOME STANDARD and CRITERIA

Pain is absent or controlled as evidenced by:

• Verbalization of decrease in pain severity
• Increase in activities of daily living
• Demonstration of distraction methods during painful episode
• Demonstration of noninvasive pain relief measures

NURSING INTERVENTIONS

• Employ arterial positioning (if not contraindicated), using 6-inch shock blocks at head of bed to achieve leg dependency

- Minimize tissue oxygen demands by limiting activity
- Avoid activities that promote vasoconstriction (e.g., cigarette smoking, exposure to cold)
- Avoid restrictive clothing such as antiembolism stockings
- Administer analgesics per physician's prescription, and ascertain degree of relief by questioning patient
- Provide emotional support and use comfort measures such as touch, massage, music, and diversion
- Teach distraction methods, such as counting items in the room, listening to music with earphones, or guided imagery
- Teach noninvasive pain relief measures such as relaxation techniques, massages, or warm or cold compresses (as preferred or recommended)

■ **NURSING DIAGNOSIS**

Patient and/or family anxiety, related to insufficient knowledge about impending surgery.

OUTCOME STANDARD AND CRITERIA

Anxiety is reduced or absent as evidenced by:
- Asking questions to enhance knowledge of impending surgical procedures
- Verbalization of adequate knowledge of surgical procedures
- Verbalization of appropriate concerns and fears

NURSING INTERVENTIONS
- Encourage patient and family to explore concerns with nursing staff preoperatively (e.g., fear of death, limb loss, pain, potential complications)
- Assess patient and family readiness to learn and reinforce preoperative teaching, reviewing perioperative routines and specific surgical plans (individually for each patient)
- Orient patient and family to critical care setting and explain routine procedures
- If appropriate, teach patient leg and foot exercises to help promote venous return while at bed rest postoperatively, and breathing exercises to minimize pulmonary compromise. These exercises allow some control of recuperative process

■ **NURSING DIAGNOSIS**

Altered tissue perfusion, related to surgery.

OUTCOME STANDARD AND CRITERIA

Tissue perfusion is improved as evidenced by:
- Palpable pulse(s)
- Improved ABI
- Intact motion and sensation
- Warm, pink limb

NURSING INTERVENTIONS
- Assess pulses hourly for 24 hours, then every 4 hours, also Doppler pressure (may require physician order) in affected extremity
- Assess sensory and motor function of lower extremities

- Provide adequate hydration to assure normovolemia and avoid hypotension
- Monitor vital signs hourly for 24 hours, then every shift unless directed otherwise
- Inspect affected limb for evidence of severe swelling, which may impede blood flow through the graft
- If marked edema develops, elevate foot off bed slightly and apply elastic bandage from foot to thigh (surgeon's order), *provided adequate arterial circulation has been restored*
- Record bilateral circumferential measurements of ankle, calf, and thigh daily
- Report any sudden change in tissue perfusion (e.g., loss of palpable pulse; acute nonincisional pain; change in color, motion, sensation) to physician immediately

HIGH-RISK NURSING DIAGNOSES

Many patients undergoing lower extremity arterial bypass surgery also have concomitant cardiopulmonary dysfunction as well as pain and impaired mobility. Thus, other possible high-risk nursing diagnoses might include:

- High risk for decrease in cardiac output related to myocardial ischemia or infarction subsequent to surgical or anesthetic stress
- High risk for impairment of gas exchange related to altered tissue perfusion secondary to preexisting chronic obstructive pulmonary disease, general anesthesia, pain, and/or immobility
- High risk for activity intolerance related to incisional pain
- High risk for infection related to compromised circulation or skin disruption from surgery

Astute nursing assessment and management of patients with lower extremity arterial occlusive disease affords the critical care nurse the challenge of recognizing and preventing disastrous events that might threaten the viability of an ischemic limb, as well as the opportunity to facilitate recuperation and minimize complications in the vascular surgical patient.

Lower Extremity Venous Disease

Normal Venous Anatomy and Physiology

Prior to the seventeenth century, blood was thought to be produced in the liver and receive natural, vital, and animal spirits from other organs. William Harvey was the first to theorize that blood actually *circulates* through a system of blood vessels, the beginning and end point being the beating heart, with arteries functioning to carry oxygenated blood to all body cells and veins providing a return route for deoxygenated blood and waste products.

Histologically, the walls of veins are similar to those of arteries; they too have intimal, medial, and adventitial layers. The primary differences are that in veins there is less medial elastic tissue and the medial and adventitial layers are less clearly defined. Veins are capacitance vessels, capable of "storing" a tremendous volume of blood because of their relatively large diameter.

Major venous pathways parallel those of similarly named arteries (Figure 25-11). Nearly all veins have valves permitting unidirectional flow toward the heart. The exceptions to this rule are those veins in the visceral venous system which drain blood to the liver for purification before it returns to the heart. In addition to returning blood to the heart, the venous system also functions to regulate vascular capacity and to maintain thermoregularity.

In the lower extremity there are three major systems of veins: superficial veins, communicating or perforating veins, and deep veins. The *superficial veins* course in the subcutaneous tissue layer and generally have fewer valves than deep veins. Examples of superficial veins in the leg include the greater and lesser saphenous vessels. The entire superficial system can be sacrificed, as in ligation and stripping procedures, without leading to signs and symptoms of ve-

nous insufficiency. *Communicating or perforating veins* connect the superficial and deep systems. Valves in these vessels permit flow from the superficial to the deep system only. *Deep veins* course deeply within the leg musculature and are unquestionably the most functionally important vessels. They are normally responsible for at least 90% of venous outflow from the leg. Examples of deep veins in the leg are the femoral and popliteal veins.

Pathophysiology

The most common type of venous dysfunction is thrombosis, a narrowing or obstruction of venous outflow by intravascular clot formation. The terms *thrombosis* and *thrombophlebitis* are often used interchangeably, although thrombophlebitis involves a noninfectious inflammatory component in addition to intraluminal clot formation.

A frequent site of intravenous thrombus formation is the valve cusps. Venous stasis in these cusps allows for accumulation and adherence of platelets and fibrin. Once initiated, the thrombus enlarges and eventually occludes the vessel lumen. If the thrombus only partially obstructs the lumen, it becomes covered by smooth endothelium *(recanalization)* and the process stops. It is also possible that the thrombus may dislodge and embolize distally in the venous circuit and migrate back to the heart and into the pulmonary arterial circulation *(pulmonary embolism)*. If the thrombus does not become detached, it will become firmly adherent to the vein wall within 24 to 48 hours, and the body's intrinsic fibrinolytic system will gradually lyse the clot.

Thrombophlebitis can occur in either the superficial or the deep venous systems, but its consequences are more severe with deep vein involvement. Virchow, in 1846, identified three major elements promoting the development of venous thrombosis: hypercoagulability, venous stasis, and intimal damage, which have come to be known as *Virchow's triad*. Common clinical causes of these elements are outlined in the upper box on p. 626. Risk factors associated with the development of deep venous thrombosis are listed in the lower box on p. 626. Review of these factors quickly identifies the marked risk of deep vein thrombosis (DVT) in critically ill patients.

Superficial venous thrombosis is usually a self-limiting problem and is treated with conservative measures, which include elevation, application of moist heat, and administration of antiinflammatory agents such as aspirin. Antibiotics may also be prescribed if an infectious component is suspected.

Deep vein thrombosis may lead to two significant sequelae: pulmonary embolism and postphlebitic syndrome. *Pulmonary embolism* (PE) is the most acute

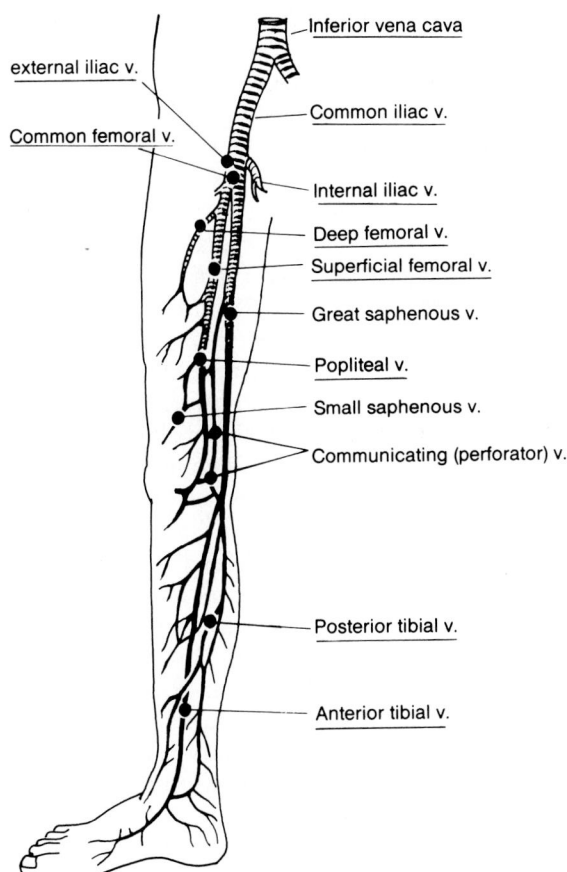

Figure 25-11   Major venous pathways of the lower extremity.

Inferior vena cava
external iliac v.
Common femoral v.
Common iliac v.
Internal iliac v.
Deep femoral v.
Superficial femoral v.
Great saphenous v.
Popliteal v.
Small saphenous v.
Communicating (perforator) v.
Posterior tibial v.
Anterior tibial v.

Virchow's Triad

Hypercoagulability
  Blood dyscrasias (such as antithrombin III deficiency)
  Trauma
  Advanced malignant disease
  Estrogen therapy
  Systemic infection
  Cigarette smoking
Venous stasis
  Heart disease, especially congestive heart failure
  Dehydration
  Immobility
  Incompetent vein valves
Intimal damage
  Trauma
  Infection
  Venipuncture
  IV infusion of irritant solutions

Risk Factors Associated with Development of Deep Vein Thrombosis

Prolonged bed rest
Cancer, especially pancreatic or prostatic
Advanced age
Obesity
Congestive heart failure
Previous venous disease
Pelvic surgery
Pregnancy, postpartum state
Lower extremity trauma

consequence of DVT and is potentially lethal. Pulmonary embolism occurs in over 650,000 patients annually and is fatal in approximately 38% of symptomatic patients.

The pathophysiological effect of pulmonary embolism depends on the size of the obstructing clot and becomes significant when more than 25% of the pulmonary arterial circulation is occluded. With 25% to 30% occlusion, pulmonary artery pressure rises, indicating impending heart failure. Cardiac output remains normal until occlusion reaches or exceeds 50%. It is critical to keep in mind, however, that preexisting cardiac or respiratory insufficiency contributes significantly to premature cardiac failure. In addition to these hemodynamic effects, pulmonary emboli can also exert mechanical effects such as potential dysrhythmias as the clot traverses the right side of the heart, bronchial artery dilatation, and decreased pulmonary blood flow.

The risk of PE is least when DVT is confined to the calf veins and increases proportionally with proximal propagation of the clot. Iliofemoral DVT is associated with a significant incidence of PE.

Postphlebitic syndrome, also known as *venous insufficiency,* is a chronic consequence of DVT. It results from permanent valvular incompetence secondary to valve destruction by the clot. The consequences of chronic venous insufficiency, most significantly venous ulceration, are infrequently encountered by critical care nurses and are therefore beyond the scope of this discussion.

Data Acquisition

History and Physical Assessment. The clinical presentations of superficial and deep vein thrombophlebitis are markedly different. Superficial thrombophlebitis presents as a local inflammatory response, with erythema and tenderness in a localized area. The affected vein may be palpable as a subcutaneous cord. The most common sites of superficial thrombophlebitis are the upper extremity veins subsequent to intravenous infusions, and the saphenous system of the lower extremities. Deep vein thrombophlebitis most commonly affects the major venous pathways in the lower extremity and is usually unidirectional. With DVT there are often systemic signs of inflammation such as low-grade fever. The most common clinical findings are generalized edema and resultant intense pain in the involved extremity.[45] Edema results from obstruction to venous outflow with venous engorgement and fluid transudation from the capillary bed into the extravascular tissue.

Additionally, the patient with DVT may exhibit a positive *Homans' sign* (sharp muscular calf pain on dorsiflexion), asymmetry in leg circumference, and/or a positive *Pratt's sign* (pain resulting from compression of the calf against the tibia). These findings are much less reliable, however.

The patient with PE may present clinically with an acute event leading to cardiac failure and death, but lesser degrees of PE may also present in patients who are asymptomatic or those with chest pain and dyspnea. In addition, tachypnea and tachycardia are common. Unexplained restlessness and apprehension, especially in a high-risk patient, should alert the examiner to the possibility of PE. Hemoptysis may or may not be present. Pleuritic chest pain may develop from pulmonary infarction. Recurrent small pulmonary emboli may lead to pulmonary hypertension and compromise of right ventricular heart function. With a massive PE, acute cor pulmonale, decreased cardiac output, hypoxemia, and shock develop.

Noninvasive Diagnostic Procedures. The noninvasive tests previously used to detect deep vein thrombophlebitis in clinical practice were impedance plethysmography, phleborrheography, and Doppler venous evaluation. Each of these tests has inherent shortcomings, with different degrees of specificity and sensitivity according to the location of the thrombus and the experience of the examiner. However, a promising noninvasive procedure is duplex scanning. This imaging technique consists of brightness (B-mode) ultrasound, which provides high-resolution images, and pulsed Doppler, which elucidates blood flow characteristics within a vein or artery.[46] The accuracy of this procedure has been heralded as approximately 100% when used by skilled personnel.[47] It provides clinicians with both anatomic (B-mode ultrasound) and hemodynamic information (Pulsed Doppler) similar to the data obtained by venography. Patients are placed in reverse Trendelenburg position for this procedure. Duplex screening has a very low risk and can be repeated in a serial fashion to monitor a thrombus.

The gold standard of diagnostic tests for DVT remains contrast venography. Positive findings on venogram include filling defects, sharp termination of a column of contrast, and/or nonfilling of the deep vein system.

Several screening tests are commonly employed for patients with suspected pulmonary embolism. Laboratory evaluation includes analysis of arterial blood gases (ABGs), which usually signify a decreased PO_2 (<80 mmHg) and decreased PCO_2 secondary to hyperventilation. Serum enzymes may be analyzed to differentiate symptoms from those of a myocardial infarction (MI). Increased serum lactate dyhydrogenase (LDH) may be indicative of pulmonary infarction. An ECG is also routinely employed, again to differentiate between PE and acute MI. Chest x-rays, especially when used in conjunction with other studies, may help to rule out other possible causes of symptoms, such as pneumonia or pleural effusion.

Radionuclide lung scanning is a useful screening technique. The primary value of this test is that a normal perfusion scan virtually rules out a PE if done within 8 hours of the onset of symptoms. The specificity of perfusion lung scanning is increased when combined with a ventilatory component. In addition to the injection of labeled albumin, the patient inspires xenon gas. A mismatch between the ventilation and perfusion scans (e.g., adequate ventilation with absence of gas exchange in the vasculature) is highly suggestive of PE. However, the ventilation component requires the cooperation of the patient and may be difficult or impossible to perform in some critically ill patients.

Invasive Diagnostic Procedures. Pulmonary arteriography remains the only conclusive diagnostic test for PE. This involves the injection of radiopaque contrast material into the pulmonary artery under fluoroscopy. It is considered diagnostic if an intraluminal filling defect can be identified or if there is sharp cutoff of lobar or segmental vessels.

Medical Management

The goals of therapy for DVT and PE include prophylaxis, management during the acute phase, and long-term anticoagulation. The aim of prophylaxis is to reduce all elements of Virchow's triad: hypercoagulability, venous stasis, and intimal damage. This can be achieved by such measures as active or passive exercise for patients at bed rest, early ambulation whenever possible, leg elevation, use of graduated compression stockings, treatment with pneumatic compression boot devices, and administration of prophylactic minidose subcutaneous heparin in high-risk patients.[48]

Management during the acute phase of DVT and PE involves administration of anticoagulants, as well as symptomatic relief methods. Continuous intravenous heparin is the treatment of choice for both DVT and PE. The goal of therapy in DVT is to prevent propagation of the deep vein thrombus and to minimize the risk of embolization. The goal of therapy in PE is to treat the underlying cause and to prevent recurrent embolism. Heparin acts directly on both the intrinsic and extrinsic coagulation pathways, by inhibiting thrombin-mediated conversion of fibrinogen to fibrin. It also interferes with the action of several clotting factors and potentiates the actions of antithrombin III, an intrinsic anticoagulant. The goal of treatment is prolongation of the activated partial thromboplastin time (APTT) to 1½ to 2½ times control (in seconds). Heparin does not dissolve the clot; however, the thrombus is lysed by the body's intrinsic fibrinolytic agents, which have more recently been employed to lyse extensive DVT or massive PE.[49]

Symptomatic relief methods for DVT include strict bed rest until acute symptoms subside, leg elevation, and application of warm, moist heat. With PE, strict bed rest with intensive care unit monitoring is preferable. Invasive hemodynamic monitoring via pulmonary artery catheter provides valuable information with respect to cardiac function. Cardiopulmonary support with administration of digitalis to improve myocardial contractile function and administration of oxygen may be indicated. Additionally, use of antiembolization stockings assists in promoting venous outflow.

Long-term oral anticoagulation with warfarin sodium (Coumadin) is recommended for at least 6 months following acute DVT or PE, the goal of therapy being prevention of recurrence. Warfarin inhibits synthesis of vitamin K-dependent clotting factors by the liver by competitively interfering with vitamin K. Treatment with oral anticoagulants is initiated concurrently with heparin, and an overlap of 3 to 5 days

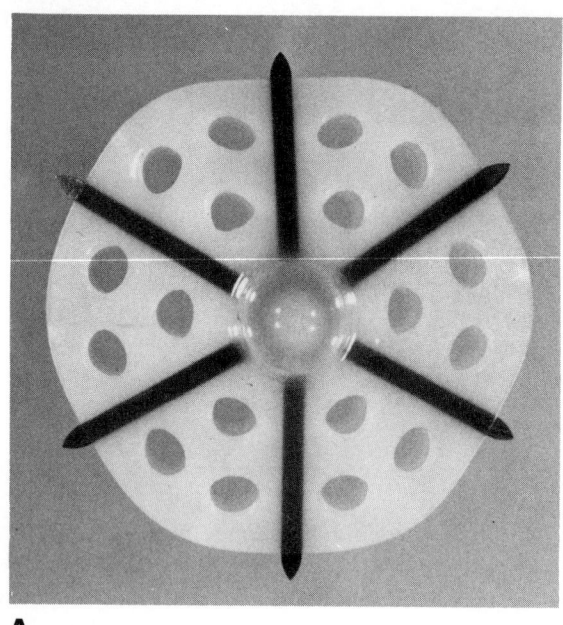

A

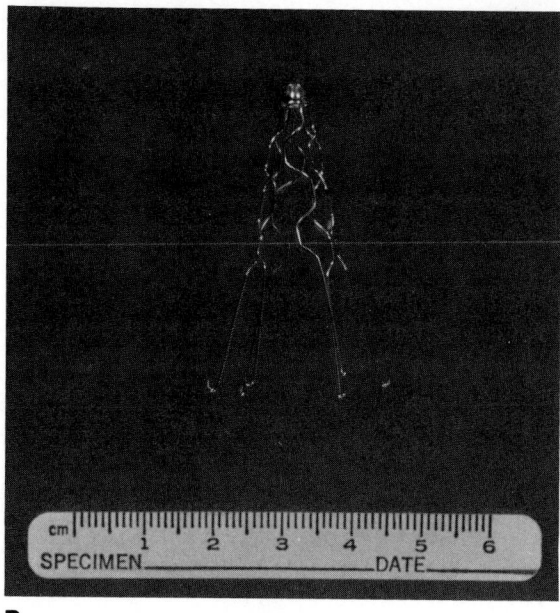

B

Figure 25-12   *A,* Mobin-Uddin intracaval "umbrella" filter. *B,* Kimray-Greenfield intracaval filter.

is often necessary to ensure the therapeutic effectiveness of warfarin. The goal of treatment is prolongation of the prothrombin time (PT) to 1½ to 2½ times control (in seconds).

Surgical Management

Only rarely is surgery indicated as a treatment for deep vein thrombosis—most often to protect a patient from initial or recurrent pulmonary embolism when conventional anticoagulation is contraindicated or has failed. Surgical options include pulmonary embolectomy and interruption of the inferior vena cava (IVC). Pulmonary embolectomy requires major thoracic surgery and is often undertaken as a "last resort" life-saving attempt, since the majority of patients suffering massive PE are hemodynamically unstable.

Extravascular interruption of the IVC involves abdominal surgery. A partitioning Teflon clip (Adams-DeWeese clip) can be applied to the cava which effectively partitions the lumen, preventing passage of large emboli. Caval clipping is sometimes done prophylactically during other abdominal surgical procedures (such as cholecystectomy or hysterectomy) in high-risk patients.

If patients are too ill to undergo abdominal surgery, an intravascular filter device can be inserted under local anesthesia in the radiology suite, using fluoroscopic control. The device, attached to a loading catheter, is threaded into the right internal jugular vein in the neck and positioned in the IVC just distal to the renal veins. The device is released from the catheter and lodged securely in place. It functions as a sieve, permitting filtration of emboli without ob-

struction of venous outflow. The two most commonly used intracaval filter devices are the Mobin-Uddin "umbrella" and the Kimray-Greenfield filter (Figure 25-12).

NURSING MANAGEMENT OF DEEP VENOUS THROMBOPHLEBITIS AND PULMONARY EMBOLISM

In nearly every patient cared for in an intensive care setting, be it medical or surgical, there are one or more factors that place the person at risk for the development of DVT and subsequent threat of PE. Prevention is the cornerstone of treatment. However, early recognition and reporting of the signs and symptoms of these pathophysiological processes facilitate prompt intervention, which may avert life-threatening consequences.

Nurses in the critical care setting routinely care for patients who are at high risk for the development of DVT and/or PE. They also provide care to those who are acutely symptomatic from PE. Therefore, a sound knowledge base regarding prophylaxis and treatment of these processes is an essential nursing skill. The nursing diagnoses and plans of care outlined below are applicable to these problems.

HIGH-RISK NURSING DIAGNOSIS

High risk for altered health maintenance, related to insufficient knowledge of anticoagulant therapy and signs and symptoms of complications.

OUTCOME STANDARD AND CRITERIA

Health maintenance is normal as evidenced by:
- Ability to seek help as needed or ask questions to maintain healthy state
- Verbalization of signs and symptoms that need to

be reported to health care team
- Verbalization of health behaviors needed to manage thrombophlebitis
- Verbalization of signs and symptoms of anticoagulant therapy complications

NURSING INTERVENTIONS
- Assess knowledge of thrombophlebitis and pulmonary embolism
- Instruct patient regarding activities and situations that promote vasoconstriction, such as smoking and cold temperatures
- Instruct patient to report signs and symptoms of pulmonary embolism, such as sudden chest or shoulder pain, cough with hemoptysis, restlessness, or increasing anxiety
- Instruct patient regarding active and passive ROM while on bed rest
- Instruct patient to report side effects of anticoagulant therapy such as signs of bruising or bleeding
- Help patient to evaluate personal limitations that affect health maintenance
- Help patient to develop behaviors that support health maintenance

The following nursing interventions are aimed at supporting the medical plan of care for the patient at high risk for pulmonary embolism due to deep venous thrombosis:
- Administer anticoagulant medication per physician order—usually IV bolus of heparin sodium followed by continuous infusion, utilizing regulatory infusion pump
- Monitor PTT as evidence of therapeutic effectiveness of heparin: regulate heparin dosage according to physician's order
- Monitor body secretions (e.g., urine, stool, nasogastric aspirate if any) for occult blood
- Monitor and document results of invasive hemodynamic tests, notifying physician of deteriorating arterial blood gas results, worsening pulmonary hypertension, persistent dysrhythmias, or hypotension

VASCULAR TRAUMA

Vascular trauma related to motor vehicle accidents, gunshot wounds, or the use of sharp instruments,[50] is a common injury seen in emergency departments. These vascular injuries can be categorized as blunt or penetrating trauma and are discussed in greater detail in conjunction with the associated effect of compartment syndrome.

Categories

Blunt Trauma

Vascular injuries caused by blunt trauma are commonly associated with motor vehicle accidents. The blunt force may directly injure a vessel, or injury may

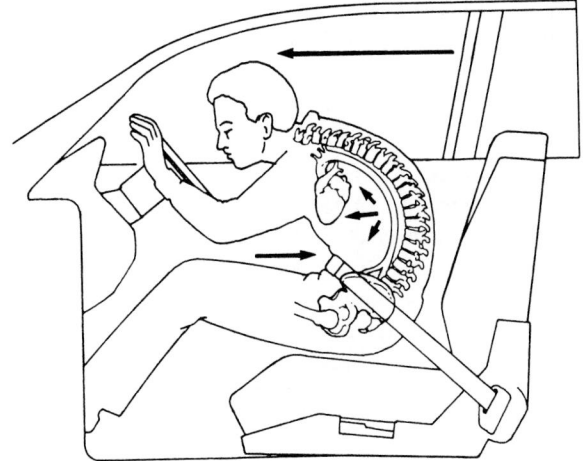

Figure 25-13 Forces present at impact.

be caused by the shearing force of rapid deceleration.[51] Automobile accidents in which the victim has not worn a seat belt may cause direct blunt injury to the chest and abdomen with resulting injuries such as cardiac contusion, fractures to the sternum and ribs, flail chest, hemothorax and pneumothorax, and injury to the liver or spleen.[50] Nevertheless, the seat belt has been implicated as a factor in the development of both direct and deceleration injuries involving the thoracic and abdominal aorta.

Direct force injuries occur when the aorta is squeezed between the seat belt and the spine. In deceleration injuries, the gravitational forces of the abrupt cessation of motion from the impact causes a tearing force in two directions within the aorta. The seat belt compresses the descending aorta, which is a column of blood under pressure, resulting in backflow and distention of the aortic arch. This tension is thought to cause rupture of the ascending aorta. The seat belt also compresses the aorta and abdominal contents into the pelvis which further stretches the aorta and may cause intimal damage of the vessel[52,53] (Figure 25-13).

Penetrating Injury

Most penetrating injuries are caused by sharp instruments or low-velocity bullets which limit the damage to the wound tract. High-velocity missiles produce widespread damage to surrounding tissues. Severe soft tissue injury can occur with high-velocity missiles and with low-velocity missiles at close range. Victims of automobile accidents commonly have multiple injuries that include fractures and dislocations.[51] Vascular wounds are frequently the result of fractures especially near the joint where the vessels are relatively fixed and vulnerable to shear forces. Posterior dislocations of the knee are likely to injure the popliteal artery and vein.[54]

Data Acquisition

Physical Assessment

The assessment of a patient with vascular injuries may be complicated by the multiple injuries present, and the evaluation of respiration and circulation with standard resuscitation measures should be implemented initially. Brink[55] has classified patients with vascular injuries into three categories. Category 1 patients have obvious life-threatening injuries, category 2 patients have obvious injuries that may be threatening to a limb or an organ, and category 3 patients have injuries near major blood vessels but with no obvious direct injury.[55] Patients in category 1 must receive immediate surgery to control bleeding. Clinical features of injuries to major vessels include (1) cardiac arrest with a presentation of asystole or electrical-mechanical dissociation, (2) persistent shock, (3) cardiac tamponade, (4) wide mediastinum, or (5) recurring hemothorax. Patients in categories 2 and 3 require further evaluation to determine the treatment modality most appropriate for the injury.[50]

In extremity injuries, assess for the "six P's" of arterial insufficiency—pain, pallor, pulselessness, paresthesia, paralysis, and poikilothermia (coldness).[56] Menzoian and associates[57] have found a significant correlation between certain clinical findings and the confirmation of significant vascular injury. The presence of a bruit or thrill, signs of distal ischemia, absence of pulses, active hemorrhage, neurological deficit, and hematoma correlate positively with vascular injury at the time of surgery.

Diagnostic Procedures

The chest x-ray may demonstrate widening of mediastinum or capping of the apical pleura in patients with major vessel injury. Computed tomography (CT) or nuclear magnetic resonance imaging (MRI) may further delineate disruption of major vessels within the thorax or abdomen in the presence of blunt trauma.[50,51,58]

X-rays of the injured extremity are obtained to confirm fractures.[54,57] Doppler sound and Doppler ankle/brachial index assessment of the extremity in patients with absent or diminished pulses provide confirmation of abnormality and a baseline for ongoing care. A decrease in ankle/brachial index and an abnormal arterial waveform may indicate significant arterial injury.[51,56]

In the stable patient, arteriography helps to identify and confirm arterial injury as well as to delineate the extent of injury. When patients are at risk from active bleeding or significant ischemia, immediate surgical intervention is advocated. For patients with an injury to surrounding vessels but with no specific clinical signs of arterial injury, arteriography is advocated.[51,56]

Intraarterial digital subtraction angiography (DSA) may further clarify vascular injuries, uses less contrast material, is faster, uses smaller catheters, and is less expensive than conventional arteriography. However, DSA involves more complicated equipment and greater technical assistance, can only be used to identify a small area of injury, and requires a compliant patient.[51]

Medical Management

Initial treatment of patients with vascular trauma includes advanced cardiac life support resuscitation measures and protection of the cervical spine. Once the patient has been assessed, further diagnostic interventions may be employed, and patients with Brinks category 1 or 2 are taken to surgery. Antibiotic therapy is initiated preoperatively, especially for patients with penetrating wounds. Anticoagulant therapy is generally contraindicated in the trauma patient, but careful administration of a heparin infusion may be required to prevent clot formation in associated vessels which may occlude collateral blood supply to an extremity.[51]

Major Vessels

In patients in whom major chest vessel injury has occurred, the mortality and morbidity are high.[58] In those patients who present to the hospital, immediate resuscitation may be needed or there may be time for arteriography or computed tomography. Aortic disruption is treated emergently with control of bleeding and surgical intervention as described earlier.

Major vein injury of the superior or inferior vena cavae or the subclavian vein requires fluid resuscitation, but intravenous access should not be placed in the injured extremity since these fluids may infuse into the chest cavity.[51] Pneumatic antishock garments may be used effectively to manage hypotension in the patient with abdominal and pelvic injuries. Major venous vessels can be repaired by lateral suture technique, end-to-end anastomosis, or interposition vein grafts.[51]

Lower Extremity Injury

Injuries of the lower extremities frequently involve arteries, veins, and nerves because of their close proximity to each other. Approximately one fifth of lower extremity arterial injuries involve the femoral arteries.[51,54,56,57] The superficial femoral artery is one of the most frequently injured because it lies near the distal femur and therefore is vulnerable to injury from fractures. Popliteal artery injuries result from posterior dislocation of the knee.[51,54,56,57]

Obvious fractures should be stabilized before surgery to control bleeding.[51] Frank bleeding is controlled by a compression dressing or direct digital pressure. Orthopedic injuries are repaired after vascular integrity is established. External fixation of the fracture is advocated by Menzoian et al. for postoperative monitoring of soft tissue injury, arterial flow, and neurological function.[51]

Arterial injuries may be repaired by many techniques including simple suturing of lacerations, end-to-end anastomosis, and interposition bypass grafts. Saphenous veins are used when available, but when injury is extensive, synthetic graft materials may be used.[51,54,56,57] Once the artery is repaired, intraoperative arteriography is performed to assure patency of the vessel and define any technical problems of the procedure.[51,54,56,57]

When the patient's condition allows, venous injuries should be repaired. Venous ligation may be necessary when other multiple injuries and the patient's condition do preclude repair. Venous repair may decrease soft tissue edema and improve arterial perfusion.[51,54,56,57]

Soft tissue injury is associated with trauma, particularly blunt trauma, and high-velocity penetrating injuries.[50,51] Edema of skeletal muscle and soft tissue in areas contained within compartments may lead to increased pressure and the development of ischemia known as *compartment syndrome*. Fasciotomy of the extremity is indicated to prevent compartment syndrome or for the relief of increased compartment pressure.

Complications

Postoperative complications following vascular trauma may be categorized as early and late and as having local or systemic effects. Early local complications are bleeding, thrombosis of the repaired vessel, spasm of the vessel leading to ischemia, and reperfusion edema which may lead to compartment syndrome.[50,51] Systemic effects of these local complications may be related to the effects of reperfusion syndrome.[51] Late complications include graft infection, false aneurysm formation, arteriovenous fistulae, and posttraumatic pain syndrome.[50,51,58]

Early Complications

Bleeding may occur from the use of anticoagulation, coagulopathies from the multiple areas of trauma, or the extensive administration of blood products.[51] A specific site of bleeding within the vessel or anastomosis is the most common factor in bleeding complications; it is treated by reexploration of the vessel.

Thrombosis of the vasculature may be due to the technical aspects of the surgical procedure or spasm of the vessel.[50,51] Soft tissue injury and fractures increase the incidence of thrombosis.

When perfusion is restored to an ischemic area, the capillaries are more permeable and there is an increase in flow which results in both intracellular and extracellular edema.[51] In injury to the lower extremities where there is limited space to allow for edema, an increase in pressure cannot be relieved. The pressure increase promotes the development of compartment syndrome.[51,54,57]

Reperfusion to an ischemic extremity also may stimulate systemic effects. As perfusion is restored, the buildup of acidic metabolites and potassium excreted from necrotic muscle is flushed through the body. The resultant metabolic acidosis and hyperkalemia stimulate dysrhythmias and hypotension. With the ischemia of muscle, myoglobin is released into the systemic circulation following reperfusion. Myoglobin in combination with acidosis leads to a precipitate obstruction within the renal tubules. Alkalinization of the urine and significant diuresis prevent the progression to acute tubular necrosis.[51]

Late Complications

Vascular graft infections are generally related to contamination at the time of surgery and may present months to years following the original surgery. The circumstances surrounding the need for surgery, specifically contamination due to multiple injuries, increase the likelihood of infection. The infection may stimulate thrombosis or the development of a false aneurysm within the vessel. Treatment of the infected graft may include replacement of the vascular graft, debridement of the surrounding tissue, antibiotic therapy, or revascularization by using grafts to bypass infected tissue.[51]

Aneurysms and false aneurysms may develop when the extent of vessel disruption is underestimated. Aneurysms present as pulsatile masses which are usually painless and without symptoms of distal ischemia. A murmur may be heard over the aneurysm. As the aneurysm enlarges, compression of nerves proximal to the aneurysm develops.[50,51]

Arteriovenous (AV) fistulas may be associated with false aneurysms or may be caused by penetrating injuries to nearby arteries and veins. A continuous, machinery-type murmur over the fistula, evidence of venous hypertension, and varicosities in the area are typical symptoms of AV fistulas. In large fistulas, there is contrasting warmth over the region of the fistula with distal coolness. AV fistulas between the aorta and the vena cavae cause high-output heart failure since there is shunting of large volumes of arterial blood into the right atrium.[50,51] Treatment of AV fistulas is based on the size and location of the fistula. Small distal fistulas may be ligated while large proximal fistulas require restoration of continuity of both artery and vein.[50,51]

Posttraumatic pain syndrome generally occurs in the lower extremity following trauma. Symptoms of posttraumatic pain syndrome may vary but include severe burning pain, sympathetic dysfunction which may lead to vasodilation or vasoconstriction, delayed functional recovery, and trophic changes. Surgical sympathectomy is an effective treatment of this pain syndrome.[51]

COMPARTMENT SYNDROME

Compartment syndrome is described as a progressive process resulting from increased pressure within a limited anatomic space which compromises circulation, viability, and function of the tissue within that space.[59,60] Compartments are made up of muscle, nerves, and blood vessels surrounded by inelastic tissue, specifically skin, fascia, and/or bone. Compartments within the extremities are particularly vulnerable to compartment syndrome. The most common sites are the four compartments of the lower leg (Figure 25-14).[61]

Pathophysiology

Increasing pressure within the compartment may be due to a decrease in compartment size such as premature closure of fascial defects; an increase in compartment contents (edema or bleeding); or external pressure from casts, dressings, or pneumatic antishock garments.[60] The physiological effects of compartment syndrome begin with compression of the venous capillary beds. This leads to an increase in venous hydrostatic pressure and an increase in interstitial fluid volume. As this process continues, the increased pressure compromises arteriolar flow and stimulates spasm. Arterial flow is diminished and ischemia results. Factors that increase the potential for the development of compartment syndrome are shock, hypotension, reperfusion following trauma, and decreased oncotic pressure as may result from burns.[62]

The amount of injury is based on the degree of injury and the duration of ischemia experienced. Initial symptoms may develop within 2 hours of the injury; ischemia lasting 4 to 6 hours may cause irreversible tissue damage.[62] If untreated, necrosis of the muscle results in contractures, a nonfunctional extremity, and possibly amputation. Systemic effects of muscle necrosis include metabolic acidosis, hyperkalemia, renal dysfunction, and sepsis.

Data Acquisition

Physical Assessment

The symptoms of compartment syndrome reflect the increased pressure and its effects within the area. Hypoesthesia and deep, throbbing, unrelenting pain disproportionate to the degree of injury and elicited with passive stretching of the muscles involved are early indicators of muscle tissue hypoxia. Extension and flexion of the toes and inversion and dorsiflexion of the foot should be assessed in the lower extremity and extension, flexion, abduction, and adduction of the fingers should be assessed in the upper extremity to elicit increased pain and weak movement significant in compartment syndrome. In general, changes in pulses, temperature, and color of the skin are unreliable indicators of compartment syndrome.[63]

Diagnostic Procedures

Many invasive methods are available to determine intracompartment pressures, including the placement of a needle, wick, slit catheter, or continuous infusion device. Critical values vary with the technique used, but pressures greater than 40 mmHg signal significant pressures within the compartment. Venograms and arteriograms may be used to rule out other causes of pain, and Doppler studies act as an adjunct to the clinical signs of compartment syndrome.[64]

Medical Management

Treatment of compartment syndrome is by fasciotomy. An incision is made through the skin, subcutaneous tissue, and fascia to allow room for expansion of underlying muscle. Following fasciotomy, open wounds are packed with dressings soaked in normal saline to provide moisture to the tissues and maintained until secondary closure occurs or the area receives a skin graft. Frequent neurovascular assess-

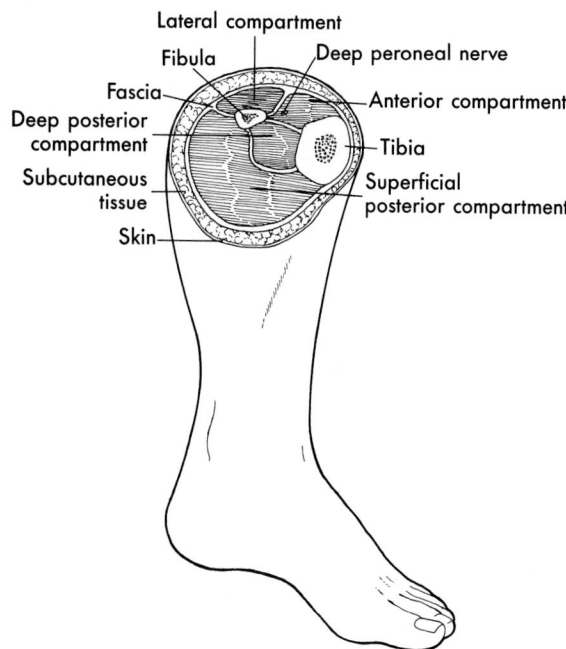

Figure 25-14 Muscle compartments of the lower extremity.

ments of the distal extremity are required to assess that adequate circulation is maintained.[60]

Nursing Management

Nurses play a critical role in the early detection and treatment of compartment syndrome. Neuromuscular findings in compartment syndrome include (1) pain greater than anticipated from clinical situation, most pronounced with passive stretching of muscles in the involved extremity; (2) hypesthesia in nerves within the compartment; (3) muscular weakness; and (4) increased muscle tension.[65]

Neuromuscular and circulatory assessment should continue in the postoperative period. Following surgical treatment by fasciotomy, the nurse must also provide meticulous wound care, keeping the exposed muscle moistened with normal saline or ¼ strength (isotonic) povidone-iodine soaked gauze. It is critical that the muscle not be allowed to dry out. If muscle necrosis develops, the surgeon should be notified, since the risk of bone and soft tissue infection increases. Surgical debridement of necrotic muscle may be necessary.

REFERENCES

1. Auerbach, O., & Garfinkel, L. (1980). Atherosclerosis and aneurysm of the aorta in relation to smoking habits and age. *Chest, 78,* 805-809.
2. Norrgard, O., Angquist, K., & Johnson, O. (1985). Familiar aortic aneurysms: Serum concentrations of triglyceride, cholesterol, HDL-cholesterol and VLDL and LDL-cholesterol. *British Journal of Surgery, 72*(2), 113-116.
3. Reilly, J. M., & Tilson, M. D. (1989). Incidence and etiology of abdominal aortic aneurysms. *Surgical Clinics of North America, 69,* 705-711.
4. Cole, C. W., et al. (1989). Abdominal aneurysms: Consequences of a positive family history. *Canadian Journal of Surgery, 32,* 117-120.
5. Dobrin, P. (1989). Pathophysiology and pathogenesis of aortic aneurysm. *Surgical Clinics of North America, 69,* 687-703.
6. Donaldson, M. C., Rosenburg, J. M., & Buckham, C. A. (1985). Diagnosis of ruptured abdominal aortic aneurysm. *Connecticut Medicine, 49*(1), 3-6.
7. Kouchoukos, N. T., & Karp, R. B. (1983). Aneurysms of the ascending aorta. In W. W. L. Glenn (Ed.), *Thoracic and cardiovascular surgery* (4th ed.). Norwalk, CT: Appleton-Century-Crofts.
8. Eagle, K. A., & DeSanctis, R. W. (1988). Diseases of the aorta. In E. Braunwald (Ed.), *Heart disease: A textbook of cardiovascular medicine* (3rd ed.) (pp. 1548-1562). Philadelphia: Saunders.
9. Baum, P. L. (1982). Abdominal aortic aneurysm? This patient takes AAA care. *Nursing, 12,* 34-41.
10. Wheat, M. (1985). Acute dissection of the aorta. In K. McCauley, A. Brest, & D. McGoon (Eds.), *McGoon's cardiac surgery: An interprofessional approach to patient care.* Philadelphia: Davis.
11. Hammond, B. B. (1982). The patient with an acute aortic dissection: Assessment and management. *Critical Care Nurse, 2*(2), 46-52.
12. Axiotis, C. A. (1985). Dissecting thoracic aortic aneurysm perforating the esophagus and masquerading as peptic ulcer disease. *The Royal Society of Medicine, 78,* 160-161.
13. Borner, N., Erbel, R., Braun, B., et al. (1984). Diagnosis of aortic dissection by transesophageal echocardiography. *American Journal of Cardiology, 54,* 1157-1158.
14. Finnerty, F. A., Jr. Treatment of hypertensive emergencies. *Heart Lung, 10,* 275-284.
15. Lindsay, J., Jr., DeBakey, M. E., & Beall, A. C., Jr. (1982). Diseases of the aorta. In J. W. Hurst, R. B. Logue, C. E. Rackley, et al. (Eds.), *The heart: Arteries and veins.* New York: McGraw-Hill.
16. Gordon, M. (1982). *Nursing diagnosis: Application to theory and practice.* New York: McGraw-Hill.
17. Porter, J. M., Taylor, L. M., Jr., & Baur, G. M. Drugs in vascular surgery. In W. S. Moore (Ed.), (1983). *Vascular surgery: A comprehensive review.* New York: Grune & Stratton.
18. Smith, C. D., & McKendry, R. J. (1982). Controlled trial of nifedipine in the treatment of Raynaud's phenomenon. *Lancet, 2,* 1299-1301.
19. Porter, J. M., Taylor, L. M., Jr., & Baur, G. M. Non-atherosclerotic vascular disease. In W. S. Moore (Ed.), (1983). *Vascular surgery: A comprehensive review.* New York: Grune & Stratton.
20. Fielding, J. E. (1985). Smoking: Health effects and control. *New England Journal of Medicine, 313,* 491-498.
21. Gordon, M. (1991). *Manual of nursing diagnosis.* St. Louis: Mosby–Year Book.
22. Harkonen, S., & Kjellstrand, C. M. (1977). Exacerbation of diabetic renal failure following intravenous pyelography. *American Journal of Medicine, 63,* 939-946.
23. Eisenberg, R. L., Bank, W. O., & Hedgock, M. W. (1981). Renal failure after major angiography can be avoided with hydration. *American Journal of Radiology, 136,* 859-861.
24. Imparato, A. M., Kim, G. E., Davidson, T., et al. (1975). Intermittent claudication: Its natural course. *Surgery, 78,* 795-799.
25. Coffman, J. D. Disease of the peripheral vessels. In P. B. Beeson, W. McDermott, & J. B. Wyngaarden (Eds.), (1979). *Cecil's textbook of medicine* (15th ed.). Philadelphia: Saunders.
26. Coffman, J. D. (1979). Drug therapy: Vasodilator drugs in peripheral vascular disease. *New England Journal of Medicine, 300,* 713-717.
27. Porter, J. M., Cutler, B. S., Lee, B. Y., et al. (1982). Pentoxifylline efficacy in the treatment of intermittent claudication: Multicenter controlled double-blind trial with objective assessment of chronic occlusive arterial disease patients. *American Heart Journal, 104*(1), 66-72.
28. Nunnelee, J. D. (1988). Medications used in vascular patients. In V. A. Lahey (Ed.), *Vascular nursing* (pp. 169-183). Philadelphia: Saunders.

29. Block, P. C., Myler, R. K., Stertzer, S., et al. (1981). Morphology after transluminal angioplasty in human beings. *New England Journal of Medicine, 305,* 382-385.

30. Eagan, J. S. (1989). Lasers: Applications in cardiovascular atherosclerotic disease. *Critical Care Nursing Clinics of North America, 1*(2), 311-326.

31. Ford, K. A. (1990). Laser assisted angioplasty in the patient with peripheral vascular disease. *Journal of Vascular Nursing, 8*(3), 6-8.

32. Wright, J. G., et al. (1989). Laser angioplasty for limb salvage: Observations on early results. *Journal of Vascular Surgery, 10*(1), 29-37.

33. Ginsburg, R. (1985). Percutaneous transluminal laser angioplasty for treatment of peripheral vascular disease. *Radiology, 156*(3), 619-624.

34. Rosenscheim, U., et al. (1990). Ultrasonic angioplasty in totally occluded peripheral arteries. *Circulation, 82*(4), III-20. (Abstract)

35. Goldhaber, S. Z., et al. (1988). Randomized controlled trial of recombinant tissue plasminogen activator versus urokinase in the treatment of acute pulmonary embolism. *Lancet, 2*(8606), 293-298.

36. Bell, W. R., & Meek, A. G. (1979). Current concepts: Guidelines for the use of thrombolytic agents. *New England Journal of Medicine, 301,* 1266-1270.

37. Porter, J. M., & Taylor, L. M. (1985). Current status of thrombolytic therapy. *Journal of Vascular Surgery, 2,* 239-249.

38. Anderson, C. (1991). Angioscopy. *Journal of Vascular Nursing, 9*(2), 8-11.

39. Doyle, J. E. (1984). The person with lower extremity arterial occlusive disease. In C. E. Guzzetta, & B. M. Dossey (Eds.), *Cardiovascular nursing: Bodymind tapestry.* St. Louis: Mosby.

40. Fellows, E. (1991). Vascular graft research: Endothelial cell seeding of synthetic bypass grafts. *Journal of Vascular Nursing, 9*(2), 12-14.

41. Cranley, J. J., & Haffner, C. D. (1982). Revascularization of the femoropopliteal arteries using saphenous vein, polytetrafluoroethylene, and umbilical vein grafts: Five- and six-year results. *Archives of Surgery, 117,* 1543-1550.

42. LoGerfo, F. W., & Coffman, J. D. (1984). Current concepts: Vascular and microvascular disease of the foot in diabetes. Implications for foot care. *New England Journal of Medicine, 311,* 1615-1619.

43. Bensen, J. L., & Karmody, A. M. (1987). In-situ artery bypass. *AORN Journal, 45*(1), 40-55.

44. Leather, R. P., & Veith, F. J. (1989). In-situ vein bypass. In H. Haimovici (Ed.), *Vascular surgery: Principles and technique* (pp. 517-525). East Norwalk, CT: Appleton & Lange.

45. Menzoian, J. O., Sequeira, J. C., Doyle, J. E., et al. (1983). Therapeutic and clinical course of deep vein thrombosis. *American Journal of Surgery, 146,* 581-585.

46. Kohler, T. R., & Strandness, D. E. (1988). Duplex scanning of peripheral arteries: Practical application. In J. J. Bergan, & J. S. T. Yao (Eds.), *Arterial surgery:*

New diagnostic and operative techniques (pp. 437-439). Orlando, FL: Grune & Stratton.

47. Nussbaum, M. S., et al. (1987). *The Mont Reid handbook* (pp. 304-337). Chicago: Year Book.

48. Kakkar, V. (1990). Prevention of venous thrombosis and pulmonary embolism. *American Journal of Cardiology, 65,* 50C-54C.

49. Bell, W. R. (1982). Thrombolytic therapy—a new realistic approach in treatment of thromboocclusive vascular disease. *Surgery, 92,* 913-914.

50. Perry, M. O. (1985). Vascular injuries. In G. T. Shires, (Ed.), *Principles of trauma care* (3rd ed.). New York: McGraw-Hill.

51. Menzoian, J. O., Cantelmo, N. L., Wright, J. G., et al. (1992). Vascular trauma. In J. Loscalzo, M. A. Creager, & V. J. Dzau (Eds.), *Vascular medicine* (pp. 1145-1172). Boston: Little, Brown.

52. Randhawa, M. P. S., Jr., & Menzoian, J. O. (1990). Seat belt aorta. *Annals of Vascular Surgery, 4,* 370-377.

53. Van De Wal, H. J. C. M., Draaisma, J. M. T., Vincent, J. G., et al. (1990). Rupture of the subdiaphragmatic inferior vena cava by blunt deceleration trauma: Case report. *Journal of Trauma, 30*(1), 111-113.

54. Drost, T. F., Rosemurgy, A. S., Proctor, D., et al. (1989). Outcome of treatment of combined orthopedic and arterial trauma to the lower extremity. *Journal of Trauma, 29*(10), 1331-1334.

55. Brink, B. E. (1977). Vascular trauma. *Surgical Clinics of North America, 57,* 189-196.

56. Rutherford, R. B. (1988). Diagnostic evaluation of extremity vascular injuries. *Surgical Clinics of North America, 68,* 683-691.

57. Menzoian, J. O., Doyle, J. E., Cantelma, N. L., et al. (1985). A comprehensive approach to extremity vascular trauma. *Archives of Surgery, 120,* 801-805.

58. Mattox, K. L. (1988). Thoracic great vessel injury. *Surgical Clinics of North America, 68,* 693-703.

59. Shah, P. M., Wapnir, I., Babu, S., et al. (1989). Compartment syndrome in combined arterial and venous injuries of the lower extremity. *American Journal of Surgery, 158,* 136-141.

60. Ross, D. (1991). Acute compartment syndrome. *Orthopaedic Nursing, 10*(2), 33-38.

61. Proehl, J. A. (1988). Compartment syndrome. *Journal of Emergency Nursing, 14*(5), 283-290.

62. Lagerstrom, C. F., Reed, R. L., Rowlands, B. J., et al. (1989). Early fasciotomy for acute clinically evident posttraumatic compartment syndrome. *American Journal of Surgery, 158,* 36-39.

63. Larson, M., Leigh, J., & Wilson, L. R. (1986). Detecting compartmental syndrome using continuous pressure monitoring. *Focus on Critical Care, 13*(5), 51-56.

64. Heppenstall, R. B., Sapega, A. A., Izant, T., et al. (1989). Compartment syndrome: A quantitative study of high-energy phosphorous compounds using 31P-magnetic resonance spectroscopy. *Journal of Trauma, 29*(8), 1113-1119.

65. Mravie, P. J., & Massey, D. M. (1992). Compartment syndrome. *Journal of Vascular Nursing, 10*(1), 9-12.

Cardiac Surgery

Susan L. Stewart

Cynthia O'Sullivan

Joan Vitello-Cicciu

Mary-Michael Brown

During the last two decades, a great many cardiac surgical procedures, both reparative and reconstructive, have been evaluated. Specific operations for valvular heart disease are discussed in Chapter 24. This chapter is devoted to coronary artery bypass graft (CABG) surgery and to a brief discussion of surgery for septal defects that the critical care nurse may encounter in adult patients.

CORONARY ARTERY BYPASS SURGERY

Coronary artery bypass graft (CABG) surgery evolved when cardiac catheterization enabled physicians to evaluate coronary anatomical abnormalities. In addition, cardiac catheterization for the first time allowed surgeons to evaluate the effects of surgical procedures.[1] Before the advent of cardiac catheterization, numerous operative interventions, such as thoracic sympathectomy, epicardial abrasion, and placement of vascularized pedicles on the surface of the heart, were attempted from 1900 to 1960. None of these procedures was shown to provide sustained benefit, and they were often associated with a high operative mortality. The first successful surgery for coronary artery disease is usually credited to Rene Favalaro and his associates. In 1967, Favalaro's group used saphenous vein grafts to bypass obstructed coronary vessels and thus successfully revascularized ischemic myocardium. Since that time, CABG surgery has become one of the most commonly performed operations in the United States. More than 350,000 such procedures have been performed in the United States annually since 1988.[2]

In concept, the procedure for coronary artery bypass surgery is a relatively straightforward technique. A conduit of the patient's tissue is connected to the aorta and anastomosed to the coronary artery distal to the site of blockage. Unlike medical therapy, which generally attempts to reduce myocardial oxygen demands, CABG surgery increases blood flow to the myocardium thereby improving MVo_2, but it is not a cure for the underlying atherosclerotic disease process. The major goals of CABG surgery are to relieve symptoms, prolong survival, and improve the quality of life. However, much controversy exists concerning the degree to which surgical coronary revascularization actually achieves these goals. This is especially true with continued improvements in pharmacological therapy and medical alternatives. Nonetheless, sophisticated surgical techniques, generally low operative mortality, and data demonstrating improvement in patient symptoms and longevity have established surgical coronary revascularization as an acceptable, and in some cases preferred, treatment for certain patients with coronary artery disease.

Indications

The criteria used to select patients for surgical myocardial revascularization are the subject of continued debate. Patients are generally carefully chosen on the basis of certain clinical, coronary arteriographic, and hemodynamic data. Improvement in longevity and relief of symptoms are the ultimate goals of surgical intervention.

Longevity Improvement

For most patients the major issue concerning the treatment of coronary artery disease is longevity. Statistics regarding the effects of CABG surgery on survival are especially meaningful to patients without severe chronic angina who fear a possible premature death.

In an attempt to identify objective criteria for coronary revascularization, several studies have described the long-term survival of patients with certain anatomical coronary lesions managed surgically or medically. In general, a stenosis of greater than 70% to 75% of the arterial lumen is considered significant,[3] and lesions in the more proximal portions of the coronary arteries are considered more lethal than distal blockages because they jeopardize larger areas of myocardium. Probably the most straightforward, undisputed indication for coronary artery bypass surgery is arteriographic documentation of left main coronary artery stenosis greater than 50%, regardless of symptoms. Numerous investigations, including the V. A. Cooperative Study[4] and the large European Coronary Study Group,[5] have shown a significant increase in longevity when these patients are managed surgically rather than medically. These same studies, along with the Coronary Artery Surgery Study (CASS),[3] documented that patients with triple-vessel coronary artery disease (CAD) and decreased ejection fractions who undergo CABG surgery have significantly improved survival rates at 5 years as compared to patients treated medically. The indications for surgery in patients with triple-vessel disease and normal left ventricular function have been less clearly delineated. Although the European Study (1980) found an improved 5-year survival when these patients were managed surgically, the CASS study (1983) found no difference in 5-year survival of patients in this group managed medically or surgically. The CASS study (1983) demonstrated no difference in longevity in patients with double- or single-vessel disease managed with medicine or surgery. However, the CASS 10-year follow-up study revealed two subgroups of patients with mild to moderate angina with or without a recent myocardial infarction (MI) who should have a clear surgical advantage: patients with proximal left anterior descending (LAD) disease greater than or equal to 70% with less than a 50% ejection fraction (EF), and patients with triple-vessel CAD with less than 50% EF.[3] The European Study found a better survival curve in patients with double-vessel disease that involved the proximal left anterior descending coronary artery who were treated surgically rather than medically.

Symptom Relief

The most frequently cited indication for surgical intervention is disabling angina that is unrelieved by medical management.[6,7] Numerous studies have documented the superiority of surgical treatment over medical therapy in reducing symptoms.[7,8] Angina is abolished in 60% to 70% of patients, and 90% to 95% of patients have some symptomatic improvement following CABG surgery.[7,9] Although interrup-

tion of nerve fibers, intraoperative infarction of isochemic myocardium, and a placebo effect have all been postulated as contributing to the reduction in symptoms, thallium perfusion scanning has demonstrated that a majority of patients with improvement in symptoms exhibit increased myocardial blood flow following CABG surgery.[10] Selection of patients based on symptoms is open to much variation, however. The amount of angina that is disabling is extremely subjective and dependent on the patient's lifestyle. Further, medical management may not be maximal because of patient noncompliance or differences in physician protocols. Despite these discrepancies, severity of symptoms is an important surgical consideration.

Chronic Stable Angina

In patients with chronic stable angina who are at increased risk due to the extent of their coronary disease and left ventricular dysfunction, older age, and associated disease states (both cardiac and noncardiac), CABG surgery may prolong survival when compared to medical therapy alone.[6,7] Operative mortality has also declined substantially. For patients at low risk, medical therapy is warranted initially, followed by surgery if symptoms worsen or ischemia increases.[6,7]

Unstable Angina

A related indication for coronary revascularization is unstable angina. Patients with angina of new onset that progresses rapidly in intensity and severity, patients with sudden acceleration of previously stable angina, or patients with pain at rest are considered to have unstable angina.[7,11] Patients who develop angina 1 week to 3 months after an acute myocardial infarction are also considered to be in this group. Although hospitalization and aggressive medical management (including intraaortic balloon counterpulsation) are the initial treatments of choice for patients with unstable angina, urgent catheterization and surgery are indicated when angina or signs of ischemia persist.[7,11,12] Studies have documented low operative mortality and significant relief of symptoms when this group is treated with surgical intervention,[7] although operative mortality has been reported at approximately twice that of patients with stable angina preoperatively.[13]

Other Indications

Medical intervention is the usual treatment of choice in the patient with an uncomplicated MI,[6] but for patients with postinfarction angina, CABG surgery is advocated within 30 days of the MI.[14] Coronary revascularization in patients with evolving myocardial infarction has been attempted at some institutions in an effort to limit infarct size and preserve left ventricular function. The most beneficial results are achieved in patients with subendocardial rather than transmural infarcts, and occur when revascularization is accomplished within the first 6 hours of symptoms.[15] However, the high operative mortality associated with this group of surgical candidates must be weighed against the ease of administration, availability, and success of thrombolytic techniques.[11] Current data suggest that urgent operation is indicated for the postmyocardial infarction patient who develops significant congestive heart failure from acute rupture of the ventricular septum or papillary muscle,[7,16] and for patients who develop symptoms such as congestive heart failure, angina, or systemic emboli from a left ventricular aneurysm.[17] When percutaneous transluminal coronary angioplasty (PTCA) results in coronary dissection, emergency CABG surgery is indicated. However, this complication is associated with a significantly greater risk of operative death and perioperative infarction than elective CABG.[18]

Risks

Operative mortality of 1% or less has been reported in the majority of patients undergoing CABG surgery.[19] Certain factors, however, have been associated with significantly higher surgical mortalities and include left ventricular dysfunction, emergency operation, increasing age, female sex, hemodynamic instability, associated mitral valve incompetence, the number of diseased vessels, and incomplete revascularization.[19]

Before the development of hypothermic cardioplegia, severe left ventricular dysfunction was considered a contraindication to CABG surgery.[1] With recent improvements in myocardial preservation, studies have documented a significant reduction in operative mortality and improvement in symptoms in some patients with ejection fractions as low as 20%. In particular, patients with ventricular dysfunction whose primary symptom is angina may have ischemia with a viable myocardium. These patients have been shown to benefit significantly from surgical revascularization.[3] However, when low ejection fractions are associated with chronic congestive heart failure (in the absence of a ventricular aneurysm), CABG surgery may not be beneficial.[20] Preoperative congestive heart failure was identified as the factor associated with the greatest operative mortality in patients undergoing CABG surgery at Cleveland Clinic from 1980 to 1982.[20]

Emergency operation, incomplete revascularization at the time of surgery, and an abnormal preoperative electrocardiogram have been associated with high operative mortality. Further, women in this study had a significantly higher operative risk than men (1.9% versus 0.7%), which is thought to be related to smaller vessel size in females.[20] Women generally tend to have a higher operative risk, which may be related to patterns of later surgical referral during the course of their disease process than occurs in men.[21]

Surgical treatment of coronary artery disease in the elderly is becoming increasingly acceptable. As the U.S. population has aged, the mean age of the CABG surgical patient has increased. Reports have indicated that patients in their seventh and eighth decade have undergone surgical coronary revascularization with relatively low operative mortality (2%), increased long-term survival, and reduction in angina.[22,23] Therefore, age per se does not appear to be a contraindication for surgery. However, investigators have documented a high incidence of neurological complications and/or behavioral changes following CABG surgery in patients over the age of 70.[24] Therefore, the presence of cerebrovascular disease or significant carotid artery stenosis may present especially great risk in the elderly CABG patient.

Patients with diffuse narrowing of the coronary vessels, poor distal runoff, and significant obstructions in intramyocardial vessels have been described as poor surgical candidates.[7] All these factors have been associated with reduced graft flow and possible subsequent graft closure. However, studies indicate that coronary revascularization is being successfully performed on patients with more diffuse coronary atherosclerosis.[25] The long-term result of surgical intervention in these patients is yet to be documented.

Although not a contraindication, obesity has been linked with an increase in complications following CABG surgery including leg and sternal wound problems, dysrhythmias, extended cardiopulmonary bypass time, difficulty in weaning from mechanical ventilation, and perioperative MI. In addition, recurrent angina and further weight gain postoperatively are not uncommon.[26]

Obviously, the decision regarding surgical intervention in coronary artery disease must be individualized. Numerous factors concerning the patient's clinical, physiological, and psychological state must be considered. Potential benefits of surgery are carefully weighed against operative risk.

Choice of Conduits

A variety of conduits have been used in coronary revascularization, including the radial and splenic arteries and the cephalic and basilic veins, but the material now in most common use is the saphenous vein from the leg, or the internal thoracic artery (ITA). Although the ITA has been associated with longer operative, aorta cross-clamp, and cardiopulmonary bypass times and increased chest tube drainage during the immediate postoperative period, no appreciable increases in operative morbidity, as compared to the saphenous vein graft (SVG), have been reported.[27] The ITA has also been used successfully in patients greater than 70 years.[28] Bilateral ITA grafts have not been associated with an increased incidence of sternal wound problems in nondiabetic patients as compared to single ITA grafts or SVGs.[29] Coronary revascularization using the greater saphenous vein still has many advantages, including expendability, ease of procurement, usual proportionate size, adequate length, and relative durability under arterial pressures. Because it can be harvested and inserted quickly, it is often used as a conduit following failed PTCA and for acute ischemia with left main disease.[30]

With the vein graft in reverse position so that the venous valves do not obstruct blood flow, one end is sutured to a small opening made in the ascending aorta, and the other end is attached to an opening in the coronary artery distal to the atherosclerotic obstruction (Figure 26-1). In this manner, a new conduit for blood flow is established between the aorta and the ischemic myocardium. The "sequential" or "jump" graft is an increasingly popular variation of this "single bypass" procedure. In this technique, a single vein graft segment is attached to more than one coronary artery (Figure 26-2). The vein graft has one attachment to the aorta but bypasses more than one diseased vessel. The advantages of this procedure include increased distal runoff, fewer proximal anastomoses per bypass graft, and better utilization of

available vein length.[31] So far, equivalent patency rates have been reported for single and sequential grafts, but theoretically, sequential grafts may increase long-term patency by establishing a higher rate of flow through the proximal portions of the graft.[25] However, possible kinking of this longer-type graft is a danger, and a proximal occlusion jeopardizes more than one coronary bypass location.[31]

The most frequently used alternative to the aortocoronary saphenous vein bypass is the internal mammary artery (IMA) graft. This procedure involves dissecting the internal thoracic artery (ITA), ligating it from the chest wall, and anastomosing its end to the coronary artery. Blood flow to the ischemic myocardium is thus established via the normal internal mammary artery circulation (Figure 26-3). This technique has gained renewed interest because of studies[32,33] demonstrating higher long-term patency of IMA grafts (88.5% at 1 year; 84.1% at 10 years) compared to saphenous vein grafts (76% patency at 1 year; 52% at 10 years). According to one study, 50% of all coronary revascularization procedures performed involve the use of IMA grafts.[20] Other advantages cited by proponents of the IMA graft include the need for only one anastomosis, less size disparity between graft and coronary artery, and the avoidance of a leg incision.[1] However, the internal mammary artery can be used only to vascularize vessels on the anterior surface of the heart. It requires extensive dissection and a longer operating time,[1] and has been associated with a slightly increased incidence of postoperative bleeding and pulmonary as well as wound complications.[27]

Another arterial conduit that has been receiving renewed interest for use with CABG surgery is the

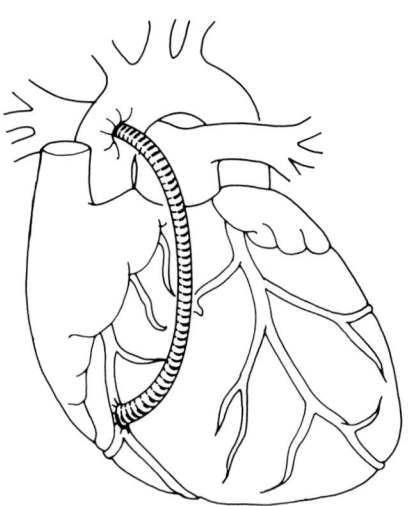

Figure 26-1 Aortocoronary artery saphenous vein bypass graft.

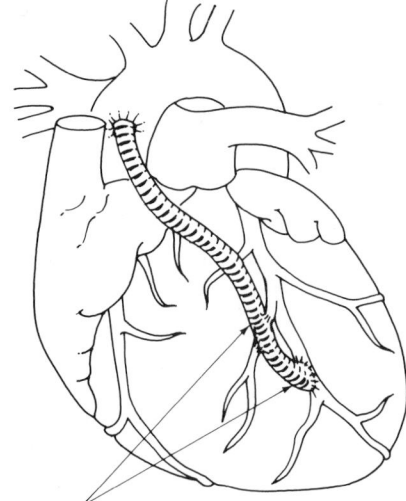

One saphenous vein, two anastamoses

Figure 26-2 Aortocoronary artery saphenous vein "sequential" bypass graft.

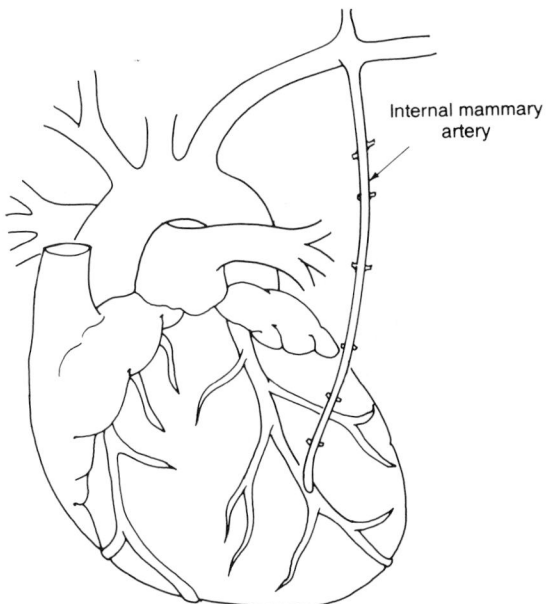

Internal mammary
artery

Figure 26-3   Internal mammary artery coronary artery
bypass graft.

gastroepiploic artery (GEA). Although long-term results are not available, it does not appear to be affected by atherosclerotic changes.[34] Other advantages
are that it may be harvested at the same time as the
ITA and SVG,[35] and may help avoid the use of bilateral ITA, which has been associated with sternal
wound complications in diabetic patients.[36] It is often
used as a free graft but may also be used in situ
(although the latter method limits its availability for
various lesions), both with very good results.[37,38]

Although only preliminary results are available,
successful grafting using a nonbiological polytetrafluoroethylene (PTFE) graft, especially during active
infarction and ischemia, has been reported.[39] Also,
the bovine ITA graft has been used experimentally.[40]
Both of these methods show promise for use in patients who have severe varicose veins and unsuitable
or previously utilized internal thoracic arteries, or for
emergency operations.[39,40]

A troublesome problem during CABG surgery is
the coronary artery with multiple obstructions, or a
stenosis that is inaccessible on the surface of the heart.
In an attempt to provide more complete myocardial
revascularization, the use of intraoperative transluminal coronary angioplasty in the operating room is
presently being attempted. Some studies suggest that
selective intraoperative angioplasty may be an adjunct
to effective coronary revascularization.[41,42] Efforts are
also under way to investigate the removal of focal
coronary atherosclerotic obstructions by carbon
dioxide and argon, and excimer laser. Data from current studies show promise that laser therapy during
cardiac surgery may ablate coronary artery lesions.[43,44] The future may hold exciting advancements
in myocardial revascularization techniques.

Procedure

Coronary artery bypass surgery is most commonly
performed via a median sternotomy incision. Cardiopulmonary bypass (CPBP) is used to arrest the heart
during the most technically difficult part of the surgery, the anastomosis of the bypass grafts to the coronary arteries. Patients are routinely monitored
throughout the procedure with an arterial line, pulmonary artery catheter, continuous electrocardiogram, and urinary catheter placed prior to surgery.
After CPBP is discontinued, atrial and, frequently,
ventricular epicardial pacing wires are placed on the
anterior heart and tunneled through the chest wall
where they are sutured to the skin. The wires are then
accessible for use in cardiac pacing and electrocardiography. Prior to closure of the incision, mediastinal chest tubes are routinely placed within the pericardium and beneath the sternum (although the exact
placement may vary). A pleural chest tube is usually
needed after an internal mammary bypass graft. The
chest tubes evacuate air and drainage, and most important, aid in monitoring mediastinal bleeding and
preventing cardiac tamponade. Because of the length
of anesthesia and the frequently associated respiratory dysfunction, CABG patients routinely remain intubated for 12 or more hours following surgery.

Cardiopulmonary bypass is used almost exclusively in open cardiac operations and has a significant
impact on patient outcome. Nursing care of the coronary artery bypass patient requires an understanding
of the conduct of CPBP and its potential physiological
effects.

Cardiopulmonary Bypass

Cardiopulmonary bypass is a technique in which
blood is diverted away from the heart and lungs into
a machine (the heart–lung machine) that substitutes
for the ventilatory and pumping functions of these
organs. In 1953 Gibbon performed the first successful
cardiac operation in which the patient was totally
supported by CPBP.[45] Until this time, heart surgery
was limited to closed, quickly performed procedures
such as valve commissurotomy. The introduction of
cardiopulmonary bypass made it possible to repair
intracardiac defects under direct vision.

CPBP has been used to sustain patients (especially
newborn infants) with severe but potentially reversible respiratory distress, and in patients undergoing
operations on the thoracic aorta. By far the most
common use of CPBP, however, is to perform the

function of the heart and lungs during cardiac surgery, and provide a motionless "empty" organ on which to carry out delicate surgical maneuvers.

The heart–lung machine drains blood from the heart, oxygenates it, and pumps it into the body. The perfusion apparatus consists of cannulas, reservoirs, pumps, filters, and an oxygenator.

Blood is diverted from entering the heart by a single catheter placed in the right atrium or by catheters placed separately in the inferior and superior vena cava.[45,46] An arterial cannula placed in the ascending aorta (or less commonly in the femoral artery) directs blood from the heart–lung machine to the patient. A small catheter is inserted into the aortic root so that cardioplegia solution may be administered for myocardial preservation. In some cases a venting catheter may be passed into the left ventricle (directly or through the left atrium or pulmonary artery). The blood returning to the left heart during bypass via the thebesian veins and bronchial circulation can cause elevation of intraventricular pressure. Significant left ventricular distention is associated with a decrease in subendocardial blood flow and an increase in pulmonary vascular pressures, thus potentially contributing to postoperative cardiac and pulmonary dysfunction. Many surgeons do not routinely use the left ventricular venting catheter because of the danger of introducing air emboli with this device, and because of studies demonstrating the questionable necessity of this intervention.

Components of Bypass System

Reservoirs. A reservoir is used to collect venous blood from the patient. The height of this reservoir below the level of the right atrium determines the blood flow from the patient by gravity. A smaller reservoir chamber is used to collect blood suctioned from the operative field (cardiotomy suction reservoir). This blood is then returned to the CPBP circuitry and the patient. Another reservoir contains cardioplegia solution.

Pumps. Two types of CPBP circuit pumps are the (1) nonocclusive roller and (2) impeller centrifugal rotating cone. The arterial pump is used to propel blood through the system. The flow pattern produced is a flat, nonpulsatile waveform. This pulseless flow pattern is clearly a major deviation from normal physiological conditions. For many years extensive efforts focused on producing the normal physiological pulse contour during CPBP because it was believed that this would improve the distribution of blood flow and thus reduce postoperative organ dysfunction. Evidence suggests that pulsatile flow compared to non-pulsatile perfusion results in lower peripheral vascular resistance, increased oxygen uptake, and reduced lactate buildup.[46] Several studies have also demonstrated

increased urinary output and creatinine clearance during pulsatile perfusion, as well as lower renin and vasopressin levels. Pulsatile pumps, however, are more complex than roller pumps and, therefore, more difficult to operate. Further, pulsation through the CPBP circuit may damage blood cells by jet effects or may induce shearing of atherosclerotic plaques. At present, nonpulsatile flow is not thought to be associated with intolerable subsystem distortions during routine CPBP procedures. Therefore, roller pumps and nonpulsatile flow are used in essentially all cardiac surgical operations.[45,47]

Filters. Current methods of CPBP result in the production and release of numerous particulate, fat, and gaseous emboli. These can potentially adversely affect the performance of any organ subsystem. The use of blood filters within the CPBP circuit has resulted in major reductions in the quantity and size of emboli and reduced postoperative complications from this mechanism. It has been extensively documented that the greatest and most frequent source of emboli is generated from the cardiotomy suction system. Blood returning from this system, referred to as field aspirated blood, has been shown to contain calcium fragments, suture, fat, fibrin, and other debris. Filtration of the cardiotomy return blood is therefore viewed as essential. Blood filters may also be used within the arterial line of the CPBP circuit to further reduce air and particulate matter returning to the patient.

Oxygenators. Oxygenation of venous blood diverted from the patient's right atrium occurs in the oxygenator of the CPBP circuit. Two types of oxygenators (Figure 26-4) are presently used to perform the gas exchange function of the lungs. The *bubble oxygenator* accomplishes this oxygen interchange by bubbling oxygen through a vertical column of blood. Thus, a thin venous blood layer is in direct contact with finely dispersed gas bubbles. Concentration gradients cause oxygen to diffuse out of the bubble into the blood and carbon dioxide to diffuse from the blood to the bubble. In *membrane oxygenators*, blood and gas are not in direct contact but are separated by a semipermeable membrane. Oxygen diffuses from the gas compartment through the membrane into the blood compartment, and carbon dioxide diffuses in the opposite direction. This design most closely simulates the human lung. Controversy exists concerning the superiority of one type of oxygenator over the other.[45,46] Bubble oxygenators are the most simple to use. However, the direct blood–gas interface has been shown to cause more trauma to blood cells. Membrane oxygenators appear to cause less trauma to both formed and unformed blood elements, but these devices are more difficult and time-consuming to use. Several studies have shown that when bypass time is

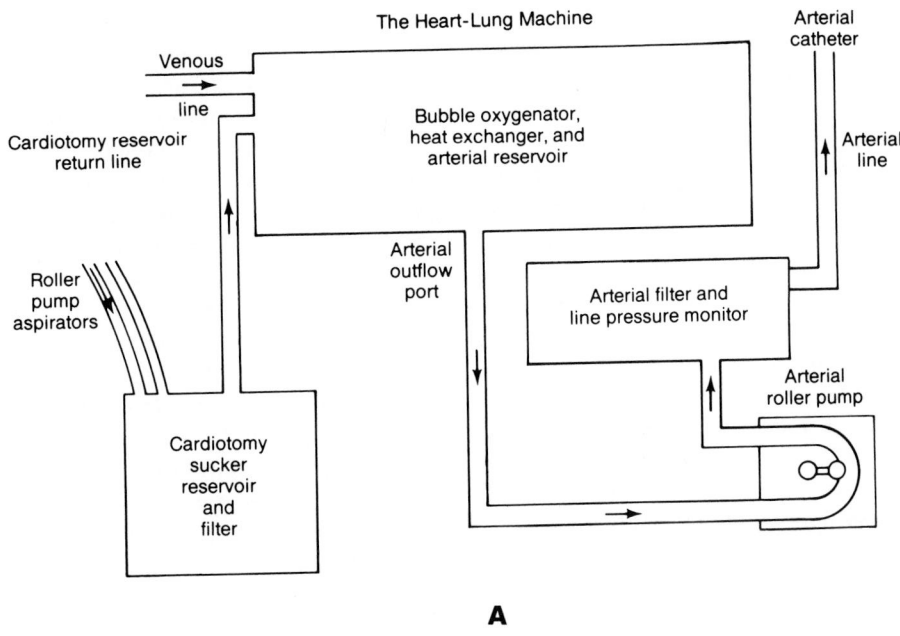

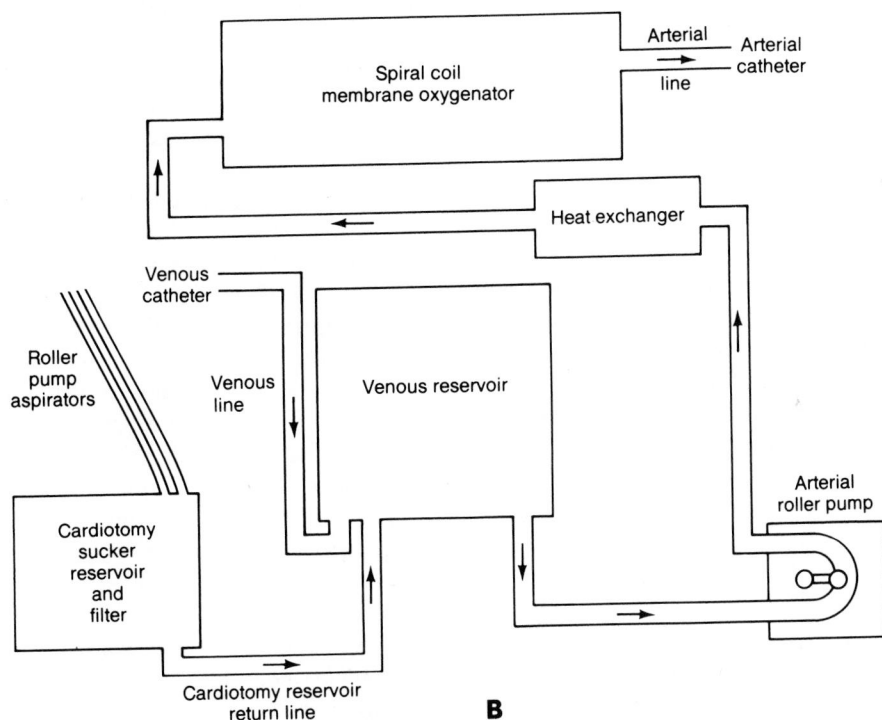

Figure 26-4 *A,* Diagram of CPBP setup with a bubble oxygenator. *B,* Diagram of a CPBP setup with a membrane oxygenator.

Modified from Edmunds, L., & Stephenson, L. (1991). Cardiopulmonary bypass for open heart surgery. In W. W. L. Glenn (Ed.), *Thoracic and cardiovascular surgery* (4th ed.). Norwalk, CT: Appleton & Lange.

less than 3 hours the amount of trauma to blood elements is not significantly different between bubble and membrane oxygenators.[45]

Adjunct Techniques. Despite improvements in equipment, the CPBP machine falls short of reproducing the normal functions of the heart and lungs. To circumvent this problem, several adjunct techniques are used to assure adequate total body perfusion and preservation of organ function during extracorporeal circulation. An explanation of these related factors is important in understanding the physiological effects of CPBP.

Hypothermia. A commonly employed adjunct to CPBP is the use of systemic hypothermia. Metabolic processes are slowed as body temperature is lowered. Hypothermia provides for a margin of safety and helps reduce the occurrence of oxygen debts during extracorporeal circulation. It has been demonstrated that the metabolic rate is reduced approximately 7% for each 1° C lowering of body temperature. Generally, hypothermia is induced by cooling the bloodstream via a heat exchanger located in the venous, or more commonly on the arterial, inflow side of the heart-lung machine. This "core cooling" is more effective than surface cooling because the organs with the best perfusion and highest oxygen requirements are cooled most rapidly and completely.[48]

The exact level of perfusion hypothermia employed varies with the specific requirements of the surgical procedure. Most commonly, temperatures of 15° to 20° C are suggested.[45] More profound hypothermia (as low as 18° C) has been used with total circulatory arrest in neonates and infants undergoing intracardiac repair of complex anomalies. Although hypothermia greatly reduces metabolic demands, it is not without untoward effects. The rise in blood viscosity that occurs when the body temperature is lowered may result in sluggish capillary and organ blood flow. Further, hypothermia causes oxygen to be more tightly bound to hemoglobin and therefore less available to the tissues. Rewarming of the patient is achieved by circulating warm water through the same heat exchanger. Although normal blood temperature is reestablished before CPBP is terminated, areas of the body that receive relatively low proportional blood flow may remain hypothermic. Body temperature may tend to drop in the first few hours after bypass as temperature throughout the body equilibrates.

Hemodilution. Before CPBP is initiated, the heart-lung machine must be filled with a priming solution to remove air from the circuit and to provide adequate volume to fill the bypass apparatus and augment the patient's vascular compartment. In the early days of cardiac surgery, large amounts of banked blood were used to prime the circuitry. At present, virtually all cardiac surgery is performed with the use of a nonblood priming solution. The use of colloid and crystalloid nonblood priming solution significantly reduces the patient's hematocrit (hemodilution). The optimal hematocrit during CPBP is controversial, but 20% is a commonly accepted level for patients less than 65 years old.[45] Although the patient's blood is maximally diluted at the onset of CPBP, the diluent tends to be lost from the perfusate, both in the interstitial space and the urine, as extracorporeal circulation continues.[46] Thus, the hematocrit tends to rise progressively throughout perfusion but usually remains low (30%) in the immediate postoperative period unless transfusions are given. Although the lowered hematocrit reduces the oxygen-carrying capacity of the blood, decreases colloidal osmotic pressure, and may contribute to interstitial edema, the numerous advantages of hemodilution outweigh these factors. Most notably, hemodilution lowers blood viscosity and vascular resistance, thus counteracting the deleterious effects of hypothermia and improving capillary blood flow.[46] Hemodilution also decreases trauma to blood cells, thus reducing hemolysis and platelet denaturation. Postoperative renal and pulmonary dysfunction have been shown to be lower when hemodilution rather than blood priming solution is used. A decrease in postoperative bleeding has also been cited with hemodilution.[48] Finally, the decreased demand on limited blood bank supplies, as well as the decreased risk of transfusion reaction, hepatitis, and HIV transmission give further support to the use of the hemodilution technique.

Heparin. Studies have shown indirect evidence that the Hageman factor (factor XII) is activated almost immediately after the start of CPBP by the massive contact of blood with nonbiological surfaces.[49] Heparin, therefore, is routinely administered immediately prior to and throughout the course of CPBP to inhibit factors V, IX, XI, XII, and thrombin. Because of the wide variation in individual responses to heparin, the activated clotting time (ACT) is measured frequently during bypass to guide heparin administration. Heparin must be neutralized by protamine at the termination of CPBP, prior to closure of the chest, to assure adequate hemostasis.

Blood Flow. The goal of CPBP is to maintain near-normal cardiac output while the patient is being supported. Theoretically, perfusion rates should equal the basal conditions in adults, calculated as a cardiac index of 3 L/min/m² with an oxygen uptake of 125 ml/min/m². However, factors such as cannula size, intravascular volume changes, and altered venous return make the maintenance of these blood flow rates somewhat difficult throughout extracorporeal perfusion. Such high flows would also considerably increase blood trauma.[46] Data indicate that the basic flow rate of 2.0 to 2.4 L/min/m² ensures acceptable perfusion during CPBP.[45,49] Although oxygen-carrying capacity of blood is reduced by hemodilution, total body oxygen consumption is lowered by hypothermia; therefore, the body's metabolic demands can be met at these lowered perfusion rates.

With the start of CPBP, perfusion pressure tends to fall sharply but after a brief period begins to rise. Perfusion pressures generally stabilize between 55 to 75 torr.[45] At flow rates of 2.4 L/min/m² and with the use of hypothermia and hemodilution as described, the mean arterial pressure level is usually well tolerated. Research data suggest that sustained mean perfusion pressures below 50 mmHg are associated with higher complication rates (especially cerebral complications).[45,46] Lower perfusion pressures may have especially untoward consequences in patients with high resistance atherosclerotic obstructions (common in the elderly). However, high pressures must also be avoided. Mean arterial pressures greater than 90 to 100 mmHg may increase the incidence of intracerebral bleeding in the heparinized patient. Mean arterial pressure during bypass is controlled between 60 to 80 mmHg with added volume or pharmacological agents as indicated. Experience has demonstrated that CPBP can be conducted safely at flow rates of 2.4 L/min/m², and with a mean arterial pressure of 55 to 70 mmHg up to 4 to 6 hours without major deleterious effects.[48]

Myocardial Preservation. Exclusion of the heart from circulation during CPBP provides a relatively bloodless field on which to perform delicate surgical procedures. However, extracorporeal circulation interrupts normal myocardial blood flow. Preservation of myocardial function during CPBP is crucial to the patient's survival after open heart surgery. Steps must be taken to preserve myocardial tissue and assure adequate cardiac function following the operative procedure. Specifically, interventions must be aimed at assuring a balance between myocardial oxygen demand and supply. Three techniques in particular have enjoyed widespread use: coronary perfusion, global ischemic arrest with topical cooling, and hypothermic cardioplegia.

One of the major advances in cardiac surgery was the development of hypothermic potassium cardioplegia in the 1970s. The best and most consistent myocardial preservation during CPBP has been achieved with this technique, which is currently the preferred technique of cardiac surgeons. The goals of chemical cardioplegia are to stop the heart safely and prevent significant myocardial damage. Although the exact composition of cardioplegic solutions varies, they all have some elements in common. Concentrations of potassium, magnesium, or procaine are used to cause immediate electromechanical asystole when infused through the coronary arteries into the myocardium. This immediate arrest has been shown to eliminate the large energy expenditures associated with ventricular contraction, thus maintaining the integrity of the myocardial cell membrane.[46] Use of cold solutions (around 4° C) lowers myocardial temperature and significantly reduces metabolic requirements, thus protecting against ischemic damage during interruption of coronary blood flow. The addition of blood and/or glucose to the cardioplegia solution assures some energy supplies to the myocardium at this time. Buffers are often added to the solution to optimize pH; calcium and steroids may be used for myocardial membrane stabilization; and osmolarity is controlled to minimize myocardial edema.

The conduct of CPBP with cardioplegic myocardial protection generally includes the following routines, although some variations are common. A loading heparin dose is administered. The aorta and right atria are cannulated. Flow through the CPBP circuit is established with concomitant lowering of body temperature. Following adequate systemic cooling (15° to 20° C), the aorta is cross-clamped. The cardioplegic cannula is inserted into the ascending aorta. At this point the heart is arrested and cooled by infusing cold cardioplegic solution (4° C) into the aortic root via the cardioplegic cannula. If aortic regurgitation is present, selective cannulation of the coronary ostia is used to assure delivery of cardioplegia. The perfusion of the previously described cardioplegic solution into the coronary arteries causes immediate electromechanical asystole. One or more thermistors are usually inserted into the left ventricle and myocardial temperatures are lowered to 15° to 20° C.[45]

Iced saline solution is instilled into the pericardial cavity to provide further myocardial cooling. At this point, with the heart arrested and a myocardial temperature of 15° C, the distal anastomoses of the coronary artery grafts are completed. Myocardial hypothermia is maintained throughout this part of surgery by intermittently infusing cardioplegia into the aortic root, and by injecting the solution into each new graft as the distal anastomoses are sutured.[46] When all distal anastomoses are completed, air is carefully evacuated from the heart, and the aorta is unclamped. The heat exchanger is set to begin rewarming the patient, and any proximal vein graft anastomoses are completed. In the majority of patients cardiac activity returns promptly, but ventricular fibrillation can be easily converted with direct defibrillation.

Once the patient is rewarmed, the CPBP cannulas

are removed, and protamine is given to reverse the effects of heparin. It is at this critical point that the heart resumes its normal workload and any ischemic damage is evident. Although use of hypothermic cardioplegia has been credited with significant reduction in operative mortality,[20] evidence suggests that a more subtle form of intraoperative myocardial damage may still occur.[50] Further research may elucidate more effective methods of assuring myocardial preservation during CPBP.

Physiological Effects of Cardiopulmonary Bypass. Patient responses to extracorporeal perfusion are extremely complex, and potentially involve all body functions. To care effectively for the CABG patient, the critical care nurse needs to understand the potential problems associated with cardiopulmonary bypass. A review of data from research reveals alterations in virtually all physiological subsystems following CPBP. Table 26-1 presents research findings regarding the effects of CPBP and the potential postoperative problems often associated with those effects. It is evident that care of the patient who has undergone extracorporeal perfusion constitutes a major challenge in the acute care setting.

Postoperative Considerations

Because of the potential effects of CPBP on all body systems, the postoperative CABG surgery patient offers a major challenge in the critical care setting. Potential problems commonly encountered in the postoperative phase are related to the operative procedures and the effects of CABP. This section highlights the most predominant concerns.

Several studies have documented a significant decrease in left ventricular ejection fraction and cardiac index in as many as 90% of patients 2 hours after CABG surgery.[51,52,53] Thus, transient left ventricular dysfunction may be common following coronary revascularization. The frequency of decreased cardiac output (CO) in the postoperative CABG patient makes it a problem of major importance. Many factors may adversely affect the performance of the heart following cardiac surgery. The most important include the extent of preoperative cardiac dysfunction,

TABLE 26-1   **Postoperative Effects of Cardiopulmonary Bypass in Patients Receiving CABG Surgery**

Effects of CPBP	Potential Problems
ENDOCRINE SYSTEM	
Catecholamine release	
Epinephrine 10 × baseline and norepinephrine 4 × baseline at 2-4 post-CPBP	Elevated systemic vascular resistance as much as 44.6% in 75% of post-CPBP patients
Elevated renin, angiotensin, and aldosterone levels	Hypertension occurs in 33% of post-CABG patients
Increase in antidiuretic hormone 30-40 × baseline during CPBP, returns to normal in 2-3 days	Excess sodium and water retention, and potassium excretion
Decreased ACTH levels and decreased cortisol response during CPBP	Danger of steroid inadequacy
Increased T_4 levels, decreased T_3 levels, and decreased TSH response	Danger of thyroid insufficiency
Elevated blood glucose levels and depressed insulin response	Ketoacidosis
	Hyperosmolar, hyperglycemic, nonketotic acidosis
ELECTROLYTES	
Dilution of serum potassium	Hypokalemia
Large potassium losses in the urine	Hypokalemia
Intracellular potassium shifts	Hypokalemia
Use of potassium cardioplegia	Hyperkalemia
Defective intracellular transport of glucose and potassium	Hyperkalemia
Dilution of serum sodium	Hyponatremia
Decreased urinary excretion of sodium, most marked on postoperative day 2	Hypernatremia
Dilution of serum calcium and intracellular calcium shifts	Hypocalcemia
Dilution of serum magnesium and intracellular magnesium shifts	Hypomagnesemia
Magnesium losses in the urine	Hypomagnesemia

Adapted from Stewart, S. (1985). The physiologic effects and nursing implications of cardiopulmonary bypass. Unpublished master's thesis, Boston University, Boston.

Effects of CPBP	Potential Problems
IMMUNE SYSTEM	
Exposure to multiple sources of pathogens	Lethal infections in general (pulmonary, mediastinal, urinary, blood) 1.1% of cardiac surgery patients die from postoperative infections
Decreased complement and immunoglobulin levels for up to 1 week	
Suppression of the reticuloendothelial system	Mediastinitis occurs in 1.5% of cardiac surgical patients
Impaired phagocytosis and function of leukocytes	A total body inflammatory reaction (?) "post-perfusion syndrome"
Release of complement anaphylotoxins	
COAGULATION SYSTEM	
Dilution, absorption, and destruction of coagulation factors in the CPBP circuit	Life-threatening hemorrhage occurs in 5% to 25% of post-CPBP patients
Heparin rebound after neutralization with protamine	
Platelet counts reduced by 30% and platelet function impaired for 3-5 days	
THE HEART	
Emboli, inadequate perfusion, inadequate myocardial cooling, and ventricular fibrillation may all contribute to myocardial ischemia and/or necrosis	Reported incidence of perioperative myocardial infarction varies from 5% to 20%
	Release of capillary damaging enzymes, lowered colloid osmotic pressure, high coronary perfusion pressures, and distention of the left ventricle contribute to myocardial edema
	Reperfusion injury (mechanism poorly understood)
Low postoperative cardiac output; up to 90% of patients show a decrease in ejection fraction 2 hours post-CPBP	
RENAL SYSTEM	
Decreased renal blood flow and decreased glomerular filtration rate	Oliguric renal failure found to occur in 1.5% of post-CPBP patients
Microemboli to renal vasculature	
Damage to RBCs with release of hemoglobin	
FLUIDS	
Increased total body water	Total body hypervolemia
Increased extravascular fluid	Interstitial edema and possible organ dysfunction
Decreased intravascular volume	Intravascular hypovolemia
GASTROINTESTINAL SYSTEM	
Catecholamine release and "stress response"	Gastrointestinal bleeding
Coagulation defects	Incidence of less than 1%
Emboli to pancreatic vasculature	Acute pancreatitis
Complement activation	Incidence estimated at 1.6% with a mortality of 86%
Emboli to intestinal vasculature	Intestinal ischemia or infarction
Low perfusion state	
PULMONARY SYSTEM	
Complement activation, air and particulate emboli all contribute to alveolar–capillary membrane damage	Increased interstitial lung water
	Atelectasis
Hemodilution decreases colloid osmotic pressure and may contribute to interstitial pulmonary edema	Respiratory insufficiency
Minimal circulation to lung parenchyma during bypass may result in decreased surfactant production	
Alterations of ventilatory patterns during bypass (deflation, static inflation, or intermittent inflation) may contribute to atelectasis	
CENTRAL NERVOUS SYSTEM	
Cerebral particulate emboli (especially fat emboli) and air emboli	Stroke (occurs in approximately 2% of post-CPBP patients)
Alterations in cerebral blood flow (especially with perfusion pressures less than 50 torr)	Transient motor deficits (occurs in approximately 0.3% of post-CPBP patients)
Systemic heparinization	Cerebral hemorrhage

the stress of the surgical intervention (anesthesia, CPBP, and surgical manipulation), and any uncorrected cardiovascular pathology.[53]

Cardiac Rhythm Disturbance

Heart rate and rhythm are important postoperative considerations in the management of CABG patients. Some postoperative cardiac rhythm disturbance (SVT) occurs in up to 30% cardiac surgery patients.[54] Supraventricular dysrhythmias, sinus bradycardia, sinus tachycardia, various degrees of heart block, junctional rhythms, AV dissociation, ventricular dysrhythmias, and transient bundle branch blocks have all been reported.[51,54,55] Several electrophysiological screening tests have been devised to identify patients at risk of developing postoperative dysrhythmias so that therapy can be directed appropriately. For example, Lowe and associates[56] used a low-amperage electric current to stimulate the right atrium intraoperatively and successfully identified those patients who then developed atrial fibrillation postoperatively. Because the development of dysrhythmias tends to extend the length of stay in the critical care unit, diagnostic methods such as this one may become routine in the future.[56]

Epicardial pacing wires are frequently used for the recognition and treatment of rhythm disturbances and to augment cardiac output in the postoperative cardiac surgery patient. Prior to closure of the sternum, pacing wires are commonly loosely sutured to the right atrial epicardium. Sometimes ventricular wires are attached as well. These wires are then tunneled out through the anterior chest wall in the soft tissue below the sternum. In the event of a slow rhythm or heart block that compromises hemodynamics, the wires can be connected to a pacemaker generator for cardiac pacing. Pacing the heart at a rate slightly faster than the patient's spontaneous rate may also suppress atrial or ventricular ectopic beats and augment cardiac output. Further, atrial tachydysrhythmias or recurrent ventricular tachydysrhythmias can frequently be terminated by overdrive pacing. The use of epicardial pacing wires was examined in a prospective study and found to be needed most in older patients, patients who had sustained a recent MI, and those who had received postoperative diuretics.[57]

Atrial pacing wires are also useful in distinguishing supraventricular from ventricular dysrhythmias. Tracings that reveal enhanced atrial activity can be obtained by an atrial electrogram (AEG). A unipolar atrial electrogram requires only one atrial pacing wire and records both atrial and ventricular activity. The bipolar AEG usually records only atrial activity and requires two atrial pacing wires. The AEG provides a quick and safe method for interpreting dysrhythmia

such as atrial fibrillation, atrial flutter (Figure 26-5), and premature atrial and ventricular contractions in the postoperative CABG surgery patient. See Chapter 21 for further discussion.

Stroke Volume Alterations

In addition to heart rate and rhythm, stroke volume is another important postoperative determinant of cardiac output. Optimizing stroke volume requires management of its three determinants: preload, afterload, and contractility.

Preload. The postoperative CABG patient may experience alterations in *preload* for numerous reasons. The most obvious of these is fluid loss, which often occurs from postoperative bleeding or urinary diuresis.

Studies indicate that post-CBPB urinary diuresis may be brisk, especially when dilute hyperosmolar priming solutions are used during the pump run.[58] Further, despite obvious postoperative interstitial edema, many cardiac surgery patients exhibit a decrease in intravascular volume for several days after the operation.

The profound vasoconstriction following CPBP and frequently documented low preoperative blood volumes in patients with coronary artery disease may result in significant hypovolemia in these patients as rewarming and vasodilation occur in postoperative period. Some mediastinal bleeding following cardiac surgery is expected. However, chest tube drainage greater than 2 ml/kg/hr, 2 or more hours following surgery, is usually considered abnormal.[55] Coagulation abnormalities may occur from numerous effects of CPBP. These must be identified and treatment aimed at the specific defect. Mediastinal bleeding may be treated with autologous blood (autotransfusion) or banked blood according to practitioner preference. The Transfusion Practice Committee of the American Association of Blood Bank recommends the following transfusion support in patients undergoing coronary artery bypass grafting:[59]

1. Institutions with CABG programs should establish a multidisciplinary approach to use a combination of interventions aimed at minimizing homologous blood exposure.
2. The practice of prophylactically infusing plasma and platelets is of no benefit and should not be used because of the increased risk to the patient.
3. Designated blood donations of first-degree relatives carry an associated risk of contributing to graft-versus-host disease and should not be used.
4. Crystalloid or colloid solutions do not carry the potential for transmission of infection and are therefore recommended for support of intravascular volume.

Bleeding into the pericardial space may also result

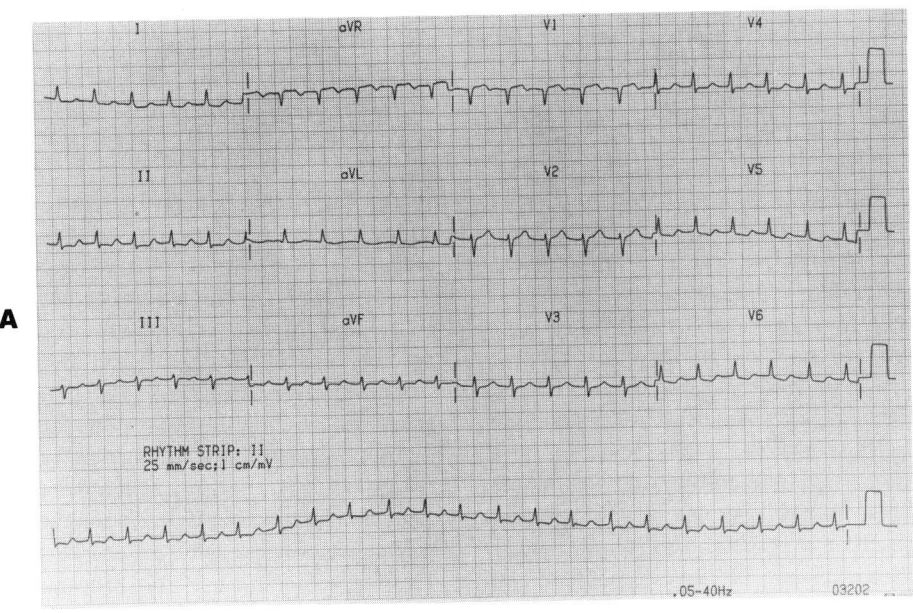

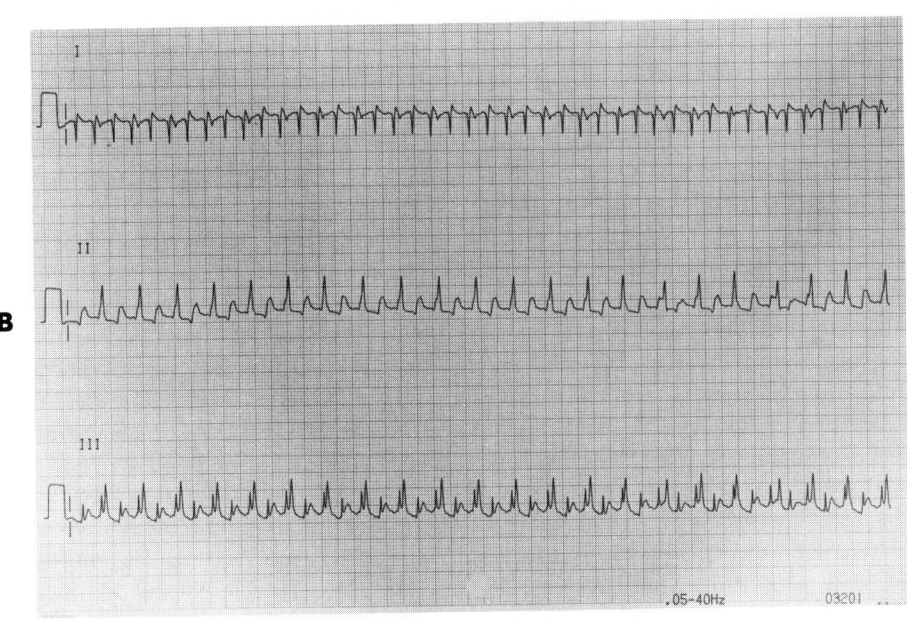

Figure 26-5 *A,* Conventional surface 12-lead ECG in a 59-year-old man (CABGx3) who was 10 hours postoperative.
B, Atrial electrogram obtained simultaneously with above surface ECG which revealed atrial flutter with 2:1 conduction
in bipolar lead (lead I) and unipolar leads (leads II and III).

in cardiac tamponade. The increased volume and
pressure within the pericardial space prevents adequate filling of the heart, reduces preload, and results
in significant reductions in cardiac output. Assessment and immediate intervention is necessary to avoid
life-threatening sequelae.

Afterload. Numerous factors predispose the post-
CABG patient to significant elevations in systemic
vascular resistance (SVR) and blood pressure, which
are clinical determinants of afterload. These factors
include the effects of CPBP, pain, agitation, shivering,

hypoxia, hypercarbia, and withdrawal of anithyper-
tensive medications. Studies have shown that in the
early postoperative period, hypertension has occurred
in 36% of patients following coronary artery bypass,
and the majority of postoperative cardiac surgery patients have exhibited a significant elevation in systemic vascular resistance.[60] Such increases in afterload
may critically intensify myocardial oxygen demands
and significantly reduce cardiac output. As well as
these effects on cardiac function, hypertension may
cause disruption of fresh suture lines (especially aor-

totomy or coronary anastomoses), or result in cerebral bleeding in patients with widespread atherosclerotic changes.

Contractility. Despite optimization of heart rate, preload, and afterload, numerous factors can adversely affect the postoperative cardiac inotropic state. These include advanced preoperative myocardial disease, the effects of CPBP, operative trauma, and incomplete surgical repair. Postoperative hypoxemia, severe acid–base or electrolyte imbalances, or negative inotropic drugs may further reduce myocardial contractility in the postoperative CABG patient. Finally, any impairment in myocardial contractility may be further exacerbated by an ischemic event. Despite present myocardial preservation techniques during CPBP, perioperative myocardial infarction is expected in the range of 2.5%.[11]

Respiratory Problems

Respiratory problems such as atelectasis constitute the most frequent complication after all types of thoracic and cardiac operations,[46] leading to impaired gas exchange.[57] Gas exchange is frequently impaired in the postoperative cardiac surgical patient for several reasons. As outlined under Cardiopulmonary Bypass, numerous effects of extracorporeal perfusion cause alveolar–capillary membrane injury, increasing the amount of interstitial lung water. In the presence of damaged alveolar capillary membranes, any elevations of left heart filling pressure (PAWP or LAP) may cause further extravasation of fluid and increased pulmonary interstitial fluid. These and other factors related to CPBP result in areas of atelectasis in the lung. Low postoperative hemoglobin levels related to hemodilution may contribute to impaired gas exchange by lowering the oxygen-carrying capacity of red blood cells. Further, anesthesia, sedation, pain, and immobility may lead to hypoventilation and further exacerbate atelectasis. All of these factors contribute to impairment in oxygen and carbon dioxide gas exchange in the postoperative CABG patient.

Neurological Problems

Another postoperative consideration is the incidence of stroke or transient motor deficits following CPBP, which has been reduced to 2% or less. A more frequently encountered problem has been behavioral changes following cardiac surgery which range from mild confusion to frank psychosis. Manifestations of delirium appear around 3 to 5 days after surgery.[61] The condition is first apparent when a patient makes an inappropriate remark or has a dramatic outburst. It is believed that factors contributing to the syndrome of delirium include advanced age, severe preoperative cardiac dysfunction, a history of psychiatric illness,

sleep deprivation, and prolonged intensive care unit stay.[61] Treatment for postoperative delirium consists of haloperidol or other sedatives. It has been noted that in the sleep-deprived patient, once sleep has been achieved, the delirium will resolve.[66]

Another neurological complication affecting cardiac surgery patients is brachial plexus injuries believed to be caused by excessive sternal retraction during surgery and manifested as ulnar or median neuropathy. Ulnar neuropathy is exhibited by numbness of the small finger and ring finger of the affected extremity. Median neuropathy is depicted as motor weakness to the muscles of the forearm and hand. The patient may first be made aware of this deficit by an inability to grasp a cup or utensil. Both of these neuropathies tend to occur on the third or fourth postoperative day with more left-sided involvement than right-sided.[62]

SEPTAL DEFECT SURGERY
Atrial Septal Defect

An atrial septal defect (ASD) is an abnormal opening that can occur almost anywhere in the atrial septum. An ASD usually causes left-to-right shunting of blood with eventual right ventricular volume overload, high pulmonary artery blood flow, and a murmur.

Adults in whom congenital ASD is diagnosed often present with effort intolerance, easy fatigability, recurrent respiratory infections, and supraventricular dysrhythmias.[63] Echocardiography, cardiac catheterization, and cineangiography verify the presence of an ASD. Mitral and tricuspic valve incompetence may accompany an ASD as may systemic arterial hypertension.

The size and location of the ASD dictate the type closure. Cardiopulmonary bypass is instituted, and a simple continuous suture technique is used for a small ASD, whereas a large ASD may require a Dacron or pericardial patch.

Postoperatively, nursing care includes usual nursing measures employed with cardiac surgical patients, and assessment for development of a new murmur, abnormally high mixed venous oxygen levels, and atrial dysrhythmias. Most patients receive Coumadin on postoperative day 2 and for approximately 8 to 12 weeks to minimize thrombus formation and emboli. Those patients who develop atrial fibrillation receive Coumadin for life.[63] The hospital mortality for patients undergoing an ASD repair is close to zero.[63]

Ventricular Septal Defect

A ventricular septal defect (VSD) is an abnormal opening that can occur anywhere along the ventricular septum. In adult patients, a VSD is most often a rupture in the anterior or apical portion of the ventricular septum as a consequence of a myocardial infarction.[63] A new murmur in a patient who is hospitalized for a myocardial infarction must be investigated as a possible VSD.

The chest roentgenogram of a patient with a VSD reveals large pulmonary blood flow. The pulmonary artery catheter is used to determine if abnormally high pulmonary artery oxygen values are present, indicating left-to-right shunting of blood. Additional studies include cardiac catheterization to confirm the presence of a left-to-right shunt; coronary arteriography to determine which coronary arteries require grafting; and, if the patient's condition permits, left ventriculography to ascertain the number and location of defects.

Intraoperatively, a patch of pericardially lined Dacron is used to close the defect.[63] Any ventricular aneurysm is excised or repaired.

Postoperatively, the patient will undergo intraaortic balloon counterpulsation and will be at high risk for dysrhythmias and low cardiac output states. All other nursing measures described in the care of the pre- and postoperative cardiac surgical patient are warranted when caring for the patient with a VSD repair.

Morbidity and mortality are contingent on the patient's preoperative hemodynamic stability and on the timeliness of the repair. For stable patients, deferring surgery for 2 to 3 weeks is indicated, whereas in patients in cardiogenic shock, VSD repair is urgent.[63]

NURSING MANAGEMENT: PREOPERATIVE

Cardiac surgery involves the potential for alterations in all body systems. The extensiveness of the procedure and the implications of surgery on the heart may cause tremendous psychological stress for the patient as well. Although each patient's care must be planned individually, certain interventions are necessary for all patients in the preoperative phase.

First, the nurse should perform and document a complete nursing history using Gordon's or another framework and physical examination on admission. This will enable the nurse to obtain a baseline profile, determine any present abnormalities and potential changes, and formulate collaborative diagnoses as well as nursing diagnoses.

Second, the nurse should monitor for and document any clinical signs of compromised organ function preoperatively. In particular, this assessment should include the following data:

Neurological: Decreased LOC, neurological deficits, weakness, impaired verbal response

Cardiovascular: Heart rate and rhythm disturbances,

heart sounds, unequal blood pressure in both arms, decreased or absent peripheral pulses, edema, neck vein distention, and bruits

Respiratory: Breath sounds, tachypnea

Renal: Diminished urinary output

Gastrointestinal: Abdominal distention, absent bowel sounds

Immunological: Temperature, localized infections

The nurse should also ensure that all diagnostic tests are completed and any abnormalities reported to the surgeon, including ECG, chest x-ray, arterial blood gases, CBC, electrolytes, coagulation profile, BUN and creatinine, cardiac enzymes, liver profile, and urinalysis.

In addition, the nurse will need to monitor the patient's response to medical interventions aimed at minimizing postoperative complications. These may include treatment of preoperative edema, pulmonary hygiene, or electrolyte and other pharmacological interventions. The nurse must instruct the patient in effective deep breathing and coughing exercises, and leg exercises to prevent postoperative pneumonia and venous stasis.

Some anxiety concerning the operative procedure and postoperative recovery is a universal response to cardiac surgery. This anxiety may range from mild to extremely high. Again, each plan of care must be individual. One source of anxiety for the cardiac surgical patient is lack of knowledge concerning pre- and postoperative events. A possible intervention that deserves attention is to encourage the patient in the preoperative period to elicit the relaxation response. In an experimental study by Leserman and associates,[64] patients who practiced the relaxation response both before and after surgery had a reduction in psychologic tension. The authors also concluded that eliciting the relaxation response may reduce the incidence of supraventricular tachycardia (SVT), anger, and tension. Much of nursing's role is to educate the patient and family or significant others. In the past most of this teaching was done in the inpatient setting; however, the trend today is to provide some information on an outpatient basis, which has been found to be effective.[65]

After all these aforementioned interventions have been accomplished, a plan of care should be formulated. Because most patients and their families exhibit some degree of fear concerning the operative procedure, a universal nursing diagnosis pertaining to preoperative cardiac surgical patients and families is fear related to perceptions of surgery and inadequate knowledge of events surrounding surgery and postoperative course.

■ NURSING DIAGNOSIS

Patient and family fear, related to impending surgery and inadequate knowledge of events surrounding surgery and postoperative course.

OUTCOME STANDARD AND CRITERIA

Fear is reduced or absent as evidenced by:

- Ability to verbalize specific fears regarding coronary artery bypass surgery
- Demonstration of appropriate problem-solving techniques to alleviate fears
- Verbalization of adequate knowledge of surgical and postoperative events

NURSING INTERVENTIONS

- Assess patient's and family's previous experiences with major surgery, stress levels, coping mechanisms, fears, and support systems
- Assist patient and family in recognizing and acknowledging specific fears
- Design an individual teaching plan based on the patient's and family's knowledge of the operative procedure and events, and their readiness to learn
- Assist the patient and family in identifying signs that indicate increased fear, such as increased pulse, respirations and blood pressure, sweating, and changes in voice pitch or voice tremors
- Allow for continuity or consistency of nursing personnel to enhance trust and familiarity with nursing staff so as to minimize fears associated with unfamiliar environment
- Provide the patient and family with time to ask questions and follow through with accurate and realistic answers. Encourage the patient and family to verbalize their fears with specific questions, such as, "What worries do you have?"
- Offer realistic support and encouragement rather than vague comments, such as, "Everything will be okay."

NURSING MANAGEMENT: POSTOPERATIVE

Although the complex care of cardiac surgical patients involves a concerted team effort, the safety with which the patient can be conducted through the immediate postoperative phase is conditional upon the astute assessment and interventional skills of the critical care nurse.

Postoperative nursing care focuses on identifying actual and high-risk problems and preventing complications. Nursing interventions are based on an accurate, ongoing patient assessment as well as comprehensive nursing history and preoperative data base.

In the immediate postoperative phase, cardiac dysrhythmias or decreased cardiac output often result in decreased tissue perfusion. The critical care nurse should be concerned with preoperative myocardial function (especially pulmonary wedge pressure, ejection fraction, and cardiac index) as well as obtaining a detailed account of operative events in order to anticipate altered tissue perfusion.

■ NURSING DIAGNOSIS

Altered tissue perfusion, related to a decrease in cardiac output secondary to (1) cardiac dysrhythmias, (2) inappropriate preload status, (3) increased afterload, and/or (4) depressed myocardial contractility.

OUTCOME STANDARD AND CRITERIA

Tissue perfusion will improve as evidenced by:

- Normal sinus rhythm without any hemodynamically compromising dysrhythmias
- Cardiac index greater than 2.5 L/min/m², systolic BP greater than 90 mmHg, CVP and PAWP within patient's normal limits and absence of signs of hypovolemia, hemorrhage, hypervolemia, or cardiac tamponade
- Systolic BP less than 140 but greater than 90, diastolic BP less than 90 but greater than 60, calculated SVR less than 1,400 dyn/sec/cm⁵
- No clinical signs of hypotension, urinary output not less than 30 ml/hr, no signs of cool clammy skin, no diminished peripheral pulses, and warm, dry extremities with capillary refill less than 4 seconds

NURSING INTERVENTIONS

- Monitor the patient's ECG continuously with high and low alarms set and QRS volume on to detect any changes in heart rate or rhythm
- Document (with ECG) and report any changes in heart rate and/or rhythm and associated clinical response (BP, CI, peripheral pulses)
- Monitor for and report any factors that may contribute to dysrhythmias in the cardiac surgical patient, such as acidosis, alkalosis, hypoxia, hypokalemia, or hyperkalemia
- Institute measures to warm the postoperative hypothermic patient because a low core body temperature may contribute to bradydysrhythmias
- Administer pain medication, offer the patient explanations and reassurance, and provide the patient with comfortable positioning to minimize sympathetic stimulation and catecholamine outpouring which may contribute to dysrhythmias
- Be prepared to treat a hemodynamically compromising dysrhythmia immediately by having cardioverter/defibrillator readily available (for treating ventricular fibrillation, ventricular tachycardia, or SVT) and pharmacological agents on hand, especially atropine, for bradydysrhythmias
- Appropriately administer any ordered pharmacological treatment, monitoring the patient's response and untoward side effects. In particular, this may include:

  Lidocaine: Intravenous (IV) bolus at 1 mg/kg for ventricular dysrhythmias, then administer a continuous infusion at 1 to 4 mg/min, followed by an additional 0.5 mg/kg IV bolus 5 to 10 minutes after the initial dose if ectopy still present. IV bolus should not exceed 3 mg/kg

    Verapamil: 0.075 to 0.15 mg/kg IV over 2 to 3 minutes for SVT (up to 10 mg)

    Atropine: 0.5 mg IV repeat at 5-minute intervals. Total dose not to exceed 2.0 mg

    Adenosine: 6 mg rapid IV push and repeat 12 mg at 2-minute intervals two times, if needed, to convert or diagnose SVT

- Identify presence of atrial and/or ventricular temporary epicardial pacing wires and assure these are securely attached to external pulse generator with functioning batteries and with ordered settings
- Be prepared to initiate temporary pacing or change settings as directed by physician
- Document supraventricular dysrhythmias by atrial electrocardiogram
- Prevent microshock and associated dysrhythmias by covering any exposed pacing wires with rubber gloves, using only grounded electrical equipment in room, and avoiding contact with any electrical equipment and the patient simultaneously
- Monitor all hemodynamic and clinical parameters for signs of hypovolemia, which include low PAWP, PAP, and CVP; increased HR; decreased BP and CI; weak peripheral pulses; cool, pale skin; and fluid output greater than intake
- While the hypothermic patient is being warmed, monitor all the above parameters every 5 minutes and be prepared to administer volume replacement as the patient's temperature rises and the vascular bed dilates, producing a relative hypovolemia
- Monitor all hemodynamic and clinical parameters for signs associated with bleeding and hemorrhage, which include chest tube drainage greater than 2 ml/kg/hr, 2 or more hours following surgery; bloody oozing from incisions or catheter sites; hematuria; bloody nasogastric drainage; abnormal clotting studies; decreased hemoglobin and hematocrit values
- Be prepared to administer blood products, coagulation factors, or protamine sulfate appropriately as ordered
- Monitor all hemodynamic and clinical parameters for signs of hypervolemia, which may include increased PAWP, PAP, and CVP; crackles; peripheral edema; jugular venous distention; and fluid volume intake in excess of output
- Report any of the above signs of hypervolemia and administer pharmacological agents appropriately as ordered. These may include:

    Furosemide or other diuretic agents given to increase urinary output and decrease intravascular fluid volume and preload

    Nitroglycerin given by continuous intravenous infusion at rates up to 200 to 300 mg per minute to dilate the venous vascular bed and thus lower preload by decreasing venous return

- Position the hypervolemic patient in Fowler's position to aid in decreasing venous return
- Minimize fluid administration in the hypervolemic patient by concentrating intravenous medications in minimal fluid volume
- Monitor all hemodynamic and clinical parameters for signs of cardiac tamponade, which may include elevated and equalized CVP, PAD, LAP, and PAWP; decreased cardiac index; jugular venous distention; cool, clammy skin; diminished peripheral pulses; pulsus paradoxus; muffled heart sounds; sudden cessation of chest tube drainage
- Milk chest tubes every 15 to 30 minutes per physician order to maintain patency and prevent tamponade, but refrain from vigorous stripping of chest tubes, which may exacerbate bleeding problems because of high pressures produced by stripping[66]
- Monitor blood pressure continuously and immediately report a sustained systolic BP above 140 mmHg, or a mean arterial pressure above 90 mmHg
- Calculate systemic vascular resistance (SVR) every hour in the immediate postoperative period and report SVR greater than 1,400 dyn/sec/cm^5
- Monitor for clinical signs of peripheral vasoconstriction such as cool, pale, mottled extremities and sluggish capillary refill
- Administer pain medication and provide patient with comfortable positioning, reassurance, and emotional support to minimize catecholamine outpouring associated with discomfort and emotional stress which would further elevate SVR
- Institute measures to rewarm the hypothermic cardiac surgical patient with elevated SVR to decrease peripheral vasoconstriction. This may include warm blankets, blood warmers for transfusions, use of hypothermia blankets, or rewarming lights, and also increasing the temperature of the room
- Be prepared to administer afterload-reducing drugs appropriately. In particular, this may include sodium nitroprusside, a potent peripheral vasodilator administered via continuous intravenous infusion at a rate of 0.5 up to 8.0 μg/kg/min
- Monitor for and maintain optimum preload and afterload as outlined above to enhance cardiac contractility and decrease myocardial oxygen demands
- Monitor hemodynamic and clinical parameters for signs of impaired myocardial contractility, which may include CI less than 2.5 L/min/m^2; hypotension; tachycardia; crackles; cool, clammy skin;

weak peripheral pulses; low urine output; and lethargy or restlessness

- Monitor for signs of myocardial ischemia, which may include ST segment elevation or depression on ECG, elevated CK-MB isoenzymes, and patient complaints of angina-like chest pain
- Institute measures to reduce myocardial oxygen demands wherever possible. These may include providing for a quiet, restful environment; treating pain expediently; offering comfort measures and emotional support to the patient; and timing procedures and interventions to allow for periods of rest between events
- Discontinue rewarming interventions when the patient's temperature is within 1 to 2 degrees of normal (98.6° F) to prevent temperature elevation which further increases myocardial oxygen demands
- Expediently report and treat shivering, hypertension, tachycardia, and fever, which all increase myocardial oxygen demands
- Provide for optimal myocardial oxygen supply by monitoring for and reporting hypoxemia by arterial blood gases or hematocrit values less than 30, and expediently reporting and treating hypotension and hemodynamically compromising dysrhythmias
- Monitor for and report abnormalities that may further compromise myocardial contractility, such as acidosis or electrolyte imbalances
- Administer positive inotropic agents as ordered to enhance myocardial contractility and thus improve cardiac output. These may include:

  Dopamine: A chemical precursor of norepinephrine, given by continuous intravenous infusion. This drug acts on different receptors at varying infusion rates. Between 1 and 2 µg/kg/min exerts dopanergic effects and increases renal and mesenteric blood flow. Between 2 and 10 µg/kg/min stimulates β_2 receptors, thus enhancing myocardial contractility and heart rate. Over 10 µg/kg/min causes more alpha stimulating effects resulting in vasoconstriction, rise in BP, and increased afterload[64]

  Dobutamine: Direct beta-adrenergic receptor stimulator given by continuous infusion at rates of up to 10 µg/kg/min. Mainly enhances cardiac contractility with little vasoconstriction and less arrhythmogenesis than dopamine

- Administer intravenous nitroglycerin as ordered to optimize myocardial oxygen supply. Nitroglycerine has been shown to dilate coronary arteries, increase coronary collateral blood flow, and relax areas of coronary artery spasm. Thus, this drug may be effective in treating or preventing myocardial ischemia in the cardiac surgery patient

■ **NURSING DIAGNOSIS**

Impaired gas exchange, related to atelectasis.

OUTCOME STANDARD AND CRITERIA

Gas exchange is adequate as evidenced by:

- Patient's arterial blood gases show PO_2 greater than 60 with an O_2 saturation above 90%; PCO_2 between 35 to 45; and pH of 7.35 to 7.45
- Patient's respiratory rate is less than 20 with no use of accessory muscles
- Patient's breath sounds are not decreased in lung fields with no crackles, rhonchi, or wheezes
- Patient exhibits no cyanosis
- Sputum remains clear

NURSING INTERVENTIONS

- Monitor hemodynamic and clinical parameters for signs of hypoxia, which may include increased respiratory rate, use of accessory muscles of respiration, tachycardia, hypertension, confusion or restlessness, and low arterial PO_2
- Institute measures to mobilize and remove secretions as well as open closed alveoli. These include turning and positioning the patient every 2 hours, endotracheal suctioning as necessary followed by manual hyperinflation of the lungs, and head of bed elevated to promote diaphragmatic excursion
- Administer pain medication to decrease splinting and hypoventilation by the patient. Instruct the patient in use of a pillow or blanket to support the incisional area in order to increase comfort during deep breathing, coughing, and movement, and thus improve alveolar ventilation
- Monitor for signs of other complications which may further compromise gas exchange. These may include:

  Pulmonary edema: Crackles, elevated PAWP, elevated PAP, frothy pulmonary secretions

  Pneumothorax or hemothorax: Decreased or absent breath sounds, high peak inspiratory pressures, tracheal deviation

  Pulmonary embolus: Chest pain, hemoptysis, elevated PAP, cyanosis

  Gastric distention: Large, firm abdomen; absence of bowel sounds; diminished bilateral basilar breath sounds

- Follow extubation with use of incentive spirometry and deep breathing exercises every 1 to 2 hours
- Begin progressive patient ambulation as soon as possible postoperatively. This usually means getting the patient out of bed the day following surgery after removal of the endotracheal tube and pulmonary artery catheter

■ **NURSING DIAGNOSIS**

Patient anxiety, related to pain, feelings of helplessness, or lack of knowledge regarding the progress of events, routines, and/or equipment.

Anxiety is a common response to cardiac surgery. In the postoperative period, the patient is faced with numerous potential sources of emotional stress. The median sternotomy and leg incisions (CABG surgery), the presence of an endotracheal tube and chest tubes, and relative immobility because of equipment, are all obvious sources of discomfort. It is well accepted that pain (discomfort) and anxiety can create a vicious cycle. Pain produces anxiety, which intensifies the pain, which results in greater anxiety.

During the period of endotracheal intubation, the patient's difficulty with communication may heighten feelings of helplessness and anxiety. Dependency on machines and medical staff may intensify the patient's fears of permanent disability and death, which, along with lack of knowledge regarding the progress of events, routines, equipment, and normal feelings, may also contribute to emotional stress.[67]

Failure to alleviate or minimize anxiety may lead to adverse physiological sequelae. The outpouring of catecholamines owing to the stress response can result in tachycardia, hypertension, and peripheral vasoconstriction, all of which increase myocardial oxygen demands and may have untoward hemodynamic consequences in the patient with coronary artery disease.

OUTCOME STANDARD AND CRITERIA

Anxiety is reduced or absent as evidenced by:
- Verbalization of effective ways of dealing with anxiety
- Verbalization or demonstration of a decrease in anxiety as evidenced by decreased respiratory and heart rate, tremors, shakiness, voice or pitch changes
- Increased ability to deal with problems and to concentrate

NURSING INTERVENTIONS
- As the patient wakes up in the intensive care unit, the nurse should use a calm, controlled voice, offer frequent explanations, reorienting the patient to place, time, and events, including reminders that the operation is over
- Explain to patient why he or she is unable to talk (endotracheal tube in place). Take time to develop a mode for patient communication during intubation. This may include providing the patient with a writing pad and pen, or using lip reading, or having the patient form letters with his or her fingers. Assure patient that a nurse is always within sight, and establish a method for patient to signal need for nurse's attention
- Encourage the patient to communicate sources of discomfort and assess the patient continuously for nonverbal cues of pain. In general, this may include

facial grimacing, stiffness or reluctance in moving in bed, and splinting of body parts. Sympathetic nervous system responses are common when pain is of low or moderate intensity; pallor, tachycardia, increased BP, dilated pupils, increased respiratory rate, and skeletal muscle tension. When pain is more severe, parasympathetic responses may predominate: pallor, diminished heart rate, hypotension, nausea, vomiting, weakness, and prostration[55]
- Provide the patient with pain medication, antianxiety medications, comfortable positioning, and other comfort measures such as mouth care
- Encourage the patient to make some decisions in his or her care, even in the intensive care unit, to minimize feelings of loss of control and helplessness. This may be as simple as having the patient decide which side to turn to or how high to elevate the head of the bed
- Orally communicate signs of progress to the patient and inform him or her of the next step in recovery

■ NURSING DIAGNOSIS

Family anxiety, related to feelings of helplessness and lack of knowledge regarding the patient's condition and expected course of events.

The cardiac surgical patient is not an isolated individual, but the member of a family unit. The anxiety and stress of the surgical event are felt by the patient's significant others. The family is faced with the threat of loss of a loved one, feelings of helplessness in the intensive care environment, and lack of knowledge regarding the patient's condition and expected course of events. In recent years several studies have described the needs of relatives of the critically ill patient.[68,69,70] Rodgers' study looked specifically at needs of families of the cardiac surgery patient in the initial postoperative period.[69] Although the order of rank was slightly different, in the three studies, eight of the top ten ranked needs of families were identical. The box on p. 654 lists a compilation of the highest ranking needs.

The AACN's *Standards for Nursing Care of the Critically Ill* emphasizes that the nursing care of CABG patients must include assessment and intervention in family needs.[71]

OUTCOME STANDARD AND CRITERIA

Anxiety is absent or reduced as evidenced by:
- Verbalization of questions and concerns that contribute to the onset of anxiety
- Decrease in such behavioral symptoms such as difficulty expressing oneself, selective inattention, indecisiveness, restlessness, and irritability
- Verbalization of decreased anxiety

NURSING INTERVENTIONS
- Take time to elicit questions and concerns from family members. Offer the family honest, simple

---

The Highest Ranked Needs of Families of Critically Ill Patients

To feel there is hope

To feel that hospital personnel cared about the patient

To have my questions answered honestly

To know that I would be called at home for a change in the patient's condition

To have specific facts concerning the patient's progress

To know the patient's chances of recovery (prognosis)

To have explanations given that I could understand

To receive information about the patient's condition once a day

Compiled from Leske,[70] 1986; Rodgers,[69] 1983; Molter,[68] 1979.

---

explanations of events and equipment

- Encourage family members to address questions and concerns to physicians and reiterate the physician's explanations whenever necessary
- Offer the family members reassurance whenever possible. Make sure a phone number where the family can be reached is available at the patient's bedside
- Verbally communicate signs of the patient's progress to family members
- Assist the family in communicating with the patient utilizing the methods established above

ADDITIONAL NURSING CONSIDERATIONS

Numerous other potential clinical problems may apply to the cardiac surgical patient. Nursing care must focus on monitoring for and identifying any postoperative abnormality in neurological functioning. Further, interventions directed at reorienting the patient to time, place, and person; providing for periods of uninterrupted sleep; allowing time for family–patient interaction; and providing the patient with familiar objects, sights, and sounds (radio, pictures from home) may help to decrease the incidence of psychological complications in the postoperative period.

The incidence of infection following CPBP is a concern in the postoperative period. Meticulous handling of all invasive lines and incisions, as well as monitoring for signs of infection, are vital nursing interventions in the postoperative surgical patient. A discussion of sternal wound infection is beyond the scope of this chapter. The reader is referred to reference 72 for a detailed review of this subject.

The incidence of acute renal failure following CPBP is low. However, nursing care must include scrupulous monitoring of fluid intake and output, as well as monitoring of serum BUN and creatinine levels.

There are numerous sources of emboli during CPBP. The postoperative surgical patient must be carefully assessed for any evidence of such a complication.

Identification of postoperative ileus, return of bowel sounds, and effective gastric decompression are important collaborative considerations in the cardiac surgical patient. Additionally, consideration must be given to the patient with prior history of peptic ulcer disease. The administration of antacids may be needed in the postoperative phase for these patients. Another consideration is the changing population of cardiac surgical patients. Older, sicker, and second-time patients are being seen in critical care units following CABG surgery. The risks associated with a second bypass operation almost double those of a first bypass operation.[11] These patients also are at increased risk for many of the complications discussed in this chapter.

CARDIAC REHABILITATION

Medical, surgical, and nursing management of the cardiac surgical patient is incomplete without discussion of rehabilitation. Despite successful treatment or repair of the initial cardiac abnormality, many patients become unnecessarily incapacitated, do not return to work, and report depression and a poor quality of life.

Cardiac rehabilitation is defined as "the process of actively assisting the known cardiac patient to achieve and maintain his optimal state of health."[71] The ultimate goal is to enable the cardiac patient, largely by his or her own endeavors, to regain preillness capabilities or make adjustments necessary for an active, productive life. The key concept here is assisting the patient to function at the highest level compatible with his or her disease. To achieve this goal, rehabilitative efforts must be holistic in design and must involve a team approach that includes the patient himself or herself. The actual composition of the cardiac rehabilitation team varies widely from program to program, but an ideal list might include the following: cardiac patient and family, attending physician, primary nurse, cardiac rehabilitation clinical nurse specialist, cardiologist, physical therapist, occupational therapist, social worker, dietician, vocational rehabilitation counselor, chaplain, psychologist or psychiatric clinical nurse specialist, and pharmacist.

Although cardiac rehabilitation principles and techniques have largely developed from care of patients recovering from myocardial infarction, the approach can be applied successfully to patients recovering from surgical procedures such as CABG, septal repair, coronary angioplasty, valvular repair, or cardiac transplantation.

Cardiac rehabilitation programs are commonly divided into three phases. The two major components of these phases are progressive physical activity or exercise, and patient and family education and counseling. Each phase is characterized by slightly differing objectives.[72,73,74]

Phase 1: Hospitalization (7 to 10 days)
"Early or in-hospital phase"
Objectives: Minimize deleterious effects of bed rest and immobility, and provide education to adequately prepare patient for discharge.

Phase 2: Convalescence (6 to 10 weeks)
"Therapeutic or restorative phase"
Objectives: Cardiac conditioning or training to pre-event levels (e.g., MI), reinforcement of patient education, and psychological support.

Phase 3: Long-term (following completion of phase 2)
"Maintenance phase"
Objectives: Retention of previous training, and stimulation of further progress.

Discussion of a total cardiac rehabilitation program is beyond the scope of this text. However, the critical care nurse must have a basic understanding of concepts relating to phase 1 of rehabilitative care of the cardiac patient. To be most effective, rehabilitation efforts must begin at the time of admission. In particular, the critical care nurse can be invaluable in minimizing the untoward effects of bed rest, preventing deconditioning, and decreasing the patient's anxiety to promote learning and adaptation. Refer to references 73 through 75 for a more detailed discussion concerning cardiac rehabilitation.

REFERENCES

1. Chaux, A., & Matloff, J. M. (1990). A historical perspective of cardiac surgery. In R. J. Gray, & J. M. Matloff (Eds.), *Medical management of the cardiac patient*. Baltimore: Williams & Wilkins.

2. American Heart Association. (1991). *Heart and stroke facts*. Dallas: Author.

3. Chaitman, B. R., et al. (1990). Coronary Artery Surgery Study (CASS): Comparability of ten year survival in randomized and randomizable patients. *Journal of the American College of Cardiology, 16*(5), 1071-1078.

4. Takaro, T., Hullgren, H., & Lipton, M. (1976). The VA cooperative randomized study of surgery for coronary arterial occlusive disease: Part 2. Subgroup with significant left main lesions. *Circulation, 54*(Suppl III), III-107.

5. European Coronary Surgery Study Group. (1980). Prospective randomized study of coronary artery bypass surgery in stable angina pectoris. Second interim report by the coronary surgery study group. *Lancet, 2,* 491-495.

6. Gersh, B. J., et al. (1989). Coronary bypass surgery in chronic stable angina. *Circulation, 79*(Suppl.) I-46-I-59.

7. Matloff, J. M. (1990). Current indications for surgery. In R. J. Gray, & J. M. Matloff (Eds.), *Medical management of the cardiac surgical patient*. Baltimore: Williams & Wilkins.

8. Rahimtoola, S. (1981). Coronary artery bypass for chronic angina—1981: A perspective. *Circulation, 65,* 225-241.

9. Smith, H., Frye, R., & Piehler, J. (1983). Does coronary bypass surgery have a favorable influence on the quality of life? *Cardiovascular Clinics, 13* 253-264.

10. Ritchie, J., et al. (1977). Thallium-201 myocardial imaging before and after coronary revascularization: Assessment of regional myocardial blood flow and graft patency. *Circulation, 56,* 830-936.

11. ACC/AHA Task Force Report. (1991). Guidelines and indications for coronary artery bypass surgery. *Journal of the American College of Cardiology, 17*(3), 543-589.

12. Franki, W. C. (1990). A comparison of coronary artery bypass surgery and percutaneous transluminal coronary artery in treatment of coronary artery disease: Part 2. *Modern Concepts of Cardiovascular Disease, 59*(7), 37-42.

13. Kaiser, G. C. (1989). Myocardial revascularization for unstable angina pectoris. *Circulation, 79*(Suppl. 6), I-60-I-67.

14. Kouchoukos, N. T., et al. (1989). Coronary artery bypass grafting for postinfarction angina pectoris. *Circulation, 79*(Suppl. 6), I-68-I-72.

15. DeWood, M. A., et al. (1989). Medical and surgical management of early Q wave myocardial infarction: Part 1. Effects of surgical reperfusion on survival, recurrent myocardial infarction, sudden death, and functional class at 10 or more years of follow-up. *Journal of the American College of Cardiology, 14,* 65-77.

16. Harold, J. G. et al. (1987). Mitral valve replacement early after myocardial infarction: Attendant risk of left ventricular rupture. *Journal of the American College of Cardiology, 9,* 277-282.

17. Cosgrove, D. M., et al. (1989). Ventricular aneurysm resection: Trends in surgical risk. *Circulation, 79*(Suppl. 6), I-97-I-101.

18. Naunheim, K. S., et al. (1989). Emergency coronary artery bypass grafting for failed angioplasty: Risk factors and outcome. *Annals of Thoracic Surgery, 47*(6), 816-822.

19. Kirklin, J. W., et al. (1989). Summary of a consensus concerning death and ischemic events after coronary artery bypass grafting. *Circulation, 79*(Suppl., Pt. 2), I-81-I-91.

20. Cosgrove, D., et al. (1984). Primary myocardial revascularization: Trends in surgical mortality. *Journal of Thoracic and Cardiovascular Surgery, 88,* 673-684.

21. Kahn, S. S., et al. (1990). Increased mortality of women in coronary artery bypass surgery: Evidence of referral bias. *Annals of Internal Medicine, 112,* 561-567.

22. Mullany, C. J., et al. (1990). Early and late results after isolated coronary artery bypass in 159 patients aged 80 years and older. *Circulation, 82*(Suppl. 5), IV-229-IV-236.

23. Merrill, W. H., et al. (1990). Cardiac surgery in patients age 80 years or older. *Annals of Surgery, 211*(6), 772-775.

24. Townes, B. D., et al. (1989). Neuro-behavioral outcomes in cardiac operations. A prospective controlled study. *Journal of Thoracic and Cardiovascular Surgery, 98*(5, Pt. 1), 774-782.

25. Lytle, B., & Loop, F. (1985). Elective coronary surgery. In K. McCauley, A. Brest, & D. McGoon (Eds.), *McGoon's cardiac surgery: An interprofessional approach to patient care.* Philadelphia: Davis.

26. Prasad, U. S., et al. (1991). Influence of obesity on the early and long term results of surgery for coronary artery disease. *European Journal of Cardiothoracic Surgery, 5*(2), 67-72.

27. Sethi, G. K., et al. (1991). Comparison of postoperative complications between saphenous vein and internal mammary artery grafts to left anterior descending artery. *Annals of Thoracic Surgery, 51*(5), 733-738.

28. Azariades, M., et al. (1990). Five-year results of coronary bypass grafting for patients older than 70 years: Role of internal mammary artery. *Annals of Thoracic Surgery, 50*(6), 940-945.

29. Loop, F. D., et al. (1990). J. Maxwell Chamberlain Memorial paper. Sternal wound complications after isolated coronary artery bypass grafting: Early and late mortality, morbidity, and cost of care. *Annals of Thoracic Surgery, 49*(2), 179-186.

30. Grondin, C. M., et al. (1989). Coronary artery bypass grafting with saphenous vein. *Circulation, 79*(Suppl.), I-24-I-29.

31. Ruel, G. (1984). Revascularization of the ischemic myocardium. In D. Cooley (Ed.), *Techniques in cardiac surgery.* Philadelphia: Saunders.

32. Grondin, C., Campeau, L., Lesperance, J., et al. (1984). Comparison of late changes in internal mammary artery and saphenous vein grafts in two consecutive series of patients 10 years after operation. *Circulation, 70*(Suppl. I), I-208-I-212.

33. Lytle, B., Loop, F., Cosgrove, D., et al. (1985). Long term (5 to 12 years) serial studies of internal mammary artery and saphenous vein coronary bypass grafts. *Journal of Thoracic and Cardiovascular Surgery, 89,* 248-258.

34. Foster, E. D., & Kranc, M. A. T. (1989). Alternative conduits for aortocoronary bypass grafting. *Circulation, 79*(Suppl. I), I-34-I-39.

35. Mills, N. L., & Everson, C. T. (1989). Right gastroepiploic artery bypass. *Annals of Thoracic Surgery 47*(5), 706-711.

36. Mills, N. L., & Everson, C. T. (1991). Techniques for use of the inferior epigastric artery as a coronary bypass graft. *Annals of Thoracic Surgery, 51*(2), 208-214.

37. Ramstrom, J., et al. (1990). Myocardial revascularization with three native in situ arteries. Gastroepiploic

and bilateral internal mammary artery grafting. *Scandinavian Journal of Thoracic of Cardiovascular Surgery, 24*(3), 177-180.

38. Suma, H., et al. (1991). Does use of gastroepiploic artery graft increase surgical risk? *Journal of Thoracic and Cardiovascular Surgery, 101*(1), 121-125.

39. Suma, H., et al. (1991). Bovine internal thoracic artery graft. Successful use of urgent coronary bypass surgery. *Journal of Cardiovascular Surgery, 32*(2), 268-270.

40. Hartman, A. R., et al. (1991). Emergency coronary revascularization using polytetrafluoroethylene conduits in patients in cardiogenic shock. *Clinical Cardiology, 14*(1), 75-78.

41. Roberts, A., et al. (1983). Comparison of early and long term results with intraoperative balloon catheter dilatation and coronary artery bypass grafting. *Journal of Thoracic and Cardiovascular Surgery, 86,* 435-440.

42. Caralps, J. M., Crexells, C., Aris, A., et al. (1984). Combined aortocoronary bypass and intra-operative transluminal angioplasty in left main coronary disease. *Annals of Thoracic Surgery, 37,* 291-294.

43. Blanche, C., et al. (1991). Excimer laser angioplasty during aortocoronary bypass grafting. *Annals of Thoracic Surgery, 51*(4), 670-672.

44. Ollivier, J. P., et al. (1990). Intraoperative coronary artery endarterectomy with excimer laser. *Journal of Thoracic and Cardiovascular Surgery, 100*(4), 606-611.

45. Blanche, C., Matloff, J. M., & McKay, D. (1990). Technical aspects of cardiopulmonary bypass. In R. J. Gray, & J. Matloff (Eds.), *Medical management of the cardiac surgical patient.* Baltimore: Williams & Wilkins.

46. Litwak, R., & Giannelli, S. (1982). Open intracardiac operations employing extracorporeal circulation. In R. Litwak, & R. Jurado (Eds.), *Care of the cardiac surgical patient.* Norwalk, CT: Appleton-Century-Crofts.

47. Henze, T., Stephen, H., & Sonntag, H. (1990). Cerebral dysfunction following extracorporeal circulation for aortocoronary bypass surgery: No differences in neuropsychological outcome after pulsatile versus nonpulsatile flow. *Thoracic and Cardiovascular Surgeon, 38*(2), 65-68.

48. Guyton, R., Williams, W., & Hatcher, C. (1990). Techniques of cardiopulmonary bypass. In J. W. Hurst, R. C. Schlant, C. E. Rackley, et al. (Eds.), *The heart* (7th ed.). New York: McGraw-Hill.

49. Davies, G., Sobel, M., & Salzman, E. (1980). Elevated plasma fibrinopeptide A and thromboxane B_2 levels during cardiopulmonary bypass. *Circulation, 61,* 808-814.

50. Kirklin, J. W., Blackstone, E. H., & Kirklin, J. K. (1988). Cardiac surgery. In E. Braunwald (Ed.), *Heart disease* (3rd ed.). Philadelphia: Saunders.

51. Roberts, A., Spies, S., Sanders, J., et al. (1981). Serial assessment of left ventricular performance following coronary artery bypass grafting. *Journal of Thoracic and Cardiovascular Surgery, 81,* 69-84.

52. Phillips, H., Carter, J., Okada, R., et al. (1983). Serial changes in left ventricular ejection fraction in the early

hours after aortocoronary bypass grafting. *Chest, 83,* 28-34.

53. Jansen, K. J., & McFadden, P. M. (1986). Post-operative nursing management in patients undergoing myocardial revascularization with internal mammary artery bypass. *Heart Lung, 15,* 48-54.

54. Gray, R. C., & Mandel, W. J. (1990). Management of postoperative arrhythmias. In R. C. Gray, & J. M. Matloff (Eds.), *Medical management of the cardiac surgical patient.* Baltimore: Williams & Wilkins.

55. Markmann, P., & Wallace, P. (1985). Nursing care in the intensive care unit. In K. McCauley, A. Brest, & D. McGoon (Eds.), *McGoon's cardiac surgery: An interprofessional approach to patient care.* Philadelphia: Davis.

56. Lowe, J. E., et al. (1991). Intraoperative identification of cardiac patients at risk to develop postoperative atrial fibrillation. *Annals of Surgery, 213*(5), 388-391.

57. Vitello-Cicciu, J., et al. (1987). Profile of patients requiring the use of epicardial pacing wires after coronary artery bypass surgery. *Heart Lung, 16*(3), 301-305.

58. Utley, J., & Stephens, D. (1983). Fluid balance during cardiopulmonary bypass. In J. Utley (Ed.), *Pathophysiology and techniques of cardiopulmonary bypass.* Baltimore: Williams & Wilkins.

59. Goodnough, L. T., et al. (1990). Guidelines for transfusion support in patients undergoing coronary artery bypass grafting. Transfusion Practice Committee of the American Association of Blood Banks. *Annals of Thoracic Surgery, 50*(4), 675-683.

60. Jones, E. L., et al. (1982). Clinical factors influencing survival and adequacy of revascularization after coronary bypass operation. *International Journal of Cardiology, 2,* 109-123.

61. Gray, R. J. (1990). Cognitive and psychological changes. In R. J. Gray, & J. M. Matloff (Eds.), *Medical management of the cardiac surgical patient.* Baltimore: Williams & Wilkins.

62. Gray, R. J. (1990). Normal convalescence. In R. J. Gray, & J. M. Matloff (Eds.), *Medical management of*

the cardiac surgical patient. Baltimore: Williams & Wilkins.

63. Kirklin, J. W., & Barrett-Boyes, B. G. (1988). *Cardiac surgery: Morphology, diagnostic criteria, natural history, techniques, results, and indications.* New York: Churchill Livingstone.

64. Leserman, J., et al. (1989). The efficacy of the relaxation response in preparing for cardiac surgery. *Behavioral Medicine, 15*(3), 111-117.

65. Lepczyk, M., Raleigh, E. H., Rowley, C. (1990). Timing of preoperative patient teaching. *Journal of Advanced Nursing, 15*(3), 300-306.

66. Duncan, C., & Erikson, R. (1982). Pressures associated with chest tube stripping. *Heart Lung, 11,* 166-171.

67. Belitz, J. (1983). Minimizing the psychological complications of patients who require mechanical ventilation. *Critical Care Nurse,* May-June, 42-46.

68. Molter, N. (1979). Needs of relatives of critically-ill patients: A descriptive study. *Heart Lung, 8,* 332-339.

69. Rogers, C. (1983). Needs of relatives of cardiac surgery patients during the critical care phase. *Focus on Critical Care, 10,* 50-55.

70. Leske, J. (1986). Needs of relatives of critically-ill patients: A follow-up. *Heart Lung, 8,* 332-339.

71. American Association of Critical-Care Nurses. (1989). *Standards for nursing care of the critically ill.* St. Louis: Reston.

72. Norris, S. O. (1989). Managing postoperative mediastinitis. *Journal of Cardiovascular Nursing, 3*(3), 52-65.

73. Wenger, N. K., & Fletcher, G. F. (1990). Rehabilitation of the patient with atherosclerotic coronary heart disease. In J. W. Hurst, R. C. Schlant, C. E. Rackley, et al. (Eds.), *The heart* (7th ed.). Philadelphia: Saunders.

74. Lanoue, A. (1986). Cardiac rehabilitation. In B. Yee, & S. Zorb (Eds.), *Cardiac critical care nursing.* Boston: Little, Brown.

75. Sivarajan, E. (1990). Cardiac rehabilitation: Activity and exercise program. In S. Underhill, S. Woods, E. Sivarajan, et al. (Eds.), *Cardiac nursing.* Philadelphia: Lippincott.

PART FIVE

Pulmonary Patient Care Problems

27

Pulmonary Anatomy and Physiology

Thomas S. Ahrens

Glenda Nelson

As life evolved from simple single-celled organisms, the problem of gas exchange became increasingly complex. Whereas in an aqueous environment oxygen could diffuse into, and carbon dioxide diffuse out of, the organism, the addition of subsequent layers of cells to form tissues increased the distance between the aqueous environment and the centers of gas exchange. It soon became imperative that some method of gas transport occur to permit atmospheric oxygen to reach and carbon dioxide to leave the internal milieu of the organism. The process of gas exchange in the human being is marvelously complex; we may begin to gain an understanding of its perturbations by examining the process from both anatomical and physiological standpoints.

ANATOMY

Upper Airway

Assuming a normal tidal volume of 500 to 700 ml and a normal respiratory rate of 15 per minute, approximately 10,000 L of air each day must pass in and out of the lungs; this same volume first is modified as it enters the nose and mouth. As air passes into the nose, it divides through the left and right nasal passages separated by the nasal septum. At the back of the nasopharynx these two passages merge into one. Within the nasal passages are the turbinates, which have a rich blood supply and may swell or shrink as environmental conditions dictate. The airway is lined with ciliated epithelium and mucous glands that help to trap particles and contaminants in the air.

The major function of the nasal mucosa is to modify the atmospheric air. This process includes heating, absorption of noxious gases, humidification, and fil-

tration. By the time the air has reached the posterior nasopharynx, it is within a few degrees of body temperature and saturated with water vapor. Water-soluble gases such as sulfur dioxide are readily absorbed in the nasopharynx, and many large particles are filtered within the passage. Thus, the initial few centimeters of the respiratory tree are responsible for the majority of cleansing, humidification, and warming of air that reaches the lungs.

As air passes through the pharynx it enters the larynx and from there the trachea. The entire upper airway may contribute to resistance in airflow at different points because of variability in diameter. For example, because of the high collapsibility of the nasopharynx, inspiratory airflow is limited to a maximum of approximately 2 L per second through the nose; this is in contrast to maximum inspiratory flows of about 10 L per second through the mouth. Constriction in the airway may also occur in the oral pharynx when obstructed by the base of the tongue as in obstructive sleep apnea, or in the larynx from vocal cord paralysis.

Tracheobronchial Tree

Air passes through the nose and mouth into the oral pharynx, through the larynx, and into the trachea, the largest of the *conducting airways*. These include the trachea which bifurcates into two mainstem bronchi, which in turn divide into approximately seven divisions of smaller bronchi. These bronchi lose their cartilage as they branch into bronchioles. After about 20 divisions, respiratory bronchioles can be identified along whose circumference are situated the sites of gas exchange. Alveolar ducts are noted after about 23 divisions from the trachea; these lead directly into the alveoli, whose major function is that of gas exchange.

As each airway branches from the trachea to the smallest terminal bronchioles, the diameter of each division becomes progressively smaller. However, the total cross-sectional area at each division increases, so that the velocity of gas decreases as the airstream moves to the periphery of the lung.

The conducting airways do much more than simply conduct air from the outside world to the interior; they are lined with cells which may secrete mucus, immunoglobulins, and other substances, and they may dilate and contract in response to the tone of the smooth muscle contained in their walls.

At the very end of the conducting airways distal to the end of a terminal bronchiole lies the *terminal respiratory unit*. This may consist of an *alveolar duct* with one or more *alveolar sacs* containing individual *alveoli*.

The alveolus may be thought of as the final respiratory chamber. It is typically 250 μm in size, and each person may have 300 million alveoli. The total surface area of alveoli is approximately 80 m², of which the great majority (about 80%) is covered with pulmonary capillaries. The surface area exposed to the atmosphere within the lung is 40 times as great as the surface area of the skin, so that the lung provides us with our greatest area of direct contact with the atmosphere.

The surface of the alveolus is where the exchange of gases takes place between the environment and the organism. The epithelium of the alveolus consists of *type 1* cells or *squamous pneumocytes*, or *type 2* cells or *granular pneumocytes*. It is believed that the type 2 cells are responsible for secretion of *surfactant*, which is a lipoprotein material vital in maintaining the lung in an uncollapsed state. The alveolar surface abuts directly on the capillary surface to provide a region over which oxygen and carbon dioxide can pass to and from the blood through capillary and alveolar endothelium, alveolar airspace, and atmosphere.

In summary, as the flow of gas moves from the atmosphere into the lungs, it passes through the nasal and oral pharynx. From there, air enters the larynx, then the trachea, and then moves down the left and right mainstem bronchi. Inspired air then travels through seven divisions of cartilaginous bronchi, through a dozen more divisions of noncartilaginous conducting airways, and into the terminal respiratory units, which contain respiratory bronchioles, alveolar ducts, and alveoli. Gas can then move from the alveolus across the epithelium and into the pulmonary capillary where it may be carried throughout the body.

Pulmonary Vasculature

There are two circulations to the lungs: the pulmonary and bronchial circulations. The *pulmonary circulation* returns venous (unoxygenated) blood to the lungs for exchange of oxygen and carbon dioxide. The *bronchial circulation* provides the lung with its own supply of oxygen and nutrients.

The main pulmonary artery arises from the outflow tract of the right ventricle and divides into the left pulmonary artery which runs posteriorly, and the right pulmonary artery which runs anteriorly. The pulmonary arteries generally follow the route of the tracheobronchial tree. The proximal pulmonary arteries are elastic, whereas the smaller arteries which accompany the bronchioles have a thin muscular coat. The *pulmonary arterioles* are the smallest branches of the pulmonary arterial system. These arterioles lead directly into the *pulmonary capillaries*. As blood emerges from the pulmonary capillaries, it enters the *pulmonary veins*. Pulmonary veins eventually merge into several main veins to return oxygenated blood to the left atrium of the heart. The major function of the pulmonary veins is to serve as a reservoir of blood for the left atrium and the left ventricle.

In contrast to the pulmonary arterial circulation, the bronchial circulation supplies the lungs with oxygenated blood for nutrition of the pulmonary nerves and ganglia, arteries and veins, pleura and connective tissue. The right lung is supplied by a right intercostal artery which originates from the right subclavian or internal mammary artery; the bronchial supply to the left lung originates from the aorta. Unlike the pulmonary arterial circulation which receives the entire cardiac output, only 1% or 2% of the cardiac output is distributed to the lung via the bronchial circulation.

Lymphatic Vessels

As blood flows through the pulmonary capillaries, some of the plasma is filtered into the interstitium of the lung, where it is collected into lymphatic channels and ultimately returned to the general circulation. One of the major functions of the pulmonary lymphatics is the removal of interstitial fluid. Although most of the filtered fluid returns through lymphatics that run through the lung parenchyma, another set of lymphatic vessels returns lymph over the surface of the lung within the pleura. When interstitial lymphatic vessels become enlarged through increased fluid filtration such as may occur with pulmonary edema, they may be identified as horizontal linear opacities (Kerley B lines) on the chest radiograph. Normal lymph flow has been estimated in humans at 20 ml/hr, increasing to 200 ml/hr during pulmonary edema. In conditions where the major lymphatic drainage through the thoracic duct is blocked, lymph may back up through the lymphatics to form a pleural effusion composed of lymph; this is called a *chylous effusion*.

Nerve Supply to the Lungs

The major nerve supplies to the lungs are carried by the vagus nerve and by thoracic sympathetic ganglia. The vagus returns information to the central nervous system from several receptors within the lung, including stretch receptors, irritant receptors, and J receptors.

Stretch receptors may respond to lung inflation or increased lung volume with bronchodilatation, tachycardia, and decreased systemic vascular resistance. *Irritant receptors* may be responsible for wheezing, bronchoconstriction, and cough after being stimulated by pulmonary edema and chemical or mechanical irritation. *J receptors* are believed to result in laryngeal constriction, hypotension, and bradycardia when stimulated by embolism or pulmonary edema.

Other responses of the lung such as pulmonary hypertension from hypoxia or bronchoconstriction may occur in the absence of any nervous system input and may be caused by local responses of the lung to a variety of stimuli.

Lung parenchyma contains no pain fibers, and procedures such as transbronchial biopsy need no anesthetic. However, blood vessels and pleura are pain sensitive, and pathways include predominantly intercostal nerves and thoracic ganglia.

Muscles of Respiration

When there is no muscular activity of the respiratory system or when the patient is completely paralyzed, the thorax is in the position of passive end-expiration, and the lung volume is said to be at *functional residual capacity* (FRC). Any changes in the volume of the lungs or thorax from this position require active contraction of the respiratory muscles.

The *diaphragm* is the major muscle of respiration. It is shaped like a dome and contracts in a downward and forward position, pulling the lungs open and increasing their volume. As inspiration proceeds, the volume in the thorax increases and the abdomen appears to enlarge in an anteroposterior dimension, because the abdominal contents are compressed by the diaphragm. Additional inspiratory muscles include the *scaleni*, the *sternocleidomastoideus*, and the *external intercostals*, all of which help to pull the ribs upward to increase the volume of the thorax.

Normally, expiration is passive. In other words, no active muscle contraction is needed to expel air from the lungs. Rather, the elastic recoil of the lung returns the lung to its original volume after cessation of inspiratory muscle activity. Expiration may be aided by active contraction of the *rectus abdominis, iliocostalis lumborum,* and *intercostales interni*, all of which may aid in depressing the ribs to decrease the volume of the thorax, and contracting the abdominal wall to press the abdominal contents back up into the chest.

The diaphragm receives its nerve supply from the phrenic nerves which arise from the third, fourth, and fifth cervical segments of the spinal cord. Most of the other accessory respiratory muscles are innervated from thoracic and lumbar segments. For this reason, lower cervical or thoracic injuries may completely paralyze the accessory muscles, while action of the diaphragm is preserved.[1]

PHYSIOLOGY

Ventilation and Mechanics of Breathing

Lung Volumes

To understand how the anatomical components of the respiratory system interact in health and disease, it is important to be familiar with the physiological concepts applied to breathing. As mentioned in the previous section, the column of air from atmosphere to alveolus is continuous; however, for conceptual purposes it is helpful to divide this air into different compartments.

Total lung capacity (TLC) is the total volume of gas contained in the respiratory system, including gas contained in the upper airway, conducting airways, and alveoli. To measure TLC directly, it would be necessary to empty all the gas from the respiratory system. Since this is not possible in humans, a method is employed which introduces a known quantity of gas such as helium. By allowing the helium to equilibrate throughout the respiratory system, one can then measure the concentration of helium in an expired sample and calculate the total quantity of gas that must be present to produce this final concentration.

If one takes a deep breath and inhales maximally to TLC, the total amount of gas that is expelled on a forced expiration is termed the forced *vital capacity* (VC). This can be measured by exhaling into a calibrated spirometer that measures the amount of gas exhaled. The amount of gas that remains in the respiratory system after a vital capacity maneuver is the *residual volume* (RV). Normally, we do not breathe from total lung capacity to residual volume; instead we take a submaximal inspiration and submaximal exhalation. This amount of air, which is normally inhaled and exhaled during quiet breathing, is called the *tidal volume* (V_T). This, too, can be measured spirometrically. The amount of gas remaining in the respiratory system at the end of a quiet exhalation is called the *functional residual capacity*.

The accumulated tidal volume for 1 minute is the *minute ventilation* ($\dot{V}_E$). Alternatively, one may measure the minute ventilation and then divide by the respiratory frequency (F) to obtain the tidal volume.

Alveolar Ventilation and Dead Space

Just as the structure of the respiratory tract changes from upper airway to the alveoli, so does its function. One way to describe these differences in function is to separate the tidal volume into the portions that are involved in gas exchange (*alveolar ventilation*, or V_A), and those areas that merely conduct the air but are not involved in gas exchange (*dead space*, or V_D).

$$V_T = V_D + V_A$$

The upper airway, trachea, major bronchi, and smaller conducting bronchioles are considered *anatomical dead space*, whereas respiratory bronchioles and alveoli all contribute to the alveolar ventilation. Normally, approximately 150 ml, or about one third of the tidal volume, occupies dead space and does not participate in gas exchange. In disease states, however, not all of the anatomic gas-exchanging units may be functioning. For example, emphysema or obliterative vascular disease may cause a loss of the ability of respiratory bronchioles to exchange gas. Under these conditions, structures that would normally participate in alveolar ventilation contribute functionally to dead space; their volume is referred to as *physiological dead space*. Dead space increases when ventilation occurs in excess of blood flow. The concept of ventilation/perfusion relationships, which explains dead space and other gas exchange abnormalities, is presented later in this chapter.

Physiological dead space in normal subjects is almost equal in volume to anatomical dead space and is frequently expressed as the ratio of dead space to tidal volume (V_D/V_T). Normal values for V_D/V_T are about 0.33 (one third of the tidal volume).

In practice, the physiological dead space/tidal volume ratio may be measured simply by drawing a sample of arterial blood and measuring the P_{CO_2}, and by collecting the patient's expired gas in a Douglas bag or other similar device for several minutes. By withdrawing a sample of mixed expired air in the bag and obtaining the partial pressure of carbon dioxide, one can calculate the dead space/tidal volume ratio in the following manner:

$$V_D/V_T = (P_{a}CO_2 - P_{E}CO_2)/P_{a}CO_2$$

where $P_{E}CO_2$ equals the partial pressure of carbon dioxide in the mixed expired air.[2]

Resistance and Compliance

With an appreciation of how the respiratory muscles inflate the lung, it is also important to understand the factors that impede air movement. *Elastic resistance* is the tendency of the lungs to oppose stretching because of frictional and elastic properties of the connective tissue of the lung. Abnormalities of the chest wall or abdominal cavity such as ascites or bony deformity may also oppose inflation of the lung.

An additional form of resistance to airflow is offered by *airway resistance*. When gas flow through the airways is strictly laminar, the resistance of the airways is expressed by Poiseuille's law:

$$R = \frac{8nl}{\pi r^4}$$

This law demonstrates that the major components of resistance to airflow are the radius of the airway *(r)*, the length of the airway *(l)*, and the viscosity of the gas *(n)*. In most clinical situations (during laminar flow) the major determinants of resistance are airway caliber and length. Since resistance is a function of the radius to the fourth power, airway caliber is more important than length. For example, halving of the radius will increase the resistance by 16 times. High peak pressures seen on a ventilator during inspiration may result from bronchospasm, mucous plugging, or airway edema, all of which increase airway resistance. The airway resistance *(R)* may be roughly estimated by dividing the change in pressure between peak (P_{max}) and pause (P_{plat}) values by the airflow *(Q)* at that point:

$$R = \frac{P_{max} - P_{plat}}{Q}$$

Airflow may be determined by reading the value set on the ventilator or by dividing the delivered tidal volume by the inspiratory time. In general, the greater the difference between peak inspiratory and lowest expiratory pressure, the greater the airway resistance. The less the difference between the pressures, the greater the share of compliance in accounting for pressures observed during mechanical ventilation.

The resistance to inflation under conditions of no airflow is described by the concept of *compliance*. Compliance refers to the distensibility of a structure in terms of its volume and pressure. For example, a patient with highly compliant lungs will be able to take a large breath without developing high pressures across the lung. In contrast, a patient who may have low compliance from adult respiratory distress syndrome or pulmonary edema will require much higher pressures to distend the lung to the same degree. Changes in compliance may be demonstrated clinically by determining the static pressures on the ventilator at the end of an inspiration in relation to the volume of inspired gas. *Static compliance* (C_{stat}) of the respiratory system may be calculated by dividing the change in volume (ΔV) by the change in pressure (ΔP):

$$C_{stat} = \frac{\Delta V}{\Delta P} = \frac{\text{Tidal volume}}{P_{plat} - P_{end\text{-}expiration}}$$

The change in volume may be obtained by knowing the tidal volume set on a respirator; the change in pressure may be obtained by subtracting starting pressure ($P_{end\text{-}expiration}$), usually zero or atmospheric, but may be more when the patient is receiving positive end-expiratory pressure) from the pause pressure at the end of an inspiration (P_{plat}). Note that airway resistance is a factor only during airflow, and when there is no flow, then none of the airway pressure results from resistance. Compliance, on the other hand, has nothing to do with flow, or how fast the volume is changed, but rather describes how "stretchable" the respiratory system is. Clearly, in critically ill patients both resistance and compliance play a role in ventilator management.

Distribution of Gas within the Lungs

As air moves into the respiratory system, it must all pass through the trachea. The velocity of gas moving in and out of the trachea is relatively great; as the conducting airways branch through subsequent divisions, the total cross-sectional area gradually increases. At first, this might seem surprising, since the airways become progressively narrower. However, even though the airways narrow, there are more of them so that the total area increases. As a result, the velocity of gas moving at any point in the respiratory system decreases from the trachea toward the alveoli. Near the alveoli, the velocity of gas approaches zero; in fact, at the level of the alveoli there is really no mass movement of gas in and out. Instead, diffusion of gas in the alveoli accounts for exchange of oxygen and carbon dioxide.

The distribution of gas to all parts of the lung is not uniform, because of gravitational and anatomical forces. In an upright position, the alveoli in the apices of the lung are relatively open and distended; since pressure changes during breathing are smallest in that portion of the lung, relatively little ventilation is distributed to the upper regions. In contrast, near the bases of the lung, the alveoli are subject to greater changes in pressure; most of the ventilation is distributed to the bases. Most critically ill patients are supine, so that the situation is somewhat different, but the same general principles apply: The anterior or uppermost portions of both lungs are not as well ventilated as are the posterior or dependent portions.

Small airways are very flexible, and some of them may collapse as lung volume decreases while gas still remains in the alveoli. The lung volume at which a significant portion of alveoli contain trapped air is known as the *closing volume*. In normal persons, this occurs well below functional residual capacity, so that all the alveoli remain open during quiet breathing. In disease states such as obesity, obstructive lung disease, or adult respiratory distress syndrome (ARDS), these alveoli may tend to close more readily so that some air trapping may occur even during normal breathing. For this reason, the semi-Fowler's position may be beneficial for the obese patient with respiratory difficulty. The closing volume may be measured in the pulmonary function laboratory with the single-breath nitrogen test; this is not widely available, and is not practical in critically ill patients.

Regulation of Ventilation

Of all the muscular functions that are vital to life, two of the most critical are the beat-to-beat contraction of the heart and the regular rhythm of the respiratory muscles. Of course, the automatic contraction of muscles throughout the body is necessary for maintenance of basic functions. The respiratory system, however, is unique. The muscles of respiration are entirely composed of voluntary, striated muscle, yet their control is automatic.

The regulation of ventilation cannot be explained by a single mechanism. Rather, many different mechanisms may come into play at different times to exert influence on breathing. Unfortunately, we do not yet have a complete understanding of this complex and multifaceted system. Some of the major components that contribute to the regulation of breathing include:
- The integrity of neurons in the medulla
- Reciprocal innervation between inspiratory and expiratory neurons in the pons
- Acid–base status
- The state of wakefulness

Many texts describe the apneustic and pneumotaxic pontine respiratory centers, which control the innate respiratory rhythm and inhibition of inspiration. However, the nervous control of respiration is considerably more complex than such explanations imply. It is not simply the result of interaction of two discrete centers in the brainstem. Nevertheless, the central nervous system controls the basic rate and rhythm of regular breathing. This basic rhythm may be influenced by a variety of voluntary and involuntary factors.

Modification and fine-tuning are achieved in large part by peripheral and central chemoreceptors. The *peripheral chemoreceptors* monitor arterial oxygen, carbon dioxide, and hydrogen ion concentration. The *carotid bodies* are the peripheral chemoreceptors which exert the major influence on the respiratory system. They receive a tremendous blood flow relative to their weight and are capable of responding to changes in arterial blood-gas tension within several seconds. Discharge from their afferent nerves (which follow the glossopharygeal nerve) may occur with a decrease of arterial P_{O_2} below about 60 mmHg. The carotid bodies may also respond to a decrease in pH, an increase in temperature, low perfusion, or chemical stimulation by substances such as nicotine, cyanide, or carbon monoxide.

The *central chemoreceptors* are found along the ventrolateral surface of the cerebral medulla. They are stimulated by changes in P_{CO_2} or pH. However, hypoxemia, which stimulates the carotid body, may have no effect on central chemoreceptors, or may even depress respiratory rate and volume. The central chemoreceptors are the strongest influence on respiration. A small change in Pa_{CO_2} levels produces a direct change in breathing. For example, an increased Pa_{CO_2} produces an increase in respiratory drive.

Other factors that can affect the pattern and extent of ventilation include pulmonary stretch reflexes, the inflation reflex, and the cough reflex. Additionally, baroreceptors in the carotid sinus and aortic arch may respond to a drop in blood pressure by signaling an increase in rate and depth of respiration. This reflex may be clinically evident in patients in shock who hyperventilate in response to low cardiac output.

In critically ill patients an additional factor must be considered: the effect of drugs on the control of ventilation. Commonly used stimulant drugs include aminophylline, which causes an increased sensitivity to P_{CO_2} and may induce hyperventilation. CNS depressants such as anesthetic agents and sedatives may depress the ventilatory response and cause severe respiratory depression in both volume and frequency.[3]

Pulmonary Blood Flow

The lungs are the only organs in the body that receive the entire cardiac output. Venous blood that drains the lower portions of the body returns via the inferior vena cava, and blood that drains the upper portions of the body returns via the superior vena cava into the right atrium. During diastole, blood flows from the right atrium through the tricuspid valve into the right ventricle. As systole begins, blood moves from the right ventricle through the pulmonic valve into the main pulmonary trunk. Since there is no net gain or loss of blood volume from the pulmonary or systemic circulation, the blood flow through the pulmonary artery must be the same as the blood flow through the aorta. Interestingly, the pressures are much lower in the pulmonary circula-

tion than in the systemic circulation, even though the blood flows are equal. This is because the pulmonary circulation offers a much lower resistance to blood flow than does the systemic circulation.

The concept of *pulmonary vascular resistance* is analogous to the concept of airway resistance; the major determinants of vascular resistance include vessel length, radius to the fourth power, and viscosity. Just as in the airways, caliber is the major determinant of resistance in the blood vessels. In the circulation, however, viscosity may also play a role, as when the hematocrit is high from chronic hypoxemia. In this condition, the elevated hematocrit causes greater resistance in the pulmonary circulation, and pulmonary vascular pressures may be increased.

The factors that determine pulmonary vascular caliber are complex, but several of them may be considered separately. First, the level of perfusion of the pulmonary vascular system may affect its resistance. For example, under conditions when blood volume is very low, as in hemorrhagic shock, the pulmonary vascular system may not be distended enough to open all the pulmonary capillaries. Those pulmonary capillaries which do not participate in blood flow remain closed and thereby decrease the total cross-sectional area of the pulmonary vascular tree. As blood volume is replaced and cardiac output increases, more of these pulmonary capillaries will open and begin to participate in blood flow through the lungs. This concept of opening pulmonary capillaries by increasing blood flow is called *recruitment*.

Increasing pulmonary blood volume may lower pulmonary resistance in another way. As blood volume and cardiac output increase, pulmonary capillaries may distend with blood, resulting in a larger radius. Since resistance falls as a function of increasing radius, distending pulmonary capillaries will cause a decrease in pulmonary vascular resistance. Although most physiologists believe that recruitment is the major process of decreasing pulmonary vascular resistance with increasing flow, *distention* may also be an important factor.

Second, the state of lung inflation may affect the caliber of pulmonary capillaries. As the lung is progressively inflated, it enlarges in all dimensions. This results in a stretching of pulmonary capillaries along their length. More important, it results in a squeezing of the pulmonary capillaries between inflated alveoli. As the lung is inflated and as alveolar pressure increases, the pulmonary capillaries are progressively squeezed so that their radius decreases. Thus, high levels of lung inflation are associated with an increased pulmonary vascular resistance, whereas lower lung volumes are associated with lower pulmonary vascular resistance.

Third, the pulmonary vessels may respond with active constriction to a variety of stimuli. In humans, the most potent stimulus for pulmonary vasoconstriction is hypoxemia. This is usually evident at a PO_2 of less than 60 mmHg. *Hypoxemic pulmonary vasoconstriction* is an important factor in many disease processes, including pulmonary hypertension from chronic obstructive lung disease and high-altitude pulmonary edema. In addition to hypoxemia, acidosis may cause elevated pulmonary artery pressures from pulmonary vasoconstriction.

Fourth, other factors may influence the caliber of pulmonary capillaries. For example, pulmonary edema may lead to the accumulation of fluid in the interstitium. Fluid accumulation may increase so that pulmonary capillaries are compressed, thereby increasing pulmonary vascular resistance.

Finally, a variety of destructive and obliterative disease processes may increase pulmonary vascular resistance. These include pulmonary embolism, which decreases the total cross-sectional area of the pulmonary vascular tree by occluding several of its major branches; and emphysema, which increases pulmonary vascular resistance in large part by reducing the number of available pulmonary capillaries.

Pulmonary vascular resistance may be calculated in a manner entirely analogous to that for airway resistance. Since resistance is a function of pressure and flow, a pulmonary artery catheter provides the means for estimating pulmonary vascular resistance. Flow may be determined from obtaining a cardiac ouput (CO) by thermodilution; pressure may be determined by subtracting the pulmonary capillary wedge pressure (PCWP) from the mean pulmonary artery pressure (MPAP):

Pulmonary vascular resistance =

$$\frac{MPAP - PCWP}{Cardiac\ output} \times 80$$

Mean pulmonary artery pressure may be estimated by the following formula:

$$PAD + \left(\frac{PAS - PAD}{3}\right)$$

where
PAD = pulmonary artery diastolic pressure
PAS = pulmonary artery systolic pressure

Pulmonary blood flow is influenced by several factors, including the amount of blood that is returned to the heart (venous return), the function of the heart, and pulmonary vascular resistance. These are similar to the factors of preload, contractility, and afterload, respectively, that are applied to the study of left ventricular physiology.

The distribution of blood to the lungs is not uniform; the effects of gravity cause increased blood flow in the lower portions of the lung relative to the upper portions. In an upright person, this means that there may be little or no pulmonary blood flow to the apices of the lung, with most of the blood flow going to the bases. Most critically ill patients are in the supine position, so that the blood flow to the apical region is similar to that to the bases of the lungs. However, the lowest portions of the lung, that is, the dependent or posterior regions of the lung, receive more blood flow than the anterior portions, because of the effects of gravity.[4]

Matching of Ventilation and Perfusion

From the foregoing discussion it is evident that neither ventilation nor blood flow is distributed uniformly throughout the lung; rather, different parts of the lung receive different amounts of ventilation ($\dot{V}$) and blood flow ($\dot{Q}$).

In areas of the lung that receive similar amounts of blood flow and ventilation, we say that there is good *ventilation/perfusion matching*. In such areas of the lung, gas exchange is most efficient, since carbon dioxide diffuses out of pulmonary arterial blood to the alveolus, and oxygen brought in from the atmosphere diffuses into the blood. Other areas of the lung, however, may demonstrate *ventilation/perfusion inequality*, resulting in less efficient gas exchange.

At one extreme, we may imagine the situation where ventilation is maintained to alveoli but no blood flow passes through the pulmonary capillaries. This may result from vascular occlusion with pulmonary emboli, low cardiac output, hypoxemic vasoconstriction, or gravity. Under these conditions, ventilation is wasted, since it does not allow exchange of gases through the pulmonary vasculature. Recall that this concept of wasted ventilation was referred to as physiological dead space. In fact, physiological dead space represents one extreme of ventilation/perfusion inequality; when the ratio of ventilation to perfusion is extremely high, physiological dead space is the result.

At the other end of the spectrum are lung units with low ventilation/perfusion ratios. Clinical examples of this situation include mucous plugging or obstruction of a bronchus by a tumor or foreign body. Under this condition, pulmonary arterial blood, which contains low levels of oxygen and high levels of carbon dioxide, is exposed to poorly ventilated alveolar air containing low PO_2 and high PCO_2. Thus, hypoxemic and hypercarbic blood is returned to the left side of the heart for distribution to the systemic arterial circulation. When blood perfuses an area of lung with essentially no ventilation, we say the blood is "shunted" past the lung. The PO_2 is more readily affected by intrapulmonary shunts than by the $PaCO_2$. In clinical practice, intrapulmonary shunts account for almost all the reasons for a decrease in PaO_2 levels.

The approximate fraction of shunted blood relative to total blood flow ($\dot{Q}s/\dot{Q}T$) may be estimated from the following formula:

$$\dot{Q}s/\dot{Q}T = \frac{(CcO_2 - CaO_2)}{(CcO_2 - C\overline{v}O_2)}$$

where $\dot{Q}s$ equals the flow of shunted blood, $\dot{Q}T$ equals the total cardiac output, CcO_2 equals the oxygen content in pulmonary capillary blood, CaO_2 equals the oxygen content in arterial blood, and $C\overline{v}O_2$ equals the oxygen content in mixed venous blood. Arterial and venous oxygen contents may be calculated by measuring the hemoglobin and obtaining blood gas samples from a peripheral artery and from the pulmonary artery catheter.

Pulmonary capillary oxygen content may be calculated by assuming that pulmonary capillary blood becomes perfectly equilibrated with alveolar air; to calculate the oxygen content, one uses the alveolar PO_2 calculated from the alveolar air equation (see below). In normal persons, approximately 2% of the total cardiac output is shunted. Patients with the most severe form of ARDS may show shunt fractions of 50%. Measurement of $\dot{Q}s/\dot{Q}T$ is not always practical due to the need for $S\overline{v}O_2$ and $P\overline{v}O_2$ values. Estimates of intrapulmonary shunts may be used instead of actually measuring the $\dot{Q}s/\dot{Q}T$. Common estimates of $\dot{Q}s/\dot{Q}T$ include the PaO_2/FiO_2 ratio, PaO_2/PAO_2 ratio, and PAO_2-PaO_2 gradient. These estimates are limited in accuracy but may be useful in providing approximations of $\dot{Q}s/\dot{Q}T$ values. Table 27-1 gives normal values for each of the estimates of $\dot{Q}s/\dot{Q}T$.[5]

The least accurate of the $\dot{Q}s/\dot{Q}T$ estimates is the A-a gradient. The other estimates are similar in accuracy, although the PaO_2/FiO_2 is the easiest to calculate.

Another estimate of $\dot{Q}s/\dot{Q}T$ is the clinical shunt equation (Table 27-1). This method assumes a

$CaO_2-C\overline{v}O_2$ difference and may be more accurate than the other estimates. It is slightly more difficult to compute.

Between the two extremes of $\dot{V}/\dot{Q}$ disturbances, a wide spectrum of ventilation–perfusion inequality may occur, resulting in intermediate problems in gas exchange. Thus, the pulmonary venous blood that returns to the left atrium is a mixture of blood from different areas of the lungs with differing ventilation/perfusion ratios. When we obtain a sample of arterial blood for oxygen and carbon dioxide analysis, we measure the overall function of the lung, and the arterial value represents a kind of average of the gas-exchanging function of the lung as a whole. The concept of ventilation–perfusion imbalance in disease states will be discussed in a subsequent section.

Another important concept in ventilation/perfusion ratios concerns the zones of the lung (Figure 27-1). In a normal upright individual, pulmonary arterial pressure may be insufficient to reach the very top of the lungs; thus, no blood flow is distributed to these areas. The result is physiological dead space. This is referred to as *zone 1*. Just below zone 1, pulmonary artery pressure may be high enough to perfuse pulmonary capillaries. However, alveolar pressure is high enough to cause partial collapse of the pulmonary capillaries, because alveolar pressure is higher than pulmonary venous (or left atrial) pressure. In this condition, it is the relationship between pulmonary artery pressure and alveolar pressure that determines how much blood flow will be delivered to that lung segment. This condition is called *zone 2*. Below zone 2, pulmonary venous pressure is increased because of gravity, and will be greater than alveolar pressure. Here the difference in pressure between pulmonary artery and pulmonary vein (or left atrium) will determine how much blood flow is delivered. This condition is known as *zone 3*.[6]

In the supine patient, zone 1 is normally not encountered, because pulmonary artery pressure is sufficient to perfuse all areas of the lung. The use of

TABLE 27-1   Estimates of the Intrapulmonary Shunt

Estimate Measure	Formula	Clinically Normal Levels
Alveolar–Arterial Gradient	$PAO_2 - PaO_2$	Less than 20 torr on room air; level increases with increasing FiO_2
Arterial/Alveolar Ratio	PaO_2/PAO_2	Greater than 60%
PaO_2/FiO_2 Ratio	PaO_2/FiO_2	Greater than 286
Respiratory Index	$\dfrac{PAO_2 - PaO_2}{PAO_2}$	Greater than 1
Clinical Shunt	$\dfrac{CcO_2 - CaO_2}{CcO_2 - CaO_2 + 3.5}$	3.5 – 5.0 cc/dl

KEY: PAO_2 = alveolar oxygen tension; PaO_2 = arterial oxygen tension; CcO_2 = pulmonary capillary oxygen content; CaO_2 = arterial oxygen content.

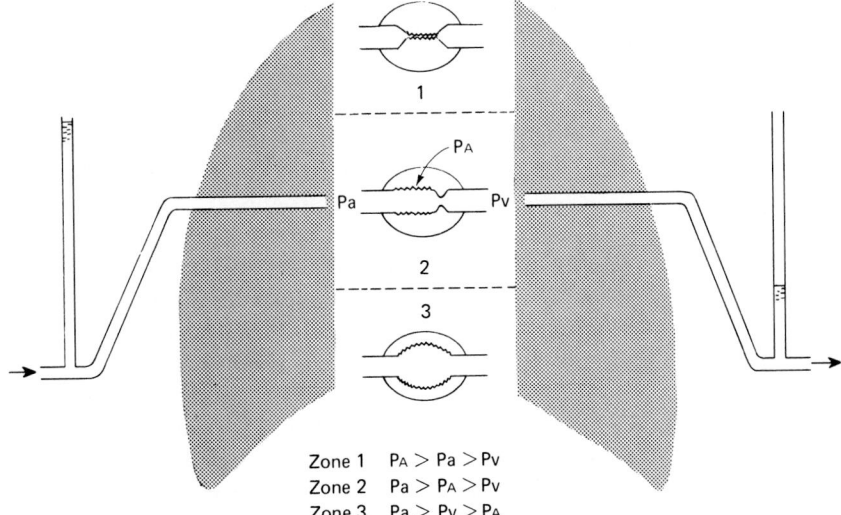

Zone 1 $P_A > P_a > P_v$
Zone 2 $P_a > P_A > P_v$
Zone 3 $P_a > P_v > P_A$

Figure 27-1   Model to explain the distribution of pulmonary blood flow based on pressures affecting the capillaries. The lung is divided into three zones depending on the magnitude of the pulmonary arterial, alveolar, and venous pressures. The lines separating the zones are not topographically precise.

From West, J. B. (1988). The use of radioactive materials in the study of lung function. In A. P. Fishman (Ed.), *Pulmonary diseases and disorders*. New York: McGraw-Hill. Used by permission of the publisher.

positive end-expiratory pressure (PEEP) in critically ill patients, however, may result in alveolar pressures that are sufficiently high to collapse pulmonary capillaries and prevent perfusion of certain segments of the lung. In actual practice, positive end-expiratory pressure is well known to increase the physiological dead space in the lung by this mechanism. The clinical significance of an increased zone 1 is twofold: (1) An increased V_T will be necessary to maintain gas exchange; (2) pulmonary artery catheter readings can be altered.

EXCHANGE AND TRANSPORT OF OXYGEN AND CARBON DIOXIDE

Review of Gas Laws

A basic understanding of the physical behavior of gases is necessary to understand the normal and altered physiology of the respiratory system. The ideal gas law states that pressure, volume, and temperature have fixed relationships. What this means is that one cannot change one of these factors without altering the other in a predictable way. The quantitative relationships between volume, pressure, and temperature have been defined by basic gas laws.

Boyle's Law

$$P_1 \times V_1 = P_2 \times V_2 \text{ (at constant temperature)}$$

Since the product of pressure and volume is constant, then an increase in pressure must be accompanied by a decrease in volume. Similarly, if one increases the volume of a gas, then the pressure must decrease.

Charles' Law

$$\frac{V_1}{T_1} = \frac{V_2}{T_2}$$

An increase in temperature must be accompanied by an increase in volume. Alternatively, if the volume of a gas is to increase, then the temperature must rise.

By combining the above equations we obtain the general gas law:

$$P \times V = R \times T$$

where R is a constant. These equations are used to correct the volume of gas collected under one set of conditions but measured under another. For example, lung volumes are reported at body temperature, but the spirometer which measures the gas is at room temperature. To correct, we may use Charles' law to multiply the volume in the spirometer (V_1) by the ratio of body temperature (T_2) to ambient temperature (T_1) (in degrees Kelvin):

$$V_2 = V_1 \times \frac{T_2}{T_1}$$

Dalton's Law of Partial Pressure

This law states that the total pressure of a volume of gas equals the sum of the *partial pressures* of each individual gas in the gas mixture. For example, room air at sea level has a pressure of 760 mmHg (about 30 inches of mercury, or about 1,000 cm of water), and contains 21% oxygen and 79% nitrogen (carbon dioxide and water vapor contents are negligible). To determine the partial pressure of oxygen, we multiply the concentration (frequently expressed as FiO_2) by the total pressure. Thus, the partial pressure of oxygen in room air at sea level is 760 mmHg times 21%, or 158 mmHg. *Tension* is another word for partial pressure.

Henry's Law

When gases are exposed to a liquid, some of the gas will dissolve in the liquid. The amount of gas that moves into the liquid depends on two factors: the partial pressure of the gas over the liquid, and the solubility of the gas in the liquid. The solubility of the gas in the liquid is determined by the chemical composition of the particular gas and the liquid; the partial pressure may be determined by the total pressure and the concentration of the gas (Figure 27-2).

A common example of Henry's law is demonstrated when a bottle of carbonated beverage is opened. Before the cap is removed, a relatively large quantity of carbon dioxide is dissolved in the liquid because the pressure within the bottle is high. When the cap is removed, the pressure falls to atmospheric, and dissolved gas from the liquid moves out into the atmosphere. It is this partial pressure of gas moving out of a liquid phase that is measured when one obtains a sample of blood for blood gas analysis. The results are written as PaO_2 for the arterial partial pressure of oxygen, and $PaCO_2$ for that of carbon dioxide.

Diffusion of Gases

Diffusion of gas refers to the transfer of molecules of gas from an area of high partial pressure to an area of lower partial pressure. Unlike other examples of gas movement we have considered up to this point, there is no bulk movement of gas. Rather, there is random movement of molecules, without a total pressure gradient between one area of diffusion or another. For example, if we were to open a bottle of 100% oxygen in room air, the total pressure inside the bottle and outside the bottle would each be 760 mmHg. However, because the partial pressure of oxygen inside the bottle (760 mmHg) is higher than the partial pressure outside the bottle (158 mmHg, or 760×0.21), the gas in the bottle diffuses out of the mouth of the bottle by random movement of the molecules. Diffusion will continue to occur until the partial pressure of oxygen inside the bottle is equal to that outside the bottle. It should be noted that there is another gradient for diffusion, namely the diffusion of nitrogen from outside the bottle to inside the bottle. Here, the relevant partial pressures are 602 mmHg outside (760 mmHg $\times$ 0.79) to 0 mmHg inside the bottle.

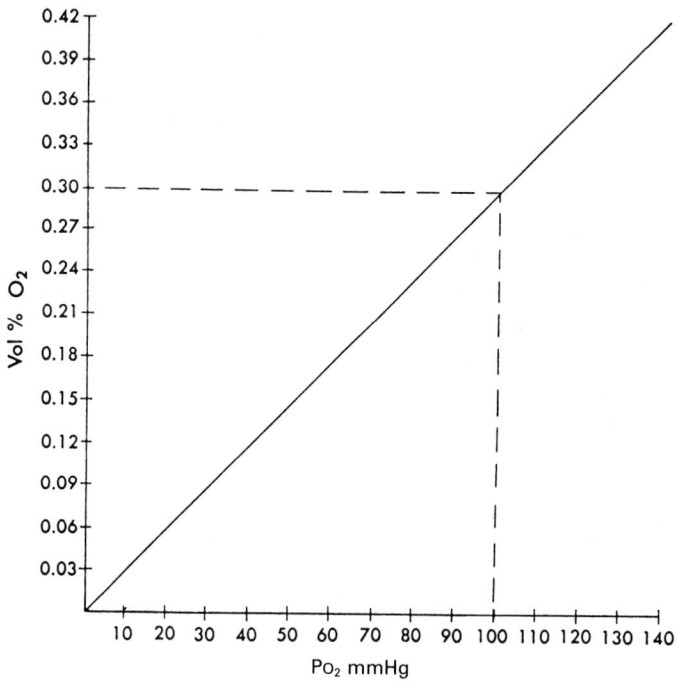

Figure 27-2   The relationship between the number of milliliters of oxygen dissolved in blood and its consequent partial pressure is linear. Each 0.003 ml of oxygen dissolved in 100 ml of blood (vol % of O_2) exerts a pressure of 1 mmHg. The dashed line emphasizes the fact that arterial blood, with an average PO_2 of 100 mmHg, has 0.3 ml of oxygen dissolved in each 100 ml.

From Scanlan, C. L., Spearman, C. B., Sheldon, R. L., et al. (1990). *Egan's fundamentals of respiratory care* (5th ed.). St. Louis: Mosby–Year Book.

Quantitative aspects of diffusion are demonstrated by a modification of Fick's law:

$$\text{Diffusion} = \frac{A}{T} \times D \times (P_1 - P_2)$$

where A is the total area over which the gas diffuses, T is the thickness of the area over which the gas diffuses, P_1 and P_2 are partial pressures of the gas on the two sides, and D is a diffusion constant which is related to the solubility and molecular weight of the gas. From simple inspection of this equation, it can be seen that increases in area, decreases in thickness, and increase in pressure difference between the two sides will all increase diffusion.

In the alveoli, fresh gas from the atmosphere mixes by diffusion with venous gas coming into the alveolus from the pulmonary capillaries. The gas then must diffuse through a pathway that includes the alveolar epithelium and basement membrane; the pulmonary interstitium, which includes collagenous and elastic fibers; and the pulmonary capillary endothelium and basement membrane; the total thickness is about 0.5 μm. Once the gas has reached the capillary, it has a very short distance to travel before reaching the red blood cell, because the diameter of the capillary is very narrow, and the red blood cell must squeeze through it in order to pass. Thus, the red cell surface is almost in contact with the pulmonary capillary wall. The final pathway of diffusion into the blood includes the distance from the periphery to the interior of the red blood cell, which is about 2.5 μm.

Under normal circumstances, the diffusion of oxygen and carbon dioxide is accomplished very rapidly. It takes only a fraction of a second for the partial pressures of oxygen and carbon dioxide to become nearly equal in the capillary and alveolus. This is important because, at rest, blood moves through the capillary at a fixed rate, and there must be sufficient time for diffusion to occur before the red blood cell leaves the pulmonary capillary. The red blood cell spends an average of 0.75 second within the pulmonary capillary, and diffusion is nearly complete by about 0.25 second. Under certain conditions, discussed below, abnormalities of the diffusion process may prevent the red blood cell from reaching equilibrium with alveolar gas by the time it leaves the capillary.[2]

Transport of Oxygen and Carbon Dioxide in the Blood

With an understanding of the behavior of gases according to physical gas laws, we must now consider the unique property of hemoglobin in its relationship to the oxygen-carrying capacity of blood.

Hemoglobin is a molecule composed of a ferri-chrome and a globin or protein portion. Each hemoglobin molecule can bind four atoms of oxygen near its iron-containing ring. This unique property of hemoglobin allows much more oxygen to be carried in a given volume of blood than could be carried by dissolved oxygen alone. To gain an appreciation for the enormous capacity of hemoglobin to carry oxygen, we may perform some simple arithmetic estimates of the *oxygen content* of blood with and without hemoglobin.[6]

The amount of oxygen dissolved in blood, as described by Henry's law, is a function of the partial pressure of oxygen and the solubility of oxygen. To calculate the amount of dissolved oxygen, we can multiply the factor 0.0031 by the partial pressure of oxygen in millimeters of mercury. For example, with a PO_2 of 100 mmHg, the amount of dissolved oxygen would equal 0.0031×100, or 0.3 ml of oxygen for every 100 ml of blood. This quantity of oxygen is insufficient to sustain life.

Each gram of hemoglobin, when fully saturated with oxygen, can carry 1.34 ml of oxygen. To calculate the oxygen-carrying capacity of 100 ml of blood one needs to know how much hemoglobin is present and how saturated it is with oxygen. The concentration of hemoglobin (in grams per 100 ml) is multiplied by 1.34, and that number is multiplied by the percent saturation. For example, in someone with a hemoglobin concentration of 10 g/100 ml and fully saturated hemoglobin, the amount of oxygen carried by the hemoglobin would be equal to 1.34×10, or 13.4 ml of oxygen per 100 ml of blood. Clearly, the amount of oxygen carried by fully saturated hemoglobin at a PO_2 of 100 mmHg is over 30 times the amount carried in the dissolved form. The total amount of oxygen carried by a quantity of blood is known as the *oxygen content*, and is the sum of the dissolved and hemoglobin-bound oxygen. The factors that affect the oxygen content include the PO_2 in the blood, the hemoglobin concentration, and the percent saturation of hemoglobin (Hb):

$$O_2 \text{ content} = (\text{Hb in grams} \times 1.34 \times \% \text{ sat}) + (0.0031 \times PO_2)$$

As one might imagine, when the PO_2 is extremely high (above about 150 mmHg), then the hemoglobin is completely saturated with oxygen; in other words, all four binding sites on each hemoglobin molecule are occupied with an atom of oxygen. When the PO_2 is very low, then many of the binding sites on the hemoglobin will be unoccupied. The precise relationship between partial pressure of oxygen (PO_2) and the number of binding sites occupied by oxygen atoms is described by the *oxygen–hemoglobin dissociation curve*. This is not a simple relationship but follows a

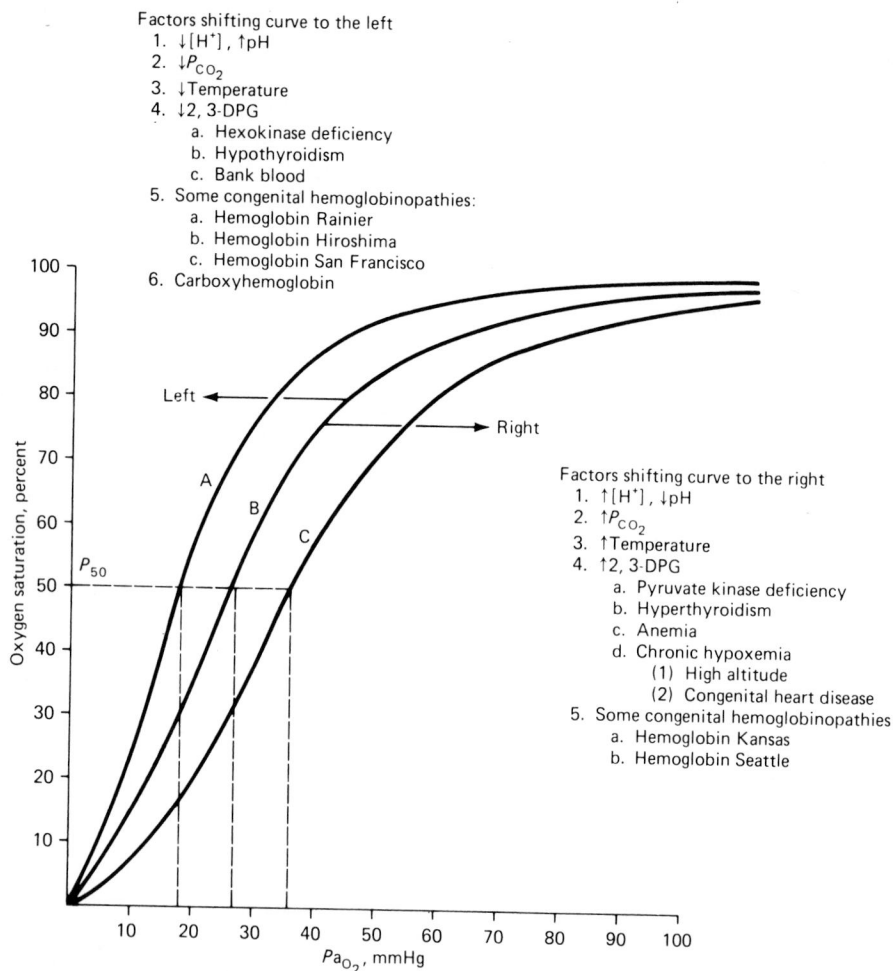

Factors shifting curve to the left
1. ↓[H⁺], ↑pH
2. ↓P_{CO_2}
3. ↓Temperature
4. ↓2, 3-DPG
   a. Hexokinase deficiency
   b. Hypothyroidism
   c. Bank blood
5. Some congenital hemoglobinopathies:
   a. Hemoglobin Rainier
   b. Hemoglobin Hiroshima
   c. Hemoglobin San Francisco
6. Carboxyhemoglobin

Factors shifting curve to the right
1. ↑[H⁺], ↓pH
2. ↑P_{CO_2}
3. ↑Temperature
4. ↑2, 3-DPG
   a. Pyruvate kinase deficiency
   b. Hyperthyroidism
   c. Anemia
   d. Chronic hypoxemia
     (1) High altitude
     (2) Congenital heart disease
5. Some congenital hemoglobinopathies:
   a. Hemoglobin Kansas
   b. Hemoglobin Seattle

Figure 27-3 Factors affecting hemoglobin's affinity for oxygen. Curve B is the standard oxyhemoglobin dissociation curve. Factors that result in a shifting of this curve either to the left or to the right are represented by curves A and C, respectively.

sigmoid shape as shown in Figure 27-3.

Several aspects should be emphasized regarding the relationship between the partial pressure of oxygen and the percent saturation of hemoglobin. First, at partial pressures of oxygen above about 60 mmHg, the hemoglobin is more than 90% saturated with oxygen. This means that even large increases in PO_2 will not be able to further increase the amount of oxygen carried by hemoglobin, because all the binding sites are already occupied. The amount of dissolved oxygen, however, will increase as a function of increasing the PO_2 as described earlier (Figure 27-4).

Second, once the PO_2 falls below 60, the amount of oxygen carried by the blood decreases significantly. For example, when the PO_2 falls from 60 mmHg to 40 mmHg, the saturation of hemoglobin may fall from 90% to 75%. By substituting into the equation

for oxygen content above, one can see that this represents a decrease in oxygen content of about 15%.

Third, the relationship between PO_2 and hemoglobin saturation is not absolute; it may be affected by several common clinical conditions. Factors that are said to decrease the affinity of hemoglobin for oxygen (shift the hemoglobin–oxygen dissociation curve to the right) include fever, acidosis, elevated PCO_2, and elevated 2,3-diphosphoglycerate (2,3-DPG). Factors that tend to increase the affinity of hemoglobin for oxygen (shift the hemoglobin–oxygen dissociation curve to the left) include hypothermia, alkalosis, low PCO_2, and decreased 2,3-DPG.

Carbon dioxide is transported differently from oxygen in the blood. It may be found in three forms: in the form of *bicarbonate*, in a *dissolved* form, and in *combination with proteins*. Dissolved carbon dioxide behaves very much like dissolved oxygen, except

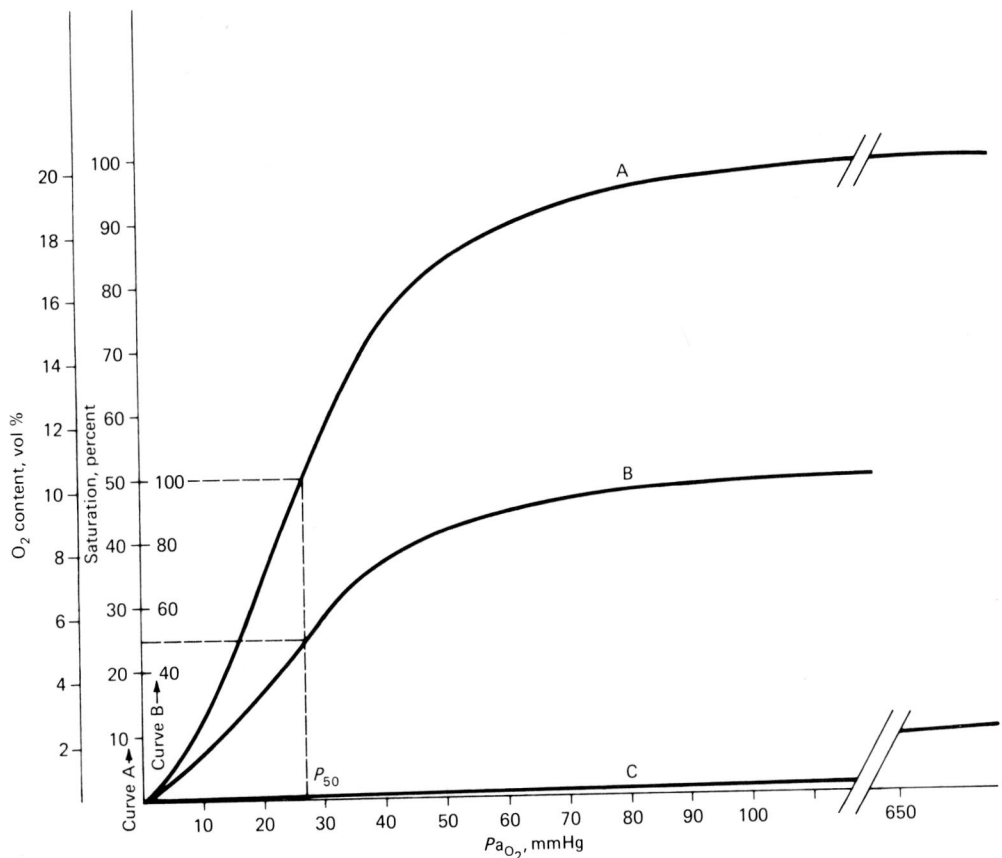

Figure 27-4 The oxyhemoglobin dissociation curve. Curve *A* shows the standard oxyhemoglobin dissociation curve formed when hemoglobin is exposed to air containing increasing amounts of oxygen. Plotted on the ordinate are both percent saturation of hemoglobin and hemoglobin oxygen content (15 g Hb per 100 ml of blood). The abscissa is the Pa_{O_2} value. Curve *B* is a similar plot for a patient with anemia (7.5 g Hb per 100 ml of blood). Notice how the sigmoid shape, percent saturation, and the P_{50} value are unchanged; but the maximum oxygen content is one half of the normal situation. Line *C* represents the dissolved oxygen. Note that oxygen content increases linearly with increasing oxygen tensions but that the total amount is very small compared with the oxygen carried by hemoglobin.

that carbon dioxide is 20 times more soluble in blood than is oxygen. As a result, almost 10% of the entire carbon dioxide content in the blood is carried in the dissolved form.

Bicarbonate is formed by the combination of carbon dioxide with water to form carbonic acid, H_2CO_3. In plasma, carbon dioxide and water combine very slowly, but in the red blood cell the presence of the enzyme *carbonic anhydrase* speeds the reaction considerably (Figure 27-5). Carbonic acid then dissociates to hydrogen ion, H^+, and bicarbonate ion, HCO_3^-. Because of the permeability characteristics of the cell membrane, HCO_3 may diffuse out, but H^+ remains within the cell. To maintain electrical neutrality, chloride diffuses into the cell from the plasma. Some of the hydrogen ion produced from the dissociation of carbonic acid combines with reduced hemoglobin; oxygenated hemoglobin is less able to com-

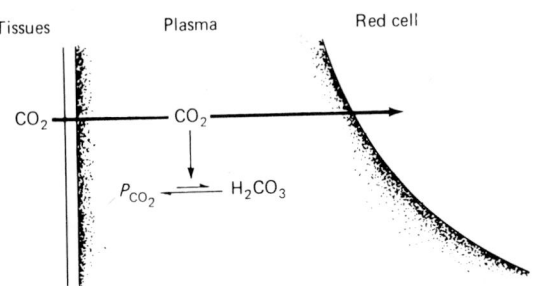

Figure 27-5 Carbon dioxide–carbonic acid relationship in plasma; 5% of the CO_2 entering the blood remains in plasma. Most of this exists as dissolved CO_2 since the chemical reaction $H_2O + CO_2 \rightarrow H_2CO_3$ is very slow; therefore, measuring P_{CO_2} is equivalent to measuring H_2CO_3 concentration.

From Shapiro, B. A., Harrison, R. A., Cane, R. D., et al. (1989). *Clinical application of blood gases* (4th ed.). St. Louis: Mosby–Year Book.

bine with hydrogen ion. This increased ability of deoxygenated blood to help with CO_2 transport is known as the *Haldane effect*.

Carbon dioxide may combine with proteins to form carbamino compounds. The most important protein that combines with carbon dioxide is hemoglobin. Unoxygenated hemoglobin is capable of binding more carbon dioxide than is fully saturated hemoglobin. Thus, consumption of oxygen in the periphery and unloading of oxygen atoms from the hemoglobin molecule increase the ability of hemoglobin to combine with carbon dioxide for removal to the lungs.

In arterial blood, 90% of the total carbon dioxide content is carried in the form of bicarbonate. Only about 5% is carried in the form of carbamino compounds and another 5% as dissolved CO_2.

Recall that the relationship between oxygen content (expressed as hemoglobin saturation) and the partial pressure of oxygen was described by the sigmoid relationship of the oxygen hemoglobin dissociation curve. In a similar manner, we can portray the relationship between carbon dioxide content and partial pressure of CO_2 by means of the CO_2 content curve. Unlike the sigmoid hemoglobin–oxygen dissociation curve, the CO_2 content curve is linear over the entire physiological range. What this means is that increases in partial pressure of CO_2 will increase the total CO_2 content. This is not the case with oxygen content, where increasing P_{O_2} above 60 mmHg has little effect on increasing the content of oxygen.

The normal mixed venous P_{CO_2} is about 45 mmHg, in contrast to the normal arterial P_{CO_2} of 40 mmHg. The increased carbon dioxide that results from cellular metabolism is returned to the lungs in mixed venous blood, where it is removed by alveolar ventilation. Approximately 10,000 mEq of carbonic acid are excreted every day through the lungs.

Oxygen Delivery

Even a very high oxygen content will be of no help to the patient if sufficient delivery of that oxygen to the tissues is not accomplished. *Oxygen delivery* may be calculated according to the following equation:

$$O_2 \text{ delivery} = O_2 \text{ content} \times \text{cardiac output}$$

From inspection of this equation, we can see that oxygen delivery must be increased either by increasing the oxygen content or by increasing the blood flow, or both. Conversely, it should be recognized that oxygen delivery may be severely compromised by an inadequate cardiac output, even though the O_2 content may be completely normal.

When cardiac output falls, as in cardiogenic shock, several internal regulatory mechanisms are called into play to protect vulnerable organs, including regulation of the distribution of blood flow. In shock states, blood flow to less vital areas such as the skin and gut is decreased to maintain blood flow to more vital structures such as the brain and heart.

Oxygen Consumption

The major purpose of the respiratory and cardiovascular systems is the transport of gases to and from the atmosphere and tissues for energy production. As oxygenated blood moves through the arterial tree, it does so in arteries and arterioles of successively decreasing caliber, finally entering the systemic capillaries which supply oxygenated blood to the tissues. The tissues and organs of the body may differ very widely in their demands for oxygen (Table 27-2). For example, the heart and brain require high amounts of oxygen for normal functioning, whereas the kidney and skin require very little. To some degree, these variations are accounted for by internal regulation of blood flow to specific areas as their needs for oxygen dictate. However, regional differences in blood flow do not entirely meet the demands of individual organs. Thus, some tissues extract more oxygen over a period of time than do others since they require more oxygen.

If oxygen is delivered to a tissue at a certain rate (oxygen delivery), and oxygen is extracted from the blood supply at a constant rate (oxygen consumption), then by simple arithmetic a certain amount of oxygen will remain in the venous blood. This relationship may be expressed by the Fick equation:

O_2 consumption

$$= O_2 \text{ delivered} - O_2 \text{ remaining}$$
$$= (\text{cardiac output} \times \text{arterial } O_2 \text{ content})$$
$$- (\text{cardiac output} \times \text{venous } O_2 \text{ content})$$

The two commonly performed measurements of oxygen in the venous blood are the mixed venous oxygen

TABLE 27-2   Oxygen Extraction by Various Organs and Their Characteristic Venous Oxygen Tensions

Organ	Arteriovenous Oxygen Content Differences, vol %	$P\bar{v}_{O_2}$, mmHg
Heart	11.4	23
Muscle	8.4	34
Brain	6.3	33
Splanchnic	4.1	43
Kidney	1.3	56
Skin	1.0	60

Adapted from Finch, C. A., & Lenfant, C. (1972). Oxygen transport in man. *New England Journal of Medicine, 286*, 407.

saturation ($S\bar{v}O_2$) and the mixed venous PO_2 ($P\bar{v}O_2$). Unfortunately, we are unable to measure the individual oxygen consumption of different tissues; this would require a sampling of venous blood draining each of the tissues in which we were interested. However, we may measure the venous oxygen tension of the entire patient.[5]

The measurement of mixed venous PO_2, or mixed venous oxygen saturation, is commonly performed by placing a catheter in the pulmonary artery. Many critical care units routinely use fiberoptic pulmonary artery catheters that continuously measure $S\bar{v}O_2$ levels. Since the blood in the pulmonary artery is a mixture of the venous blood draining all the tissues, it is an indication of the overall state of oxygen extraction of the patient. The mixed venous PO_2 and $S\bar{v}O_2$ thus reflects the balance between overall oxygen delivery and oxygen extraction. Areas or organs that have relatively greater proportion of delivery, or relatively greater oxygen extraction, will contribute a greater portion to the mixed venous PO_2 and $S\bar{v}O_2$.

In general, a mixed venous PO_2 of 40 mmHg and $S\bar{v}O_2$ between 0.60 and 0.75 are normal. $P\bar{v}O_2$ values less than 40 and $S\bar{v}O_2$ values less than 0.60 are low and may indicate an imbalance between oxygen delivery and utilization. We may rewrite the Fick equation to better examine those factors that influence the mixed venous O_2 content (or mixed venous PO_2);

$$\text{Mixed venous } O_2 \text{ content} = \text{arterial } O_2 \text{ content} - \frac{O_2 \text{ consumption}}{\text{Cardiac output}}$$

First, the overall oxygen consumption may be increased. This is seen during generalized hypermetabolic states such as hyperthyroidism, fever, seizures, trauma, etc. Second, a low mixed venous PO_2 and $S\bar{v}O_2$ may result from inadequate arterial oxygen content, such as during hypoxia from a variety of causes, anemia, or shift in the hemoglobin–oxygen saturation curve. Third, low mixed venous O_2 may occur from decreased cardiac output. This is because less O_2 is delivered over a time when the cardiac output is low, so that less O_2 will remain in the venous blood if O_2 consumption does not change.[7]

Cellular Respiration

One of the most important aspects of respiration is also one of the most poorly understood, in part because of its inaccessibility: the uptake of oxygen by tissues and cells. The final pathway for oxygen is the diffusion out of the capillary into the tissues, cells, and organelles. Estimates of the PO_2 necessary to maintain cellular energy stores within mitochondria are as low as 1 mmHg!

Although the basic processes that govern diffusion

of oxygen into and diffusion of carbon dioxide out of tissues are no different from those described above, we are somewhat hampered in our further understanding by our inability to measure tissue or cellular PO_2. Factors that may influence the diffusion of oxygen from capillaries into the tissues include the density of capillaries in a given tissue, the blood flow through the capillaries, and the oxygen extraction by the tissues. It may be that these are the factors that are most disturbed in clinical examples of sepsis, shock, and ischemia. Unfortunately, it is at the tissue and cellular level that we are least successful in our therapy. Thus, most therapeutic efforts are aimed at increasing total oxygen delivery through increasing cardiac output or oxygen content.

Several controversial theories exist regarding the assessment of cellular oxygenation. Currently, most prevalent theory proposes a critical oxygen delivery ($\dot{D}O_2$) point. According to this theory, a critical level of oxygen delivery exists whereby oxygen delivery and consumption are independent of each other. Once the critical oxygen delivery point is exceeded, oxygen consumption becomes dependent on oxygen delivery. Clinically, this point is detectable by continuously measuring both oxygen delivery and consumption (Figure 27-6). It may be possible to detect this point by monitoring $S\bar{v}O_2$ values. For example, if the oxygen delivery increases, the $S\bar{v}O_2$ should improve if oxygen consumption is independent of oxygen delivery. If oxygen consumption is dependent on oxygen delivery, $S\bar{v}O_2$ values will not improve as oxygen delivery increases.

However, identifying cellular oxygenation problems remains exceedingly difficult. Newer technologies such as magnetic resonance imaging and position emission tomography may eventually identify cellular oxygenation more specifically. At present, however, cellular oxygenation assessment remains difficult.

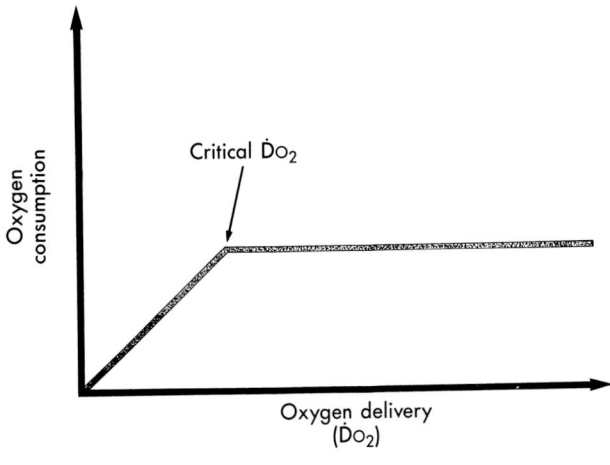

Figure 27-6 Critical oxygen delivery point.

Blood Gas Analysis

When a sample of blood is sent to the laboratory for blood gas analysis, the partial pressures of oxygen and carbon dioxide are measured by exposing the sample to oxygen and CO_2 electrodes. Actually, the electrode is separated by a thin membrane from the blood itself, so that the oxygen diffuses from the blood into the solution surrounding the electrode. The amount of current passed across the electrode is proportional to the P_{O_2}.

Carbon dioxide tension is measured somewhat differently. The CO_2 electrode is in reality a pH electrode which is surrounded by a bicarbonate buffer separated from the blood. As CO_2 diffuses from the blood into the buffer around the electrode, the pH of the buffer changes. This is measured by the electrode and the results are reported as P_{CO_2}.

It is important to remember that blood gas analysis can tell us only the partial pressures of the gases within the blood sample, and may not reflect the oxygen content. Remember that oxygen content is a function not only of the partial pressure of oxygen but of the hemoglobin concentration and the affinity of that hemoglobin for oxygen as well (saturation).

Normal oxygen tensions are dependent upon the age of the patient. In general, normal oxygen tensions are between 80 and 100 mmHg; normal P_{CO_2} lies between 35 and 45 mmHg. Normal pH values range from 7.35 to 7.45. When submitting a sample of blood for blood gas analysis, it is important also to record the patient's temperature. Recall that an increase in temperature will shift the hemoglobin dissociation curve to the right, while a decrease may shift it to the left. Calculations of hemoglobin saturation are available on most blood gas machines, and take into account the normal position of the oxygen–hemoglobin dissociation curve, with subsequent corrections for the patient's temperature, pH, and P_{CO_2}.

Mixed venous blood is often sent for blood gas analysis as well. Normal mixed venous blood has a P_{O_2} of about 40 mmHg, and a P_{CO_2} of 45 mmHg.

ABNORMALITIES OF GAS EXCHANGE

The process of normal gas exchange depends on the coordination and interaction of many factors, as can be appreciated from the foregoing sections. In this section, we will examine in detail abnormalities of gas exchange. These will include problems in oxygenation and problems with carbon dioxide.

It is important to clarify certain terms. *Hypoxia* is the condition of insufficient oxygen availability at the cellular level. *Hypoxemia* may be defined as an abnormally low partial pressure of oxygen. *Ischemia* refers to inadequate oxygenation because of insufficient flow of oxygen-containing blood to a local area; when blood flow is inadequate for the entire patient,

this is sometimes referred to as circulatory hypoxia. *Hypercarbia* refers to elevated partial pressure of carbon dioxide.

Hypoxia

Before explaining each type of hypoxia in more detail, it is important to consider hypoxia in general.

The body's oxygen stores are small, and all humans are dependent upon a continuing and virtually uninterrupted supply of oxygen, since only about a 5-minute supply exists. The organs, however, vary in their susceptibility to sustained hypoxia, with the brain being one of the most sensitive structures. As mentioned previously, tissue oxygen tensions cannot be measured directly, and, therefore, indirect methods of assessing the state of tissue oxygenation must be used. In the absence of an adequate mitochondrial oxygen supply, metabolic activity through the usual aerobic pathway ceases, and the less efficient anaerobic pathway is utilized. This pathway produces lactic acid as a metabolic end product and yields a metabolic acidosis that can be identified by a large anion gap and an elevated blood lactate level. Therefore, lactic acidosis is presumptive evidence of tissue hypoxia. The box below shows some of the parameters commonly evaluated in the assessment of tissue hypoxia.

Hypoxemic Hypoxia

Hypoxemic hypoxia is, in essence, inadequate tissue oxygenation (hypoxia) that is caused by a de-

---

Assessment of Tissue Hypoxia

1. Evidence of anaerobic metabolism:
   Lactic acidosis
2. Evidence of altered perfusion:
   Tachycardia
   Hypotension
   Changes in skin color and temperature
   Changes in capillary filling
3. Evidence of organ dysfunction:
   Cerebral: altered sensorium
   Myocardial: low cardiac output
   Renal: decreased urine output
4. Assessment of oxygen delivery:
   Pa_{O_2}
   Hemoglobin concentration
   Arterial blood oxygen content
   Oxyhemoglobin dissociation curve
   Cardiac output
   Regional blood flow characteristics
5. Invasive parameters:
   Mixed venous oxygen tension ($P\overline{v}_{O_2}$)
   Mixed venous oxygen saturation ($S\overline{v}_{O_2}$)
   Arteriovenous oxygen content difference

creased arterial blood oxygen tension (hypoxemia). The decreased PaO$_2$ may come from one or more of the abnormalities in the process of respiration. It is one of the most common causes of tissue hypoxia encountered in clinical practice. A detailed discussion is presented in the next section.

Anemic Hypoxia

Anemic hypoxia is deficient tissue oxygenation resulting from a decrease in arterial blood oxygen content. This deficiency may result either from a decrease in the amount of hemoglobin present (i.e., anemia) or from a decrease in the ability of hemoglobin to hold oxygen (e.g., carboxyhemoglobin, methemoglobin). Recall these equations:

Oxygen content = oxygen combined with Hb + oxygen dissolved in plasma

$$\text{Oxygen content (vol \%)} = (\text{hemoglobin} \times 1.34 \times \% \text{ saturation}) + (\text{PaO}_2 \times 0.003)$$

As previously discussed, the amount of oxygen dissolved in the blood is small, owing to the low solubility of oxygen (solubility coefficient = 0.003 vol %/mmHg). Even with a patient breathing 100% oxygen (which at sea level would produce a maximum PaO$_2$ of 650 mmHg), the total contribution from dissolved oxygen is less than 2 vol % (i.e., 650 × 0.003). The low carrying capacity from the PaO$_2$ is one major reason blood gas assays are of minor value in assessing oxygen delivery.

Hemoglobin is responsible for the majority of the oxygen carried by the blood. The oxygen-carrying capacity of 15 g of hemoglobin is 20.1 ml. This value must be multiplied by the hemoglobin saturation to get the actual amount of oxygen combined with hemoglobin.

In Table 27-3, notice that the total oxygen content of the blood in a normal person with a hemoglobin concentration of 15 g/100 ml (and a saturation of 97.5%) equals 19.9 vol %, of which 19.6 vol % is

oxygen carried by hemoglobin and only 0.3 vol % is dissolved oxygen.

In the anemic patient (with a hemoglobin concentration of 7.5 g/100 ml), the oxygen content is decreased to 10.1 vol %, of which 9.8 vol % is oxygen combined with hemoglobin. If the anemia is severe enough to result in an inadequate supply of oxygen to the tissues (relative to oxygen demand), then anemic hypoxia results. In clinical practice this seldom occurs, since the body will respond to a severe anemia by increasing the cardiac output, thereby increasing tissue oxygen delivery per unit of time. If this is still not adequate to meet the oxygen demand, then "high output failure" supervenes. It is therefore more common to see anemia contributing to overall hypoxia, as in a setting that combines anemia with hypoxemia, low arterial saturation, and a low cardiac output from congestive heart failure.

Carbon Monoxide. Another type of "anemic" hypoxia results from the inactivation of hemoglobin by carbon monoxide. Carbon monoxide and oxygen bind to hemoglobin at exactly the same site; the two molecules are, in effect, in competition for these hemoglobin-binding sites. However, since carbon monoxide has a much stronger affinity for hemoglobin (some 210 times stronger), it is bound more avidly and held tighter. To use the magnet analogy, hemoglobin is not only an oxygen magnet but a carbon monoxide magnet as well. In fact, it is a much stronger carbon monoxide magnet, and if given a choice between the two molecules, it will combine with carbon monoxide every time. In this way, carbon monoxide produces a "functional" anemia, since it occupies potential oxygen-binding sites. It is convenient to discuss carbon monoxide's effect on hemoglobin as the equivalent reduction in the amount of hemoglobin that is available to combine with oxygen. Therefore, a carboxyhemoglobin level of 10% means there is 10% less hemoglobin available to combine with oxygen.

The ambient levels of carbon monoxide are usually

TABLE 27-3   **Calculation of Oxygen Content**

Patient	Measured Values			Calculated Values (vol %)			
	Hb, g/100 ml	PaO$_2$, mmHg	O$_2$ Saturation, %	O$_2$ Capacity of Hb*	O$_2$ Combined with Hb†	Dissolved O$_2$‡	Total O$_2$ Content§
Normal	15.0	100	97.5	20.10	19.6	0.30	19.9
Anemia	7.5	100	97.5	10.05	9.80	0.30	10.1
Hypoxemia	15.0	50	83.5	20.10	16.79	0.15	16.94

*Step 1: Oxygen capacity of Hb (vol %) = Hb (g/100 ml) × (1.34 ml O$_2$/g Hb).
†Step 2: Oxygen combined with Hb (vol %) = Hb (g/100 ml) × 1.34 (mL O$_2$/g Hb) × saturation (%).
‡Step 3: Oxygen dissolved in plasma (vol %) = PaO$_2$ (mmHg) × 0.003 (vol %/mmHg).
§Step 4: Total oxygen content (vol %) = step 2 + step 3.

quite low, but tobacco smokers and people in some urban environments may develop high levels of carbon monoxide in the blood. For example, heavy cigarette smokers may achieve carboxyhemoglobin levels as high as 15%, and persons with carbon monoxide poisoning (accidental or otherwise) attain levels that are much higher.

The danger level of carbon monoxide in the blood depends to a certain extent on the individual. A normal person may tolerate levels as high as 40% with only a headache, nausea, and vomiting; but above 50%, seizures and coma appear. The lethal level of carbon monoxide is usually between 67% and 70%. However, a patient with severely compromised cardiac function could experience more difficulty with lower levels of carbon monoxide in the blood; a 20% carboxyhemoglobin level may prove fatal. In each case, tissue hypoxia resulting from a decreased oxygen content of the blood is the mechanism whereby carbon monoxide produces its ill effects.

Circulatory Hypoxia

Circulatory hypoxia is an example of deficient tissue oxygenation that results from a decrease in blood supply. As noted earlier, oxygen delivery is a function of both oxygen content and blood flow. Blood flow may be generally decreased (i.e., decreased cardiac output), or it may be deficient in one region. Examples of the latter include local obstructions to arterial blood flow, as in peripheral arterial lesions from advanced arteriosclerotic disease or from direct arteriovenous connections that bypass the systemic capillary bed, and therefore result in a decrease in tissue capillary blood flow. Note that circulatory hypoxia is strictly a cardiovascular phenomenon and need not be accompanied by arterial hypoxemia or a decrease in blood oxygen content.

Low cardiac output is perhaps the most common cause of tissue hypoxia, and may be due to numerous conditions. Therapy is aimed at the underlying cause. Oxygen therapy would be expected to have only minimal benefits if the arterial blood oxygen content were otherwise normal, since the problem is in the delivery of that oxygen.

The effect of regional blood flow abnormalities depends upon the severity of the ischemia and the particular vascular bed involved. In this way, a decrease in blood flow to a small portion of the brain (as may result from an intracerebral thrombosis or hemorrhage) may lead to severe consequences, as may a relatively small vascular thrombosis in a major coronary artery. Prolonged hypoxia in these circumstances may lead to actual cell death and necrosis (infarction).

Finally, various types of direct arteriovenous (AV) communications may occur and lead to tissue hypoxia by diverting blood away from the capillary bed. Examples include deliberate creation of AV fistulas in patients with renal disease undergoing hemodialysis; patients with cirrhosis of the liver who have abnormal AV communications in the skin and viscera (including the lung); fistulas that form as a result of trauma or infections; and rare inherited or congenital lesions as in the Osler-Weber-Rendu syndrome. This type of regional blood flow abnormality only rarely results in clinically significant tissue hypoxia.

Hypoxia from Increased Hemoglobin Affinity for Oxygen

Tissue hypoxia may occur despite a normal PaO_2, adequate arterial oxygen content, adequate cardiac output, and sufficient local vascular perfusion. In this instance, enough oxygen is delivered to the tissues; but because of an increase in hemoglobin's affinity for oxygen, the O_2 is more tightly bound and therefore released more reluctantly in the tissues. This was previously described as a shift to the left in the oxyhemoglobin dissociation curve. Figure 27-3 lists some of the possible causes. Although the basic mechanism is a decrease in oxygen delivery to the tissues, fundamental differences allow for a clear separation between this phenomenon and the other causes of decreased oxygen delivery: hypoxemic hypoxia, anemic hypoxia, and circulatory hypoxia.

Clinically, this mechanism should be kept in mind when dealing with patients who have undergone massive transfusions with old bank blood, in which supplies of 2,3-diphosphoglycerate (2,3-DPG) are depleted. Various congenital hemoglobinopathies may result in a left-shifted oxyhemoglobin dissociation curve, but these are not compatible with life if they lead to significant tissue hypoxia.

Histotoxic Hypoxia

Histotoxic hypoxia refers to hypoxia that occurs as a result of the inability of the tissues to utilize oxygen. As in the case of hypoxia from increased hemoglobin affinity for oxygen, the parameters of tissue oxygen delivery are all normal; the abnormality is in oxygen utilization. The classic example of this type of hypoxia is cyanide poisoning. Detailed investigations of these patients reveal a decrease in oxygen consumption, an increased mixed venous oxygen tension, and a decreased arteriovenous oxygen content difference.

Table 27-4 is a quantitative comparison between the four classic types of hypoxia. The values presented are only approximate and are rounded off for illustrative purposes. In the normal situation, note the parameters of oxygen delivery (arterial blood oxygen

TABLE 27-4 **A Quantitative Comparison between the Four Classic Types of Hypoxia**

| | Arterial | | | | Venous | | | A–V O_2 Content, Difference, vol % | O_2 Consumption, cm³/min | Cardiac Output, L/min |
	O_2 Capacity, vol %	Hb Saturation, %	O_2 Content, vol %	Pao_2, mmHg	Hb Saturation, %	O_2 Content, vol %	$P\bar{v}o_2$, mmHg			
Normal	20	95	19	100	70	14	40	5	250	5.0
Hypoxemic hypoxia	20	75	15	_50_	55	11	30	4	250	7.0
Anemic hypoxia	_10_	95	9.5	100	65	6.5	35	3	250	9.3
Circulatory hypoxia	20		19	100	50	10	27	9	225	_2.5_
Histotoxic hypoxia	20	95	19	100	85	17	60	2	_150_	7.5

Note: The primary abnormality in each of the four types is underlined.

capacity, saturation, content, and tension; and cardiac output) and oxygen utilization (oxygen consumption; mixed venous blood, oxygen saturation, content, and tension; and arteriovenous oxygen content difference). In hypoxemic hypoxia, the *primary abnormality* is a decreased Pao_2, which results in a decreased hemoglobin saturation and O_2 content; but O_2 capacity and O_2 consumption are normal. Cardiac output is increased to assure adequate oxygen delivery. Values in venous blood are decreased in proportion to the arterial hypoxemia, and the A/V oxygen content difference is near normal. In anemic hypoxia, the primary abnormality is a decrease in O_2 capacity, with a normal Pao_2. Note the compensatory increase in cardiac output (which is necessary if O_2 delivery is to remain normal in the face of a decreased arterial blood O_2 content). Circulatory hypoxia, in the example shown, has a decrease in cardiac output as the primary abnormality responsible for the hypoxia. Note that the arterial blood values are all normal, but the mixed venous blood reflects the effects of increased oxygen extraction and the A/V oxygen content difference is widened. Finally, histotoxic hypoxia has as its primary insult a decreased oxygen consumption. Therefore, starting with normal arterial blood parameters, the mixed venous blood reflects this lack of oxygen extraction, and the A/V organ content difference is narrowed.[8]

Hypoxemia

The Oxygen Cascade

The concept of the oxygen cascade is helpful in differentiating many of the causes of hypoxemia. It is referred to as a *cascade*, because of each successive step along the pathway of movement of oxygen from atmosphere to the blood, the Po_2 falls in steps (Figure 27-7). To begin, we may calculate the partial pressure of oxygen in room air according to Dalton's law:

$$PBo_2 = Pb \text{ (barometric pressure)} \times Fio_2$$

where Fio_2 is equal to the fraction of inspired oxygen, and PBo_2 is the partial pressure of oxygen in the atmosphere. Substituting normal values:

$$PBo_2 = 760 \times 0.21$$
$$= 160 \text{ mmHg}$$

When room air enters the airway, it is humidified with water vapor. This gas has a partial pressure (Pio_2) of 47 mmHg at body temperature. Since we must now account for this additional gas added to the total mixture at barometric pressure, we must subtract this value from barometric pressure and recalculate our partial pressure of oxygen within the airway:

$$Po_2 = (760 - 47) \times 0.21$$
$$Po_2 = 713 \times 0.21$$
$$Po_2 = 150 \text{ mmHg}$$

As saturated air moves into the alveolus, it encounters an additional gas: carbon dioxide, which is produced by the body and added to alveolar air. Thus, our first approximation of alveolar Po_2 (Pao_2) can be represented by:

$$Pao_2 = Pio_2 - Paco_2$$
$$Pao_2 = 150 - 40$$
$$Pao_2 = 110 \text{ mmHg}$$

This equation is not entirely accurate because oxygen and carbon dioxide pressures are not static in the alveolus. Instead, oxygen is continually being taken

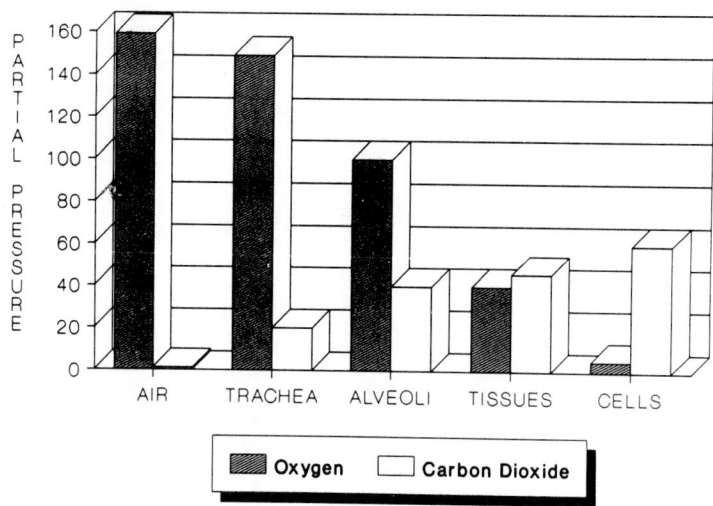

Figure 27-7   Diffusion "cascades" for oxygen and carbon dioxide.
From Scanlan, C. L., Spearman, C. B., Sheldon, R. L., et al. (1990). *Egan's fundamentals of respiratory care* (5th ed.), St Louis: Mosby—Year Book.

up by the capillaries and carbon dioxide is continually being delivered into the alveolar air. For this reason, we include a factor known as the respiratory quotient, R, to correct for this decreased pressure of oxygen and increased pressure of CO_2. This is practically done by assuming a normal respiratory quotient of 0.8 for average conditions:

$$PA_{O_2} = PI_{O_2} - \frac{PA_{CO_2}}{R}$$
$$= 150 - \frac{40}{0.8}$$
$$= 150 - 50$$
$$= 100 \text{ mmHg}$$

This is a simplified form of the *alveolar air equation*. Note that at a constant PI_{O_2}, increases in carbon dioxide tension would lower the PA_{O_2}: decreases in carbon dioxide tension will increase the PA_{O_2}. This reciprocal relationship will be discussed in a subsequent section under causes of hypoxemia.

Once the tension of oxygen within the alveolus is known, the next thing to be considered is the tension of oxygen in pulmonary arterial blood. The concept of the *alveolar–arterial O_2 gradient* has frequently been employed to describe the imperfect transfer of gas from alveolus to capillary. As mentioned, other methods exist to describe gas transfer between the alveoli and capillaries, such as the arterial/alveolar (a/A) ratio and the Pa_{O_2}/FI_{O_2} ratio. Both are more accurate in estimating the problem in gas transfer between the alveoli and capillaries than the A-a gradient. Although several factors may impede perfect equilibration between the alveolar oxgyen and arterial oxygen, the most common one is a low ventilation/perfusion ratio. In normal people breathing room air, about 10 to 20 mmHg is lost in transferring oxygen from the alveolus to the capillary. In the critically ill patient with marked lung dysfunction, the difference between alveolar and arterial levels can be greatly increased.[9]

Adequacy of Oxygenation

Even though a young person may have a predicted Po_2 of 90 mmHg, a measured Po_2 of 80 mmHg may not reflect any serious underlying disorder (of course, even a mildly abnormal test may indicate subclinical disease and may need to be investigated). In terms of actual oxygenation, however, there is little difference between a Po_2 of 80 and 90 mmHg. This is because the oxygen content is not very different in blood that has a Po_2 of 80 mmHg from that with a Po_2 of 90 mmHg, since the amount of dissolved oxygen is nearly the same and because the saturation of hemoglobin is not different.

On the other hand, even a normal or greater than normal Po_2 may be present in light of severely impaired oxygenation. This is because, once again, the oxygen delivery content must be considered. For example, in a severely anemic patient, the Po_2 may be normal, but because there may be only half the hemoglobin normally available, there will only be half the oxygen content normally available. Similarly, a patient with severe cardiac failure may have a normal hemoglobin and a normal Po_2, but a marked reduction in oxygen delivery because of the low cardiac output. In this situation, oxygenation of the tissues could be severely impaired even though oxygen content is normal.

Thus, the question of adequate oxygenation needs to be answered in light of adequate oxygen supply to meet the body's demands. Assessing the adequacy of oxygen supply remains a pressing problem in critical-care medicine. The best overall method to judge the adequacy of oxygen delivery is to observe the function of the various organ systems (see Table 27-3).[10]

Abnormal mentation, confusion, sleepiness, hallucinations, and other signs of CNS dysfunction may result from inadequate oxygen delivery to the brain. The brain is very intolerant of hypoxia, and it may sustain irreversible neuronal damage within minutes of interruption of oxygen supply. Evidence of inadequate oxygen supply to the heart is suggested by angina pectoris, congestive heart failure, papillary muscle dysfunction, and dysrhythmias or even myocardial infarction. Abnormal oxygen delivery to the skin can be seen in livedo reticularis, a condition in which the skin is mottled with a blue or purple discoloration from ischemia. The liver may show evidence of insufficient oxygenation in a variety of ways, the most serious of which is "shock liver," in which serum transaminases are markedly elevated; global liver dysfunction may be present with elevated bilirubin, alkaline phosphatase, and depressed synthetic function demonstrated by prolonged partial thromboplastin and prothrombin times, and decreased serum albumin. The mesenteric circulation may be impaired during severe hypoxia or ischemia, resulting in abdominal pain or bowel infarction. Renal and endocrine manifestations of hypoxia include decreased glomerular filtration rate and increased secretion of antidiuretic hormone and hyponatremia.

In the critically ill patient, additional methods are employed to assess overall oxygenation. One of these is the measurement of serum lactate. Under hypoxic conditions, cellular metabolism results in an accumulation of lactic acid, which is then released into the blood. One example of lactate accumulation that does not indicate disease is severe exercise. During exercise to near exhaustion, blood flow to the working muscles is insufficient to keep up with energy production, so that the muscles turn to anaerobic metabolism and lactate production to meet their energy needs; this is an example of local ischemia resulting in lactate production. When oxygen delivery to the entire body is depressed, lactate may accumulate and be measured in the blood. Lactate levels greater than approximately 2 mmol per liter suggest inadequate oxygen delivery, and lactate levels greater than 20 mmol per liter may imply poor chance of recovery.[11]

The mixed venous PO_2 and $S\bar{v}O_2$ are also used as indicators of adequate oxygen delivery. If the oxygen demand remains constant and oxygen consumption does not change, then a decrease in oxygen delivery will result in a decreased venous content. Normal mixed venous PO_2 is about 40 mmHg, corresponding to a saturation of approximately 75%. A mixed venous PO_2 of 30 to 40 mmHg and $S\bar{v}O_2$ below 0.60 suggest inadequate oxygen delivery, and a mixed venous PO_2 below 30 mmHg and $S\bar{v}O_2$ below 0.50 suggest severe depression in oxygen delivery.

It should be emphasized that although it is a laudable goal to maximize oxygen delivery, we still have much to learn about the interpretation of mixed venous PO_2 and the relationship between oxygen delivery and oxygen consumption. For example, it has been suggested that in septic shock, tissue extraction of oxygen might be impaired; since less oxygen is extracted by tissues, the mixed venous PO_2 and the $S\bar{v}O_2$ will be increased. In this situation, the mixed venous PO_2 and $S\bar{v}O_2$ may be better indicators of oxygen utilization than oxygen delivery. Currently, this author considers the mixed venous PO_2 and the $S\bar{v}O_2$ to be useful adjuncts to other clinical estimates of adequacy of oxygenation.

Mechanisms of Hypoxemia

Aerohypoxia. Aerohypoxia may be defined as a low arterial PO_2 that results from a decreased partial pressure of oxygen in the inspired gas mixture. This situation is most frequently encountered during travel to high altitude, since barometric pressure decreases as one ascends. For example, barometric pressure at the top of Mount Everest (where the altitude is 29,000 feet) is 235 mmHg. Therefore, the partial pressure of oxygen in the atmosphere on the top of Mount Everest is $235 \times 0.21 = 49$ mmHg; this is in contrast to the partial pressure of oxygen at sea level, which is approximately 160 mmHg.

Another example of decreased barometric pressure is travel in commercial airliners. Cabins of these aircraft may be pressurized to only about 7,000 feet, corresponding to a barometric pressure of somewhere around 600 mmHg; the inspired partial pressure of oxygen would be correspondingly reduced. One other situation which is fortunately quite rare, but which may account for aerohypoxia, is the inadvertent substitution of inappropriate gas mixtures in a controlled setting, such as during anesthesia or mechanical ventilation. Administration of nitrous oxide instead of oxygen, for example, may result in aerohypoxia by decreasing the fractional concentration of inspired oxygen.

The treatment of aerohypoxia is straightforward: Increasing the concentration of oxygen will correct the difficulty.

Hypoventilation. We have already described minute ventilation as the total amount of gas that moves in and out of the lungs in 1 minute; reduction in this minute ventilation may have predictable results. First,

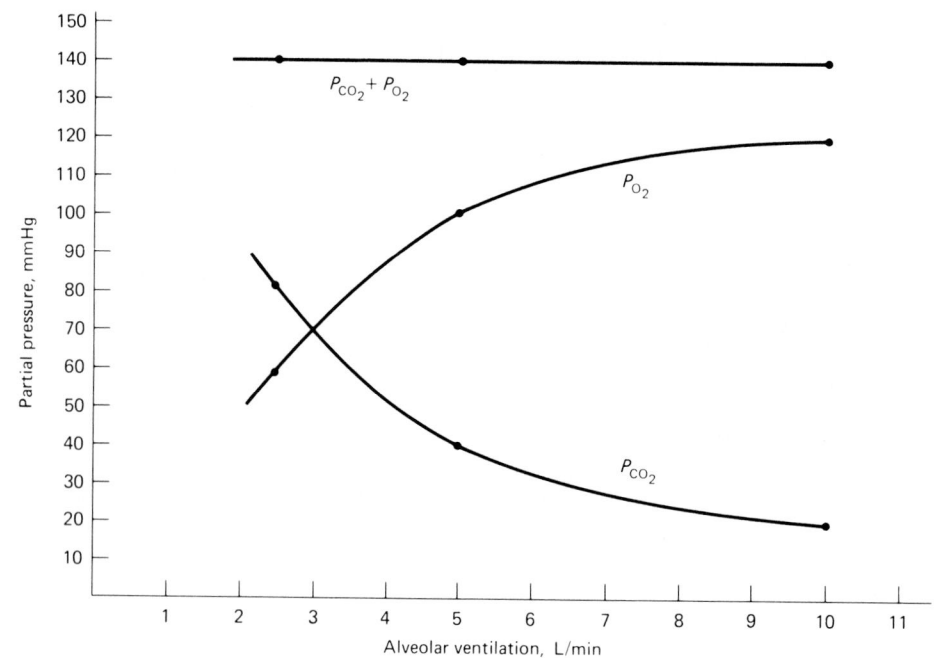

Figure 27-8   Normal alveolar ventilation. $\dot{V}A$ is approximately 5 L/min and corresponds to a P_{CO_2} of 40 mmHg (the P_{CO_2} here may be either PA_{CO_2} or Pa_{CO_2}, since carbon dioxide is readily soluble). Under these conditions, the normal P_{O_2} is approximately 100 mmHg (the P_{O_2} here is the PA_{O_2}, as Pa_{CO_2} is expected to be slightly lower, owing to the $D(A\text{-}a)O_2$ and oxygen's low solubility). Note that by halving $\dot{V}A$, the P_{CO_2} doubles, and the P_{O_2} falls accordingly, but the P_{CO_2} and P_{O_2} total remains close to 140 mmHg. Similarly, by increasing $\dot{V}A$, P_{CO_2} falls, and P_{O_2} rises, but the total remains close to 140 mmHg. Hypoxemia due solely to hypoventilation displays this feature. If other mechanisms of hypoxemia are operative, then the P_{CO_2} and Pa_{O_2} total will be less than the predicted 140 mmHg. (Compare this approximation to the $D(A\text{-}a)O_2$ calculation.)

since oxygen is continually removed from the alveoli into the blood, insufficient oxygen from the atmosphere will be delivered to renew the gas being absorbed in the alveoli, so that the partial pressure of oxygen within the alveoli will decrease. Secondly, carbon dioxide, which is normally removed from the alveolus by ventilation, will continue to accumulate (Figure 27-8). The hallmark of hypoxemia resulting from hypoventilation, then, is an elevated partial pressure of carbon dioxide. In fact, an elevated partial pressure of carbon dioxide may be used to define hypoventilation (see the box on p. 683).

A common clinical problem is presented by the patient who develops hypoxemia and an elevated P_{CO_2}. The question arises: Is this patient's hypoxemia all attributable to hypoventilation? To answer this question, one has simply to use the alveolar air equation.

As we have seen, aerohypoxia results from a decreased PI_{O_2}; hypoxemia from hypoventilation results from an increased P_{CO_2}. Other causes of hypoxemia result from an increase in the alveolar–arterial O_2 difference. A clinical example may illustrate this point.

Suppose a patient's blood gas studies show a P_{O_2} of 65 mmHg and a P_{CO_2} of 60 mmHg while breathing

room air. We wish to know if the hypoventilation, that is, the elevated P_{CO_2}, alone may account for the low P_{O_2}. To answer this question, we substitute into the alveolar air equation:

$$Pa_{O_2} = PI_{O_2} - \frac{Pa_{CO_2}}{R} - (A\text{-}a)O_2 \text{ difference}$$

We know that the PI_{O_2} is approximately 150 mmHg, and we assume that the $(A\text{-}a)O_2$ difference is normal, that is, about 10 mmHg. Substituting into the equation:

$$Pa_{O_2} = 150 - \frac{60}{0.8} - 10$$
$$Pa_{O_2} = 150 - 75 - 10$$
$$Pa_{O_2} = 65$$

Thus, we would predict that with a normal $(A\text{-}a)O_2$ difference and a normal inspired oxygen tension, an elevation in the P_{CO_2} to 60 mmHg would result in a P_{O_2} of 65 mmHg. We conclude that hypoventilation alone accounts for the observed blood gases.

Hypoventilation most often occurs in association with chronic obstructive pulmonary disease. Patients with bronchitis are especially prone to elevated P_{CO_2} from a variety of causes. First, because of increased

Hypoxemia Due to Hypoventilation

I. Pathophysiology:

    Hypoxemia always accompanied by hypercarbia ($\uparrow$ Pa_{CO_2})

II. Etiology:

    A. Hypoventilation with normal lungs:

        1. Damage to or depression of the brain's respiratory center:

            Head trauma

            Strokes

            CNS depressant drugs

        2. Neuromuscular defects in the respiratory apparatus:

            Myasthenia gravis

            Guillain-Barré syndrome

            Polio

            Spinal cord injuries

            Botulism

            Tetanus

            Neuromuscular blocking drugs

    B. Hypoventilation with abnormal lungs:

        1. Obstructive airways disease (asthma, chronic bronchitis, and emphysema)

        2. Loss of elasticity of pulmonary parenchyma (emphysema)

        3. Restrictive lung diseases (e.g., kyphoscoliosis, morbid obesity)

III. Diagnosis:

    By arterial blood gases

    Hypoxemia with a $\uparrow$ Pa_{CO_2} and a normal $D(A-a)O_2$

IV. Therapy:

    Improve oxygenation by increasing alveolar ventilation

    Specific therapy depending upon the specific etiology

airway resistance, they must work harder to maintain an adequate minute ventilation; if they cannot sustain the increased work of breathing, then they lower their minute ventilation, resulting in CO_2 retention. Second, the increased work of breathing may cause the respiratory muscles to produce increased quantities of CO_2, placing a greater demand on the minute ventilation. Finally, patients with a variety of lung diseases have an increased dead space-to-tidal volume ratio (V_D/V_T), leaving less available tidal volume for alveolar ventilation. Since a greater part of each breath ventilates dead space, there is less opportunity for CO_2 to be removed from the alveolus.

A diagnosis of hypoxemia from hypoventilation may indicate some problem other than intrinsic lung disease. In other words, there may be no problem in gas exchange of the lungs, but rather a problem in regulating ventilation to remove carbon dioxide. Hypoxemia from hypoventilation is treated by correcting the cause of the hypoventilation. In practice, this may involve reversal of sedative drugs, stimulation of respiration, or mechanical ventilatory support.

Diffusion Abnormalities. Although the process of diffusion is an important part of gas exchange within the lungs, it is unlikely that a simple derangement in the pathway for diffusion of oxygen is responsible for most instances of clinical hypoxemia. One of the reasons for this is that the lung has much reserve with respect to diffusion. Under normal conditions diffusion is complete by about 0.25 second, but the red blood cell spends another 0.5 second (0.75 second total) within the pulmonary capillary. In addition, the pathway for diffusion involving the alveolar–capillary interface is relatively short in the overall pathway, which includes the alveolar air space, endothelial and epithelial membranes, capillary plasma, and the interior of the red blood cell. In general, it is safe to say that diffusion impairment alone (as measured by the diffusing capacity for carbon monoxide) is of little significance in the hypoxemic, critically ill patient.

There are several conditions, however, under which diffusion impairment may significantly contribute to hypoxemia (see box on p. 684). One of these is exercise. During exercise cardiac output is greatly increased, so that the velocity of blood traversing the pulmonary capillaries is increased; therefore, the amount of time spent in a pulmonary capillary by each red blood cell is shortened. If some abnormality of diffusion is already present, then increases in cardiac output might result in insufficient time for equilibration within the pulmonary capillary (Figure 27-9). In fact, this is commonly seen when one measures arterial oxygen tension during exercise in patients with interstitial lung disease. Other causes of local increases in blood flow could also cause hypoxemia in the setting of a diffusion impairment, such as a pulmonary embolus. One might imagine that a pulmonary embolism in one portion of the lung might divert blood to another, resulting in a local increase in velocity of blood and insufficient time for equilibration.

Another situation in which diffusion impairment may play a role in clinically observed hypoxemia is in aerohypoxia. When inspired oxygen tensions are decreased, such as at high altitude or in a pressurized airplane cabin, then the gradient for gas diffusion may be decreased; the result would be a prolongation of the time needed to reach equilibrium within the pulmonary capillary, and hypoxemia due to a diffusion problem.

More commonly, processes that lead to marked diffusion abnormalities and thickening of the alveolar–capillary membrane also result in widespread ventilation–perfusion inequality. Most of the hypoxemia observed in these conditions, which include sar-

Hypoxemia Due to Diffusion Abnormalities

I. Pathophysiology:
   A. Increased diffusion pathway—prevents equilibrium between alveolar oxygen and pulmonary capillary blood, so that the blood exiting the capillary is hypoxemic
   B. Decreased diffusion area—destruction of membrane surface area available for diffusion and loss of pulmonary capillary bed

II. Etiology:
   A. Increased diffusion pathway:
      1. Accumulation of fluid—e.g., congestive heart failure and pulmonary edema
      2. Accumulation of collagen in the pulmonary interstitium—e.g., idiopathic pulmonary fibrosis, sarcoidosis, and collagen-vascular disease
   B. Decreased diffusion area:
      1. Pulmonary resection
      2. Destructive lung diseases—e.g., emphysema and obliterative pulmonary vascular diseases

III. Diagnosis:
   A. History and physical findings compatible with the primary diagnosis
   B. Laboratory:
      1. PFTs reveal decreased DL_{CO}, exercise arterial blood gas measurements reveal arterial desaturation
      2. Chest x-ray compatible with interstitial fibrosis, emphysema, etc.

IV. Treatment:
   A. Oxygen administration
   B. Evaluation of need for home oxygen therapy

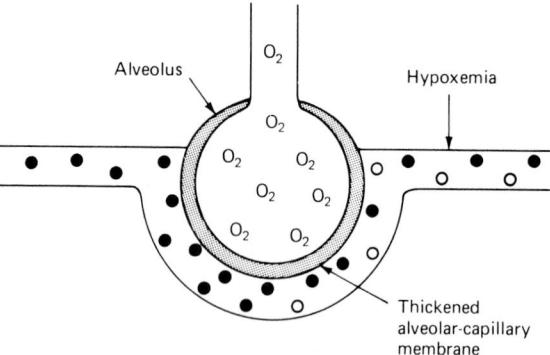

Figure 27-9 Schematic representation of a diffusion defect. Note the marked thickening of the alveolar-capillary membrane. Hypoxemia results because a red blood cell traversing this capillary does not have sufficient time to establish equilibrium with the alveolar oxygen.

coidosis; interstitial fibrosis; collagen vascular diseases of the lung, including scleroderma and lupus erythematosis; and other similar disorders, results from uneven distribution of ventilation and perfusion. The decreased diffusion capacity seen in emphysema may be a result of destruction of functioning alveoli, so that the interface between the alveolar and the pulmonary capillary surface is disrupted. This may be thought of as a decrease in the total area over which diffusion may occur. Nevertheless, hypoxemia in patients with emphysema is more a result of ventilation-perfusion inequality than diffusion problems.

Because it is technically difficult to measure the diffusing capacity for oxygen, clinical pulmonary function laboratories measure the diffusing capacity for carbon monoxide. In addition to the length and cross-sectional area, the pulmonary blood volume is another important factor that may affect the diffusing capacity for carbon monoxide. In fact, conditions that cause a high pulmonary blood volume result in a measurably increased diffusion capacity; conditions that cause a decreased pulmonary blood volume result in a decreased diffusing capacity. Furthermore, the hemoglobin concentration may also affect diffusing capacity. Elevation in hemoglobin results in an increased diffusing capacity, whereas anemia may result in a decreased diffusing capacity.

Hypoxemia due to impairment in diffusing capacity may be readily corrected by administration of 100% oxygen. This is because when pure oxygen is administered, the PO_2 in the alveoli rises to very high levels. Since one of the factors that determine diffusion is the partial pressure gradient, diffusion is greatly facilitated by increasing the partial pressure of oxygen in the alveolus to very high levels.

Ventilation–Perfusion Imbalance. This is the most common cause of hypoxemia. It is the main mechanism accounting for hypoxemia occurring in such diverse conditions as pulmonary embolism, chronic obstructive lung disease, pneumonia, and interstitial lung disease (see box on p. 685).

For the entire lung, the overall ventilation/perfusion ratio is about 0.8. This is because normal alveolar ventilation is approximately 4 L per minute, and normal pulmonary blood flow (cardiac output) is about 5 L per minute; thus, the ratio of ventilation to perfusion is 4 to 5, or 0.8. To reach this average, it is clear that the average ventilation/perfusion ratio for each of the lungs' 300 million alveoli is 0.8. In actuality, however, some alveoli have ventilation/perfusion ratios that are greater, and some have ventilation/perfusion ratios smaller than 0.8.

As you will recall from preceding sections, there is greater blood flow to the lung bases primarily because of the effect of gravity. Similarly, the greater propor-

Hypoxemia Due to $\dot{V}/\dot{Q}$ Mismatching

I. Pathophysiology:
- A. Low $\dot{V}/\dot{Q}$ units, with perfusion in excess of ventilation, result in hypoxemia because the blood traversing these units is not fully oxygenated.
- B. Low $\dot{V}/\dot{Q}$ units may result from partial obstruction of airways by foreign bodies, secretions, edema, inflammation, bronchospasm, etc.

II. Etiology:
- A. Obstructive airway disease:
    - Chronic bronchitis
    - Emphysema
    - Asthma
- B. Restrictive lung disease:
    - Obesity
    - Kyphoscoliosis
    - Interstitial lung disease
- C. Pulmonary vascular disease

III. Diagnosis:
- A. History—look for clues to the above diagnoses.
- B. Physical exam—abnormal chest wall motion, abnormal distribution of breath sounds, bronchospasm.
- C. Laboratory data—arterial blood gases with hypoxemia and a widened $D(A-a)O_2$; characteristic change on CXR, PFTs, and $\dot{V}/\dot{Q}$ scan.

IV. Treatment:
- A. Administer supplemental oxygen.
- B. Identify the underlying cause.
- C. Specifc therapy varies depending upon the specific etiology.

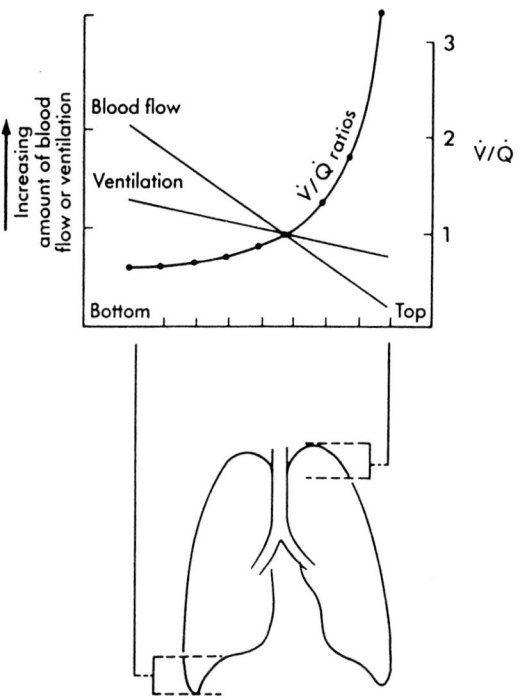

Figure 27-10   Changes in $\dot{V}/\dot{Q}$ ratios in the upright lung. At the top of the lung, ventilation is greater than perfusion, resulting in high $\dot{V}/\dot{Q}$ ratios. From the top to the bottom of the lung, there is a progressive increase in both ventilation and perfusion. Since blood flow increases more than ventilation, the $\dot{V}/\dot{Q}$ ratios decrease and are lowest at the bottom of the lung.

From Martin, L. (1987). *Pulmonary physiology in clinical practice: The essentials for patient care and evaluation.* St. Louis: Mosby–Year Book.

tion of ventilation is to the bases of the lungs. Figure 27-10 portrays this relationship and emphasizes another fact: Blood flow increases out of proportion to the increase in ventilation as one moves toward the dependent portions of the lung, so that the ventilation/perfusion ratio decreases at the lung bases.

Lung units with high ventilation/perfusion ratios are normally found at the apex of the lung; this is because blood flow is relatively low or even absent in the upright position at the apex of the lungs, whereas ventilation is only modestly reduced compared to the bases. Pulmonary capillary blood returning from apical portions of the lung has a high PO_2 and low PCO_2. However, such units have little effect on arterial blood gas findings, since blood flow is so low that they contribute a relatively small volume of blood toward the final composition of mixed arterial blood. In areas where ventilation is extremely high in proportion to blood flow, or where blood flow

is practically zero, physiological dead space is the result.

Figure 27-11A demonstrates the effect of units with high and low ventilation/perfusion ratios on the mixed arterial blood oxygen tension. Figure 27-11A portrays the normal situation in which ventilation and perfusion are matched. Figure 27-11B demonstrates a unit with a high ventilation/perfusion ratio resulting from a decreasing blood flow. Although this ventilation contributes to dead space ventilation, there is little effect on the arterial blood gas tension, because there is little blood flow from such units. Figure 27-11C demonstrates a unit with a low ventilation/perfusion ratio because of partial collapse of the airway. In this example, unoxygenated mixed venous blood enters the unit from the pulmonary artery and passes through the capillary without becoming saturated with oxygen. The result is that relatively unoxygenated blood from this low ventilation–perfusion unit mixes with the blood from the remainder of the lung, resulting in hypoxemia.

Abnormalities in ventilation/perfusion matching

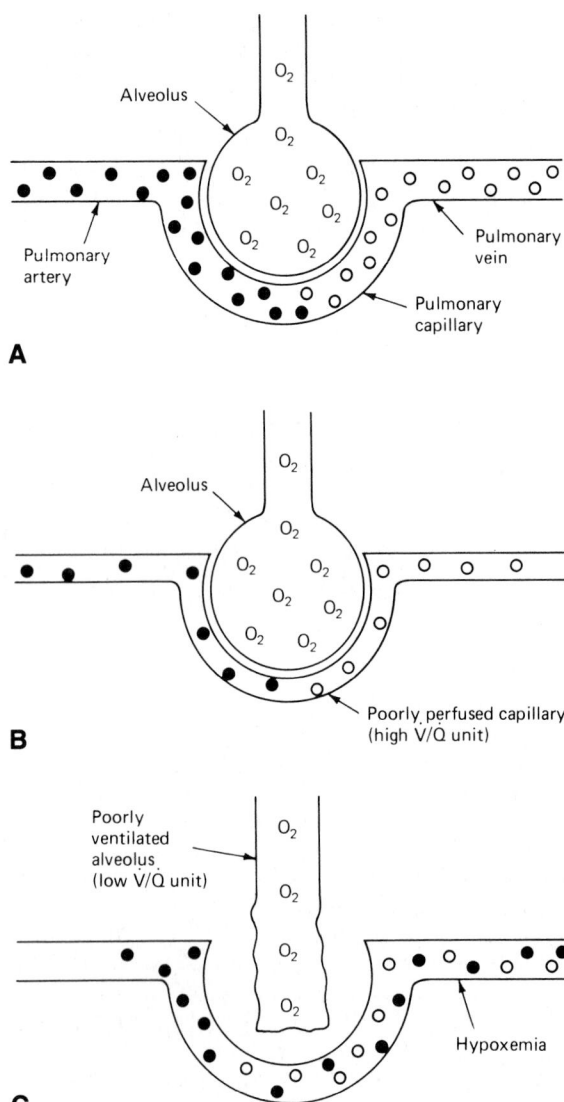

Figure 27-11   Schematic representation of a normal alveolar–capillary unit, *A*, a high $\dot{V}/\dot{Q}$ unit, *B* and a low $\dot{V}/\dot{Q}$ unit, *C*. See text for explanation. The illustration depicts oxygen (O_2) in the airways and the ventilated alveoli; deoxygenated venous blood in the pulmonary artery entering the alveolar–capillary unit (represented by the solid circles); and oxygenated blood (represented by the open circles) emerging from the alveolar–capillary unit and entering the pulmonary vein on the way back to the left side of the heart. Notice how low $\dot{V}/\dot{Q}$ units cause hypoxemia by failing to normally oxygenate all the blood that flows through these areas.

may occur from a variety of pulmonary diseases. Airway secretions, edema, or inflammation such as are seen in bronchitis or asthma will cause the alveoli distal to those airways to be underventilated. Interstitial lung diseases, including idiopathic pulmonary fibrosis, may be characterized by unevenness in ventilation/perfusion matching, resulting in hypoxemia.

Hypoxemia is a common finding in acute pulmo-

nary embolism, and usually results from ventilation–perfusion inequality. As one envisions an embolism lodged in a pulmonary artery, blood flow would be interrupted but ventilation would be maintained to that area of the lung. The result would seem to be an area of dead space. However, blood flow would now be directed away from one portion of the lung into another, with a reduction in the ventilation/perfusion ratio. Furthermore, the elaboration by the embolus of chemical mediators may result in changes in ventilation and perfusion ratios in the embolized areas of the lung.

If one analyzes the problem of hypoxemia in a patient with ventilation–perfusion imbalance by using the alveolar air equation, the result is that the a/A and PaO_2/FiO_2 ratios are decreased. A low ventilation/perfusion ratio is the major cause of the reduced (a/A) and PaO_2/FiO_2 ratios.

Hypoxemia related to ventilation–perfusion inequality is treated by the administration of oxygen. Since, by definition, there is still some ventilation present to areas of low ventilation/perfusion ratios, increasing the inspired oxygen tension will result in an increased partial pressure of oxygen in the alveolus. Thus, an improvement in oxygenation to the blood perfusing these units will be the result. Returning to Figure 27-11C we can see that if the partially collapsed alveolus were filled with a large number of O_2 molecules, then the unoxygenated blood entering this unit would become normally oxygenated, with relief of the hypoxemia.

Shunting

We have previously referred to shunting as one extreme of ventilation–perfusion imbalance, that is, the extreme where ventilation is zero. Thus, mixed venous blood is shunted past the lung without becoming oxygenated and is returned directly to the heart for mixing in the arterial tree, resulting in hypoxemia (see box on p. 687).

Shunts may be divided into anatomical and physiological types (Figure 27-12). An *anatomical shunt* is present in normal persons, comprising approximately 2% of the cardiac output. It is the result of the blood flow through bronchial, pleural, and thebesian veins that drain directly into the arterial circulation. Their presence is part of the reason that the alveolar–arterial oxygen gradient exists in normal subjects.

Pathological shunts may occur as congenital arteriovenous fistulas, from trauma, from cirrhosis of the liver, or in the heart. Tetralogy of Fallot and Eisenmenger's syndrome are examples of right-to-left shunting through the heart. Perhaps a more common form of intracardiac shunting may be observed in patients with high pulmonary artery pressures, in

Hypoxemia Due to Shunting (R→L)

I. Pathophysiology:
   A. Hypoxemia results from venous admixture when deoxygenated, mixed venous blood bypasses functional alveolar–capillary units and mixes with normally oxygenated blood in the systemic circulation.
   B. Shunts may be either anatomical or physiological.

II. Etiology:
   A. Anatomic shunts: blood bypasses the alveolar–capillary unit
      1. Normal anatomical shunts—bronchial, pleural, thebesian veins
      2. Intrapulmonary shunts—e.g., pulmonary AV fistulas
      3. Intracardiac shunts—e.g., tetralogy of Fallot, Eisenmenger's syndrome
      4. Other pathological shunts—e.g., shunts associated with neoplasms
   B. Physiological shunts: blood shunted through nonfunctional alveolar–capillary units
      1. Alveolar collapse—e.g., atelectasis, pneumothorax, hemothorax, pleural effusion
      2. Alveoli filled with a foreign material—e.g., pulmonary edema, pneumonias, ARDS

III. Diagnosis:
   A. Hypoxemia with a normal or decreased Pa_{CO_2} and a widened $D(A-a)O_2$
   B. 100% O_2 test: widened $D(A-a)O_2$ persists, shunt may be estimated

IV. Treatment:
   A. Oxygen administration has little effect.
   B. Proper therapy depends upon the specific etiology.

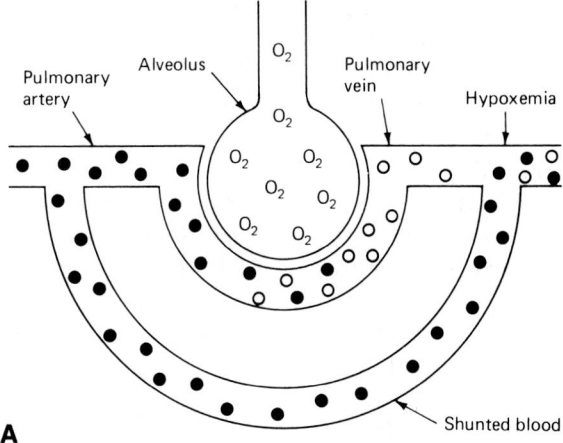

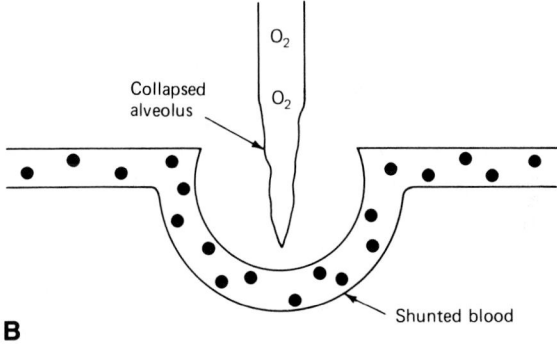

Figure 27-12 Schematic representation of the two main types of shunts. An example, *A*, of an anatomical shunt, illustrated as an anomalous communication between a pulmonary artery and a pulmonary vein. These shunts occur normally in the chest (bronchial, pleural, and thebesian veins) and are seen in a variety of pathological conditions. A physiological shunt, *B*, caused by $\dot{V}/\dot{Q}$ unit with intact blood flow but no ventilation because of a totally collapsed alveolus ($\dot{V}/\dot{Q}$ ratio of zero). In both instances, the shunted blood is not exposed to oxygen and, therefore, emerges from the lung as unaltered venous blood.

whom the foramen ovale may become patent and allow right atrial blood to pass directly into the left atrium, bypassing the lungs.

Physiological shunts occur at the alveolar level. They may occur, for example, as the result of total alveolar collapse in association with atelectasis, obstruction from a tumor, or from a pneumothorax or pleural effusion. Additionally, physiological shunting may occur in alveoli that are open but are filled with fluid, as in pulmonary edema. Pneumonia represents a condition in which alveolar spaces may be filled with inflammatory exudate, and ARDS may result in alveoli filled with proteinaceous material.

The degree of hypoxemia that results from a shunt depends upon two factors: the severity or degree of shunting (usually expressed as a percentage of the total cardiac output) and the oxygen content of the shunted blood. This latter point should be stressed further.

Let us take the example of a patient with pneumonia and sepsis. Because of the pneumonia, our patient has a 10% shunt. The following day, it is noted that the patient's cardiac output has fallen dramatically, and that her atrial hypoxemia has worsened even though there is no change on the x-ray and no change in administered oxygen. The explanation may be that, because of a decreased cardiac output, less oxygen has been delivered to the tissues. Since the oxygen consumption has remained the same, there is less oxygen remaining in the blood after consumption by the body; the result is a decreased mixed venous PO_2 or $S\bar{v}O_2$. As this mixed venous PO_2 and $S\bar{v}O_2$ with a lower oxygen tension and lower oxygen content moves through the 10% shunt, it mixes with arterial blood and worsens the degree of hypoxemia. In other words, even though the degree of shunting has not changed, the composition of the blood passing through the shunt has changed, altering the arterial oxygen tension.[10]

The shunt equation that was previously discussed may be used to calculate the degree of shunting. One needs to know the oxygen content of mixed venous blood, the oxygen content of arterial blood, and oxygen content of pulmonary capillary blood (one assumes that capillary PO_2 equals alveolar PO_2; the alveolar oxygen tension must be calculated from the alveolar air equation). A rough estimate of degree of shunting is provided by the following rule: With a patient breathing 100% oxygen for 15 minutes, an arterial blood gas sample is drawn, and the PO_2 in the sample is compared to the normal value of 650 mmHg. For every 50 mmHg that the patient's arterial PO_2 falls below the normal value of 650, a 2.5% shunt is present. For example, if the observed PO_2 under such conditions is 450 mmHg, then this represents 4 decrements of 50 mm below the target value of 650, corresponding to a $4 \times 2.5 \times 10\%$ shunt.

In contrast to diffusion abnormalities and ventilation–perfusion imbalances, the administration of oxygen would be expected to have no effect on shunt. This is because the shunted blood has no opportunity to come into contact with gas-exchanging tissues. Thus, although the administration of high oxygen levels would be expected to increase alveolar PO_2, shunted blood would be unaffected. Although increasing alveolar PO_2 may increase the saturation in blood draining normal units, there will be little overall effect on the arterial blood, since the blood is already 95% saturated with oxygen. Thus, the lack of response to administration of 100% oxygen defines the presence of anatomical or physiological shunt.

Since administration of oxygen has little effect on hypoxemia resulting from shunting, one must look to other methods for treating pulmonary shunts. The treatment of shunts lies in the treatment of their underlying causes. Thus, attention must be focused on proper treatment of pneumonia, pulmonary embolism, ARDS, or some other primary etiological factor.

Additionally, the effect of a shunt, though not the magnitude, may be decreased by ensuring adequate cardiac output and thereby preventing a decrease in the mixed venous PO_2. Positive end-expiratory pressure may also decrease the shunt by increasing lung volume and recruiting additional alveoli for gas exchange.

REFERENCES

1. Murray, J. F. (1986). *The normal lung* (2nd ed.). Philadelphia: Saunders.
2. West, J. B. (1990). Respiratory physiology—the essentials. Baltimore: Williams & Wilkins.
3. Milhorn, D. E., & Eldridge, F. L. (1986). Role of ventrolateral medulla in regulation of respiratory cardiovascular systems. *Journal of Applied Physiology, 332,* 1.
4. Russell, J. A., Ronco, J. J., Lockhat, D., et al. (1990). Oxygen delivery and consumption and ventricular preload are greater in survivors than in nonsurvivors of the adult respiratory distress syndrome. *American Review Respiratory Disease, 1441,* 659.
5. Shumaker, P. T., & Cain, S. M. (1987). The concept of a critical oxygen delivery. *Intensive Care Medicine, 13,* 223.
6. Cain, S. M. (1986). Assessment of tissue oxygenation. *Critical Care Clinics, 2,* 537.
7. Astiz, M. E., Rackow, E. C., Kaufman, B., et al. (1988). Relationship of oxygen delivery and mixed venous oxygenation to lactic acidosis in patients with sepsis and acute myocardial infarction. *Critical Care Medicine, 16,* 655-658.
8. Weg, J. G. (1991). Oxygen transport in adult respiratory distress syndrome and other acute circulatory problems: Relationship of oxygen delivery and oxygen consumption. *Critical Care Medicine, 19,* 650-657.
9. Ahrens, T. S., & Rutherford, K. (1987). The new pulmonary math: Applying the a/A ratio. *American Journal of Nursing, 87*(3), 337A-340H.
10. Cane, R. D., Shapiro, B. A., Templin, R., et al. (1988). Unreliability of oxygen tension–based indicies in reflecting intrapulmonary shunting in critically ill patients. *Critical Care Medicine, 16,* 1243.
11. Lorenz, A. (1989). Lactic acidosis: A nursing challenge. *Critical Care Nurse, 9,*(4), 64-73.

28

Pulmonary Data Acquisition

Thomas S. Ahrens

CHEST TOPOGRAPHY

A basic understanding of the topography of the chest is essential in assessing lung function, since a working knowledge of the location of organs within the chest and structures of the thorax is important in distinguishing between normal and abnormal findings. It is important to remember that there are normal variations in structure among individuals.[1]

The bony thorax consists of the sternum, ribs, and vertebral column. The sternum includes the manubrium, body, and xiphoid process. The manubriosternal junction is called the *angle of Louis*, a reference point for locating the second costal cartilage and for measuring central venous pressure. There are 12 pairs of ribs. The first seven are individually connected to the sternum. The eighth, ninth, and tenth ribs are joined together by a common cartilage and attached to the sternum. The eleventh and twelfth ribs are not connected to the sternum and are called *floating ribs* (Figure 28-1).

The lungs in midinspiration are located from the first rib anteriorly to approximately the seventh rib and from the first rib posteriorly to approximately the tenth vertebra or tenth intercostal space. This is demonstrated in Figure 28-2 by the lung diagram area with the vertical lines. The lung in deep inspiration (represented in the same figure by the dotted inferior lung area) descends approximately 2.5 cm anteriorly, 5 cm posteriorly, and 7.5 cm laterally to fill the pleural cavity and part of the costophrenic sinus.

The lungs are relatively symmetrical. The right lung has three lobes: upper, middle, and lower. The

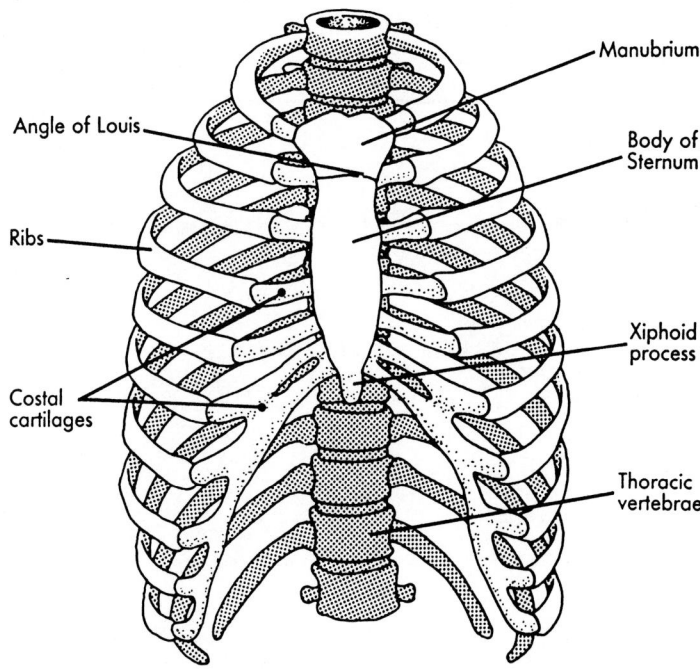

Figure 28-1 Chest cage. Ribs arch around from vertebral column joining sternum through cartilaginous extensions.

From Scanlan, C. L., Spearman, C. B., Sheldon, R. L., et al. (1990). *Egan's fundamentals of respiratory care* (5th ed.). St. Louis: Mosby–Year Book.

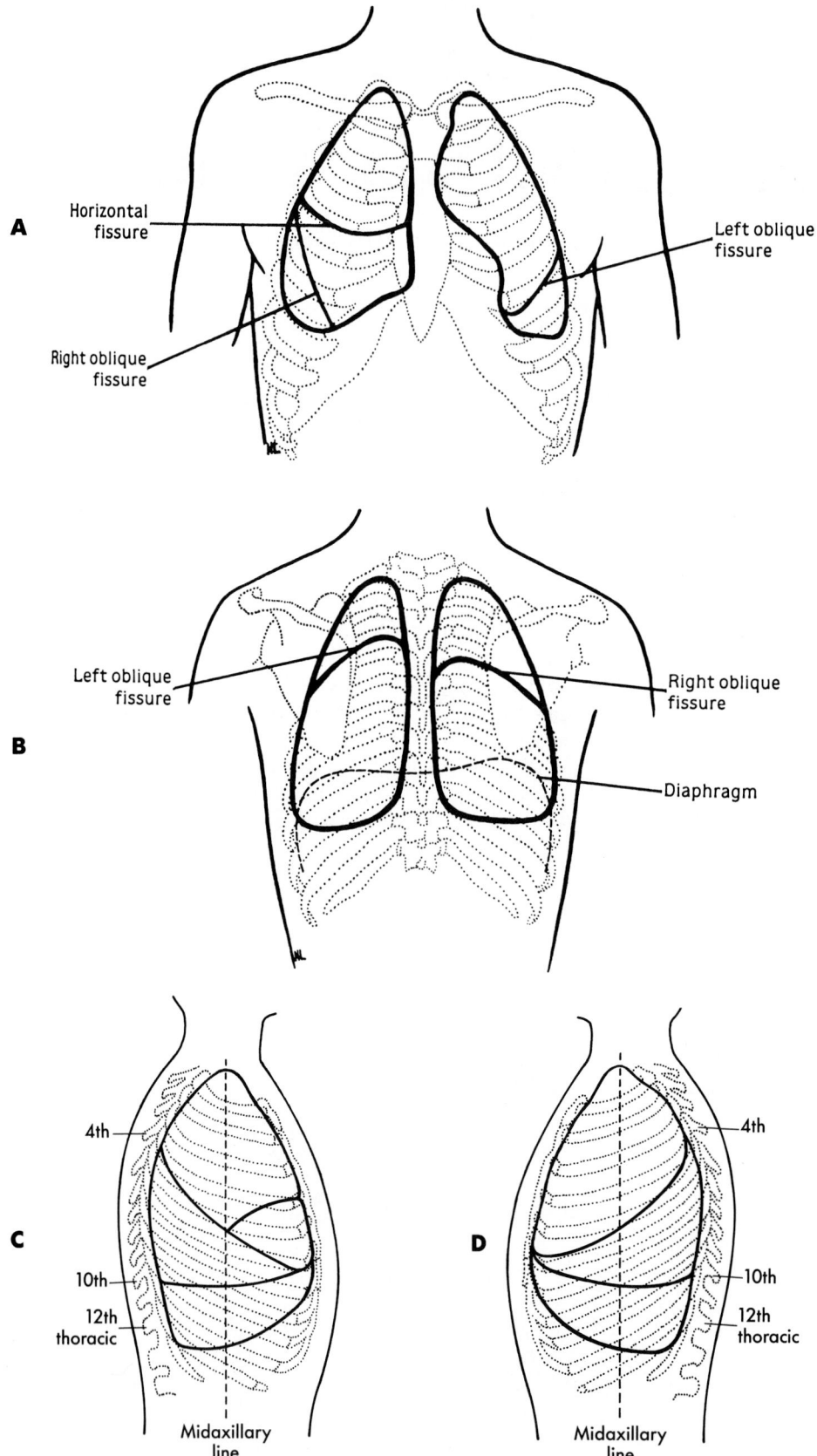

Figure 28-2   *A,* Topographic position of lung fissures on anterior chest. *B,* Topographic position of lung fissures on posterior chest. *C* and *D,* Lateral views of the fissures.

left lung has two lobes: the upper and lower; however, the lingular segment of its upper lobe corresponds to the middle lobe of the right lung. Each lobe is separated from the others by natural divisions of the lung called *lobar fissures*. The major or oblique fissure separates the upper and lower lobes bilaterally. The fissure is located posteriorly at approximately T3 or 4, extends to the fifth rib laterally at the midaxillary line, and around to the sixth intercostal space anteriorly. The minor or transverse fissure divides the mid-

dle and upper lobes of the right lung and is located at the fourth intercostal space anterior to the midaxillary line at the fifth rib (see Figure 28-2).

Each lung is further divided into segments. See Figure 28-3 for the distribution of the lobar bronchi, their segmental branches, and the pulmonary segments. The *mediastinum* contains such structures as the heart, trachea, major bronchi, lymphatic structures, great vessels, thymus, and esophagus. Figure 28-4 shows the surface projection of the heart and

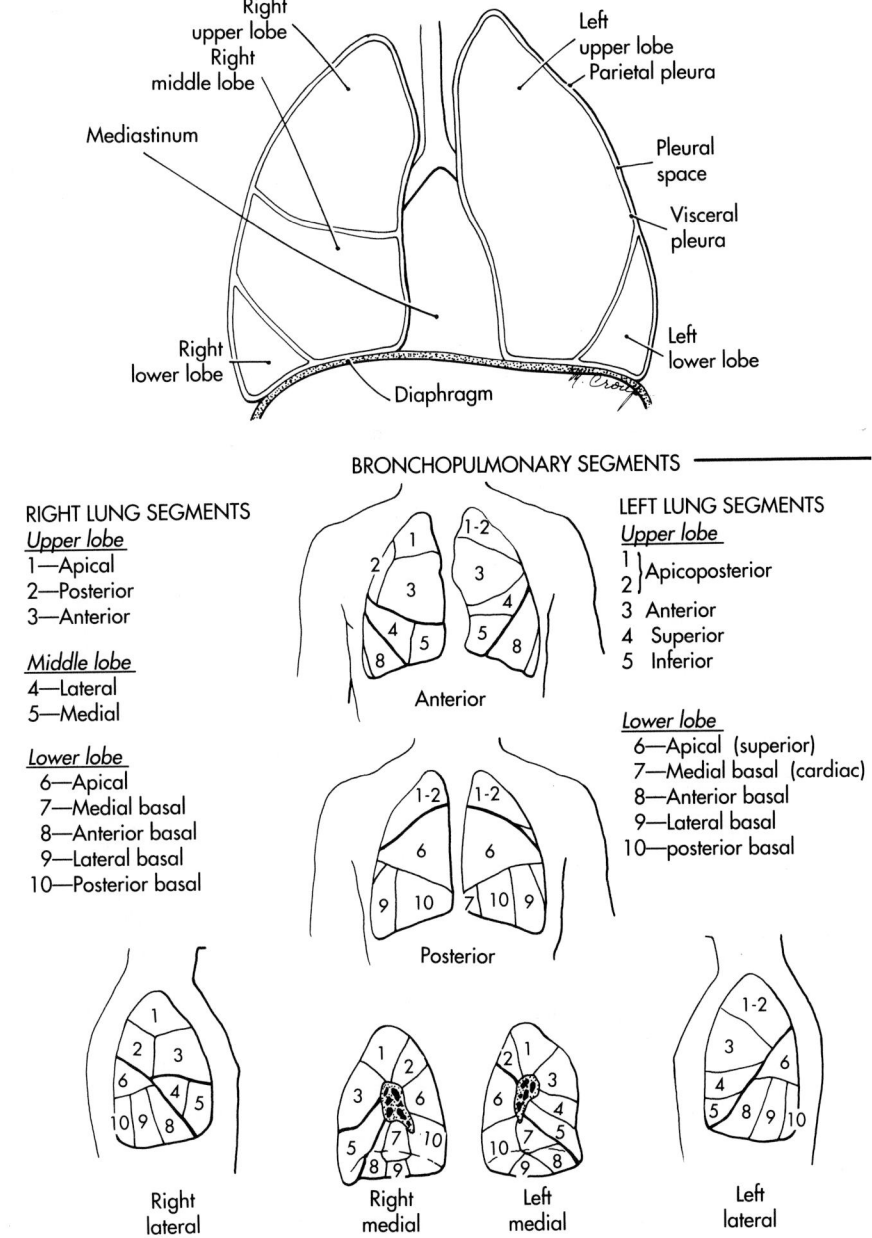

RIGHT LUNG SEGMENTS
Upper lobe
1—Apical
2—Posterior
3—Anterior

Middle lobe
4—Lateral
5—Medial

Lower lobe
6—Apical
7—Medial basal
8—Anterior basal
9—Lateral basal
10—Posterior basal

LEFT LUNG SEGMENTS
Upper lobe
1
2 } Apicoposterior
3 Anterior
4 Superior
5 Inferior

Lower lobe
6—Apical (superior)
7—Medial basal (cardiac)
8—Anterior basal
9—Lateral basal
10—posterior basal

Figure 28-3 Thoracic cavity and bronchopulmonary segments.

From Price, S. A., & Wilson, L. M. (1992). *Pathophysiology: Clinical concepts of disease processes* (4th ed.). St. Louis: Mosby–Year Book.

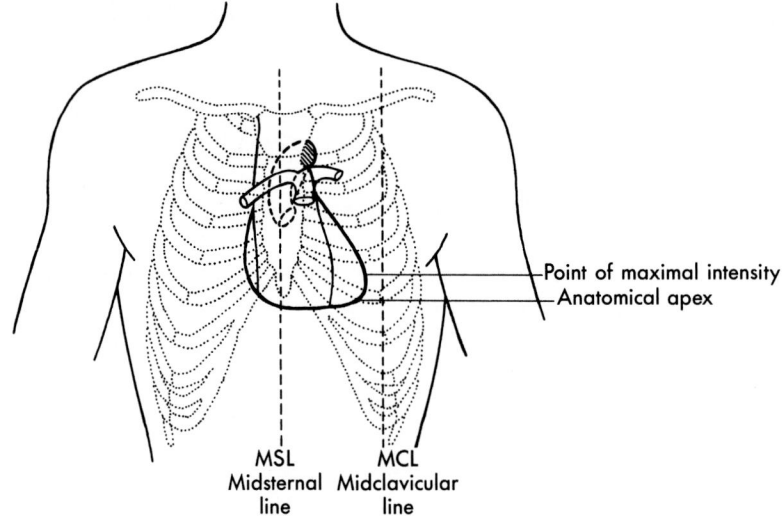

Figure 28-4 Surface projection of the heart and large vessels.

large vessels. The right border of the heart is normally located 1 cm lateral to the right sternal border edge. It extends from the third rib superiorly down to the fifth intercostal space inferiorly. The left border begins superiorly at the third rib or third intercostal space approximately 1 cm lateral to the left sternal edge. It continues down diagonally to the sixth rib, approximately 5 cm from the left sternal border or 7 to 9 cm from the midsternal line.

Other areas of note anatomically are the diaphragm, liver, stomach, and spleen, as shown in Figure 28-5. The diaphragm is a dome-shaped projection in the lower thoracic cage and is located (on mid-expiration) at the fifth intercostal space on the right hemithorax and the sixth rib on the left hemithorax. The liver lies beneath the right diaphragm, with the superior border located at about the fifth rib, and extends downward to the eleventh rib.

The stomach normally contains an air bubble of variable size that yields a percussion sound of tympany. The tympanic sound is usually heard in the upper portion of the stomach under the left diaphram and behind the sixth, seventh, or eighth intercostal space.

The spleen is located under the left lateral thoracic wall and extends down from the ninth to the eleventh rib.

PHYSICAL ASSESSMENT

The techniques used in assessing lung function are inspection, palpation, percussion, and auscultation. Adequate examination of the thorax and lungs can best be achieved with the patient in a sitting position and unclothed from the waist up, if possible. Adequate lighting is essential.

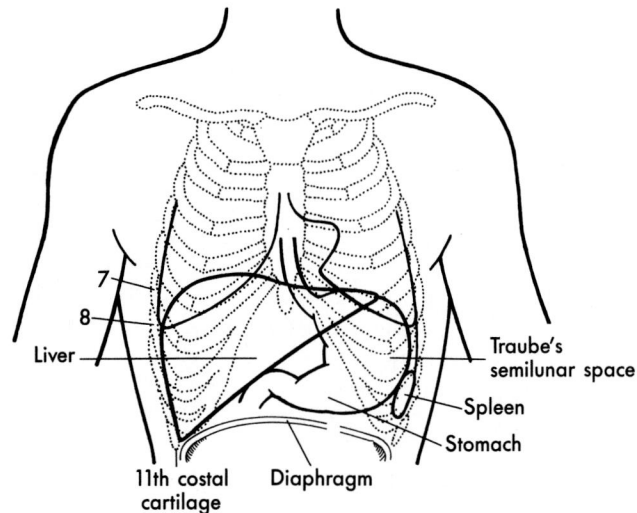

Figure 28-5 Surface projections of the diaphragm, liver, spleen, and stomach.

In critical care settings, optimal positioning is frequently difficult to achieve. Most patients have limited mobility and may not be able to sit upright. Even if they are able to sit upright, the examination should not take place immediately after sitting since the lungs are in the process of adjusting to a new position. Gravity-dependent crackles, for example, may change after sitting upright in comparison to lying down.

If the patient cannot sit for prolonged periods, the examination should be conducted with the patient in the most comfortable position, and the position used should be noted.

Inspection

The quality, rate, depth, and pattern of respiration should be observed visually. Men and children usually

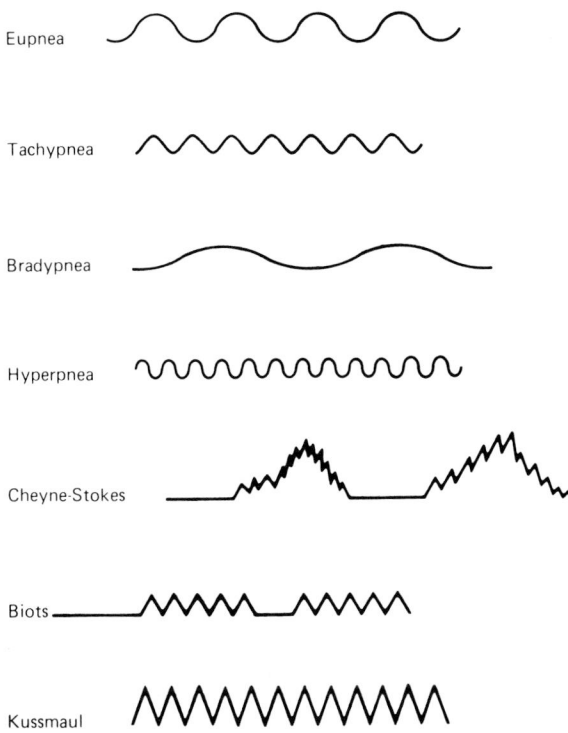

Eupnea

Tachypnea

Bradypnea

Hyperpnea

Cheyne-Stokes

Biots

Kussmaul

Figure 28-6   Abnormalities in rate and pattern of respiration.

breathe diaphragmatically, whereas women often breathe thoracically or costally. Patients who appear to have labored respiration should be observed for use of accessory muscles of respiration (sternocleidomastoids, trapezii) and also for supraclavicular retraction.

There are many abnormal patterns of respiration (Figure 28-6). The ratio of respiratory rate to heart rate is normally 1:4. Impedance to air inflow is frequently identified by the presence of laryngeal stridor or retraction of the intercostal spaces during inspiration. Prolonged expiratory times signify outflow impedance.

The thoracic cage is normally shaped like a truncated cone with the transverse diameter larger than the anteroposterior (AP) diameter. In addition, the thoracic spine is slightly convex and makes a perpendicular line with the floor. Abnormalities of size and contour are referred to as barrel chest, kyphosis, scoliosis, kyphoscoliosis, pigeon breast, and funnel breast. These deformities have the potential of interfering with thoracic expansion; therefore, the existence of such deformities should be noted.

Barrel chest is characteristically seen in patients with chronic emphysema. The AP and transverse diameters increase in size, giving a circular appearance to the cross section of the thorax. The constantly increased lung volume in emphysema is believed to cause the chest to become barreled; thus, little motion of the chest appears evident during the respiratory cycle.

Kyphosis is an exaggeration of the normal posterior convexity of the thoracic spine. The condition may be caused by senile osteoporosis, ankylosing spondylitis, Paget's disease, or acromegaly.

Scoliosis is a lateral curvature of the thoracic spine resulting in an S-shaped formation. This abnormality causes one shoulder to be raised and the hip to be lowered. This deformity may result from polio, congenital deformities, thoracoplasty, spinal tumor, or muscular disorders.

Kyphoscoliosis is a deformity in which both kyphosis and scoliosis are present. The significance of this clinical entity is that the thoracic cavity may be so reduced that there is a decreased lung volume, which may severely compromise respiratory and cardiac function.

Pigeon breast, or pectus carinatum, is an abnormality of the thorax usually caused by rickets in childhood. During the active process of rickets, the upper ribs soften and bend inward. This forces the sternum forward, increasing the AP diameter and diminishing the transverse diameter.

Funnel breast, or pectus excavatum, is the opposite of pigeon breast. This abnormality is usually congenital and results when the softened ribs of the lower part of the sternum retract inward toward the spine and create a depressed area near the infrasternal notch. This decreases the AP diameter.

In addition to observing the size and contour of the chest, the examiner should keep in mind other abnormalities such as pulsations indicative of an aortic aneurysm, precordial lift due to cardiac enlargement, and nodules or masses of the thoracic cage. The axillary area should be examined for inflammation of hair follicles and enlarged lymph nodes.

Palpation

Palpation usually begins with assessing for symmetrical expansion of the thoracic cage during respiration. The chest is palpated, using the palmar surface of the fingers, for sensitive or painful areas, subcutaneous crepitus (air bubbles under the skin), and tactile fremitus.

To assess *respiratory excursion,* have the patient sit upright. Stand facing the patient's back and grasp the patient's lateral rib cage, placing your thumbs at approximately the level of and parallel to the tenth ribs. Then draw both hands medially, pulling the underlying skin with them to position loose skin folds between the thumbs and spine. Ask the patient to inhale deeply. Observe the outward movement of your thumbs for range and symmetry of thoracic expansion. The technique can be modified for the bedfast patient by placing the hands over the anterior surface of the thorax at the level of the lower margin of the sternum and performing the same maneuver but pulling the hands medially with the thumbs positioned together in the midline of the sternum and then instructing the patient to inhale deeply.

Tactile fremitus is the palpable vibration transmitted through the bronchopulmonary system to the chest wall when the patient makes a deep vocal sound. Using one hand over symmetrical areas or both hands over corresponding areas, place the palmar aspects of the fingers or the ulnar aspect of the hand on the chest and ask the patient to say in a deep voice, "ninety-nine" or "one, two, three." A vibratory sensation should normally be felt over lung fields.

The sensation of tactile fremitus is usually uniform over most areas of the lung. When the right main stem bronchus is closer to the chest wall, however, fremitus is increased. Fremitus is also increased in conditions of lung consolidation such as pneumonia. Decreased fremitus occurs when the bronchus is obstructed or the pleural space is occupied by fluid, air, or solid tissue, as in pleural effusion, pneumothorax, or fibrosis.

Two other areas are important in palpation as related to lung function: determining the alignment of the trachea, since misalignment denotes a shifted mediastinum; and detecting palpable lymph nodes in the axillary and supraclavicular areas, which indicate localized or generalized inflammation or malignant disease.

To palpate for tracheal alignment, ask the patient to position the head in a relaxed neutral position. Locate the trachea in the suprasternal notch. Normally, it should be in the midline, with the spaces on each side of the trachea equidistant. Tracheal deviations usually result from masses in the neck or mediastinum or from pleural or pulmonary anomalies.

Percussion

Percussion of the chest provides further information regarding the status of lung function. The technique of manual percussion over the thorax is the same as that used for percussion over other body parts, as are the names given to characteristic percussion sounds. The noisy environment of a busy intensive care unit may make this technique of physical assessment less useful than others.

In the thoracic area, a practitioner may normally elicit a variety of sounds due to the presence of different structures making up the bony thorax and various organs located within the thoracic cage (Table 28-1). Normal lung tissue, however, produces only a resonant percussion sound.

The procedure for percussion may start with the apices and progress to the posterior and lateral thorax moving from top to bottom in a systematic manner. If percussion of the anterior chest seems warranted, keep in mind the location of the heart, mediastinum, and liver.

For percussion of the apices, the patient should be in a sitting position facing the examiner. Compare the supraclavicular areas on contralateral sides and note whether the areas are symmetrical.

For percussion of the posterior thorax, the patient is positioned with arms folded over the chest; the shoulders are bent foward in a sitting position if possible. A patient who cannot sit is placed in a left then right lateral decubitus position (remember that the lying position produces dullness in some areas because of the compression of the thorax against the mattress and the body weight itself).

The procedure, regardless of position, begins at the top of each shoulder, an area overlying each lung apex. Progress downward and percuss about a 5-cm area at a time, moving to symmetrical areas of each side of the thorax posteriorly and laterally. Avoid the scapular areas and spinal column. The lateral chest is percussed with the patient's arm positioned over the head.

TABLE 28-1 **Percussion Sounds**

Note	Pitch	Intensity	Quality	Duration	Density	Examples of Location
Tympany	Very high	High	Musical	Long	More air than solid tissue	Gastric air bubble
Hyperresonance	Low	Moderately high	Slightly musical	Moderately long	More air than solid tissue	Emphysematous lung
Resonance	Moderately low	Moderate	Nonmusical	Moderate	Normal air to tissue ratio	Normal lung
Dull	Moderately high	Low	Nonmusical, muffled	Short	Fluid plus solid tissue	Liver, heart
Flat	High	Low	Soft thud	Short	Solid tissue	Bone, thigh

To measure diaphragmatic excursion, ask the patient to inspire fully and hold the breath. Percuss along the midscapular line bilaterally from top to bottom until the percussion note changes from resonant to dull. Mark the point of transition bilaterally. Then have the patient exhale fully and hold the breath. Percuss upward from the transition line to a resonant percussion note and mark the point. Measure the excursion distance between the two lines. The normal diaphragm will move bilaterally from 3 to 5 cm. A 1-cm difference in bilateral movement may indicate an abnormality.

Percussion may be very useful in the identification of a pneumothorax. The air trapped by the pneumothorax is readily heard as a tympanic or resonant noise in comparison to other areas.

Auscultation

Auscultation of the lung is a means by which the practitioner can determine the effectiveness of airflow through the airways of the lungs. The origin of breath sounds is still being debated; however, it is generally believed that breath sounds are produced by air moving through the airways while the sound is transmitted out through the chest wall. Solid matter conducts sound waves better than air. Sounds transmitted through consolidated areas of the chest wall sound louder than normal. The chest sounds of an emphysematous patient will normally be very faint, whereas a patient with a pneumonia will have increased sounds over the affected area.

Auscultation of the lungs requires a quiet environment. The patient should be seated upright in a relaxed position; however, this is often difficult in a critical care setting. Therefore, assistance may be needed to support the patient in a sitting position, or the patient may have to remain in a recumbent position and be turned to the left and right lateral positions. Regardless of the position, the lungs are auscultated over each segment from top to bottom, anteriorly, posteriorly, and laterally. Instruct the patient to breathe with the mouth open. If the patient is receiving mechanical ventilation, listen during the ventilation breath. Breathing should be normal but deep enough to move secretions, if any are present. With the diaphragm of the stethoscope pressed snugly against the skin, listen over symmetrical areas of the chest. There are three types of sounds to listen for when auscultating the lungs: breath sounds, voice sounds, and adventitious or extra sounds. Patients who are receiving mechanical ventilation should be removed from the ventilator and given gentle bag ventilation by hand to decrease extraneous noise. Nasogastric suction and chest tube suction should be temporarily clamped, whenever possible, to decrease extraneous noise.

Breath Sounds

Three types of breath sounds are heard over the normal lung, depending on the area that is being auscultated: vesicular, bronchial or tubular, and bronchovesicular. Breath sounds can be described diagrammatically, as shown in Figures 28-7 and 28-8. The upstroke denotes inspiration, and the downstroke denotes expiration. The thickness of the line represents the intensity of the sound, and the height of the angle represents the pitch.

Vesicular breath sounds are soft, low-pitched sounds normally heard over most of the lung but

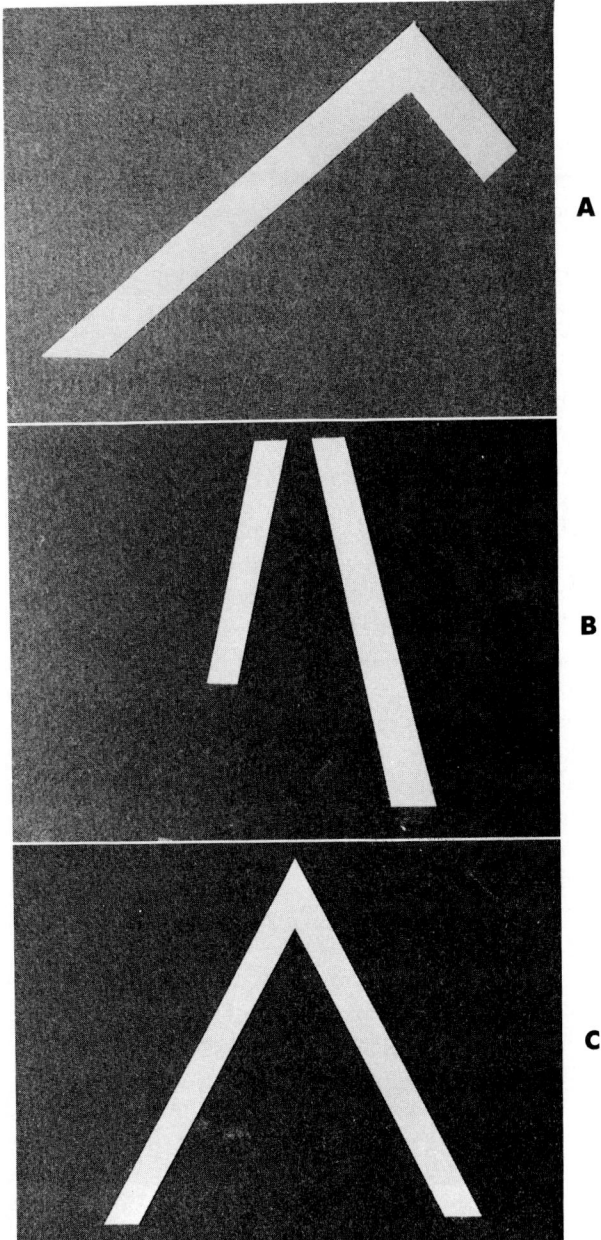

A

B

C

Figure 28-7 *A,* Vesicular breath sounds. *B,* Bronchial breath sounds. *C,* Bronchovesicular breath sounds.

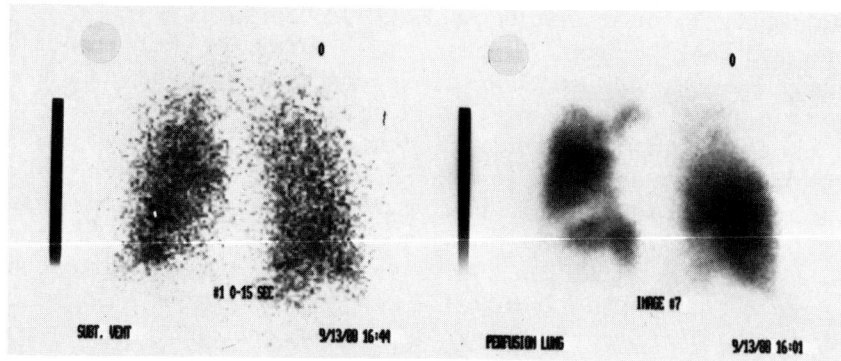

Figure 28-8   Abnormal ventilation/perfusion scan. The ventilation study (left scan) demonstrates bilateral lung filling without gross defects; however, the perfusion scan (right scan) shows multiple subsegmental perfusion defects of both lungs. These findings are highly suggestive of pulmonary emboli.

From Wilkins, R. L., Sheldon, R. L., & Krider, S. J. (1990). *Clinical assessment in respiratory care* (2nd ed.). St. Louis: Mosby—Year Book.

heard best over the lower posterior and axillary region of the chest. The inspiratory phase is most easily heard because of the increased inspiratory flow rate. The expiratory phase is short (approximately one third of the inspiratory phase) and faint because the expiratory flow is initially great, then diminishes through the expiratory cycle (see Figure 28-7).

Bronchial or *tubular* breath sounds are usually coarse, high-pitched sounds heard normally over the trachea. The expiratory phase is longer in duration than the inspiratory phase, and they are separated by a silent interval or gap. This type of sound heard elsewhere over lung tissue is indicative of extensive consolidative disease. The bronchioles are patent and are surrounded by consolidated lung tissue.

Bronchiovesicular breath sounds are a combination of bronchial and vesicular breath sounds. They are normally of moderate pitch and intensity. The inspiratory and expiratory phases are of equal duration and are normally heard near the major bronchi, below the clavicles, and between the scapulae, especially on the right. If bronchovesicular sounds are present elsewhere in the chest, early pulmonary disease should be suspected.

Voice Sounds

The types of voice sounds that are useful in diagnosing lung disease, primarily consolidation of lung tissue, are bronchophony, whispering pectoriloquy, and egophony.

Bronchophony is the transmission of louder and clearer voice sounds than one normally hears when auscultating the lungs. Listen with the stethoscope while the patient says "one, two, three" or "ninety-nine." The presence of bronchophony is indicative of consolidation.

Whispering pectoriloquy is tested for by having the patient whisper a combination of words such as "one, two, three." If there is consolidation, the whisper is clearly heard through a stethoscope. If there is no consolidation, the whisper is not heard.

Egophony is tested for by having the patient say aloud "eee." If the sound of the spoken *E* takes on a nasal quality and sounds like *A* (*E* to *A* change), consolidation is usually present.

Adventitious Sounds

Adventitious sounds are extra sounds heard in addition to breath sounds. There are basically two types of adventitious sounds: wheezes and crackles. Pleural friction rubs are an extrapulmonary sound but can be considered as an adventitious sound.

Wheezes are whistling sounds produced by airflow through narrowed tubes, resulting in severe turbulence. Wheezes occur primarily on expiration; however, with severe bronchial constriction they may be heard on inspiration.

Wheezes are referred to as a continuous sound. Wheezes can be high- or low-pitched. Low-pitched wheezes are sometimes referred to as rhonchi. Avoiding terms like rhonchi is helpful in improving communication about the meaning of a particular lung sound.

Crackles are short, discrete, popping or crackling sounds produced in the small airways. The term *rales* is sometimes used to describe crackles.[2] This term is confusing and should be avoided. Crackles are possibly due to excessive fluid in the lung or weakened airway wall strength. This difference in the origin of the crackle may be important. If the crackle is due to weakened wall strength, fluid removal is unimportant. Consequently, administering diuretics for all crackles is not appropriate.

Cardiac disease is more likely to produce excessive

TABLE 28-2   Common Respiratory Problems of Critically Ill Patients

Disease	Tactile Fremitus	Percussion	Auscultation
Consolidation (e.g., pneumonia)	Increased	Dull	Bronchial breath sounds, crackles, bronchophony, egophony, whispered pectoriloquy
Bronchitis	Normal	Resonant	Normal to decreased breath sounds, wheezes
Emphysema	Decreased	Hyperresonant	Decreased intensity of breath sounds, usually with prolonged expiration
Asthma (severe attack)	Normal to decreased	Resonant to hyperresonant	Wheezes
Pulmonary edema	Normal	Resonant	Crackles at lung bases, possibly wheezes
Pleural effusion	Absent	Dull to flat	Decreased to absent breath sounds, bronchial breath sounds and bronchophony, egophony, and whispering pectoriloquy above the effusion over the area of compressed lung
Pneumothorax	Decreased	Hyperresonant	Absent breath sounds
Atelectasis	Absent	Flat	Decreased to absent breath sounds

fluid-type crackles whereas pulmonary disease is more likely to produce crackles not responsive to fluid removal.

Pleural friction rubs are creaking, leathery, loud, dry, coarse sounds indicative of pleural irritation. They are produced by the rubbing of the inflamed surfaces of two pleural layers against one another during respiration. Pleural friction rubs are heard at the end of inspiration and the beginning of expiration. They are heard best over the lower lateral aspects of the rib cage, since this area has the greatest amount of pleural movement during breathing.

Table 28-2 presents common respiratory problems of patients in critical care units.

DIAGNOSTIC PROCEDURES
Chest X-ray

Serial chest x-rays are used to monitor progression of disease and response to treatment. Portable equipment is usually used for critically ill patients because of the difficulties associated with transportation to the radiology suite. It is important to note that chest films made with portable equipment vary in their degree of sharpness and magnification and are not considered to be images of highest quality.

Immediately prior to obtaining a chest x-ray, the critical care nurse should remove metallic objects which are in contact with the patient's thorax such as jewelry, ECG leads, safety pins, and snaps on the patient's gown and attempt to position ventilator tubing so that it does not obscure important views of the chest. The most common view obtained in patients on bed rest is the posteroanterior, in which the x-ray beam is directed toward the patient, with the film plate behind the spine.[3]

Chest x-rays can detect common pulmonary disorders as well as anatomical abnormalities. They assist in determining the location and size of a lesion, assessing pulmonary status, and verifying proper placement of an endotracheal tube or central venous catheter. It is possible for serial films to assist in the differentiation of pulmonary edema, parenchymal inflammation, and infection.

In the normal radiograph, the trachea has a tube-like appearance and is visible in the midline of the anterior mediastinal cavity. The heart is visible in the anterior left mediastinal cavity and should occupy approximately one third of the thoracic cavity. The clavicle and ribs should be evaluated for fractures or misalignment if trauma is suspected. The bronchi are usually not clearly visible but have a tubelike appearance if surrounded by consolidated tissue. The parenchyma of the lungs is usually not visible throughout the lung fields, except for fine white lines radiating from the hilum which represent the pulmonary vascular tree. The height of the diaphragm should be compared (the right side is commonly 1 to 2 cm higher than the left). The costaphrenic angles should be well defined. Changes in the appearance of the chest x-rays over time tend to be much more significant in monitoring the critically ill patient than any single film.

Pulmonary Function Tests

Pulmonary function tests (PFT) evaluate lung mechanics by measuring the volume of air a patient is able to move in and out during ventilation and estimating several lung capacities. It is essential that the patient be able to participate volitionally in a test in order to complete the full set of studies. This is fre-

TABLE 28-3 Pulmonary Function Parameters Commonly Used in Critical Care Unit

Measurement of Pulmonary Function	Implications
Tidal volume (V_T): Amount of air inhaled or exhaled during normal tidal breathing	Decreases may indicate patient fatigue or onset of parenchymal process
Minute volume (V_E): Total amount of gas breathed per minute	May indicate work of breathing, onset of metabolic rate changes, or parenchymal process
Inspiratory capacity (IC): Amount of air that can be inhaled after a normal exhalation	Decreased IC indicates restrictive lung disease; one of the parameters used to determine patient's possiblity of being weaned from mechanical ventilation
Functional residual capacity (FRC): Amount of air remaining in the lungs after a normal or tidal exhalation. This is the combined value of the expiratory reserve volume (ERV); amount of air that can be exhaled after a normal exhalation and residual volume (RV); amount of gas remaining in the lungs at all times	Decreased FRC is the hallmark of adult respiratory distress syndrome (ARDS). Increased FRC reflects overdistention of the lungs, which may result from chronic obstructive pulmonary disease (COPD) or excessive use of positive end-expiratory pressure
Forced vital capacity (FVC): Dynamic measure of amount of gas exhaled after maximal inspiration	Decreased FVC indicates resistance to expiratory flow as in COPD
Forced expiratory volume (FEV): Amount of air exhaled in the first, second, and third second of FEV maneuver, as indicated by number, e.g., FEV_1	May be prolonged in COPD. Improved FEV_1 following administration of beta blockers may indicate a degree of bronchospasm that prohibits further administration of the drugs

quently not possible in the critically ill patient, and selected subtests may have to suffice.

PFTs help to determine whether an abnormality is functional or restrictive, to assess the level of dysfunction, and to assess the effectiveness of specific medications such as bronchodilators, as well as the side effects of other drugs such as beta blockers. They also help to assess the timeliness of weaning from mechanical ventilation. A full set of PFTs consists of spirometry, gas diffusion, and diffusing capacity (Table 28-3).

Ventilation/Perfusion Scanning

These two complementary tests involve the inhalation and the intravenous injection, respectively, of a radiopaque material. Both produce images of the agent's distribution throughout the lung, revealing abnormal patterns of ventilation or perfusion. Although these tests are useful in a variety of disorders, they are most commonly used to diagnose pulmonary emboli in the critically ill patient. The results are expressed in terms of probability, and more invasive tests such as pulmonary angiography can validate the diagnosis (see Figure 28-8).

Pulmonary Angiography

This invasive test involves x-ray examination of the pulmonary circulation after injection of a radiopaque iodine contrast material through a catheter inserted into the pulmonary artery or one of its branches. It allows visualization of the pulmonary

vascular bed and measurement of pressures at various sites during catheter insertion, as well as determination of cardiac output and pulmonary vascular resistance. Because of the attendant risks, this test is restricted to identifying defects in pulmonary vascular perfusion such as thrombi, aneurysms, and blood vessel displacement. It is used to confirm symptomatic pulmonary embolism (Figure 28-9) when lung scans show no abnormalities, especially in the patient for whom anticoagulant therapy carries a particularly high risk. It also assists in the preoperative evaluation of pulmonary circulation in patients with congenital heart disease. Complications of pulmonary angiography include allergic reaction, arterial occlusion, ventricular arrhythmias, and myocardial perforation.

Direct Laryngoscopy

This technique allows direct visualization of the larynx through the use of a fiberoptic laryngoscope passed through the mouth or nose and pharynx. The larynx is observed at rest and during phonation. Laryngoscopy is performed to detect lesions, strictures, or foreign bodies of the larynx. It may also be used in conjunction with a biopsy to distinguish laryngeal edema from response to radiation or tumor and to examine the condition of the larynx following prolonged endotracheal intubation.

Bronchoscopy

The direct visualization of the trachea and tracheobronchial tree is now commonly performed by

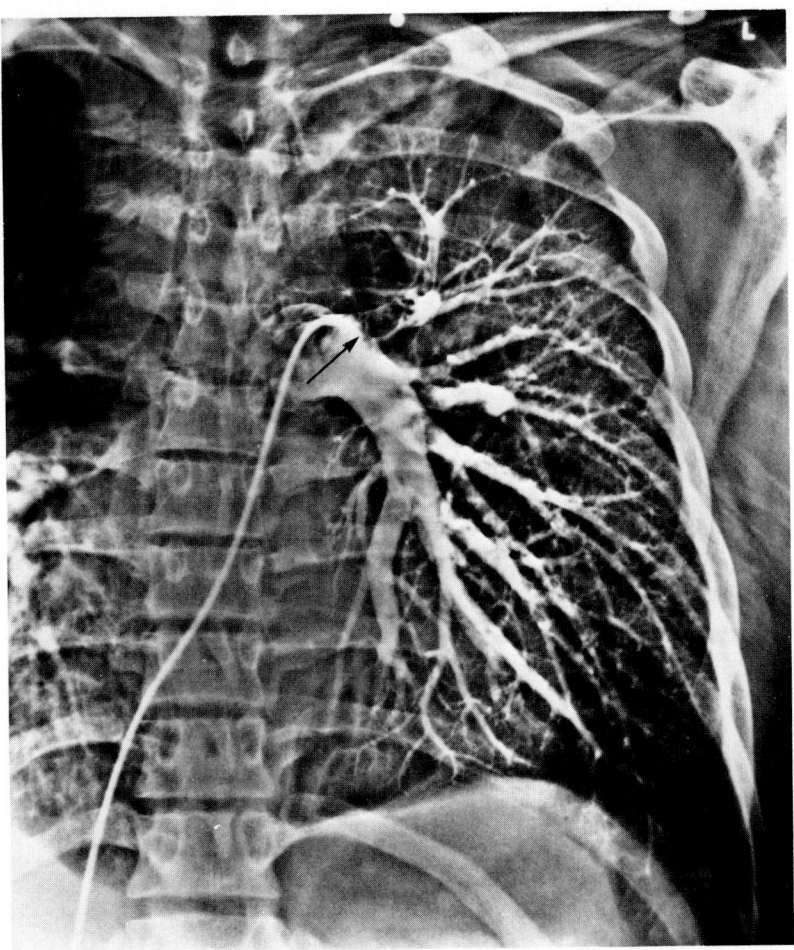

Figure 28-9   Abnormal pulmonary angiogram. The radiograph demonstrates a large clot in the pulmonary vascular tree. A small amount of dye was able to slip around the clot and outline the embolus (arrow).
From Wilkins, R. L., Sheldon, R. L., & Krider, S. J. (1990). *Clinical assessment in respiratory care* (2nd ed.). St. Louis: Mosby–Year Book.

the fiberoptic bronchoscope. Its diagnostic value lies in the visual examination and identification of potential tumor, obstruction, or foreign body in the tracheobronchial tree, which aids in the diagnosis of carcinoma, interstitial pulmonary disease, and pulmonary infection by allowing procurement of a specimen for microbiological and cytological examination. It can also assist in locating a bleeding site or in determining the cause of a poorly functioning intubation.

Therapeutic benefits of a bronchoscopy include removal of a foreign body or mucus plug, treatment of atelectasis, drainage of an abscess, and improvement in bronchial clearance.[4] Bronchoscopic findings are always correlated with radiographic, cytological, and clinical data.

End-tidal Carbon Dioxide Monitoring (PetCO₂)

PetCO₂ monitoring has been advocated for use in clinical settings because of its correlation with arterial CO₂ (PaCO₂) values. PetCO₂ is correlated with PaCO₂ because of the method by which carbon dioxide is eliminated during expiration. Initial expiration contains gas primarily from the major airways and is therefore low in carbon dioxide. As airflow becomes more heavily influenced by lower airways, carbon dioxide levels increase. Theoretically, at the end of expiration, gases are coming from alveolar levels (Figure 28-10). Alveolar carbon dioxide levels determine arterial carbon dioxide values. Therefore, end-expiration (end-tidal) carbon dioxide values approximate arterial carbon dioxide values.[5]

In normal persons, the correlation with PetCO₂ and PaCO₂ is relatively good. The PetCO₂ almost always is slightly less (about 1 to 4 mmHg) than PaCO₂ values. In some disease states, particularly those with large dead space, the correlation is less accurate. To use PetCO₂ values safely, the clinician must first establish that a good correlation exists between PetCO₂ and PaCO₂. If this correlation is present, then the

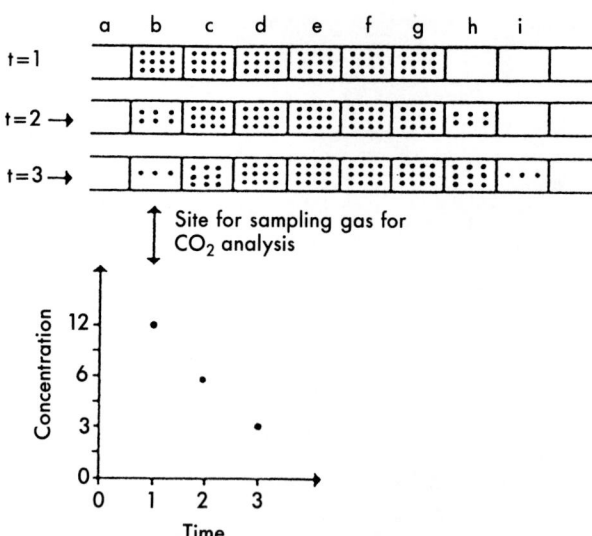

Figure 28-10 Movement of carbon dioxide in a tube. Diagrammatic representation of how a capnogram is generated. At time t = 1, a tube consisting of segments *a* through *i* contains carbon dioxide in segments *b* through *g*. At time t = 2, half a segment of fresh gas is pushed into segment *a*, half of which is pushed into segment *b*, and so on. The process is repeated at time t = 3. Carbon dioxide concentration is analyzed in segment *b* at times t = 1, t = 2, and t = 3 and the data are plotted. Connecting the points of the plot with a line generates a capnogram.

From Gravenstein, J. S., Paulus, D. A., & Hayes, T. J. (1989). *Capnography in clinical practice.* Boston: Butterworths.

$PetCO_2$ can be used as an indicator of changing $PaCO_2$ values. However, the $PaCO_2-PetCO_2$ difference may be the most useful application of $PetCO_2$. The greater the $PaCO_2-PetCO_2$ difference, the larger the physiological dead space in the lungs. Since dead space can change, either through a reduction (improvement) or enlargement (worsening), monitoring the $PaCO_2-PetCO_2$ difference may be an improved clinical indicator of pulmonary function.

Pulse Oximetry (SpO_2)

SpO_2 allows for the noninvasive estimation of oxyhemoglobin in the arteries (SaO_2). SpO_2 use has increased to the point where it is used on almost all critically ill patients with pulmonary involvement. SpO_2 values usually overestimate SaO_2 values by about 2% to 5%, depending on the degree of skin pigmentation and abnormal hemoglobin. However, as long as normal levels of dysfunctional hemoglobin (such as carboxyhemoglobin) are present, SpO_2 values are usually very accurate. The value of pulse oximetry is twofold: (1) It allows for the monitoring of intrapulmonary shunts, the most common reason for a decreased PaO_2 and SaO_2;[6] (2) SpO_2 allows for manipulation of oxygen (FiO_2) and positive pressure (PEEP) therapy without the need for blood gases mea-

surements.[7] As long as the SpO_2 is maintained at levels greater than 0.92 or 0.93, SaO_2 values are probably near 0.90. SaO_2 values near 0.90 are consistent with adequate levels of oxyhemoglobin.[8] Adjustments in FiO_2 and PEEP can occur safely, if SpO_2 values are greater than 0.92 or 0.93. (Some clinicians prefer to compare the SpO_2-SaO_2 difference directly rather than assuming a 2% to 5% SpO_2-SaO_2 difference. This can be done by measuring SaO_2 in the laboratory and comparing the result with the SpO_2.) Pulse oximetry, while not perfect, is a vast improvement in the assessment of oxyhemoglobin. Formerly, crude assessment signs such as cyanosis were required.[9,10,11]

Transcutaneous Oxygen Monitoring ($TcPO_2$)

$TcPO_2$ monitoring allows for continuous noninvasive assessment, through the use of an electrode placed on the skin, of the minute-to-minute changes that can occur in oxygen levels. The electrode has a heating unit to warm the skin, causing capillaries to dilate and thereby increasing blood flow. The monitor measures the amount of oxygen diffusing through the skin, which sometimes correlates with arterial oxygen levels. In neonates the correlation is high, making it possible to monitor the effect of treatment on oxygenation and avoid episodes of hypoxemia. The correlation in adults is less reliable, but the result is helpful in certain conditions.

REFERENCES

1. Bates, B. (1991). *A guide to physical examination* (5th ed.). Philadelphia: Lippincott.
2. Loudon, R., & Murphy, R. L. H. (1984). Lung sounds. *American Review of Respiratory Disease, 130,* 663.
3. Sanchez, T. (1986). Fundamentals of chest x-ray interpretation. *Critical Care Nurse, 6,* 41-63.
4. Burton, G., & Hodgkin, J. E. (1991). *Respiratory care* (3rd ed.). Philadelphia: Lippincott.
5. St. John, R. E. (1989). Exhaled gas analysis: Technical and clinical aspects of capnography and oxygen consumption. *Critical Care Nursing Clinics of North America, 1,* 669-680.
6. Rutherford, K. A. (1989). Principles and application of oximetry. *Critical Care Nursing Clinics of North America, 1,* 649-657.
7. King, T., & Simon, R. H. (1987). Pulse oximetry for tapering supplemental oxygen in hospitalized patients. *Chest, 92,* 713-716.
8. Tremper, K. K., & Barker, S. J. (1989). Pulse oximetry. *Anesthesiology, 70,* 98-108.
9. Martin, L., & Khalil, H. (1990). How much reduced hemoglobin is necessary to generate central cyanosis. *Chest, 97,* 182.
10. Comroe, J. H., & Bothelho, S. (1947). The unreliability of cyanosis in the recognition of arterial anoxemia. *American Journal of Medical Science, 214,* 1.
11. Carroll, P. L. (1988). Cyanosis: The sign you can't count on. *Nursing 88, 18,* 50.

29

Respiratory Disorders

Thomas S. Ahrens

All respiratory disorders have the potential to impair pulmonary function through their impact on either alveolar ventilation ($\dot{V}$) or perfusion ($\dot{Q}$) in the lungs. The term *ventilation/perfusion ($\dot{V}/\dot{Q}$) ratio* is used to describe how respiratory disorders affect pulmonary function. Under normal circumstances, ventilation at the alveolar level is nearly matched by blood flow to the alveoli. When ventilation is reduced relative to blood flow, an abnormality called a low $\dot{V}/\dot{Q}$ ratio exists. When blood flow is reduced relative to alveolar ventilation, a high $\dot{V}/\dot{Q}$ ratio exists. Low ventilation/perfusion ratios (also termed intrapulmonary shunts or $\dot{Q}s/\dot{Q}T$) tend to produce problems with maintaining adequate PaO_2 and SaO_2 levels. High ventilation/perfusion ratios (also termed physiological dead space or $\dot{V}_D/\dot{V}_T$) are more likely to interfere with $PaCO_2$ levels. Either or both types of $\dot{V}/\dot{Q}$ disturbance can be present in respiratory disorders. Regardless of the type of respiratory disorder, the clinical impact of the disorder is directly related to the degree of disturbance caused in the $\dot{V}/\dot{Q}$ ratio.

If the type of $\dot{V}/\dot{Q}$ abnormality is understood, assessment and treatment measures can be more appropriately implemented. Respiratory disorders causing primarily low $\dot{V}/\dot{Q}$ ratios are assessed by measures of intrapulmonary shunting and PaO_2/SaO_2 analysis. Therapies are directed at improving ventilation relative to blood flow. Respiratory disorders causing primarily high $\dot{V}/\dot{Q}$ ratios are assessed by measures of dead space analysis and $PaCO_2/pH$ relationships. Treatments focus on improving blood flow relative to ventilation.

As the different types of respiratory disorders are presented, the reader should keep in mind the type of $\dot{V}/\dot{Q}$ disturbance present. The first category of respiratory disorders presented, parenchymal lung disorders, is perhaps the best illustration of disturbances in $\dot{V}/\dot{Q}$ ratios. This category describes a large number of respiratory disorders that interfere with ventilation and perfusion. Some disorders interfere more with ventilation than perfusion, such as ARDS, pneumo-

nias, and pulmonary edema. Others interfere more with perfusion to the lung, as described in the section on pulmonary perfusion. Regardless of the disorder, they all alter the $\dot{V}/\dot{Q}$ relationship and will have a characteristic impact on blood gases and clinical symptoms.

PARENCHYMAL LUNG DISORDERS
Adult Respiratory Distress Syndrome (ARDS)

Catastrophic respiratory failure of sudden onset may occur in patients with previously normal or healthy lungs who sustain any one of a variety of pulmonary or systemic insults that cause diffuse injury to the lung. The initial insult may be any one of a diverse group of injuries, yet the histological response of the lung, regardless of the insult, is virtually identical. The fact that the lung has a characteristic clinical, physiological, and pathological response to acute injury, regardless of etiology, allows the critical care practitioner to group a variety of illnesses that have one or more common phases under the singular heading of ARDS.[1,2,3]

The absence of a single causative event and the lack of any specific diagnostic test for ARDS necessitate the use of a descriptive definition for this syndrome. The following constellation of pulmonary responses characterize ARDS:

- *Clinical:* Dyspnea, tachypnea, tachycardia
- *Radiological:* Diffuse bilateral pulmonary infiltrates (an "alveolar pattern" or "white out")
- *Physiological:* Decreased pulmonary compliance (i.e., increased "stiffness" of the lungs), impaired oxygen diffusion across alveolar capillary membrane (i.e., decreasing arterial oxygen tension nonresponsive to "standard" oxygen therapy)
- *Pathological:* Interstitial edema, intra-alveolar exudation, hemorrhage, microemboli, and hyaline membrane formation

The clinical hallmarks of this variety of respiratory failure include an initial insult, such as massive hemorrhage and hypovolemic shock, and a latent period during which pulmonary function appears normal, followed by respiratory decompensation. Initially the patient is tachypneic and dyspneic; the arterial oxygen tension decreases in spite of standard oxygen therapy. The arterial carbon dioxide tension is low initially ($Paco_2$ below 40 torr*) but rises rapidly in spite of the tachypnea as the respiratory insufficiency progresses.

The use of the term *ARDS* should not obscure the fact that the initial insult and mechanism of pulmonary injury vary widely. Therapy should be focused on two areas: supportive therapy to treat the secondary alterations in pulmonary function and maintain the patient, and treatment of the initiating or causal insult. Some of the causal factors seen in medical and surgical settings that are related to the development of ARDS are listed in the box to the right.

Advances in emergency medical care during the Vietnam war period allowed for prolonged survival of trauma victims who previously would have died on the battleground. Two of the most notable advances were (1) rapid treatment and recovery from initial shock and trauma, and (2) rapid evacuation within 15 to 20 minutes to sophisticated treatment centers. Observations made during World War II were confirmed and extended to include development of respiratory failure after a posttraumatic latent period of 12 to 48 hours. One reason for the apparently increasing incidence of ARDS over the years has been improvements in medical therapy and technology that facilitate the victim's survival of severe initial insults that lead to ARDS.

Pathology

Although ARDS may have a variety of causes, the pathological changes are remarkably consistent. On gross examination at autopsy the lungs are heavy, congested, and hemorrhagic and have the appearance of liver. Such lungs sink when placed in water. Generally there is not a significant amount of secretions in the large airways, nor is there visible obstruction of the major vessels.

Frequently cited findings in ARDS include thickened alveolar walls, interstitial edema, intraalveolar edema, and hemorrhage. Focal atelectasis is present. Congestion, plugging of small arterioles with fibrin and debris, and partial or even complete disruption of portions of the pulmonary vascular bed occur. Migration of the cellular material into the alveoli may be noted. Localized areas of aveolar wall necrosis and an increased number of pulmonary macrophages may be seen.

Hyaline membranes are also noted on microscopic

---

*A torr is a unit of pressure that is equivalent to 1 mmHg under standard conditions.

Factors Related to Development of ARDS
Aspiration of gastric contents
Drug ingestion and overdose
Hydrocarbon ingestion
Trauma and hemorrhagic shock
Near drowning
Smoke and gas inhalation
Disseminated intravascular coagulation
Septic shock
Fat and air embolism
Severe pneumonitis (viral and other)
Oxygen toxicity
Postperfusion (cardiopulmonary bypass)
Anaphylaxis
Uremia
Hemorrhagic pancreatitis
Head injury
Homologous blood transfusion

examination. They are probably formed from transudated plasma proteins and can increase the alveolar capillary membrane to 50 to 100 times its normal thickness. These membranes form a formidable barrier to gas diffusion.

Etiology

The support and management of all ARDS patients are similar yet vary somewhat according to the etiology. Mortality rates range from 20% to 50%. A successful outcome depends upon recognition and treatment of all contributing factors. For example, the critically ill patient with multisystem trauma may have ARDS, fat embolism, sepsis, and posttraumatic pancreatitis as active problems. It is important to consider all possible contributing problems to facilitate proper management (see the box above).

The lung exhibits a limited number of responses to injury. ARDS is one type of response to a severe insult. Knowledge of the mechanisms of pulmonary injury is largely inferred rather than directly observed, with the exception of direct trauma and aspiration. It can also be assumed that some systemic response mediating the lung injury is present, since not all patients having similar insults develop ARDS. The nature of this response is unclear.

It is generally accepted that a period of pulmonary hypoperfusion is associated with the origin of most cases of ARDS. The precise mechanism by which this hypoperfusion develops into ARDS has not been fully identified, but it probably involves intravascular coagulation with subsequent thromboembolism within the pulmonary microvasculature (Figure 29-1). It has now been proved that in ARDS of all causes the initial

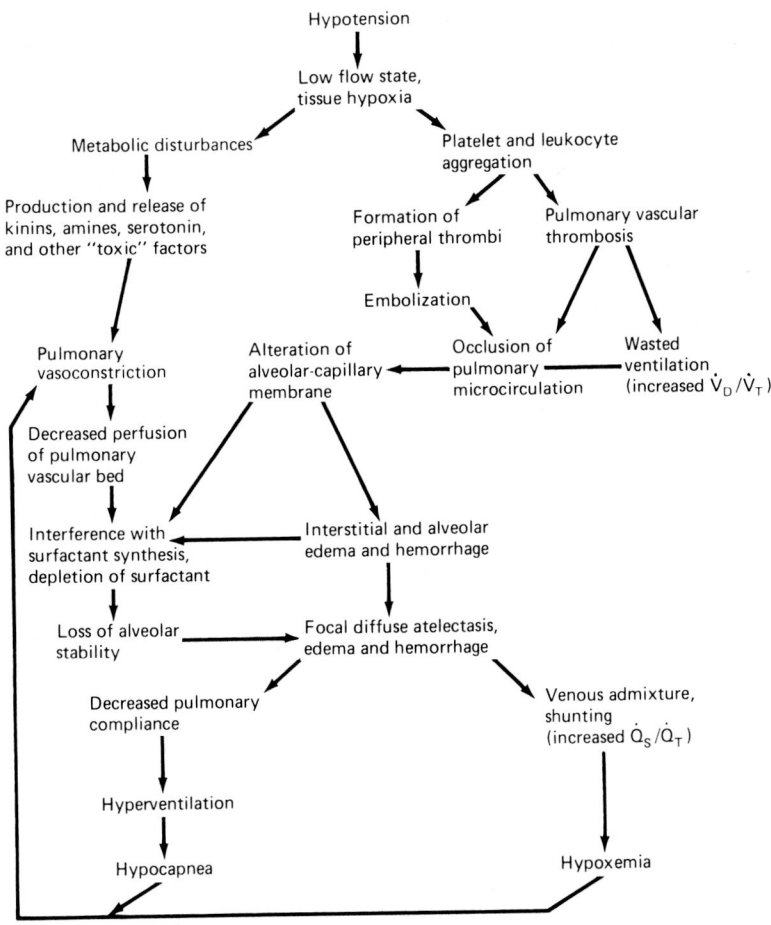

Figure 29-1 Pathogenesis and pathophysiology of ARDS.

Adapted from Lake, K., & Rumsfeld, J. (1991). The adult respiratory distress syndrome (shock lung). In G. G. Burton, G. N. Gee, & J. E. Hodgkins (Eds.), *Respiratory care; a guide to clinical practice.* Philadelphia: Lippincott.

injury is to the capillary endothelium; however, there are many known mediators of lung injury which, if they do not initiate the syndrome, perpetuate it (see the box to the right).

Intravascular coagulation can develop from a variety of causes. Transfusion with mismatched blood, with resulting hemolysis, is a significant cause. Other complications of shock states that lead to intravascular coagulation are tissue trauma mobilizing tissue thromboplastin, bacterial toxins through platelet aggregation with the release of thromboplastin, ischemia from endothelial cell damage, the release of tissue thromboplastin, and acidosis. Systemic microvascular obstruction with microemboli results in decreased tissue perfusion, progressive metabolic acidosis, and a secondary increase in coagulability.

Following resuscitation of the patient in a shock state, flow in the microcirculation is reestablished and the products of peripheral intravascular coagulation are flushed into the systemic circulation and carried to the vascular bed of the lungs. The filtering action of the pulmonary vascular bed removes gross and

---

Mediators Associated with ARDS

Coagulation products
Complement products
Platelets and platelet activating factor
Prostaglandins
Histamine
Bradykinin
Serotonin
Polymorphonuclear leukocytes
Tumor necrosis factor

---

microscopic clots. Unstable circulating clots fragment until the microcirculation of the lung is reached. Stasis here in the microcirculation invites further thrombosis because of endothelial cell damage distal to the emboli.

Thromboemboli cause pulmonary damage via at least two mechanisms: (1) release of potent bronchoconstrictors and venoconstrictors, and (2) mechanical obstruction of blood flow. Vasoactive amines such as serotonin and histamine are released from platelet microemboli and produce microvascular constriction. Other agents, including bradykinin and catecholamines, are also released from white blood cell–platelet microaggregates and result in vasoconstriction, bronchoconstriction, and alterations in alveolar-capillary membrane permeability.

The primary target for all these forces is the alveolar–capillary membrane. Hypoxia, lactic acidosis, and intravascular clotting occur. Hypoxemia and acidemia themselves increase pulmonary artery pressure and pulmonary vascular resistance. The capillary membranes are damaged by these insults and their permeability is increased, allowing extravasation of fluids into the interstitial space. Initially the fluid is a transudate, but as the leakage increases, larger molecules such as proteins and formed blood elements leak out. Lymph channels that would normally remove this material are compressed by the extravasated fluid, further favoring interstitial fluid collection and retention (Figure 29-2).

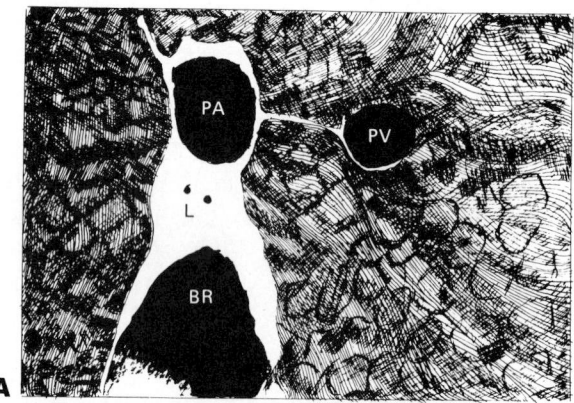

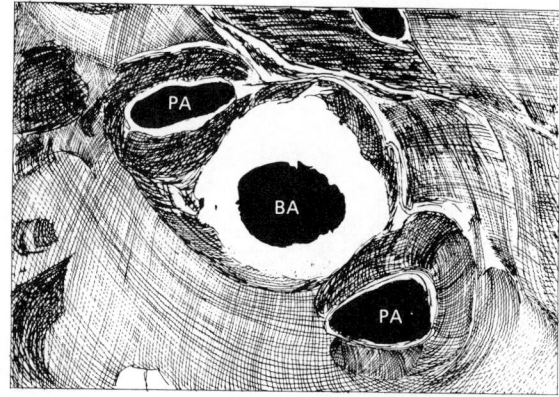

Figure 29-2 *A,* Normal lung showing bronchus (BR), pulmonary artery (PA), and pulmonary venule (PV). The only visible interstitial space (L) is between the airway and the artery in which lymph vessels are located. *B,* Massive fluid expansion of loose interstitial perivascular and peribronchial space. Note "halo" effect surrounding the pulmonary artery (PA) and the bronchial artery (BA).
Courtesy of E. F. Lenihan.

Perivascular edema and decreased capillary perfusion damage the alveolar type 2 pneumocyte, decreasing surfactant production. The alveoli become increasingly unstable and tend to collapse unless filled with fluid from the interstitium. These alveoli, in either case, cannot participate in effective gas exchange, and this area becomes a mass of interstitial and alveolar edema with hemorrhage and atelectasis.

Pathophysiology

Pulmonary function abnormalities in patients with ARDS have been well described in several review articles.[1,2,3] The primary feature of ARDS is the alteration in capillary permeability secondary to capillary endothelial injury. The injury is secondary to some other process, either in the lung or from a systemic response.

A reduction in functional residual capacity is a hallmark of this syndrome. Localization of edema fluid in the peribronchovascular interstitial space raises the normally subatmospheric pressure of the interstitial space. This reduces the transmural pressure gradient that helps to maintain patent airways. If these small airways close and remain closed, distal atelectasis and loss of lung volume occur. Lung volume also decreases as accumulating edema fluid begins to flood alveoli or as the alveoli become smaller because of the increasing surface forces.

Decreasing pulmonary compliance is another characteristic finding in ARDS. This means that greater than normal inspiratory pressure is needed to deliver he same tidal volume. This loss of compliance is directly due to increasing tissue elasticity or recoil caused by pulmonary congestion and the increasing alveolar surface forces resulting from loss or inactivation of surfactant. The decreasing compliance is indirectly a result of the overall decreasing lung volume. As compliance decreases, there is a progressive reduction in the volume of gas present in the involved lung units at functional residual capacity (FRC). If the process is severe, the volume of gas may be so small and the surface forces so great that the alveoli and/or terminal bronchioles collapse completely on deflation. When this occurs, the unit cannot reopen until a "critical opening pressure" has been exceeded during inspiration.

Hypoxemia is an invariable feature of ARDS. A large number of gas exchange units fail to contribute fully to the uptake of oxygen and elimination of carbon dioxide because of the processes described above. Alveoli that receive blood flow but no ventilation are sites of intrapulmonary shunting ($\dot{Q}s/\dot{Q}T$). In other areas where there is vasoconstriction and microembolization, "wasted" ventilation ($\dot{V}_D/\dot{V}_T$) exists. The net result over the entire pulmonary bed is $\dot{V}/\dot{Q}$ mismatching and hypoxemia.

A reflex increase in cardiac output and alveolar minute ventilation occurs to compensate for the hypoxia and resultant acidosis. However, the lowered $PaCO_2$ from hyperventilation increases both airway resistance and oxygen consumption and decreases dynamic compliance. All these effects contribute to additional pulmonary dysfunction. Increased inspiratory effort is needed to open previously closed alveoli. The increased inspiratory effort increases venous return to the right side of the heart, yet the total volume of the pulmonary circulatory bed is decreased because of coagulopathy and increased resistance. This causes further extravasation of fluid and formed elements into the interstitial space. As osmotically active particles leak through the damaged endothelial membrane and into the interstitial space, more water is drawn to them and the lungs become stiffer. The increased oxygen consumption required by the increased work of breathing is far too costly in the presence of progressive hypoxemia.

The role of the central nervous system in ARDS has been suggested by many neurosurgeons. A model has been described in which cerebral hypoxia initiates the sequence by interfering with hypothalamic cellular metabolism. Descending sympathetic fibers are activated which pass through the cervical spinal cord and on to the vessels of the lung. The importance of these neurogenic factors is still unclear. Some head-injured patients without pulmonary or other major extracranial injuries show ventilation/perfusion disorders.

Data Acquisition

Recognition of ARDS in the late stages is relatively easy, yet diagnosis in the early, subtle stages is difficult unless members of the health care team are alert to its development in susceptible patients. Early diagnosis helps to avoid compounding the problem by mishandling oxygen, mechanical ventilation, and other therapeutic tools.

During the initial shock phase, therapeutic interventions are directed toward converting the low-flow state to a high-flow state by administration of the appropriate fluids, blood products, or both to reverse the hypotension.

There may be few or no pulmonary symptoms at this time and for the next 12 to 48 hours. Early symptoms include dyspnea, restlessness, and/or cough. Dyspnea, however, may not appear early in the young, healthy patient who can double or triple minute ventilation with ease. The initial finding in mechanically ventilated patients may be an increase in the peak inspiratory pressure necessary to deliver a given tidal volume (evidence of decreasing pulmonary compliance).

Abnormal findings on physical examination indicate that the disease process has already progressed beyond the early stages. Evidence of increased work of breathing such as hyperpnea, noisy respirations at a rapid rate, and intercostal and supracostal retraction may be noted. Cyanosis will be present if there is adequate capillary perfusion and more than 5 g of reduced hemoglobin. Pallor will be seen if perfusion is poor. Tachycardia, diaphoresis, and decreased mentation are seen frequently once the syndrome has progressed. Initially chest auscultation is normal, but crackles, wheezes, and bronchial breath sounds may be heard as the syndrome progresses to the later stages. Physical findings related to the underlying etiology, such as skin, conjunctival, and retinal changes in fat embolism and singed nasal hairs in pulmonary burns, should be sought.

Tests of gas exchange and pulmonary mechanics are useful in evaluating and managing ARDS. The hallmark of this syndrome remains a lowered arterial oxygen tension that is unresponsive to increased concentrations of inspired oxygen. A more exact method of evaluating this is by calculating the intrapulmonary shunt ($\dot{Q}s/\dot{Q}T$), or estimating the shunt with oxygen-derived variables such as the arterial/alveolar or the PaO_2/FiO_2 ratio, or the clinical shunt equation.

Normal persons breathing spontaneously have shunt fractions of less than 6%, and $\dot{Q}s/\dot{Q}T$ fractions of less than 10% in patients receiving mechanical ventilation reflect a normal cardiopulmonary system. Until recently, an FiO_2 of 100% was used to calculate "true shunt." In critically ill patients, the "physiological shunt" (which includes areas of low $\dot{V}/\dot{Q}$) is now considered more clinically meaningful when calculated at an FiO_2 of 50% to 60%. In either case, the following guidelines are useful for evaluation of shunt fractions on ventilator patients:

1. A calculated shunt greater than 30% is generally considered incompatible with prolonged spontaneous ventilation.
2. Calculated shunts between 20% and 30% are considered compatible with spontaneous ventilation so long as the cardiovascular reserves are adequate and the status of the central nervous system and hepatorenal system are acceptable.
3. Calculated shunts less than 20% are considered compatible with prolonged spontaneous ventilation.

Alveolar ventilation remains high until late in the course of ARDS. A $PaCO_2$ of 35 to 45 torr in a very dyspneic, hypoxemic patient is not "normal," and when it does occur, it suggests that the seriously compromised lungs are no longer able to increase alveolar ventilation in response to hypoxemia and other stimuli.

The pH normally rises as $PaCO_2$ falls (respiratory alkalemia). Failure to rise indicates that metabolic acidemia is present. In the presence of shock and hypoxemia, this is most commonly the result of lactic acidosis, which can be confirmed by directly measuring serum lactate levels.

Tests of pulmonary mechanics show decreasing static and dynamic compliance. There is also a decrease in lung volumes, particularly FRC.

There is a real need for a sensitive test that can detect ARDS in an early phase when fluid is beginning to collect in the lung. Tests that measure lung water directly would obviously be desirable and might be a means for early diagnosis. A number of techniques have been used, but at this time none have proved their applicability to the clinical diagnosis of ARDS.

The radiological picture of this syndrome is the result of movement of fluid out of the injured alveolar capillary into the interstitium and later into the alveolus. There must be a large increase in lung water before the chest roentgenogram becomes abnormal. The lungs frequently appear normal in the early stages of ARDS, although a considerable degree of microatelectasis may be present. Subtle findings such as thickened or blurred margins of bronchi or vessels may be seen first. Except for the absence of left ventricular enlargement, the roentgenogram of ARDS may be difficult to distinguish from that of cardiogenic pulmonary edema. Proper resolution demands films of good quality with sufficient contrast and good detail.

The first changes of fine reticulation progress to give the lung a ground glass appearance. A typical air-space alveolar pattern may be seen as fluid leaks into the alveoli. Terminally, when consolidation is seen, there may be few recognizable air spaces; at this point the term *white lung* is applicable.

There are no sensitive practical means for early detection of ARDS. Detectable changes are probably the result of significant water accumulation in the lung. Therefore, relatively minor alteration in tests of pulmonary function of patients who are at risk of ARDS should receive special attention. Early endotracheal intubation and mechanical ventilation should be considered as soon as abnormalities occur.

Figure 29-3 shows by means of x-rays the progress of a 35-year-old man who was admitted with a gunshot wound through the right lobe of the liver. The bullet involved the base of the right lung. After admission to the hospital, the patient appeared well and breathed room air spontaneously. PaO_2 was 67 torr and $PaCO_2$, 34 torr; pH was 7.42.

Three days later, after developing severe respiratory failure, the patient was transferred to another institution. He had been given massive doses of diuretics and concentrated albumin solution and was receiving assisted mechanical ventilation (AMV) with a positive end-expiratory pressure (PEEP) of 10 cmH_2O. Dopamine was needed to maintain blood pressure, and pancuronium was given because ventilation could not be synchronized with AMV. The PaO_2 was 48 torr and the $PaCO_2$, 42 torr; pH was 7.12 on FiO_2 of 1.0. Lactate level was 5.6 mmol/L, and the patient was oliguric.

The final x-ray was made 8 hours after the patient was admitted to the second institution. He had received 2 U of whole blood and 4 L of crystalloid and was now receiving 26 cmH_2O PEEP; intermittent mandatory ventilation (IMV) rate was six breaths per minute; FiO_2 was 0.5 torr; PaO_2 was 92 torr and $PaCO_2$, 43 torr; the pH was 7.37; the lactate level was 2 mmol/L. The patient was producing copious pink frothy sputum from the endotracheal tube and was nursed face down so that pulmonary edema fluid could be allowed to drain. He was not given suction during the first 36 hours after admission, because secretions were being washed out by the pulmonary edema fluid. Circulatory integrity returned in 36 hours, when the patient had normal renal function. He required some ventilatory support for another 5 days. By then he had returned to his admission weight, having voided the extra fluid given during resuscitation.

Patients with fully developed ARDS invariably require mechanical ventilation. The decision as to when to intervene with ventilatory support in patients with minor pulmonary function abnormalities suggesting ARDS may be difficult. Early intubation and ventilation are recommended because of the previously described cycle of edema, decreasing lung volume, and the appearance of hypoxia, leading to more edema and more volume loss, contributing to further hypoxia.

Endotracheal intubation should be performed initially. The widespread use of high-volume, low-pressure cuffs on endotracheal tubes has sufficiently decreased the rate of tracheal complications from these tubes so that today tracheostomy is not normally required unless prolonged mechanical ventilation is anticipated.

When mechanical ventilation is initiated in ARDS, tidal volumes of 10 to 15 ml per kilogram of body weight should be used. Volumes in this range are more effective in reducing or preventing atelectasis. When large tidal volumes are used with continuous positive pressure ventilation (CPPV), alveolar hyperventilation may be seen. Since a low $PaCO_2$ has been shown to decrease cardiac output and increase oxygen consumption as well as airway resistance, it is important to keep the $PaCO_2$ in the range of 35 to 45 torr. Additional mechanical dead space may be added to the ventilator circuit to achieve this, or the respiratory rate may be decreased, provided the patient can be assisted to breathe synchronously with the machine. One would not want to decrease tidal volume in order

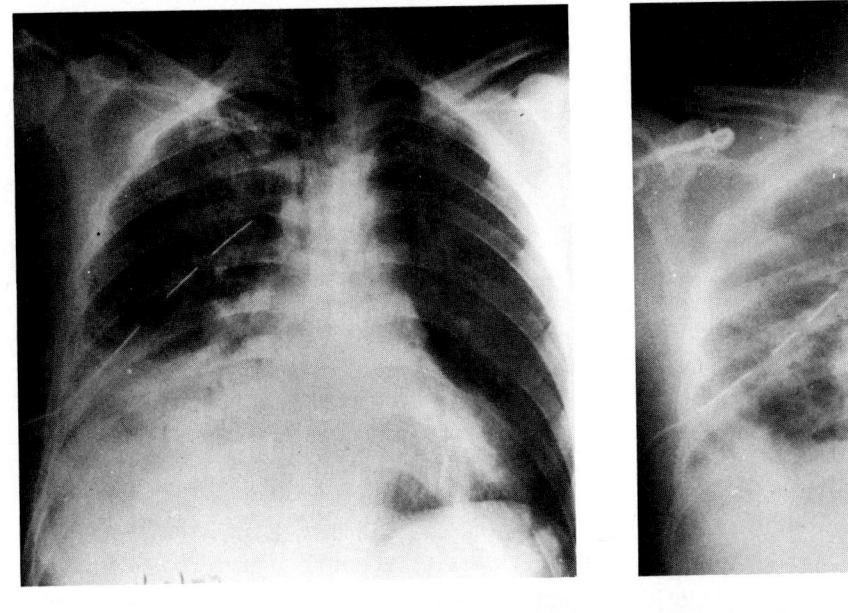
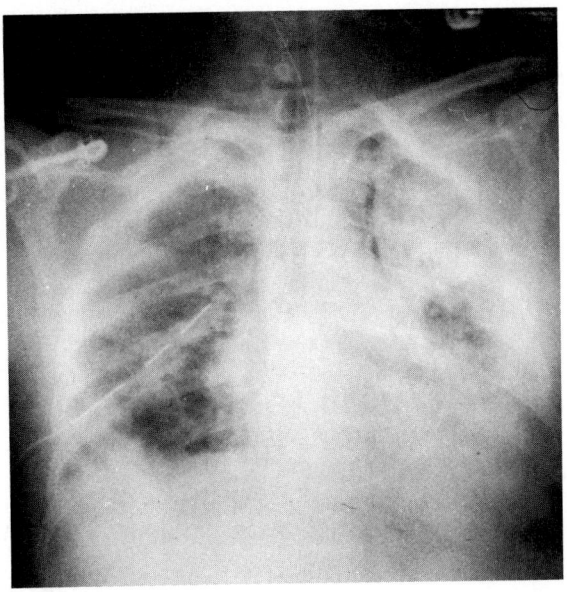
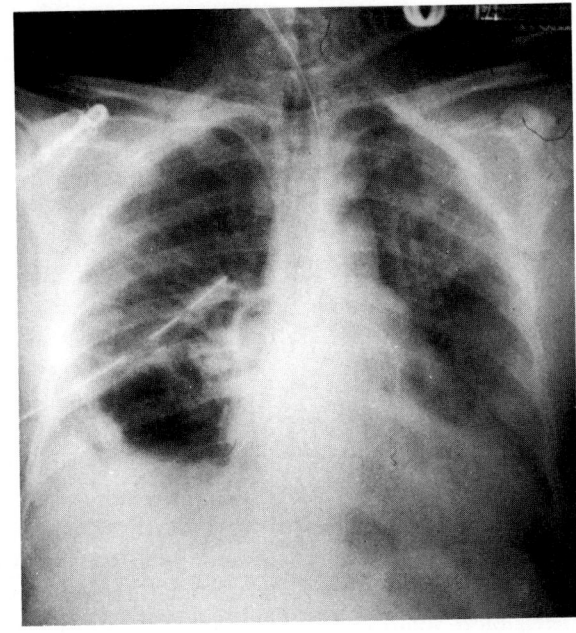

Figure 29-3 Chest x-rays of 35-year-old man with a gunshot wound through the right lobe of the liver. The bullet tract involved the base of the right lung. *A,* After admission to the hospital, patient was breathing room air spontaneously and appeared well. *B,* Three days later, after developing severe respiratory failure, the patient was transferred to another institution. *C,* Patient 8 hours after admission, having received 2 U of whole blood and 4 L of crystalloid. PEEP and IMV had begun.

to relieve the hyperventilation in these patients because of the atelectatic nature of the syndrome.

Many patients with ARDS are restless and tachypneic, which causes them to be overventilated when receiving CPPV and to breathe out of phase with the ventilator. Sedation should be used to avoid these problems; usually intermittent small intravenous doses of morphine or a benzodiazepine (e.g., Versed) are sufficient. A neuromuscular blocking agent such

as curare or pancuronium (Pavulon) may be helpful to completely paralyze and control a restless patient. Patients who are receiving such agents are paralyzed but fully awake and aware of their surroundings. Sedatives should be given in conjunction with these drugs.

The use of CPPV with PEEP has a well-documented role in the treatment of patients with ARDS. PEEP augments the reduced lung volumes seen in ARDS by producing a constantly positive distending pressure in the airways and alveoli. Intrapulmonary shunting is reduced because alveoli remain open and gases are available for diffusion throughout the respiratory cycle. The improved ventilation to gas exchange units that were previous sites of shunting or marked $\dot{V}/\dot{Q}$ abnormalities increases arterial P_{O_2} and reduces the aveolar–arterial difference. PEEP also physically expands alveoli and exerts gas pressure against the transudating fluid in the alveoli so that the volume of fluid that previously filled the lumen forms a layer on the alveolar surface wall through which gas diffusion can occur.

The use of PEEP with CPPV has certain limitations because of hazards associated with combining these two therapies. PEEP adds more pressure to the already high mean intrathoracic pressures needed to mechanically inflate stiff lungs with positive pressure. This high pressure is transmitted, in part, to the pleural space and great veins of the chest. Added pressure can compress these vessels and reduce venous return to the right side of the heart, thereby reducing cardiac output. This can lead to poor tissue perfusion and lactic acidosis. Pulmonary vascular resistance is also increased, which increases the work of the right ventricle in pumping blood into the normally low-resistance pulmonary bed. PEEP in excess of 15 cmH$_2$O has seldom been successful with CPPV.

The cardiac effects of PEEP are modified by its use in conjunction with spontaneous ventilation (continuous positive airway pressure, or CPAP) or with IMV. The combination of PEEP therapy with CPAP or IMV may enhance the therapeutic potential of PEEP in ARDS (increased transpulmonary pressures) while reducing detrimental cardiovascular effects (control of intrapleural/mean intrathoracic pressure).

Patients requiring PEEP therapy for severe ARDS have an increased incidence of barotrauma when compared with a mixed population of intensive care unit (ICU) patients receiving mechanical ventilation without PEEP. This increase in barotrauma, however, is due to the severity of the parenchymal disease rather than to the level of PEEP therapy. It is now accepted that there are no absolute contraindications to the use of PEEP in ARDS.

The development of a flow-directed thermodilution catheter and cardiac output computer has allowed direct measurement of mixed venous and systemic arterial blood gases, central venous pressure, and pulmonary artery wedge pressure for monitoring cardiovascular compromise. This information is necessary to determine the relations between PEEP, intrapulmonary shunt, and cardiac output.

The availability of bedside monitors that perform hemodynamic and oxygenation calculations allows long and tedious mathematical calculations to be done accurately and rapidly. Cardiac function can be evaluated by preload, the degree to which the myocardium is stretched before contraction; contractility; and afterload, the resistance against which the blood is expelled. Preload is reflected by the pulmonary artery wedge pressure and central venous pressure. Contractility is evaluated in terms of the measured cardiac output and heart rate as well as the calculated left ventricular stroke work index and stroke volume. Afterload is obtained from calculations of pulmonary and systemic vascular resistance. The effects of ventilatory support can be evaluated along with their effects on the cardiovascular circuit and appropriate interventions instituted to support the cardiovascular system during ventilatory therapy.

The goal of PEEP therapy in ARDS is to reduce the physiological shunt enough so that adequate arterial oxygen content (adequate hemoglobin content plus adequate arterial P_{O_2}) is achieved without significant compromise of cardiac output while potentially detrimental alveolar oxygen concentrations are avoided.

Intensivists at some major centers use the techniques previously described to treat the patient to achieve a calculated intrapulmonary shunt of 20% or less. Other groups treat to achieve a P_{O_2} greater than 60 to 70 torr at an F_{IO_2} of less than 0.50. Regardless of blood gas values, should the patient exhibit signs of labored breathing, anxiety, or unexplained restlessness, inadequacy in the amount of mechanical ventilatory support being supplied should be considered.

Invasive cardiovascular monitoring is initiated whenever potential cardiovascular compromise is anticipated or when levels of PEEP greater than 15 cmH$_2$O are applied. Pulmonary wedge pressure, which reflects left ventricular filling pressure, should be kept as low as possible to avoid increases in extravascular lung water. This is achieved by giving red cells or fluids as bolus IV infusions in an amount sufficient to maintain a reasonable cardiac output for the particular patient. Support of the cardiovascular function with fluid infusions or pharmacological agents is necessary only if the ventilatory support needed to achieve adequate pulmonary function decreases the usual pumping ability of the heart.

Medical Management

Fluid replacement in ARDS is an extremely controversial topic. The question focuses on the choice of colloids or crystalloids for fluid volume replacement. It has been proposed that intravascular volume should be replaced with colloids, since the major intravascular force keeping fluid within the capillaries is the protein osmotic pressure. Administration of colloids, then, would keep the protein osmotic pressure within the vascular space from diminishing. However, a rapid equilibration of protein concentrations between vascular and interstitial spaces undoubtedly occurs when the capillary endothelium is leaky, and the oncotic pressure gradient across the capillary wall would thus be lost. The administration of colloids and the rapid exudation of protein into the interstitium may actually make the situation worse, since protein-rich fluid is cleared slowly from the interstitium and alveoli. Some physicians fear that resuscitation with colloids might increase lung water more than resuscitation with crystalloids. There is no clear-cut experimental evidence favoring either crystalloids or colloids for fluid replacement.

Crystalloid solutions have several practical advantages. They are effective, readily available, and inexpensive. Colloids, on the other hand, are expensive and limited in supply. In the absence of documented therapeutic benefits, crystalloid solutions appear preferable, since they can adequately replenish intravascular volume and restore functional extracellular fluid volumes. It seems reasonable to consider crystalloids early in the course of ARDS when the increase in permeability is greatest. Later, if the serum protein concentration is low, colloid solutions may be used. However, appropriate fluids must be used to maintain optimal cardiac output while instituting PEEP.

Successful employment of any regimen utilizing mechanical ventilation is dependent upon a knowledgeable and highly skilled nursing staff. They must understand the principles of mechanical ventilation and the interpretation of arterial blood gases and must have a high level of expertise in physical assessment, techniques of pulmonary toilet, and proper maintenance of cuffed endotracheal tubes. The nurse must also know how to assist in emergency procedures when indicated (e.g., development of bradycardia, emergency insertion of chest tube). If monitoring of the patient with a flow-directed thermodilution catheter is employed, the nurse must be familiar with care of the catheter and insertion site, must have visual recognition of the various pressure waveforms, and must be cognizant of the basic interpretation of numerical values associated with pulmonary artery and wedge pressures.

When perfusion of one lung is a major concern in addition to ventilation, beds that allow for maximal changes in patient position are desirable (see Figure 29-4 and the box to the right). A patient with unilateral pulmonary disease can be positioned so that the diseased lung is elevated and the unaffected lung is in the dependent position. Both ventilation and perfusion will be preferentially delivered to the unaffected lung, resulting in less perfusion of nonven-

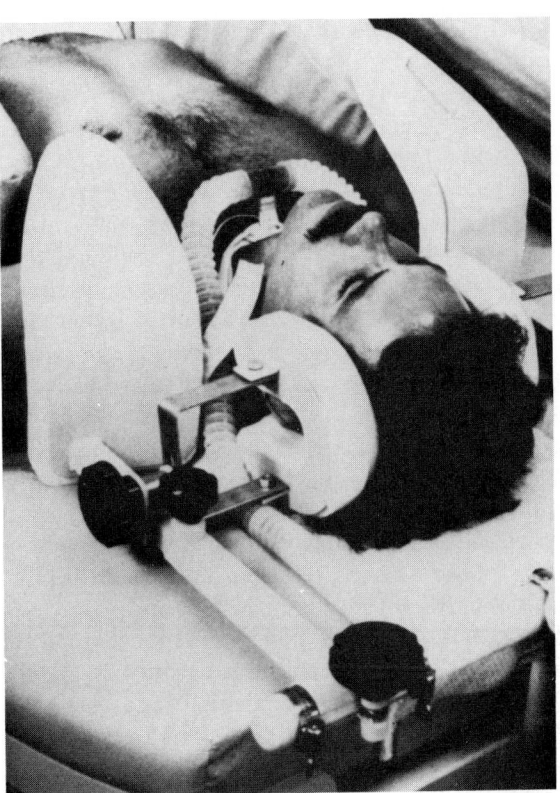

Figure 29-4 The Rotorest bed enables the critical care practitioner to care for the patient who requires sophisticated mechanical ventilation with greater ease and patient comfort and offers a number of clinical advantages over conventional beds.

Pulmonary Benefits of Beds Allowing Numerous Patient Positions

Mobilize secretions
Provide for continuous postural drainage
Decrease shunt by preferential positioning
Facilitate selective suctioning
Make possible x-ray through table surfaces
Stabilize ventilator tubing
Facilitate maintenance of chest tubes
Give comfortable positioning for percussion and postural drainage
Eliminate disadvantages of prone positioning
Provide access for CPR or airway maintenance

---

tilated areas in the diseased lung and producing a decreased intrapulmonary shunt and decreased microvascular pressure in that lung, all of which favor the egress of fluid.

Several indexes are available for the determination of adequate tissue oxygenation, although individual values are useful only in conjunction with others. Arterial PO_2 is accessible but provides little useful information, since it reflects oxygenation of blood that has not yet reached the peripheral tissues. A more precise estimate of tissue oxygenation is the correlation of arterial P_{O_2} with the mixed venous P_{O_2} and $S\bar{v}_{O_2}$. Most tissues compensate for inadequate oxygen delivery by increasing their extraction of oxygen from arterial blood, thus widening the difference in oxygen content between arterial and venous blood and decreasing mixed venous P_{O_2} below the normal 40 torr. Serum lactate levels will also rise as a result of the metabolic acidosis produced by poor oxygenation.

Infection may produce or complicate the picture of ARDS. When infection is suspected, aggressive efforts should be made to identify the specific etiological agent. This can usually be accomplished by Gram's stain and culture of aspirated tracheal secretions with sensitivity determinations. If more vigorous effort is needed, fiberoptic bronchoscopy can fairly easily be performed in patients receiving mechanical ventilation. Using the fiberoptic bronchoscope makes possible the use of a brush biopsy and bronchial lavage of localized areas. Needle aspiration and, rarely, open-lung biopsy may be required. Once an organism has been identified, appropriate therapy can be initiated according to the usual principles of antibiotic therapy.

Viral Pneumonia

Early descriptions of viral pneumonia were often confused by the presence of secondary bacterial pneumonias. Since bacterial pneumonias can be controlled with antibiotic therapy, the pathological changes of viral pneumonia within the lung are now being identified.[4] In fulminating cases the alveoli are filled with fibrin, fluid, red blood cells, and macrophages. These patients have profound hypoxemia, often relatively unimproved by oxygen administration, and should be treated like ARDS patients. Prognosis is grave, and fortunately, these cases are less common. Far more common are cases of patchy areas of viral pneumonitis, occurring during an influenzal infection and not extensive enough to cause severe arterial desaturation. In fact, presenting signs and symptoms are less severe than the roentgenogram would suggest. Diseases that suppress the immune system (e.g., AIDS) predispose patients to unusual pneumonias, including viral pneumonias.

Although a viral pneumonia may be suspected clinically, the diagnosis is usually made retrospectively using serological studies. Pneumonia complicating viral influenza is commonly bacterial, although in the 1957 pandemic, fatal cases were recorded as resulting from purely viral pneumonia.

Pneumonia due to varicella virus may complicate severe chickenpox in adults and among adults constitutes 38% of the varicella cases. Predisposing factors include chronic illness, steroid treatment, and treatment with antimetabolic drugs. Pulmonary symptoms begin 2 to 5 days after vesicle eruption. Severe respiratory distress, cough, chest pain, and frequently hypoxemia and hemoptysis are typical, although milder cases also occur. Pleural friction rub, pleural effusion, and radiological shadows have been described on the ipsilateral side in patients with intercostal herpes zoster, also thought to be caused by the varicella virus.

In addition to influenza and varicella viruses, measles and cytomegalovirus are the most commonly involved organisms in viral pneumonia.[5] Whenever the viral pneumonia is severe, it rapidly progresses to a clinical picture of ARDS and should be treated as previously described.

Aspiration Pneumonia

Aspiration of acid gastric contents often causes a widespread, severe chemical pneumonitis with diffuse alveolar filling. Aspiration pneumonia actually occurs in three different forms: acute aspiration pneumonia (septic pneumonitis, or Mendelson's syndrome), chronic aspiration pneumonia, and lipoid pneumonia.

Acute aspiration pneumonia is caused by the aspiration of gastric contents, primarily hydrochloric acid. It is extremely severe and can be fatal. Predisposing conditions include trauma, burns, general anesthesia, comatose states, and the presence of nasogastric or endotracheal tubes. There is characteristically a latent period between aspiration and the onset of respiratory distress. Diagnostic findings are similar to those described with ARDS. The chest roentgenogram initially shows bilateral patchy pulmonary edema. Treatment is the same as described for ARDS. The use of corticosteroids in acute aspiration pneumonia, as in ARDS, is controversial.

Chronic aspiration pneumonia is a localized consolidation of dependent portions of the lungs or of the bilateral midzones due to repeated aspiration of small quantities of infected pharyngeal secretions. It is particularly common in persons who abuse alcohol or drugs and in patients who are obtunded. Nasogastric and endotracheal tubes as well as swallowing defects and hiatus hernias are common predisposing factors. Infecting organisms are usually anaerobes or gram-negative bacilli; necrosis and abscess formation are common.

Lipoid pneumonia (oil granuloma) results from aspiration of such substances as milk, mineral oil, or oily nose drops. It presents radiologically as a chronic consolidation resembling carcinoma.

Radiation Pneumonitis

Radiation therapy to or near the lungs may result in acute radiation pneumonitis and/or radiation fibrosis. The reaction is limited to the area that has been irradiated, and, therefore, the condition is usually severe only when the irradiation is bilateral. The effect varies with the radiation dosage, the proportion of lung that has been irradiated, and the rate of administration. It is more likely to occur in thin persons. It usually develops within a month or two after the initiation of therapy and appears on the roentgenogram as a soft, fluffy alveolar infiltrate. There is an associated loss of lung volume and the characteristic picture of an air bronchogram. Radiation fibrosis is a chronic restrictive abnormality that usually follows but may develop independently of radiation pneumonitis. The affected area of lung becomes small and firm, and the mediastinum may be shifted to the involved side with elevation of the hemidiaphragm. Cor pulmonale occurs if the process is sufficiently extensive.

Cardiogenic Pulmonary Edema

It is beyond the scope of this discussion to consider cardiogenic pulmonary edema in any depth. Like ARDS (noncardiac pulmonary edema), it is the result of excessive accumulation of lung water. In this case the cause is a failing left ventricle or excessive administration of intravenous fluids. Increased left atrial pressure increases hydrostatic pressure in the pulmonary capillary bed. The lung's lymphatics, which can normally handle moderately increased fluid loads with minimal increases in interstitial fluid accumulation, are overwhelmed. The increased intravascular hydrostatic pressure causes an increase in net filtration pressure. The capillary endothelium remains intact, but fluid transudates from the capillary into the interstitium and eventually into the alveolus. One major difference between ARDS and cardiogenic pulmonary edema is the loss of capillary endothelial integrity in ARDS. If the capillary endothelium remains intact in cardiogenic pulmonary edema, one would expect the fluid migrating into the alveoli to remain a transudate without the proteinaceous material seen in ARDS. In fact, when pulmonary edema fluid is due to high filtration pressures, the protein concentration of tracheal fluid is usually less than one-half that in plasma. In noncardiac pulmonary edema the alveolar fluid protein composition is much higher and similar to that of circulating plasma.

Severe cardiogenic pulmonary edema may be treated as described for ARDS, but with particular attention to cardiovascular functioning. Treatment includes optimizing preload, contractility, and afterload.

Oxygen Toxicity

The advent of outer space and underwater exploration has necessitated the development of new perspectives on oxygen exposure. As long as humans were restricted to life at or near sea level, the term FIO_2 was adequate to quantify oxygen exposure. This term reflects the fraction of total inspired gas that is pure oxygen. However, when humans are exposed to oxygen under hyperbaric conditions (increased barometric pressures), they develop oxygen toxicity at a lower FIO_2. Alternatively, under hypobaric conditions (lowered barometric pressures), oxygen toxicity does not develop even at a very high FIO_2. The term PIO_2 was developed to give a better index of exposure. It represents the partial pressure of inspired oxygen and is calculated by a formula that takes atmospheric pressure into consideration:

$$PIO_2 = (P_B - 47) \times FIO_2$$

P_B is barometric pressure, and 47 represents the partial pressure of water vapor at body temperature. The PIO_2 is used to determine oxygen toxicity.

The term *atmosphere of oxygen* allows PIO_2 to be expressed in terms of atmospheric pressure. This term is calculated as

$$\text{Atmosphere of oxygen} = \frac{PIO_2}{760}$$

where 760 represents atmospheric pressure at sea level.

Oxygen is a drug, and like any other drug, its toxicity is determined by host tolerance, effective dose, and duration of exposure. Host tolerance is difficult to assess. There is tremendous species variation in response to oxygen. There is a great deal of variation between individual humans and, at times, in the same individual. Corticosteroids, hypercarbia, and hyperthermia may facilitate the development of oxygen toxicity, and this may have some clinical significance, since most critically ill patients experience at least one if not all of these conditions in the critical care unit.

Intermittent exposure seems to be the strongest minimizing factor in oxygen toxicity. This is an excellent area for research. However, at present, critical care practitioners are already using PEEP and CPAP to keep oxygen exposure as low as possible while maintaining adequate tissue oxygenation. It would be a gross error in judgment to jeopardize tissue oxygenation intermittently for the purpose of minimizing oxygen toxicity.[6]

Clinical symptoms of early oxygen toxicity include tracheobronchitis beginning in the area of the carina, cough, and inspiratory pain. In the late stages of this phase, dyspnea may develop.

The late phase of oxygen toxicity affects the alveolar unit. It has been reported to develop after short-term (24 hours) exposure to 50% O_2 at 1 atm.

During this phase, noncardiogenic interstitial and later alveolar pulmonary edema develop. The clinical picture is the same as described for ARDS.

The end stage of oxygen toxicity is one of progressive consolidation and fibrosis of the lung. If the patient's total exposure to oxygen is within the toxic range and a compatible clinical picture is present, the diagnosis of oxygen toxicity can be made. Detection of this condition is valuable because, while it is potentially lethal, the chance for complete recovery exists once O_2 levels are reduced below toxicity level.

The pathological picture of oxygen toxicity is the same as that described for ARDS. The earliest changes are an exudative phase including capillary endothelial cell damage and loss of membrane integrity, interstitial edema, alveolar hemorrhage, and destruction of type 1 pneumocytes. Following the death of the type 1 alveolar cells, the basement membrane is exposed and covered with fibrin and cellular debris, leading to the formation of a hyaline membrane.

The proliferative phase that follows includes hyperplasia of type 2 pneumocytes. The alveoli become lined with these abnormal cells, and fibroblasts proliferate in the interstitium. Once this stage occurs, recovery is unlikely and permanent fibrosis of the interstitium is probable.

Hypoxemia is a frequent occurence in critically ill patients; its damage is usually rapid, often irreversible, and sometimes fatal. Pulmonary oxygen toxicity is uncommon, variable in onset, and slow in developing. As previously stated, a patient should not be subjected to tissue hypoxia for the purpose of preventing oxygen toxicity. The best approach seems to be the judicious use of oxygen therapy to treat hypoxemia and tissue hypoxia without overtreating and needlessly exposing the patient to excessive amounts of the drug. PEEP and CPAP should be used to the extent possible to avoid subjecting the patient to an FiO_2 greater than 0.40 to 0.50.

Near Drowning

Submersion injuries are classified as drowning or near drowning. The *drowning* victim is one who dies within 24 hours, while *near-drowning* victims survive for more than 24 hours.[7] Both injuries can be further classified as *wet,* when aspiration has occurred, or *dry,* when damage has been caused by asphyxiation without aspiration. In the dry group, intact laryngeal reflexes probably cause laryngospasm, thus preventing aspiration. The wet group are more likely to have been obtunded and to have experienced aspiration.

The type of injury seen in near-drowning victims depends on the toxicity of the fluid aspirated, the temperature, the nature of contaminants in the water (e.g., bacteria, protozoa, algae, sand) which may have

been aspirated, and the duration of hypoxia. Differences are present between aspiration of seawater (3.5% NaCl) and hypotonic fresh water. The clinical picture, however, from a treatment perspective, is similar for both. Every near drowning is a response to a unique set of contaminants and environmental circumstances. Many submersion injuries are preceded or accompanied by other primary events such as myocardial infarction, seizures, and spinal cord or head injuries due to a dive into shallow water. Near-drowning victims brought in for resuscitation should be carefully studied for other primary pathological conditions.

Hypothermia also has a dramatic impact in the near-drowning victim. Body temperature falls rapidly following submersion, since the thermal conduction properties of water are 32 times greater than those of air. Death before drowning may occur in healthy persons swimming in cold water. Cold water immersion causes hyperventilation, which may result in hypocapnia, disorientation, and possible loss of consciousness, leading to drowning.

Hypothermia also increases blood viscosity, slowing flow through the coronary arteries and other vessels. Shifting of the oxyhemoglobin dissociation curve to the left increases the affinity of hemoglobin for oxygen and decreases oxygen unloading.

The hypoxemia after human submersion is caused by a combination of interstitial and alveolar pulmonary edema similar to that previously described for ARDS. There is damage to pulmonary capillaries, decreased surfactant, and a hyaline membrane type of formation by proteinaceous material. There is a decrease in pulmonary compliance, increased dead space, and increased intrapulmonary shunt. Ventilation and perfusion are mismatched, and there is an increased alveolar–arterial oxygen difference.

When first seen, victims of submersion injury may show a variety of symptoms ranging from crackles and wheezes to cardiac arrest. A few may be relatively asymptomatic but proceed to develop ARDS within the next 24 hours. All patients with a history of significant submersion should have medical observation for at least 24 hours.

Therapeutic efforts for the pulmonary manifestations of near drowning are the same as those described for ARDS. The objectives of increasing lung volumes and matching ventilation with perfusion can be accomplished by the use of mechanical support with IMV ventilation, PEEP, and circulatory support when needed. Mask CPAP may prove beneficial in patients who are hypoxemic but can maintain a normal $PaCO_2$. Mask CPAP should not be used in patients who are obtunded or unconscious because of the hazard of vomiting and aspiration.

There are reports of survival after prolonged submersion and cardiac arrest in very cold water. One report describes a submersion and cardiac arrest lasting approximately 40 minutes that was followed by survival without significant residual neurological deficits. In such cases the decrease in metabolic rate, cellular metabolism, and oxygen consumption in the central nervous system and heart may have prevented damage from hypoxia. Resuscitation should be attempted in the hypothermic drowning victim even though prolonged submersion may have occurred.

Families and friends of near-drowning victims require a great deal of psychological support from critical care unit personnel. Near drowning represents the extremely sudden onset of critical illness for which family members are totally unprepared. They have not had time to develop any coping mechanisms and certainly will be in the very earliest stages of the grieving process. ICU personnel should also be sensitive to the possibility that extreme guilt may plague the family members of these patients. If the victim is a small child, the parents may carry unrealistic amounts of guilt regarding supervision of the child. Regardless of the known circumstances surrounding the submersion incident, if family members or friends of the patient exhibit behavior indicating that they are having difficulty coping with the situation, an appropriate referral to a chaplain, psychiatric social worker, or psychologist should be initiated.

Acquired Immune Deficiency Syndrome (AIDS)

AIDS is characterized by the development of multiple severe opportunistic infections and rare neoplasms in previously healthy persons. The population at significant risk to date includes homosexual males, bisexuals, Haitians, intravenous drug abusers, recipients of large amounts of blood replacement products, and oncologic and transplant patients receiving immunosuppressive therapy, although the prevalence in the heterosexual population is increasing. Characteristic disorders seen in the AIDS patient include depressed blastogenesis, lymphopenia with a selective decrease in T cells, and a marked depletion of T4 cells as compared with T cells.

Patients with AIDS usually have had one or more episodes of serious respiratory illness that required hospitalization. Most patients exhibit signs of opportunistic infections, and the initial manifestation of the disease is usually pulmonary.[8] The most common pulmonary pathogen is *Pneumocystis carinii*, alone or in combination with cytomegalovirus. Bouts of *Pneumocystis carinii* pneumonia have been successfully treated by trimethoprim-sulfamethoxazole (Bactrim, Septra) or pentamidine isethionate. This is the only AIDS-related pulmonary disease in which suc-cessful treatment has been documented. Respiratory disease (ARDS) is the most common cause of death, and in most patients, additional unsuspected pulmonary disease is diagnosed on autopsy—most commonly cytomegalovirus pneumonitis.

Patients with pulmonary manifestations of AIDS complain most frequently of dyspnea and fever and exhibit bilateral diffuse pulmonary infiltrates on chest x-ray. Often tachypnea, fever, and dyspnea are more impressive than the radiographic findings. Bronchoscopic findings indicate a positive diagnosis in 70% to 80% of cases.

At present, only a minority of the infectious complications of AIDS can be successfully treated. The necessity for endotracheal intubation and mechanical ventilation is a grave prognostic sign; few patients with it survive to leave the hospital. Only a high index of suspicion, prompt diagnosis, and early treatment offer a prolonged, high-quality period of continued life for the AIDS victim.

Drug Overdose and Head Injury

Drug overdose and head injury produce, on rare occasions, a devastating form of acute hemorrhagic pneumonitis. The effect of some agents, such as barbiturates, is to depress other system functions. Indirect effects on the lung may give rise to management problems in the recovery period.

Pathophysiology

Cerebral hypoxia has been indicated as a possible major cause for acute respiratory failure. This would account for the condition arising in head injury and the apnea or hypoventilation of drug overdose. The hypoxia and hypocapnia noted as early as the time of admission of patients with severe head injury may reflect increased intrapulmonary shunting and may progress to ARDS. Although pulmonary edema is an uncommon clinical problem in these patients, studies have suggested that extravascular lung water may be increased.

Acute hypoxia at the time of injury or with the intravenous injection of an excessive dose of narcotics (*mainlining*) has been suggested as a possible cause of pulmonary failure. If a patient has a respiratory arrest, the resulting hypoxia gives rise to a massive sympathetic discharge, with a marked augmentation of cardiac output. At the same time, the pulmonary vascular resistance is much increased by hypoxia and possible acidemia. Consequently, there is an extremely high pulmonary artery pressure. This hypertension damages the pulmonary arterioles enough to allow considerable extravasation of blood. When the airway and ventilation are restored, the circulation returns to normal, but the lungs have been severely damaged. By the time the patient is being cared for and life-saving maneuvers have been started, the noxious effects of hypoxia have seemingly vanished and the subsequent respiratory distress is labeled as an idiosyncratic reaction to narcotics or pulmonary edema due to head injury.

Aspiration pneumonitis is another possible cause of failure in comatose patients who are not properly positioned and whose airways are not secured. Frequently it goes unrecognized because gastric juice with low pH often is clear, watery, and free from bile.

Medical Management

Head injury provides a special set of difficulties. The balance of adequate hydration of the body to maintain the circulation without causing cerebral edema makes the combination with acute respiratory failure particularly dangerous. High pressures from mechanical support of the lung can increase intracranial pressure. There appears to be no universally acceptable answer. Mild hyperventilation, which reduces cerebral edema, in combination with sufficient mechanical support of the lungs to maintain an arterial oxygen tension above 70 torr, with an inspired oxygen fraction of 40% to 45%, would seem a reasonable compromise. The use of IMV to minimize intrathoracic pressure that might be transmitted as venous pressure would also seem desirable. Monitoring cardiovascular and intracranial pressures may be helpful in determining the balance of therapy to reduce cerebral edema.

Drug overdose provides a lesser problem, in that volume loading and standard therapy for acute respiratory failure can be more easily managed without damaging the patient. Hydration should be just sufficient to maintain cardiac and renal function. If a low-output low-pressure state develops, inotropic support is permissible but is associated with a higher mortality.

In general, the basic principles of mechanical support of the lungs in both head injury and overdose patients are not rendered invalid by the patient's primary condition.

Atelectasis

One of the most common respiratory disorders in the critically ill patient is atelectasis. It may also be one of the most preventable complications of any hospitalized patient. By definition, *atelectasis* is collapse of alveoli or diminution of volume of lung units. Although it is a frequent complication of upper abdominal surgery, atelectasis may be caused by compression of lung tissue, as by tumors, effusions, pneumothorax, hemothorax and empyema, as well as by any condition that decreases the inspiratory effort of the patient. This collapse may be lobar or segmental but is most often randomly spread throughout the lung (patchy atelectasis).

Pathophysiology

Three factors have been implicated in the collapse of alveoli: airway obstruction (*resorptive atelectasis*), ineffective ventilation, and decreased surfactant levels. Resorptive atelectasis results when gas is unable to reach alveoli because of obstruction. A mucous plug or foreign body, aspirated matter, or tumor material can decrease ventilation to the alveoli. Once obstruction occurs, the gas distal to it is absorbed into the circulation because oxygen tension in the pulmonary arteries is lower than that in the alveoli. Thus, oxygen diffuses from the area of greater to that of lower concentration. The higher the concentration of oxygen in the alveoli, the faster the absorption rate; thus, the higher the FiO_2 of inspired gas at the time of the obstruction, the faster the alveolar collapse.

Obstruction of the larger lobar and segmental branches most certainly leads to collapse of lung tissue distal to it. However, atelectasis beyond this level is probably not caused by obstruction. Collateral ventilation usually permits passage of gas into the obstructed alveoli. Thus, resorptive atelectasis does not occur even with complete obstruction of peripheral airways unless underlying disease has prevented collateral ventilation.

Ineffective ventilation is probably the main factor in postoperative atelectasis. Studies have shown that constant tidal volumes lead to decreased lung volume, decreased compliance, and increased shunting. This collapse of alveoli is reversible by hyperinflation of the lung. Upper abdominal surgery may cause "splinting" during breathing, thereby lowering tidal volumes. Stasis of secretions due to ineffective coughing further reduces the amount of gas available for gas exchange. In addition to these conditions, compression by space-occupying lesions of the chest decreases the number of ventilated alveoli.

Surfactant, which has the property of lowering surface tension to prevent collapse, may be a significant factor in atelectasis. Decreased surfactant levels are thought to be a factor in promoting collapse of lung units. It has yet to be established whether these low levels are the cause or the result of atelectasis. It seems highly probable, however, that decreased blood flow decreases surfactant level.

Data Acquisition

Mild atelectasis is often asymptomatic, but with inadequate treatment the atelectatic areas may enlarge and lead to symptoms of hypoxemia. Acute onset of obstruction is marked with dyspnea, restlessness, and tachycardia. With extensive involvement, cyanosis may be evident. Structures in the mediastinum may shift toward the affected side when a collapse of a major portion of the lung occurs.

Generally, crackles are heard on auscultation unless major collapse causes diminished or absent sounds. Characteristically, the blood gases show a decreased PaO_2 and normal or decreased $PaCO_2$; the levels are dependent on the extent of shunting and the respiratory rate. Patchy atelectasis may be exhibited on chest x-ray as bilateral radiopaque areas. Massive involvement may be demonstrated roentgenographically by increased density at the hilus and extending peripherally. The hemidiaphragm may be elevated on the affected side.

With persistent atelectasis, signs of pneumonia may be seen. Increased temperature, dyspnea, tachycardia, and cyanosis are generally evident. The accumulated secretions are a good medium for growth of bacteria.

Medical Management

Compression atelectasis is usually relieved once the precipitating cause is removed (e.g., drainage of effusion, removal of tumor), while hyperinflation of the lung will aid in opening atelectases of other causation. It has been suggested that deep breathing may stimulate surfactant mobilization.

Once atelectasis is present, secretions should be removed by coughing, endotracheal suctioning, or therapeutic bronchoscopy, if necessary. The best treatment is prevention. This task rests with the nurse or respiratory therapist and should never be overlooked. Preoperative teaching of coughing and deep breathing is essential to maintain efficient postoperative performance.

Frequent position changes, early ambulation, and vigorous chest physiotherapy are mandatory with any patient at risk for atelectasis. Humidification and adequate hydration will keep secretions loose and enhance expectoration. Good nutrition is a vital part of therapy to prevent muscle atrophy, which can reduce inspiratory effort. The more chronic the atelectasis, the more vigorous these measures should be.

In the intubated patient, the use of high tidal volumes and/or PEEP can help keep alveoli open. Instillation of saline for irrigation during suctioning may loosen secretions and enhance removal. Bronchodilators and mucolytic agents may also prove useful.

Prophylactic measures should be instituted in all critically ill patients to prevent atelectasis. Position changes and chest physiotherapy are required for any patient for whom bed rest is prescribed. Coughing and deep breathing are to be encouraged at routine intervals, since they are considered the first line of defense in prevention and treatment of atelectasis.

Bacterial Pneumonia

Bacterial pneumonia is a consolidative inflammation caused by pathogenic microorganisms. It is a major source of additional morbidity and mortality in the critically ill patient.

The radiographic picture of bacterial pneumonia shows an alveolar filling pattern that is soft, fluffy, and poorly demarcated. If an entire lobe is involved, an air bronchogram may be the most outstanding marker. Lobular bacterial pneumonias are usually primary processes and not complications of preexisting disease. They present with an acute onset of fever, cough, dyspnea, chest pain, and hypoxemia.

Some bacterial pneumonias present radiographically as bronchopneumonia, with multiple poorly defined areas of alveolar consolidation involving one or both lungs. Organisms presenting in this fashion include *Streptococcus, Hemophilus influenzae, Pseudomonas, Serratia, Proteus, Escherichia coli,* and the anaerobes. *Staphylococcus* may produce a pattern of bronchopneumonia, particularly if the route of infection is hematogenous. Bronchopneumonias are often secondary to other predisposing conditions such as immunosuppressive therapy or diseases (e.g., AIDS). The clinical criteria for pneumonia include leukocytosis, fever, purulent tracheobronchial secretions, and previously undetected infiltrates observed on chest x-ray. Pulmonary infection is commonly acquired through inhalation. Nosocomial bacterial pneumonia is most often associated with *Klebsiella, Staphylococcus aureus, Pseudomonas aeruginosa,* and *Escherichia coli.* It is usually distributed throughout the lung in a lobar or segmental pattern. A single lobe or segment is usually affected, although multiple areas of disease may appear simultaneously, especially with *Staphylococcus.* Bronchoalveolar lavage may be useful in identifying the causative organism in bacterial pneumonias.[9]

Up to 60% of ICU patients may develop pneumonia, depending on the severity of their underlying disease. Specific etiological diagnosis is commonly lacking because specimens tend to be contaminated by oropharyngeal secretions. Significant predisposing factors in the development of nosocomial pneumonias include (1) concurrent antibiotic treatment, which predisposes the patient to colonization with resistant gram-negative bacilli of the oropharynx; (2) aspiration of oropharyngeal or gastric secretions; (3) bypassing of normal respiratory clearance mechanisms and subsequent implantation of bacteria onto alveolar surfaces; and (4) hematogenous spread to the lungs from distant foci.

Initial therapy of bacterial pneumonia is determined by Gram's stain of the sputum and later by culture. Antibiotic coverage may be started on the basis of the stain and modified later when culture results with antibiotic sensitivities are obtained. Dosage should be calculated as indicated on the package insert for *serious* infection and should be adjusted according to pre- and postadministration serum levels.

Prevention, not treatment, should be the primary approach to nosocomial bacterial pneumonias in critically ill patients. Scrupulously sterile technique when using respiratory therapy equipment and during suctioning of patients is necessary. A program of infection control surveillance is essential in the modern critical care unit.

NURSING MANAGEMENT: CASE STUDY

A 68-year-old male is admitted to the critical care unit with acute shortness of breath. He has a medical history of congestive heart failure which has been under control in the recent past. His level of consciousness has decreased in the past hour, and he presently has a total Glasgow Coma Score of 8. He is intubated and placed on mechanical ventilation with the following settings:

Mode	Assisted Mandatory Ventilation
Vt	800 cc
RR	12
FiO_2	0.80
PEEP	+5

The physician believes the patient may have aspirated some GI contents during the intubation. The following laboratory data are available:

PaO_2	67 torr
$PaCO_2$	32 torr
pH	7.35
HCO_3	21 mEq
Hemoglobin	11 g/dl

■ NURSING DIAGNOSIS

Impaired gas exchange, related to low ventilation/perfusion ratio.

OUTCOME STANDARD AND CRITERIA

Gas exchange will be normal as evidenced by:
- Acceptable PaO_2 and SaO_2 levels without oxygenation and ventilation support

NURSING INTERVENTIONS

- Provide mechanical ventilation and oxygenation support as prescribed
- Use pulse oximeter to monitor changes in FiO_2 and PEEP
- Assess intrapulmonary shunt through PaO_2/FiO_2, a/A ratio or other measures of intrapulmonary shunt estimates

- Assist with airway protection through suctioning as indicated
- Observe for signs of barotrauma (pneumothorax) secondary to mechanical ventilation and PEEP therapy
- Monitor position changes with pulse oximeter to determine if any position has better $\dot{V}/\dot{Q}$ relationships. Position changes can range from supine to prone
- Monitor need for rest or sedation through pulse oximetry. Note activities that cause a decrease in pulse oximeter readings
- Monitor impact of therapies on the $\dot{V}/\dot{Q}$ ratio to determine which therapies are most effective
- Assess the need for mechanical ventilation by monitoring weaning parameters
- Assess impact of changes in $\dot{Q}s/\dot{Q}T$ on oxygen delivery and cellular oxygenation through use of $S\bar{v}O_2$ values, lactate levels, and changes in cardiac output

■ NURSING DIAGNOSIS

Impaired gas exchange, related to high ventilation/perfusion ratio.

OUTCOME STANDARD AND CRITERIA

Gas exchange will be normal as evidenced by:
- Maintenance of acceptable $PaCO_2$ and pH levels without ventilatory support

NURSING INTERVENTIONS

- Assess effect of increased physiological dead space on work of breathing by measuring respiratory rate and minute ventilation
- In consultation with respiratory therapist, measure carbon dioxide production (VCO_2) to differentiate increased dead space from increased VCO_2 as a cause for increased respiratory efforts
- Use end-tidal CO_2 values ($PetCO_2$) to establish the $PaCO_2$–$PetCO_2$ difference. Use this difference to establish the severity of increases in physiological dead space. If the difference is small (less than 5 torr), $PetCO_2$ may be a reliable estimate of $PaCO_2$ values
- Assess need for mechanical ventilation through daily assessment of spontaneous breathing capability

■ NURSING DIAGNOSIS

High risk for altered nutrition, related to inability to eat.

OUTCOME STANDARD AND CRITERIA

Nutritional intake meets metabolic requirements as evidenced by:
- Stable or increased weight
- Adequate protein reserves

NURSING INTERVENTIONS

- Measure or estimate caloric requirements through exhaled gas analysis or body size
- Collaborate with dietary consultants to maintain

adequate caloric and substrate intake
- Assess most appropriate route for maintaining nutritional support

RESTRICTIVE LUNG DISORDERS
Lung Abscess

Lung abscess is a pyogenic lesion of the lung parenchyma giving rise to a cavity. Most often it is attributed to the aspiration of foreign material into the respiratory tract. It may also arise systemically by hematogenous spread or may follow a lung infarct. Obstruction of the bronchioles and stasis of secretions contribute to the infection.

An aspiration abscess may be seen in any condition leading to a suppression of the cough reflex, including anesthesia, head injury, diabetic coma, drug overdose, epileptic or alcoholic coma, and near drowning. A detailed history should be sought from patients in whom lung abscess is suspected, since any one of these conditions can be found in up to 70% of the cases (Table 29-1). Oral infections such as pyorrhea or infected tonsils may be unrecognized causes of abscess formation if the debris is aspirated.

Tumors that cause abscess formation are usually malignant, the most common malignant type being bronchial carcinoma (squamous cell type). These tumors are likely to become infected and cause obstruction of lung segments by acting like a foreign body, causing stasis of secretions. Any patient with a diagnosis of lung abscess and no history of aspiration should undergo diagnostic testing for carcinoma. Very often chest therapy and antibiotics clear the abscess while the tumor remains undetected.

Necrosis of consolidated areas seen in bacterial pneumonia predisposes to abscesses. These cystlike sacs distend with inspired air and can easily burst into the pleura, causing collapse of the lung tissue. This mechanism is seen more frequently in children than adults because of the thin, less tough wall of the pleura in children.

Pathophysiology

The site of the abscess is determined by the position of the body during aspiration. The aspirate will travel to the most dependent region of the lung. Thus, in a supine patient the foreign material will move into the right lung (recall the anatomic angle of the right mainstem bronchus). From the right bronchus, material usually moves into the posterior segment of the upper lobe or superior segment of the lower lobe.

Fibrous granulation tissue usually forms around most of the abscess while it becomes embedded in the parenchyma. The abscess may extend toward the pleural cavity but rarely ruptures into it. Pleuritic pain and pleural effusion due to irritation of the pleural space by the granulation tissue may occur. The abscess fills with pus, and the now granulated portion often erodes into a bronchus, causing the drainage of foul-smelling pus into the trachea. If the pleuritic pain is not significant, the aspiration of pus is often the first sign of abscess formation. The expectoration of the pus may lead to partial healing and cavity formation. However, inadequate drainage and chest therapy can lead to multiple small abscesses within the lung.

Data Acquisition

The onset of symptoms may be insidious or acute. Typically, general malaise and fever with or without pleuritic pain are seen. Over a number of days, fever with temperature spikes persists, pleuritic pain is evident, and dyspnea may be seen, depending on the size of the abscess and its effect on lung tissue. The presence of foul-smelling pus in tracheal aspirate or

TABLE 29-1   **Common Causes of Lung Abscess**

Aspiration Abscess	Malignant Abscess	Pulmonary Embolus	Infection
Alcoholism	Necrotic bronchial carcinoma	Pulmonary infarct infection	Pneumonia
Anesthesia	Bronchial obstruction and stasis of secretions	Septic emboli	Pyogenic bacteria (notably *Staphylococcus aureus*)
Oversedation	Head and neck malignant tumor	Fragments from bacterial endarteritis	Defective ciliary action
Coma (diabetic, epileptic, drug overdose, cerebrovascular accident)			Inefficient expectoration
Oral infection			Infected cyst
Food or foreign body			Necrotic lesion
Laryngeal palsy			Subdiaphragmatic infection (usually liver)
Carcinoma of esophagus ("spillover" aspiration)			Open chest wound

expectoration clarifies the diagnosis. Purulent drainage may be blood-tinged owing to bronchial erosion. Unfortunately, the symptoms are like those of pneumonia, and often the initial diagnosis is incorrect. For this reason, the history is most important.

Physical examination shows a dullness to percussion and decreased or absent breath sounds with intermittent pleural friction rub, depending on the extent of abscess formation and its proximity to the pleural space. Crackles may be present but are not definitive. Chest x-ray shows areas of consolidation that may indicate other disease entities. It is not until a fluid level is evident, usually indicating communication with the bronchus, that the diagnosis can be narrowed down to either empyema with bronchopleural fistula or a lung abscess.

Medical Management

The initial evaluation of the patient must determine the presence of anaerobic or aerobic pyogenic organisms. Early bronchoscopy may be desirable, followed by appropriate anaerobic and aerobic antibiotic therapy. Although the culture report should be followed closely to determine sensitivity, flora is usually mixed. In general, however, the antibiotic therapy should be changed according to clinical findings, not bacterial culture changes, when deterioration of the patient is noted.

The use of therapeutic bronchoscopy for drainage is somewhat controversial. Diagnostically, bronchoscopy can be used to rule out carcinoma or foreign body. It can also be useful in locating the site of the draining bronchus, thereby aiding positioning to facilitate drainage. Some clinicians believe that bronchoscopy should be reserved for those patients in whom other treatment brings no improvement. It can be used to aspirate the abscess and to obtain specimens for diagnostic purposes. The fear of spreading infection to other parts of the lung, however, often deters clinicians from performing bronchoscopy.

The need for surgical treatment is rare but has been reported. The indications for surgery are (1) failure of the abscess to diminish in size, (2) continued toxicosis and sepsis, (3) suspicion of cancer, and (4) recurrent infection. Once the visceral and parietal pleura have become inflamed and pleural symphysis has occurred, surgery can be performed. Open drainage is the most common form of surgical intervention. The use of a double-lumen endotracheal tube is advocated to prevent spillage of the drainage to uninfected areas of the lung. Successful percutaneous drainage (*pneumonotomy*) has been reported. A cleansing bronchoscopy should be performed on both lungs after surgery is completed.

Pleural Effusion

The potential space between the visceral and parietal pleura is lined with a thin layer of fluid that constantly changes with the motion of the lungs. There are two types of fluid passage, classified according to the presence or absence of protein. Protein usually enters the pleural space by leaking from the pleural capillaries and is drained by the lymphatic system. Protein-free fluid flows from the parietal pleura via systemic capillaries into the pleural space and is absorbed into the visceral pleura by the pulmonary capillaries. This mechanism is dependent upon hydrostatic and colloid osmotic pressures across the space.

Systemic capillary hydrostatic pressure (parietal pleura) is higher than the pulmonary capillary pressure (visceral pleura), with colloid osmotic pressure the same in both systems. The pleural space has an osmotic pressure below that of the two capillary systems it separates. Thus, the hydrostatic pressure in the systemic capillaries, coupled with negative pleural pressure, forces the movement of fluid from the parietal pleura into the pleural space. Conversely, the higher colloid osmotic pressure in the pulmonary capillaries results in a shift of fluid into the visceral pleura from the pleural space (Figure 29-5). Since this movement of fluid is dependent on the various pressures, any hemodynamic changes in the cardipulmonary system will be reflected in the formation and absorption of fluid in the pleural space.

Pathophysiology

A pleural effusion is excess fluid in the pleural space. It is usually thought of as a sign of disease, not a disease entity in itself. Effusions are classified as transudate or exudate, with the distinction between them based on protein content.

Transudates are usually produced when there is a disturbance in the flow of protein-free fluid in the pleural space. Thus, the protein content in transudates remains normal or less than 3 g/dl. Pleural transudate is usually clear or pale yellow with a specific gravity of less than 1.015 and is usually bilateral. It is often termed *hydrothorax*.

Exudates usually result from disease of the pleural surface, due to either increased permeability of capillaries with resultant leakage of proteins or an obstruction in the lymphatic system inhibiting drainage of proteins. Therefore, the protein content in exudates is high, usually more than 3 g/dl. The specific gravity is increased (more than 1.016) because of the increased protein. The exudate is often dark yellow or amber and is usually unilateral.

Table 29-2 gives a partial list of the causes of pleu-

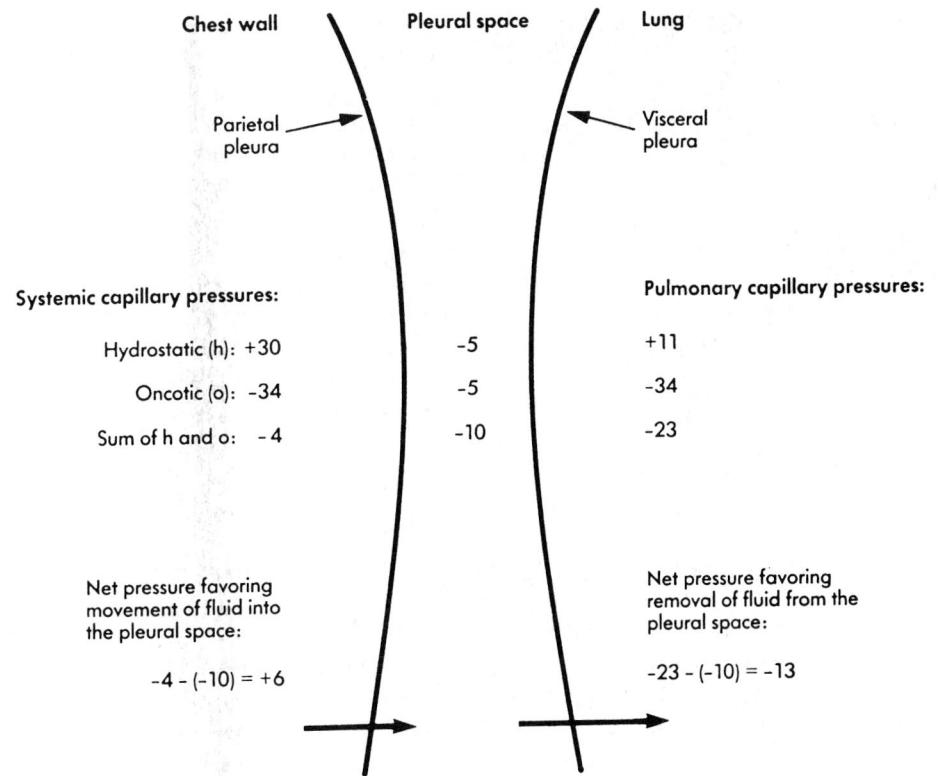

Figure 29-5 Normal pleural fluid movement. A physiological balance between the systemic and pulmonary capillaries provides for continuous movement of fluid from parietal pleura capillaries into the pleural space and then into visceral pleura capillaries. All pressures are in cmH_2O. Pressures that tend to force fluid out of the capillaries are shown by a plus sign (+); pressures that act to hold fluid in the capillary or pleural space are assigned a minus sign (−). There is a net +6 cmH_2O pressure favoring fluid movement into the pleural space. In this diagram the surfaces are shown apart, but in healthy people they touch, separated only by a thin (and radiologically invisible) film of pleural fluid.
From Martin, L. (1987). *Pulmonary physiology in clinical practice: The essentials for patient care and evaluation.* St. Louis: Mosby–Year Book.

ral effusion categorized as exudate or transudate. It is necessary to differentiate the type of effusion in order to determine the cause. Transudates, since they are not caused by pleural disease, do not usually require the extensive diagnostic follow-up that is often needed for exudates.

A number of tests for pleural fluid are available to differentiate exudates from transudates and to diagnose the cause of exudates. Besides determination of the color, the amount of protein, and the specific gravity, other tests include the differentiation of serum and pleural lactic acid dehydrogenase and protein levels, red cell count, white cell count with differential, pleural fluid cytological study (for malignant cells), glucose and amylase levels, pH, and culture with bacteriological stains.

Data Acquisition

Pleural effusions usually show a restriction of chest wall expansion on the affected side if the effusion is large. Dullness to percussion and absent or decreased

breath sounds over the area are noted. If the effusion is infected or purulent, temperature elevation may be present. Dyspnea is common in a rapidly accumulating effusion, whereas chronic or slow accumulation may cause no respiratory distress.

Chest x-ray abnormalities may be undetectable if the effusion is small (less than 100 ml). Larger effusions are seen as dense opacities. A level of fluid may be observed in a gravity-dependent position; thus, if the patient lies on the affected side prior to x-ray, fluid may be seen in the lateral chest wall.

Medical Management

Any pleural effusion should be subjected to a diagnostic tap (thoracentesis). Chemical, cytological, and bacteriological analyses may yield valuable information to determine cause.

The position of the patient during the procedure is important to prevent the occurrence of pneumothorax or hemothorax. A good position for a lateral or posterior tap is for the patient to sit on the edge

TABLE 29-2 Causes of Pleural Effusions

Exudates	Transudates
Malignancy	Congestive heart failure
Carcinoma	Hypoproteinemic states, including:
Mesothelioma	
Lymphoma	Nephrotic syndrome
Infection	Liver cirrhosis
Parapneumonic	Pneumothorax
Tuberculosis	Atelectasis
Fungal	Pulmonary embolism (some
Viral	cases)
Collagen-vascular	Peritoneal dialysis
Systemic lupus	Meigs's syndrome (benign
Rheumatoid arthritis	ovarian tumor)
Pulmonary embolism	
(some cases)	
Pancreatitis	
Subphrenic abscess	
Uremia	
Asbestosis	
Chylothorax	
Traumatic hemothorax	
Esophageal rupture	
Drug-induced effusion	
Postradiation therapy	
Sarcoidosis	
Idiopathic (undiagnosed)	

From Martin, L. (1987). *Pulmonary physiology in clinical practice.* St. Louis: Mosby–Year Book.

of the bed and lean forward onto an overbed table. The skin is cleaned with iodophor or iodine solution and anesthetized with local anesthetic. A tap requires insertion of the needle into the intercostal space along the upper surface of the lower rib. The presence of fluid confirms entrance into the pleural space. Usually no more than 1,000 ml of fluid should be drained rapidly, and even less if the patient exhibits signs of respiratory distress. A pleural biopsy is also recommended at this time.

Recurrent pleural effusions present a management problem. Effusions from bronchial carcinoma and from metastatic tumors of extrathoracic origin fall into this category. Often a malignant effusion reaccumulates shortly after it is aspirated. Attempts are made to eliminate or reduce the number of recurrent effusions. The use of nitrogen mustard instilled in the pleural space has been reported to slow down the rate of effusion. Pleurodesis using iodized talc in an aerosol produces similar results.

The nurse must be aware of the conditions that precipitate effusions. Since malignant disease carries a high incidence of fluid accumulation, those patients being diagnostically evaluated for lung cancer should have frequent chest auscultation. Any decreased or absent sounds, as well as signs of dyspnea, should be reported at once.

Kyphoscoliosis

Kyphoscoliosis is an orthopedic problem that may severely impair respiratory and cardiovascular function. *Scoliosis* is curvature of the spine laterally (twisted); *kyphosis* is curvature forward. This spinal deformity usually starts in adolescence as scoliosis and later becomes kyphotic. The condition may rarely be due to Pott's disease (tuberculosis of the spine), in which the kyphosis is more pronounced, or it may be due to poliomyelitis or rickets, or to osteoporosis in the aged. Unfortunately, the majority of cases are designated idiopathic.

Pathophysiology

The impairment of respiratory function results from distortions in the shape of the lung and the rib cage which prevent normal expansion. If there is a cone-shaped distortion, compression of the lung by the chest wall is usually more severe at the bases, with atelectasis and bronchopneumonia common findings. Overexpansion of the upper lobes may be evident. Rigidity of the chest wall is common with advancing age.

This rigidity of the chest wall and compression of the lung decrease the vital capacity, tidal volume, and alveolar ventilation and increase the work of breathing. The atelectasis alters the ventilation/perfusion $(\dot{V}/\dot{Q})$ ratio to increase shunting. The resultant hypoxemia and hypercapnia are pronounced in severe cases.

Constriction of the pulmonary vessels, primarily due to the compression of the chest cavity, may lead to pulmonary hypertension. The vascular resistance may be elevated from the effects of hypoxia, and the right ventricle may fail from continually forcing blood through the compromised pulmonary vasculature. The resultant right-sided heart failure and the ventilatory compromise are the usual cause of death.

Data Acquisition

The main clinical signs in a patient with severe kyphoscoliosis are similar to those in cor pulmonale. Severe dyspnea and rhonchi are often present in the late stages of the disease. Lung volumes reveal decreased tidal volume, minute volume, vital capacity, functional residual capacity, and expiratory reserve volume. Arterial blood gas analysis reveals decreased PaO_2, increased $PaCO_2$, and decreased pH due to effects of progressive respiratory failure.

Pitting edema of the extremities is noted if the patient is in right heart failure. Chest x-ray interpretation is often difficult because of poor positioning.

Radiological findings consistent with pneumonia and atelectasis are present.

Medical Management

Initial management of the deformed chest wall in children is by correction of the chest wall by body casts. Some increase in vital capacity has been achieved. Operative procedures may be effective.

Ventilatory support is necessary for patients with acute respiratory failure from infection. High peak-inspiratory pressure may be useful in improving the compliance of the chest wall, thereby improving lung compliance. The relation betweeen lung compliance and the amount of peak-inspiratory pressure is under investigation.

Treatment of kyphoscoliosis is purely symptomatic. Management of congestive heart failure and respiratory failure are described elsewhere in this book. Long-term therapy is similar to that of bronchitis. Recurrent infections, a common complication, are treated with antibiotics.

OBSTRUCTIVE LUNG DISORDERS

Asthma

The term *asthma* is used to describe a recurrent, reversible airway obstruction with prolonged expiratory length, air trapping during attacks, ventilation/perfusion mismatching, increased intrapulmonary shunting, cough, and tenacious sputum. The obstruction may be so mild that the patient experiences dyspnea only on exertion or so severe and prolonged that it results in respiratory failure or even death by asphyxiation. Symptoms may be intermittent with normal pulmonary function between attacks or may cause chronic debilitation from compromised pulmonary function.

The acute obstruction of asthma is a reversible process involving spasm of the smooth muscle in the bronchial walls. As the episode progresses, mucus from the lumina of the bronchi, together with edematous inflammation of the mucosa, further narrows the airways. The resultant ventilation/perfusion mismatch produces arterial hypoxemia.

Preventive care has decreased the morbidity associated with asthma in recent years, while more appropriate use of medications and respiratory therapy has improved the mortality associated with severe attacks.

Pathophysiology

Asthma reflects a hyperactive response of the bronchial airways to a variety of factors including extrinsic allergens. It is manifested by widespread airway narrowing that changes in severity either spontaneously or with treatment. It has long been known that immediate hypersensitivity, mediated by immune globulin E (IgE), plays an important role in this syndrome.

Some clinicians identify a subgroup known as intrinsic asthma, or asthmatic bronchitis. This type of asthma is not mediated by IgE. Emotions and their impact on the sympathetic and parasympathetic nervous systems play a role in this process. Also, chronic obstructive pulmonary disease (COPD) usually has a bronchospastic component that can be considered intrinsic asthma.

A theory called *beta blockade* suggests that an imbalance exists in the normal sympathetic and parasympathetic nervous innervation of the airways. Beta-adrenergic (β_1 and β_2) receptors in the airways are responsible for bronchial smooth muscle relaxation when stimulated by cyclic adenosine monophosphate (cAMP). When β_2 stimulation does not occur, cAMP is lower, and bronchoconstriction occurs. Cardiopulmonary blood vessels are also supplied with β_1 receptors. Stimulation of these receptors produces vasoconstriction and undesirable side effects, including tachycardia, possibly dysrhythmias, and blood pressure alteration.

Without beta stimulation, bronchoconstriction occurs in response to a variety of stimuli including hyperventilation, extreme temperature and humidity changes, emotional disturbances, infection, and the classic "allergic" response to extrinsic allergens.

In some persons, upper airway irritation may cause bronchoconstriction by stimulation of the vagus nerve. This parasympathetic stimulation may also enhance mucus secretion and be responsible for the cough and hyperventilation that accompany bronchospasm. Parasympathetic blockade using atropine may initially appear to be advantageous because it dries bronchial secretions, but it is contraindicated because of the increased risk of bronchial plugging. Parasympathetic and sympathetic forces create two opposing systems, then, with parasympathetic stimulation encouraging bronchospasm while sympathetic stimulation of both alpha and beta receptors favors bronchial relaxation.

Chemical mediator substances such as histamine, slow-reacting substance of anaphylaxis, prostaglandins, serotonin, and bradykinin also influence the degree of bronchoconstriction. Stimulation of mast cells in the pulmonary submucosa causes them to release these mediators, producing bronchoconstriction and/or vasodilatation. The mediators are inhibited by cAMP. In addition to its effect on smooth muscle, β_2 stimulation induces bronchial relaxation. Figure 29-6 shows the effects of alterations in sympathetic and parasympathetic influence on the development of bronchospasm, as well as the effect of mast cell mediator substances.

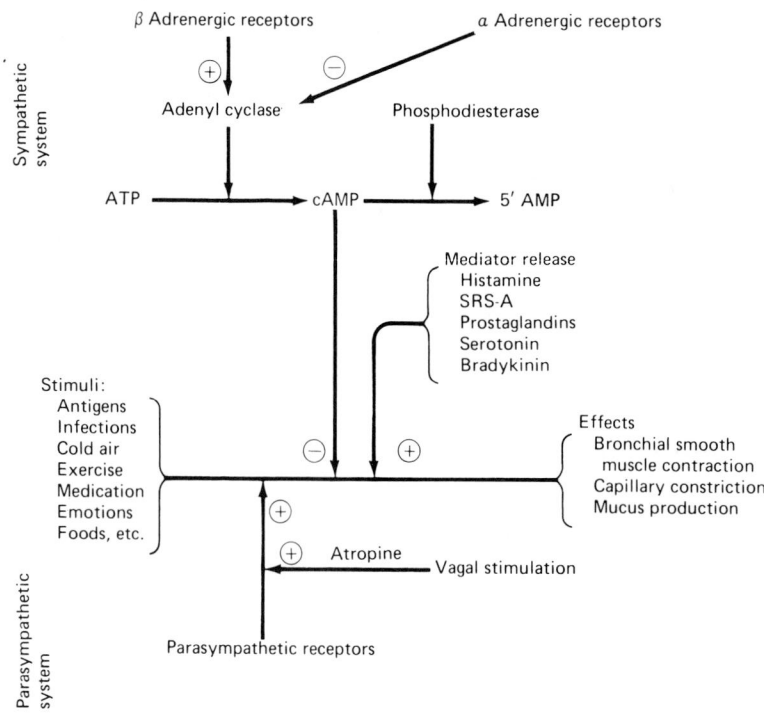

Figure 29-6 Sympathetic and parasympathetic influences on the development of bronchospasm.

It is important to remember that severe broncho-spasm involves more than just bronchoconstriction. Bronchial wall edema and mucus hypersecretion also contribute to pathophysiological changes during asthmatic crisis.[9]

Once bronchospasm has developed, a variety of events follow, as shown in Figure 29-7. Marked pulmonary hyperinflation may result. Total lung capacity may increase by up to 30%, and residual volume is markedly increased. An overinflated lung is stiff, and compliance is low, and this increases the work of breathing. The patient then begins to perceive dyspnea, a hallmark of asthma attack. This process is aggravated by anxiety and a reflex hyperventilation.

As a result of hyperventilation, $PaCO_2$ is usually low during an attack. If severe bronchospasm persists, however, the patient tires and cannot maintain hyperventilation. $PaCO_2$ rises to normal and finally becomes elevated. Excessive sedation or narcotic administration decreases ventilatory drive and can hasten decompensation during an asthma attack. Decreasing overall ventilation combined with ventilation/perfusion mismatching leads to hypercapnia, and mechanical ventilation is needed to maintain the patient.

Accumulation of secretions in airways leads to cough, which may stimulate more bronchospasm. Bronchial hygiene and maintenance of adequate hydration are important in controlling the problems associated with accumulation of secretions.

Hypercapnia is a late sign noted only in severe and prolonged asthma attacks. Hypoxemia is the common blood gas abnormality, resulting from the shunt created by uneven ventilation and perfusion. Oxygen therapy is needed to treat the hypoxemia, but assisted ventilation is necessary if the $PaCO_2$ starts to rise.

In *status asthmaticus,* the patient is severely distressed from the dyspnea and exhaustion. The patient is often unable to maintain adequate oxygenation and becomes cyanotic. Severely elevated intrathoracic pressures may interfere with venous return to the right ventricle; cardiac output falls, and vascular collapse may ensue. Dehydration due to fluid loss from hyperventilation may also contribute to impaired venous return. Cor pulmonale occurs late, when the situation is desperate. Tachycardia indicates the stress placed on the cardiovascular system. A pulse rate greater than 120 in a patient who has not taken alpha-adrenergic stimulating drugs (e.g., epinephrine) signifies the need for urgent measures.

Data Acquisition

The signs and symptoms of asthma reflect the distal airway obstruction and interference with gas exchange. The primary symptom is dyspnea. The patient has difficulty forcing air out of the lungs and frequently wheezes in the attempt. Prolongation of expiration is audible on auscultation.

Cough is another symptom of bronchospasm in asthma. As the attack progresses, the cough becomes

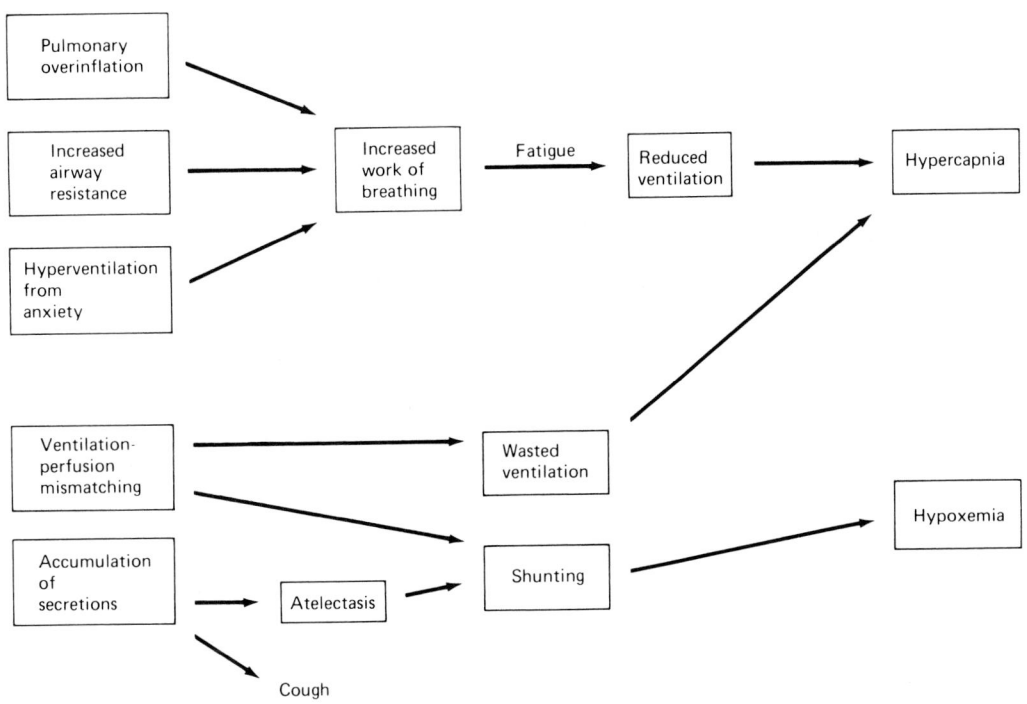

Figure 29-7 Consequences of bronchospasm.

productive, dyspnea and wheezing increase, and the patient may speak only in short phrases. Preferential body position is seated, with forward tilt of the upper torso, arms braced, shoulders held high, and chest distended with little movement. There is retraction of the suprasternal notch and intercostal spaces.

In a very severe attack there may be so little air movement in the chest that a wheeze is not audible. Coughing is virtually impossible. The chest is hyperresonant, and breath sounds are diminished. Heart tones are distant.

The pulse is rapid and thready. In severe episodes, the pulse may be paradoxical, with diminished volume on inspiration. This is from decreased filling of the right atrium due to decreased lung compliance, itself a result of pulmonary overdistention and high intraalveolar pressures. The patient becomes hypoxemic, cyanotic, and lethargic or unresponsive. Asphyxia is imminent unless the symptoms are reversed. The term *status asthmaticus* denotes the point in the course of asthma at which the bronchospasm can no longer be relieved by bronchodilators.

The duration of an asthma attack is variable. It may last 30 minutes to 1 hour and be terminated by the use of medication, or it may last for days or weeks. The frequency of attacks is even more variable. Some patients have a single attack once or twice a year, while others are in chronic respiratory distress with frequent acute exacerbations.

The exact point at which patients in acute asthmatic attack will tire, become severely hypoxemic,

and lose consciousness is unpredictable. Some patients are in status asthmaticus almost as soon as symptoms begin, but more commonly this condition occurs when there is a delay between the onset of symptoms and administration of medication. Patients receiving continuous high-dose therapy are more likely to present in status asthmaticus in the emergency room than those receiving seasonal or no medications.

The main abnormality in asthma is airway obstruction. Pulmonary function tests show decreased expiratory gas flow, including forced expiratory volume in 1, 2, and 3 seconds (FEV_{1-3}) and forced vital capacity (FVC). Functional residual capacity (FRC) is increased because of air trapping behind the bronchioles that have contracted in spasm during expiration. Pulmonary function usually improves after inhalation of a bronchodilator, indicating reversibility of the obstruction. During a symptom-free period, the pulmonary function studies may be completely normal.

Radiology is not extremely valuable in asthma. During an asthma attack, the chest film may show hyperinflation, identified by a low diaphragm. The heart may be long and narrow and the peripheral vessels poorly visualized. The film is more beneficial if taken during expiration, since the lowered diaphragm is more obvious. The main object in chest radiographs is to exclude the presence of other conditions or complications, especially pneumothorax. Secondary infections may sometimes be detected, and impacted mucus may be suspected from segmental collapse.

Medical Management

Precipitating factors in asthma attacks are identifiable by careful history taking, and many are readily avoidable. Asthmatic persons should avoid bronchial irritants, promptly treat respiratory infections, and avoid drugs capable of inducing bronchospastic reactions, such as propranolol.

When a few specific allergens cause a large fraction of asthmatic episodes, hyposensitization injections may be helpful. This therapy induces the formation of IgG antibodies, which block antigen binding with IgE, although this is probably not the sole mechanism. In an unknown manner, hyposensitization also reduces IgE levels, at least in some cases. Unfortunately, hyposensitization is prolonged, expensive, and only partially effective.

Cromolyn sodium is an effective preventive agent in some asthmatic patients. This drug is not a bronchodilator but apparently blocks the release of chemical mediators of bronchospasm from the bronchial mucosa (Figure 29-8). It is administered as a propelled

powder from a hand-held inhaler and occasionally causes bronchial irritation on contact. Cromolyn sodium should not be given once bronchospasm has begun.

Vigorous bronchial hygiene is essential during periods of asthmatic exacerbation to keep airways clear and minimize ventilation/perfusion mismatching. Adequate fluid intake is necessary to prevent dehydration from hyperventilation and to liquefy secretions.

Inhaled bronchodilators should be used but not abused. Metaproterenol (Alupent) and albuterol (Proventil, Ventolin) are commonly used bronchodilators. They are relatively selective β_2 agents and are particularly useful in bronchospastic patients who are hypoxemic and who have tachycardia or underlying coronary artery disease. Metaproterenol is claimed to have fewer cardiac stimulatory side effects than drugs like isoproterenol. β_1 side effects of metaproterenol are probably as common as those of isoproterenol. Terbutaline (Brethine) has a higher β_2/β_1 ratio than either isoproterenol or metaproterenol and has negligible alpha activity. Oral administration of this drug has a marked tendency to produce muscular

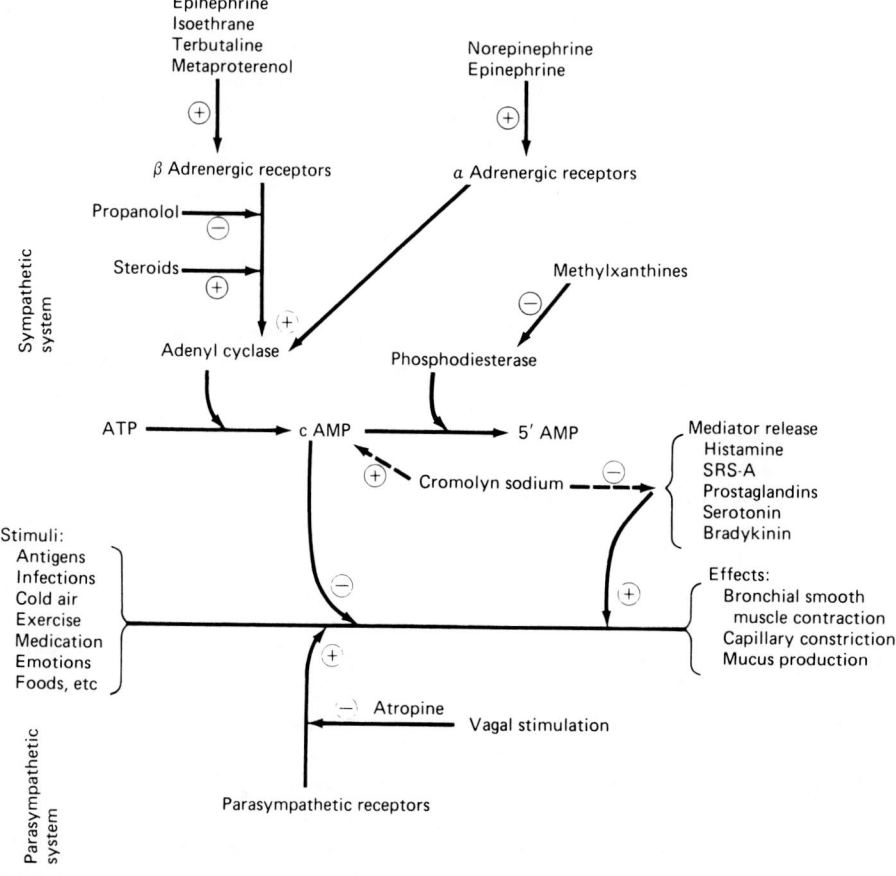

Figure 29-8   Interaction of pharmacological agents with mechanisms of asthmatic bronchospasm.

tremor and nervousness. Subcutaneous injections of terbutaline in doses of 0.125 to 0.25 mg, which may be repeated 30 minutes later, have proved useful in the critical care setting. No more than 0.5 mg should be given in a 4-hour period. Beclomethasone (Vanceril) is a metered inhaled corticosteroid preparation which delivers 50 μg per puff. Investigations suggest that use of up to 2 mg per day is without significant steroid effect. Most asthmatic patients do well on smaller doses, and many steroid-dependent patients have been transferred from oral preparations, which cause Cushing's syndrome, to safer aerosol therapy.

The beneficial actions of corticosteroids in asthma are not fully understood, but the following actions are believed to be of significant benefit: (1) prevention of antibody-antigen reaction by inhibition of antibody formation, (2) inhibition of formation or storage of mediators such as histamine, and (3) inhibition of nonspecific inflammatory processes. Steroids potentiate sympathomimetic drugs, probably by acting on β_2 receptors to produce smooth muscle relaxation and increase circulating levels of cAMP. The antiinflammatory steroids (glucocorticoids) are beneficial in status asthmaticus of any cause.

Prednisone and prednisolone are oral corticosteroid agents suitable for maintenance use. They are similar to hydrocortisone but more potent. During acute exacerbations they may be given in large doses of 40 to 70 mg per day for 5 to 7 days, titrated down to a maintenance dose of 5 to 20 mg per day. Cushing's syndrome can develop with prolonged use. Many asthmatic patients do well on alternate-day dosage schedules, which decrease the incidence of unwanted side effects. In cases of status asthmaticus in the critical care unit, intravenous hydrocortisone (Solu-Cortef) can be given as 250 to 500 mg initially, followed by 100 to 250 mg every 3 hours.

Patients with bronchospasm benefit greatly from any drug with bronchodilator capability. Epinephrine, 0.2 to 0.5 ml of 1:1,000 solution by subcutaneous injection, was formerly used extensively, though now its use has been largely supplanted by methylxanthines (aminophylline) and inhaled drugs. Epinephrine has α, β_1, and β_2 effects and, thus, in addition to being a potent bronchodilator, has unwanted cardiovascular and nervous system effects. It is dangerous to use in patients with underlying cardiac disease, especially the elderly.

Isoproterenol was once the most popular bronchodilator and is one of the most potent β_2 stimulators but is rarely used now. It also has strong β_1 actions and carries a risk of dangerous inotropic and chronotropic cardiac stimulation. The β_1 cardio-stimulatory effects of isoproterenol and its short duration of action are notable disadvantages compared

with newer, more selective β_2 agents.

Methylxanthines are still popular drugs used to treat bronchospasm, although they are controversial in the treatment of acute bronchospasm. They inhibit phosphodiesterase activity, thereby preventing breakdown of cAMP and favoring bronchial relaxation. Theophylline has many additional beneficial effects, including an increase in cardiac output, decrease in venous pressure, dilatation of pulmonary vascular bed, and improved renal circulation and cerebral stimulation.

The most serious common side effect of theophylline and its derivatives is increased gastric secretion, peptic irritation, and gastric bleeding. This is more common in oral preparations but is also a function of the blood level of the drug. Optimal therapeutic blood levels are close to toxic levels, and intermittent dosage may result in serum peak levels in the toxic range. Hepatic metabolism and renal excretion of the drug are often impaired, and for all these reasons, periodic serum drug levels should be monitored (preferably daily) in critically ill patients. Gastric pH should be monitored whenever possible, and the use of antacids is recommended to minimize gastric complications.

Aminophylline is a synthetic theophylline derivative that is 20 times more soluble in water and can therefore be administered intravenously, whereas theophylline cannot. A loading dose of 5 to 6 mg/kg in an average adult who has not recently taken aminophylline is recommended. This is followed by 0.3 to 0.9 mg/kg/hr via slow intravenous drip.

Treatment priorities for the patient in status asthmaticus with hypoxemia and increasing $PaCO_2$ are as follows: (1) oxygen inhalation via mask with patient breathing spontaneously or with manually or mechanically assisted ventilation; (2) normalization of pH when necessary (pH less than 7.20) with IV bicarbonate, preferably in an intravenous drip titrated to maintain a desired arterial pH; (3) pharmacological management of bronchospasm as described above; (4) supportive measures such as bronchial hygiene and fluid therapy; and (5) tracheal intubation, curarization, and sedation, used with controlled ventilation. If mechanical ventilation becomes unavoidable, the patient must be sedated and probably paralyzed to avoid fighting the ventilator because of the high risk of pneumothorax and cardiac arrest. A pleural chest drainage apparatus should be readily available on standby. The use of PEEP can be dangerous if large areas of the lung are already atelectatic because of overdistention of already open lung units. The decision regarding the time at which to intubate may be a difficult one. The combination of respiratory distress and rising $PaCO_2$ in the asthmatic patient in-

TABLE 29-3   Pulmonary Function Profiles of Obstructive Pulmonary Diseases

Disease	Elastic Recoil	Static Compliance	Airway Resistance	Residual Volume/ Total Lung Capacity	Bronchodilator Response
Bronchitis	Normal	Normal	↑	Normal to ↑	+
Asthma	Normal (↓ in acute attack)	Normal (↑ in acute attack)	↑		+ +
Emphysema	↓	Normal	Normal	↑	0

dicates patient fatigue, and mechanical ventilation is necessary to prevent the development of severe respiratory failure.

Chronic Bronchitis

Chronic bronchitis is a syndrome arbitrarily defined as cough with sputum production during at least 3 consecutive months in at least 2 consecutive years.

Pathophysiology

The primary abnormality in this process is mucosal swelling, inflammation, and hypertrophy with excessive production of thick, tenacious secretions in the airways. There is an increase in the size and number of mucus-secreting glands, which are overflowing with mucus. In the smaller bronchi and bronchioles, excessive numbers of mucus-producing goblet cells are found in the epithelial lining layer. Along the epithelial surface there is denuding of cilia in random fashion. Several inhalants have been implicated as causative agents in the development of chronic bronchitis, the most common of which is cigarette smoke. Other pollutants, such as oxides of nitrogen and sulfur dioxide, have been shown to diminish ciliary activity and stimulate hypersecretion of mucus. Patients with chronic bronchitis should be encouraged to stop their cigarette habit and examine their work environment for possible pollutants. Chronic bronchitis has some response to treatment, unlike emphysema.

Data Acquisition

Expiratory prolongation is notable on physical examination, as in the emphysematous patient. During acute exacerbations, inspiration may also be prolonged because of occlusion of airway lumina by secretions. Percussion is usually normal, and auscultation will reveal crackles and wheezes. The sounds are usually loud and are caused by secretions in the airways. Peripheral edema, hepatomegaly, and cyanosis are present in the patient with severe bronchitis and pulmonary hypertension (cor pulmonale).

On pulmonary function testing, flow rates during both expiration and inspiration may be reduced, al-though the reduction is more pronounced on expiration. Patients with this condition have normal elastic recoil (in contrast to patients with emphysema) and relatively normal diffusing capacities. Air trapping is consistent and depends on the severity of airway obstruction (Table 29-3).

Patients with chronic bronchitis are sometimes referred to as "blue bloaters" because they are cyanotic, hypercapneic, and have right ventricular failure with peripheral edema. They are cyanotic and edematous because of the secondary cor pulmonale. All these changes are related to the severity of the disease process and the amount of ventilation/perfusion mismatch (primarily intrapulmonary shunt).

Medical Management

Treatment for chronic bronchitis is aimed at airway clearance and prevention of infection. Brochodilator therapy to control any bronchospasm present (previously described) and adequate hydration are essential. Mucolytics are controversial relative to their effectiveness. Patients often have renewable prescriptions at local pharmacies and begin themselves on ampicillin or other effective antibiotic whenever they note a change in sputum color or tenacity. There is controversy over whether the use of continuous antibiotic therapy for prophylaxis is of any value. Corticosteroids and hyposensitization therapy are of no value. Chest physiotherapy is helpful for airway clearance.

Emphysema

Pulmonary emphysema involves the enlargement of the distal terminal bronchioles with alveolar fragmentation and destruction of the alveolar septa. Lung elasticity (elastic recoil) is progressively lost. Airway support is lost in emphysema because of the loss of parenchymal tissue, which normally give structural support to the bronchioles and alveolar ducts. The terminal airways collapse during expiration. Patients with emphysema also tend to retain secretions and develop repeated infections easily.

Approximately 80% of patients with chronic obstructive pulmonary disease have centrilobular emphysema in addition to chronic bronchitis. The major areas of destruction are the respiratory bronchioles. Another form of emphysema, *panlobular* or *panacinar,* is primarily caused by alveolar fragmentation. The most common cause of this emphysema is cigarette smoking. Also implicated are certain atmospheric pollutants such as oxidants, certain dusts, and cadmium vapors. One form of panlobular emphysema results from a genetic deficiency of the enzyme α_1-antitrypsin. The enzyme inactivates proteases from white blood cells which, when not inactivated, destroy lung parenchyma.

Pathophysiology

Ventilation, diffusion, and perfusion are all altered in emphysema. Ventilation is regionally decreased because of loss of elastic recoil, poor support of terminal airways, gas trapping, and poor alveolar gas mixing in the involved areas.

Pulmonary diffusion is reduced because of a loss of alveolar surface area and pulmonary vasoconstriction. Hypoxemia and pressure from adjacent distended alveoli may decrease perfusion to normal alveoli, further reducing capillary blood volume and decreasing diffusing capacity.

The perfusion abnormality is one in which hypoxemia causes generalized pulmonary artery constriction, shunting blood away from even relatively normal areas of lung.

Cor pulmonale usually occurs during exacerbations of the disease, late in its course, probably owing to pulmonary hypertension produced by hypoxia, against which the right ventricle must pump. The ventricle, which normally pumps against low resistance, dilates.

Data Acquisition

A barrel chest deformity is characteristic of advanced emphysema. There is kyphosis, increased anteroposterior diameter, horizontal ribs, wide subcostal angles, and flat, immobile diaphragms. Hyperresonance to percussion, decreased breath sounds, and restricted chest wall movement are present. If crackles are present, they will be heard bilaterally at the bases, particularly in patients with cyanosis. Cor pulmonale, hepatomegaly, and peripheral edema may be present in severe cases. Prolongation of expiration is pronounced, and accessory muscles of respiration are used. The patient elects to sit upright with arms braced in the "emphysematous habitus." Heart sounds may be difficult to hear.

The chest roentgenogram typically shows a lowlying diaphragm, overexpansion, and a long, narrow heart. The lung fields are hyperlucent, with pronounced vessels and diminished peripheral vascular markings. The lateral view may show flattened diaphragms and an increased retrosternal air space. Sometimes bullae can be identified by fine, hairlike margins and lack of vascular supply.

Pulmonary function testing shows increased residual volume (RV). The increased ratio of RV to total lung capacity (TLC) reflects expiratory airway collapse and airway trapping. Expiratory flow rates (FEV_{1-3}) are decreased because of loss of elastic recoil.

Arterial blood gas analysis usually shows hypoxemia; CO_2 retention may or may not be present. Patients who maintain good ventilation/perfusion matching (the "pink puffers") can maintain blood gases fairly well until late in the disease.

Medical Management

Emphysema is an irreversible disease for which care is only supportive, with the exception of lung transplantation. Improved activity performance and decreased morbidity have been demonstrated in patients who participate in pulmonary rehabilitation programs. Pursed-lip breathing adds a form of expiratory retard to the patient's spontaneous respiration and may improve gas distribution. Most patients find that it eases their dyspnea.

Home oxygen is useful for patients who cannot maintain a $PaCO_2$ greater than 55 torr when breathing room air. Low-flow (1 to 2 L/min) oxygen at night is currently used to relieve pulmonary hypertension from hypoxemia and prevent secondary polycythemia.

Chronic obstructive pulmonary disease (COPD) is a combination of emphysema and chronic bronchitis with a varied component of bronchospasm. Emphysema, like chronic bronchitis, can usually be managed with controlled oxygen therapy, chest physiotherapy to clear airways, bronchial hygiene, antibiotics to treat infection, and cardiovascular support. Low-flow oxygen by nasal cannula is usually used to treat the patients. When $PaCO_2$ is chronically elevated, breathing drive is regulated by hypoxemia. Oxygen should be carefully monitored to avoid excessive exposure of the patient, which might result in respiratory depression. Flow rates of 2 to 4 L/min are usually appropriate. The FiO_2 varies since it is determined by the tidal volume of room air the patient also inhales. Oxygen by Venturi-principle face mask allows more precise administration of oxygen when necessary. Endotracheal intubation and mechanical ventilation are avoided if at all possible because of the high risk of complications and additional morbidity.

Criteria for endotracheal intubation and mechanical ventilation vary, but most agree that if $PaCO_2$ increases above normal levels for that patient, and if acidemia and hypoxemia with mental obtundation are present, there is a need for more aggressive pulmonary support.

Continuous mechanical ventilation may impede venous return to the right side of the heart and therefore cardiac output. This occurs more commonly in patients with COPD, since their highly compliant lung tissue conducts the increased mean intrapulmonary pressure to the heart and great vessels with ease. Intermittent mandatory ventilation (IMV) can be successfully used in these patients. IMV offers the advantages of less influence on venous return as well as avoidance of the alkalemia, hypokalemia, and cardiac dysrhythmias seen upon rapid reduction of $PaCO_2$ on continuous mandatory ventilation.

Weaning may occur with IMV, since it essentially begins with the onset of mechanical ventilation. The patient does not need to "relearn" breathing and retrain respiratory muscles when IMV is used. IMV eliminates the fear and anxiety experienced by many patients with abrupt removal of the ventilator during conventional weaning. This is particularly significant for this group of patients, since anxiety increases their dyspnea and may increase bronchospasm, making weaning more difficult and very emotionally traumatic.

Psychosocial Aspects of COPD

The relation between the psychological and physical is closer, perhaps, in COPD than in most other chronic diseases. Many patients deal with their disease in one of two ways, and both are maladaptive. Some patients, when experiencing excitement, anxiety, or emotions like anger, become more active and hyperventilate. This adds strain to their already maximally functioning cardiopulmonary systems, and they become dyspneic. This dyspnea creates more anxiety, and a vicious cycle ensues.

A second group of patients, possibly those who have observed the relation between their emotions and dyspnea, begin to fear emotion. They use mental defense mechanisms of isolation, denial, and depression to accomplish this. Nurses should assess these mechanisms in assessing these patients and to adjust the plan of care accordingly.

The patient's family also needs special support. With this disease complex, the best they can hope for is extension of life and maximization of present level of function. They live from stage to stage of the disease with no hope for cure. They frequently feel helplessness, fear, guilt, and anger. They usually feel so guilty about their feelings of anger that they fre-

quently overprotect the patient. This definitely deters the patient from maximizing the level of functioning. The family of the COPD patient needs and deserves support from the medical and nursing staff. Referral to the psychiatric social worker or staff psychologist may be indicated.

PERFUSION LUNG DISORDERS
Pulmonary Thromboembolism

Pulmonary thromboembolism (PTE) is a common condition that complicates hospitalization today. The term is used to describe a blockage of a portion of the pulmonary arterial system by a blood clot arising from the systemic veins. Two factors concerning PTE should be considered. First, its incidence can be reduced if awareness of the high-risk factors predisposing to PTE leads to prophylactic treatment; and second, misdiagnosis is frequent because of the nonspecific signs and symptoms.

The incidence of PTE is estimated to be 650,000 annually, with a 30% mortality. The most common type of embolus is that arising in a peripheral vein. It is usually a result of deep vein thrombosis (DVT) in the lower part of the body, notably the calf and the plantar, common femoral, and superficial femoral veins.[10]

Three contributing factors predispose to thrombus formation: stasis, or reduction of blood flow; intercurrent illness; and vessel wall damage. Venostasis still remains a leading cause of DVT. Prolonged bed rest, immobility due to old age or muscular weakness, and obesity may decrease blood flow. Long operative procedures in which cardiac output is reduced, such as CABG and neurosurgery, decrease limb perfusion. Myocardial infarction, atrial fibrillation, and congestive heart failure also decrease cardiac output. A history of any of these factors should alert those managing critically ill patients to the increased possibility of PTE.

Changes in coagulation factors as a cause of thrombus formation have been under investigation. Studies have shown that there is an increased incidence of venous thrombosis and PTE during pregnancy and in women taking oral contraceptives. Estrogens are known to promote coagulation and increase platelet aggregation. It is also believed that coagulation changes may precipitate thrombus formation in the postoperative period and after abrupt discontinuation of anticoagulation therapy. Damage to the endothelial wall of a vessel may be precipitated by venostasis, trauma, sepsis, or major body burns. Thrombus formation is enhanced by platelet adhesiveness and the release of serotonin. Both hypercoagulability and vessel wall injury are factors in thrombus formation, although they are usually seen in conjunction with venostasis. It is still uncertain whether they may cause thrombosis without accompanying stasis.

Pathophysiology

The formed thrombus can dislodge and travel through the circulation to rest in the pulmonary artery. Although the thrombus may dislodge spontaneously, the more common mechanism is the jarring of the clot from the vessel wall by mechanical forces. These forces include sudden standing, usually during initial ambulation, or changes in the rate of blood flow due to a Valsalva maneuver.

Smaller emboli tend to lodge in the distal branches of the pulmonary artery at the periphery of the lung. The severity of emboli is greater when a large number of small emboli travel to the lungs simultaneously or one large embolus blocks a larger vessel. The subsequent obstruction of blood flow in the pulmonary circuit has both respiratory and hemodynamic consequences.

Initially, the number of perfused alveoli decreases, thereby increasing dead space or "wasted ventilation." Recall that ventilatory dead space results from lack of perfusion of ventilated alveoli. This yields a high ventilation/perfusion ($\dot{V}/\dot{Q}$) mismatch.[11] Because no gas exchange can take place, bronchoalveolar hypocarbia results (decreased alveolar CO_2). Hypocarbia contracts the bronchial smooth muscle, causing bronchoconstriction and alveolar shrinking. This constriction leads to maldistribution of ventilation and increased airway resistance and, thus, increases the work of breathing. The constrictive response may be viewed as a protective measure, since the amount of wasted ventilation is reduced. The inspired air is propelled into perfused alveolar units rather than into the alveoli in which perfusion cannot take place. This mechanism is not enough, however, to normalize the $\dot{V}/\dot{Q}$ ratio.

Another mechanism that leads to alveolar collapse is the reduction of surfactant. Cessation of blood flow probably leads to reduced surfactant levels. This reduction may be due to the anoxic effects on the mitochondria of the alveolar type 2 cells which produce surfactant. Atelectasis as an end result of bronchoalveolar constriction and decreased surfactant levels usually occurs 24 to 48 hours after obstruction to blood flow.

Hemodynamic consequences seem to depend on the extent of pulmonary blood flow obstruction and the cardiopulmonary status prior to the episode. The primary consequence of obstruction is an increase in pulmonary vascular resistance. The right ventricle must maintain enough pressure to propel blood through this resistance; thus, an increase in pulmonary artery pressure (PAP) is seen. If this pulmonary hypertension is severe enough, the right ventricle will fail. Tachycardia and decreased cardiac output are frequently seen at this stage. Frequently, PTE is not totally obstructive, and the cardiopulmonary responses may be only slight.

There is evidence that humoral responses (e.g., release of serotonin from platelets surrounding the PTE) may be involved in the constrictive response of the bronchioles and terminal lung units. This does not necessarily involve the areas affected by the embolus and often involves functioning alveoli. Thus, one sees perfusion with little or no ventilation because of the constriction of the alveoli. This may lead to areas of atelectasis and shunting, possibly explaining the arterial hypoxemia frequently seen in PTE. Another factor contributing to increased shunting is pulmonary hypertension. The main response is the decrease in diffusion of gases in the lung. Thus, three main factors lead to ventilation/perfusion mismatching in PTE. One is the dead space effect of alveoli ventilated but not perfused because of the obstruction of blood flow from the thrombus. Another is the shunting of blood past nonventilated alveoli that have collapsed from atelectasis. A third response is no ventilation and no perfusion seen in silent units.

Pulmonary infarction as an end result of PTE is relatively uncommon. In most instances in which infarct develops, there is underlying pulmonary disease that has already impaired pulmonary circulation or increased pulmonary congestion, as seen in cardiac failure. It is characterized by marked consolidation, usually from hemorrhage, and is frequently associated with pleuritic pain from pleurisy or effusion. The infarct may necrotize and become infected, forming a lung abscess. Healing of involved lung usually results in some degree of pulmonary fibrosis.

Data Acquisition

One of the factors contributing to the misdiagnosis of PTE is the vagueness of the signs and symptoms. In general, sudden onset of dyspnea is the most common complaint. Unless the embolus is severe, this may be the only symptom. Massive PTE may produce chest pain, the origin of which is unclear. Tachycardia and increased intensity of the pulmonary S_2 heart sound can be found if pulmonary hypertension is present. Other less frequent findings include nonspecific crackles, mild temperature elevation, gallop rhythm, and possibly signs of phlebitis. Hypotension with peripheral vasoconstriction and accompanying cyanosis may be evident.

When pulmonary infarct has occurred, the symptoms are usually more specific. Cough, hemoptysis (usually seen as blood-tinged sputum), and pleuritic pain are relatively common. There may be signs of consolidation, pleural effusion, and infection of the infarct. Bronchial breathing, pleural friction rub, and high fever are classic signs. It must be remembered that pulmonary infarct is *not* a common complication of PTE; therefore, the presence of these signs is rare.

Laboratory tests are usually not specific for PTE but are useful adjuncts to rule out other pulmonary disease. Leukocytosis is rare except in cases of infarction but may differentiate a diagnosis of pneumonia. Analysis of arterial blood gases is ambiguous, although hypoxia, hypocarbia, and respiratory alkalosis are common changes. $PaCO_2$–$PetCO_2$ difference is widened because of increased dead space. The main point to keep in mind is that arterial blood gas changes may help to confirm the diagnosis of PTE; however, normal arterial blood gas levels do not rule it out.

Chest x-ray and ECG findings are also vague. A normal chest x-ray, frequently seen, does not exclude the diagnosis of PTE. The changes, if any, are subtle but may include the following:

1. Differences in the diameter of normally equal size vessels, due to the fact that if one vessel is blocked the other may have to accommodate pulmonary blood flow.
2. Abrupt cessation of a vessel due to obstruction.
3. Shadow from a clot with no blood flow distally.
4. Abnormal radiolucency due to absent or decreased blood flow (Westermark's sign).
5. Diaphragmatic elevation.

ECG changes usually do not occur unless there is extensive embolization. A tall peaked T wave, ST changes from right ventricular strain, and tachycardia may be present.

The use of radionuclide scanning can assist with the diagnosis. Once there is a suspicion of an embolus, based on a history of risk factors and any of the laboratory tests, a *lung perfusion scan* is usually done by injecting aggregates of serum albumin labeled with a radioactively tagged substance. The indicator is mixed in the heart and distributed with blood flow to the lungs. Thus, scanning of the anterior, posterior, and lateral views of the lung can show the overall distribution of blood. A normal perfusion scan can rule out PTE. However, abnormal scans are seen in a multitude of pulmonary and cardiac diseases and do not establish the presence of PTE with absolute certainty. An abnormal perfusion scan that conforms to a lobe or segment increases the probability of embolism.

A *ventilation lung scan* determines the distribution of gas in the alveoli by detection of a radiolabeled gas. A defect in the ventilation lung scan that matches the perfusion is usually not seen in PTE unless infarction has occurred, and this can be demonstrated on chest x-ray. If there is no ventilation defect in the nonperfused area, the likelihood of PTE increases. However, if doubt persists, a pulmonary angiogram should be obtained if operative intervention is contemplated.

Pulmonary angiography is considered the definitive test for diagnosis of PTE. The technique involves the injection of radiopaque dye into the pulmonary artery. The presence of a filling defect or "cutoff" of an artery confirms the diagnosis. It should be noted that small peripheral emboli may not be seen by angiography, but these rarely cause symptoms of breathlessness or the usual consequences of embolism.

From this discussion, it is easily concluded that the diagnosis of PTE is not a simple task. Anyone presenting with breathlessness warrants a detailed history specifically designed to ferret out risk factors. Prolonged bed rest, obesity, and cardiac failure are all significant findings. A history of recent hip fracture, malignant disease, pregnancy, use of oral contraceptives, burns, trauma, respiratory failure, or surgery should raise the question of possible pulmonary embolism. Although some of the reasons why these conditions precipitate PTE are still unknown, they merit consideration.

Medical Management

Treatment should include two main objectives: anticoagulation to prevent further thrombosis and cardiopulmonary supportive therapy. Continuous intravenous heparin remains the drug of choice for anticoagulant therapy. A coagulation profile should be drawn before heparin is administered.

An initial loading dose of 2,000 to 3,000 U of heparin may be given. Usually, 800 to 1,200 U/hr is adequate to maintain proper anticoagulation. Periodic determinations of anticoagulant levels are necessary, twice per day initially and then once per day. Partial thromboplastin time (PTT) should also be elevated to 2 to 2.5 times normal (i.e., 50-80 seconds). The activated partial thromboplastin time (APTT) should be at least 1.5 times the control (i.e., 20-35 seconds).

Heparin therapy should be continued for approximately 7 to 10 days. However, this depends on a number of factors. When ambulation can be started, the extent of the venostasis and the preexisting condition of the patient should be considered before the therapy is discontinued. As long as the patient remains on prolonged bed rest, a significant risk factor, heparin therapy should be continued. For example, the patient with acute respiratory failure and sepsis may require bed rest for longer periods, which predisposes to more thrombus formations. The transition from heparin to oral anticoagulants may be made as soon as the patient is up and about. Prothrombin time (PT) is used to determine the dosage of warfarin needed to maintain anticoagulation. The length of time anticoagulants are needed depends on the existence of factors that predispose the patient to thrombosis.

Supportive therapy is required to maintain cardiopulmonary function. Oxygen administered by nasal cannula or endotracheal tube may be needed to maintain adequate oxygenation. The use of inotropics and pressors to maintain cardiac output has proved effective. Volume loading may be used to increase pulmonary blood flow to previously unperfused segments. The increased and more evenly distributed flow has implications for increased arterial saturation.

The use of thrombolytics such as streptokinase, urokinase, and tissue-type plasminogen activator (tPA) for massive PTE with severe hemodynamic consequences has been advocated. Definitive studies have shown streptokinase and urokinase to produce earlier reduction of obstruction and more rapid restoration of hemodynamic properties than heparin alone. Streptokinase is a secretory protein of hemolytic streptococci that is thought to activate plasminogen, a fibrinolytic enzyme precursor. Its effect should be noticed after 24 hours of administration. Adverse reactions are bleeding and a low-grade fever. Urokinase, also an activator of plasminogen, is an enzyme found in human urine. Its maximum effect should be seen in 12 to 24 hours.

Thrombolytic therapy should be followed by heparin/warfarin therapy to prevent further thrombosis and embolization. It appears that these substances can be used in massive PTE for those patients in whom surgical therapy is contraindicated.

Although the need for surgical intervention has decreased because of better pharmacological agents, surgery may be necessary for those patients with massive pulmonary embolus (usually 50% obstruction). Patients in whom conventional therapy has been ineffective, those who exhibit life-threatening complications, or those in whom anticoagulant therapy is contraindicated may require surgical intervention. Pulmonary embolectomy for these patients requires documentation by pulmonary angiography and the use of a cardiopulmonary bypass apparatus.

The intracaval "umbrella" is useful in preventing further PTE. The umbrella may be placed under local anesthesia and is associated with a reduced mortality. The Greenfield filter (Figure 29-9) is an example of an antithrombus "umbrella" device. It has proved to be safe, economical, and effective and is rapidly becoming the method of choice because of its relatively

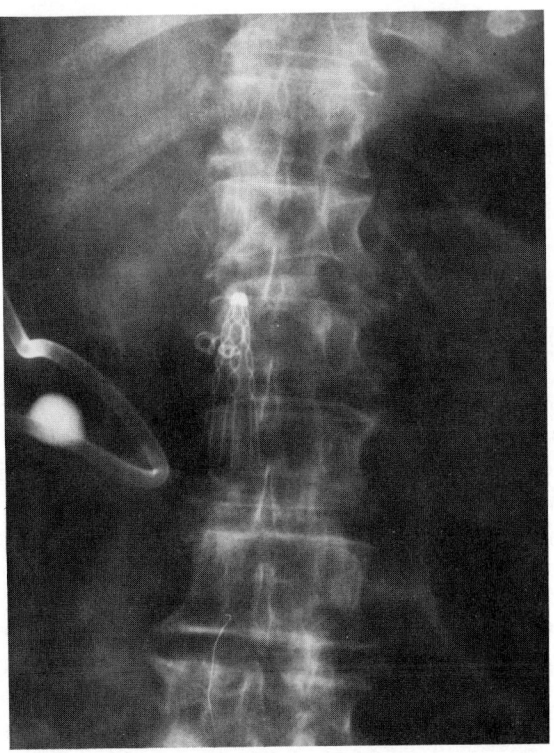

Figure 29-9   Greenfield filter can be seen positioned in the inferior vena cava. Foreign body seen in the right flank is a nephrostomy tube.

low rate of complete caval occlusion.

Many clinicians believe that the main emphasis in the treatment of PTE should be prevention of deep vein thrombosis. Increased use of venous Doppler studies is indicated in any high-risk PTE group for early detection of thrombus formation. Low-dose heparin therapy appears to be the most promising prophylactic measure. Studies have also been conducted using warfarin and aspirin. Minidose heparin therapy has resulted in few bleeding problems and no significant rise in clotting times or PTT.

Nonpharmacological methods used to prevent thrombus formation are early ambulation, use of elastic stockings, leg elevation, and use of various exercise machines. It has not been proved that these methods significantly reduce the incidence of deep vein thrombosis, particularly in the high-risk patient. Intraoperative passive range of motion and the use of intermittent compression of the leg seem to retard venostasis and show promising results.

Clearly, clinical suspicion and the identification of high-risk factors in PTE are necessary for prevention. Once the predisposing factors are identified, prophylactic therapy may be instituted. The nurse must be aware of the subtle changes in patient status that might indicate PTE or deep vein thrombosis. Any slight change in heart rate and breathing pattern in a high-risk patient should initiate an investigation for PTE. Preoperative teaching of range of motion exercises and their rationale should be instituted with patients. Postoperative exercises and early ambulation should be carried out routinely. The dangers of prolonged sitting and crossed legs should be explained, particularly to the patient prone to thrombosis. The key to management of PTE patients is prevention and early detection.

Air Embolus

Entrance of air into the circulatory system under appropriate conditions can result in the same pathological changes as are found with solid-particle emboli. Pathological conditions leading to symptomatic air embolus include intravenous infusion, tubal insufflation, pneumoperitoneum, uterine douches, surgical treatment of the neck, neurosurgical procedures, open heart surgery, retroperitoneal air injection, irrigation of nasal sinuses, chest trauma, and rapid decompression. It has been estimated that 10 to 100 ml of air can be lethal and lesser amounts can lead to frothing in the circulatory system. The symptoms are as much a function of rate of air entry into the circulation as of the absolute amount of air.

Because venous pressure can reach levels below atmospheric pressure, air entering the bloodstream enters mainly through the venous system. Under such circumstances, if the venous system is open to the atmosphere, air enters the circulation. Any portion of the venous system positioned above the level of the heart reaches a subatmospheric pressure and poses a threat of air embolus if the venous system is opened. Surgery of the neck, venous catheterization, and use of the sitting position in neurosurgery risk the entrance of air into the patient's venous system when a vein is perforated. An added risk is encountered during surgery near the major venous sinuses of the brain because their rigid walls fail to collapse when opened and large amounts of air can rush in.

Postcardiac surgery air embolus may develop if air has been trapped in the right or left side of the heart during surgery. The air in the left side poses a more serious problem, not only of myocardial ischemia but of the possibility of air passage through the aorta to the cerebral circulation. Air should be vented from the heart before cardiopulmonary bypass is discontinued.

In air embolism that follows insertion of a central venous pressure (CVP) line, air has been found to have entered via an opening in the catheter system, most commonly through a disconnected or broken CVP line. A catheter tip placed in the superior vena cava or right atrium is in a venous system that is subatmospheric during inspiration. Therefore, any part of the catheter system open to the atmosphere presents an opening for an inrush of air during inspiration. Catheters placed in veins of the neck may also give rise to air embolus because of negative venous pressure when the head is in the upright position.

Although the role of subatmospheric venous pressure in causing air embolism has been emphasized in the foregoing discussion, instances of increased air pressure as a cause have been reported. Chest trauma, tubal insufflation, and pneumoperitoneum may cause an entrance of air into the venous system because of the increase in air pressure relative to venous pressure. In chest trauma, lung damage may result when communication is established between the venous system and bronchi. Forced expiration or mechanical ventilation can force air into the open venous system, resulting in air embolus. Tension pneumothorax can produce similar results.

Similar to air embolus is gas embolus, which occurs frequently in deep sea divers and persons exposed to increased atmospheric pressure. Under high atmospheric pressure, increased amounts of hydrogen, oxygen, and nitrogen are dissolved in the bloodstream. If the ascent to lesser atmospheric pressure is too rapid, the three gases come out of solution. The hydrogen and oxygen are reabsorbed, but the nitrogen remains out of solution and portions coalesce, possibly forming large nitrogen bubbles that may obstruct the vascular tree. Clotting of small blood vessels may occur because of activation of a clotting cascade downstream of the bubbles and loss of plasma volume with hemoconcentration, due to transcapillary leakage of plasma water. Hyperbaric chambers are used to reverse this process.

Data Acquisition

Air may enter the venous system at a slow infusion rate or as a large bolus. A small, slow infusion during normal respiration has been shown to initiate a gasp reflex, causing a large amount of air to be sucked into the veins. Signs and symptoms usually vary with the amount of air pulled into the venous system. It is believed that slow infusion of air results in decreased peripheral resistance and that the physiological changes seen are due to pulmonary vasculature changes.

ECG changes include a peaking of P waves and, later on, ST depression. When cardiovascular deterioration has been established, a churning noise ("mill wheel murmur") may be heard on auscultation. Central venous pressure gradually rises during slow infusion of air, while pulmonary artery pressure (PAP) increases early. At low infusion rates, blood pressure decreases and pulse increases. Signs of shock may be seen as peripheral resistance decreases.

With a bolus of air, cardiovascular collapse occurs because of an air obstruction in the heart. The rise in PAP is not seen, probably because the circulatory collapse can occur within seconds and the air is not pumped into the pulmonary artery.

Medical Management

Since air embolism can be fatal within minutes, complete resuscitative methods should be initiated immediately. The patient should be placed on the left side in a head-down position (Durant's maneuver). This allows the air bubbles to float to the right atrium and away from the pulmonary artery. Positioning may not prove effective or in cases of large air embolism, since inflow to the right side of the heart is also obstructed. Intracardiac aspiration of air may be achieved through a subclavian or central line positioned in the right atrium. Success, however, depends on early detection and rapid aspiration. Large amounts of air can remain in the right side of the heart once clotting of blood has begun.

Air can also be removed from the right side of the heart by external cardiac massage. The probable mechanism is a forcing of air out of the heart into the pulmonary circulation, fragmenting into smaller air bubbles.

Clinicians should be aware of the potentially lethal effects of air embolus whenever penetration of the venous system is contemplated. Proper positioning and the use of detection devices may aid in reducing overall mortality. During insertion of a central venous catheter, the patient should be placed in the head-down position, to increase venous pressure and prevent the sucking in of air. This technique also applies when treating patients with penetrating lung wounds. Positioning the patient with the laceration below the level of the right atrium may decrease the likelihood of air entering the system.

The use of a Doppler ultrasound apparatus during neurosurgical procedures has been advocated to detect the presence of air embolus. With a clear, patent system and the transducer at the level of the right atrium, even minute bubbles of air can be detected. The Gardner antigravity suit (a circumferential pneumatic pressure suit) has been used to decrease postural hypotension, thereby increasing venous pressure and preventing air embolus. Its use, however, remains controversial.

Fat Embolus

A complex and highly debated entity is fat embolization. This is a condition characterized by microembolization (usually 10 to 40 μm) of fat, resulting in obstruction of blood flow and inflammatory reactions around the vessels affected. Fractures of the long bones and major soft tissue trauma are the leading causes of fat embolus syndrome—thus the high incidence of the syndrome in the young and vigorous and the elderly.[12] Occasionally, embolization follows osteomyelitis, cardiopulmonary bypass, burns, poisoning, pancreatitis, and renal transplantation. Characteristically, larger emboli lodge in the pulmonary vasculature, while the smaller globules travel through the circulation to other parts of the body.

The incidence of pathological fat emboli is far greater than their clinical manifestation. Embolization is often not heralded by clinical symptoms but is rather an incidental pathological finding in trauma patients who die of other causes.

Fat emboli arise from the marrow of the injured bone and subcutaneous tissue where fat globules enter the venous circulation through ruptured veins, being drawn into the veins because of the difference in pressure in the damaged marrow and the venous system. The fat globules are in the form of neutral fat (saturated) and fatty acids (unsaturated). After the initial injury, the release of fat globules may continue intermittently, depending on the amount of patient manipulation. This theory is supported by the high incidence of fat emboli following long bone fracture and the fact that fat found in the lungs has been found to resemble marrow fat.

A chemical theory suggests that emboli are also formed from fat emulsions in the plasma. It is theorized that plasma lipids, in a hypercoagulable state, form with platelets and embolize. This process is probably triggered by the leakage of a small amount of fat from the marrow. The fact that other causes of fat emboli besides fractures have been described tends to support this theory.

Pathophysiology

The majority of emboli rest in the pulmonary vasculature. However, a small portion pass through the lungs and enter the circulation. The mechanism for the passage is still controversial. One theory suggests that a large number of emboli reach the lungs simultaneously and the lung is unable to filter all of them. Another cites local alveolar capillary dilatation or the effects of shunting, which allow emboli to pass through into the circulation. These emboli can travel to the brain, heart, kidney, skin, posterior pituitary, and eye.

The obstruction of pulmonary blood flow accounts for the number of alveoli ventilated but not perfused (alveolar dead space). However, the effects on the pulmonary vasculature and alveoli are probably similar to those described in ARDS. Intraalveolar hemorrhagic edema may be associated with rupture of the capillaries. Parenchymal damage is frequently seen and is probably caused by local lipolysis and decreased surfactant production, which are in turn related to edema and cessation of blood flow. The hypoxemia frequently seen in fat embolism is primarily due to shunting. This may be a result of three factors: considerable atelectasis from the intraalveolar hemorrhage or inflammatory edema; precapillary shunting; and alveolar capillary dilatation, which allows an accelerated blood flow, inhibiting oxygenation of hemoglobin molecules.

Systemic fat emboli are usually liquid-deformable and may partially or temporarily obstruct vessels. As emboli penetrate the capillaries, they break into smaller globules; this probably explains why systemic emboli are smaller than those found in the lung. Frequent passage through the circulation and the lungs make the emboli small enough to be eventually removed by phagocytosis. As the fat is broken down by lipases in plasma and macrophages, fatty acids are released which cause an inflammatory reaction.

Although there may be petechial eruption in the white matter of the brain, the main effects are from obstruction of smaller arteries in the gray matter, causing infarcts which may or may not be hemorrhagic. In the heart there may be areas of fatty degeneration, although symptoms are mild, if they exist at all, and the condition is reversible. Petechiae can also appear in the kidneys but have not been proved to cause tubular necrosis or renal failure. Fat emboli can cause blind spots in the eyes which resolve with no ill effects. Microemboli may be visualized in the retinal vessels. Skin rash, usually seen on the anterior chest and shoulders and in the axillae, is probably the result of embolization of the capillaries in the dermis. It has been suggested that thrombocytopenia may induce this petechial eruption, but this has not been definitely proved. Petechiae often appear in the conjunctivae of the eyelids.

Data Acquisition

Although severe fat emboli may develop rapidly and progress to coma and death, most clinical cases are asymptomatic and remain undiagnosed. Emboli reach the lung within minutes, and early signs of hypoxemia may be evident. Most patients have a PaO_2 of 60 to 70 torr on admission following a long bone fracture. However, a more fulminant respiratory picture may develop, with PaO_2 levels below 60 torr, along with the clinical signs of systemic emboli.

Classic symptoms can develop hours to 4 days after injury. Besides mild hypoxemia, subtle mental changes may appear in the first 24 hours. Changes in patient behavior, slight disorientation, and increases in pulse and temperature may be early warning signs. If the embolization is partial, any of the cerebral,

pulmonary, or skin rash effects may be absent. These symptoms usually disappear in about a week with adequate treatment.

More severely affected patients exhibit severe respiratory compromise similar to ARDS. Petechial rash usually appears within 24 hours. Cerebral effects culminate in coma and death, most likely due to brainstem infarction.

Other findings include fat in the sputum due to leakage into the alveoli, lipuria, decreased hematocrit readings related to trapping of red cells, thrombocytopenia, and ECG changes. Elevated serum lipase levels appear about the third day after injury and may be a guide to prognosis.

Medical Management

Prevention of fat emboli following trauma and long bone fracture should be of prime concern when handling fracture patients initially. Care should be taken to splint the fracture as soon as possible and to avoid overmanipulation. The use of pneumatic tourniquets during elective surgery on long bones has been advocated to minimize the possibility of fat reaching the lungs.

The use of oxygen is clearly beneficial. It is thought that oxygen administration, besides correcting the hypoxemia, may inhibit passage of emboli through the lungs. Mechanical ventilation and the use of PEEP are required with severe respiratory compromise.

Heparin, aprotinin (Trasylsol), dextran, and corticosteroids have all been advocated. However, these therapies, with perhaps the exception of steroids, are no longer used.

Nursing care of any patient following long bone fracture or trauma involves recognition of the subtle changes seen with fat emboli. The baseline admission data should include a thorough neurological assessment and evaluation of arterial blood gases. Any slight change in these parameters may indicate the beginning of a fat embolus syndrome.

CHEST TRAUMA
Pulmonary Contusion

Pulmonary contusion is usually characterized by damage to the lung parenchyma that results in localized edema and hemorrhage. It is often associated with more acute trauma (e.g., pneumothorax or hemothorax) and may go unnoticed until the hypoxic effects cause severe respiratory distress. Pulmonary contusion was widely recognized during World War II as "blast injury," caused by underwater detonation of high explosives or other forms of shock wave compression of the chest wall.

High-speed automobile accidents are presently a leading cause of lung contusion resulting from deceleration of the chest wall as it strikes the steering wheel. The contusion may be the result of direct force (the anterior portion of the lung striking the steering wheel), or a contrecoup effect of the posterior lung bouncing back against the rib cage. Blunt chest trauma and shotgun and high-velocity missiles often give rise to the same parenchymal damage. Because of the large number of automobile accidents and handgun injuries, clinicians should be alert to the possibility of pulmonary contusion.

Pathophysiology

Rapid compression and decompression by a high-pressure wave causes parenchymal damage, hemorrhage, and edema. It is thought that the initial injury compresses the thoracic cavity and diminishes its size. The increase in intrathoracic pressure then compresses the lung, damaging the parenchyma. When decompression occurs, the lung springs back, causing rupture of the capillaries and the subsequent hemorrhage.

The degree of the pathological change varies with the severity of the contusion. Less severe trauma usually produces focal areas of hemorrhage, while more

severe injury can cause a firm purple lesion. The initial blow produces capillary damage and hemorrhage. The results of this hemorrhage and the vicious cycle effects are summarized in Figure 29-10. The vascular damage from cellular debris is similar to the mechanism described in the section dealing with ARDS. In pulmonary contusion, the cellular debris from cell damage also contributes to the collapse of the alveoli. If the patient has multiple trauma, fat embolism is a likely additional cause of pulmonary failure. Review the section on ARDS for a more complete description of the pathophysiological changes.

Data Acquisition

The recognition of pulmonary contusion presents problems. Often contusion is sustained without penetrating trauma to the chest. It has been observed that the more severe contusions are found in cases with no associated rib fractures. A temporary deformity of the rib cage may compress the lung, or the acceleration–deceleration effect may cause the lung to strike the rib cage.

On the other hand, contusions associated with fractured ribs and flail chest often go unnoticed. It is

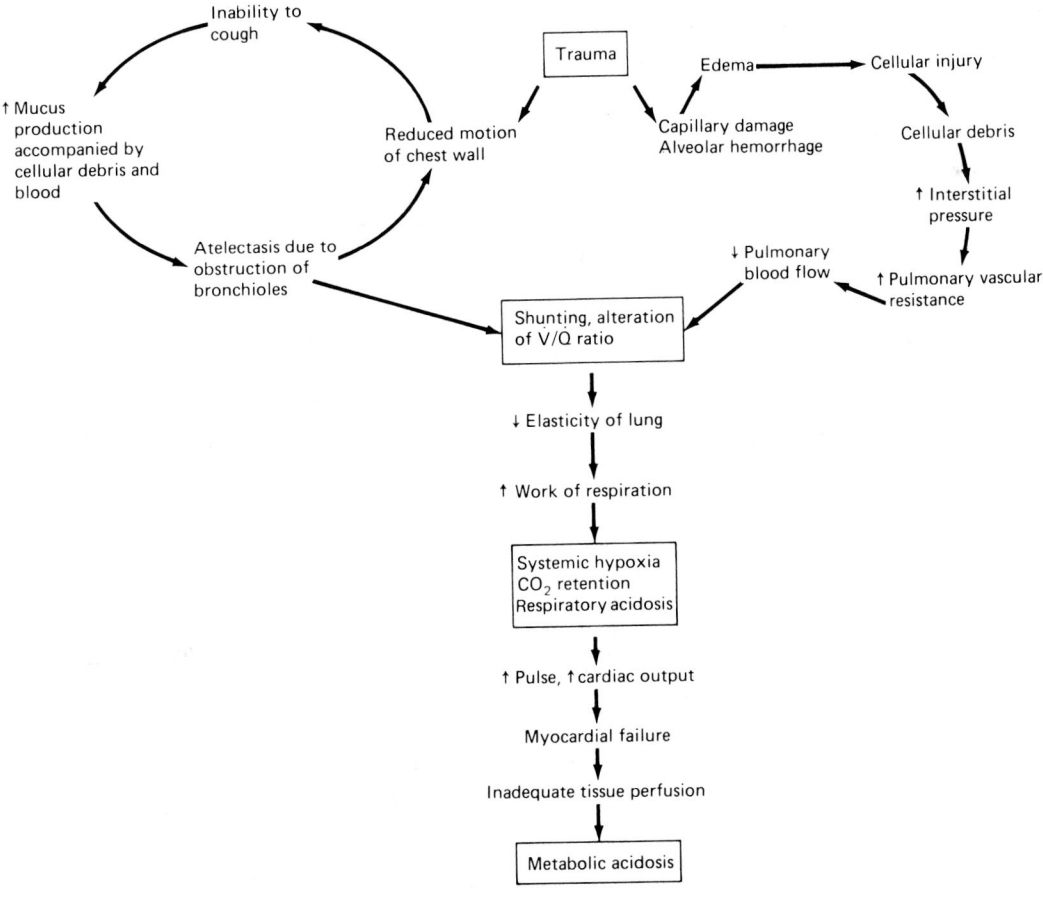

Figure 29-10 Pathophysiology of pulmonary contusion.

probable that the hypoxic effects seen in flailing are primarily due not to the free-floating ribs but rather to the underlying contusion. This is discussed further in the section dealing with flail chest.

Another problem with the diagnosis of pulmonary contusion is the poor correlation of the initial signs and symptoms and the initial chest x-ray with the extent of the injury. A number of reports have shown that contusion may not appear clinically for 2 to 24 hours after chest injury, with a lag of 4 to 6 hours frequently found between the time of injury and an abnormal chest x-ray. The appearance of an abnormal roentgenographic pattern also does not correlate well with the extent of the injury. The less severe contusion may reveal patchy areas of ill-defined infiltrates which can progress to well-defined opacities. In its severest form, the classic *white lung* may be seen. One of the more promising diagnostic tests is computed tomography (CT) and potentially others, such as magnetic resonance imaging.[13] CT is generally more useful than other tests in identifying the severity of the contusion.

Pulmonary contusion can be classified as mild, moderate, or severe. Physical symptoms vary accordingly. Patients with mild contusions usually present with tachypnea, tachycardia, and blood-tinged secretions. They cannot cough effectively, probably because of the chest pain associated with the initial trauma. Crackles may be heard on chest examination. Arterial blood gas measurements may reveal a slightly decreased PaO_2 on room air and a decreased $PaCO_2$ due to tachypnea.

If the contusion is more severe, the tachypnea, tachycardia, and crackles persist. Secretions become more copious, and frank blood may become evident. The patient is unable to clear the secretions. Severe hypoxemia and CO_2 retention with a progressively worsening a/A ratio indicate severe respiratory failure. Chest x-rays usually exhibit some abnormal findings at this stage, but they often do not correlate with the extensive damage.

Medical Management

The primary goals in treatment of pulmonary contusion are early diagnosis, maintenance of a patent airway, and adequate oxygenation by maintenance of lung function. Because of the frequent lack of symptoms and confirmation of the extent of injury, the suspicion of contusion should be entertained in any chest trauma. Close observation of the patient for 24 to 48 hours is highly desirable to detect signs of increased respiratory insufficiency. Once flail chest, pneumothorax, and/or hemothorax are corrected, the a/A ratio should improve. Any subsequent signs of hypoxemia most likely indicate the presence of a contusion.

Mild contusion may be treated without ventilatory support. Oxygen by mask with good humidification may be all that is needed until signs of adequate oxygenation are seen. Vigorous chest physiotherapy and nasotracheal suctioning may be beneficial in helping to clear secretions. If these methods are not sufficient, therapeutic bronchoscopy may be used. Adequate relief of pain is needed to facilitate coughing and deep breathing.

Bacterial culture and sensitivity tests of sputum should be obtained periodically, since the damaged lung may be susceptible to infection. Broad spectrum antibiotics have not proved useful prophylatically, so coverage should be adjusted according to culture reports.

In patients with mild contusions, damage may be expected to resolve rapidly (3 to 4 days). However, there is a danger in diagnosing a mild contusion and treating without ventilatory support. Misdiagnosis of a contusion as mild is a distinct possibility when diagnosis is based on initial chest x-ray findings and presenting symptoms. The patient must be closely observed for signs of increasing hypoxemia as the extent of the disease becomes more apparent.

The more severe contusions require ventilatory support. Since many clinicians consider lung contusions in their severest form a disorder similar to ARDS, the ventilatory management is based on similar principles. Controlled mandatory ventilation or intermittent mandatory ventilation is necessary. The use of positive end-expiratory pressure is adjusted according to the criteria described for ARDS. Review the section on ARDS for nursing and medical management of pulmonary contusion in its most severe form.

Flail Chest

Paradoxical movement of the chest wall during respiration is known as *flail chest*. It is observed when the ribs are broken in two or more places, leaving them free-floating in the chest cavity. Flailing is frequently seen after blunt chest trauma or may occur iatrogenically during overzealous cardiopulmonary resuscitation. In the latter case, the anterior rib fracture is often associated with costochondral separation.

Pathophysiology

The multiple rib fractures incurred during crushing injuries cause the chest wall to lose its continuity. During inspiration, atmospheric pressure exceeds intrathoracic pressure on the affected side, causing the chest wall to move inward. Conversely, on expiration, intrathoracic pressure exceeds atmospheric pressure, causing the chest wall to move outward until the thorax contracts. Reduced pulmonary ventilation results.

The patient experiences pain and an inability to cough effectively. The increased work of breathing associated with noncompliant lungs, along with the lack of ventilated alveoli beneath the affected ribs, leads to atelectasis and hypoxemia. It should be noted that since flail chest from crushing injury is often associated with other pulmonary complications, including pulmonary contusion, pneumothorax, and hemothorax, the diagnosis of flailing should include a search for these other disorders.

Data Acquisition

The most apparent sign of flail chest is the paradoxical movement of part of the chest wall, although tissue swelling, chest wall hematoma, or poor inspiratory effort by the patient may mask this sign. Pain may be severe and increase with movement. The patient is usually short of breath, tachypneic, or tachycardic. If the flailing is related to other pulmonary injury or myocardial contusion, hypotension and cyanosis may be evident. Chest x-ray is useful in diagnosing rib fractures and the presence of underlying pulmonary trauma but *not* the presence or absence of flailing.

Medical Management

The main emphasis in treatment of flail chest is stabilization of the chest wall. Formerly this was accomplished by sandbagging the flail segment, chest wall traction with towel clips, or manual pressure during exhalation. The increase in atelectasis due to pressure on the chest wall has led many clinicians away from this type of management. Generally, if adequate oxygenation can be maintained with a manual inflation bag until ventilatory support can be established, mechanical stabilization is not necessary.

The concept of using controlled mechanical ventilation for treatment of flailing was common until a few years ago. Modes of support have included intermittent positive pressure breathing, control ventilation with PEEP, and, more recently, intermittent mandatory ventilation (IMV) with PEEP. However, the most recent emphasis is to provide adequate pain management and avoid unnecessary mechanical ventilation.

Allowing the patient to breathe spontaneously with some ventilator support (IMV) and positive pressure has some advantages. The patient receiving controlled ventilation may build up subatmospheric intrathoracic pressure trying to breathe spontaneously, thus increasing pain and the potential for dislodging ribs. With the use of IMV and PEEP, the patient does not "fight" the ventilator and the pressure needed to generate a breath is minimized.

The effects of flail chest may be due not to the orthopedic problem but rather to the tissue damage.

It was originally thought that PEEP improved oxygenation by reducing flailing. However, a number of clinicians believe that the hypoxemia is due to underlying pulmonary contusion, atelectasis, and the increased work of breathing. The fractured ribs and flailing may initiate the problem, but the contusion is probably responsible for the continued hypoxic effects.

Pain medication should be administered according to patient need. The use of mechanical ventilation should not rule out pain medication but can reduce the amount needed. Pain, tachypnea, and tachycardia may increase oxygen consumption and defeat the purpose of ventilation. Morphine sulfate, in controlled doses, is enough to control pain without depressing respiration.

Pneumothorax

The entry of air into the pleural space with partial or complete collapse of the lung is defined as *pneumothorax*. Pneumothorax can be classified as closed or noncommunicating (simple); tension; and open or communicating (sucking wound). Since the severity, pathophysiology, and management of these conditions are different, they are discussed here separately. Normally the pleural space is potential rather than actual, occupied by only a thin film of fluid. Any disruption in this "traction" on the lung can cause serious effects on ventilation.

Simple or Closed Pneumothorax

The incidence of pneumothorax in patients sustaining blunt chest trauma has been reported to be as high as 50%. Automobile accidents, high falls, blows to the chest, and blast injuries are leading causes. Frequently the pneumothorax is a result of lung lacerations from fractured ribs. When there are no associated fractures, it may be a result of compression at the height of inspiration when alveolar pressure is high. A blow to the chest increases the pressure, causing rupture of the alveoli, escape of air, and collapse of lung tissue.

Spontaneous pneumothorax can be due to the rupture of an emphysematous bleb, cystic lung disease, pulmonary carcinoma, or tuberculosis. Iatrogenic causes include subclavian venous catheter insertion, intracardiac injection, thoracentesis, or positive pressure ventilation. Simple, or closed, pneumothorax has been so classified because of its self-sealing effect. Once the air has entered the pleural space, the lung seals and prevents further leakage. Pneumothorax may be small (<15%), moderate (15% to 60%), or large (>60%).

Although pneumothorax usually produces symptoms, some patients are totally asymptomatic. In general, the greater the extent of the collapse, the more pronounced the symptoms. The presence of underlying pulmonary disease, however, may produce severe symptoms with even a small pneumothorax. Chest x-ray is helpful in establishing the presence of a small collapse or the extent of a larger one.

Shortness of breath and restlessness are classic signs. Chest pain radiating to the back, face, abdomen, and shoulders may be caused by stretching of the parietal pleura. The larger the collapse, the more likely are signs of increasing hypoxemia and inability to maintain adequate ventilation.

Inspection reveals decreased or absent motion of the chest wall and a tracheal shift toward the unaffected side. Subcutaneous emphysema is often present, particularly in the larger pneumothorax. Absent or decreased breath sounds and hyperresonance to percussion are common.

The treatment of closed pneumothorax is dependent upon the severity of the lung collapse and respiratory compromise. A small collapse may be followed by daily chest x-rays. One can expect the lung to reexpand at a rate of approximately 1.25% of the area per day. If the size continues to increase, insertion of a chest tube is the treatment of choice.

Symptomatic pneumothorax mandates the release of air. A chest tube is inserted into the second or third intercostal space at the midclavicular line. If at all possible, the patient should be in the upright or semi-upright position. This helps to ensure that the underlying lung falls away from the chest wall. The skin should be cleansed with iodine or povidone-iodine, and sterile gloves should be used. After a 1- to 2-cm skin incision, the chest tube is inserted using a trocar or hemostat. When the chest tube is connected to underwater seal drainage, the presence of bubbling confirms the escape of air. The tube should be sutured into place and all tubing connections tightened or taped to prevent disconnection. A chest x-ray is taken after the procedure and repeated daily to monitor the reexpansion of the lung.

In caring for the patient with chest tubes connected to underwater seal drainage, one golden rule should be observed: chest tubes generally should not be clamped unless changing the drainage system. The effects of tension pneumothorax from pressure build-up are far more damaging than the effects of an open pneumothorax from disconnection of the underwater seal. In the event of a bottle break or crack, the chest tube may be submerged in a bottle of sterile water until new equipment is available.

Pneumothorax is often associated with underlying pulmonary disease. Chest physiotherapy may still be done with the patient in a modified postural drainage position (flat) so long as the underwater seal remains intact and the water seal is below the level of the heart. Pain may inhibit vigorous physiotherapy, and therefore, the patient should be premedicated and percussed for shorter periods more frequently. Once the chest tube is inserted, the patient may be turned from side to side. Care must be taken to prevent kinking of the tubing when turning the patient toward the affected side.

Recurrent or chronic pneumothorax may require additional therapy. Thoracotomy with decortication is reserved for those who have had multiple attempts at reexpansion of the lung. The procedure involves stripping of the parietal pleura from the apex of the lung to allow the visceral pleura to adhere to the chest wall. The mediastinal and diaphragmatic pleura are left intact. The leak in the lung may be repaired or resected during the procedure. Recurrence is relatively rare.

Tension Pneumothorax

Blunt chest trauma may also precipitate a tension pneumothorax. Although controlled mechanical ventilation, when used with positive end-expiratory pressure, has been associated with tension pneumothorax, the use of intermittent mandatory ventilation has reduced this occurrence. It is possible that the incidence of tension pneumothorax in severe pulmonary disease is related to the frequency of high peak pressures during lung inflation.

As air increases in the pleural space, tension increases. If the tear does not seal, a one-way valve effect may be produced, allowing air to enter during inspiration but not to escape during exhalation. The intrapleural pressure, if not relieved, compresses the vena cava, causing decreased diastolic filling of the right ventricle, with a fall in cardiac output. The cardiovascular collapse is coupled with the compression of the unaffected lung because of intrathoracic pressure. The combination of decreased cardiac output and decreased ventilation is soon fatal unless immediate action is taken.

The patient with a tension pneumothorax is usually in marked respiratory distress. Tachypnea, cyanosis, tachycardia, and hypotension accompanied by restlessness and agitation are immediate danger signs. Subcutaneous emphysema is almost always present. If the patient is intubated, there is usually difficulty in ventilating manually because of high intrathoracic pressure. The shift of the trachea and mediastinum to the opposite side is acute, and breath sounds are absent. Often the affected side of the chest wall expands because of intrathoracic pressure.

Tension pneumothorax is an emergency situation, and treatment must not be delayed for any reason. Cardiopulmonary resuscitation for cardiovascular collapse is often ineffective until the tension inside the chest cavity is relieved. Insertion of a chest tube is the treatment of choice. If equipment for thoracotomy is not immediately available, a large-bore needle and syringe may be inserted into the second intercostal space to temporarily relieve the pressure. Because of the incidence of lung perforation from needle aspiration, this method should be used carefully. The use of a spring-loaded needle has been advocated. This needle has a sharp edge for insertion which springs back, leaving a blunt-end needle for escaping air. The use of this device has produced no evidence of lung perforation. These techniques, however, are only temporary measures; chest tubes should be inserted as soon as available.

Routine management is the same as that for simple pneumothorax. A functioning chest tube does not preclude the use of PEEP. If positive pressure ventilation is required for respiratory failure, it should be maintained once the chest tube is inserted and functioning, even if the lung collapse was caused by the PEEP. The persistent air leakage will be relieved by the chest tube until the mechanical ventilation is no longer needed.

Open or Communicating Pneumothorax

Penetrating trauma to the chest wall causes the atmospheric air to have direct access to the pleural cavity, causing an open, sucking wound. Common causes are gunshot and stab wounds, although any defect of the chest wall can cause the open communication. Surgical intervention in the chest may also precipitate an open pneumothorax.

This injury involves the bulging inward of the affected lung during inspiration and an outward movement during exhalation. The affected lung's air is soon depleted, and it is unable to expand because of free air movement from outside into the pleural space. The unaffected lung receives air from the trachea *and* from the affected lung during inspiration. During expiration, air is exhaled into the trachea and into the unaffected lung. Thus, this lung is moving deoxygenated air in and out, increasing functional dead space and causing carbon dioxide retention.

The most obvious sign of an open pneumothorax is the chest wall defect. The patient is usually in respiratory distress, tachycardic, and dyspneic. Subcutaneous emphysema is often present and expanding. Immediate action is needed to close the defect. Sterile gauze can be used until petroleum gauze can be secured with adhesive over the wound. Chest tube insertion is necessary to expand the affected lung once the open air port has been sealed. When the patient is stabilized, surgical intervention may be necessary to explore and debride the wound. Irrigations with saline and broad spectrum antibiotics have been recommended.

Patients with open pneumothorax require close observation both pre- and postoperatively. Besides the pneumothorax, a hemothorax from a penetrating wound is possible. Infection from the instrument used to inflict the wound may precipitate empyema or pyopneumothorax (collapse of the lung from pus). Both of these complications may develop 24 to 48 hours after trauma.

Hemothorax

Hemothorax is collapse of the lung from the accumulation of blood in the pleural space (Figure 29-11). Blunt and penetrating chest trauma, as well as the iatrogenic causes previously indicated, may give rise to bleeding. The heart, lungs, great vessels, or any of the chest wall vessels are common sources of rupture. Usually this bleeding is self-limiting because of low pulmonary arterial pressure, thromboplastin in the lungs, and compression of the site of bleeding by the pool of blood already accumulated.

Hemothorax has two main debilitating effects. First, the pool of blood causes the collapse of alveoli; second, the amount of blood loss can lead to hypovolemia. Severity of the condition depends upon the amount of lung tissue displacement and the amount and rate of blood loss.

Loss of less than 400 ml of blood may cause little or no change in the patient's condition. Chest x-ray may show a loss of the acute costophrenic angle and a hazy appearance over the lower chest. Patients with

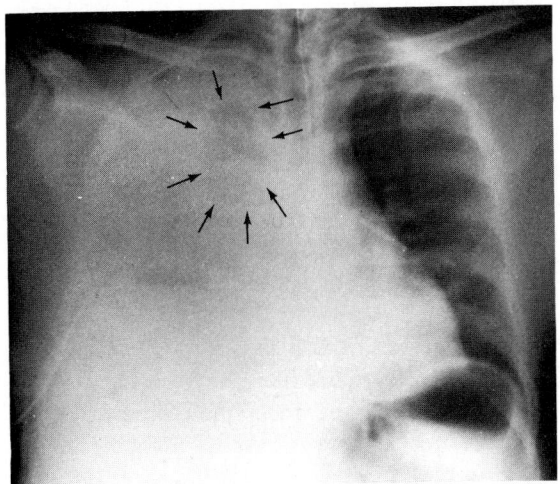

Figure 29-11   Chest x-ray of 32-year-old male following attempted right subclavian catheterization. Opacification of the right side of the chest is seen, with some mediastinal shift to the left. Arrows indicate collapsed right lung. At thoracotomy to control hemorrhage, 3 L of clotted blood was removed from the right pleural cavity and no bleeding point was found. The patient made a full recovery.

larger losses usually exhibit the classic signs of shock: pallor, tachycardia, hypotension, and restlessness, together with dyspnea and a tightness in the chest. Breath sounds range from diminished to absent, and there is dullness on percussion. Chest x-ray is useful in diagnosing the extent of fluid loss but may often be eliminated because of the severity of the shock.

The preferred treatment for self-limiting hemothorax is chest tube insertion. The patient should be in the upright or semiupright position when the chest tube is inserted in the fifth or sixth intercostal space at the midaxillary line. This helps alleviate the risk of puncturing a high-lying diaphragm, spleen, liver, or colon.

Massive hemothorax necessitates fluid administration for resuscitation. If the bleeding is not self-limiting, thoracotomy for repair of the site is necessary.

REFERENCES

1. Campbell, G. S., & Cone, J. B. (1991). Adult respiratory distress syndrome. *American Journal of Surgery, 161,* 239-42.
2. Petty, T. L. (1990). Acute respiratory distress syndrome (ARDS). *Disease a Month, 36,* 1.
3. Shoemaker, W. C. (1989). Pathophysiology and fluid management of postoperative and post traumatic ARDS. In W. C. Shoemaker, S. M. Ayres, A. Grenvik, et al. (Eds.), *Textbook of critical care.* Philadelphia: Saunders.
4. Ramsey, K. M. (1990). Viral pneumonias. A diagnostic and therapeutic challenge. *Postgraduate Medicine, 88,* 49-50.
5. Scheld, W. M. (1991). Developments in the pathogenesis, diagnosis and treatment of nosocomial pneumonia. *Surgery, Gynecology and Obstetrics, 172,* 42-53.
6. Bravo-Cuellar, A., Ramos-Damian, M., Puebla-Pérez, A. M., et al. (1990). Pulmonary toxicity of oxygen. *Biomedicine and Pharmacotherapy, 44,* 435-437.
7. Beyda, D. H. (1991). Pathophysiology of near-drowning and treatment of the child with a submersion incident. *Critical Care Nursing Clinics of North America, 3,* 273-280.
8. Kovacs, J. A. (1990). Advances in the diagnosis of pneumocystis carinii pneumonia. *AIDS Clinical Review, 10,* 129-147.
9. Reiss, T. F., & Ahmad, M. (1991). Asthma: Current strategies for treatment. *Cleveland Clinic Journal of Medicine, 58,* 161-169.
10. Dehring, D. J., & Arens, J. F. (1990). Pulmonary thromboembolism: Disease recognition and patient management. *Anesthesiology, 73,* 146-164.
11. Shapiro, B. A., Harrison, R. A., Cane, R. D., et al. (1989). *Clinical application of blood gases.* Chicago: Yearbook Medical.
12. Levy, D. (1990). The fat embolism syndrome. A review. *Clinical Orthopaedics and Related Research, 261,* 281-286.
13. Wagner, R. B., & Jamieson, P. M. (1989). Pulmonary contusion. Evaluation and classification by computed tomography. *Surgical Clinics of North America, 69,* 31-40.

30

Mechanical Support of Ventilation

Thomas S. Ahrens

TYPES OF MECHANICAL VENTILATORS

Many different mechanical ventilators are currently available, and these machines vary in their capabilities. For the sake of simplicity, ventilators are classified here according to the mechanism most often employed to terminate the inspiratory phase.

Volume-cycled Ventilators

The volume-cycled (or volume-preset) ventilators terminate inspiration after delivering a preset volume of gas. These ventilators will deliver the desired volume regardless of the pressure required to do so. The volume remains the same unless excessively high peak airway pressures are reached. To prevent potential lung damage due to high peak-inspiratory pressures, all volume-preset ventilators have an adjustable safety release mechanism. The safety release pressure is set manually at about 10 cmH$_2$O above the peak-inspiratory pressure. All commonly used ventilators can perform volume-cycled ventilation. Newer ventilators, such as the Puritan-Bennett 7200, Siemens Servo C, and Bourns Bear 5, can perform additional modes of ventilation (Figure 30-1).[1]

The inspiratory time is determined by adjusting the flow rate of the gas to be delivered. The more rapid the flow of gas, the shorter the inspiratory time. Conversely, the slower the flow rate, the longer the inspiratory time. Expiratory time is determined by setting a respiratory rate. Thus, if inspiratory time is adjusted and a certain number of breaths are to be given per minute, the remaining time is available for expiration. For example, if the tidal volume is preset for 1,000 cc and the respiratory rate is 10 per minute, this allows 6 seconds for each respiratory cycle. If the flow rate is adjusted so that inspiration of the desired tidal volume occurs in 2 seconds, then 4 seconds remains for expiration.

Many models of volume-cycled ventilators have a built-in oxygen selector and can be adjusted to deliver any concentration of oxygen from 21% to 100% (Figure 30-2). However, because of variable accuracy, the concentration should be checked by means of a reliable oxygen analyzer.

Generally, the volume-cycled ventilators are more powerful than other types and more useful when ventilating patients with "stiff" lungs, such as patients with adult respiratory distress syndrome. The ventilator will continue to deliver a constant tidal volume regardless of the changes in airway resistance or in compliance of the lungs and thorax. Time-cycled ventilators, such as the Siemens Servo, achieve volume ventilation by a timing mechanism.

Pressure-cycled Ventilators

The pressure-cycled (or pressure-preset) ventilators, such as the newer ventilators listed earlier and some older ventilators (Puritan-Bennett PR-2 and Bird Mark VII), terminate inspiration upon achieving a preset pressure. Gas flows to the patient until the preset pressure is reached throughout the system: the ventilator, tubing, and the patient's airways. When this pressure is reached, the gas flow is terminated, and the patient passively exhales. Many pressure-cycled ventilators have some means of adjusting the gas flow rate, the sensitivity of the ventilator's response to the patient's own inspiratory effort, and the respiratory frequency initiated by the machine.

One of the greatest disadvantages of pressure-cycled ventilators is that varying resistance interferes with gas flow, since flow is a function of pressure and resistance. This resistance causes a change in tidal volume, since volume is a product of flow and time. Thus, the delivered volume varies as resistance varies. If resistance does not vary appreciably, as in a young drug-overdosed patient, this ventilator may be used. However, it is inappropriate for patients with chang-

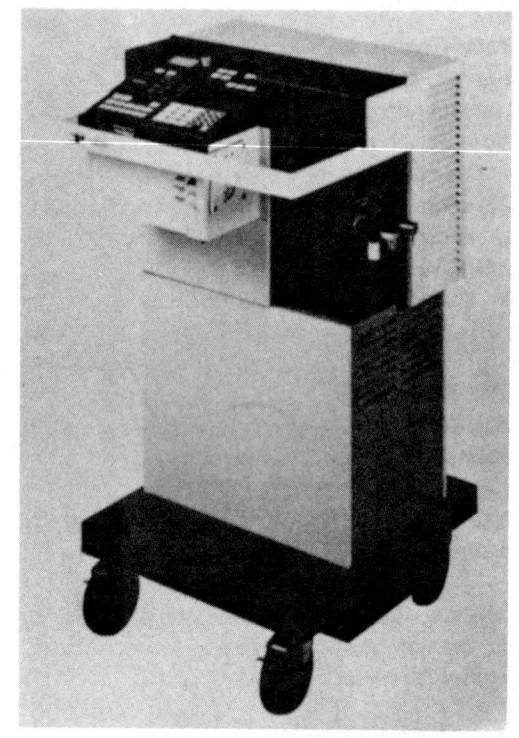

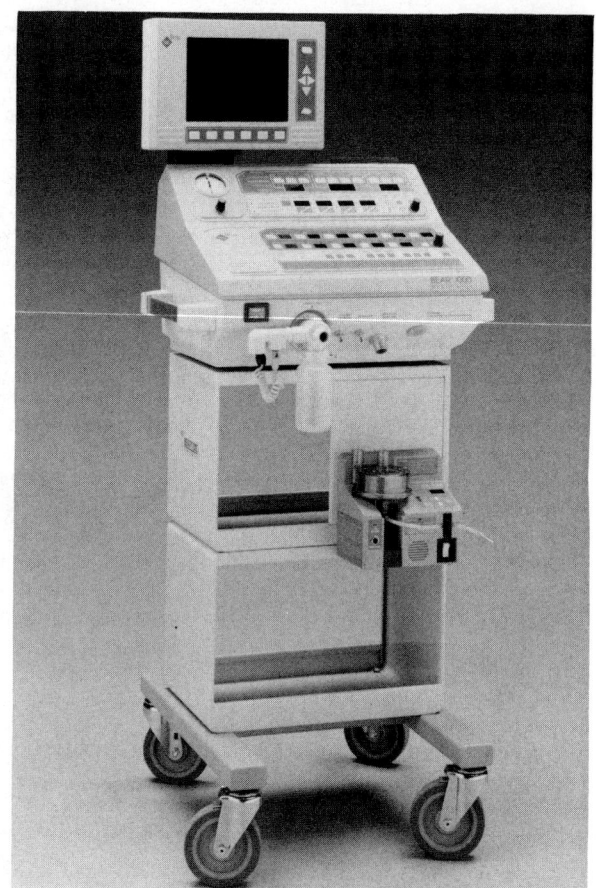

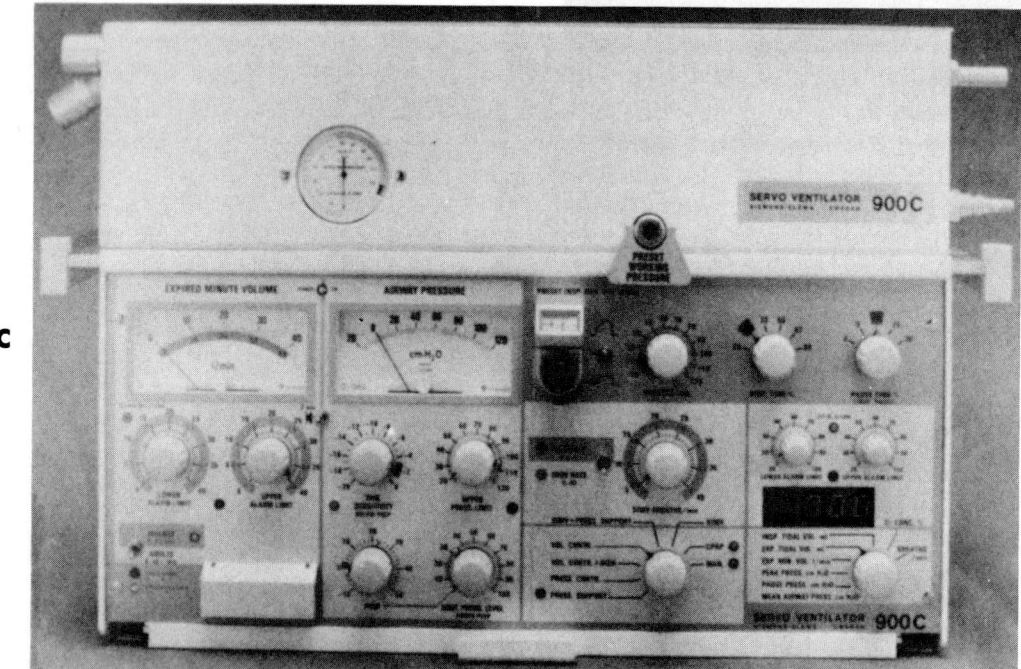

Figure 30-1 Current ventilators can perform multiple modes of ventilation, including pressure- and volume-cycled modes.

A, Puritan-Bennett 7200 microprocessor ventilator shown with optional pedestal and compressor.

Courtesy Puritan-Bennett Corporation, Kansas City, MO.

B, Bear-2 adult volume ventilator.

Courtesy BEAR Medical Systems, Inc., Riverside, CA.

C, Siemens Servo Ventilator 900C.

Courtesy A. B. Siemens-Elema, Solna, Sweden. From Dupuis, Y. (1992). *Ventilators: Theory and clinical applications* (2nd ed.). St. Louis: Mosby—Year Book.

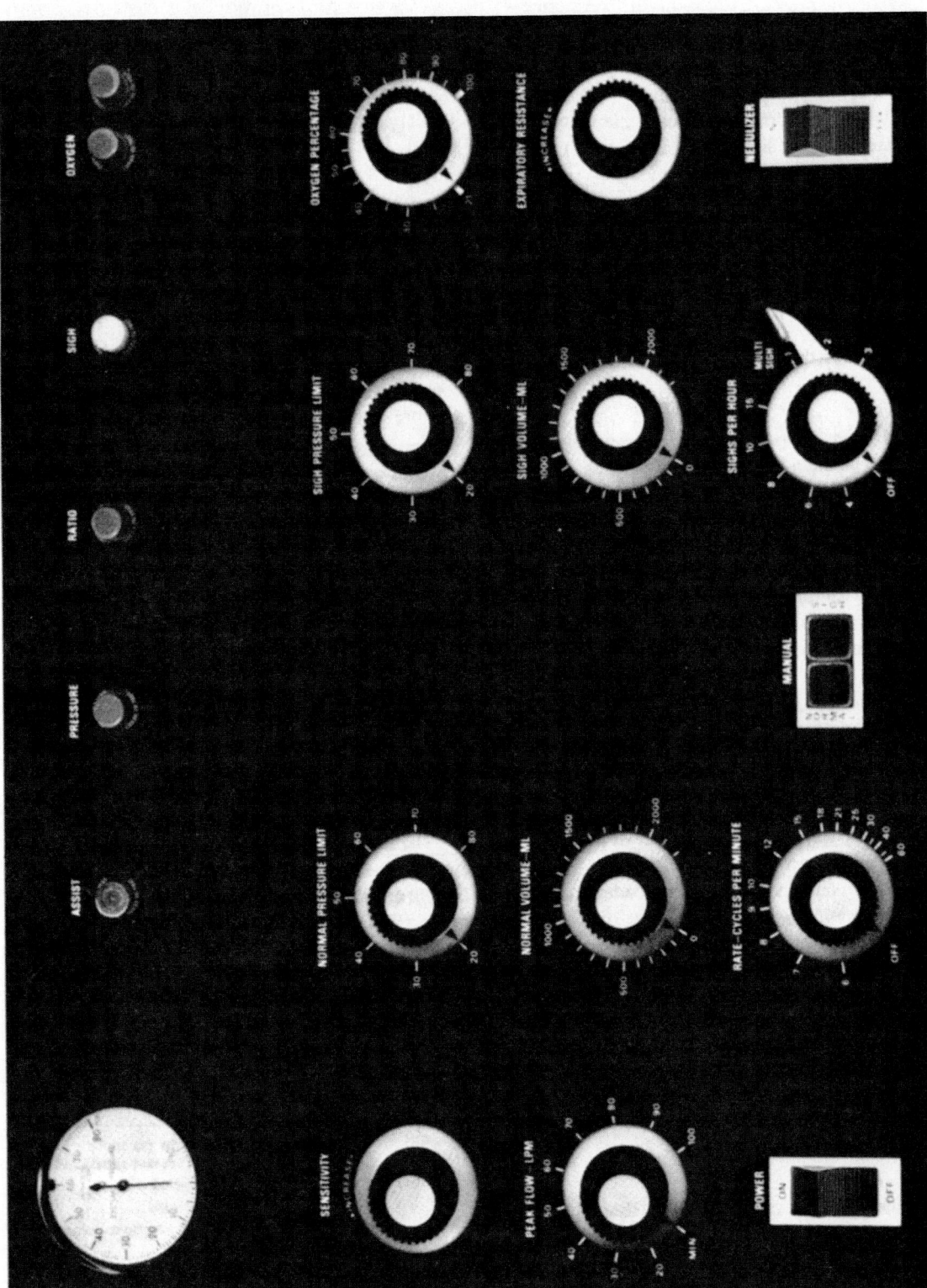

Figure 30-2 Control panel of early Bennett MA-1 ventilator. Fraction of inspired oxygen (FiO₂) can be regulated between room air (21%) and 100%.
From Dupuis, Y. (1992). *Ventilators: Theory and clinical applications.* (2nd ed.). St. Louis: Mosby–Year Book.

ing pulmonary resistance, as in acute bronchospasm and in postoperative states. These patients would receive varying volumes with each breath.

The relatively low pressure capability (top effective peak pressure is 30 to 40 cm from a 50-lb/in² source) is another disadvantage of pressure-cycled ventilators. A patient with very stiff lungs may need a pressure of 80 cm to deliver an adequate tidal volume. However, many clinicians may prefer to ventilate at lower airway pressures but prolong the inspiratory phase (pressure-controlled inverse ratio ventilation). The lower airway pressures, even in acutely ill patients, may avoid barotrauma which occurs with high airway pressure.

A recent application of pressure ventilation is in weaning patients from mechanical ventilation. This application of pressure support is presented in the section Modes of Ventilation.

External Body Ventilators

The external body ventilators assist the patient's spontaneous ventilatory effort by applying intermittent subatmospheric ("negative") pressures to the trunk of the body. For example, the body tank ventilator, or iron lung, may be of value for the patient whose vital capacity is reduced to a value just below that needed for spontaneous ventilation. However, it is large, noisy, restrictive, and rarely seen in critical care settings.

Another example of this class of ventilator is the cuirass, which functions similarly to the iron lung. This is a rigid shell that covers only the thorax and abdomen. A disadvantage is the difficulty in attaining and maintaining a tight seal.

Body ventilators are seen primarily in chronic care settings. The critical care nurse may see these ventilators if a patient is using one at home and develops an exacerbation, requiring an ICU admission.

MODES OF VENTILATION

Several modes of mechanical ventilation are employed in the care of the critically ill today, including controlled mandatory ventilation, assisted mandatory ventilation, intermittent mandatory ventilation, pressure support ventilation, and high-frequency jet ventilation. A variety of terms may be used to describe these basic modes.[2,3]

Controlled Mandatory Ventilation (CMV)

CMV totally regulates the patient's breathing. A set rate, tidal volume, or minute volume is dialed into the ventilator, which cycles automatically regardless of the patient's ability to breathe. This type of ventilation guarantees a set minute ventilation for the patient who cannot breath spontaneously. It is used for totally paralyzed and/or apneic patients (such as those with neuromuscular dysfunction, severe brain damage, spinal cord injuries, drug overdose, or status asthmaticus). In critical care settings, CMV is not a commonly employed mode of ventilation.

For the patient who is able to initiate a breath, this type of ventilation becomes difficult to manage. Many patients "fight" the ventilator and require paralysis and sedation in order to maintain adequate ventilation without additional work of breathing or risk of cardiovascular compromise or barotrauma.

The respiratory rate and tidal volume should be regulated by the $PaCO_2$ and pH. Alkalemia due to a falling $PaCO_2$ is a problem and often requires a reduction in the ventilator delivered rate or volume.

The cardiovascular effects of CMV include decreased venous return and cardiac output. These can be related to both mechanical factors and alkalemia.

Assisted Mandatory Ventilation (AMV)

AMV, also referred to as assist/control ventilation, allows the patient to trigger a breath from the ventilator. The ventilator can be set to detect the patient's inspiratory effort and initiate inspiration. Once the patient triggers the ventilator, gas flow will be delivered to the patient until a preset tidal volume, pressure, or time limit has been reached. Should the patient stop triggering the ventilator, the control mode will take over at a preset rate. This method allows patients to initiate ventilation at their own rate but maintains a desired rate should the patient become apneic.

The advantage of AMV over CMV is that the patient can breathe at a rate in excess of the ventilator-delivered rate. The arguments to support this type of ventilation are based on patients' use of their own muscles to initiate the breath. Theoretically, there is a period when intrathoracic pressure decreases transiently before the ventilator delivers the tidal volume, thereby enhancing venous return and cardiac output. However, many clinicians dispute this theory, arguing that when the patient triggers, the ventilator will respond instantly, thereby mimicking CMV with its resultant cardiovascular effects.

As in CMV, the $PaCO_2$ and pH are used to determine the tidal volume and respiratory rate. Patients may require sedation, particularly if they are breathing too rapidly for the ventilator to complete a cycle.

Intermittent Mandatory Ventilation (IMV)

IMV allows the patient to breathe spontaneously from a gas reservoir while still receiving periodic mechanical hyperinflations. In this manner the patient's own spontaneous minute ventilation is augmented to a desired level by machine-delivered breaths. The sum of mechanical and spontaneous ventilation provides adequate alveolar minute ventilation. IMV is widely advocated for weaning, although many clinicians employ it from the start of mechanical ventilation. Although studies differ regarding which mode of ventilation is best, IMV is widely used beyond weaning from mechanical ventilation.

There are numerous advantages to IMV. As mechanical ventilation is reduced, the weaning process is facilitated. The patient has been spontaneously breathing during the entire course of therapy and gradually assumes the total responsibility for ventilation. It is not necessary to relearn breathing. IMV reduces the necessity for paralysis. Sedation, although it can be used with IMV, may be needed less often than with CMV.

The alkalemia seen in patients on AMV is diminished in patients on IMV, since these patients breathe spontaneously most of the time and mechanical ventilation is supplied only as needed. Some clinicians believe IMV is best utilized in patients with respiratory rates below 30 breaths per minute. Oxygen consumption is likely to increase with a faster respiratory rate. AMV, with its larger tidal volumes in comparison to patient-generated volumes, generally reduces the respiratory rate better than IMV.

Mechanically supplied breaths under positive pressure increase dead space (V_D/V_T), worsening the ventilation/perfusion ratio in patients whose primary disease process is characterized by $\dot{V}/\dot{Q}$ mismatching. The use of fewer machine-delivered breaths by employing IMV minimizes this effect.

The introduction of IMV has also helped to lower the incidence of pulmonary barotrauma. The mean intrathoracic pressures are lower, since the high-pressure mechanically delivered breaths come less frequently and intrathoracic pressure is lower during spontaneous breathing.

A slight variation on IMV is synchronized intermittent mandatory ventilation. In this mode the ventilator delivers its mandated breath in synchronization with the patient's own inspiration. Virtually all ventilators operate in this synchronized manner.

IMV rate is determined by patient need on the basis of three criteria: (1) the pH should be maintained within normal limits, (2) the spontaneous respiratory rate should be 30 or less, and (3) the $PaCO_2$ should be maintained at the patient's normal level. This is particularly useful in patients with chronic obstructive pulmonary disease, who usually maintain high $PaCO_2$ while metabolically compensating to maintain a normal pH.

Pressure Support Ventilation (PSV)

PSV has become popular for weaning from mechanical ventilation. Although it could be used as a primary mode of ventilation, its limitations have generally directed PSV toward weaning only.[4]

PSV provides ventilator-delivered breathing that is based on a pressure-limited cycle. Because the cycle is initiated by a patient-generated breath, the ventilator can augment the patient's own breathing. In patients with a low tidal volume, PSV supplementation may assist in weaning.

PSV can also help overcome the airway resistance imposed by the endotracheal tube and ventilator. Low levels of PSV, usually less than 10 cmH_2O, will generate a small tidal volume that may compensate for the work required to initiate the ventilator breath.

PSV can be combined with other forms of ventilation. For example, IMV can be programmed to incorporate PSV with spontaneous breaths, since PSV alone generally requires patient-generated breathing efforts. Therefore, a safe mode of ventilation must either incorporate a back-up ventilator rate (with IMV) or use a ventilator with an apnea mode that will convert to a programmed ventilator rate and volume if a period of apnea is detected.

The use of PSV for weaning and overcoming work of breathing may be valuable in patients with borderline pulmonary function and respiratory muscle strength.

High-frequency Jet Ventilation (HFJV)

HFJV abandons the theory that alveolar ventilation can occur only when tidal volume exceeds anatomical dead space, the premise of all other types of ventilation. The method employed is relatively simple, much like "panting" ventilation in the dog. The jet ventilator delivers low tidal volumes (100 to 300 ml) at rapid rates (60 to 100 breaths per minute). Gas is delivered from a pressurized source through a valve into a narrow cannula placed in the endotracheal tube. The patient is also connected to a volume ventilator usually set for continuous positive airway pressure. As the jet stream is propelled into the tube, surrounding gases are entrained and propelled down the trachea. Exhalation is passive, and the inspiratory time (or ON time) is 33%, yielding a 1:2 inspiration/expiration ratio. Humidification is accomplished in two ways: the entrained gases are humidified via the cascade on a volume ventilator (used in conjunction with the jet), and an infusion of normal saline into a port of the endotracheal tube (which exits just above and in front of the injector catheter tip) humidifies the jet gases.

Studies have suggested that HFJV provides low

mean and peak airway pressures, lowers the incidence of barotrauma when high peak pressures are needed on conventional ventilation, decreases cardiovascular compromise, and facilitates weaning. Reports about the validity of these claims still conflict. Research is continuing in the areas of its usefulness in cardiovascular surgery and neurosurgery, in augmenting pulmonary toilet and mucus clearance, and in ventilatory support during cardiopulmonary resuscitation. This type of ventilation has shown promise in tracheoesophageal fistulas, bronchopleural fistulas, and oropharyngeal, laryngeal, and tracheal surgery.

ADJUNCTS TO MECHANICAL VENTILATION

Positive End-expiratory Pressure (PEEP)

PEEP is positive resistive pressure applied to exhalation. This distending pressure in the airways and alveoli keeps small airways open throughout the entire ventilatory cycle (Figure 30-3). It increases functional residual capacity (or the volume of gas left in the alveoli at the end of exhalation) and eliminates the need to achieve a critical pressure during inspiration to reopen closed alveoli (commonly called *alveolar recruitment*). For these reasons, PEEP has been deemed essential in improving gas exchange and pulmonary function.

The clinical goal of PEEP is fourfold: (1) a PaO_2 greater than 60 to 70 torr,* (2) arterial hemoglobin saturation (SaO_2) greater than 0.90, (3) FiO_2 of 0.5 or below, and (4) no significant decrease in cardiac

*A unit of pressure equal to 1 mmHg.

output. It is commonly accepted that any patient receiving mechanical ventilation should receive low-level physiological PEEP (5 cmH_2O). PEEP should be increased or decreased in increments of 3 to 5 cm H_2O while the patient is monitored for improvement in PaO_2 and SaO_2 without a decrease in cardiac output. If a cardiac output measurement is unavailable, decreases in blood pressure or increases in heart rate may suggest a decline in cardiac output.

Complications associated with the use of PEEP include cardiovascular compromise and pulmonary barotrauma. The cardiovascular compromise can be corrected by administration of intravenous fluid or, in rare cases, inotropic or pressor agents. Levels below 10 cmH_2O rarely require inotropic or pressor therapy. The use of a flow-directed balloon catheter is warranted when high levels of PEEP are used to monitor fluid administration and inotropic support. Pulmonary barotrauma has been significantly reduced by the use of PEEP in conjunction with IMV rather than with CMV or AMV. The incidence of pneumothorax is increased with PEEP levels above 20 cmH_2O. This condition may be corrected by insertion of a chest tube.

Continuous Positive Airway Pressure (CPAP)

CPAP is PEEP applied to a spontaneously breathing patient and has the same physiological effect of increasing functional residual capacity. It is useful in patients who require a positive distending pressure to maintain oxygenation but do not require mechanical

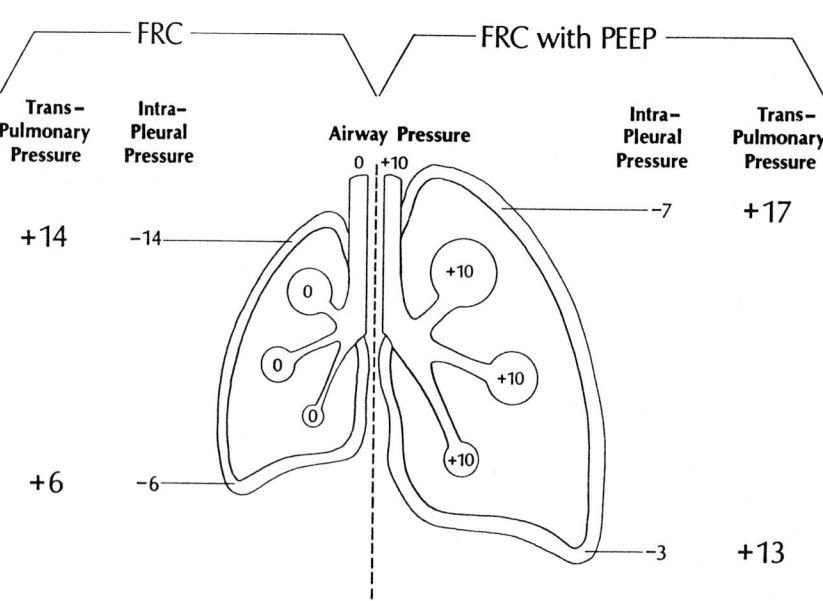

Figure 30-3 Positive end-expiratory pressure (PEEP) distends small airways, facilitating gas exchange and allowing for a reduction in FiO_2.

From Shapiro, B. A., Harrison, R. A., Kacmarek, R. A., et al. (1991). *Clinical application of respiratory care* (4th ed.). St. Louis: Mosby–Year Book.

ventilation. The term *expiratory positive airway pressure* has also been used to describe this adjunct, since the spontaneous inspiration of the patient results in negative pressure and the expiration results in positive pressure. The physiological effects are the same.

Inverse Ratio Ventilation (IRV)

When extreme hypoxemia is present and is resistant to FiO_2 and PEEP therapy, IRV may be employed. IRV is a mode of ventilation that reverses the normal inspiratory and expiratory times. Instead of a short inspiration and long expiration, the ventilator delivers a long inspiration and short expiration. The changing of the inspiratory/expiratory (I/E) ratios is the basis for successful improvement in hypoxemia with IRV.[5]

Normal I/E ratios on mechanical ventilation are about 1:4 (1 second for inspiration, 4 seconds for expiration). The total expiratory cycle time is about 5 seconds, giving a respiratory rate of about 12 (60/5) per minute. In IRV, the I/E ratio is brought closer together initially until inspiration and expiration are about equal (I/E of 1:1). Blood gases are monitored to ensure that adequate time is allowed for CO_2 to escape during expiration. Cardiac output (or heart rate and blood pressure) is monitored to ensure that no loss of blood flow occurs.

The I/E ratio can be reversed to levels of about 2:1, usually not much more than this. Once near this point, further increases generally are not helpful.

When IRV is used, pressure control ventilation is normally employed as a maneuver to keep mean airway pressure as low as possible. Also, since IRV may be uncomfortable, sedation and paralysis are usually necessary.

MEDICAL MANAGEMENT

Mechanical ventilation must be initiated whenever the patient's ventilatory function fails to maintain an adequate pulmonary blood gas exchange. It is emphasized that the clinical observation or measurement of pulmonary function (ventilation) does not reflect the adequacy of gas exchange (respiration). Arterial blood gas (ABG) determinations are essential to confirm a suspicion of impending acute ventilatory failure.

The clinical goals of mechanical ventilation are (1) to provide the pulmonary system with the mechanical power to maintain physiological ventilation, (2) to manipulate the ventilatory pattern and airway pressures for the purpose of improving the efficiency of ventilation and/or oxygenation, and (3) to decrease myocardial work by diminishing the work of breathing and improving ventilatory efficiency.

Ventilators are generally set to provide a fairly high tidal volume of approximately 10 to 15 ml per kilogram of body weight at a relatively low respiratory rate of 10 to 14 breaths per minute and an FiO_2 below 0.5. Final adjustments of the mechanical ventilatory pattern ultimately depend on blood gas analysis. The physician should prescribe ventilator settings, sedation, and weaning parameters as guidelines for the nurse or therapist who routinely provides patient care.

The effectiveness of any life support system depends upon the patency of the airway. Endotracheal tubes, including nasotracheal, orotracheal, and tracheostomy tubes, are used to eliminate any soft tissue or laryngeal obstruction. A nasal tube may be preferred for long-term intubation because (1) it is easier to stabilize, (2) it is easier to suction (longer catheters may be necessary), and (3) it is better tolerated by the alert patient. One disadvantage of nasotracheal intubation is that the tube diameter is limited by the nostrils and turbinates and meticulous care must be given to prevent pressure necrosis. Also, significant septal deviation may cause encroachment on the lumen of the tube, which does not affect ventilation but prevents the suction catheter from passing readily.

Many respiratory problems, particularly those due to retained secretions, can be resolved during the 48 to 72 hours of the more conservative endotracheal intubation if vigorous treatment is given. However, if prolonged ventilatory support is anticipated, tracheostomy may be performed at any convenient time following initial intubation. There are no specific criteria for the appropriateness of endotracheal versus tracheostomy airway management. Endotracheal tubes have been safely left in place for more than 2 weeks. However, each clinical encounter must be decided on an individual basis. The primary concern is to prevent laryngeal trauma and granuloma. If successful weaning has not been achieved after 2 weeks, many physicians elect to perform a tracheostomy unless extubation is likely in the next few days.

NURSING MANAGEMENT

Coordination of care rendered to the critically ill patient is the responsibility of the nurse. Respiratory care given to the patient receiving mechanical ventilation can be performed by a nurse, a respiratory therapist, or a combination of the two. Who is responsible for respiratory care and ventilator maintenance in a particular institution is less important than who is coordinating that care. The nurse and the therapist must be aware of all treatments given to the patient and the response to those treatments. It is the nurse's responsibility to ensure that the patient is receiving the care necessary for a successful outcome. Teamwork and cooperation are essential.

Working nursing diagnoses are described with individual disease entities, but the two diagnoses discussed below are appropriate for any patient receiving mechanical ventilation regardless of the disorder.

■ NURSING DIAGNOSIS

Ineffective airway clearance, related to placement of endotracheal tube.

OUTCOME STANDARD AND CRITERIA

Airways are clear as evidenced by:

* Loose secretions
* Absence of retained secretions

NURSING INTERVENTIONS

* Provide humidification
* Suction prn
* Reposition patient from side to side and to prone, every 1 to 2 hours
* Chest physiotherapy every 4 hours
* Medicate prn to prevent "fighting" the ventilator
* Assess ABG and pulse oximeter levels prn

It is imperative that the gas delivered through an artificial airway be 100% humidified at body temperature. Effective airway humidification may be accomplished by incorporating a heated humidifier into the ventilator so that the air reaching the patient's airway (37° C) is 100% saturated with water vapor. The humidifier must be heated because an air mixture passing through water at room temperature is only 20% to 30% saturated when it is heated to body temperature in the tracheobronchial tree.

Humidifying devices and connecting tubing must be inspected at regular intervals. Condensed water within the tubing may either obstruct airflow or empty into the trachea. Condensed water should never be returned retrogradely to the sterile humidifier.

The intubated patient has an ineffective cough reflex and may not exert a large intrathoracic pressure against a closed glottis; therefore, secretions must be suctioned from the airway. Tracheal suctioning should not be performed on a routine schedule; "every half-hour" may be too often for one patient and not often enough for another. Needless suctioning produces unnecessary tracheal irritation and should be avoided. Since secretions can be suctioned only from the main stem of the bronchi, it is essential that they be mobilized from the more distal regions by a regular schedule of patient repositioning.

The patient should be informed of the suctioning procedure. The ventilator tubing should be disconnected after the inspiratory phase of respiration (if an in-line suction catheter is not in place). When disconnected, the ventilator end of the tubing should be placed so that it does not become contaminated.

High concentrations of oxygen should be administered for several inspirations prior to and immediately following tracheal aspiration. Most new ventilators have a computer function key that allows for the administration of 100% oxygen for a prescribed time (e.g., 2 minutes). If the ventilator being used does not have this function, either the oxygen concentration on the ventilator should be turned temporarily to 100%, or "bag" ventilation should be instituted. A PEEP valve should be used on the bag when appropriate.

Strict adherence to sterile suctioning techniques is mandatory. Many hospitals have converted to closed suction systems to reduce the likelihood of infections and to aid in maintaining arterial oxygen levels. In addition, the nurse should, regardless of technique used, employ universal precautions against contamination by any body secretions. Patients who require mechanical ventilation are generally debilitated and, therefore, more susceptible to infection. In addition, the placement of a tube in the airway greatly reduces the normal protective and defense mechanisms of the lungs. The catheter, about one half the inner diameter of the tube, should be gently guided, not pushed or shoved, into the trachea. Suction is not applied while the catheter is being inserted. Lung collapse is possible if an excessive vacuum exists. For this reason, suctioning should not be done for longer than 8 to 12 seconds, and the negative pressure should not be greater than 150 cmH_2O (for adults). Since each aspiration period lowers the Po_2, it is unwise to make a second attempt at suctioning without first reoxygenating the patient. It is possible that oxygen tensions below 50 torr potentiate dysrhythmias, and reported cases of cardiac arrest during or following tracheal suctioning are well substantiated in the literature. All ventilator patients must have continuous electrocardiographic monitoring, and the monitor must be observed during the suctioning procedure.

The patient's position in bed determines which portions of the lungs are ventilated and perfused. Stasis of secretions in the bases and periphery of the lungs is enhanced by the frequently observed supine semi-Fowler's position. In this position it is difficult, if not impossible (particularly with positive pressure ventilation), for secretions to ascend from the bases of the lungs to the main stem of the bronchi where they can be reached by the aspirating catheter. Right and left lateral positioning, with the head of the bed gradually lowered, is tolerated by most patients receiving mechanical ventilation.

An optimum time to suction is just prior to a position change. The patient's head should be turned at the same time as the rest of the body and kept in alignment. Extreme care must be taken to avoid twisting, hyperextending, or hyperflexing the neck, since these maneuvers traumatize the trachea. Arm and leg exercises are essential to maintain muscle tonus and joint range of motion. A program of breathing retraining and strengthening exercises should begin as soon as possible for patients with chronic airway obstruction. Deconditioning may be reduced and exercise tolerance increased by various arm and leg exercises, which should be synchronized with the breathing pattern while the patient is being assisted by the ventilator. Thus, "weaning" is easier to accomplish.

As soon as medically stable, the patient should sit in a chair, even if only for brief periods, since this produces both physiological and psychological improvement. Continuous ventilatory assistance should not interfere with the patient's freedom out of bed. For patients receiving long-term treatment, a walker can be equipped with a small ventilator to allow early ambulation.

A patient who is "fighting" the ventilator is restricting the respiratory cycle by actively "pushing out" while the machine is "pushing in." This dramatically decreases alveolar ventilation and increases intrathoracic pressure, consequently decreasing venous return and cardiac output. Patients who "fight" the ventilator are usually hypoxemic, underventilated, or uncomfortable because of pain or anxiety.

The individual clinical situation determines the frequency and timing of ABG studies. It generally takes about 5 to 20 minutes for a blood gas steady state to be reached after a ventilator adjustment, and the stability of the clinical situation should be assured before performing the arterial puncture. Generally, blood gas measurements are unnecessary if a pulse oximeter is present and the parameters to be monitored include only the PaO_2 and SaO_2. If pH and $PaCO_2$ values are desired, a blood gas measurement is necessary.

In this era of cost containment, the abuse of ABG testing has received considerable attention. In the initial phases of respiratory decompensation numerous ABG measurements should be necessary to achieve an optimal ventilatory state. Once the patient is stabilized, however, routine ABG measurements should be eliminated. Determination of PaO_2 values can largely be eliminated through monitoring of pulse oximetry levels. Indications for evaluating ABGs depend on the patient's clinical presentation. Certainly the patient whose vital signs are stable, who is alert and oriented and appears comfortable, or whose SpO_2 values are stable, does not require frequent ABG measurement. ABG evaluation every 4 hours or every shift is unnecessary when the ventilatory status is stable.

A Wright respirometer or the ventilator-displayed breathing parameters may be used to monitor the

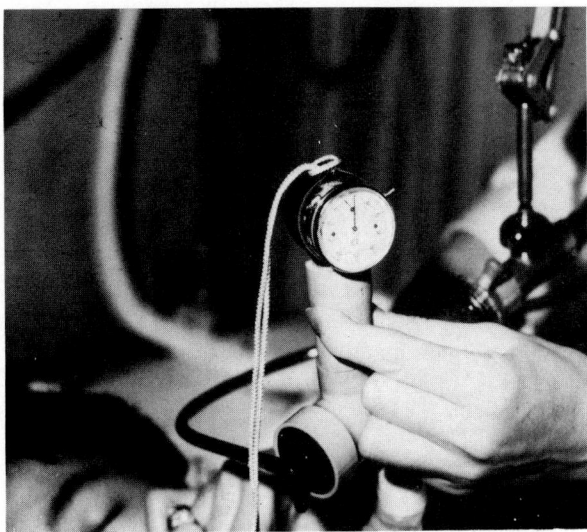

Figure 30-4   Wright respirometer is used to measure expired volume in patient on ventilator.

tidal volume and minute ventilation, thereby ascertaining the stability of the mechanical ventilation (Figures 30-4 and 30-5). Frequent checking of the ventilator alarms and oxygen delivery is essential.

■ NURSING DIAGNOSIS

Anxiety, related to inability to communicate (endotracheal tube placement) and sensory overload and/or deprivation.

OUTCOME STANDARD AND CRITERIA

Anxiety is absent or reduced as evidenced by:
• Expression that anxiety is absent or reduced
• Absent or reduced manifestations of anxiety

NURSING INTERVENTIONS

As the treatment of conditions that once were rapidly fatal has become more successful, the patient requiring ventilatory assistance is exposed to much longer periods of uncertainty, general emotional distress, sensory deprivation, and monotony. The ventilators and monitors with their buzzers and flashing lights surround the patient like sentinels. Flow sheets chronicling the numerous physiochemical variables dangle from the bed and from every available hook. But the tears, pain, loneliness, fear, helplessness, and despair cannot be measured or computed. How easy it is to neglect the patient's emotional well-being because of the pressing demands to take care of the more tangible and task-oriented duties!

One of the most frustrating problems the patient experiences is communication. At a time when the patient's ability to breathe has reached a crisis point, a tube is passed between the vocal cords, thereby preventing speech. The need of the patient to communicate is intensified; the ability to do so is severely

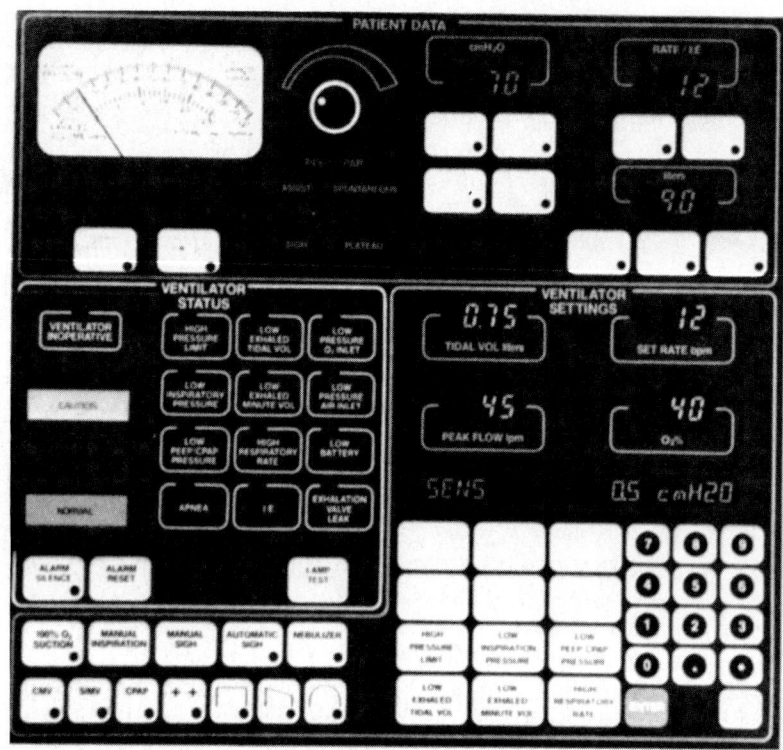

Figure 30-5 Control panel of Puritan-Bennett 7200 microprocessor ventilator.
From Dupuis, Y. (1992). *Ventilators: Theory and clinical applications* (2nd ed.). St. Louis: Mosby–Year Book.

compromised. A Magic Slate or pencil and paper may be used. The intravenous apparatus should be placed, if possible, in the nonwriting arm.

It is ironic that a patient suffering sensory overload may at the same time be deprived of the sensory perceptions needed for orientation. Artificial elimination of the day and night sequence, sleep deprivation, and almost constant bombardment by strange and obtrusive auditory and visual stimuli can produce severe behavioral disturbances. Every effort should be made to organize care in such a way as to permit the patient to have disturbance-free rest periods during the day and quiet nights, interrupted only when absolutely necessary for clinical evaluation or treatment.

Orientation may be enhanced by windows, a visible clock, and a large wall calendar (with each day marked off as it passes). The family should be encouraged to talk about their activities, the news, and weather to help the patient keep in touch with reality. Many patients, of course, will not be able to respond, but they *can* hear and use the information to prevent confusion and disorientation. Family members should be encouraged to visit the patient, touch or hold the patient's hand, and participate in routine care whenever or however possible. The sight of a familiar object may relieve some of the anxiety produced by unfamiliar and frightening surroundings. Background music interrupts the rhythmic monotony of ventila-

tors cycling and monitors beeping and helps to relieve tension in both patients and staff.

Sitting in a chair frequently bolsters a patient's morale, and orientation is enhanced if eyeglasses, dentures, and hearing aids are returned to the patient as soon as practical. Combing the hair should not be overlooked. Patients receiving long-term ventilation require activities and frequent stimulation. The family, volunteers, recreational therapists, and physical therapists should all be involved.

WEANING

Modern respiratory care has demonstrated that the majority of patients appropriately committed to and maintained on mechanical ventilation readily tolerate its discontinuance when their disease process has been reversed. The criteria for weaning from mechanical ventilation are approximately the reciprocals of the indications for which ventilatory support was initiated. Since ventilatory support is primarily used for patients with profound gas transport abnormalities, its use may be discontinued only after therapy has been directed to correcting the pathophysiological alteration. The ventilator does not cure; it is simply a temporary support system that "buys time" for correction of the underlying situation that precipitated its use in the first place. It is essential that other physiological problems be minimized before the weaning

TABLE 30-1   **Weaning Parameters**

MECHANICAL EFFICIENCY TESTS	
Vital capacity	>10 ml/kg of body weight
Tidal volume	>2 ml/kg
Respiratory rate	<35 breaths/min
Peak negative pressure	>−20 cmH$_2$O
Minute ventilation	5-10 L/min
TESTS OF OXYGENATION	
Pao$_2$	>60 torr on <0.4 Fio$_2$
Spo$_2$	>92% on <0.4 Fio$_2$
$\dot{Q}$s/$\dot{Q}$T	<15%
Pao$_2$/Fio$_2$ ratio	>200
a/A ratio	>25%
TESTS OF VENTILATION	
$\dot{V}_D$/$\dot{V}_T$	<60%
pH	7.35-7.45
Paco$_2$	<45 torr except in patient who chronically retains Paco$_2$. Then, whatever level is necessary to achieve a normal pH.

process begins. Acid–base abnormalities, electrolyte, imbalances, fever, anemia, infection, hypotension, dysrhythmias, and nutritional problems should be corrected and stabilized prior to weaning. As in the discharge or transfer process, preparation for weaning should be implicit in the start of intubation and mechanical ventilation. Monitoring and correcting other problems during the course of therapy greatly facilitates the weaning process. Once it has been established that the patient is physiologically capable of independence from the ventilator, the weaning process should be directed toward psychological aspects.

Several physiological tests have been established to serve as guidelines for determining the patient's readiness for ventilator discontinuation. These tests measure mechanical capabilities and effective oxygenation (Table 30-1). The clinician must be careful not to base weaning on a single parameter such as blood gases. Both mechanical abilities (e.g., tidal volume, vital capacity, minute ventilation, and peak inspiratory effort) and gas exchange must be assessed before beginning the weaning process.

With the patient who has been on mechanical ventilation for a short period (less than 36 hours), abrupt cessation of the ventilator may be successful. If a patient meets all the weaning criteria and has no underlying nutritional or respiratory muscle alterations, mechanical ventilation can be quickly terminated. The patient can be given a "T-piece" and monitored

for 30 to 60 minutes. If this initial trial is successful, the patient can be extubated.

The majority of patients wean quickly and successfully, but some patients will not meet the weaning parameters or will fail the weaning trial. In this group, one of three methods of weaning can be attempted:[6]

1. *AMV with T-piece trials:* In this mode of weaning, the patient is placed on brief periods of T-piece (spontaneous) breathing combined with periods of AMV. The goal of this mode is to exercise the respiratory muscles and then let the muscles rest, much the same way a standard exercise program works. The period of time without ventilation should be based on assessments by the nurse and respiratory therapist of the patient's tolerance of spontaneous breathing. Patient tolerance is defined as maintaining good gas exchange, acceptable respiratory rates (<35 breaths per minute), and stable hemodynamics.

2. *IMV:* In IMV weaning, the ventilator support is gradually removed, allowing for increased patient-supported breathing. The IMV rate is reduced according to patient tolerance. When an IMV of about 4 is reached, along with good patient tolerance, extubation can occur.

3. *Pressure support ventilation:* PSV weaning is done in much the same manner as IMV. The pressure support is gradually reduced according to patient tolerance. When the PSV level is about 5 cmH$_2$O, extubation can usually take place. PSV or the spontaneous breathing component of assist/control weaning can be used. Theoretically, low PSV levels (about 5 to 10 cmH$_2$O) can help overcome airway resistance from the endotracheal tube and ventilator circuit.

Prolonged ventilatory assistance leads to respiratory muscle weakness and seriously interferes with the patient's ability to breathe alone when the ventilator is disconnected. The incorporation of some weaning technique that allows for patient-initiated breathing as soon as it is clinically feasible (not when ventilator discontinuance is considered) may decrease the time of ventilator support and the weaning process.

Premature and unsuccessful attempts at weaning have adverse psychological effects on the patient; therefore, it is of utmost importance that the patient be both physically and psychologically prepared for ventilator discontinuation. When the ventilator is discontinued, the patient should be in a sitting position, and humidified 40% oxygen should be readily available by mask.

When it is clinically advisable to remove the airway, the oropharynx and trachea should be suctioned and "bagged" with oxygen between suctioning attempts to prevent hypoxia. As the tracheal cuff is slowly deflated, the patient is given one big breath via the bag. As the tube is gently removed, the patient's automatic response is either to exhale forcibly or to cough up any remaining secretions lodged in the vicinity of the cuff.

Following both ventilator discontinuation and airway removal, the patient should be observed for signs of respiratory insufficiency (increased respiratory rate, increased pulse, diaphoresis). Deep breathing and coughing exercises should be started immediately.

COMPLICATIONS

Obviously, all complications cannot be avoided, but if a specific complication can be successfully treated, it may also be prevented.

Tracheal Tube Complications

Prolonged intubation may promote laryngeal trauma and massive gastric distention. Right mainstem intubation may produce alveolar hyperventilation, atelectasis, and/or pneumothorax. Herniation of the cuff over the distal end of the tube causes airflow obstruction. Tracheal ischemia and necrosis are not as common today with the use of high-volume, low-pressure "floppy" cuffs. The intermittent deflation of these cuffs has no proven advantage in preventing mucosal necrosis. Any routine of inflation and deflation generally leads to careless reinflation and possibly higher cuff pressures. It is generally agreed that it would be optimal to have a high-volume cuff that could maintain an adequate seal at a resting tracheal mucosal pressure of 15 mmHg. The low-volume, high-pressure cuffs should *not* be used. The intraarterial pressure in blood vessels within the adult tracheal wall is approximately 30 mmHg, and the high-pressure cuffs are capable of exceeding pressures of 300 mmHg.

Ventilator Malfunctions

Some of the potentially serious ventilator malfunctions include mechanical breakdown, overheating of the inspired air, inadequate nebulization, and alarm failure. A common error with older ventilators in the suctioning procedure was neglecting to turn the alarm system back on following suctioning. All new ventilators have alarms that cannot be turned off for more than 1 to 2 minutes. If a patient's tubing becomes disconnected while the alarm is shut off, the result can be catastrophic. A patient receiving continuous ventilatory support should always have qualified personnel in attendance. When the alarm sounds, it does not identify the nature of the problem but merely indicates that something is wrong. The source of the alarm should be promptly identified and cor-

rected (e.g., tubing disconnected, high pressure). If the source of the problem cannot be found, the patient should be immediately ventilated with a self-inflating manual resuscitator (bag).

The excessive-pressure alarm usually indicates that the patient needs to be suctioned or an obstruction is present somewhere in the system. A slow rise in the pressure required to deliver a constant volume may indicate decreasing pulmonary compliance (pulmonary edema due to fluid overload). A low-pressure alarm usually signifies a leak in the system such as disconnection from the ventilator. A frequent site is the humidifier after it has been filled with sterile water and the lid has not been connected tightly. A segment of tubing may also be disconnected, particularly after the patient has been moved.

Nosocomial Infection

Patients requiring ventilatory support are often debilitated and have a lowered resistance to infection. Endotracheal tubes bypass the normal upper airway defense mechanisms. Aerosol therapy is a common source of nosocomial infection, because *Pseudomonas* and other gram-negative bacteria thrive in such hot, wet environments. For this reason, all parts of the ventilatory equipment that come in contact with the patient should be changed at least every 48 hours. Meticulous attention to details of good respiratory care techniques, sterile procedures, and frequent hand washing will minimize the incidence of nosocomial infections. Sputum examination should be performed routinely.

Intubation prevents the patient's nose and throat from warming and humidifying the inspired gas; therefore, heat and humidity must be continuously provided to the upper airway. The lack of humidity promotes drying and retention of secretions, which may obstruct airways and result in atelectasis and pneumonia.

Barotrauma

Barotrauma means injury as a result of pressure. Patients receiving continuous ventilatory support are subjected to high positive pressures in the lungs which may produce pneumothorax, pneumomediastinum, or subcutaneous emphysema. A common cause for pneumothorax is "ball-valving." This phenomenon occurs in an area of the lung that can accept air during inspiration but cannot expel it during expiration, because bronchial tubes enlarge on inspiration but may close with expiration. As this sequence persists, air collects in this particular lung zone, pressure builds up, and rupture occurs. Pneumothorax in a patient receiving mechanical ventilation can be detected by an abrupt rise in peak-inspiratory pressure for the same tidal volume delivered. In patients with chronic airway obstruction, barotrauma frequently results from overdistention. Some investigators contend that there is no longer any place for the sigh in modern ventilatory management, except that a single manually activated sigh may be a useful physical therapy adjunct.

Auto-PEEP

The phenomenon of "auto-PEEP" occurs when inadequate expiration time is allowed. This phenomenon is common in patients with rapid respiratory rates or obstructive lung disease. In both these conditions, there is not enough time for expired air to escape during exhalation. The result is a trapping of air and pressure in the lung, creating a PEEP-like effect. Assessment for auto-PEEP is important in any patient who is breathing rapidly or who has lung disease, since it is not easily detected without special measurement (Figure 30-6). Undetected auto-PEEP can worsen barotrauma and reduce cardiac output.

Hypotension

Positive-pressure ventilation can reduce cardiac output by decreasing venous return to the heart, particularly if the patient is hypovolemic. This adverse effect on venous return can be minimized if the expiratory phase is long enough to allow venous return during this period to compensate for the decrease that occurs during inspiration. An expiratory time that is 30% longer than inspiratory time will usually stabilize cardiovascular hemodynamics; however, marked hypotension may occur if the patient is hypovolemic or is receiving PEEP therapy.

REFERENCES

1. Kacmarek, R. M., & Meklaus, G. J. (1990). The new generation of mechanical ventilators. *Critical Care Clinics, 6,* 551-578.
2. Weilitz, P. B. (1989). New modes of mechanical ventilation. *Critical Care Nursing Clinics of North America, 1,* 689-695.
3. Matthay, M. A. (1989). New modes of mechanical ventilation for ARDS. How should they be evaluated? *Chest, 95*(6), 1175-1177.
4. St. John, R. E., & Lefrak, S. S. (1990). Alternate modes of mechanical ventilation. *AACN Clinical Issues in Critical Care Nursing, 1,* 248-259.
5. Thairatt, R. S., Allen, R. P., & Abertson, T. E. (1988). Pressure controlled inverse ratio ventilation in severe adult respiratory failure. *Chest, 94,* 755.
6. Geisman, L. K. (1989). Advances in weaning from mechanical ventilation. *Critical Care Nursing Clinics of North America, 1,* 697-705.

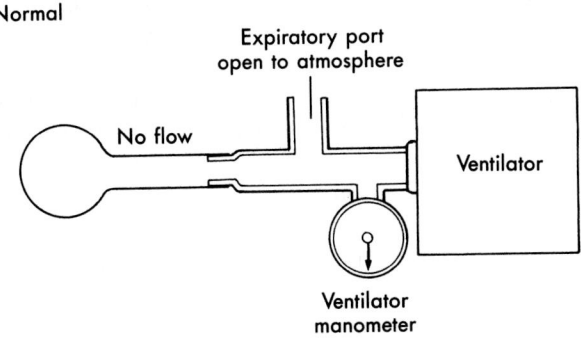

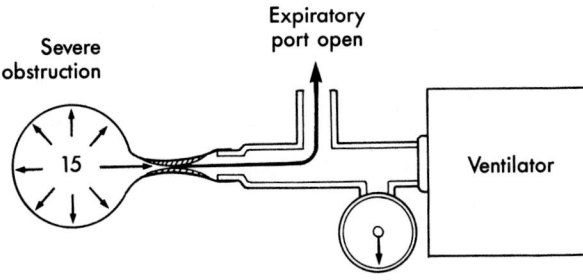

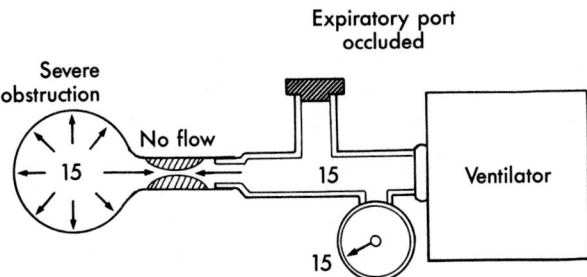

Figure 30-6 Measurement of "auto-PEEP."

PART SIX

Neurological Patient Care Problems

31

Neurological Anatomy and Physiology

Pamela H. Mitchell

The nervous system is the most fundamental and the most complex of all the physiological systems. It is the primary system that allows us to interact with our environment—to function simultaneously at the most basic level of survival and the highest level of creativity. Because of its complexity in integrating multiple aspects of physical and cognitive function, knowledge of its structures is not enough. Care of the patient with disorders of the nervous system must be built upon an understanding of the relationship between the structures damaged by the injury, disease, or pathophysiological process and the human function served by those structures.

STRUCTURAL AND FUNCTIONAL INTERRELATIONSHIPS

This chapter is organized to present the nervous system in two ways. First, an overview of the basic human functions and anatomical correlates is presented. Then the structural–functional correlates are discussed on the basis of the four gross divisions of the nervous system structures (neuroaxis approach). This organization is intended to help the reader appreciate both the vertical integration of human functions at all levels of the nervous system and the horizontal integration of higher order and reflex aspects of function within each anatomical compartment. Figure 31-1 shows the relation between the vertical (functional) and the horizontal (neuroaxis) approaches to understanding functional neuroanatomy. Such an organization is helpful in focusing initial assessment parameters on those functions most at risk when the injury is at a specific location such as the thoracic spinal cord. On the other hand, understanding that a given function—perception of pain, for example—is integrated at several anatomical levels helps to avoid focusing care planning on only the human responses predicted by the local area of injury.

The gross anatomical divisions of the nervous sys-

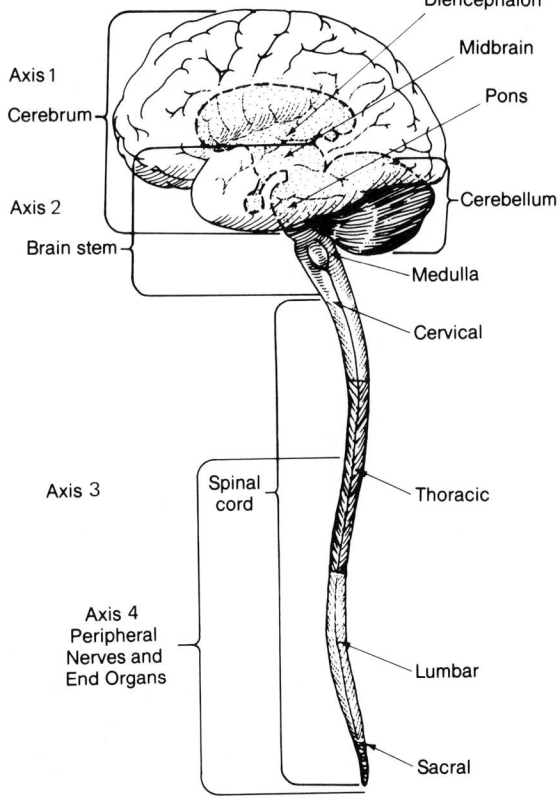

Figure 31-1 The neuraxis related to human functions.
Adapted from Langley, L. L., Telford, I. R., & Christensen, J. B. (1980). *Dynamic anatomy and physiology* (5th ed.). New York: McGraw-Hill.

tem are the central nervous system and the peripheral nervous system. The *central nervous system* (CNS) comprises the brain, brainstem, and spinal cord. The *peripheral nervous system* comprises the cranial and spinal nerves. The autonomic nervous system, which is frequently considered separately, includes parts of the central and peripheral nervous systems.

Microscopically, the nervous system consists of

support structures called *neuroglial* cells and the basic nerve cell, or *neuron*. The glial cells, which support, protect, and nourish the neurons, include astrocytes, oligodendroglia, microglia, and ependymal cells. The astrocytes are located between the blood vessels and neurons, restricting the passage of substances into the central nervous system. The oligodendroglia synthesize and maintain myelin. The microglia serve as phagocytes. The ependymal cells, which line the ventricular system and the central canal of the spinal cord, play a major role in cerebrospinal fluid production. The peripheral neuroglia are found in ganglia and along nerve trunks.

The *neuron* is the structural, genetic, and functional unit of the nervous system. It is composed of a cell body, dendrites, and axons. The *cell bodies*, or gray matter, are located in layers on the surface of the brain, or *cortex*, and in groups deeper within the brain; cell bodies are also found in the brainstem and spinal cord and certain other locations.

Dendrites are short receptor fibers that receive impulses and conduct them to the cell body. *Axons* are the myelinated long fibers that transmit impulses away from the cell body. Within the central nervous system, the axons form the white matter. The *myelin sheath* is a semifluid protein and lipid substance surrounding the axon and providing insulation. *Schwann cells* form a delicate membrane that surrounds the myelin sheath of the peripheral nerve fibers. Within the central nervous system, groups of axons with a common origin that travel alongside each other constitute a *tract*.

Vertically organized, the nervous system comprises four *functional* systems: (1) consciousness/mentation, (2) movement, (3) sensation, and (4) integrated regulation. These systems have both reflex and higher order components. Reflex components are the sensory or receptor mechanisms and the output or effector mechanisms. Higher order components consist of mechanisms that interpret incoming sensory information and integrate and initiate motor output.

Horizontally, the nervous system can be subdivided into four axes: Axis 1: the cerebral hemispheres, which include the diencephalon and basal ganglia; Axis 2: the brainstem and cerebellum; Axis 3: the spinal cord; and Axis 4: the peripheral nerves and the end organs they innervate. Each axis contains aspects of more than one functional subsystem. For example, the cerebral hemispheres mediate arousal, mentation, higher order movement, sensation, and integrative regulatory functions.

Finally, the discussion of functional anatomy and physiology must take into account the structures that protect, support, and nourish the nervous system. Disease or injury that damages these structures will have profound functional effects, often affecting the entire nervous system, not any single localized structure.

FUNCTIONAL ANATOMY AND PHYSIOLOGY

Basic human functions that allow us to interact normally with the environment include becoming aroused, thinking, moving, feeling, and performing such basic regulatory functions as breathing, eating, and circulating the body fluids. All these functions are organized by the nervous system and can be subsumed into four basic functions: consciousness, mentation, movement, sensation, and integrative regulation. Each function is organized vertically when the nervous system structure is considered as a whole. Each requires some kind of *sensory input* and *motor output*, which is received from and transmitted to the periphery (limbs, head, viscera). In addition, each function requires mechanisms to interpret and process the information for appropriate storage or response. Such processing may occur in the spinal cord or brainstem at a lower order, or *reflex* level, or may occur in the cerebral hemispheres as a higher order type of processing. In this section, the anatomical structures are described at each level of processing the four functional systems. Table 31-1 summarizes the anatomical correlates for these functional systems.

Consciousness/Mentation

Clinical definitions of consciousness (as contrasted with metaphysical or spiritual definitions) involve two components: arousal and self-awareness. Because the component of self-awareness blends with the functions of cognition, it is useful to consider the functions of consciousness and mentation (or cognition) together when discussing anatomical correlates. The *reticular activating system*, or RAS (Figure 31-2), is the anatomical substrate for the function of arousal or behavioral activation. The RAS is a functional system composed of the reticular formation and its projections to the thalamus and cerebral hemispheres. The *reticular formation* is a group of neurons and their connecting axons located in the central core of the brainstem, ascending from the pyramids of the medulla and ending at the thalamus. These neurons project fibers to the thalamus and all areas of the cerebral cortex, alerting the cerebral hemisphere to incoming stimuli. Because the reticular structures are tightly packed in the brainstem, very small lesions in the central brainstem can cause loss of arousal (or consciousness). In contrast, the diffuse nature of the projections in the cerebral hemispheres requires considerably larger lesions or bilateral lesions to disrupt arousal at the level of the hemispheres.

The reticular core contains the cell bodies that synthesize the monoamines responsible for the chemical

TABLE 31-1   Neuroanatomical Correlates of Fundamental Human Functions

Function	Anatomical Correlate
Consciousness	
Arousal	Reticular activating system, brainstem reticular formation, diffuse projections to thalamus and cortex, diencephalon
Self-awareness	Cerebral hemispheres
Mentation	
Memory	Limbic system, cortex; ascending activation via reticular activating system and thalamic projection system
Affect	Limbic system
Language (spoken, read, written)	Left cerebral hemisphere
Spatial perception	Right hemisphere
Problem solving	Cerebral hemispheres
Movement	
Head	
Seeing (eye movement)	Cranial nerves III, IV, VI; brainstem internuclear pathways; cerebellum
Chewing	Cranial nerves V, VII, XII
Swallowing	Cranial nerves IX, X, XII
Speaking	
Articulating	Cranial nerves VII, IX, XII and cerebellum
Phonating	Cranial nerve X
Body	
Walking	Motor cortex, basal ganglia
Activities of daily living	Pyramidal and extrapyramidal systems, cerebellum
Coordination	Cerebellum
Sensation	
Seeing (vision)	Cranial nerve II
Smelling	Cranial nerve I
Tasting	Cranial nerves VII and IX
Hearing	Cranial nerve VIII
Balance	Cranial nerve VIII and posterior columns of spinal cord
Feeling	
Pain, temperature	Spinal cord: spinothalamic tracts, anterolateral tracts; cerebral hemispheres: thalamus
Touch, position	Spinal cord: posterior columns; cerebral hemisphere: sensory cortex
Discrimination, higher sensation	Cerebral hemisphere: sensory cortex
Integrative regulation	
Breathing	Motor cortex, medullary inspiratory/expiratory centers; peripheral chemoreceptors and stretch receptors; diaphragm: C3, 5; intercostal muscles: T2-T11
Circulation	Hypothalamus; cranial nerve X, sympathetic ganglia (heart and lungs); cervical ganglia (head and upper extremities); T2, 6 (thorax); T5-10 (abdomen); T11-L2 (lower extremities and pelvis); craniosacral parasympathetic ganglia; postganglionic sympathetic, parasympathetic fibers
Temperature control	Hypothalamus; dermatomal cutaneous sympathetic and parasympathetic fibers
Ingestion/digestion	Medial temporal lobe, hypothalamus, midbrain, pons, visceral parasympathetic via cranial outflow; sacral via pelvic nerve; sympathetic via lower thoracic ganglia
Elimination	Medial frontal lobe; paracentral gyrus, hypothalamus, midbrain, pons, S2-4 pelvic, pudendal, perineal, hypogastric nerves
Sexual response	Limbic system, preoptic hypothalamus, spinal reflex centers (T11-L2, S2-4); pelvic, pudendal, perineal, and hypogastric nerves
Affect (emotional expression)	Limbic system, hypothalamus, visceral and cutaneous sympathetic and parasympathetic effectors, musculoskeletal and proprioceptive reflexes

Adapted from Mitchell, P. H., Cammermeyer, M., Ozuna, J., et al. (1984). *Neurological assessment for nursing practice.* Englewood Cliffs, NJ: Reston.

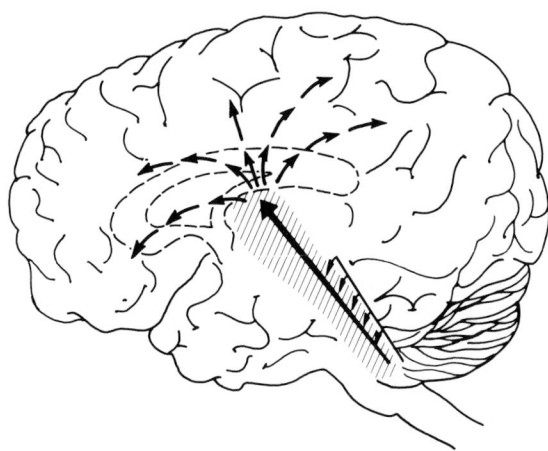

Figure 31-2 The reticular activating system. The small arrows represent multiple sensory inputs at the level of the brainstem; the large arrows are projections to the cortex.

transmitters between neurons of not only the arousal system but also the motor system, pain transmission, affective states, and a number of basic vegetative responses. Norepinephrine pathways arise in the locus ceruleus (medial brainstem) and are implicated in the normal cycling between REM and non-REM sleep. Serotonin pathways begin in the raphe nucleus of the lower brainstem and are important in cycling between wake and sleep and among sleep stages.

The self-awareness component of consciousness is a summation of a number of mentation, or cognition, functions of the cerebral hemispheres. Although the brain functions as a whole in human interaction with the environment, a number of anatomical areas are known to be crucial to the normal functioning of such mental activities as memory; production and understanding of language; and recognition of shapes, faces, and space. These areas are contained in both surface and deep structures of the cerebral hemispheres.

Cerebral Hemispheres

The cerebral hemispheres are paired structures that are most highly developed in primates, including humans. Each hemisphere consists of gray matter (neuronal cell bodies), found primarily in the cortex and the basal ganglia; and white matter, or myelinated fiber tracts that connect the numerous functional areas of the hemispheres. *Association fibers* connect areas within the same hemisphere; transverse fibers called *commissures* connect symmetrical areas between the two hemispheres. *Projection fibers* connect the cerebral cortex with deeper brain structures, brainstem, and spinal cord. The *corpus callosum* is the commissural fiber tract that connects the two hemispheres.

The surfaces of the brain contain grooves known

as *fissures* and *sulci*. The fissures (the larger grooves) mark the boundaries between lobes of the brain; the sulci are smaller grooves that serve as landmarks to identify areas within lobes. The convolutions of the brain between the sulci are known as *gyri*. Figure 31-3 shows the relation of fissures, sulci, and gyri to the lobes of the hemispheres.

The *longitudinal fissure* separates the cerebral hemispheres. Each hemisphere is subdivided into lobes, which are separated by deep sulci or fissures. The *central sulcus (fissure of Rolando)* marks the boundaries of the frontal and parietal lobes, whereas the *fissure of Sylvius* separates the temporal from the parietal and frontal lobes. The *parietooccipital fissure* separates the occipital from the parietal and temporal lobes. The *limbic system* is a paired collection of structures on the medial portion of the hemispheres. Structures commonly considered part of the limbic cortex include the cingulate gyrus, the hippocampus, the amygdala, the inferior medial frontal lobe, and the fiber tracts connecting these structures.

Several cognitive functions with identifiable anatomical correlates are disrupted in conditions requiring critical care. These functions include memory, production and understanding of language, emotional expression, spatial perception, and generalized information processing (thinking, problem solving).

Memory

The medial temporal lobes are crucial to the storage of short-term memory and perhaps to the retrieval of longer-term memory. Damage to the hippocampal gyrus and mammillary bodies of the hypothalamus is associated with impaired storage of short-term memories. There appears to be hemispheric specialization with regard to memory functions, with the left hippocampus and medial temporal lobe being more important to storage of verbal information and the corresponding areas in the right medial hemisphere mediating memory for faces, shapes, and spatial information. No specific brain location has been isolated for long-term memory, suggesting that the brain as a whole is involved in storage of long-term information.

Language

Language is a system of spoken and written symbols and involves more than just the ability to make sounds and form words. In most people, the left cerebral hemisphere is critical in the production and understanding of language. *Broca's area*, the third convolution (gyrus) of the frontal lobe, is important in initiating the oral movements necessary for speech. The person with lesions of Broca's area cannot easily produce words (although the ability to move the mouth is unimpaired) but can understand speech.

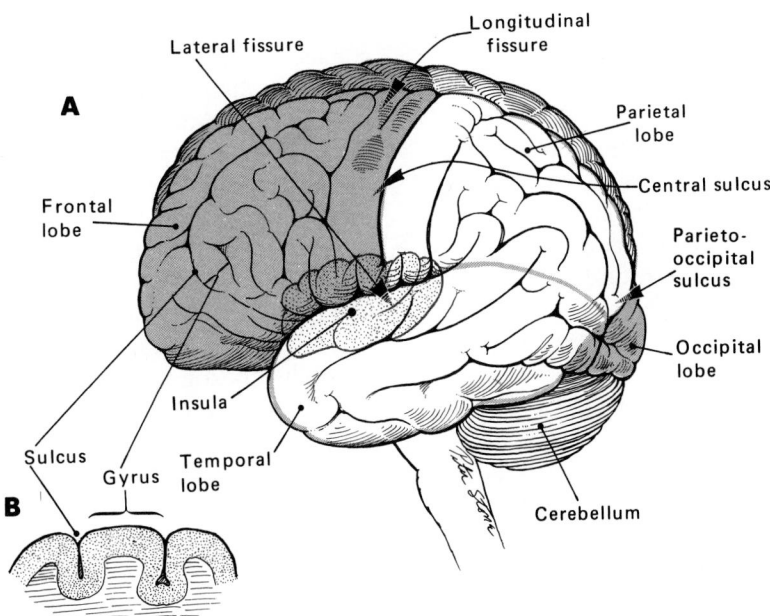

Figure 31-3   *A,* Lateral view of the cerebrum. *B,* A portion of the cortex in cross-section.
From Langley, L. L., Telford, I. R., & Christensen, J. B. (1980). *Dynamic anatomy and physiology* (5th ed.). St. Louis: Mosby.

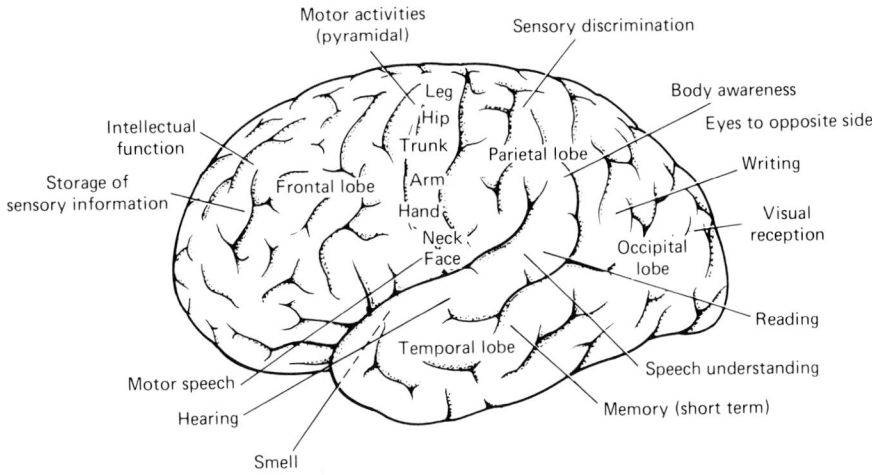

Figure 31-4   Localized functional areas of the cerbral cortex.

The areas necessary to understanding spoken language are *Wernicke's area* (posterior, superior left temporal lobe) and the primary auditory area in the superior temporal lobe. These areas are shown in Figure 31-4. Comprehension of written language requires an intact visual area (posterior and medial occipital lobe) as well as intact communication with Wernicke's area.

Affect

The frontal lobes and subcortical structures of the limbic system (hippocampus, cingulate gyrus, septum, and amygdala) interact to produce affective behavior. The frontal lobes appear to inhibit more primitive or undifferentiated emotional responses that are integrated by the limbic system. Thus, persons with generalized brain damage or those with medial frontal lobe damage may exhibit wide swings of emotion or have difficulty modulating emotional expression.

Spatial Perception

Recognition of the relation of objects in space, of shapes, and of other persons is mediated in most people more by the right cerebral hemisphere than the left. The right parietal lobe is crucial in appreciating the three-dimensional nature of objects, locating oneself in space, and appreciating that the right side of the body is one's own. The recognition of faces is more impaired by lesions of the right hippocampus than by those of the left.

Complex Cognitive Functions

Complex cognitive functions such as problem solving, decision making, and judgment cannot be easily localized to any "center" in the brain. These activities require numerous coordinated processes of memory, recognition of pattern, and so forth. Damage to any part of the brain can impair the efficiency and quality of these operations. Thus, many different lesions may result in irritability, distractibility, and difficulty in processing multiple inputs simultaneously.

Movement

The motor system is subdivided into the pyramidal and extrapyramidal systems. The pyramidal system is composed of the cells of the precentral gyrus of the frontal lobes and several tracts that descend through the internal capsule to the brainstem and spinal cord. It is the system serving voluntary muscle movement. The corticomesencephalic tract terminates in the brainstem at the motor nuclei of cranial nerves III (oculomotor), IV (trochlear), and VI (abducens). The corticobulbar tract terminates at the motor nuclei of cranial nerves V (trigeminal), VII (facial), IX (glossopharyngeal), X (vagus), XI (spinal accessory) and XII (hypoglossal). Fibers forming the corticospinal tract arise from each hemisphere, pass through the posterior limb of the internal capsule, and descend through the brainstem. The majority cross over (de-cussate) to the opposite side of the medulla to form the lateral corticospinal tract (Figure 31-5). These fibers terminate at the different spinal cord segments and synapse with the anterior horn cells. The fibers that do not decussate descend as the anterior corticospinal tract and synapse directly with neurons in the spinal cord.

Motor impulses which originate in the prefrontal gyrus, are transmitted by the corticospinal tract to the efferent cranial and spinal fibers and on to the periphery (Figure 31-6). The pyramidal system primarily regulates skilled motor activities of the distal extremities and the skeletal musculature of the head and neck. The cerebral cortex has several *suppressor areas* which inhibit movements of the musculature when they are stimulated. Eye movements are influenced by suppressor areas in the frontal and occipital lobes. The motor speech area is located in the posterior-inferior aspect of the frontal lobe, with the main language center being located in the left hemisphere. Motor speech is also influenced by the facial (VII), glossopharyngeal (IX), vagus (X), and hypoglossal (XII) nerves.

The extrapyramidal system is composed of the ba-sal ganglia and a complex network of tracts which connect the cerebral cortex, basal ganglia, cerebellum, brainstem, and spinal cord. Many circuits and feedback loops within and between the structures provide the interaction and constant influence over the parts of the cerebral cortex that give rise to the descending motor tracts, both pyramidal and extrapyramidal. The activity of the lower motor neurons of the peripheral nervous system is under the influence of the extrapyramidal system.

The extrapyramidal spinal tract either facilitates or inhibits flexor and extensor activities. The net result of extrapyramidal activity is maintenance of muscle tone, control of gross skeletal muscle activities, control of rhythmic movements such as running and walking, and control of head and trunk movements related to maintaining an upright position.

The cerebellum and the related fibers that provide connections with the basal ganglia and the reticular formation coordinate muscle activities and time muscle contractions to facilitate smoothness and accuracy (synergy). Intent and performance are correlated, providing for error control. The cerebellum also provides a "braking" or damping function to enable movements to be stopped where intended. The cerebellum receives sensory input from a number of afferent fibers which assist in maintaining equilibrium and the control of spinal reflex movements (see Figure 31-6).

Impulses from visual, auditory, vestibular, tactile, and proprioceptive stimuli, as well as input from the cerebral cortex, reach the cerebellum, where rapid correlation and integration take place. The cerebellum then transmits impulses that modify motor commands to voluntary muscles.

Impulses from the basal ganglia and cerebellum are first transmitted to the thalamus, where they are modified and integrated before being transmitted to the cerebral cortex. Impulses from the facilitory and inhibitory reticular nuclei are transmitted by the reticulospinal tracts to the anterior horn motor nuclei. When facilatory impulses are transmitted to extensor muscles, reciprocal impulses are transmitted to inhibit flexor muscle activity, with the effect being extensor facilitation and flexor inhibition. When inhibitory impulses predominate, lower motor neurons transmit impulses to inhibit muscle activity. There is normally a balance of facilatory and inhibitory impulses at the lower neuron level so that muscle tone is maintained.

Sensation

The sensory system consists of afferent peripheral nerves; the spinothalamic tracts and dorsal columns of the spinal cord; tracts within the brainstem; the thalamus; and the frontal, parietal, temporal, occipital, and limbic lobes.

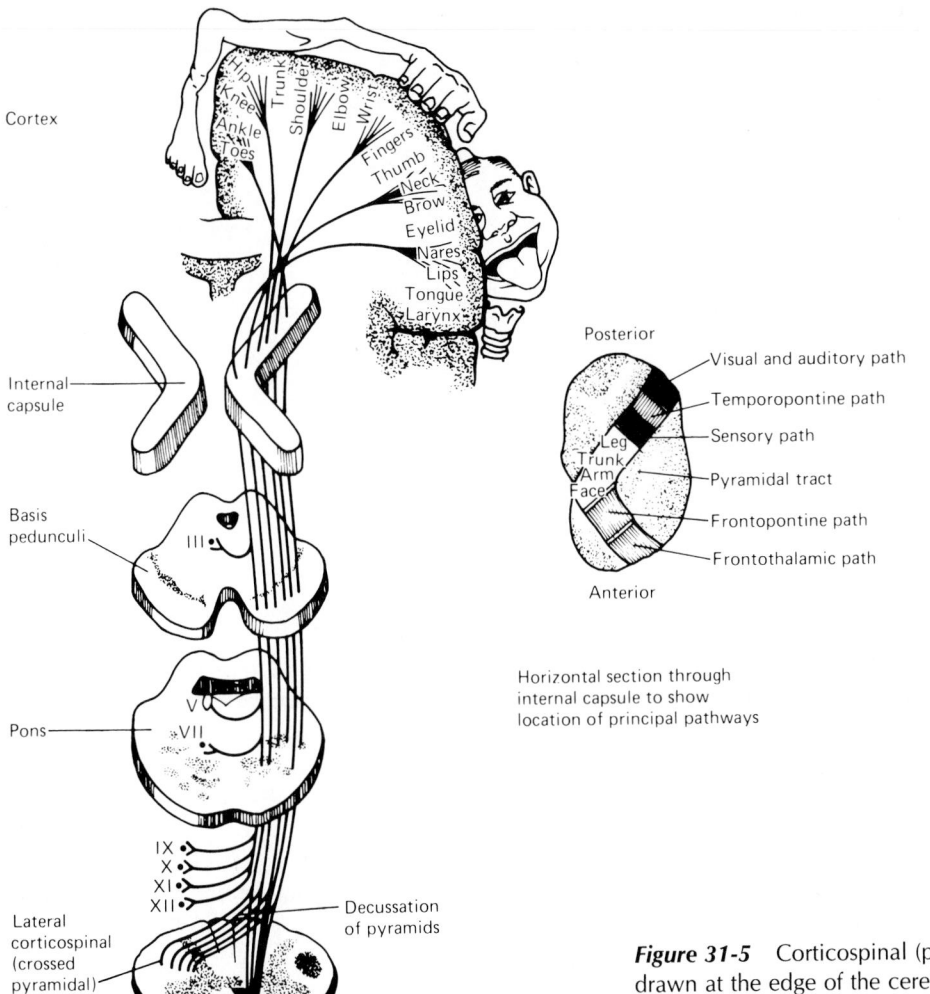

Cortex

Internal
capsule

Basis
pedunculi

Pons

Lateral
corticospinal
(crossed
pyramidal)
tract

Spinal
cord

Decussation
of pyramids

Anterior
cortico-
spinal (direct
pyramidal) tract

III

V

VII

IX
X
XI
XII

Hip
Knee
Trunk
Shoulder
Ankle
Elbow
Toes
Wrist
Fingers
Thumb
Neck
Brow
Eyelid
Nares
Lips
Tongue
Larynx

Posterior

Visual and auditory path

Temporopontine path

Sensory path

Pyramidal tract

Frontopontine path

Frontothalamic path

Leg
Trunk
Arm
Face

Anterior

Horizontal section through
internal capsule to show
location of principal pathways

Figure 31-5 Corticospinal (pyramidal) tract. The figure drawn at the edge of the cerebral hemisphere depicts the amount of surface area on the cortex assigned to the motor function of each body part.

From DeGroot, J. (1991). *Correlative neuroanatomy and functional neurology* (21st ed.). Los Altos, CA: Appleton & Lange.

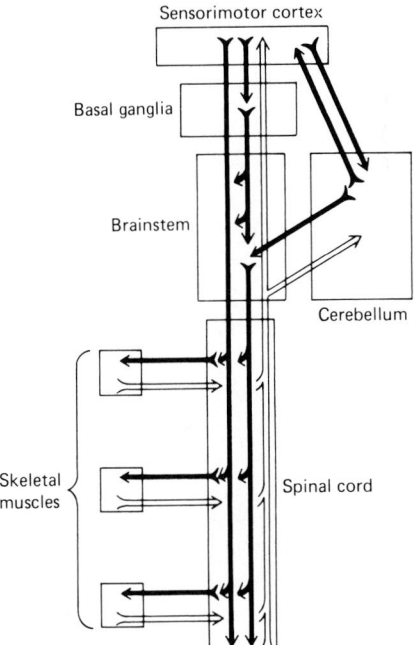

Sensorimotor cortex

Basal ganglia

Brainstem

Cerebellum

Skeletal
muscles

Spinal cord

Figure 31-6 Schematic representation of the motor system. Suprasegmental (pyramidal tract) influences are represented by the arrows connecting the motor cortex (axis 1), brainstem (axis 2), and spinal cord (axis 3). Segmental pathways (lower motor neuron) are shown by the arrows between spinal cord and skeletal muscles (axis 4). The cerebellum (axis 3) has no direct connections to cortex or spinal cord but serves to coordinate the entire system.

From Mountcastle, V. (Ed.). (1980). *Medical physiology* (14th ed.). St. Louis: Mosby.

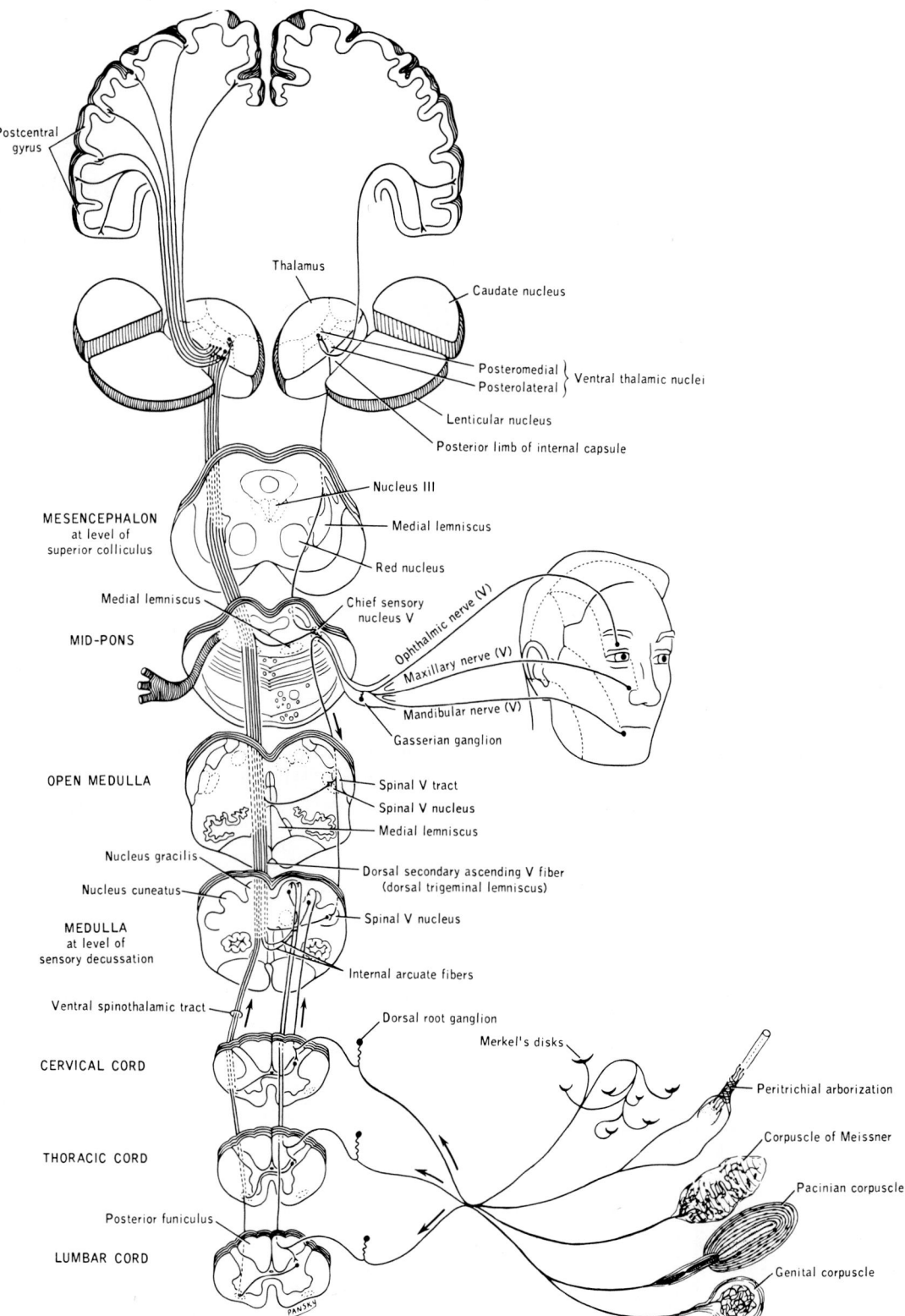

Figure 31-7   Sensory pathways. The pathway for the transmission of light touch is shown. Note that input from peripheral nerves serving the head and face is at the brainstem level. Touch sensory fibers from the trunk, arms, and legs travel upward in the posterior funiculus and join head and face fibers in the brainstem in the medial lemniscus.

From House, E. L., Pansky, B., & Siegel, A. (1979). *A systematic approach to neuroscience* (3rd ed.). New York: McGraw-Hill.

The cranial nerves transmit highly specialized sensations to the central nervous system. The olfactory nerves transmit the sense of smell. The optic nerves receive and transmit visual input. The acoustic nerves transmit sound by the cochlear branch and the sense of equilibrium by the vestibular branch. Taste is transmitted by the glossopharyngeal and facial nerves.

The superficial sensations of crude touch, pain, and temperature of the eye and face are transmitted into the brainstem by the trigeminal, facial, and vagus nerves. The cutaneous receptors for the superficial sensations of the body are located in specific anatomical areas known as *dermatomes*, which correspond roughly to the peripheral distribution of the sensory spinal nerve fibers. The superficial sensations are transmitted to the spinal cord by the posterior spinal nerve roots, where they synapse, pass immediately to the contralateral spinothalamic tract, and are transmitted to the thalamus and cerebral cortex.

The deep, more complex sensations of pressure, position *(proprioception)*, vibration, fine touch, and deep pain are transmitted by the posterior spinal nerve roots to the dorsal column to ascend to the level of the medulla oblongata, where the fibers cross to the opposite side and extend to the thalamus and cerebral cortex (Figure 31-7).

The reticular formation integrates all sensory input prior to transmission to higher levels. The stimulation of the reticular formation in the upper brainstem produces impulses that lead to cortical arousal and contribute to conscious awareness.

All the lobes of the cerebral hemispheres have specific areas to receive sensory impulses and other areas to integrate this information and enable it to be understood (see Figure 31-4). The frontal lobe functions include reception of the sense of smell, storage of information for memory, abstract thought processes, judgment, and other higher intellectual functions.

The activities of the parietal lobes consist primarily of sensory discrimination and bodily awareness for the side of the body contralateral to each lobe. Awareness of size, shape, and texture of objects; the relationship of body parts; two-point discrimination; and localization of other sensations are parietal lobe functions. A center for perceiving the meaning of speech is located in the dominant hemisphere parietal lobe.

The occipital lobes are primary visual receiving and understanding areas. The temporal lobes are primarily auditory and olfactory reception areas; however, the hippocampal gyrus receives the sensory input associated with memory and bodily awareness. The limbic structures process and sort information as well as supply information for storage; therefore, learning and memory for recent events are under the influence of the limbic system.

Integrative Regulation

Integrative regulation refers to the functional system that regulates basic survival functions. In order for mammals to adapt and survive in their environments, they must be able to carry out a large number of functions quite automatically. A regulatory system is one that maintains and adjusts physiological stability without conscious effort from the organism. The autonomic nervous system is usually thought of as the primary regulator in humans. However, it is only one participant in a truly integrated process. Neurons of the regulatory system must receive sensory stimuli (from the peripheral and autonomic sensory nerves), interpret the stimuli at several reflex and conscious levels, coordinate multiple inputs, transmit motor responses to the somatic, neuroendocrine, and autonomic motor systems, and provide feedback about the state of the end organ.

Basic regulatory functions include breathing, circulation, temperature control, ingestion/digestion, elimination, and sexual and emotional expression. Sensory input to each system is via the peripheral nerves (spinal nerves, cranial nerves, or autonomic nerves). Interpretation of sensory input occurs at several levels: spinal cord, brainstem, hypothalamus, limbic cortex, and possibly the cerebellum. Motor output may be voluntary or reflexly controlled. The cerebral cortex mediates voluntary control, while the sympathetic and parasympathetic systems mediate reflex control. All the integrated regulatory subsystems have control at four levels: (1) voluntary control at the cerebral cortex, (2) central reflex control at the hypothalamus and limbic system, (3) autonomic reflex control at the brainstem and spinal cord, and (4) peripheral control at the end organ. Disorders that disrupt nervous system functioning at any of these levels have the potential to disturb several integrated regulatory functions. Figures 31-8 and 31-9 show the relation of the cranial nerves and the autonomic nervous system to regulatory functions.

The sympathetic and parasympathetic systems are the primary effectors of integrated regulatory activity. The hypothalamus is the major cerebral hemisphere regulator of these two systems. The anterior and medial nuclei of the hypothalamus excite parasympathetic activity, causing sweating, decrease in the rate and force of cardiac contractions, and pupil constriction. The posterior and lateral nuclei excite sympathetic activity, causing vasoconstriction, increased rate and force of cardiac contractions, increased respirations, and inhibition of peristalsis. Pupillary dilation occurs passively when parasympathetic input is removed, and vasodilatation occurs passively when sympathetic stimulation is removed. The physical expression of "fight or flight" emotion, which in-

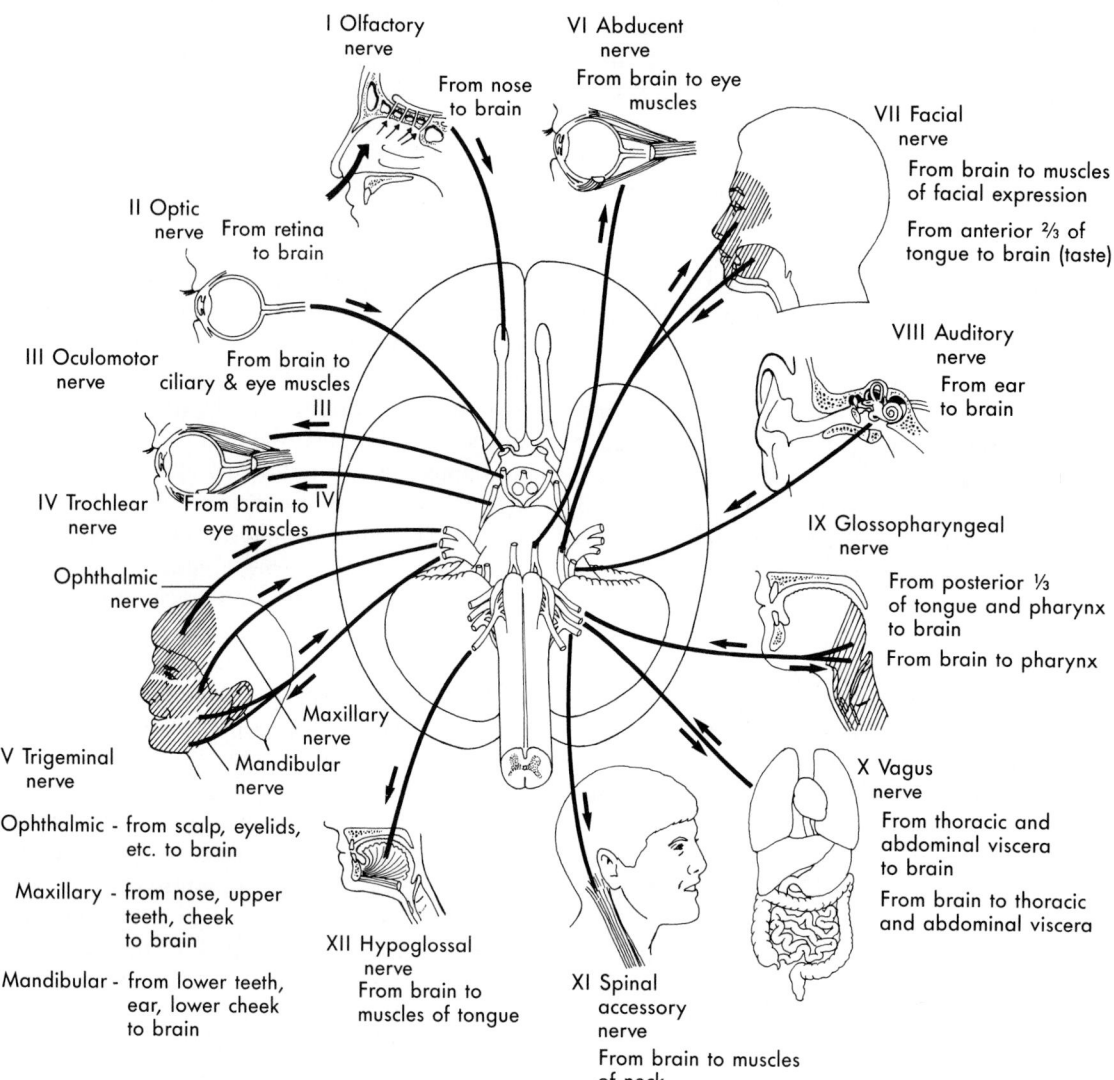

Figure 31-8   The cranial nerves. Cranial nerves I through VII and XI serve somatic motor and sensory functions. Cranial nerves IX, X, and XII provide motor and sensory input to a variety of integrated regulatory functions.

cludes accelerated heart rate, elevated blood pressure, flushing or pallor of the skin, sweating, gooseflesh, dry mouth, and gastrointestinal disturbances, is a reflection of autonomic activities that are modulated by the hypothalamus.

The hypothalamic nuclei regulate body temperature. The parasympathetic activities of sweating and vasodilatation lower the body temperature. Shivering and vasoconstriction, which are sympathetic activities, help elevate body temperature. The regulation of eating, drinking, emptying the urinary bladder, defecation, and sexual activity is under the influence of the hypothalamic structures and the sympathetic and parasympathetic fibers.

The supraoptic nuclei of the hypothalamus and its neuronal connections with the posterior pituitary are referred to as the *neurohypophysis* (see Chapter 37). The neurohypophysis regulates body water metabolism by producing, storing, and releasing antidiuretic hormone (ADH; also called vasopressin). ADH is produced by the hypothalamic nuclei and transferred to the posterior pituitary for storage. Capillaries in the supraoptic nuclei monitor the osmolality of the blood. The secretion of ADH by the posterior pituitary is either stimulated or inhibited on the basis of the existing osmolality. Increased osmolality and a reduction of extracellular volume, which stimulate the pressure receptors in the hypothalamus, cause the posterior pituitary gland to release ADH. The presence of ADH in the blood promotes increased water reabsorption from the distal convoluted tubules of the kidney, thereby limiting the volume of water lost in

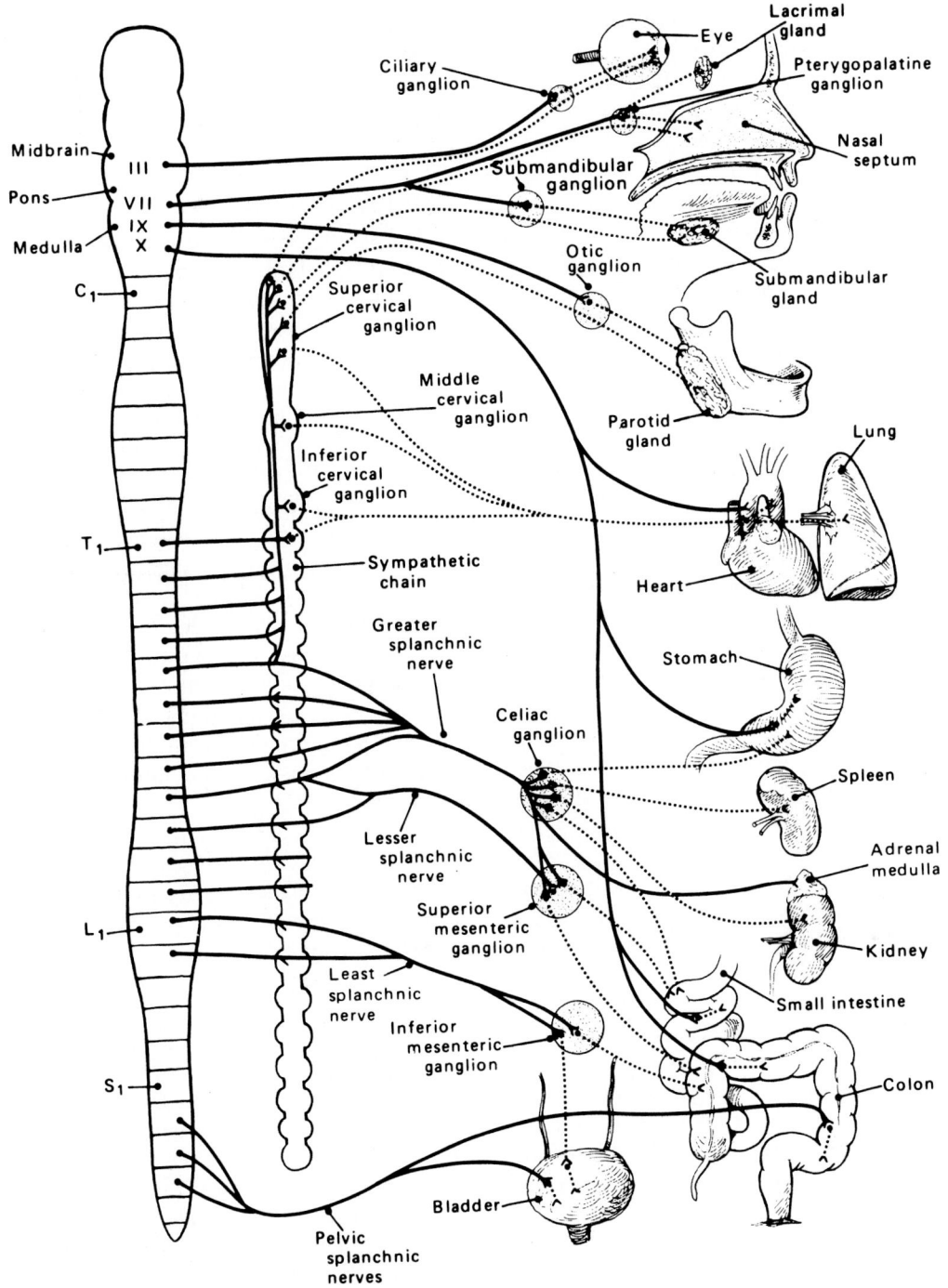

Figure 31-9 The autonomic nervous system, schematic drawing. Only one of the two sympathetic chain ganglia is shown.

From Langley, L. L., Telford, I. R., & Christensen, J. B. (1980). *Dynamic anatomy and physiology* (5th ed.). St. Louis: Mosby.

the urine. The return to normal osmolality is further assisted by the hypothalamic structures, since stimulation of the hypothalamus by a state of increased osmolality brings with it a feeling of thirst.

Breathing

Voluntary control of breathing involves the abdominal and thoracic muscles via the motor cortex, with cerebellar influence on coordination of breathing. Reflex control occurs in the pons and medulla in response to changes in the pH of blood and tissues. Spinal reflexes include innervation of the phrenic nerve to the diaphragm at spinal cord levels C3 to C5 and innervation to the intercostal muscles at levels T1 through T11. The rate and rhythm of automatic breathing is regulated in the cerebral hemispheres.

Circulation

Individuals can regulate heart rate and blood pressure voluntarily through biofeedback, suggesting that a mechanism exists for higher control of circulatory functions; however, the anatomical site for such control is unknown. Homeostatic control of blood pressure and heart rate is regulated via centers in the pons and medulla. Hypothalamus and brainstem nuclei regulate sympathetic and parasympathetic cardiovascular responses to a variety of stimuli. The anterior hypothalamus and parasympathetic nuclei in the brainstem decrease heart rate, decrease cardiac output, decrease AV bundle conduction, and perhaps constrict coronary arteries. Cranial nerve X (vagus) is the primary efferent for hypothalamic mediation of parasympathetic response.

Posterior hypothalamic nuclei, with efferents to the reticular core and to the sympathetic spinal ganglia, form the pathway for sympathetic control of circulation. Norepinephrine, the postganglionic neurotransmitter for the sympathetic system, functions to increase peripheral resistance, increase the rate and force of cardiac contraction, and increase myocardial blood flow.

Temperature Control

Thermoregulation can be cortically controlled via conscious decisions to seek warmer or cooler environments. Both the sensory and motor cortex, as well as whole brain decision processes, are involved in such control. Cerebral reflex control is centered in the hypothalamus, which is thought to function as a thermostat. Heat-losing mechanisms are regulated by the anterior hypothalamic nuclei, which stimulate parasympathetic activities such as sweating, panting, and vasodilatation. Heat production mechanisms are controlled by the posterior hypothalamus and lead to vasoconstriction, shivering, and increased metabolism.

The spinal reflexes control the autonomic functions necessary to implement hypothalamically signaled activities such as reflex constriction or dilatation of skin vessels, piloerection (gooseflesh), and increased respiration.

Ingestion/Digestion

The act of chewing and swallowing is a movement function, as discussed earlier. However, the movement of food through the alimentary tract and its digestion is a more automatic and regulatory function. This function is mostly reflex, mediated by the cranial nerves involved in chewing and swallowing and the autonomic systems of the gut. These cranial nerves include V (chewing, sensation to the inside of the mouth), VII (salivation, lip movement, taste), IX (sensation to the pharynx, upward movement of the pharynx, salivation, taste, gag reflex), X (swallowing, glottis closure, peristalsis, digestive stimulation), and XII (tongue movement). The vagus (cranial nerve X) is parasympathetic to the digestive tract and facilitates normal movement of food through the gut (Table 31-2). The splanchnic nerves arise from the thoracic ganglia and serve as sympathetic innervation to the gut. These fibers intermingle with the parasympathetic divisions of the vagus in the autonomic plexus in the abdomen.

Elimination

Bowel and bladder evacuation are presumed to have similar anatomical correlates, although the innervation of the bowel has not been as clearly identified, particularly in terms of cerebral level controls. Cortical control of bladder evacuation is found in the medial portions of the motor and sensory cortex, as shown in Figure 31-10. The sensory areas serve perception of the fullness of the bladder, and the motor areas allow voluntary initiation and inhibition of voiding (*micturition*). Fibers from these areas synapse with inhibitory neurons in the pons and inhibit the detrusor muscle of the bladder, thereby inhibiting reflex emptying of the bladder. Motor pathways from the midbrain-pontine micturition centers synapse in the interomedial gray area and the anterior horn cells of the sacral spinal cord (levels S2 through S4) and connect higher level voluntary and reflex control with spinal reflex control. Sensory input to the reflex arc at the sacral cord comes from the sensory stretch receptors in the bladder via the dorsal root of the spinal cord. The end organ is the urinary bladder, which has three muscles innervated by this system: the trigone, the detrusor, and the striated muscle of the urethra. The *trigone* is a triangular muscle that is continuous with the ureters. It is surrounded by the *detrusor,* a smooth muscle. When the detrusor contracts, it pulls away from the trigone and urine pas-

TABLE 31-2   **Summary of Cranial Nerve Functions**

Number and Name	Brainstem Level	Type	Major Functions
I Olfactory	None	Sensory	Smells
II Optic	None	Sensory	Sees (central and peripheral vision)
III Oculomotor	Midbrain	Motor	Moves eyes, elevates upper eyelid
		Parasympathetic	Constricts pupil
IV Trochlear	Midbrain	Motor	Moves eyes downward and inward
V Trigeminal	Pons to cervical cord	Sensory	Feels: touch, pain, temperature
			Jaw and eye muscle proprioception
		Motor	Masticates
VI Abducens	Pons	Motor	Abducts the eyes
VII Facial	Pons	Motor	Closes eyelids, muscles of facial expression
		Parasympathetic	Secretes: glands of mouth and eyes
		Sensory	Tastes (anterior two thirds of tongue)
VIII Acoustic	Pons and medulla	Sensory	
Vestibular branch			Equilibrates
Cochlear branch			Hears
IX Glossopharyngeal	Medulla	Motor	Moves pharyngeal muscles
		Parasympathetic	Secretes saliva: parotid glands
		Sensory	Feels: pharyngeal and posterior tongue
X Vagus	Medulla	Motor	Moves pharynx and larynx
		Parasympathetic	Visceral activities
		Sensory	Pharyngeal and laryngeal sensation, taste
XI Spinal accessory	Medulla	Motor	Moves: pharynx (accessory to vagus), sternocleidomastoid, and trapezius
XII Hypoglossal	Medulla	Motor	Moves tongue

sively flows from the bladder into the urethra. Relaxation of the detrusor allows the muscle to come back together and close off the urethra. The *striated muscle* in the urethra allows passage out of (but not into) the urethra. Parasympathetic motor output to the bladder is carried via the pelvic nerve to the detrusor muscle, sympathetic output via the inferior mesenteric ganglion to the detrusor, and voluntary motor output via the pudendal nerve to the urethra (see Figure 31-10).

Lesions that interrupt this circuit in the cerebral cortex and midbrain/pons area create a condition called *uninhibited bladder.* The functional outcome is a sense of urgency and inability to postpone voiding. Lesions in the cord itself may create a condition called *reflex bladder,* in which there is no sensation of fullness or voluntary control but the bladder remains able to empty reflexly when full. Lesions of the sacral cord or of the peripheral nerves serving the bladder may interrupt the reflex emptying mechanism.

The regulatory system for bowel evacuation is presumed to be similar to that for bladder evacuation with respect to cortical and midbrain/pontine levels of voluntary and inhibitory control of the anal reflex.

The internal and external anal sphincter reflexes are mediated at the spinal cord at the S2 through S4 levels. The anal sphincter is striated muscle and is served by the pudendal nerve, which is innervated from cord levels S1 through S4. The lower bowel is supplied by parasympathetic fibers from the pelvic plexus. Socially uninhibited bowel emptying can be seen in degenerative brain disorders. Reflex emptying of the bowel can be achieved in patients with spinal cord lesions above the level of the sacral reflex arcs. Lesions of the sacral cord or of the peripheral nerves serving the bowel reflex can produce a flaccid anal sphincter and decreased colonic peristalsis, with resulting constipation and overflow diarrhea.

Sexual Response

Human sexual response encompasses three phases: desire, excitement, and orgasm. The *desire phase* is essentially a cognitive/affective response thought to be mediated by the limbic system and the preoptic nuclei of the hypothalamus. This phase can be lost in damage to the brain; conversely, it can remain as a source of sexual pleasure when spinal cord damage disconnects the physical sensations from the fantasy or cerebral aspects of sexuality.

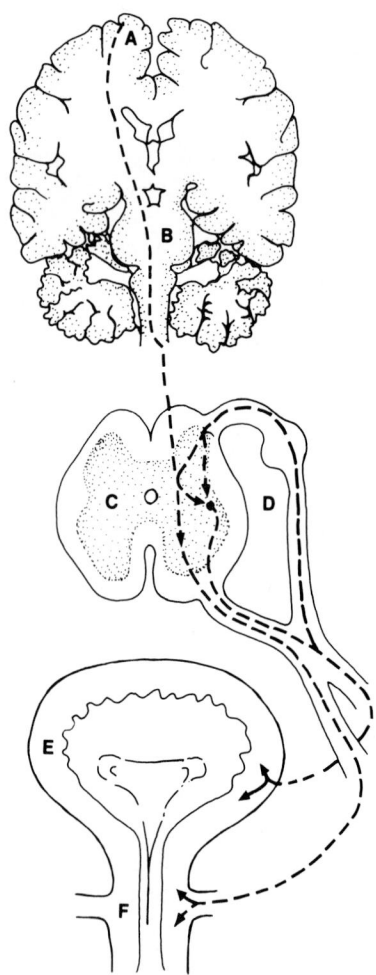

Figure 31-10   Integrated regulation of bladder: evacuation at four levels of the neuraxis. The medial frontal cortex (A) appreciates the sensation of a full bladder and works together with the pontine inhibitory center (B) to inhibit reflex bladder contractions. Spinal cord reflexes occur in the sacral cord (C), receiving sensory input from autonomic peripheral nerves (D) and sending motor signals to smooth muscle in the bladder (E) and striated muscle in the urethra (F).

The *excitement phase* is mediated by reflex vasodilatation of genital blood vessels. Arteriolar dilatation is mediated by spinal cord levels T11 through L2 and S2 to 4. The vasocongestion is primarily parasympathetic. Penile and clitoral erection and vaginal lubrication are the physical indicators of this response. The thoracolumbar area is believed to be more responsive to input from the limbic system and cortex, while the sacral centers are stimulated by tactile input to the genitals. Thus, reflex erection can be stimulated even when the higher regulatory centers are functionally disconnected by spinal cord injury.

The phase of orgasm is mediated by the pudendal sensory fibers for input to the cord and motor output from the T11 through L2 levels.

Emotional Response

Emotional experience is not only a psychological state but has motor and autonomic components as well. We feel with our "guts" as much as with our minds. The limbic system is considered to be the major neuroanatomical correlate of emotion. The major tracts connecting portions of the limbic cortex converge on the hypothalamus, activating several effector systems that serve the visceral and motor component of emotion. Stimulation of the anterior hypothalamus not only activates the parasympathetic nervous system but also reduces movement and metabolism. Depression of affect is accompanied by a whole constellation of effects involving conservation of energy and withdrawal from activity. Conversely, stimulation of the posterior hypothalamus produces energy-using defensive patterns. The affect may be anger or aggression, with much motor activity and sympathetic visceral responses. Ordinarily there is automatic balance between activation and conservation, but it is speculated that many affective disorders are caused by a loss of the ability of the limbic system to maintain affective balance. Disorders that directly damage the limbic system or its connections with the neocortex and hypothalamus may be expected to alter emotional control and experience.

FUNCTIONAL ANATOMY RELATED TO THE NEURAXIS

The usual approach to neuroanatomy is to describe the functions of the divisions of the nervous system. It is useful to be able to overlap both approaches described in this chapter: to know the anatomic correlates of a given human function and to know the function or level of a function mediated by each of the major axes of the nervous system.

Axis 1: Cerebral Hemispheres

The cerebral hemispheres, also called the *encephalon*, are the most recent evolutionary development of the nervous system. They are the last part of the nervous system formed by the embryo and continue to develop after birth. Their major functions are to perceive and interpret incoming sensory stimuli and to initiate voluntary activity in response to such stimuli. They are also critical to the cognitive functions that allow us to learn, to plan, and to create. The cerebral hemispheres serve the most complex and highest level of information processing in the nervous system. The self-awareness component of consciousness is mediated only in the cerebral hemispheres, as is mentation. Initiation and voluntary control of movement and of integrated regulatory functions occur here, as do conscious awareness and interpretation of sensation and emotion.

For purposes of this discussion, axis 1 is considered to consist of the hemispheres themselves, the basal ganglia, and the diencephalon. Some authorities place the diencephalon within the hemisphere axis, and some group it with the brainstem. Because its structures contribute to complex perception and integration, it is placed in axis 1 in this discussion.

The cerebral hemispheres consist of the medial and lateral cerebral cortex and the connecting association fibers, as described earlier in this chapter. The limbic cortex and its connections with the neocortex, thalamus, and hypothalamus are considered part of the cerebral cortex. The limbic cortex is often called *paleocortex* ("old" cortex) in recognition of the earlier embryological development of this medial cortex and its persistence in more "primitive" levels of mammalian phylogenetic development. The term *neocortex* ("new" cortex) refers to those collections of cell bodies on the convexities or lateral surfaces of the brain. The neocortex develops somewhat later in the embryo than does the limbic cortex.

The term *diencephalon* ("between brain") refers to the thalamus, hypothalamus, subthalamus, and epithalamus. These structures are collections of cell bodies through which all sensory, motor, and integrative regulatory information passes between neocortex and brainstem/spinal cord. Together, these structures form key relay points in perceiving and processing information before it is interpreted by higher cortical centers. The thalamus is located on either side of the third ventricle. The hypothalamus is a collection of paired nuclei (cell bodies) surrounding the inferior third ventricle and extending from the level of the optic chiasm to the midbrain.

The *basal ganglia* are paired subcortical gray structures located adjacent to the internal capsule (Figure 31-11). The structures that make up the basal ganglia are the caudate nucleus, the putamen, the globus pallidus, and the amygdala. These structures, along with important connections to the substantia nigra in the brainstem and the cerebellum, are critical in the initiation and maintenance of coordinated automatic movements.

Axis 2: Brainstem and Cerebellum

The brainstem consists of the midbrain, the pons, and the medulla oblongata. The midbrain is composed of fibers that connect the diencephalon with the lower brainstem and cerebellum. The substantia nigra and the red nucleus are located in the midbrain. The nuclei of cranial nerves III (oculomotor) and IV (trochlear) are located in the midbrain. The midbrain is located in the tentorial notch.

The pons lies in the front of the cerebellum. Fibers that connect to the underlying spinal cord pathways pass through the pons. The nuclei of cranial nerves V (trigeminal), VI (abducens), VII (facial), and VIII (acoustic) are located in the pontine area.

The medulla oblongata is a pyramid-shaped structure that connects the pons with the spinal cord at the level of the foramen magnum. Tracts that connect the cerebral cortical areas with the spinal pathways cross in the medulla. The nuclei of cranial nerves IX (glossopharyngeal), X (vagus), XI (spinal accessory), and XII (hypoglossal) are located in the medulla.

The cerebellum consists of a midline portion, the *vermis*, and two lobes or hemispheres. Each cerebellar hemisphere contains an outer cortex of gray matter, a core of white fibers, and central nuclei. It is located directly below the occipital lobes and is covered by the tentorium.

The reticular formation is located in the central

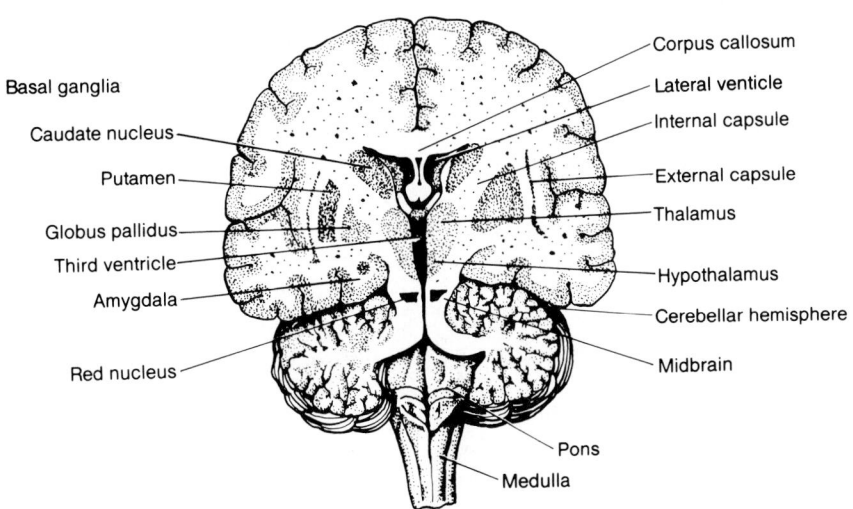

Figure 31-11   Coronal secretion of the cerebrum with basal ganglia, cerebellum, and posterior view of brainstem.

core of the brainstem, ascending from the medulla to the midbrain, with projections to the diencephalon and neocortex. All sensory input to the brainstem is relayed through the reticular formation, and the cell bodies for the monoamine neurotransmitters are located in the formation.

The functions served by axis 2 are maintenance of arousal and normal sleep–wake cycles, reflex level coordination, and integration of motor and sensory information. The cranial nerve nuclei in the midbrain, pons, and medulla serve the reflexes involved in the functions of moving the eyes, chewing, swallowing, and making sounds. Inhibitory and excitatory nuclei in the pons and medulla are part of the systems regulating breathing, circulation, and elimination. Parasympathetic output to the head, neck, and thorax is mediated from the brainstem nuclei. Finally, the coordination of voluntary movement is mediated by the cerebellum, whose only connection to the cerebral hemispheres is via the brainstem.

The brainstem is the passageway between the spinal cord and the cerebral hemispheres, and it is a relatively small structure. Therefore, the fibers relaying sensory and motor information, the primary cranial nerve, and the regulatory nuclei are closely packed together. Consequently, relatively small lesions in the brainstem can disrupt many functions: arousal, movement, sensation, and inhibitory control of regulatory functions. Lesions of the cerebellum affect coordination not only of movement but also of autonomic motor output. Further, because of the proximity of the cerebellum to the vital regulatory centers in the pons, expanding lesions of the cerebellum may threaten breathing and circulation by compression of the pons.

Axis 3: Spinal Cord

The spinal cord is a cylindrical structure that joins the brainstem at the level of the foramen magnum and ends at the L1-L2 vertebral level. The upper cervical cord segments correspond to the same vertebral level, whereas cord segments from C8 and below correspond to the vertebral level above each segment. For example, the C3 cord segment lies opposite vertebra C3, but the T1 cord segment lies above vertebra T1 (Figure 31-12).

The spinal cord consists of central gray horns which form an H shape (Figure 31-13). The gray matter is surrounded by columns of white matter which are fiber tracts. The size and shape of the spinal cord, the relative proportion of gray and white matter, and the configuration of the gray matter vary by segmental level. The cervical cord is the largest in diameter. The cervical and lumbar segments contain a greater proportion of gray than of white matter because of the larger number of neurons used to con-

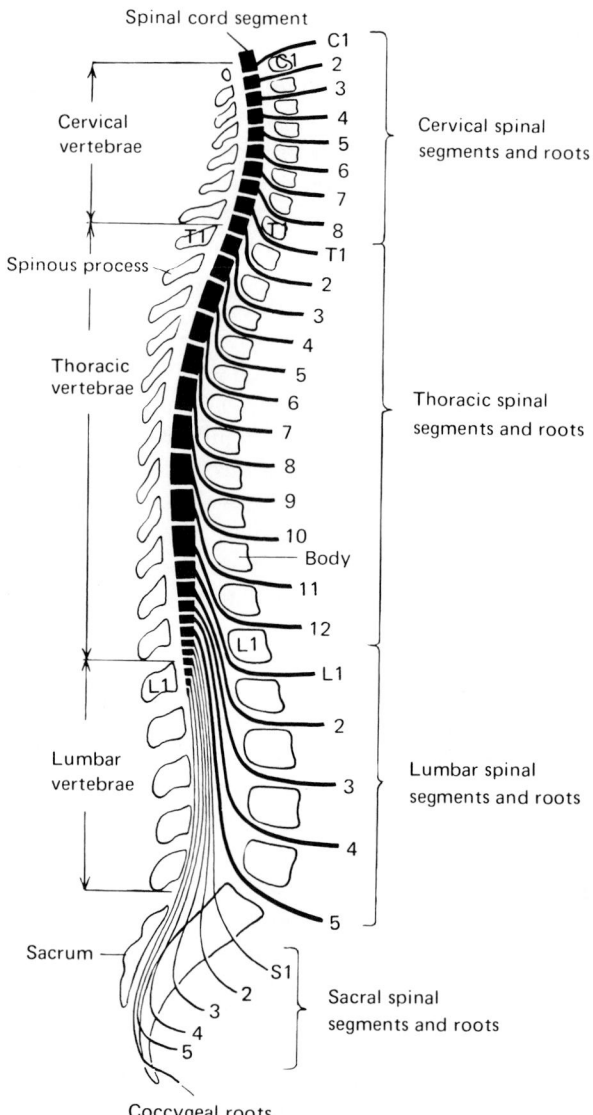

Figure 31-12   The relation of the spinal cord segments and spinal nerves to the vertebral column.
From Noback, C. R., & Demarest, R. J. (1991). *The human nervous system* (4th ed.). New York: McGraw-Hill.

trol the upper and lower extremities. The spinal cord is divided into left and right halves by a posterior sulcus and an anterior fissure. The halves are connected by commissures of gray and white matter.

The anterior, or *ventral*, horn contains the cell bodies of anterior (motor) nerve roots. The posterior, or *dorsal*, horn contains cells on which posterior (sensory) nerve roots terminate. Lateral horns of gray matter in the thoracolumbar area contain cells that give rise to sympathetic fibers of the autonomic nervous system. Interomedial gray matter in the cord, segments S2 through S4, gives rise to parasympathetic fibers.

The white matter is subdivided into groups of

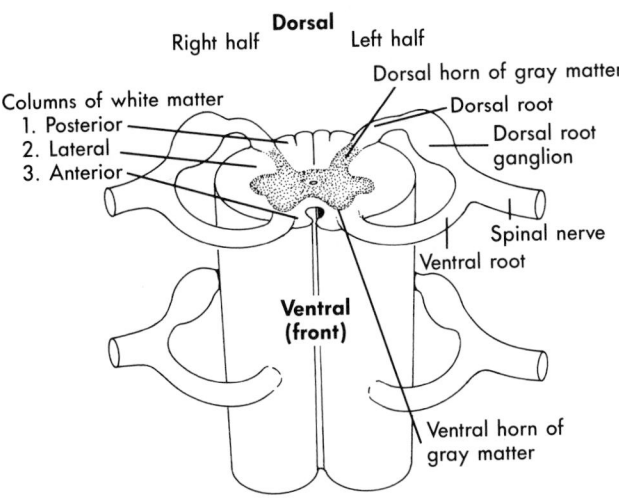

Figure 31-13   A segment of the thoracic spinal cord seen in cross section. Neurons serving the autonomic ganglia and nerves are located in the gray matter between the dorsal and ventral horns.

tracts that ascend and descend the spinal cord. The major tracts are located posteriorly and anteriorly. The posterior tracts *(dorsal columns)* and the anterior and lateral spinothalamic tracts conduct sensory impulses upward to the thalamus and the cerebral cortex. The lateral (corticospinal, pyramidal) tracts conduct motor impulses to the anterior horn cells.

Thus, it is clear that the functions of the spinal cord are to transmit motor and sensory information between the brain and the muscles and internal organs. The major functional outcome of damage to the spinal cord is to interrupt this flow of information. Information to and from the muscle or end organ at a given level of the spinal cord will not be impeded by damage to the cord *above* that level. In other words, the spinal reflex arc will be intact, and the local reflex will be unimpaired. However, inhibitory control from the higher axes (brainstem and hemispheres) will not be received, nor can sensory information from the local level reach the cerebral hemispheres. The functional outcome of such a situation is uninhibited motor and autonomic reflexes in response to local sensory stimuli. Spasticity and autonomic dysreflexia are examples of such outcomes in the case of spinal cord injury.

Axis 4: Peripheral Nerves and End Organs

The functional unit in axis 4 consists of the end organ (viscera, sensory receptor, or muscle), the sensory neuron and peripheral nerve transmitting information to the spinal cord, and the motor neuron and motor peripheral nerve transmitting information to the end organ. Interruption at any of the three components of the functional unit disrupts the reflex arc and thereby disrupts the function at the level of the

end organ. As with the spinal cord axis, the primary functions served are movement, sensation, and integrated regulation, but the functional outcome is loss of not only the observable or felt function but also the spinal reflex component. For example, peripheral motor neuropathy, like spinal cord injury, may result in inability to walk. However, in peripheral neuropathy, the paralysis is flaccid (disruption of the reflex), whereas in spinal cord injury the paralysis is spastic because reflexes are not inhibited. The person with spastic paralysis may be able to use the spasticity for stability during transfer to a wheelchair, whereas the person with flaccid paralysis will need to adopt a method of transfer that does not necessitate weight bearing by the feet.

The peripheral nerves comprise the cranial nerves (peripheral from the brainstem), the somatic nerves (from the spinal cord), and the autonomic ganglia and postganglionic fibers.

Cranial Nerves

The cranial nerves are considered part of the peripheral nervous system. There are 12 pairs of cranial nerves (see Figure 31-8). The names and numbers of the cranial nerves, as well as their functions, are listed in Table 31-2.

Cranial nerves I (olfactory) and II (optic) are unlike the other 10 in that they extend to become tracts that connect with structures within the cerebral hemispheres. In contrast, cranial nerves III through XII originate from nuclei (collections of neurons) that are located either superficially or deep within the brainstem structures. Cranial nerve I arises from the olfactory bulb and extends under the frontal lobes to penetrate the frontal and temporal lobes, where it becomes part of the limbic system. Cranial nerve II arises from the inner retinal layer of the eye and extends posteriorly to enter the intracranial cavity. The optic nerves join at the optic chiasm, which lies above the pituitary gland. The optic tracts and radiations then extend posteriorly to areas of the occipital lobe.

Cranial nerves III through XII extend peripherally to the eye muscles, face, ear, and pharynx. Cranial nerve X (vagus) extends down the neck into the thorax and the abdomen. Cranial nerve XI extends to the muscles of the neck and shoulders with minor input to the larynx. Parasympathetic fibers of the autonomic nervous system extend peripherally with the oculomotor, facial, glossopharyngeal, and vagus cranial nerves.

Somatic Peripheral Nerves

Distributed along the spinal cord are 31 pairs of spinal nerves: 8 cervical, 12 thoracic, 5 lumbar, 5 sacral, and 1 coccygeal. Each segment of the spinal cord has posterior (dorsal) nerve roots with ganglia

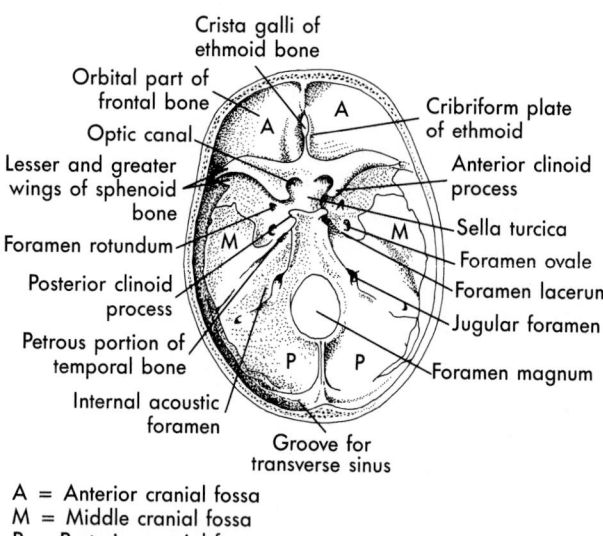

Crista galli of ethmoid bone
Orbital part of frontal bone
Optic canal
Lesser and greater wings of sphenoid bone
Foramen rotundum
Posterior clinoid process
Petrous portion of temporal bone
Internal acoustic foramen
Groove for transverse sinus
Cribriform plate of ethmoid
Anterior clinoid process
Sella turcica
Foramen ovale
Foramen lacerum
Jugular foramen
Foramen magnum

A = Anterior cranial fossa
M = Middle cranial fossa
P = Posterior cranial fossa

Figure 31-14 The bones that form the floor of the cranial cavity.

and anterior (ventral) nerve roots (see Figure 31-14), which exit the vertebrae through the intervertebral foramina and join to form the spinal nerves. The large bundle of lumbosacral nerve roots that descend from the end of the cord are referred to as the *cauda equina*. The cervical nerves exit at the corresponding vertebral level. All other spinal nerves exit one or two vertebral levels below the vertebra having the same number. The spinal nerves join peripherally to form plexuses. The cervical and brachial plexuses supply the upper extremities; the lumbar and sacral plexuses supply the lower extremities. The plexuses divide to form the various peripheral nerves. The peripheral nerves frequently have motor and sensory fibers intermingled.

Autonomic Nervous System

The autonomic nervous system receives higher level control from the hypothalamus and descending pathways within the brainstem and spinal cord. A series of ganglia and small nerve fibers constitute the peripheral portion of the system. The hypothalamus receives axons from the anterior and inferior portions of the frontal lobes. Fibers leave the hypothalamus and descend to groups of cells in the brainstem and spinal cord. The autonomic fibers are distributed with the cranial and spinal peripheral nerves to the visceral organs (see Figures 31-8 and 31-9).

The autonomic nervous system consists of the parasympathetic and sympathetic divisions, which differ anatomically, functionally, and pharmacologically. The peripheral autonomic fibers that originate in the cranial and sacral areas make up the parasympathetic division. Peripheral sympathetic fibers orig-

inate in the thoracic and lumbar areas (see Figure 31-9). Each visceral organ controlled by the autonomic nervous system has both parasympathetic and sympathetic innervation.

All autonomic fibers extend to synapses in ganglia after leaving their points of origin in the central nervous system. The sympathetic preganglionic fibers extend to a chain of paired ganglia located along the vertebral column. Most presynaptic fibers are short. The postsynaptic fibers are usually long and must travel the remaining distance to the organs they innervate. Sympathetic fibers are distributed to the head, neck, thorax, abdomen, and pelvic areas in conjunction with thoracolumbar spinal nerves.

Parasympathetic fibers extend to ganglia located adjacent to the organs they innervate. Thus, their presynaptic fibers are long and their postsynaptic fibers short. Parasympathetic fibers are not as widely distributed as the sympathetic fibers.

The adrenal medulla, unlike other viscera, is innervated directly by presynaptic fibers. The cells of the adrenal medulla are derived from nerve tissue and constitute a modified sympathetic ganglion.

SUPPORTIVE AND PROTECTIVE STRUCTURES OF THE CENTRAL NERVOUS SYSTEM

The structures that encase, support, and protect the delicate, semisolid nervous system include the bones of the skull, the vertebral column, and the three meningeal layers.

Skull

The roof of the cranial cavity, or *calvaria*, covers the superior aspects of the brain. The calvaria consists of the frontal, the occipital, and the paired parietal and temporal bones, which are fused at suture lines. The floor of the cranial cavity consists of a group of bony structures that have many ridges and grooves (Figure 31-14). The floor conforms to the shape of the base of the brain and is divided into three fossae: anterior, middle, and posterior. The anterior fossa contains the frontal lobes. The middle fossa contains parts of the temporal lobes, the upper brainstem, and the pituitary gland. The posterior fossa contains the brainstem and the cerebellar hemispheres. A number of small openings, or *foramina*, are located in the base of the skull to permit paired blood vessels and cranial nerves to enter and leave the intracranial cavity. There is also a large opening, the *foramen magnum*, where the brainstem connects to the upper cervical spinal cord.

The bones that form the cranial cavity are composed of three layers: the outer solid layer (outer table), the middle spongy layer (diploe), and the inner solid layer (inner table). The construction of the skull provides for great strength with economy of weight and insulation. The thickest parts of the skull are the midfrontal and midoccipital bones; the thinnest parts are the temporal bones. The inner table, which lies over the convexity of the brain, is very smooth and contains grooves in which the branches of the middle meningeal arteries are located. The viability of the skull is maintained by thin layers of periosteum which are attached to the inner and outer tables. Periosteum contains blood vessels that nourish the bone and osteoblasts that maintain its strength and density.

Vertebral Column

The vertebral column consists of 7 cervical, 12 thoracic, 5 lumbar, 5 sacral, and 4 fused coccygeal vertebrae (Figure 31-15). The vertebrae are joined by several ligaments and intervening disks which provide flexibility and stability. The vertebral column supports the skull and forms a spinal canal that surrounds and protects the spinal cord, spinal nerves, and underlying structures. The spinal canal extends for the length of the vertebral column and conforms to the spinal curvatures and to the variations in size of the spinal cord. The vertebrae are progressively larger down to the sacrum and then become smaller. The diameter of the spinal canal is greatest in the cervical region.

The first and second cervical vertebrae are highly specialized. The first cervical vertebra, or *atlas*, is joined to the base of the skull. The second cervical vertebra, or *axis*, forms a pivot around which the atlas rotates the skull. The remaining cervical, thoracic, and lumbar vertebrae have typical characteristics. Each vertebra consists of a body, a vertebral arch,

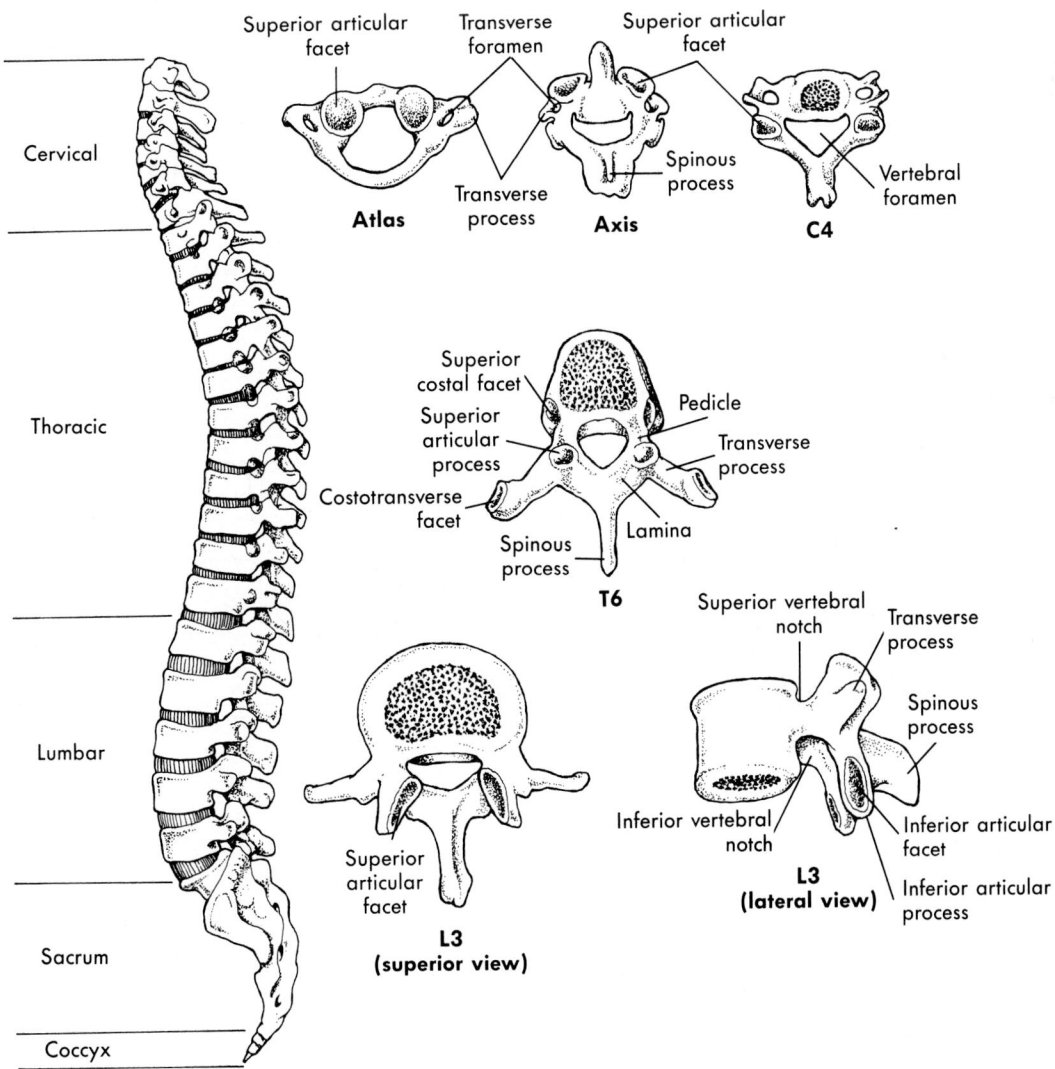

Figure 31-15   The vertebral column with individual vertebrae.

and several processes for muscular and articular attachments. The vertebral body is located anteriorly and consists of a spongy bone which gives strength and supports weight. The vertebral arch lies posterior to the body and completes the formation of the spinal canal. The arch is composed of pedicles and lamina. A spinous process projects posteriorly, and transverse processes project laterally from the vertebral arch.

Each vertebral arch has several articulating processes which permit motion between adjacent vertebrae. The vertebral notches in each pedicle form an intervertebral foramen that permits passage of the spinal nerves and associated blood vessels. Each of the transverse processes of the cervical vertebrae have foramina that form a passageway for the vertebral arteries, veins, and sympathetic nerves.

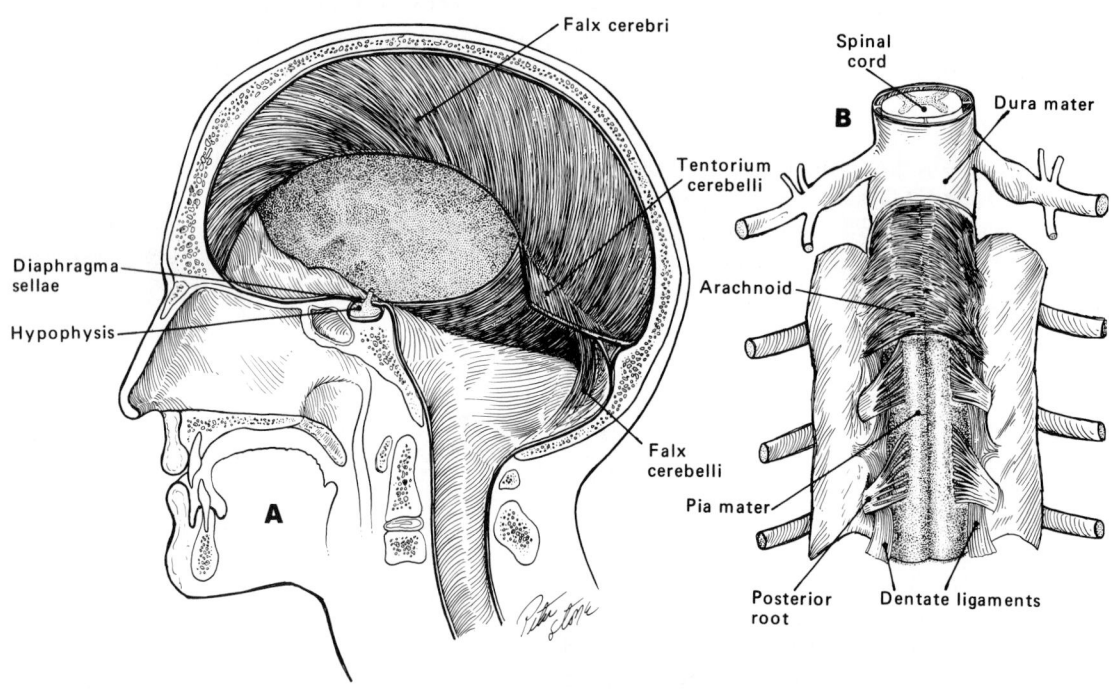

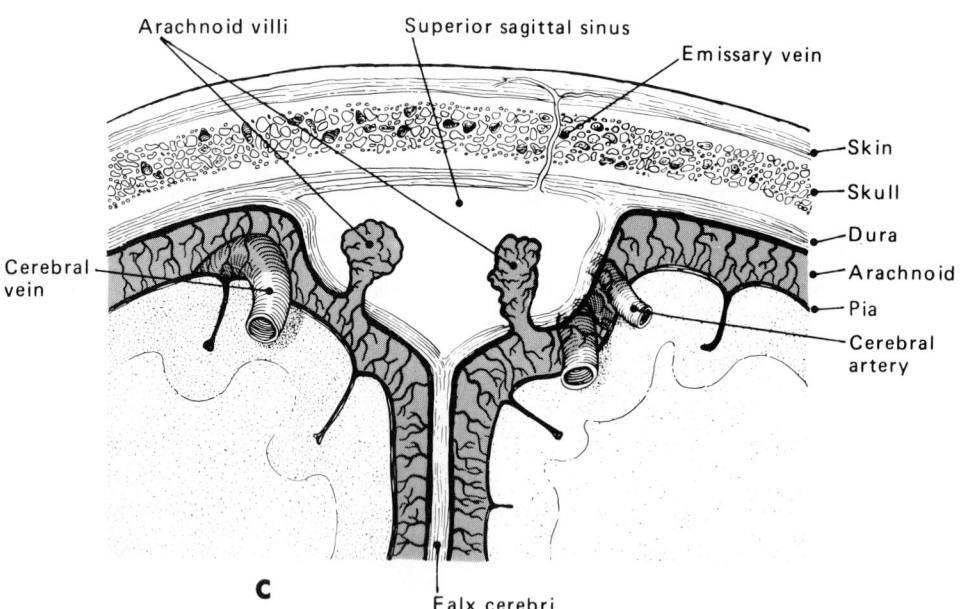

Figure 31-16   The meninges: *(A)* Extensions of the dura mater in the cranial cavity, sagital view. *(B)* The dura and arachnoid sheath the spinal nerves at their origin. The dentate ligament separates dorsal from ventral roots and adheres to the dura. *(C)* Coronal section through the superior sagittal sinus. Note also the layers of bone between the skin and dura.

From Langley, L. L., Telford, I. R., & Christensen, J. B. (1980). *Dynamic anatomy and physiology* (5th ed.). St. Louis: Mosby.

An intervertebral disk, which acts as a cushion, separates the adjacent vertebral bodies. The disk is composed of a central cartilaginous core, the *nucleus pulposus,* which is surrounded by a fibrous capsule, the *anulus fibrosus.* A series of strong, fibrous, overlapping ligaments connect the vertebrae with each other and with the cranium. The ligaments allow safe smooth movement of the head, protection from trauma, and stability and motion at the articulating processes. Additional support of the thoracic vertebrae is provided by the rib attachments.

Meninges

The brain and spinal cord are protected, supported, and surrounded by three layers of meninges (Figure 31-16). The outer layer, or *dura mater,* consists of thick, tough connective tissue. The cranial dura forms an envelope that lines the inside of the skull and is firmly attached to it, serving as a periosteum. Folds of dura divide the intracranial cavity into four compartments. The horizontal dural fold that forms the roof over the posterior fossa is known as the *tentorium.* The occipital and posterior temporal lobes are located directly above the tentorium. The cerebellar hemispheres are located under the tentorium in the *infratentorial compartment.* The dural fold that separates the cerebellar hemispheres is called the *falx cerebelli.* The supratentorial compartment is divided by a midline dural fold, the *falx cerebri,* which separates the cerebral hemispheres. Venous sinuses (channels draining blood from the brain) are located between the layers of dura at the posterior-superior and basal parts of the skull.

The spinal dura is a continuation of the cranial dura. The dura surrounds the spinal cord from the foramen magnum to the level of the second sacral vertebra, where it terminates as the dural sac. The spinal dura is not attached to the vertebrae. Extensions of the dura surround the spinal nerve roots, forming dural root sleeves.

The *pia mater* is the inner vascular membrane that adheres to the surface of the brain and spinal cord. Folds of pia form part of the choroid plexus, support the superficial blood vessels that penetrate the central nervous system, and provide support for the spinal cord. Tissue bands, the *dentate ligaments,* which attach the spinal cord to the dura, are formed by the pia. At the end of the cord, the pia forms the *filum terminale,* which merges with the dura and is attached to the coccyx.

The *arachnoid* (from the Greek word for cobweb) is the delicate, spiderweb-like membrane between the dural and pial layers. The arachnoid surrounds the surface of the brain without following its contour, surrounds the spinal cord, and extends along the roots of the cranial and spinal nerves. The combined pial and arachnoid membranes are referred to as the *leptomeninges.*

There is a potential space between the dura and the arachnoid, the *subdural space.* Vessels cross this area with little support. The space between the arachnoid and the pia mater, the *subarachnoid space,* is filled with cerebrospinal fluid. The depth of the subarachnoid space varies. The space is narrow over the convexity of the cerebral hemispheres. At the base of the brain and around the brainstem, the space widens to form large cisterns. The largest cistern, the *cisterna magna,* is located between the medulla and the inferior surface of the cerebellum. A lumbar cistern located at the end of the spinal cord contains sacral nerve roots.

Tiny projections of meninges, *arachnoid granulations,* protrude into the large venous sinuses formed by the dural layers such as the *superior sagittal sinus* (see Figure 31-16). The cerebrospinal fluid that is contained in the subarachnoid space is transferred into the venous sinuses as a result of hydrostatic pressure. The arachnoid granulations are permeable and permit one-way flow of cerebrospinal fluid, plasma proteins, and serum albumin into the venous blood.

NUTRITIVE AND METABOLIC SUPPORT OF THE CENTRAL NERVOUS SYSTEM

The nutritional and metabolic needs of the central nervous system are met by the cerebrospinal fluid and the ventricular and circulatory systems.

Ventricular System

The ventricular system is located within the brain substance. It consists of four communicating compartments: two lateral ventricles and a third and a fourth ventricle (Figure 31-17). Each of the lateral ventricles is a cavity within the cerebral hemispheres that communicates with the third ventricle by an intraventricular foramen, the *foramen of Monro.* Each lateral ventricle has a body and the anterior (frontal), inferior (temporal), and posterior (occipital) horns.

The third ventricle is a thin, centrally located cavity surrounded by the thalamic structures. The third ventricle is connected to the fourth ventricle by a narrow channel, the *aqueduct of Sylvius,* which is located in the midbrain. The fourth ventricle is an angular cavity located posterior to the pons and medulla and anterior to the cerebellum; it extends to the central canal of the upper cervical cord. Three foramina connect the fourth ventricle with the subarachnoid spaces.

Cerebrospinal Fluid

Cerebrospinal fluid (CSF) is a clear, colorless liquid that contains small amounts of protein, glucose, and cells and a large amount of sodium chloride. CSF cushions the central nervous system against trauma,

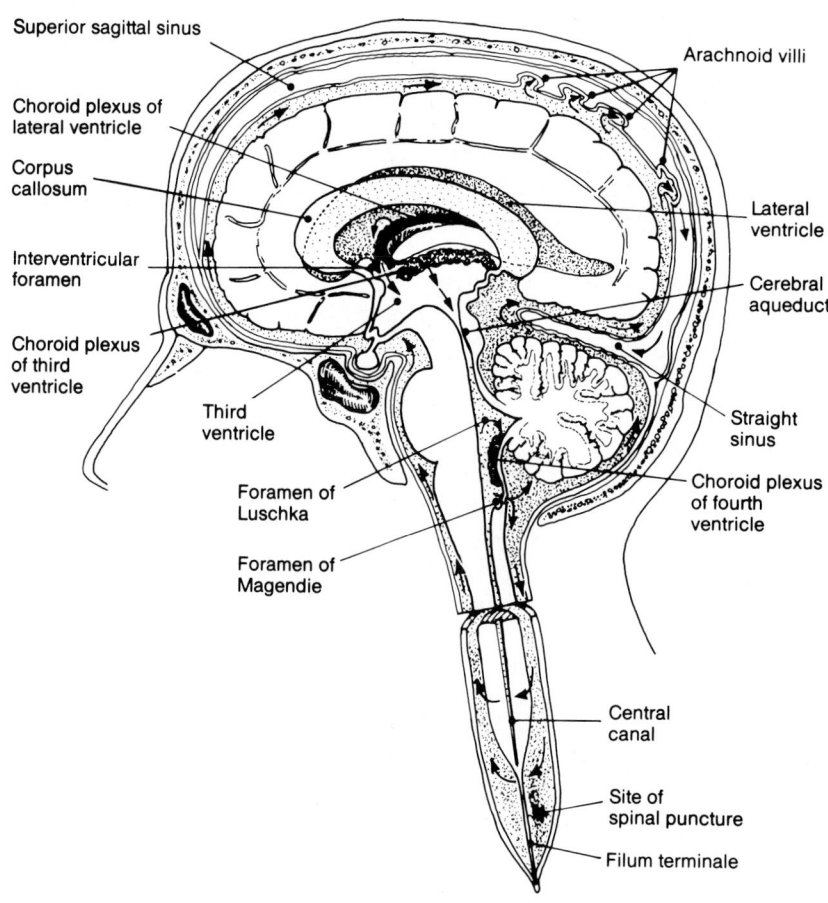

Superior sagittal sinus

Choroid plexus of lateral ventricle

Corpus callosum

Interventricular foramen

Choroid plexus of third ventricle

Third ventricle

Foramen of Luschka

Foramen of Magendie

Arachnoid villi

Lateral ventricle

Cerebral aqueduct

Straight sinus

Choroid plexus of fourth ventricle

Central canal

Site of spinal puncture

Filum terminale

Figure 31-17 Lateral view of the ventricular system. Arrows show direction of flow of CSF: choroid plexus of lateral ventricles to third ventricle, through cerebral aqueduct to fourth ventricle; into subarachnoid space via foramina of Luschka and Magendie; within spinal canal and over brain; and reabsorbed in arachnoid villi of subarachnoid space of brain.

From Langley, L. L., Telford, I. R., & Christensen, J. B. (1980). *Dynamic anatomy and physiology* (5th ed.). St. Louis: Mosby.

provides nutrition, removes waste products of neuronal metabolism, and assists in maintaining a relatively constant intracranial pressure. The pressure of the CSF at the lumbar cistern is 10 to 15 cmH_2O in the recumbent position or 0 to 10 mmHg in the cerebral ventricle.

CSF is formed principally in the lateral and third ventricles by a network of capillaries, the *choroid plexus*. Active transport mechanisms, the expenditure of energy, and osmotic pressure combine to produce about 500 to 600 ml of CSF per day. The CSF circulates from the lateral ventricles through the foramen of Monro into the third ventricle, through the aqueduct of Sylvius into the fourth ventricle, and into the cranial and spinal subarachnoid spaces, where it is returned to the venous system. The total volume of CSF in the ventricular system and the subarachnoid spaces at any given time is approximately 140 ml, of which less than half is in the ventricular system.

Brain Barrier System

The activity of the central nervous system is dependent upon the physical and chemical environment. The brain barrier system is a complex network of structures that provide a stable environment by regulating the transport of chemical substances between the plasma, the cerebrospinal fluid, and the brain. A barrier exists between the bloodstream and the brain, between the bloodstream and CSF, and between CSF and the brain. The barrier system includes the capillary endothelium, the pial-glial membrane, astrocytes, ependymal cells, the choroid plexus, and the arachnoid membrane.

Circulatory System

The metabolic demands of the central nervous system for oxygen and glucose are high in comparison with other body organs. The brain consumes approximately 20% of the total body oxygen requirement. The oxygen is used for the oxidation of glucose, which is the major source of energy. The constant delivery of oxygen and glucose via the bloodstream is maintained by a complex network of arteries.

Cerebral Circulation

The brain receives blood from the paired carotid and vertebral arteries, which fill from the aortic arch. The carotid arteries supply 80% of the total cerebral flow, and the vertebral arteries supply the remaining 20%. The internal carotid arteries supply the anterior and middle parts of the cerebral hemispheres. The vertebral arteries join to form the basilar artery. The vertebral-basilar arteries supply the posterior parts of the cerebral hemispheres, the brainstem, and the cerebellum. Blood flows from the internal carotid and vertebral-basilar arteries into a ring of anastomotic vessels, the *circle of Willis,* which is located at the base of the brain (Figure 31-18). The circle of Willis consists of an anterior communicating artery and paired anterior cerebral, internal carotid, posterior communicating, and posterior cerebral arteries. The posterior arteries are the major branches of the basilar artery.

Each cerebral artery supplies a specific region of the brain. The anterior cerebral arteries supply the medial surface of the frontal and parietal lobes. The middle cerebral arteries supply the lateral surfaces of the cerebral hemispheres and provide penetrating arteries to supply deeper structures such as the internal capsule, basal ganglia, and thalamic nuclei. The posterior cerebral arteries supply the medial and inferior surfaces of the occipital and temporal lobes.

The venous drainage of the brain consists of a network of fine veins which drain into superficial and deep veins. The superficial veins pass over the surface of the brain, pass through the subarachnoid space, and empty into the venous sinuses in the margins of the dura. The paired deep cerebral veins also drain into the venous sinuses. Blood then drains into the superior and inferior sagittal sinuses, into the cavernous sinuses, through the transverse sinuses, and into the internal jugular veins. The venous sinuses are usually distended and do not collapse. Cerebral veins and sinuses do not have valves.

The vascular system regulates the resistance of the arterioles so as to maintain a constant cerebral blood flow, regardless of the pressure in the systemic arteries. This property of maintaining constant flow is known as *autoregulation.* When systemic blood pressure drops or rises precipitously outside the range of 50 to 150 mmHg mean arterial pressure, autoregulation does not compensate and cerebral blood flow passively follows systemic pressure. Autoregulation functions poorly when intracranial pressure is ele-

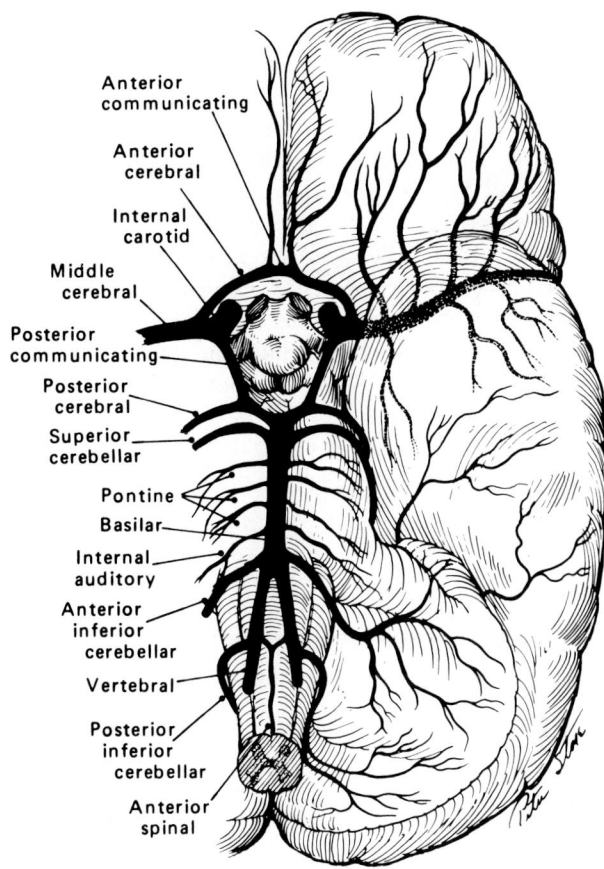

Figure 31-18 Arteries of the brain, seen from the base. The circle of Willis, at the center, joins branches of the basilar and internal carotid arteries. The vertebral arteries provide the main supply of blood to the spinal cord.

From Langley, L. L., Telford, I. R., & Christensen, J. B. (1980). *Dynamic anatomy and physiology* (5th ed.). St. Louis: Mosby.

vated beyond 25 to 30 mmHg. Physiological factors that alter cerebral blood flow, independent of systemic blood pressure, include the partial pressure of oxygen and carbon dioxide in the plasma. Marked hypoxemia (PaO_2 less than 60 mmHg) or hypercarbia ($PaCO_2$ more than 40 mmHg) increases cerebral blood flow through vasodilatation of cerebral arterioles.

Spinal Cord Circulation

The spinal cord receives its blood supply from descending branches of the vertebral arteries and multiple radicular arteries. The vertebral arteries give rise to the anterior spinal artery and the posterior spinal arteries. The radicular arteries enter the spinal canal through the intervertebral foramen and divide into anterior and posterior radicular arteries. The anterior spinal arteries join to form a single midline vessel, which is joined by anterior radicular arteries to supply the anterior and lateral parts of the spinal cord. The pair of posterior spinal arteries descends the posterior surface of the spinal cord and receives blood from the posterior radicular arteries to supply the posterior third of the spinal cord. The cervical cord segments are supplied primarily by branches of the vertebral arteries. The radicular arteries are the major source of blood supply to the thoracic and lumbar spinal cord segments.

A complex network of intradural and extradural veins provides for the venous return from the spinal cord. The distribution of the spinal veins is similar to that of the spinal arteries. Since the spinal veins have no valves, venous blood may flow directly into the systemic venous system.

BIBLIOGRAPHY

Gilman, S. (1992). *Manter and Gatz's essentials of clinical neuroanatomy and neurophysiology* (8th ed.). Philadelphia: Davis.

Kandel, E. R., & Schwartz, J. H. (Eds.). (1991). *Principles of neural science* (3rd ed.). New York: Elsevier.

Mitchell, P. H., Cammermeyer, M., Ozuna, J., et al. (1984). *Neurological assessment for nursing practice.* Englewood Cliffs, NJ: Reston.

Snell, R. S. (1992). *Clinical neuroanatomy for medical students* (3rd ed.). Boston: Little-Brown.

32

Neurological Data Acquisition

Pamela H. Mitchell

Data regarding the neurological status of critically ill patients are gathered for a variety of purposes. These purposes include:

1. Diagnosis of the disease producing the critical illness
2. Monitoring of psychophysiological status to detect change (improvement or worsening)
3. Determination of the patient's ability to participate in care and treatment regimens
4. Determination of the patient's capacity to respond to demands of the care environment

Data collected for purposes 1 and 2 are used to guide medical diagnosis and intervention. Data collected for purposes 2, 3, and 4 are used to guide nursing diagnosis and intervention. Because so many areas of critical care nursing practice and critical care medicine are collaborative, critical care nurses must understand the purposes of medical diagnostic procedures and be skillful in using the neurological history and examination data from both medical and nursing perspectives.

The medical history, neurological examination, and neurodiagnostic tests are directed toward diagnosing the underlying disease and monitoring change in the patient's pathophysiological state. Serial assessments by the critical care nurse contribute to the data used for the medical diagnosis and are crucial in monitoring change in pathophysiological states, particularly in early detection of deteriorating status. Additionally, the nursing history, interpretation of the physical examination, and monitoring assessments are used to determine the patient's ability to respond to the demands of the physical and psychosocial environment and to participate in the care and treatment regimen.

This chapter describes two major categories of data used directly or indirectly by critical care nurses in monitoring status and determining nursing therapies for persons critically ill with neurological disorders: (1) the history and physical assessment, which includes the patient interview and physical examination, and (2) diagnostic procedures, which include invasive and noninvasive radiological, electrophysiological, and biomechanical studies.

HISTORY AND PHYSICAL ASSESSMENT

The most common method of acquiring data about the patient's problem and its cause is direct interview and examination, with subsequent serial directed assessments that are compared to the baseline established at the initial examination. In neurological disorders, the presence or absence of change in symptoms and the pattern and rapidity of change are often crucial in establishing the correct medical diagnosis. For example, the physician's differentiation of an intracranial hemorrhage from an embolic stroke is based, in part, on the worsening course associated with hemorrhage versus the static course of a completed embolic stroke.

It is the physician's responsibility to perform the initial neurological examination to establish the baseline for medical diagnosis. It is neither necessary nor appropriate for the critical care nurse's examination to substitute for the medical examination. What is necessary is that the critical care nurse establish a baseline against which to measure change in neurological status for the purpose of monitoring status, evaluating changing ability to adapt to environment demands, and evaluating ability to participate in care.

Consequently, the most useful form of the examination for both physician and nurse is likely to be what is termed the *directed examination*—directed toward patients' presenting symptoms or toward detecting the most likely complications of the disorder. Such directed examination is different from the more comprehensive and detailed neurological examination outlined in physical assessment textbooks and commonly performed by neurologists and neurosurgeons when patients come to their offices or clinics.

The critical care nurse may employ a directed examination to detect such life-threatening changes in neurological status as those associated with potential brain herniation. Alternatively, a directed examination may be used to determine a patient's ability to tolerate environmental demands from such care activities as hygiene and position change and to determine the extent to which the patient can or should participate in care. In this section, attention is directed to the interpretation of findings related to nursing diagnosis and monitoring as well as to interpretation that contributes to medical diagnosis and the monitoring of pathophysiological states.

The medically focused neurological examination detects evidence of the location and nature of neurological disease through indirect evaluation of the *structures* of the nervous system: cerebral hemispheres (mental status), cranial nerves, motor system (including cerebellum), sensory system, and reflexes. The nursing-focused examination detects evidence of self-care deficit and ability to adapt physiologically to environmental demands by evaluating *functions* of the nervous system: consciousness, mentation, movement, sensation, and integrated regulation (see Chapter 31 for the structures that serve these functions). Because of the interdependence of medical and nursing diagnosis in the critical care setting, it is appropriate and efficient to organize the examination and record the findings according to the medical format—that of central nervous system structures. Both nursing diagnoses and collaborative problems can be identified from the data, regardless of whether they are gathered structurally or functionally (Table 32-1).

History

The history is the interview phase of data collection. The neurological focus is used to determine whether the presenting problem is related to a nervous system disorder and to detect neurological deficits coexisting with the primary problem that may influence care and recovery.

Because of the acute nature of many problems which precipitate admission to the critical care setting, it is common for the history to be obtained from a variety of data sources, including:

Ambulance or emergency medical technician (EMT) field notes and oral report
Physician's admission history and examination
Patient, if alert enough
Family or significant other
Old medical records if this is a readmission

If the patient was transported by ambulance or medical aid unit, the EMT notes provide valuable baselines of level of consciousness, movement, and basic vegetative functions (breathing, circulation) prior to arrival in the critical care or emergency setting. The initial physician's history should provide either brief or detailed data regarding the initial problem, rapidity of onset, precipitating and ameliorating factors, and course of symptoms. In addition, there will be at least a brief review of examination parameters: mental status, cranial nerves, motor and reflex status.

When such a physician's neurological history and notes are available, the critical care nurse need not repeat them but rather should proceed to interview the patient or family regarding aspects of neurological functioning that will form the database for nursing diagnosis: namely, how the presenting problem has affected the patient's ability to:

Breathe, maintain blood pressure, eliminate wastes (integrated regulation)
Remain aroused and alert, sleep normally (consciousness)
Follow directions, respond to confusing environments, think and solve problems (mentation)
Eat, swallow, move, care for self (movement)
See, hear, protect eyes and skin, appreciate pain (sensation)

If the situation is emergent or the patient's condition is rapidly deteriorating (or has the potential to do so), the history is deferred, and a directed monitoring examination is the first priority.

TABLE 32-1 **Comparison of Structural and Functional Approaches to Neurological Examination**

Structural	Level of Neuraxis	Functional
Purpose: to determine CNS location and nature of disease or pathophysiological state		Purpose: to determine alterations in ability to perform normal human functions and tolerate environmental demands
Mental status	Axis 1	Consciousness/mentation
Cranial nerves	Axis 2	Movement, sensation
Motor/cerebellar system	Axis 2, 3	Movement
Sensory system	Axis 1-3	Sensation
Reflexes	Axis 3, 4	(Included in movement/sensation)
	Axis 1-4	Integrated regulation

Neurological Examination

As indicated earlier, the initial and subsequent monitoring examinations are not the detailed, comprehensive neurological examination conducted in a clinic or office. Rather, the examination provides a baseline for evaluating change in neurological status and capacity for self-care. Therefore, only selected portions of the examination in each category are needed to detect predicted or unexpected changes in status. A moderately detailed neurological examination requires that a patient be able to follow directions. If the patient cannot, because of either confusion or decreased arousal, an approach must be used that evaluates reflex responses to stimuli, such as that described in Chapter 33 (section on brain herniation).

Consciousness/Mentation

This functional category assesses general behavior, level of consciousness, intellectual performance, affective behavior, and language.

General behavior is assessed by determining the appropriateness of gestures, facial expressions, attitudes toward self and others, and general appreciation of what is happening. In the intensive care setting, inappropriate responses may be related to medications, anxiety, and the sensory overload of the setting as well as to underlying neurological disease.

The level of consciousness comprises arousal and awareness. *Arousal* is determined by responsiveness to auditory, visual, or tactile stimuli. *Awareness* is reflected in orientation to self, environment, and others in the environment. It is tested by asking the patient who and where he or she is and the day and date or month and year. Operational definitions of levels of consciousness correspond to observable responses to verbal or painful stimuli:

Awake and alert: opens eyes spontaneously, follows commands, oriented to self, to environment, and to others in environment

Decreased arousal: may open eyes spontaneously or to stimuli; may follow commands; confused verbal responses

Obtunded: opens eyes only to stimuli; may follow commands; confused or inappropriate responses to verbal stimuli

Stupor: opens eyes to painful stimuli; appropriate motor responses to painful stimuli, confused or inappropriate verbal responses

Comatose: does not open eyes to painful stimuli; does not follow commands; no intelligible verbal response

The specific assessment for signs of brain herniation in patients with altered consciousness is discussed in Chapter 33.

Brainstem Function

Brainstem nuclei (collections of neurons) control a variety of functions essential to regulation of primary survival functions: breathing, circulation, and temperature control, for example. Important protective reflexes are mediated by brainstem nuclei and their sensory and motor cranial nerves. For example, airway protection is determined by the gag and swallow reflexes; eye protection is mediated by the corneal reflex (sensory cranial nerve V) and the blink reflex (motor output through cranial nerve VII). Finally, information about the functioning of the cranial nerves originating between the midbrain and the pons provides important information regarding impending brain herniation in patients with a decreased level of consciousness (see Chapter 33).

The cranial nerves that should be repetitively assessed include III, IV, VI (extraocular movements and pupillary reflex); VII (facial symmetry); and IX, X, and XII (gag, swallow). Others are repetitively assessed when the presenting problem or subsequent consequences suggest a problem with functions mediated by those nerves. Table 32-2 summarizes clinically practical tests for each of the cranial nerves and clinical problems that may be seen with abnormal findings.

The cranial nerves are peripheral nerves. Strictly speaking, cranial nerves I and II are not true nerves but rather fiber tracts of the brain itself. The true cranial nerves all arise from nuclei in the brainstem. The motor portion arises deep in the anterior brainstem in motor nuclei that are analogous to the anterior horn cells of the spinal cord. The sensory input from cranial nerves may synapse with sensory ganglia just outside the brainstem (for example, the geniculate ganglion of cranial nerve VII) or with sensory nuclei in the dorsal portion of the brainstem (cranial nerve V, for example).

The *olfactory nerve* (cranial nerve I) serves the sense of smell. *Anosmia* is the absence of the sensation of smell, and *hyposmia* is a decrease in sensitivity to smell. Decreased smell is usually associated with nasal disorders rather than neurological problems. However, a tumor, meningitis, subarachnoid hemorrhage, or head injury can disrupt or destroy the olfactory nerve endings and thus impair smell. Hallucinations of smell may indicate lesions of the temporal lobe, where olfactory stimuli are interpreted.

The sense of smell is tested by having the patient close the eyes and occlude one nostril, then the other, and identify the scent while the examiner passes aromatic substances under the nose. Commonly used scents include coffee, cinnamon, and vanilla. Irritative substances, such as ammonia or oil of peppermint, test the response of cranial nerve V rather than cranial nerve I.

Functional problems associated with anosmia include inability to detect, by smell, warnings of environmental danger such as fire or gas leak. Pleasure in eating may be diminished because the olfactory contribution to the taste of food is lost.

The *optic nerve* (cranial nerve II) carries impulses from the retina to the optic chiasm. From here the impulses go to areas in the cerebral cortex where visual images are recognized and interpreted. Lesions causing disorders can occur anywhere from the eyeball to the occipital cortex. Two aspects of vision are commonly tested: visual acuity and visual fields. In addition, an ophthalmoscope is used to examine the retina, optic disk, vessels, and macula.

Visual acuity is easily tested in the critical care unit with a newspaper or magazine. The patient, wearing

TABLE 32-2   Clinically Practical Methods of Testing Cranial Nerve Functions and Interpretation of Problems Associated with Dysfunctions

Cranial Nerve	Function	Tested by	Interpretation of Abnormal Function
I Olfactory	Senses smells	Aromatic substance (coffee, soap), not irritants (ammonia, oil of peppermint)	*Disease:* Sphenoid ridge tumors, shearing trauma after head injury, meningeal inflammation *Functional effects:* Decreased appreciation of taste; safety hazard (cannot smell smoke, escaping gas, etc.)
II Optic	Sees	Acuity: pocket Snellen, size of headline patient can read Optic disk: fundoscopy Fields: confrontation	*Disease:* Optic nerve damage, increased intracranial pressure, field cuts indicate damage from optic radiation *Functional effects:* Safety hazard with decreased acuity, field cuts, cannot appreciate objects at sides of field; may confuse environmental cues
III Oculomotor	Moves eyes medially and up and down; constricts pupil	Extraocular movements, pupillary size and equality and symmetry of response to light shined in eyes	*Disease:* Unilateral pupillary change indicates uncal herniation; ptosis may indicate herniation, primary brainstem disorder, Horner's syndrome, or myasthenia gravis *Functional effect:* Diplopia
IV Trochlear	Moves eyes down and in	Tested with III and VI	*Disease:* Paralysis of superior oblique muscle alone indicates lesion in brainstem nucleus *Functional effect:* Diplopia on upward gaze
V Trigeminal	Sensation for face, scalp, cornea, and nasal and oral cavities; moves jaw	Ability to sense pinprick and cotton wisp over face; ability to clench teeth together	*Disease:* Tumor of cerebellopontine angle or acoustic neuroma, tetanus, myasthenia gravis; ALS *Functional effects:* Potential for corneal abrasion; difficulty with chewing
VI Abducens	Moves eyes medially	Tested with III and IV	*Disease:* Isolated sixth nerve paralysis associated with diabetic neuropathy, aneurysms *Functional effect:* Diplopia on medial gaze

TABLE 32-2   **Clinically Practical Methods of Testing Cranial Nerve Functions and Interpretation of Problems Associated with Dysfunctions—cont'd**

Cranial Nerve	Function	Tested by	Interpretation of Abnormal Function
VII Facial	Controls facial expression, also tastes (anterior two thirds of tongue)	Ability to smile, frown, close eyes tightly; distinguish flavors—salt, sweet, sour, and bitter (front of tongue)	*Disease:* Paralysis of entire half of face indicates lesion in brainstem nucleus or peripheral nerve; weakness or paralysis of lower half of face indicates lesion in motor cortex *Functional effects:* Embarrassment over asymmetric facial appearance; some loss of clarity of speech sounds formed with lips; potential for corneal abrasion due to inability to close eye; loss of enjoyment of eating due to diminished taste
VIII Acoustic	Hears; maintains equilibrium	Ability to detect sounds in each ear; oculocephalic reflex in unconscious patients	*Disease:* Neural deafness; loss of oculocephalic reflex indicates loss of brainstem function between VIII and III, IV, VI *Functional effects:* Difficulty interpreting auditory environment; vertigo and nausea if vestibular function impaired
IX, X Glossopharyngeal, vagus	Controls gag and swallow reflexes, visceral regulation, palatal articulation	Palatal elevation, swallow and gag reflexes, glottal and palatal sounds—tested as unit	*Disease:* Brainstem lesions at level of medulla; peripheral lesions along course of nerves or muscle supplied by them *Functional effects:* Choking, aspiration, change in phonation (hoarseness) dysarthria
XI Spinal accessory	Shrugs shoulders, turns head	Ability to shrug shoulders, turn head against resistance	*Disease:* Supranuclear lesions from stroke, dystonias; brainstem lesions in syringomyelia; basal skull fracture, meningitis may affect the peripheral portion *Functional effects:* Pain, fatigue and deformity from hypertrophy of sternocleidomastoid; difficulty maintaining head posture with paralysis
XII Hypoglossal	Moves tongue; tastes (posterior third of tongue)	Ability to protrude tongue, push tongue against cheek; lingual sounds	*Disease:* Motor neuron disease creates wasting, cortical lesions cause spasticity *Functional effects:* Bilateral disorders—dysarthria affecting labial and lingual sounds; dysphagia due to difficulty moving bolus of food

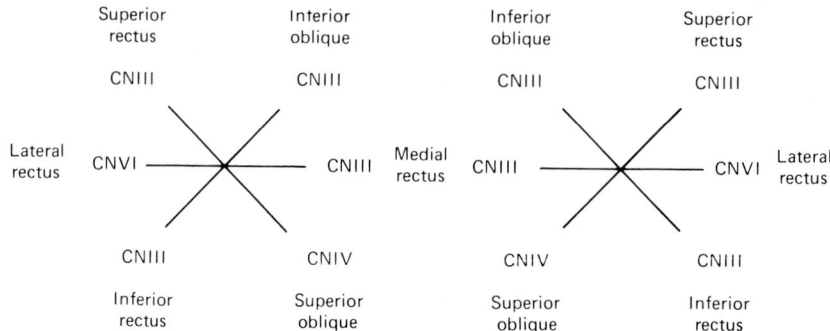

Figure 32-1   Cardinal positions of gaze with corresponding cranial nerves and muscles.

glasses if they are normally worn, is asked to read with one eye at a time, covering the other with a patch. It is important first to determine a patient's ability or lack of ability to read, since this will affect not only the test but the patient's ability to participate fully in the program of treatment. For example, instructions regarding activities or consent forms for procedures may be given to the patient to read. Certain cerebral disorders such as a cerebrovascular accident also may alter the ability to read and/or to interpret written items.

Visual field testing, when done in the unit, uses the confrontation method. Each eye is evaluated separately as the examiner stands an arm's length from the patient. The patient is asked to close (cover with the hand) the right eye and look with the left eye at the examiner's nose. A wiggling finger is steadily brought in from the periphery until the patient sees it. The finger should be an equal distance between the examiner and the patient except when approaching temporally, when the examiner must start behind the patient. This maneuver is performed for all quadrants and then repeated with the other eye. If a defect is found, the configuration is determined by retesting and sketching the defect. Normally, the patient will see an object 60° nasally, 50° upward, 90° temporally, and 70° downward.

The *oculomotor* (cranial nerve III), *trochlear* (cranial nerve IV), and *abducens* (cranial nerve VI) nerves have similar functions and are usually examined together. These three cranial nerves act together in controlling the ocular muscles to ensure that the eyes remain parallel through all movements. In addition, the oculomotor nerve controls the muscle that elevates the upper lid and innervates the constrictor muscle of the pupil. A lesion of these nerves may produce diplopia (double vision) because of weakness of the ocular muscles and deviation of the eyeball from a parallel position. Ptosis of the eyelid and sustained pupillary dilatation indicate possible problems with the oculomotor nerve. Before testing, inspect the po-

sition of the upper eyelids with the patient gazing directly at you. Observe for ptosis and for any lower lid sagging, which may indicate weakness of the orbicularis oculi muscle.

To evaluate extraocular movements, ask the patient to follow your finger through the six cardinal positions of gaze (Figure 32-1). Pause during lateral and upward gaze to observe for nystagmus. Also observe for any deviation from normal conjugate movements and for the relation of the upper lid to the eye globe. The upper lid normally overlaps the iris slightly as the gaze moves upward from the downward position. This overlapping may not occur if the patient has hyperthyroidism.

The pupils are evaluated for size, equality, and the pupillary light reflex. Shine a light directly into one pupil and observe for constriction. This is called the *direct light response*. Again shine a light in one pupil and observe the response in the other pupil. This is called the *consensual light response*. Failure of pupillary response to light is an important sign of possible oculomotor lesions. Test accommodation and convergence by having the patient focus at a distance and then follow your finger as you bring it in toward the patient's nose. Note convergence of the eyes and the pupillary constriction as the pupil accommodates. Loss of the accommodation-convergence reflex may result from a lesion of cranial nerve III (oculomotor).

The ophthalmoscopic examination, not an easy task, is undertaken to add to the store of knowledge about the critically ill patient. It is not a routine part of the nursing examination. This examination should be conducted in a darkened room. The technique of using the examiner's right hand and right eye to test the patient's right eye and the examiner's left hand and left eye for the patient's left eye should be observed. The ophthalmoscope should be set at the diopter setting best suited to the examiner's needs. A setting of zero diopters is neutral (it does not converge or diverge light rays). A plus diopter (black numbers) setting is used for a farsighted patient and a minus diopter (red numbers) for the nearsighted patient. The procedure is as follows:

Place your thumb on the patient's brow and have the patient focus on a spot at a distance somewhere over your shoulder. Approach gradually from a distance of about 15 inches and a position 15° lateral to the patient's direct line of vision. Shine the light on the pupil, noting the red reflex and any lens opacities. Move in until you are touching the thumb of your opposite hand (which is on the patient's brow) with the ophthalmoscope. You should now be viewing the optic disk, which is a red-orange, smooth, round or vertically oval structure. If the disk is not yet in view, follow a blood vessel until you locate it. Observe the disk for color, shape, margin clarity, and the physiological cup (a bright area in the center of the disk). Note the disk/physiological cup ratio; also observe any pigmented rings or crescents around the disk. Observe the vessels for distribution in all four quadrants. Follow the vessels from the disk to the margin of the fundus, observing for occlusion, arteriolar or venous nicking, and abnormal size. Veins are normally larger and darker and pulsate; arterioles are smaller and brighter and do not pulsate (Figure 32-2). Examine the general background, noting pigmentation appropriate to individual coloring (the darker the skin, the darker the fundus). Observe also for hemorrhages, "cotton wool" patches, exudates, and retinal edema. Now evaluate the macula and the fovea with the patient looking directly into the light. The macula is two to three disk diameters temporally from the disk, and the fovea is in the center of the macula (see Figure 32-2).

The most important abnormalities which are found on fundoscopic examination are hyperemic (pinker) disks, disk atrophy (pale with blurred edges), or papilledema (choked or swollen disk). The first signs of papilledema may be the absence of retinal vein pulsation or enlargement and an increase in the

size of retinal veins as compared with the arterioles. Abnormal arteries may be thickened and pulsating. Optic atrophy may be related to diseases that affect the optic nerve, such as syphilis. Papilledema, which is secondary to fairly long-standing increased intracranial pressure, may also cause optic atrophy.

Changes in visual acuity, the appearance of the optic disk, or eye movements can be indicators of expanding brain mass, as discussed in detail in Chapter 33. In addition, patients who have less emergent changes in visual acuity or eye movement may experience a number of functional problems associated with these abnormal findings.

Loss of visual acuity for either near or far distance is common, particularly as people age. Patients who are used to wearing glasses for distance may become disoriented in the intensive care unit when they cannot see clearly what is happening. Similarly, patients with dysfunction of cranial nerves III or IV may experience diplopia. The functional consequence of diplopia may be nausea or a predisposition to sensory deprivation and disorientation.

The *trigeminal nerve* (cranial nerve V) mediates general sensation, including perception of pain, temperature, and touch for the entire face (except the angle of the jaw) and for the scalp to the vertex. It also mediates sensation for the cornea, the mucous membranes of the paranasal sinuses, and the nasal and oral cavities. The sensory divisions are the ophthalmic, the maxillary, and the mandibular. The motor portion of the nerve controls the jaw reflex and the muscles of mastication.

The trigeminal nerve is tested by determining the patient's ability to perceive pain (pinprick) and touch (cotton wisp) over the face and anterior scalp. The oral and nasal cavities are tested only if there is reason to expect problems with this nerve. The corneal reflex is tested by having the patient look up and straight ahead while the examiner approaches from the side with a fine wisp of cotton. The examiner touches the cornea lightly, avoiding the eyelashes. A less invasive way to test the ophthalmic portion of the nerve is the *lash test*. The patient's eyes may be closed or open. The examiner gently touches the eyelashes. A blink indicates that the eye protective reflex is present.

The motor portion is tested by having the patient clench the teeth while the examiner palpates the temporal and masseter muscles. The muscles should be symmetric and the examiner should not be able to open the patient's clenched jaw.

Dysfunction of the trigeminal nerve is most commonly caused by a tumor at the cerebellopontine angle, often an acoustic neuroma. Loss of the corneal reflex may indicate primary brainstem damage or brainstem compression due to brain herniation.

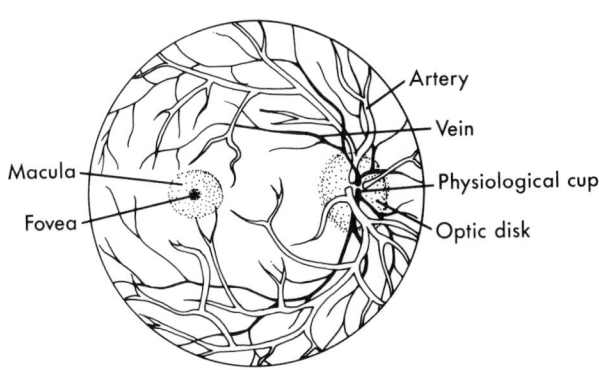

Figure 32-2　Optic disk, macula, and retinal vessels as viewed through an ophthalmoscope.

Weakness of the jaw musculature may be due to primary neuromuscular junction disease (tetanus, botulism, myasthenia gravis) or motor neuron disease (amyotrophic lateral sclerosis).

Functional problems associated with loss of sensation to the cornea include a potential for corneal abrasion. Loss of sensation from the maxillary and mandibular divisions (local dental anesthesia is an example of a temporary loss of sensation from peripheral branches of these divisions) may produce a potential for injury to the mucous membranes of the cheek or to the tongue. Difficulty in chewing results from damage to the motor portion of the nerve.

The *facial nerve* (cranial nerve VII) innervates all the muscles of facial expression. The sensory portion mediates taste from the anterior two thirds of the tongue and carries fibers that innervate the lacrimal, submaxillary, and sublingual glands. The motor portion is tested by having the patient look up and wrinkle the forehead (frontalis muscle); close the eyes tightly and resist the examiner's efforts to open them (orbicularis orbis muscle); and smile, whistle, and show the teeth (lower face muscles). Facial asymmetry at rest should be noted.

The sensory portion of this nerve is rarely tested as a routine part of the nursing examination. The neurologist's record of the initial examination will indicate whether the patient had presenting symptoms suggesting dysfunction of cranial nerve VII. Change in this initial symptom can be tested by having the patient protrude the tongue while the examiner touches each side with a moist applicator dipped in one of four test substances: salt, sugar, sour, or bitter. The tongue should not be withdrawn into the mouth until the substance is identified.

Facial paralysis may be due to lesions of any part of the nerve or cranial nerve nuclei. True cranial nerve facial paralysis is referred to as *peripheral* facial paralysis. Paralysis includes both the forehead and lower facial muscles. The facial "droop" following a lesion of the cerebral motor cortex involves only the lower face; it does not affect forehead wrinkling and eye closure. Tumors of the cerebellopontine angle are a common cause of progressive or permanent peripheral facial paralysis. Permanent paralysis may also be seen after removal of large acoustic neuromas (cranial nerve VIII) that also wrap around cranial nerve VII.

Functional problems associated with dysfunction of cranial nerve VII include difficulty in speaking clearly due to inability to move the lips symmetrically, and a potential for eye injury due to incomplete closure of the eyelids. In addition, the patient may find the facial appearance embarrassing.

The *acoustic nerve* (cranial nerve VIII) has two divisions: the *cochlear,* which mediates hearing, and the *vestibular,* which controls balance, position, and spatial orientation.

To test the cochlear portion the examiner whispers or rubs two fingers together next to each ear and determines what the patient heard. Alternatively, a vibrating tuning fork may be held next to each ear.

If there are hearing losses, the physician may use Weber's and Rinne's tests to determine whether the loss is due to physical sound conduction or neural causes. *Weber's test* involves placing a vibrating tuning fork on the vertex of the skull and asking the patient whether the sound is heard equally in both ears or more to one side or the other. Equal perception is normal. Sensorineural loss in one ear will cause the sound to be perceived better in the other ear. Conversely, if there is a conduction defect (wax, fluid, or middle ear disorder), the sound will be perceived as loudest on the side of the impaired conduction. In *Rinne's test,* a vibrating tuning fork is held on the mastoid process behind one ear. When the patient indicates that the sound is no longer heard, the tuning fork is held directly beside the ear. The sound should still be heard beside the ear, since air conducts sound waves longer than bone. The normal air/bone conduction ratio is approximately 2:1. Sensorineural hearing loss impairs both air and bone conduction, whereas conduction defects impair only the ability to detect sound conducted through the air.

The vestibular portion of the acoustic nerve is tested in nonemergent situations by the physician if the patient has a history of vertigo or ataxia. The *cold caloric test* is used for this determination, if indicated. The patient is placed in the supine position, with the head tilted forward 30°. The examiner inspects the ear otoscopically to ascertain that the eardrum is intact and then introduces 5 to 10 ml of ice water into the ear canal. The normal reaction in the conscious patient is nystagmus, with the quick component to the side opposite the stimulated ear. Vertigo, nausea, and vomiting are common reactions in the conscious patient.

In the critical care setting, the vestibular portion of the acoustic nerve is stimulated in the unconscious patient to determine the intactness of brainstem pathways between the vestibular and ocular cranial nerves. Either the oculocephalic reflex or the oculovestibular reflex may be used to stimulate the vestibular nerve.

The *oculocephalic reflex,* commonly referred to as the "doll's head" or "doll's eye" maneuver, is mediated afferently by the vestibular portion of cranial nerve VIII and efferently by cranial nerves III and VI. The reflex is tested by rapidly rotating the patient's head to one side and observing the eye movements (Figure 32-3). If the reflex is intact ("doll's eyes" pres-

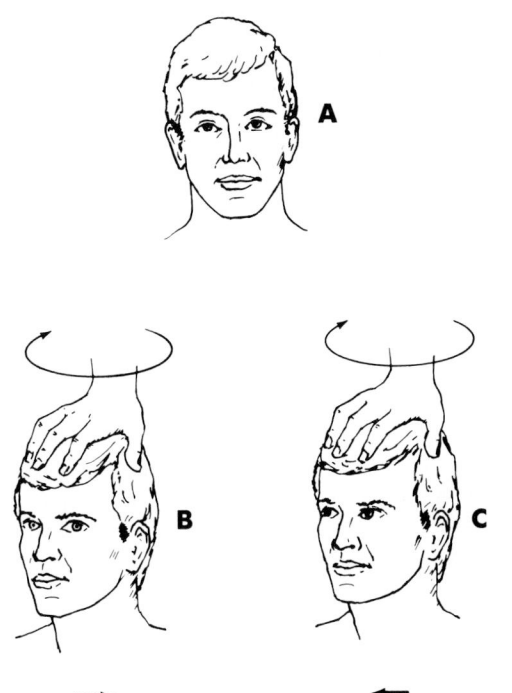

Figure 32-3 Oculocephalic reflex. *A,* Moving the unconscious patient's head to the right moves the eyes initially to the left if the reflex is present *(B).* If the reflex is absent *(C),* eyes will move to the right along with the head.

ent), the eyes appear to remain in the initial position and then slowly turn to the direction in which the head was rotated. If the reflex is not intact ("doll's eyes" absent), the eyes will move with the head as though fixed in place. The reflex is present in all persons with intact brainstems during sleep. It cannot be elicited in the awake person because conscious fixation of the eyes overcomes the reflex. In altered consciousness the presence of the reflex indicates that the brainstem function is intact between cranial nerves VIII and III.

The *oculovestibular reflex* is mediated by the same set of cranial nerves. This reflex is tested as described earlier (cold caloric test) with either warm or cold water in the ear canal. The oculovestibular reflex is preserved somewhat longer than the oculocephalic in brain dysfunction. Therefore, when the oculocephalic reflex is lost, the physician may wish to perform caloric stimulation to determine whether any function remains in the reflex pathway.

As described in Chapter 33, loss or change in these reflexes is an important indicator of brain herniation. From a functional perspective, loss of either the oculocephalic or the oculovestibular reflex suggests that cranial nerve function may be lost one level below as well. It should therefore be assumed that the patient does not have adequate function of cranial nerves IX and X and thus the airway is not protected through the gag and cough reflexes.

The *glossopharyngeal* and *vagus nerves* (cranial nerves IX and X) are usually considered together. The glossopharyngeal mediates taste from the posterior third of the tongue, innervates the carotid sinus and the carotid body, and supplies general sensation to tonsillar and pharyngeal mucous membranes. The vagus nerve innervates all thoracic and abdominal visceral organs, the larynx, the pharynx, and the palate and conveys numerous sensory impulses from the walls of the digestive tract, heart, and lungs.

Clinically testable functions include the gag reflex, swallowing, and the sensation of taste. Pharyngeal function is tested by having the patient say "aah" and watching the soft palate and uvula. The soft palate should rise symmetrically and promptly. The gag reflex is tested by touching the posterior wall of the soft palate. The soft palate should contract and the uvula retract simultaneously. Swallowing is tested by giving the alert patient ice chips or water to swallow. If consciousness is impaired, the neck over the larynx is stroked to stimulate reflex swallowing of secretions. If the gag reflex is impaired in an unconscious patient, it should be assumed that swallowing is also abnormal.

The *spinal accessory nerve* (cranial nerve XI) supplies the sternocleidomastoid muscle and the upper part of the trapezius muscle. The muscles are examined for atrophy. Strength is tested by having the patient shrug the shoulders against the examiner's resistance (trapezius) and turn the head to each side against resistance (sternocleidomastoid). The most common cause of sternocleidomastoid weakness is trauma to the neck. Weakness of this muscle may make it difficult for the patient to support the head unaided.

The *hypoglossal nerve* (cranial nerve XII) innervates the tongue musculature. It is tested by inspecting the tongue for fasciculations (fine tremors), wasting, and lack of power or mobility. The examiner observes the patient's protruded tongue for deviation and wasting. Fasciculations are best observed when the tongue is resting inside the mouth. Strength is examined by having the patient alternately push the tongue against each cheek, against the resistance of the examiner's finger. Bilateral weakness of the tongue (or paralysis) may occur in amyotrophic lateral sclerosis and in myasthenia gravis. Unilateral weakness may be associated with neck trauma, extensive neck surgery, or brainstem lesions (tumors or stroke). Difficulty in speaking clearly or in manipulating food in the mouth and swallowing may be a functional outcome of tongue weakness.

Motor Function

The motor system includes those components of the nervous system concerned with the initiation, maintenance, and control of movements of the body. Skeletal abnormalities, joint swelling or pain, a decreased range of motion, and disturbances in posture and balance are sought, and strength and mass of specific muscle groups are evaluated. The abbreviated motor examination used in detecting brain herniation is described in Chapter 33.

Functional outcomes of motor system dysfunction depend upon whether the neurological lesion is at the suprasegmental, segmental, or myoneural junction level of the motor system. Terms commonly used to describe lesions of the suprasegmental level are *upper motor neuron lesion, corticobulbar lesion, corticospinal lesion, pyramidal lesion,* and *long tract lesion.* Terms used to describe the segmental level are *lower motor neuron lesion, final common pathway lesion, anterior horn cell lesion,* and *ventral horn cell lesion.* The myoneural junction is the end point of the motor segment and is included here because the functional outcome of dysfunction at this level is somewhat different from that for the spinal or peripheral portion of the motor segment. Differing functional effects of lesions at the three levels are shown in Table 32-3.

Examination of motor function includes determination of muscle strength and mass, including symmetry of strength, tone, presence of involuntary movements, coordination, gait, and balance. Gait and balance cannot be tested in the patient confined to bed; only limited aspects of coordination can be tested

in such a patient. Patients with altered consciousness may be examined primarily in terms of response to simple stimuli, and only the most gross motor function can be tested.

In the alert patient who is able to follow directions, assessment of strength and mass begins with inspection of the major muscle groups of the arms, legs, and trunk for any differences in size. If differences in mass are seen or suspected, the limb girth should be measured. Reduced size of one limb may indicate segmental motor function loss.

Strength is tested on a scale of 0 to 5, defined as follows:

0 No muscle contraction
1 Flicker or trace of voluntary muscle contraction
2 Active movement with gravity eliminated
3 Active movement against gravity but not against resistance
4 Active movement against gravity and resistance but not full strength
5 Full power against examiner's resistance

Examination of the strength of the upper extremities proceeds systematically along major muscle groups, from the proximal to the distal. A number of the maneuvers used to test strength are described below.

The deltoid and trapezius (abduction strength in the shoulder) are tested by having the patient push the upper arm against resistance. The biceps are tested by having the patient flex the forearm against the upper arm and resist the examiner's attempt to straighten the elbow. Wrist flexion and extension

TABLE 32-3 **Clinical Signs of Disrupted Motor Function at Three Levels of the Nervous System**

Level	Clinical Signs	Examples of Causative Disorders
Suprasegmental	Weakness or paralysis of voluntary movement Increased muscle stretch reflexes; reflex arc intact (after "spinal shock") Some muscle atrophy secondary to disuse EMG normal	Spinal cord lesions such as trauma, infarct, tumor, and hemorrhage
Segmental	Weakness or paralysis of voluntary movement Decreased or absent muscle stretch reflexes (reflex arc disrupted) Marked muscle atrophy secondary to denervation (↓ trophic factors) EMG changes: fibrillation, giant polyphasic action potentials (denervation supersensitivity)	Brainstem lesions affecting cranial nuclei: tumors, infarct, hemorrhage Cerebellopontine angle tumors compressing cranial nerves Polyneuropathies such as Guillain-Barré syndrome, alcoholic polyneuropathy, diphtheritic polyneuropathy, and toxic chemical polyneuropathy
Myoneural junction	Weakness or paralysis of voluntary movement Muscle stretch reflexes intact No muscle atrophy EMG diminished: muscle able to contract when directly stimulated. Pattern of ↓ contraction varies with disorder	Chronic: myasthenia gravis (may have acute episodes of life-threatening myasthenic or cholinergic crisis); Eaton-Lambert syndrome (myasthenic symptoms associated with carcinoma) Acute: botulism, curare, succinylcholine, "nerve gas," organophosphate insecticides

(flexor and extensor carpus radialis and carpus ulnaris) are tested by having the patient alternately flex and extend the wrist against resistance.

General strength of the proximal arm muscles is tested by having the patient close the eyes and hold both arms out, palms up. The examiner observes for downward drifting of either arm and pronation of the hand. The appearance of either is termed *pronator drift* and indicates a problem in the suprasegmental motor system. The *new* appearance of the sign in a patient with a potentially expanding lesion in the brain indicates brain shift or compression. Patients with old hemiparesis from stroke, neurosurgery, or old head injuries may demonstrate pronator drift as a continuing sign of residual neurological deficit.

The intrinsic muscles of the hands are screened by testing finger strength and grip. Abduction of the fingers is tested by having the patient spread the fingers and thumbs and resist the examiner's attempt to push the fingers together. Grip is tested by having the patient hold the first two fingers of the examiner's hands while the examiner attempts to pull away. Both maneuvers test the function of the intrinsic muscles and the three nerves serving the hands (the ulnar, radial, and medial nerves). If weakness exists, the physician may wish to test the muscles individually. Nurses in specialized or expanded roles that require such testing should consult one of the neurological examination textbooks in the references for the technique.

Trunk strength is difficult to assess directly, as the major truncal muscles are those assisting respiration. However, the examiner can note whether a sitting patient is able to maintain the erect posture. Maintaining sitting posture is a function of the strength of the paraspinal muscles. Rising to a sitting position is a function of the strength of the abdominal muscles.

The lower extremities are evaluated in the following manner: Have the supine patient raise first one knee and then the other and resist your attempts to push the knee to the chest. This action tests the iliopsoas muscle. Have the patient extend the legs and resist your attempts to flex the knee. This tests the quadriceps. Have the patient flex the knee and resist your attempts to extend it. This tests the hamstring muscles. Have the patient dorsiflex the foot and resist your attempts to overcome the flexion. This tests the tibialis anterior muscle. Have the patient hold the knees tightly together while you attempt to open them. This tests the thigh abductor muscles. Have the patient hold the knees apart while you attempt to push them together. This tests the gluteus minimus and medius muscles. Have the patient stand on the toes. This tests flexion of the foot, while standing on the heels tests extension of the foot.

Muscle tone is tested by passively putting a limb through full range of motion. *Tone* refers to the re-

sistance detected by the examiner. Reduced tone may be caused by diseases of the cerebellum and by lower motor neuron diseases; since normal resistance is slight, decreased tone may be difficult to detect. Increased tone is much easier to detect and is classified as spastic, resulting from upper motor neuron lesions, or rigid, as in lesions of the basal ganglia. *Spasticity* affects certain muscle groups differently. For example, with upper motor neuron lesions, the flexors in the arms and extensors in the legs are most affected. These are the antigravity muscles where most muscle spindles are located. *Rigidity,* as in Parkinson's disease, is demonstrated in the heightened tone of all flexor muscles, resulting in flexed posture.

The most common involuntary movement is the rhythmic movement known as *tremors.* Tremors resulting from diseases affecting the basal ganglia, such as Parkinson's, exist during relaxation and are called *rest tremors.* Tremors associated with cerebellar diseases are characteristically seen when the patient attempts to perform an activity.

Chorea is another type of involuntary movement and is characterized by rapid, jerky, irregular, and purposeless contractions of random muscle groups followed by immediate relaxation. The basal ganglia are affected. The best-known choreas are Huntington's and Sydenham's.

Disturbances in *coordination* can be indicative of cerebellar disorders. The following activities are useful in detecting a lack of coordination:

Have the patient pat the knee rapidly, alternating the back of the hand with the palm. Have the patient rapidly pat one hand against the palm of the other hand. Have the patient rhythmically touch the tip of the nose with the index finger with the eyes open, then closed. In cerebellar disease, the movements in these tests are slowed and nonrhythmic and may "hang." With hemiplegia, movements are just slow and stiff.

Have the patient quickly and consecutively touch the tip of the thumb to each finger of the same hand. These movements are slowed and inaccurate in cerebellar disease, whereas in certain movement disorders, such as Parkinson's disease, the movement is slowed and loses the amplitude of tapping.

Have the patient quickly and smoothly move the finger back and forth between the nose and the examiner's finger. With cerebellar disease, the hand deviates and may miss the target.

The only test of lower extremity coordination that can be performed by the bedridden patient is the heel-to-shin test. Have the patient run the heel of one foot down the shin of the other leg in a straight line while not looking. Cerebellar disease will cause irregular deviations of the heel to either side.

Since standing and walking properly require adequate muscle strength, coordination, proprioception, vestibular function, and vision, gait and stance may well have been implicitly included in the evaluation of these functions. The observation of simple walking reveals much; for example, in hemiparesis the normal rhythmic arm swinging is reduced on the side of the hemiplegia.

Gait is evaluated by having the patient walk heel to toe down a straight line and walk briskly around a chair. Cerebellar disorders cause the patient to walk with a wide base and to stagger or reel laterally. Hemiplegia causes circumduction of the leg, with a stiff knee and extended ankle, while a bilateral spastic paresis of the leg produces scissoring of the knees.

If any difficulty with coordination or gait has been noted, *Romberg's test* should be performed. This test differentiates cerebellar from sensory ataxia. The patient stands with feet close together and eyes first open, then closed. Increased swaying and falling occurs with closed but not open eyes in persons with an impairment of proprioception. Cerebellar disease may result in swaying but not falling with the eyes open or closed, and in unilateral vestibular disorders, the patient tends to fall to the ipsilateral side.

Sensory Function

The sensory system conveys information to the central nervous system about the status of the body surface and its surrounding environment, about the position of the body and its extremities in space, and about the status of the internal organs. When evaluating the sensory system, great care must be taken to listen carefully and record accurately the patient's reporting, because sensory interpretation is extremely subjective. The patient's responses to touch and pain, temperature sensation, proprioceptive (motion and position) sensation, vibratory sensation, and cortical sensory functions are elicited on the examination. Specific patterns of sensory loss result from specific lesions; therefore, the sensory loss demonstrated may be highly diagnostic.

Superficial pain is tested by lightly pinpricking over the body in a symmetrical fashion. Particular attention should be paid to any suspected or stated area of sensory loss or deficit such as numbness or tingling. When in doubt about the reliability of the response, alternate the sharp point with the dull end of the pin. The dull end acts as a control; it does not test pain perception. If decreased sensation is found, determine the margins of the suspect area. When making a survey of the body in the absence of problems, be sure to compare each side with the other.

Deep pain is tested by squeezing the Achilles tendon, squeezing the calf muscles, and/or applying firm pressure on the sternum. Deep and superficial pain are carried in the same central pathways, and there-

fore, lesions affecting one response will usually affect the other.

Temperature perception pathways are closely related to those for pain and usually do not need testing if pain perception is normal. Always test the temperature response if there is any impairment of pain perception. Test tubes filled with hot and cold water are used, applying them alternately over the body and asking the patient to distinguish between them.

Touch is evaluated by using a cotton wisp or a soft brush and stroking corresponding parts of the entire body. Ask the patient to respond when touch is perceived. Touch is usually intact, even with severe involvement of sensory areas, because of the many multiple pathways. If defects are found, however, determine the area of loss by defining margins. Drag the cotton wisp over the area of decreased sensation until margins of sensation can be defined; then record your findings.

Proprioception, or *motion and position sense*, is tested in every extremity by using passive motion and asking the patient to identify the position with eyes shut. Have the patient state when the movement begins and whether the extremity is up or down or how it is pointed. Position sense is best tested on the thumbs, fingers, and toes. Position sense is always lost distally first in organic lesions; so if perception is intact in the distal extremities, there is generally no need to test the more proximal portions.

Vibratory sense is tested by placing a vibrating tuning fork against any bony prominence of each extremity—ankle, toe, thumb, or wrist—and asking the patient to tell you when the vibration stops. As with position sense, vibratory perception is initially lost distally.

Cortical sensory perception can occur only if the higher cerebral centers of integration, those beyond the thalamus, are intact. The primary sensory modalities are evaluated first in order to be sure they are intact. For example, a peripheral nerve injury affecting the hand would alter perception of objects placed in the hand but not necessarily indicate a cortical deficit.

Cortical sensory perception is tested in the following ways. *Stereognosis* is the perception of objects through touch. Test each hand with the eyes closed by placing a button, key, coin, or other familiar object in the hand and asking for identification. Two-point discrimination is determined by using the points of a calibrated compass on the fingertip and asking the patient to tell you when one and two points are felt. Normally, two points can be distinguished when the points are 0.3 to 0.6 cm apart. The number of centimeters of separation required to distinguish two points is important. The average distance on the palms and soles is 1.5 cm; on the dorsum of the hand,

TABLE 32-4 **Spinal Segment, Stimulus/Site, and Expected Response of Deep Tendon and Superficial Reflexes**

Reflex	Spinal Segment	Stimulus/Site	Expected Response Observed	Palpated
Biceps	C5, C6	Biceps tendon	Flexion at the elbow	Contraction of biceps
Triceps	C7, C8	Triceps tendon above elbow	Extension at elbow	Contraction of triceps
Brachioradialis or supinator	C5, C6	Radius, 1-2 in above wrist	Flexion and supination of forearm	
Abdominal	T8, T9, T10 (above umbilicus) T10, T11, T12 (below umbilicus)	Abdomen; stroke the four abdominal quadrants toward the umbilicus	Contraction of abdominal muscle, and umbilicus deviates toward stimulus	
Cremasteric	L1, L2	Upper thigh; scratch inner aspect	Testicle elevates on stimulated side; absence of response suggests corticospinal tract lesion at or below L1-L2	
Patellar or knee	L2, L3, L4	Patellar tendon	Extension of knee	Contraction of quadriceps
Achilles or ankle	S1, S2	Achilles tendon	Plantar flexion at ankle	
Plantar	L4, L5, S1, S2	Lateral aspect of sole of foot from heel to ball and curving across ball	Plantar flexion of toes and foot (dorsiflexion of big toe with fanning of other toes—*Babinski response*)	

3 cm is average; and on the shin, 4 cm is usually necessary. *Double simultaneous stimulation* is the appreciation of two simultaneous touches on symmetrically opposite sides of the body. This requires normal cortical function. All the above responses are designed to test cortical sensory perception and are affected by lesions of the sensory cortex.

Reflexes

Deep tendon reflexes are best elicited by having the patient relax. The examiner then positions the limb in a manner that slightly stretches the muscle and strikes a brisk blow with a reflex hammer over the tendon insertion of the muscle. The two sides of the body are compared for equality of response. Reflexes are usually graded on a 0 to 4+ scale.

4+   Very brisk, hyperactive, and may indicate disease
3+   More brisk than average but may well be normal
2+   Average or normal response
1+   Decreased response
0   No response

In addition to the deep tendon reflexes, three superficial reflexes are usually tested: the abdominal reflex, the cremasteric responses, and the plantar reflex. Reflexes, generally speaking, tend to be increased in suprasegmental neuron disease and decreased in segmental disease. Table 32-4 shows the expected response, stimulus, site of stimulation, and corresponding spinal segments of commonly tested deep tendon and superficial reflexes.

DIAGNOSTIC PROCEDURES AND MONITORING

The physician may use a variety of radiological, electrophysiological, and laboratory techniques to aid in the diagnosis and monitoring of the neurological disease process. The nurse's understanding of these studies serves two purposes. First, the nurse can prepare the patient and family for what the patient will experience during the diagnostic examination and can help them understand the purpose and meaning of the tests and their findings. Second, the nurse can use the results of many of the studies to supplement physical examination findings in determining patient responses to the neurological problem and the critical care environment. For example, if the brainstem evoked potential examination shows intact auditory pathways for an unresponsive patient, the nurse can plan to protect the patient from noise or unguarded conversations within the patient's hearing.

Laboratory Studies

The most common diagnostic tests are the blood and cerebrospinal fluid (CSF) analyses used in the differential diagnosis of neurological disorders. Examination of serum electrolytes helps sort out metabolic from cerebral sources of altered consciousness, for example. Screening of urine and serum for toxic substances helps determine whether unexplained coma results from drug overdose or trauma. The majority of such studies are routine for all patients in critical care units. Table 32-5 summarizes normal values for constituents of serum and CSF and the major neurological implications of abnormalities.

Radiological Studies

Only a few decades ago, relatively few radiological studies were available for diagnosing and following neurological disorders. With the advent of computer technology and very short half-life radioisotopes, the means to investigate both structures and functions of the living nervous system are increasing exponentially.

Examination of Nervous System Structures

Plain Films. The most common radiological studies to show the structures of the nervous system are *plain films of skull and spine*. A variety of views of the skull and spine are used to detect fractures, in the case of trauma, or bony erosion suggestive of underlying tumors. Skull and spine films are important in ruling out fractures of the face, orbit, and spine in patients who have sustained injuries in motor vehicle accidents or other forms of trauma. Any patient who has sustained a head injury should be assumed to have an associated cervical spine injury until the latter has been ruled out by adequate films of the entire cervical spine. Table 32-6 describes nursing implications of abnormal findings on skull and spine films.

Computed Tomography (CT) and Magnetic Resonance Imaging (MRI). Computed tomography (CT), also known as computed axial tomography or computer-assisted tomography (CAT), of the brain and spine and magnetic resonance imaging (MRI), or nuclear magnetic resonance (NMR), are two technologies that have revolutionized diagnostic imaging in neurological disorders. Both technologies allow remarkably clear noninvasive visualization of brain and spinal cord structures. In many cases, the ability to see evidence of stroke, tumors, intracranial bleeding, and aneurysms enables the physician to avoid the use of invasive radiological examinations such as angiograms or myelograms.

Computed tomography uses many thousands of x-ray beams, successively directed at horizontal "slices" of the skull or spine. With the assistance of a computer, the attenuation of the beams by the differing densities of bone, blood, and cerebral (or spinal) gray and white matter is measured and shown as a clear image of the brain (or spinal cord) in horizontal sections. Radiation exposure is approximately the same as that from a plain skull film.

Magnetic resonance imaging is actually a biophysical rather than a radiographic technique. Instead of using ionizing radiation, MRI uses a powerful magnetic field to provide data for computer imaging of the nervous system. The patient is placed in the magnetic field, and a specific radio frequency pulse is introduced into the field. This pulse causes the hydrogen ion nuclei (protons) of tissue cells to realign their axes. When the pulse is removed, the protons return to their original alignment, and the changes in radio frequency energy that were absorbed and then emitted by the tissues are analyzed by computer. The image that is constructed is based on the fact that different types of CNS tissue emit different energies.

MRI distinguishes more clearly between gray and white matter and gives better identification of white matter lesions than CT scanning. Images can be made in several planes (coronal, axial, and sagittal). In addition, because bone does not produce artifacts in MRI, clearer images can be obtained of lesions involving the posterior fossa, brainstem, and spinal cord. CT scanning is superior to MRI in detecting trauma, intracranial hemorrhage, and bony abnormalities and in verifying suspected disk herniation. MRI takes longer than CT, and therefore, movement artifact is a greater problem in MRI. Thus, CT is the better method in acute trauma, where time is crucial, and for patients who are confused or unable to cooperate.[1,2,3]

No health hazards have yet been demonstrated from the magnetic field or radiofrequency pulses in persons who have no implanted magnetic devices.[1,3] Personnel and patients with magnetic implants such as postoperative clips for hemostasis, aneurysms, and intracranial bypass; cardiac pacemakers; internal cardioverter/defibrillators; and insulin pumps should not be near the MRI unit since the magnetic field may dislodge these devices or interfere with their function.

TABLE 32-5   Neurological Implications of Abnormalities in Serum and CSF

	Average Values*		Implications
	Cerebrospinal Fluid	Serum	
Osmolarity, mosm/L	295	295	Lethargy, confusion, seizures may be precipitated by hypo- or hyperosmolarity (<200; >350 mosm)
Sodium, mEq/L	138	138	↓ Na⁺ may be result of excess parenteral fluid administration or inappropriate ADH secretion; major electrolyte contributing to osmolarity
Potassium, mEq/L	2.8	4.1	Cardiac dysrhythmias and muscle weakness may occur when K⁺ is outside normal range
Calcium, mEq/L	2.4	5.2	Tetany with hypocalcemia; weakness and lethargy with hypercalcemia
Magnesium, mEq/L	2.7	1.9	Tremor, weakness, tetany with hypomagnesia; weakness and confusion with hypermagnesia
Chloride mEq/L	124	101	↓ CSF with TB meningitis; ↓ Na⁺ and Cl in adrenoleukodystrophies
Bicarbonate, mEq/L	23	23	Patterns of blood gases, bicarbonate, pH, chloride useful in differentiating metabolic and respiratory acidosis
Carbon dioxide, mmHg	48	38 (arterial)	Lethargy, confusion, tremors with marked hypercarbia; circumoral tingling, numbness of fingers and toes with hypocarbia
Ammonia, μg/dl	30	70	Hyperammonemia found in a variety of inherited metabolic disorders; in Reye's syndrome, hepatic encephalopathy
Urea, mmol/L	4.7	5.4	↑ Renal failure, uremic encephalopathy
Creatinine, mg/dl	1.1	1.6	↑ Renal failure; ↑ in some infantile metabolic disorders
Phosphorus, mg/dl	1.6	4.0	↑ Organophosphate insecticide poisoning; muscle weakness and paralysis
Total lipid, mg/dl	1.25	876	Serum lipids ↑ in some lipid storage diseases; ↓ serum levels of high-density lipoproteins associated with cerebrovascular disease
Glucose, mg/dl	>45	90	Confusion, coma with hypoglycemia; coma with hyperglycemia and hyperosmolarity; ↓ CSF glucose in bacterial meningitis, TB meningitis
Lactate, mEq/L	1.6	1.0	Metabolic acidosis
Total protein, mg/dl	15-50	6.5-8.4	↑ CSF with tumor, infection, demyelinating disease, polyneuropathy
Gamma globulin, % of total	3% to 12%	18%	CSF proportion ↑ in multiple sclerosis, subacute encephalitis, Guillain-Barré disease

* Average values from Adams, R. D., & Victor, M. (1989). *Principles of neurology* (3rd ed.). New York: McGraw-Hill.

The left box on p. 797 summarizes precautions that must be taken with regard to the magnetic field of the MRI.

Plain x-ray films can be made at the bedside of critically ill patients, but CT and MRI scans cannot. Therefore, the critical care nurse may be directly involved in ensuring continuity of monitoring and care in the radiology department for the neurotrauma pa-

tient. CT scanning is much more readily available than MRI in almost all centers that have critical care units. It is the preferred imaging technique for suspected hemorrhage or trauma and in patients unable to cooperate. Transporting the critically ill patient to the scanner requires excellent teamwork among nursing, radiology, and often respiratory therapy personnel in managing portable monitoring equipment,

TABLE 32-6   **Nursing Implications of Abnormal Skull and Spine X-rays**

Finding	Significant Results	Nursing Implications
SKULL X-RAYS		
Fracture	Elevation, depression	Establish baseline neurological and vital signs; head injury with associated concussion, contusion, or laceration of brain requires frequent monitoring
	Relationship to other structures (e.g., parietal occipital)	Be alert to signs and symptoms indicating increased intracranial pressure
		Hemorrhage from blood vessels in immediate area possible, e.g., epidural hematoma from parietal fracture along meningeal artery; requires neurological assessment
		Prevent further contamination, infection
		Use loose dressings; do not try to prevent drainage
Calcifications	Tumor (glioma)	Shifts in pineal body may be first documentation of midline shift caused by mass effect
	Old hematoma	
	Pineal body, choroid plexus	Listen for bruits of carotid arteries, and intracranially over eye, temporal bone
	Degenerative changes	
	Vascular abnormalities	
	Endocrine disorders	
	Systemic diseases	
Deformities enlarged size, separating sutures	Osteitis deformans	Note condition of anterior fontanel; bulging may indicate increased intracranial pressure (normally closed at 18 months)
	Hydrocephalus	
	Tumor growth	
Erosion of bone	Underlying or invading tumor, e.g., erosion of sella turcica with pituitary tumor	Monitor electrolytes, intake and output, and specific gravity of urine, serum and urine osmolalities, essential in pituitary tumor
		Erosion may cause CSF leaks; check draining fluids (especially clear) for glucose with a Diastix to differentiate from mucous membrane secretions and blood
SPINE X-RAYS		
Fracture	Level of fracture	Immobilize suspect region; rule out cervical injury before extending, flexing neck
	Soft tissue changes	Maintain traction
	Relationship to other structures (e.g., spinal cord, nerve root level)	Correlate level of injury with clinical findings; look for evidence of ascending deficits
		Take additional precautions during transfer by restricting movement and positioning
		Ensure patient safety and immobilization by safety belts, immobilization, and protecting against drops, bumps, and collisions
Subluxations	Interlocking of facets	Notify physician if patient relates sensation of change in traction, "popping," or cracking (may indicate unlocking of facets)
Congenital abnormalities	E.g., spina bifida	Monitor neurological and vital signs in comparison to baseline findings
Degenerative changes	E.g., arthritis	
Bony erosions	Invading or underlying tumor	Report any tissue or fluid leaks

From AANN. (1984). *Core curriculum for neuroscience nursing* (Vol. 1, pp. 136-137). Park Ridge, IL: Author; and AANN. (1990). *Core curriculum for neuroscience nursing* (3rd ed.) (p. Vc2). Chicago: Author.

Patient Precautions in MRI Scanning

Information for the patient: The scan takes about 30 to 60 minutes and the patient must lie absolutely still, because movement will interfere with the ability of the computer to receive clear signals from the scanner. All metal objects should be removed prior to the scan (such as watch, rings, clothing with snaps, zippers, metal parts)

Contraindications to MRI scanning
  Inability to lie still
  Metal implants:
    Aneurysm vascular clips
    Orbital prosthesis anchors
    Cardiac pacemakers
    Hemostatic metal clips
    Intracranial bypass clips
    Metal ear prostheses
    Internal cardioverter/defibrillators
    Metal cardiac valves
    TENS units, insulin pumps
  Traumatic metal residuals (such as bullets, shrapnel)
Metals that are not contraindicated:
  Tantalum
  Dental alloys (tooth fillings)
  Many joint prostheses
  Vascular stents

Protocol for CT or MRI Transport from Critical Care Unit

1. Determine exact time patient is to be scanned. Patient should never wait in radiology department for procedure.
2. Notify respiratory therapy.
3. Check transport pack for appropriate medications and supplies.
4. Attach transport monitoring equipment; zero, calibrate, and set alarms. Minimal monitoring required: ECG, BP, ICP.
5. Administer osmotic diuretic and/or sedation if required.
6. Unplug all equipment (IV infusion pumps, pulse oximetry, bed).
7. Set up patient on transport ventilator or, if not available, Ambu bag with 100% O_2.
8. Transport patient to radiology department with head of bed elevated.
9. Transfer patient to CT or MRI table.
10. Arrange monitoring equipment so it can be visualized from control room. Check alarm status.
11. Perform rapid neurological assessment. Medicate patient as necessary.
12. Begin scanning patient.
13. Continue to observe patient and monitor parameters.
14. Transfer patient back to bed and return to unit.

From Marshall, S. B., Marshall, L. F., Vos, H. R., et al. (1990). *Neuroscience critical care* (p. 132). Philadelphia: Saunders.

---

maintaining ventilation during transport, restoring mechanical ventilation in the radiology department, and ensuring optimal therapeutic positioning throughout. It is essential that the critical care nurse accompany the patient throughout the procedure. The box above to the right outlines a protocol for transport of a critically ill patient for CT or MRI.

The nurse can prepare patients who are awake for the need to lie as still as possible and should inform them that people will leave the room during the scanning period but will be able to see them and all the monitors. Patients having MRI scanning will hear rhythmic knocking sounds as the radiofrequency generator is turned on and off.

Angiography and Myelography. The blood vessels may be visualized by angiography and the spinal canal by myelography, radiological techniques that employ a radiopaque contrast media. Their use in detecting tumors or other space-occupying lesions of the CNS has diminished with the advent of CT and MRI scanning. However, they are still valuable and have not yet been replaced in determining the patency of cerebral and spinal vessels, the presence and location of aneurysms and arteriovenous malformations, and the presence of obstruction to the cerebrospinal fluid

flow. MRI scanning is rapidly gaining favor in detecting spinal disk herniation, very small aneurysms, and intraluminal vascular clots.[2,3]

In *angiography*, the contrast medium (radiopaque dye) is injected into the artery via a percutaneous needle or cannula, and sequential x-ray films are taken as the medium flows through the vessels. Thus, the extracranial and intracranial vessels can be visualized in the arterial, arterial–capillary, and venous phases. Patient risks include an approximate 1% chance of vasospasm, embolism, or thrombosis in the territory of the catheterized artery. Allergic reaction to the contrast medium may occur, as well as hematoma or hemorrhage at the site of the cannula or needle puncture. Patients often experience an unpleasant sensation of warmth and burning during injection of the medium and may develop headache or nausea. A nursing care plan for patients undergoing cerebral angiography is shown in Table 32-7.

Digital subtraction angiography involves intravenous rather than intraarterial injection of contrast medium. Digital computer processing is then used to enhance the x-ray image of the cervical and intracra-

TABLE 32-7 **Patient Care Plan: After Cerebral Angiography**

Patient Problem	Expected Outcome	Management
Circulatory compromise due to hematoma, edema, spasm, thrombosis, embolism, blood loss	Absence of neurological deterioration Absence of seizures Verbalizes changes in sensory function, e.g., temperature, tingling Absence of bleeding, swelling Distal/extremity pulses present Extremity color and temperature within normal limits Vital signs stable	Record condition of puncture site and distal pulses prior to and following procedure Monitor neuro/vital signs and check distal pulses and site frequently during 48 hours postprocedure, e.g., q15min × 1 hour; q30min × 4 hours; qh × 4 hours Be aware of changes in patient's agitation LOC (clue to B/P) Check limb size, temperature, sensory level distal to site Check pressure dressing for occlusion of artery, bleeding, and swelling Apply ice pack to site immediately postprocedure, 2-4 hours Minimize activity level × 24 hours Position extremity to relax muscle Avoid flexion at site
Discomfort/pain at puncture site	Minimal discomfort/pain	Apply ice pack to site Position of comfort Medicate as ordered Activity to comfort level after 24 hours
Compromise of adjacent structures a. Tracheal compression carotid sinus sensitivity due to carotid puncture	Absence of airway obstruction/ stridor Temporal pulse present Absence of bradycardia, syncopes, hypotension	Check temporal pulse, B/P, apical pulse Observe for neck swelling, facial color, trachial deviation, and respiratory effort (stridor)
b. Brachial artery/nerve/plexus compression due to brachial/ axillary puncture	Radial pulse present Arm sensation and movement present	Observe for pale, cold, pulseless hands Check radial pulses Position of comfort, usually elevated Check procedural record for sensory changes due to local anesthesia Observe arm sensation and movement
c. Femoral artery/nerve compression due to femoral puncture	Pedal pulse present Leg sensation and movement present Blood pressure stable	Check procedural record for sensory changes due to local anesthesia Measure limb size Check for absence of bleeding into thigh and abdominal cavity Check and record distal pulses Observe for sensory and movement changes Avoid hip flexion
d. Pneumothorax due to subclavian puncture	Absence of respiratory distress Breath sounds present bilaterally	Observe for respiratory distress and changes in respiratory pattern Check breath sounds
e. Spasm/compression due to vertebral artery puncture	Absence of visual deficits	Observe for visual deficits, e.g., cortical blindness, hemianopsia Provide reassurance to patient (event may be transient)
f. Renal failure due to radiopaque dye, femoral approach	Urinary output at least 30 ml/hr	Observe intake and output × 24 hours Encourage fluids, e.g., 600 ml × 8 hours Adequately hydrate patient preprocedure Check renal function tests If nausea and vomiting persist, request IV therapy

From AANN. (1984). *Core curriculum for neuroscience nursing* (Vol. 1, pp. 155-156). Park Ridge, IL: Author.

nial vessels. Large volumes of intravenous fluid may be used; thus, this examination is contraindicated if there is concomitant cardiac failure.

Myelography involves the injection of radiopaque contrast medium into the spinal subarachnoid space in order to visualize the spinal canal and surrounding spaces. The contrast dye is injected via a spinal needle inserted percutaneously into the lumbar spinal canal. The x-ray table is tilted to move the contrast medium along the subarachnoid space. Water-based contrast (e.g., metrizamide) is lighter than CSF and will tend to move higher in the spinal canal, whereas oil-based contrast (e.g., iophendylate) is heavier than CSF and will move to the lower portion of the canal. Oil-based media are not absorbed and must be removed at the end of the procedure, while water-based media may or may not be removed. If water-based contrast is used and allowed to be absorbed, it may act as an osmotic diuretic because of its large-molecule structure. Seizures may occur if water-based contrast reaches the cranial subarachnoid space.

Radionuclide Scintigraphy. Radioisotope scanning of brain and cranial or spinal bone is used to visualize tumors, subdural hematomas, inflammatory masses, and some vascular lesions. Radioactive isotopes of technetium are most commonly used and are injected intravenously, with subsequent scanning of brain or bone by a gamma camera. This device detects uptake of the injected radioisotope and continuously displays its accumulation and distribution, with photographs taken at intervals. Cerebral or bone lesions that disrupt the blood–brain barrier or are highly vascular will take up more radioisotope than normal tissue. The half-life of the radioisotopes is quite short, and the dosage is low; thus, the radiation hazard to patient and personnel is minimal. Radiology personnel should follow standard precautions in handling radioactive materials. Nursing personnel in the patient's unit are not at risk for radiation hazard.

Examination of Cerebral Function

The preceding radiological studies make it possible to visualize neural structures. The technique called *positron emission tomography (PET)* makes it possible to visualize the brain as it is actively working—i.e., the metabolic functioning of different portions of the cerebral hemispheres. Radioactively marked nuclides (tracers) of substances such as oxygen, glucose, nitrogen, and carbon are inhaled or injected. These substances readily cross the blood–brain barrier and are used by metabolically active tissues. They emit positrons, which, when activated by electrons, emit gamma rays. A computerized detection system identifies the gamma rays and measures their intensity. The device then creates a tomographic image that indicates the areas of highest metabolic activity. The half-life of the nuclides is extremely short; thus, there is little exposure of staff or patients to radiation.

Differences in metabolic patterns have been found between normal brains and those of people with such disorders as Alzheimer's disease, schizophrenia, and perhaps Parkinson's disease. PET scanning has also been useful in localizing epileptic foci and in following the course of acute cerebral ischemia.[4,5] Because of its cost and the need to have a cyclotron on site to make the isotopes, PET scanning is still largely a research tool at specialized medical centers. Although PET scanning offers simultaneous measurement of regional cerebral blood flow (rCBF), metabolism, and biochemistry, its expense and technological requirements render it unavailable at most centers. *Single photon emission tomography* (SPECT) is more widely used. SPECT measures only rCBF, but since blood flow is linked to metabolism, it offers an indirect measure of brain metabolic activity. Readily available radioisotopes are used to provide the photons, which are measured by a rotating gamma camera.[3,6]

Neurophysiological Studies

Neurophysiological studies are based on the existence of electrical properties in functioning neural tissues. The voltage discharged from the firing of motor fibers, cortical neurons, and peripheral nerve fibers is amplified and measured. These values and patterns of electrical activity are then compared with normal patterns to help determine the location of disordered nervous system functioning.

The *electroencephalogram* (EEG) is the oldest and most widely used of the neurophysiological techniques. It is most commonly used to detect seizure activity in the brain and to measure sleep stages. In the critical care unit, the EEG may be used to monitor status epilepticus and to verify brain death. Portable units can be brought to the bedside for monitoring in the unit. Electrodes are placed on the patient's scalp or, more rarely, subdermally. Movement of eyelids, face, or body will create artifacts, and such movement should be noted on the paper recording.

EEG monitoring is increasingly used intraoperatively during a variety of neurosurgical procedures. In cerebral vascular surgery, changes in the EEG pattern provide quick evidence of compromised cortical function and ischemia. Direct recording of the cortex (electrocorticography) is often used in localizing epileptic foci during epilepsy surgery.

Evoked potentials involve computer averaging of the electrical activity evoked in the cerebral cortex and subcortical relay sites by stimulation of sense organs or peripheral nerves. Ordinarily it is not possible to distinguish the neural response to such sensory input from the background brain activity that is seen in the EEG. However, computer averaging of the signals makes possible the enhancement of such small inputs to visualize distinctive waveforms for auditory, visual, and somatosensory stimuli. Normal waveforms that correspond to specific subcortical and cortical structures have been defined, as have the normal latencies (time needed to reach specified sites).[7]

Visual evoked potentials (VEPs) are tested by having the patient watch a rapidly changing geometric design while the potentials are recorded from surface electrodes plated on the scalp. Visual potentials are also called *pattern reversal electrical potentials* (PREPs) or *visual evoked responses* (VERs). VERs can be recorded in the unresponsive patient by using a flashing light as the stimulus. This test is used to determine whether lesions are in the visual pathways or the visual cortex.

Auditory evoked potentials (AEPs) are also called *brainstem auditory evoked responses* (BAERs). Multiple click stimuli are presented to each ear via earphones, and the latency and shape of the waveform at the brainstem and cortical levels are evaluated. Brainstem auditory evoked potentials are preserved under anesthesia and in drug overdose and often in traumatic head injury, provided the brainstem auditory pathways are not injured. Although the presence of normal AEPs in a comatose patient does not mean the patient processes information into long-term memory at the cortex, it does mean that the pathways for hearing are intact. AEPs are used in many centers to help localize lesions and, in some cases, to follow the course of recovery from trauma.

Somatosensory evoked potentials (SEPs or SSEPs) are recorded from the scalp after electrical stimulation of selected peripheral nerves (usually the median, peroneal, or tibial). Once the nerve has been located, subsequent electrical stimulation is very low level and painless. Alterations in normal latency and waveform help differentiate lesions of the peripheral nerves from those of the subcortical and cortical central sensory pathways. SEPs have been found useful in following the course of recovery from spinal cord injury and are often used in helping confirm the diagnosis of multiple sclerosis.[7]

Electromyography (EMG) records the electrical activity of muscle fibers at rest and during movement. This activity can be recorded from groups of muscle fibers by electrodes placed on the surface of the skin. This type of recording is used primarily in biofeedback and relaxation training rather than for differential diagnosis of motor unit diseases. In neurodiagnostic EMG, a coaxial needle is inserted into the muscle. The needle acts as an electrode and records the electrical activity of the muscle fiber. Action potentials are observed during muscle contraction, and their shape and firing rate are used to determine the presence or absence of denervation of muscle fibers, myopathies, and myotonias. The frequent moving and reinsertion of the needles makes this an uncomfortable procedure for the patient.

EMG is also used for nerve conduction studies in diagnosing lesions of peripheral nerves. A peripheral nerve is stimulated electrically, and the time between action potentials at the stimulating and the recording electrodes is determined. The sensation is that of repetitive muscle twitching, which may become muscle spasms for some patients, and sometimes mild electrical shock.

Biophysical Studies

A number of studies that may be conducted in the critical care unit or during neurosurgery depend upon physical principles such as conduction of sound through tissue and fluid or dispersion of tracers in cerebral circulation.

Ultrasound studies use the principle that sound waves are deflected at different speeds from structures of differing densities. The *echoencephalogram*, or *echogram*, uses this principle to detect displacement of midline cranial structures as an indirect indication of mass lesions in the cranium. The ready availability of CT scanning, which can more specifically identify the location and nature of the mass lesion, has decreased the use of echograms considerably.

Carotid artery imaging by Doppler and B-mode scanners is the most common use of ultrasound in neurological and neurosurgical patients. Doppler and B-mode scanners emit ultrasound waves, which are reflected off red blood cells, vessel walls, and muscles that surround the vessels. In Doppler scanning, the velocity of blood flow is measured from sound waves reflecting from the red blood cells. Variations in velocity are interpreted as evidence of narrowed or patent arteries. B-mode scanning combines the Doppler estimates of velocity with images created by differing reflection of ultrasound waves from the structures in the neck and the pulsations of the carotid arteries to produce an image of the lumen of vessels during blood flow. Both examinations are noninvasive. A transducer about the size of the head of an electric razor is placed on the patient's neck, over the common carotid artery. The sounds of the pulsating vessel can be clearly heard.

More recently, Doppler ultrasound has been used to image intracerebral vessels with the *transcranial Doppler*. Vasospasm in subarachnoid hemorrhage patients can be detected early by this method.[3,8,9]

Oculoplethysmography is a noninvasive technique for estimating carotid flow and ultimately cerebral circulation by measuring pressure in the ophthalmic artery. The ophthalmic artery is supplied by the internal carotid artery, as is the cerebral circulation. The test may be used in the diagnosis of carotid artery disease and in follow-up after carotid endarterectomy. In flow oculoplethysmography, the pulsation from the ophthalmic artery (internal carotid circulation) arriving at the eyes (detected through an eye-cuplike device) and at photoelectric detectors on the ears (external carotid circulation) are compared. Any differences are considered evidence of reduced flow. Postprocedure nursing care consists in preventing or detecting corneal abrasion from the eyecup or from rubbing the eyes before the anesthetic eyedrops wear off.

Cerebral blood flow is measured by using the Fick principle to calculate the transit time of a tracer substance. Whole-brain cerebral blood flow is measured by using nitrous oxide as a tracer and measuring the time it takes for a systemic arterial blood sample to appear in the internal jugular venous circulation. Because this method gives only blood flow in the whole brain, rather than flow in different regions of the brain, it is less useful in detecting localized problems than methods of detecting regional cerebral blood flow.

Regional cerebral blood flow is most often measured in centers with large clinical research programs, as it requires elaborate detection equipment. Radioactive isotope tracers are either injected (in the carotid artery or intravenously) or inhaled and detected by external collimeters mounted around the patient's head. The flow in any given region is computed from the rate of clearance of the tracer from the brain region directly under each detector. The direct intracarotid injection gives the most accurate flow, since the radioisotope is exhaled before being recirculated to the brain. Nursing observation for hematoma or evidence of cerebral emboli (see Chapter 33) is essential after measurement of regional cerebral blood flow by direct carotid injection. Intravenous and inhalation techniques are safer and relatively noninvasive, but these procedures disperse the tracer to all body tissues and thus distort the brain clearance curve somewhat.

Surgical Diagnostic Procedures

Craniotomy is the ultimate neurosurgical diagnostic procedure to confirm what has been hypothesized from preliminary studies. However, a number of minor surgical procedures may be used in the intensive care unit to add to the diagnostic testing or to monitor the patient's progress through invasive measurement of physiological variables.

Lumbar and *cisternal puncture* are invasive procedures that may be used to obtain cerebrospinal fluid for diagnostic analysis, to inject dye for myelography, to administer antibiotics or antitumor agents directly into the CSF or, more rarely, to measure intracranial pressure. If increased intracranial pressure is suspected, pressure should be measured by one of the cranial methods (see below) rather than by lumbar puncture. In existing intracranial hypertension, there is a high risk of brain herniation if fluid is removed from the lumbar space, thereby creating a pressure differential between spinal and cranial cavities. Cisternal puncture is used only by experienced physicians, and only when spinal block makes it necessary to obtain CSF samples above the block or to administer medications intrathecally to the cervical spinal area. The obvious danger of cisternal puncture is inadvertent puncture of the medulla.

The most common site for lumbar puncture is at the L3-L4 vertebral interspace. The spinal cord ends at about L1-L2 and, therefore, is not likely to be entered. However, in infants and young children the cord may extend to the L3-L4 interspace, so the L4-L5 interspace is recommended in children. Some patients may have a headache following lumbar puncture and will benefit from lying flat after the procedure. Nursing observation to detect brain herniation is imperative for any patient in whom there is concern about intracranial hypertension.

Skull trephination by either twist drill (small-diameter drill bit) or burr hole (larger-diameter drill bit) may be done in patients in whom extradural or subdural bleeding is suspected. Although CT scanning allows the neurosurgeon to visualize hemorrhage, the radiological procedure requires considerable time for transporting the patient and performing the scan. Many neurosurgeons believe that they can alleviate pressure on the brain more quickly by using trephination to locate and remove the clot and then transporting the patient to the operating room for location and cauterization of the bleeding vessels.

Intracranial pressure may be diagnosed and monitored by cannulation of a cerebral ventricle (ventriculostomy) or by recording the pulsations of the dura or subarachnoid space. Intracranial pressure monitoring is discussed in Chapters 4 and 33.

REFERENCES

1. Bydder, G. M., Steiner, R. E., Young, I. R., et al. (1982). Clinical NMR imaging of the brain: 140 cases. *American Journal of Roentgenology, 139,* 215.
2. Earnest, F., Baker, H. L., Kispert, D. B., et al. (1984). Magnetic resonance imaging vs. computed tomography: Advantages and disadvantages. *Clinical Neurosurgery, 32,* 540-573.
3. Marshall, S. B., Marshall, L. F., Vos, H. R., et al. (1990). *Neuroscience critical care* (pp. 115-146). Philadelphia: Saunders.

4. Phelps, M. E., Schelbert, H. R., & Mazziota, J. C. (1983). Positron computed tomography for studies of myocardial and cerebral function. *Annals of Internal Medicine, 98,* 339-359.

5. Thomas, D. G. T., Gibbs, J. M., & Wise, R. J. S. (1984). Use of positron emission tomography scanning in cerebral ischemia. *Clinical Neurosurgery, 32,* 51-69.

6. Podrecka, I., Suess, E., Goldenberg, G., et al. (1987). Initial experience with technetium-99m Hm-PAO SPECT. *Journal of Nuclear Medicine, 28,* 1657-1666.

7. Greenberg, R. P., & Ducker, T. B. (1982). Evoked potentials in the clinical neurosciences. *Journal of Neurosurgery, 56,* 1-18.

8. Aaslid, R., Markwalder, T. M., & Nornes, H. (1982). Noninvasive transcranial Doppler ultrasound recording of flow velocity in basal cerebral arteries. *Journal of Neurosurgery, 57,* 769-774.

9. Grolimund, P., Seiler, R. W., Aaslid, R., et al. (1987). Evaluation of cerebrovascular disease by combined extracranial and transcranial Doppler sonography. Experience in 1039 patients. *Stroke, 18,* 1018-1024.

33

Neurological Disorders

Pamela H. Mitchell

Neurological and neurosurgical disorders often present a bewildering array of disease entities to practicing nurses. For the critical care nurse, the patient is in danger of rapid deterioration in neurologic condition. Because the central nervous system regulates all other body systems, neurologic disease and trauma often complicate and initiate multisystem problems. How, then, can order be brought to the confusion and mystery that so often surround "neuro"?

Although the disorders that can affect nervous system functioning are numerous, the mechanisms by which they threaten life, their effects on the human responses that underly multisystem functioning, and their effects on the human responses that affect a person's ability to care for self are reasonably circumscribed. Thus, the concepts that clinicians must understand to provide informed care for critically ill persons with neurological dysfunction are few.

This chapter discusses two concepts: (1) the common underlying pathophysiological states that represent major threats to life or to stable multisystem functioning and (2) the categories of human response accompanying those pathophysiological states. Each of these categories is presented in relation to major diseases or conditions patients bring to critical care units.

LIFE-THREATENING NEUROPATHOPHYSIOLOGICAL STATES

Of the many disorders that may affect the central and peripheral nervous systems, a relatively small number are life-threatening. The three major ways in which these disorders threaten life are by disruption of consciousness, disruption of ventilation secondary to loss of movement but not of consciousness, and neurally induced multisystem failure.

This chapter discusses these life-threatening clinical problems that disrupt consciousness: brain edema and swelling, intracranial hypertension, subarachnoid hemorrhage and cerebral vasospasm, brain herniation syndromes, and seizures and status epilepticus.

Life-threatening motor and sensory dysfunctions that affect ventilation but not consciousness are usually caused by extracerebral disorders that affect the brainstem, spinal cord, peripheral nerves, or motor unit. Such disorders include: spinal cord injury, myasthenia gravis, and Guillain-Barré syndrome.

Multisystem failure follows cerebral damage to hypothalamic regulation of autonomic functions or disruption of input to the peripheral sympathetic system. Head injury, spinal cord injury, and meningoencephalitis may lead to multisystem failure.

States That Disrupt Consciousness

Trauma, ischemia, and metabolic or infectious injury to the central nervous system are ultimately translated into a few pathophysiological states that seriously threaten life. Much of the medical and nursing care of patients who are critically ill with neurological disorders is directed at reversal, stabilization, or symptom management of these pathophysiological states. Therefore, specific clinical problems, associated nursing diagnoses, and relevant collaborative and independent nursing interventions are discussed for each category of pathophysiological state.

Clinical problem is used in Carpenito's terminology to mean a physiological or pathophysiological disturbance of functioning that is managed collaboratively by nursing and one or more other disciplines (one usually being medicine).[1] *Collaborative interventions* are those that require the protocol or "order" of another discipline to initiate but require considerable nursing judgment to execute. A *nursing diagnosis* is the statement of an existing or highly potential health problem or pathophysiological state for which intervention may be independently managed by nursing. Many current statements of nursing diagnoses applicable to critically ill patients overlap with statements of clinical problems or pathophysiological states as defined above. These are included and identified when appropriate in this chapter.

Brain Hyperemia and Brain Edema

Brain swelling is a generalized pathophysiological process that has the potential to disrupt consciousness. Almost any severe insult to the cerebral hemispheres may disrupt vasomotor regulation, cellular metabolism, or the integrity of cell membranes sufficiently to affect the autoregulation of blood flow to the brain or the amount of water in the gray and white matter.[2] *Brain swelling* is a net increase in *any* of the brain fluid compartments (intravascular, intracellular, or extracellular), whereas *brain edema* is defined as a net increase in the intracellular or extracellular *water content* of the brain.[3,4] The two most common sources of brain swelling are (1) an increase in the intravascular volume, or *hyperemia,* and (2) an increase in extracellular or intracellular water volume, or *edema.*[5]

Brain hyperemia is most commonly seen in the first hours following head injury but may also occur in the first hours following craniotomy if manipulation of the cerebral vessels results in vasomotor paralysis. Hyperemic brain swelling thus represents a temporary failure of autoregulation. Cerebral arterioles continually constrict or dilate in response to fluctuations in blood pressure in order to maintain constant cerebral blood flow. Trauma or surgical manipulation may disrupt this vasomotor stability. The excess fluid in the cerebral cavity is contained entirely within the cerebral vessels and does not represent excess brain water, as in brain edema.

Brain hyperemia is evident on CT scan as an increase in overall density (blood being read as denser than brain tissue) and is found in as many as 70% to 90% of patients with acute head injury.[6,7,8] Clinically, rapid and massive brain swelling may be manifested as intracranial hypertension (increased intracranial pressure).

A similar process has been seen in the initial hours following experimental spinal cord injury, with initial vasoconstriction and subsequent vasomotor paralysis.[9] The volume of the spinal cord is increased by virtue of an increase in the volume of blood contained in the intramedullary vessels, just as the volume of blood in the cranial vessels increases the overall volume of the cranial cavity. The functional effects of spinal cord swelling are manifested in changes in motor and sensory function rather than changes in consciousness.

As indicated earlier, central nervous system edema is a state reflecting a net increase in the water content of the CNS. The water is found either between neurons (extracellular, interstitial) or within neurons (intracellular). Neural edema has been divided into three classes: vasogenic, cytotoxic, and interstitial (hydrocephalic).[3,7,10]

Vasogenic edema is the most common of the brain edemas and results from disruption of the blood–brain barrier. The barrier between the systemic blood (in capillaries) and brain tissue is formed by the tight junctions of the endothelial cells that line the capillaries. Normally, only water and very small molecules pass through these junctions into the cerebral interstitial spaces. It is thought that the tight junctions may open in brain injury, owing to endothelial cell shrinkage, or that cytoplasmic transport of protein molecules across the endothelial cells increases, perhaps secondary to the presence of free oxygen radicals or other perioxidation by-products.[3,10] The end result is an increase in water content between cells as the hydrostatic pressure in the capillaries causes fluid to flow passively across the capillary membrane and into the interstitium of the brain. White matter accumulates more of the fluid than gray matter because it is less resistant to flow. Reabsorption takes place primarily via the glial cells of the white matter. The disorders in which vasogenic edema is most commonly seen include trauma, tumors, heavy metal encephalopathies, and infectious processes such as meningitis and abscesses.

Cytotoxic edema is an intracellular process, most commonly seen in disorders in which the intracellular sodium-potassium pump fails. The cell thus loses the ability to maintain an osmotic gradient in relation to the extracellular fluid, and water passively flows into the cell to restore osmotic equilibrium. Astrocytes, which constitute a large percentage of the brain cells in the white matter, are the primary site of cytotoxic edema. In addition, endothelial cells exhibit an increased permeability to water and add a component of vasogenic edema to the picture. Hypoxia, ischemia, Reye's syndrome, hypoosmolality, and a variety of neuronal poisons are all conditions in which cytotoxic edema may occur.[11]

Cytotoxic edema may also occur in head injury as a secondary injury due to inadequate cerebral blood flow or inadequate glucose delivered to the brain. Hypoxia, intracranial pressure sufficient to decrease cerebral perfusion pressure, or systemic hypotension are examples of states that could lead to cellular ischemia, with cytotoxic edema as a marker of secondary injury. The cellular mechanisms dependent on ATP rapidly fail, allowing water and Ca^{2+} into the cell as the membrane pumps fail. The Ca^{2+} then triggers a cascade of events that damage the cell, including lipolysis, release of prostaglandin metabolites, and generation of free oxygen radicals. Thus, a potentially reversible edema becomes associated with irreversible damage to basic cellular mechanisms.[4,10,11]

Because edema-based brain swelling reflects an overall increase in water, CT scan will show *decreased* density, since water is seen by the x-rays as less dense than either blood or brain tissue. Most commonly, the area of decreased density surrounds a focal lesion (tumor, hematoma, etc.), but it may also be diffuse.

Interstitial, or *hydrocephalic, edema* is seen only as a long-term consequence of obstructive hydrocephalus and is not of primary concern in the critical care setting. It is believed to be due to diffusion of ventricular fluid into the spaces around the cerebral ventricles secondary to the hydrostatic pressure of increasing fluid in the obstructed ventricles.[10]

The net result of either hyperemic brain swelling or brain edema may be intracranial hypertension due to a net increase in the volume of either blood or water in the intracranial cavity. Therefore, the associated nursing diagnoses and medical management are discussed later, with that clinical problem. However, it is useful to differentiate the source of the intracranial hypertension as either hyperemia or edema.

Brain swelling due to hyperemia may occur within minutes or hours of injury to the CNS, whereas brain swelling due to edema is a slower process, commonly manifested in 24 to 72 hours following trauma or surgery. Both hyperemia and edema may be clinically manifested by changes in level of consciousness or by intracranial hypertension, but the time course and CT findings help differentiate the source of the clinical symptoms. This differentiation becomes important in medical therapy, since the treatment of vasogenic edema involves removing water while the treatment of hyperemia is intended to constrict vessels.

Hyperemia and edema of the spinal cord are believed to contribute to secondary injury by interfering with adequate blood flow to the cord. The associated problems and nursing diagnoses vary with the level of the spinal cord affected and are discussed later with disorders that affect ventilation and multisystem function.

Intracranial Hypertension

Many textbooks describe signs of transtentorial herniation as if they were also signs of increased intracranial pressure. Although rapidly increasing intracranial pressure may cause transtentorial herniation, it need not do so and furthermore cannot do so by itself. The purpose of this section is to separate what is known about increased intracranial pressure from its potentially life-threatening outcome in transtentorial herniation.

Pathophysiology. The neurocranium, or brain case, contains three basic substances—brain tissue, blood, and cerebrospinal fluid—within a nearly inexpandable cranial cavity. Expansion of the volume of any one of these three elements requires adjustment of the volumes of the other two in order to maintain intracranial pressure at a steady level. This principle is known as the *Monro-Kellie doctrine.* Experimental work with nonhuman primates has demonstrated that there is considerably more compensatory reserve in the intracranial cavity than was previously believed. Up to a point, expansion of any of the three elements can be compensated for by contraction of the other two components of the intracranial space.

When an intracranial mass expands or when cerebrospinal fluid (CSF) flow is blocked and fluid accumulates, some CSF will be expressed from the cranial cavity to accommodate the expanded volume. Intracranial pressure (ICP) remains nearly constant so long as the volume of CSF or intravascular blood displaced is nearly equal to the volume of tissue or fluid added to the cranial compartment. This effect is illustrated in the flat portion of the volume–pressure curve shown in Figure 18-1 in Chapter 18. In this flat portion, additions to intracranial volume do not result in appreciable changes in pressure.

Displacement of intracranial fluid volume can occur in three ways: decrease in rate of formation of CSF, slight increase in rate of CSF reabsorption, and displacement of CSF into the spinal sac. In slowly growing brain masses, these compensatory mechanisms may be sufficient to maintain nearly normal ICP for some time.

Eventually, however, the limits of volume displacement are reached; volume is added at a rate greater than displacement, and ICP rises. Note on the steep portion of the volume–pressure curve that continued additions to volume result in disproportionately greater rises in pressure. This relation of change in pressure to change in volume ($\Delta P/\Delta V$) is termed *elastance.* Elastance is the inverse of *compliance* ($\Delta V/\Delta P$), a term used to describe pressure–volume relationships in the lung. In the case of intracranial pressure, high elastance (synonymous with low compliance) implies a large change in pressure with a small change in volume. Any disorder that increases brain mass, decreases absorption of CSF, or blocks the flow of CSF increases intracranial pressure. Common examples of these disorders are summarized in Table 33-1.

Increase in Brain Mass. The most obvious example of an increase in brain mass is an intracranial tumor. Most tumors are relatively slow-growing and thus increase ICP at relatively slow rates. Generally, it is only late in the course of tumor growth that cranial contents are so displaced that ICP rises rapidly. Tumor growth or brain displacement may obstruct CSF pathways and thus create more rapid rise in ICP.

Hemorrhage, into either the brain substance or the subdural and epidural layers, acts as a mass lesion. Although the hemorrhage is not brain tissue, the effect is the same as expansion of the brain tissue itself. The growing mass of blood acts as a rapidly expanding

TABLE 33-1 Causes of Intracranial Hypertension

Functional Cause	Examples of Disorders
↑ Brain mass	Hyperemic brain swelling
	Edematous brain swelling
	Cerebral tumor
	Intracranial, extradural, and intradural hemorrhage
↓ CSF reabsorption	Subarachnoid hemorrhage
	Meningitis
Blockage of CSF circulation	Cerebral tumor
	Brain herniation
	Chronic hydrocephalus
	Normal-pressure hydrocephalus
	Ventricular tumor

lesion, creating volume–pressure curves like the classic one shown in Figure 18-1.

Subdural hematomas are of two types, acute and chronic. Acute subdural hematomas may result from head trauma, bleed relatively rapidly from dural-cortical bridging veins, and result in acute brain herniation. Chronic subdural hematoma is more often associated with lesser or even unremarkable blows to the head, bleeds at a slower rate, and grows more from the coalescence of fibrous membranes and breakdown products of blood. It acts more like a slow-growing tumor in terms of ICP changes.

Head injury does not always cause increased ICP. If the trauma leads to hematoma, intracranial hemorrhage, significant brain swelling, or alterations in CSF pathways, intracranial pressure may increase. As many as 60% to 70% of head-injured patients in highly specialized neurosurgical critical care units have been reported to have diffuse brain injury. However, only 30% to 50% of these patients have increased ICP, depending upon the level of ICP accepted as the upper limit of normal and the specialized nature of the critical care unit from which the study comes. Many of these patients are comatose and exhibit signs of brainstem dysfunction attributable to their injury rather than to increased intracranial pressure.[7,8]

Another cause of increasing brain volume affecting ICP is brain swelling. If the whole brain is hyperemic or if a portion of the brain (for example around a tumor, infarct, or contusion) is rapidly becoming edematous, compensatory volume displacement may be insufficient to maintain normal ICP. Reye's syndrome, a metabolic disorder of children, is a classic example of massive cytotoxic and vasogenic brain edema with concomitant intracranial hypertension. Others include hypoxic-ischemic brain edema and edema following massive hemispheric infarction.

Alteration in CSF Absorption and Flow. The volume of CSF can increase by three means: an increase in production, a decrease in absorption, or a blockage of flow. Increase in production can occur with tumors of the choroid plexus, which are relatively rare. In the populations seen in critical care, decrease in absorption and blockage of flow are the most common factors in CSF volume change.

Cerebrospinal fluid is produced in the choroid plexus of the lateral ventricles, flows downward through the third and fourth ventricles, exits the ventricles through the foramen of Magendie, is collected in the cisterns at the base of the brain, and then cir-

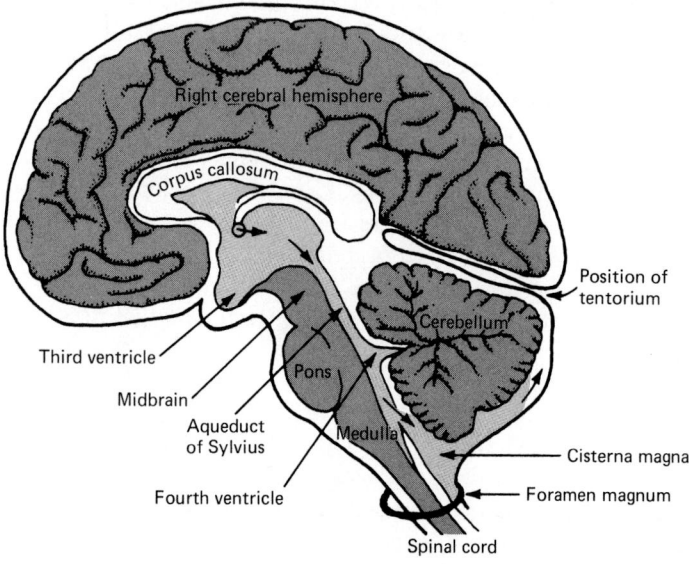

Figure 33-1 Normal flow of cerebrospinal fluid. Cerebrospinal fluid is formed in the choroid plexus and flows caudally through the lateral to fourth ventricles. It exits the ventricular system at the cisterna magna and flows up over the surface of the brain, to be reabsorbed over the convexities. A large portion of the CSF is held in the spinal dural sac as well.

culates upward to be reabsorbed over the convexities of the brain. Cerebrospinal fluid also circulates through the subarachnoid space of the spinal cord, passing to and from the basal cisterns. This movement of CSF is shown in Figure 33-1.

Any disorder that affects the meninges can alter reabsorption. Infections such as meningitis can alter CSF reabsorption by covering the meninges with exudate. More commonly, the breakdown of fibrin and blood products after subarachnoid hemorrhage "coats" the meninges and prevents reabsorption. The CSF can still circulate, since the pathways are not blocked, but it cannot be reabsorbed; cranial volumes of CSF increase secondary to malabsorption. This condition is called *communicating hydrocephalus*. Up to 20% of patients with subarachnoid hemorrhage have communicating hydrocephalus at least temporarily. Only about 10% require permanent shunt procedures to control ICP. Studies suggest that changes in ICP previously attributed to hydrocephalus may actually be due to a combination of hydrocephalus and vasospasm.

Blockage of CSF pathways produces *noncommunicating hydrocephalus*. The most common blockage of CSF pathways related to brain herniation occurs at the aqueduct of Sylvius (see Figure 33-1). As the brain herniates over the tentorium, the outflow from the third to the fourth ventricle is blocked. Herniation of cerebellar tonsils into the foramen magnum can block the basal cisterns. When elastance is high (when the patient is on the steep part of the volume–pressure curve), even temporary obstruction to CSF flow at the basal cisterns or at the entry to the spinal subarachnoid space may leave sufficient CSF in the cranial cavity to precipitate an increase in ICP.

Increase in Cerebral Blood Volume. The volume of blood in the normal brain is regulated in such a way that it is relatively constant despite changes in arterial blood pressure through a fairly wide range (mean arterial pressures from 50 to 170 mmHg). Consequently, in normal circumstances, cerebral blood volume contributes little to ICP. However, in the injured brain and in the brain in which tissue or CSF volumes are already increased, small changes in cerebral blood volume may lead to large changes in ICP.

Causes of altered cerebral blood volume may be (1) vasodilatation, (2) passive transmission of arterial blood pressure if autoregulation is lost, and (3) decrease in venous outflow.

Hyperemic brain swelling is a persistent state of vasodilatation that increases overall blood volume in the brain. Transient dilatation of cerebral resistance vessels occurs markedly with hypercapnia (almost on a millimeter-by-millimeter basis), with hypoxemia (PaO_2 less than 50 mmHg), and if the patient is exposed to volatile anesthetics such as halothane or nitrous oxide. Arterial pulsations are transmitted to the cerebral cavity most forcibly when mean arterial pressure exceeds 170 mmHg. Such pressures may be reached in normal persons while straining at stool and in the afterphase of the Valsalva maneuver. When intracranial pressure exceeds about 30 mmHg, autoregulation of cerebral blood volume is lost, and arterial pressure is passively transmitted to the cerebral circulation. With continuous ICP monitoring at such times, one finds greater amplitude of ICP pulse pressure and more marked arterial waveforms (dicrotic notch). Such arterial pulsations can produce a "water hammer" effect on brain cells, which may account for the permanent brain damage seen in such conditions as chronic hydrocephalus.

Finally, cerebral blood volume is increased if venous return is obstructed. This can happen with increases in intrathoracic pressure, as during the Valsalva maneuver or during positive end-expiratory pressure (PEEP) in respiratory therapy. Flexion of the neck and extreme head rotation have been demonstrated to obstruct the internal jugular vein and potentially compress basal CSF cisterns.

Measurement of Intracranial Pressure. Intracranial pressure monitoring research has demonstrated repeatedly that the presence of increased ICP cannot be reliably inferred from clinical signs and symptoms. In a patient at risk for intracranial hypertension, the only reliable means to determine whether it exists is to measure the ICP continuously.

There are many means of measuring ICP. The oldest and least reliable is single measurement of CSF pressure in the spinal sac during lumbar or cisternal puncture. Not only are single measurements useless in determining ongoing intracranial dynamics, but also any disorder that blocks free flow of CSF from cranial to spinal cavity invalidates the spinal pressure as a reliable estimate of intracranial pressure.

In a pioneering study conducted in the 1960s, intraventricular pressure was monitored continuously in over 100 patients with space-occupying lesions. This study led to ICP monitoring becoming commonplace in critical care units throughout the world. ICP may be measured by direct cannulation of a cerebral ventricle (usually a lateral ventricle), by pulsations in the subarachnoid space (via a "screw" or "bolt" threaded into the skull), by pulsations of the dura (epidural transducer), or by pulsations of the brain tissue (intraparenchymal). (See Chapter 4.) Pulsations of the CSF tissue or of the meninges are then converted to electrical signals and displayed by means of a graph or printout, or on a computer screen. These methods of ICP measurement (ventricular, subarachnoid, intraparenchymal, and epidural) are highly correlated linearly, although the actual values obtained tend to be lower with epidural recording.

In addition to continuous electronic monitoring, some institutions use external ventriculostomy shunts as indices of ICP. An intraventricular cannula is connected to a pressure reservoir external to the patient, and CSF is continuously drained against positive pressure. For example, if the surgeon wishes to maintain ICP at about 10 cmH$_2$O (about 8 mmHg), the pressure reservoir is set 10 cm above the zero ICP reference point (usually taken at the external auditory meatus). Whenever pressure inside the ventricle reaches or exceeds 10 cmH$_2$O, CSF drains into the reservoir. A manometer can be set up in such a system for intermittent measurement of ventricular fluid pressure. *Any manometer system must be considered as only an indication of ICP.* Manometers damp the rapid oscillations of ICP that are normally seen with heart rate and respiration. At rapid oscillation, the pressure measured in a manometer is likely to be falsely low by an undefined amount.

Ideally, ICP is expressed in millimeters of mercury to facilitate calculation of perfusion pressure. It will be recalled that cerebral perfusion pressure (CPP) reflects the mean arterial blood pressure (MABP) minus the mean intracranial pressure (MICP):

$$CPP = MABP - MICP$$

Normal ICP is generally accepted as 0 to 10 mmHg. Miller and colleagues[12] make a strong case for using 10 mmHg as the upper limit of normal. They cite numbers of patients with high elastance whose resting ICP was between 10 and 15 mmHg. In other words, though the resting ICP remained relatively "normal," addition of a small volume of fluid precipitated a marked rise in ICP. ICP values of 20 mmHg and over are uniformly regarded as elevated. Values greater than 40 mmHg are considered seriously elevated. Note that with an ICP of 40 mmHg and an MABP of 90 mmHg, CPP would be only 50 mmHg, barely adequate to sustain neuronal perfusion. Ranges of ICP are shown in Table 33-2. CPP normally ranges from 70 to 90 mmHg, with EEG changes evident experimentally when CPP drops below 45 mmHg.[13]

TABLE 33-2 **Ranges of Intracranial Pressure (Supratentorial Cavity)**

	mmHg	mmH$_2$O
Normal	0-10	0-136
Possibly elevated	11-15	150-204
Elevated	>15	>200
Moderately elevated	>20	>270
Markedly elevated	>40	>500

There is increasing clinical evidence that the level of CPP is the best predictor of outcome in severe head injuries and that uniformly poor outcomes are associated with CPP of less than 40 mmHg.[14,15] Most clinicians attempt to maintain a CPP no lower than 50 to 60 mmHg.

Medical Management of Intracranial Hypertension

There is no single therapy for intracranial hypertension. The ideal medical therapy would be to remove the cause of the increased ICP. When this cause is a mass lesion or a tumor that blocks CSF flow, such surgical therapy is definitive. Unfortunately, the majority of critically ill patients with intracranial hypertension do not have such lesions. Large series of head injury cases from specialized critical care settings in several countries indicate that patients with surgically treatable lesions make up 25% to 58% of all head-injured patients.[6,12,16,17]

For those patients who do not have surgically remediable lesions, the aim of medical therapy is to control intracranial hypertension and maintain adequate cerebral perfusion in order to protect the brain from secondary injury. Secondary injury is neuronal ischemia or hypoxia beyond that induced by the primary brain insult. Medical therapies can be categorized as pharmacological, mechanical, or systemic. These therapies and their proposed mechanisms of function are summarized in Table 33-3. The pharmacological and mechanical measures used to control ICP have multisystem effects. Consequently, careful attention must be paid to the fluid and electrolyte, respiratory, and cardiac status of the patient in whom these therapies are used.

Pharmacological therapies consist of hyperosmotic agents, corticosteroids, sedatives, and muscle-paralyzing and anesthetic agents. Hyperosmotic agents such as mannitol and glycerol draw fluid out of brain tissue by increasing the osmolality of the blood. Such agents depend upon an intact blood–brain barrier to prevent diffusion of the large molecules into the brain itself. Agents such as urea can cross the blood–brain barrier, equilibrate with brain interstitial fluid, and thus cause a rebound increase in ICP some hours after administration. The lesser ability of mannitol to diffuse across membranes is the factor behind the relatively low incidence of rebound effect in its use.[18] The usual dose is 0.5 to 1.0 g/kg, given as a bolus. The concomitant use of furosemide (Lasix) potentiates the duration of effect of mannitol. Repeated use of mannitol can lead to continuously elevated serum osmolality, with attendant risk of seizures, renal failure, and serious fluid and electrolyte imbalance. Consequently, urine output, serum electrolytes, and osmolality must be monitored frequently in patients receiving mannitol. Serum osmolality should be main-

TABLE 33-3　Medical Therapies Commonly Used in Uncontrolled Intracranial Hypertension

Medical Therapy	Proposed Mechanism	Nursing Responsibility
ICP >20-25 mmHg FOR >5 MIN Hyperventilation	Vasoconstriction: ↓ cerebral vasodilatation and thus cerebral blood volume	Maintain $Paco_2$ of 27-30 mmHg; may hyperinflate prior to noxious stimuli
Drain CSF against positive pressure (10-20 cmH$_2$O)	↓ CSF volume	Maintain positive pressure to avoid ventricular collapse; prevent infection with aseptic technique
Osmotic diuretics (mannitol, sometimes urea, glycerol); loop diuretics (furosemide)	↓ Brain water (may affect CSF formation)	Monitor serum osmolality; do not give if >315 mosm. Monitor electrolytes, particularly Na^+ and K^+. Monitor intake and output
ICP STILL >20-25 mmHg DESPITE ABOVE Sedation: diazepam (Valium), morphine (dose and combination vary with physician preference)	↓ Response to environmental stimuli; morphine may affect cerebral metabolism	Monitor respiration (sedation depresses rate if patient not receiving controlled ventilation). Monitor blood pressure (BP), maintain normotension. Pupillary response may be constricted by morphine
Muscle paralyzing agents (pancuronium)	↓ Motor response; prevents Valsalva, isometric muscle contractions that ↑ BP; prevents posturing	Protect patient from assumption that lack of movement means lack of hearing; protect eyes; prevent immobility complications. Careful observation of pupillary changes (dilatation), which may be only sign of seizures, herniation
Anesthetic agents: short-acting barbiturates, lidocaine	↓ Cerebral metabolism; topical lidocaine ↓ cough response to suctioning	Barbiturates: monitor cardiac output, BP, maintain normotension, temperature (therapy induces poikilothermia), urinary output; may monitor EEG; only evidence of seizures is sudden pupillary dilatation. Lidocaine in bolus may induce seizures

tained below 315 to 320 mosm.

Corticosteroids, particularly dexamethasone (Decadron) and methylprednisolone (Solumedrol), are frequently given to control ICP. Although the efficacy of corticosteroids on the edema surrounding tumors is well established, there is no similar evidence for the value of corticosteroids in brain edema secondary to head injury. Prospective double-blind studies have not shown any differences in outcome or level of ICP in patients treated with placebo, low-dose steroids, or high-dose steroids.[19,20,21] Some argue, however, that the high doses used in clinical studies (up to 3.0 mg/kg of dexamethasone) are not high enough to demonstrate the effect seen in laboratory studies and that corticosteroids exert their helpful effects by inhibiting lipid perioxidation rather than by glucocorticoid properties.[10,22] Although steroids are often implicated as the cause of gastrointestinal bleeding in head trauma patients, the incidence of gastrointestinal bleeding, hyperglycemia, and infection has not been demonstrated to be greater in steroid-treated patients than in those given placebo.[19,20,22]

Sedating agents such as morphine sulfate and benzodiazepines (chiefly diazepam) are often given to reduce responsiveness to environmental stimuli and thereby maintain ICP at a more even level. It is also thought that morphine may exert a direct effect on cerebral metabolism and thereby on cerebral blood volume. Muscle-paralyzing agents are intended to reduce decerebrate posturing and other sustained muscle contractions that serve to increase blood pressure and thus increase cerebral blood flow in the nonautoregulating brain. The most common agent used is pancuronium (Pavulon), because of its relatively short duration of action and thus ease of reversal. Because all muscles are paralyzed, including those of respiration, this drug is used only in mechanically ventilated patients. It is crucial to remember that this drug is not a CNS sedative; a patient will *appear* unresponsive because motor output is lost but may be completely aware of what is occurring in the environment.

Anesthetic agents often used in the control of ICP include barbiturates and lidocaine. Barbiturate coma has fluctuating popularity in controlling intracranial hypertension that has been unresponsive to other therapies. Decreased mortality has been shown in some uncontrolled studies in patients with uncontrollable ICP treated with pentobarbital or thiopentone. However, controlled studies comparing high-dose barbiturates to similar treatment without barbiturates have not shown any difference in long-term outcome in either head injury or postcardiac arrest.[24,25,26] A variety of short- and long-acting barbiturates are used, with the aim of maintaining serum levels at about 3 to 5 mg/dl. The mechanism of action in head injury is not clear. Current hypotheses include a direct vasoconstrictive effect on cerebral vessels, reduction of cerebral blood flow secondary to decreased cerebral metabolism, and amelioration of cerebral edema secondary to reducing formation of free oxygen radicals. Barbiturate coma requires complete supportive care of the comatose, ventilated patient. In addition, monitoring of arterial blood pressure, cardiac output, and pulmonary wedge pressure is needed in view of the systemic effects of barbiturates on cardiac output and blood pressure. Hypotension (due to reduced cardiac output) is a serious potential problem with this therapy, since it can compromise CPP.

Lidocaine is often used topically to reduce the ICP response to suctioning and has also been found to reduce ICP over a sustained time when given in intravenous boluses.[27] Like all anesthetics, lidocaine has the potential to induce seizures and depress respirations and cardiac rhythms. Consequently, these parameters must be monitored when lidocaine is used on a prn basis.

Mechanical therapies include the use of hyperventilation and drainage of CSF. Assisted ventilation, with hyperventilation to maintain $PaCO_2$ at around 27 to 30 mmHg, is commonly used to control ICP. It should be recalled that increases in $PaCO_2$ act as potent vasodilators and thus increase cerebral blood volume. Conversely, a decrease in $PaCO_2$, as in hyperventilation, acts to constrict cerebral vessels. The very low $PaCO_2$ levels formerly used (20 to 25 mmHg) may induce cerebral ischemia and are no longer commonly prescribed.

Continuous or intermittent drainage of CSF is particularly indicated when the cause of intracranial hypertension is increased production or blocked circulation of CSF. It is of little value in brain hyperemia or in edema. Indeed, in such cases, drainage of CSF may lead to ventricular collapse and loss of all opportunity to monitor ventricular fluid pressure. CSF drainage does not change the shape of the volume–pressure curve—that is, does not change elastance.[28] Absolute pressure can be reduced, thus improving cerebral perfusion pressure temporarily. Drainage against positive pressure is the safest way to prevent ventricular collapse. Rapid removal of CSF and ventricular collapse can cause the brain to pull away from the dura, rupturing bridging veins and perhaps adding subdural hematoma to the patient's problems.

Systemic support refers to general medical therapies that maintain blood pressure and adequate ventilation. Since cerebral perfusion pressure is clearly the *key* factor in survival and ultimate outcome in patients with severe head injuries, it is critical to maintain adequate systemic blood pressure. In patients with normal CT scans at admission who ultimately develop intracranial hypertension, abnormally low blood pressure is one of the few predictive factors.[8,28,29] Medical therapies for patients with dysrhythmias, hypotension, and adult respiratory distress syndrome are discussed in Chapters 10, 7, and 29, respectively.

NURSING MANAGEMENT OF INTRACRANIAL HYPERTENSION

Intracranial hypertension is a clinical problem that coexists with a number of medical diagnoses (Table 33-1). Nursing implementation of the medical therapies described above requires considerable knowledge and independent judgment. For example, when intracranial pressure is rising, the nurse must decide whether to give or withhold mannitol on the basis of the osmolality. Management of the blood pressure and prevention of infection are part of the judgment nurses use in caring for patients in barbiturate coma. In addition, nurses have been trying to delineate a nursing diagnosis that indicates the complexity of the independent nursing judgment and management required in the care of patients with intracranial hypertension.

A number of diagnostic labels have been proposed for nursing diagnoses associated with the clinical problem of intracranial hypertension, including potential for secondary brain injury, decreased cerebral perfusion pressure, alteration in cerebral tissue perfusion, and decreased intracranial adaptive capacity.[30,31] The diagnosis *decreased intracranial adaptive capacity* is used in this chapter because it can be defined in terms of clinically recognizable indicators and can be managed independently by nurses. (See also

Chapter 18.) Decreased cerebral perfusion pressure is itself an indicator for this diagnosis; altered cerebral tissue perfusion cannot be verified clinically; and potential for secondary brain injury is a clinical problem that encompasses more than just intracranial hypertension.

Decreased intracranial adaptive capacity is caused by the failure of normal intracranial compensatory mechanisms and is manifested by repeated disproportionate increases in ICP in response to a variety of noxious and other stimuli. Thus, the patient with intracranial hypertension whose ICP is increased 5 to 10 mmHg above baseline for 3 minutes or longer with turning, suctioning, or verbal stimuli is manifesting decreased intracranial adaptive capacity. The intracranial system is unable to compensate for the transient increases in cerebral blood volume, systemic blood pressure, or trapped CSF that accompany these activities, and thus, ICP increases markedly with small changes in input to the system. Nursing management of patients with this diagnosis has two major goals: to reduce adaptive demand and to increase adaptive capacity. Activities that accomplish these goals are described below.

Not every patient with intracranial hypertension has decreased adaptive capacity, nor is it desirable to wait until those with the diagnosis have marked and potentially harmful increases in ICP with ordinary care activities. Therefore, it is useful to identify patients at high risk for the diagnosis and institute nursing management that decreases adaptive demands and increases adaptive capacity.

Patients with any disorder that is associated with intracranial hypertension (Table 33-1) are potentially at risk for decreased intracranial adaptive capacity. Those with CT evidence of brain hyperemia or edema with decreased or absent visualization of ventricles are at even higher risk. In the presence of trauma or cerebral disorders that produce brain swelling, the absence of visible ventricles and compression of the basal cisterns both indicate loss of the major intracranial compensatory mechanism—the CSF ventricular and spinal spaces that increase CSF capacity. The presence of hypotension adds to the risk factors.

If ICP is not monitored electronically, it must be assumed that patients with the above risk factors have high potential for both the clinical problem, intracranial hypertension, and the nursing diagnosis, decreased intracranial adaptive capacity. If the patient has an ICP monitor, the clinical problem of intracranial hypertension will be evident, and several pieces of clinical data more easily identify the patient who is at high risk for the nursing diagnosis of decreased intracranial adaptive capacity. These risk factors have

been identified from clinical research and include:[31]
Repeated large and sustained increases in ICP in response to a nursing maneuver (>10 mmHg above baseline for >3 minutes)
Abnormal volumetric challenge response
Any two of the following: ICP >20 mmHg, CPP <50 mmHg, wide-amplitude ICP tracing

A single disproportionate response to a nursing care activity or environmental demand is somewhat predictive of further such increases.[31] Volumetric challenges may be either a roughly reversible challenge such as brief bilateral compression of the external jugular veins (reduces venous return, thus leaving more blood in the cranial vessels), or a controlled addition of a small bolus of saline to the ventricles. A noticeable increase in ICP in response to bilateral compression or an ICP increase that is at least twice the volume of fluid injected is considered abnormal. Volumetric challenges are usually under supervision of the patient's physician and thus provide additional but not integral information related to the nursing diagnosis.

NURSING MANAGEMENT OF DECREASED INTRACRANIAL ADAPTIVE CAPACITY

As noted earlier, the goals of nursing interventions for the diagnosis *decreased intracranial adaptive capacity* are to reduce adaptive demands (activities that increase cerebral blood volume or CSF volume) and increase adaptive capacity (activities that improve cerebral compliance). Concomitant with these independent activities are those involved in collaboratively managing the medical therapies for the basic clinical problem of intracranial hypertension. The outlines below summarize nursing care for both the nursing diagnoses and the clinical problems in patients with intracranial hypertension, then further expand on the nursing interventions according to precipitating factor and mechanisms involved.

■ NURSING DIAGNOSIS

Decreased intracranial adaptive capacity, related to inadequate or failing normal compensatory mechanisms.

- *Defining Characteristics:* Repeated disproportionate rises in ICP with environmental stimuli
- *Clinical Indicator:* Repeated sharp increases in ICP with stimuli (≥10 mmHg, above baseline ≥3 minutes)
- *Risk factors:* ICP ≥20 mmHg, CPP <50 mmHg; wide-amplitude ICP trace; high elastance or low compliance

OUTCOME STANDARD AND CRITERIA

Intracranial adaptive capacity will be improved as evidenced by:

- Absence of sustained (>3-minute) increases in ICP following nursing care activities
- CPP maintained at >50 mmHg

GENERAL NURSING INTERVENTIONS

Demand on intracranial adaptive capacity can be reduced by spacing activities, turning patient slowly, and reducing environmental stimuli.

Adaptive capacity will be increased by:

- Positioning patient's head for maximum venous return
- Use of medical therapies such as sedation or osmotic diuretics prior to known noxious stimuli

SPECIFIC NURSING INTERVENTIONS

Precipitating activity: Passive or active turning in bed. *Mechanisms:* Decreased venous outflow secondary to head flexion or rotation; increased BP with Valsalva; arousal response:

- Maintain patient's head and neck in neutral position throughout turn
- Use turning sheet or turning bed for exceptionally labile patients
- Premedicate with prn sedation or muscle relaxants in labile patients

Precipitating factor: Decerebrate or decorticate posturing. *Mechanism:* Increased BP secondary to isometric muscle contraction:

- Use slow, sustained movements
- Premedicate with pancuronium or muscle relaxants prior to movement

Precipitating activity: Head rotation or flexion. *Mechanisms:* Decreased venous outflow, possibly transient occlusion of CSF outflow to spinal sac:

- Maintain patient's head in neutral position with small pillows
- Do not allow head to flex during patient positioning
- Cervical collar may be useful

Precipitating factor: Bowel evacuation. *Mechanisms:* Increased intrathoracic pressure and BP secondary to Valsalva; in conscious patients, isometric muscle contractions involved in using bedpan:

Prevent constipation: use stool softeners, adequate fluids, prn suppositories.

Precipitating factor: Coughing. *Mechanism:* Increased intrathoracic pressure and BP; stimulated by suctioning, endotracheal tube, PEEP:

- Firmly secure endotracheal tube to prevent movement in trachea
- Minimize suction time (<10 seconds); no more than two suction passes
- Maintain head-up position (15° to 30°) to increase venous outflow unless CPP drops in head-up position
- Use lidocaine prn endotracheally prior to suctioning in particularly labile patients; pancuronium may be used also

Precipitating factor: Sensory stimuli (touch, conversation, noise). *Mechanism:* Possibly increased or decreased ICP; increase may be secondary to arousal or startle response; mechanism of decrease not clear:

- Approach all patients as if they hear and process sensory stimuli
- Warn patient prior to touching; stroke slowly and firmly
- Minimize loud noises in environment
- Use stimuli that are associated with decreased ICP for the individual patient

■ **NURSING DIAGNOSIS**

Pain (headache), related to CSF pulsations and effect of mass lesion on pain-sensitive dural structures.

- *Defining Characteristics:* Restlessness, verbalization of head pain

NURSING INTERVENTIONS

- Decrease adaptive demands as described above to minimize transient increases
- Medicate with nonnarcotic analgesics on regular basis
- Maintain patient in head-up position

COLLABORATIVE PROBLEM

High risk for inadequate cerebral perfusion, related to decreased adaptive capacity.

- *Defining Characteristics:*

CPP ≤50 mmHg even transiently with given environmental stimuli

Highest risk in patients with systemic hypotension and intracranial hypertension

NURSING INTERVENTIONS

- Monitor ICP and systemic arterial blood pressure (SABP)
- Reduce demands on intracranial system as above

COLLABORATIVE PROBLEM

High risk for transtentorial brain herniation, related to decreased adaptive capacity.

- *Defining Characteristics:*

Rapid, persistent increase in ICP despite usual efforts to control

Sudden expansion of intracranial mass, evident by CT or ultrasound

Highest risk in patients with active intracranial bleeding

NURSING INTERVENTIONS

- Monitor ICP and SABP
- Monitor for signs of brain herniation (changes in level of consciousness, pupil equality, motor signs)

Nursing activities that represent adaptive demands are those that have been systematically identified as influencing ICP: prone position; turning in bed; endotracheal suctioning; use of bedpan; rapid shift in position; head rotation; conversation about prognosis, pain, and condition; and cumulative nursing care activity, regardless of nature.[31,32] Modifications of nursing care relevant to patients at risk for decreased intracranial adaptive capacity can be inferred from the mechanisms influencing ICP.

Nursing activities that increase cerebral blood volume should be avoided. Any activity that increases systemic arterial pressure may increase cerebral blood volume when autoregulation has failed. In the injured brain, this failure of autoregulation may occur at a point far below the limits in the normal brain. Activities known to increase MABP include coughing, Valsalva maneuver, and isometric muscle contractions. Frequent decerebrate posturing is particularly troublesome in this regard. Any tactile stimulus in the course of care may stimulate such posturing, and pancuronium (Pavulon) or phenothiazines (Thorazine) may be necessary to reduce it.

Cerebral blood volume can also be increased by obstruction to venous outflow. Head rotation obstructs jugular venous return, as does the Valsalva maneuver. Moderate elevation of the head (15° to 30°) improves venous outflow and can be shown to decrease ICP. When patients are turned, special care should be paid to the position of the head to avoid forward, backward, and lateral neck flexion and head rotation.

Prone position probably increases ICP by a combination of abdominal compression and jugular compression from head rotation. Fortunately, with assisted ventilation and mechanical aids to prevent skin breakdown, the use of the prone position is not crucial for the critically ill patient.

Suctioning can produce hypoxemia, leading to vasodilatation and increased blood pressure related to coughing. Although suctioning is often noted to increase ICP, careful attention to minimizing the suction period, no more than two passes of 10 seconds each, and pretreatment with oxygen can minimize but not completely prevent many of the increases seen with uncontrolled suction.[33,34]

Positioning the patient to prevent obstruction of CSF flow is important. CSF flow obstruction due to a pathological condition is beyond the control of the nurse, but the body position of the patient can create transient obstruction to CSF flow. Head rotation and neck flexion and extension not only obstruct venous outflow but probably briefly obstruct free passage of CSF between cranial and spinal dural sacs. In the patient with high elastance, even small amounts of CSF trapped in the cranial cavity can increase ICP. The supine position is most likely to create forward neck flexion, whereas lateral positions with the head in neutral position allow free flow of CSF into the spinal sac.

The mechanisms underlying increases and decreases in ICP seen with turning the patient in bed are not clear. Obstruction of CSF flow between cranial and spinal sacs, blood pressure waves secondary to rapid movement, and stimulation of decerebrate posturing are among the possibilities. Not all patients have an increase in ICP with turning. Patients with decreased adaptive capacity manifested by response to other maneuvers are at highest risk. Several studies have shown minimal ICP and CPP response to turning in patients with a baseline ICP below 15 mmHg and in those who have no increase with the initial turn in a sequence.[31] Cumulative effects of nursing activities have not been demonstrated consistently in nursing studies. It is likely that the patients who demonstrate a cumulative increase in ICP with a series of nursing care activities are those with decreased adaptive capacity, and that such a cumulative increase is not seen with all patients.

Independent nursing interventions are aimed primarily at decreasing adaptive demands by modifying procedures such as turning and suctioning, but some specific activities can be used to increase adaptive capacity. In patients with communicating hydrocephalus, the elevated head position or side-lying position may increase adaptive capacity by improving venous return or CSF flow. Careful timing of medical pharmacological therapies such as mannitol may increase compliance before a known noxious stimulus occurs and may also increase adaptive capacity. Finally, there is some evidence that interpersonal activities such as stroking and soothing verbal communication reduce ICP, at least in some children. The mechanism is unknown, but it may be speculated that such activities improve intracranial adaptive capacity.

These nursing management measures are designed to minimize or prevent frequent transient increases in ICP in the patient with intracranial hypertension. Despite careful nursing management, it is possible for the intracranial pressure to rise steeply in response to basic pathophysiological processes. In such cases, it is necessary to use the medical protocol to reduce ICP and maintain CPP. Nursing measures should never be substituted for the medical protocol in such situations.

Subarachnoid Hemorrhage and Cerebral Vasospasm

Another pathophysiological state that is a source of sudden or gradual deterioration in level of consciousness or general neurological function is cerebral vasospasm following subarachnoid hemorrhage. Subarachnoid hemorrhage may occur spontaneously in persons with uncontrolled hypertension or it may result from head trauma that ruptures cerebral arterioles, particularly in the vertebrobasilar system, or from rupture of saccular aneurysms in the intracranial circulation, particularly in the circle of Willis.

Vasospasm is defined in this context as a narrowing of the arteries of the circle of Willis and its major branches that is verified by angiography. Since angiography is not routinely performed in patients with subarachnoid hemorrhage without neurological deficit, the true overall incidence is unknown. However, a number of reports are available documenting vasospasm in patients with subarachnoid hemorrhage who develop new neurological deficits and who have not had fresh bleeding from their aneurysm. These reports suggest that the incidence of neurological deficit attributable to vasospasm in aneurysm patients ranges from 21% to 50%.[35,36,37] The extent of symptomatic vasospasm in posttraumatic subarachnoid hemorrhage is difficult to determine, because the initial injury often substantially impairs consciousness and neurological function. Some angiographic series are available, however, and the incidence of angiographic vasospasm has been estimated at 20% or more in trauma patients as well.[7,17]

Cerebral vasospasm is more common following subarachnoid hemorrhage in patients with intracranial hypertension, severe initial neurological deficits, and large collections of blood in the basilar cisterns on CT scan. The presence of intraventricular hemorrhage is not predictive of vasospasm.[35,37,38] For reasons not yet clearly understood, the presence of blood in the subarachnoid space stimulates intense constriction of cerebral vessels. It is thought that over time, this constriction leads to inadequate cellular respiration of the vessel, a subsequent inflammatory reaction, impairment of the normal regulation of muscle relaxation by Ca^{2+}, swelling of the intima, and endothelial damage. A variety of vasoactive substances, such as serotonin, prostaglandins, and catecholamines, have been postulated as initiators of the vasoconstriction. The subsequent intimal swelling is believed to contribute to ischemia by increasing vessel resistance and decreasing blood flow. The end result of sustained vasospasm is reduction of flow to brain cells in the distribution of the involved artery, ischemia, and ultimately cerebral infarction.

Cerebral vasospasm is most likely to occur 4 to 12 days after the subarachnoid hemorrhage and should be suspected in any patient with a ruptured aneurysm or head trauma who begins to deteriorate neurologically. A CT scan can quickly rule out fresh bleeding or acute communicating hydrocephalus as the source of new changes in consciousness.

Medical Management of Subarachnoid Hemorrhage and Vasospasm

Medical management of subarachnoid hemorrhage from aneurysm varies considerably. Some neurosurgeons restrict fluid intake, induce systemic hy-

potension, and delay surgical repair of the aneurysm as long as possible to allow time for reduction of brain swelling, while others operate early to reduce the chance of rerupture of the aneurysm and use calcium channel blockers and volume expansion to reduce vasospasm.[37] The antifibrinolytic agent aminocaproic acid (Amicar) is used by some physicians to prevent clot lysis and thus rerupture of the aneurysm while waiting for surgery. Antifibrinolytics have been shown to lower the incidence of rebleeding, but they are also associated with a higher likelihood of vasospasm and with other complications related to abnormal clotting, such as deep venous thrombosis and pulmonary embolism.[37] Current research supports early surgery, subarachnoid clot removal, and calcium channel blockers as the most effective regimen.[35,37]

Nursing Management of Subarachnoid Hemorrhage and Vasospasm

Nursing management in this clinical problem is collaborative with medical management. The clinical problem is the potential for vasospasm and permanent neurological deficit. The desired outcome is early detection of vasospasm and improvement of cerebral perfusion. Initial action consists of knowledgeable monitoring of clinical status, particularly for subtle changes in level of consciousness and motor or reflex status. A protocol should be in effect that allows for prompt CT scanning to rule out fresh bleeding and institution of hypervolemic and hypertensive therapy. Nursing monitoring of neurological, hemodynamic, respiratory, and ICP status is crucial in titrating this therapy to the point of neurological improvement without inducing pulmonary edema.

Pharmacological therapies are aimed at preventing vasospasm or at reducing ischemia if vasospasm has occurred. Calcium channel blockers such as nimodipine and nicardipine have been shown to reduce ischemic deficits when compared to placebo.[35,37] Once vasospasm has occurred, hypervolemic and hypertensive therapy is directed at increasing CPP in the hope of improving cerebral microcirculation in the ischemic area. Intracranial pressure is monitored and reduced if necessary via ventricular drainage and osmotic diuresis. Intravascular volume is expanded with intravenous crystalloids and colloids to maintain a pulmonary artery wedge pressure of approximately 18 to 20 mmHg, with recommended hematocrit reading of 30% to 40%. If the neurological status does not improve, controlled hypertension is induced with vasopressors, raising the blood pressure to the level that will effect improvement in neurological status or until the systolic pressure is in the range of 180 to 200 mmHg. Bradycardia and diuresis may occur reflexly with this regimen and are managed with atropine to maintain the heart rate at 80 to 120 beats per minute.[37,38]

Brain Herniation Syndromes

Observation for brain herniation syndromes is undoubtedly the most commonly taught neurological assessment procedure in nursing. Yet the pathophysiology and the nature of what the nurse is attempting to prevent are often left unclear. Brain herniation is usually discussed under increased intracranial pressure, without a clear distinction between the two. Syndromes of central and uncal herniation are addressed as if they were one, and cerebellar herniation is rarely described at all. The following presentation is an attempt to clarify the situation. The widely accepted Plum and Posner classification of herniation syndromes is used here to place syndromes in categories by functional anatomy.[39]

Herniation refers to the protrusion of an organ through a natural or accidental opening in the wall of its cavity. In the brain, herniation is the protrusion of a portion of the brain through the openings or linings of the cranial cavity. Although the incisure or notch of the tentorium (Figure 33-2) is the best known of these natural openings, herniation can also occur under the falx cerebri and through the foramen magnum. Three distinctive syndromes may result: (1) that of cingulate lobe herniation, which involves movement laterally under the falx cerebri; (2) the syndrome of central or uncal transtentorial herniation (through the incisure); and (3) the syndrome of cerebellar herniation, which takes place either upward through the incisure or downward through the foramen magnum.

Each of these involves displacement of brain through or around openings in the lining of the cranial cavity. Each produces a distinctive syndrome by virtue of displacement, distortion, or necrosis of specific brain tissue.

Transtentorial Herniation. For all practical purposes, cingulate herniation can be considered with transtentorial syndromes, since any condition that creates cingulate herniation is likely to produce transtentorial herniation also. The unifying and essential feature of cingulate-tentorial syndromes is the rostral–caudal, or literally "head-to-tail," nature of their progression. They are caused by any of a variety of expanding mass lesions above the tentorium. Anything that acts as a mass in the relatively closed cranial cavity and which is growing will eventually push aside and distort brain tissue. Eventually, the expanding brain will seek a relief valve by herniating through the few openings available—around the falx, through the tentorium, or through the foramen magnum. The numerous conditions that can lead to an increase in brain mass and brain herniation are listed in Table 33-4. The most obvious is a brain tumor. Similarly, the clot from an intracerebral hemorrhage acts as a mass, and as an expanding one if hemorrhage continues. General or local brain edema also increases the mass of the brain. Trauma, contusions, thrombotic and embolic stroke, hypoxia, and metabolic and infectious processes can create areas of focal or general edema.

Although many of the conditions listed in Table 33-4 may lead to increased intracranial pressure, it is important to remember that intracranial hypertension by itself does not inevitably lead to herniation unless the cause of the elevated pressure is also a cause of mass effect (for example, massive brain edema). Herniation may also be secondary to intracranial hypertension if pressure is rising very rapidly or if there are

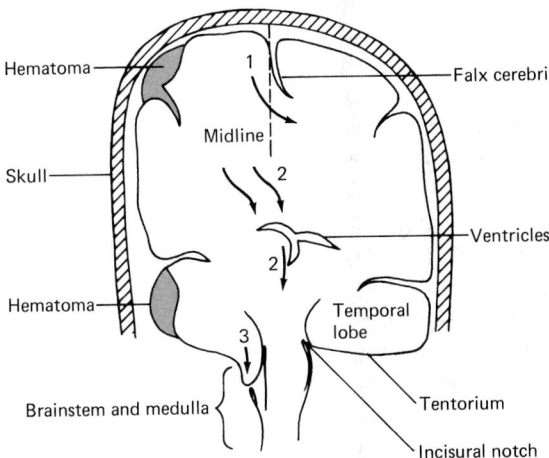

Figure 33-2 Three types of supratentorial herniation. Cingulate herniation (1) occurs when the falx cerebri is displaced. Central herniation (2) is the downward movement of the brain, displacing the ventricles. Uncal herniation (3) involves compression of the midbrain and brainstem by the herniating tip of the temporal lobe.

Based on Moidel, H., et al. (Eds.). (1976). *Nursing care of the patient with medical-surgical disorders* (2nd ed.). New York: McGraw-Hill.

TABLE 33-4 Symptoms of Brainstem Compression Caused by Brain Herniation

Symptoms	Cause of Brain Herniation
Diminished consciousness; coma (with inability to communicate and to protect airway)	Head injury, e.g., contusion leading to subdural or epidural hematoma; intracranial hemorrhage
Respiratory alkalosis/acidosis from impaired breathing patterns	Cerebral edema from head trauma, tumor, metabolic or fluid–electrolyte disturbance (e.g., Reye's syndrome)
Decerebrate/decorticate rigidity	
Intracranial hypertension (may coexist)	

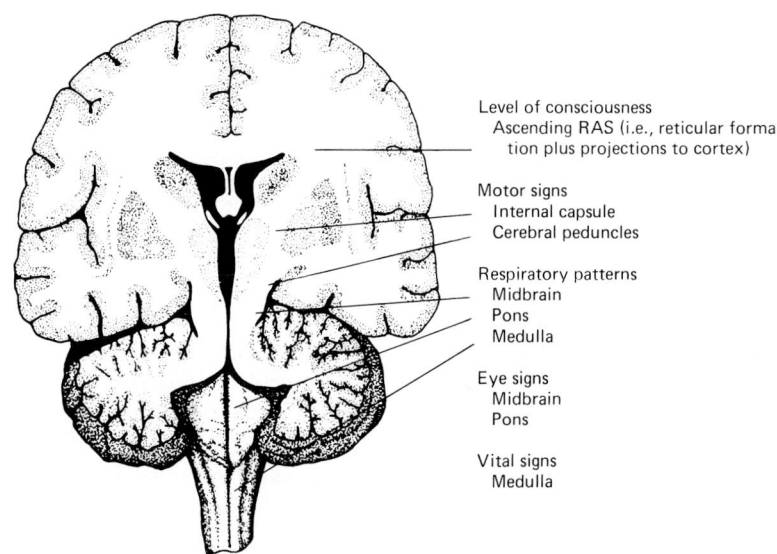

Level of consciousness
  Ascending RAS (i.e., reticular forma-
    tion plus projections to cortex)

Motor signs
  Internal capsule
  Cerebral peduncles

Respiratory patterns
  Midbrain
  Pons
  Medulla

Eye signs
  Midbrain
  Pons

Vital signs
  Medulla

Figure 33-3 Categories of brain function that may be affected by brain herniation as it reaches the levels shown. Courtesy of George McNeil.

pressure differentials between supratentorial and infratentorial compartments.

Astute observation of changing neurological function can not only aid in early detection of progressing herniation but also help the experienced clinician determine the area of brain still functioning. This last is crucial to detecting further deterioration once consciousness has been lost. It is also central to protecting the patient against complications resulting from an absence of defenses such as gag and corneal reflexes.

The purposes of assessment in conditions that place the patient at high risk for brain herniation are (1) to detect progressing brain herniation, (2) to determine the level of brain functioning, and (3) to determine the extent of protective care required. Although Chapter 31 provides a review of general neuroanatomy and physiology, pertinent functional neuroanatomy is presented here to aid in understanding how signs and symptoms relate to the brain function impaired. Although all nurses know the general signs of herniation ("neurocheck"), there is frequently an overreliance on signs of brainstem dysfunction (pupils) through failure to appreciate the rostral–caudal nature of herniation.

Because of the widespread influence of the ascending reticular activating system, changes in the level of consciousness are the earliest and often most subtle signs of progressing brain dysfunction. In central and transtentorial herniation, changes in respiratory pattern and motor function closely follow alterations in consciousness. Conjugate eye movements, equal pupil size, and pupil reactivity change when brain function is disrupted at the level of the midbrain (at approximately the same level as the tentorial incisure).

The rostral–caudal pattern of brain herniation generally progresses through five categories of brain function. Inspection of Figure 33-3 shows that these functions correspond roughly to anatomical levels of the brain. To determine whether the patient is getting better or worse and at what level the brain is functioning, the practitioner must routinely evaluate all five categories. The categories of brain function, in descending order, are level of consciousness, motor function, respiratory patterns, eye function (movements and pupillary reaction), and vital signs.

Level of Consciousness. Consciousness, arousability, and orientation to self and environment are governed by the reticular activating system (RAS). This system originates in the brainstem and ascends to influence the cerebral cortex (see Chapter 31). Because it is widespread, disturbances at many levels affect consciousness. Although changes in level of consciousness clearly indicate that brain function is disrupted, knowing the level of disruption requires information from the other assessment parameters, particularly motor function and eye movements. Nevertheless, a change in consciousness is a clear indication that brain function is further disrupted.

Many schemes have been proposed to quantitate consciousness and to construct a terminology consistent among medical centers. Probably the most useful measure is a very simple one, the *Glasgow Coma Scale* (Table 33-5). It was devised to systematically record neurological function in a multi-institutional study of the outcomes of head injury. In the coma scale, consciousness is evaluated with respect to three kinds of response to stimuli: eye opening, verbal response, and motor response. A sample assessment record is shown in Figure 33-4.

TABLE 33-5 Glasgow Coma Scale

Category of Response	Appropriate Stimulus	Response	Score
Eyes open	Approach to the bedside	*Spontaneous*	4
	Verbal command	*To speech.* Eyes open to name or to command	3
	Pain (pressure on the proximal nail bed)*	*To pain.* Does not open eyes to previous stimuli but does to pain	2
		None. Does not open eyes to any stimulus	1
Best verbal response	Maximum arousal. Painful stimulus may be needed	*Oriented.* Converses; knows who he or she is and where, year and month	
		Confused. Converses but disoriented in one or more spheres	4
		Inappropriate words. Without sustained conversation; words disorganized or inappropriate (for example, cursing)	3
		Incomprehensible. Makes sounds (moaning, for example) but no recognizable words	2
		None. No sound even with painful stimuli	1
Best motor response	Verbal command (for example: "Raise your arm; hold up two fingers")	*Obeys command*	6
	Pain (pressure on the proximal nail bed)	*Localizes pain.* Does not obey but "finds" offending stimulus and attempts to remove it	5
		Flexion-withdrawal.† Flexes arm in response to pain, without abnormal flexion posture	
		Abnormal flexion. Flexes arm at elbow and pronates, making a fist	3
		Abnormal extension. Extends arm at elbow, usually adducts and internally rotates arm at shoulder	2
		None	1

* Produces least interrater variability.
† Added to the original scale by many centers.

The kind of stimulus required and response obtained are rough measures of arousability. If a verbal stimulus does not produce measurable response (eye opening, verbal response, obeying command), a painful stimulus is employed. Points can be assigned to each level of response and a coma score obtained. Provided that instruction is given, a high degree of interrater reliability can be achieved by different levels of staff assessing the same patient. Any change of two points or more on the total coma score is likely to represent a real improvement or deterioration.[40] A number of publications are available for instructing staff on use of the scale.[41,42,43]

When recorded in conjunction with data regarding respiratory pattern, symmetry and type of motor response, pupillary response, and eye movements, the coma scale allows one to see graphically any progression toward brain herniation and to judge the level at which the brain is functioning. This last not only allows the physician to better diagnose the nature of the disorder causing progressive brain dysfunction but also allows the nurse and physician to recognize early the need to protect functions dependent upon brainstem reflexes such as coughing, gagging, and swallowing.

Motor Function. Evaluation of motor response brought the most consistent ratings in testing the reliability of the Glasgow Coma Scale. However, best

Neurological Assessment Record

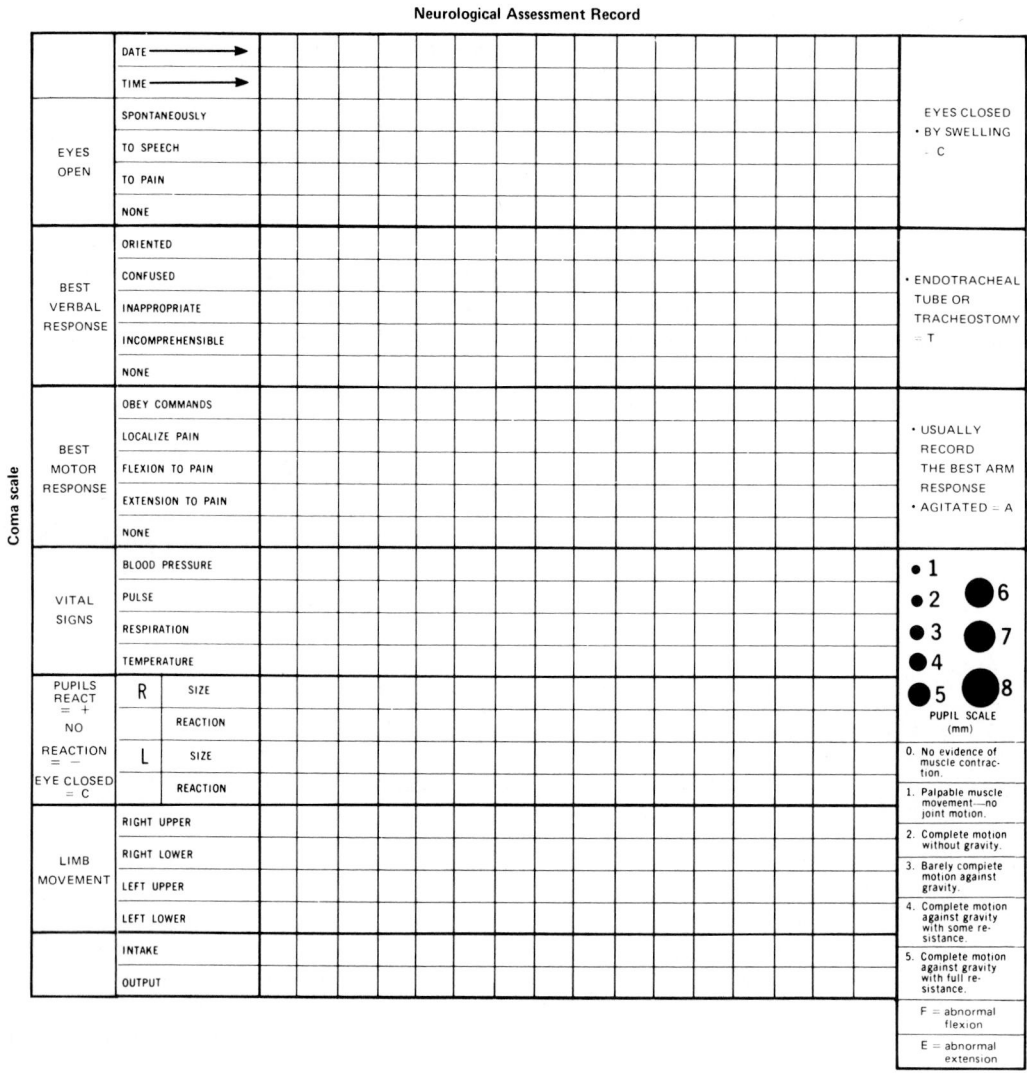

Figure 33-4   Neurological assessment record employing the Glasgow Coma Scale (reduced from original size). A suggested operational definition of coma is a score of 7 or less (no eye opening, no comprehensible verbal response, no motor response to command). Dysphasic patients cannot be scored on the verbal section; a note is made on the observation record of dysphasia or mechanical impediment to speech, such as endotracheal tube or tracheostomy.

motor response to stimulation is only one aspect of motor function that must be considered in determining whether brain function is worsening.

Motor function should be evaluated serially and systematically in relation to the following areas: type of response to verbal or painful stimuli, tone and strength, symmetry of response, and presence of pathological reflexes.

The ability to obey a command to perform a motor act is one measure of how well consciousness and voluntary movement are integrated. Impairment of consciousness (operationally defined as inability to follow a motor command) requires use of a painful stimulus. A variety of painful stimuli are employed to elicit motor response, but the Glasgow group found

pressure applied to the proximal nail bed to provide the most reproducible motor response.

A number of terms have evolved to describe motor response, some related to the "appropriateness" of response to pain, others to the presumed anatomical deficit causing abnormal reflex response (for example, *decerebrate* and *decorticate*). Such terms are open to a range of subjective interpretation and are not as helpful in identifying a rostral–caudal pattern of deterioration as the operationally defined responses of the Glasgow Coma Scale. The coma scale defines "best" motor response in relation to consciousness per se. Response on both sides of the body (symmetry of response) must also be compared.

The type of stimulus applied (verbal, then painful

if there is no response to verbal) and the nature of the response are noted. At the highest level of integration, the patient follows a verbal command, for example, "Hold out both arms." With some impairment of consciousness, a painful stimulus may need to be applied. If there are functioning motor tracts (corticospinal and corticobulbar), the patient will attempt to remove the painful stimulus. Pathological motor responses are evident in flexion and extension at the elbow in response to painful stimuli. These responses imply functional disconnection of the inhibiting influences of the cerebral cortex on motor tract synapses deep in the hemisphere and midbrain. Appearance of these abnormal postural reflexes spontaneously or in response to pain indicate that transtentorial herniation is impending or may already have occurred. *Decerebrate* and *decorticate posture* (or simply *posturing*) are terms commonly used in reference to these pathological postural reflexes.

The appearance of an extensor plantar reflex *(Babinski's sign)* implies dysfunction of the corticospinal tract anywhere from the cortex to the anterior horn cell in the spinal cord. The appearance of this abnormal reflex as a new finding does not help localize the dysfunction, but it does indicate deterioration of brain function in the patient at risk for herniation.

Strength and tone of muscles must be evaluated in conjunction with type of motor response. Motor fibers are fairly widely distributed at the cortex but converge into a relatively tight bundle deep in the hemisphere. Because fibers from the upper extremities are lateral in the corticospinal bundle until they reach the internal capsule, pressure from an expanding hemispheric lesion may cause subtle weakness before consciousness is markedly impaired. Such weakness tends to affect the proximal rather than distal muscles of the upper extremity. Thus, simply testing strength of hand grip may not detect early onset of weakness. *Pronator drift* is a subtle early sign of proximal weakness. It can be noted by asking the patient to hold out both arms with palms up (thus simultaneously testing ability to obey commands). If drift (and therefore proximal weakness) is present, the affected arm drifts downward slightly, with the wrist and hand pronating. Such a finding implies dysfunction of motor tracts in the opposite hemisphere. If the patient cannot follow commands, both arms may be lifted simultaneously and then dropped. The weaker one will fall to the bed more rapidly. Absence of spontaneous movement on one side of the body also implies disruption of motor tracts in the opposite hemisphere.

Weakness or paralysis may become bilateral when herniation has progressed to the midbrain level for anatomical reasons. The cerebral peduncles, which carry corticospinal tract fibers, join the brainstem at the midbrain. The fibers course downward in the lateral aspects of the brainstem before they cross in the pyramid of the medulla and continue down the spinal cord to innervate the side of the body opposite to the hemisphere in which they arose.

An expanding mass that has distorted tissue sufficiently may push the midbrain across the midline, compressing structures between the midbrain and the tentorium on the side opposite the expanding mass. This will be disclosed by the appearance of bilateral decerebrate posturing and ocular abnormalities in a patient in whom these signs have previously been unilateral. If herniation cannot be reversed at this point in adults, it is likely to be irreversible.

Abnormal postural and cutaneous reflexes may become bilateral with distortion of the brain higher in the hemispheres. The level of brain function cannot be identified and subsequent irreversibility of herniations estimated from signs of a single system alone. Table 33-6 summarizes the constellation of findings at three levels of brain function and the implications for reversibility.

Respiratory Patterns. Plum and Posner carefully documented the correlations between patterns of respiration and level of brain function.[39] These are useful in detecting decrease in level of brain function with brain herniation (Figure 33-5).

Cheyne-Stokes respiration is characterized by a pattern of crescendo–decrescendo breathing followed by apnea. This pattern represents disturbance of deep-hemispheric function bilaterally and is differentiated from periodic apnea of brainstem origin by the regularity of the hyperpneic-apneic pattern. Cheyne-Stokes breathing occurs physiologically because of abnormally increased central ventilatory response to carbon dioxide (hyperpneic phase). The hyperventilation reduces arterial carbon dioxide to the point where breathing is no longer stimulated and apnea results. Arterial partial pressure of carbon dioxide, building during apnea, finally exceeds the respiratory stimulation threshold and restarts the oscillating cycle. The overreaction involved in this control of breathing has been compared to the overcompensation of the drunk driver for the normal variations of movement of the car.

Metabolic disorders usually affect all parts of the nervous system equally and are the most common cause of the bilateral hemisphere dysfunction manifested by Cheyne-Stokes respiration. Such respiration is also seen in patients with bilateral cerebral infarct or hypertensive encephalopathy (implying bilateral lesions) and during non-REM sleep in some persons with chronic respiratory disease and some with prolonged circulation time (cardiac failure). However,

TABLE 33-6 **Transtentorial Herniation Syndromes at Various Brain Levels**

Cortex, Hemisphere: Signs of Early Brain Shift*	Diencephalon: Signs of Later Brain Shift†	Midbrain: Signs of Herniation‡
Subtle changes in consciousness: ↑ stimulus required to elicit eye opening, verbal response Ability to follow commands usually intact	↓ Consciousness: Painful stimulus required for arousal Does not follow commands	Unresponsive to verbal stimuli Abnormal posturing to painful stimuli
Motor changes: Unilateral pronator drift *Gegenhalten* (↑ tone) may be present	Motor changes (usually unilateral): ↑ tone May be hemiplegic; may show motor change ipsilateral to lesion if brain has shifted across midline	Abnormal motor posturing Flexor/extensor posturing May show motor change
Eye signs: Pupils equal, and reactive to light (PERL) intact; extraocular movements (EOM) intact	Eye signs: PERL and EOM intact to "doll's eye" maneuver Spontaneous "roving" disconjugate gaze may occur	Eye signs: Pupils unequal, unresponsive to light unilaterally or bilaterally Loss of oculocephalic reflex unilaterally or bilaterally
Respirations unremarkable	Respirations may be Cheyne-Stokes or hyperventilatory	Respirations hyperventilatory

* Reversible if mass lesion can be treated.
†Reversible.
‡May be reversible if herniation does not proceed to pons.

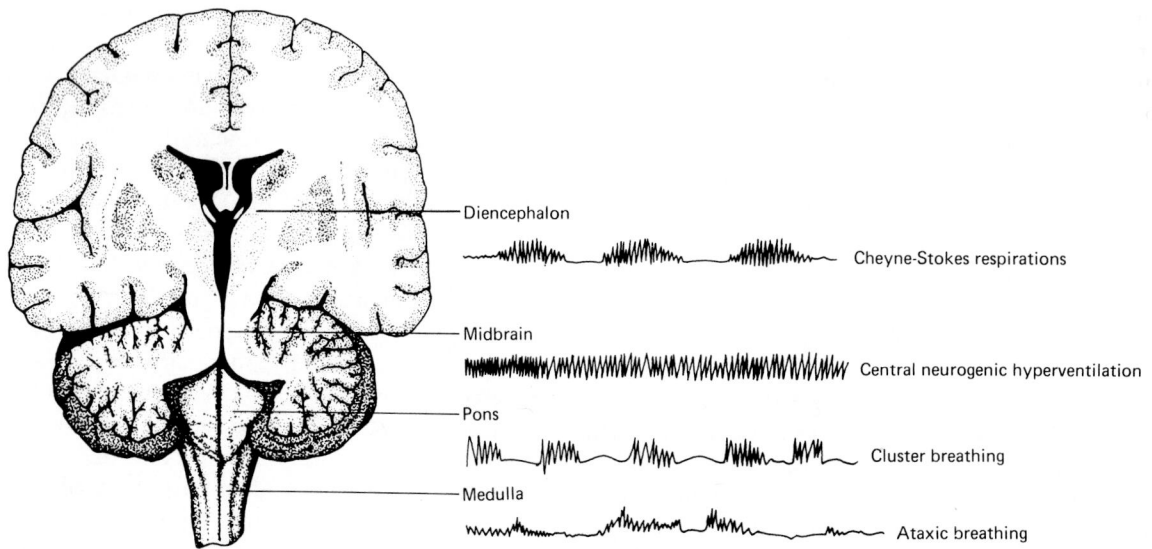

Figure 33-5 Respiratory patterns correlated with brain function level. As the influence of higher areas is removed through ischemia or compression, characteristic breathing patterns are found.

the appearance of Cheyne-Stokes respiration in a patient at risk for transtentorial herniation signals deteriorating brain function and imminent herniation. Because the appearance of this pattern seems to require bilateral dysfunction of the internal capsules, concurrent changes in motor functions would be expected.

The manner in which a focal mass lesion can cause bilateral deep hemisphere dysfunction leading to

Cheyne-Stokes respiration can be inferred from Figure 33-5. Expansion of the right hemisphere lesion and surrounding edema may initially compress structures in that hemisphere and produce focal findings on the opposite side of the body. Further expansion leads to additional swelling and eventually movement of brain tissue from one hemisphere across the midline with subsequent downward displacement of structures in both hemispheres.

Other abnormal breathing patterns occur with brainstem and medullary dysfunction. These patterns are useful in determining whether neurological status is deteriorating or improving once consciousness is lost. They must be used along with other signs of midbrain and brainstem functioning.

Central neurogenic hyperventilation is a pattern of deep, regular, and rapid hyperpnea. It occurs with dysfunction of the *tegmentum,* or central portion of the brainstem, usually between the lower midbrain and pons. Since arterial oxygen tension is normal in patients with "true" central neurogenic hyperventilation, the physiological explanation must be an abnormally low threshold for stimulation by carbon dioxide.

Pontine-medullary breathing patterns include *ataxic* breathing (sometimes called *Biot's respiration*) and *cluster* breathing (see Figure 33-5). Both are forms of periodic breathing, with frequent periods of apnea. Reciprocal firing of inspiratory and expiratory neurons in the medulla is impaired. Since the medulla is well below the tentorium, such patterns occur only in well-established herniation and portend a poor prognosis. Posterior fossa lesions that cause herniation of brainstem and posterior fossa contents *upward* through the tentorium may produce ataxic breathing. Rapidly expanding posterior fossa lesions leading to herniation of cerebellar tonsils into the foramen magnum are more likely to produce respiratory arrest. Posterior fossa lesions include those of the cerebellum, the fourth ventricle, and the area where the cerebellar fibers join the pons.

Eye Signs. Pupillary reaction and ocular motility are important clues to the state of brain structures at the level of the tentorium. Cranial nerve III controls pupillary reactivity and elevation of the eyelid. Its nucleus is in the midbrain. The nerve itself courses between the posterior cerebral and superior cerebellar arteries and passes out of the brainstem through the incisure. Consequently, pressure from a herniating temporal lobe can produce unilateral pupillary dilatation, oval pupil, and/or ptosis before the midbrain is compressed sufficiently to alter ocular motility. The parasympathetic fibers of cranial nerve III are in the outermost portion of the nerve bundle. Paralysis of these parasympathetically mediated functions (pupillary constriction and eyelid elevation) follows compression of the nerve against the incisure or the posterior cerebral artery. The appearance of unilateral pupillary dilatation in a patient with head trauma or suspected mass lesion is a definitive sign that herniation is occurring and constitutes a neurosurgical emergency. In patients who are in therapeutic barbiturate coma or paralyzed with pancuronium, pupillary dilatation will be the *only* sign of herniation.

The *pupillary light reflex* is mediated by parasympathetic fibers that constrict the pupil when light stimulates the optic nerve. The reflex can be interrupted by structural damage at several points: the optic nerve, diencephalic nuclei (pretectal), midbrain nuclei (Edinger-Westphal), cranial nerve III itself, and the ciliary ganglion (just dorsal to the eye). In tentorial herniation, damage to cranial nerve III at the incisure or compression of the midbrain are the most likely reasons pupils lose their reactivity to light. Preservation of the light reflex in coma is an important clue that the cause is metabolic (for example, drug overdose or uremia) rather than structural. A strong light and magnifying glass may be necessary to determine with certainty that the pupillary light reflex is or is not present.

Because ocular motility is controlled by brainstem structures, eye movements provide important clues to the level of brain function. When consciousness is depressed, changes in eye movements may provide the only clues that brain function is deteriorating because of transtentorial herniation. Symmetry of eye movements and presence or absence of oculocephalic reflexes are evaluated; these eye movements not only provide clues to the level of brain functioning but also yield information regarding the body's ability to protect the airway and vital functions such as respiration.

Eye movement is controlled by cranial nerves III, IV, and VI. Even in the unconscious patient, in whom voluntary control of eye movement cannot be tested, spontaneous roving eye movement may occur. In general, if brainstem function is intact, these eye movements will be conjugate and full, indicating that all three of the cranial nerves are functioning. Cranial nerve III controls all eye movement except lateral movement and downward movement when the orbit is rotated internally. (In patients lacking voluntary control, the function of cranial nerve IV can rarely be observed.) Although cranial nerve III also controls pupillary constriction and eyelid elevation, changes involving movement of the eye are apt to occur later than those controlling pupils and eyelid elevation. Consequently, changes in pupil size may be observed before the onset of disconjugate gaze. Although disconjugate gaze is evidence of abnormally functioning brainstem structures, in the comatose patient it cannot help localize damage; instead, the oculocephalic reflex is employed.

The *oculocephalic reflex,* commonly referred to as *doll's eye phenomenon,* is mediated afferently by the cranial nerve VIII and efferently by the cranial nerves III and VI. This reflex may be tested by rapidly rotating the head to one side and observing the eye movements. If the reflex is intact, when the head is rotated the eyes appear to remain in the initial position and then slowly turn in the direction to which the head is rotated (*doll's eyes present*). If the reflex

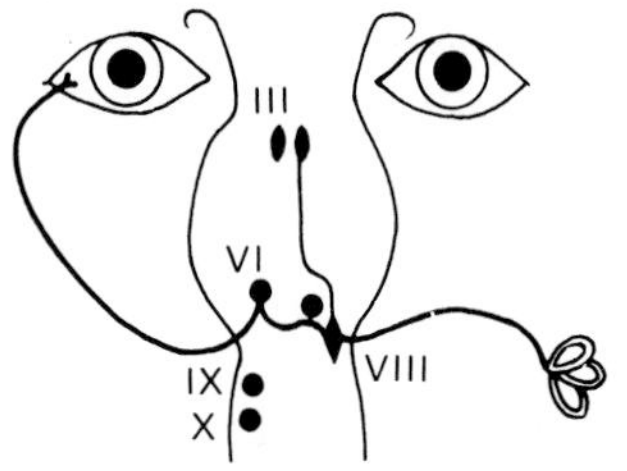

Figure 33-6 Protective reflexes: anatomical relation of ocular movements (cranial nerves III and VI) to swallow, gag, and cough reflexes (cranial nerves IX and X). Cranial nerve VIII is the afferent limb of the oculocephalic reflex.

is not intact, the eyes move with the head as though fixed in place *(doll's eyes absent)*. (See Chapter 32 for discussion of the reflex.)

The oculocephalic reflex is elicited by head movement that moves fluid in the semicircular canal, stimulating the vestibular portion of cranial nerve VIII. The vestibular impulses pass through the brainstem to the nuclei of the cranial nerves III and VI, thereby eliciting the eye movement seen. The neural connections are shown in Figure 33-6. The reflex is present in all persons with intact brainstems during sleep. In an awake person, the reflex cannot be elicited because the eyes will be fixed upon objects and the reflex overcome. In altered states of consciousness, the presence of the reflex indicates that the brainstem function is intact between cranial nerves VIII and III.

The oculovestibular reflex is mediated by the same set of cranial nerves. It is stimulated directly by irrigation of the ear with either hot or cold fluid, a procedure commonly called *caloric stimulation*. Although the two reflexes use the same afferent and efferent pathways, the oculovestibular reflex is preserved somewhat longer in brain dysfunction than the oculocephalic reflex. Thus, when the oculocephalic reflex is absent, the physician may wish to use caloric stimulation to determine whether the reflex pathway has indeed been lost. These tests are described in Chapter 32.

Testing the oculocephalic and oculovestibular reflexes appears to have prognostic value for comatose patients who have suffered structural brain damage and for patients who have suffered metabolic brain damage other than barbiturate overdosage. In large studies of brain-injured patients and patients in metabolic coma, investigators found that the absence of oculovestibular reflexes for periods longer than 24 hours correlated strongly with either death or vegetative existence.[17,44] It must be emphasized that this correlation does *not* apply to patients with a drug overdose, particularly barbiturate overdose. These substances depress the entire central nervous system but do not appear to cause irreversible metabolic

damage. Thus, the absence of oculovestibular reflexes in these patients does not by itself imply a poor prognosis.

Tests of eye movement symmetry and oculocephalic reflexes have two major uses by critical care nurses: (1) to detect further rostral–caudal deterioration in patients who have lost consciousness and (2) to determine the need for protective care of the airway.

In the patient who is already unresponsive to verbal and painful stimuli, the appearance of disconjugate eye movements or the change from present to absent oculocephalic reflexes indicates that the brain is functioning at a lower anatomical level than before. Cranial nerves III and VI are at the level of the tentorium, and VIII is nearly at the level of the medulla. Consequently, disappearance of oculocephalic reflexes or a sudden asymmetry of eye movement in response to head rotation indicates that brainstem function is seriously compromised and that tentorial herniation is occurring. Furthermore, it warns that the airway is in imminent danger. As shown in Figure 33-6, cranial nerves IX and X are innervated just caudal to cranial nerve VIII. These cranial nerves are important in the cough and gag reflexes. Thus, impairment of intrinsic airway protection is predicted by loss of brain function just rostral to the pons. The absence of oculocephalic reflexes or change in their function thus indicates the need for endotracheal intubation and for particular attention to pooling of secretions in the patient's airway and to suctioning.

Vital Signs. Vital signs—blood pressure, pulse, respiratory rate—are frequently listed among high-priority observations in the critically ill neurological patient. However, as Figure 33-3 clearly indicates, the structures that mediate these functions are low in the brainstem and the medulla. Consequently, sustained major change in these functions occurs late in the process of transtentorial herniation. Reliance upon changes in vital signs to *detect* impending herniation is unwise, because these changes occur too late to protect the patient and prevent herniation. Fluctuating vital signs may well reflect fluctuating levels of intracranial pressure.

Blood pressure is mediated at a reflex level in the medulla. Although the classic *Cushing triad* is often referred to as a sign of increasing intracranial pressure and/or impending transtentorial herniation, it really is a sign of imminent death. The classic triad consists of increasing systolic blood pressure, decreasing diastolic blood pressure, and bradycardia. The mechanism for this triad of symptoms appears to be ischemia and pressure upon medullary brain structures. Although there may well be gradual increases in systolic blood pressure in patients with herniation and fluctuating periods of bradycardia, the presence of the triad is the terminal event in both experimental and clinical studies of the phenomenon. Waiting for the triad to appear before doing anything is waiting much too long! As indicated earlier in this chapter, respiratory patterns can provide clues to the level of brain still functioning, but absolute respiratory rate is both notoriously inaccurate and not particularly helpful.

Uncal Herniation. Herniation of the *uncus,* or medial portion of the temporal lobe, may occur in connection with central herniation or by itself with intracranial or epidural lesions of the temporal lobe (see Figure 33-2). Epidural hematoma from a lacerated middle meningeal artery often produces classic uncal herniation, whereas a unilateral intracerebral hematoma may produce a combined central-uncal herniation as the expanding hemisphere pushes the uncus over the tentorial incisure.

The major difference in clinical presentation of central and uncal syndromes is the point at which pupillary changes occur relative to change in consciousness and movement. Because the uncus is at the level of the tentorium, pure uncal herniation may present with rapid changes in motor function and pupillary equality nearly simultaneous with deterioration of consciousness. Although differentiating the type of syndrome is not critical to evaluating impending herniation, the nurse should be alert to patients particularly at risk for the uncal syndrome and be prepared to mobilize neurosurgical help immediately upon change in neurological status. Such patients include those with linear skull fractures of the temporal bone (high risk of lacerating the middle meningeal artery) and those postcraniotomy patients who have had temporal lobe surgery, with subsequent risk of postoperative localized edema.

Cerebellar Herniation. Not only can the brain be displaced downward through the tentorial incisure but also, as already mentioned, the contents of the posterior fossa can herniate upward through the incisure. The contents of the posterior fossa consist mainly of the cerebellum, the nerve trunks connecting the cerebellum to the pons, and the cranial nerves that exit the brainstem at the pons. Downward displacement drives the structures toward the foramen magnum. Abrupt herniation into the foramen magnum impinges upon the medulla and is fatal.

Because the cerebellum lies just posterior to pontine-medullary structures mediating respiration, expansion of posterior fossa contents may be heralded by ataxic respirations or apnea. Upward herniation of posterior fossa contents may compress the brainstem at the midbrain, thereby impairing consciousness, pupillary reflexes, and eye movements. Pupils are likely to be constricted and nonreactive because of compression of ocular sympathetic pathways as they pass through the pons as well as compression of parasympathetic fibers of cranial nerve III. The upward-herniating subtentorial brain accounts for direct compression of this nerve.

Patients at high risk for acute upward herniation are those with lesions that have the potential for *rapid* expansion: cerebellar hemorrhage and occipital skull fracture with attendant risk of epidural or subdural bleeding. Patients with cerebellar abscesses and tumors are ultimately at risk for herniation if the disease process is not arrested. However, such lesions usually expand slowly, and the brain can compensate for the relative compression ischemia for a remarkably long time. In contrast, in rapidly expanding lesions the process is too fast for the brain to compensate for the attendant ischemia and compression.

Medical and Nursing Management. Potential for brain herniation is a clinical problem, managed collaboratively by nursing and medicine. The problem may be managed at the level of primary prevention by any concerned health professional or member of the general public. Early detection of the problem is a major goal of intensive-care monitoring by both physicians and nurses. Physicians carry primary responsibility for definitive therapy of treatable lesions that are precipitating brain herniation (for example, expanding epidural hematoma). Both physicians and nurses have collaborative responsibilities in maintaining and monitoring the pharmacological and supportive therapy regimens that reduce brain mass in nonsurgical conditions causing brain herniation.

It behooves all critical care professionals to take an active part in community education aimed at primary prevention. Head trauma sustained in motorcycle, bicycle, automobile, and home accidents accounts for a substantial portion of the patients in any intensive or trauma unit who are at risk for brain herniation. Uncontrolled hypertension is the primary cause of intracerebral and cerebellar hemorrhage. All health professionals have a role in educating the public regarding proper use of helmets on bicycles and motorcycles and seat belts in automobiles. The National High Blood Pressure Education Program has identified a major role for nurses in both education and early detection of hypertension.

The preceding discussion has been aimed largely at secondary prevention, or the early detection of an existing disorder, which prevents further complications. If herniation can be detected before it has become irreversible, the opportunity for effective medical therapy is greatly enhanced. Computed tomography (CT scan) is frequently used upon admission or upon appearance of focal or diffuse brain damage signs to determine whether a mass lesion exists. In some cases, echoencephalography may be performed at the bedside to detect brain shift.

If a mass lesion is found to be the cause of deteriorating neurological function, removal of the mass becomes the major aim of medical care. For example, evacuation of a subdural hematoma or evacuation and ligation of the bleeding artery in epidural hematoma removes the expanding mass lesion and allows the brain to assume its normal relationships. Hypertonic agents such as mannitol and urea may be given prior to emergency craniotomy in the hope of shrinking a swollen brain and "buying time" to get the patient to the operating room. If herniation is secondary to focal or general cerebral edema, removal of the cause becomes more difficult. In such cases, symptomatic treatment of the edema and resultant increased intracranial pressure may be pursued until the brain's healing processes have reversed the edema. It must be emphasized that the use of such agents as mannitol, urea, glycerol, corticosteroids, and barbiturates is aimed at controlling intracranial pressure secondary to swelling and edema.

In severe brain swelling, surgical decompression may be used in the hope that herniation will be reversed or averted long enough for reparative processes to shrink the swollen brain. A flap of bone is removed, and the dura may be incised to allow the expanding brain a place to expand other than through the tentorium. Needless to say, care must be taken not to place external pressure on the surgical dressing over the exposed dura mater.

Nursing monitoring for the clinical problem of potential for brain herniation has already been described. Several nursing diagnoses associated with this problem are common to many brain-injured patients. Chief among these are complete physical immobility related to coma and potential for injury related to inability to protect cornea, airway, and skin. Nursing interventions for these diagnoses are basic to care of the immobilized, unresponsive patient and are outlined in the section on head injury under Neurotrauma, later in this chapter.

Seizures

By definition, generalized seizures and focal seizures that become general affect the functioning of the whole brain and thereby disrupt consciousness. A generalized seizure is the result of uncontrolled neuronal discharge in the brain. In a seizure, neurons begin to discharge uninhibitedly, recruit other nearby neurons, and thus excite a "storm" of electrical activity in the brain. The discharge may arise from deep in the central core of the brain, immediately disrupting consciousness through excess activity in the reticular activating system. Other generalized seizures may arise from focal areas of hyperactive neurons, whose uncontrolled discharge spreads to central structures and becomes general. Both the typical *grand mal*, or major motor seizure, and *petit mal*, or "absence attacks" of children, are generalized seizures. Electroencephalography during such a seizure shows excessive electrical activity over the entire brain. Clinically, consciousness is disrupted in both types of seizure, but excessive motor activity is characteristic of grand mal episodes, while arrest of motor activity (but not loss of tone) is characteristic of the typical petit mal of childhood. In addition, the typical EEG pattern, although general in both, is quite different in petit mal and in grand mal.

Most seizures are idiopathic, that is, without identifiable cause. However, in critically ill patients, they are likely to stem directly from an identifiable disorder that primarily or secondarily affects the patient's brain. Metabolic disorders, by altering the acid–base and fluid environment of the brain, effectively lower membrane potential and, thus, the threshold for seizures. Both hypertonicity and hypotonicity of brain fluid can lead to seizures by altering the normal electrochemical balance on each side of the cell membrane.

Trauma can predispose the patient to seizures. The underlying cause is not well understood. Seizures immediately following trauma may be related to cellular membrane instabilities associated with vasogenic edema or lactic acidosis and respiratory alkalosis secondary to neurogenic hyperventilation. Seizures of later onset (or true posttraumatic epilepsy) may be related to cell membrane injury from oxygen free radicals that are liberated in response to focal or diffuse traumatic brain hemorrhage.[45] In the immediate posttraumatic period, the most effective treatment for seizures is to correct the underlying structural, metabolic, or respiratory problems. Anticonvulsants have been shown to be effective in controlling these immediate seizures but not in preventing delayed posttraumatic epilepsy. Some speculate that experimental antioxidants (for example, superoxide dismutase or 21-aminosteroids) may prevent posttraumatic epilepsy as well as improve neurological outcome following head trauma.[10,45]

The primary clinical problem associated with seizures in critically ill patients is potential for secondary brain damage related to uncontrolled seizures. This is a clinical problem that must be managed collaboratively by nurses, physicians, and sometimes respiratory therapists. The metabolic requirement of brain cells during epileptic discharge far exceeds that of resting or normally active brain cells. Even focal seizures (epileptic discharge confined to a small area of the brain) increase overall cerebral metabolism, and generalized seizures increase cerebral metabolic requirements severalfold. Most often, cerebral blood flow increases sufficiently to deliver oxygen and substrate to the cells. Therefore, investigators now believe that the primary cause of cell death is breakdown of internal cellular metabolic machinery.[46] The major goal of care is absence of neuronal damage, and the expected outcomes are detection of generalized seizures and rapid control of generalized seizures. Management to achieve these outcomes consists of (1) monitoring for signs of focal or generalized seizures, (2) institution of predetermined protocols to manage seizures if they occur, and (3) nursing measures to protect the patient from physical injury during a seizure.

Monitoring to detect focal and generalized seizures is made more difficult in many critically ill neurological patients at high risk for focal and generalized seizures because the protocols for management of brain swelling, intracranial hypertension, and respiratory insufficiency mask motor manifestations of seizures. Thus, patients who are artificially ventilated and paralyzed with pancuronium have little or no motor response to focal or generalized motor seizures. Depending upon the serum level of pancuronium, these patients may show only minor twitching or only a sudden marked increase in level of ICP (secondary to increase in cerebral blood flow to meet the flow needs of excessive cellular activity) and sudden dilatation of pupils. The attending physician may elect continuous EEG monitoring to detect recurrent seizure activity in such patients.

Because the injured brain is more vulnerable to secondary injury from excessive neuronal activity, seizures must be stopped rapidly. The pharmacological protocol used most commonly includes a short-acting benzodiazepine (diazepam or lorazepam) to stop the seizure, followed by a loading dose and then maintenance doses of a longer-acting anticonvulsant (most commonly phenytoin or phenobarbital). Dosages and nursing observations are discussed later under Status Epilepticus.

Nursing management is collaborative in monitoring and carrying out the drug protocol in the event of seizures. Further nursing intervention is required for the nursing diagnosis of potential for physical injury, which is present in any patient suffering generalized seizures. Goals of care are to maintain an adequate airway and prevent aspiration and to prevent injury to soft tissues and bones. Interventions to protect the airway include:

1. Positioning the patient in the lateral position.
2. Use of an oral airway or endotracheal tube.
3. Oropharyngeal suctioning to keep the mouth free of secretions that could be aspirated.
4. Prevention of bone and soft tissue injury by taping pillows or commercially available pads to the bed rails and loosening any limb restraints that may be in place.

Injury to teeth is best prevented by *avoiding* the use of padded tongue blades.

Status Epilepticus. A patient who is having seizures from any acute or chronic cause may develop status epilepticus, but it is more common in those with epilepsy whose brain cells have become regulated by anticonvulsants. The sudden withdrawal of these, either deliberately or by forgetting medication, renders all the brain cells hyperexcitable, thereby leading to seizure activity among epileptic foci cells. Neurochemical changes in the cellular fluid around these cells then render neighboring cells more excitable and lead to generalized seizures.

Grand mal status epilepticus is an absolute emergency! Continual seizures prevent brain cells from restoring metabolic processes between firing. Patients in grand mal status epilepticus whose seizures cannot be controlled die of brain exhaustion with definite evidence of metabolic and structural neuronal death. Investigators have demonstrated that prevention of muscular activity during continual seizures in baboons neither protected the brain nor prevented death.[46,47] Electroencephalography demonstrated that continual seizure activity occurred even though the motor manifestations were prevented by curare and even though respirations and blood pressure were supported. In both baboons and rats, neuronal damage was greatest in the neocortex and hippocampus.

In addition to the protective care described above, critical care nurses should be prepared to institute anticonvulsant therapy for a patient in status epilepticus. The time necessary for a physician to arrive, evaluate the situation, and initiate therapy may be sufficient for large numbers of brain cells to be irreparably damaged. Therefore, the nurse should be able to (1) recognize status epilepticus and (2) initiate a standard protocol determined in advance by the critical care staff. A typical protocol is shown in the box on p. 826.

A typical generalized seizure lasts 20 to 40 seconds, with recovery of consciousness within 30 minutes. Generalized status epilepticus is thus defined as seizure activity that exceeds usual time. Specifically, status epilepticus is a single seizure lasting longer than 15 to 20 minutes, or a series of seizures over 20 to 30 minutes in which the patient fails to regain consciousness between seizures.

Treatment of generalized status epilepticus follows the same steps involved in any emergency: attention to airway and breathing, steps to diagnose the un-

Protocol for Management of Status Epilepticus

1. Obtain adequate airway.
2. Establish diagnosis: 15 to 20 min of generalized motor seizure or 20 to 30 min of overlapping seizures without regaining consciousness.
3. Establish intravenous line.
4. Draw blood for laboratory studies: glucose, electrolytes, CBC, calcium, BUN, toxicology screen, liver enzymes, anticonvulsant serum levels.
5. Administer anticonvulsant therapy:*
   a. Benzodiazepine:
      Diazepam (Valium)—5-10 mg over 5-10 min, repeated at 15 min if needed, not to exceed 30 mg total. Be prepared for mechanical ventilation in the event of respiratory arrest.
      Alternative drug: Lorazepam (Ativan)—4-8 mg IV over 2 min; repeated at 10 min if needed. Be prepared for respiratory arrest.
   b. Phenytoin (Dilantin):
      Initial dose: 20 mg/kg no faster than 50 mg/min. Monitor ECG.
      Stop drug if ST segment widens.
      Maintenance dose: 250 mg IV every 4 hours to total of 1 g in first 24 hours.
6. If seizures are not stopped with initial one or two drugs, phenobarbital IV, paraldehyde IV, barbiturate, or general anesthesia may be considered.

*Adult dosages.

derlying cause, protective care while the seizures persist, and definitive treatment. Establishment of an adequate airway is, as always, of prime importance. At the same time, oxygen should be administered by prongs or mask. If the patient does not have an artificial airway already in place, one should position the patient on his or her side and insert an oral airway. An endotracheal tube may ultimately be required if the seizures prove difficult to control.

Because most status epilepticus seen in critically ill patients is a symptom of an underlying structural or metabolic pathology, determination of the primary cause is crucial to long-term therapy. If an intravenous line is not already established in the patient, one should be established as soon as airway patency is attended to. At this time, blood should be drawn for laboratory tests, including blood glucose, serum osmolality, and serum electrolytes. It is often the case that correction of the underlying metabolic deficit (for example, hypoglycemia or hyperosmolality) will end the seizures.

Among the drugs used to control repetitive seizures, the initial drug of choice is most commonly *diazepam* (Valium), given intravenously. Diazepam

may be given to adults in doses of 5 to 10 mg over 5 to 10 minutes, repeating as necessary at 15-minute intervals but not exceeding 30 mg for a total dose. In children, the dose should be 0.25 to 0.4 mg/kg over 2 minutes with a maximum of 5 to 10 mg per bolus and 30 mg per episode.[48] Alternatively, 5 mg/min may be administered by intravenous drip, using nonabsorptive tubing.[49] Diazepam is a short-acting anticonvulsant with a rapid onset of action. Large doses can depress, or even arrest, respirations. Therefore, a slow rate of administration is crucial, and equipment to ventilate the patient manually should be readily available.

Lorazepam (Ativan) is a benzodiazepine that is often used instead of diazepam. It has a longer duration of action and somewhat less sedating activity. Respiratory depression and respiratory arrest are potential side effects, just as with diazepam.[50]

Following the initial dose of benzodiazepine to rapidly control the seizures, *phenytoin* (Dilantin) is given for longer-term anticonvulsant effect. It is preferable to phenobarbital in persons with central nervous system disorders because it has much less sedating effect in large doses than phenobarbital. Phenytoin is given initially as an intravenous loading dose (15 to 20 mg/kg for both children and adults) at a rate no greater than 50 mg/min in adults and 3 mg/min per kilogram in children. The maximum dose in 24 hours is 1 g. Phenytoin crystallizes when standing in solution and therefore should be given intravenously in a bolus, directly into the cannula, rather than mixed in a hanging solution. It is never appropriate to give phenytoin intramuscularly; tissue absorption and, therefore, serum levels are unpredictable by this route, and crystallization in tissues has been demonstrated.

Phenytoin has potentially dangerous side effects on cardiac rhythm, particularly in elderly patients and in those with heart disease. Therefore, the ECG should be monitored when phenytoin is used in status epilepticus. Indications for immediate discontinuance of the drug are hypotension, widening of the QRS complex, prolongation of the PR or QT intervals, and depression of T waves.

If a benzodiazepine and phenytoin are not successful in controlling the seizures, *amobarbital* or *phenobarbital* is often given intravenously, in a dose of 5 to 10 mg/kg and a rate of 30 mg/min in children and 9 mg/kg at 50 mg/min in adults, with total dose not to exceed 1 g for either. Potential side effects to be monitored include sedation, hypotension, respiratory depression, and cardiac arrest.

Paraldehyde may be added if these drugs fail to control the seizures. Rectal administration of paraldehyde is no longer recommended, as the rate of absorption is unpredictable. Paraldehyde is given intravenously in a solution of 4 ml of paraldehyde in 100 ml of normal saline at 3.75 ml per kilogram of solution (0.15 ml per kilogram of the drug) over 60 minutes, to a total not to exceed 100 to 125 ml of solution. Paraldehyde dissolves plastics and, therefore, must be mixed and administered in glass containers. It will deteriorate to acetic acid upon exposure to the air, so must be mixed fresh for each administration. Pulmonary edema and hepatic and renal toxicity are potential side effects.

If all else fails, general anesthesia by barbiturate (pentobarbital) or inhalation may be used to stop the seizures. Such therapy requires continuous EEG monitoring to determine whether the brain seizure activity has ceased.[51] Patient care is otherwise identical to that for patients with uncontrollable ICP under barbiturate coma.

States That Disrupt Ventilation but Not Consciousness

The disorders commonly seen that may produce respiratory problems include high cervical spinal cord injury, polyneuropathies (such as Guillain-Barré syndrome), and motor unit disorders, such as myasthenia gravis, botulism, and tetanus. In these states the respiratory problem is secondary to loss of motor function rather than to loss of consciousness and ability voluntarily to protect the airway.

Disorders of this kind disrupt human functioning in all basic aspects of self-care except mentation and consciousness. Survival and the quality of life after recovery are vitally dependent upon skilled and knowledgeable nursing care.

Motor loss from extracerebral causes can threaten life if it involves sensory or motor reflexes that protect the airway or if innervation of respiratory musculature is depressed or lost. Thus, relevant nursing diagnoses include (1) ineffective airway clearance, related to loss of airway protective reflexes; and (2) ineffective breathing patterns, related to paralysis or weakness of respiratory muscles.

NURSING MANAGEMENT

■ NURSING DIAGNOSIS

Ineffective airway clearance, related to loss of airway protective reflexes.

OUTCOME STANDARD AND CRITERIA

Airways are clear as evidenced by:
- Absence of rhonchi/gurgles or localized wheezes after cough
- Reduction of peak airway pressure at some ventilator settings

The gag, swallowing, and cough reflexes that protect the airway are integrated in the brainstem, at the medullary segment. Cranial nerves IX, X, and XII are the peripheral nerves carrying motor and sensory fibers to and from the structures involved in these functions. Table 33-7 summarizes the anatomical structures involved.

NURSING INTERVENTIONS: EVALUATION OF AIRWAY PROTECTION

Since airway protection is dependent upon the reflexes that serve gag, cough, and swallowing, ongoing monitoring and assessment of the adequacy of these functions is important. In contrast to the patient with cerebral involvement who is at risk for inadequate airway protection, the patient with extracerebral motor problems is usually conscious. Consequently, the nurse can evaluate speech, facial movement, and head and shoulder movement to assess closely related cranial nerve function. Finally, the nurse must know which patients are at risk for loss of airway protection and evaluate potential loss of protection in light of general motor functioning.

Patients who are at risk for airway problems and who may be seen in critical care include those with myasthenia gravis (particularly after thymectomy, during intercurrent illness, or in myasthenic or cholinergic crisis), those with polyneuropathy involving upper extremities and/or cranial nerves, those with poliomyelitis (involving brainstem motor neurons), and those with brainstem stroke or contusion. The last group of patients may be unconscious if the re-

TABLE 33-7 **Nerve Fibers and Skeletal Muscles Involved in Protecting the Airway**

Function	Afferent Fibers, Cranial Nerve No.	Efferent Fibers, Cranial Nerve No.	Muscle(s)
Gag	IX (glossopharyngeal)	IX, X (vagus)	Stylopharyngeus, soft palate, pharynx
Swallow	IX (posterior ⅓ of tongue; pharynx, larynx)	X	Pharynx, soft palate
	X (epiglottal taste buds)	XII (hypoglossal)	Tongue
Cough	X (pharynx, larynx, trachea, bronchial tree)	X, to respiratory center (medulla) and then to periphery via:	Soft palate, larynx, glottis
		(1) Phrenic nerve (C4-C5)	Diaphragm
		(2) Intercostal nerves (T1-T11)	Intercostal

TABLE 33-8 **Critical Evaluation in Myasthenia Gravis**

Vital capacity	Maximum expiratory volume following maximum inspiration, measured in liters by spirometer
Swallowing	Measured subjectively by asking the patient to identify the type of substance or diet thought possible to swallow at the time:

	0—nothing	3—pureed soft	
	1—saliva	4—soft	
	2—liquids	5—regular diet	

Ptosis	Documented according to the following scale (with the patient looking straight ahead): 1—Unable to open eye, none of iris visible 2—Lids open, some of lowermost iris visible 3—Lower half of pupil visible 4—All of pupil visible, none of uppermost iris visible 5—All of pupil visible, some of uppermost iris visible
Diplopia	Measured subjectively by asking the patient to move eyes through their extreme range of motion and identify positions in which diplopia is experienced

Adapted from Blount, M., Kinney, A., & Luttrell, N. (1982). Myasthenia gravis and the Guillain-Barré syndrome. In D. L. Nikas (Ed.), *The critically ill neurosurgical patient.* New York: Churchill Livingstone; and Blount, M., Kinney, A. B., & Stone, M. (1979). Plasma exchange in the management of myasthenia gravis. *Nursing Clinics of North America, 14,* 173-190.

ticular activating system is involved. Cranial nerves IX, X, and XII are most crucially involved in protecting the airway. Evaluation of the function of adjacent cranial nerves helps detect potential problems before aspiration has occurred. Table 33-7 describes cranial nerves in relation to the functions served.

Important questions to consider in evaluating lower cranial nerve function are the following:

- Is the quality of speech changing or becoming nasal, slurred, or "thick-tongued"?
- Is the volume of speech decreasing?

In regard to swallowing:

- Is food or fluid coming back through the nose (indicating palatal weakness)?
- Does the patient choke on nonviscous substances such as water?
- Can the patient swallow his or her own saliva?
- Is there pooling of secretions in the mouth of the conscious person?

In testing swallowing, it should be remembered that water is the most difficult substance to swallow—more difficult than saliva. Therefore, if the nurse is concerned that the patient may aspirate the test substance, ice chips rather than water should be used.

In ascending polyneuropathies, upper extremity function and movement of head and neck may be affected before the cranial nerves serving airway protection. Therefore, changes in the strength and symmetry of head turning, neck flexion, and extension are important cues to evaluate swallow, gag, and cough more frequently in patients with such changes. These evaluations of cranial nerve function are not relevant to the patient with cervical spine injury (unless there is associated head injury), because any spinal cord injury compatible with life is below the cranial nerves.

In myasthenia gravis, changes in muscular function may occur very rapidly, within minutes. Therefore, for these patients, airway protection and respiratory status must be evaluated frequently. Any slurring or nasality of speech or increased ptosis of eyelids serves as a cue to evaluate swallowing and cough and vital capacity as often as every 5 minutes if changes are occurring rapidly.[52] Such variables are summarized in Table 33-8.

Of the disorders used as examples in this section, only brainstem stroke and contusion are stable lesions. Once the initial damage has occurred, symptoms tend to remain the same or diminish. The other disorders (polyneuropathies and disorders of neuromuscular transmission) may become progressively worse and often involve respiratory musculature as well. In these disorders, potential for ineffective airway clearance and potential for ineffective breathing pattern must be evaluated together. They should be evaluated as frequently as the vital signs. Any deterioration occurring in any of the functions is an important cue to increase the frequency of evaluation. The nurse *must intervene* if the patient cannot swallow saliva, if gag or cough reflex or both are markedly diminished or lost, if food and fluid regurgitates through the nose, or if vital capacity is less than one third of the predicted normal (or 600 cm^3 in the "average" adult). The combination of bulbar dysfunction and decreased vital capacity puts the patient at particular risk of both aspiration and respiratory failure.

Collaborative management consists of placement of a cuffed endotracheal or tracheostomy tube (depending upon anticipated length of dysfunction) to prevent aspiration of saliva and a nasogastric, esophageal, or gastric feeding tube. Reintroduction of oral feeding requires careful nursing monitoring.

■ NURSING DIAGNOSIS

Ineffective breathing patterns, related to dysfunction of respiratory musculature.

OUTCOME STANDARD AND CRITERIA

Breathing pattern is normal or improved as evidenced by:

- Normal respiratory rate, depth, timing, and rhythm
- Absence of inspiratory retractions/nasal flaring
- Absence of accessory muscle use
- Synchronous motion of thorax and abdomen during inspiration
- Absence of grunting and/or abdominal end-expiratory contraction
- Presence of normal bilateral breath sounds

Decreased movement of air due to disordered respiratory musculature may be life-threatening. Muscles important to breathing are the diaphragm and the intercostal muscles. In health, the diaphragm is the primary muscle of inspiration. The internal and external intercostal muscles assist in deep inspiration. Expiration is a passive process. The motor neurons of the diaphragm receive impulses from the phrenic nerve, which emerges from spinal nerve C4, with some input from C3 and C5. Spinal nerves T1 to T11 innervate the intercostal muscles.

Thus, spinal cord lesions at C5 and above will affect both diaphragmatic and intercostal musculature. Lesions below C5 will allow diaphragmatic movement but paralyze the intercostals. During the period of spinal shock, a patient with a lesion of the midthoracic region is able to voluntarily depress the diaphragm and thus take a breath. The ability to inspire maximally is lost because the intercostal muscles are paralyzed. When reflexes return, spasticity of the intercostal muscles aids in maximal chest expansion.

Respiratory musculature can also be affected by peripheral polyneuropathies, which impair both voluntary and reflex movement by demyelination of the motor component of the reflex arc. Myasthenia gravis and other disorders of neuromuscular transmission interfere with respiratory movement by blocking transmission at the myoneural junction. The intense muscular spasms of tetanus can also interfere with respiration by preventing full expansion of the chest.

NURSING INTERVENTIONS: EVALUATION OF RESPIRATORY FUNCTION

In patients at risk for ineffective breathing patterns due to respiratory musculature failure, function can be evaluated by measuring vital capacity serially, measuring blood gas values, and observing respiratory effort. Secondary clues to impending respiratory distress are increasing anxiety and fear of going to sleep. Patients at risk include those with spinal cord lesions above T6, those with polyneuropathies with trunk and upper extremity weakness, and those with generalized myasthenia gravis, particularly postoperative

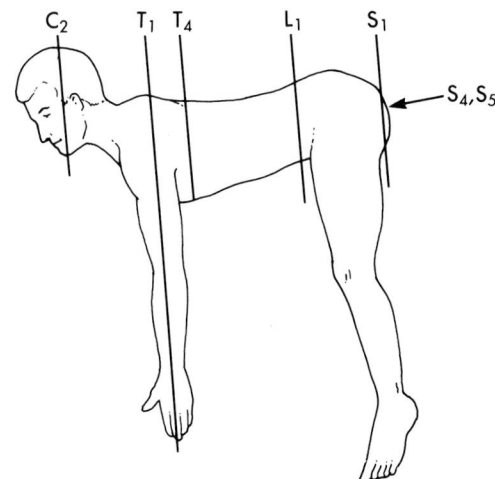

Figure 33-7 Representation of demarcating sensory dermatomes in the quadruped human. The quadruped figure illustrates the extension along the arms and legs of the dermatomes dividing the the thoracic and lumbar spine.

patients and those with intercurrent illness.

Since spinal cord sensory roots follow skin dermatomes, and since most traumatic lesions of the cord involve both motor and sensory pathways, the level of cord injury can be roughly estimated by *mapping sensory dermatome levels*. Figure 33-7 depicts schematically important dermatome levels in the quadruped human. The figure is shown in quadruped fashion to aid in appreciation of the extension of sacral and thoracic dermatomes along arms and legs.

Critical dermatomes in terms of functional outcome are shown. T1 extends from about the level of the scapula along the arm and is the upper limit of the intercostal nerves. T4 is approximately at the nipple line. Patients with lesions slightly below T4 will probably have adequate voluntary respiratory function, while those with lesions at T4 and above require frequent evaluation of respiratory function and may need ventilatory assistance. The functional significance of other dermatomes is discussed later under multisystem problems. Although most of the severe polyneuropathies involve greater motor than sensory loss, sensory dermatomes may be of some value in determining the level of peripheral nerve loss in symmetric polyneuropathy. Sensory dermatome evaluation is of no value in disorders of neuromuscular transmission (such as myasthenia gravis), since the disturbance is entirely at the neuromotor junction.

Although much more sophisticated measures of pulmonary function are available, bedside evaluation of *vital capacity* remains an important tool in serially evaluating respiratory status in neurological disorders. The bedside spirometer is easily used with the conscious patient and provides an immediate measure, without the time lag inherent in blood gas measurement. A single measurement of vital capacity is not as useful as a series, compared with the predicted normal for a person that size. Continually decreasing vital capacity indicates a patient who is losing respiratory muscle function and may need respiratory assistance. As a rule of thumb, patients with vital capacity below one third of normal (or below 600 cm^3) require assisted ventilation. A decrease in tidal volumes or vital capacity in a patient with spinal cord injury indicates extension of the injury (because of edema or bleeding into the cord). Such decreases may be expected in a patient with ascending polyneuropathy or worsening myasthenia gravis.

Measurement of *partial pressure of dissolved gases* in the blood is important in evaluating the overall respiratory status of patients with severe motor disorders but is not to be relied upon in determining the need for assisted ventilation in disorders characterized by rapid deterioration. For example, in myasthenia gravis, a patient may move from intact respiratory status to complete loss of voluntary respiratory effort in 20 minutes. Although polyneuropathies such as Guillain-Barré syndrome have a somewhat slower time course, waiting for the determination of arterial blood gases may delay respiratory assistance unnecessarily. Blood gas values may be more appropriately used to guide decisions regarding respiratory assistance in more stable lesions such as spinal cord injury. Secondary evaluative cues may be helpful. The nurse may observe respiratory effort or a patient's anxiety about going to sleep. Such secondary cues should prompt the nurse to initiate measurement of vital capacity and blood gases and to increase the frequency of evaluation.

Management of ineffective breathing pattern is collaborative among physicians, nurses, and respiratory therapists. The expected outcomes are (1) early detection of ineffective breathing pattern, (2) maintenance of adequate oxygenation with mechanical ventilation, and (3) restoration of effective breathing patterns without mechanical ventilation in patients whose lesions allow independent breathing.

Monitoring is the primary management strategy for early detection of insufficient respiratory effort and is described above. Assisted or controlled mechanical ventilation is generally necessary when vital capacity is less than 33% of expected normal or when blood gases are abnormal.

Care of patients on assisted ventilation is described in Chapter 30. Secondary nursing diagnoses that apply to patients with neurologically induced respiratory muscle failure include fear or anxiety, related to ineffective breathing; complete physical immobility; and impaired verbal communication, related to presence of endotracheal tube.

PSYCHOSOCIAL CONSIDERATIONS

Although the pathological processes that cause extracranial life-threatening motor dysfunction are quite different, they all can lead to severe immobilization in a person who is fully alert and aware of what is happening. The patient with Guillain-Barré syndrome lives with paralysis creeping upward rather rapidly; the patient with tetanus experiences growing stiffness, culminating in suffocating muscular spasm; the person with myasthenia never knows whether the next dose of medication can be swallowed, or worse, whether breathing will be possible from hour to hour. Finally, the patient with a cervical spine injury is transformed suddenly from a healthy active person to a person who cannot even breathe. Coupled with these devastating changes in body image and function are the frightening sights and sounds of critical care. Many of these patients have only the ceiling or floor to look at and can only imagine the worst about what is happening.

The reactions of most persons with acute, life-threatening illnesses follow a similar pattern: fear, denial, anger, depression, and resolution. In critically ill patients, one is most likely to see alternating fear, anger, and denial. While few patients deny that they cannot move at the moment, most deny that this situation will be permanent. Such denial probably has both physiological and psychological protective value during critical illness. It is appropriate to support the patient's hope for complete recovery in such disorders as Guillain-Barré syndrome and diphtheritic polyneuropathy, as this is consistent with the natural history of the disorders. False hope should not be offered the patient with an apparent complete spinal cord injury; neither should the patient be forced to abandon denial of the injury's severity. With modern rehabilitative techniques, most persons with spinal cord injuries can expect to lead an independent life. A study of the attitudes of nurses toward spinal cord–injured patients suggests that critical care nurses were the most pessimistic compared to intermediate care and rehabilitation nurses.[53] This pessimism probably reflects exposure to these patients during their bleakest time and may make it difficult for critical care nurses to offer sincere hope to them.

Coupled with the abrupt change in lifestyle and the patient's reasonable fears about survival is the difficulty of communicating inherent in tracheostomy and assisted ventilation. It is crucial to invent some means of communication that allows more than yes and no answers whenever possible. (See Chapter 15.) If the patient has any strength in the mouth, a letter board and mouthstick can be used to point out phrases and individual letters. Some patients have been able to use Morse code through eye blinks or small finger taps. As the patient stabilizes, sophisticated computer technology can be operated by breath or head movements.

Fear can express itself in both anger and incessant requests for nurse attention. Firm limits regarding what the nurse can and cannot do and when may help provide a sense of security for the patient, *provided* the nurse is consistent in letting the patient know what to expect and consistently follows through. It is important to remember that increased anxiety may reflect respiratory insufficiency as well as psychological response to injury.

Patients with severe extracranial motor dysfunction may spend long periods in critical care if ventilatory assistance is required. Consequently, the axiom that rehabilitation begins in critical care is certainly true with these patients. Skin care to prevent pressure sores, passive range of motion to prevent contractures, and attention to psychological needs are second only to measures to preserve life.

■ NURSING DIAGNOSIS

Impaired gas exchange, related to pulmonary embolism.

In addition to the direct effect of motor loss on respiratory musculature, patients immobilized from motor disorders are at increased risk for pulmonary embolism from deep vein thrombosis. Although there is disagreement in the literature regarding the incidence of deep vein thrombosis in spinal cord–injured patients and others with neurologically induced immobility, studies that report a low incidence rely on clinical signs rather than the more accurate plethysmography or ^{125}I-labeled fibrinogen studies to detect thrombosis. Clinical signs have been shown to miss both thrombosis and pulmonary embolism in the most widely studied groups, postoperative patients and patients after myocardial infarction. The few studies published that used appropriate techniques to detect thrombosis show an incidence that ranges from zero in patients with spinal fracture but no paralysis to as high as 75% to 100% in paralyzed spinal cord–injured persons.[54,55] The rate of pulmonary embolism in spinal cord–injured patients has been shown to be as high as 9% or 10%, with up to 3% mortality.[54,55,56,57] Management of pulmonary embolism is a collaborative problem, involving the ventilation/perfusion mismatch engendered by the embolism. Refer to Chapter 29 for discussion of medical therapy for pulmonary embolism.

Multisystem Dysfunction and Failure

Since the central nervous system integrates the input to the autonomic nervous system at both the cerebral and spinal cord levels, general injury to the diencephalon, brainstem, or spinal cord can interfere with autonomic and endocrine regulation of numerous body systems.

Cerebral regulation of the autonomic and endocrine systems occurs at the level of the diencephalon, with the hypothalamus the major integrator of input to the pituitary releasing hormones and of the preganglionic level of the sympathetic nervous system. Regulation of temperature, metabolic rate, blood pressure, and fluid balance all have important hypothalamic and pituitary inputs. Cranial regulation of the parasympathetic nervous system occurs in the brainstem.

Thus, patients with diffuse damage from head injury, intracranial hemorrhage, global hypoxia, or massive cerebral edema are all at risk for multisystem dysfunction secondary to abnormal cranial regulation of vegetative functions.

Clinical Problems Associated with Autonomic/Endocrine Dysfunction

The clinical problems stemming from disordered endocrine and autonomic control that may be manifested in such patients include hyperosmolar and hypoosmolar states, hyperthermia, catabolic state, coagulation disorders, and ventilation/perfusion mismatch (shunting).

Hyperosmolar and Hypoosmolar States. The most common source of hyperosmolar and hypoosmolar states is inappropriate management of parenteral fluids.[58] However, diabetes insipidus and syndrome of inappropriate antidiuretic hormone are potential neuropathological causes of the fluid and electrolyte imbalance problems that may be seen in patients with diffuse head injury, diencephalic stroke, or parasellar tumors or in those who have had pituitary surgery.

Diabetes insipidus is caused by an inability to produce antidiuretic hormone (ADH; vasopressin), with resultant polyuria and, if untreated, subsequent dehydration, hemoconcentration, and hypovolemia. Diabetes insipidus is characterized by urine output in excess of fluid intake, hypotonic urine (specific gravity 1.001 to 1.005 and urine osmolality 50 to 150 mosm/kg), and normal or increased serum sodium.[58,59] The conscious patient experiences excessive thirst. Nonketotic hyperglycemia is a second source of a hyperosmolar state, with subsequent osmotic diuresis. It may be seen in patients with occult diabetes but more commonly is the result of excessive mannitol, high-protein tube feedings, or corticosteroids. The common treatment of a hyperosmolar state includes replacement of urinary losses plus insensible losses with dextrose and water, rather than saline. Administration of vasopressin may be necessary to control the diuresis.

In contrast, *syndrome of inappropriate antidiuretic hormone (SIADH)* is caused by excessive production of ADH, resulting in low urine output compared with fluid intake, hypertonic urine (increased urinary sodium, urine osmolality higher than serum osmolality, and decreased serum sodium and serum osmolality of <280 mosm/kg).[58] Treatment of the hypoosmolar state consists of fluid restriction titrated by monitoring of urinary sodium and serum osmolality. Some investigators advocate adding hypertonic saline. Over-rapid correction of the hyponatremia can lead to central pontine myelinolysis.[7]

Careful nursing monitoring of fluid balance, electrolytes (both urine and serum), and osmolality is essential in the prevention or early detection of iatrogenic sources of fluid–electrolyte imbalance in these patients. The majority of critically ill patients with neurological disorders are comatose or too confused to express their thirst and thus meet their own fluid intake needs. Therefore, only careful monitoring and analysis of intake and output and urine and serum electrolytes will prevent serious fluid imbalance.

Hyperthermia. Hyperthermia is a second problem that may stem from failure of CNS regulatory mechanisms in patients with severe head injuries, hypothalamic stroke, or hypothalamic damage from any source. Infection must be ruled out before assuming that fever in neurological and neurosurgical patients is of hypothalamic origin. Respiratory and urinary tract infections are the most common sources of fever in neurological disorders.

Patients undergoing therapeutic barbiturate coma may become *poikilothermic*—i.e., take on the temperature of the environment—because of the action of barbiturates on central temperature regulation.[60] Therefore, it may be necessary to use artificial warming or cooling to maintain the patient's core temperature at 33° to 39° C.[60]

Catabolic State. Controversy exists regarding the extent to which neural trauma, as compared with trauma from all causes, induces a catabolic state. The bulk of evidence suggests that head trauma, at least in the first week after injury, increases metabolism to a greater degree than is seen after surgery or non-CNS trauma. The net effect is high nitrogen excretion in the urine, extremely high caloric need, and rapid muscle wasting when caloric needs cannot be met nutritionally.

The catabolic state is a collaborative problem and is best managed by close teamwork of nutritionists, physicians, and nurses. Ordinary intravenous fluids cannot deliver more than about 600 kcal per day, far short of the estimated 3,500 kcal needed to maintain body weight during hypermetabolism after head in-

jury. Therefore, the goal of nutritional regimens for severely head–injured patients is to provide calories via dextrose in water intravenously for as short a time as possible, advancing to enteral feedings via nasogastric tube as soon as the patient has adequate bowel tones. If enteral feeding is not possible, total parenteral alimentation is necessary. A common nutritional goal is 3,500 kcal per day, with 20 g of nitrogen per day. Caloric needs increase in the presence of fever and continuous spontaneous movement. Corticosteroids used in the treatment of intracranial pressure also increase nitrogen excretion and impair cellular response to insulin. The most rational nutritional regimen is tailored to the metabolic needs of the individual patient and coordinated by a skilled nutritionist.[61,62]

Coagulation Disorders. Coagulation disorders, specifically disseminated intravascular coagulopathy (DIC), may occur in any multiply injured patient, including those with head and spinal cord injury as part of their multiple trauma. The incidence of abnormal coagulation increases markedly with the severity of head injury, although not every patient with abnormal coagulation develops DIC.[17] Heparin is the treatment of choice in DIC, as outlined in Chapter 42. However, neurosurgical patients with DIC receiving heparin must be monitored exceptionally carefully because of the possibility of precipitating an intracranial hemorrhage.

Ventilation/Perfusion Mismatch. Ventilation/perfusion mismatch, or shunting, is a common finding in patients following head injury, massive cerebral ischemia, and intracranial hemorrhage.[63] There is continuing discussion regarding the comparative extent to which this reflects impaired central regulation of sympathetic input to the pulmonary vasculature rather than systemic problems that influence the pulmonary disorder.

There is experimental evidence that severe CNS injury can create massive sympathetic nervous system discharge, leading to constriction of pulmonary vessels, increased hydrostatic pressure in the pulmonary vasculature, subsequent extravasation of fluid into the interstitium and alveoli, and finally, pulmonary edema or adult respiratory distress syndrome (ARDS). Although frank neurogenic pulmonary edema is rarely seen, the presence of some degree of shunting in a large proportion of head-injured patients has led a number of researchers to propose that neural as well as systemic factors are responsible.

In addition, neurally injured patients are frequently in coma and thus unable to protect the airway from aspiration of oral and gastric secretions; may have concomitant chest trauma or multiple fractures that predispose them to fat embolism; and are at high risk for pulmonary embolism from deep vein thrombosis. Treatment of ARDS and pulmonary emboli is discussed in Chapter 29. Positive end-expiratory pressure (PEEP) is a common therapy in ARDS and other pulmonary disorders. It has the potential to increase intracranial pressure in high-risk patients because of its effect on intrathoracic pressure. However, a number of investigations have shown that PEEP can be used safely in neurosurgical patients if the head is kept elevated at 30° and PEEP is maintained at about 10 cmH₂O.[23]

Multisystem Disorders Typical of Acute Spinal Cord Injury and Polyneuropathy

Multisystem failure may also occur following injury or disease of the spinal cord, which is a primary integrator of peripheral autonomic nervous system function. The following discussion of multisystem problems is most pertinent to acute spinal cord injury. Since polyneuropathies may also have an autonomic neuropathy component, it is applicable to patients with polyneuropathies as well. The effects on the respiratory system have already been discussed. Multisystem effects are summarized in Table 33-9.

Cardiovascular Effects. The cardiovascular effects are related primarily to loss of sympathetic outflow below the level of injury. A period of spinal shock occurs for some time after injury, in which somatic and autonomic reflex activity is lost. Although autonomic demyelination is not the rule in polyneuropathy, it can occur and present similar systemic problems.

Monitoring of cardiac rate and rhythm should be instituted in patients with cervical cord injury to detect serious dysrhythmias or bradycardia that would impair cardiac output. Hypotension is usually time-limited and self-regulating. However, if associated injuries are causing bleeding or sequestration of fluid in third spaces, cautious volumetric and colloid replacement may be used. Care must be exercised not to put the patient into pulmonary edema through overzealous fluid replacement.

Thermoregulatory Effects. Difficulties with temperature regulation are related to loss of peripheral vasodilatation and constriction. Again, the higher the lesion, the less ability the body has to regulate temperature by constriction and dilatation of skin vessels. The patient becomes *poikilothermic*, that is, takes on the temperature of the environment. Instead of being able to regulate the core temperature through vasodilatation to lose heat through the skin or vasoconstriction to conserve heat, the vessels of the patient in spinal shock remain dilated. Most commonly, the functional result is that body temperature drops, particularly in air-conditioned units. However, in extremely warm weather, hyperthermia may result because the patient cannot sweat below the level of the lesion and further dilatation of skin vessels cannot occur. The patient's environment must be regulated to maintain core temperature. If hypothermia is serious, it may be necessary to monitor core temperature by means of tympanic membrane or esophageal temperature. Usually rectal or oral electronic measurements are sufficient to indicate trends in temperature. In no case should touch or skin temperature be relied upon to monitor the patient's temperature. The patient may be warmed by blankets, by increasing the room temperature, or by electrical heating devices or may be kept cool by fans or other cooling devices. It is imperative to remember that the patient cannot feel these devices and cannot sense when there is danger of thermal or cold injury.

Visceral Effects. Most visceral innervation is from the sympathetic outflow. The efferents leave the spinal cord in the thoracolumbar spine, between T1 and L1 to 2. Heart, lungs, tracheobronchial tree, viscera, peripheral blood vessels, bowel, and bladder all receive their sympathetic innervation from the thoracolumbar sympathetic ganglia. Parasympathetic innervation of these organs is from the vagus nerve (medulla) and, that of the bladder, rectum, and penis from the pelvic plexus (sacral spinal nerves). Consequently, any lesion of the thoracic or cervical cord will interrupt cardiovascular function and the function of most of the viscera. The higher the lesion, the greater the disruption of autonomic function.

The viscera will not cease functioning entirely, because they also receive parasympathetic input. However, the parasympathetic input is unbalanced and will tend toward quiescence. For example, paralytic ileus occurs because motility depends upon the balance of sympathetic and parasympathetic activity. Cardiac and lung function do not cease, because of intrinsic rhythmicity in the heart and because vagal input is still intact. However, bradycardia and dysrhythmias may occur because the vagal influence is unopposed. In addition, with a cervical lesion, hypotension may occur because there is no sympathetic outflow to maintain peripheral vascular resistance. Cardiovascular reflexes that adjust blood pressure to postural changes are impaired in such cases, and hypotension may manifest itself whenever the patient's position is changed, even from side to side. Finally, added to the risk of deep vein thrombosis due to immobility is that from decreased peripheral vascular tone and thus increased tendency to stasis of blood. Absence of muscle tone impairs venous return and

TABLE 33-9 Relation of Brainstem and Spinal Segments to Critical Functions in Acute and Long-term Spinal Disorders

Muscles	Brainstem or Spinal Segment	Dermatome Reference Points	Acute Dysfunctions	Functional Ability if Lesion Persists
Soft palate, pharyngeal, tongue	Medulla (CN IX, X, XII)	—	↓ Gag, swallow leading to choking, aspiration	Swallowing with retraining if reflex returns; may need permanent esophagostomy
All below trapezius, sternocleidomastoid	C2	Back of head	Total loss of respiration and movement from shoulder down (such patients now survive with speedy prehospital care)	Requires permanent respirator; can shrug shoulders, turn head (CN XI), and use all cranial nerves
Diaphragm	C3, 4, 5	Ear, neck, clavicle to wrist	↓ Or absent diaphragmatic as well as intercostal respiratory effort, high risk of hypotension, hypothermia, ileus, atonic bladder, skin breakdown	Can move head, shrug shoulders, breathe with intercostals (after reflexes return); experimental use of phrenic nerve stimulation
Deltoid, biceps	C6	Lateral third of arm, shoulder to thumb	↓ Respiratory function (diaphragm intact, without intercostals); risk for hypotension, hypothermia, ileus, atonic bladder, skin breakdown	Can move head, shoulders; breathe independently but with ↓ reserve; flex elbow, feed self with prosthesis; use electric wheelchair
Latissimus, serratus, pectoralis, radial wrist extensors	C7	Dorsal midarm to digits 1 or 2 (dorsal and palmar)	↓ Respiratory function (without intercostals); risk for hypotension, hypothermia, atonic bladder, ileus, skin breakdown	Some rolling over; can flex elbow, feed self with hand devices; sit up; self-propel adapted wheelchair
Triceps, finger extensors and flexors	C8	Medial third of arm including digits 3 and 4	↓ Respiratory function; risk of hypotension, hypothermia, ileus, atonic bladder, skin breakdown	Can feed self with devices, roll over, sit up, transfer, dress, toilet, move in bed unassisted
Hand intrinsics, ulnar, wrist, and fingers	T1	Midpectoral (T4 at nipple line)	↓ Respiratory function; risk of hypotension, hypothermia, ileus, atonic bladder, skin breakdown	Independent eating, moving in bed, toilet, use of wheelchair, respiratory reserve
Upper intercostals, upper back	T6	Two segments below nipple, three segments above umbilicus (T10)	Ileus, atonic bladder, skin breakdown; low risk of hypotension and hypothermia	Normal respiratory reserve; independent in all of above; can stand with bracing
Abdominals, thoracic extensors	T12	Between umbilicus (T10) and inguinal fold (L1)	Atonic bladder, fecal retention	Can ambulate with bracing; reflex bowel and bladder (true of all lesions above sacral cord)

Note: All patients with lesions above T6 have high risk for hypotension and hypothermia/hyperthermia because of interruption in sympathetic outflow. These same persons are at increased risk for autonomic hyperreflexia in the rehabilitation period. All lesions above the lumbar level carry high potential of paralytic ileus; all persons with lesions above sacral cord have atonic bladder and anal sphincter during the acute phase. Lesions above the sacrum convert to reflex, and bladder and bowel are uninhibited when reflexes return. Those with sacral lesions are most apt to retain atonic bladder and bowel secondary to absent reflexes.

contributes to both hypotension and venous thrombosis.

Loss of gastrointestinal motility may manifest itself in paralytic ileus. The nurse should not wait for distention and vomiting before assessing gastrointestinal function. Any patient with a sensory loss above T8 (output to the splanchnic plexus) is at risk for decreased gastric motility. As Figure 33-7 shows, L1 is just above the inguinal crease. Thus, patients with lesions between the inguinal fold and umbilicus (and above) should be evaluated for ileus.

Bowel sounds should be assessed regularly and low nasogastric suction begun if they are decreased or absent. Gastrointestinal bleeding from stress ulcers occurs in up to 20% of patients. Pain may be absent, and tarry stools may be the only manifestation.

Bowel and bladder evacuation are impaired by a variety of lesions above the sacral cord. Most sympathetic and parasympathetic input is from the lumbar and sacral plexuses. Therefore, almost any cord injury or polyneuropathy affecting the lower extremities can be expected to involve the bowel and bladder. Until reflexes return, the bladder will fill and distend just as the bowel does. Periodic release of urine with intermittent or continuous catheterization will be necessary. Nasogastric suction and intravenous feeding will be required until bowel sounds return. If feces are present in the rectum, manual removal or gentle enemas may be needed until rectal reflexes return. The presence of rectal reflexes can be determined by inserting a gloved finger into the rectum. The rectal sphincter will contract on the finger if the reflex is present.

Integumentary Effects. The integument is at high risk for breakdown in the paralyzed patient. Loss of sympathetic tone, diminished trophic influence of motor nerves, and paralysis combine in a paralyzed limb or body to bring about a more rapid breakdown of skin under pressure. Studies in both animals and humans have demonstrated histological evidence of tissue destruction within 1 to 2 hours of sustained pressure in normal tissue; this time is shortened by as much as half in paralyzed tissue. In the person with either segmental or suprasegmental motor loss, mechanical devices that vary pressure over body surfaces and frequent change of position are imperative from the moment of admission.

Skin breakdown can also occur in the severely immobilized patient with myasthenia gravis but is not so rapid as in disorders of the central or peripheral nerves. Sepsis secondary to pressure sores was the major cause of death in spinal cord injury prior to the development of modern spinal cord injury centers. It remains one of the major sources of disability and hospitalization.

NEURAL DISORDERS THAT ALTER CONSCIOUSNESS, VENTILATION, AND MULTISYSTEM REGULATION

The preceding portions of this chapter have been focused on pathophysiological states common to many neural disorders and the clinical problems and nursing diagnoses common to these states. The remaining section of the chapter is organized around neurological diseases and disorders that are frequently seen in critically ill patients. Since so many of the human responses are common to many disorders, relevant nursing diagnoses and clinical problems are presented in tables with cross-referencing to the first description of appropriate protocols and nursing interventions. Five categories of disorder account for the majority of critically ill patients with nervous system disease: neurotrauma, cerebrovascular disorders, neurosurgical procedures, infectious disorders, and autoimmune and neurotoxic disorders.

Neurotrauma

Head and spinal cord injuries are the primary kinds of neurotrauma that lead to hospitalization in critical care units. The annual incidence of head and spinal cord injury is estimated at over 2 million, with close to 500,000 requiring hospital admission. Nearly 25 billion dollars is spent yearly on acute and chronic care of persons so injured.[77]

Since both head and spinal cord injury stem from motor vehicle accidents and falls, such as those in diving, skiing, and skateboarding, such neurotrauma is largely preventable.[64] All health professionals share a responsibility for community and individual education regarding means to prevent such accidents. Legislation and personal decisions regarding the use of seat belts, automobile air bags, proper sports training and techniques, and alcohol-free driving are all means of reducing the number of head and spinal cord injuries.

Head Injury

Head injury is a catch-all term for a large number of medical diagnoses related to trauma involving the skull and brain. A common operational definition requires a blow to the head and altered consciousness, no matter how brief. Minor head injuries are considered to be those in which the loss of consciousness is less than 20 minutes and in which the Glasgow Coma Score is 13 to 15. Major, or severe, head injuries are operationally defined as those with Glasgow Coma Scores of 8 or less. (Several combinations of responses are possible, but commonly these patients open their eyes only to pain, do not follow directions, may have abnormal movements, and utter no comprehensible sounds or only inappropriate words.)

Head injury serious enough to require critical care results from a blow to the head, often delivered at high speed. There may be focal injury consisting of contusions and hematomas at the site of the blow, the opposite side of the brain (contrecoup injury), and where the brain hits the rough projections on the underside of the skull. Rupture of small and large vessels may result in subdural and epidural hematomas, which act as mass lesions, and subarachnoid hemorrhage, which releases blood into the cerebrospinal fluid. In addition, the dissipation of energy throughout the brain tissue often results in diffuse tearing of nerve fibers. Such widespread diffuse damage is often associated with a long-term vegetative state and is now known to be the source of what used to be called primary brainstem damage.

Pathophysiological responses to these structural injuries include brain swelling and edema, increased intracranial pressure, and transtentorial herniation. Focal or generalized motor seizures may develop as early sequelae (during the first week) or late sequelae (up to 2 years after injury) to the injury. Hypothalamic damage or ischemic responses to intracranial hypertension may initiate alterations in temperature regulation, coagulation disorders, cardiac dysrhythmias, hyper- and hypoosmolar states, and increased metabolism.[65,66]

Medical and Nursing Management. Table 33-10 summarizes the medical protocols and nursing diagnoses commonly applicable to patients with acute head injury.

Spinal Cord Injury

Spinal cord injury resulting from dislocated fracture, contusion, or direct injury to the cord may result in functional transection of the spinal cord at any level, with concomitant multisystem dysfunction during the initial phase of spinal shock. Injuries at C6 and above impair ventilation by disrupting neural input to the diaphragm. Injuries between C6 and T11 impair the ventilatory function of the intercostal muscles.

The overall U.S. incidence of spinal cord injury is estimated at 3 per 100,000 persons annually, with 72% of new injuries occurring in males in the 15- to 24-year age group. The overwhelming preponderance of spinal cord injuries in this group is the result of motorcycle and automobile accidents. The second most susceptible group is elderly adults, with the injuries resulting from falls.

In experimental studies of the pathological changes occurring from blows to the spinal cord, there is an initial phase of 15 to 30 minutes in which neurons and vessels appear normal, followed by a massive release of vasoactive neurochemicals with subsequent cord swelling and then ischemia. Eventually neurons in the cord die and are replaced by glial cells or by cavities.[9] The degree to which cell death occurs de-

TABLE 33-10 Medical and Nursing Management of Severe Head Injury

Collaborative Diagnosis	Common Medical Protocol	Nursing Diagnosis	Outcome Standard	Nursing Interventions
Potential for brain swelling and intracranial hypertension	Hyperventilation, corticosteroids, mannitol	High risk for decreased intracranial adaptive capacity	No sustained increases in ICP (>10 mmHg over baseline for 5 or more minutes) with activity	1. Monitor for disproportionate charge in ICP with activity. Assess electrolytes, osmolality. 2. Position patient carefully. 3. Institute drug protocols to decrease ICP prior to nursing activities. 4. Use kinetic bed or turning sheets to minimize tactile stimulation.
Potential for brain herniation	Surgical decompression; hypertonic agents		Herniation is detected early	1. Monitor and assess neurological status, particularly level of consciousness.
High risk for hypermetabolism (alteration in nutrition, less than body requirements)	Tube feeding; hyperalimentation if needed		Optimal weight is maintained	1. Monitor bowel sounds and institute enteral feeding as soon as they return. 2. Coordinate nutritionist referral as needed. 3. Monitor osmolarity, electrolytes.

TABLE 33-10 **Medical and Nursing Management of Severe Head Injury—cont'd**

Collaborative Diagnosis	Common Medical Protocol	Nursing Diagnosis	Outcome Standard	Nursing Interventions
High risk for hypo- or hyperosmolar state	See text under Multisystem Dysfunction and Failure		Serum osmolality is normal	1. Monitor electrolytes, osmolarity, urine specific gravity.
		Complete physical immobility, related to coma	Complications of immobility are prevented as exhibited by absence of skin, thrombotic, embolic, or ileus complications	1. Change patients position frequently, with careful monitoring of ICP response. 2. Give passive range-of-motion exercises. 3. Use antiembolic stockings or pneumatic compression boots to prevent thrombosis. 4. Monitor bowel activity and prevent constipation.
		High risk for injury, related to coma: skin breakdown, corneal abrasion	Skin remains intact or improved; no corneal abrasions occur	1. Change patient's position frequently. 2. Give good skin care. 3. If patient cannot close eyes, use eyedrops every 1 to 2 hours; patch eyes periodically.
		High risk for ineffective breathing patterns, related to coma: atelectasis	Breath sounds are normal	1. Monitor blood gases, respiratory status. 2. Turn frequently, deep breathe.
		High risk for injury, related to hyperarousal	Acquired injury is absent	1. Pad bed rails. 2. Use sheepskin-type bedding to prevent sheet burns.
		Impaired family coping, related to severity of injury	Family coping is effective	1. Provide information as appropriate; inform promptly about status changes. 2. Facilitate family contacts with physician and social worker. 3. Assure family it is permissible to take time for themselves if indicated. 4. Facilitate family–patient interaction.

termines the completeness of the functional transection of the cord. Sensory and reflex input from intact cord distal to the injury cannot reach the brain, and motor and autonomic output from the brain and brainstem cannot reach the periphery past the injured area. The effects of functional transection on ventilation and multisystem function are described fully in the earlier section, Multisystem Dysfunction and Failure.

Initial management of acute spinal cord injury is collaborative, involving emergency medical techni-cians, emergency room nurses, and physicians. The primary goal of management in the field and upon arrival at the acute care hospital is to *minimize the extent of spinal cord trauma.* The primary intervention is immobilization and stabilization of the fracture and spinal cord.

Although critical care nurses are not often the first to attend to the newly spinal-injured patient, they should understand the principles of movement and transfer of such patients from the moment of injury, which are crucial to prevention of further damage to spine or cord. Nothing is more tragic than for a patient to come to the hospital with a fractured spine and with moving extremities and to leave paraplegic or quadriplegic after inexpert transfer from bed to x-ray to bed.

At the scene of the accident or at the first contact with the patient, the possibility of a spinal injury must always be kept in mind. *Patients with head injury, particularly if unconscious, must be presumed to have cervical spine injury until proved otherwise by an x-ray that visualizes all eight cervical vertebrae.* Approximately 10% to 15% of head-injured patients have associated cervical spine injuries. In the conscious patient, reported pain over any portion of the spine, parathesias or decreased sensation in the trunk or extremities, or difficulty in moving extremities is presumptive evidence of spinal injury. The patient should be transported as if spinal injury were present until this is definitively ruled out by x-ray. Until x-rays have been taken and read, the patient should remain on the emergency vehicle stretcher. Each additional transfer of the patient with an unstable fracture increases the chances of cord compression.

Any patient with a suspected spinal injury must be transported supine on a hard, flat surface. The hard surface is sufficient in itself to immobilize the thoracic and lumbar spine. In suspected cervical spine injury, the head must be in neutral position, with lateral immobilization by sandbags and preferably a stiff cervical collar. Wide tape or cloth extending over the forehead and to the spine board will help prevent forward flexion. The major objective of neck immobilization is to *prevent flexion, extension, and rotation of the cervical spine.* Figure 33-8 shows one method of manually immobilizing the neck while allowing maximum visualization of all cervical vertebrae during x-ray.

Transfer of the patient from one surface to another should not be started until a person skilled and trained in such transfers is present to act as team leader. A patient with an unstable fracture will never be harmed by remaining on an emergency vehicle stretcher but may be permanently paralyzed by improper transfer from it to an emergency room or nursing unit bed. Transfer of the patient with cervical spine injury requires at least four persons: three to support the body and maintain perfect alignment with the head, which is immobilized by the fourth person. The best method of stabilizing the head is to use a cervical traction halter. One hand exerts a gentle cephalad pull on the ties of the halter and the other is used under the occiput to support the head and neck in neutral alignment. Transfer of the patient with thoracic or lumbar injury is similar but does not require traction and immobilization of the neck.

If there is an unstable fracture or fracture dislo-

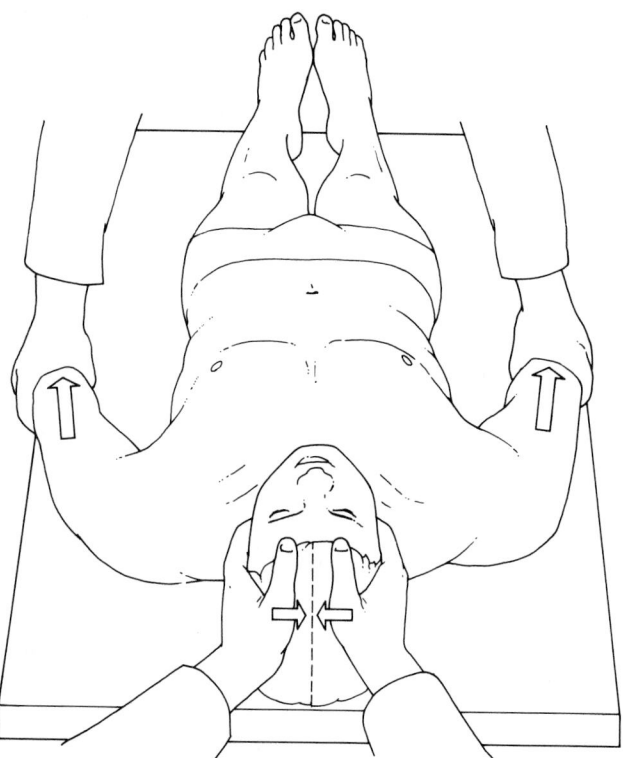

Figure 33-8 A technique for immobilizing the head and exerting gentle manual traction during x-ray of a patient with suspected cervical spine injury.

cation, the neurosurgeon or orthopedic surgeon usually applies skeletal traction in the form of skull tongs. The patient in skeletal traction is then maintained on the nursing unit in a standard bed, Stryker frame, or kinetic bed. Cleansing of the insertion sites daily or twice daily and application of antibiotic ointment are useful in preventing local infection around the tongs.

Medical Management. Ongoing medical management varies considerably according to physician preference. High-dose methylprednisolone (30 mg/kg initial bolus with a 5.4 mg/kg/hr infusion) over the next 23 hours started within 8 hours of injury has become standard practice in many centers, based on a multicenter randomized controlled trial showing significant neurological improvement in patients so treated compared to placebo or naloxone.[67] This therapy is believed to be effective by stabilizing cell membranes through inhibition of lipid peroxidation and membrane lipolysis.

A number of other experimental techniques such as perfusion of the cord with hypothermic solutions, myelotomy, and osmotic diuretics have been tried in attempts to reduce the secondary cord injury from swelling. No controlled trials have been conducted to evaluate these therapies adequately.

Low-dose heparin, aspirin, dipyridamole (Persantine), and calf compression have all been recommended to prevent deep-vein thrombosis and pulmonary embolism.[55,57] However, no adequately controlled trials have been conducted to satisfactorily answer the question of whether the risk of heparinization is justified, given the relatively low rate of morbidity and mortality despite a high rate of deep-vein thrombosis in these patients.[57] Gastric suction and intermittent or continuous catheterization are routinely ordered in managing paralytic ileus and neurogenic bladder.

Nursing Management. Nursing management is collaborative with medicine in minimizing the extent of cord damage, preventing multisystem complications, and monitoring for extension of the injury. The functional problems faced by the spinal cord–injured patient relative to the level of cord injury are summarized in Table 33-9; the primary potential nursing diagnoses can be inferred from those problems and include the following:

Ineffective breathing, related to respiratory muscle dysfunction

Impaired gas exchange, related to pulmonary embolism (from deep vein thrombosis)

Multisystem dysfunction, related to spinal shock: positional hypotension, bradycardia, paralytic ileus, atonic bladder with urinary retention, poikilothermia

Complete self-care deficit, related to level of paralysis

Impairment of skin integrity, related to immobility and decreased trophic factors in paralyzed tissue

Grief response, related to abrupt change in lifestyle

Nursing intervention combines monitoring with specific actions for common problems. Monitoring is critical in early detection of extension of injury or development of multisystem failure. Knowledge of the level of spinal injury from the x-ray findings plus mapping of sensory dermatomes and motor ability will enable the nurse to focus observation on those problems most likely to occur for each patient. The primary nursing diagnoses and management strategies are summarized in Table 33-11.

Sensory level can best be mapped by beginning in areas that are known to be anesthetic and moving upward, asking the patient to indicate when a pricking pin feels sharper. This level should be marked on the skin to note a baseline and aid in determining whether the level of injury is extending. Swelling and intracord hemorrhage in the first hours after injury may extend the level of damage both up and down the cord. Muscle testing uses the 0 to 5 scale described in Chapter 32, with zero indicating no flicker of contraction and 5 indicating full resistive strength. The minimum tests necessary to adequately monitor change in motor function following spinal cord injury are:[68]

Testing of shoulder shrug
Raising arms, flexing and extending elbows, dorsiflexing and extending wrists
Pinch strength of thumb and index finger
Hip, knee, and ankle extension and flexion
Abdominal and anal reflexes

Cerebrovascular Disorders

The majority of cerebrovascular disorders, transient ischemic attacks, and strokes do not necessitate critical care. However, massive hemispheric stroke, intracerebral hemorrhage, aneurysmal subarachnoid hemorrhage, and some brainstem strokes can impair consciousness or ventilation sufficiently to necessitate intensive nursing care. Further, current therapies for vasospasm secondary to subarachnoid hemorrhage require intensive technological monitoring. Concentration of all stroke patients in critical stroke units has not been found to have any advantages over having a knowledgeable stroke team available to patients on the general units.[70]

Cerebrovascular accident, or stroke, is not a single entity but rather a category of cerebrovascular disease that leads to sudden or rapidly progressive nonconvulsive neurological deficit. Stroke is the third leading cause of death in the United States, second only to coronary artery disease and cancer. The annual U.S. incidence of stroke is falling, but remains around 2 million, with 155,000 deaths. Over half of all patients hospitalized for neurological disease have had acute strokes.

Cerebrovascular accidents or strokes are characterized by progressive or abrupt focal neurological deficits that result from ischemia or infarction of the brain tissue supplied by a particular cerebral artery and its branches. The specific neurological deficits depend on the function of the portion of the brain supplied by that arterial distribution. The internal carotid and its branches supply the anterior portion of the brain, including most of the cerebral cortex. The structures supplied by the carotid and its major branches include the frontal lobes, motor cortex, sensory cortex, auditory cortex, and optic radiations. Branches of the anterior circulation penetrate into the medial surface of the brain and supply the hippocampus, basal ganglia, and internal capsule (radiations of the motor fibers from motor cortex to brainstem). Thus, ischemia or infarction of the anterior distribution of the cerebral blood supply can impair the functions of movement, sensation, speech, cognition and vision, depending upon which brain area is infarcted. Consciousness is not commonly altered in anterior circulation stroke unless there is bilateral hemispheric damage, hemorrhage into the intracerebral ventricles, or brain shift and swelling from large intracerebral hemorrhage or infarct.

TABLE 33-11 **Medical and Nursing Management of Acute Spinal Cord Injury**

Collaborative Clinical Problem	Common Medical Protocol	Nursing Diagnosis	Outcome Standard	Nursing Interventions
Ineffective breathing pattern with cervical or high thoracic injury	Assisted ventilation if needed; respiratory therapy		Breathing pattern is adequate for respiratory demands	1. Monitor respirations, blood gases, and vital capacity. 2. Assist patient in coughing. 3. Give deep breathing exercises. 4. Position for comfort and enhanced respiratory excursion.
Impaired gas exchange secondary to pulmonary embolism	May or may not use prophylactic low-dose heparin	High risk for impaired gas exchange	Hypoxemia is absent or reduced	1. Apply antiembolic stockings. 2. Monitor for sudden change in respiratory status. 3. Administer oxygen. 4. Position patient for maximum oxygenation (e.g., normal area dependent).
Potential for secondary injury due to displacement or fracture	May include immobilization, frame bed, traction, cervical tongs, etc.; may use corticosteroids to prevent cord edema	High risk for secondary injury	Extension of injury does not occur	1. Give scrupulous attention to maintaining alignment of neck and back during transfer or turning.
Potential for multisystem dysfunction related to spinal shock	Nasogastric decompression for ileus, urinary catheter for atonic bladder		Multisystem dysfunction does not occur	1. Monitor for return of bowel sounds. 2. Use intermittent or continuous catheter. 3. Monitor for hypotension and bradycardia, particularly that stimulated by positioning change or suctioning. 4. Monitor temperature, maintaining environment that keeps patient normothermic.

TABLE 33-11 **Medical and Nursing Management of Acute Spinal Cord Injury—cont'd**

Collaborative Clinical Problem	Common Medical Protocol	Nursing Diagnosis	Outcome Standard	Nursing Interventions
		Alteration in skin integrity, related to immobility and paralysis	Skin is intact or improved as indicated by normal color, texture, and turgor and absence of ulcers or lesions	1. Change patient's position every 2 hours and inspect all skin surfaces. 2. Use kinetic bed if possible to help prevent skin breakdown and atelectasis. 3. Assure adequate nutrition. 4. Use elbow and heel protectors. 5. Apply lotion to dry skin; select soaps and bathing according to skin condition.
		Potential alteration in comfort, related to immobility, paresthesia, inability to scratch self	Pain, itching, and other sources of discomfort are absent as verbalized by patient	1. Assist patient in scratching, etc., as needed. 2. Give pain medication as needed for incisional pain if laminectomy or spinal fusion is done. 3. Change patient's position frequently. 4. Provide diversional activities if appropriate. 5. Provide sensory and procedural information prior to techniques.
		Potential grief response, related to sudden change in lifestyle	Grief response is adaptive as indicated by effective coping mechanisms and decision making	1. Listen to patient's expressions of anger or denial. 2. Focus on short-term goals and achievements. 3. Provide as much control for patient as possible in choices about ongoing care. 4. Foster support by family, clergy, and others considered significant by patient.

The vertebral arteries provide the posterior circulation of the brain, which supplies the brainstem, medial surface of the occipital lobe, diencephalon, and cerebellum. Ischemia or infarction of this distribution can affect the functions of visual perception, movement (via brainstem motor tracts or cerebellar control of coordination), cranial nerves, or control of breathing. Consciousness is generally preserved unless there is infarction of the reticular formation in the pons or midbrain, pressure on the brainstem from cerebellar hemorrhage and swelling, or subarachnoid hemorrhage into the basal cisterns.

Ischemia and infarction may occur in the cerebral circulation from occlusive emboli and thrombi, from rupture of microaneurysms into the brain parenchyma (hypertensive intracerebral hemorrhage), or from rupture of saccular (Berry) aneurysms into the subarachnoid space (subarachnoid hemorrhage). Strokes from any cause become life-threatening if they alter consciousness or ventilation. Therefore, the following discussion of nursing diagnoses and clinical problems in stroke relates only to those life-threatening problems likely to be seen in critical care.

Intracerebral Infarct or Hemorrhage

Strokes from emboli or thrombi rarely cause coma unless an entire hemisphere is infarcted and massive swelling ensues.[39] However, intracerebral hemorrhage from the anterior or posterior circulation often causes coma. Posterior circulation hemorrhage into the diencephalon creates coma by direct effects on the reticular activating system, whereas anterior circulation hemorrhages are more likely to alter consciousness as a result of brain shift from mass effect or secondary swelling. Cerebellar hemorrhage (posterior circulation) may cause coma by direct compression of the brainstem from the expanding mass or by upward herniation of the cerebellum through the tentorium.

Medical management of intracerebral or intracerebellar hemorrhage consists of definitive diagnosis of hemorrhage versus large infarct by computed tomography or magnetic resonance scan, supportive therapy to prevent secondary brain injury, and, if surgically feasible, evacuation of the hematoma. Evacuation of hemorrhages into the basal ganglia and of cerebellar hemorrhage is often followed by rapid clinical improvement. Hemorrhage into the third ventricle may require ventricular shunting. Hemorrhage into the midbrain-upper pons is manifested by both coma and absence of spontaneous breathing or markedly abnormal breathing patterns and is not benefited by surgical therapy.

Nursing management of patients with completed hemorrhagic stroke that impairs consciousness is nearly identical to that for the patient with impaired consciousness from any other disorder affecting the cerebral hemispheres. The principal potential nursing diagnoses and collaborative clinical problems include:

Brain herniation (transtentorial for intracerebral hemorrhage, upward for cerebellar hemorrhage)

Ineffective airway clearance

Intracranial hypertension

Complete self-care deficit

Complete physical immobility, with potential for multiple secondary injury: skin breakdown, atelectasis, corneal abrasion, deep vein thrombosis, renal calculi

Multisystem dysregulation: hyper- or hypoosmolarity, poikilothermia, cardiac arrhythmias

Relevant nursing management is summarized in the earlier section on head injury.

Brainstem Stroke

The posterior cerebral circulation supplies the brainstem, which in turn regulates the function of the cranial nerves and basic vegetative functions, such as swallowing, breathing, and control of blood pressure. Further, all motor and sensory fibers pass through the brainstem enroute to the cortex from the periphery.

The majority of brainstem strokes impair one or more focal neurological functions but do not threaten life. However, when airway protection, automatic control of breathing, or the muscles of respiration are impaired, the patient requires ventilatory support and critical care nursing. Infarction or hemorrhage of the caudal anterior pons (basis pontis) spares the reticular formation but impairs all the cranial nerve nuclei from IX through XII, interrupts all motor output, and produces what is known as the *locked-in syndrome*. The patient is fully alert but unable to speak or move except for the eyes. Nursing diagnoses for such patients include:

Ineffective airway clearance, related to paralysis of palate and pharynx

Potential for inadequate gas exchange, related to paralysis of intrinsic muscles of respiration (phrenic nerve may remain intact)

Complete physical immobility, related to flaccid paralysis of lower face and total body, with potential for multiple secondary complications: skin breakdown, atelectasis, subluxation of shoulders, renal calculi, constipation or impaction, urinary tract infection

Complete self-care deficit

Potential for inadequate nutrition, related to inability to swallow

Inadequate verbal communication, related to paralysis of speech structures

Fear, related to inability to communicate alertness

Subarachnoid Hemorrhage

Subarachnoid hemorrhage and cerebral vasospasm were discussed earlier under States That Disrupt Consciousness. Subarachnoid hemorrhage is classified as a type of stroke and most often occurs following rupture of saccular (Berry) aneurysms in relatively young people. A smaller number of subarachnoid hemorrhages occur when vessels rupture into the subarachnoid space in head trauma or in older people with hypertension, presumably from microaneurysmal rupture into the subarachnoid space rather than into the brain parenchyma. The severity of neurological deficit following aneurysm rupture is somewhat indicative of prognosis and surgical risk. The grading system of Hunt and Hess is commonly used to quantify such risk and deficits:[71]

0 Unruptured aneurysm

I   Asymptomatic or minimal headache, slight nuchal rigidity

Ia Fully alert, no meningeal signs, but fixed neurological deficit

II   Moderate to severe headache, nuchal rigidity, perhaps cranial nerve palsy but no other neurological deficit

III Drowsiness, confusion, or mild focal neurological deficit

IV Stupor, moderate to severe hemiparesis, perhaps early decerebration, vegetative disturbances

V   Decerebrate rigidity, vegetative dysfunction, deep coma

Several mechanisms have been proposed to account for the changes in level of consciousness noted with subarachnoid hemorrhage. Initially, intracranial pressure increases sharply, which may account for changes in consciousness with rupture. Sustained coma usually indicates extensive bleeding into the brain parenchyma or ventricles. Changes in level of consciousness several days after the initial rupture may indicate rerupture of the clot, cerebral vasospasm, or increasing ICP secondary to communicating hydrocephalus.

A number of disturbances in integrated regulatory functions (vegetative functions) occur in patients with subarachnoid hemorrhage, including cardiac dysrhythmias, hyper- and hypoosmolality, and sometimes unexplained fever. Since the majority of saccular aneurysms occur in the circle of Willis, it is postulated that the sudden ejection of blood under high pressure directly injures the hypothalamus or that the accumulation of blood in the basal cisterns interferes with hypothalamic function.

Medical Management. Medical management of subarachnoid hemorrhage varies widely in physician preference. Control of hypertension in patients with hypertensive hemorrhage is crucial to prevent further episodes. In patients with saccular aneurysms, the goal is to prevent secondary brain injury following the initial bleeding and to obliterate the aneurysm to prevent rebleeding. Achieving this goal is complicated by two factors: the state of the injured brain following initial rupture and the fact that about 20% of aneurysm patients have multiple aneurysms.

There is considerable controversy among neurosurgeons regarding the best timing for surgery to obliterate aneurysms and the supportive therapy to prevent rebleeding and vasospasm prior to surgery. However, the International Cooperative Study on the Timing of Aneurysm Surgery has clearly shown the advantage of early surgery in preventing morbidity and mortality associated with rebleeding.[7,37,72]

Despite the variety of medical and surgical therapies attempted in aneurysmal subarachnoid hemorrhage, the mortality and morbidity remain high, with deaths within 3 months ranging from 40% to 50%.

Nursing Management. Nursing management is collaborative with medical management in monitoring for rebleeding (peak incidence 7 to 15 days) and vasospasm (4 to 7 days after bleeding), supporting systemic physiological function, and preventing secondary brain injury. In centers that use hypervolemic and hypertensive therapy to prevent vasospasm, nursing monitoring and knowledgeable titration of fluid volume and hypertensive therapy in accordance with neurological status is crucial. Nursing has primary responsibility for creating an environment that minimizes rebleeding in situations where early surgery is not feasible. Typical aneurysm precautions are designed to prevent emotionally or physically induced sudden increases in blood pressure that could rupture the newly formed clot or additional aneurysms.[73]

Nursing diagnoses and clinical problems that may arise in patients with aneurysmal subarachnoid hemorrhage are summarized in Table 33-12.

Neurosurgical Procedures

In most critical care units, the majority of patients with nervous system disorders are likely to be there for monitoring following neurosurgical procedures. It is common for patients to be closely observed in intensive care for 24 hours or so after craniotomy,

TABLE 33-12 **Nursing and Medical Management of Aneurysmal Subarachnoid Hemorrhage**

Collaborative Clinical Problem	Common Medical Protocol	Nursing Diagnosis	Outcome Standard	Nursing Interventions
High risk for vasospasm	Hypervolemic and hypertensive therapy; may add vasopressors			1. Monitor neurological status, particularly level of consciousness. 2. Monitor ICP and institute protocols to reduce ICP if needed. 3. Monitor hemodynamic status, titrating volume expansion to maintain pulmonary artery wedge pressure of 18 to 20 mmHg, hematocrit reading of 30% to 40%. 4. If neurological status is not improved, add vasopressors according to protocol to increase blood pressure, titrated to point of neurological improvement.
		Self-care deficit, related to altered consciousness and neurological grade (see text for grading system)	Activities of daily living (feeding, bathing, toileting) are performed to the maximal level of independence with assistance	1. Encourage patient participation in self-care (feeding, hygiene) as ability permits, but caution against straining and isometric muscle contraction, which increase blood pressure. 2. Develop appropriate rest/activity schedule. 3. Teach family assistive techniques.

carotid endarterectomy, cervical laminectomy, and hypophysectomy. The primary complications being monitored for include brain swelling, intracranial or intracord bleeding, ventilatory insufficiency, and fluid and electrolyte imbalance following pituitary surgery. The potential nursing diagnoses are discussed below in relation to the category of neurosurgical procedure. Relevant nursing observations and management are discussed earlier in this chapter in the sections on head injury and spinal cord injury, under Neurotrauma.

Supratentorial Craniotomy

Supratentorial craniotomy refers to all neurosurgical procedures in the cranium above the level of the tentorium. Craniotomy may be performed to remove intracranial tumors, hematomas, arteriovenous malformations, epileptic foci; to clip aneurysms in the anterior circulation; or to create focal lesions in the thalamus. The primary complications that may ensue are intracerebral bleeding and brain swelling, either of which may lead to intracranial hypertension, altered consciousness or, if severe, transtentorial brain herniation. Focal deficits related to ischemia or infarction of the areas involved in the surgical procedure may also occur.

Therefore, the primary potential clinical problems for which these patients are at risk include intracranial hypertension secondary to brain swelling (24 to 72 hours after surgery) and transtentorial brain herniation secondary to intracranial bleeding (first 24 hours). The potential concomitant nursing diagnoses are decreased consciousness with resultant self-care deficit and physical immobility, skin breakdown related to lack of position change during surgery, and alteration in comfort (headache, related to craniotomy).

Primary management consists of careful monitoring of neurological status as described under Brain Herniation Syndromes and often monitoring of intracranial pressure (described under Intracranial Hypertension). Dexamethasone is commonly given to control postoperative brain edema, and antiembolic stockings are used to prevent deep vein thrombosis. Atelectasis is a potential problem, as with all postoperative patients, and preventive management is complicated by the detrimental effect of coughing on intracranial pressure. Deep breathing alone will maintain open alveoli, and it is unnecessary to stimulate these patients to cough.

Infratentorial Craniotomy

Craniotomy in the posterior fossa (below the tentorium) is used to remove cerebellar tumors and hemorrhages and acoustic neuromas and other tumors of the brainstem, cranial nerves, or cerebellopontine angle. The primary complications stem from the potential for swelling or bleeding in a small space that is immediately adjacent to the brainstem structures that control airway protection, breathing, motor coordination, and many cranial nerve functions.

The potential clinical problems that must be monitored for include respiratory arrest secondary to medullary compression or tonsillar herniation, decreased consciousness secondary to upward herniation, and aspiration secondary to loss of gag reflex. Concomitant potential nursing diagnoses include corneal injury, related to loss of corneal reflex; inadequate verbal communication, related to dysarthria; and self-care deficit, related to ataxia or dysmetria. Respirations and level of consciousness must be carefully monitored, and serial assessment of cranial nerve functioning (particularly corneal, gag, swallow, and articulation) must be performed. The onset of hiccups is an ominous sign of medullary involvement.

Patient positioning is designed to protect the surgical site and avoid flexion and extension of the neck, which might increase pressure in the posterior circulation and brainstem. The patient should be turned like a log, with support to the head and neck. Coughing and Valsalva maneuver should be avoided to prevent sudden increases in systemic blood pressure. Suctioning, if necessary to remove oral secretions, should be gentle and should avoid stimulating the cough reflex. Deep breathing is sufficient to prevent atelectasis. Aspiration can be prevented by scrupulous oral hygiene and careful testing of gag and swallow reflexes prior to allowing oral feeding.

Cerebrovascular Surgery

Vascular procedures involving the cerebral circulation may involve both vascular and neurological surgeons. Patients thought to benefit from cerebrovascular surgery are those with transient ischemic attacks who have demonstrable stenosis of the carotid artery or its major branches. Most authorities recommend against surgery when stenosis is not symptomatic. When the stenosis is in the extracranial carotid circulation, endarterectomy is the procedure of choice, with the surgical objective of restoring normal flow and removing the plaque, which is a source of emboli. The ultimate goal is prevention of a completed stroke (or additional strokes if one has already occurred).

The major potential clinical problems are embolic stroke during or following surgery, oozing or frank hemorrhage at the incision site on the artery secondary to preoperative and intraoperative heparinization, respiratory distress due to hematoma or edema at the operative site, and peripheral cranial nerve injury. Nursing monitoring is directed to early detection of incipient stroke, inadequate airway (from hematoma compressing trachea), and cranial nerve injury. Serial neurological examination, involving comparison with preoperative status, is essential. Stroke is best detected by recurrent examination of movement, speech, visual fields, and sensation contralateral to the side of the surgery. Hematoma at the operative site can be detected by observing the neck for swelling and tracheal deviation and by listening for stridor and labored respirations. Cranial nerve assessment should focus on the nerves that traverse the neck, such as the recurrent laryngeal, vagus, accessory, and hypoglossal. Speech clarity, swallowing, head and shoulder strength, facial symmetry, and pulse rate are important parameters for serial assessment.

Intracranial-extracranial (IC-EC) bypass surgery is sometimes used to bypass the stenosis when it is in an intracranial vessel and therefore inaccessible for endarterectomy. Most commonly, the superficial temporal artery is anastomosed to the middle cerebral artery, using microsurgical techniques. A multicenter randomized trial showed no benefit of this surgery over conservative medical therapy. However, many of these procedures continue to be done, and a number of surgeons still believe there is a subset of patients who benefit from them.[74]

Potential clinical problems include cerebral ischemia secondary to vasospasm and lost patency of the anastomosis, hemorrhage at the anastomosis secondary to preoperative heparinization, and seizures secondary to exposure of the cortex. Nursing monitoring for cerebral ischemia has been described earlier. Monitoring of blood pressure and maintenance of normotension are important, to prevent loss of patency of the anastomosis and perhaps also to prevent spasm, as is frequent monitoring of the pulse at the anastomosis site, to detect early signs of loss of patency. The patient should not lie on the operative site or use restrictive eyeglasses or head bands, to avoid compressing the anastomosis.

Infectious Disorders

Central nervous system infections that may require intensive nursing care include generalized inflammation of the cortex, white matter, and meninges (encephalitis); generalized infection or inflammation of the meninges alone (meningitis); and focal infection of the brain (brain abscess).

Encephalitis

Encephalitis is an acute inflammation of the brain proper (cortex, white matter, and meninges) that is most commonly viral. Because viruses must reproduce *within* the host's cells, viruses that gain access to the CNS have the potential to create serious, irreparable damage to brain tissue. The most common cause of viral encephalitis is herpes simplex type 1 (estimated at 100 to 1,000 cases annually in the United States). Other causative viruses include arboviruses (eastern and western equine and St. Louis encephalitis, also called *sleeping sickness,* and a variety of togaviruses seen only in Asia and the Pacific); enteroviruses (polio virus, echovirus, coxsackie virus); other herpesviruses that cause encephalitis only in immunocompromised hosts (Epstein-Barr virus, cytomegalovirus, and varicella-zoster virus); and a variety of other systemic viruses, the most important of which are the viruses of rabies, mumps, and measles. More rarely, bacterial, fungal, and protozoan infections may invade the brain and cause encephalitis.

The viruses or other causative organisms gain access to the brain via the bloodstream or peripheral nerves, particularly in patients who are rendered susceptible by immunosuppressive therapy, immunodeficiency diseases (AIDS, combined immunodeficiency of children), systemic debilitation, or an immune system stressed by other infectious disease. A nonexudative inflammation occurs, often with degeneration and destruction of neurons by the invading virus, demyelination, and subsequent necrosis, hemorrhage, and cavitation. Infectious organisms vary in their capacity for tissue destruction.

The symptoms reflect the involvement of the whole brain, and particularly the predilection of the viruses for the temporal lobe. Behavioral changes, including

personality change, delirium, uninhibited behavior, and restlessness, are common, occurring in up to 85% of patients. Dysphasia occurs in 67%, seizures in 67%, autonomic dysfunction in 60%, and movement problems, particularly ataxia, in 40%. There may be localized motor deficits (hemiparesis, cranial nerve deficits) in as many as 85%.[75]

Medical therapy of encephalitis depends upon clear diagnosis of the causative agent. Brain biopsy is frequently necessary to specifically identify the virus, and initial treatment is based on presumptive diagnosis, pending serological testing. There are no specific therapies for the majority of viruses that cause encephalitis, and primary prevention of such viral infections as poliomyelitis, measles, and mumps by immunization is the only viable approach. In the event of encephalitis from these agents, supportive therapy that maintains vital functions and protects the patient from injury while the body's immune functions attempt to destroy the virus is all that can be offered.

Specific antiviral therapies have been developed for herpes simplex type 1; acyclovir sodium, 30 mg/kg daily, is the drug of choice. Even with this drug, mortality remains high (28%, compared with 54% before the advent of acyclovir). Acyclovir has been found to achieve a better rate of survival than vidarabine and a lower incidence of neurological residual deficits (62% with deficits treated with acyclovir versus 87% with vidarabine).[7,76] Clearly, even when treated, herpes encephalitis has a high mortality and morbidity. Mortality is also high in eastern equine encephalitis (more than 50%), with a high incidence of neurological sequelae; these are lower in western equine and St. Louis encephalitis (3% and 2% to 20%, respectively, depending upon age).[76]

Meningitis

Meningitis is an inflammation of the leptomeninges that does not invade the brain parenchyma. Some infections involve both the meninges and the parenchyma; such a disorder is classified as *meningoencephalitis.* Meningitis can be caused by viruses, in which case it is called *aseptic meningitis;* or by bacteria—*purulent meningitis.*

The most common viruses causing aseptic meningitis are enteroviruses: coxsackie virus and echovirus. Prior to the development of an adequate vaccine, poliovirus was the most common cause of meningitis and encephalitis. Aseptic meningitis may have a sudden onset or may follow a prodromal phase of "flu," fever, sore throat, and gastrointestinal symptoms. Fever, drowsiness, frontal headache, stiff neck, and perhaps paresthesias are common. No specific therapy is available, but recovery is usually complete, and patients with aseptic meningitis are not seen in critical care units. Purulent meningitis, however, may produce serious and life-threatening symptoms, particularly if the cranial nerves protecting the airway are involved and if acute brain swelling (and thus increased ICP) occurs.

Organisms gain access to the meninges via the bloodstream in systemic bacteremia; directly when the dura has been torn by injury; by nasopharyngeal venules that communicate with the meninges; and by direct spread from adjacent foci of infection as in sinusitis or brain abscess. Bacterial meningitis is preceded by upper respiratory tract infection, otitis media, or pneumonia in the majority of cases attributed to *Haemophilus influenzae, Neisseria meningitidis,* and *Streptococcus pneumoniae.* Gram-negative bacillary meningitis (*Escherichia coli, Enterobacter, Klebsiella, Proteus, Serratia,* and *Pseudomonas*) is usually seen only in immunosuppressed patients, infants, and patients with advanced cancer. Meningococcal meningitis *(N. meningitidis)* occurs in outbreaks in crowded situations and is the only meningitis to require fecal and oral precautions prior to achieving adequate antibiotic levels, as well as prophylactic treatment of contacts.

As with encephalitis, specific medical therapy depends upon identification of the causative organism. Fortunately, therapy for bacterial diseases is better developed than that for viral disorders, and early specific treatment often results in resolution of the meningitis with little or no neurological residual. Large doses of antibiotics are given intravenously, to ensure an adequate level in the CNS. Penicillin G is the antibiotic of choice for the majority of organisms. Gram-negative organisms may require third-generation cephalosporins. Intrathecal administration is sometimes necessary.[7,76]

Brain Abscess

Brain abscess is a localized area of bacterial encephalitis, usually caused by direct extension of bacteria from infected sinuses or mastoids or of organisms that have entered the brain from a traumatic wound or via the bloodstream in septicemia, bacterial endocarditis, or lung abscess. Because they are localized and act as space-occupying lesions, brain abscesses mimic tumors or hematomas. Diagnosis is usually made on the basis of epidemiological evidence for a source of infection and a characteristic ring around the abscess on CT scan. Medical therapy is initially conservative, with antibiotics appropriate to the suspected or confirmed organism. If the abscess is encapsulated, craniotomy may be performed to drain it.

Nursing Management. Although the initiating organisms and thus the specific drug therapy differ, the potential human responses common to all three infectious processes described are (1) alterations in consciousness, behavioral control, movement, and multisystem regulation; and (2) injury related to coma and seizures. Because the whole brain is involved, the potential disruption in function is widespread, as in acute head injury.

Alterations in consciousness may range from decreased arousal to hyperarousal. Because all three pathological processes have the potential to increase intracranial pressure or act like a mass lesion, potential brain herniation is a clinical problem common to all.

Nursing management has a strong monitoring component, including monitoring to detect signs of brain herniation; monitoring intracranial pressure and adaptive capacity (see Table 33-10); monitoring for signs of cranial nerve dysfunction, particularly as it affects airway and eye protection and protection from injury during seizures; and monitoring for multisystem regulatory problems such as SIADH, DIC, and septic shock.

Management relevant to airway protection, protection from injury, and multisystem failure is discussed under Neurotrauma, as is the care for the patient with decreased arousal. Nursing care related to seizures is discussed under Seizures, earlier in this chapter.

Hyperarousal is a common manifestation of meningeal and brain parenchymal irritation. The patient with abnormally increased arousal has a high potential for injury from random movements, for nutritional deficit related to increased caloric expenditure, and for skin breakdown due to rubbing on sheets. Common interventions consist of padding the bed with bolsters and lining it with sheepskin to prevent skin abrasions and bruises. The patient who no longer needs intravenous lines or monitoring lines but still requires close observation to prevent injury may be moved to an intermediate care unit, with a floor bed used to avoid falls. Caloric intake is increased via tube feeding or oral feeding, and all staff should take special care to orient the patient continually to the environment and to maintain as quiet and nonstimulating an environment as possible.

Autoimmune and Neurotoxic Disorders

Several disorders of autoimmune and neurotoxic origin alter ventilation and movement without impairing consciousness and may be sufficiently severe to require intensive care. Myasthenia gravis, Guillain-Barré syndrome, and multiple sclerosis with respiratory involvement are all disorders in which the body is believed to direct its immune processes, normally used to combat foreign tissue, against its own nervous system. The body makes antibodies to muscle acetylcholine receptors in the case of myasthenia gravis, against central myelin in multiple sclerosis, and against peripheral nerve myelin in Guillain-Barré syndrome.

Neurotoxic disorders include those, such as botulism and tetanus, that are caused by endogenous neurotoxins produced by invasion or ingestion of anaerobic organisms and those resulting from exogenous toxins such as organophosphates.

Guillain-Barré syndrome is a disorder of the peripheral nerves in which the myelin degenerates, presumably in response to autoimmune processes following a viral infection. It is generally characterized by ascending motor, more than sensory, loss and becomes life-threatening if it involves the muscles of respiration and the peripheral portion of the cranial nerves that protect the airway. Consciousness is fully preserved in Guillain-Barré patients, but they may be able to communicate with others only by moving the eyes. Generally, the Schwann cells regenerate and restore the myelin over several weeks; thus, full recovery is possible. Expert nursing care is critical to prevent secondary complications that interfere with that recovery. Nursing diagnoses and nursing care are essentially the same as for a patient with high cervical cord injury, except that the paralysis is flaccid (rather then becoming spastic after spinal shock) and that the patient often has sensory function and may thus be in considerable discomfort from the immobility.

Myasthenia gravis and the neurotoxic disorders are primarily disorders of the myoneural junction. The nerve terminal of the motor axon releases packets of acetylcholine, or *quanta*. These quanta bind to receptors on the membrane of the muscle fiber and create end-plate potentials, which eventually summate and produce an action potential and contraction of the muscle fiber. Deficits in firing may occur because too little acetylcholine is released (as is thought to occur in botulism); because acetylcholinesterase clearance in the synaptic cleft is inhibited with resultant fatigue of the receptors (as in organophosphate poisoning); or because receptor sites are too few (as is thought to be the case in myasthenia gravis) or are occupied by another neurochemical. The end result of these differing pathological processes is the same: muscular weakness or paralysis, which becomes worse with repetitive stimulation, and depression of reflexes.

Myasthenia Gravis

Myasthenia gravis is a disorder that challenges both patient and professional staff when control is unstable. It can be highly unpredictable and may rapidly become unstable, thus requiring astute nursing monitoring. Although patients suffering from ascending polyneuropathy (Guillain-Barré syndrome) may increasingly lose function over a period of days, the patient in myasthenic or cholinergic crisis may lose ability to protect the airway in *less than one hour*. Furthermore, it is often difficult to determine whether increasing weakness is secondary to too little medication (myasthenic state) or too much medication (cholinergic state).

Clinically, the patient with myasthenia experiences increasing weakness with continued effort and weakness of specific muscle groups. Some patients have weakness only of the extraocular muscles, with continual or intermittent diplopia and ptosis. Others may have primarily head and upper extremity weakness, and still others may have involvement of all extremities as well as the head and neck.

The onset is bimodal, with women more often affected between 20 and 30 years and men between 50 and 60 years. Spontaneous remissions occur, although remission is more likely following thymectomy in young women. The critical care nurse is most likely to care for a person with myasthenia who has lost or is at high risk of losing the ability to protect the airway because of myasthenic crisis (severe weakness with decreasing response to medication), cholinergic crisis (severe weakness plus cholinergic signs due to overdosage with medication), or thymectomy. Myasthenic crisis may be directly related to increased demands upon the patient's system, such as severe illness or surgical procedures unrelated to the myasthenia, or may be of unknown cause.

Anticholinesterase drugs are the most common treatment for myasthenia; pyridostigmine bromide (Mestinon) is the most widely used. Neostigmine (Prostigmin) is shorter-acting and less used for maintenance; however, it can be given parenterally and may be used more often in acute situations. Edrophonium chloride (Tensilon) is an extremely short-acting anticholinesterase used diagnostically. All anticholinesterase agents act to prevent acetylcholinesterase from chemically breaking acetylcholine in the synaptic cleft into acetate and choline. Such chemical breakdown of the acetylcholine ends depolarization of the muscle membrane and allows the muscle to repolarize and thus be ready for another action potential. Since the number of receptor sites is reduced in myasthenia, prolongation of depolarization allows somewhat longer firing of fewer fibers and thus increased muscle contraction. Obviously, excessive prolongation of depolarization can *increase* the weakness if further nerve impulses are unable to initiate further action potentials; consequently, muscle weakness can result from too much anticholinesterase medication as well as from too little. Although the drug treatment of myasthenia may dramatically improve the patient's ability to carry on daily tasks, it does not alter the basic disorder. Plasmapheresis, the exchange of the patient's plasma for plasmalike solution, temporarily affects the disease process by removing autoantibodies.

Patients in the neurology units of a hospital may be well enough to administer their own anticholinesterase drugs, but those who are critically ill most often must rely upon the nurse for this. It cannot be overemphasized that timing is crucial. A delay of 15 to 20 minutes can make the difference between a patient who has sufficient strength to swallow the medication and one who does not. Any patient at risk or in crisis has the potential for rapid changes in condition and rapid changes in strength. Since excess medication is one cause of increasing weakness, the nurse is frequently in the position of having to decide whether increasing weakness is from too little or too much medication. If it is from too much, the next dose must be omitted. Unfortunately, the clinical presentation of myasthenic and cholinergic crisis are so similar that even the most experienced clinicians may have difficulty making this differentiation.

Although both situations produce increasing weakness in the patient, the timing of such weakness is one clue to the cause. Weakness due to myasthenia is apt to come at about the time of onset of action of the medication, whereas weakness due to excess medication usually occurs within the duration of action of the drug. The presence of abdominal cramps, salivation, diarrhea, and muscle fasciculations accompanied by increased weakness are also highly suggestive of cholinergic (drug excess) rather than myasthenic state. If the increasing weakness is clearly drug-related, the next dose must be omitted to prevent precipitation of life-threatening cholinergic crisis. However, it is often difficult to tell whether the weakness is related to too much or too little anticholinesterase drug. In such cases, the physician will often elect to perform an *edrophonium test*. If weakness is due to excess drug, the weakness will become even worse and often be associated with cramping with the addition of edrophonium, whereas the clinical condition will improve if the weakness is secondary to too little anticholinesterase. Because edrophonium is a rapid-acting, short-duration drug, both worsening and improvement in condition are transient. The nurse must be prepared to administer atropine sulfate to reverse the anticholinesterase effect and to suction or even ventilate the patient if the edrophonium test precipitates a cholinergic crisis. However, used judiciously, the test can often prevent crisis by distinguishing between the two states before dysphagia and bulbar weakness are pronounced.

Prevention of Neurotoxic Disorders

The life-threatening motor problems caused by tetanus, botulism, and diphtheritic neuropathy are totally preventable by prevention of the basic disorders. Table 33-13 summarizes the sites of action, critical care problems, and management of these disorders in relation to the endotoxins that attack the nervous system. It is evident that once the endotoxin has been made in the body, there is little in the way of definitive treatment. Expert nursing care is the key to the survival of patients until the endotoxin is no longer being formed and the body can heal itself. How much better for the patient to have been appropriately immunized or for the food to have been properly prepared in the first place! Both diphtheria and tetanus are completely preventable by appropriate immunization in childhood, with booster doses for tetanus at 10-year intervals. Toxoid boosters may be given to persons previously immunized and exposed to diphtheria and to those who sustain a contaminated injury (tetanus).

Botulism most commonly occurs following the ingestion of food containing botulinus toxin. Improperly cooked home-canned foods are the most common source. The best prevention for botulism is to follow canning directions carefully, especially for nonacid foods. Many recommend boiling home-canned nonacid foods prior to eating as an additional precaution.

Nursing Management

Nursing management of patients with polyneuropathies and of those with autoimmune and neurotoxic disorders of the myoneural junction is quite similar, even though the pathological conditions differ. The primary potential nursing diagnoses are:
Inadequate airway clearance
Inadequate breathing pattern
Total self-care deficit, related to complete immobility
Fear and anxiety, related to decreasing ability to
  breathe and fear of dying
Inadequate nutrition, related to inability to swallow
  safely

TABLE 33-13   **Comparison of Sites of Action, Critical Problems, and Management of Movement Problems Caused by Endotoxins**

Endotoxin	Site of Action	Effect	Management
Tetanus: tetanospasmin made by *Clostridium tetani*	Local effect on muscle. Major effect is to interfere with spinal inhibitory neurons	Sustained muscle contraction; rigidity, stiffness progressing to paroxysmal spasms without loss of consciousness. Death may occur from apnea, suffocation, secondary spasm of glottal muscles and respiratory muscles. Circulatory collapse possible	Single-dose antitoxin (no effect on established symptoms but prevents further endotoxin production). Tracheostomy if having spasms; minimal manipulation, sedation, minimal stimulation; nursing care crucial in maintaining quiet environment. Constant monitoring. Curare if spasms uncontrollable; requires total life support
Diphtheritic neuropathy: endotoxin from *Corynebacterium diphtheriae*	Membrane of Schwann cell of proximal peripheral nerve and dorsal root ganglion. Demyelination occurs	Weakness, paralysis of muscles affecting cranial nerves 1-2 weeks after infection; spinal peripheral nerves about 7-10 weeks after infection. Usually descending weakness of bulbar muscles, arms, legs	Symptomatic; antitoxin ineffective once neuropathy established (affects about 20% of patients). Expert nursing care; detection of bulbar symptoms early; tracheostomy if necessary. Prognosis good for recovery if well supported in acute phase
Botulism: botulinus toxin from *Clostridium botulinum*	Neuromuscular junction; interferes with release of acetylcholine	Weakness, paralysis of bulbar, systemic, and smooth muscles	Expert supportive nursing care; may require complete respiratory, alimental support; symptoms may fluctuate, requiring frequent evaluation

Discomfort, related to preservation of sensation with total immobility

Pain, related to severe muscle spasms in tetanus

Nursing monitoring and management relevant to these problems were discussed earlier under States That Disrupt Ventilation but Not Consciousness.

REFERENCES

1. Carpenito, L. J. (1991). *Nursing diagnosis: Applications to clinical practice* (3rd ed.). Philadelphia: Lippincott.
2. Butterworth, J. F., & DeWitt, D. S. (1989). Severe head trauma: Pathophysiology and management. *Critical Care Clinics, 5*(4), 807-820.
3. Klatzo, I. (1985). Brain oedema following brain ischaemia and the influence of therapy. *British Journal of Anaesthesia, 57,* 18-22.
4. Miller, J. D. (1991). Basic intracranial dynamics. In R. A. Minns (Ed.), *Problems of intracranial pressure in childhood* (pp. 1-12). New York: Cambridge University Press.
5. Miller, J. D. (1985). Head injury and brain ischaemia. *British Journal of Anaesthesia, 57,* 120-130.
6. Gennarelli, T. A., Spielman, G., Langfitt, T. W., et al. (1982). Influence of the type of intracranial lesion on outcome from severe head injury. *Journal of Neurosurgery, 56,* 26-32.
7. Marshall, S. B., Marshall, L. F., Vos, H. R., et al.

(1990). *Neuroscience critical care: Pathophysiology and patient management.* Philadelphia: Saunders.

8. Narayan, R. K., Kishore, P. R. S., Becker, D. P., et al. (1982). Intracranial pressure: To monitor or not to monitor? *Journal of Neurosurgery, 56,* 650-659.

9. Janssen, L., & Hansebout, R. R. (1989). Pathogenesis of spinal cord injury and newer treatments. *Spine, 14*(1), 23-32.

10. Hall, E. D. (1989). Free radicals and CNS injury. *Critical Care Clinics, 5*(4), 793-805.

11. Murdoch, J., & Hall, R. (1990). Brain protection: physiological and pharmacological considerations: Part 1. The physiology of brain injury. *Canadian Journal of Anaesthesiology, 37,* 663-671.

12. Miller, J. D., Becker, D. P., & Ward, J. D. (1977). Significance of intracranial hypertension in severe head injury. *Journal of Neurosurgery, 47,* 503-517.

13. Graham, D. (1985). The pathology of brain ischaemia and possibilities for therapeutic intervention. *British Journal of Anaesthesia, 57,* 3-17.

14. McGraw, C. P., & O'Conner, C. (1986). Analysis of the intracranial responses to mannitol and furosemide. In J. D. Miller, G. M. Teasdale, J. O. Rowan, et al. (Eds.), *Intracranial pressure VI* (pp. 601-604). Berlin: Springer.

15. Tsutsumi, H., Ide, K., Mizutani, J., et al. (1986). The relationship between intracranial pressure, cerebral perfusion pressure and outcome in head injured patients: The critical level of CPP. In J. D. Miller, G. M. Teasdale, J. O. Rowan, et al. (Eds.), *Intracranial pressure VI* (pp. 661-666). Berlin: Springer.

16. Marshall, L. F., Smith, R. W., & Shapiro, H. M. (1979). The outcome with aggressive treatment in severe head injuries: Part 1. The significance of intracranial pressure monitoring. *Journal of Neurosurgery, 50,* 20-25.

17. Jennett, B., & Teasdale, G. (1981). *The management of head injuries.* Philadelphia: Davis.

18. Pollay, M., Fullenwider, C., Roberts, P. A., et al. (1983). Effect of mannitol and furosemide on blood-brain osmotic gradients and intracranial pressure. *Journal of Neurosurgery, 59,* 945-950.

19. Cooper, P. R., Moody, S., Clark, W. K., et al. (1979). Dexamethasone and severe head injury: A prospective double-blind study. *Journal of Neurosurgery, 51,* 307-316.

20. Kaktis, J., & Pitts, L. H. (1980). Complications associated with megadose steroids in head-injured patients. *Journal of Neurosurgical Nursing, 12,* 166-171.

21. Pitts, L. H., & Kaktis, J. (1980). The effect of megadose steroids on ICP in traumatic coma. In K. Shulman, A. Marmarov, J. Miller, et al. (Eds.), *Intracranial pressure IV* (pp. 638-642). Berlin: Springer.

22. Braughler, J. M., & Hall, E. D. (1985). Current applications of "high-dose" steroid therapy for CNS injury. *Journal of Neurosurgery, 62,* 806-810.

23. Londrini, S., Monfolivo, M. D., Pluchino, F., et al. (1989). Positive end-expiratory pressure in supine and sitting positions: Its effect on intrathoracic and intracranial pressures. *Neurosurgery, 24,* 873-877.

24. Brain Resuscitation Clinical Trial I Study Group. (1986). Randomized clinical trial of thiopental loading in comatose survivors of cardiac arrest. *New England Journal of Medicine, 314,* 397-403.

25. Ward, J. D., Becker, D. P., Miller, J. D., et al. (1985). Failure of prophylactic barbiturate coma in the treatment of severe head injury. *Journal of Neurosurgery, 62,* 383-388.

26. Yano, M., Ikeda, Y., Kobayashi, S., et al. (1986). The outcome with barbiturate therapy in severe head injuries. In J. D. Miller, G. M. Teasdale, J. O. Rowan, et al. (Eds.), *Intracranial pressure VI* (pp. 769-773). Berlin: Springer.

27. Hall, R., & Murdoch, J. (1991). Brain protection: Physiological and pharmacological considerations: Part 2. The pharmacology of brain protection. *Canadian Journal of Anaesthesiology, 37,* 762-777.

28. Miller, J. D. (1975). Volume and pressure in the craniospinal axis. *Clinical Neurosurgery, 22,* 76-105.

29. Selig, J. M., Klauber, M. R., Toole, B. M., et al. (1986). Increased ICP and systemic hypotension during the first 72 hours following severe head injury. In J. D. Miller, G. M. Teasdale, J. O. Rowan, et al. (Eds.), *Intracranial pressure VI* (pp. 675-679). Berlin: Springer.

30. American Nurses' Association and American Association of Neuroscience Nurses. (1986). *Neuroscience nursing practice: Process and outcome criteria for selected diagnoses.* Kansas City, MO: ANA.

31. Mitchell, P. H. (1986). Intracranial hypertension: Influence of nursing care activities. *Nursing Clinics of North America, 21,* 563-576.

32. Magnaes, B. (1976). Body position and cerebrospinal fluid pressure: Part 1. Clinical studies on the effect of rapid postural changes. *Journal of Neurosurgery, 44,* 687-697.

33. Rudy, E. B., Turner, B. S., Baun, M., et al. (1991). Endotracheal suctioning in adults with head injury. *Heart Lung, 20,* 667-674.

34. Parsons, L. C., & Shogan, J. S. O. (1984). The effect of endotracheal tube suction/manual hyperventilation procedure on patients with severe closed head injuries. *Heart Lung, 13,* 372.

35. Adams, H. P. (1990). Calcium antagonists in the management of subarachnoid hemorrhage: A review. *Angiology, 4,* 1010-1016.

36. Heros, R. C., & Korusue, F. (1989). Hemodilution for cerebral ischemia. *Stroke, 20,* 423-427.

37. Ausman, J. I., Diaz, F. G., Malik, G. M., et al. (1989). Management of cerebral aneurysms: Further facts and additional myths. *Surgical Neurology, 32,* 21-35.

38. Heros, R. C., & Korusue, F. (1989). Hemodilution for cerebral ischemia. *Stroke, 20,* 423-427.

39. Plum, F., & Posner, J. B. (1980). *The diagnosis of stupor and coma* (2nd ed.). New York: Davis.

40. Teasdale, G., Knill-Jones, R., & Van der Sande, J. (1978). Observer variability in assessing impaired con-

sciousness and coma. *Journal of Neurology, Neurosurgery and Psychiatry, 41,* 603-610.

41. Jones, C. (1979). Glasgow coma scale. *American Journal of Nursing, 79,* 1551-1553.

42. Teasdale, G. (1975). Acute impairment of brain function: Part 1. Assessing the "conscious level." *Nursing Times, 71,* 914-917.

43. Teasdale, G., & Galbraith, S. (1975). Acute impairment of brain function: Part 2. Observation record. *Nursing Times, 71,* 972-973.

44. Born, J. D., Albert, A., Hans, P., et al. (1985). Relative prognostic value of best motor response and brain stem reflexes in patients with severe head injury. *Neurosurgery, 16,* 595-601.

45. Willmore, L. J. (1990). Post traumatic epilepsy: Cellular mechanisms and implications for treatment. *Epilepsia, 31*(Suppl. 3), S67-S73.

46. Simon, R. P. (1985). Physiologic consequences of status epilepticus. *Epilepsia, 26*(Suppl. 1), 558-566.

47. Treiman, D. M., Walton, N. Y., & Kendrick, C. (1990). A progressive sequence of electroencephalographic changes during generalized convulsive status epilepticus. *Epilepsy Research, 5,* 49-60.

48. Lovely, M. P., & Ozuna, J. (1982). Status epilepticus. In D. L. Nikas (Ed.), *The critically ill neurosurgical patient.* New York: Churchill Livingstone.

49. Bell, H. E., & Bertino, J. S. (1984). Constant diazepam infusion in the treatment of continuous seizure activity. *Drug Intelligence and Clinical Pharmacy, 18,* 965-970.

50. Lacey, D. J., Singer, W. D., Horwitz, S. J., et al. (1986). Lorazapam therapy of status epilepticus in children and adolescents. *Journal of Pediatrics, 108,* 771-774.

51. Lowenstein, D. H., Aminoff, M. J., & Simon, R. P. (1988). Barbiturate anesthesia in the treatment of refractory status epilepticus. *Neurology, 38,* 395-400.

52. Blount, M., Kinney, A. B., & Luttrell, N. (1982). Myasthenia gravis and the Guillain-Barré syndrome. In D. L. Nikas (Ed.), *The critically ill neurosurgical patient.* New York: Churchill Livingstone.

53. Leinart, B. (1979). Attitudes of nurses toward spinal cord injury patients. *ARN (Journal of the Association of Rehabilitation Nurses), 4*(1), 7-9.

54. Chu, D. A., Ahn, J. H., Ragnarsson, K. T., et al. (1985). Deep venous thrombosis: Diagnosis in spinal cord injured patients. *Archives of Physical Medicine and Rehabilitation, 66,* 365-368.

55. Myllynen, P., Kammonen, M., Rokkanen, P., et al. (1985). Deep venous thrombosis and pulmonary embolism in patients with acute spinal cord injury: A comparison with nonparalyzed patients immobilized due to spinal fractures. *Journal of Trauma, 25,* 541-543.

56. Cerrato, D., Ariano, C., & Fiacchino, F. (1978). Deep vein thrombosis and low-dose heparin prophylaxis in neurosurgical patients. *Journal of Neurosurgery, 49,* 378-381.

57. Sugarman, B. (1985). Medical complications of spinal cord injury. *Quarterly Journal of Medicine* (New Series 54), *213,* 3-18.

58. Saul, T. G. (1983). Intensive care of the brain-injured patient. *Critical Care Quarterly, 5*(4), 82-89.

59. Raimond, J., & Taylor, J. W. (1986). *Neurological emergencies: Effective nursing care.* Rockville, MD: Aspen.

60. Shapiro, H. M. (1985). Barbiturates in brain ischaemia. *British Journal of Anesthesia, 57,* 82-95.

61. Deutschman, S. S., Konstantinides, F. N., Raup, S., et al. (1986). Physiological and metabolic response to isolated closed head injury. *Journal of Neurosurgery, 64,* 89-98.

62. Robertson, C. S., Clifton, G. L., & Goodman, J. C. (1985). Steroid administration and nitrogen excretion in the head-injured patient. *Journal of Neurosurgery, 63,* 714-718.

63. Sanford, S. (1982). Respiratory complications of intracranial disorders. In D. L. Nikas (Ed.), *The critically ill neurosurgical patient.* New York: Churchill Livingstone.

64. McGuire, A. (1986). Issues in the prevention of neurotrauma. *Nursing Clinics of North America, 21,* 549-554.

65. Gardner, D. (1986). Acute management of the head-injured adult. *Nursing Clinics of North America, 21,* 555-562.

66. Nikas, D. L. (1986). Resuscitation of patients with central nervous system trauma. *Nursing Clinics of North America, 21*(4), 693-704.

67. Bracken, M. B., Shephard, M. J., Collins, W. F., et al. (1990). A randomized, controlled trial of methylprednisolone or naloxone in the treatment of acute spinal cord injury. *New England Journal of Medicine, 322,* 1405-1411.

68. Metcalf, J. A. (1986). Acute phase management of persons with spinal cord injury: A nursing diagnosis perspective. *Nursing Clinics of North America, 21,* 589-598.

69. American Association of Critical-care Nurses. (1990). *Outcome standards for nursing care of the critically ill.* Laguna Niguel, CA: Author.

70. Norris, J. W., & Hachinski, V. (1985). Acute stroke units: A reappraisal. *Current Concepts of Cerebrovascular Disease (Stroke), 20*(6), 31-33.

71. Hunt, W. E., & Hess, R. M. (1968). Surgical risk as related to time of intervention in the repair of intracranial aneurysms. *Journal of Neurosurgery, 28,* 14-20.

72. Adams, H. P., Kassell, N. F., Torner, J. C., et al. (1981). Early management of aneurysmal subarachnoid hemorrhage: A report of the cooperative aneurysm study. *Journal of Neurosurgery, 54,* 141-145.

73. Lee, K. (1980). Aneurysm precautions: A physiologic basis for minimizing rebleeding, *Heart Lung, 9,* 336-343.

74. Goldring, S., Zervas, N., & Langfitt, T. (1987). The extracranial-intracranial bypass study: A report of the committee appointed by the American Association of Neurological Surgeons to examine the study. *New England Journal of Medicine, 316,* 817-820.

75. Hirsch, M. S. (1985). Acute viral central nervous system diseases. In E. Rubenstein, & D. D. Federman (Eds.), *Scientific American Medicine,* Section 7, XXVII, 1-5.

76. Simon, H. B. (1986). Immunizations and chemotherapy for viral infections. In E. Rubenstein, D. P. Federman (Eds.), *Scientific American Medicine,* Section 7, XXXIII, 12-15.

77. U.S. Public Health Service. (1989). Interagency head injury task force report. Washington, DC: USPHS.

PART SEVEN

Renal Patient Care Problems

34

Renal Anatomy and Physiology

Charold L. Baer

"The chief functions performed by the kidney we know; how the kidney performs them remains a comparative mystery. The extreme complexity of this gland, with its various tubules and cells, has always attracted and baffled physiologists and histologists, so that today we are in some respects less certain of the methods of renal secretion than we seemed to be some years ago." To some clinicians, H. MacLean's assertion seems to reflect the current status of knowledge surrounding the renal system, but MacLean made it in 1921! Fortunately, the knowledge that has been amassed from research over the years has been assimilated into clinically applicable information. Thus, clinicians are now able to decipher the intricate functions of the renal system in maintaining the homeostatic composition of the internal environment of the human body. Such comprehension enables the clinician to monitor the function of the renal system so as to intervene appropriately to prevent insult or to minimize the deleterious effects of dysfunction. These interventions are important in any patient population, but particularly so in critically ill individuals who are already compromised by multisystem dysfunction. This discussion provides an overview of renal anatomy and physiology to assist in the clinical decision making required to provide quality care to critically ill individuals.

ANATOMY

Renal anatomy can be divided into the following components for discussion: a general description, the gross structure, the nephron, vasculature, the lymphatic system, and innervation.

General Description

The normal adult kidney is approximately 11 cm long, 2.5 cm thick, and 5 cm wide. It weighs between 120 and 170 g, and the combined weight of both kidneys constitutes 0.4% of the total body weight. As depicted in Figure 34-1, the kidneys are located retroperitoneally in the lumbar area with the right kidney positioned slightly lower than the left because of the liver mass that lies above it. The left kidney is slightly longer than the right and lies closer to the midline. When an individual is in the supine position, the kidneys lie between the 12th thoracic and 3rd lumbar vertebrae. In the erect position, however, or when an individual takes a deep inspiration, the kidneys descend toward the iliac crest. Likewise, when an individual is in the Trendelenburg position, the kidneys ascend to the level of the 10th and 11th intercostal spaces. Clinically, it is important to note that the kidneys move with respiration or position changes. Thus, when assisting with a renal biopsy or educating a patient about this procedure, it is important to explain why the patient is asked to take a deep breath and hold it. This specific action stabilizes the kidney in one position and facilitates obtaining the biopsy specimen.

The kidneys, as illustrated in Figure 34-2, are surrounded by several layers of protective coverings, including the true or fibrous capsule, perirenal fat, renal fascia, and pararenal fat. These coverings and adipose layers provide stability and a protective cushion of tissue to insulate the kidneys from injury due to impact. The innermost layer, the true or fibrous capsule, is a smooth, white, thin, resistant, glistening membrane that encases the renal parenchyma, or functional tissue. The next layer of covering is the perirenal fat, which is an adipose capsule that surrounds the kidney and is located within the renal fascia. The renal fascia, a sheet or band of two layers of fibrous tissue, is the third layer, and the fourth layer of covering is the pararenal fat, which is retroperitoneal adipose tissue that lies outside the renal fascia.

Gross Structure

The kidney has both lateral and medial margins with the lateral margin facing toward the side of the body and the medial margin being directed toward

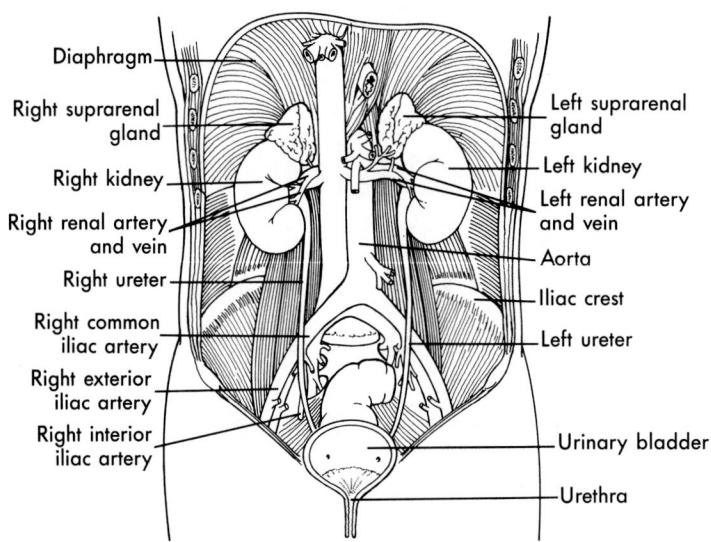

Figure 34-1   An anterior view of the location of the kidneys.

Adapted from an original painting by Frank H. Netter from *The atlas of human anatomy.* © 1989, by Ciba Geigy Corp.

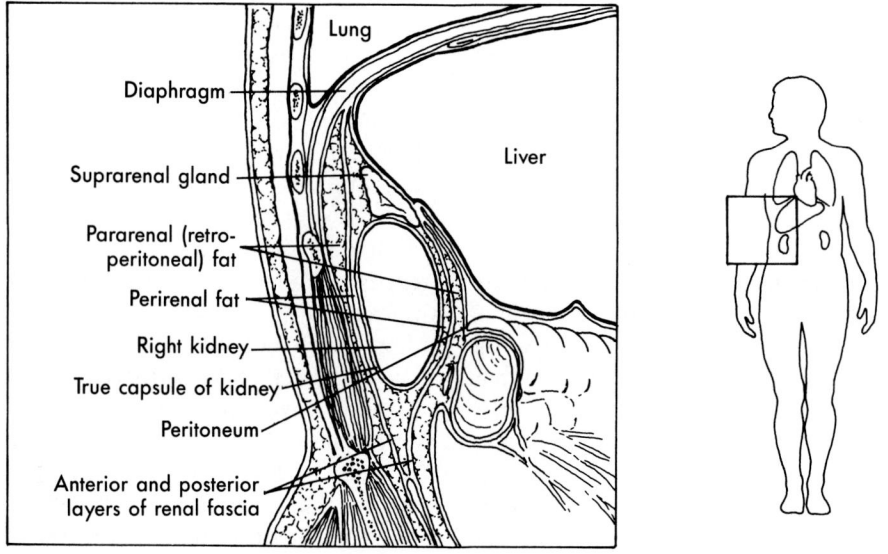

Figure 34-2   A saggital section illustrating the various coverings of the kidney.

Adapted from an original painting by Frank H. Netter from *The atlas of human anatomy.* © 1989, by Ciba Geigy Corp.

the midline of the body. Located at the medial margin is the hilus or hilum, which is the indentation of the kidney where blood and lymph vessels enter and the ureter emerges. The hilus leads to the renal sinus, a spacious cavity filled with adipose tissue, the minor and major calices, the renal pelvis, and the ureter. The renal sinus is surrounded by parenchyma. The minor calices receive urine from the papillary ducts of the pyramids and join to form the major calices which empty into the renal pelvis. The renal pelvis receives all of the urine and conducts it toward the emerging ureter.

Figure 34-3 depicts the renal parenchyma, which consists of a cortex and a medulla. The cortex, or outermost layer, is approximately 1 cm wide and is composed of cortical arches, the columns of Bertin, and the medullary rays of Ferrein. The cortical arches are areas of tissue that separate the medullary pyramids from the surface of the kidney; the columns of Bertin are areas of tissue that separate the medullary pyramids from each other. The medullary rays of Ferrein are long, delicate processes that emerge from the bases of the pyramids and enter the cortex. There are about 20,000 rays in each kidney, and each ray represents a lobule.

The medulla, or inner zone of the kidney, is approximately 5 cm wide and contains the pyramids, papillae, and papillary ducts of Bellini. The pyramids

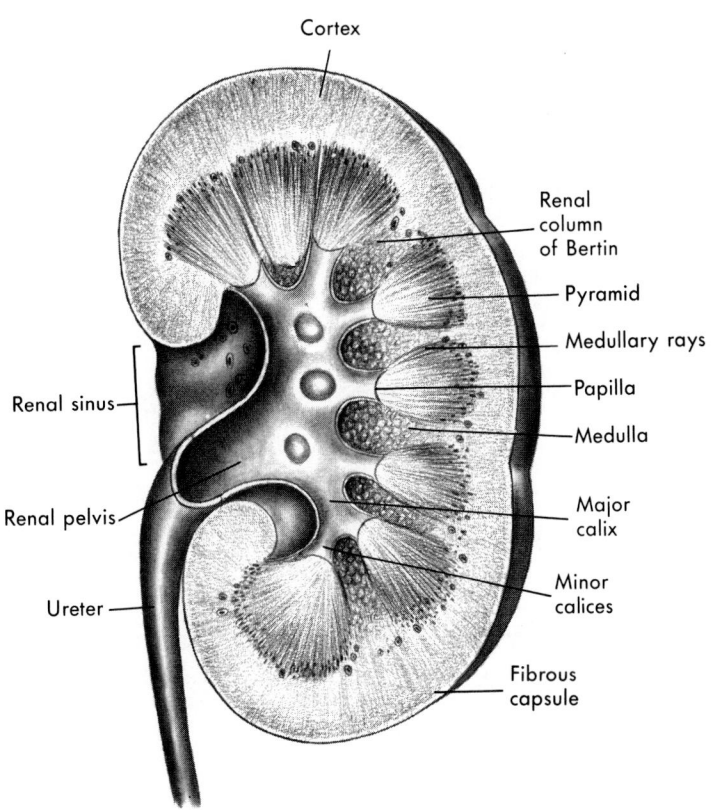

Figure 34-3   The gross internal structure, or parenchyma, of the kidney.
Modified from Thompson, J. M., McFarland, G. K., Hirsch, J. E., et al. (1989). *Mosby's manual of clinical nursing* (2nd ed.). St. Louis: Mosby–Year Book.

are conical structures with the bases lying parallel to the surface of the kidney and the apices, or papillae, directed toward the renal sinus. There are about 18 pyramids per kidney. The papillary ducts of Bellini are the radial striations in the pyramids that represent the collecting ducts. The papillary ducts empty into the papillae through small pores.

The Nephron

The nephron, illustrated in Figure 34-4, is the functional unit of the kidney. There are approximately 1 to 3 million nephrons in each kidney. Anatomically, the nephron is a tubular structure composed of a renal corpuscle and a tubular system. About 85% of the nephrons are cortical and have short loops of Henle. The other 15% are juxtamedullary and have very long loops of Henle. The juxtamedullary nephrons are major components in the physiological process of concentrating urine.

The renal corpuscle, depicted in Figure 34-5, is composed of the glomerulus and Bowman's capsule. The glomerulus is a skein of minute blood vessels that filter the blood. The walls of the glomerulus are lined with endothelium that has a pore diameter of 500 to 1,000 Angstrom. Thus, large molecules such as protein are retained in the plasma, while other smaller molecules pass through the glomerular capillaries and

enter Bowman's capsule. Other components of the glomerular walls include (1) the mesangium, a thin membrane that supports the capillary loops; (2) the basement membrane, which provides structural support, has a negative charge, and participates in the process of filtration; and (3) the visceral epithelium, which forms the outer layer of the glomerulus and the inner layer of Bowman's capsule and contains podocytes, or footlike processes, with fenestrations (openings) to facilitate the movement of the filtrate from the glomerulus through Bowman's capsule.

Bowman's capsule is a concave epithelial sac that surrounds the glomerulus and receives the filtrate from the glomerular capillaries. Structurally, Bowman's capsule is part of the tubular system. The walls of the capsule are composed of a basement membrane, a layer of parietal epithelium, and a layer of visceral epithelium which is shared with the glomerular capillaries.

The renal corpuscle has two poles, one vascular and the other urinary. The afferent arteriole enters the renal corpuscle, and the efferent arteriole emerges from the renal corpuscle at the vascular pole. The tubular system emerges from the renal corpuscle at the urinary pole. The tubular system, as depicted in Figure 34-4, is composed of the proximal convoluted tubule, the loop of Henle, the distal convoluted tu-

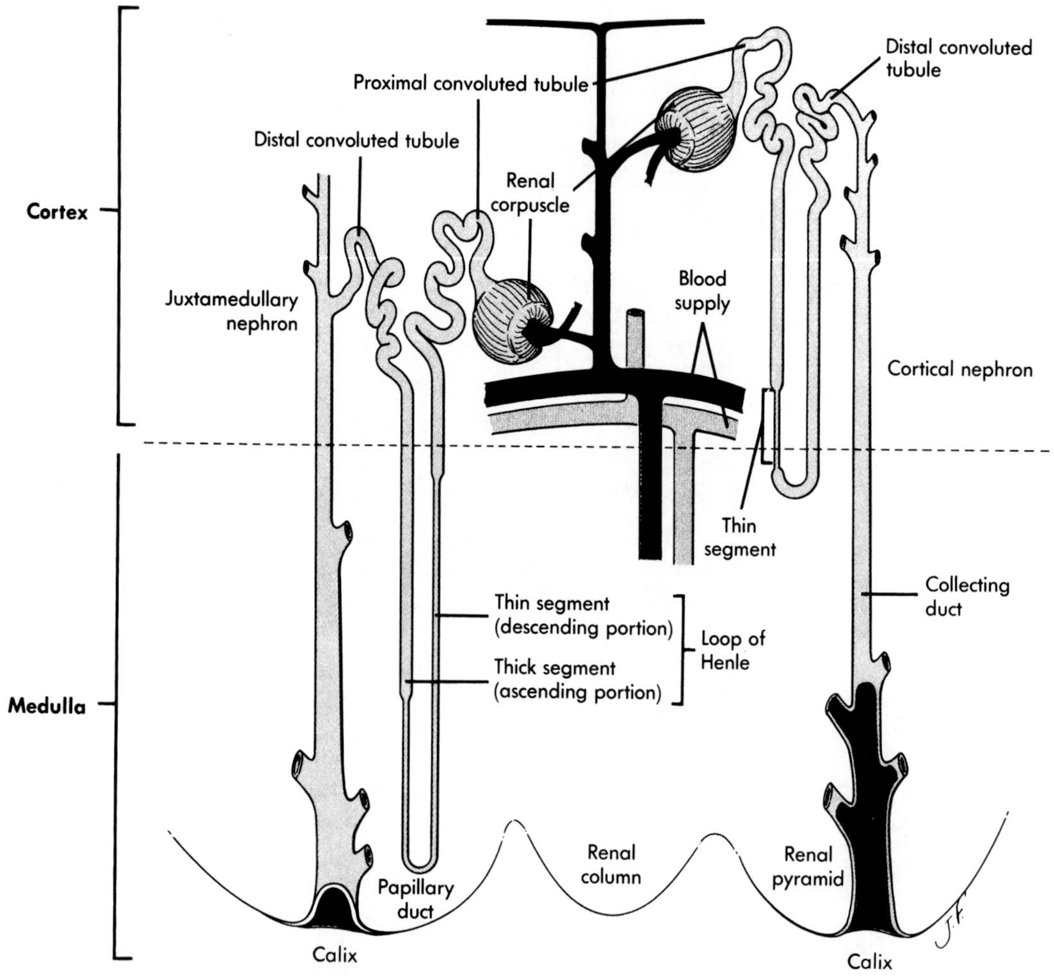

Figure 34-4   The nephron, or functional unit of the kidney.

Modified from Seeley, R., Stephens, T., & Tate, P. (1989). *Anatomy and physiology*. St. Louis: Mosby–Year Book.

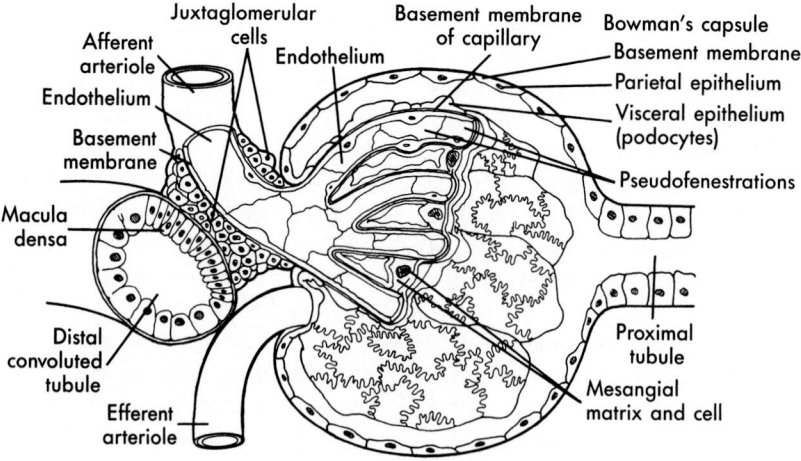

Figure 34-5   The renal corpuscle.

Adapted from an original painting by Frank H. Netter from *The CIBA collection of medical illustrations*. © 1979, by Ciba Geigy Corp.

bule, and the collecting ducts in addition to Bowman's capsule. The proximal convoluted tubule is composed of columnar cells which have numerous mitochondria that provide energy for the active transport of solutes. In addition, the lumenal surface is lined with hundreds of microvilli, also called the *brush border,* that increase the overall reabsorptive capacity of the tubule. Thus, the majority of the substances that are reabsorbed by the tubular system are reabsorbed in the proximal convoluted tubule. The proximal convoluted tubule straightens and narrows to form the loop of Henle.

The loop of Henle is composed of squamous cells, which have few organelles and a few short microvilli, along its thin descending limb. The thin ascending limb widens, and the cells are cuboidal, with more organelles and microvilli. The distal convoluted tubule emerges from the thick ascending limb of the loop of Henle. This distal convoluted tubule is composed of columnar cells which have numerous mitochondria and few microvilli. The mitochondria supply the energy required for the active transport of solutes, as well as the synthesis of ammonia and the acidification of the urine.

The collecting ducts are composed of several cell types depending upon their location within the kidney. In the cortex and outer medulla, the collecting ducts are composed of cuboidal cells and change to columnar cells as they reach the papillae. The collecting ducts also have fewer mitochondria and microvilli than the other components of the tubular system. Several collecting ducts join and then open into the papillary ducts of Bellini.

Anatomically, urine flow progresses as follows: (1) blood enters the afferent arteriole; (2) blood flows through the glomerulus where it is filtered; (3) the filtrate passes through podocytes into Bowman's capsule; (4) the filtrate then progresses through the tubular system, beginning with the proximal convoluted tubule, then the loop of Henle, then the distal convoluted tubule, and finally through the collecting duct; (5) from the collecting duct, the filtrate empties through the papillary ducts of Bellini, out the papillae, and into the minor calices; (6) the filtrate then flows into the major calices and the renal pelvis; (7) from the renal pelvis, it enters the ureter and is conducted by peristaltic action to the bladder; and finally, (8) the filtrate is stored in the bladder until the micturition process is initiated and completed, when it is excreted as urine.

Renal Vasculature

The kidneys receive 20% to 25% of the cardiac output, or 1,200 ml/min under normal circumstances. In general, the body's total blood supply circulates through the kidneys approximately 12 times per hour. Approximately 90% of the renal blood supply circulates through the cortex, while 10% circulates through the medulla. The blood supply to the kidneys originates from the renal arteries that branch from the abdominal aorta. The left renal artery is shorter than the right. As depicted in Figure 34-6, each renal artery enters the kidney at the hilus and then subdivides into five segmental arteries. The five segmental arteries are labeled according to the areas of the kidney to which they supply blood. They include the superior segmental artery, the anterior superior segmental artery, the anterior inferior segmental artery, the posterior segmental artery, and the inferior segmental artery. The segmental arteries subdivide into interlobar arteries, depicted in Figure 34-7, which travel parallel to the sides of the pyramids

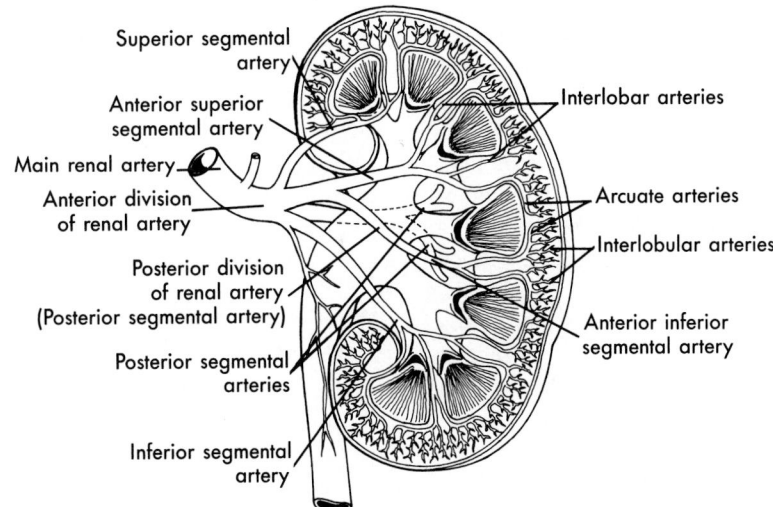

Figure 34-6   The subdivisions of the renal artery.

Adapted from an original painting by Frank H. Netter from *The atlas of human anatomy.* © 1989, by Ciba Geigy Corp.

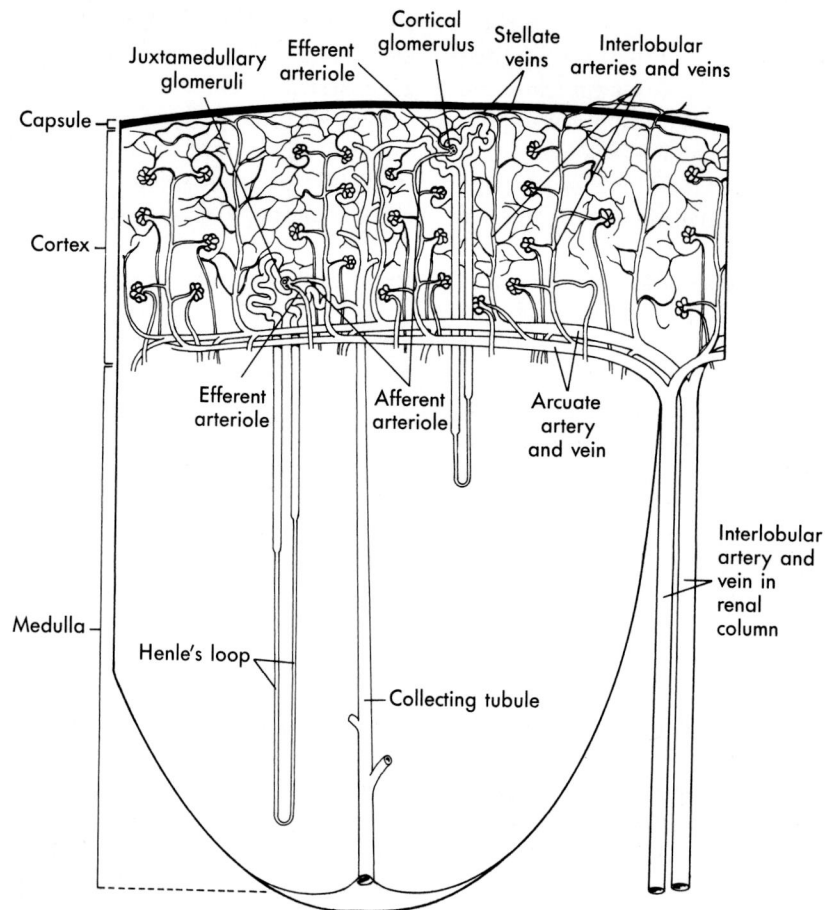

Figure 34-7 The vasculature of the renal parenchyma.

Adapted from an original painting by Frank H. Netter from *The atlas of human anatomy.* © 1989, by Ciba Geigy Corp.

in the medulla. At the junction of the medulla and cortex, the interlobar arteries change direction 90° and travel along the bases of the pyramids as arcuate arteries. The arcuate arteries branch into interlobular arteries in the cortex and the interlobular arteries subdivide to form the afferent arterioles of the glomeruli.

The afferent arterioles branch to form the capillary network of the glomerulus and then reunite to form the efferent arterioles. The efferent arteriole of a cortical glomerulus is smaller in diameter than the afferent arteriole; it supplies blood to the peritubular capillaries surrounding the proximal and distal convoluted tubules and the loop of Henle. It also supplies the peritubular capillaries of the juxtamedullary proximal and distal convoluted tubules. The efferent arteriole of a juxtamedullary glomerulus is the same diameter or slightly larger than the afferent arteriole and forms the vasa recta which are located in the medulla. The vasa recta are hairpin-shaped capillaries that parallel the long loops of Henle of the juxtamedullary nephron. The vasa recta are an important

contributing factor to the countercurrent exchange process that facilitates urine concentration.

The venous system of the kidney parallels the subdivisions of the arterial system, with the exception of the segmental arteries. Thus, the blood from the peritubular capillaries drains into the interlobular veins which drain into arcuate veins, then into interlobar veins, and finally into one of the four to six trunks of the renal vein. In addition, there are stellate veins that drain the subcapsular plexus and then flow into the interlobular veins. The renal vein exits the kidney at the hilus and joins the inferior vena cava.

Lymphatic System

The kidney has a rich lymphatic network that is composed of two basic plexuses. The first is a subcapsular plexus that drains the outer cortex and freely anastomoses with a perinephric system in the adipose and other tissue surrounding the kidney. The second plexus drains the inner cortex through a series of channels that follow the interlobular, arcuate, and interlobar vessels. This plexus exits the kidney at the hilus. Both plexuses drain into the lateral aortic and paraaortic nodes and then into the thoracic duct.

Innervation

The kidney is innervated from many sources, including branches from the celiac plexus, thoracic nerves, upper lumbar splanchnic nerves, and the intermesenteric and superior hypogastric plexus. The branches from these several origins converge to form an open meshed plexus around the renal vessels. It is from this renal plexus that the intrinsic renal nerves originate. Although the kidney is innervated with both parasympathetic and sympathetic fibers, the sympathetic fibers predominate.

PHYSIOLOGY

The renal system maintains homeostasis of the internal environment of the body through the following general functions: (1) regulation of the volume, concentration, and pH of the body fluids; (2) detoxification and elimination of waste products; (3) regulation of blood pressure; (4) regulation of erythropoiesis; and (5) vitamin D metabolism. These general functions are dependent upon several physiological mechanisms and processes of the nephron including glomerular filtration, clearance principles, tubular transport processes, tubular reabsorption, tubular secretion, maximal tubular transport capacity, electrolyte regulation, water regulation, hydrogen ion regulation, blood pressure regulation, erythropoiesis regulation, and vitamin D metabolism. Essentially, the nephron produces a protein-free filtrate at the glomerulus that consists of about 94% water and 6% solute. This filtrate is then modified by selective tubular reabsorption and secretion and finally excreted as urine.

Glomerular Filtration

Glomerular filtration is the process of ultrafiltering the blood as it flows through the kidney. Normally about 20% of the plasma that enters the glomerular capillaries is filtered into Bowman's capsule. This amount is known as the *filtration fraction*. Approximately 180 liters of filtrate are produced daily with 99% of this volume being reabsorbed. The glomerular filtration rate (GFR) is dependent upon three factors: the permeability of the glomerular capillaries, vascular pressure, and the net or effective filtration pressure. The permeability of the glomerular capillaries is a reflection of porousness and surface area. Vascular pressure is related to fluid volume, peripheral resistance, position changes, exercise, and emotion. Increases and decreases in vascular pressure directly affect renal blood flow and, thus, glomerular filtration rate. The net, or effective, filtration pressure is the force that drives the fluid and small molecular solutes through the glomerular capillary walls into the lumen of Bowman's capsule. The effective filtration pressure, depicted in Figure 34-8, is the difference between those forces that facilitate and those that oppose glomerular filtration. The glomerular intracapillary hy-

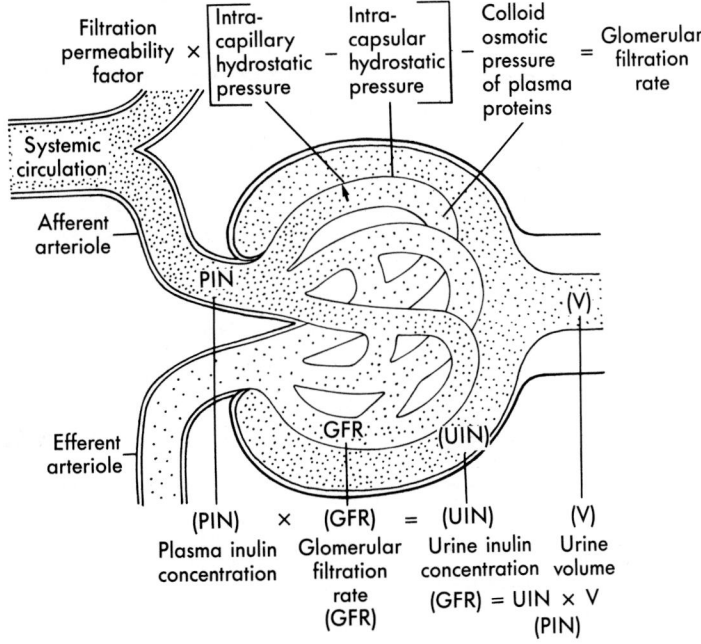

$$\text{Filtration permeability factor} \times \left[\text{Intracapillary hydrostatic pressure} - \text{Intracapsular hydrostatic pressure} \right] - \text{Colloid osmotic pressure of plasma proteins} = \text{Glomerular filtration rate}$$

$$\underset{\substack{\text{Plasma inulin}\\\text{concentration}}}{(PIN)} \times \underset{\substack{\text{Glomerular}\\\text{filtration}\\\text{rate}\\(GFR)}}{(GFR)} = \underset{\substack{\text{Urine inulin}\\\text{concentration}}}{(UIN)} \quad \underset{\substack{\text{Urine}\\\text{volume}}}{(V)}$$

$$(GFR) = \frac{UIN \times V}{(PIN)}$$

Figure 34-8 Effective glomerular filtration pressure.

Adapted from an original painting by Frank H. Netter from *The CIBA collection of medical illustrations.* © 1979, by Ciba Geigy Corp.

drostatic pressure facilitates glomerular filtration, while the glomerular intracapillary colloid osmotic pressure and the intracapsular hydrostatic pressure of Bowman's capsule oppose glomerular filtration. The normal values for these pressures are:

Glomerular intracapillary hydrostatic pressure, 50 mmHg

Glomerular intracapillary colloid osmotic pressure, 25 mmHg

Intracapsular hydrostatic pressure of Bowman's capsule, 10 mmHg

Thus, the effective filtration pressure can be computed as:

$$50 \text{ mmHg} - 25 \text{ mmHg} - 10 \text{ mmHg} = 15 \text{ mmHg}$$

The normal glomerular filtration rate is determined by administering a diagnostic substance such as inulin, a fructopolysaccharide that is filtered by the glomerulus but is neither metabolized, reabsorbed, nor secreted by the tubules, and then measuring the amounts of the substance that appear in the plasma and the urine. These data are then used with the following formula to calculate the glomerular filtration rate:

$$GFR = \frac{\text{Urinary inulin} \times \text{urine volume (ml/min)}}{\text{Plasma inulin}}$$

The glomerular filtration rate is normally about 120 ml/min but can vary for any specific individual and is usually higher for males than females.

Clearance Principles

The concept of clearance is important in understanding renal function. *Clearance* is defined as the volume of plasma that is cleared of a dissolved substance by the kidneys per unit of time, usually 1 minute. It is calculated using the formula:

Clearance of the substance =
$$\frac{\text{Urinary substance} \times \text{urine volume (ml/min)}}{\text{Plasma substance}}$$

The clearance of a specific substance is dependent upon how the substance is handled by the tubular system, which is governed by four basic principles.

The four basic clearance principles are:

1. If a substance such as inulin is filtered by the glomerulus and not reabsorbed or secreted by the tubules, then the clearance of the substance is equal to the glomerular filtration rate.
2. If a substance such as sodium or calcium is filtered by the glomerulus and is partially or completely reabsorbed by the tubules, then the clearance of the substance is less than the glomerular filtration rate.
3. If a substance such as paraaminohippurate (PAH) is filtered by the glomerulus and secreted by the

tubules, then the clearance of the substance is greater than the glomerular filtration rate.
4. If a substance such as potassium or uric acid is filtered by the glomerulus and then both reabsorbed and secreted by the tubules, then the clearance of the substance may be equal to, greater than, or less than the glomerular filtration rate, depending upon the reabsorption and secretion rates.

Urea clearance is dependent upon dietary protein intake, endogenous protein catabolism, hepatic conversion, glomerular filtration rate, and back diffusion along the tubule. In states of diuresis when flow rates are greater than 2 ml/min, the filtrate is hypotonic, and back diffusion is limited, so the clearance of urea is increased. In such states, urea clearance equals about 60% of the glomerular filtration rate. In states when flow rates are less than 2 ml/min, the filtrate is more concentrated, and more urea is present. Thus, there is more opportunity for urea to back diffuse, decreasing its clearance. The back diffusion of urea is important because it provides solute for the medullary interstitium and assists in concentrating urine.

Creatinine clearance is the best measure of glomerular filtration rate because of creatinine's relatively constant rate of production and excretion. Creatinine originates from the metabolism of creatine and phosphocreatine, substances that are present primarily in skeletal muscle. Thus, because muscle mass does not vary rapidly, the rate of production of creatinine is relatively constant. Likewise, because creatinine is neither reabsorbed nor secreted by the tubules, the rate of creatinine excretion is also fairly constant, which makes it an ideal substance to use in measuring renal function, or glomerular filtration rate. Creatinine clearance is calculated using the following formula:

Creatinine clearance =
$$\frac{[\text{Urinary creatinine} \times (\text{Urine volume/unit of time})]}{\text{Plasma creatinine}}$$

The average normal value for creatinine clearance is approximately 120 ml/min, but the rate varies with muscle mass. Thus, males tend to have slightly higher than average values, and females tend to have slightly lower than average values.

Tubular Transport Processes

The transport processes involved in tubular function are either active or passive. *Active transport* requires cellular or metabolic energy to move substances against a concentration or electrochemical gradient. Substances that are moved by active transport in tubular functions include sodium, potassium, glucose, amino acids, calcium, phosphate, urate, sulfates, and lactates. *Passive transport* does not require energy because substances move in accordance with a concentration or electrochemical gradient. Substances that move by passive transport in tubular function include water, urea, chloride, and some bicarbonates and phosphates. The passive movement of water in accordance with a concentration gradient (i.e., from an area of lower solute concentration to an area of higher solute concentration) is called *osmosis*. The passive movement of solute in accordance with a concentration gradient (i.e., from an area of higher concentration to an area of lower concentration) is called *diffusion*.

Tubular Reabsorption

Tubular reabsorption is the process of moving substances from the filtrate in the tubular lumen back into the plasma via the capillaries. Approximately 99% of the glomerular filtrate is normally reabsorbed, primarily in the proximal convoluted tubules. Some reabsorption also occurs in the loop of Henle, the distal convoluted tubule, and the collecting ducts, depending upon the requirements of the body.

Tubular Secretion

The process of tubular secretion is the movement of substances from the plasma in the peritubular capillaries to the filtrate in the tubular lumen. Substances that are normally secreted by the tubules include metabolic by-products, hydrogen ions, ammonium, uric acid, and potassium.

Maximal Tubular Transport Capacity

The transport processes involved in tubular reabsorption and secretion are governed by saturation kinetics. The saturation limitation of the tubules is referred to as the maximal tubular transport capacity, or T_m. T_m is defined as the point at which the tubular membrane transport mechanism, or carrier, that is responsible for moving a substance becomes saturated with the substance and cannot accept or convey more. When T_m is attained for the reabsorption of a substance, a substance that is normally reabsorbed is instead excreted. Likewise, when T_m for the secretion of a substance is attained, a substance that is normally secreted and excreted will instead by retained in the plasma. The T_m is different for each substance that is influenced by tubular functioning. In addition, the T_m for specific substances also varies among individuals. Thus, although averages have been determined for the T_m for a specific substance, those values vary widely among the general population.

Electrolyte Regulation

One of the renal system's primary general functions is that of regulating the electrolyte composition of the internal environment.

Sodium

Approximately 99% of the total filtered load of sodium is reabsorbed by various parts of the nephron, leaving only about 1% to be excreted in the urine. The reabsorption occurs as follows: 65% to 70% in the proximal convoluted tubule, 20% to 25% in the loop of Henle, 6% to 8% in the distal convoluted tubule, and 1% to 2% in the collecting duct. The reabsorption of sodium is an active process that is dependent upon the Na^+/K^+–dependent ATPase pumps that exist at the basolateral component of the peritubular membrane. Factors that enhance sodium reabsorption include a decreased glomerular filtration rate, aldosterone secretion, glomerulotubular balance, the redistribution of blood from the cortical to the juxtamedullary nephrons, increased peritubular capillary oncotic pressure, and, to a lesser extent, the serum sodium concentration, catecholamine secretion, and prostaglandin secretion. Factors that enhance sodium excretion include an increased glomerular filtration rate, decreased aldosterone secretion, and atrial natriuretic hormone, also known as third factor.

Sodium reabsorption is an important process because it also facilitates the reabsorption of other substances. Not only does sodium act as a cotransport carrier for some substances and a countertransport carrier for others, but it also facilitates diffusion and osmosis by altering the transtubular membrane potential. Thus, substances such as chloride, phosphate, bicarbonate, urea, and water are more easily reabsorbed.

Potassium

Most of the potassium (K^+) that is filtered at the glomerulus is reabsorbed in the proximal convoluted tubule. Of the filtered load of potassium, about 70% is actively reabsorbed in the proximal tubule, 20% is passively reabsorbed in the loop of Henle, and the remaining 10% is delivered to the distal tubule. Further active reabsorption can occur in the distal tubule and collecting duct, depending on the level of potassium in the body. The primary activity of the distal tubule, however, is the active or passive secretion of potassium. This distal tubular secretion, the main regulator of renal potassium excretion, is influenced by the following factors: increased aldosterone secretion; increased sodium delivery to the distal tubule; decreased hydrogen ion secretion; increased amounts of nonreabsorbable anions such as phosphate, sulfate, and bicarbonate; increased urinary flow rates; increased potassium intake; and diuretic therapy.

Chloride

The regulation of chloride is dependent upon the acid–base balance of the body fluids and aldosterone secretion. In general, the regulation of chloride is very similar to that of sodium, primarily because the two ions are coupled in many of the reabsorption, secretion, and transport processes, thus maintaining electrical neutrality. In most instances, chloride ion movement is passive and depends on active sodium transport. There are, however, two sites in the tubular system where this dependent relationship does not exist. The first site is the proximal tubule, where chloride reabsorption and excretion are dependent upon hydrogen ion secretion rather than on sodium transport. Thus, the degree of proximal tubular acidification determines the amount of chloride that is reabsorbed and excreted. The nature of this relationship is such that an increase in hydrogen ion secretion in the proximal tubule results in a compensatory increase in chloride excretion in response to an increase in bicarbonate reabsorption. The second site is in the loop of Henle, where chloride ion transport may be more active than passive. Consequently, chloride movement is less dependent on sodium transport in this portion of the tubule.

The influence of aldosterone on chloride regulation is secondary to its effect on sodium and water reabsorption. Aldosterone acts on the distal tubule and collecting duct to increase the reabsorption of sodium. As sodium is actively reabsorbed, water and chloride are also passively reabsorbed. Thus, there is increased reabsorption of sodium, chloride, and water.

Calcium

The regulation of calcium (Ca^{2+}) varies according to dietary intake. The tubular management appears to be similar to that of sodium. There are such clear similarities that it has been suggested by more than one expert that there may be a common transport pathway for the two ions. Unfortunately, such a common pathway has yet to be delineated. Of the 60% to 65% of the non-protein-bound calcium load that is filtered, about 55% is reabsorbed in the proximal tubule, about 30% is reabsorbed in the loop of Henle, and about 12% is reabsorbed in the distal tubule. The remaining 3% is excreted by the kidneys. The renal excretion of calcium is increased by the following factors: increased effective arterial pressure, most diuretics, hypercalcemia, hypophosphatemia, thyrocalcitonin, growth hormone, thyroid hormone, glucocorticoids, and acidosis. Those factors that decrease the renal excretion of calcium include decreased effective arterial volume, thiazide diuretics, hypocalcemia, hyperphosphatemia, vitamin D, parathyroid hormone, and alkalosis.

Phosphate

The renal excretion of phosphate is dependent primarily upon the serum phosphate concentration and parathyroid hormone. These two factors affect renal excretion by determining the amount and rate at which phosphate can be reabsorbed by the kidney. About 70% of the filtered phosphate is reabsorbed in the proximal tubule and 25% in the distal tubule. This reabsorption is dependent on the tubular maximal reabsorptive capacity that is established by parathyroid hormone.

The renal excretion of phosphate is increased by the following factors: parathyroid hormone, acute fluid volume expansion, hyperphosphatemia, thyrocalcitonin, glucagon, metabolic acidosis, hypokalemia, and diuretics that function by acting on the proximal tubule. The renal excretion of phosphate is decreased by vitamin D, growth hormone, insulin, hypophosphatemia, and a decrease in fluid volume.

Magnesium

The renal excretion of magnesium is the primary determinant of magnesium balance in the body. Reabsorption of 70% to 80% of the non-protein-bound filtered magnesium occurs in all parts of the tubule, but probably to a greater extent in the distal portion. The reabsorption is regulated by T_m, which seems to be equal to the filtered load of magnesium that is present at normal plasma concentrations of magnesium. Therefore, even small increases in extracellular magnesium surpass the T_m and increase the renal excretion of magnesium. Factors other than hypermagnesemia that increase the renal excretion of magnesium include: extracellular fluid volume expansion, especially with saline solutions; diuretic agents including osmotic diuretics; renal vasodilatation; hypercalcemia and hypercalciuria; thyrocalcitonin; alcohol ingestion; thyroid hormone; growth hormone; increased sodium intake; acute metabolic acidosis; chronic mineralocorticoid effect; and phosphate depletion. Factors that decrease the renal excretion of magnesium are hypomagnesemia, parathyroid hormone, and decreased extracellular fluid volume.

Bicarbonate

The plasma bicarbonate levels are regulated primarily by the renal reabsorption and regeneration of bicarbonate as a result of hydrogen ion secretion. About 80% to 90% of the bicarbonate that is filtered by the glomerulus is reabsorbed in the proximal convoluted tubule. The remaining 10% to 20% is reabsorbed in the distal tubule and collecting duct. In addition, the kidney regenerates bicarbonate that has been used to buffer nonvolatile acids in the extracellular fluid. Thus, the amount of bicarbonate that is reabsorbed and regenerated is roughly equivalent to the amount of hydrogen that is excreted as titratable acid and ammonium. Factors that increase the renal excretion of bicarbonate include extracellular fluid

TABLE 34-1   **Summary of the Renal Regulation of Specific Substances**

Substance	Amount Filtered	Amount Excreted	% Reabsorbed
Sodium, mEq/L	25,000	50-200	>99
Potassium, mEq/L	720	40-120	80-95
Chloride, mEq/L	19,500	50-200	>99
Calcium, mEq/L	450	5-12	>99
Phosphate, mEq/L	360	20-70	80
Magnesium, mEq/L	270	2-18	90
Bicarbonate, mEq/L	4,500	0	100
Water, L	180	0.5-3.0	98-99
Glucose, g	180	0	100
Urea, g	56	28	50

volume expansion, hypophosphatemia, decreased PCO_2 levels, hyperkalemia, hyperchloremia, decreased secretion of adrenocorticoid hormone, and parathyroid hormone. Factors that decrease the renal excretion of bicarbonate include extracellular fluid volume contraction, hypokalemia, hypercalcemia, increased PCO_2 levels, hypochloremia, and increased secretion of adrenocorticoid hormone.

The renal regulation of electrolytes is summarized in Table 34-1 according to the average amounts filtered, reabsorbed and excreted daily. Water, glucose, and urea have been added to the table to facilitate comparisons.

Water Regulation

The regulation of water is accomplished by two processes: hormonal control and the countercurrent mechanism. Hormonal control involves the osmoreceptor–antidiuretic hormone (ADH) system; the countercurrent mechanism involves the countercurrent multiplication and exchange systems.

Hormonal Control

The osmoreceptor–ADH system responds to alterations in the osmolality of the body fluids of as little as 1% to 2%. The response begins with the osmoreceptors that regulate the release of ADH. The *osmoreceptors* are specialized neurons located in or near the supraoptic nuclei of the anterior hypothalamus. These neurons contain fluid chambers filled with intracellular fluid, and they continuously emit nerve impulses. The fluid chambers respond specifically to changes in the extracellular fluid concentration. When the osmolality of the extracellular fluid decreases, making it hypotonic to the fluid in the chambers, water enters the fluid chambers to reestablish equilibrium between the two fluids. The influx of water causes the fluid chambers to swell, resulting in a decreased rate of impulse discharge. This means that fewer impulses are transmitted from the osmoreceptors in the supraoptic nuclei through the pituitary stalk to the neurohypophysis to promote the release of ADH. Thus, less ADH is secreted, and diuresis occurs to reestablish the normal osmolality of the extracellular body fluid.

When the extracellular fluid osmolality increases, the reverse of the process occurs. The increase in osmolality creates extracellular fluid that is hypertonic to the fluid in the chambers. Water then leaves the fluid chambers and flows into the extracellular fluid, shifting the system toward equilibrium. This efflux of water results in a shrinking of the fluid chambers and an increase in the rate of impulse discharge to the neurohypophysis. The net effect is an increased secretion of ADH, less urine volume and a subsequent dilution of the extracellular fluid, thus reestablishing a normal osmolality.

Antidiuretic hormone, or *arginine vasopressin,* is synthesized in the supraoptic and paraventricular nuclei of the hypothalamus and is stored as granules in the posterior pituitary. It is secreted into the blood according to the rate of impulses transmitted from the osmoreceptors to the neurohypophysis. The rate of impulse generation is also influenced by the action of venous, cardiac, and arterial baroreceptors. Once ADH is in the blood, it circulates to the kidneys and acts on the distal tubules and collecting ducts to increase water reabsorption. Thus, the more ADH is secreted, the more water is reabsorbed.

The Countercurrent Mechanism

The *countercurrent mechanism* utilizes the juxtamedullary nephrons with their long hoops of Henle and occurs within the renal medullary interstitium. It is composed of two processes: countercurrent multiplication and countercurrent exchange.

The *countercurrent multiplication* process occurs in the medullary interstitium via the loop of Henle and is the mechanism that enables the body to excrete urine with an osmolality higher than that of serum. The process facilitates this phenomenon by creating a hypertonic interstitial fluid from the generation of multiplying osmotic gradients through the active transport of sodium chloride from the impermeable ascending limb of the loop of Henle. The hairpin shape of the loop of Henle enhances the process by altering the osmotic gradient at the loop and stimulating the increased transport of sodium and chloride to reestablish the effective 200 mosm gradient. The net effect is an increase in the osmotic gradient along the entire length of the loop, thus multiplying the total osmolality.

The *countercurrent exchange* process is the maintenance component of the countercurrent mechanism. This process involves the hairpin-shaped *vasa recta,* blood vessels that are looped around the tubules in the renal medullary interstitium. The vasa recta minimize the loss of solute from the interstitium by passive diffusion, thus maintaining the osmotic gradients necessary for the countercurrent multiplication process.

Both of these processes involved in the countercurrent mechanism are significantly affected by the secretion of ADH. Antidiuretic hormone increases the permeability of the renal collecting ducts to water, which assists in producing an osmotically concentrated urine. It also assists in maintaining the hypertonic medullary interstitium by decreasing the rate of blood flow through the vasa recta of the medulla.

Movement through the Nephron

Water enters the nephron in the isotonic glomerular filtrate and moves to the proximal convoluted tubule where 70% is passively reabsorbed. The filtrate that leaves the proximal convoluted tubule remains isotonic. In the loop of Henle, an additional 10% to 20% of the water is reabsorbed, and the filtrate that leaves is hypotonic. The distal convoluted tubule, in the presence of ADH, is responsible for reabsorbing another 10% to 15% of the water, and the filtrate exists either as a hypotonic or an isotonic solution. An additional 1% of the water is reabsorbed in the collecting duct, in the presence of ADH, and the filtrate that leaves is hypertonic. At this point, the filtrate is in the final form of urine to be excreted from the body.

Hydrogen Ion Regulation

The renal system regulates hydrogen ion concentration in body fluids through the following five processes illustrated in Figure 34-9: (1) hydrogen ion secretion; (2) sodium reabsorption; (3) bicarbonate reabsorption; (4) excretion of titratable acids, or acidification of phosphate salts; and (5) ammonia synthesis. These processes occur in the proximal and distal convoluted tubules and are catalyzed by *carbonic anhydrase,* an enzyme that is present in the luminal border of the tubule. Within the tubular cell, depicted in Figure 34-9*A,* carbon dioxide and water combine in the presence of carbonic anhydrase and form carbonic acid. The carbonic acid dissociates into a hydrogen ion and a bicarbonate ion. The hydrogen ion is actively secreted into the tubular lumen in exchange for the active reabsorption of sodium from the luminal fluid into the plasma. The bicarbonate ion is passively reabsorbed into the plasma. In the tubular lumen, the secreted hydrogen ion combines with a filtered bicarbonate ion to form carbonic acid, which dissociates into water and carbon dioxide in the presence of carbonic anhydrase. The carbon dioxide is

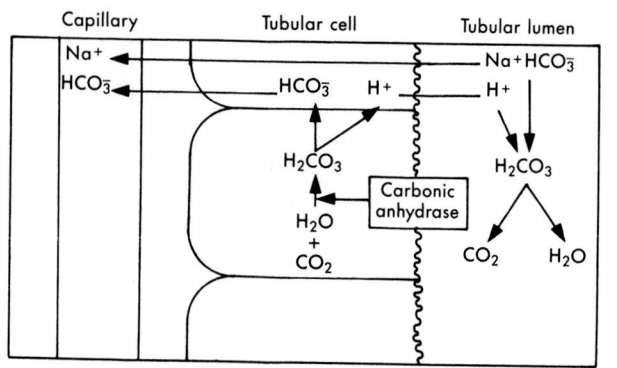

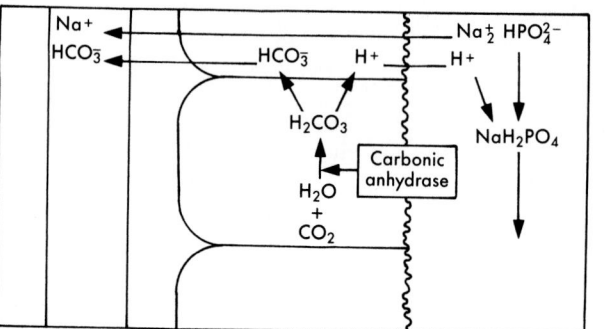

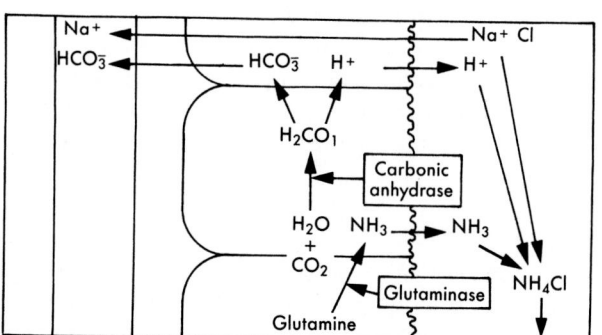

Figure 34-9 *A, B, C,* The processes involved in the renal regulation of hydrogen ions.

then reabsorbed and further utilized by the body, and the water is either reabsorbed or secreted. Overall, for every filtered bicarbonate ion that combines with a secreted hydrogen ion, a new bicarbonate ion is generated and reabsorbed.

Hydrogen ions are also buffered by other substances in the tubular lumen including phosphate and ammonia. The use of phosphate to buffer hydrogen ions is called the *excretion of titratable acids* (Figure 34-9*B*). This process involves the same activities within the tubular cell as were previously discussed. The changes occur in relation to the buffering agent that is present in the luminal fluid. In this case, the luminal fluid contains a disodium monohydrogen phosphate that rapidly loses a sodium ion in exchange for the secreted hydrogen ion. The monosodium monohydrogen phosphate then combines with the secreted hydrogen ion to form the acid, monosodium dihydrogen phosphate, that is excreted in the urine.

The buffering of hydrogen ions for excretion using ammonia is a similar type of process (Figure 34-9C). The processes that occur in ammonia synthesis are the same as those already discussed. However, in addition, the tubular cells also synthesize ammonia from glutamine in the presence of glutaminase. The ammonia is passively secreted into the luminal fluid where it accepts a secreted hydrogen ion to form ammonium. Ammonium is nondiffusible and is excreted in the urine.

Blood Pressure Regulation

The concept of renal regulation of blood pressure has two components, autoregulation and systemic regulation. *Autoregulation* refers to the ability of the kidneys to maintain a constant rate of intrarenal blood flow even when the mean arterial pressure varies between 80 and 180 mmHg. The autoregulation mechanism involves two intrarenal components that alter the intrarenal vascular resistance to maintain a relatively constant renal blood flow and glomerular filtration rate. These components are the myogenic mechanism and tubuloglomerular feedback. The *myogenic mechanism* involves the active contraction of vascular smooth muscle in response to increased stretch (dilation). It probably is caused by an influx of calcium across the plasma membrane into the smooth muscle cells in response to the stretching of cell walls.

The *tubuloglomerular feedback mechanism* primarily affects glomerular filtration rate and, secondarily, renal blood flow. This autoregulation mechanism responds to an increase in arterial pressure via detecting increases in fluid flowing through the macula densa. The macula densa then stimulates the secretion of a vasoconstrictor agent from the cells in the juxtaglomerular apparatus. The vasoconstrictor agent produces vasoconstriction which increases the vascular resistance and opposes the overall increase in filtration rate and blood flow.

Thus, the intrarenal autoregulation mechanism functions to maintain constancy in the rates of renal blood flow and glomerular filtration. Fluctuations do occur, but these changes are of a lesser magnitude than would be expected if autoregulation were not operative. In addition, it appears that autoregulation is functional only at mean arterial pressures greater than 70 mmHg; therefore, it cannot deter the ischemic changes that are likely to occur at lower arterial pressures.

The renal regulation of systemic blood pressure involves: (1) plasma sodium balance; (2) renin–angiotensin activity; (3) sympathetic nerve stimula-tion; and (4) prostaglandin, thromboxane, and kinin activity. The first of these factors, the plasma sodium balance, is regulated by selective tubular reabsorption and secretion. Since the direct effect of sodium on arterioles is vasoconstriction, maintaining an appropriate balance is essential for regulating blood pressure.

The renin–angiotensin system also participates in systemic blood pressure control. This system involves the juxtaglomerular apparatus of the nephron. The juxtaglomerular apparatus is composed of the macula densa, which is located at the point where the afferent and efferent arterioles touch the distal convoluted tubule; the granular cells of the afferent arteriole; the efferent arterioles; and the extraglomerular mesangium. As is illustrated in Figure 34-10, when the extracellular fluid volume is decreased, the intrarenal baroreceptors located in the granular cells sense the pressure change and increase the secretion of renin. The macula densa also responds to the decrease in volume and stimulates the granular cells to secrete renin. *Renin* is a proteolytic enzyme that acts as a catalyst on a plasma protein called angiotensinogen and converts it to angiotensin I. As angiotensin I circulates through the lungs, it is altered by angiotensin-converting enzyme to form angiotensin II. Angiotensin II is a hormone that constricts peripheral vessels, thus increasing overall peripheral resistance and blood pressure. Angiotensin II also stimulates the adrenal cortex to secrete aldosterone, which increases the amount of sodium and water retained and thereby increases vascular volume and pressure.

Sympathetic nerve stimulation also participates in regulating blood pressure. When the extracellular fluid volume is decreased, the lower arterial pressure is detected by the carotid sinus and aortic arch baroreceptors, and the sympathetic nervous system is stimulated. Stimulation of the sympathetic nervous system increases the activity of the renal sympathetic nerves, an alpha-adrenergic response, with concomitant increases in constriction of the renal arterioles. This vasoconstriction decreases renal blood flow and glomerular filtration rate, indirectly increases renin secretion, and enhances sodium and water retention, thereby raising overall arterial pressure. Sympathetic nerves that terminate in the area of the granular cells of the juxtaglomerular apparatus also assist in this process by exerting a direct stimulatory effect on renin secretion via a $beta_1$-adrenergic response.

Prostaglandins, thromboxane A_2, and kinins also influence the renal regulation of systemic blood pressure. The prostaglandins and thromboxane A_2 are vasoactive metabolites of arachidonic acid, which is released from membrane-bound phospholipids by the enzyme phospholipase A_2. The prostaglandins, PGE_2

TABLE 35-2   **Renal-related Information to Be Documented in a General Systems Review—cont'd**

Body System	Information to Be Elicited	Clinical Significance
Gastrointestinal	Anorexia	Uremia
	Nausea and vomiting	Uremia
		Electrolyte imbalances
	Constipation or diarrhea	Fluid volume changes
		Electrolyte imbalances
	Guaiac positive stools	Uremia
Renal and urological	See Table 35-1.	
Genitoreproductive	Difficulty achieving or maintaining an erection	Uremia
	Decreased libido	Uremia
	Infertility	Uremia
Musculoskeletal	Joint pain	Fluid volume excess
		Uremia
		Electrolyte imbalances
	Gout	Increased uric acid
	Muscle pain	Electrolyte imbalances
		Uremia
	Restlessness	Uremia
	Cramps	Uremia
		Electrolyte imbalances
Endocrine	Tetany	Electrolyte imbalances
	Thirst	Diabetic nephropathy
Hematopoietic	Fatigue	Uremia
	Malaise	Uremia
	Anemia	Uremia
	Bleeding	Uremia

Listening to bowel sounds to determine motility can validate the presence of electrolyte imbalances that might be reflective of renal dysfunction. The hyperkalemic state that often accompanies renal failure is reflected by intestinal hyperactivity and an increased frequency and loudness of bowel sounds in all quadrants.

If an individual has a previously created vascular access site, it is important to auscultate that site frequently to determine its continued patency. In most instances, a bruit can be detected. The presence of a bruit at a vascular access site is a normal finding and should be documented as such. If a bruit is not audible, it is possible that the vessels are occluded and the site is no longer functional. Early detection of alterations in patency is essential to reestablish normal function in the vascular access site.

Palpation and Percussion

Palpation and percussion of the kidneys are done in the lower portion of the upper right and left quadrants of the abdomen and in the flank areas. Because of other anatomical structures, only the lower pole of the right kidney is usually palpable. Anterior palpation is done to determine changes in the size of the kidney, while flank area palpation at the costovertebral angle is done to elicit pain resulting from an infective process. Percussion of the kidneys provides data related to changes in kidney size, as well as the presence of perinephric areas of fluid accumulation. Overall, however, the clinician will not find the physical examination to be particularly helpful in assessing the renal system. Its utility is probably most pronounced in detecting congenital or chronic pathological conditions. Fortunately, other diagnostic techniques yield similar data.

DIAGNOSTIC PROCEDURES

The physiological functions of the renal system influence the internal environment of the body to such an extent that any dysfunction is relatively quickly evident in diagnostic data. Such data are acquired principally via three mechanisms: laboratory assessments, noninvasive procedures, and invasive procedures.

Laboratory Assessments

Data obtained from the laboratory analyses of serum and urine samples provide information that is essential for assessing renal function. The most significant laboratory data are obtained from specific studies of renal function, serum analysis, and urinalysis.

Renal Function Studies

The best measure for evaluating renal function is urinary creatinine clearance which is calculated using the following formula:

$$U_c \times V/P_c = C_{cr}$$

In this formula, U_c equals the concentration of creatinine in the urine, V equals the volume of urine per unit of time, P_c equals the concentration of creatinine in the plasma, and C_{cr} equals creatinine clearance. Creatinine clearance is an estimate of glomerular filtration rate and is measured in ml per minute. It is determined by multiplying the urinary creatinine concentration times the urine volume in ml per minute and dividing that number by the plasma creatinine concentration. Given the following set of patient data: U_c = 125 mg/100 ml, V = 288 ml/24 hr, P_c = 12.5 mg/100 ml, the patient's creatinine clearance would be calculated as:

$$(125 \text{ mg/100 ml} \times 288 \text{ ml/1,440 min/24 hr})/ \\ 12.5 \text{ mg/100 ml} = 2 \text{ ml/min}$$

Because a normal creatinine clearance is about 120 ml/min, this calculated creatinine clearance is consistent with renal dysfunction.

Creatinine clearance is the best measure of renal function because creatinine is a metabolic by-product of creatinine or phosphocreatinine in the muscles. Levels of creatinine produced by the body remain relatively stable because individuals do not usually alter muscle mass rapidly. Since the levels are usually stable, they promptly reflect alterations in the renal system. Unfortunately, however, creatinine clearance values are not often readily available or practical for use in assessing the critically ill individual because they require a 24-hour urine sample for accurate calculation. The second best measure of renal function, serum creatinine, is consequently used, followed closely by the serum blood urea nitrogen (BUN) level. The BUN, however, is the less reflective of these two serum values, because it is easily influenced by other factors such as catabolism, bleeding, and volume depletion. Urine volume is also not a good measure of renal function. Many individuals evidence a nonoliguric or polyuric renal failure. Thus, they have renal dysfunction but excrete large volumes of fluid that lack the appropriate quantities of solutes and waste products. Patterns of urine output are more reflective of renal perfusion states than they are of renal function and, therefore, must be documented. The clinician, however, must be clear in noting that patterns of urine output reflect renal perfusion rather than renal function.

Tubular function is often cursorily estimated by evaluating the concentrating and diluting capacity of the kidneys. Additional factors, such as ADH level, are involved in the concentrating and diluting processes of the kidneys, so the degree of function can only be approximated rather than accurately quantified. An individual's maximum urine concentrating ability is determined by restricting the fluid intake for at least 16 hours. After such a restriction, a normal response is the excretion of urine with an osmolality in excess of 800 mosm/kg and a specific gravity of greater than 1.024. Abnormal results require additional testing involving more prolonged periods of fluid restriction or the administration of pitressin. Urine dilution capacity tests are usually so dependent upon other factors that they involve too many confounding variables to be accurately interpreted. Thus, such tests are not frequently conducted in clinical settings unless there are very specific reasons.

Serum Analysis

Alterations in renal function are rapidly reflected in an individual's serum laboratory values. To acquire the most accurate data about the renal system, these laboratory values should be monitored at least daily. More frequent monitoring may be necessitated by the patient's status. The serum laboratory values that are most helpful in assessing the renal system are displayed in Table 35-3. The eclectic normal ranges for those values and their usual deviations in renal dysfunction are also included.

Urinalysis

As the end product of renal function, the urine also provides useful data for assessing the renal system. For those data to be valid, however, the urine specimen must be appropriately collected and stored or preserved. An aliquot voided specimen is usually sufficient for most laboratory analyses. Culture and sensitivity studies, however, require at least a clean catch midstream specimen. An aliquot voided specimen is also not appropriate for studies requiring larger quantities of urine for analysis. Once a specimen is obtained, it should either be sent to the laboratory within 1 hour of voiding, or it should be refrigerated. Urine that remains at room temperature for longer than 1 hour undergoes subtle changes that alter its composition. For example, red blood cells hemolyze, and urea decomposes to ammonia as the urine remains stagnant outside the bladder. These changes could produce spurious laboratory values. Table 35-4 displays the urine values typically used for assessing the renal system, their eclectic normal ranges,

TABLE 35-3 Serum Laboratory Values for Assessing the Renal System

Substance	Normal Range	Deviation in Renal Dysfunction
Sodium	136-146 mEq/L	↑ or normal, but varies
Potassium	3.5-5.5 mEq/L	↑
Chloride	96-106 mEq/L	↑, but varies
BUN	9-20 mg/dl	↑
Creatinine	0.7-1.5 mg/dl	↑
Phosphorus	2-4.5 mg/dl	↑
Uric acid	3-7 mg/dl	↑
CO_2 combining power	24-28 mEq/L	↓
Magnesium	1.6-2.2 mEq/L	↑ or high normal
Alkaline phosphatase	5-13 King-Armstrong units	↑
Osmolality	280-295 mosm/kg H_2O	↑, but varies
Hematocrit	40% to 50%	↓
Hemoglobin	12-16 g/dl	↓
WBC	4,000-10,000/mm³	Varies

TABLE 35-4 Urine Values for Assessing the Renal System

Parameter or Substance	Normal Range	Deviation in Renal Dysfunction
Amount	1,200-1,500 ml	↓, but varies
Specific gravity	1.003-1.030	↓, but varies
pH	5.0-8.0	↑, but varies
Glucose	0	Normal or ↑
Protein	0-<150 mg/24 hr	Normal or ↑
Creatinine	1.0-1.6 g/24 hr	↓
Osmolality	500-1,200 mosm/kg H_2O	↓
Sodium	50-130 mEq/L	Normal or varies
Potassium	20-70 mEq/L	↓
Chloride	50-130 mEq/L	↓
Magnesium	2-18 mEq/L	↓
Phosphorus	1 g/24 hr	↓ or varies
Urea	10-20 g/L	↓
RBC	1,000,000/24 hr (Addis counts)	Varies
WBC	2,000,000/24 hr (Addis counts)	Varies
Casts	100,000/24 hr (Addis counts)	Varies
Bacteria	<100,000 organisms/ml	Varies

and their deviations in renal dysfunction. However, specific renal disorders may significantly alter the urine values from those that are expected.

In addition to the urine laboratory values, other characteristics of the urine should be noted. Those characteristics include color, clarity, odor, and abnormal constituents, often called *sediment*. The color of the urine can reveal important information, but it needs to be viewed within the total context of patient care. Therapeutic and diagnostic agents can alter urine color. Thus, the clinician must be aware of all possible factors that are likely to alter urine color. Table 35-5 lists the range of colors in the urinary rainbow, their etiologies, and the potential clinical significance.

The clarity of the urine can also provide valuable assessment data. Normal voided urine is usually clear. Cloudiness, or turbidity, can suggest the presence of microscopic substances such as pus, blood, epithelial cells, protein, chyle, sperm, prostatic fluid, fat, bacteria, urates, or phosphates.

Freshly voided urine usually has a mild, slightly aromatic odor resulting from the presence of ammonia. Concentrated urine usually has a stronger, more pungent odor, whereas infected urine has a definite malodorous scent. The odor of the urine can be

TABLE 35-5 **Urinary Color Variations**

Variation	Etiology	Clinical Significance
Light yellow	Anxiety	Normal dilute urine
	Diabetes mellitus	Pathological polyuria
	Diabetes insipidus	Pathological polyuria
	Nephrogenic diabetes	Pathological polyuria
	Hypervolemia	Normal dilute urine
Yellow	Urochrome	Normal
	Nitrofurantoin	Normal
Amber	Hypovolemia	Normal concentrated urine
	Hypercatabolism	Normal increased urochrome
	Riboflavin	Normal
	Pregnancy	Normal increased urochrome
	Carotenoids	Normal
Orange	Pyridium	Normal therapeutic
	Azulfidine	Normal therapeutic
	Bilirubin	Normal or pathological
	Bile pigments	Normal or pathological
Red	Hemoglobin	Pathological
	Myoglobin	Pathological
	Porphyrin	Pathological
	Aniline dye	Normal
	Beets	Normal
	Erythrocytes	Normal or pathological
	Urates	Pathological
Brown to black	Hemoglobin	Pathological
	Methemoglobin	Pathological
	Hemogentisic acid	Pathological
	Erythrocytes	Normal or pathological
	Melanin	Pathological
	Methyldopa	Normal therapeutic
	Mercury poisoning	Pathological
	Lead poisoning	Pathological
	Phenol	Pathological
	Phenylpyruvic acid	Pathological
	Levodopa	Normal therapeutic
Green-blue	Methylene blue	Normal
	Indigo blue	Normal
	Pseudomonas	Pathological
Purple	Stagnant porphyrin	Pathological
White	Phosphates	Normal or pathological
	Lipiduria	Pathological
	Chyle	Pathological

influenced by specific foods or pathological processes. Classic examples include the aromas produced in the urine as a result of ingesting asparagus or those accompanying diabetic ketoacidosis or phenylketonuria.

Abnormal constituents or sediment may be present in the urine. These constituents include cells, crystals, casts, and bacteria. The presence of a small quantity of these constituents may be normal, but often their detection heralds a pathological event. The presence of excessive numbers of red, white, or tubular cells almost always indicates a pathological condition. Likewise, the presence of excessive numbers of bacteria typically indicates an infective process. Crystals are present in normal urine, and the type of crystal is dependent upon the pH of the urine. Crystals that indicate pathology include cystine, leucine, tyrosine, and sulfonamide. *Casts*, or cylindrical masses of agglutinated material that reflect the shape of the tubular lumen, are usually indicative of pathology. Most casts are composed of the Tamm-Horsfall mucoprotein in combination with other components. For

TABLE 35-6   **Urinary Casts and Associated Pathological Conditions**

Type of Cast	Potential Condition
Red cell	Vasculitis
	Glomerular disease
	Cortical necrosis
	Acute tubular necrosis
White cell	Acute parenchymal inflammation
	Acute parenchymal infection
Epithelial cell	Acute tubular necrosis
	Interstitial nephritis
	Acute glomerulonephritis
	Chronic glomerulonephritis
Granular	Acute tubular necrosis
	Interstitial nephritis
	Acute glomerulonephritis
	Chronic glomerulonephritis
	Chronic renal disease
	Any proteinuric state
Broad, waxy	Chronic renal disease
Broad	Chronic renal disease
	Recovery phase of acute tubular necrosis
Fatty	Nephrotic syndrome
	Proteinuric states

example, hyaline casts, which are often documented in normal urine, are composed of Tamm-Horsfall mucoprotein, albumin, and immunoglobulins. Other casts have varying compositions and are more clinically significant. Table 35-6 lists the most frequently occurring urinary casts and the related potential pathological conditions.

Noninvasive Procedures

Paramount among the noninvasive diagnostic procedures for assessing renal function are measuring intake and output daily, obtaining daily weights, and integrating data from x-ray films. As simple as these assessment procedures are, opportunities for errors exist. Because accuracy is important, it is essential that the appropriate, calibrated measuring devices be used to obtain the amounts of urine, rather than estimates. In addition, baseline values must be established for the individual, measurement patterns must be compared, and intake and output measurements must be validated by accurate daily weights. Body weight may not correlate precisely with intake and output measurements. The clinician should recall that there are about 500 ml in a pound and should factor an individual's insensible losses into the process. The two measurements should then closely coincide.

An x-ray of the kidneys, ureters, and bladder (KUB) is frequently used to assess the renal system.

This plain film of the abdomen is taken with the patient in a supine position and is used to evaluate the size, shape, position, and possible areas of calcification of the kidneys. The KUB is usually performed before any other radiological procedures are conducted.

Radiological Procedures

Other diagnostic procedures provide specific data that are necessary to complete the total assessment of the renal system. These procedures include: excretory urography, computed tomography (CT scan), nephrosonography, nephrotomography, renal angiography, renal scan, and renal biopsy. The following general interventions are important for any individual who is undergoing these diagnostic procedures:

1. Explain the procedure to the individual, emphasizing the individual's responsibilities during the procedure.
2. Reinforce the explanations that have been previously provided by other health care team personnel concerning the procedure.
3. Complete any preparatory activities required for the procedure.
4. Provide appropriate fluids to assist the individual in maintaining an adequate hydration state before and after the procedure.
5. Assist with the procedure whenever possible or necessary.
6. Monitor the individual for any complications after the procedure.
7. Document the individual's response to the procedure.

Excretory Urography

Excretory urography, or intravenous pyelography (IVP), is a major component of any renal or urological evaluation. It was first performed in 1929 but did not become popular as a diagnostic tool until the mid-1950s when an appropriate, relatively nontoxic, iodinated contrast medium became available. The purpose of excretory urography is to visualize the renal parenchyma, calices, pelves; the ureters; and the bladder to obtain information regarding the size, shape, position, and function of the kidneys. The patient voids to empty the bladder and then assumes a supine position. Contrast medium is injected intravenously, and films of the kidneys and bladder are taken at 5, 10, and 15 minutes. The first minute after injection of the contrast medium is termed the *nephrographic stage*; the time between 3 and 5 minutes after injection is called the *pyelographic stage*. These two stages represent the expected length of time needed for the contrast medium to move through the anatomical structures of the kidney.

Major potential problems associated with the IVP include a hypersensitivity reaction and acute renal dysfunction. Any individual with preexisting renal disease, multiple myeloma, diabetes, or hypovolemia is at high risk for developing acute renal failure after excretory urography. Special clinical considerations include observing the patient for a hypersensitive reaction, which occurs in about 10% of the patients; monitoring the injection site for a postinjection hematoma; and assessing the patient's continuing renal function.

Computed Tomography

Since its inception in the 1970s, computed tomography (CT scanning) has earned a significant place in assessment of the renal system. Its accuracy in diagnosing renal masses has made it a major contributor in clinical settings. The purpose of the CT scan is to visualize the renal parenchyma to obtain information about the presence and appearance of lesions such as cysts, masses, calculi, obstruction, congenital anomalies, and abnormal accumulations of fluid. The patient assumes a supine position and is reminded that at various times during the 40-minute scan it will be necessary to hold his or her breath for a short time. A contrast medium may or may not be injected intravenously, and x-rays are taken at 10° intervals for a complete 180° rotation. The information is transmitted to a computer that creates an image of the kidney and calculates its density.

The major potential problem with the CT scan is a hypersensitivity reaction if a contrast medium is used. Special clinical considerations include monitoring the patient's renal function, observing the patient for a hypersensitivity reaction or postinjection hematoma, and reassuring patients who may encounter claustrophobic sensations while they are undergoing scanning.

Nephrosonography

Nephrosonography, which is an ultrasonographic evaluation of the kidneys, has been gaining wider acceptance since it was introduced in the early 1970s. Basically, nephrosonography is a noninvasive means of visualizing the renal parenchyma, calices, and pelves, as well as the ureters and bladder to obtain information about the size, shape, position, and internal structures of these organs and the perirenal tissue. It is also used to assess and localize urinary obstructions and abnormal accumulations of fluid. Many clinicians recommend it for differentiating hydronephrosis, acute renal failure, or posttransplant complications. It also has a high degree of reliability and accuracy in distinguishing cysts and cystic masses from solid masses. The patient assumes either a sitting or prone position. An ultrasound probe, called a transducer, is moved over the patient's body. It emits and receives inaudible, high-frequency sound waves that reflect off the kidney and are transformed into an image that is projected onto a screen. No potential problems or special clinical considerations have been identified for nephrosonography. Its limitations are related to the inability of the sonic beam to penetrate gas or bone. Spurious results may sometimes occur.

Nephrotomography

The form of renal x-ray called a nephrotomogram was first introduced in the 1950s. It did not become popular until the mid-1960s, when its utility for differentiating between cystic and solid masses was demonstrated. In general, nephrotomography is used to visualize "slices," or layers of the renal parenchyma, calices, and pelves to obtain information regarding tumors, cysts, lacerations, or areas of nonperfusion. A more recent role for nephrotomography is the identification of renal masses that might have otherwise been missed. Plain x-ray films of the kidneys are first obtained. The arm-to-kidney circulation time of a contrast substance is calculated. A loading dose of contrast medium is injected intravenously, followed by a second dose. Another x-ray of the kidneys is obtained at the predetermined circulation time, and tomograms ("slices") of the kidneys are taken at 1-cm intervals. The major potential problems associated with nephrotomography are a hypersensitivity reaction and hematoma at the injection site. The special clinical considerations include monitoring the patient for these problems.

Renal Angiography

Visualization of the renal vascular system by means of injected contrast medium, *renal angiography*, has been in use since the late 1920s. The advent of less toxic contrast media and more rapid film changers in the 1950s added to its diagnostic value. In recent years, less invasive techniques have replaced angiography to some extent. Its principal current uses are preoperative delineation of renal masses, defining intravascular tumor extensions, preoperative donor transplant evaluation, postoperative transplant recipient evaluation, assessment after blunt trauma, and diagnosis of renovascular hypertension. Renal angiography is used to visualize the arterial tree, capillaries, and venous drainage of the kidney to obtain information regarding the presence of tumors, cysts, stenoses, infarction, aneurysms, hematomas, lacerations, and abscesses. The patient assumes a supine position under the fluoroscope. After a local anesthetic has been administered to the catheter insertion site, a catheter is inserted via the femoral artery to the aorta. A contrast medium is injected via the catheter, and films of the kidney are obtained during the arterial, nephrographic, and venous phases of filling. When the procedure is completed, the catheter is withdrawn, and a pressure dressing is applied to the site. The patient remains on bed rest for 12 to 24 hours after angiography.

The major potential problems include a hypersensitivity reaction, hemorrhage at the catheter insertion site, and acute renal dysfunction due to nephrotoxicity from the contrast medium. Special clinical considerations include offering the patient additional fluids to maintain adequate hydration, observing the patient for a hypersensitivity reaction, monitoring the patient's renal function, monitoring the insertion site for bleeding or a hematoma, and encouraging the patient to maintain bed rest for the prescribed length of time.

Renal Scan

The renal scan, or radionuclide imaging of the renal system using gamma scintigraphy, has been widely used in diagnosis because it provides dynamic study data regarding pathology or pathophysiology. Different radiopharmaceutical agents are used depending upon the patient and the diagnostic need. In general, the renal scan is used to determine renal function by visualizing the appearance and disappearance of radioisotopes within the kidney. It also provides some anatomical and vascular information but may be less definitive than other procedures because of poorer resolution. The main indications for using a renal scan appear to be (1) a documented sensitivity to a radiocontrast medium; (2) diminished renal function that increases the hazards associated with excretory urography; (3) posttransplant evaluation; (4) the need for additional renal function data; and (5) specific types of suspected lesions, such as renovascular hypertension, trauma, abscesses, cysts, and obstructive uropathies.

The patient assumes a prone or other designated position, and a radioisotope is injected intravenously. Sequential views are obtained to illustrate the uptake and excretion of the radioisotope by the kidney. The major potential problems associated with the renal scan are hypersensitivity reactions and postinjection hematomas. The special clinical considerations include monitoring for these complications.

Renal Biopsy

Renal biopsy has been used successfully for over 35 years. It is usually performed to obtain data for a histological diagnosis to determine the extent of disease, the appropriate therapy, and the possible prognosis. The major indications for performing a renal biopsy include persistent proteinuria or microscopic hematuria, nephrotic syndrome, prolonged oliguric acute renal failure, systemic lupus erythematosus, glomerulonephritis, and posttransplant deterioration or rejection. The contraindications include a patient unable to cooperate, a bleeding disorder, uncontrolled hypertension, a documented renal mass or cysts, infection, and, in some cases, a solitary kidney or documented uremia.

The biopsy can be performed using either a percutaneous approach, usually done in the fluoroscopy or ultrasound laboratory, or an open approach which is accomplished in the operating room. The percutaneous method is preferred and used whenever possible. After appropriate prerequisite diagnostic tests have been completed, the patient's clotting time, prothrombin time, and platelet count are assessed. The patient assumes a prone position with the area to be biopsied slightly elevated using a support. The area is cleansed and anesthetized, and an exploratory needle is inserted (while the patient holds his or her breath) to determine depth and position. The area is anesthetized again, if necessary, and the biopsy needle and obturator are inserted while the patient holds his or her breath. The obturator is extracted, replaced with the cutting prongs, and a tissue sample is obtained. The prongs, tissue, and needle are removed, and the patient is instructed to breathe normally. Gentle pressure is applied to the site followed by a compression bandage. The patient remains on bed rest for 24 hours.

The major potential problem postbiopsy is hemorrhage, which is usually evidenced by gross hematuria. This complication occurs in about 5% of patients and usually subsides after the patient remains on bed rest for 24 hours. Other complications that may occur include a perirenal hematoma, visceral lacerations of adjacent organs, and infection. The special clinical considerations include observing for hemorrhage and a hematoma at the site, observing the patient's urine for hematuria, monitoring the patient's vital signs frequently, encouraging the patient to remain on bed rest for 24 hours, assessing the patient periodically for flank pain, and offering increased amounts of fluid to maintain a dilute urine to prevent intrarenal clot formation.

BIBLIOGRAPHY

American Nephrology Nurses' Association. (1991). *Core curriculum for nephrology nursing* (2nd ed.). Pitman, NJ: A. J. Jannetti.

Brenner, B. M., Coe, F. L., & Rector, F. C. (1987). *Clinical nephrology*. Philadelphia: Saunders.

Bricker, N. S., & Kirschenbaum, M. A. (1984). *The kidney: Diagnosis and management*. New York: Wiley.

Cleigh, J. S., Stenzel, K. H., & Rubin, A. L. (1981). *Manual of clinical nephrology.* Boston: Martinus Nijhoff.

Flamenbaum, W., & Hamburger, R. J. (1982). *Nephrology: An approach to the patient with renal disease.* Philadelphia: Lippincott.

Franklin, S. S. (1981). *Practical nephrology.* New York: Wiley.

Graff, L. (1983). *A handbook of routine urinalysis.* Philadelphia: Lippincott.

Hamburger, R. J., Crosnier, J., & Grunfeld, J. P. (1979). *Nephrology.* New York: Wiley.

Reiley, P. J. (1984). Assessing renal and urologic function (Chap. 2); Implementing the diagnostic workup (Chap. 3). In *Renal and urologic disorders.* Springhouse, PA: Springhouse.

Richard, C. J. (1986). *Comprehensive nephrology nursing.* Boston: Little, Brown.

Rosenfield, A. T., Glickman, M. G., & Hodson, J. (1979). *Diagnostic imaging in renal disease.* New York: Appleton-Century-Crofts.

Schrier, R. W. (1990). *Manual of nephrology: Diagnosis and therapy* (3rd ed.). Boston: Little, Brown.

Stein, J. (1980). *Nephrology.* New York: Grune & Stratton.

36

Acute Renal Failure

Charold L. Baer

Providing care for a critically ill individual with multisystem involvement is a demanding task. The challenge is heightened as additional body systems become dysfunctional or as previously altered systems exert an exaggerated effect on an individual's physiological functioning. Such is the case when the renal system becomes dysfunctional and can no longer maintain a homeostatic internal environment. The additive effect is that the individual's overall adaptive capacities are severely compromised and more intensive therapeutic interventions are required to sustain life and restore optimal health. Thus, the challenge for the clinician is magnified and must be met with an appropriate set of responses. This chapter is designed to provide the clinician with a database sufficient for responding to the challenge posed by the insult of acute renal failure.

DEFINITION

Technically, acute renal failure is defined as an abrupt diminution or cessation of renal function. From a clinical perspective, however, it is more relevant to define acute renal failure in terms of what the individual is likely to experience during the course of the pathophysiological process, that is, in terms of onset, duration, and prognosis.

Onset

The onset of acute renal failure is usually very sudden and is characterized by either anuria, oliguria, or polyuria.

Anuria designates a urine volume of less than 100 ml per 24 hours.

Oliguria refers to a urine volume of 100 to 400 ml per 24 hours.

Polyuria describes a urine volume in excess of 400 ml per 24 hours that accompanies a diagnosed state of acute renal failure.

The oliguric state is most frequently encountered in acute renal failure. Polyuria, or nonoliguric acute renal failure, occurs much less frequently, but its incidence appears to be increasing, particularly in relation to the nephrotoxic etiologies. Individuals with non-oliguric acute renal failure may excrete in excess of 1.5 liters of fluid per day, but the fluid is deficient in the solutes and waste products that normal urine contains. Anuria is the least frequently occurring of the urine volume states in acute renal failure, and total anuria is rare. The documentation of an anuric state should raise the possibility of an obstruction as the etiology. In those instances, all anatomical and mechanical conduits must be investigated to verify their patency.

Phases

Acute renal failure is a short-term, relatively self-limiting pathological condition that usually persists for about 10 to 25 days. During that time, the individual traverses through four distinct phases of the clinical course of the disease process, including onset, oliguria or anuria, diuresis, and convalescence. Table 36-1 summarizes each phase according to its definition, time span, renal blood flow and oxygen consumption, urine volume, and filtration clearance.

Onset Phase

The onset phase encompasses the period extending from the occurrence of the precipitating event until the beginning of the change in urine output, usually either oliguria or anuria. This phase usually lasts from less than 1 day to 2 days and marks the initiation and progression of the deterioration of normal renal function. During this phase, renal blood flow and oxygen consumption decrease to about 25% of normal, urine volume decreases to 20% of normal, and filtration clearance decreases to 10% of normal. The end of this phase usually heralds the onset of significant systemic clinical signs and symptoms of acute renal failure, which are reflective of the chemical imbalances in the internal environment.

Oliguric–Anuric Phase

This phase is the period during which the individual's urine volume remains diminished, usually at

TABLE 36-1   **Phases of Acute Renal Failure**

Phase	Definition	Time Span	Renal Blood Flow and O$_2$ Consumption, % of Normal	Urine Volume, % of Normal	Filtration Clearance, % of Normal
Onset	The period from the precipitating event to the beginning of the oliguria or anuria	0-2 days	25	20	10
Oliguric–anuric	The period during which the urine volume remains less than 400 ml/24 hr	8-14 days	25	5	10
Diuretic					
Early	The period when the urine output becomes greater than 400 ml/24 hr until the laboratory values stop rising	10 days	30	150	10
Late	The period from when the laboratory values begin to decrease until they stabilize		50	200	50
Convalescent	The period from the stabilization of laboratory values until totally normal renal function occurs	4-6 months	100	100	100

From Schoengrund, L., & Balzer, P. (1985). *Renal problems in critical care.* New York: Wiley.

levels less than 400 ml per day. The duration of this phase is usually 8 to 14 days. During this phase, renal blood flow and oxygen consumption remain at 25% of normal, urine volume usually decreases even further to about 5% of normal, and filtration clearance remains at 10% of normal. It is clinically significant that the longer an individual remains in the oliguric-anuric phase, the poorer is the prognosis for recovery. The potential deterioration in the prognosis is directly related to the increased risk for fluid and electrolyte imbalances and other complications that the individual may encounter during this time.

Diuretic Phase

The diuretic phase lasts for about 10 days and consists of two stages, early diuresis and late diuresis. The *early stage* of diuresis includes the period when the urine output increases sufficiently to surpass the oliguric level of 400 ml per day and the laboratory values stabilize. During this stage, renal blood flow and oxygen consumption increase to about 30% of normal, urine volume increases to 150% of normal, and filtration clearance remains at 10% of normal. The improvement in renal blood flow and overall urine volume accounts for the stabilization of laboratory values, while the lack of improvement in filtration clearance explains why those values do not begin to approach more normal levels.

The *late stage* of diuresis is marked by the beginning of the normalization of the laboratory values,

and it extends until they reach a stable level. The level of stability achieved in this stage, however, is usually higher than the individual's normal level. During this stage, renal blood flow and oxygen consumption continue to increase to about 50% of normal, urine volume peaks to about 200% of normal, and filtration clearance increases to 50% of normal. This stage manifests a significant improvement in renal function but not a return to normal renal function. Indeed, during this stage the individual continues to be susceptible to fluid and electrolyte imbalances as well as other complications. Some clinicians consider the individual's vulnerability at this stage to be equivalent to that in the oliguric stage.

Convalescent Phase

The convalescent phase encompasses the remaining recovery time for the individual and usually lasts for 4 to 6 months. This phase begins with the stabilization of the laboratory values and extends until they return to a totally normal level for the individual. The return to normal may indicate the resumption of 100% of normal renal function, or it may signal a return of only 97% to 99% of normal function. Usually the 1% to 2% degree of residual renal impairment is not clinically significant. Those who are most likely to experience a residual impairment, however, are individuals with already declining renal function, such as the elderly or those with previously existing renal disease.

Nonoliguric Acute Renal Failure

The foregoing phases depict the classic progression of an episode of oliguric acute renal failure but fail to delineate the course of the disease process for nonoliguric acute renal failure. In the case of nonoliguric acute renal failure, the time frame is more variable and may be shorter, and fewer factors need to be assessed. Urine volume may not be a useful parameter, but analysis of urinary constituents reveals essential information. Indeed, analysis of the progression of the alterations in both the urine and serum laboratory values yields the most clinically useful information.

Prognosis

The prognosis for returning to normal or optimal renal function after an episode of acute renal failure is very good for 50% to 60% of patients. In the other 40% to 50% of patients, about two thirds will continue to experience difficulty and will ultimately develop chronic renal failure, and the remaining third will die because of a delay in seeking health care, complications secondary to the acute renal failure episode, or clinical mismanagement. A major responsibility of the critical care nurse in caring for patients with acute renal failure is to be sufficiently knowledgeable and competent to recognize complications and avert mismanagement. This task is becoming more and more complex. Opportunities for compromised individuals to develop acute renal failure appear to be increasing. Thus, even though significant advances have been made in the therapeutic management of individuals with acute renal failure, the overall statistical outcomes have not kept pace. Mortality rates per 100,000 that were documented 25 years ago remain unchanged.

Etiology

Acute renal failure can be precipitated by numerous clinical conditions. The etiologies of acute renal failure are usually classified as (1) prerenal, (2) postrenal, or (3) parenchymal (intrarenal), depending upon where in the kidney they exert their pathophysiological effects. These classifications and corresponding examples of clinical conditions are delineated in Table 36-2. The *prerenal* etiologies include

TABLE 36-2   Etiologies of Acute Renal Failure

Classification	Examples of Clinical Conditions
PRERENAL	
Hypovolemia	Vascular loss—hemorrhage
	Gastrointestinal loss—vomiting, diarrhea
	Renal loss—diuretic abuse, osmotic diuresis associated with diabetes
	Integumentary loss—burns, diaphoresis
Cardiovascular failure	Myocardial infarction
	Tamponade
	Vascular pooling—sepsis
	Vascular occlusion—thrombosis, embolism
POSTRENAL	
Obstruction	Ureteral—fibrosis, calculi, crystals, clots, accidental ligation
	Bladder—neoplasms
	Urethral—stricture, prostatic hypertrophy
PARENCHYMAL	
Glomerulonephritis	Acute poststreptococcal, systemic lupus erythematosus, Goodpasture's syndrome, bacterial endocarditis
Vasculitis	Periarteritis, hypersensitivity angiitis
Interstitial nephritis	Acute pyelonephritis, allergic nephritis, hypercalcemia, uric acid nephropathy, myeloma of the kidney
Renal vascular disease	Renal artery occlusion, renal vein thrombosis
Acute tubular necrosis	
Postischemia	Hypovolemia, cardiogenic shock, endotoxic shock
Nephrotoxins	Heavy metals, organic solvents, glycols, antibiotics, anesthetics, radiographic contrast media
Pigments	
Hemoglobin	Intravascular hemolysis—transfusion reactions, toxic hemolysis
Myoglobin	Rhabdomyolysis—trauma, muscle disease, seizures, severe exercise, prolonged coma

From Schoengrund, L., & Balzer, P. (1985). *Renal problems in critical care.* New York: Wiley.

conditions that induce acute renal failure by interfering with renal perfusion. *Postrenal* etiologies encompass conditions that induce acute renal failure by obstructing the flow of urine. *Parenchymal* etiologies are conditions that induce acute renal failure by directly insulting functioning kidney tissue. In general, conditions of the prerenal and postrenal type, which are often referred to as secondary renal problems, can often be reversed. With early detection and prompt corrective interventions, acute renal failure may be averted in some individuals. Parenchymal etiologies, which are usually referred to as primary renal problems, are more difficult to detect and are often not reversible. Consequently, parenchymal problems frequently initiate or precipitate acute renal failure.

Pathophysiology

The pathophysiology of acute renal failure is usually initiated by either (1) hypoperfusion or an ischemic episode accompanied by subsequent alterations in cellular metabolism, or (2) a nephrotoxic insult. The process involves five specific mechanisms: (1) in-

creased intrarenal vasoconstriction, (2) cellular edema, (3) decreased glomerular capillary permeability, (4) intratubular obstruction, and (5) the back leak of glomerular filtrate. Whether, when, and to what extent these mechanisms are actually operating during acute renal failure remains controversial. There appears to be some consensus that any or all of these mechanisms may be operative in any individual at some specific time, thereby causing oliguria.

Figure 36-1 depicts the pathophysiological processes involved in acute renal failure, beginning either with hypoperfusion accompanied by altered cellular metabolism or with a nephrotoxic substance. Hypoperfusion leads to decreased renal blood flow and ischemia, thereby activating the renin–angiotensin system, which induces increased intrarenal vasoconstriction. This vasoconstriction further decreases renal blood flow, thereby reducing glomerular blood flow and causing cellular insult to the renal tubules. Because glomerular blood flow is reduced, glomerular capillary pressure and permeability are also reduced, lowering the glomerular filtration rate and leading to

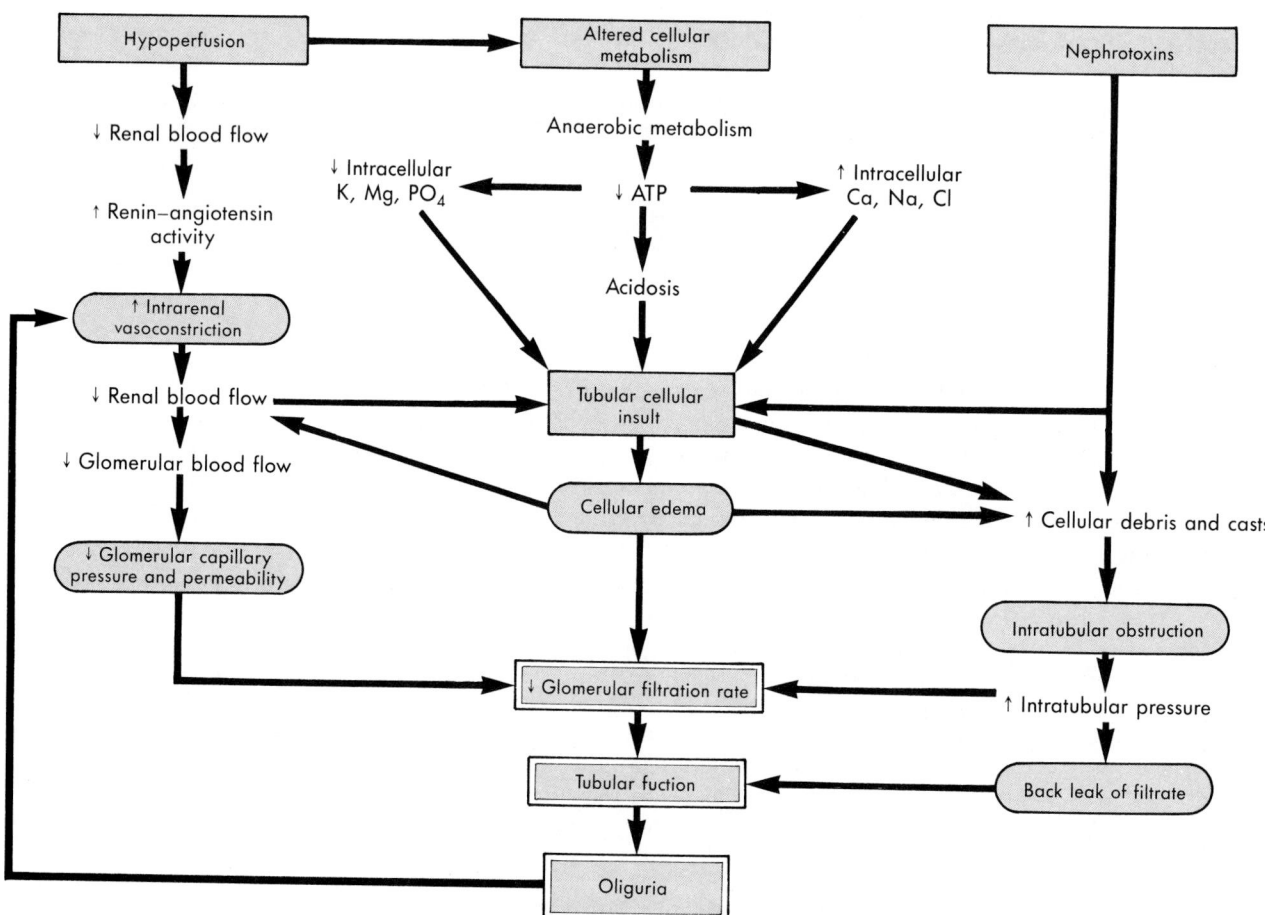

Figure 36-1 The pathophysiology of acute renal failure.

tubular dysfunction and oliguria. Not only does the diminution of tubular function cause oliguria, but it also exacerbates the intrarenal vasoconstriction, further compromising renal blood flow and perpetuating the dysfunction.

Hypoperfusion or ischemia alters cellular metabolism by converting the aerobic metabolism to anaerobic metabolism in which less adenosine triphosphate (ATP) is produced and acidosis develops. Without the energy usually supplied by ATP, the cell membrane and its ion pumps cannot function normally to pump sodium out of the cell or accumulate potassium. Also, chloride enters the cell as depolarization occurs. Calcium ATPase is also decreased so intracellular calcium increases. The overall result is a decrease in intracellular potassium, magnesium, and phosphate and an increase in intracellular calcium, sodium, and chloride. The abnormal composition of the intracellular solutes together with acidosis damage the cellular structures of the tubules. The increase in cellular solutes also facilitates cellular edema which further decreases renal blood flow and glomerular filtration rate and leads to decreased tubular function and oliguria.

The amount and degree of cellular damage resulting from hypoperfusion depends somewhat on the length of the ischemic episode. Data suggest that an ischemic episode of 25 minutes' duration or less causes reversible, mild injury, whereas ischemia lasting 40 to 60 minutes causes more severe damage. In addition, it appears that renal blood flow does not return to normal promptly during reperfusion after an ischemic event. This continued decrease in blood flow, accompanied by the formation of oxygen free radicals, further damages the cells. Damaged tubular cells and cellular edema result in the accumulation of necrotic endothelial cells and other cellular debris as casts, which can obstruct the lumen of the tubule. This intratubular obstruction increases the intratubular pressure, which decreases glomerular filtration rate and leads to tubular dysfunction and oliguria. In addition, the tubular damage usually alters the tubular basement membrane, permitting the glomerular filtrate to leak out of the tubular lumen and back into the plasma via the peritubular capillaries. This back leak of filtrate is a component of the tubular dysfunction that results in oliguria.

Nephrotoxins, such as heavy metals, contrast media, pharmacological agents, microbial by-products, and circulating inflammatory mediators, damage the tubular cells directly. The nephrotoxic agent destroys component parts of the tubule, causing intratubular obstruction and the back leak of glomerular filtrate and the subsequent pathological alterations associated with these events. The end result is tubular dys-

function and often oliguria. In many instances, acute renal failure due to nephrotoxins is of shorter duration than that resulting from hypoperfusion. It is also more likely to be characterized by nonoliguria, rather than by oliguria.

Systemic Manifestations

Acute renal failure affects all other body systems. Thus, the clinician must be aware of all potential problems in order to prevent complications that would further compromise the patient's health state. Table 36-3 summarizes the systemic manifestations of acute renal failure according to body system and indicates the pathophysiological mechanisms underlying each manifestation. Information contained in this table provides the foundation for formulating an appropriate plan of care. The subsequent discussion focuses on a few points specific to some of the body systems.

In regard to the *vascular system*, the following alterations in the individual's *serum laboratory values* should be anticipated in acute renal failure: elevated levels of sodium (although this varies according to dilution), potassium, chloride, BUN, creatinine, phosphorus, uric acid and alkaline phosphatase levels; decreased levels of calcium and CO_2 combining power levels; a magnesium level in the high normal range. Alterations in the *urine laboratory values* vary greatly, depending on the pathophysiology involved. In general, however, the clinician might anticipate the following: decreased values of creatinine, osmolality, sodium, potassium, chloride, calcium, and phosphorus; an increase in pH; a fixed specific gravity; and normal glucose and protein levels. It is important to note the level of urinary sodium is higher than that which accompanies a prerenal state but is always less than the amount normally excreted.

An increased susceptibility to *infection* presents a major problem for an already compromised patient with acute renal failure. Not only is the individual less able to combat infection, but he or she is now more likely to develop infection because of the repeated invasive procedures needed to maintain and sustain life. The clinician must be ever vigilant regarding the potential for infection because sepsis is the leading cause of death in individuals experiencing acute renal failure.

The *gastrointestinal* symptoms of anorexia, nausea, and emesis associated with acute renal failure increase the likelihood of a catabolic state due to insufficient caloric intake. The more catabolic the individual becomes, the more unexcretable waste products accumulate in the individual's serum, accelerating the uremic state.

The *gastrointestinal bleeding* that occurs due to

TABLE 36-3   **Systemic Manifestations of Acute Renal Failure**

System	Manifestation	Pathophysiological Mechanisms
Vascular	Fluid overload	↓ Excretion
	Electrolyte imbalances	↓ Excretion
	Metabolic acidosis	↓ Hydrogen ion secretion
		↓ Sodium ion reabsorption
		↓ Bicarbonate ion reabsorption and generation
		↓ Excretion of phosphate salts or titratable acids
		↓ Ammonia synthesis and ammonium excretion
	Hypertension	Fluid overload
		↑ Sodium retention
		Inappropriate activation of the renin–angiotensin system
Cardiac	Congestive heart failure	Fluid overload
		Hypertension
	Dysrhythmias	Electrolyte imbalances, especially hyperkalemia, hypocalcemia, and variations in sodium
	Pericarditis (seen more frequently in patients with chronic renal failure)	Uremic toxins
		↑ Pericardial membrane permeability
	Peripheral or systemic edema	Fluid overload and ↑ hydrostatic pressure (an associated ↓ osmotic pressure ↑ the degree of edema)
		Right ventricular dysfunction
Hematopoietic	Anemia	↓ Erythropoietin secretion
		Loss of red blood cells through the GI tract, mucous membranes, or dialysis
		↓ Red blood cell survival time due to uremic toxins
		Burr cells are produced by a hypertonic serum due to uremic toxins
		Uremic toxins interfere with folic acid action
	Alterations in coagulation	Platelet dysfunction due to uremic toxins
		Hypocalcemia could contribute but rarely does because of the metabolic acidosis
	↑ Susceptibility to infection	↓ Neutrophil phagocytosis and chemotaxis due to uremic toxins
Respiratory	Pulmonary edema	Fluid overload
		↑ Pulmonary capillary permeability
		Left ventricular dysfunction
	Pneumonia or pneumonitis	Thick, tenacious oral secretions due to ↓ fluid intake
		A weakness, lethargy, and depressed cough reflex due to uremia
		↑ Pulmonary macrophage activity
		Fluid overload
	Kussmaul respirations	↑ Rate and depth of respirations to ↓ CO_2 in the body and compensate for the metabolic acidosis
Gastrointestinal	Anorexia, nausea, and emesis	Uremic toxins
		Decomposition of urea in the GI tract releasing ammonia that irritates the mucosa
	Stomatitis and uremic halitosis	Uremic toxins
		Decomposition of urea in the oral cavity releasing ammonia
	Gastritis and bleeding	Uremic toxins
		Decomposition of urea in the GI tract releasing ammonia that irritates the GI mucosa producing small ulcerations
		↑ Capillary fragility
	Bowel problems	Uremic toxins
	Diarrhea	Hypermotility due to electrolyte imbalances, especially hyperkalemia
	Constipation	Hypomotility due to electrolyte imbalances, ↓ fluid intake, ↓ activity, and ↓ bulk in the diet

From Schoengrund, L., & Balzer, P. (1985). *Renal problems in critical care.* New York: Wiley.

TABLE 36-3   **Systemic Manifestations of Acute Renal Failure—cont'd**

System	Manifestation	Pathophysiological Mechanisms
Neuromuscular	Drowsiness, confusion, coma, and irritability	Uremic toxins produce a uremic encephalopathy
		Metabolic acidosis
		Electrolyte imbalances
	Tremors, twitching, and convulsions	Uremic toxins produce a uremic encephalopathy
	Peripheral neuropathy (Stages 2 and 3 are rare in patients with acute renal failure)	↓ Nerve conduction, both motor and sensory, due to uremic toxins
	Stage 1: Restless leg syndrome and paresthesias	
	Stage 2: Motor involvement leading to footdrop	
	Stage 3: Paraplegia	
Psychosocial	↓ Mentation, ↓ concentration, and altered perceptions (even to the point of frank psychoses)	Uremic toxins produce a uremic encephalopathy
		Electrolyte imbalances
		Metabolic acidosis
		Tendency to develop cerebral edema
Integumentary	Pallor	Uremic anemia
	Yellowness	Retained urochrome pigment is excreted through the skin
	Dryness	↓ Secretions from oil and sweat glands due to uremic toxins
	Pruritic	Dry skin
		Calcium and/or phosphate deposits in the skin
		Effects of uremic toxins on nerve endings
	Purpura and ecchymoses	↑ Capillary fragility
		Platelet dysfunction
	Uremic frost (seen only in terminal or severely critically ill patients)	Urea or urate crystals are excreted through the skin
Endocrine	Glucose intolerance (usually not clinically significant)	Peripheral insensitivity to insulin due to uremia
		Prolonged insulin half-life due to ↓ renal metabolism
Skeletal	Hypocalcemia	Hyperphosphatemia due to ↓ renal excretion
		↓ GI reabsorption due to ↓ renal conversion of vitamin D
	Osteodystrophy	↑ Osteoclastic activity in response to an ↑ secretion of PTH
	Soft tissue calcification	Deposition of calcium phosphate crystals in soft tissue and other structures
Reproductive	Infertility	↓ Sperm production and ↓ ovulation due to uremia
	↓ Libido	A combination of the pathophysiological and psychological effects of uremia

uremia is an oozing of blood rather than a full-blown hemorrhagic state. Bleeding can progress to the hemorrhagic level, but in most individuals it remains as a continuous small loss of blood. Thus, its significance clinically is not in its contribution to anemia but instead in its ability to accelerate the uremic process. As the gastrointestinal bleeding continues, some of the blood is reabsorbed and metabolized by the body. Because blood is a protein, its metabolism further increases the amount of unexcretable nitrogenous waste products in the body and enhances the individual's already uremic state.

Uremic individuals experience clinically significant alterations in their *mental processes.* They often respond more slowly to questions and directives, tend to have difficulty remembering the instructional components of their care, and may view invasive procedures as threatening.

The yellow coloration seen in the *skin* of uremic individuals is due to the retention of urochrome pigment and its excretion through the skin. Urochrome pigment normally gives urine its yellow color. When the individual is not excreting much urine, the pigment accumulates and seeks other excretory pathways. Uremic yellowness differs from the yellowness that accompanies hepatic dysfunction (jaundice) in two ways: it is less brilliant, and it does not affect the sclerae of the eyes.

CLINICAL ASSESSMENT

The clinical assessment of the individual with acute renal failure is a systematic process that follows the same format and includes the same components used in assessing any critically ill patient. The specific components of the assessment process as it relates to an individual experiencing acute renal failure are detailed in Chapter 35, Renal Data Acquisition. This discussion will focus only on the differential diagnosis of prerenal oliguria and intrarenal acute renal failure.

Clinically it is important to distinguish between prerenal oliguria and intrarenal acute renal failure. The therapeutic interventions for these two altered renal states differ markedly, and, thus, they are not interchangeable. Table 36-4 displays the parameters used by clinicians to differentiate between prerenal oliguria and intrarenal acute renal failure.

Of the parameters in the table, the urine sodium is most frequently used by clinicians. This measurement has great practical value. In prerenal or hypoperfusion states, the kidneys respond to the influence of aldosterone and ADH by maximally conserving or reabsorbing sodium and water. Thus, a small amount of very concentrated urine with a high specific gravity, high osmolality, and low sodium is excreted. Although sodium is maximally reabsorbed, the urine remains concentrated due to the presence of urea and other solutes. In instances of intrarenal acute renal failure, however, the damage to the tubular cells is such that dysfunction occurs and substances cannot be appropriately reabsorbed. The result is a small amount of urine with a fixed specific gravity and osmolality that is similar to that of the plasma and a higher than normal sodium concentration.

Two other values in Table 36-4 are frequently used to differentiate between prerenal oliguria and intrarenal acute renal failure: the fractional excretion of sodium and the renal failure index (RFI). These two values offer more precise quantifications of tubular function than do the other suggested measurements. The fractional excretion of sodium (FE_{Na}) is the percentage of filtered sodium that actually appears in the urine. The value for this parameter is calculated using the following formula:

$$FE_{Na}\% = (U_{Na}/P_{Na})/(U_{Cr}/P_{Cr}) \times 100$$

Using this formula, the percentage of fractional sodium that is excreted is determined by dividing the urine sodium by the plasma sodium and further dividing that number by the quotient derived from dividing the urine creatinine by the plasma creatinine. The resulting number is then multiplied by 100 to convert it to a percentage. A value for FE_{Na} of less than 1% is consistent with a prerenal or hypoperfusion state, while a value greater than 1% indicates intrarenal acute renal failure. In normal individuals, the value is also less than 1%.

The renal failure index (RFI) is a derivative of the formula for the fractional excretion of sodium. It expresses the urinary sodium concentration as a function of the ratio of the urine/plasma creatinine concentration using the following formula:

$$RFI\% = U_{Na}/(U_{Cr}/P_{Cr}) \times 100$$

In other words, the RFI is a percentage that is determined by dividing the urine sodium by the quotient of the urine creatinine divided by the plasma creati-

TABLE 36-4   **Differential Assessment Parameters for Prerenal Oliguria and Intrarenal Acute Renal Failure**

Clinical Parameter	Prerenal Oliguria	Intrarenal Acute Renal Failure
Creatinine clearance	15-80 ml/min	<5 ml/min
Urine volume	>400 ml/24 hr	<400 ml/24 hr *or* >400 ml/24 hr
Urine sodium	<20 mEq/L	>30 mEq/L
Urine specific gravity	>1.015	1.010
Urine osmolality	>500 mosm/kg H_2O	<350 mosm/kg H_2O
Urine sediment	Normal with minimal casts	Cellular debris, various types of casts
Serum BUN to creatinine ratio	>10	10
Urine to serum creatinine ratio	>20	<20
Urine to serum osmolality ratio	>1.2	<1.2
Fractional excretion of sodium	<1%	>1%
Renal failure index	<1%	>1%

nine and multiplying that value by 100. An RFI of less than 1% is consistent with a prerenal or hypoperfusion state, while a value greater than 1% indicates intrarenal acute renal failure.

Therapeutically, the value of differentiating between these two clinical entities is essential. For example, in prerenal or hypoperfusion states, the aim is to correct the underlying volume depletion. Because there is no intrarenal renal damage, the kidney usually responds well to the therapeutic intervention of volume replenishment, and urine output and serum chemistry values fairly rapidly return to normal. However, in cases of intrarenal acute renal failure, volume replenishment is usually not indicated. Instead, therapeutic interventions must focus on correcting the alterations that were produced by the inability of the dysfunctional kidneys to maintain a homeostatic internal environment.

NURSING MANAGEMENT

In providing care for an individual experiencing acute renal failure, the critical care nurse functions as a collaborative member of a multidisciplinary health care team. The patient will require many kinds of assistance throughout the course of the disease. The box below lists some of the nursing diagnoses that are likely to be identified for the patient in acute renal failure. The list is not all encompassing, nor is

it sufficiently specific to be applied to any individual patient. Instead, it presents an overview of the problems the critical care nurse may encounter in caring for a patient experiencing acute renal failure. It is obvious from the length of this beginning list of diagnoses that priorities for care must be established. Thus, this discussion focuses on the seven nursing diagnoses that appear to be most important for sustaining the patient during this very vulnerable period. A basic plan of care using the seven priority nursing diagnoses is presented below. The nursing interventions include independent, interdependent, and dependent functions without differentiation. Monitoring and intervening functions are presented separately. The *monitoring functions* assist the clinician in collecting additional data for use in the ongoing assessment process. Monitoring functions can assist in defining problems, but they do not alter an individual's state. *Intervening functions*, when implemented by the clinician, should lead to a change in the individual's clinical state.

■ NURSING DIAGNOSIS

Fluid volume deficit or excess and altered electrolyte and acid–base balance, related to renal dysfunction.

OUTCOME STANDARD AND CRITERIA

Fluid, electrolyte, and acid–base balance is maintained or reestablished as evidenced by:

Nursing Diagnoses Related to Acute Renal Failure

Anxiety/fear, related to the disease process, therapeutic interventions, and uncertainty of the prognosis

Alterations in bowel elimination: diarrhea or constipation, related to fluid and electrolyte imbalances, dietary and fluid restrictions, and decreased activity

Alterations in breathing patterns, related to fluid, electrolyte, acid–base imbalances, and uremic toxins

Alterations in cardiac output: decreased, related to fluid, electrolyte, and acid–base imbalances, dysrhythmias, uremic pericarditis, and pericardial effusion

Alterations in comfort: pain, related to the effects of uremic toxins on peripheral sensory nerves

Alterations in comfort: nausea and vomiting, related to the effects of uremic toxins on the stomach

Alterations in comfort: pruritus, related to the uremic toxins and the deposition of calcium phosphate crystals in the skin

Alterations in electrolyte and acid–base balance, related to renal dysfunction

Ineffective family coping, related to the critically ill state of the family member, the disease process, the uncertain prognosis, and the therapeutic interventions

Fatigue, related to the anemia resulting from a deficient production of erythropoietin and the effects of fluid, electrolyte, and acid–base imbalances

Fluid volume deficit, related to fluid loss during diuresis or dialysis

Fluid volume excess, related to fluid retention during the oliguric–anuric phase

Ineffective individual coping, related to the overwhelming disease process

Potential for infection, related to altered immune processes, uremic toxins, and invasive lines and procedures

Potential for injury, related to platelet dysfunction due to uremic toxins

Knowledge deficit regarding the course of the disease, the therapeutic regimen, and the prognosis

Alterations in nutrition: less than body requirements, related to dietary restrictions and an altered metabolic state

Alterations in oral mucous membranes, related to the effects of the uremic toxins

Sensory/perceptual alterations, related to the effects of the uremic toxins on the central nervous system

Impaired skin integrity, related to the effect of uremic toxins

Alterations in thought processes, related to the effect of uremic toxins on the central nervous system

- A balanced fluid intake and output, minus insensible loss
- A body weight within 2 lb of the individual's dry weight
- Stable vital signs within the normal range, or consistent with the individual's baseline values
- A central venous pressure reading of between 5 and 8 cmH$_2$O
- Normal skin moisture, turgor, texture, and elasticity
- Normally hydrated oral mucous membranes
- Normal muscle strength
- Normal bowel sounds and fecal excretory patterns
- Negative Chvostek's and Trousseau's signs
- An intact skeletal system
- Serum laboratory values within the normal ranges for the individual
- Arterial blood gas values within the normal parameters for the individual

NURSING INTERVENTIONS

Monitoring Functions

- Monitor intake and output patterns at least every 4 hours.
- Monitor weight daily.
- Monitor serum laboratory values, especially BUN, creatinine, and potassium, at least daily.
- Monitor arterial blood gas values as dictated by patient's clinical state.
- Monitor urinary laboratory values at least daily during the diuretic phase.
- Monitor vital signs at least every 2 hours.
- Perform a complete cardiovascular assessment at least every 8 hours.
- Assess apical and peripheral pulse differences to monitor for dysrhythmias at least every 2 hours.
- Perform a complete respiratory assessment at least every 8 hours.
- Perform a complete neurological assessment at least every 8 hours.
- Monitor for clinical signs of cerebral edema at least every 4 hours.
- Monitor Chvostek's and Trousseau's signs at least daily.
- Monitor the characteristics and constituents of the urine, especially color, odor, pH, specific gravity, protein, and glucose, at least daily.

Intervening Functions

- Maintain all prescribed fluid and electrolyte restrictions, usually very similar to those displayed in Table 36-5.
- Administer all prescribed fluids and pharmacological agents precisely, particularly those used to treat hyperkalemia as suggested in Table 36-6.
- Institute seizure precautions.
- Administer any necessary blood transfusions prior

TABLE 36-5 Daily Dietary Requirements and Restrictions in Acute Renal Failure

Dietary Component	Recommended Daily Amount
Water	400-600 ml plus the urine output
Calories	35-50 kcal/kg
Protein	0.5-1.5 g/kg
Sodium	500-1,000 mg
Potassium	20-50 mEq
Phosphate	700 mg or less
Calcium	800-1,200 mg
Carbohydrate	Unrestricted
Fats	Variable

Daily water-soluble vitamin supplements will also be required.
From Hartshorn, J., Lamborn, M., & Noll, M. L. (Eds.). (1992). *Introduction to critical care nursing.* Philadelphia: Saunders.

to or during dialysis if possible.
- Prepare the patient for dialysis or institute hemofiltration as prescribed.

■ **NURSING DIAGNOSIS**

Decreased cardiac output, related to alterations in preload, afterload, contractility, or heart rate/rhythm.

OUTCOME STANDARD AND CRITERIA

Adequate cardiac output is maintained as evidenced by:

- Stable vital signs within the appropriate range for the individual
- Normal skin color, texture, turgor, and temperature
- A relaxed, sedate body posture and behavior
- A cardiac rhythm and rate that is consistent with the individual's fluid and electrolyte status

NURSING INTERVENTIONS

Monitoring Functions

- Assess apical pulses at least every 4 hours to detect dysrhythmia.
- Perform a total cardiovascular assessment at least every 8 hours.
- Monitor fluid balance at least every 2 hours.
- Monitor electrolyte balance at least daily.

Intervening Functions

- Maintain all prescribed fluid and electrolyte restrictions.
- Administer all prescribed fluids and pharmacological agents precisely.
- Prepare the patient for dialysis or institute hemofiltration as prescribed.

■ **NURSING DIAGNOSIS**

High risk for infection, related to compromised immune processes.

OUTCOME STANDARD AND CRITERIA

Infection is absent as evidenced by:

- Stable vital signs that are consistent with the base-

TABLE 36-6   Treatment Approaches for Hyperkalemia

Approach	Methods	Efficacy
Reduce the body potassium content	↓ Potassium intake	May ↓ plasma and total body potassium content over time
	↑ Fecal excretion of potassium using cation exchange resins such as Kayexelate	Takes hours to be effective but will eventually ↓ both plasma and total body potassium content
	↑ Renal excretion of potassium by using mineralocorticoid agents, ↑ salt intake, or using diuretic agents	Any of these would be effective in ↓ both plasma and total body potassium content if the individual has normal renal function
	Dialysis	↓ Plasma and total body potassium content within 4 to 6 hours
Shift the potassium intracellularly	Administer glucose and insulin intravenously	↓ Plasma potassium for about 2 hours, but has no effect on total body potassium content
	Administer an alkali such as sodium bicarbonate	↓ Plasma potassium for a short time but has no effect on total body potassium content
Antagonize the cellular membrane effect	Administer calcium salts	Has no effect on either plasma or total body potassium content
	Administer hypertonic sodium salts	Has no effect on either plasma or total body potassium content

From Hartshorn, J., Lamborn, M., & Noll, M. L. (Eds.). (1992). *Introduction to critical care nursing*. Philadelphia: Saunders.

line values for the individual, especially body temperature
- An activity level that is consistent with the individual's usual expenditure of energy
- Either a normal, intact integumentary system, or normal coloration, turgor, texture, temperature, and odor, and decreasing size of any interruptions in the integument
- Cognitive clarity and responsiveness that is consistent with the individual's baseline
- Normal breath sounds upon auscultating the lungs
- A chest x-ray that reveals no consolidation or infiltration
- A micturition pattern that is consistent with the individual's baseline
- Negative culture results for all body secretions and wound areas
- A white blood cell count and differential that is consistent with the individual's baseline

NURSING INTERVENTIONS
Monitoring Functions
- Assess the environment, visitors, and personnel who care for the individual to decrease the possible cross contamination that can occur.
- Assess all interruptions in the integument at least every 8 hours.
- Monitor all vital signs at least every 4 hours.
- Auscultate breath sounds at least every 4 hours.
- Assess cognitive clarity at least every 2 hours.

- Monitor the results of all laboratory and diagnostic tests at least daily.
Intervening Functions
- Avoid invasive instrumentation and manipulation whenever possible.
- Implement positive preventive pulmonary maintenance therapies, such as turning, coughing, deep breathing, incentive inspirometry, and suctioning at least every 2 hours.
- Maintain an anabolic state by providing or administering the appropriate nutrients and calories, consistent with the restrictions prescribed.
- Administer nutritional supplements, such as vitamins, as prescribed.

■ NURSING DIAGNOSIS
Altered nutrition, related to gastrointestinal manifestations of acute renal failure.

OUTCOME STANDARD AND CRITERIA
Nutritional intake meets metabolic requirements as evidenced by:
- A dry body weight (clinically defined as that weight below which the signs and symptoms of hypotension occur) that is consistent with the individual's age, height, and body frame size
- A caloric intake that is appropriate for the individual's age, height, weight, body frame size, energy expenditure and pathophysiological state, usually in excess of 2,500 calories to prevent additional catabolism

- Anthropometric measurements that are consistent with the individual's physical stature, such as mid-arm circumference of greater than 26.3 cm, a mid-arm muscle circumference of greater than 22.8 cm, and a triceps skin fold of greater than 11.3 mm
- Integument, hair, nails and mucous membranes that are consistent with the individual's pathophysiological state in terms of turgor, texture, intactness, and degree of hydration
- Energy level that is consistent with the individual's pathophysiological state
- Cognitive clarity that is consistent with the individual's pathophysiological state
- Serum laboratory values that are either normal or consistent with the individual's pathophysiological state
- Other serum laboratory values that are either consistent with the individual's pathophysiological state, or within the following ranges:

  Total protein: 6-8 g/dl
  Albumin: 3.5-5.5 g/dl
  Transferrin: 205-375 mg/dl
  Triglycerides: 40-150 mg/dl
  Cholesterol: 150-250 mg/dl
  Iron: 75-175 mg/dl
  Vitamin B_{12}: 180-1,000 pg/dl
  Folic acid: 1.8-9 ng/dl

NURSING INTERVENTIONS
Monitoring Functions

- Monitor body weight and caloric intake at least daily.
- Obtain anthropometric measurements at least weekly.
- Monitor the integument, hair, nails, and mucous membranes at least daily.
- Assess activity and energy level at least daily.
- Assess cognitive clarity at least every 4 hours.
- Monitor the serum laboratory values at least daily.
  Intervening Functions
- Provide an oral or enteral diet that contains the essential nutrients but maintains the prescribed restrictions.
- Assist with oral hygiene 10 minutes before the ingestion of food.
- Remove all noxious stimuli from the individual's environment.
- Provide at least 30 minutes of rest time before the ingestion of food.
- Provide small, frequent feedings at times the patient has selected for ingestion.
- Structure the time of food ingestion to be a social event by inviting family members or others to join the patient.
- Establish competitive goals for the patient to achieve regarding the ingestion of food.
- Administer pharmacological agents, vitamin supplements, and nutritional supplements as prescribed.
- Administer hyperalimentation precisely as prescribed.

■ **NURSING DIAGNOSIS**

High risk for impaired skin integrity, related to integumentary manifestations of acute renal failure.

OUTCOME STANDARD AND CRITERIA

Skin is intact, or integrity is improved as evidenced by:

- An intact integument that has the color, odor, texture, turgor, temperature, elasticity, and degree of moistness that is consistent with the patient's pathophysiological state
- Verbalizations by the patient regarding the status of the integument

NURSING INTERVENTIONS
Monitoring Functions

- Assess the skin at least daily.
- Monitor fluid and nutritional intake at least daily.
  Intervening Functions
- Assist the patient in bathing at least daily using a nonirritating, nondrying, non-lanolin-based substance, such as an oil- or oatmeal-based substance, or sodium bicarbonate bath water.
- Apply nonlanolin, light-oil-based lubricating lotions at least every 4 hours to decrease pruritus.
- Trim the patient's nails at least weekly to prevent abrasions or infection due to scratching.
- Provide additional perineal care twice a day using a mild cleansing agent and water.
- Implement an hourly turning or movement schedule.
- Perform active (or assist the patient in performing passive) range of motion activities at least every 4 hours.
- Implement adjunct therapies such as a foam or other special type of mattress, protective padding, sheepskin pads, and massage to assist in decreasing pressure and friction at various points on the integument.
- Handle and manipulate all edematous tissues gently and carefully.
- Administer pharmacological agents as prescribed to assist in controlling pruritus.
- Provide fluids and nutritional substances that are consistent with the prescribed restrictions.
- Prepare the individual for dialysis as prescribed.

■ **NURSING DIAGNOSIS**

Altered thought processes, related to neuromuscular manifestations of acute renal failure.

OUTCOME STANDARD AND CRITERIA

Effective cognition is maintained or restored as evidenced by:

- Verbal demonstration of the individual's orientation to person, place, and time

- Appropriate eye contact during interactions
- Clear, coherent, logical, appropriately paced communication patterns
- Affect, mannerisms, and gestures that are consistent with the individual's baseline and/or pathophysiological state and appropriate for the interaction
- Levels of concentration and participation that are consistent with the individual's pathophysiological state
- Verbal responses or questions that are indicative of an understanding of the content of the interaction
- Participation in activities that directly relate to the content of the interaction
- Serum laboratory values that are consistent with the individual's pathophysiological state

NURSING INTERVENTIONS

Monitoring Functions

- Assess level of orientation at least every 4 hours.
- Assess eye contact, communication patterns, gestures, mannerisms, level of concentration, and degree of participation during each interaction.
- Assess verbal responses and questions during each interaction.
- Monitor activities after each interaction.
- Monitor serum laboratory values at least daily.

Intervening Functions

- Establish a therapeutic rapport with the patient.
- Structure the interactions so that they are brief and focused.
- Use repetition to reinforce key points during the interaction.
- Assist the patient in differentiating the types of stimuli that are encountered during the interaction.
- Prepare the patient for dialysis as prescribed.

■ NURSING DIAGNOSIS

Knowledge deficit, related to incomplete information about illness and therapy.

OUTCOME STANDARD AND CRITERIA

The individual is an informed participant in the health care process as evidenced by:

- Appropriate verbalizations and questions regarding the disease process and the health care regimen
- Cooperation with and participation in the health care regimen

NURSING INTERVENTIONS

Monitoring Functions

- Assess the content of the patient's verbalizations and questions at least daily.
- Monitor the degree of cooperation and participation in the health care regimen.

Intervening Functions

- Provide specific, factual information about the pathophysiological disease process, its impact on the individual, its progression and prognosis, and its prescribed therapeutic regimen.
- Reinforce verbally or in writing the information

that is provided as appropriate, or at least daily.
- Include family members in the educational process so that they are also aware of the facts and can reinforce the information with the patient.
- If appropriate, arrange for a former patient who has experienced acute renal failure to talk with the individual.

MEDICAL MANAGEMENT

The therapeutic management strategies employed when caring for a critically ill patient experiencing acute renal failure are designed to meet eight general goals:

1. To correct the primary disorder causing the renal dysfunction, if possible
2. To prevent infection
3. To treat fluid imbalances
4. To treat electrolyte imbalances
5. To treat acid–base imbalances
6. To maintain the patient in an anabolic state
7. To treat any symptomatic anemia
8. To treat the systemic uremic symptoms

In general, a "three-D" approach is used to meet these goals, including the components of *d*ietary (nutrition) management, *d*iuretic therapy, and *d*ialysis therapy. These components are usually instituted aggressively and early in the course of the disease process.

Dietary Management

The general goals of dietary management are to minimize uremic toxicity, minimize fluid and electrolyte imbalances, and maintain adequate nutrition and an anabolic state. The importance of this strategy should not be underestimated. Critically ill patients with acute renal failure who have a positive caloric balance have a much higher survival rate than those with a negative balance. These findings are substantiated by the known sequence in which an inadequate caloric intake leads to increased protein catabolism and thereby accelerates the formation and accumulation of uremic toxins. In addition, catabolic processes are enhanced in renal failure because the average metabolic rate for individuals in this state is about 20% greater than normal. Also, dialysis therapy contributes to protein catabolism and further increases the patient's nutritional needs. The loss of amino acids and water soluble vitamins via the dialysate constitutes another mechanism for depleting nutritional stores.

The *daily* nutritional requirements for an individual experiencing acute renal failure include:

Caloric intake: 35 to 50 kcal/kg of ideal body weight (IBW)

Protein intake: 0.5 to 1.5 g/kg of IBW, 75% to 80% of which is of high biological value and contains all of the required essential amino acids

Sodium intake: 0.5 to 1 g
Potassium intake: 20 to 50 mEq
Calcium intake: 800 to 1,200 mg
Fluid intake: equal to the volume of the individual's
   urine output, plus an additional 600 to 1,000 ml
In addition, multivitamins, including the vitamin B complex and vitamin C, folic acid, and occasionally an iron supplement might also be prescribed to replace the water-soluble vitamins and other essential elements lost during dialysis.

If the patient is unable to ingest or tolerate an oral nutritional intake that is adequate to maintain an anabolic state, hyperalimentation may be prescribed. Aggressive hyperalimentation therapy will supply nonprotein glucose calories, specific essential amino acids, fluids, specific electrolytes, and essential vitamins sufficient to create a more stable internal environment. Such an internal environment helps to prevent further catabolism, negative nitrogen balance, muscle wasting, and other uremic complications. It also enhances the patient's regenerating capacity of the renal tubules and improves resistance to infection and ability to combat other multisystem dysfunctions. To facilitate the aggressive use of hyperalimentation, aggressive, early dialysis therapy is also required.

Diuretic Therapy

The cost/benefit ratio of using diuretic agents in the management of acute renal failure remains controversial. It appears that both osmotic and loop diuretics may be effective in decreasing the initial insult to the renal system *if* they are given promptly at the onset of oliguria. Diuretic therapy is thought to increase renal blood flow, glomerular filtration rate, and intratubular pressure while decreasing the possibility of tubular obstruction and dysfunction. It is possible, however, that diuretics only increase urine volume without affecting glomerular filtration rate or tubular function. This action could easily further compromise the already damaged kidneys. Only the osmotic or loop acting types of diuretics will appreciably increase glomerular filtration rate and renal blood flow. In addition, if the patient has a glomerular filtration rate of less than 20 ml/min, only the loop acting agents and saluretics are likely to induce diuresis.

Dialysis Therapy

Renal replacement therapy is the ultimate supportive and therapeutic measure for managing acute renal failure. Without some form of mechanical substitute for renal function, the patient is unlikely to sustain life during the dysfunctional episode. Thus, dialysis therapy is usually initiated early in the course of the renal failure to maintain the individual's serum creatinine below 10 mg/dl and BUN below 100 mg/ dl. The early institution of dialysis therapy assists in creating an internal biochemical environment that deters the complications associated with uremia. It also increases the range of other therapeutic measures that can be employed to assist the individual in adapting to this major physiological stress. The facets of dialysis therapy that the clinician should be familiar with include vascular access, hemodialysis, and continuous arteriovenous hemofiltration.

Vascular Access

An adequate, easy access to the bloodstream is essential for the implementation of any renal replacement therapy. The access must provide high rates of blood flow for the replacement therapy to be effective. Three mechanisms are used to obtain access to the vascular system for renal replacement therapy: temporary venous catheters, arteriovenous shunts, and arteriovenous fistulas. Temporary catheters and arteriovenous shunts are typically selected because they can be used immediately and are less permanent than the arteriovenous fistula.

A *temporary venous catheter* is usually inserted into either the subclavian, jugular, or femoral vein. The typical temporary access device has either a single or double lumen and is designed to be used only for short-term renal replacement therapy during acute or crisis situations. Examples of such devices are the Hickman, Uldall, Hemocath, and Shaldon catheters.

An *arteriovenous shunt* consists of a surgically implanted extracorporeal apparatus that connects an artery with a vein. Once the apparatus is in place, it can easily be opened or, in some cases, punctured to provide access to the bloodstream. Several types of shunts are currently available, but the most popular seems to be the Quinton-Scribner shunt, which is made of Silastic and Teflon and consists of two lengths of tubing joined by a connector. Each length of tubing has three portions. The first portion is implanted in the vessel and lies beneath the skin; the second portion is a steplike gradation that emerges from the plane of the vessel upward to exit onto the skin through a puncture wound; and the third portion is external and lies flush with the skin. Access to the vascular system is obtained by removing the connector and attaching dialysis tubing directly to the arterial and venous lines of the shunt.

It is important to protect the vascular access site and monitor it at least hourly. In addition, an extremity with an arteriovenous shunt or fistula in place is rarely used for drawing blood specimens or obtaining blood pressure measurements. Such activities could produce pressure changes within the altered vessels that could lead to clotting or rupture. In either case, the loss of the access site could be imminent.

Hemodialysis

Dialysis therapy is based on the principles of osmosis, diffusion, and filtration as they relate to the movement and transport of fluid and electrolytes within the body. *Osmosis* is the movement of fluid or water molecules across a semipermeable membrane from an area of lesser solute concentration to an area of greater concentration until the concentrations of solute are equal on both sides of the membrane. *Diffusion* is the movement of solute molecules across a semipermeable membrane from an area of greater solute *concentration* to an area of lesser solute concentration. Diffusion continues until equilibrium is established across the membrane. *Filtration* is the movement of fluid across a semipermeable membrane from an area of greater *pressure* to an area of lesser pressure.

Osmosis, diffusion, and filtration are influenced by many factors, including the size of the pores of the semipermeable membrane, the size of the solute molecules, the existing osmotic concentrations and pressure gradients, the temperature of the solution, and the rate of blood flow in the body. The size of the pores of the membrane and the size of the solute molecules determine which substances can be transported. Concentration and pressure gradients determine the extent to which transport processes can occur. The gradients are sustained by the high rate of blood flow in the body. As the blood flows through the body, it continuously replaces the dialyzed blood with undialyzed blood. The undialyzed blood has very high concentrations of solutes, thus maintaining the established gradients. The temperature of the solution influences the velocity of the molecular movement and, thus, affects the transport rate. An increase in the temperature of a solution will increase the rate of the transport processes that occur within the solution.

Hemodialysis is the therapy most frequently used to replace the function of the kidneys during managing acute renal failure. *Hemodialysis* is the separation of solutes by differential diffusion through a celluloid membrane positioned between the individual's blood and the dialysate solution. An additional dimension of hemodialysis is that it is extracorporeal, meaning that it occurs outside the patient's body.

The major advantages of hemodialysis are that it requires only 4 to 6 hours per session, is very efficient, and corrects biochemical disturbances quickly. It has several disadvantages:

Special staff education and training are required to implement the therapy.

Acute fluid and electrolyte imbalances can occur rapidly.

An individual could easily hemorrhage or exsanguinate during the therapy.

There is a risk of contracting hepatitis as a result of the therapy.

The equipment is expensive, and machine availability may be a problem at any specific time.

The potential complications associated with hemodialysis therapy include sepsis or clotting of the shunt, catheter, or fistula; hemorrhage; hypovolemia; acute electrolyte imbalances; air emboli; and disequilibrium syndrome. The contraindications most frequently cited include hemodynamic instability, insufficient blood volume (hypovolemia), an inadequate vascular access site, and the unavailability of the appropriate equipment. At present, hemodialysis is usually employed unless the patient's hemodynamic status is so compromised that flow rates are insufficient for the therapy to be successful. In many intensive care units, however, hemofiltration may be selected for temporary renal replacement, to be followed by hemodialysis when the patient has been stabilized.

Hemofiltration

Continuous arteriovenous hemofiltration (CAVH) is a convective mode of blood cleansing controlled by the patient's hydrostatic pressure, wherein large volumes of fluid exchange account for virtually all solute removal. As a convective mode it is not dependent on concentration or particle size. It may actually mimic the function of the kidney more closely than hemodialysis, but it is much less efficient in removing small molecules.

Among the advantages of CAVH are that it removes solutes gradually, carries a lower risk of hemodynamic instability than hemodialysis, and provides increased flexibility in fluid administration therapy. It also requires only minimal heparinization and can be used to maintain a metabolically stable state. It is relatively inexpensive, and minimal staff education is required to implement the therapy. It appears to be ideal for physiologically unstable patients. The disadvantages of CAVH are that it is not very efficient in removing solutes, the individual must remain in bed during the entire course of therapy, and it requires at least mild anticoagulation.

The potential complications associated with CAVH include: (1) depletion syndrome, which results in the loss of vitamins, amino acids, and other substances; (2) acid–base imbalances; (3) fluid and electrolyte imbalances; (4) hemorrhage due to anticoagulation or disruption of the filter or tubing; (5) infection; (6) rupture or leakage of the filter; (7) clotting in the filter; and (8) loss of the vascular access site. CAVH is contraindicated in patients with a systolic blood pressure lower than 60 mmHg, a hematocrit greater than 45%, or the inability to tolerate high volumes of fluid exchange.

Prevention

The best way to address acute renal failure is to prevent its occurrence. Some measures that will assist in deterring the onset of acute renal failure include:

1. Maintaining an adequate hydration state at all times, but especially preoperatively and prior to excretion urography
2. Maintaining renal perfusion by appropriately administering the prescribed agents, which might include:

   Vasoactive agents that will increase renal blood flow, such as acetylcholine

   Low doses of dopamine, isoproterenol, kinins, prostaglandins, or calcium antagonists

   Volume expanders such as saline and mannitol; and loop acting diuretics

3. Continuously monitoring the duration, dosage, and combinations of antibiotics administered to the patient
4. Maintaining a continuous assessment of the patient's renal function

When preventive measures are aggressively implemented, the individual has an enhanced chance of eluding acute renal failure with all of its concomitant impact. Unfortunately, priorities of care may require the deferral of such measures, in which case acute renal failure may ensue, increasing the complexity of the patient's therapeutic management.

BIBLIOGRAPHY

Baer, C. L. (1990). Acute renal failure. *Nursing 90, 20*(6), 34-39.

Baer, C. L. (1992). Acute renal failure. In J. C. Hartshorn, M. Lamborn, & M. Noll (Eds.), *Introduction to critical care*. Philadelphia: Saunders.

Baer, C. L., & Lancaster, L. E. (1992). Acute renal failure. *Critical Care Nursing Quarterly, 14*(4), 1-21.

Bennett, W. M. (1983). Management of acute renal failure in sepsis—clinical considerations. *Circulatory Shock, 11*(3), 261-267.

Bergstrom, J. (1989). Toxicity of uremia: Physiopathology and clinical signs. *Contributions to Nephrology, 71*, 1-9.

Brenner, B. M., Coe, F. L., & Rector, F. C. (1987). *Clinical nephrology*. Philadelphia: Saunders.

Brenner, B. M., & Lazarus, J. M. (1988). *Acute renal failure* (2nd ed.). New York: Churchill Livingstone.

Burke, T. J., Burnier, M., Langberg, H., et al. (1986). Renal response to shock. *Annals of Emergency Medicine, 15*, 1397-1400.

Burke, T. J., & Schrier, R. W. (1983). Ischemic acute renal failure—pathogenetic steps leading to acute tubular necrosis. *Circulatory Shock, 11*(3), 255-259.

Butt, K. M. H. (1983). Angioaccess. In W. Drukker, F. M. Parsons, & J. F. Maher (Eds.), *Replacement of renal function by dialysis* (2nd ed.) (pp. 171-185). Boston: Martinus Nijhoff.

Collins, A. J., Keshaviah, P., Ilstrup, K. M., et al. Clinical comparison of hemodialysis and hemofiltration. *Kidney International, 28*(S17), S18-S22.

Eknoyan, G., & Knochel, J. P. (1984). *The systemic consequences of renal failure*. Orlando, FL: Grune & Stratton.

Finn, W. F. (1990). Diagnosis and management of acute tubular necrosis. *Medical Clinics of North America, 74*(4), 873-891.

Goldstein, M. S. (1983). Acute renal failure. *Medical Clinics of North America, 67*(6), 1325-1341.

Golper, T. A. (1985). Continuous arteriovenous hemofiltration in acute renal failure. *American Journal of Kidney Diseases, 6*(6), 373-386.

Harper, J. (1990). Rhabdomyolysis and myoglobinuric renal failure. *Critical Care Nurse, 10*(3), 32-34, 36.

Irwin, B. C. (1979). Hemodialysis means vascular access and the right kind of nursing care. *Nursing 79, 9*(10), 48-53.

Kramer, P. (1985). *Arteriovenous hemofiltration*. Berlin: Springer-Verlag.

Lancaster, L. E. (1984). *The patient with end stage renal disease* (2nd ed.). New York: Wiley.

Lancaster, L. E., & Baer, C. L. (1985). The pathophysiology of acute renal dysfunction. In L. Schoengrund, & P. Balzer (Eds.), *Renal problems in critical care* (pp. 21-46). New York: Wiley.

Lawyer, L. A., & Velasco, A. (1989). Continuous arteriovenous hemodialysis in the ICU. *Critical Care Nurse, 9*(1), 29-32, 34-35, 38-41.

Maher, J. F. (Ed.). (1989). *Replacement of renal function by dialysis* (3rd ed.). Kluwer Academic Publishers.

Mandal, A. K., Lightfoot, B. O., & Treat, R. C. (1983). Mechanisms of protection in acute renal failure. *Circulatory Shock, 11*(3), 245-253.

Mitch, W. E., & Klahr, S. (1988). *Nutrition and the kidney*. Boston: Little, Brown.

Nahman, N. S., & Middendorf, D. F. (1990). Continuous arteriovenous hemofiltration. *Medical Clinics of North America, 74*(4), 975-983.

Norris, M. K. G. (1989). Acute tubular necrosis: Preventing complications. *Dimensions of Critical Care Nursing, 8*(1), 16-26.

Paradiso, C. (1989). Hemofiltration: An alternative to dialysis. *Heart Lung, 18*(3), 282-290.

Porush, J. G. (1986). New concepts in acute renal failure. *American Family Physician, 33*(3), 109-118.

Price, C. A. (1989). Continuous arteriovenous ultrafiltration: A monitoring guide for ICU nurses. *Critical Care Nurse, 9*(1), 12-14, 17-19.

Ronco, C., Brendola A., Bragantini, L., et al. (1985). Continuous arteriovenous hemofiltration. *Contributions to Nephrology, 48*, 70-88.

Schoengrund, L. (1985). Nursing management of the patient with acute renal failure. In L. Schoengrund, & P. Balzer (Eds.), *Renal problems in critical care* (pp. 47-67). New York: Wiley.

Schrier, R. W. (1992). *Renal and electrolyte disorders* (4th ed.). Boston: Little, Brown.

Strupp, T. W. (1988). Postshock resuscitation of the trauma victim: Preventing and managing acute renal failure. *Critical Care Nursing Quarterly, 11*(2), 1-9.

Thurau, K. (1983). Pathophysiology of the acutely failing kidney. *Clinical Experience in Dialysis and Apheresis, 7*(1,2), 9-24.

Waltzer, W. C., & Rapaport, F. T. (1984). *Angioaccess— principles and practice.* Orlando, FL: Grune & Stratton.

Whittaker, A. A. (1985). Acute renal dysfunction: Assessment of patients at risk. *Focus on Critical Care, 12*(3), 12-17.

Wilkins, R. G., & Faragher, E. B. (1983). Acute renal failure in an intensive care unit: Incidence, prediction, and outcome. *Anaesthesia, 38*(7), 628-634.

Wills, M. R. (1990). Effects of renal failure. *Clinical Biochemistry, 23,* 55-60.

Winkelman, C. (1985). Hemofiltration: A new technique in critical care nursing. *Heart Lung, 14*(3), 265-271.

Wolfson, M. (1987). Nutritional support in acute renal failure. *Dialysis and Transplantation, 16*(9), 493, 496.

PART EIGHT

Endocrine Patient Care Problems

37

Endocrine Anatomy and Physiology

Teresa Choate Loriaux

Functional integrity of the human organism requires that physiological balance be maintained and complex processes be precisely regulated. Many of these processes are controlled by the endocrine system, which regulates growth and development; fluid and electrolyte metabolism; carbohydrate metabolism; reproduction; pregnancy; and lactation. This chapter discusses the structural and functional categories of hormones as well as the mechanisms by which they exert their effects. Its primary focus is on hormones and hormonal mechanisms most relevent to the critical care setting. A list of endocrine glands and their locations is given in Table 37-1.

HORMONES: THE PHYSIOLOGICAL EFFECTORS

Hormones can be classified into four categories based on structure: proteins, amines, iodothyronines, and steroids.[1] The box on p. 907 provides a complete list of the hormones and their chemical classification.

Structural Classification

Proteins

Proteins (polypeptides) can be subdivided into small peptides, peptides, and glycoproteins. Protein hormones are synthesized in the same way as other proteins: transcription, translation, transport, and maturation.[2] When a "signal" peptide (a short amino acid chain) is attached to the peptide hormone, it is referred to as a *preprohormone*. The signal peptide facilitates entry into the endoplasmic reticulum. The signal peptide is then cleaved off and the remaining structure is a *prohormone*. Prohormones are stored in the Golgi apparatus of the cell or secreted into the extracellular fluid where the final chemical modulations take place. Less than 1 hour is required for peptide hormone synthesis and secretion.[3]

Amines

The amines are synthesized from the amino acid tyrosine in nerves and the adrenal medulla. Amine hormones include the catecholamines norepinephrine and epinephrine, dopamine, and melatonin. Norepinephrine is formed from phenylalanine and tyrosine through the actions of enzymes present in adrenergic nerve endings. Epinephrine is synthesized by the methylation of norepinephrine by enzymes found only in the adrenal medulla. Thus, norepinephrine is secreted from adrenergic nerve endings, and both epinephrine and norepinephrine are released from the adrenal medulla.[1]

Iodothyronine

The iodothyronines are thyroxine (T_4) and triiodothyronine (T_3). Dietary iodide is oxidized to iodine in the thyroid follicle and attached to tyrosine by a process known as organification. Monoiodotyrosine (MIT) or diiodotyrosine (DIT) is produced depending on whether one or two molecules are added to the tyrosine. Thyroxine (T_4) is formed when two DIT molecules are coupled, and triiodothyronine (T_3) is formed when a DIT molecule combines with an MIT molecule. The actions of T_4 and T_3 are discussed later in the section on the thyroid gland.

Steroids

All steroid hormones are derived from cholesterol and all have the same cyclopentanoperhydrophenanthrene core. Steroid hormones include the glucocorticoids, mineralocorticoids, androgens, estrogens, and progestins. The adrenal cortex secretes glucocorticoids (cortisol) and mineralocorticoids (aldosterone). The testes and ovaries secrete the androgen testosterone, the estrogen estradiol (E_2), and the progestin progesterone.[2]

TABLE 37-1   **Location and Function of the Endocrine Glands**

Gland	Location	Function
PITUITARY (HYPOPHYSIS)	Cranial cavity sella turcica	
Anterior lobe (adenohypophysis)		Functional integrity and responsiveness of thyroid gland via **TSH**, adrenal cortex via **ACTH**, gonads via **FSH**, **LH**
		Anabolism, growth via **GH**
		Lactogenesis via **prolactin**
Posterior lobe (neurohypophysis)		Milk ejection via **oxytocin**
		Maintenance of free water balance via **ADH**
THYROID	Neck, one lobe on each side of trachea	Control of metabolic rate via T_4, T_3
PARATHYROID (FOUR)	Neck, one in each corner of thyroid gland	Maintenance of serum calcium level via **PTH**
ADRENAL (TWO)	Upper poles of kidneys (retroperitoneal space)	
Adrenal cortex	Zona fasciculata	Production of **glucocorticoids;** enables physiological stress response
	Zona glomerulosa	Production of **mineralocorticoids;** maintenance of extracellular fluid volume via **mineralocorticoids**
	Zona reticularis	Production of adrenal androgens; masculinization via **adrenal androgens**
Adrenal medulla	Interior portion of gland	Augmentation of sympathetic nervous system "fight or flight" response via **catecholamines**
ENDOCRINE PANCREAS (ISLETS OF LANGERHANS)	Abdomen: pancreas	Glucose uptake, energy storage via **insulin**
		Glucose release, energy substrate mobilization via **glucagon**
PINEAL	Cranial cavity (below third ventricle)	Function unclear; secretes **melatonin**
THYMUS	Mediastinum	Development, maturation of T cells via **thymosin**

Mechanisms of Hormone Action

Once secreted, hormones enter the circulation and exert their influence on an organ that contains specific receptors that can bind to the particular hormone involved. There are two kinds of receptors: membrane bound receptors (located on the outside of the cell) and soluble or cytosol receptors (located in the cell interior). The catecholamines and polypepide hormones bind to membrane receptors. The steroid and thyroid hormones bind to cytosol receptors. Cytosol receptors interact with the nucleus directly. Membrane receptors interface with the nucleus by way of a *second messenger*. There are several second messengers, including cyclic AMP (cAMP), cyclic GMP (cGMP), calcium, and phosphoinositol. Each of the second messengers activates one or more intracellular proteins that act directly on the nucleus. Cytosol receptors, often binding with the hormone, bind directly to *regulatory elements* on the genes to modulate gene transcription.[4] The mechanisms of hormone action for membrane bound receptors and cytosol receptors are shown in Figure 37-1.

Regulation and Feedback Mechanisms

Hormones can be released at a relatively constant rate (T_4); in a pulsatile fashion, as are adrenocorticotropic hormone (ACTH), luteinizing hormone (LH), and follicle stimulating hormone (FSH); or according to a particular rhythm (circadian, diurnal). Factors influencing hormone secretion include central nervous system stimuli, other hormones (trophic hormones), and physiological responses such as changes in circulating levels of glucose or electrolytes.[2] Regulation of hormone secretion may involve more than one of these mechanisms. One example is insulin secretion which changes in response to increased glucose, sympathetic nervous system stimulation, and/or cortisol secretion.

Negative feedback provides another regulatory mechanism for certain hormonal secretion. Negative

Classification of Hormones

AMINES
Dopamine
Norepinephrine
Epinephrine
Melatonin

IODOTHYRONINES
Thyroxine (T_4)
Triiodothyronine (T_3)

PEPTIDES
Insulin
Glucagon
Atrial naturetic factor (ANF)
Growth hormone (GH)
Human placental lactogen (HPL)
Prolactin (PRL)
Parathyroid hormone (PTH)
Calcitonin
Adrenocorticotropic hormone (ACTH)
Secretin
Cholecystokinin (CKK)
Gastric-inhibitory (GIP)

SMALL PEPTIDES
Vasopressin
Oxytocin
Melanocyte-stimulating hormone (MSH)
Thyrotropin-releasing hormone (TRH)
Gonadotropin-releasing hormone (GnRH)
Somatostatin (SRIF)
Angiotensins

GLYCOPROTEINS
Follicle-stimulating hormone (FSH)
Luteinizing hormone (LH)
Chorionic gonadotropin (CG)
Thyroid-stimulating hormone (TSH)
Proopiomelanocortin (POMC)

STEROIDS
Estrogens (E_2 and E_3)
Progesterone (P)
Testosterone (T)
Dihydrotestosterone (DHT)
Glucocorticoids
Aldosterone
Cholecalciferol (vitamin D)

Adapted from Jordan, R., & Kohler, P. (1990). Principles of endocrine physiology. In J. Stein (Ed.), *Internal medicine* (3rd ed.). Boston: Little, Brown.

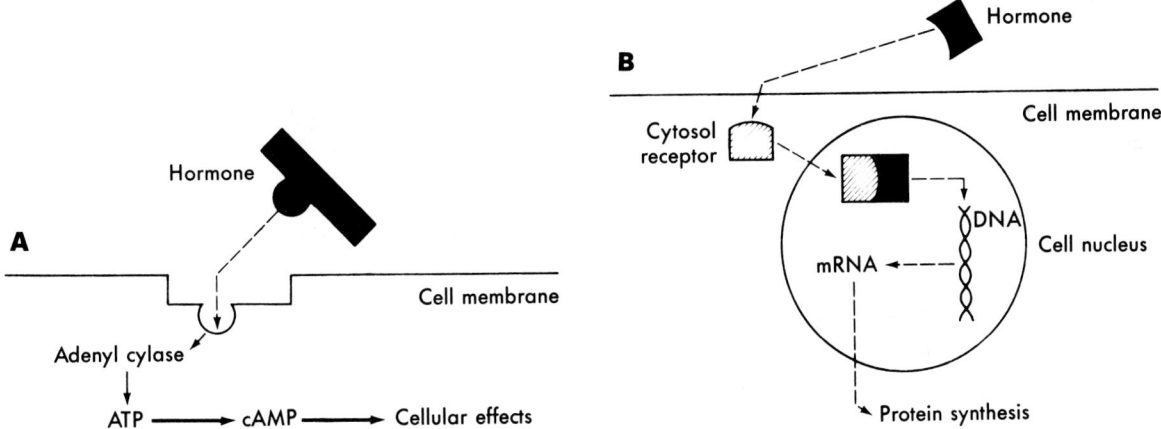

Figure 37-1   The mechanisms of hormone action. *A*, Membrane-bound receptor is on the outside of the cell and requires a "second messenger", cAMP activation. *B*, Cytosol receptors are inside the cell and communicate directly with the nucleus.

feedback occurs when a rise in a hormone's level depresses its own stimulating factor, resulting in decreased hormone production and secretion. Negative feedback is improtant, for example, in regulating the hypothalamus–pituitary–target organ axis.[5]

Functional Categories

The endocrine hormones can be classified as hypothalamic hormones, pituitary hormones, and target gland hormones.

Hypothalamic Hormones

The releasing and inhibiting hormones are synthesized by the hypothalamus. Their only target is the anterior pituitary gland. Six hormones have been identified:

1. Corticotropin-releasing hormone (CRH)
2. Thyrotropin-releasing hormone (TRH)
3. Growth hormone–releasing hormone (GRH)
4. Growth hormone–inhibiting hormone (somatostatin, or SRIF)

5. Prolactin-inhibiting hormone, or PIH
6. Gonadotropin-releasing hormone (GnRH) (dopamine or dopamine-related)

The hormonal relationships between the hypothalamus and anterior pituitary gland are summarized in Figure 37-2.

Pituitary Hormones

The anterior pituitary gland secretes six trophic hormones: adrenocorticotropic hormone (ACTH), thyroid-stimulating hormone (TSH), follicle-stimulating hormone (FSH), luteinizing hormone (LH), growth hormone (GH), and prolactin (PRL). Trophic hormones are necessary for the growth and development of the tissues to which they are targeted: a gland (such as the thyroid by TSH), an organ (such as the breast by PRL), or specific tissues (such as the epiphyses by GH.) Each of the trophic hormones is discussed in the section on the anterior pituitary gland.

Trophic hormone secretion is directly influenced by hypothalamic releasing and inhibiting hormones. Blood levels of target gland hormones also influence trophic hormone secretion. As the blood level of a target gland hormone increases, the secretion rate of the anterior pituitary trophic hormones decreases; thus target gland hormones exert negative feedback upon further trophic hormone release. Negative feedback also operates at the hypothalamic level with regard to the secretion of releasing hormones.

Target Gland Hormones

Target hormones are gland specific in origin; that is, they are secreted by the gland in which their synthesis occurs. Examples of target gland hormones include cortisol, the thyroid hormones T_3 and T_4, antidiuretic hormone (ADH), prolactin, estrogen, and testosterone. Their targets are perfused by the general circulation and are defined by the presence of receptors capable of responding to the particular structure of the hormone.

Control over the secretion of target hormones is complex. The autonomic nervous system directly affects the release of some target hormones (e.g., catecholamines); the hypothalamus indirectly affects others via releasing hormones and the pituitary trophic hormones. Figure 37-3 shows the stimulation, inhibition, and feedback relationships between the hypothalamus, pituitary, and target gland hormones. Specific information about each target hormone can be found in the section discussing the relevant endocrine gland.

ENDOCRINE GLANDS
Hypothalamus

The regulation of the endocrine system is influenced by the central nervous system. The brain communicates with endocrine glands via the hypothalamus, a small area of the brain located beneath the thalamus and surrounding the third ventricle. The hypothalamus and pituitary gland are connected by the pituitary stalk, which is composed of capillaries and neural connections. The hormones produced by the hypothalamus reach the pituitary gland by traveling through the vasculature referred to as the hypophyseal-portal circulation. Figure 37-4 presents a diagram of the anatomical relationship between the hypothalamus and pituitary gland.

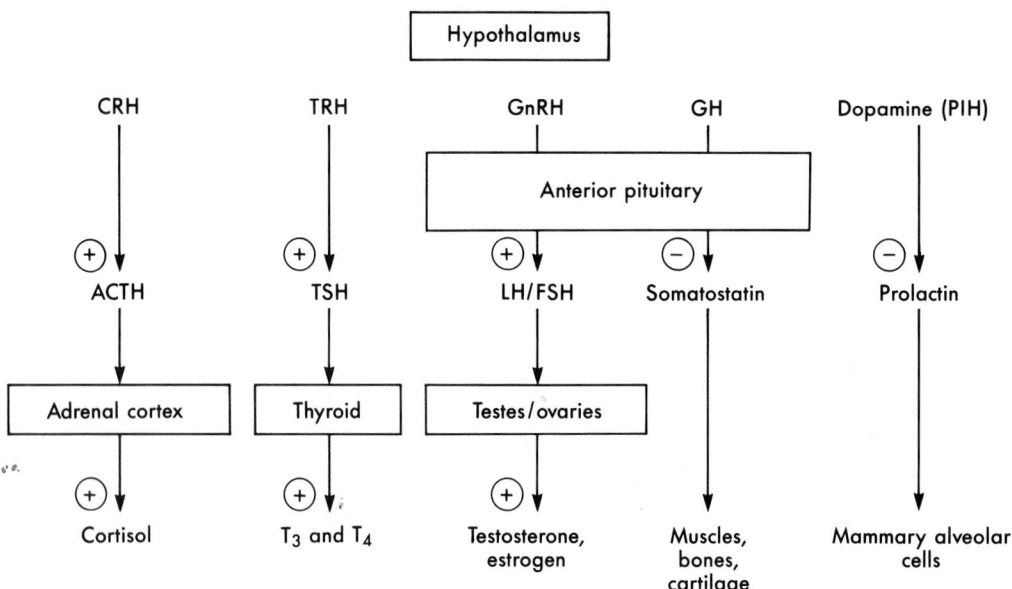

Figure 37-2   Normal relationships between the hypothalamus and anterior pituitary gland. + = stimulation; − = inhibition.

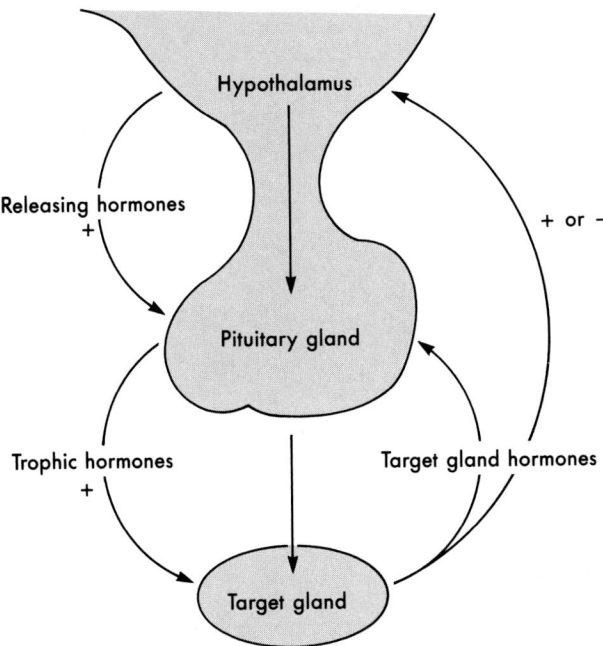

Figure 37-3   Stimulatory and inhibitory feedback relationships between the hypothalamus, pituitary, and target gland hormones. + = stimulating effect; − = inhibiting effect.

The hypothalamus plays a major role in regulating endocrine and autonomic nervous system function. It affects body temperature, sleep, appetite, thirst, blood pressure, gastrointestinal motility, growth, and response to pleasure and pain.[5] This chapter discusses the hypothalamus as it relates to endocrine control.

Anterior Pituitary Gland

The pituitary gland (hypophysis) is a peanut-sized organ located in the sella turcica. The anterior pituitary (or adenohypophysis) is composed of three kinds of granular secretory cells, connective tissue, and a dense vascular network. The vascular network of the anterior pituitary enters the gland as a continuation of the portal capillary network in the pituitary stalk. After extensive winding among the secretory cells, it empties into the general circulation. The dense vasculature of the anterior pituitary provides the anatomical basis for the interaction between the hypothalamus and the anterior pituitary. Not only does it allow the anterior pituitary secretory cells to be bathed in blood that contains releasing and inhibiting hormones from the hypothalamus, but it also allows anterior pituitary hormones to be readily delivered to the general circulation.[6]

The six hormones secreted by the anterior pituitary gland are TSH, ACTH, GH, and PRL, and the gonadotropins LH and FSH.

Thyroid-stimulating hormone supports thyroid gland function and stimulates the release of T_3 and T_4. Without TSH, the thyroid gland atrophies. If excessive TSH is present, enlargement of the gland, or goiter formation, occurs.

Adrenocorticotropic hormone regulates the adrenal cortex. In the absence of ACTH, the adrenal gland atrophies and becomes incapable of synthesizing and secreting adequate quantities of glucocorticoids.

Luteinizing hormone stimulates the testes to secrete testosterone and the ovary to secrete estradiol and progesterone. *Follicle-stimulating hormone* is necessary for granulosa cell growth and development. Granulosa cells nurture the developing egg.

The gonadotropin secretory pattern responds directly to the secretory patern of hypothalamic GnRH; LH and FSH are both secreted in pulses at roughly 90-minute intervals. Steroid "feedback" alters the amplitude and frequency of these pulses, leading to the characteristic pattern of gonadotropin secretion across the reproductive cycle. Estrogen negative feedback is exerted at the level of the pituitary to alter pulse amplitude. Testosterone and progesterone negative feedback is exerted mainly at the level of the hypothalamus to alter pulse frequency.

Prolactin is a lactogenic hormone that stimulates milk production by the mammary alveolar cells. Prior estrogen and progesterone "priming" is necessary for full effect. The secretion of prolactin is suppressed by dopamine from the hypothalamus. Estrogen enhances prolactin secretion through a mechanism not fully understood. The rising estrogen levels of pregnancy cause increased prolactin secretion. By 8 days after parturition, serum prolactin returns to nonpregnant levels. Suckling increases prolactin secretion during this period, but the response progressively declines.

Growth hormone is produced by the anterior pituitary. It acts as an anabolic agent to promote growth and development at the tissue level by acceleration of amino acid transport into cells and stimulation of intracellular protein synthesis. A peptide substance known as *somatomedin, or insulin-like growth factor 1* (IGF-1), appears to mediate many of these effects.[7]

Bones are also affected by growth hormone and, like muscle and cartilage, increase in mass under its influence. Linear growth of long bones occurs at the epiphyseal growth plates. Growth hormone promotes long-bone lengthening until fusion or closure of the epiphyseal plates occurs. This closure marks the termination of puberty.

The secretion of GH, like that of ACTH, follows a diurnal pattern that is determined by a hypothalamic "clock." Growth hormone secretion peaks at night and in association with the onset of non−rapid eye movement (non-REM) sleep.

The interplay between GRH and somatostatin results in wide fluctuation in growth hormone plasma concentrations. Somatostatin, a 14 amino acid poly-

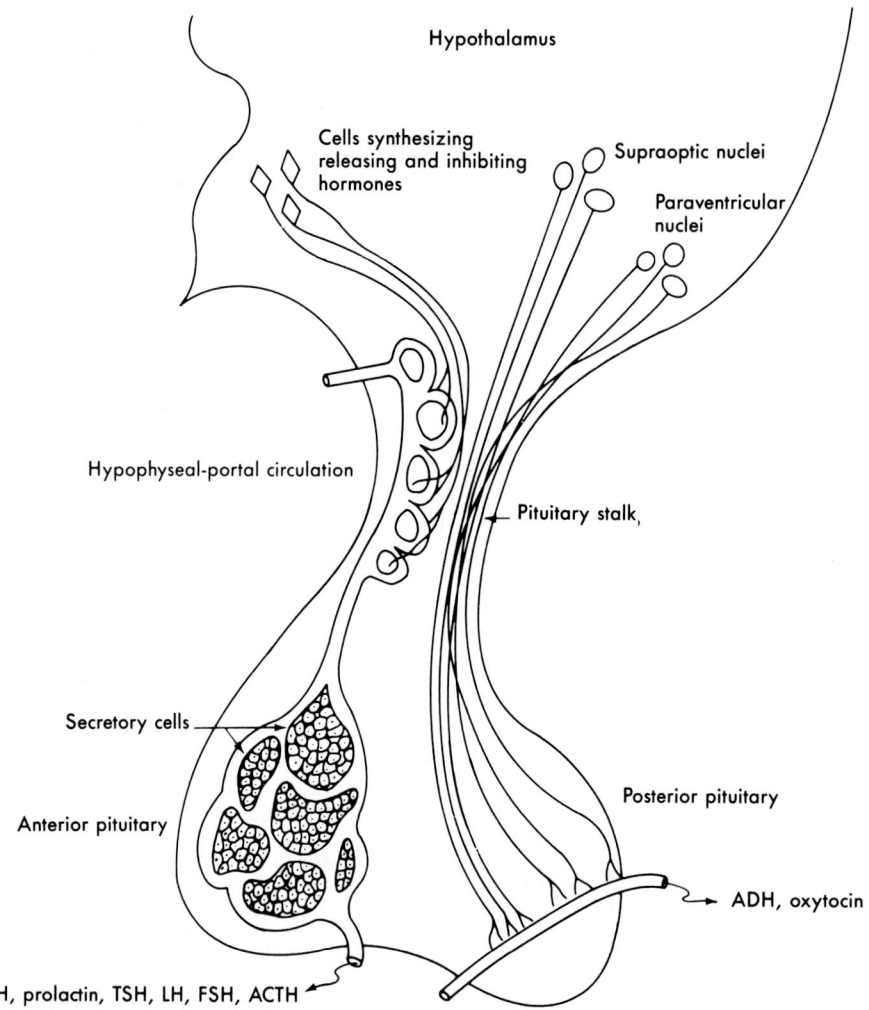

Figure 37-4   Anatomical relationship between the hypothalamus and pituitary gland.

peptide hormone, is a hypothalamic inhibitor of growth hormone secretion.[7]

Stimuli for the secretion of growth hormone include stress, exercise, hypoglycemia, and amino acid "loads" such as a high-protein meal. Growth hormone responds to these stimuli by mobilizing free fatty acids to create a readily available energy pool that reverses an insufficiency of energy. At the same time, it facilitates amino acid transport into the cells for tissue synthesis, sparing amino acids from hepatic gluconeogenesis. A schematic representation of hypothalamic–anterior pituitary hormonal interrelationships is shown in Figure 37-4.

Posterior Pituitary Gland

The posterior pituitary gland (neurohypophysis) secretes oxytocin and antidiuretic hormone (ADH, or vasopressin). Both of these hormones are synthesized in cell bodies located in the supraoptic and paraventricular nuclei of the hypothalamus. Axons from these cells combine and form the hypothalamic–hypoph-

yseal tract (or pituitary stalk) connecting the hypothalamus and the posterior pituitary gland (see Figure 37-4). These hormones are secreted in response to stimuli sensed at the hypothalamic level.[5]

Oxytocin stimulates the secretory ducts of the breast to eject milk. It does not influence milk synthesis. Milk ejection is initiated by nipple stimulation. Genital stimulation and intense emotions can also initiate the milk ejection reflex.

Oxytocin causes contraction of uterine smooth muscle and is secreted during labor. It may play a role in the initiation of labor, but this role has yet to be defined.[5]

Antidiuretic hormone (also known as vasopressin) acts to retain free water, an "antidiuretic" effect. It acts on the distal tubules and collecting ducts of the kidney where it increases tubular permeability. This allows water to follow the osmotic gradient out of the tubules into the surrounding hypertonic interstitium and, thus, be reabsorbed. This dilutes the osmotic toxicity of the body fluids.[5]

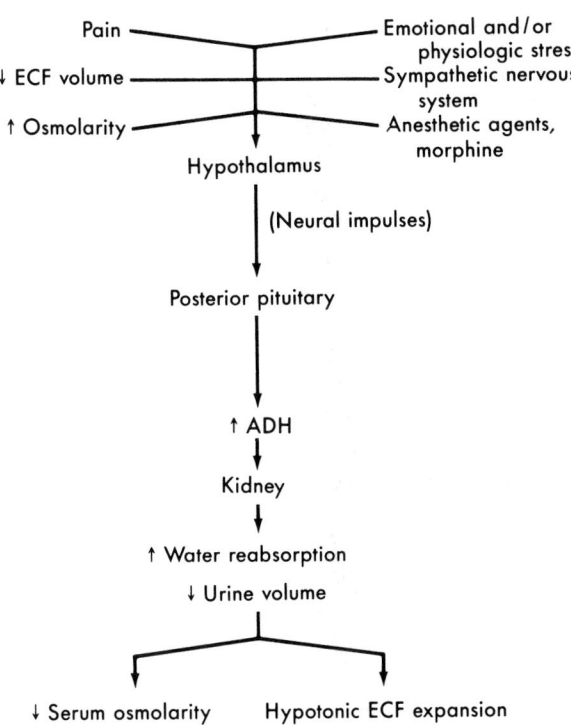

Figure 37-5   Stimuli affecting ADH secretion.

When ADH secretion is low, urine volume is high, and urine concentration decreases. The osmotic pressure of blood is increased. Osmoreceptors in the hypothalamus sense this, and ADH secretion is stimulated. Water is retained and osmolarity returns to "normal." When water is present in excess, hypothalamic osmoreceptors suppress ADH secretion leading to dilute urine and hemoconcentration.

Secretion of ADH is also affected by extracellular fluid volume. Stretch receptors in the great vessels sense extracellular volume. When volume is decreased, ADH secretion is increased. When volume is increased, ADH secretion is reduced. These receptors are extremely sensitive. They can stimulate an increase in ADH secretion in response to the volume shift associated with a change in body position from recumbent to upright.

Other stimuli increasing ADH secretion include pain, emotional or physical stress, sympathetic nervous system activation, and a variety of pharmacological agents including anesthetics, morphine, and barbiturates.[8] Alcohol decreases ADH secretion. A schematic representation of the stimuli modulating ADH secretion is shown in Figure 37-5.

Thyroid Gland

The thyroid gland embraces the trachea just below the larynx. An isthmus connects the lobes on either side of the trachea. The thyroid gland is made up of follicles that synthesize the iodine-containing thyroid hormones that regulate metabolic rate. Thyroxine (T_4) contains four iodine molecules; triiodothyronine (T_3) contains three. Parafollicular cells between the follicles synthesize calcitonin. Calcitonin has no clearly defined role in human physiology but has been shown to be involved in calcium regulation and bone metabolism in other species. Normal rates of thyroid hormone synthesis require the gland to concentrate 120 µg of iodine each day. Because the concentration of iodine in the blood is low, the blood flow through the gland must be high.[9]

T_4 and T_3 increase metabolic rate and stimulate oxygen consumption by most of the cells of the body. Their secretion is under the control of pituitary TSH secretion, which is regulated by hypothalamic TRH. The feedback regulation of thyroid hormone secretion is achieved mainly by T_3 and T_4.[10] These hormones block the TSH-stimulating effect of TRH.

Parathyroid Glands

The four parathyroid glands reside in the four poles of the thyroid gland. The secretory cells of the parathyroid glands, known as chief cells, secrete parathormone (PTH). PTH increases the serum level of ionized calcium by a direct resorptive effect on bone. In addition, PTH stimulates renal reabsorption of calcium and renal production of 1,25-dihydroxycholecalciferol, or active vitamin D, which enhances calcium absorption from the gut.[5]

Adrenal Glands

There are two adrenal glands, one next to each kidney. The gland is composed of cortex and medulla.

Adrenal Cortex

The adrenal cortex surrounds the medulla and secretes three steroid hormones: cortisol, aldosterone, and dehydroepiandrosterone (DHEA).

Cortisol is the primary glucocorticoid secreted in humans. It regulates the metabolism of carbohydrates, fats, and proteins. The secretion of cortisol is dependent upon ACTH from the anterior pituitary and CRH from the hypothalamus. Cortisol secretion is increased in stress, but the reasons for this and the subsequent effects are unknown. See the discussion of ACTH under Anterior Pituitary Tropic Hormones for a discussion of this topic. A schematic representation of the hypothalamic–pituitary–adrenal axis is presented in Figure 37-6.

Aldosterone is the primary mineralocorticoid in the human. Mineralocorticoids maintain extracellular fluid volume through the conservation of sodium and the excretion of potassium. Aldosterone secretion is regulated by the renin–angiotensin system. Renin is an enzyme released by the juxtaglomerular apparatus of the kidney in response to a decrease in extracellular

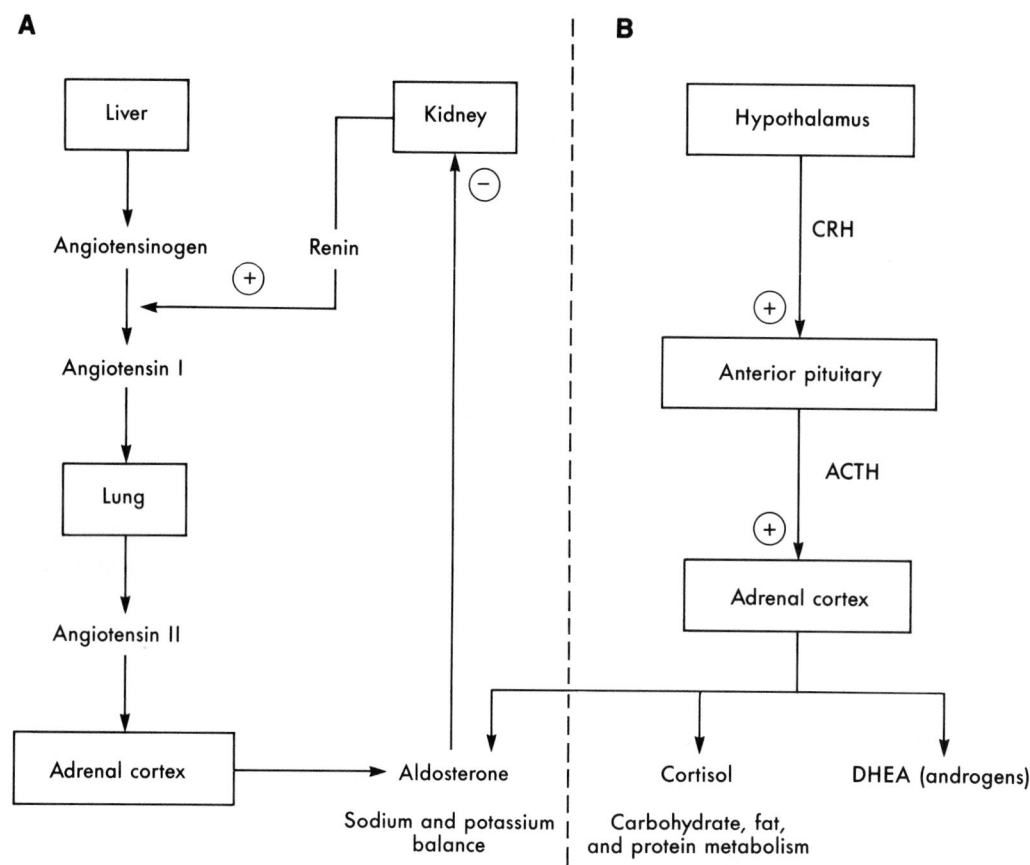

Figure 37-6   *A,* The renin–angiotensin system and *B,* the hypothalamic–pituitary–adrenal axis.

fluid volume perceived by sensors in renal afferent arterioles. Angiotensinogen from the liver is converted to angiotensin I by renin. Angiotensin I is converted to angiotensin II by converting enzymes in the lung. Angiotensin II stimulates the adrenal cortex to produce aldosterone, leading to an expansion in extracellular fluid volume that inhibits further renin secretion. (Figure 37-6 provides a schematic representation of the renin–angiotensin system and the hypothalamic–pituitary–adrenal axis.) Aldosterone is nonessential except in conditions of deficient salt intake. Its primary site of action is the proximal renal tubule where it exchanges sodium ions for potassium and hydrogen ions.[11]

The adrenal cortex also produces adrenal androgens. These are not hormones but are the precursors of the true androgens such as testosterone. Dehydroepiandrosterone (DHEA) is produced in large amounts in response to ACTH secretion by the anterior pituitary gland. DHEA has no known effect in man.[12]

Adrenal Medulla

The adrenal medulla secretes epinephrine and norepinephrine. These catecholamines serve a critical role in the physiological preparation to meet or cope with an emergency. Stimuli known to enhance catecholamine secretion include hypoxemia, hypoglycemia, cold, hemorrhage, and emotional stress provoked by frightening or unfamiliar situations. Factors regulating sympathoadrenal catecholamine secretion are shown in Figure 37-7.

Epinephrine relaxes bronchiolar smooth muscle, causing the bronchioles to dilate and, thereby, facilitating maximum ventilation. Both catecholamines increase the force and rate of myocardial contraction. *Norepinephrine* induces vasoconstriction in most, if not all, organs. Epinephrine induces vasodilation in skeletal muscles, the central nervous system, the myocardium, and the liver. In the presence of both catecholamines, total peripheral resistance to blood flow is decreased, but delivery of oxygen to many less vital organs is decreased because of decreased perfusion.

The metabolic effects of catecholamines are profound. They increase metabolic rate. The mechanisms involved in the catecholamine-induced increase in metabolic rate are not precisely known but are thought to involve increased glycogenolysis in skeletal muscle (producing hyperglycemia) and increased hepatic oxidation of lactic acid. Lactic acid production is a function of norepinephrine-induced vasoconstriction and decreased oxygen delivery to less vital cells

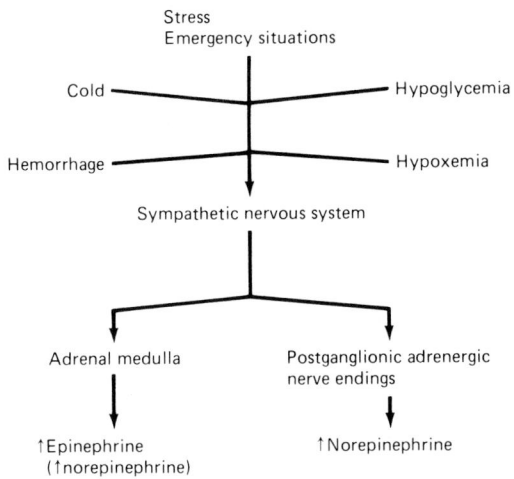

Figure 37-7   Control of catecholamine secretion.

leading to dependence on anaerobic metabolism.[12]

Epinephrine and norepinephrine are central nervous system neurotransmitters. Vigilance in the form of alertness and attentiveness is increased by catecholamines. Epinephrine is also thought to play a role in the genesis of anxiety and fear.

Endocrine Pancreas

The endocrine component of the pancreas is small but mighty. It constitutes about 2% of the total pancreatic mass and is composed of clusters of endocrine cells called *islets of Langerhans,* or pancreatic islets. There are three types of cells in these islets: alpha, beta, and delta cells. Alpha cells constitute about 20% of the cells and secrete *glucagon.* Beta cells constitute about 75% and secrete *insulin.* Delta cells make up the remainder and supplement hypothalamic secretion of somatostatin. Somatostatin inhibits secretion of insulin and glucagon from beta and alpha cells, respectively.[5]

Insulin and glucagon are major factors in the regulation of carbohydrate, protein, and fat metabolism. Insulin increases the storage of glucose, fatty acids, and amino acids. Glucagon mobilizes glucose and breaks down or converts stored fat and protein into utilizable energy sources. These two hormones are antagonists, so their secretory patterns are generally reciprocal. The overall status of energy stores at any given time reflects the ratio of insulin to glucagon. When a balanced diet is being consumed, the insulin/glucagon ratio is 2:1, indicating a net tendency toward storage. Fasting decreases the insulin/glucagon ratio leading to catabolism and weight loss.

Insulin

Insulin increases glucose uptake in most cells but not in pancreatic beta islet cells, brain, renal tubules, intestinal mucosa, or red blood cells. The mechanism involves facilitation of glucose transport across cellular membranes. Insulin also increases free fatty acids and net protein synthesis by preventing the action of enzymes necessary for their breakdown and increasing amino acid transport into cells. Insulin also decreases hepatic glucose output and stimulates glycogenesis in liver and skeletal muscle.

Insulin secretion is regulated by blood glucose concentration. Glucose entry into beta cells is not affected by insulin. Thus, changes in glucose level are rapidly sensed by these cells. When blood glucose levels are low, insulin secretion is inhibited. When blood glucose levels are high, insulin secretion is stimulated. The subsequent decrease in blood glucose removes the stimulus for insulin secretion. This feedback mechanism operates with great precision and results in a close parallel between blood glucose and insulin levels.[14]

The presence of keto- and amino acids in the serum can increase insulin secretion by a mechanism that has not been defined. Insulin increases synthesis of protein, thus preserving amino acids from being used as cellular energy sources. Serum ketones reflect fatty acid breakdown, and insulin reverses this process.

The secretion of insulin in response to intravenous infusion of glucose and amino acid is less than that induced by oral ingestion of the same substances. This difference can be attributed to the action of a hormone secreted by the intestinal mucosa, *gastric inhibitory peptide* (GIP). In the presence of glucose or fat, secretion of GIP rises. GIP inhibits stomach motility and stimulates pancreatic insulin secretion. The gastrointestinal tract produces several hormones having similar effects: cholecystokinin, secretin, gastrin, and mucosal glucagon. Glucagon is discussed in detail in the section that immediately follows.

Epinephrine and sympathetic stimulation prevent insulin secretion. Other factors inhibiting insulin secretion include thiazide diuretics, diazoxide, and somatostatin. Several hormones, including glucocorticoids and growth hormone, impair insulin action.

Glucagon

Glucagon is secreted principally by the alpha cells but also by mucosal cells of the gastrointestinal tract. Glucagon increases hepatic glycogenolysis and gluconeogenesis and promotes fat breakdown. Blood glucose is elevated by glucagon, leading to an increase secretion of insulin. Insulin facilitates tissue uptake of the released energy sources. Glucagon in large quantities also exerts an inotropic effect on the myocardium, but the effect is minor in comparison with its role in metabolism.[14]

A variety of stimuli affect glucagon secretion. These include catecholamines, glucocorticoids, and exercise. Amino acids can also stimulate glucagon secretion. Glucagon secretion assures normal blood glucose levels, while insulin promotes the use of these substances for tissue synthesis. Glucagon facilitates the protein-sparing and the storage effects of insulin in this way.

The secretion of glucagon in response to orally ingested amino acids is greater than that induced by intravenous administration of the same substances. The presence of protein in the gastrointestinal tract stimulates the secretion of cholecystokinin and gastrin from mucosal cells, and both these substances increase glucagon secretion from the alpha cells as well as from the intestinal mucosa.[14]

Glucagon secretion is inhibited by hyperglycemia. This inhibition is dependent upon insulin. Alpha cells are unable to react to elevated blood glucose levels unless insulin first promotes glucose transport into alpha cells. When blood glucose levels are low, glucagon increases blood glucose and insulin. Glucagon secretion is inhibited by somatostatin. A schematic representation of the control of energy metabolism by the pancreas is presented in Figure 37-8.

Pineal Gland

The pineal gland is located at the midline of the cranial cavity just under the third ventricle. During infancy the pineal gland is large, but by puberty it has atrophied considerably. The function of the pineal gland and its secretory product, *melatonin*, is not well understood but is the subject of much research related to biological rhythms.

Secretion of melatonin is modulated by light and dark. The rhythmic production of melatonin is lowest during daylight and highest during hours of darkness. In blind individuals, "free-running" 24-hour cycles occur that are indifferent to light and darkness. Some investigators believe that jet lag can be attributed to the need to readjust melatonin rhythm after travel across time zones. Melatonin is also believed to decrease self-reported alertness and increases sleepiness. Some researchers hypothesize that melatonin has a role in seasonal affective disorder (SAD), a psychological disturbance related to environmental light and dark.

Thymus Gland

The thymus gland is located in the mediastinum and is the primary organ of the lymphatic system. It is composed of two lobes. Its largest dimensions are seen at puberty, but by old age it has largely been replaced by fat.

The function of the thymus is vital to the development of the immune defense mechanism. This function is essentially completed early in life and, thus, unaffected by later involution. Soon after birth the thymus affects maturation of fetal lymphocytes that

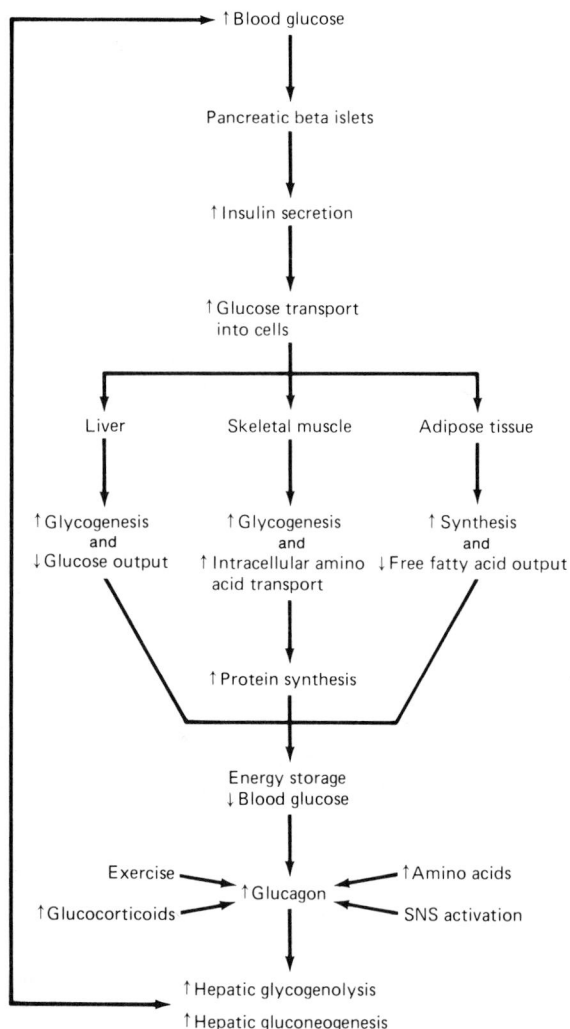

Figure 37-8   Control of energy metabolism by the endocrine pancreas.

then migrate and accumulate in splenic lymph nodes and lymphatic tissues.[15]

The thymus secretes a hormone known as *thymosin*. Thymosin is involved in the development and maturation of T cells which play a vital role in cellular immunity (see Chapter 43). T cell activation provides the primary defense against viral invasion but also leads to rejection of transplanted tissue.

Thymosin administration enhances immune defenses, presumably by increasing the number or activity of T cells. Its use in immunosuppressed patients (such as those undergoing chemotherapy or radiation therapy for malignant disease) can increase resistance to systemic infection. It can help in the body's defense against malignant processes in that tumor cells are known to contain foreign antigens. Theoretically, if T cells could be sufficiently activated, they could destroy these cells.[15]

REFERENCES

1. Jordan, R. M., & Kohler, P. O. (1990). Principles of endocrine physiology. In J. H. Stein (Ed.), *Internal medicine* (3rd ed.). Boston: Little, Brown.

2. Baxter, J. D. (1992). Principles of endocrinology. In J. B. Wyngaarden, & L. H. Smith (Eds.), *Cecil textbook of medicine* (18th ed.) (pp. 1252-1267). Philadelphia: Saunders.

3. Becker, K. L. (1990). General principles of endocrinology. In K. Becker (Ed.), *Principles and practice in endocrinology and metabolism* (pp. 2-80). Philadelphia: Lippincott.

4. Boyd, A. E., III, Jordan, R. M., & Kohler, P. O. (1986). Disorders of the hypothalamus and anterior pituitary. In P. Kohler (Ed.), *Clinical endocrinology* (pp. 11-52). New York: Wiley.

5. Drass, J. A., Loriaux, T. C., & Solomon, B. (1992). Endocrine and metabolic systems. In J. Thompson, G. K. McFarland, J. E. Hirsch, et al. (Eds.), *Mosby's manual of clinical nursing* (pp. 876-967). St. Louis: Mosby—Year Book.

6. Frohman, L. A. (1992). Neuroendocrine regulation and its disorders. In J. B. Wyngaarden, & L. H. Smith (Eds.), *Cecil textbook of medicine* (19th ed.) (pp. 1215-1224). Philadelphia: Saunders.

7. Frohman, L. A. (1992). The anterior pituitary. In J. B. Wyngaarden, & L. H. Smith (Eds.), *Cecil textbook of medicine* (19th ed.) (pp. 1224-1238). Philadelphia: Saunders.

8. Moses, A. M., Streeten, D. H. P. (1986). Disorders of the hypothalamic-neurohypophyseal system. In P. Kohler (Ed.), *Clinical endocrinology* (pp. 53-72). New York: Wiley.

9. Jackson, I. M. D., & Cobb, W. E. (1986). Disorders of the thyroid. In P. Kohler (Ed.), *Clinical endocrinology* (pp. 73-166). New York: Wiley.

10. Larsen, P. R. (1992). The thyroid. In J. B. Wyngaarden, & L. H. Smith (Eds.), *Cecil textbook of medicine* (19th ed.) (pp. 1248-1271). Philadelphia: Saunders.

11. Tyrell, J. B., & Baxter, J. D. (1992). Disorders of the adrenal cortex. In J. B. Wyngaarden, & L. H. Smith (Eds.), *Cecil textbook of medicine* (19th ed.) (pp. 1271-1291). Philadelphia: Saunders.

12. Loriaux, D. L. (1990). The adrenal glands. In K. Becker (Ed.), *Principles and practice in endocrinology and metabolism* (pp. 92-246). Philadelphia: Lippincott.

13. Loriaux, D. L., & Cutler, J. B., Jr. (1986). Diseases of the adrenal glands. In P. Kohler (Ed.), *Clinical endocrinology* (pp. 167-238). New York: Wiley.

14. Kahn, C. (1990). Disorders of fuel metabolism. In K. Becker (Ed.), *Principles and practice in endocrinology and metabolism* (pp. 1032-1248). Philadelphia: Lippincott.

15. Hall, N. R., & Goldstein, A. L. (1990). The endocrine thymus. In K. Becker (Ed.), *Principles and practice in endocrinology and metabolism* (pp. 1351-1356). Philadelphia: Lippincott.

38

Endocrine Data Acquisition

Teresa Choate Loriaux

Evaluation of endocrine function is one of the most formidable challenges in nursing practice. The effects of endocrine dysfunction are pervasive and multidimensional. Assessment of endocrine function requires comprehensive data collection and interpretation. The interactive and overlapping nature of endocrine functions complicates the differential determination of alterations in glandular responses, secretion patterns, and consequences. Compounding the complexity is the inability to visualize the glands themselves. Recognition of altered glandular structure and function depends on understanding the diffuse and delicate balance between various glands and other body systems.[1] In the critical care setting, recognition of endocrine dysfunction is essential; the potential consequences of inadequate treatment are severe and life-threatening, but most endocrine disorders can be treated effectively once recognized. This chapter provides information to guide the critical care nurse in the acquisition of data as it relates to clinical endocrinology.

Endocrine dysfunction involves two types of disorders: hyperfunction and hypofunction. *Hyperfunction* is caused by increased hormone activity; *hypofunction* is caused by deficient hormone action. Because of the interrelated nature of the endocrine system, hyper- and hyposecretory syndromes can be caused by dysfunction of a particular gland, altered secretion of the trophic hormones for that gland, or an altered response to the hormone itself. *Primary dysfunction* refers to a disorder of the gland. *Secondary dysfunction* refers to an altered trophic hormone secretory pattern. *Resistance* refers to an altered response to the hormone.[2] Some disorders of hormone excess or deficiency are readily apparent through clinical manifestations (e.g., Cushing's syndrome), but others require careful laboratory testing for diagnosis (e.g., adrenal insufficiency).

NURSING ASSESSMENT

History

The history begins with a full account of why treatment has been sought or is being rendered. It is important to elicit the nature and onset of symptoms; the location, duration, quality, and severity of the symptoms; and aggravating or alleviating factors. Patient perceptions and correlations between the symptoms and sleep, activity, emotional state, and food intake are significant. All prescription and nonprescription medications and previous medical and surgical procedures should be noted.[3]

Changes in weight, thirst, appetite, bowel habits, and volume or frequency of urination are important general indicators of health status. Energy changes and the pattern of sleep and its ability to restore energy are important. Muscle tremors, palpitations, intolerance to heat, and insomnia may suggest hyperthyroidism. Cold intolerance and somnolence may suggest hypothyroidism.[4] Because some endocrine disorders have a hereditary pattern, family history of diabetes, thyroid disorder, hypertension, cardiac or renal disease, and cancer should be noted.

Physical Examination

The general nature of the endocrine system mandates a systematic approach to the physical examination. The suggested approach generally follows a head-to-toe framework. A generalized endocrine nursing assessment guide is provided in the box on p. 918.

Vital Signs

Measurement of heart and respiratory rate, blood pressure, and temperature is the first step in the physical examination. Sinus tachycardia and dysrhythmias such as atrial fibrillation or paroxysmal atrial tachycardia can be associated with hyperthyroidism. Slowed pulse rates can reflect hypothyroidism.[5]

The character and rate of respiration should be described. Rapid deep *Kussmaul respiration* is a hallmark finding in diabetic ketoacidosis, which is often accompanied by an odor of acetone to the breath.

Blood pressure should be measured in both arms and checked for postural change. Hypertension with a widened pulse pressure commonly accompanies hyperthyroidism. Elevated blood pressure is a frequent

Endocrine Nursing Assessment Guide

GENERAL OBSERVATIONS

Body size and stature
Body proportions (upper body/lower body ratio)
Weight
Height

RESPIRATORY ASSESSMENT

Rate per minute
Regularity
Breath sounds
Breath smell (acetone, sweetness)
Kussmaul respirations
Dyspnea
Laryngeal stridor

CARDIOVASCULAR ASSESSMENT

Heart rate and rhythm
   Palpitations, dysrhythmias
Blood pressure lying, sitting, & standing
   Pulse pressure
   Orthostatic changes
Body temperature
   Cool/warm to touch
   Moist/dry to touch
   Night sweats
   Bruisability

FOOD AND FLUID INTAKE

Appetite
Recent weight gain/loss
Nausea/vomiting
Food cravings (salt?)
Polydipsia
Polyphagia
Insulin history
Ulcer disease

ELIMINATION

Fecal
   Bowel sounds/abdominal distention or hardness
   Frequency of defecation
   Characteristics of stool
   ↑ GI motility
Urinary
   Frequency of urination
   Characteristics of urine (color, concentration)
   Polyuria
   Nocturia
   Recent ↑ or ↓ in urine volume
   History of renal pain or calculi
   History of urinary tract infections

NEUROMUSCULAR

Weakness
Fatigue
Dysesthesia

Paresthesia
Tremors/spasms
Paralysis
Carpal tunnel syndrome
Fractures/osteoporosis
Seizures
Coordination
Reflexes
Syncope/dizziness
Anxiety
Speech (slurred, pressured)
Vision changes (visual fields, acuity, exophthalmos)
Hearing changes
Thought processes: memory loss, confusion, cognition
Trousseau's sign
Chvostek's sign

SKIN

Pigmentation
Turgor and elasticity (thinning?)
Hair growth
   Body hair distribution (pubic, axillary, facial)
   Coarse, thinning, baldness
Fat distribution
   Central, supraclavicular, dorsocervical
Striae (note color)
Capillary fragility (easy bruisability)
Nails
Mucous membranes
Myxedema
Acropachy
Acanthosis nigricans
Multiple lipomas
Skin tags

SLEEP/REST

Hours per night
Difficulty falling asleep/waking
Early morning awakening
Nightmares
Circadian variations (shift work, etc.)

REPRODUCTION

Onset of puberty
Onset of menarche, thelarche
Menstrual history: regularity, flow, pain, amenorrhea,
   oligomenorrhea, dysmenorrhea, menopause
Voice changes
Changes in hair growth
Libido
Galactorrhea
Impotence
Fertility
Exogenous hormones and drug use (birth control pills,
   steroids, alcohol, prescription and nonprescription
   drugs, including recreational drugs)

finding in Cushing's syndrome, hyperaldosteronism, and pheochromocytoma. Hypotension, frequently with postural exaggeration, occurs in adrenocortical insufficiency. Hyperglycemic osmolar diuresis associated with both diabetic ketoacidosis and nonketotic hyperosmolar states can lead to extracellular volume depletion and to sustained and postural hypotension.

Temperature elevations can accompany hyperthyroidism and adrenocortical insufficiency. Hypothermia, on the other hand, is characteristic of myxedema and is a frequent finding in diabetic ketoacidosis.[5]

General Observations

As the physical examination is initiated, obvious signs of endocrine dysfunction should be noted. Stature should be examined first. Excessive secretion of growth hormone before epiphyseal closure of the long bones leads to gigantism. After epiphyseal closure, excessive growth hormone causes acromegaly, a disorder associated with enlargement of the nose, jaw, tongue, and soft tissues of the hands and feet. In hypothyroidism, mucopolysaccharide infiltration can cause facial swelling and puffiness around the eyes. Features look coarse and eyebrows appear thinned.[3,6]

Cushing's syndrome is accompanied by weight gain and central obesity. Characteristic are a moon face, buffalo hump, pendulous abdomen, and thin limbs.[7]

Skin

Normal pigmentation reflects racial and ethnic background and is characteristically greater on the face, the backs of the hands, the areolae, and the genitalia. All pigmentation intensifies during pregnancy. Significant hyperpigmentation suggests adrenocortical insufficiency. Carotinemia, a yellow tinge, is associated with hypothyroidism. Jaundice can be differentiated from carotinemia by inspecting the sclerae. Only jaundice produces yellowing of the sclerae.

Petechiae, excessive bruising, evidence of poor wound healing, and striae ("stretch marks"), especially on the abdomen, may indicate Cushing's syndrome. Dry scaly skin often accompanies hypothyroidism. Hyperthyroidism is characteristically associated with smooth, flushed-appearing diaphoretic skin.

The condition of the hair can also suggest endocrine dysfunction. Coarse, dry hair, especially with evidence of hair loss, can accompany hypothyroidism. In hyperthyroidism, the hair tends to feel smooth, soft, and fine. Unusual hair loss can also signal chronic adrenocortical insufficiency and pituitary or parathyroid disorders.

In women, excessive hair or hair in abnormal locations such as on the face, chest, or abdomen, is called *hirsutism*. It suggests Cushing's syndrome or the presence of excessive androgens.

The nails also can mirror endocrine function. Pitting can be associated with hypoparathyroidism. Nails separated from nail beds, *onycholysis*, is a frequent finding in hyperthyroidism. Thickened, brittle, and friable nails can indicate hypothyroidism. Pigmented, darkened nails can signal adrenocortical insufficiency.

Finally, skin turgor should be assessed. Poor turgor can reflect dehydration, a feature of diabetes insipidus, diabetic ketoacidosis, and nonketotic hyperglycemic hyperosmolar states. Edema can occur in thyroid disorders. Acute and severe hyperthyroid states can lead to high output heart failure. In hypothyroidism, pericardial effusion can lead to congestive heart failure.

Head

A flat or dull expression, especially coupled with coarse features and puffy eyes, suggests hypothyroidism. An overalert to anxious expression can mean hyperthyroidism.

Retracted upper eyelids with protruding eyeballs are hallmarks of *exophthalmos*; an appearance of continuous staring. It results from an autoimmune-mediated inflammation of the retroorbital contents, and it is characteristic of hyperthyroidism.

Visual field defects or cranial nerve dysfunction can be associated with a pituitary tumor. If double vision (diplopia) is reported, cranial nerve dysfunction should be suspected. Conjugate gaze should be maintained, and eye movements should be smooth. Nystagmus should be noted. The patient should be asked to raise the eyebrows, close the eyes tightly, puff the cheeks, show the teeth, frown, and smile. Muscle contraction on both sides of the face should be equal (see also Chapter 32).

A nasal speculum is used to check the patency of the nasal canals. Signs of inflammation, reddened mucous membranes, and discharge can indicate infection. Highly inflamed nasal passages can reflect use of cocaine, an agent that can mimic endocrine dysfunction.

The lips and tongue should be evaluated for symmetry and color. An enlarged tongue can indicate myxedema; asymmetry can reflect a pituitary lesion. Malformed or pitted teeth can occur in hypoparathyroidism. As previously noted, an acetone or fruity odor to the breath is associated with diabetes mellitus.

Neck

The endocrine evaluation of the neck focuses on the thyroid gland. Unlike other glands, assessment of the thyroid gland involves inspection. The neck should be inspected for signs of thyroid enlargement (goiter) or asymmetry. Swallowing will often highlight the gland. Any reported difficulty with swallowing or hoarseness should be noted.

The normal thyroid gland is usually not palpable unless the patient has a thin neck. To palpate the thyroid gland, have the patient flex the neck slightly to relieve tension on the sternocleidomastoid muscles. Changes in the isthmus can be palpated by placing the index and middle fingers just below the cricoid cartilage on one side. Ask the patient, still with neck flexed, to turn the head slightly to the side being palpated and swallow. Repeat the procedure for the other side. Changes in the lobes of the gland can be detected by displacing the thyroid cartilage slightly to first one side and then the other. With the cartilage thus displaced, the space between the sternocleidomastoid and cartilage can be palpated.[4]

The thyroid should be auscultated when enlargement or nodules are formed. A bruit can often be heard in hyperthyroidism. To distinguish a bruit from a venous hum, ask the patient to stop breathing momentarily; then, while compressing the jugular vein on the same side as the lobe being auscultated, listen to first one lobe and then the other. Compression of the jugular will remove a venous hum but not a bruit.[5]

Abdomen

With the patient in a supine position, examine for contour, bulges, striae, and discolorations. Normal abdominal contour is flat; a protuberant contour can reflect hypothyroidism or Cushing's syndrome. Striae result from stretching of the skin. Typically, young or new striae are bright pink or blue, whereas longstanding ones tend to be silvery pink. Purple striae are characteristic of Cushing's syndrome.[7]

Bowel sounds should be auscultated and frequency, pitch, and duration noted. Normal bowel tones occur at 5- to 10-second intervals, are low-pitched, and last roughly 1 to 5 seconds. Decreased or absent bowel sounds are common in hypothyroidism and pheochromocytoma. Hyperactive, high-pitched sounds are common in hyperthyroidism.

All four quadrants of the abdomen should be palpated to ascertain the presence of tenderness, masses, or enlarged organs. An enlarged liver due to fatty infiltration can result from poorly controlled diabetes. Upper abdominal tenderness, sometimes severe, accompanies acute pancreatitis and can be followed by the acute onset of diabetes. A mass near the kidneys can be pheochromocytoma or adrenal cancer.

DIAGNOSTIC PROCEDURES

Many diagnostic tools are available for assessing endocrine function. Radioimmunoassay (RIA) allows the direct measurement of most hormones. Radio-

graphic procedures such as computed tomography (CT) allow determination of the size and structure of selected tissues.[8] Radioactive iodine uptake allows some measure of thyroid function and architecture.

Laboratory Studies

Laboratory studies used to assess endocrine function fall into three categories: measurement of basal serum or plasma hormone levels, measurement of urine levels of a hormone or its metabolite, and measurement of hormonal regulation through stimulation and suppression tests. Typically, abnormalities in standard laboratory screens provide the stimulus for the use of tests from one or more of these categories. For example, an increased cholesterol in a blood chemistry test can prompt the measurement of free T_4 to rule out hypothyroidism. Similarly, hypochloremia noted in a routine electrolyte screen may prompt 24-hour measurement of urinary aldosterone to determine whether primary hyperaldosteronism is present. Elevated BUN and creatinine levels in a blood chemistry test can lead to an ACTH stimulation test to evaluate adrenal function.[1,8]

Pituitary Function

Pituitary function is most commonly assessed by measuring the plasma levels of target hormones and the relevant trophic hormones. Assessment of anterior pituitary function thus involves measurements relating to adrenocorticotropic hormone (ACTH), thyroid stimulating hormone (TSH), luteinizing and follicle stimulating hormones (LH and FSH), growth hormone (GH), and prolactin (PRL). Antidiuretic hormone (ADH) and oxytocin are measured to evaluate posterior pituitary function.

Hyperpituitarism most commonly is reflected by excessive secretion of one or more anterior pituitary hormones. Elevations usually involve PRL, GH, or ACTH, and, rarely, TSH, FSH, or LH. Hypopituitarism, on the other hand, most commonly is reflected in decreased levels of GH, FSH, LH, TSH, ACTH, or PRL. Panhypopituitarism and deficiency of all anterior pituitary hormones can occur but is extremely rare and usually accompanies glandular destruction such as hemorrhage into a tumor or glandular infarction.[9,10]

Radioimmunoassays are available to measure plasma levels of all anterior pituitary hormones. Absolute values must take into account the diurnal secretion patterns of several hormones. Table 38-1 lists normal values of anterior pituitary hormones along with the stimulation or suppression tests most commonly used to detect anterior pituitary dysfunction.[8,9]

Laboratory evaluation of posterior pituitary function focuses on antidiuretic hormone (ADH) or va-

TABLE 38-1   **Laboratory Assessment of Anterior Pituitary Hormones in Adults**

Hormone	Normal Value	Stimulation Test/Normal Value	Suppression Test/Normal Value
Growth hormone (GH)	*Men:* 0-5 ng/ml *Women:* 0-7 ng/ml	Arginine stimulation: *Men:* GH rise to >7 ng/ml *Women:* GH rise to >10 ng/ml	Glucose loading: GH suppression to <3 ng/ml
ACTH	8 A.M.: <40 pg/ml 4 P.M.: 10-50 pg/ml	None	None
Thyroid-stimulating hormone (TSH)	1-7 µg/ml	None	None
Prolactin (PRL)	2-30 ng/ml	None	None
Luteinizing hormone (LH)	*Women:* Follicular phase: 5-25 mIU/ml Ovulatory phase: 35-150 mIU/ml Luteal phase: 5-25 mIU/ml Postmenopausal: 30-200 mIU/ml *Men:* 6-25 mIU/ml	None	None
Follicle-stimulating hormone (FSH)	*Women:* Follicular phase: <25mIU/ml Ovulatory phase: <35 mIU/ml Luteal phase: <25 mIU/ml Postmenopausal: >30 mIU/ml *Men:* <25 mIU/ml	None	None

TABLE 38-2   **Laboratory Assessment of ADH**

Parameter	Normal Value	Increased in:	Decreased in:
Serum ADH	1-5 pg/ml	SIADH, hyperthyroidism, adrenal insufficiency, hemorrhage or shock, stress, pain	Diabetes insipidus
Serum osmolality	280-295 mosm/kg	Diabetes inspidus, ketotic and nonketotic hyperglycemic states, hypercalcemia	SIADH, excessive water intake
Water-deprivation test	Urine flow decreased to <0.5 ml/min; urine osmolality >800 mosm/L	Diabetes insipidus: decreased concentration ability	

sopressin. Direct measurements of serum and urine ADH are possible but rarely used. Instead, evaluation of ADH centers on serum osmolality and water deprivation or loading tests. Table 38-2 summarizes values and findings for the assessment of ADH.[11,12]

Thyroid Function

Radioimmunoassays and stimulation and suppression tests are used to assess thyroid function. Free T_4 is the most useful measurement. Because "free hormone" levels are the active fraction, adjustment for changes in protein levels and protein-binding concentrations, is unnecessary. Free T_4, coupled with a measurement of TSH, characterizes the functional capacity of the thyroid gland (see also Chapter 37).[13] Table 38-3 summarizes normal laboratory values and findings in thyroid evaluation.

Parathyroid Function

Radioimmunoassay measurement of serum parathormone (PTH) is a fundamental part of an evaluation of parathyroid function. It is necessary, how-

TABLE 38-3 Laboratory Assessment of Thyroid Function

Parameter	Normal Value	Increased in:	Decreased in:
Thyroxine (T_4)	5-12 µg/dl	Thyrotoxicosis, acute thyroiditis, pregnancy	Hypoparathyroidism, chronic debilitating illness
Triiodothyronine (T_3)	80-230 ng/dl	Thyrotoxicosis, pregnancy	Severe acute illness, trauma, malnutrition
Thyroid stimulating hormone (TSH)	1-7 µIU/ml	Primary hypothyroidism	Secondary hypothyroidism (anterior pituitary hypofunction), thyrotoxicosis

ever, to measure serum calcium simultaneously as normal parathyroid secretion of PTH is controlled by the serum calcium.[8] Table 38-4 summarizes laboratory findings used to evaluate parathyroid function.

Adrenocortical Function

Both RIA measurement of blood and urine hormone levels and stimulation and suppression tests are used to evaluate function of the adrenal cortex. Urinary studies, including free urinary cortisol, are also employed to evaluate overall adrenocortical production. Urinary free cortisol is the best test to differentiate patients with Cushing's syndrome from normal subjects. Measurement of serum ACTH is used to define the cause of the elevated cortisol products. Table 38-5 summarizes laboratory values and findings in adrenocortical evaluation.[7,14,15]

Adrenomedullary Function

Laboratory evaluation of the adrenal medulla involves direct measurement of plasma and urine catecholamines. Urinary vanillylmandelic acid (VMA) is also measured. Urinary VMA, a catecholamine metabolite, is influenced by diet, strenuous exercise, and stress, and can be somewhat nonspecific.[8,15] Table 38-6 summarizes laboratory values and findings used in evaluation of the adrenal medulla.

Endocrine Pancreas Function

Most laboratory studies involved in evaluation of the endocrine pancreas focus on measurement of glucose in blood or urine. Common tests used to measure serum glucose include random samples after fasting and 2 hours after eating a meal (postprandial). Glucose tolerance tests are also commonly performed when diabetes is suspected. This test provides what may be the most sensitive and accurate evaluation of carbohydrate metabolism. In glucose tolerance testing, a loading dose of glucose is administered orally after 3 days of high-carbohydrate diet and an overnight fast. For the next 3 hours, plasma and urine glucose levels are monitored at frequent intervals to assess insulin secretion and glucose metabolism.[8]

In persons known to be diabetic, the glycosylated hemoglobin test helps to assess average glucose levels over time. Glucose molecules attach to hemoglobin normally by a process called glycosylation. Since the lifespan of red blood cells is 120 days, measurement of glycosylated hemoglobin provides an "average" glucose level over the lifespan of the red blood cell.[16]

Serum insulin and glucose are correlated in hypoglycemia. These data can help differentiate between glucocorticoid deficiency, hepatic disease, and hypoglycemia due to insulinoma or hyperplasia of the pancreatic islet cells.[8,16]

Urinary tests for glucose include copper reduction (Clinitest) and glucose oxidase (Tes-Tape, Clinistix) procedures. They can be used for self-testing. Both tests produce standardized color reactions either by reduction of copper in a hot alkaline solution with subsequent formation of a colored precipitate or by sequential enzymatic oxidation of glucose. Glucose oxidase tests are generally more accurate for glucose because the reagent strips contain specific enzymes. Similarly, strips impregnated with sodium nitroprusside, an agent specific for acetoacetic acid, allow self-testing for ketones.[3,16] Table 38-7 summarizes laboratory values and findings used to assess function of the endocrine pancreas.

Radiographic and Nuclear Imaging Tests

Radiographic and nuclear imaging tests used in endocrine evaluation include x-rays, computed tomography (CT), arteriography, ultrasonography, and nuclear isotope studies (radionuclide scintigraphy). Generally, one or more of these procedures are used to confirm suspected anatomical glandular changes such as hypo- or hyperplasia, cyst, neoplasm, or glandular destruction.[8]

Thyroid evaluation frequently employs a nuclear isotope scan and ultrasonography. Measuring the thyroid uptake of radioactive iodine (^{131}I uptake) can help distinguish between the different causes of hyperthyroidism. The test involves external monitoring

TABLE 38-4　Laboratory Assessment of Parathyroid Function

Parameter	Normal Value	Increased in:	Decreased in:
Parathyroid hormone (PTH)	163-347 pg/ml (depends on serum calcium)	Hyperparathyroidism	Parathyroid trauma, para- thyroidectomy
Calcium	Serum: 8.2-10.5 mg/dl Ionized serum: 4.5-5.5 mg/dl Calculated ionized: 3.9- 4.8 mg/dl	Hyperparathyroidism, metastatic bone tumors, nonparathyroid PTH- secreting tumors (lung, breast, kidney)	Hypoparathyroidism, al- coholism, chronic renal disease, malabsorption syndrome
Phosphates	*Child:* <7 mg/dl or 4.1 mEq/L during periods of rapid bone growth *Adult:* 2.5-4.5 mg/dl or 1.8-2.6 mEq/L	Hypoparathyroidism, non- endocrine hypocal- cemia, renal insuffi- ciency or failure	Hyperparathyroidism, nonendocrine dysplasia

TABLE 38-5　Laboratory Assessment of Adrenocortical Function

Parameter or Test	Normal Value	Increased in:	Decreased in:
Cortisol	8 A.M.: 8-20 μg/dl 4 P.M.: 4-10 μg/dl	Adrenocortical hyper- function, stress, pregnancy	Adrenocortical hypo- function, Cushing's syndrome (ACTH independent)
ACTH	8 A.M.: <140 pg/ml 4 P.M.: 10-50 pg/ml	Primary adrenal insuf- ficiency, stress	Hypopituitarism, ad- renal hypofunction
Aldosterone	A.M. Supine: 5-10 ng/dl A.M. Upright: 9-60 ng/dl Value increases × 2-4 with low sodium diet	Primary and secondary hyperaldosteronism, nephrotic syndrome	
Urinary free cortisol (UFC)	*Men:* 10-85 μg/dl *Women:* 10-90 μg/dl	Cushing's syndrome	
Urinary 17-hydroxycorti- costeroids	*Men:* 2-12 mg/24 hr *Women:* 2-12 mg/24 hr	Adrenal hyperfunction, hyperthyroidism	Adrenal hypofunction, hypopituitarism, hypothyroidism
Urine aldosterone	3-19 μg/24 hr	Primary and secondary aldosteronism, se- vere stress	Adrenal hypofunction
ACTH stimulation test (25 U via IV bolus)	Cortisol >20 μg/dl 30-45 min after bolus		Adrenal insufficiency
Dexamethasone suppres- sion test	Overnight screening: cortisol <5 μg/dl		Cushing's syndrome, depression

of radioactivity to measure the accumulation of ^{131}I in the thyroid gland. Thyroid scans can provide data about glandular size, uniformity of iodine uptake, and overall metabolic function of the gland. Gray-black regions on the scan, referred to as "hot spots," indicate hyperfunction. "Cold spots" indicate hypofunction and may be associated with tumor. Ultrasonography can be used to distinguish between cysts and nodules of the thyroid gland.[4] Ultrasonography is also useful in studies of the size, contour, and texture of the pancreas and parathyroid glands.

CT and magnetic resonance imaging (MRI) scans of the pituitary have replaced x-rays of the sella turcica. They are also useful in adrenal evaluation. Small, hard-to-locate tumors of the adrenal glands such as the pheochromocytomas are often discernible by CT or MRI scan.

TABLE 38-6 Laboratory Assessment of Adrenomedullary Evaluation

Parameter	Normal Value	Increased in:*
Serum catecholamines	Supine, resting: Epinephrine: 0-150 μg/L Norepinephrine: 100-200 μg/L	Pheochromocytoma
Urinary vanillylmandelic acid	1.8-7 mg/24 hr	Pheochromocytoma, neuroblastoma, ganglioblastoma, physiological and emotional stress, muscle disorders

* Decreases in parameters not found in any pathological condition.

TABLE 38-7 Laboratory Assessment of Endocrine Pancreatic Function

Parameter	Normal Value	Increased in:	Decreased in:
Plasma glucose	Fasting: 70-120 mg/dl; 2 hr Postprandial: <145 mg/dl	Diabetes mellitus, Cushing's syndrome, acromegaly, stress	Hypoglycemia, adrenocortical insufficiency, malnutrition, alcoholism
Glucose tolerance	Plasma glucose at 30 min: <160 mg/ml, normal at 2 hr; no urine sugar	Diabetes mellitus	
Serum insulin	<30 μIU/ml	Insulinoma, insulin resistance	Diabetes mellitus
Glycosylated hemoglobin	<7.8%	Hyperglycemia, poorly controlled diabetes mellitus	Hemolytic states due to hemoglobin loss as opposed to decreased production
Urine copper reduction (Clinitest)	Negative	Color changes indicate glycosuria in diabetes mellitus, adrenal and thyroid dysfunction	
Urine glucose oxidase (Tes-Tape, Clinistix)	Negative	Color changes indicate glycosuria in diabetes mellitus, adrenal and thyroid dysfunction	
Urine ketone	Negative	Color changes indicate ketonuria and reliably reflect serum ketone levels; ketonuria occurs in uncontrolled diabetes mellitus and starvation	

REFERENCES

1. Baxter, J. D. (1992). Principles of endocrinology. In J. B. Wyngaarden, & L. H. Smith (Eds.), *Cecil textbook of medicine* (18th ed.) (pp. 1252-1267). Philadelphia: Saunders.
2. Becker, K. L. (1990). General principles of endocrinology. In K. Becker (Ed.), *Principles and practice in endocrinology and metabolism* (pp. 2-80). Philadelphia: Lippincott.
3. Solomon, B. L., Loriaux, T. C., & Drass, J. A. (1992). Endocrine and metabolic systems. In J. Thompson, G. K. McFarland, J. E. Hirsch, et al. (Eds.), *Mosby's manual of clinical nursing* (pp. 876-967). St Louis: Mosby–Year Book.
4. Jackson, I. M. D., & Cobb, W. E. (1986). Disorders of the thyroid. In P. Kohler (Ed.), *Clinical endocrinology* (pp. 73-166). New York: Wiley.
5. Larsen, P. R. (1992). The thyroid. In J. B. Wyngaarden, & L. H. Smith (Eds.), *Cecil textbook of medicine* (19th ed.) (pp. 1248-1271). Philadelphia: Saunders.
6. Frohman, L. A. (1992). The anterior pituitary. In J. B. Wyngaarden, & L. H. Smith (Eds.), *Cecil textbook of*

medicine (19th ed.) (pp. 1224-1238). Philadelphia: Saunders.

7. Loriaux, D. L., & Cutler, J. B., Jr. (1986). Diseases of the adrenal glands. In P. Kohler (Ed.), *Clinical endocrinology* (pp. 167-238). New York: Wiley.

8. Jordan, R. M., & Kohler, P. O. (1990). Laboratory diagnosis in endocrinology. In J. H. Stein (Ed.), *Internal medicine* (pp. 2088-2103). Boston: Little, Brown.

9. Boyd, A. E., III, Jordan, R. M., & Kohler, P. O. (1986). Disorders of the hypothalamus and anterior pituitary. In P. Kohler (Ed.), *Clinical endocrinology* (pp. 11-52). New York: Wiley.

10. Robertson, G. L. (1990). The endocrine brain and pituitary gland. In K. Becker (Ed.), *Principles and practice in endocrinology and metabolism* (pp. 92-246). Philadelphia: Lippincott.

11. Frohman, L. A. (1992). Neuroendocrine regulation and its disorders. In J. B. Wyngaarden, & L. H. Smith (Eds.), *Cecil textbook of medicine* (19th ed.) (pp. 1215-1223). Philadelphia: Saunders.

12. Moses, A. M., & Streeton, D. H. P. (1986). Disorders of the hypothalamic-neurohypophyseal system. In P. Kohler (Ed.), *Clinical endocrinology* (pp. 53-72). New York: Wiley.

13. Wilber, J. F. (1991). The current status of the TRH test. *The Endocrinologist, 1,* 45-48.

14. Loriaux, D. L. (1990). The adrenal glands. In K. Becker (Ed.), *Principles and practice in endocrinology and metabolism* (pp. 92-246). Philadelphia: Lippincott.

15. Tyrell, J. B., & Baxter, J. D. (1992). Disorders of the adrenal cortex. In J. B. Wyngaarden, & L. H. Smith (Eds.), *Cecil textbook of medicine* (19th ed.) (pp. 1271-1291). Philadelphia: Saunders.

16. Kahn, C. R. (1990). Disorders of the fuel metabolism. In K. Becker (Ed.), *Principles and practice in endocrinology and metabolism* (pp. 1032-1248). Philadelphia: Lippincott.

39

Endocrine and Diabetic Disorders

Teresa C. Loriaux

Janice A. Drass

Endocrine crises, although rare, are dramatic. When they occur, either as primary pathological events or in conjunction with other critical illnesses, prompt recognition and intervention are vital.

In this chapter, eight endocrine conditions and three diabetic comas are discussed: diabetes insipidus, syndrome of inappropriate antidiuretic hormone secretion, pituitary tumors, thyroid storm, hypothyroid crisis or myxedema coma, hypoparathyroidism, acute adrenal insufficiency, and pheochromocytoma; and hyperglycemic, hypoglycemic, and hyperosmolar comas. Pathophysiology, medical therapies, and nursing diagnoses and interventions are discussed for each condition. Some background anatomy and physiology and specific data acquisition information are integrated into the discussion of each condition; for greater detail, refer to Chapters 37 and 38.

ENDOCRINE DISORDERS

Diabetes Insipidus

Diabetes insipidus (DI) is caused by insufficient antidiuretic hormone (ADH, or vasopressin). ADH is secreted by the posterior pituitary gland. *Osmoreceptors* in the hypothalamus alter impulse generation to the posterior pituitary in response to changes in body tonicity or osmolality. Increased osmolality leads to release of ADH from the posterior pituitary. ADH secretion leads to retention of free water, thereby decreasing plasma osmolality.

Errant sensing of water overload can occur in cerebral inflammatory conditions and cerebral edema. Direct damage to the hypothalamus, the hypothalamic–hypophyseal tract, or the posterior pituitary can also produce DI, as can acute traumatic head injury, craniotomy, cerebral infarct, and metastatic or infiltrative lesions.[1]

Diabetes insipidus can also be nephrogenic in origin. In contrast to neurogenic DI, nephrogenic DI results from decreased renal responsiveness to ADH.

Diabetes insipidus can also be pharmacologically induced. Lithium and demeclocycline decrease renal responsiveness to ADH, whereas phenytoin inhibits ADH secretion.

The primary clinical problem of DI is polyuria. Hypotonic, dilute urine is excreted in large volumes— as much as 10 to 12 L per day. The excessive urinary free water loss depletes total body water and sets the stage for hyperosmolality. Fortunately, in the presence of an adequate thirst mechanism and ability to obtain and drink water, the likelihood of significant free water loss is small.

Chronic DI is uncommon. Most often, DI is related to surgical or traumatic injury of the hypothalamus, and polyuria characteristically lasts for 1 to 6 days.

Patients who are unable to respond to thirst or for whom perception of thirst is diminished are vulnerable to dangerous and potentially lethal hyperosmolality. Depressed levels of consciousness are frequent in patients unable to perceive or respond to thirst. These patients may require tube feeding or total parenteral hyperalimentation to meet nutritional needs. Unfortunately, many of the solutions used in these therapies are hypertonic, so these interventions can potentiate the existing risk of severe water deficit resulting from insufficient ADH.

Medical Management

The goal in treating DI is maintenance of normal water balance and osmolality. Fluid and hormone replacement therapy are the mainstays of medical treatment. Oral fluids are the preferred replacement. When oral fluids cannot be given, IV fluids should be set to provide a urine output of 2,400 ml per day.

Desmopressin (DDAVP), and aqueous vasopressin (Pitressin) are the two commonly used hormone replacement agents. *Desmopressin* is a synthetic form of antidiuretic hormone. It has become increasingly popular because it has markedly fewer side effects than other forms of vasopressin. It is supplied in 2.5 ml vials containing 100 μg desmopressin per ml; the daily dose ranges from 5 to 20 μg. Desmopressin is administered intranasally by means of a calibrated catheter supplied with each vial. Side effects are rare but include headache, abdominal cramps, and nausea.[2] The DDAVP daily dose should be adjusted according to urine output achieved with IV fluid replacement minus insensible losses.

Aqueous vasopressin is a water-soluble pituitary extract containing 20 U/ml of arginine vasopressin. It is usually administered subcutaneously in doses of 5 to 10 U. Its onset of action occurs in about 1 hour, and it has a duration of 3 to 4 hours.[2] It can also be administered by slow intravenous drip, but if it is, an infusion control device, electrocardiographic monitoring, and frequent recording of vital signs are recommended. Side effects include water intoxication leading to hyponatremia, irritability, and in the worst circumstance, seizures.

NURSING MANAGEMENT

In critically ill patients, diabetes insipidus most commonly accompanies cerebral insult, whether iatrogenic as a complication of surgical procedures or resulting from traumatic injuries or inflammatory processes. Nursing care must combine interventions designed to manage the effects of real and potential neurological compromise with those needed to manage the effects of insufficient ADH. Refer to Chapter 33 for discussion of nursing care for patients with neurological disorders.

The primary nursing diagnosis in diabetes insipidus is actual or potential fluid volume deficit, related to excessive fluid loss. An additional nursing diagnosis, sleep pattern disturbance related to polydipsia and nocturia, is applicable in alert, ambulatory patients.

■ NURSING DIAGNOSIS

Actual or potential fluid volume deficit, related to excessive urinary fluid loss.[3]

OUTCOME STANDARD AND CRITERIA

The targeted outcome is an adequate fluid volume as indicated by:[4]
- Stable daily weights
- Balanced intake and output
- Normal filling pressures (CVP, PAWP)
- Absence of postural hypotension
- Normal urine volumes (less than 3 L/day)
- Restoration of urine and serum osmolarity

NURSING INTERVENTIONS

Nursing management begins with early identification of patients at risk for actual or potential fluid volume deficit related to excessive urinary fluid loss. All patients unable to perceive or respond to thirst are vulnerable. That vulnerability is exaggerated by tube feedings, parenteral hyperalimentation, and either a history of or current administration of lithium, demeclocycline, or phenytoin, because, as noted earlier, the first two agents decrease renal responsiveness to ADH, whereas the third inhibits ADH secretion. In addition, any patient with a history of ongoing vasopressin replacement therapy is at risk.

Ongoing assessment centers on hydration status. Meticulous recording of body weight and of intake and output are necessary for accurate determination of trends. Urine specific gravity and plasma and urine osmolality should be recorded. In early untreated DI, urine volumes can approach 2 L/hr, and body weight can decrease dramatically without adequate fluid replacement. Characteristically, urine specific gravity is less than 1.003 and urine osmolality less than 500 mosm/kg. In contrast, plasma osmolality exceeds 295 mosm/kg. Laboratory studies reveal hemoconcentration and hypernatremia.[5]

Physical examination of the patient with fluid volume deficit related to excessive urinary loss reveals signs of water deficit or dehydration. Skin turgor is decreased, and mucous membranes appear dry and even cracked. If the condition is prolonged or untreated, signs of extracellular fluid volume depletion appear. Postural or orthostatic hypotension progresses to sustained hypotension; tachycardia also occurs and can presage impending hypovolemic shock.

Nursing interventions include administration of fluids (oral and intravenous) and pharmacological agents. During the hormone replacement process, continued vigilance needs to be directed at hydration status. Water intoxication and fluid overload can occur as a complication of aggressive replacement therapy.

Patients receiving tube feedings or parenteral hyperalimentation pose additional nursing challenges. Many of the solutions used are hypertonic. Enteric preparations can produce an osmotic fluid gradient into the gastrointestinal tract, with a net inward flow of body water. This water influx produces gastrointestinal distention, one of the most powerful stimuli to increased motility. Consequent diarrhea then worsens free water loss. Nursing interventions for patients receiving enteral alimentation include addition of supplemental water to hypertonic preparations to decrease the potential for significant osmotic influx of water into the gastrointestinal tract. Controlling the rate of administration of enteral solutions to avoid rapid delivery of large volumes can also decrease gastrointestinal distention and the likelihood of diarrhea.

Parenteral hyperalimentation involves infusion of a large glucose load, potential hyperglycemia, spilling of glucose into the urine, and initiation of osmotic diuresis. If the condition is allowed to progress, extracellular volume and water depletion compound the initial hyperosmolar state. With patients receiving parenteral hyperalimentation, even optimal vasopressin replacement may be inadequate. Free water availability is decreased, and body water that is available follows the strongest osmotic gradient. The presence of high levels of renal tubular glucose results in physiological competition for water between the tubular and interstitial spaces. In these situations, additional nursing interventions must be directed at monitoring and managing serum and urine glucose levels.

Finally, nursing interventions should be directed at preserving and promoting skin integrity and moist mucous membranes. Frequent adjustments in position, massage, and supplemental padding for bony pressure points should all be employed. Providing ice chips if the patient can take them or swabbing the mouth with a lubricant can be helpful.

Syndrome of Inappropriate ADH (SIADH)

The syndrome of inappropriate ADH (SIADH) is characterized by aberrant or sustained ADH effect in the face of hypotonic expansion of body fluids. Ingested water is not excreted. Hypotonic volume expansion increases glomerular filtration. Excessive sodium is excreted in the urine, leading to a progressive decline in body sodium. The result is a varying degree of absolute body sodium depletion, water retention, and a consequent marked decrease in serum sodium.[6]

SIADH occurs in many situations. Water retention and hyponatremia can appear postoperatively as a result of anesthetic agents, stress response, and medications such as morphine. Positive pressure ventilation can also promote increased ADH secretion through alteration of the pressure relationships involved in pulmonary volume-sensing mechanisms.

In congestive heart failure, cirrhosis of the liver, nephrosis, and interstitial sodium shifts and edema are often compounded by water retention. In these situations, ADH secretion is "inappropriate" and exaggerates and complicates the initial disease.[6]

Cerebral disease can also lead to inappropriate secretion of ADH. Intracranial lesions are thought to produce this effect by one of three possible mechanisms: (1) allowing "escape" of the hormone because of structural damage to the posterior pituitary, (2) producing an irritated focus that stimulates the posterior pituitary to release ADH, and/or (3) stimulation of the sympathetic nervous system due to cerebral hypoxia.

Intrathoracic disease can also interfere with ADH secretion. In these situations, it is thought that the neural pathways that normally translate and transmit messages regarding body fluid volume to the hypothalamus are disrupted. Normal suppression of ADH secretion fails, and ADH secretion is inappropriately increased. Intrathoracic metastatic lesions can also secrete ADH. Bronchogenic, prostatic, and pancreatic cancers can also secrete ectopic ADH.

Medical Management

When SIADH results from malignant disease, surgical resection, radiation, or chemotherapy is indicated. In SIADH associated with intracranial, pulmonary, myocardial, and hepatic or renal disease, treatment is directed at specific precipitating pathological processes. Regardless of cause, and even if the syndrome is thought to be transient, the goal of medical interventions is to restore normal free water balance.

Free water intake is restricted, and overall fluid intake is based on urine output plus insensible loss. In severe hyponatremic states, hypertonic sodium chloride infusions, intravenous furosemide or osmotic diuretics such as urea or mannitol can be used to promote water excretion.[5]

NURSING MANAGEMENT

Nursing therapies in providing care for patients with SIADH center on the goal of restoring fluid and electrolyte balance. The primary nursing diagnosis in SIADH, actual or potential fluid overload, is discussed below.

■ NURSING DIAGNOSIS

Actual or high risk for fluid volume excess, related to compromised regulatory mechanisms (excessive secretion of ADH).

OUTCOME STANDARD AND CRITERIA

Fluid intake approximates output and body weight returns to normal as evidenced by:

- Serum and urine osmolality within normal limits
- Relief of signs of water intoxication
- Alertness and orientation to surroundings
- Normal deep tendon reflexes and gastrointestinal motility

NURSING INTERVENTIONS

Nursing management begins with aggressive monitoring and identification of patients at risk for SIADH (see the box on p. 930). Ongoing assessment focuses on the status of fluid and electrolyte balance. Deliberate and sequential evaluation involves careful monitoring of intake and output, consistent recording of daily weights, and monitoring of urine and serum osmolality (urine >150 mosm/L, serum <285 mosm/L), and serum sodium (less than 135 mEq/L). Generally, unless the condition is complicated by cirrhosis or nephrosis, extracellular volume in SIADH is adequate, and blood pressure is normal with minimal postural or orthostatic changes. Dilutional hyponatremia is present due to the retention of free water. Hence, edema is not a characteristic feature of this disorder.[2]

Physical examination reveals nonedematous weight gain due to intracellular fluid excess. Early in the course of SIADH, neurological signs of water intoxication are subtle and include a decrease in level of consciousness, headache, fatigue, and weakness. Later, sensorium changes can include confusion, irritability, a sense of impending doom, restlessness, sluggish deep tendon reflexes, and seizures. Anorexia, nausea, and vomiting can also be present, reflecting the effect of hyponatremia on the gastrointestinal tract.

Nursing interventions include fluid restriction, electrolyte supplementation, and management of the neurological and gastrointestinal effects of water intoxication. Because fluid intake is restricted, the patient's environment should be controlled to limit access to fluids. Patient and visitor compliance must be assessed after the nurse has explained the nature and purpose of fluid restrictions. Similarly, the basis for behavior changes should be explained. Frequent reorientation of the patient may be required in the event of water intoxication.

Constipation can occur from the combined effects of restricted fluid intake, decreased activity, and decreased gastrointestinal motility related to hyponatremia. Enemas, if needed, should not be of the tapwater type because of the risk of water absorption.

With confusion, weakness, and the potential for seizure activity, safety measures should be instituted. Side rails should be kept up and padded if hyponatremia is severe; the bed should be kept in the lowest position, and the patient should not get up unattended. Environmental confusion should be minimized.

Finally, nursing care should be provided to limit the effects of immobilization. Frequent position changes, deep breathing, aggressive skin care, and graduated activity need to be instituted.

Pituitary Tumors

Pituitary tumors can produce ACTH (Cushing's disease), prolactin (amenorrhea-galactorrhea), GH (acromegaly), TSH, and the gonadotropins. One third of all pituitary tumors are prolactin-secreting adenomas. Tumors that secrete TSH or gonadotropin comprise less than 5% of pituitary tumors.

The clinical manifestations of a pituitary tumor depend upon its size, its encroachment on surrounding structures, and the hormones it secretes or fails to secrete. Headache is a common symptom in patients with pituitary tumors. When pituitary tumors invade the hypothalamus, temperature regulation, appetite, thirst, and sleep can be altered. Diabetes insipidus also can occur. Large pituitary tumors can affect cranial nerves III, IV, V, and VI. Visual field defects that can occur when the tumor compresses the optic chiasm include the loss of red perception, bitemporal hemianopsia, superior bitemporal defect, and scotoma. These visual field defects can progress with tumor growth. Hemorrhage into a pituitary tumor can cause severe headache, an increase in visual disturbances, cranial nerve palsy, and signs of increased intracranial pressure leading to listlessness and coma.

In adults, the hypersecretion of growth hormone by a pituitary tumor causes acromegaly. In children, excessive growth hormone secretion can lead to gigantism. Manifestations of acromegaly include enlargement of kidneys, heart (with subsequent cardiac abnormalities), spleen, and liver. Soft tissue growth enlarges the hands (ring size), feet (shoe size), and tongue (speech changes) and leads to coarsening of facial features (pronounced cheeks and jaw). Changes in bone and teeth are often recognized first by the family dentist. The anti-insulin effects of GH lead to glucose intolerance.

The most common pituitary tumor is the prolactinoma. Clinical manifestations include galactorrhea, amenorrhea or impotence, decreased libido, and visual field disturbances. Large tumors can cause hypothyroidism and adrenal insufficiency. Bromocryptine is the usual treatment.[7]

Excessive production of ACTH leads to Cushing's disease. Pituitary tumors secreting gonadotropins occur primarily in males. Clinical manifestations include visual impairment and signs of hypogonadism.

Medical Management

The radiographic techniques of computed tomography (CT scan) and magnetic resonance imaging (MRI) have made it possible to visualize tumors less than 3 mm in diameter. Radioimmunoassay (RIA) enables careful management of the various hormone levels that can be elevated or suppressed by a pituitary tumor.[8] Diagnostic procedures may include examination of GH, ACTH, prolactin, cortisol, and TSH levels.

Bromocryptine, a dopamine agonist, is the preferred treatment for prolactinoma and can often be used to treat acromegaly. Surgical removal of the pituitary tumor, transsphenoidal microadenomectomy, is generally employed for acromegaly and Cushing's disease. Indications for hypophysectomy include visual field deterioration, hydrocephalus, Cushing's syndrome, acromegaly, and pituitary apoplexy. Transsphenoidal hypophysectomy is contraindicated during a nasal or sphenoid sinus infection.

The pituitary gland is usually approached via the transsphenoidal route, which provides direct access to the sella turcica. Surgery is performed with the patient in a sitting position. An incision is made in the upper gum line and a nasal speculum provides access to the sphenoid sinus and floor of the sella turcica. This surgical approach is relatively safe, avoids entering the cranium, and leaves no visible surgical scar. After the tumor has been resected, the opening in the sella is packed with a muscle graft.

When tumor size or shape or an abnormal anatomy of cerebral blood vessels prevents surgical access via the transsphenoidal route, a transfrontal craniotomy can be performed. Medical and nursing management is usually the same as for a patient undergoing a craniotomy (see Chapter 33).

NURSING MANAGEMENT

The most common postoperative complication of hypophysectomy is diabetes insipidus: 40% of patients develop transient diabetes insipidus, which usually resolves within 3 months. However, 10% of patients develop persistent diabetes insipidus and may require life-long vasopressin replacement (usually in the form of intranasal DDAVP). Nursing management of diabetes insipidus should include monitoring urine volume, ensuring adequate fluid replacement, and administering vasopressin.

Patients should be observed carefully for signs of infection, particularly meningeal signs. Rhinorrhea

suggests a cerebrospinal fluid (CSF) leak and should be tested. Frequent assessment for visual changes should be performed.[7]

Postoperative care includes the maintenance of nasal packing and a moustache dressing for 2 to 3 days after surgery. To avoid displacement of the packing and muscle graft, the patient should be instructed to avoid blowing the nose, sneezing, coughing, or bending over at the waist (head lowered). Tooth brushing should be restricted for 2 weeks; oral hygiene can be performed with a saline or a half-strength peroxide solution flavored with mouthwash.

Nursing management of the patient undergoing transsphenoidal surgery requires understanding about the surgical approach, the hormonal effects of the tumor, the postoperative care needed to prevent and respond to surgical complications, and the need for hormonal replacement following surgery.

■ NURSING DIAGNOSIS

Knowledge deficit, related to lack of understanding of diagnosis and surgical procedure.

OUTCOME STANDARD AND CRITERIA

The patient will have adequate knowledge for self-care as indicated by verbalization of expected procedures and alterations in ADLs.

NURSING INTERVENTIONS

Patient teaching should include explanations of diagnostic tests and procedures and the indication for transsphenoidal surgery. Preoperative instruction also should include the postoperative restrictions: no brushing teeth for 2 weeks after surgery and alternatives for oral care; avoidance of sneezing, coughing, and blowing the nose; potential fluid restrictions. Nasal packing causes some discomfort and makes it necessary to breathe through the mouth. Lips should be moisturized to prevent cracking while mouth breathing is necessary. Patients should be warned to expect a decrease in sense of taste and smell for a few months following surgery.

HIGH-RISK NURSING DIAGNOSIS

High risk for fluid volume deficit, related to possible onset of diabetes insipidus.

OUTCOME STANDARD AND CRITERIA

The patient will not experience undetected diabetes insipidus as evidenced by documented fluid balance assessment.

NURSING INTERVENTIONS

Urine should be tested for osmolality, and serum electrolytes and osmolality should be monitored. Urine specific gravity can be used to monitor the patient's ability to concentrate urine. Intake and output should be carefully measured and documented.

■ NURSING DIAGNOSIS

Knowledge deficit, related to need for hormonal replacement.

OUTCOME STANDARD AND CRITERIA

The patient will have adequate knowledge for self-management of hormonal replacement and emergency procedures as evidenced by verbalization and return demonstration of procedures.

NURSING INTERVENTIONS

Depending on residual pituitary function following surgery, the patient may need to replace hydrocortisone, vasopressin, gonadotropins, estrogen, or testosterone. These needs depend upon surgical outcome and the patient's reproductive choices. Patient teaching includes the dosage, schedule, and route of administration. If the patient requires hydrocortisone replacement therapy, self-injection must be demonstrated by the patient prior to discharge. An emergency identification bracelet should be provided indicating the need for hydrocortisone in the event of trauma. A wallet card can provide diagnosis, medications, and emergency phone numbers (including health care provider). Patients should be instructed to carry an emergency hydrocortisone injection kit, and family members or significant individuals should be included in the teaching.

Thyroid Storm

Hyperthyroid crises (thyrotoxic crisis, thyroid storm) is an emergency state that occurs in untreated or inadequately treated patients with hyperthyroidism. It is precipitated by febrile illness; physiological stress such as injury, surgery, diabetic ketoacidosis, or toxemia of pregnancy; and psychological trauma. The mechanism is unclear.

The most common cause of hyperthyroidism is Graves' disease. Thyroid hormone–induced increases in metabolic rate promote development of a negative nitrogen balance because protein and fat are catabolized to meet increased energy needs. Characteristics of Graves' disease include weight loss and heat intolerance, both of which reflect the effect of increased metabolic rate. *Exophthalmos*, or bulging ocular orbits, is a hallmark of Graves' disease. It reflects inflammatory disease of the retrobulbar tissues.[9]

Other causes of hyperthyroidism include hyperfunctioning thyroid adenomas (often called *hot nodules*), toxic multinodular goiter, early granulomatous thyroiditis, TSH-producing pituitary adenomas, thyroid carcinomas, and ingestion of excessive amounts of thyroid hormone. In all these conditions, hyperthyroidism can lead to clinical findings that include nervousness and tremors; warm, pink skin; hyperthermia; increased pulse and pulse pressure; and increased urine output. Potentiation of catecholamines in neurotransmission with increased excitability of peripheral reflexes is probably the basis for the nervousness and tremors. Warm, pink skin reflects activation of heat-dissipating mechanisms (vasodilation), necessary because the increased metabolic rate produces hyperthermia. Increased pulse rate and pressure and increased urine output reflect compensatory increases in cardiac output and glomerular filtration.

High-output cardiac failure can occur if compensatory increases in cardiac output are inadequate to maintain tissue perfusion. Hyperthyroid persons are vulnerable to liver failure. Hepatic glycogen stores are chronically depleted in an attempt to meet increased metabolic needs. Such glycogen depletion increases susceptibility to hepatic injury and degeneration.[10]

Thyrotoxic crisis was once thought to be caused by a sudden increase in circulating thyroid hormone, presumably due to exacerbation of underlying hyperthyroidism. Laboratory studies, however, have not found levels of thyroid hormones during thyroid storm to be significantly higher than those characteristic of the hyperthyroid state. It may be that an abrupt but transient release precipitates thyrotoxic crisis.[10]

An alternative precipitatory theory is the basis for the alternate name *decompensated thyrotoxicosis* often applied to thyrotoxic crisis. According to this hypothesis, crisis occurs when peripheral tissues are no longer able to respond to elevated circulating levels of thyroid hormones. Catecholamines are potentiated by thyroid hormones, and prolonged adrenergic influence could certainly predispose tissues to decompensation.[9] In crisis states, cardiac exhaustion is a prominent feature, and heat can no longer be effectively dissipated. Since thyrotoxic crisis often occurs with or shortly after febrile illness and other stress reactions, the decompensation theory for the crisis state seems plausible.

Clinical findings in thyrotoxic crisis are similar to those of hyperthyroidism but are more severe. Hyperthermia can be extreme and cardiac and gastrointestinal decompensation pronounced. Tachycardia is marked and unrelenting and is frequently accompanied by congestive failure and angina. Hyperdefecation and vomiting are also common.

Medical Management

Treatment for hyperthyroidism is either ablative (radioactive iodine or surgery) or nonablative (antithyroid pharmacological agents). Two thionamides, propylthiouracil (PTU) and methimazole (MMI), are used to treat hyperthyroidism. These agents block organification of iodine, thereby decreasing formation of thyroid hormones. PTU is administered orally, initially 100 mg three times a day. As levels of thyroid hormone normalize, the dose is decreased to 50 to 200 mg daily in equally divided doses. MMI has 10 times the potency of PTU, and the usual starting dose is 10 mg three times a day. MMI has a longer half-life than PTU. One dose of 5 to 10 mg daily often suffices for chronic long-term therapy.[9] PTU is frequently preferred over MMI in thyrotoxic crisis because it blocks peripheral conversion of thyroxine to T_3. PTU is administered orally, by nasogastric tube if necessary, 300 mg every 6 hours. In conjunction with PTU, iodine is administered to inhibit thyroid hormone release. Saturated solution of potassium iodide (SSKI) contains about 50 mg of iodine per drop; in crisis states it is given orally, 10 drops every 8 hours, beginning shortly after the first dose of PTU. As an alternative, sodium iodide may be given intravenously 1 to 2 g per day.[10]

Since thyroid hormones have a prolonged half-life, blocking synthesis and release of new hormone is not sufficient in crisis states; the effects of circulating hormone must also be decreased. Sympatholytic agents, most commonly propranolol in doses of 1 to 3 mg IV or 20 to 40 mg PO every 2 to 4 hours, are indicated unless there is a history of asthma or congestive failure independent of the thyrotoxic state.[10] Reserpine or guanethidine can also be used.[10]

To facilitate the blockade of T_4 to T_3 conversion established with PTU, 2 mg dexamethasone PO are given every 6 hours. Digitalis preparations are often used to relieve congestive failure and antipyretics to control body temperature. High-calorie nutritional support, frequently with supplemental vitamin B complex, is provided, as is intravenous fluid therapy. Levels for both caloric and fluid intake are significantly above normal levels because of the need to respond to extreme hypermetabolism.

NURSING MANAGEMENT

Nursing care in thyrotoxic crisis must combine interventions addressing precipitating factors with those necessary because of the profound hypermetabolic emergency state. Frequent multisystem evaluation is necessary, including cardiac, respiratory, neurological, and gastrointestinal assessments.

HIGH-RISK NURSING DIAGNOSIS

Altered nutrition: high risk for less than body requirements, related to hypermetabolism.

Focused assessment addresses nutritional and metabolic status. Appetite and food intake are typically increased, but the patient nonetheless loses weight. Mild hyperdefecation occurs, reflecting autonomic hyperactivity and the effect of thyroid hormones on intestinal motility.

Reflective of catabolism, anthropometric measurements frequently fall at 90% of reference levels or below for midarm circumference, midarm muscle circumference, and triceps skinfold thickness. Muscle weakness is present, and muscle wasting is often visible. Rapid protein turnover leads to soft, fine hair (*lanugo*) and friable nails; frequently the free margin

of the nails is lifted from its base (*onycholysis*).

Serum proteins, particularly albumin, may be decreased. Other hematologic findings may include neutropenia, lymphocytosis, anemia, and increased red cell mass due to the excessive demand for oxygen.[5]

OUTCOME STANDARD AND CRITERIA

The desired outcome is adequate nutritional intake to meet metabolic demands as evidenced by:[4]
- Normal serum protein
- Stabilized weight
- Normal serum transferrin and iron-binding capacity

NURSING INTERVENTIONS

Nursing interventions focus on the provision of a diet high in calories, protein, and carbohydrates. This includes administration of glucose-rich infusions and monitoring for appropriate glucose metabolism. Serum and urinary glucose must be monitored. Hyperglycemia can occur from increased glycogenolysis, impaired insulin secretion, and insulin resistance associated with elevated glucocorticoids and the physiological stress response. Frequent feedings should be provided to counteract losses from bowel hypermotility. Foods known to increase peristalsis (including coffee, tea, and colas) should be avoided. Visitors should be encouraged to supply favorite foods and beverages. A dietary consultation should be obtained to assure well-balanced, nutritionally sound meals. Daily weight and caloric consumption should be monitored and carefully recorded.[3]

In administering pharmacological agents, hypermetabolism should be kept in mind. Because of the greatly increased metabolic rate, drug turnover and degradation are accelerated; above-normal dosages given at shorter intervals than usual may be required.

■ NURSING DIAGNOSIS

Impaired thermal regulation, related to insufficient heat dissipation.

In thyrotoxic crisis, hypermetabolism is pronounced and tissue decompensation, most notably cardiac exhaustion, impairs effective heat dissipation. Nursing assessment should include body temperature. Cardiovascular assessment reveals an increased systolic blood pressure, widening of pulse pressure, tachycardia, and dysrhythmias. Flushed, moist skin is common and heat intolerance profound. Fever may approach 41.1° C (106° F) and can be triggered by minor infections.

OUTCOME STANDARD AND CRITERIA

Body temperature is within normal limits (36.6° to 37.5° C or 97.8° to 99.4° F).

NURSING INTERVENTIONS

Nursing interventions center on fever reduction. Antipyretic agents, usually acetaminophen, are administered. Aspirin is not recommended in thyrotoxic crisis because it displaces thyroid hormone from its carrier protein, thereby increasing free hormone levels. Hypothermal blankets, tepid baths, fans, and ice packs over major vessels are also used. Cooling methods should be tapered at 38° C (100.4° F).

■ NURSING DIAGNOSIS

Sleep pattern disturbance, related to insomnia.

Elevated thyroid hormone levels directly impair sleep. Insomnia is a frequent problem. Non-REM and REM sleep debts may develop from an inability to obtain adequate sleep. Non-REM sleep debts lead to physical fatigue and malaise; in thyrotoxic crisis these effects no doubt exaggerate the effects of muscle weakness. REM debts may induce disorientation, suspiciousness, and withdrawal; paranoia and even hallucinations can occur in severe deprivation (see Chapter 13).

OUTCOME STANDARD AND CRITERIA

Sleep is adequate as evidenced by:
• Absence of fatigue and malaise
• Alertness and orientation to surroundings

NURSING INTERVENTIONS

Nursing therapies center on minimizing fatigue by providing frequent uninterrupted rest periods. Attention must also be given to promoting a restful environment, enhancing patient comfort and promoting relaxation through back rubs and position changes, and ensuring patient privacy.

■ NURSING DIAGNOSIS

Impaired gas exchange, related to dyspnea.

Elevated thyroid hormone levels increase peripheral tissue oxygen consumption. Increased demand, coupled with intercostal muscle weakness and resultant dyspnea, produces the potential for impaired gas exchange. In thyrotoxic crisis, increased oxygen demand is further exaggerated by extreme hypermetabolism. Additional respiratory compromise is caused by cardiac failure and pulmonary edema. Respiratory failure may occur.

OUTCOME STANDARD AND CRITERIA

Gas exchange is adequate as evidenced by:
• Normal respiratory rate
• Absence of dyspnea, cyanosis, or restlessness
• Normal arterial blood gas levels

NURSING INTERVENTIONS

Nursing interventions include serial assessments of pulmonary function. Arterial blood gases should be monitored and breath sounds auscultated regularly. Patient activity needs to be paced to conserve energy and allow for uninterrupted rest periods.

■ NURSING DIAGNOSIS

Sensory/perceptual alterations: overload, related to hypersensitivity to the environment.

Increased thyroid hormone levels and potentiation of catecholamines lead to excessive adrenergic activity. Hypersensitivity to the environment is manifested by exaggerated alertness, inability to relax and, frequently, overreaction to almost all stimuli. In thyrotoxic crisis, hypersensitivity is pronounced; patients often have a shortened attention span and are agitated and nervous. REM sleep deprivation can compound symptoms by adding suspiciousness and paranoia. Delirium and emotional lability may progress to psychosis.[5]

OUTCOME STANDARD AND CRITERIA

Response to sensory/perceptual stimuli is appropriate as evidenced by:
• Orientation to time, place, person
• Accurate descriptions of the environment

NURSING INTERVENTIONS

Nursing interventions center on providing structure, consistency, and simplicity in care activities. The scope of the environment should be limited; a private room is desirable. External stimuli should be minimized to avoid distraction and confusion.

Frequent, even repetitive, reassurances and calm explanations are needed. The number of caregivers and the frequency of instructions should be limited to minimize confusion. Safety measures should be instituted if the patient is delirious; side rails should be kept up and the bed maintained in the lowest position. The patient should not be allowed to get up without assistance.

COLLABORATIVE PROBLEMS
• Altered cardiac output, related to excessive demand
• Decreased cardiac output, related to dysrhythmias

Thyroid hormones increase metabolic rate and stimulate oxygen consumption throughout the body. Demand on cardiac function is thus increased in hyperthyroid states. Thyroid hormones also directly affect the myocardium. Palpitations, tachycardia and tachydysrhythmias (typically atrial fibrillation and paroxysmal atrial tachycardia), systolic hypertension, and increased pulse pressure are common findings. In thyrotoxic crisis these findings are often accompanied by angina and signal impending myocardial failure and decompensation.[10] Acute pulmonary edema and anasarca may develop. In the elderly, as well as those patients with preexisting cardiovascular disease, signs of cardiovascular compromise may dominate the clinical presentation in thyrotoxic crisis.

NURSING INTERVENTIONS

Nursing interventions include administration of agents to control cardiac dysrhythmias. Rhythm disturbances frequently are refractory until the effects of thyroid hormones have been blocked. Sympatholytic agents are also administered. Their effects must be monitored carefully, especially if the patient has a history of asthma or congestive heart failure. Ongoing cardiac assessment requires dynamic monitoring of heart rate and rhythm and blood pressure.

Myxedema Coma

Myxedema coma is the extreme of hypothyroidism and represents a life-threatening emergency. It can be precipitated by infection, trauma, critical illness, exposure to cold, or administration of sedatives, anesthetics, narcotics, or psychotropic drugs. It can also be caused by insufficient thyroid hormone replacement after thyroidectomy or ablative therapy, traumatic injury to the thyroid gland, or chronic or autoimmune thyroiditis.

In hypothyroidism without crisis, the effect of insufficient thyroid hormone levels is reflected in the clinical findings: decreased metabolic rate, weight gain, and intolerance of cold. Reflexes and mentation are frequently slowed. Cutaneous accumulations of water and protein–polysaccharide compounds occur as a result of slowed metabolism and protein synthesis. A puffy appearance and a nonpitting edema provide the basis for referring to adult hypothyroidism as myxedema.

With the onset of myxedema coma, all symptoms of hypothyroidism are exaggerated. Hypothermia is so pronounced that thermometer malfunction is often suspected. Hypercarbia and hypoventilation are common and probably reflect the effects of reduced ventilatory capacity due to interstitial accumulations of mucopolysaccharides, lesions in the respiratory muscles, and decreased responsiveness in the central nervous system respiratory center.[10] Decreased myocardial contractility leads to severe hypotension and bradycardia. Level of consciousness is significantly depressed, and frank coma can develop. Hypoglycemia occurs, probably reflecting the effect of decreased caloric intake in the obtunded state and decreased gluconeogenesis due to hypometabolism. Mild to severe dilutional hyponatremia also accompanies myxedema coma. A decreased glomerular filtration rate and superimposed SIADH are the most likely causes.[10]

Medical Management

Thyroxine (T_4) (Synthroid, levothyroxine) is usually used for hormone replacement in myxedema crisis. It is given intravenously (2 μg/kg over 5 to 10 minutes), followed by 100 μg IV daily. This approach must be used with extreme caution in the presence of cardiac disease. Oral administration of thyroid hormone replacement is inappropriate in myxedema crisis because of the likelihood of ileus and poor gastrointestinal absorption. As clinical improvement begins, the IV dose is gradually adjusted downward, and oral replacement is resumed.

Respiratory acidosis and hypercarbia are treated by intubation and mechanical ventilation. Hypotension is treated by volume expansion, hormone replacement, and glucocorticoids if necessary. Pressor agents are usually avoided because the risk of cardiac dysrhythmias and myocardial decompensation with increased peripheral resistance. Glucose-containing fluids are administered intravenously on the basis of serum glucose values. Hypotonic solutions and free water are avoided, however, because of the risk that the hyponatremia will be worsened.[12]

NURSING MANAGEMENT

Nursing care in myxedema coma involves interventions directed at reversal of the precipitating event and the acute thyroid hormone deficiency. Frequent nursing assessment focusing on cardiac, respiratory, and neurological function as well as hydration and metabolic status is required.

■ **NURSING DIAGNOSIS**

Impaired gas exchange, related to decreased ventilatory capacity.

OUTCOME STANDARD AND CRITERIA

Hypoxia and hypercapnia are absent or reduced as evidenced by arterial blood gas levels within normal ranges.

NURSING INTERVENTIONS

Assessment addresses adequacy of ventilation and oxygenation and focuses on potential for respiratory depression. Initially, mechanical ventilatory support may be needed to control respiratory acidosis. Serial pulmonary auscultation to ensure optimal ventilation of all lung fields and monitoring of arterial blood gases are required. When the patient no longer needs mechanical ventilatory assistance, serial monitoring of lung sounds and blood gases is important, as are frequent repositioning and encouragement of deep breathing. Decreased ventilatory capacity occurs from interstitial accumulations of mucopolysaccharides and compromised respiratory musculature. Decreased responsiveness of the central nervous system respiratory center leads to continuing vulnerability to respiratory insufficiency as the crisis state is reversed and peripheral oxygen demands increase.

Pharmacological agents with a potential for respiratory depression are to be avoided. Delayed metabolism and degradation of agents in the myxedematous state should be considered when calculating dosages. Lower doses may be indicated.

■ **NURSING DIAGNOSIS**

Hypothermia, related to decreased metabolic rate.

OUTCOME STANDARD AND CRITERIA

Body temperature is within normal limits as described earlier.

NURSING INTERVENTIONS

Hypothermia is profound in myxedema coma as a result of severe hypometabolism. Generally, the lower the temperature, the worse the prognosis. Nursing interventions to raise body temperature are needed. It is essential, however, that efforts be gradual. Rapid rewarming can place an excessive or sudden demand on an already compromised and depressed myocardium by increasing peripheral oxygen requirements and decreasing vascular tone. Room temperature should be increased (75° F) and extra blankets provided. Warming lights and externally warmed blankets may be used. Core body temperature must be monitored frequently. Arterial blood gases should be monitored. Laboratory studies should include serum electrolyte, BUN, creatinine, and glucose.

■ NURSING DIAGNOSIS

Fluid volume excess, related to decreased cardiac output and impaired regulatory mechanisms.

Insufficient thyroid hormone in myxedema coma leads to depressed cardiovascular function, decreased glomerular filtration, and impaired free water clearance. Congestive failure may alter intrathoracic pressure relationships and cause concurrent SIADH, with aggravation of total body water excess. Nursing assessment centers on evaluation of cardiac and respiratory status and hydration.

Assessment involves careful monitoring of intake and output, consistent recording of daily weights, and monitoring of urine and serum osmolality and serum sodium. Clinically, physical examination reveals weight gain without edema because fluid excess is intracellular.

Monitoring for actual or potential water intoxication includes neurological assessment. Complaints of headache, fatigue, and weakness and a deteriorating level of consciousness are associated with early water intoxication. In myxedema coma, however, these signs can be obscured by the existing depressed level of consciousness. The sluggish deep tendon reflexes, confusion, agitation and restlessness, and sense of impending doom that accompany pronounced water intoxication (SIADH) may also be masked.

OUTCOME STANDARD AND CRITERIA

Fluid volume is adequate as evidenced by:
- Absence of pulmonary congestion and acute dyspnea
- Normal filling pressures and serum and urine osmolarity

NURSING INTERVENTIONS

Seizures may occur in severe hyponatremia; therefore, nursing interventions should ensure patient safety. Padding of side rails and keeping the side rails up and the bed in the lowest position are indicated. Other measures include vigorous skin care, frequent repositioning, and provision of padding over bony pressure points.

Nursing interventions include careful administration of fluid as well as diuretics and glucose. The treatment goal is to reverse dilutional hyponatremia and restrict free water intake.

If seizures are present or hyponatremia is severe, hypertonic sodium chloride solutions with concurrent furosemide can be used. Osmotic diuretics are generally not indicated in myxedema coma because the mobilization of excessive free water from the intracellular space poses too great a risk for cardiac decompensation. Infusion control devices help ensure delivery of appropriate amounts of fluid.

If the patient is capable of ingesting oral fluids, the nature and purpose of water restrictions should be explained. Although occasional ice chips can be provided, they must be included in the intake measurement. Access to fluid must be prevented. Frequent mouth care can help the patient tolerate water restrictions.

Glucose-containing infusions provide caloric intake. Extreme hypermetabolism lowers nutritional requirements. Nonetheless, because hypoglycemia often occurs in myxedema coma, nursing interventions should include glucose monitoring.

As the patient improves and oral intake resumes, the potential for impaired bowel function must be considered. Low-calorie, well-balanced meals high in fiber should be supplied. Constipation, abdominal distention, and paralytic ileus can occur in extreme hypothyroid states. Nursing interventions should include assessment of gastrointestinal function. Bowel sounds should be auscultated and abdominal girth measured. If constipation occurs, enemas can be instituted. Tap-water enemas, however, should not be used because of the potential for free water absorption from the colon.

COLLABORATIVE PROBLEM

Decreased cardiac output, related to depressed myocardial function.

An insufficiency of thyroid hormone decreases myocardial contractility. Hypotension and bradycardia may be severe. Thus, assessment focuses on the adequacy of cardiovascular function. Continuous electrocardiographic and hemodynamic monitoring is indicated. The ECG is likely to show low voltage and prolongation of the QT interval. Clinically, heart sounds may be distant, and pericardial effusion may occur. Chest x-rays typically reveal cardiomegaly.[8]

NURSING INTERVENTIONS

Nursing interventions include consistent serial monitoring of cardiovascular response as thyroid hormone replacement is provided and body temperature rises. Hormone replacement and correction of hypothermia may increase myocardial demand and precipitate tachydysrhythmias, ischemia with angina, and congestive failure. Hypotension is usually treated with volume expansion, glucocorticoid support, and thyroid hormone replacement. Pressor agents are generally avoided because of the risk of dysrhythmias, excessive stimulation of the depressed myocardium, and increased peripheral resistance.

Hypoparathyroidism

Hypoparathyroidism occurs when the parathyroid glands fail to produce an amount of parathyroid hormone sufficient to maintain normal serum calcium levels. This can seriously compromise cardiac, respiratory, and skeletal muscle function.

Hypoparathyroidism can result from ischemia; damage to or inadvertent removal of parathyroid tissue during neck surgery for thyroid or other disorders; or damage to the gland from neoplasms, autoimmune processes or infiltrative diseases. Hypomagnesemia (as in chronic alcoholism and malabsorption syndromes) can also cause parathormone insufficiency because decreased magnesium levels interfere with parathyroid hormone. Pseudohypoparathyroidism is a genetic disorder characterized by peripheral resistance to the actions of parathormone.[11]

An insufficiency of parathormone increases renal calcium loss and decreases renal phosphate excretion; generally, there is a reciprocal relationship between serum ionized calcium and phosphate levels. Along with the ensuing hypocalcemia, mild metabolic alkalosis also develops because bicarbonate excretion is decreased. Other effects of parathormone insufficiency exaggerate the impact of increased renal calcium excretion and include a decrease in bone resorption, vitamin D activation, and gastrointestinal calcium absorption.

Clinically, the findings associated with hypoparathyroidism reflect hypocalcemia. Even minor reductions in serum calcium increase neuromuscular excitability and cause muscle tremors and cramps. Numbness and tingling in the extremities and circumoral area may occur.

With severe reductions in serum calcium, tetany, or muscle twitching and spasm without effective contraction, and generalized tonic-clonic seizures may develop. Two hallmarks of the disorder are:
A positive *Chvostek's sign,* or unilateral twitching and muscle spasm of the upper lip in response to a supramandibular finger tap over the parotid gland
A positive *Trousseau's sign,* or carpopedal spasm in response to inflation of a blood pressure cuff.

Diarrhea, abdominal cramps, and biliary colic are also common. Spasm in the bronchial and laryngeal musculature can produce laryngeal stridor, wheezes, and labored breathing. In an extreme form, tetany of the respiratory musculature results in respiratory arrest.

Hypocalcemia also directly impairs cardiac func-

tion. Bradycardia with first- and second-degree blocks can progress to cardiac arrest. Myocardial contractility is also decreased, and this decrease can lead to a decrease in cardiac output and blood pressure. Electrocardiographic changes include prolongation of the ST and QT intervals. Low prothrombin levels are also seen in hypocalcemia.[11]

Medical Management

In chronic hypoparathyroidism, supplemental oral calcium and vitamin D are required. Many calcium supplements are available: calcium lactate (8 g = 1 g calcium), calcium gluconate (10 g = 1 g calcium), or calcium carbonate (2.5 g = 1 g calcium). Generally, 1 to 3 g of calcium is the daily dosage.[11]

Vitamin D supplement is provided either by administering 50,000 to 100,000 IU of vitamin D daily or by using a daily dosage of 0.25 to 0.50 μg of 1,25-dihydroxyvitamin D. The latter is preferred in documented hypoparathyroidism because conversion of vitamin D to the active form is impaired in parathormone insufficiency.

In acute hypoparathyroid states manifested by significant hypocalcemia, signs of pronounced neuromuscular excitability, and cardiac or respiratory compromise, calcium is provided intravenously. Typically, 10 ml of a 10% calcium gluconate solution is infused over 10 minutes. Sustained infusions involving 10 to 15 mg per kg over 4 to 8 hours can also be used. Serial monitoring of serum calcium is a fundamental element of medical treatment.[11]

NURSING MANAGEMENT

Hypoparathyroidism in critically ill patients is often associated with surgical procedures involving the neck or ablative treatment of the thyroid. It can occur in the immediate postoperative period or develop over time. Nursing management begins with identification of patients at risk for hypoparathyroidism.

COLLABORATIVE PROBLEM

Decreased cardiac output, related to hypocalcemia.

Hypocalcemia in hypoparathyroidism profoundly affects the myocardium; nursing assessment centers on evaluation of cardiovascular status. Electrocardiographic monitoring is needed to detect and evaluate changes in the ST and QT intervals, heart rate, and rhythm. Hemodynamic monitoring can be used to evaluate cardiac output in severe hypocalcemia. Vital signs should be assessed serially at a frequency appropriate to the patient's condition. Because hypocalcemia causes insensitivity to digitalis, it is important to continue to monitor cardiovascular status after serum calcium levels rise to prevent digitalis toxicity. Intake and output and daily weights should be monitored as part of the evaluation of cardiac function.

NURSING INTERVENTIONS

Nursing interventions include administration of fluids and calcium replacement preparations in collaboration with physician prescriptions. Infusion control devices should be employed to ensure an appropriate rate of administration of fluid and calcium. Overly rapid infusion of calcium solutions can enhance the effect of cardiac glycosides and lead to cardiac arrest. Finally, regular assessment of intravenous line patency is needed to avoid tissue necrosis caused by calcium extravasation.

When the patient is able to eat, a high-calcium diet should be instituted, and high-calcium snacks should be available.

■ **NURSING DIAGNOSIS**

Impaired mobility, related to increased neuromuscular excitability.

Increased neuromuscular excitability with a likelihood of spasm, tetany, and cramping accompany hypoparathyroidism-induced hypocalcemia. Assessment focuses on neuromuscular status. Serial checking for positive Chvostek's and Trousseau's signs as described earlier is indicated. The presence of paresthesias, numbness, or tingling should be determined.

OUTCOME STANDARD AND CRITERIA

Mobility is increased as evidenced by:
- Ability to perform purposeful and desired movements[4]
- Absence of pain, spasms, and tetany

NURSING INTERVENTIONS

Nursing intervention is directed toward preventing spasm and tetany and improving activity tolerance. Assistance with moving and repositioning should be provided gently and at a pace determined by the patient. Positions that might promote or aggravate muscle spasm by putting pressure on motor nerves should be avoided: the legs should not be crossed, and care should be taken to prevent overcompression of the arms when the patient is in the side-lying position. Moist heat can help prevent spasms, and passive or limited active range of motion exercises may decrease the discomfort associated with numbness and tingling. Finally, providing frequent rest periods and minimizing demands are important to avoid fatigue.

Seizure activity can occur with profound hypocalcemia. Safety measures must be instituted: side rails should be padded and kept in the upright position. The bed should be kept in the lowest position. Anticonvulsant medications should be immediately available.

■ **NURSING DIAGNOSIS**

Alterations in thought processes or moods. Hypocalcemia is often associated with mood changes, irritability, and depression.

Nursing assessment focuses on changes in mood and thought processes, symptoms of depression, and evaluation of current coping skills and support systems.

OUTCOME STANDARD AND CRITERIA

The patient will exhibit normal thought processes as evidenced by:
- Clear communication
- Participation in care as appropriate

NURSING INTERVENTIONS

Nursing interventions include reassurance about the temporary nature and basis of these changes. Providing an accepting, quiet environment and anticipating comfort needs can be helpful in promoting effective patient coping. The nurse should limit environmental stimuli and explain extraneous and unfamiliar occurrences.

Acute Adrenal Insufficiency

Chronic adrenal insufficiency is either primary or secondary in nature. Primary chronic adrenal insufficiency occurs with bilateral destruction of the glands. Secondary chronic adrenal insufficiency involves disorders of the hypothalamic–pituitary axis and resultant impaired secretion of adrenocorticotropic hormone (ACTH)[12] (see Chapter 37). Addisonian or adrenal crisis is an emergency characterized by the syndrome of cardiogenic shock.

Glucocorticoid deficiency also leads to water retention, hypoglycemia, and failure to respond to norepinephrine from adrenergic nerve endings. The latter condition promotes vascular dilatation and hemodynamic collapse. Mineralocorticoid deficiency compounds the problem by allowing excessive renal sodium excretion, extracellular volume depletion, and potassium retention. Clinically, the findings include hyponatremia, hypoglycemia, hypotension, hypovolemia, and hyperkalemia. Hyperthermia may also be present but does not always occur and is poorly understood.

Medical Management

Chronic adrenal insufficiency is treated with glucocorticoid replacement. Mineralocorticoid replacement may also be used but is not always necessary because glucocorticoids exert some mineralocorticoid effect and, in combination with an elevated salt intake, may suffice.

Hydrocortisone should be given in a dose of 12 to 15 mg/m². If mineralocorticoid replacement is needed, 0.1 to 0.2 mg fludrocortisone is given orally, once a day.

If superimposed acute illness is present, especially involving fever or potential extracellular volume depletion as with vomiting or diarrhea, replacement doses of glucocorticoids are at least doubled. Vomiting within an hour after ingestion of the replacement dose cancels the dose, and readministration is required. In severe illness, the replacement dose of glucocorticoids may be more than doubled.[12]

Adrenal crisis requires supraphysiological doses of replacement glucocorticoids and rapid volume restoration. Blood samples are obtained for measurement of glucose, electrolytes, and cortisol, but treatment is initiated immediately without waiting for results if there is clinical suspicion of adrenal crisis. An intravenous bolus of 100 mg of hydrocortisone succinate, hydrocortisone phosphate, or an equivalent is followed by either repeat doses every 6 to 8 hours or continuous infusion. Intravenous mineralocorticoid preparations are not available, but large doses of hydrocortisone coupled with volume restoration generally correct hypotension. If hypotension remains a problem even with glucocorticoid and fluid replacement, volume expanders may be used.[14]

Fluid replacement in adrenal crisis should be aggressive. Glucose-containing physiological saline is used at the outset. There may be a deficit of several liters, and fluid replacement must be rapid. Typically, the first liter is infused within 60 minutes, followed by 1 to 2 L over the ensuing 4 to 8 hours.[12]

NURSING MANAGEMENT

Nursing management of patients with acute adrenal insufficiency begins with recognition of those at risk for crisis. Patients with chronic Addison's disease can develop adrenal crisis during periods of stress associated with critical illness. Overwhelming sepsis, especially involving mennigococci, staphylococci, pneumococci, streptococci, or *Haemophilus influenzae*, can precipitate adrenal crisis, as may hemorrhagic disorders and leukemic crisis. Finally, intense and prolonged critical illness has been known to trigger adrenal crisis in persons with no prior history of adrenal insufficiency. In this circumstance, stress-induced hypothalamic secretion of CRH and pituitary secretion of ACTH overstimulate the adrenal cortex. Glandular decompensation results and is often accompanied by internal decompensation, hemorrhage, and glandular destruction.[5]

The development of headache or abdominal, leg, and back pain can indicate an impending adrenal crisis in the patient with adrenal insufficiency. The patient should be encouraged to report the onset of pain immediately.

Hydrocortisone replacement administered parenterally and comfort measures should be initiated. Pain should subside with glucocorticoid replacement.

■ NURSING DIAGNOSIS

Fluid volume deficit, related to mineralocorticoid deficiency.

Insufficient mineralocorticoid activity in adrenal crisis leads to excessive renal sodium excretion and extracellular volume deficiency. Ongoing nursing assessment must center on evaluation of hydration status. Assessment includes careful monitoring of intake and output, consistent recording of daily weights, and monitoring for adequacy of central and peripheral perfusion. Blood pressure and heart rate should be monitored closely. Postural changes in both parameters should also be evaluated. Continuous electrocardiographic monitoring is indicated; a shortened PR interval may result from insufficient glucocorticoids. Hemodynamic monitoring may provide useful data regarding cardiac output, atrial filling pressure, and peripheral vascular resistance, all of which are decreased in acute adrenal crisis as a result of decreased vascular tone (glucocorticoid insufficiency) and hypovolemia (mineralocorticoid insufficiency).

OUTCOME STANDARD AND CRITERIA

Fluid volume is restored as evidenced by:
- Normal filling pressures
- Absence of postural hypotension

NURSING INTERVENTIONS

Nursing interventions include administration of glucocorticoid (hydrocortisone), mineralocorticoid (fludrocortisone), and volume replacement. As deficiencies are corrected, the patient should be carefully monitored. Fluid replacement must be rapid. If not carefully administered and monitored, this may result in cardiovascular overload.

Improvement is usually dramatic and rapid. As the patient is stabilized, glucocorticoid dosages are decreased and administered orally. Fludrocortisone can also be administered orally. Similarly, fluid intake is encouraged. The patient should be encouraged to consume food and fluids high in sodium and low in potassium. Intake and output should be monitored. Nursing interventions to minimize nausea, vomiting, and diarrhea should be employed to maintain nutrition and fluid balance. The patient should be encouraged to change position gradually to avoid fainting caused by orthostatic hypotension.

Pheochromocytoma

A pheochromocytoma is a chromaffin tissue tumor that secretes epinephrine and norepinephrine. The tumors may be single or multiple, wherever chromaffin tissue is present. Chromaffin tissue is widespread in utero. After birth, however, most cells degenerate and disappear. The chromaffin tissue that remains is found predominantly in the adrenal medulla but also occurs less often in the paraspinous ganglionic regions of the abdomen and pelvis. The vast majority (95%) of pheochromocytomas occur in the adrenal medulla, the remainder in the abdomen and pelvis.[15]

The adrenal medulla is best characterized as an extension of the sympathetic nervous system. Its secretion of epinephrine and norepinephrine normally occurs with sympathetic activation. Physiologically, glandular catecholamine secretion reinforces the sympathetic "flight or fight" response. The medulla secretes both catecholamines, but proportionally more epinephrine than norepinephrine.[8] The physiological effects of both catecholamines are widespread and profound (see Chapter 37).

Secretion by pheochromocytomas results from sympathetic nervous system activation, but unlike the normally functioning adrenal medulla, pheochromocytomas secrete epinephrine and norepinephrine autonomously as well. The tumors typically secrete both catecholamines, although tumor activity is not consistent. When hyperglycemia and hypermetabolism are prominent features, epinephrine is probably the more plentiful catecholamine. In situations characterized by hypertension of a fairly sustained nature, norepinehrine is likely to be the predominant catecholamine in the tumor.

Classically, pheochromocytoma is associated with paroxysmal and labile hypertensive episodes. One mechanism postulated for these episodes describes bursts of epinephrine from the tumors as the initiating event. The resultant decrease in peripheral resistance, coupled with hypovolemia (see below), dramatically reduces blood pressure and leads to sympathetic activation. The subsequent release of norepinephrine from vascular adrenergic nerve endings leads to vasoconstriction and hypertension. Presumably, the tumor's epinephrine content is depleted by the initial burst, and despite both adrenomedullary and tumor stimulation with sympathetic activation, norepinephrine-mediated vasoconstriction dominates while synthesis and replenishment of tumor epinephrine content is restored. This mechanism is consistent with other findings associated with hypertensive episodes. Dizziness, fainting, snycopal episodes, flushing, warmth, and palpitations probably reflect the effects of epinephrine-induced peripheral vasodilatation and myocardial stimulation.[14]

Tachydysrhythmias, angina, cardiomegaly, and catecholamine myocardiopathy all occur with pheochromocytomas and are thought to reflect the effect of excessive catecholamines on the heart. Congestive heart failure from cardiomyopathy may ensue.

Hyperglycemia and hypermetabolism reflect the metabolic consequences of excessive catecholamine levels, effects that undoubtedly contribute to the polyuria and subsequent hypovolemia associated with pheochromocytoma. Diaphoresis is often profuse. Weight loss, weakness, and fatigue are common in patients with pheochromocytomas and reflect the effect of the general catabolic condition. Anorexia and nausea, common gastrointestinal responses to sympathetic nervous system activation, further aggravate these findings.[14]

Headache almost always accompanies hypertensive events with pheochromocytomas. Although the mechanism is not clear, additional central nervous system manifestations are associated with pheochromocytomas, including tremulousness, anxiety, agitation, and, infrequently, psychosis.[15]

Medical Management

Definitive treatment of pheochromocytoma requires excision of the tumor(s). Prior to surgery, specific preparation is required. Generally, the goals of presurgical treatment are to reduce or eliminate hypertension and/or hypertensive attacks and their associated symptoms and to institute adrenergic blockade to prevent precipitation of an extreme crisis state caused by bursts of catecholamine secretion from the tumor(s) under the influence of anesthesia and surgical manipulation.

Phenoxybenzamine, a noncompetitive inhibitor of norepinephrine, is usually used to provide alpha-adrenergic inhibition. Although the faster-acting agent prazosin has also been used, it tends to be associated with a greater incidence of symptomatic postural hypotension.

Typically, the initial dosage of phenoxybenzamine is 10 mg administered every 12 hours. Every 2 days thereafter the dosage is increased by 10 mg a day to achieve a recumbent, resting blood pressure that is within normal range and is not associated with symptomatic postural hypotension. That dosage is then continued for approximately 1 week. If catecholamine myocardiopathy has led to heart failure, longer preparatory phenoxybenzamine treatment may be used in an attempt to optimize myocardial function preoperatively.[15]

When alpha-adrenergic blockade is ineffective in controlling hypertension or when medication side effects limit its usefulness, a norepinephrine synthesis blocker such as metyrosine can be tried. This agent inhibits the enzyme tyrosine hydroxylase and has been found to reduce the synthesis of norepinephrine to less than half the pretreatment rate. The initial dosage of 250 mg twice a day is gradually increased, according to patient tolerance, to up to 500 mg four times per day. Metyrosine depletes levodopa and dopamine in the central nervous system, however, and side effects tend to be pronounced. Excessive sedative effects and parkinsonian symptoms are frequently reported and often disabling.[15]

Tumors that secrete large amounts of epinephrine tend to be associated with a high incidence of tachydysrhythmias. Beta-adrenergic blocking may also be a part of surgical preparation for patients with such symptoms. Agents commonly employed include propranolol and metoprolol. Dosage is typically adjusted to maintain a resting heart rate of 100 beats per minute or less.[15]

NURSING MANAGEMENT

Patients with pheochromocytoma are encountered in the critical care setting during severe hypertensive crises or for postoperative care following excision of the tumor(s). Occasionally, patients are also admitted for monitoring or evaluation of undiagnosed hypertension or syncope. In these patients, the possibility of pheochromocytoma is often considered only after all other potential causes have been ruled out.

When the cause of hypertension is not clear, obtaining a urine sample for catecholamine measurement is a simple and relatively inexpensive way to obtain useful diagnostic data (see Chapter 38). If hypertension is episodic, obtaining such a sample during or shortly after blood pressure elevations is crucial. Because 24-hour levels of urinary catecholamine metabolites have a wide range of normal values, bursts of secretion can be masked in a 24-hour sample. Sometimes correlation of the urinary content of catecholamine by-products with clinical findings gives the only laboratory clue to the presence of a pheochromocytoma.

■ NURSING DIAGNOSIS

Alteration in peripheral, myocardial, and cerebral tissue perfusion, related to catecholamine effects.

Epinephrine and norepinephrine exert profound direct and indirect effects on peripheral circulation. Norepinephrine induces pronounced peripheral vasoconstriction with increased systemic vascular resistance, increased cardiac workload, and peripheral ischemia. Epinephrine, on the other hand, induces vasodilataion and decreased peripheral resistance. With untreated pheochromocytomas, either sustained or episodic hypertension may occur. In addition, pronounced hypotension, exaggerated by postural and position changes, may also occur as a result of epinephrine-induced vasodilatation and varying degrees of hypovolemia. Thus, in the periphery, either sustained ischemia or alternating periods of vasoconstriction and vasodilatation may be found.

The effect of catecholamines on the myocardium can indirectly influence tissue perfusion. Both catecholamines increase heart rate, epinephrine to a much greater extent than norepinephrine. In addition, catecholamine myocardiopathy may lead to a decrease in cardiac output and potential congestive heart failure.

Nursing management of patients with pheochromocytoma begins with assessment of cardiovascular effectiveness and hydration status. Serial monitoring should include vital signs, checks for postural changes in blood pressure and heart rate, and continuous electrocardiographic monitoring. In the presence of sustained hypertension or severe episodic attacks, indwelling arterial monitoring may be instituted and requires careful serial monitoring. Intake, output, and daily weights should be recorded, as should urine specific gravity. Tissue turgor should be assessed. Lung and heart sounds should be auscultated to monitor for development of congestive failure.

The patient with sustained or episodic hypertension is at risk of myocardial ischemia or infarction and cerebral vascular accidents. Thus, ongoing assessments should include evaluation of chest pain and neurological function and serial monitoring of orientation, level of consciousness, peripheral strength, and presence and symmetry of reflexes and motor function.

OUTCOME STANDARD AND CRITERIA

Adequate and/or improved perfusion of the peripheral, cerebral, and myocardial tissues as evidenced by:

- Absence of peripheral ischemia and edema
- Absence of peripheral cyanosis, especially in the extremities
- Normal sensorium
- Reduced angina

NURSING INTERVENTIONS

Primary nursing interventions involve administration of fluid (oral and intravenous) and medications for adrenergic blocking. Alterations in cardiovascular function and fluid balance should be recorded as fluid and drugs are administered. Symptomatic postural hypotension with syncope and fainting may accompany administration of adrenergic blocking agents, and existing congestive heart failure or a predisposition to it may be aggravated by over-rapid correction of hypovolemia.

Postoperatively, undersensitized alpha-adrenergic receptors may predispose previously hypertensive patients to profound hypotension in the presence of even minor degrees of hypovolemia. Volume expanders, isotonic fluids, and blood products must be administered carefully to ensure support for circulating volume without producing undue demand on the heart.

Nursing interventions must also be directed at eliminating stimuli known to evoke autonomous tumor secretion. Both nicotine and caffeine can precipitate catecholamine discharge from pheochromocytomas; smoking, chewing tobacco, and drinking caffeine-containing substances (coffee, tea, cola drinks) should, therefore, be prohibited. Sudden or pronounced changes in activity level or position, especially assumption of a posture that compresses the abdomen, should be avoided to decrease the risk of stimulating catecholamine release from pheochromocytomas. Activities should be graduated and moderate and significant exertion prevented. Position changes should be made gradually, and positions requiring the patient to bend over or draw the knees upward should be avoided. Abdominal palpation should not be performed if pheochromocytoma is suspected. Potentially constricting or tight clothing or restraints should not be employed.

The Valsalva maneuver should also be avoided, as it has been known to precipitate tumor secretion. Patients need to be taught how to move about in bed without holding their breath; assistance should be provided in changing position; and constipation should be prevented.

■ **NURSING DIAGNOSIS**

Alteration in nutrition: less than body requirements, related to increased metabolic rate secondary to excessive catecholamines.

Excessive levels of catecholamines, as with untreated pheochromocytomas and especially those that secrete predominantly epinephrine, lead to a general catabolic state and weight loss. Compounding the catabolic condition are catecholamine-induced gastrointestinal responses that impair ability to eat and interest in eating. Under the influence of catecholamines, sphincters throughout the gastrointestinal tract close and blood flow to the tract decreases.[1] The resulting ischemia and spasm may produce nausea, vomiting, and anorexia.

OUTCOME STANDARD AND CRITERIA

Nutritional intake meets metabolic requirement as evidenced by:[4]
• Stable weight
• Positive nitrogen balance
• Adequate wound healing
• Adequate protein reserves

NURSING INTERVENTIONS

Nursing interventions center on the need to increase caloric intake and reverse the effects of catabolism. Glucose-containing infusions may be necessary for patients unable to tolerate oral food intake. In such instances, serum and urinary glucose should be monitored. Preoperatively, hyperglycemia is likely as a result of catecholamine-induced increases in glycogenolysis and insulin resistance. When glucose-rich solutions are used, hyperglycemia can become pronounced and require insulin administration. Control of serum glucose is also important to prevent the additive effect of osmotic diuresis on the potential for fluid depletion secondary to the often profuse diaphoresis (see below) and polyuria.

Postoperatively there is a risk of hypoglycemia. Sudden decreases in levels of circulating catecholamines can inhibit glycogenolysis. With removal of catecholamine-induced insulin resistance, blood glucose may fall significantly. Tachycardia, cold clammy skin, diplopia, or complaints of shakiness or "internal" tremors should prompt evaluation of serum glucose.

For patients able to eat, frequent small meals and high-calorie snacks should be provided. A dietary consultation may also be helpful to ensure adequate intake of vitamins and minerals and appropriate calorie intake. Intake and serial calorie counts should be carefully recorded. Stool softeners, dietary fiber, and adequate fluids may help minimize effort associated with bowel evacuation.

■ **NURSING DIAGNOSIS**

Anxiety and fear, related to sympathetic nervous system activation by excessive catecholamine secretion.

Untreated pheochromocytomas secrete catecholamines autonomously as well as in conjunction with sympathetic nervous system activation. With bursts of catecholamine secretion, hypertension is often accompanied by palpitations, severe headaches, profuse diaphoresis, and sometimes intense anxiety and fear *(panic syndrome)*.

OUTCOME STANDARD AND CRITERIA

Anxiety will be reduced or eliminated to the degree possible in light of the exaggerated stress response as evidenced by:
• Expressed reductions in feelings of anxiety, fear, and apprehension
• Expressed feelings of psychological support

NURSING INTERVENTIONS

The patient's immediate environment should be kept as quiet and restful as possible. Explanations and reassurances should be offered frequently and consistently. Interventions to promote comfort are important in reducing anxiety in this patient population. Keeping lights dimmed during hypertensive attacks and providing analgesics will help decrease the discomfort of headaches. Offering frequent assistance with hygiene and keeping the room cool and well ventilated may also help to relieve discomfort from diaphoresis during hypertensive periods. Additional blankets and bed clothing should be provided after hypertensive attacks to prevent chills from diaphoresis. Nursing interventions to minimize evaluation of tumor secretion as described earlier are also important for reducing and preventing the resultant states of anxiety and fear.

DIABETIC DISORDERS

Diabetes mellitus affects an estimated 5.8 million people in the United States. An additional 4 to 5 million Americans are thought to be affected with undiagnosed diabetes. It is a chronic condition characterized by insufficient insulin secretion or resistance to insulin in peripheral tissues. Common manifestations include abnormalities in carbohydrate, fat, and protein metabolism. Diabetes is not just one disease; rather, it is a genetically heterogeneous group of disorders that have in common glucose intolerance. Both genetic and environmental conditions have been implicated in the etiology of diabetes. The prevalence of diabetes in the United States is 6.6% in persons over age 18. The prevalence is highest in nonwhite Americans and increases with age.[16]

Classification

In 1979 a new classification for diabetes mellitus with five categories was established by the National Diabetes Data Group and endorsed by the American Diabetes Association (Table 39-1).

Type I, or *insulin-dependent diabetes mellitus* (IDDM), includes those disorders historically referred to as juvenile, ketosis-prone, or brittle diabetes. Those affected are typically young, lean, and dependent on exogenous insulin to prevent ketoacidosis and death. The precise causation is unclear, but studies have implicated pancreatic beta islet cell damage due to viral illness, toxic chemicals, or autoimmune processes. Genetic predisposition may also be involved; there is an association between type I diabetes and specific HLA antigens on chromosome 6. Roughly 10% of all diabetic patients are in the type I category.[17]

Type II, or *non-insulin-dependent diabetes mellitus* (NIDDM), is the most common type and includes disorders traditionally referred to as adult or maturity onset diabetes. Those affected are usually over 30 and obese and do not consistently need insulin therapy to prevent or control hyperglycemia. Unless exposed to significant stress, such as occurs with infectious processes, surgery, or trauma, type II diabetic patients are not prone to ketosis because very small amounts of endogenous insulin will prevent ketoacidosis even in the presence of hyperglycemia.

Endogenous insulin levels may be decreased, normal, or elevated in type II diabetes. In addition, tissue sensitivity to insulin is decreased, and binding of insulin to cell receptors is abnormal because fewer receptors are present and because an intracellular postreceptor defect exists. The etiology of type II diabetes has not been precisely defined, but a genetic predisposition in combination with environmental factors is thought to be involved. Those with type II disease make up 90% of all persons with diabetes.[18]

Stress may contribute to the development of both types of diabetes. The physiological response to a physical or emotional threat, including critical illness, involves the secretion of hormones that antagonize insulin action. Epinephrine, cortisol and other glucocorticoids, growth hormone, and glucagon all induce hyperglycemia and catabolism (see Chapter 37). Prolonged stress may lead susceptible persons to develop diabetes as a function of system exhaustion.

Impaired glucose tolerance is a condition in which serum glucose levels are higher than normal but not high enough to be considered diagnostic for diabetes mellitus.[19] *Gestational diabetes* results from the increased hormonal and glucose load associated with pregnancy. Gestational diabetes occurs in approximately 2% of pregnancies. Its occurrence not only increases perinatal complications but also predisposes those affected to residual and subsequent alterations in glucose metabolism. Of the women experiencing gestational diabetes, 30% to 40% develop overt diabetes mellitus 5 to 10 years after parturition.

Pathophysiology

Common to all types of diabetes is either a relative or an absolute lack of insulin and, therefore, an inability to respond to glucose stimulation. Without insulin, glucose cannot be appropriately used by insulin-dependent tissues; that is, cellular "starvation" occurs despite an elevated serum glucose. Compensatory secretion of catabolic hormones is stimulated in an attempt to meet cellular energy needs. As a result, hyperglycemia is aggravated, and cellular starvation continues.

Systemic effects of sustained hyperglycemia reflect direct effects of persistent alterations in carbohydrate metabolism. The critically ill patient with preexisting diabetes may exhibit a variety of long-term complications as a result of poorly controlled diabetes. Sustained, increased circulating levels of glucose cause sorbitol to accumulate in Schwann cells in the nervous system. The resultant myelin damage leads to the development of neuropathies. Attachment of glucose to proteins in the capillary basement membranes of the eyes and kidneys leads to retinopathy and nephropathy related to membrane thickening and damage. Altered carbohydrate and fat metabolism in diabetes accelerates progression of arteriosclerotic changes in both large and small vessels. Increased incidence of fatty plaques and increased prevalence of advanced lesions with calcified, ulcerated, or occluded vessels leads to arterial and cardiovascular compromise.[19]

Cardiovascular disease accounts for roughly 70% of deaths in the diabetic population.[19] Changes in large and small vessels occur more frequently and at an earlier age in the presence of diabetes. Both type I and type II diabetes predispose to acute myocardial infarction. Silent MIs are more common in patients with diabetes. Diabetic neuropathies can block the sensation of pain; therefore, cardiac ischemia and damage can occur without symptoms. In addition, coronary vessel sclerosis can lead to dysrhythmias such as sinoatrial and atrioventricular blocks.

Critical illness is in itself stressful. Blood glucose may be increased by the physiological response to stress, making control more difficult. In addition, for diabetic patients who use blood glucose–lowering medication, hypoglycemia poses a special risk. Pre-

TABLE 39-1 **Types of Diabetes Mellitus**

Current Name	Clinical Characteristics	Diagnostic Criteria
CLINICAL CATEGORIES		
Type I: insulin-dependent diabetes mellitus (IDDM)—formerly called juvenile diabetes (JD), juvenile-onset diabetes (JOD), ketosis-prone diabetes, brittle diabetes	Patients have little or no endogenous insulin and need injections to preserve life. New patients may be of any age but are usually young; they often have islet-cell antibodies. Causes may be genetic, environmental, or acquired, probably involving abnormal immune responses	**Diabetes Mellitus in Nonpregnant Adults:** A. Classic symptoms of diabetes—e.g., polyuria, polydipsia, ketonuria, rapid weight loss plus random blood glucose >200 mg/dl *or* B. Elevated fasting glucose on at least two occasions ≥140 mg/dl *or*
Type II: non-insulin-dependent diabetes mellitus (NIDDM)—formerly called adult-onset diabetes (AOD), maturity-onset diabetes (MOD), ketosis-resistant diabetes, stable diabetes, maturity-onset diabetes of youth (MODY)	Except during infection or other stress, patients rarely develop ketosis. They vary in amount of endogenous insulin and may need injections to avoid hyperglycemia. New patients may be of any age but are usually over 30. Most are obese. NIDDM is thought to be caused by genetic susceptibility plus environmental factors	C. Fasting glucose less than B above but sustained elevated glucose during the OGTT* on more than one occasion. Both the 2-hour sample and some other sample taken between administration of the 75-g glucose dose and 2 hours later must be ≥200 mg/dl **Diabetes Mellitus in Children:** A. Classic symptoms of diabetes—e.g., polyuria, polydipsia, ketonuria, rapid weight loss plus random blood glucose ≥200 mg/dl *or*
Diabetes mellitus associated with other conditions or syndromes—formerly called secondary diabetes	These patient's diabetes is accompanied by conditions known or suspected to cause the disease, including pancreatic or hormonal disease, drug or chemical toxicity, abnormal insulin receptors, or certain genetic syndromes	B. In asymptomatic individuals, both an elevated fasting glucose of >140 mg/dl and a sustained elevated glucose during the OGTT on more than one occasion. Both the 2-hour sample and some other sample taken between administration of the glucose dose (1.75 g/kg ideal body weight, up to a maximum of 75 g) and 2 hours later should be >200 mg/dl
Impaired glucose tolerance (IGT) Type a: nonobese Type b: obese Formerly called asymptomatic diabetes, chemical diabetes, subclinical diabetes, borderline diabetes, latent diabetes	Glucose levels are between those of normal people and diabetics. Patients have above-normal susceptibility to atherosclerotic disease. Renal and retinal complications generally do not become significant	**IGT in Nonpregnant Adults (mg/dl):** Diagnosis of impaired glucose tolerance in this population is restricted to those who have all of the following: Fasting blood glucose <140 mg/dl and 2-hour oral glucose tolerance test plasma glucose result of >140 mg/dl and a sample between administration of the glucose dose and 2 hours later ≥200 mg/dl
Gestational diabetes (GDM)—formerly called gestational diabetes	This classification is retained for women whose diabetes begins (or is recognized) during pregnancy. They have an above-normal risk of perinatal complications. Their glucose intolerance may be transitory, but it frequently recurs	**Gestational Diabetes** Two or more of the following, after a 100-g glucose dose, must be met or exceeded: Fasting 105 mg/dl 1 hours 190 mg/dl 2 hours 165 mg/dl 3 hours 145 mg/dl

* OGTT = oral glucose tolerance test.
Modified from Ames Division, Miles Laboratories, Inc., Elkhart, IN. (1979). *Diabetes: 28*(Dec):1979.

TABLE 39-1 **Types of Diabetes Mellitus—cont'd**

Current Name	Clinical Characteristics	Diagnostic Criteria
STATISTICAL RISK CATEGORIES		
Previous abnormality of glucose tolerance (prevAGT)—formerly called latent diabetes, prediabetes	Despite a history of hyperglycemia, these patients now have normal glucose metabolism	Normal glucose levels in adults: Fasting <115 mg/dl OGTT: Fasting <115 mg/dl Midpoint <200 mg/dl 2 hours <140 mg/dl
Potential abnormality of glucose tolerance (PotAGT)—formerly called potential diabetes, prediabetes	Even though they have never had glucose intolerance, these patients are judged relatively likely to become diabetic. Persons with diabetic family members or evidence of islet-cell antibodies, mothers of babies who weighed more than 9 lb at birth, Pima indians, and the obese	

cipitous or significant decreases in blood glucose may extend a preexisting or evolving infarct or even cause an infarct in susceptible persons.

All diabetic persons are predisposed to infections. Hyperglycemia alters resistance by impairing phagocytosis and slowing granulocytic activity.[20] The most common manifestations are urinary tract and skin infections. Fever associated with the infectious response can aggravate hyperglycemia by stimulating adrenal medullary secretion of epinephrine and adrenal cortical secretion of cortisol. Not surprisingly, infections are often the precipitating events for hyperglycemic states such as nonketotic hyperglycemic hyperosmolar coma or diabetic ketoacidosis.[20]

The Diabetic Patient with Critical Illness

Medical Management

Individuals in the critical care setting may have preexisting diabetes or develop diabetes during the course of acute illness. The main goals of therapy are: (1) to control blood glucose; and (2) to prevent hypoglycemia, protein catabolism, and electrolyte disturbances. Pharmacological and nonpharmacological therapies are used to achieve these goals. The critically ill diabetic will require close monitoring and frequent adjustment of pharmacological therapy to achieve these goals.

Acute and critical illness in persons with insulin-dependent diabetes mellitus can significantly increase insulin requirements. Sliding scale doses of regular insulin may be administered every 4 to 6 hours on the basis of blood glucose values. Depending on the patient's medical condition and health status, insulin may be administered by subcutaneous, intramuscular, or intravenous injection. Intravenous injection is pre-

ferred in acutely ill patients when absorption and circulatory uptake of subcutaneous or intramuscular injections are unpredictable.

Once the patient is stable, diet, exercise, and medication doses will need to be individually prescribed in preparation for discharge to home. For a complete discussion on the medical management of diabetes, the reader is referred to a more extensive source.

Patients with type II diabetes mellitus who have not required insulin prior to illness may need exogenous insulin to control hyperglycemia during episodes of acute and critical illness. Human insulin is indicated to decrease the likelihood of antibody production and allergy in the event that exogenous insulin is required intermittently.

Surgery poses a special challenge to critical care management of the diabetic patient. A number of different insulin regimens are used for diabetics undergoing surgery, but most involve either subcutaneous insulin and intravenous dextrose fluids to cover the insulin or combined insulin/dextrose intravenous infusions.

Nursing Management

Nursing care for critically ill patients with diabetes must focus on frequent and ongoing multisystem assessment, titration/administration of pharmacological blood glucose—lowering agents, and provision of nutrient sources. Bedside blood glucose monitoring is required and offers the advantage of rapid, accurate, easy-to-obtain results. Frequency and timing of blood glucose monitoring should be individually determined based on the patient's needs and goals of therapy. Early recognition of hypoglycemia, excessive hyperglycemia, protein catabolism, and electrolyte disturbances is essential. In addition, the critical care nurse may need to provide appropriate care to manage existing long-term diabetic complications such as peripheral vascular changes and diabetic retinopathy. The reader is referred to a more extensive source for a complete discussion of nursing management of diabetes mellitus. The remainder of the chapter will focus on three types of diabetic coma.

Diabetic Coma Classification

Diabetic emergencies manifested by coma can be precipitated in both undiagnosed and known diabetic patients during critical illness. All diabetic comas are life-threatening emergencies. Reversal requires prompt and appropriate therapy. There are three types of diabetic coma:

1. Hyperglycemic coma due to *diabetic ketoacidosis* (DKA), which is associated with severe insulin deficiency.
2. *Hypoglycemic coma* (low blood glucose) resulting from administration of excessive insulin or other hypoglycemic agents.
3. Hyperglycemic coma due to mild to moderate insulin deficiency, referred to as *hyperglycemic hyperosmolar nonketotic syndrome* (HHNS).

Comas in diabetes can reflect a multitude of precipitating events. Loss of consciousness in a person with known diabetes mellitus should not automatically be attributed to a diabetic emergency; however, the possibility of diabetic-related coma should always be considered. Assessment should address potential causes of coma of both diabetic and nondiabetic origin.

Diabetic Ketoacidosis

Coma due to diabetic ketoacidosis (DKA) is the more common type of diabetic hyperglycemic coma. It accounts for 9% of all hospital admissions for persons having diabetes listed as the cause of admission. Although DKA is perceived as being primarily a problem of young patients, 85% of episodes occur in adults, and 80% of DKA episodes occur in patients with known diabetes mellitus; up to 20% of patients with DKA have multiple episodes. Nationally, the mortality associated with DKA ranges from 10% to 14%.[21,22,23]

DKA most commonly occurs in persons with type I diabetes who are dependent upon exogenous insulin. Any major stress, including infection, trauma, surgery, myocardial infarction, and stroke, may precipitate DKA in a diabetic person not receiving sufficient insulin. In addition, omission of insulin doses and mismanagement of sick days are common precipitating factors. Leakage or malfunction of insulin pumps can also precipitate DKA.

Pathophysiology

Diabetic ketoacidosis is a life-threatening event that is manifested by hyperglycemia, ketosis, extracellular volume depletion, electrolyte imbalance, and acidosis. Survival depends on prompt recognition and prompt treatment in a medical intensive care unit or similar setting.[17]

The pathophysiology of DKA is outlined in Figure 39-1. Relative or absolute insulin deficiency precludes a normal response to glucose stimulation. Hyperglycemia is related to inadequate glucose disposal as well as to increased glucose production as a result of inadequate blood insulin levels and increased secretion of four counterregulatory hormones (glucagon, epinephrine, growth hormone, and glucocorticoids). When blood glucose exceeds the renal threshold, glycosuria occurs. Osmotic diuresis ensues, accompanied by loss of sodium, potassium, and body water. Extracellular volume depletion rapidly follows. As hypovolemia develops, renal function diminishes and hyperglycemia worsens.

In addition, counterregulatory hormones stimulate breakdown of amino acids to provide substrate for gluconeogenesis that itself increases hyperglycemia and accounts for muscle wasting and weight loss. Counterregulatory hormones also enhance lipolysis and subsequent ketogenesis. Increased production and decreased utilization of ketones cause them to accumulate in the blood in excess of the body's excretory or buffering ability. Respiratory compensation takes the form of rapid, deep (Kussmaul) respirations as acidosis increases the respiratory drive. However, a vicious cycle ensues as muscle weakness and decreased ventilatory ability make respiratory compensation less effective. Bicarbonate and other body buffers are depleted, blood pH drops, and metabolic acidosis follows. Without reversal, coma and death may ensue.[19,23]

Data Acquisition

Initial laboratory tests for suspected DKA include evaluation of blood glucose, serum and urinary ketones, arterial blood gases, electrolytes, serum osmolality, BUN, hematocrit, and WBC. Typical findings are:[19]

- Elevated blood glucose (over 250 mg/dl, usually 250-800 mg/dl)
- Moderate to large urinary ketones or positive serum acetone
- Low arterial pH
- Low CO_2 levels
- Increased anion gap

BUN, hematocrit, and WBC are usually elevated.

Extracellular volume depletion is the most immediate life-threatening abnormality associated with

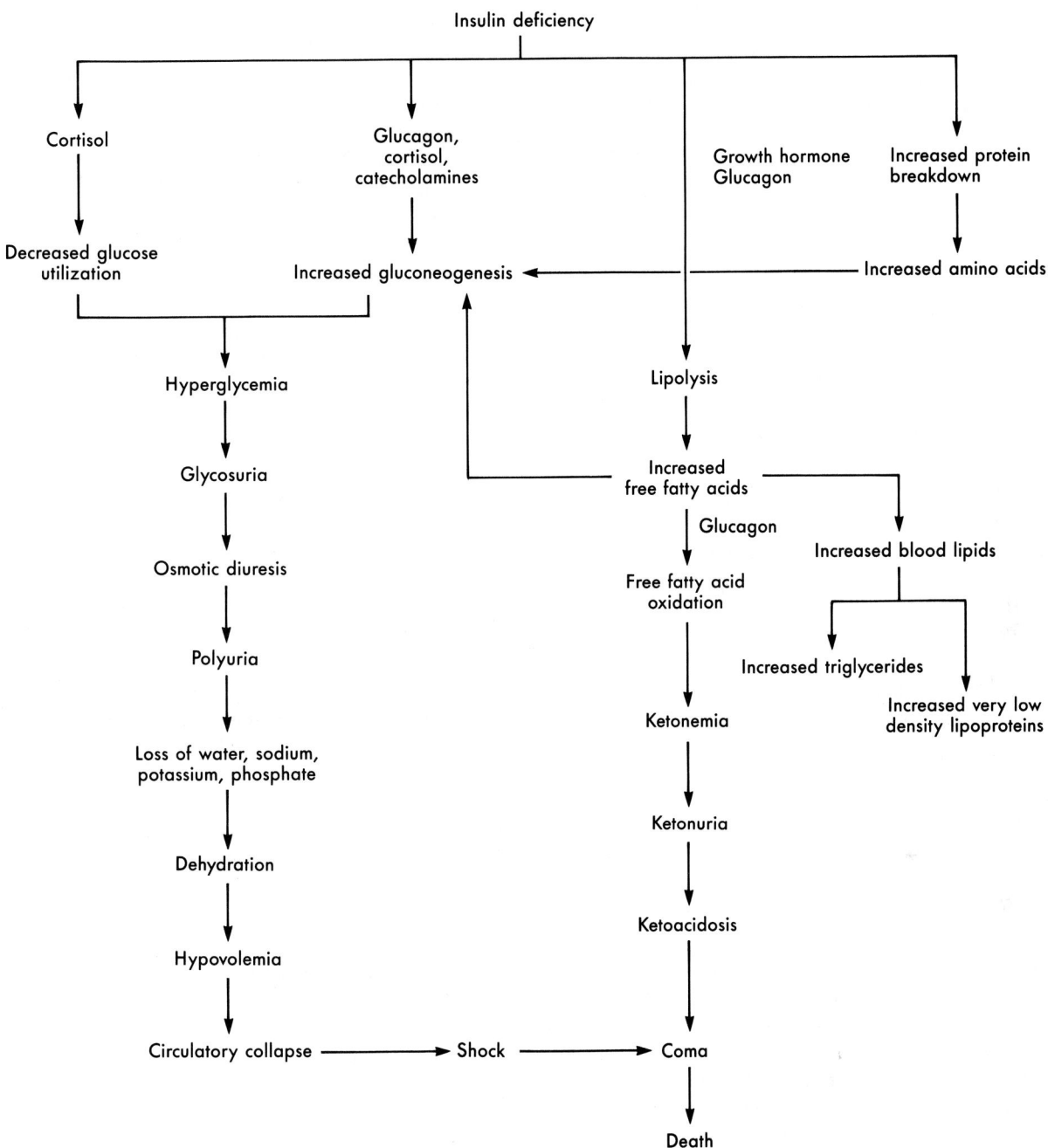

Figure 39-1 Diabetic ketoacidosis (DKA).
From Thompson J., McFarland, G. K., Hirsch, J. E., et al. (Eds.). (1992). *Mosby's manual of clinical nursing* (3rd ed.). St. Louis: Mosby–Year Book.

DKA. It manifests as tachycardia, sustained and postural hypotension, decreased pulse pressure, poor skin turgor, and dry mucous membranes. Respirations are characterized by tachypnea, Kussmaul's breathing, and acetone odor to the breath.

Although patients with DKA are always depleted in total body potassium, initial laboratory studies may show decreased, normal, or increased levels because of the catabolic state, potassium-wasting secondary to polyuria, inability of the kidneys to rapidly conserve potassium, and vomiting or diarrhea if present.[17] An ECG can be beneficial in ruling out the initial presence of hypo- or hyperkalemia. High peaked T waves are present in hyperkalemia; flattened T waves with prominent U waves are seen in hypokalemia. Other electrolytes including sodium and phosphate may also be decreased, normal, or increased on initial evaluation.[17]

Neurological status can vary from alert to deep coma. Mentation appears to correlate best with serum osmolality and not well with either blood glucose or pH levels.[19] As patient education has improved, and as self-monitoring of blood glucose has become more common, more patients are conscious when first seen. Upon admission, the history typically includes polyuria, polydipsia, weight loss, and weakness.

Nausea, vomiting, or both may be present as a result of the ketoacidotic state. Metabolic acidosis may lead to severe abdominal pain. These abdominal signs, often in association with an elevated WBC and serum amylase, may be mistakenly interpreted as evidence of an acute abdominal condition. Most often, abdominal pain disappears with rehydration and reversal of metabolic acidosis. The WBC and serum amylase levels usually return to normal with therapy. If severe abdominal pain persists, however, a surgical consultation should be obtained.[17,23]

In DKA, the presence of hypothermia is considered to be a poor prognostic sign associated with mortality of 30% to 60%.[24,25] An underlying infection should be suspected and vigorously pursued in all cases of DKA.

Medical Management

The initial goal of medical therapy should be to correct life-threatening abnormalities: extracellular volume depletion, insulin deficiency, potassium deficiency, and acidosis. In addition, the precipitating cause of DKA will need to be identified and treated and complications avoided.

Fluid replacement is a priority to restore and maintain vascular volume as well as enhance kidney function to promote excretion of excess glucose and ketones. The usual fluid deficit is between 4 and 8 L.[26] To rapidly replace the depleted circulating volume, isotonic saline is initially administered at a rate of 500 to 1,000 ml/hr for the first 2 to 4 hours. Infusion rates are then slowed to 250 to 500 ml/hr, and 0.45% normal saline may be used. Clinical and laboratory findings should guide the timing of further reductions in the rate of the infusion to 125 to 250 ml/hr. In addition, intravenous fluid should be changed to 5% dextrose or 10% dextrose when the serum glucose drops to 250 mg/dl to allow continued insulin infusion without hypoglycemia.[17,26]

Because insulin deficiency is the cause of DKA in all patients, insulin therapy is essential to successful treatment. Insulin corrects acidosis by suppressing ketone production and inhibiting lipolysis. It reduces hyperglycemia by promoting cellular utilization of glucose and by decreasing hepatic glucose production.

Only short-acting (regular) insulin should be used initially. Administering insulin intravenously is the most direct and preferred route if the infusion can be regulated. The initial bolus is 0.15 U/kg, followed by insulin infusion at a rate of 0.1 U/kg per hour of U100. If no biochemical improvement is noted within 2 to 4 hours even though intravenous lines are patent, the infusion rate may be doubled.[17,26] Glucose will be normalized more rapidly than the acidosis is corrected. Therefore, the insulin infusion should be continued until both conditions are reversed. When blood glucose falls to 250 mg/dl, the insulin infusion rate should be reduced by 50%, and 5% or 10% dextrose added to the infusion to maintain blood glucose around 250 mg/dl for the first 12 to 24 hours.[17]

Intramuscular administration of insulin is recommended *only* if there is no available method of regulating an insulin infusion. In this case, an initial bolus dose of 0.5 U/kg is usually given, followed by doses of 0.1 U/kg per hour by intramuscular injection until blood glucose is reduced to 300 mg/dl. Thereafter, doses of 0.1 U/kg should be administered intramuscularly every 2 hours as needed to maintain blood glucose around 250 mg/dl.[17]

Shortly after fluid and insulin therapy are started, serum potassium will begin to drop. Potassium replacement should be initiated within 1 to 2 hours after starting insulin therapy.[17] Once urinary output is established, potassium replacement is based on serum potassium levels. Potassium should be added to intravenous fluids in amounts ranging from 0.5 mEq/kg per hour (for serum potassium <3 mEq/L) to 0.1 to 0.2 mEq/kg per hour (for serum potassium in a range of 5 to 6 mEq/L). Serum potassium should be monitored closely. Potassium replacement should be withheld for serum potassium values greater than 6 mEq/L.

Potassium is usually replaced as potassium chloride (KCl). Potassium phosphate (K_3PO_4) may be given in limited amounts if the patient is found to have hypophosphatemia. Replacement of K_3PO_4 should not exceed 1.5 mEq/kg within 24 hours. If phosphate is given in excess, hypocalcemia may result.[17]

Routine administration of bicarbonate is not recommended in most cases of DKA when pH is greater than or equal to 7.1 because of the danger of paradoxical cerebrospinal fluid acidosis and resultant cerebral edema associated with a too rapid correction of systemic acidosis. Bicarbonate administration may be considered in severe acidosis (pH <7.0), and especially when hypotension, shock, and dysrhythmias are also present. When administered, bicarbonate should be given as an infusion of 1 to 2 mEq/kg over 2 hours, followed by a reassessment of plasma bicarbonate levels. The total amount of bicarbonate administered should not exceed 3 mEq/kg over 12 hours.[17,23]

After resolution of DKA, intensive insulin therapy

continues to be important until patients restart their usual treatment regimen, most commonly within 12 to 24 hours after admission. Subcutaneous insulin is best reinstituted before a meal and at a time that coincides with an individual's usual insulin dose. Insulin infusions can be discontinued 30 minutes after subcutaneous insulin is given. Generally, patients recovering from DKA can take food or fluids by mouth as soon as they desire. Blood glucose monitoring should continue every 4 to 6 hours to evaluate the effect of insulin on blood glucose.[17,26]

NURSING MANAGEMENT

The nursing management of critically ill patients with DKA must be directed toward managing real and potential fluid and electrolyte imbalance, administering insulin to aid in restoration of normal carbohydrate, fat, and protein metabolism; and promptly recognizing and treating systemic manifestations.

■ NURSING DIAGNOSIS

Fluid volume deficit, related to failure of regulatory mechanisms.

OUTCOME STANDARD AND CRITERIA

Fluid volume status is normal as evidenced by:
- Blood pressure and pulse within normal limits for the patient
- Balanced intake and output
- Normal electrolyte levels
- Alleviation of subjective and objective manifestations of extracellular volume depletion

NURSING INTERVENTIONS

Nursing management begins with early identification of patients at risk for acute fluid volume deficit, related to abnormal fluid loss from hyperglycemia-induced osmotic diuresis, nausea, or vomiting. In DKA, pronounced osmotic diuresis may lead to rapid depletion of extracellular volume. All patients with a history of type I diabetes who are experiencing acute or critical illness are vulnerable. Coexisting medical illness, including infection, is a common precipitating factor in the development of DKA.

Ongoing assessment centers on hydration status and prevention of complications. Fluid volume deficit, related to abnormal fluid loss, leads to signs of extracellular fluid volume depletion. Skin turgor is decreased, and mucous membranes are often parched and cracked. Extreme thirst and history of rapid weight loss are typically present.

Use of a flowsheet is essential to provide quick reference to vital parameters that can be easily followed over time in an organized manner.[19] Meticulous recordings of body weight and intake and output are necessary to accurately follow trends. Postural or sustained blood pressure decreases, especially with tachycardia, may indicate impending shock, developing as a result of fluid shifts that occur in response to volume depletion.

Hypovolemia is the most critical initial problem to be dealt with in the management of the patient with DKA. The largest practical intravenous line for rapid infusion of saline must be started and maintained throughout this critical period.[19] Treatment may lead to fluid overload if fluid replacement is too rapid. Underlying cardiac compromise exaggerates these risks. Vital signs, continuous cardiac monitoring, and auscultation of the heart and lungs need to be performed frequently to guide fluid management.[20] Monitoring should include assessment of central venous and pulmonary artery pressures, and vigilance for neck vein distention, developing peripheral edema, cardiac dysrhythmias, and crackles.

Dehydration and hyperglycemia increase the risk of hyperviscosity, abnormalities of platelet function, and increased clotting factors, all of which contribute to a tendency to hypercoagulation. The risk of thromboembolism can be reduced by taking action to prevent stasis of blood: assuring adequate hydration, providing antiembolic stockings, and performing range of motion exercises of extremities.

■ NURSING DIAGNOSIS

Impaired gas exchange, related to altered oxygen supply secondary to tachypnea.

OUTCOME STANDARD AND CRITERIA

Gas exchange is normal for the patient as evidenced by:
- Normal blood pressure and heart rate
- Normal character and rate of respirations
- Resolution of acidosis
- Alleviation of subjective and objective manifestations of impaired gas exchange

NURSING INTERVENTIONS

Kussmaul respirations are a classic finding in DKA, and result from acidosis increasing the respiratory drive to compensate for acidosis by lowering CO_2. The degree of acidosis can be assessed by monitoring blood pH, serum CO_2 and bicarbonate, and urine ketones. Other parameters to be regularly assessed include progression or regression of Kussmaul respirations, acetone or "fruity" breath, and level of consciousness.

Serial respiratory auscultation should be performed, with special attention to the adequacy of pulmonary excursion and the nature of breath sounds. The nurse should assess the patient frequently for signs of inadequate gas exchange, including tachycardia, dyspnea, skin color changes, and decreased respiratory effort. Changes in respiratory status should be reported and oxygen administered as needed. Arterial blood gases may be assessed.

Supportive measures such as ensuring an airway and insertion of a nasogastric tube should be considered in the comatose patient to maximize gas exchange and prevent aspiration pneumonia should the patient vomit.[19]

COLLABORATIVE PROBLEM

Electrolyte disturbances, related to inadequate intake of nutrients and electrolyte shifts.

OUTCOME STANDARD AND CRITERIA

Intake of nutrients and electrolytes is adequate as evidenced by:

- Electrolyte levels within normal limits

NURSING INTERVENTIONS

Acidosis and osmotic diuresis precipitate potassium and phosphate imbalance in DKA. Ongoing assessments, therefore, must include careful monitoring of parenteral infusions and monitoring for signs of electrolyte imbalance.

Initially, serum potassium may be low, normal, or high, because of the combined effects of acidosis and dehydration. With treatment and rehydration, serum potassium may decrease rapidly as potassium returns to the intracellular compartment. Cardiac dysrhythmias are likely, and continuous ECG monitoring is indicated to guide replacement therapy. Hyperkalemia is manifested by a weak, slow, and often irregular pulse. Other findings include irritability, restlessness, anxiety, abdominal cramps, weakness, nausea, vomiting, flattened P waves, tented T waves, a widened QRS interval, and a prolonged PR interval on the electrocardiographic tracing.

Once fluid replacement and insulin therapy have been initiated, nursing assessment should include monitoring for hypokalemia. Signs and symptoms associated with hypokalemia include muscular weakness, which may progress to paralysis; hypotension; anorexia; fatigue; abdominal distention; hypoactive reflexes; dizziness; paresthesias; and electrocardiographic findings, including peaked P waves, flattened T waves, prominent U waves, and ST depression. Electrolyte imbalance in hyperglycemic states can be profound, especially potassium fluctuations.[19]

As noted, coexistent phosphate depletion may be present due to decreased food intake, the catabolic state, or increased urinary excretion. However, if phosphate in the form of potassium phosphate is replaced in amounts exceeding 90 mEq/L in 24 hours, a reciprocal drop in serum calcium may lead to symptomatic hypocalcemia. Signs and symptoms of hypocalcemia include paresthesias, numbness and tingling around the mouth and in the fingers, muscle cramps, positive Chvostek's and Trousseau's signs, and, in severe cases, tetany and convulsions.[20]

■ **NURSING DIAGNOSIS**

Nutrition, altered: less than body requirements, related to inability to ingest or digest food or absorb nutrients because of biological factors.

OUTCOME STANDARD AND CRITERIA

Adequate nutrients are available to meet the body's demands as evidenced by:

- Stabilization of weight
- Body glucose levels below 250 mg/dl
- Reestablishment of regular meal and subcutaneous insulin injection patterns that are normal for the patient

NURSING INTERVENTIONS

Nursing interventions should include at least hourly beside blood sugar monitoring, urine ketone testing, and assessment of the effectiveness of insulin. The nurse will need to prepare the prescribed insulin infusion. Before the IV tubing is connected, 50 ml of the insulin infusion should be run through the tubing and discarded to saturate tubing adsorption sites.[17,19] Glucose-containing solutions are used once the blood sugar has decreased to between 250 and 300 mg/dl. At that point, the nurse should specifically assess for signs and symptoms of hypoglycemia.

Most patients recovering from DKA will be able to take food and fluids as they desire. For patients with altered levels of consciousness or altered GI motility, oral intake may be resumed as patients regain alertness and gastric peristalsis resumes. Once the usual subcutaneous injections are resumed, observations for hypoglycemia should be based on knowledge of the peak and duration of action of the insulin preparation being used.

Insulin resistance, although not common, can occur. The patency of IV tubing should be assessed regularly to assure no disruption in infusion to the patient. If the blood glucose is not decreasing despite increasingly larger doses of insulin, resistance may be responsible. Insulin sensitivity generally returns to normal after implementation of good blood glucose control.[23]

■ **NURSING DIAGNOSIS**

Impaired skin integrity, related to altered metabolic state.

OUTCOME STANDARDS AND CRITERIA

The skin is intact as evidenced by an absence of tissue disruption, wounds, or infection.

NURSING INTERVENTIONS

Nursing interventions focus on prevention, detection, and treatment of infections, as required. Infection is the most common precipitating cause of DKA. Diabetic patients commonly have underlying neuropathies and peripheral vascular compromise. Local infections may progress with few or no symptoms. Peripheral vascular compromise places the patient at risk for breakdown of tissue and slows healing once tissue disruption occurs. Documentation of wound assessment should include presence of erythema, size, drainage, and odor. Monitoring for signs and symptoms of systemic sepsis should be continuous. Depending on presenting signs and symptoms, a chest x-ray plus urine, throat, sputum and blood cultures may be obtained. Antibiotic therapy may be initiated in cases of actual and suspected infection. Infections are a major cause of mortality and morbidity for the diabetic patient. If preventive measures fail, the infection must be carefully monitored and treated.

■ NURSING DIAGNOSIS

Sensory/perceptual alteration, related to endogenous electrolyte alteration.

OUTCOME STANDARD AND CRITERIA

The patient has normal sensations and perceptions as evidenced by:
- Orientation to time, place, and person
- Electrolyte levels within normal limits
- Absence of acidosis
- Alleviation of subjective and objective manifestations of extracellular volume depletion

NURSING INTERVENTIONS

Frequent assessment of mental status is essential. As discussed under Medical Therapy, use of sodium bicarbonate to correct extracellular fluid acidosis in DKA may paradoxically increase spinal fluid acidosis and exaggerate existing alterations in level of consciousness. Cerebral edema rarely occurs but is more common in younger patients. Its development may in part be related to a too rapid decline in blood glucose. Administration of large amounts of hypotonic fluids has also been implicated, although the exact mechanism is unknown.

Meticulous monitoring of insulin infusion rates and the addition of intravenous glucose to IV fluids once serum glucose is around 250 mg/dl is essential. Early detection of potential cerebral edema is important as treatment in the early stages is much more effective than treatment in later stages.[19] Cerebral edema should be suspected whenever deterioration of consciousness occurs *after* treatment has been initiated.

Acidosis and dehydration may impair learning and concentration skills for 48 to 72 hours after a DKA crisis. Ability to concentrate, follow instructions, or engage in conversation must be monitored to assess learning readiness. Until mental recovery occurs, patient teaching should be postponed. Typically, extensive teaching including sick-day management is done after transfer from the critical care unit. Referral for psychological or psychiatric intervention should be considered in cases of recurrent DKA.

When patients are discharged from the critical care unit, the transfer summary should include information regarding the duration of diabetes, usual management, concurrent illnesses, history of the crisis event, how the patient recognized and responded to the impending crisis, and identification of family members or significant others who are available to assist with care during hospitalization and at home.

Hypoglycemic Coma

Hypoglycemia may occur in patients with a specific disease, such as an insulin-producing islet-cell tumor, or as a complication of medical therapy such as required insulin administration. About 95% of cases occur in patients with diabetes who use blood glucose–lowering medication; it is the most common acute complication in these patients. It accounts for a reported 3% to 7% of deaths in patients with type I diabetes. Although difficult to quantify precisely, hypoglycemia is generally defined as a drop in blood glucose to less than 60 mg/dl. In the diabetic patient, its occurrence is associated with a disruption in the diet–exercise–medication balance.[27]

The most common causes of hypoglycemia associated with blood glucose–lowering medication use include: (1) errors in insulin administration, dosage, or timing; (2) changes in insulin absorption; (3) diet omissions or timing errors; (4) unplanned or increased exercise; and (5) use of alcoholic beverages.[17] In addition, many common situations may predispose the individual with type I diabetes to hypoglycemia, including (1) onset of menses, (2) immediate postpartum period, and (3) presence of renal disease.[19]

Hypoglycemia in persons using oral hypoglycemic medications can be unusually severe and prolonged if the agent taken has a long half-life. The presence of liver or kidney problems or the use of a variety of medications—such as dicumarol, sulfonamides, MAO inhibitors, barbiturates, phenylbutazone, and salicylates—can lead to hypoglycemia in persons using oral hypoglycemic medications. In addition, beta-adrenergic blocking drugs mask some symptoms of hypoglycemia (tachycardia) and prevent normal recovery by impairing mobilization of substrates for gluconeogenesis.

Individuals are generally able to treat all mild and most moderate hypoglycemic reactions by themselves. Severe hypoglycemia reactions are considered medical emergencies. They are manifested by unresponsiveness, unconsciousness, and/or seizures. Initial data from the feasibility phase of the Diabetes Control and Complications Trial (DCCT) reported severe hypoglycemia occurring in 26% of intensively controlled patients compared with 9.8% of conventionally controlled patients.[28] Although all diabetic patients on glucose-lowering medications are at risk for hypoglycemia, patients with insulin-dependent diabetes are at high risk if they:

- Use intensive insulin therapy regimens
- Have autonomic neuropathy
- Have defective counterregulatory response to hypoglycemia
- Use medications that mask early warning symptoms of hypoglycemia
- Have a history of hypoglycemia unawareness
- Delay treatment of mild to moderate hypoglycemia[17]

Pathophysiology

Excessive serum insulin leads to a reduction in blood sugar and consequent hypoglycemia by (1) increasing glucose use by insulin-sensitive tissues and (2) inhibiting hepatic glucose production. Clinical symptoms of hypoglycemia (described under Data Acquisition) occur when circulating glucose is inadequate to meet tissue glucose demands. Initially, insufficient levels of circulating glucose stimulate the sympathoadrenal system, eliciting the physiological stress response. Counterregulatory hormones including glucagon, epinephrine, growth hormone, and cortisol are secreted to oppose insulin action. These four hormones enhance hepatic glucose production and decrease peripheral glucose utilization to increase circulating blood glucose levels.[27]

Catecholamines exert a major influence in counterregulation and are primarily responsible for the adrenergic or "early warning" symptoms of hypoglycemia which tend to precede changes in cortical function. If blood glucose levels continue to decline, insufficient amounts of glucose will be available to brain cells. The brain is very sensitive to low blood glucose. A decrease in glucose lowers oxygen uptake by the brain and results in the neuroglycopenic symptoms of hypoglycemia. Symptoms of hypoglycemia can be more severe and occur at higher blood glucose levels in the elderly compared to younger persons. The symptoms of hypoglycemia vary among individuals but generally not from episode to episode. Frequent or prolonged hypoglycemia can cause irreversible brain damage, including decreased intellectual functioning, impaired nerve functioning, and personality changes.

Hypoglycemia is episodic, with symptoms lasting from minutes to hours at most. In some cases, counterregulatory hormone secretion or waning of exogenous insulin action may restore normal glucose levels. In many cases, however, the individual must ingest food or fluid to raise the blood glucose level to normal; without treatment, blood glucose levels continue to decline, and severe hypoglycemia characterized by loss of consciousness, seizures, or death will ensue.[27]

Data Acquisition

Initial adrenergic symptoms of hypoglycemia mediated by epinephrine release are characteristic of *mild hypoglycemic reactions*. Symptoms include sweating, palpitations, tremors, pallor, hunger, and nervousness or irritability. Since cognitive dysfunction is not a problem, patients with hypoglycemia awareness usually recognize and self-treat mild reactions without difficulty. In persons with preexisting cardiac problems, catecholamine-induced vasoconstriction can induce tachycardia, premature ventricular ectopic beats, angina pectoris, and myocardial ischemia or infarction.

If blood glucose continues to decline, *moderate hypoglycemic reaction* characterized by both adrenergic and neuroglycopenic symptoms will develop because glucose supply to brain cells is inadequate. Symptoms include headache, decreased attentiveness, mental confusion, paresthesias, irritability, agitation, bizarre behavior, speech difficulties, combativeness, drowsiness, lethargy, and paralysis. Individuals experiencing moderate reactions may require assistance to treat these reactions.[17]

If adequate blood glucose levels are not restored, the severity of symptoms will continue to increase, and *severe hypoglycemia* will result. Severe reactions are characterized by decreased responsiveness, loss of consciousness, and seizures. Prolonged severe hypoglycemia of 4 or more hours' duration causes irreversible brain damage.[27]

Medical Management

Treatment for hypoglycemia aims to restore blood glucose levels to normal. Treatment should be initiated as soon as bedside blood glucose monitoring confirms the condition but after a blood sample for laboratory testing has been obtained.

If the patient is able to swallow, *mild reactions* should be promptly treated with 10 to 15 g of simple carbohydrate given by mouth—for example, 6 to 8 Lifesavers, chewed up; 4 oz fruit juice; 2 tablespoons raisins; or 4 oz sugar-containing soft drink. The patient should be told to rest and avoid exercise until blood sugar is restored to normal. If symptoms are still present in 10 to 15 minutes, an additional 10 to 15 g of carbohydrate can be taken. As a general rule, if the next scheduled meal is more than 1 hour away, a longer-acting snack with protein such as 8 oz of milk or half a sandwich, should be taken to prevent recurrent hypoglycemia. Patients should be allowed to resume physical activity as soon as blood glucose returns to normal.[17,19]

Moderate hypoglycemic reactions should be promptly treated with 20 to 30 g of simple carbohydrate given by mouth if the patient can swallow. Examples listed for mild reactions can be doubled in amount, and treatment should be repeated if no symptomatic improvement is noted within 10 to 15 minutes after initial treatment. An additional long-acting snack should be provided as noted above if the next planned meal is more than 1 hour away. Patients should be told to wait 10 to 30 minutes before resuming normal activities. Patients experiencing moderate reactions may need assistance in treating the reaction. Occasionally, individuals may be so uncooperative due to neuroglycopenia that glucagon by injection may be needed for treatment.[17,19]

Patients with *severe hypoglycemia* who are unresponsive, unconscious, or unable to swallow should not be given anything by mouth for the treatment for hypoglycemia since aspiration can result. Adult patients may be given 1 mg of glucagon by subcutaneous or intramuscular injection, with a second dose repeated in 15 to 20 minutes if the first injection elicits no response. Alternatively, 25 g of 50% dextrose may be given intravenously over 1 to 3 minutes. If the patient's condition does not improve within 20 minutes after dextrose administration, an additional 12.5 g should be administered intravenously. An infusion of 5% dextrose should be continued until the patient is alert enough to take oral nourishment. Once able to eat and drink, the patient should be given a 15-g simple carbohydrate snack, followed by a more substantial carbohydrate–protein snack.[17]

Diabetic patients who experience severe hypoglycemic reactions will need to have their blood glucose monitored closely for several hours to make sure that hypoglycemia does not recur. In fact, all diabetic patients experiencing hypoglycemia should be closely observed with repeat bedside blood glucose monitoring and laboratory samples to verify recovery from hypoglycemia.

NURSING MANAGEMENT

Nursing intervention for patients experiencing hypoglycemia focuses on administering substances to elevate plasma glucose; preventing injury; and educating patients, families, and significant others about causes, symptoms, treatment, and prevention of hypoglycemia.

■ NURSING DIAGNOSIS

Nutrition, altered: less than body requirements, related to inadequate intake of nutrients in diet.

Nursing assessment centers on the manifestations of acute glucose deficiency. Adrenergic or neuroglycopenic symptoms, or both, may be present. Cardiovascular findings include tachycardia with peripheral vasoconstriction due to the stress response–induced surge in catecholamine secretion. In patients with a history of myocardial compromise, continuous electrocardiographic monitoring is indicated, because angina and premature ventricular contractions may occur during hypoglycemic events. The burst of catecholamines is also thought to be the basis for complaints of shakiness, hunger, nervousness, trembling, and the typical cold, clammy diaphoresis. In addition, critically ill diabetic patients who are unable to ingest regular meals present a special challenge. Difficulty balancing nutrient intake with blood glucose–lowering medication may predispose these patients to hypoglycemia.

OUTCOME STANDARD AND CRITERIA

Intake of nutrients is sufficient to meet the body's demands as evidenced by:
- Normal blood glucose levels
- Alleviation of subjective and objective manifestations of hypoglycemia

NURSING INTERVENTIONS

Primary nursing interventions focus on obtaining both a bedside capillary blood sample and a laboratory sample for glucose testing and *immediately* administering glucose supplements. Typically, supplements are provided until consciousness returns or blood glucose returns to normal. When the critically ill diabetic patient is receiving total parenteral nutrition or tube feedings, care must be taken to assure their availability without interruption in relation to the glucose-lowering medication. Whether supplements are provided orally or intravenously, careful observation as well as frequent and serial bedside blood glucose testing should be performed to monitor patient response to therapy. A nutrition consultation may be warranted. Recurrent episodes of hypoglycemia should be analyzed and may be indicative of the need to adjust glucose-lowering medication doses.

■ NURSING DIAGNOSIS

Potential for injury, related to sensory dysfunction. Neuroglycopenic symptoms of hypoglycemia can predispose the patient to injury related to sensory dysfunction secondary to inadequate glucose to brain cells.

OUTCOME STANDARD AND CRITERIA

The patient remains free of personal injury and verbalizes the importance of safety measures such as carrying diabetic identification and a source of carbohydrate at all times.

NURSING INTERVENTIONS

Nursing assessment first should focus on identifying the patient's usual symptoms of hypoglycemia. The nurse should limit physical activity and/or mobility during episodes of hypoglycemia. Hazardous environmental factors should be reduced. Causative factors for sensory dysfunction should be discussed with the patient and the family or significant other. Recommended types and amounts of nutrients should be offered at usual times. Patient should be instructed to carry a source of simple carbohydrate and diabetic identification at all times.

If blood glucose exceeds 200 mg/dl but the pre-event level of consciousness does not return, residual neurological compromise may be present. Nursing interventions in such instances should include frequent serial neurological assessments and specific evaluation to assure adequacy of basic protective reflexes, including the gag, swallow, and cough reflexes. If these responses are compromised, measures must be instituted to protect the airway. Seizure precautions should also be instituted (see also Chapter 33).

■ NURSING DIAGNOSIS

Knowledge deficit, related to lack of exposure to health teaching and/or lack of recall.

More than 50% of diabetic patients fail to follow their prescribed diet. Lack of knowledge regarding needed alterations in nutritional intake or insulin dose for lifestyle changes is common, as is lack of knowledge regarding the medical and dietary goals of treatment.

OUTCOME STANDARD AND CRITERIA

The patient is able to verbalize knowledge for self-care as evidenced by:

- Verbalization of appropriate meal and snack patterns
- Return demonstration of blood glucose monitoring technique
- Verbalization of signs, symptoms, and treatment of hypoglycemia
- Return demonstration of correct self-preparation and administration of glucagon (if indicated)

NURSING INTERVENTIONS

The nurse should assess the patient, family, or significant other to determine the probable cause of hypoglycemia; their knowledge about etiologies and signs/symptoms of hypoglycemia; and their ability to report and intervene during hypoglycemic reactions. Nursing interventions begin with ensuring that the patient clearly understands the recommended meal plan. Reinforcement of dietary goals is needed. Similarly, education is needed to facilitate establishment of appropriate meal plan choices for lifestyle or activity changes. A dietary consultation should be initiated. Education may also be necessary to ensure that ongoing monitoring of blood glucose is accurate and that information obtained is useful for self-care decisions. Patients with hypoglycemia unawareness can be assisted to recognize subtle symptoms of hypoglycemia and will be better able to intervene rapidly to prevent severe incidents.

At the point of transfer from the critical care unit, information regarding the patient's understanding of applicable medical and dietary goals, methods of monitoring blood glucose, causes and treatment of hypoglycemia as well as recognition of early signs and symptoms of hypoglycemia should be conveyed to nursing staff who will be providing care. Similarly, the presence of sensory deficits that may impair the patient's self-care ability needs to be reviewed. Finally, involvement of family and significant others in patient education can strengthen the foundation of the teaching plan to prevent recurrence of hypoglycemia. Families and significant others of patients who experience severe hypoglycemia should be instructed on the preparation and administration of glucagon for injection. Patients must be instructed to carry both a source of simple carbohydrate and diabetes identification at all times. Recurrent or severe hypoglycemia may be indicative of the need for treatment plan revision and should be promptly reported to the patient's physician for evaluation.[19]

Hyperglycemic Hyperosmolar Nonketotic Syndrome

The condition known as hyperglycemic hyperosmolar nonketotic syndrome (HHNS) most commonly occurs in elderly patients with type II diabetes or previously undiagnosed diabetes. It occurs with equal frequency in men and women and about one sixth as often as diabetic ketoacidosis. It is life-threatening and is associated with a mortality of 20% to 40% due to delay in diagnosis, misdiagnosis, or the presence of other serious complications.[29] Thus, physiological crisis often exists long before medical help is sought. Precipitating factors may include (1) massive fluid losses, (2) infections, (3) myocardial infarction, (4) gastrointestinal hemorrhage, (5) uremia, (6) hypertonic feedings, (7) pharmacological agents, (8) inadequate or limited access to fluids, or (9) surgery or other stressors. Social isolation may be a precipitating factor in 25% to 33% of cases.[29]

Pathophysiology

HHNS is characterized by four features: (1) hyperglycemia, (2) absence of significant ketosis, (3) severe dehydration, and (4) neurological manifestations. The pathophysiology of HHNS is outlined in Figure 39-2. A precipitating event combined with a decreased insulin reserve is usually responsible for the development of HHNS. The event may be ingestion of a hyperglycemia-inducing agent (hyperalimentation, insulin-inhibiting drugs), acute exacerbation of chronic disease (typically renal or cardiovascular), or any situation that provokes a stress response. The hyperglycemia that occurs is potentiated by a de-

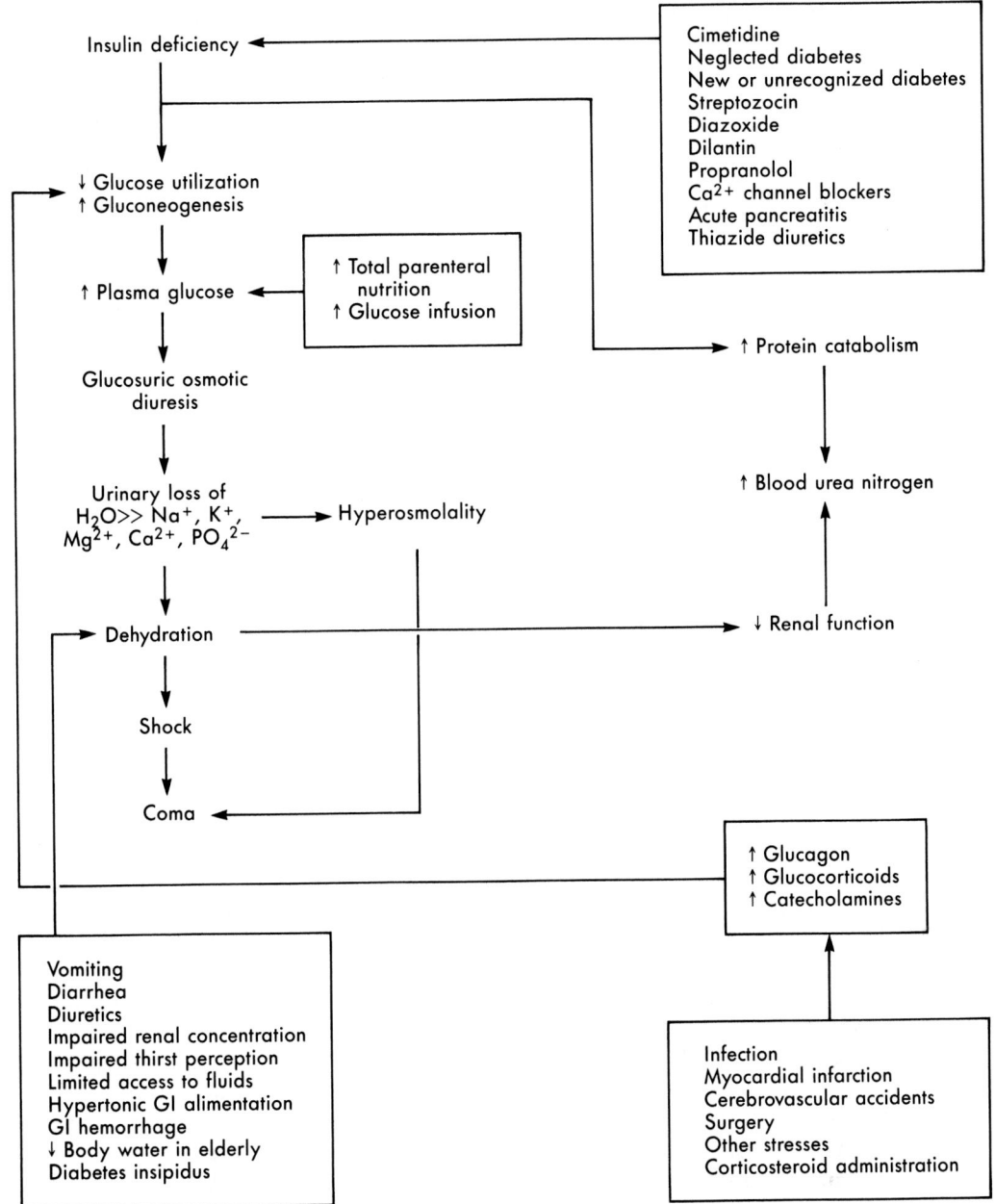

Figure 39-2   Hyperglycemic hyperosmolar nonketotic syndrome.
From Matz, R. (1988). *Clinical diabetes,* Vol. 6. New York: American Diabetes Association.

creased insulin reserve and stress-induced catechol-amine and glucocorticoid secretion. Insulin deficiency precludes cellular utilization of glucose and, in combination with counterregulatory hormones, increases hepatic glucose release resulting in severe hyperglycemia.

A comparison of diabetic ketoacidosis (DKA) and HHNS is presented in Table 39-2. Hyperglycemia is more pronounced in HHNS than in DKA. Values are typically between 600 and 2,500 mg/dl. As many as 80% of patients with HHNS have been found to have

renal function impairment. The glomerular filtration rate has been decreased by primary disease or extracellular volume depletion; the renal threshold for glucose excretion is consequently raised, and plasma glucose levels are therefore greatly elevated.[30] Because glucose is an osmotically active substance, glucosuria causes pronounced osmotic diuresis. Extracellular fluid depletion may be more pronounced in the elderly, whose kidneys are less able to concentrate urine, respond to antidiuretic hormone (ADH), and conserve body water. In addition, because elderly in-

TABLE 39-2 **Comparison of DKA and HHNS**

	DKA	HHNS
General	More acidotic, less dehydrated	Not acidotic, more dehydrated, frequently comatose
Age	Younger patient	Usually elderly
Type of diabetes	Type I	Type II
Initial lab results:		
Blood glucose	↑ 250-800 mg/dl	↑ 600-2,500 mg/dl
Plasma ketones	Positive in several dilutions	Less than large in undiluted specimen
Serum potassium	Low, normal, or high	Low, normal, or high
Serum bicarbonate	<10 mEq/L	>16 mEq/L
Blood pH	<7.35	Normal
Serum osmolality	<300 mosm/L	>350 mosm/L
Serum sodium	Low, normal, or high	Normal or high
BUN	Elevated	Markedly elevated
Anion gap	Over 12 mEq/L	10-12 mEq/L

Adapted from Kozak, G. (Ed.). (1982). *Clinical diabetes mellitus*. Philadelphia: Saunders.

dividuals have a lower total body water content compared with younger persons, they have less total water available to buffer losses. A decrease in sense of thirst or in the ability to respond to thirst may also be present. These changes in body water balance quickly lead to extracellular volume depletion and dehydration. Renal blood flow and glomerular filtration rate decrease further; BUN and creatinine increase. Oliguria and acute renal failure may occur.[29]

In contrast to diabetic ketoacidosis, HHNS is characterized by an absence of significant ketosis, perhaps because available insulin, though inadequate to control blood glucose, is sufficient to inhibit lipolysis. The absence of significant ketosis may be also attributable to low levels of free fatty acids, which are thought to be associated with reduced levels of catabolic hormone in HHNS as compared with DKA. Significant depletion of body water and marked hyperglycemia present in HHNS dramatically increase serum osmolality. In HHNS, osmolality is characterized as severe and frequently exceeds 350 mosm/L. Neurological manifestations are well correlated with the degree of osmolality and the rapidity of development. Of patients with serum osmolality greater than 350 mosm/L, 45% are comatose. In addition to an altered mental state, many patients with HHNS will have focal neurological findings that resolve after successful treatment of HHNS.[29]

Data Acquisition

Initial laboratory tests for suspected HHNS include those of blood glucose, serum and urinary ketones, electrolytes, serum osmolality, BUN, hematocrit, and WBC. Typical findings are:

- Elevated blood glucose (>600 mg/dl)
- Minimal or no ketonuria/ketonemia
- Sodium usually normal or high
- Potassium may be low, normal, or high
- Bicarbonate within normal limits
- Blood pH within normal limits
- Serum osmolality greater than 350 mosm/L

Polymorphonuclear leukocytosis is common. BUN and hematocrit are usually elevated. Hypertriglyceridemia and abnormal liver functions are present in up to one third of patients with HHNS.[29] Infrequently, anion gap acidosis may be present due to renal insufficiency. Lactic acidosis and decreased tissue perfusion may be present.

The onset of HHNS is insidious, developing typically over a period of days or weeks. Patients appear seriously ill. Extracellular volume depletion is the most immediate life-threatening abnormality associated with HHNS. Classic symptoms of uncontrolled diabetes, including polyuria, polydipsia, polyphagia, and weight loss, may be present. Body water and electrolyte loss leads to severe extracellular volume depletion manifested by sustained and postural hypotension, poor skin turgor, dry mucous membranes, tachycardia, and soft eyeballs. Sodium, potassium, calcium, chloride, phosphate, and magnesium are severely depleted. Symptoms associated with decreased electrolytes may be present. Respirations are usually shallow.

Patients with HHNS usually present with normal or elevated body temperatures. Abnormal neurological findings are common. Symptoms of HHNS are often mistaken for a cerebral vascular accident. Mental status is almost always depressed. In addition, focal neurological findings may include either focal or grand mal seizures, extensor plantar reflexes, aphasia, homonymous hemianopsia, hemisensory deficits, hemiparesis, or visual hallucinations.[29]

Medical Management

The initial goal of medical therapy should be to correct the life-threatening abnormalities: extracellular volume depletion, electrolyte imbalance, and insulin deficiency.[18] In addition, the precipitating cause of HHNS should be identified and treated, and complications avoided to the degree possible.

Fluid replacement is a priority to restore and maintain vascular volume and kidney function. Total fluid deficit in HHNS is estimated to be between 5 and 12 liters. Clinical and laboratory findings should be used to guide infusion rate determinations. Elderly patients must be hydrated with caution. Central venous pressures, pulmonary capillary wedge pressures, as well as renal function may be used to guide treatment, especially in elderly patients with known cardiovascular disease.[19]

Initially, 0.9% normal saline or a hypotonic electrolyte solution is administered at a rate of 1,500 ml/hr for the first hour; then 1,000 ml/hr for 2 hours; then 500 to 750 ml/hr for one hour. If hypotension or shock is present, rapid correction of this condition is necessary.

Crystalloid solutions or volume expanders should be administered in large volume if needed. Additionally, pressors may be used if hypotension does not respond to volume replacement efforts. Isotonic solutions should be used when serum osmolality decreases to less than 320 mosm/L. In addition, intravenous fluids should be changed to 5% dextrose in water when blood glucose drops to 250 to 300 mg/dl to allow continued insulin infusion without hypoglycemia.[29,30]

Because relative insulin deficiency is present in HHNS, insulin therapy is essential to its successful treatment. The amount of insulin needed is generally equal to or slightly less than that required for the treatment of DKA. However, in some cases, up to an 80% reduction in blood glucose has been noted following hydration and before insulin administration. In these cases, the fall in blood glucose was effected by dilution and glycosuria.

Only short-acting (regular) insulin should be used initially. Insulin reduces hyperglycemia by promoting cellular utilization of glucose and decreasing hepatic glucose production. Administering insulin intravenously is the most direct and preferred route if the infusion can be regulated. The initial bolus is usually 0.15 U/kg of regular U100 insulin, followed by an intravenous infusion at a rate of 0.1 U/kg per hour (approximately 5 to 10 U/hr). Infusion rates will usu-

ally be reduced by 50%, and 5% or 10% dextrose added to the infusion once blood glucose values reach 250 to 300 mg/dl.[29,30]

Intramuscular administration of insulin is recommended only if there is no available method of regulating an insulin infusion. In this case, an initial bolus dose of 0.5 U/kg is usually given, and followed by doses of 0.1 U/kg per hour of U100 by intramuscular injection until the blood glucose is reduced to 300 mg/dl. Thereafter, doses of 0.1 U/kg should be administered intramuscularly every 2 hours as needed to maintain blood glucose around 250 mg/dl.

Electrolyte losses are considered to be a major factor in the development of HHNS, and their replacement constitutes one of the initial goals of medical therapy. Potassium losses are attributable to the severe catabolic state and body water losses associated with HHNS. In fact, potassium losses are reported to be greater in HHNS than in DKA. Potassium replacement should be initiated within 1 hour after starting fluid replacement therapy if urine output is adequate. In the case of renal insufficiency, initial potassium replacement is based on serum potassium levels, and the infusion rate is reduced by 50% or more.[29]

The amount of potassium added to intravenous fluids depends on serum levels. If the serum level is lower than 3 mEq/L, 60 mEq are given over 1 hour. The rate of administration is then adjusted according to serum levels and ECG findings. For serum potassium levels of 4 to 5 mEq/L, infusion rates of 20 mEq per hour are used. Potassium replacement is generally withheld if serum potassium values are greater than 5 mEq/L. Hourly electrocardiogram strips may supplement laboratory analysis in monitoring potassium status. It is important to keep in mind that the magnitude of total body potassium deficit may require days to weeks to correct.[29,30] Potassium chloride is the usual replacement. If hypophosphatemia is present, potassium phosphate may be administered in doses less than a maximum of 90 mEq over 24 hours.

Magnesium deficit related to glycosuric losses may be hard to differentiate from potassium deficit because the signs and symptoms of these deficiencies are similar. If severe magnesium deficit is present, 500 ml of 20% magnesium sulfate solution may be infused over 4 to 6 hours. In a less emergent situation without renal failure, magnesium is often routinely administered in doses of 0.05 to 0.1 ml of 20% magnesium sulfate per kg, divided into two intramuscular injections.

Calcium deficits are also common, often becoming apparent within 12 hours after fluid therapy is initiated. Deficits are usually treated with 10 mEq of elemental calcium by intravenous bolus injection as needed. With successful treatment of the hyperosmolar state, all neurological abnormalities and changes usually resolve. Seizures, if present, usually do not respond to conventional anticonvulsant therapy but rather to the correction of hyperosmolarity. Thromboembolic events are considered to be a most serious complication of HHNS. Aggressive fluid replacement is essential to minimizing the risk for the development of this serious complication.[29]

After HHNS has resolved, insulin administration continues to be an important medical therapy. Once fluid balance is regained and the patient is able to take food or fluids by mouth, insulin may be given by subcutaneous injection. Subcutaneous administration of insulin is best instituted before a meal at the time of a planned insulin injection. Insulin infusions can be discontinued 30 minutes after subcutaneous insulin is given. Generally, patients recovering from HHNS can take food or fluids by mouth as soon as their level of consciousness returns to normal, provided no other medical contraindications are present.

Blood glucose monitoring should continue every 4 to 6 hours to evaluate ongoing effects of insulin on blood glucose.

Although insulin therapy may be continued for a short time after resolution of HHNS, most patients do not require long-term insulin therapy. Precipitating factors for this individual crisis must be identified and avoided in the future.

NURSING MANAGEMENT

In the critical care setting, nursing interventions involved in providing care for patients with HHNS must be directed toward management of dehydration, hyperglycemia, and altered central nervous system function. Frequent multisystem assessments must include special emphasis on cardiac, respiratory, renal, neurological, and gastrointestinal function.

Most of the applicable nursing diagnoses in HHNS are the same as those in DKA. Three additional diagnoses and their related interventions are discussed in the following paragraphs.

■ NURSING DIAGNOSIS

Fluid volume deficit, related to failure of regulatory mechanisms.

Patients at risk for fluid volume deficit, related to osmotic diuresis in HHNS, include older adults with type II diabetes or previously undiagnosed diabetes and those with underlying cardiac or renal insufficiency.

OUTCOME STANDARD AND CRITERIA

Fluid status is returned to normal as evidenced by:
- Blood pressure and pulse within normal limits for the patient
- Normal serum electrolyte levels
- Balanced intake and output
- Alleviation of dehydration

NURSING INTERVENTIONS

As in DKA, ongoing assessment in HHNS centers on hydration and prevention of complications (see also Nursing Management in section on DKA). Special attention must be directed, however, to the cardiac and renal systems. Renal assessment includes careful monitoring of intake and output and serum creatinine levels. With increasing age and microvascular changes, the renal threshold may be raised, and the kidneys may not filter excess glucose, resulting in severe hyperglycemia. The kidney's decreased ability to degrade insulin may result in a decreased requirement for insulin.

Often, it is the older adult with underlying renal or cardiac insufficiency who experiences HHNS. The underlying cardiac compromise increases the risk of overload with fluid replenishment. Frequent monitoring of vital signs and auscultation of the heart and lungs, as well as continuous cardiac monitoring, are needed to guide fluid management (see also Nursing Management in the section on DKA).

HIGH-RISK NURSING DIAGNOSIS

High risk for injury, related to sensory dysfunction.

Seizures, usually focal, occur in about 25% of patients with HHNS. The pathogenesis remains uncertain, but fluid, electrolyte, and metabolic abnormalities involved in HHNS are thought to enhance seizure activity. With treatment and return of normal osmolality, seizures tend to resolve.[29] If HHNS recurs, seizures often also recur.

OUTCOME STANDARD AND CRITERIA

The patient remains free of personal injury.

NURSING INTERVENTIONS

Nursing interventions include frequent serial neurological assessment. Seizure precautions are instituted. Anticonvulsive drugs are commonly not used because such agents are generally ineffective in HHNS and because of concern regarding inhibition of insulin release and potential for worsening the patient's condition, particularly with the use of phenytoin (Dilantin).

■ NURSING DIAGNOSIS

Knowledge deficit, related to lack of exposure to health information, cognitive limitation, or lack of recall.

OUTCOME STANDARD AND CRITERIA

Patient teaching occurs when readiness to learn is demonstrated by normal communication patterns, ordered thought process, and appropriate emotional responses. The patient and family then demonstrate appropriate knowledge for self-care.

NURSING INTERVENTIONS

Impaired learning ability from dehydration coupled with the shortness of the stay in the critical care unit dictates that extensive teaching be postponed until the patient has been transferred from the unit. At that time, the transfer summary should include information regarding the duration of the patient's disease, management of the diabetes, concurrent illnesses, history of the crisis event (including how the patient recognized it and responded), and a description of family and social support systems.

REFERENCES

1. Moses, A. M., & Streeten, D. H. P. (1986). Disorders of the hypothalamic–neurohypophyseal system. In P. Kohler (Ed.), *Clinical endocrinology* (pp. 53-72). New York: Wiley.
2. Robertson, G. L. (1990). The endocrine brain and pituitary gland. In K. Becker (Ed.), *Principles and practice in endocrinology and metabolism* (pp. 92-246). Philadelphia: Lippincott.
3. Kim, M. J., McFarland, G. K., & McLande, A. M. (1991). *Pocket guide to nursing diagnoses*. St. Louis: Mosby–Year Book.
4. American Association of Critical-care Nurses. (1990). *Outcome standards for critical care nursing*. Laguna Niguel, CA: Author.
5. Solomon, B. L., Loriaux, T. C., & Drass, J. A. (1992). Endocrine and metabolic systems. In J. Thompson, G. K. McFarland, J. E. Hirsch, et al. (Eds.), *Mosby's manual of clinical nursing* (pp. 876-967). St. Louis: Mosby–Year Book.
6. Frohman, L. A. (1992). Neuroendocrine regulation and its disorders. In J. B. Wyngaarden, & L. H. Smith (Eds.), *Cecil textbook of medicine* (19th ed.) (pp. 1215-1224). Philadelphia: Saunders.
7. Melmed, S., & Braunstein, G. D. (1990). Disorders of the hypothalamus and anterior pituitary. In J. H. Stein, W. Daly, J. D. Easton, et al. (Eds.), *Internal medicine* (3rd ed.). Boston: Little, Brown.
8. Becker, K. L. (1990). General principles of endocrinology. In K. Becker (Ed.), *Principles and practice in endocrinology and metabolism* (pp. 2-80). Philadelphia: Lippincott.
9. Jackson, I. M. D., & Cobb, W. E. (1986). Disorders of the thyroid. In P. Kohler (Ed.), *Clinical endocrinology* (pp. 73-166). New York: Wiley.
10. Wartofsky, L. (1990). The thyroid gland. In K. Becker (Ed.), *Principles and practice in endocrinology and metabolism* (pp. 263-385). Philadelphia: Lippincott.
11. Bilezikian, J. P. (1990). Hypocalcemia. In J. H. Stein, W. Daly, J. D. Easton, et al. (Eds.), *Internal medicine* (3rd ed.). Boston: Little, Brown.
12. Loriaux, D. L., & Cutler, J. B., Jr. (1986). Diseases of the adrenal glands. In P. Kohler (Ed.), *Clinical endocrinology* (pp. 167-238). New York: Wiley.
13. Baxter, J. D. (1988). Principles of endocrinology. In J. B. Wyngaarden, & L. H. Smith (Eds.), *Cecil textbook of medicine* (18th ed.) (pp. 1252-1267). Philadelphia: Saunders.
14. Loriaux, D. L. (1990). The adrenal glands. In K. Becker (Ed.), *Principles and practice in endocrinology and metabolism* (pp. 92-246). Philadelphia: Lippincott.
15. Cryer, P. E. (1992). The adrenal medulla and the sympathetic nervous system. In J. B. Wyngaarden, & L. H. Smith (Eds.), *Cecil textbook of medicine* (19th ed.) (pp. 1390-1394). Philadelphia: Saunders.
16. Bennett, P. (1990). Epidemiology of diabetes mellitus. In H. Rifkin, & D. Porte (Eds.), *Ellenberg and Rifkin's diabetes mellitus theory and practice* (4th ed.). New York: Elsevier.
17. Sperling, M. (Ed.). (1988). *Physician's guide to insulin-dependent (type I) diabetes: Diagnosis and treatment*. Alexandria, VA: American Diabetes Association.
18. Lebovitz, H. (Ed.). (1988). *Physician's guide to non-insulin-dependent (type II) diabetes: Diagnosis and treatment* (2nd ed.). Alexandria, VA: American Diabetes Association.
19. Guthrie, D. (Ed.). (1988). *Diabetes education: A core curriculum for health professionals*. Chicago: American Association of Diabetes Educators.
20. Rifkin, H., & Porte, D. (Eds.). (1990). *Diabetes mellitus theory and practice* (4th ed.). New York: Elsevier.
21. Johnson, D., Palumbo, P., & Chu, C. (1980). Diabetic ketoacidosis in a community-based population. *Mayo Clinic Proceedings, 55,* 83-88.
22. Faich, G., Fishbein, H., & Ellis, S. (1983). The epidemiology of diabetic acidosis: A population-based study. *American Journal of Epidemiology, 117,* 551-558.
23. Kreisberg, R. (1990). Diabetic ketoacidosis. In H. Rifkin, & D. Porte (Eds.), *Ellenberg and Rifkin's diabetes mellitus theory and practice* (4th ed.). New York: Elsevier.
24. Gale, E., & Tattersall, R. (1978). Hypothermia: A complication of diabetic ketoacidosis. *British Medical Journal, 2,* 1387-1389.
25. Guerin, J., Meyer, P., & Segrestaa, J. (1987). Hypothermia in diabetic ketoacidosis. *Diabetes Care, 10,* 801-802.
26. Fleckman, A. (1991). Diabetic ketoacidosis. *Practical Diabetology, 10*(3), 1-5, 8.
27. Davidson, J., Galloway, J., & Chance, R. (1991). Insulin therapy. In J. Davidson (Ed.), *Clinical diabetes mellitus: A problem-oriented approach* (2nd ed.). New York: Thieme.
28. The DCCT Research Group. (1987). Diabetes control and complications trial (DCCT): Results of the feasibility study. *Diabetes Care, 10,* 1-19.
29. Matz, R. (1990). Hyperosmolar nonacidotic diabetes (HNAD). In H. Rifkin, & D. Porte (Eds.), *Ellenberg and Rifkin's diabetes mellitus theory and practice* (4th ed.). New York: Elsevier.
30. Davidson, J. (1991). Diabetic ketoacidosis and the hyperglycemic hyperosmolar state. In J. Davidson (Ed.), *Clinical diabetes mellitus: A problem-oriented approach* (2nd ed.). New York: Thieme.

40

Hematological Anatomy and Physiology

Debra Tribett

As multicellular organisms evolved, cells lost their direct contact with the external environment. A means of transporting nutrients and wastes between the interior and exterior environments gradually took form. The circulatory system provides the interface between the internal and external environments. The heart and blood vessels are the pump and conduits, and the blood is the medium for carrying the nutrients and wastes.

This chapter focuses on the *hematopoietic system*, those structures related to the blood-making processes, and the characteristics and contributions of the constituents of the hematopoietic system to homeostasis.

PHYSIOLOGY

The principal physiological functions of the hematopoietic system are respiration, nutrition, and excretion. Blood carries the respiratory gases (oxygen and carbon dioxide), nutrients, and wastes, providing transport between all tissues and organs of the body. Because of these transport functions, the blood participates directly or indirectly in virtually all body functions. In its travels, it flows through specialized sensors located in the vasculature that selectively react to such variables as osmotic pressure, pH, temperature, and the level of certain hormones. Thus, nontransport functions in which blood participates are temperature regulation and fluid and acid–base balance. Through the process of hemostasis, the blood provides a mechanism that controls escape of blood after injury to the vascular compartment.

Components of the blood participate in the defense of the body against infectious organisms and foreign antigens creating protection through the immune response. Further discussion of this function of the blood is found in Chapter 43.

BLOOD COMPOSITION AND CHARACTERISTICS

Blood is a complex liquid tissue containing circulating cells suspended in a pale yellow liquid called *plasma*. Plasma constitutes approximately 55% of the total blood volume. It is part of the extracellular fluid of the body. The other 45% of the blood volume consists of the solid suspended cells.

Blood Volume

The total circulating blood volume in the normal adult is estimated at 75 ml/kg, or 5 L of blood for the male and 3.5 to 4.5 L in the female. Pregnancy increases the normal value for females. Assuming normal renal function, this amount is relatively constant and does not fluctuate markedly or for any length of time.

Maintaining a constant blood volume in the vascular compartment is critical because, without a minimum amount, circulation is impaired and life is endangered. A loss of 20% of the circulating volume can result in hypovolemic shock. When a person drinks a large quantity of water, the water is rather rapidly removed from the blood by the tissues or is eliminated by the kidneys. Conversely, following an episode of acute blood loss, a protective process known as *autotransfusion* occurs. Autotransfusion attempts to restore a normal circulating blood volume by allowing protein-free fluid to enter the circulation from the interstitial spaces.

Normal distribution of the blood volume in the systemic circulation includes 18% in the arteries, 6% in the capillaries, and the remaining 76% in the venules and veins. The veins act as the body's capacitance or reservoir system. They can accommodate a large volume increase with a minimal increase in venous pressure.

The pulmonary circulation contains approximately 500 ml of the total blood volume. Half of this volume is in the pulmonary capillary bed. The pulmonary arteries contain 20%, and the veins and venules contain the remaining 30%.

Plasma

Blood plasma is an extremely complex fluid containing large quantities of organic and inorganic substances dissolved in water. The solutes that make up the largest percentage (6% to 8%) of total plasma weight are the plasma proteins: albumin and globulins (alpha, beta, and gamma), and fibrinogen.

The parenchymal liver cell, the *hepatocyte,* is the main site of plasma protein synthesis. It is also the site for the production of the most of the blood proteins that are essential coagulation factors. Gamma globulins, or immunoglobulins, are the exception. These antibody proteins are synthesized by the B cell lymphocytes and plasma cells.

Serum albumin constitutes over half of the total plasma proteins. It is important to the regulation of intravascular plasma volume. Since little protein escapes from blood vessels, intravascular protein concentration is far higher than extravascular concentration. This difference in protein concentration sets up an osmotic pressure gradient that tends to bring fluid in from the interstitial space. At the arteriolar end of a capillary bed this pressure is less than the blood pressure, so there is a net movement of fluid out of blood vessels. With the drop in blood pressure at the venous end of the capillary bed, the net movement of fluid is no longer outward but inward in accordance with the osmotic pressure created by the plasma proteins.

Plasma proteins, in particular albumin, contribute to the osmotic pressure of plasma. The presence of various salts, waste products, glucose, and other crystalloids dissolved in the plasma also affect the osmotic pressure. Because the composition of the blood undergoes continual small changes, the osmotic pressure fluctuates slightly. The change in composition is due to the passage of water and dissolved nutrients and the various waste products that continually pass in and out of the blood. The osmotic pressure is maintained within physiological limits by the kidneys. The osmotic pressure of plasma averages 300 mosm per kilogram of H_2O.

If this dynamic relationship is deranged by a decrease in the plasma proteins, more fluid leaves the vessel at the arterial end than reenters at the venous end. Interstitial edema results. A decrease in plasma proteins can occur from decreased production—for example, in liver disease—or from the loss of large quantities of plasma proteins through the kidneys, as with the nephrotic syndrome.

Serum globulins (32% to 48% of serum proteins) can be subdivided into alpha, beta, and gamma fractions. The alpha fraction is associated with the transport of steroids, lipids, and bilirubin. The beta fraction is associated with transport of iron, copper, and lipoproteins. The gamma globulins and their role in immune system function are discussed in greater detail in Chapter 43.

Other plasma proteins are also involved in the coagulation process. These coagulation factors are discussed later in this chapter.

Cells of the Blood

Hematopoiesis

The principal site for *hematopoiesis,* or blood formation, is the bone marrow. The process includes cellular proliferation, division of immature stem cells, and, ultimately, the differentiation of the stem cells into mature cell types. Cells produced by the bone marrow include erythrocytes (red blood cells), leukocytes (white blood cells), and thrombocytes (platelets).

In a healthy state, hematopoiesis maintains a balance between production of new blood cells and the destruction of old blood cells. This balance requires the production of billions of cells daily. The bone marrow can increase normal production rates by five- to tenfold based on the body's needs in times of physiological stress.

Bone Marrow

The bone marrow occupies 85% of the cavities of the bones. Marrow consists of blood, hematopoietic cells, and fat. With age, hematopoietic cells are replaced with adipose tissue (fat). By age 18, the marrow-containing bones are the skull, clavicle, scapulae, sternum, ribs, vertebrae, pelvis, and the proximal ends of long bones. In normal adults, 50% of bone marrow is fat. This percentage increases to 66% by the age of 70 to 80.

All types of blood cells are derived from pluripotent stem cells located in the bone marrow. Under stimulation, stem cells have the ability to reproduce themselves and to produce the precursors to the highly differentiated cells found in the circulating blood. Each pluripotent stem cell differentiates into two types of committed stem cells. One type is defined as the *colony-forming unit—granulocyte, erythrocyte, macrophage, and megakaryocyte (CFU-GEMM).* The other is the *colony-forming unit—lymphocyte (CFU-L).*[1] The individual pathways leading to the production of each type of mature cell from its precursor cells are illustrated in Figure 40-1.

Colony-forming units for each line of specific cells are stimulated by colony-stimulating factors. *Colony-stimulating factors (CSFs)* are a group of cell-derived

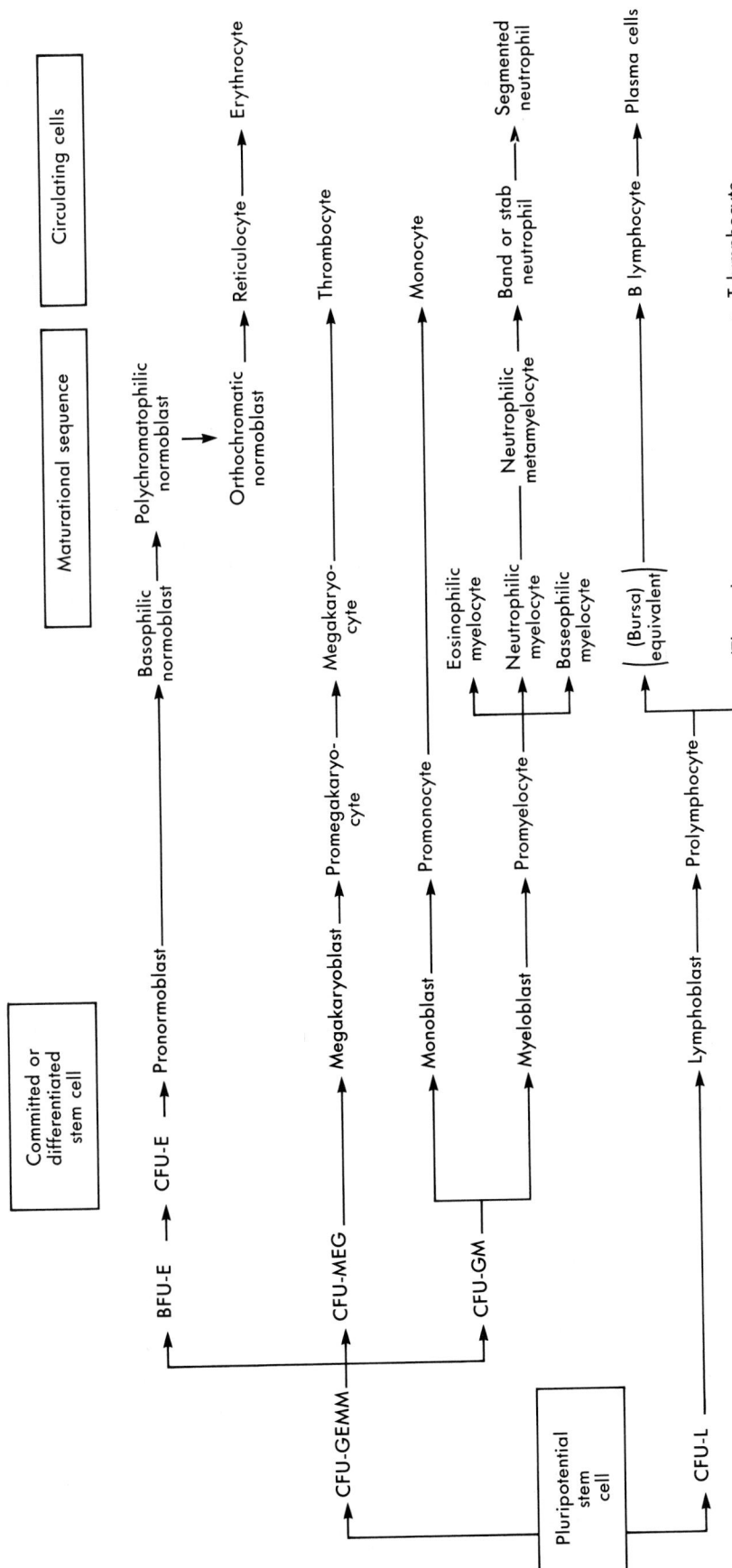

Figure 40-1   Hematopoiesis: blood cell formation and maturation.

glycoproteins that stimulate blood cell production, maturation, and function. The CSFs are synthesized from lymphocytes, macrophages, fibroblasts, and endothelial cells. They are released from their site of production, circulate in the blood, and attach to specific receptors on the cell surface of hematopoietic precursors. Specific CSFs act at different points during the differentiation of stem cells. There is overlap in their action on the colony-forming units and precursor cells. The identification of CSFs and the subsequent ability to produce recombinant forms have led to their clinical use in the stimulation of bone marrow cell production in many situations of bone marrow disease or suppression.

Erythrocytes (Red Blood Cells)

The red blood cell (RBC) is uniquely designed. The erythrocyte is a pliable biconcave disk with a thin, flexible membrane. It carries a few enzymes and hemoglobin but no nucleus. This design appears to facilitate movement through the small capillary beds and to expose more surface area for the exchange of oxygen and carbon dioxide at the tissue level. At the end of its life, the RBC is almost completely recycled.

The function of the RBC is respiration. This function is accomplished by the unique presence of *hemoglobin*. Globin is a simple protein that is attached to heme, the iron-containing pigment. Hemoglobin binds with oxygen in the capillaries of the lungs and transports it to the tissues throughout the body. In the tissue capillary bed, oxygen is exchanged for carbon dioxide, which the RBC carries back to the lungs for elimination from the body. The RBC influences oxygen transport by the concentration of hemoglobin in the blood and the regulation of the hemoglobin affinity for oxygen.

Concentration of hemoglobin determines the oxygen-carrying capacity of the blood. Each gram of hemoglobin has the ability to carry 1.34 ml of oxygen. However, the saturation of hemoglobin with oxygen is influenced by several factors. The normal concentration of hemoglobin in the blood is approximately 15 grams per 100 ml of blood.

Hemoglobin's affinity for oxygen is affected by the pH of the blood, its temperature, and the levels of intracellular 2,3-diphosphoglycerate (2,3-DPG). Hemoglobin's affinity for oxygen is lowered by acidosis, hyperthermia, and increased levels of 2,3-DPG. Alkalosis, hypothermia, and decreased levels of 2,3-DPG increase the affinity of hemoglobin to oxygen.

The partial pressure of oxygen available in the lung also influences the ability of hemoglobin to carry oxygen. As the partial pressure of oxygen increases, the amount of oxygen combining with hemoglobin increases.

Red cell production *(erythropoiesis)* takes place exclusively in the bone marrow of a normal adult. Two forms of early progenitor cells have been identified that arise from the CFU-GEMM. The more primitive is the *burst-forming unit—erythroid (BFU-E)*. It gives rise to the *colony-forming unit—erythroid (CFU-E)*. RBC production begins with the mitotic division of the pronormoblast and proceeds through three mitotic divisions taking 3 to 5 days, giving rise to the *reticulocyte*.

Erythropoietin, a glycoprotein hormone, stimulates the production of RBCs during this process. Erythropoietin is manufactured in the kidneys. It is found in high concentrations in the BFU-E. Production of erythropoietin increases in response to hypoxia. This situation can occur as a result of anemia (decreased number of RBCs) or as a result of pulmonary or cardiovascular disease impairing oxygen delivery to the tissues.

The reticulocyte stays in the bone marrow for 1 to 2 more days before being released into the circulation. In the circulating blood, reticulocytes mature into RBCs in 1 to 2 days. Normally, in the adult, fewer than 2% of circulating RBCs are reticulocytes. When the bone marrow increases production at a very rapid rate in response to body demands, increased numbers of reticulocytes appear in the circulating blood. An even greater number of immature forms of RBCs may be seen in situations of severe anemia.

To produce normal healthy RBCs, the bone marrow must have adequate substrates. These include vitamin B_{12}, folic acid, vitamin B_6, and iron. The vitamins and folic acid are obtained through dietary sources. Most of the iron used for the synthesis of hemoglobin is obtained from the recycling of senescent RBCs. However, the remainder is obtained from dietary sources.

On the surface of the RBC membrane are glycoprotein or glycolipid antigens. These antigens are inherited. There are many different types of antigens on an RBC, but the most clinically significant are the antigens that determine blood group and type. The presence or absence of A and B antigens determines the ABO blood group. D antigens, or the *Rh factor*, determine blood type. Blood is considered Rh-positive if the D antigen is present and Rh-negative if the D antigen is absent.

The serum of the adult normally contains antibodies directed to the antigen absent from the erythrocytes (Table 40-1). The most likely explanation for the presence of these natural antibodies is continual exposure to A and B antigens that are widespread in nature.

The mature RBC lives about 120 days, from the time it is released from the bone marrow until it is ultimately destroyed. Erythrocyte formation is one of the most anabolic processes in the body. Approxi-

TABLE 40-1 **ABO Blood Group System**

Blood Type	% in Population	Antigen	Antibody
A	41	A	Anti B
B	9	B	Anti A
AB	3	A & B	None
O	47	None	Anti A & B

mately 2×10^{11} erythrocytes are replaced daily.

The aging (senescent) RBC undergoes changes in its cell membrane, becoming fragile and worn. Eventually, it ruptures. Senescent RBCs are phagocytized by cells of the reticuloendothelial system, primarily in the spleen but also in the liver and bone marrow. The hemoglobin is catabolized into globin and heme. The released globin is returned to the plasma protein pool. The iron portion of the heme is returned to the stored iron pool in the liver. The biliverdin produced from heme breakdown is converted to bilirubin and bound to plasma albumin. In this state, it is known as *unconjugated* or *indirect bilirubin*. Unconjugated bilirubin is cleared from the plasma by the liver's parenchymal cells. In the liver, it is conjugated with glucuronic acid. *Conjugated bilirubin* is passed through the bile into the intestine.

The body can normally process and recycle old RBCs. However, in pathological conditions when greater numbers of RBCs are broken down or hemolyzed, the recycling efforts can be overwhelmed. Jaundice (icterus) results when production of bilirubin exceeds the liver's ability to reprocess it. Bilirubin is then deposited into the tissues, causing the yellow color of the skin, sclerae, and mucous membranes.

Leukocytes (White Blood Cells)

The leukocytes are the body's primary defense against invading organisms and foreign antigens. They are larger than RBCs and are nucleated. White blood cells (WBCs) are further classified on the basis of the unique structure of each cell type. *Granulocytes* are of three types: neutrophils, eosinophils, and basophils. *Nongranular leukocytes* are monocytes and lymphocytes.

Although WBCs are less numerous than RBCs, the blood cells of this varied group are specialized for different functions. Each type of cell and its function is discussed in greater detail in Chapter 43 as part of the review of the immune system.

Thrombocytes (Platelets)

Thrombocyte means "clot cell." Platelets do not have a nucleus and are not true cells, but they are instrumental in clot formation. They are formed by the cytoplasmic division of megakaryocytes. *Megakaryocytes* are extremely large cells present in adult bone marrow. It is estimated that each megakaryocyte is capable of producing several thousand platelets. Platelets are the smallest of the formed elements of the blood. They are tiny disk-shaped fragments capable of changing shape. The mature platelet is a complex structure and has a high rate of metabolic activity.

Platelets are often called thrombocytes because they play a key role in hemostasis. They adhere to a damaged blood vessel wall and aggregate (cluster together) to provide a mechanical barrier that prevents blood loss. In addition, they release necessary chemical coagulative substances that contribute to a more stable seal of the blood vessel by formation of a fibrin clot. Platelets of adequate number and quality are required for normal coagulation.

More than 40 different substances are released from the platelet when it is stimulated. The release reaction that follows platelet stimulation is an energy-consuming active process. Adenosine diphosphate (ADP) released from the platelet stimulates further platelet aggregation. Coagulation factors unique to platelets are also released. These factors are numbered with Arabic numbers and are different from the plasma coagulation factors designated by Roman numerals. The function of most of the eight identified platelet coagulation factors is obscure, but platelet factor 3 (PF-3) is known to be essential to clot formation, participating in two phases of the coagulation cascade reaction.

The rate of platelet production and the level of circulating platelets are believed to be controlled by a humoral hormone-like substance called *thrombopoietin*. The origin and nature of this substance are not yet known. Thrombopoietin acts on the colony-forming unit–megakaryocyte (CFU-MEG) that produce the megakaryoblast. This cell matures over 7 to 10 days into the megakaryocyte. Small fragments of its cytoplasm break off and are released from the bone marrow into the circulation as platelets.

Normally, one third of the body's platelets are sequestered in the spleen. The remaining two thirds are in the circulating blood. Circulating platelets can increase in response to exercise or the release of catecholamines into the circulatory system. This response is thought to be the result of platelet mobilization from the spleen and possibly the lungs.

Platelets normally have a life span of 7 to 14 days.[2] Approximately 10% to 15% of circulating platelets are continually being consumed in the repair of small vascular injuries that occur as a part of daily life. Those platelets not consumed in clotting reactions are removed at the end of their normal life by the spleen.

TABLE 40-2   **Blood Coagulation Factors**

Factor	Synonyms	Synthesis Site	Vitamin K–Dependent
I	Fibrinogen	Liver	No
II	Prothrombin	Liver	Yes
III	Tissue thromboplastin Tissue factor	Most body tissues	No
IV	Calcium		
V	Proaccelerin Labile factor Accelerator globulin	Liver	No
(VI)	Not assigned		
VII	Proconvertin Stable factor Serum prothrombin conversion accelerator	Liver	Yes
VIII	Antihemophilic factor Antihemophilic globulin Antihemophilic factor A Platelet cofactor 1	Endothelial cells	No
IX	Christmas factor B Plasma thromboplastin component Antihemophilic factor B	Liver	Yes
X	Stuart-Prower factor Autoprothrombin III Thrombokinase	Liver	Yes
XI	Antihemophilic factor C Plasma thromboplastin antecedent	Liver	No
XII	Hageman factor Contact factor	Obscure	No
XIII	Fibrin stabilizing factor Laki-Lorand factor Fibrinase	Megakaryocytes & possibly the liver	No

Coagulation Factors

Within the circulating blood, a small proportion of the plasma proteins are known collectively as the *clotting factors*. These proteins directly participate in the coagulation process. Over the years, considerable misunderstanding and confusion about their identification and description has developed. Several descriptive and functional names and surnames have often been used to describe the same substance. An international committee subsequently established a nomenclature of blood clotting factors (Table 40-2). Roman numerals are now used to identify the factors in the order of their discovery. This numerical sequence in no way suggests their order of reaction and participation in the coagulation process. In addition to the Roman numerals, a subscript "a" is used to indicate the active forms of each factor. For example, conversion of factor X to its active form is written $X \rightarrow X_a$.

The majority of the clotting factors are produced by the liver. Normal liver function is essential to an adequate supply of coagulation factors. Patients with liver disease often manifest coagulopathy secondary to deficient or defective coagulation factor production.

To produce factors II, VII, IX, and X, the liver requires vitamin K. These factors are referred to as vitamin K–dependent factors. Each is a glycoprotein with a specific and discrete function in coagulation. When vitamin K is deficient, regardless of the cause, the final step of biosynthesis of these factors does not occur. Precursor coagulation factors lacking calcium-binding sites are synthesized, but they do not function properly.

Coumadin administration inhibits the vitamin K–dependent biosynthesis pathway. Coumadin, therefore, produces its anticoagulant effect by interfering with the production of normal vitamin K–dependent factors.

Most coagulation factor deficiencies are thought to be inherited traits. Levels of each coagulation factor can be measured to determine its adequacy. In critically ill patients, however, most disorders of coagulation factors are acquired problems.

Each coagulation factor is essential to the coagulation process. However, detailed discussion of individual factors is limited here to those having greatest implication in critical illness.

Factor I, fibrinogen, is a glycoprotein originating in the liver. It is normally found in the bloodstream and in lymphatic fluid. The concentration of fibrinogen remains relatively constant; catabolism of fibrinogen is in a constant balance with production. The overall mechanism of fibrinogen catabolism is still under study.

Fibrinogen is an acute-phase reactant. Increased plasma levels of this protein are associated with a variety of infections, inflammation, or tissue destruction.

Fibrinogen is consumed during the coagulation process. It is converted into fibrin in the late steps of the coagulation cascade. Low levels of fibrinogen can occur during situations when the coagulation cascade is overstimulated on a large scale, for example, in disseminated intravascular coagulation (DIC).

Prothrombin, or *factor II,* is a vitamin K–dependent factor. Vitamin K deficiency caused by malabsorption, biliary obstruction, chronic diarrhea, lack of oral intake, or antibiotics may cause a deficiency in prothrombin production, leading to increased risk of bleeding in the critically ill patient.

Homogenates of normal tissues are known to markedly accelerate blood coagulation. Virtually any body tissue contains *tissue thromboplastin (factor III).* The brain, lungs, and prostate, as well as placental tissue, are particularly rich sources of tissue thromboplastin. Factor III is liberated during tissue damage. This release can initiate clot formation.

Calcium is coagulation factor IV. Approximately 50% of the calcium in the serum is ionized. Only ionized calcium can be used by the body. Only small quantities of calcium are required for normal functioning of the coagulation process. Calcium binds irreversibly with CPDA-1, the preservative used in packed RBCs. Transfusion of numerous units of banked blood can lower calcium levels and impair coagulation.

HEPATIC AND SPLENIC HEMATOPOIETIC FUNCTION

Among its many functions, the *liver* contributes to the normal activity of the hematopoietic system. Most of the coagulation proteins are synthesized by the normal liver. In cases of extreme or prolonged stress or disease of the bone marrow, the liver may become a focus for erythropoiesis. The reticuloendothelial cells of the liver assist in the removal of damaged or senescent RBCs from circulation. The liver then recycles the hemoglobin breakdown products. Bilirubin is converted into bile which aids in fat digestion. Recycled iron is also stored in the liver as ferritin until it is needed for RBC synthesis.

The *spleen* has many activities related to normal hematopoietic function. It filters the blood, removing aged or imperfect RBCs from the circulation by the process of phagocytosis. It also participates in breakdown of hemoglobin and the return of iron to the bone marrow for reuse. The spleen acts as a reservoir for one third of the circulating platelets. Although it has many important functions, the spleen is nonessential for life.

The liver and spleen are vital parts of the lymphoreticular system. The contribution of the liver, spleen and other organs to normal immune system function is addressed in Chapter 43.

HEMOSTASIS

Normally, blood is in a liquid state circulating throughout the vascular compartment. Whenever a blood vessel loses its integrity and allows the liquid blood to escape, clotting is initiated: Blood changes from its liquid state to a solid gel. The events of hemostasis or the arrest of bleeding include:

1. Vascular spasm
2. Platelet adhesion and aggregation
3. Formation of a platelet plug
4. Activation of plasma coagulation factors
5. Formation of a fibrin clot
6. Clot retraction
7. Fibrous repair of the injured vessel
8. Clot lysis

Although these steps are listed sequentially, they are closely interrelated and are occurring almost simultaneously. For ease of discussion, each of these events is presented separately.

Vascular Spasm

When a blood vessel is traumatized, the sympathetic nervous system is stimulated. Release of epinephrine and norepinephrine causes spasm of the vascular smooth muscle. The resulting vasoconstriction decreases blood loss from the damaged vessel. Vasoconstriction persists for about 10 minutes in small vessels and may last up to 30 minutes in larger vessels. If the injured vessel is small or under low pressure, vasoconstriction alone may be sufficient to achieve hemostasis. The greater the degree of trauma to the vessel, the greater the vasoconstrictive response. Therefore, crushing injury to vessels causes more spasm than a surgical incision. Also, a completely transected vessel is more likely to seal than a partially transected vessel. Permanent repair of blood vessel damage requires a hemostatic platelet plug and formation of a fibrin clot.

Disruption of the integrity of the blood vessel damages the endothelial lining. Exposure of subendothelial collagen provides a stimulus for platelets to adhere to the area. This initiates the next step in the normal coagulation process.

Platelet Activity

Platelets undergo drastic changes when they come into contact with damaged endothelium in blood vessels. The platelets immediately begin to swell and take on an irregular shape with many processes protruding from their surfaces. They become sticky, adhere to the subendothelial connective tissue, and spread to cover the damaged surface. Platelet adherence begins the formation of a mechanical plug to seal the tear in the blood vessel.

The platelets become activated and begin to release chemical substances such as ADP, prostaglandin, thromboxane A_2, and serotonin. The release of these chemicals attracts more platelets to the site forming an aggregation of platelets. Platelet aggregation normally takes place within seconds of vessel injury. The resulting mass of platelets plugs the vessel and arrests bleeding within 5 minutes of injury.

The formation of the unstable platelet plug causes the exposure of PF-3 on the platelet surface membrane. This platelet coagulation factor serves as a congregating place for the coagulation factors of the blood. Activation of these factors continues the process of coagulation to form a more stable fibrin clot at the site of injury.

Activation of Coagulation Factors

The interaction of the coagulation factors is an extremely complicated process under continuing investigation. The interaction involves the conversion of previously inert proteins into potent activated enzymes that participate in a sequential cascade reaction converting other inactive factors into activated form. This cascade hypothesis may be an oversimplification of the complex reactions, but it has been generally accepted for nearly 30 years, with modification. Figure 40-2 depicts this reaction.

The coagulation factors and their interactions that lead to fibrin formation can be divided into three distinct pathways as the intrinsic pathway, the extrinsic pathway, and the common pathway. Depending on the trigger, the coagulation cascade can be activated along either the intrinsic or the extrinsic pathway. Both of these pathways merge into the common pathway for normal hemostasis.

Intrinsic Pathway

The *intrinsic pathway* is stimulated when the blood itself or the lining of the blood vessel is damaged. It is slower to proceed than the extrinsic pathway, taking 2 to 6 minutes to cause clotting. The first step in this pathway is the activation of factor XII (Figure 40-3).

When factor XII is exposed to a negatively charged surface (e.g., collagen) it becomes activated to factor XIIa. The phenomenon of activation by contact with electronegative surfaces is termed *contact activation*. Proteolytic activation of factor XII can be caused by the substance *kallikrein*.

Factor XIIa activates factor XI. It also participates in another important reaction. With the help of a substance called *high molecular weight kininogen* (HMWK), factor XIIa converts prekallikrein to kallikrein. Kallikrein directly activates the kinin system and the fibrinolytic mechanism that will eventually break down the clot. Kallikrein helps to convert more factor XII into XIIa by proteolytic activation. The importance of HMWK, prekallikrein, and kallikrein in blood coagulation has only recently been identified.

Factor XI becomes factor XIa through the activation by factor XIIa and the cofactor HMWK. Factor XIa in turn activates factor IX. Calcium (factor IV) is necessary for activation of factor IX.

Factor IXa forms a complex with PF-3, calcium, and factor VIII. This complex functions as an enzyme to activate factor X. The activation of factor X is the beginning of the common pathway. As already mentioned, the common pathway of coagulation may also be initiated by the extrinsic pathway.

Extrinsic Pathway

The *extrinsic pathway* is activated when blood comes into contact with tissue thromboplastin (factor III). Factor III is released from traumatized tissue. This occurrence activates factor VII to factor VIIa with the assistance of calcium. Factor VIIa can stimulate the conversion of factor X into Xa. This is the point where the extrinsic pathway joins the common pathway for clot formation (Figure 40-4).

Factor VII may also be activated proteolytically by enzymes such as plasmin and kallikrein and other activated factors (XIIa, XIa, IXa). Factor III is also required for full activity.

The extrinsic pathway is the most rapid stimulation for clotting. Clotting can occur in as little as 15 to 20 seconds following severe tissue trauma.

Common Pathway

Factor X is activated by the complex enzymes that are the end products of either the intrinsic or extrinsic pathways. These two pathways merge into a final *common pathway* to clot formation (Figure 40-5). Activated factor X, factor V, calcium, and PF-3 interact to form a complex enzyme called *prothrombinase*. This enzyme binds to prothrombin (factor II) transforming it into *thrombin*. Thrombin converts fi-

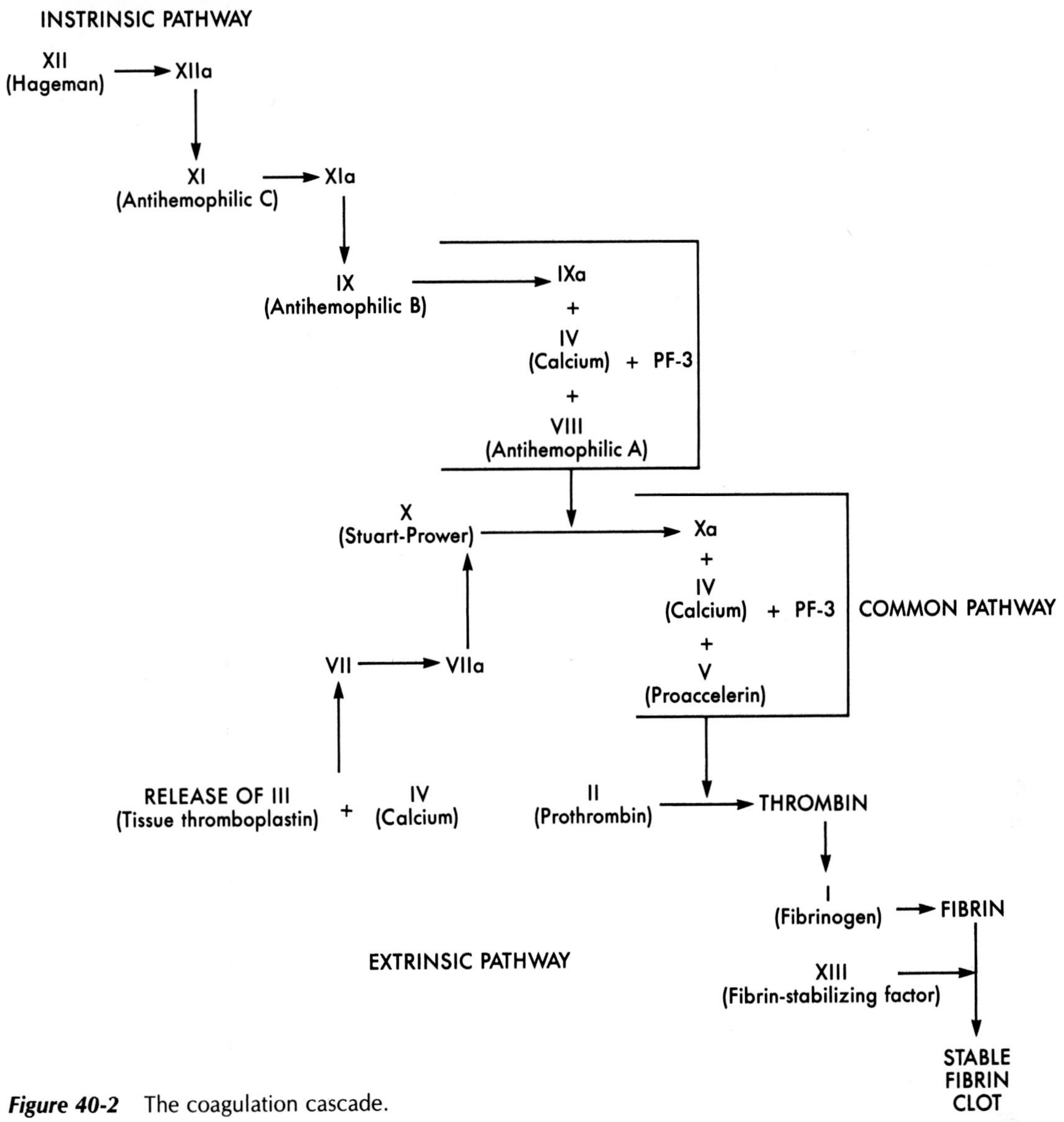

INSTRINSIC PATHWAY
XII
(Hageman)
XIIa
XI
(Antihemophilic C)
XIa
IX
(Antihemophilic B)
IXa
+
IV
(Calcium)
+ PF-3
+
VIII
(Antihemophilic A)
X
(Stuart-Prower)
Xa
+
IV
(Calcium)
+ PF-3
+
V
(Proaccelerin)
COMMON PATHWAY
VII
VIIa
RELEASE OF III
(Tissue thromboplastin)
+
IV
(Calcium)
II
(Prothrombin)
THROMBIN
I
(Fibrinogen)
FIBRIN
EXTRINSIC PATHWAY
XIII
(Fibrin-stabilizing factor)
STABLE
FIBRIN
CLOT

Figure 40-2 The coagulation cascade.

INTRINSIC PATHWAY
XII
(Hageman)
XIIa
HMWK
Prekallikrein
Kallikrein
XI
(Antihemophilic C)
XIa
IX
(Antihemophilic B)
IXa
+
IV
(Calcium)
+ PF-3
+
VIII
(Antihemophilic A)
X
(Stuart-Prower)
Xa

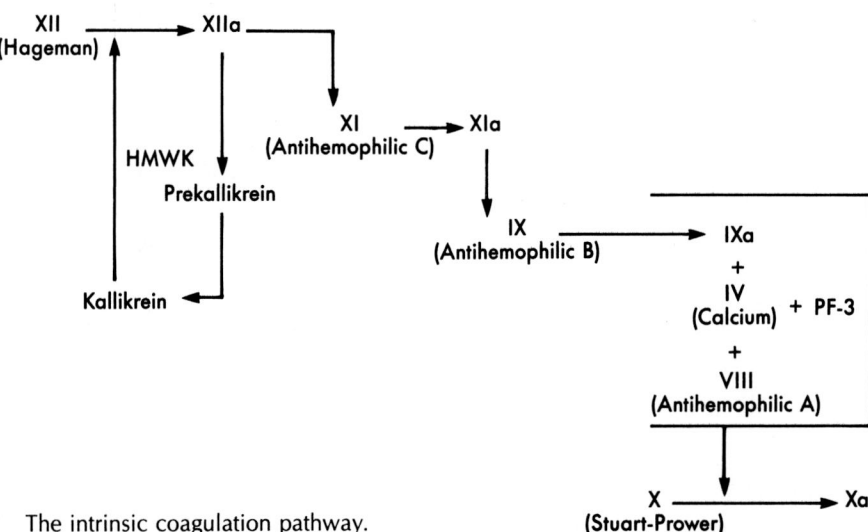

Figure 40-3 The intrinsic coagulation pathway.

EXTRINSIC PATHWAY

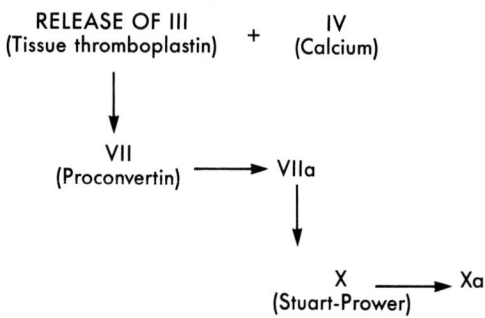

Figure 40-4   The extrinsic coagulation pathway.

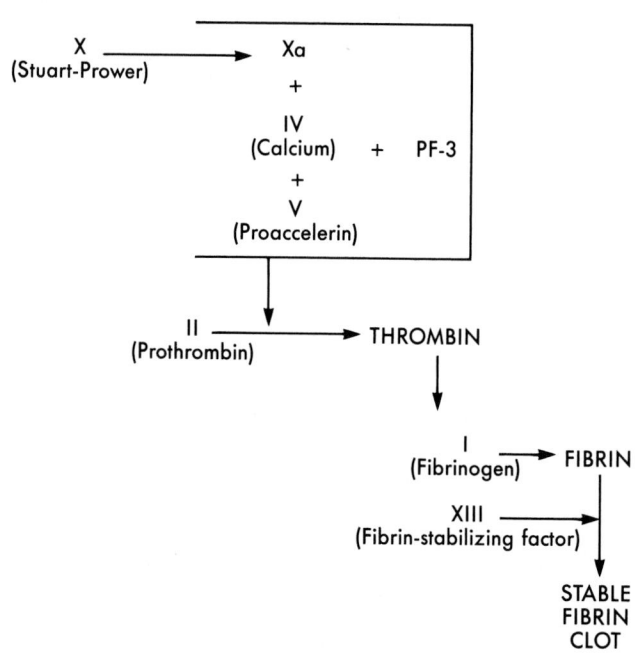

Figure 40-5   The common coagulation pathway.

brinogen (factor I) into a fibrin monomer. Fibrin polymerizes, or cross-links, to form a soluble fibrin clot. Additionally, factor XIII cross-links fibrin to form a stable or insoluble clot. The fine mesh created by fibrin traps blood cells, platelets, and plasma in the clot. The clot adheres to the site of damage to prevent further bleeding.

Clot Retraction

Within 1 hour after clot formation, the clot retracts. Platelets provide the energy required for clot retraction. They contract, shortening the fibrin strands to squeeze out serum and cells from the clot, thereby producing a smaller and denser clot and pulling the edges of the damaged vessel closer together.

Fibrous Repair

After a few hours, fibroblasts begin to invade the clot, initiating a fibrous organization. Complete fibrous organization of the clot into fibrous tissue requires about 7 to 10 days. This very effective mechanism prevents blood loss in arterioles, venules, and the capillaries of the microcirculation. However, larger veins and arteries require mechanical pressure or ligature in addition to clot formation to stop blood loss.

Fibrinolysis

The fibrinolytic system exists for the control and breakdown of blood clots. This system helps to balance hemostasis. The fibrinolytic mechanism is acti-

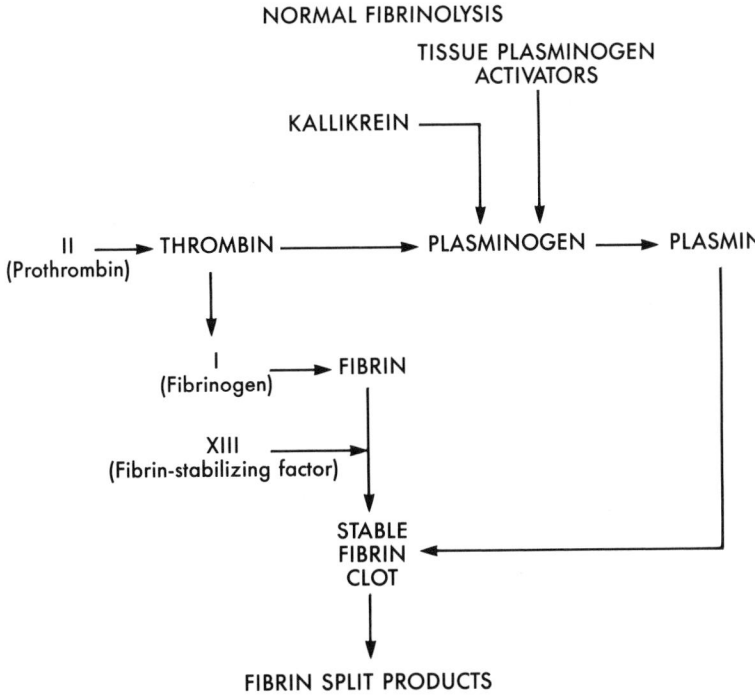

NORMAL FIBRINOLYSIS

Figure 40-6   Normal coagulation stimulates fibrinolysis.

vated within a day after clot formation. The process is initiated when factor XIIa activates kallikrein. Thrombin production also initiates clot lysis. Both of these substances act to convert the plasma precursor, plasminogen, into the proteolytic enzyme plasmin (Figure 40-6).

Additional naturally occurring activators of plasminogen are found in small amounts in the plasma. Tissue plasminogen activator (t-PA) is an important plasminogen activator released in its active form from endothelial cells. Urokinase is another plasminogen activator that is normally found in the urine. The ability to produce these substances commercially has allowed for their therapeutic use as fibrinolytic agents in a wide variety of thromboembolic disorders.

Plasminogen is incorporated into all blood clots during clot formation. It is activated into plasmin by the production of thrombin. Plasmin is released into the clot, where it begins to dissolve the fibrin strands. Fibrinolysis is caused by the action of plasmin on the fibrin clot.

As the clot is dissolved by plasmin, it releases breakdown products known as *fibrin degradation products (FDPs)* or *fibrin split products (FSPs)*. Fragments of fibrin break off as the clot is dissolved. Fragment D is one of the final products of this process.[3] The FDP have inhibitory effects on clot formation. Reticuloendothelial cells of the liver and spleen remove FDP from the blood. Removal of the fibrin clot

reestablishes blood flow through a newly healed blood vessel.

HOMEOSTATIC ANTICOAGULANT ACTIVITY

Platelet aggregation and the activation of coagulation factors constitute a threat to the body if these processes extend beyond the wound into the general circulation.[4] This does not normally occur because of homeostatic anticoagulant mechanisms that are not fully understood.

Prostacyclin is a fatty acid produced by endothelial cells and leukocytes. It inhibits platelet adhesion and aggregation and causes vasodilatation. A balance between prostacyclin production from the endothelium and thromboxane-A_2 released by platelets is thought to effect a balance that determines the reactivity of platelets to endothelium.

Blood flow past the site of clot formation helps to remove activated coagulation factors from the area. Activated factors are cleared from the blood by the action of reticuloendothelial cells. The structure of the clot itself helps to hold activated factors within the fibrin meshwork, restricting their activity to the injured area.

Physiological inhibitors of coagulation, or natural anticoagulant substances, have been demonstrated in the blood. These substances are presumed to neutralize activated coagulation factors that may enter the general circulation. Antithrombin III is an important anticoagulant. It is thought to be the major plasma inhibitor of thrombin and factor Xa, but it may inhibit every coagulation factor reaction to some degree. The action of antithrombin III is accelerated by heparin. Heparin is normally secreted in small amounts by the mast cells in the lung and liver. Alpha$_2$-macroglobin is a large molecular weight protein that inactivates several proteolytic enzymes including kallikrein, thrombin, and plasmin. Alpha$_1$-antitrypsin is a potent inhibitor of factor XIa. Protein C is a vitamin K–dependent glycoprotein synthesized by the liver. It is activated by thrombin and then shows selective activity for factors Va and VIIIa. Other such anticoagulant substances appear to exist, but their physiological significance is obscure.[5]

REFERENCES

1. Hays, K. (1990). Physiology of normal bone marrow. *Seminars in Oncology Nursing, 6*, 3-8.
2. Griffin, J. P. (1986). *Hematology and immunology concepts for nursing.* Norwalk, CT: Appleton-Century-Crofts.
3. Simmons, A. (1989). *Hematology: A combined theoretical and technical approach.* Philadelphia: Saunders.
4. Alkire, K., & Collingwood, J. (1990). Physiology of blood and bone marrow. *Seminars in Oncology Nursing, 6*, 99-108.
5. Leavell, B. S., & Thorup, O. A. (1987). *Leavell and Thorup's fundamentals of clinical hematology* (5th ed.). Philadelphia: Saunders.

41

Hematological Data Acquisition

Debra Tribett

This chapter discusses the hematological assessment of the critically ill patient. Since the signs and symptoms of hematological problems may be manifested in many organ systems, careful attention must be paid to subtle clues in the patient's history and physical assessment and to results of diagnostic laboratory tests. This chapter focuses on the assessment of erythrocyte (RBC) and thrombocyte (platelet) function and the coagulation process. The assessment of white blood cell (WBC) function and immune response is presented in Chapter 44.

Patients may be admitted to the critical care unit with a primary or a secondary hematological disorder. Even though primary hematological disorders are relatively uncommon, the critical care nurse must be aware of the impact these patient problems will have on the patient and the therapies routinely used in the critical care environment.

The critical care nurse must also be vigilant to the development of hematological dysfunction in patients with other primary problems necessitating critical care admission. The development of acquired or secondary hematological disorders is often seen in the critically ill patient. Identification of the patient at high risk for the development of hematological problems is an important part of nursing assessment. Once the high-risk patient is identified, close periodic observation must be implemented as part of the nursing care plan for this patient population.

HISTORY

In most critical care settings, with the possible exception of the emergency department, the patient's initial history and physical examination are completed before admission to the critical care unit. The critical care nurse has the advantage of reviewing this data when planning nursing care appropriate to the patient's needs.

Patient demographic data provide clues to risk factors for hematological dysfunction. The complete database should include age, gender, marital status, occupation, military service, religion, race, and ethnic background.[1] Family history should be integrated with the demographic data.

Family History

Many hematological diseases are hereditary. For example, *hemophilia* is an X-linked recessive bleeding disorder related to a specific coagulation factor deficiency. Females carry the gene, but hemophilia is a disease virtually exclusive to males.

Sickle cell anemia is a hereditary disease occurring primarily in blacks but also in persons of Mediterranean, Middle Eastern, or Asian descent. This chronic hemolytic anemia is characterized by an abnormal hemoglobin molecule. Heterozygous inheritance is usually an asymptomatic condition called *sickle cell trait*, whereas homozygous inheritance causes a severe disorder.

Thalassemia, a chronic hemolytic anemia, occurs in persons of Mediterranean ancestry. Like sickle cell anemia, it is hereditary and may take an asymptomatic heterozygous form or a symptomatic homozygous form.

Occupational History

Occupational history or military service may uncover exposure to hazardous chemicals or substances that may cause bone marrow dysfunction or hematological cancers. For example, industrial workers in chemical, paint, plastics, or rubber tire factories may be exposed to toxins leading to aplastic anemia. Health care workers and uranium miners have a common risk exposure to ionizing radiation which may also be linked to aplastic anemia. Whenever a toxin is suspected in hematological disease, the patient's daily activities and environment must be carefully reviewed. Incidental exposure to toxic chemicals may occur in significant amounts.

Lifestyle

In addition to occupation, lifestyle may contribute adversely to hematological problems. Alcoholism may affect hematological function in several ways. Alcohol may decrease the platelet count. Excessive alcohol intake can interfere with folic acid metabolism. Alcohol abusers may also have a poor dietary intake of folic acid leading to folic acid deficiency anemia. *Cirrhosis* is a disorder of the liver seen in alcoholics. As the normal tissues of the liver are replaced by fibrotic areas, the ability of the liver to produce essential coagulation factors diminishes. Factor deficiencies contribute to coagulopathy seen in these patients.

Medical History

The patient's medical history may provide additional information regarding potential or actual hematological dysfunction. The patient should be questioned regarding bleeding after injuries, dental extraction, or surgery such as tonsillectomy or circumcision. In female patients, information about menstrual periods and obstetric history should be obtained. Spontaneous hemorrhage into the skin (petechiae or ecchymoses), from mucous membranes (including epistaxis), and gastrointestinal bleeding may lead to suspicion of a platelet disorder. (See Table 41-1 for terminology associated with bleeding patterns.) Bleeding into muscles, joints, or bones may indicate a coagulation factor disorder. A number of diseases can affect the hematological system. Liver disease, uremia, systemic lupus erythematosus, or hematological malignant disease should be noted. Radiation therapy for the treatment of malignant disease is noteworthy. Radiation therapy may diminish production of blood cells by the bone marrow.

Past Surgery

Past surgical interventions may be contributing to current medical problems. Partial or total gastrec-

tomy or resection of the lower ileum may contribute to vitamin and nutrient malabsorption resulting in anemia. Cardiac surgery with mechanical valve replacement may lead to damage of RBCs and hemolytic anemia when malfunction of the valve occurs.

Diet and Nutritional Status

Dietary history is also of importance. Erythrocyte production is dependent on dietary iron, folic acid, and vitamin B_{12}. Malnourished or debilitated patients may suffer from severe anemia. If vitamin K is not obtained from dietary sources, the liver may lack sufficient quantity to produce the vitamin K–dependent coagulation factors.

Transfusion Experiences

A history of transfusion of blood or blood product should be noted. Transfusion can induce antibody formation. Platelets may be destroyed by this immune mechanism, leading to thrombocytopenia and bleeding. Any history of hemolytic or other transfusion reactions should be determined.

Current Medications

Careful attention should be given to eliciting a thorough medication history of both prescription and over-the-counter drugs. Drugs often induce or aggravate hematological disease. Many medications can interfere with hematopoiesis, hemostasis, or both. Medications commonly taken without prescription, such as aspirin and the nonsteroidal antiinflammatory agent, ibuprofen, interfere with platelet function. Many prescription drugs in a variety of categories may affect bone marrow production of blood cells. Broad spectrum antibiotic therapy may also kill vitamin K–producing organisms in the gut, thereby decreasing the availability of this vitamin for the synthesis of coagulation factors. Patients may have been receiving anticoagulant therapy (coumarin or heparin) and, therefore, may have prolonged coagulation time as a result of too high a dose of medication. Many chemotherapeutic agents given to treat malignant disease cause bone marrow suppression, thus decreasing production of all cells. Patients receiving such drugs are particularly prone to bleeding as a result of thrombocytopenia. (See Table 41-2 for drugs that affect the hematopoietic system.)

PHYSICAL ASSESSMENT

A thorough physical examination of the patient should be conducted by the physician on admission of the patient to the hospital. Coupled with the patient's history, this gives the nurse information up to the point when the patient requires admission to the critical care unit. The nurse must then perform a baseline physical assessment to establish a point of com-

TABLE 41-1 **Terminology of Bleeding Patterns**

Epistaxis	Hemorrhage from the nose
Hemarthrosis	Effusion of blood into a joint cavity
Hemoglobinuria	Presence of extracellular hemoglobin in the urine
Hemoptysis	Expectoration of bloody sputum
Melena	Black vomitus resulting from action of digestive juices on free blood in the intestinal tract
Menorrhagia	Excessive menstrual bleeding
Hematochezia	Passage of stools containing blood

TABLE 41-2 **Drugs/Agents Affecting RBCs and Platelets**

Drug/Agent	Hematological Effects
ANALGESIC	
Aspirin	Inhibited platelet function, thrombocytopenia
NONSTEROIDAL ANTIINFLAMMATORY AGENTS (NSAIDs)	
Ibuprofen	Inhibited platelet function, thrombocytopenia, hemolytic anemia, aplastic anemia
Indomethacin	Aplastic anemia, hemolytic anemia, iron deficiency anemia, thrombocytopenia
Phenylbutazone	Bone marrow depression, hemolytic anemia
ANTIDYSRHYTHMIC	
Procainamide	Hemolytic anemia, thrombocytopenia
Propranolol	Inhibited platelet function
Quinidine	Anemia, hemolytic anemia, thrombocytopenia
ANTICONVULSANT	
Carbamazepine	Aplastic anemia, thrombocytopenia
Mephenytoin	Hemolytic anemia
Phenytoin	Thrombocytopenia, pancytopenia
ANTIGOUT AGENTS	
Colchicine	Aplastic anemia, inhibited platelet function
Probenecid	Aplastic anemia, hemolytic anemia
ANTIMICROBIALS	
Amphotericin B	Anemia, thrombocytopenia
Chloramphenicol	Aplastic anemia, thrombocytopenia
Penicillins	Hemolytic anemia, thrombocytopenia
Quinine	Hemolytic anemia, thrombocytopenia, hypoprothrombinemia
Sulfonamides	Aplastic anemia, thrombocytopenia, hemolytic anemia
ANTIHYPERTENSIVES	
Captopril	Pancytopenia
Methyldopa	Inhibited platelet function, thrombocytopenia, hemolytic anemia
DIURETICS	
Chlorothiazide	Aplastic anemia, hemolytic anemia, thrombocytopenia
Furosemide	Anemia, thrombocytopenia, aplastic anemia
PSYCHOTHERAPEUTIC	
Chlorpromazine	Inhibited platelet function, hemolytic anemia
ORAL BLOOD GLUCOSE–LOWERING AGENTS	
Chlorpropamide Glipizide Glyburide	Thrombocytopenia, aplastic anemia, hemolytic anemia
OTHER AGENTS	
Insecticides	Pancytopenia
Ionizing radiation	Pancytopenia
Solvents (benzene)	Aplastic anemia

parison by which changes in patient condition may be identified. Since manifestations of hematological problems evolve or worsen over time in many organ systems, particular emphasis should be placed on frequent periodic assessment. The critical care nurse must integrate physical assessment data with the results of laboratory evaluation as discussed in that section.

Cardiopulmonary System

Changes in vital signs and hemodynamic parameters must be evaluated for indications of hypovolemia due to bleeding or as compensatory mechanisms for anemia. The respiratory system is assessed for tachypnea, exertional dyspnea, or orthopnea. The cardiovascular system is monitored for tachycardia, palpitations, the development of a systolic murmur, and orthostatic hypotension. Hemodynamic data, if available, should be monitored for signs of congestive heart failure, hypovolemic shock, or sepsis. Pericardial friction rubs or muffling of heart sounds are of particular importance because they may indicate bleeding in the pericardium or mediastinum.

Neurological System

The level of consciousness (LOC) should be monitored frequently in the critically ill patient. Impairment of LOC may result from hypoxia when a decrease in hemoglobin impairs oxygen transport to tissue. Changes in mentation, such as general malaise, drowsiness, weakness, vertigo, and headache, may be associated with anemia or may portend impending neurological disaster due to hemorrhage. Cranial nerve function, pupillary reactions, motor function, and spinal reflexes should be tested frequently in patients with bleeding tendency. Sensory disturbances, including paresthesias, numbness, or pain, may indicate formation of a hematoma that is impinging on peripheral nerves.

Integumentary System

The skin and mucous membranes reveal important clues to hematological functioning. The color of the nail beds, mucous membranes, and palmar creases can serve as a guide to hemoglobin levels, but conjunctival blood vessel patterns and color may be a more reliable index. Pallor can be a useful guideline in evaluating anemia, but it must be remembered that skin color is determined by pigment and temperature as well as by capillary blood flow. The pink color of palmar creases usually disappears at hemoglobin levels of less than 7 g/dl. Cyanosis occurs when the absolute concentration of reduced hemoglobin exceeds 5 g/dl. Cyanosis may not be seen in patients with severe anemia even when there is marked arterial desaturation. In the patient with polycythemia, ruddy color or plethora may occur on the face, conjunctivae, hands, and feet. A bronze or grayish pigmentation of the skin can be seen in patients with hemochromatosis, which is related to a marked hemolysis of RBCs. In this condition, deposition of iron-containing pigments from hemoglobin into the skin causes the discoloration.

Jaundice is usually detected if the bilirubin is 2 to 3 mg/dl. The presence of jaundice may indicate an excessive destruction of RBCs as in hemolytic anemia. Jaundice should be sought in the patient's conjunctiva and sclerae, then mucous membranes and skin. In patients with dark skin, the buccal mucosa, palms, and soles should be inspected. Jaundice is best determined in daylight.

Examination of the skin and mucous membranes

TABLE 41-3 Skin Lesions Associated with Hematological Problems

Lesion or Condition	Description
Petechiae	Small purplish, hemorrhagic spots that do not blanch with pressure; usually 1-3 mm in diameter
Ecchymosis	Variable-size macular, irregularly formed hemorrhagic area of the skin with color varying from blue-black to yellow-green; does not blanch with pressure
Purpura	Condition characterized by hemorrhages into the skin, mucous membranes, or other organs, producing skin lesions that do not disappear with pressure
Telangiectasis	Hyperemic spot due to capillary or small artery dilatation; small angioma with a tendency to hemorrhage
Spider nevus	Branched growth of dilated capillaries resembling a spider
Angioma	Form of usually benign tumor consisting principally of blood or lymph vessels
Hematoma	Blood-filled tumor

may also reveal lesions characteristic of specific bleeding problems (Table 41-3). Petechiae are usually seen in patients with platelet disorders. They occur in dependent areas. Use of blood pressure cuffs or compression devices on lower extremities may cause petechiae to develop in the thrombocytopenic patient. Ecchymoses may be seen around venipuncture sites, around invasive monitoring catheter insertion sites, or other areas where invasive procedures were performed. Removal of tape, ECG electrodes, or the suction cups from an electrocardiogram may produce ecchymoses in the patient with a bleeding tendency. In patients with dark skin, petechiae may be difficult to see except on the oral mucosal surfaces.

Close observation of the gums and mucous membranes of the mouth may reveal pallor or bleeding. The critical care nurse may observe spontaneous bleeding from oral mucous membranes or following mouth care. Suctioning procedures may also induce bleeding from upper or lower airway mucous membranes in the patient at high risk for bleeding.

The tongue may become sore in patients with pernicious anemia or vitamin deficiencies. Smoothness of the surface of the tongue may indicate vitamin B_{12} deficiency or iron deficiency anemia.

The texture of the skin may be dry and coarse, indicating iron deficiency anemia. Longitudinal striation of the nails can indicate anemia. Spoon nail, or *koilonychia,* is characteristic of iron deficiency anemia. Nail clubbing is seen in chronic hypoxia, which can also result from anemia.

Gastrointestinal System

The finding of liver or spleen tenderness or enlargement during abdominal assessment may be of hematological significance. Hepatomegaly or splenomegaly may result from congestion due to overproduction of cells, as in polycythemia, or excessive cell destruction, as in hemolytic anemia. Evidence of an enlarged spleen may also indicate a decrease in the circulating pool of platelets and an increased number of platelets sequestered in the spleen. Diarrhea, melena, or cramping should be noted because the presence of blood in the intestinal tract often acts as a cathartic. Any stomach contents obtained by nasogastric suction or vomiting, feces, or abdominal wound drainage should be routinely tested for occult blood.

Renal System

The genitourinary system should be assessed for signs of bleeding. The urine should be tested for occult blood. If hematuria is present, the urine may range from slightly smoky to bright red in color. Hemoglobinuria can result from intravascular or extravascular hemolysis. The urine is usually the color of port wine.

Musculoskeletal System

The musculoskeletal system may also indicate hematological problems. Tenderness, stiffness, or pain

in bones and joints may indicate hemorrhage into a joint capsule, increased hematopoietic activity in bone marrow, or a hemolytic sickle cell crisis.

LABORATORY AND DIAGNOSTIC PROCEDURES

Assessment of Blood Cells

Complete Blood Count (CBC)

The basic diagnostic tests for hematological functioning are the complete blood count (CBC) and the differential blood count. The CBC includes an actual count of circulating RBCs and white blood cells (WBCs), in addition to the hemoglobin and hematocrit levels.

The differential count is a measure of the total WBC count and the percentage of cells in each subcategory: neutrophils (segmented and bands), eosinophils, basophils, monocytes, and lymphocytes. A detailed presentation of aspects of WBC analysis is found in Chapter 44. Table 41-4 gives the normal values for the CBC and the clinical implications of the values. The normal values for test results will vary slightly between laboratories according to equipment and techniques used. The critical care nurse must always compare patient results with the normal values cited by the hospital's laboratory.

RBC Count

The red blood cell count is the actual number of circulating RBCs in 1 mm³ of blood. A decreased RBC count of less than 10% of normal indicates anemia, which may be due to hemorrhage, hemolysis, dietary

---

TABLE 41-4 **Complete Blood Count: Normal Values**

Parameter	Normal Values	Clinical Implications
RBCs/mm³	M: 4.6-6.2 F: 4.2-5.4	*Increased:* Dehydration, chronic hypoxia, polycythemia *Decreased:* Anemia, hemorrhage, fluid overload, leukemia, chronic renal failure
Hemoglobin, g/dl	M: 13-18 F: 12-16	
Hematocrit, %	M: 45-54 F: 36-46	
RED CELL INDICES		
MCV, μm³	81-98	*Increased:* Macrocytic anemia—aplastic hemolytic, pernicious *Decreased:* Microcytic anemia—iron deficiency, thalassemia
MCH, pg/RBC	27-32	*Increased:* Macrocytic anemia *Decreased:* Microcytic anemia
MCHC, %	32-36	*Decreased:* Hypochromic anemia, iron deficiency anemia, thalassemia
WHITE CELL COUNTS		
WBCs, thousands/mm³	5-10	*Increased:* Inflammation, infection, leukemia *Decreased:* Bone marrow suppression

problems, genetic abnormalities, or drug toxicity. An elevated RBC count may occur in persons with chronic hypoxia, adaptation to high altitudes, or polycythemia vera (a myeloproliferative process in red cell formation).

Hemoglobin and Hematocrit

Hemoglobin (Hb) assessment measures the amount of hemoglobin in the peripheral blood. Changes in hemoglobin level reflect changes in the amount present in RBCs or changes in the intravascular volume of the patient. Decreased levels are seen in anemia or in situations of fluid overload. Increased levels are seen in chronic hypoxia, for example, in chronic obstructive lung disease, adaptation to high altitudes, polycythemia, or dehydration.

The hematocrit (Hct) is the volume of packed RBCs in 100 ml (1 dl) of blood, expressed as a percentage. Low Hct is seen in hemorrhage, anemia, chronic renal failure, or fluid overload. High Hct is seen in polycythemia vera, chronic hypoxic conditions, and dehydration.

Hemoglobin and hematocrit values are assessed for evidence of hemorrhage in the critically ill patient. When these values are obtained soon after a hemorrhage they may not yet reflect the severity of the blood loss. During hemorrhage, both RBCs and plasma are lost simultaneously. Compensatory autotransfusion—the movement of the interstitial fluid into the vascular compartment—may not have taken place. Therefore, Hb and Hct may appear normal. However, once autotransfusion takes place or the patient receives fluid resuscitation with intravenous crystalloids or colloids, these two values fall, showing evidence of acute blood loss.

A simplified description of the normal relationship of RBCs, Hb, and Hct can be expressed in the following equations:[2]

$$\text{RBC count} \times 3 = \text{Hb}$$

$$\text{Hb} \times 3 = \text{Hct}$$

RBC Indices

Red blood cell indices describe the size, weight, and Hb concentration of the individual RBC. They provide information for the diagnosis of anemia.

Mean corpuscular volume (MCV) is defined as the volume of the average RBC. It is calculated by dividing the Hct by the RBC count. A decreased MCV indicates small RBCs, or microcytes. These are characteristic of iron deficiency anemia or thalassemia. An increased MCV indicates large RBCs, or macrocytes. This type of cell is seen in pernicious anemia and folic acid anemia.

The average weight or amount of Hb in a single RBC is the *mean corpuscular hemoglobin* (MCH). MCH is obtained by dividing the Hb by the RBC count. A decreased MCH is seen in hypochromic or microcytic anemia. An increased MCH is seen in macrocytic anemia.

The *mean corpuscular hemoglobin concentration,* or MCHC, is the average concentration of Hb in a single RBC. It is calculated by dividing the Hb level by the Hct. This value can only be normal or decreased because an RBC cannot contain more than the normal amount of Hb molecules. A decreased value is seen in hypochromic (pale cells) such as in iron deficiency anemia or thalassemia.

RBCs can be further examined by the laboratory for abnormalities in size, shape, or fragmentation, and for abnormal inclusions. Changes in RBC morphology can assist in the differential diagnosis of anemias or hematological conditions such as disseminated intravascular coagulation (DIC).

Reticulocyte Count

The reticulocyte count indicates bone marrow production of new RBCs. This measurement determines the percentage of immature, nonnucleated RBCs in the total RBC count. Normal values are 0.5% to 1.5% for men and 0.5% to 2.5% for women. Reticulocyte counts are normally elevated in anemia as a physiological compensation. Increased counts suggest accelerated RBC production as the bone marrow replaces lost or destroyed cells. In a patient with an otherwise normal CBC, an elevated reticulocyte count may indicate polycythemia vera.[3] A low reticulocyte count signals decreased production of RBCs by the bone marrow. This may occur in aplastic anemia, iron deficiency anemia, or bone marrow suppression following radiation or chemotherapy.

Erythrocyte Sedimentation Rate

The erythrocyte sedimentation rate (ESR) is a test that measures the rate at which RBCs settle out of an unclotted blood specimen. It is a nonspecific test that is useful for general screening. Laboratory method affects the ESR normal values. A high ESR means that the cells have settled faster. ESR gradually increases with age, and females have higher normal values than do males. The ESR is increased in pregnancy, inflammatory diseases, infection, and cancer. A decreased ESR suggests hypofibrinogenemia, sickle-cell anemia, or polycythemia.

Hemoglobin Electrophoresis

The CBC measures total Hb. More discrete testing of Hb can determine hemoglobin variants. Hemoglobin electrophoresis detects normal and abnormal Hb. Some of the variants are due to genetic traits which lead to hematological diseases, including sickle cell disease and thalassemia. This test is useful in diagnosis of anemia and hemolytic disease.

Serum Iron and Iron Binding Capacity

Iron binds with serum transferrin for transport to the bone marrow for Hb production. Transferrin is measured and expressed as the amount of iron that it binds in an index called the *total iron binding capacity* (TIBC). Serum iron and the TIBC are usually measured together. When serum iron level falls, the TIBC rises. When the serum iron level rises, the TIBC falls. These tests are useful in detecting iron deficiency anemia, blood loss, and hemolysis.

Serum ferritin is the chief iron storage protein in the body. It may be measured as the best indicator for the early detection of iron deficiency anemia. The level decreases in a parallel fashion with iron stores.

Osmotic Fragility of RBCs

An additional test that may be performed to differentiate types of anemia is the osmotic fragility test of RBCs. Fragility is tested by placing RBCs in increasingly dilute saline solutions. Fragility is increased in some hereditary anemias, hemolytic anemia, chemical toxicity, or autoimmune hemolytic anemia. Decreased fragility suggests iron deficiency anemia, thalassemia, and sickle cell anemia.

Assessment of Coagulation

Many different tests may be performed to assess the components and processes of coagulation. (See Table 41-5.)

Bleeding Time

The bleeding time is a screening test for preoperative patients and for assessing normal platelet function. Candidates for this test may be patients with a personal or familial bleeding history. A small standard incision is made in the skin and then observed at intervals to determine the time it takes for the bleeding to stop. Four different methods (Ivy, Duke, template, and modified template) may be used, and each has a different normal range. Prolonged bleeding times may be seen in thrombocytopenia; in any disorders associated with thrombocytopenia; in severe liver disease; and in severe deficiencies of factors I, II, V, VII, VIII, IX, or XI. A prolonged bleeding time with a normal platelet count indicates a platelet function disorder.

Capillary Fragility Test

A capillary fragility test measures the ability of the capillary to remain intact under increased pressure. This test is also known as a tourniquet test, positive pressure test, or the Rumple-Leede capillary fragility test. A blood pressure cuff is placed on the upper arm and inflated to a pressure halfway between the patient's systolic and diastolic pressures but not to exceed 100 mmHg. The pressure is maintained for 5 minutes. The pressure is then released, and the forearm is observed for the development of petechiae. If there are fewer than 10 petechiae, the test is normal, or negative. More than 10 petechiae represents a positive (abnormal) result.[4]

Positive results indicate a platelet defect, throm-

TABLE 41-5   Coagulation Studies

Test	Normal Value	Clinical Significance
Bleeding time	Ivy: 1-7 minutes Duke: 1-3 minutes Template: 2-8 minutes Modified template: 2-10 minutes	*Increased:* Thrombocytopenia, platelet abnormalities, aplastic anemia, DIC, severe liver disease, aspirin ingestion, anticoagulant therapy
Capillary fragility	<10 petechiae after 5 minutes	*Increased:* Platelet defect, capillary wall weakness
Platelet count	150,000-400,000/mm^3	*Decreased:* Aplastic anemia, idiopathic thrombocytopenic purpura, many drug reactions, DIC, leukemia
Prothrombin time (PT)	11-15 seconds	*Increased:* Liver disease; factor deficiencies II, V, VII, X; oral anticoagulants
Partial thromboplastin (PTT)	60-70 seconds	*Increased:* Liver disease; DIC; factor deficiencies I, II, V, VIII-XII; heparin therapy
Activated partial thromboplastin (APTT)	25-38 seconds	
Thrombin time	10-13 seconds	*Increased:* Low fibrinogen level, DIC, liver disease
Fibrinogen	200-400 mg/dl	*Increased:* Inflammatory response *Decreased:* Severe liver disease, DIC, obstetric complications
Fibrin split or degradation products	2-10 μg/ml	*Increased:* Fibrinolysis, DIC

bocytopenia; vitamin K deficiency; severe deficiencies of factor I, II, or VII; von Willebrand's disease; or DIC. Other conditions increasing capillary fragility that may also cause positive findings are measles, scarlet fever, chronic renal disease, hypertension, diabetes with coexistent vascular disease, premenstruation, or decreasing estrogen levels in women over age 40.

Platelet Count

The total platelet count provides quantitative information about thrombocytes. A decreased platelet count (thrombocytopenia) may indicate failure of bone marrow to produce platelets, sequestering of platelets by the spleen, increased destruction by antibodies or drugs, or a consumption coagulopathy such as DIC. Thrombocytopenia is associated with bleeding. A platelet count of less than 50,000/mm^3 can result in spontaneous bleeding. An increased platelet count (thrombocytosis) may occur in myeloproliferative disorders such as polycythemia vera, leukemia, and multiple myeloma. Increased platelet counts may cause increased clotting.

Prothrombin Time

The prothrombin time (PT) is a test that measures the time required for a fibrin clot to form when the extrinsic pathway for coagulation is initiated. This test does not require platelets and bypasses the intrinsic pathway for clot formation. It evaluates prothrombin; fibrinogen; and factors V, VII, and X. This is the preferred test for monitoring oral anticoagulant therapy.

The normal values vary with the method of testing. However, the most accurate reporting method compares the number of seconds it takes the patient sample to clot with a control. When patients are receiving anticoagulant therapy, the goal is to maintain the patient value at 1.5 to 2.5 times the control value. If the patient's value is greater than 2.5 times the control, bleeding is likely to occur. A prolonged PT may indicate a deficiency in fibrinogen; prothrombin; or factors V, VII, or X. Vitamin K deficiency or liver disease may also cause an abnormal PT.

Partial Thromboplastin/Activated Thromboplastin Time

The intrinsic pathway of coagulation is assessed by either the partial thromboplastin time (PTT) or the activated partial thromboplastin time (APTT). All factors except VII and XIII are evaluated. Since most congenital coagulation deficiencies occur in the intrinsic pathway, these tests are used to screen for preoperative bleeding tendency. These tests are also used for monitoring heparin therapy. The APTT uses the activator kaolin to shorten the clotting time of the patient's blood. It is a more sensitive test than the PTT and, therefore, is the more frequently used.

The PTT and APTT have different normal values reported in seconds. Therapeutic anticoagulation with heparin lengthens the results from 1.5 to 2.5 times the normal. Increased (prolonged) levels indicate factor deficiencies in V, VIII, IX, X, XI, XII, or fibrinogen; cirrhosis of the liver; vitamin K deficiency; DIC; or von Willebrand's disease.

Thrombin Time

The thrombin time provides an estimation of plasma fibrinogen levels. Thrombin is added to the patient's specimen and to a control. This quickly converts fibrinogen into a clot. The time it takes for clotting to occur in the patient's blood is compared to the control. A thrombin time of greater than 1.3 times the control may mean effective anticoagulation with heparin, or it may signify fibrinogen deficiency or defect, hepatic disease, DIC, or the use of fibrinolytics such as streptokinase or urokinase.[5]

Fibrinogen Level

Factor I (fibrinogen) levels can be directly measured in the plasma. Increased levels of fibrinogen can be seen as a result of the inflammatory response, acute infection, or collagen diseases, or in patients taking oral contraceptives. Decreased levels are seen in severe liver disease and DIC. The trend in fibrinogen level is important in critical illness. A drop in initially elevated values to normal ranges sometimes can indicate the development of a coagulopathy despite the apparently normal value.

Specific assays of each of the coagulation factors can be performed. A deficiency in one or more factors usually causes bleeding disorders. These tests are performed following other screening coagulation tests, in patients with known bleeding tendency, or with a family bleeding history.

Calcium

Although a clotting factor, calcium is measured as an electrolyte. Calcium deficits are not commonly the cause of clotting abnormalities. However, in critically ill patients who have received numerous blood transfusions, calcium levels may be of concern. The citrate preservative in banked blood binds with calcium so that it is not available in its ionized form to participate in the normal coagulation process.

Fibrin Split Products/Fibrin Degradation Products

The test of fibrin split products (FSPs) or fibrin degradation products (FDPs) is used to detect the breakdown of fibrin clot by plasmin. As plasmin lyses the clot, the fragments formed retain some anticoagulant activity. Excessive clot breakdown results in too many FSPs in the circulation, which may contribute to bleeding from multiple sites. The FSPs are elevated in DIC from the excessive fibrinolysis that occurs. Elevated levels may also be detected in obstetrical complications such as abruptio placentae, pre-eclampsia, intrauterine death or after cesarean birth, or in pulmonary embolism, active renal disease, alcoholic cirrhosis, burns, and 1 to 2 days after acute myocardial infarction. Drugs used for clot lysis (streptokinase, urokinase, t-PA) can elevate FSP levels.

The FSPs or FDPs are of different molecular weight and can be individually identified. Fragment D is one of the final products of the breakdown of fibrin. Testing specifically for the D-dimer fragment is being used as a confirmatory test for FSPs and the detection of DIC.

NONHEMATOLOGICAL DIAGNOSTIC PROCEDURES

Other diagnostic procedures may be needed to help locate and quantify bleeding in patients with hematological problems. X-rays, arteriograms, venograms, computed tomography (CT) scans, or magnetic resonance imaging may be necessary to identify sites of bleeding or thrombi. Radionucleotide scans may also be ordered to assess the function of the liver and spleen in patients with hepatomegaly or splenomegaly.

Bone marrow aspiration and needle biopsy examination yield valuable diagnostic information about blood disorders. Histological and hematological analysis of the hematopoietic tissue are useful in the diagnosis of thrombocytopenia, aplastic anemia, and leukemia; in monitoring myelosuppression; and in evaluation the effectiveness of chemotherapy. The posterior iliac crest is the preferred site for this procedure.

REFERENCES

1. Shannon-Bodner, R. M. (1990). Patient assessment: History taking and physical exam. In K. Goldberg (Ed.), *Hematologic problems.* Springhouse, PA: Springhouse.
2. Simmons, A. (1989). *Hematology: A combined theoretical and technical approach.* Philadelphia: Saunders.
3. Griffin, J. P. (1986). *Hematology and immunology concepts for nurses.* Norwalk, CT: Appleton-Century-Crofts.
4. Shaw, C. (1990). Diagnostic studies: Patient teaching, preparation, and nursing care. In K. Goldberg (Ed.), *Hematologic problems.* Springhouse, PA: Springhouse.
5. Kee, J. L. (1990). *Handbook of laboratory and diagnostic tests with nursing implications.* Norwalk, CT: Appleton & Lange.

42

Hematological Disorders

Debra Tribett

Hematological dysfunction may be the primary reason for admission to an intensive care unit, but more likely it will be a secondary complication developing in the critically ill patient. The complexity of the patient's needs and the potential for rapid changes in the condition demand that the critical care nurse pay particular attention to subtle but potentially significant changes. As the primary caregiver in the critical care setting, the nurse has a unique opportunity for continual assessment to detect the signs and symptoms in various organ systems that may indicate impending hematological emergencies. This chapter presents a wide variety of hematological disorders commonly seen in critical illness, including disorders of red blood cell function, platelets, coagulation, and fibrinolysis.

ANEMIA

The most common condition arising from hematopoietic disease is anemia. It is a clinical sign, rather than a specific disease and is characterized by a reduction in circulating red blood cells (RBCs) or hemoglobin (Hb) or both. The normal RBC count is 4.6 to 6.2 million per mm^3 in males and 4.2 to 5.4 million per mm^3 in females. Normal Hb is 13 to 18 g/dl for men and 12 to 16 g/dl for women. This corresponds to a normal male hematocrit (Hct) of 45% to 54% and female Hct of 36% to 46%. Decreases in Hb and Hct may arise from many causes. Anemia can be categorized by its etiology (see the box to the right).

The general effects of anemia can be attributed to a reduction in the oxygen-carrying capability of the blood. Tissue hypoxia occurs when oxygen is unavailable or insufficient at the cellular level for required metabolic activity. Clinical manifestations are related to the compensatory mechanisms that ensue to preserve oxygenation to the body tissues. Hypoxia has profound effects on all organ systems, but the neurological system and the cardiovascular system are particularly vulnerable.

Compensation at the RBC level consists of an increased synthesis of 2,3-diphosphoglycerate (2,3-DPG). This shifts the oxygen dissociation curve to the right, allowing easier release of oxygen to the tissues from the RBCs when anemia is present.

Another compensatory mechanism is the use of all potential collateral and capillary channels to increase tissue perfusion to vital areas at the expense of nonvital donor areas. The major donor areas for redistribution of the blood are the skin and the kidneys. Vasoconstriction and the presence of deoxygenated hemoglobin contribute to the clinical finding of pallor in the skin and mucous membranes of anemic patients. Even though the kidneys are vital organs, under normal circumstances their blood supply is far in excess of demands. So even in severe anemia, with renal blood flow reduced by almost 50%, renal function may be only mildly or moderately reduced. The benefit of reductions in blood flow to the skin and kidneys is an enhanced supply to the myocardium, brain, and muscles.

Causes of Anemia

NUTRITIONAL DEFICIENCY

Iron

Vitamin B_{12}

Folic acid

DECREASED PRODUCTION OF RBCs

Chronic illness

Aplastic bone marrow

Cancer and its therapy

HEMOLYSIS

Congenital

    Sickle cell disease

    Thalassemia

Acquired

    Immunological reaction

    Physical injury

ACUTE BLOOD LOSS

Compensatory increases in cardiac output may occur. The signs of this compensatory cardiac activity are tachycardia, the development of a systolic flow murmur, and orthostatic hypotension. A normal heart can sustain this hyperdynamic state for prolonged periods. The increase in cardiac output increases myocardial oxygen demand. High-output cardiac failure and ischemic pain may occur if coronary oxygen demands are not met, particularly if there is preexisting coronary artery disease. Cardiac output does not measurably increase in chronic anemias until the hemoglobin levels approach 7 g/dl. In acute anemia from hemorrhage, there may not be time for physiological adjustments, so the symptoms may be much more prominent.

The respiratory system compensates for anemia by increasing respiratory rate to maintain oxygenation. This mechanism accounts for tachypnea, exertional dyspnea, and orthopnea seen in the anemic patient.

The final compensatory mechanism for anemia is an increase in the rate of RBC production. This is indicated by an increase in reticulocyte count above the normal 1% of the total RBC value. The decrease in oxygen to the kidney stimulates an increase in erythropoietin production. If the bone marrow is functionally responsive, an increased number of immature RBCs (reticulocytes) will be seen in the peripheral blood. The patient experiencing increased bone marrow activity may report generalized aches and pains or sternal tenderness.

The severity of the anemic patient's symptoms depends on the speed of the onset and the duration of the anemia, the patient's metabolic demands, and the concomitant health problems. A gradual decline in RBC count or Hb by as much as 50% may be tolerated in an otherwise healthy person. If that same person suffers an acute loss of 30% of RBCs or Hb, the patient may exhibit profound shock. A patient with chronic anemia, such as occurs in the patient with chronic renal failure, will not develop severe symptoms until a very low Hb level is reached. An active person with anemia will develop symptoms earlier than a sedentary person. In a hospitalized patient, the patient may appear normal while on bed rest but develop symptoms with increased activity such as attempting to get out of bed to a chair. Concurrent medical problems affect a patient's response to anemia. A hypothyroid patient has decreased oxygen requirements and may therefore tolerate anemia better than a euthyroid patient. As mentioned earlier, patients with coronary artery disease and anemia may complain of angina when myocardial oxygen delivery is inadequate to meet the activity demands.

Patients encountered in critical care may have chronic or acute anemia. In *chronic anemia*, the blood volume is usually normal because of increased plasma volume. In *acute anemia*, particularly in the face of large volume blood loss, both volume and blood component replacement may be necessary to sustain life. Both conditions may occur concomitantly. An example of such a situation would be a patient with chronic alcoholism who is admitted with bleeding esophageal varices.

Anemia is also significant for postoperative patients and those with traumatic wounds or decubitus ulcers. Wound healing is impaired in the anemic patient because the availability of oxygen to the involved tissues is decreased.

When compensatory mechanisms cannot correct the tissue hypoxia in anemic patients, symptoms such as angina, intermittent claudication, or muscle cramps may occur. Neurological symptoms may be prominent. The patient may complain of headache, feeling light-headed, roaring in the ears (from increased cardiac output), faintness, irritability, restlessness, or depression.

Medical Management

Management of anemia is specific for its etiology. The overall goal is to identify the cause of the anemia and eliminate it if possible.[1] Maintaining adequate tissue perfusion during this period can be a challenge. In some cases, it may not be possible to eliminate the underlying cause, and long-term management of anemia is required. When the etiology of some types of anemia is not curable, death from complications of the disease or its treatment may be the ultimate outcome.

The diagnosis of anemia must first consider if the patient is truly anemic. Congestive heart failure or iatrogenic fluid overload from fluid resuscitation may cause a dilutional anemia in the critically ill patient. Dehydrated or severely burned patients may have severe anemia that is hidden by a decreased plasma volume. Analysis of trends in Hb and Hct must be correlated with the patient's volume and hemodynamic data.

The patient must be assessed for evidence of bleeding. Women of reproductive age may lose significant amounts of iron during menstruation. Gastrointestinal bleeding is a frequent cause of blood loss. In critically ill patients, one must observe for diagnostic phlebotomy as a cause for anemia. Soft tissue bleeding following surgery or trauma is another source of blood loss.

Hemolytic anemia is less common than other types of anemia and may be difficult to recognize. Patient and family history are important in the determination of inherited hemolytic anemias, such as sickle cell anemia or thalassemia. Acquired hemolytic anemia occurring intravascularly or more commonly extra-vascularly after the cells have been culled from the circulation is seen in a wide variety of critically ill patients. Hemolytic anemia induced by drugs or chemicals must be suspected in the critically ill patient receiving multiple drugs with this potential side effect.

The critically ill patient in the ICU often has several potential reasons for anemia. Most patients with active inflammatory disease or advanced malignancy have a mild to moderate anemia. A significant degree of renal, hepatic, or endocrine dysfunction also leads to anemia. Patients with immune system dysfunction or neoplasm often have anemia because the normal immune modulation or RBC production and destruction is affected.

Treatment of anemia is specific for its etiology. Detailed coverage of this subject is beyond the scope of this chapter, so concerns specific to the critically ill patient are addressed.

Nutritional Deficiencies

Normal dietary patterns are often disrupted when the patient is in the critical care unit. Patients are unable to eat a balanced diet that would ensure an intake of iron, vitamin B_{12}, and folic acid sufficient for normal RBC production. Today, more and more elderly people are being seen in critical care units. These patients may be admitted with preexisting dietary deficiencies.

Iron deficiency, often associated with an iron deficient diet, is the most common cause of anemia worldwide. Anemia from this cause is exhibited as a late sign of deficient iron stores. Blood loss from trauma, surgery, or gastrointestinal hemorrhage may cause this form of anemia in the hospitalized person. It is the only form of anemia that responds to iron replacement therapy.

Deficiency of vitamin B_{12} (cobalamin) is caused by a poor diet lacking animal products or in those who practice strict vegetarianism. It may also be related to decreased absorption, as in a deficiency of intrinsic factor secondary to partial or total gastrectomy. Parenteral administration of cobalamin is the recommended route for replacement therapy. It is low in both cost and toxicity.

Folate deficiency is seen with a poor diet, lack of vegetables, and alcoholism. Absorption may be impaired by a variety of intestinal disorders. Hemodialysis may also increase losses of folic acid. Oral therapy is satisfactory to meet most patients' needs, but a parenteral preparation may be used in the severely ill patient or in the patient unable to take oral medication.

The critically ill patient's dietary needs must often be met through the use of enteral or parenteral nu-trition. The ability of the body to utilize the nutrients, as well as the body's requirements, are affected by the systemic condition of the patient. Physical injury, trauma, burns, or sepsis increases tissue breakdown and metabolism. Greater than normal amounts of nutrients are required to maintain nitrogen and energy balance in the stressed patient. It is not clear whether stress changes the requirements for vitamins. Commercially prepared enteral feedings are designed to provide complete nutrient replacement. Total parenteral nutrition generally includes commercial preparations of adequately formulated vitamin and trace elements. It is the responsibility of the critical care team to implement these therapies to prevent or treat nutritional deficits.

Decreased Production of RBCs

Anemia of Chronic Illness. As mentioned previously, chronic illness often is associated with anemia. Treatment of the underlying cause of the disease may help alleviate the symptoms of anemia. However, it may be necessary in the critically ill patient with chronic illness to intervene with symptomatic treatments. Oxygen administration to increase oxygenation of existing RBCs and the transfusion of RBCs to restore an adequate level of Hb may be instituted.

RBC transfusion must be evaluated from a risk/benefit perspective. Transfusion has the potential risk of infection in all patients and in some patients the additional concern of fluid overload. Therefore, it is reserved for only those patients who absolutely need this intervention.

The patient with chronic renal failure is an example of an anemic patient who may tolerate a very low Hb and Hct. Blood transfusions are rarely required unless hematocrit drops below 15%.

Aplastic Anemia. The term *aplastic anemia* refers to a diverse group of severe bone marrow disorders characterized by a pancytopenia. Approximately 50% of cases are idiopathic. The remaining cases may be caused by exposure to toxic chemicals, drugs, radiation, infection, or autoimmune disorders. Aplastic anemia is rare. It usually has an insidious onset but can be dramatic in its presentation.

Idiosyncratic drug-related aplastic anemia can be caused by a wide variety of seemingly unrelated drugs. Chloramphenicol is a prototype of this group. In this variety of aplastic anemia, any drug suspected of toxicity should be discontinued.

Therapy for this patient population should be handled in a center specializing in the disease. Treatment options for these patients have included androgens, high dose corticosteroids, and antilymphocyte globulin or antithymocyte globulin. Bone marrow transplantation from a human lymphocyte antigen (HLA) compatible donor is the recommended therapy in patients under 20 who have not received previous transfusion.

Supportive care has led to the survival of patients who have aplastic anemia. Transfusions are used in patients who are not transplant candidates. They are used only when absolutely necessary in patients who are potential transplant recipients because of the risk of sensitization and subsequent graft rejection.

In addition, patients with aplastic anemia experience thrombocytopenia and leukopenia; thus, they are at risk for bleeding and the development of infection. Low platelet counts are well tolerated by these patients and therefore transfusion should be reserved for actual bleeding episodes. Implementation of precautions to prevent infection in care of these patients is important. Reverse isolation is not indicated because the patient will remain at risk for infection from their own endogenous flora.

Cancer and Its Therapy. Neoplastic infiltration of the bone marrow can occur in leukemias, lymphomas, plasma cell myeloma, and carcinoma of the breast, prostate, lung, or stomach. Replacement of the functional marrow results in anemia. Treatment to kill the tumor cells is necessary, but the therapy is also toxic to the bone marrow.

Chemotherapy and radiation for the treatment of neoplastic disease are cytotoxic to the hematopoietic stem cells. The resulting aplasia is usually reversible. Treatment for anemia in these patients may include transfusion during the nadir of their RBC counts or if the patient becomes symptomatic.

Hemolysis of RBCs

Hemolytic anemia occurs when the rate of destruction of RBCs increases, shortening their life span. It may be congenital or acquired. In congenital hemolytic anemia, the RBC has a defect in its cell membrane, enzymes, or Hb. Examples of congenital hemolytic anemia are sickle cell anemia and thalassemia. Acquired hemolytic disorders are seen in situations where noxious factors exist in the circulation causing immunological, physical, or chemical injury. For example, trauma to the RBC caused by prosthetic heart valves or cardiopulmonary bypass can lead to acquired hemolysis.

Hemolytic anemia can also be classified according to whether the hemolysis is predominantly intravascular or extravascular. The reticuloendothelial organs (liver and spleen) are the extravascular sites of RBC destruction. Most forms of hemolysis are extravascular. The severity of this form of anemia is determined by the rate of RBC destruction and the bone marrow's capacity for erythrocyte production.

Management of hemolytic anemia is largely supportive. The underlying cause must be identified in order to treat the specific problem, if possible. Improved tissue oxygenation and support of cardiovascular function are critical goals. Severely anemic patients should receive supplemental oxygen. They may be placed on bed rest to reduce demands on cardiac output. Transfusions with packed RBCs should be administered to correct hemodynamic deficits. The physician must consider the risks of transfusion. Additionally, patients with immune-mediated hemolysis are difficult to cross-match for transfusions. Maintenance of erythropoiesis in patients with chronic hemolysis requires extra quantities of folic acid and vitamin B_{12}. Splenectomy may be performed in patients whose hemolysis is predominately extravascular.

Acute Posthemorrhagic Anemia

Anemia caused by the loss of a large volume of blood may occur after trauma, surgery, gastrointestinal bleeding, or coagulopathy. It is first detected after expansion of plasma volume. In a patient on bed rest, this is generally seen within 24 hours.

The rate and volume of blood loss determine the patient's symptoms. Often patients are admitted to the critical care unit for the treatment of hypovolemia, or shock, or both; for identification of the bleeding site; and for control of the hemorrhage. Volume replacement with crystalloid and colloid solutions and RBCs is indicated.

Once the emergency has been dealt with, treatment of anemia can be initiated. Additional blood transfusion may be required, as in preparation of the patient for surgery. The use of surgical autotransfusion in cardiac, thoracic, and orthopedic procedures has been increasing. This technique allows salvage and reinfusion of the patient's own blood, eliminating some of the risks of infection associated with transfusions and postoperative anemia. Generally, the restoration of a high protein diet and iron supplementation will address the anemia in a patient with functional bone marrow once the hemorrhage has been controlled.

NURSING MANAGEMENT IN ANEMIA

The critical care nurse is often the first member of the team to learn the current laboratory values for a patient or to observe the signs and symptoms associated with anemia. Communication of these findings to the physician is one of the collaborative actions the critical care nurse performs. The nurse also institutes prescribed therapy such as oxygen, volume replacement, or RBC transfusion and evaluates the therapeutic effects of these therapies.

The nurse must use hematological data when interpreting other test results such as arterial blood gas levels (ABGs) or monitoring oxygen saturation with a pulse oximeter. The nurse must collaborate with the respiratory therapist so that both members of the team are aware of the patient's hematological status and its effect on the respiratory assessment data.

The patient's correct Hb value must be entered into the machine by the person performing arterial blood gas analysis. If this information is not provided, the ABG test results will be based on a normal Hb instead of the patient's actual value.

The nurse may experience a false sense of security when the pulse oximeter displays a value of 90% oxygen saturation. The actual oxygen content of blood that is 90% saturated with oxygen differs greatly when the Hb is only 10 g instead of a normal 15 g. The nurse must remember the individual patient's Hb level while watching the continuous display on the monitor and utilize this information when interpreting the data.

The focus of nursing care for the anemic patient in the critical care environment is related to monitoring for the compensatory cardiovascular responses and the patient's ability to tolerate the resulting increased or decreased cardiac output. In collaboration with the physician, the nurse carries out supportive therapies ordered to treat cardiovascular instability.

The nurse must assist patients in tolerating their activities of daily living and prescribed therapies with the limitations placed upon the patient by anemia. The pertinent nursing diagnosis and care plan for the patient experiencing activity intolerance related to decreased oxygen carrying capability of the blood secondary to anemia appear below.[2]

■ NURSING DIAGNOSIS

Activity intolerance, related to imbalance between oxygen supply and demand.

OUTCOME STANDARD AND CRITERIA

Prescribed activity level is tolerated as evidenced by the following during and after activity:

- Normal heart rate, heart rhythm, and blood pressure
- Subjective tolerance of activity
- No diaphoresis

NURSING INTERVENTIONS

- Set realistic goals for activity with patient
- Monitor vital signs during periods of increased activity
- Schedule activities to decrease energy expenditure
- Plan rest periods between activities and after meals
- Increase activity gradually
- Terminate activity at the onset of signs of intolerance

- Maintain supplemental oxygen therapy during activity
- Provide assistance with activities of daily living
- Teach patient self-monitoring for signs of intolerance

DISORDERS OF HEMOSTASIS

Disorders of hemostasis encountered in critically ill patients may be due to abnormalities of quantity or quality of platelets or plasma coagulation factors, use of drugs affecting the coagulation system, or damage to the vascular endothelium. Coagulopathies may be inherited or acquired. Inherited disorders, fortunately, are relatively rare. Acquired disorders are more common.

Platelet Disorders

Platelets are first to activate the process of hemostasis when a blood vessel is damaged. Bleeding associated with platelet disorders is characterized by petechiae and ecchymoses of the skin and mucous membranes. The petechiae are more numerous over dependent areas of the body because of increased venous pressure. If these grow and become confluent, large ecchymoses will occur, but petechiae still tend to be present at the margins. Bleeding differs from that observed in disorders related to plasma coagulation factors. Platelet-associated disorders are associated with a tendency to internal bleeding (cerebral, gastrointestinal, genitourinary, respiratory) as well as oozing from mucous membranes of the nose and mouth.

Quantitative Platelet Disorders

A general tendency to bleeding occurs with or without petechiae when the platelet level falls below $100,000/mm^3$. A finding of fewer platelets indicates thrombocytopenia. Platelet counts of 40,000 to $60,000/mm^3$ may lead to prolonged posttraumatic bleeding. Spontaneous hemorrhage may occur at $20,000/mm^3$. Patients with chronic long-standing thrombocytopenia can tolerate lower levels without hemorrhage. The four basic mechanisms of quantitative platelet disorders are: (1) decreased or ineffective platelet production, (2) shortened platelet survival time in the circulation, (3) splenic sequestration, and (4) intravascular dilution.

Decreased Platelet Production. Reduced platelet production may be caused by bone marrow replacement, chemical injury, or congenital disorders. Mechanical displacement of megakaryocytes in the bone marrow may be due to metastatic carcinoma, myeloma, leukemias, or lymphomas. Chemical injury to the megakaryocytes may be caused by cancer chemotherapeutic agents, alcohol, anticonvulsants, thiazide diuretics, solvents, or insecticides. Accidental or therapeutic radiation may also be responsible for decreased megakaryocytopoiesis. Rare congenital diseases such as Fanconi's syndrome, May-Hegglin anomaly, Wiskott-Aldrich syndrome, and Di-Guglielmo's disease may decrease the number of circulating platelets. Aplastic anemia, as discussed earlier in this chapter, is also an etiology for reduced platelet production.

Treatment for decreased platelet counts must be directed toward the underlying cause, if known. Supportive therapy in the form of platelet transfusions may be necessary to prevent hemorrhage.

Decreased Platelet Survival. Many drugs may cause thrombocytopenic purpura. In drug-induced thrombocytopenic purpura, bone marrow megakaryocytes are functional, but platelets are destroyed peripherally. A drug rarely induces thrombocytopenia by a direct action. Many are suspected and some have been proven to induce thrombocytopenia by an antibody-mediated immune mechanism. The drug quinidine is among the most studied in relation to this condition.[3] The drug or its derivatives or metabolites act as a hapten and form a complex with a plasma protein. The complex formed is recognized by the immune system as an antigen, and antibody is formed. When the drug is reintroduced to the system, the antibody can bind to the drug itself. The antigen-antibody complex happens to attach to platelets. Platelets coated with antibody are recognized by the reticuloendothelial system, destroyed, and thus removed prematurely from the circulation.

Therapy for drug-induced, antibody-mediated thrombocytopenia usually consists of discontinuing the drug suspected of causing the reaction. Further use of the offending agent is contraindicated. Corticosteroid therapy is recommended if the platelet count is below $30,000/mm^3$, if severe purpura exists, or if spontaneous bleeding from mucous membranes occurs. Corticosteroids inhibit the phagocytosis of the coated platelets by macrophages in the reticuloendothelial system.

Heparin is a drug frequently used in the treatment of critically ill patients. Whether administered intravenously or subcutaneously, it can induce thrombocytopenia. Two forms of thrombocytopenia seem to be associated with heparin therapy.[4] One is a mild form and the other is severe.

The more common type begins about the second or third day of heparin therapy. A mild, transient drop in platelets to $100,000/mm^3$ is seen, but spontaneous bleeding seldom occurs. The drop in platelet count is thought to be caused by increased platelet aggregation, margination, and peripheral sequestration caused by the release of adenosine diphosphate (ADP) by heparin. This condition rarely persists nor does it produce clinical signs and symptoms. Heparin therapy can be continued.

An immune mechanism is the suspected cause of the severe form of heparin-induced thrombocytopenia. Platelet counts begin to drop severely after 4 to 8 days of receiving the drug and continue to be very low until the heparin is discontinued. Heparin apparently can combine with the platelet membrane to form a hapten that stimulates antibody formation. This antibody is directed at platelet membranes and stimulates further platelet aggregation so long as heparin is present. Thrombocytopenia and resulting hemorrhage occur. Resistance to heparin also is seen. Patients experiencing this reaction may develop arterial thrombosis known as the *white clot syndrome.*

Treatment for the thrombocytopenia involves the immediate discontinuance of heparin administration, including the use of heparinized solutions for maintaining patency of intravascular devices. The platelet count usually returns to normal within 7 days. If continued anticoagulation is needed, oral therapy may be instituted. Several days may be required to reach a therapeutic level. Additional oral agents such as aspirin or dipyridamole may be used for their ability to decrease platelet aggregation. Platelet infusions have little effect on this form of thrombocytopenia.

If the white clot syndrome has occurred in conjunction with thrombocytopenia, arterial thrombus removal may be attempted. Thrombolytic agents such as streptokinase or urokinase may be employed to lyse the clot and restore perfusion to the ischemic area.

Thrombocytopenia occurring in the absence of toxic exposure or a disease associated with decreased platelets is referred to as *idiopathic thrombocytopenic purpura* (ITP).[3] In most patients with ITP, an immunological mechanism involving IgG antiplatelet antibodies is demonstrated. The spleen prematurely removes the platelets from the circulation. This has also been referred to as *autoimmune thrombocytopenic purpura.* An acute and a chronic form have been identified. Both exhibit normal production but decreased survival of platelets without splenomegaly. Therapy for ITP starts with corticosteroids and progresses to splenectomy if the drug regimen is unsuccessful. In patients who have not responded to splenectomy, immunosuppressive agents (azathioprine, cyclophosphamide, and vincristine) have had some success. High-dose intravenous gamma globulin has also been used in patients in whom splenectomy does not bring about improvement. Platelet transfusions are administered in a situation of life-threatening hemorrhage but should not be given prophylactically because they are minimally effective.

Additional causes of decreased platelet survival include acute infections, cardiopulmonary bypass, and consumption coagulopathy or disseminated intravascular coagulation (DIC). Bacterial, viral, fungal, rickettsial, and protozoan infections can all be associated with thrombocytopenia. Fortunately, only a small percentage of patients with infections develop hemorrhage from thrombocytopenia of this etiology. Patients requiring cardiopulmonary bypass are at risk for platelet activation when platelets come into contact with the surfaces of oxygenators. Currently, platelet transfusions are administered to restore hemostasis in this patient population. Both patients with infection and patients undergoing cardiopulmonary bypass, as well as many other critically ill patients, are at risk for the development of DIC. Because of the seriousness of this problem and its involvement with consumption of coagulation factors in addition to platelets, this coagulopathy is discussed in greater detail later in this chapter.

Splenic Platelet Sequestration. Any disease accompanied by splenomegaly may result in a drop in platelet count to 50,000 to 100,000/mm^3. Normally, 30% of platelets may be stored in the spleen. This figure can be as high as 90% in hypersplenism. Platelet transit time through the spleen is delayed. Splenic pooling does not require therapy unless associated with anemia. In this case, splenectomy will result in a return of both RBC and platelet counts to normal.

Dilutional Thrombocytopenia. Patients receiving massive transfusions (10 to 20 U of blood) may experience dilutional thrombocytopenia. They may also demonstrate platelet dysfunction and a coagulation defect. Platelet transfusions may be required, but administration should be based on clinical evaluation of the patient and not on platelet count alone. This patient population is also at risk for the development of DIC.

Qualitative Platelet Disorders

A normal platelet count and a prolonged bleeding time characterize patients with qualitative platelet disorders. These may be congenital or acquired defects. Congential platelet disorders such as Glanzmann's thrombasthenia and Bernard-Soulier syndrome are rare. Acquired platelet dysfunction is more common in critically ill patients as a result of drug administration or systemic disease.

Drug-induced Platelet Disorders. Three mechanisms for drug-induced suppression of platelet function have been identified: (1) Inhibition of thromboxane-A$_2$ synthesis, (2) an increased synthesis of cyclic AMP, and (3) interference of attachment of platelet aggregation agonists to binding proteins.

Nonsteroidal antiinflammatory drugs (NSAIDs) are examples of drugs interfering with thromboxane-A$_2$ synthesis. Aspirin is different from other drugs of this category in that it irreversibly inhibits the function of platelets for the rest of the normal life span. Therefore, after exposure to aspirin, it takes 5 to 10 days to restore normal platelet function by replacing the exposed platelets with new platelets produced by the bone marrow. Most patients can tolerate aspirin without developing a bleeding disorder. However, aspirin is usually avoided in the preoperative period to prevent increased bleeding and oozing during and after surgical procedures. Aspirin is used therapeutically for its antiplatelet effects in patients with coronary artery disease. Other nonsteroidal antiinflammatory drugs have reversible platelet effects and in therapeutic doses rarely affect bleeding time. However, none of the drugs in this category should be used in patients with known bleeding disorders.

Increased cyclic AMP decreases platelet function. Drugs such as prostacyclin, dipyridamole and its analogs, beta blockers, slow calcium channel blockers, and local anesthetic type antidysrhythmics cause platelet dysfunction by this mechanism of action.

Beta-lactam antibiotics are examples of the third mechanism for platelet dysfunction by interfering with attachment of platelet aggregation agonists to binding proteins. Penicillin G in high doses, carbenicillin, ticarcillin, nafcillin, and moxalactam are capable of platelet function impairment secondary to this mechanism.

The critically ill patient may receive many drugs with the potential side effect of platelet dysfunction. Suspected agents must be removed from the treatment plan if a prolonged bleeding time becomes a danger to the patient. Platelet transfusions should be limited to life-threatening situations.

Uremia. Patients with renal failure and uremia may develop a hemorrhagic disorder secondary to a defect in platelet function. Dialysis can reverse clinical and laboratory platelet defects. The administration of desarginine vasopressin (DDAVP) has also proven effective in improving platelet function in uremic patients.

Platelet Transfusion

Platelet transfusion is indicated to prevent bleeding associated with deficiencies in platelet number or function. Transfusions are generally administered to patients with platelet counts of less than 50,000/mm^3 if there is evidence of bleeding. They may be used prophylactically for patients with platelet counts of 10,000 to 20,000/mm^3. Platelets should not be administered to patients with ITP unless life-threatening bleeding is present. Prophylactic use is not recommended in massive blood transfusion or following cardiopulmonary bypass.

The usual volume of a unit of platelet concentrate is 50 to 70 ml of plasma. The dose is generally 1 unit per 10 kg of body weight or as determined by the clinical situation. A pre-transfusion platelet count should be obtained and repeated at 1 hour after transfusion to assess the therapeutic effect of the transfusion. One unit of platelets should raise the count of a 70-kg adult by 5,000/mm³.

After exposure to platelets from 20 donors, patients become alloimmunized, and the transfusions are no longer effective. This is evidenced by a lack of response in the platelet count 1 hour post-transfusion. Single-donor platelets that are HLA matched may reduce the risk of antibody formation by decreasing the number of donor exposures. HLA-matched platelets improve the patient's response only if HLA antibodies are the primary cause of platelet destruction. Patients who are undergoing immunosuppressive therapy and may be requiring platelet transfusion should be HLA typed prior to initiation of their treatment.

The risks of platelet transfusion should always be considered before initiating this therapy. Allergic or febrile reaction; transmission of hepatitis, HIV, malaria, or cytomegalovirus infections; or graft-versus-host disease are possible complications from platelet transfusions.

NURSING MANAGEMENT IN PLATELET DISORDERS/ COAGULOPATHY

The critical care nurse will often be first to detect a platelet disorder while performing routine care. Mouth care may induce oozing from the gums, or petechiae may develop from the cuff of a sphygmomanometer or the sleeve of a sequential compression device. Venipuncture sites may continue to ooze, requiring frequent dressing changes. All of these signs suggest a quantitative or qualitative platelet problem. If laboratory values are available, these clinical signs may be correlated with a platelet count and bleeding time. Detection of a problem with hemostasis must be communicated to the physician as soon as it is noted.

Since platelets perform in the earliest stages of the process of coagulation, a lack of platelets or defective platelet function can become a significant problem for the patient. In the critical care unit, many invasive procedures are used in diagnosis and treatment. The inability to form a platelet plug and trigger the coagulation process increases the danger of these procedures to the patient. Routine nursing care procedures must also be planned so as to prevent any trauma that might precipitate bleeding. Nursing care for the patient with potential for injury related to a coagulopathy follows.

Platelet transfusions are often used in critically ill patients with low platelet counts and a need for an invasive procedure. The critical care nurse must coordinate the arrival of platelets from the blood bank and their transfusion prior to the scheduled procedure, routine intravascular line change, or surgery. Close monitoring of the effects of the platelet transfusion must also be integrated into the nursing care of this patient.

The nurse must also communicate with other members of the health care team. Phlebotomists, respiratory therapists, physical therapists, and consulting physicians are among those who perform activities with potential for trauma to the patient. They must be aware of the increased risk for bleeding so that their care may be modified or postponed as indicated.

■ NURSING DIAGNOSIS

High risk for injury, related to altered hemostasis.[2,5,6]

The subjective defining characteristics for this diagnosis include:
- Pain in area of suspected bleeding such as a headache or joint pain
- Feeling of tingling or warmth in joint
- Paresthesia

The objective characteristics include:
- Petechiae
- Bruising or ecchymoses
- Purpura
- Guaiac-positive urine, stool, gastric fluids
- Mucous membrane bleeding (gingival bleeding, epistaxis, oral mucous membrane)
- Oozing from IM, IV, or venipuncture sites
- Gastrointestinal bleeding: melena or frank bleeding
- Smoky to bright red urine
- Menorrhagia
- Hematoma formation
- Acrocyanosis
- Gangrenous changes to fingertips, toes, earlobes, nose
- Changes in neurological assessment: level of consciousness, pupillary changes
- Heparin or coumarin therapy
- ETOH abuse
- Broad spectrum antibiotic therapy
- Cytotoxic drug therapy
- Pericardial friction rub
- Muffled heart sounds
- Renal failure with uremia
- Thrombocytopenia
- Prolonged PT or APTT or beyond therapeutic range if receiving anticoagulants
- Known congenital coagulopathy

OUTCOME STANDARD AND CRITERIA

Acquired injury from bleeding is absent or minimal as evidenced by:

- Absence of bleeding
- Normal coagulation studies for the individual patient's condition
- Patient return demonstration of measures necessary to prevent bleeding

NURSING INTERVENTIONS

Monitoring activities the nurse should perform include:

- Inspect all body fluids and drainage for guaiac or overt bleeding
- Review vital signs and laboratory data for signs of blood loss or shock
- Perform periodic neurological assessment with vital signs
- Auscultate heart sounds for muffling or rubs
- Review coagulation studies for significant changes or abnormal values for patient condition
- Inspect skin and mucous membranes for signs of bleeding
- Monitor and record intake and output
  Measure bloody wound drainage/weigh dressings. Count and weigh pads for menstruating women.
- Check package inserts or data for new drugs ordered for patient for side effects impairing coagulation
- Report any signs of suspected bleeding to physician
- If hematoma formation is present, measure and mark edges for comparison

Nursing activities directed at preventing trauma include:

- Oral care
  Use sponge sticks for gentle oral care.
  Avoid commercial mouthwash containing alcohol.
  Lubricate lips.
- Use electric razor or do not shave
- Implement measures to prevent constipation
- Avoid rectal temperatures, suppositories, bladder catheterization, douches, tampons
- Avoid IM injections; when necessary, use smallest needle possible
- Take BP only when necessary and inflate cuff only as high as necessary to ensure accuracy
- Avoid prolonged use of tourniquet
- Draw blood samples from arterial or venous lines to avoid venipuncture
- When applying or changing dressings:
  Use tape designed for sensitive skin.
  Remove tape gently using adhesive remover.
  Use Montgomery straps for wounds needing frequent changes.
- Pad side rails for restless patient
- Use soft restraints only when necessary
- Place sign near patient to alert personnel to patient's risk of bleeding

- When suctioning:
  Avoid nasopharyngeal route; if suctioning must be performed, use a nasopharyngeal airway.
  Do not extend suction catheter past the end of an endotracheal or tracheostomy tube.
  Avoid high negative pressure.
- Handle patient gently during turning, moving, or transport
- Use measures to prevent skin from breakdown: turning, range of motion, lubrication, air mattress, therapeutic beds, bed cradles

Nursing interventions employed to control bleeding include:

- After any invasive procedure, apply direct pressure for at least 5 to 10 minutes or until bleeding stops
- If discontinuing IV or arterial line from arm, after line is removed, raise extremity above heart level while applying pressure
- When discontinuing a central line, after line is removed and pressure is applied, raise head of bed to decrease central venous pressure
- Apply small, firm pressure dressings over sites of venipuncture or arterial puncture
- Use sandbags to immobilize limb and apply pressure to groin puncture sites after initial hemostasis has been obtained
- Use cold saline rinses for bleeding in mouth
- Apply ice pack to sites of hematoma formation or hemarthrosis
- Obtain order for use of topical thrombin for small, superficial bleeding
- Do not dislodge or attempt to remove established clots

The nurse should also teach patient, family, or significant others as the patient's condition or the situation permits:

- To recognize and report signs and symptoms of bleeding
- Use of protective measures appropriate for level of patient activity
- To wear medical alert bracelet identifying chronic problem or anticoagulation therapy
- Medications and foods to avoid
- The danger associated with removing or dislodging a formed clot

Coagulation Cascade Disorders

Both congenital and acquired causes of disorders of coagulation are seen in critically ill patients. As with other hematological problems, the critically ill patient manifests those of an acquired etiology most frequently.

Congenital Coagulation Disorders

Hemophilia. The term *hemophilia* refers to a group of X chromosome–linked recessive genetic diseases characterized by coagulation factor deficiencies or resulting from nonfunctional factors.[7] *Hemophilia A,* or classic hemophilia, is the most severe form of the disease. The patient with this form of hemophilia is lacking sufficient factor VIII. *Hemophilia B,* or Christmas disease, results from factor IX deficiency. The most rare form of the disease is *hemophilia C,* caused by factor XI deficiency.

The clinical manifestations of hemophilia vary. In all types of hemophilia, patients have abnormal bleeding. It may be mild, moderate, or severe depending on the degree of factor deficiency and the site of the bleeding. Platelet plug formation is normal; therefore, the onset of bleeding is delayed. The coagulation factor defect prevents the activation of the clotting cascade to form a stable fibrin clot. Bleeding after minor injury can persist for hours to days. Bruising, ecchymoses, and deep subcutaneous and intramuscular hematomas are frequently seen. However, petechiae and purpura do not occur. Any organ can be the site of bleeding. Hemarthrosis (blood extravasation into a joint or synovial cavity) may cause serious chronic disability. Spontaneous bleeding may occur. Exsanguination may follow injury or surgery if proper treatment is not instituted. The site of bleeding and compression of surrounding nerves, tissues, and blood vessels causes variable symptoms of pain, impaired tissue perfusion, or organ failure.

Laboratory studies in hemophilia will show a normal platelet count, bleeding time, and prothrombin level. The partial thromboplastin time is prolonged. Specific factor assays may be performed to determine the percentage of normal level present.

Treatment of the patient who is bleeding includes local measures such as application of pressure and cold to the bleeding site. Factor replacement therapy is given to correct the deficiency temporarily. For the patient with hemophilia A, the physician may order infusion of factor VIII (also known as antihemophilic factor or AHF). Cryoprecipitate can be given to replace factor VIII as well as von Willebrand's factor, fibrinogen, and factor XIII; or commercially prepared factor VIII concentrate made from large pools of donor plasma may be used. Factor VIII has a half-life of 10 to 12 hours in the circulation; therefore, therapy must be repeated two to three times a day to control a bleeding episode. Mild to moderate bleeding in hemophilia B is treated with 500 ml of fresh frozen plasma twice a day. Patients with moderate to severe hemorrhage may be given commercially prepared factor IX concentrate. Factor IX has a longer half-life than factor VIII and can be administered less frequently. Treatment is usually maintained for at least 2 days following the cessation of bleeding. Factor XI deficiency is rare and so is spontaneous bleeding in those with this defect. Fresh frozen plasma should be

given as a prophylaxis or treatment for bleeding in these patients. The half-life of factor XI is about 72 hours, so multiple transfusions are not often needed. Epsilon aminocaproic acid (EACA), an antifibrinolytic agent, may be used in hemophiliac patients who will be having dental procedures. It should not be used in conjunction with factor IX concentrates because it increases the risk of thromboembolism.[8]

As with all therapies, the treatments prescribed for control of bleeding in patients with hemophilia have potential adverse effects. Fresh frozen plasma administration carries the same risk of disease transmission (except CMV) as other blood transfusions. Allergic reactions may occur with cryoprecipitate. Administration of pooled factor preparations has an increased risk for exposure to hepatitis B and HIV infections. However, current methods for preparing commercial pooled factors have reduced this risk. Patients receiving large doses of factor IX concentrate have an increased risk for development of thromboembolism.

Von Willebrand's Disease. This disorder is an autosomal dominant or recessive inherited disease. It is due to a deficiency or abnormality of a plasma protein, von Willebrand's factor. Von Willebrand's factor is necessary for the stabilization of factor VIII in the circulation and for normal platelet adhesion to sites of vascular injury. This factor has a half-life of several hours, is very labile, and can be increased even by a vigorous Valsalva maneuver. Patients with this disease have a normal platelet count, a prolonged bleeding time, and a low factor VIII level.

Von Willebrand's disease has a wide range of clinical manifestations. It can be asymptomatic or severe enough to mimic classic hemophilia. Bleeding is usually superficial and in response to trauma. Women with this disorder have very heavy menses and postpartum bleeding problems.

Treatment for von Willebrand's disease is indicated when surgery is necessary, for severe epistaxis or menorrhagia, and for recurrent gastrointestinal bleeding. Cryoprecipitate is used because it is rich in both factor VIII and von Willebrand's factor. It should be given prophylactically immediately prior to invasive procedures. Topical measures of pressure, cold, or hemostatic agents may also be used.[9] DDAVP has also been shown to cause release of von Willebrand's factor from endothelial cells that persists for several hours. The risks associated with the administration of blood products in von Willebrand's disease is similar to that in hemophilia.

Nursing Management in Congenital Coagulopathy

The critical care unit may be used for the observation and management of patients with congenital coagulopathies after routine surgical procedures that would not normally necessitate an ICU admission. Close observation and frequent administration of blood products are easily achieved within the critical care unit. Additionally, patients with severe bleeding episodes may require the level of attention and care available from the critical care nurse.

Observation of the patient with hemophilia must include close monitoring for evidence of bleeding. The joints should be assessed to detect the development of hemarthrosis. A sensation of tingling and warmth in the joint areas signals the onset of bleeding and is followed by limited movement of the joint. Swelling will become obvious as bleeding continues. Symptoms of pain or soft tissue swelling in the joints or other body parts must be immediately assessed as active hemorrhage sites.

Depending on the location of bleeding, nursing care may include the elevation and immobilization of a bleeding site. Range of motion exercises to an affected joint should not be instituted until 48 hours after the cessation of bleeding. Application of cold compresses or ice bags may be ordered by the physician. The list of medications prescribed for the patient should not include any aspirin or other nonsteroidal antiinflammatory agents or compounds containing these drugs. Additional nursing care applicable for this patient population is included in the Nursing Diagnosis section on pp. 992-993.

Acquired Coagulation Disorders

Vitamin K Deficiency. Vitamin K is a fat-soluble vitamin that is not stored in the body. It is essential to the formation of clotting factors II, VII, IX, and X. Vitamin K is present in many plant and animal sources, so a balanced diet should provide adequate intake. It is also normally synthesized by bacterial flora in the intestinal tract. Vitamin K deficiency is rare in healthy people. In critically ill patients, it may be found in patients unable to eat an adequate diet or receiving total parenteral nutrition without vitamin K supplements, in intestinal obstruction, in malabsorption syndromes, in liver disease, and as a result of drug therapy.

Bowel sterilization regimens or the use of systemic antibiotics, in particular some third-generation cephalosporins, intereferes with vitamin K activity by disrupting intestinal flora that normally synthesize it. Vitamin K deficiency may develop within 1 to 3 weeks after intestinal synthesis is inhibited. The other drug group with significant effects on vitamin K–dependent factors is coumarin anticoagulants. These drugs are discussed in detail later in this chapter.

Vitamin K deficiency prolongs the prothrombin time (PT). If the PT is greater than two times normal, the patient will demonstrate ecchymoses, gingival bleeding, hematomas, hematuria, or melena. Oral doses of 2 to 10 mg of vitamin K should be given to patients with malabsorption of fat. Patients receiving long-term nasogastric suction or total parenteral nutrition should have vitamin K supplements included in the IV solutions. If a bleeding tendency has developed, 10 to 25 mg of vitamin K may be administered intramuscularly. However, if the bleeding tendency is great, the IV route is recommended.[10] An IV dose of 20 to 40 mg of vitamin K can be administered. The vehicle used for dilution of the drug is likely to cause an adverse reaction if the drug is administered more rapidly than 1 mg per minute via the IV route. If vitamin K is effective, the PT should begin returning to normal within 12 to 24 hours. If this dosage range does not correct the PT, then it is unlikely subsequent doses of vitamin K will be helpful.

Nursing Management in Vitamin K Deficiency

Because of the many etiologies of vitamin K deficiency, the critical care nurse may be dealing with patients in whom many primary conditions contribute to this disorder. Nursing care must be directed to the underlying condition. The nurse must be alert to the possibility of vitamin K deficiency and be observant for high-risk patients.

The nurse may be called upon to administer vitamin K replacement therapy. Because of the dangers for patient reaction to a rapid delivery of this drug, it is important to adhere to the 1 mg/min guideline previously mentioned. Close observation of the patient during the administration is essential to patient safety. Other nursing care measures for the patient with a bleeding tendency are included in the Nursing Diagnosis section on pp. 992-993.

Education regarding diet may be a long-term need of patients with vitamin K deficiency. However, the critical phase of illness may not be the best time nor the ICU the best environment for patient and family education. If patient education has not been accomplished during the ICU stay, this patient and family need must be communicated to those caring for the patient after transfer from the critical care unit.

Liver Disease

Liver disease is one of the most common causes of coagulopathies. Critical care nurses must be particularly alert for the possibility of underlying liver disease when patients have a history of alcohol abuse. Bleeding in liver disease can result from decreased synthesis of clotting factors and increased proteolytic activity caused by impairment of hepatic reticuloendothelial cells. Patients with liver disease may be unable to utilize vitamin K in the synthesis of vitamin K–dependent factors. Inadequate production of bile salts can impair digestion of food sources of this vitamin, since it is fat soluble. In patients with alcoholic liver disease, bleeding can be secondary to dietary vitamin K deficiency.

In severe liver disease, coagulation test results are usually abnormal, showing prolonged PT, prolonged PTT, and prolonged thrombin time. Fibrinogen levels are normal until the liver disease is very advanced. All clotting factors except factor VIII are typically reduced. These patients also have decreased platelet counts secondary to effects of alcohol or an enlarged spleen.

Patients with coagulopathies resulting from liver disease present treatment difficulties that depend on the severity of hepatocellular dysfunction. When these patients develop bleeding complications, factor replacement is used because the underlying disease process is often incurable. Fresh frozen plasma, cryoprecipitate, and platelet transfusions are administered if necessary. Vitamin K is also given parenterally, but if the liver cannot respond to an initial dose, it is unlikely that additional doses will have any effects. A poor prognosis is associated with failure of the PT to return to less than 1.5 times normal after vitamin K administration.

Coagulopathy is one of the many problems facing the ICU nurse when caring for the patient with liver disease. Nursing care for the patient with a coagulopathy is described on p. 992. Other nursing care measures may be geared to the management of gastrointestinal bleeding, fluid volume deficits, or shock. Because of the severity of the underlying organ failure, patients with liver disease may not survive a hemorrhagic episode. The focus of care may have to be shifted from aggressive treatment to supportive care of a dying patient and that patient's family.

Bleeding Secondary to Anticoagulant Therapy

Anticoagulant therapy is frequently used in the care of critically ill patients. Critical care nurses frequently implement heparin flushes to maintain patency of IV lines, manage continuous IV infusions of heparin for the patient with pulmonary embolism, and initiate oral anticoagulant therapy. The risk of exceeding therapeutic use of anticoagulants and the subsequent bleeding that is the most common complication of these drugs must always be considered.

Heparin. Heparin is effective immediately upon administration. It affects intrinsic and final common coagulation pathways by preventing the conversion of prothrombin to thrombin. Heparin binds with antithrombin III (AT3), allowing AT3 to enhance its normal ability to inhibit the coagulation cascade by binding active factors. Adequate AT3 is necessary for heparin to be effective.

Heparin is used to prevent and treat thromboembolism, during invasive procedures, such as cardiac catheterization, and during extracorporeal circulation. The therapeutic level of anticoagulation is achieved when the APTT is 1.5 times longer than normal. Heparin is cleared from the circulation within 2 to 4 hours after its administration.

If bleeding from heparin is minimal, it can be controlled by local measures, decreasing the dosage, or discontinuing therapy. If bleeding is severe, the antidote for heparin, protamine sulfate, may be given IV. A general starting point is 1 mg of protamine sulfate for every 100 U heparin estimated to be in the patient's circulation.

As discussed earlier in this chapter, heparin may also affect coagulation by its effects on platelets. The close monitoring of patients receiving heparin involves serial APTT studies to monitor heparin's effects on coagulation and daily platelet counts to detect thrombocytopenia.

Coumarin. Coumarin anticoagulants are used in long-term therapy for prevention of recurrent thromboembolism in patients exhibiting deep vein thrombosis, pulmonary embolism, or myocardial infarction. This drug acts by inhibiting the effects of vitamin K, thereby depressing production of the vitamin K–dependent coagulation factors. The maximum effects of the drug are not seen until 3 to 4 days after its initiation, as the clotting factors produced before coumarin was initiated must be cleared from the system.

Administration of coumarin involves balancing the drug dosage against dietary intake of vitamin K to achieve a PT about 1.5 times the normal control value. The dosage required initially may be 5 to 10 mg per day with subsequent doses adjusted according to PT values. The half-life of this drug is about 35 hours.

It is not uncommon for patients receiving the therapeutic range of anticoagulation to exhibit some mild bleeding from the gums, trace hematuria, or purpura from minor trauma. If the patient is overanticoagulated these symptoms become more serious, and the patient is at risk for gastrointestinal, genitourinary, or intracranial bleeding. If severe bleeding occurs, it may be treated with fresh frozen plasma as a source of vitamin K–dependent factors. Vitamin K may be administered IV. Administration of more than 5 mg of vitamin K intravenously will make the patient resistant to coumarin. Giving small doses of vitamin K together with fresh frozen plasma while monitoring the PT is one strategy for correcting the PT to the therapeutic range without total suppression of the anticoagulant state.

Nursing Management in Anticoagulant Therapy

Nursing care required by the patient receiving anticoagulants includes monitoring and prophylactic care, management of acute bleeding episodes, and providing patient and family education regarding self-care and home management of continuous therapy. Nursing care for the patient with a coagulopathy is presented on p. 992.

Specific points to remember during heparin therapy include the need to assess the most recent APTT before administering a dose of heparin. The time an APTT was drawn in relationship to an intermittent heparin dose is also an important part of the interpretation of the result. Heparin comes in different strengths for use in different situations. Double-checking the dosage and strength of heparin with another nurse prior to its administration is a safe nursing practice. A supply of protamine sulfate should be readily available to the ICU nurse whenever a patient is receiving heparin therapy. Close monitoring of the patient's laboratory values and dosage administration should prevent overanticoagulation, but in case of an untoward event, the antidote for heparin should be available. Close monitoring of the patient receiving heparin also includes circulatory assessments for arterial thrombus formation. This is particularly important in a patient who is exhibiting a dropping platelet count.

When preparing to give a dose of coumarin to a patient, the nurse must be aware of the patient's most recent PT results to determine whether the patient is within therapeutic range. Consultation with the physician may be needed to adjust the dosage of coumarin. The patient treated with coumarin must receive extensive preparation regarding diet and safety precautions before leaving the hospital. Initiation of patient education may begin in the critical care unit, based on the readiness of the individual to learn. If not completed while in the ICU, it must be referred to the nurses and dietitian caring for the patient prior to discharge.

Bleeding Secondary to Thrombolytic Therapy

The therapeutic use of fibrinolytic or thrombolytic agents in critical illness has significantly increased, particularly in suspected myocardial infarction. Thrombolytic agents are plasminogen activators that convert plasminogen to the active enzyme plasmin. Plasmin degrades fibrin and additionally fibrinogen, factor V, and factor VIII. Degradation of fibrin produces fibrin split products which have an anticoagulant effect. These effects increase the risk of bleeding in patients who receive thrombolytic agents.

Streptokinase and urokinase administration usually results in a systemic fibrinogen degradation or lytic state. Tissue plasminogen activator (t-PA) is more clot-selective in its effects than the other two products. Anisoylated plasminogen streptokinase ac-

tivator complex (APSAC) is a streptokinase–human plasminogen combination. It is inactive on administration but activates after fibrin binding, resulting in semiselectivity for clots. It has a more prolonged thrombolytic activity than streptokinase. None of these agents can differentiate between a pathogenic clot and a protective hemostatic clot.[11] Heparin infusion and antiplatelet therapy are often instituted in addition to a thrombolytic agent to prevent reocclusion after successful lysis of a clot. These drugs increase the risk of bleeding from mechanisms previously described.

Surface bleeding from venous or arterial access sites and after femoral artery catheterization is most common. Internal bleeding from the gastrointestinal or genitourinary tract or retroperitoneal bleeding from posterior femoral artery puncture can occur. Intracranial bleeding, although rare, is the most serious form of internal bleeding that may result from thrombolytic therapy.

Patient selection for thrombolytic therapy must identify those patients in whom existing hemostatic clots are most likely to be present and those who are at high risk of severe hemorrhagic complications. Thrombolytic therapy is contraindicated for patients with a history of cerebrovascular accident, recent (within 2 months) intracranial or intraspinal surgery or trauma, intracranial neoplasm, arteriovenous malformation or aneurysm, severe uncontrolled hypertension, active internal bleeding, or a history of bleeding diathesis. For patients with many other conditions, the risk of bleeding must be weighed against the benefit of the thrombolytic therapy.

Baseline CBC and coagulation data should be obtained before therapy is initiated. Coagulation study specimens obtained during treatment will not accurately reflect the patient's condition. After completion of drug infusions, fibrinogen levels may be decreased, PT and PTT prolonged, and levels of fibrin split products (FSPs) or fibrin degradation products (FDPs) increased in response to clot lysis.

Medical measures to prevent bleeding patients who are candidates for fibrinolytic therapy include thorough screening and patient selection. Noncompressible sites such as the subclavian and internal jugular veins should be avoided when selecting sites for central venous access. If femoral artery cannulation is necessary, care must be taken to prevent posterior wall puncture and subsequent retroperitoneal bleeding. Consideration may be given to the prophylactic use of antiulcer therapy to prevent gastrointestinal bleeding. Also, obtaining blood type and screen specimens prior to therapy may save time should transfusion therapy be needed to treat hemorrhage.

Control of surface bleeding, should it occur, can

usually be accomplished by direct pressure over a site for 30 minutes or until bleeding stops. A firm pressure dressing should be applied to the site. If the site is the femoral artery, the usual post–cardiac catheterization precautions are indicated: immobility, minimal elevation of the head of the bed, and assessment of the groin and distal pulse every 15 minutes. Any internal bleeding causing significant blood loss or hemodynamic compromise warrants discontinuing an infusion of a thrombolytic agent. Volume replacement to prevent shock and administration of blood products to correct coagulation deficits may be needed.

Nursing Management in Thrombolytic Therapy

The care of the patient receiving thrombolytic therapy is based on the location and severity of the thrombosis and is beyond the scope of this chapter. Only the nursing care related to the potential for bleeding is presented.

Although it is the physician's role to diagnose a thrombosis and order therapy, the nurse must be aware of the contraindications for such therapy. Collection of a complete database assists in the identification of risk factors for bleeding and conditions limiting the use of thrombolysis.

The nursing care plan presented on p. 992 is applicable to this patient population. However, some specific modifications in care are associated with the administration of thrombolytic agents. All intravenous or arterial line accesses must be initiated before therapy is begun. If an arterial line has not yet been placed, establishing an IV site suitable for blood sampling is advisable to minimize the need for venipuncture. This IV site would also be available should the need arise for emergency infusion of drugs or blood products. If unsuccessful venipuncture attempts have been made, these sites must be closely observed for clot lysis after the drug administration has occurred. If an arterial or venous puncture must be performed after therapy has been initiated, pressure must be applied for 30 minutes or until bleeding stops. Therefore, no vascular access site that is not directly compressible should be employed. Direct pressure should be followed with a firm pressure dressing to maintain hemostasis. Discontinuation of an arterial or venous line should be avoided until 24 hours after the end of the thrombolytic administration to allow blood coagulation factors to approach normal.

Frequent assessment during the treatment for detection of surface bleeding or signs of internal bleeding is an important nursing role. Neurological assessment should accompany vital sign assessment to detect evidence of intracranial bleeding. If the patient has undergone cardiac catheterization or arteriography, the arterial puncture site and the distal pulse of the involved extremity must be frequently assessed. If the femoral artery has been cannulated, the patient must be assessed for signs of retroperitoneal bleeding, such as complaints of low back pain and muscle weakness or numbness in the lower extremities. Vital signs and laboratory test results should be monitored for evidence of hemorrhage, hypovolemia, or shock.

Disseminated Intravascular Coagulation (DIC)

This acquired coagulopathy always arises as a secondary complication of a wide variety of underlying patient conditions. Possible etiologies of DIC are listed in Table 42-1. No common factor for the conditions triggering DIC has been identified. DIC may occur after excessive platelet aggregation, from simulation of the extrinsic pathway by release of tissue thromboplastin, or through damage to the vascular endothelium causing intrinsic pathway activation.

The term *disseminated* refers to the involvement of all aspects of the coagulation process, not to coagulation throughout the body. Although DIC can occur as a generalized systemic process, it can also be localized. DIC may be chronic, as in some oncological disorders, or acute.[12] Critically ill patients most often exhibit an acute, generalized form of DIC.

DIC occurs when the normal coagulation cascade is overstimulated so that excessive thrombin circulates systemically, overwhelming the normal capability of antithrombins. Thrombin can activate fibrinogen, leading to deposition of fibrin in the microvasculature. Thrombin also initiates fibrinolysis by converting plasminogen into plasmin. Rapid clot formation depletes existing platelets and coagulation factors faster than these components of coagulation can be produced. Fibrinolysis releases fibrin degradation products (FDPs) from the clots; these anticoagulants are normally cleared by the reticuloendothelial system, but overproduction overwhelms the system. Circulating levels of these anticoagulant substances rise.

The inappropriate accelerated systemic stimulation of normal coagulation causes a paradoxical clinical situation: thrombosis of the microcirculation with concurrent hemorrhages from a variety of sites (Figure 42-1). Inappropriate microvascular clotting causes tissue ischemia that leads to infarction, and organ dysfunction. Depletion of coagulation factors together with active fibrinolysis prevents a stable hemostatic clot from forming after injury to the vasculature. The patient bleeds from both old and new sites.

The clinical presentation of DIC varies greatly, according to the underlying primary condition. Although the body system affected by thrombosis produces symptoms of organ failure, it is usually the symptoms of bleeding that stimulate an investigation

TABLE 42-1   Common Etiologies of Disseminated Intravascular Coagulation

Category	Associated Conditions
Shock	Septic, hypovolemic, cardiogenic
Infection	Gram-negative, gram-positive, viral, rickettsial, protozoal
Tissue trauma	Burns, crushing injury, surgical operations, extracorporeal circulation, acute hypoxia, heat stroke, snakebite
Obstetrical complications	Abruptio placentae, eclampsia, retained dead fetus, abortion, amniotic fluid embolus, placenta previa
Malignant disease	Leukemia; solid tumor of the prostate, pancreas, lung, colon, stomach, or breast
Immunological reactions	Incompatible transfusion, allograft rejection, immune complex disease
Cardiovascular crisis	Myocardial infarction, pulmonary embolism, dissecting aneurysm

and diagnosis of DIC. The location and extent of tissue damage and the severity of the bleeding determines the manifestation of symptoms.

An early sign is obvious bleeding or oozing from multiple sites such as the oral mucous membranes, vascular access sites, or surgical wounds. Even old puncture sites may begin to bleed. Petechiae, ecchymoses, or hematomas may form. Hematuria, hemoptysis, and gastrointestinal or intracranial bleeding can occur. A major hemorrhagic episode may take place causing the onset of hypovolemic shock.

Multisystem organ failure may result from the deposition of clots in the microcirculation. The patient may develop acute tubular necrosis when the kidneys are affected. Adult respiratory distress syndrome (ARDS) may occur secondary to the fibrin in the pulmonary capillary bed. When the gastrointestinal tract is affected, abdominal pain and diarrhea are seen. Changes in mental status, confusion, or seizures indicate central nervous system involvement.

The skin can be a most impressive visible example of thrombosis, reflecting the process that is occurring

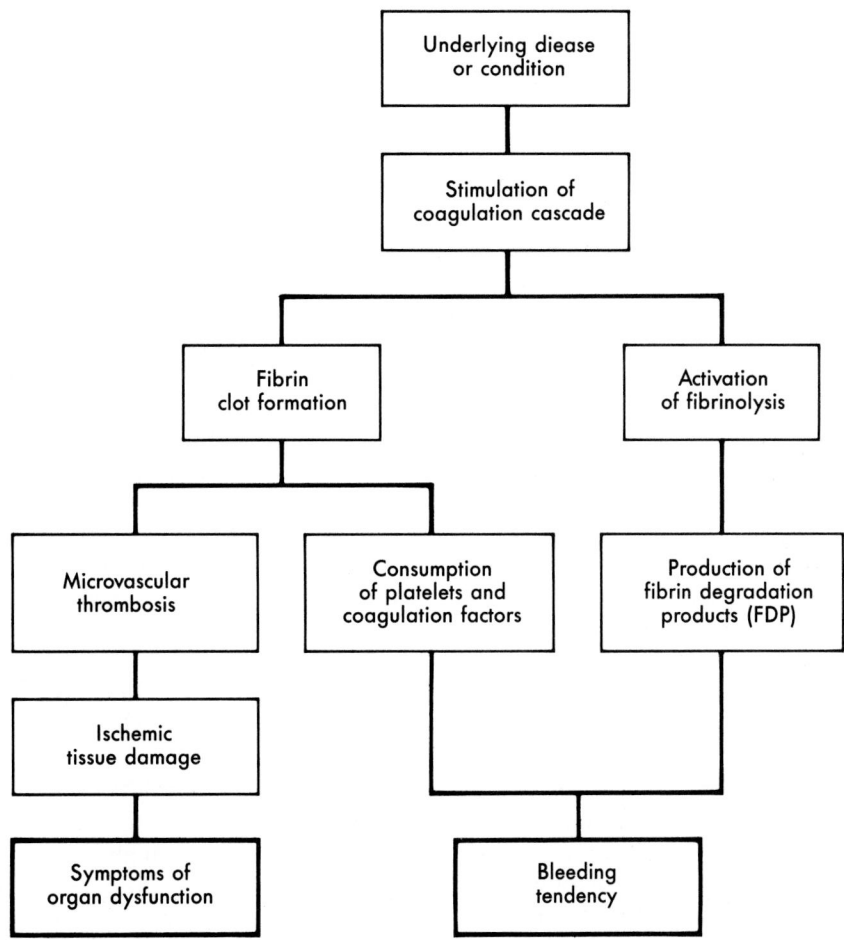

Figure 42-1   Pathophysiology of disseminated intravascular coagulation.

TABLE 42-2 **Laboratory Findings in DIC**

Platelet count	↓
PT	Prolonged
APTT	Prolonged
Thrombin time	Prolonged
Fibrinogen	Normal or ↓
Factor V	↓
Factor VIII	↓
Fibrin degradation products	↑
D-dimer	↑
Antithrombin III	↓
Schistocytes	Present

internally in other organs. Patients may develop gray to purple discoloration of the skin with sharp, irregular lines of demarcation on the toes, fingers, lips, nose, and ears. This acrocyanosis can progress to focal areas of gangrene.

Diagnosis of DIC is based on the clinical presentation and circumstances of the patient, rather than on laboratory data. No single test is diagnostic for DIC. If the patient has liver disease, it may be particularly difficult to make a diagnosis because of the liver's role in production of coagulation factors. Table 42-2 lists the laboratory findings seen in DIC.

A drop in platelet count is apparent in most cases of DIC as platelets are activated early in the clotting cascade. Fibrinogen is consumed by the coagulation process. Interpretation of the fibrinogen level must consider the magnitude of change in the level, as well as a comparison of the patient's value to normal. Some patients have an elevated fibrinogen level due to their underlying condition (pregnancy, sepsis, neoplasia). In these cases, a significant drop in a previously elevated fibrinogen level may signal the presence of DIC. As clotting factors are depleted, prolongation of the PT and APTT will be seen in addition to decreases in specific factor levels.

Excessive fibrinolysis increases the levels of fibrin split or degradation products. The D-dimer test is used to confirm an elevated FDP in DIC.[13] The level of antithrombin III is diminished because it binds the excessive thrombin in an attempt to block thrombin's effect on fibrinogen. Schistocytes appear on the peripheral blood smear when red blood cells are damaged by the fibrin obstructing the microcirculation.

Medical management of DIC is directed at the patient's underlying disease or condition. Once the primary problem is resolved, normal coagulation will be restored if the patient's liver and bone marrow are functional. If and until the underlying condition can be managed, the patient in DIC remains a medical management challenge.

Transfusion therapy is indicated to replace coagulation factors and blood loss due to hemorrhage. Packed RBCs and platelets are used to replace losses. Fresh frozen plasma provides all clotting factors and naturally occurring antithrombins and can contribute to volume replacement. Infusion of cryoprecipitate helps to replace fibrinogen and factor VIII. If vitamin K deficiency accompanies DIC, supplementation is needed so the liver can produce coagulation factors.

The use of heparin therapy in treating DIC remains controversial. Heparin is given in low doses for its ability to work with antithrombin III to neutralize circulating thrombin. Heparin can also serve as an anticoagulant to prevent further thrombosis in the microvasculature and prevent platelet aggregation. It will not dissolve existing clots, but by slowing additional coagulation, it buys time for the body to replenish its clotting factors. No randomized controlled studies have conclusively proven the efficacy of heparin in treating acute DIC. Heparin infusions are used in the management of chronic DIC when there is evidence that thrombosis is producing organ dysfunction. Use of low-dose heparin and replacement of antithrombin III is a newer speculative therapy in acute DIC.

Epsilon aminocaproic acid (EACA) is no longer recommended for the treatment of DIC.[12] The fibrinolytic inhibitor action of preventing lysis of the microthrombi and decreasing release of FDP also slows the clearance of the thrombi from the occluded capillaries. Serious complications of worsening thrombosis can occur from this drug.

Medical management of DIC must be individually adjusted to the underlying condition of the patient. It may include support of the cardiovascular system with hemodynamic monitoring, aggressive volume replacement, and inotropic support. The respiratory system must be supported to prevent hypoxia and acidosis. This may require intubation and mechanical ventilation. Medical interventions must be directed toward oxygen systems manifesting signs of dysfunction. Because DIC is a secondary complication associated with a serious primary problem, mortality is estimated at greater than 50% despite vigorous treatment.

Nursing Management in DIC

Critical care nurses must identify the high-risk patient and maintain a high level of suspicion for the development of DIC. Thorough, frequent assessments of the critically ill patient for detection of organ system dysfunction and covert bleeding are responsibilities of the nurse. Little can be done to prevent the onset of DIC, but early detection may improve patient outcome. Communication of abnormal findings to the physician facilitates medical intervention for the underlying cause.

The nursing care plan for the patient with a coagulopathy described on p. 992 is applicable to DIC. Because DIC is a secondary complication to an existing patient problem, many invasive therapies may have been instituted or proposed. Every nursing care activity must be reevaluated for its necessity and risk for trauma. Routine care of patients such as oral care, back rubs, and taking vital signs bring risks of bleeding to the patient with acute DIC. Nurses often take pride in maintaining a neat and clean patient. However, in DIC it is not safe to remove clotted blood and constant oozing saturated dressings, tapes, and bed linens. Families may also interpret the presence of blood on the patient or dressings as signs of inadequate care. The patient and family must receive information appropriate to their level of understanding about the nature of the bleeding problem and the need to modify routine care.

Thrombosis of the microcirculation causes pain. Depending on the degree and location of the thrombosis, pain may be localized or widespread. Medication ordered for pain should not be given by injection or suppository. The medication should not have known side effects that impair the normal coagulation process.

When acrocyanosis is present from thrombosis of the capillary bed in the skin, prevention of trauma to these areas is important. Although gangrene may occur, the nurse must attempt to maintain the integrity of the involved areas. Prevention of pressure on the affected areas is critical. Creative yet secure methods for stabilizing tubes that may be present in the patient's nose and mouth must be used. Separating the toes with lamb's wool and use of a bed cradle to keep bed linen pressure from the feet may be necessary. Pressure on the ears must be considered when turning and repositioning the patient.

DIC shock and multisystem organ dysfunction may combine to create a dismal outcome for the critically ill patient. The critical care nurse must support the patient and family in their decisions to continue aggressive therapy or to forego further interventions. Providing emotional support to the dying patient and their family and friends may be the ultimate form of nursing care provided to the patient with DIC.

REFERENCES

1. Keitt, A. S. (1988). Introduction to the anemias. In J. B. Wyngaarden, & L. H. Smith (Eds.), *Cecil textbook of medicine* (Vol. 1) (18th ed.). Philadelphia: Saunders.

2. American Association of Critical-Care Nurses (Eds.). (1990). *Outcome standards for nursing care of the critically ill.* Laguna Niguel, CA: AACN.

3. Marcus, A. J. (1988). Hemorrhagic disorders: Abnormalities of platelet and vascular function. In J. B. Wyngaarden, & L. H. Smith (Eds.), *Cecil textbook of medicine* (Vol. 1) (18th ed.). Philadelphia: Saunders.

4. Baldwin, D. R. (1989). Heparin-induced thrombocytopenia. *Journal of Intravenous Nursing, 12,* 378-382.

5. Dressler, D. K. (1989). Disseminated intravascular coagulation. In K. T. Von Rueden, & C. A. Walleck (Eds.), *Advanced critical care nursing: A case study approach.* Rockville, MD: Aspen.

6. McNally, J. C., Stair, J. C., & Sommerville, E. T. (Eds.). (1985). *Guidelines for cancer nursing practice.* New York: Grune & Stratton.

7. Shelton, B. K. (1990). Acquired coagulation disorders: Thrombocytopenia, DIC, and other problems. In K. Goldberg (Ed.), *Hematologic problems.* Springhouse, PA: Springhouse.

8. Mosher, D. F. (1988). Disorders of blood coagulation. In J. B. Wyngaarden, & L. H. Smith (Eds.), *Cecil textbook of medicine* (Vol. 1) (18th ed.). Philadelphia, Saunders.

9. Shelton, B. K. (1990). Congenital coagulation disorders. In K. Goldberg (Ed.), *Hematologic problems.* Springhouse, PA: Springhouse.

10. Bang, N. U. (1989). Diagnosis and management of bleeding disorders. In W. C. Shoemaker, S. Ayres, A. Grenvik, et al. (Eds.), *Textbook of critical care* (2nd ed.). Philadelphia: Saunders.

11. Kline, E. M. (1990). Pharmacologic review of thrombolytic agents. *Critical Care Nursing Clinics of North America, 2,* 613-626.

12. Bang, N. U. (1989). Diagnosis and management of thrombosis. In W. C. Shoemaker, S. Ayres, A. Grenvik, et al. (Eds.), *Textbook of critical care* (2nd ed.). Philadelphia: Saunders.

13. Bell, T. N. (1990). Disseminated intravascular coagulation and shock. *Critical Care Nursing Clinics of North America, 2,* 255-267.

PART TEN

Immunological Patient Care Problems

43

Immunological Anatomy and Physiology

Debra Tribett

The human body is constantly exposed to an environmental barrage of millions of microorganisms. The immune system provides a defense against this hostile external environment and protects against internal threats to the body's integrity. The body employs both natural defenses and acquired, adaptive defenses in its attempts to protect itself from harm. Natural defenses are nonspecific mechanisms either present at birth or developed in the course of maturation. If natural defenses allow a foreign substance to invade and subsist in the body, an acquired adaptive mechanism is called into action. This is the *immune response*, which, unlike natural defenses, specifically recognizes and destroys the foreign substance.

The anatomy of the immune system is diffuse, involving structures often attributed to other body systems. It consists of the white blood cells (lymphocytes), their chemical products, and the tissues and organs where they reside.

The functions of the immune system are designed to maintain and preserve the integrity of the biological self of the host. It identifies and destroys foreign invaders such as bacteria, viruses, or fungi. Additionally, it assists in the removal of damaged or senescent body cells by acting as a scavenger. A third action is the surveillance for cells that do not conform to the normal genetic code of the host and participation in their subsequent destruction.

Compared to what we know of other body systems, our knowledge of this complex system and its activities is very new and continually evolving. The immune system is being implicated as a major contributor to the pathophysiology of many problems that commonly occur in critically ill patients, such as sepsis, septic shock, adult respiratory distress syndrome (ARDS), and multisystem organ failure. A thorough understanding of the structure and function of the immune system is essential for critical care nurses because the treatment of many diseases has begun to include the therapeutic manipulation of the immune system.

CELLS OF THE IMMUNE SYSTEM
White Blood Cells (Leukocytes)

Leukocytes, or white blood cells (WBCs), are the mobile units of the body's immune system. These cells are produced in the bone marrow. They are larger than red blood cells (RBCs) and are less numerous. Normally, 5,000 to 10,000/mm³ of these cells are circulating within the vascular system, and many more are marginated along the walls of blood vessels and sequestered in other structures of the immune system.

The WBCs are grouped into two major categories based on their nucleus structure: granulocytes and nongranulocytes. Each group contains different cells with specialized functions. *Granulocytes,* also known as *polymorphonuclear leukocytes,* are divided into three cell types: neutrophils, eosinophils, and basophils. *Nongranulocytes,* or *mononuclear cells,* are the monocytes and lymphocytes (Figure 43-1).

Pluripotent stem cells of the bone marrow differentiate into two types of colony-forming units. The type called colony-forming unit—granulocyte, erythrocyte, macrophage, and megakaryocyte (CFU-GEMM) produces the granulocytes (neutrophils, eosinophils, and basophils). The type called colony-forming unit—lymphocyte (CFU-L) gives rise to monocytes and lymphocytes.

Colony-forming units for each line of specific cell types are stimulated by colony-stimulating factors (CSFs). These cell-derived glycoproteins stimulate blood cell production, maturation, and function. Specific CSFs act at different points during the differentiation of stem cells; their action on CFUs and pre-

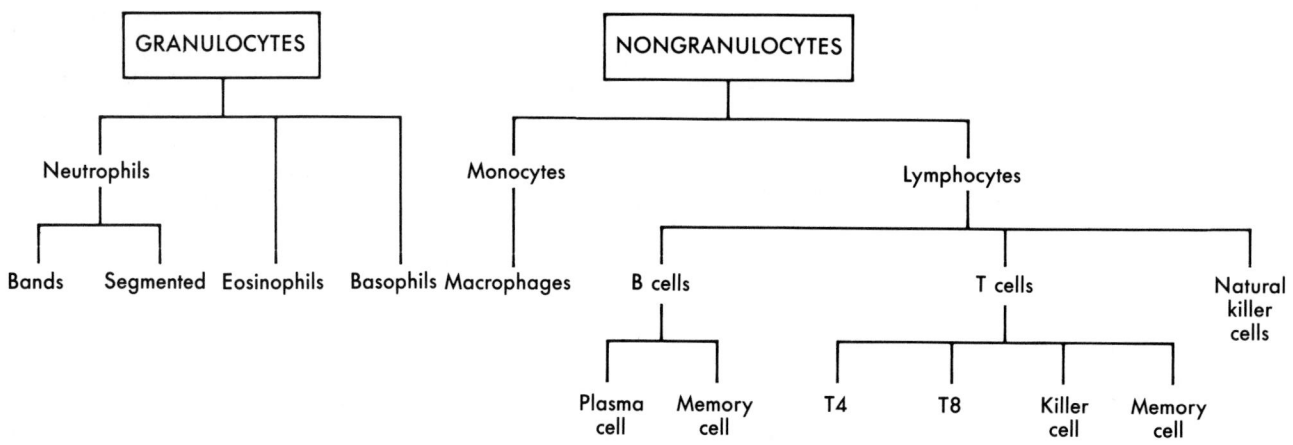

Figure 43-1   Types of leukocytes or white blood cells.

cursor cells overlaps. Identification of CSFs and the ability to produce recombinant forms have led to their clinical use in the stimulation of bone marrow cell production in situations of bone marrow disease or suppression.

Granulocytes

Neutrophils

Neutrophils are the most numerous of the granulocytes. They make up 60% to 70% of all WBCs in the peripheral blood of normal adults. These cells are the first to respond and the most numerous types of cells to arrive at the site of tissue injury or disease and function as a nonspecific phagocyte.

The neutrophil is produced in the bone marrow, where it matures before being released into the circulation. This process takes approximately 10 days. Neutrophils are subdivided into two categories based on the appearance of their nuclei. The mature, *segmented neutrophils*, or "segs," constitute the majority (56%) of circulating WBCs. Immature neutrophils, called bands, are normally 3% to 6% of WBCs.

Once released into the circulation, neutrophils can no longer replicate. Their circulating half-life is about 6 to 8 hours. They then leave the blood and travel to the tissues. Neutrophils do not recirculate to the bone marrow.

The process that draws the neutrophils to the tissue sites in need of their services is called *chemotaxis*. Inflammation and bacterial proliferation liberate serum chemicals called *chemotaxins* through a complex process thought to involve the activated complement system, lymphocytes, the neutrophils themselves, as well as bacteria and their products.

In the tissues, neutrophils seek out invading microorganisms (primarily bacteria) and damaged or senescent cells and destroy them through phagocytosis. During *phagocytosis*, a neutrophil engulfs, kills,

and digests the target cell. The neutrophil dies as a result of this process. Dead neutrophils contribute to the formation of pus.

The process of phagocytosis is complex and not fully known. Apparently, a mature neutrophil can destroy several bacteria before its cytoplasmic granules containing lysosomal enzymes are exhausted or it is overwhelmed by toxins produced during the process of phagocytosis. During phagocytosis, the neutrophil exhibits a *respiratory burst* of oxygen consumption in which superoxide, hydrogen peroxide, and hydroxyl radicals are produced. These substances are toxic to the target of the neutrophil but also to surrounding normal tissues. Investigators are exploring the association of neutrophil activation with host injury as a possible mechanism of pathophysiological conditions such as ARDS.

When the need for phagocytosis increases, the bone marrow is stimulated to release increased numbers of neutrophils into the blood, a condition called *neutrophilia*. The increased demand for neutrophils causes the release of immature bands into the circulation, increasing the percentage of this form of neutrophil in the circulation. Neutrophilia occurs in association with any activity or process that increases the level of epinephrine, ACTH, or adrenal corticoids in the bloodstream. Such diverse conditions as foreign protein injection, excessive exercise, blood loss, and excessive fatigue all lead to neutrophilia. The increased capillary blood flow resulting from the vasodilating effects of epinephrine flushes out sequestered leukocytes and mobilizes them to the defense of insulated body tissue. Conditions that increase cardiac output, such as hyperthyroidism, may also lead to neutrophilia.

An insufficiency of neutrophils in the blood is referred to as *neutropenia*. This state places the individual at risk for the development of infection, particularly from bacteria. The risk is greatest when the total neutrophil count is below 1,000/mm³. Neutropenia is associated with pathological conditions of hematological malignancy, aplastic anemia, and treatment with cytotoxic drug regimens. Even though infected, the neutropenic patient may lack evidence of pus at an infected site due to the lack of neutrophils to participate in phagocytosis.

Eosinophils

Eosinophils mature in the bone marrow for 3 to 6 days before they are released into the circulation. They have a circulating half-life of about 30 minutes, before migrating to the tissues. Like neutrophils, they do not recirculate to the bone marrow; however, their tissue half-life is 12 days. The mucosal surfaces of the respiratory and gastrointestinal tracts contain large numbers of eosinophils, which are eliminated from the body through these surfaces.

The mature eosinophil constitutes 1% to 4% of the total number of leukocytes in the normal adult. Although physically larger than neutrophils, eosinophils are weaker in their phagocytic activity. Their specific function is not certain. They do participate in the ingestion of immune complexes and possibly the inactivation of mediators of acute allergic responses. The granules in their cytoplasm contain substances toxic to parasites, so they participate in the body's defense against this type of organism.

An elevated level of eosinophils, or *eosinophilia*, is seen during an allergic response. Increased numbers of eosinophils migrate to the cells at the site of allergic inflammation. The gastrointestinal and respiratory mucosa are common entry points for foreign protein substances; the normal presence of eosinophils in these areas suggests that they defend against invasion at these sites.

Basophils

Fewer than 1% of circulating leukocytes are basophils. These cells have no phagocytic activity. Little is known about their formation or distribution. Basophils have been likened to mast cells, which are fixed cells located near capillary beds. Both types of cells degranulate during acute allergic reactions, releasing heparin, histamine, serotonin, and bradykinin into the bloodstream.

Nongranulocytes

Monocytes

The largest of the nongranular leukocytes are the monocytes, which comprise 2% to 6% of the total circulating WBCs. After release from the bone marrow, monocytes circulate for 1 to 2 days. They migrate to tissues throughout the body and mature into

macrophages. Unlike the granulocytes, macrophages can divide. Monocytes in the lungs are called *alveolar macrophages;* those in the liver are called *Kupffer cells:* in the spleen, lymph nodes, or peritoneum they are called macrophages. These tissue macrophages form the basis of the reticuloendothelial defense system. They are involved in the removal of damaged or senescent cells, cellular debris, and in the removal of abnormal or tumor cells. Macrophages may live for months to years unless they are destroyed in the phagocytic process.[1]

Macrophages are capable of phagocytizing large foreign particles and cell fragments. They can ingest larger particles and five times as many particles as neutrophils. An important function of the macrophage is to phagocytize necrotic tissue in chronic infections. These phagocytes contain substances that are bactericidal; that is, they are capable of destroying bacteria before they can multiply and destroy the phagocyte. Macrophages are second (after neutrophils) to respond to an area of inflammation and respond in lesser numbers. These phagocytes are consumed in the process of clearing cellular debris and, like neutrophils, contribute to the formation of pus.

Macrophages participate in the nonspecific removal of invading nonself microorganisms. During this phagocytosis, the macrophage identifies the invader as nonself, processes it, and presents the invading microorganism to the T4 helper lymphocyte. This initiates a specific immune response by the lymphocytes to aid in the destruction of the invader and future protection of the body.

The macrophage produces and releases chemical substances called *cytokines* that communicate with other cells of the immune system and modulate body responses to microorganisms. Interleukin-1 (IL-1) is one of the cytokines produced. It is a known *pyrogen*, leading to the development of fever. When processing viruses, the macrophages produce interferon. These and other cytokines are discussed at length later in this chapter.

Lymphocytes

The lymphocytes are produced in the bone marrow and travel to other parts of the body for differentiation and maturation into distinct subsets of cells responsible for the specific immune response of the body. Together all lymphocytes comprise 20% to 35% of the total WBC count. Lymphocytes follow a recirculating pathway between the blood, lymph, lymph nodes, and the bone marrow (Figure 43-2). Recirculating lymphocytes "patrol" or survey the entire body for invading antigens, but most of their work is performed in the peripheral tissues where most of them reside. Lymphocyte subsets include B

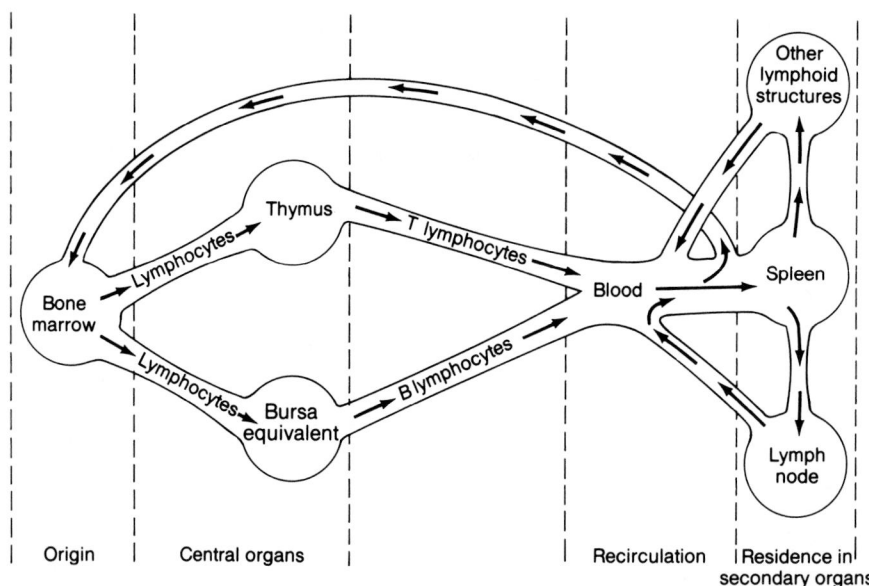

Figure 43-2 Lymphocyte developments and circulation patterns.

cells, T cells, and natural killer (NK) cells. Lymphocytes participating in the immune response replicate themselves into clones specific to the microorganism invading the host.

B Cells (B Lymphocytes). Between 10% and 15% of the total lymphocyte count are B cells. B cells in humans are thought to mature in the bone marrow. Other species have a bursa tissue that performs this function. After leaving the bone marrow, the B cells migrate preferentially to the spleen. The life expectancy of a B cell is about 16 days.[2]

The B cells are responsible for *humoral immunity*. Their major function is to produce antibodies, or *immunoglobulins* (Ig). Each B cell has a genetic specificity for one type of invading antigen and will react to the antigen by producing antibody against it. Production of antibody mediates humoral immunity. This immune response protects the host primarily against infection by bacteria and viral invasion. Humoral immunity can be transferred by plasma to another host.

The B cell must differentiate into a plasma cell before it is capable of producing Ig. The plasma cell becomes an Ig factory with the ability to produce Ig of different types or categories. Plasma cells remain fixed in reticuloendothelial organs. Some B cells exposed to antigens develop into *memory B cells* which store information about the initial antigen–antibody reaction. During subsequent exposure to the same antigen, memory B cells can initiate a rapid protective antibody response by the host.

The chemical structure of an immunoglobin molecule consists of two heavy chains and two light

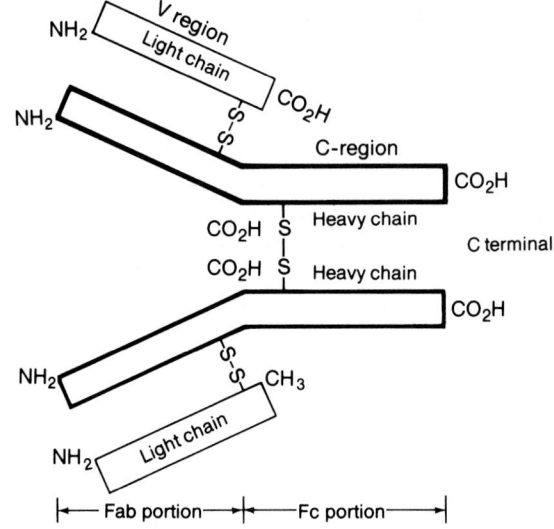

Figure 43-3 Structure of immunoglobin. The Fab portion is variable and confers specificity for antigen attachment. The Fc portion is constant.

chains held together by disulfide bonds in a Y-shaped structure. The Y portion of the molecule, a highly variable sequence of amino acids called the *Fab portion*, confers specificity for antigen binding. The other end of the molecule is constant and is called the *Fc portion*. The Fc portion will attach to any cell with an Fc receptor (Figure 43-3). Antibodies (Ig) bind specifically to the antigen that promoted their synthesis, forming an *antigen–antibody complex* that can then be destroyed by phagocytosis.

The Fc end of the Ig molecule has a fixed sequence of amino acids that remains constant within a category of antibody. The plasma cell produces five different categories of antibody: IgM, IgG, IgA, IgE, and IgD. Each category has its own specific functions and characteristics (Table 43-1).

T Cells (T Lymphocytes). The majority (80%) of lymphocytes are T cells. After production in the bone marrow, T cells travel to the thymus gland where they are differentiated into distinct subsets. These subset cells emerge and migrate to peripheral lymphoid tissue. T cells lie in wait for exposure to foreign substances and participate in the circulating pool of white blood cells. T cells are responsible for the cell-mediated immunity of the body. *Cell-mediated immunity* protects the host from intracellular organisms such as viruses, fungi, and parasites, and it inhibits the development of abnormal (tumor) cells. In patients undergoing organ transplantation, cellular immunity causes graft rejection.

Subsets of T cells may be identified by their different *surface proteins*, or *markers*, that allow for the different functions of the cells. Following exposure to an antigen, the T cell is activated: it enlarges proliferates into one of four subsets of T lymphocyte: T4 or helper/inducer cells, T8 or suppressor cells, cytotoxic T cells, and memory T cells. Normally, there are twice as many T4 cells as T8 cells.

T lymphocytes induce other components of the immune response. They are cytotoxic through their production of *lymphokines*, which are cytokines produced by lymphocytes. The release of lymphokines also modulates the activity of the immune system to activate or suppress the specific immune response.

Natural Killer Cells. A third type of lymphocyte that is neither a T cell nor a B cell comprises 5% to 10% of the total number of lymphocytes. These large granular lymphocytes, or natural killer (NK) cells, are cytotoxic. These cells function nonspecifically, without prior sensitization; tumor cells and cells infected by viruses are their targets. The NK cells appear to have no memory function.[3] Natural killer cells are currently under investigation as a potential therapy for some types of cancer. NK cells that have been incubated with the lymphokine interleukin-2 for this purpose are called *lymphokine-activated killer cells,* or *LAK cells.*

Cytokines

Cytokines are protein substances produced predominantly by the monocytes or macrophages and the T cells. However, they are also produced by diverse tissue at many sites throughout the body. They are somewhat like hormones but are chemically active at much lower concentrations. Cytokines provide a chemical communication system between the cells of the immune system to modulate the inflammatory and immune responses in the body. These chemical mediators are important to normal homeostasis and to the body's response to injury.

At one time, these chemical mediators were assigned several names on the basis of origin. Those produced by monocytes were called monokines. Those produced by lymphocytes were called lymphokines. As knowledge about the immune system grew, it became evident that production and function of these substances overlapped. The term *cytokine* refers to this entire category of mediator proteins. Table 43-2 summarizes the cytokines, their origin, and their predominant functions.

Cytokines are being very actively studied. Some are believed to have potentially helpful effects in compromised immune function or cancer. Other studies are exploring cytokines to identify mediators responsible for such common critical care problems as septic shock and multisystem organ failure. Further discussion of cytokines is included in the section of this chapter pertaining to specific immune responses.

TABLE 43-1 **Classes and Characteristics of Immunoglobins (Antibodies)**

Class	Characteristics
IgM	First immunoglobin produced after exposure to a new antigen (primary response)
	Fixes complement
	Present in serum
IgG	Produced after repeated exposure to antigen (secondary response)
	Mediates agglutination and opsonization of antigens
	Major constituent of commercial immunoglobins
	Present in serum and intercellular fluids
	Only immunoglobulin transferred across the placenta
IgA	Provides body surface protection by preventing surface attachment of organisms
	Major component of secretions: saliva, tears, bronchial, intestinal, breast milk
	Transported across mucous membrane with secretions
IgE	Provides subsurface protection
	Mediates immediate hypersensitivity (anaphylactic) reactions
	Elevated in allergic and certain parasitic diseases
	Present in serum and intercellular fluids
IgD	Function unknown at this time
	Found on the surface of B lymphocytes; may act as a receptor
	Not detected in the serum

TABLE 43-2   Cytokines

Name	Source	Principal Action/Effect
Interleukin-1 (IL-1)	Monocytes	Induces fever
	Macrophages	Activates T4 cells
	Neutrophils	Enhances T cell proliferation
	B lymphocytes	Stimulates bone marrow to release granulocytes
	Endothelial cells	Stimulates myelopoiesis via colony-stimulating factors
Interleukin-2 (IL-2)	Activated T4 cells	Immunostimulant
		Enhances T4 proliferation and differentiation
		Stimulates T8 proliferation
		Augments NK cell function
Interleukin-3 (IL-3)	Activated T4 cells	Stimulates all classes of myeloid precursors
Interleukin-4 (IL-4)*	Activated T4 cells	Differentiates B cells into plasma cells
Interleukin-6 (IL-6)†	Activated T4 cells	B cell proliferation
		Induces fever
Macrophage chemotactic factor (MCF)		
Macrophage inhibition factor (MIF)		
Macrophage activation factor (MAF)	T4 cell	Enhance/induce phagocytosis
Leukocyte chemotactic factor (LCF)		
α-Interferon	Monocytes	Defense against viruses
		Prevents tumor growth
		Augments NK function
γ-Interferon	T cells	Enhances cytotoxicity
	NK cells	Induces T cell growth, differentiation, and function
		Augments NK function
		Activates macrophages
Granulocyte macrophage colony-stimulating factor (GM-CSF)	T cells	Stimulates production of granulocytes and macrophages
	Macrophages	
	Endothelial cells	
Granulocyte colony-stimulating factor (G-CSF)	Monocytes	Stimulates production of granulocytes
	Fibroblasts	Enhances neutrophil function
Tumor necrosis factor (TNF)	Monocytes	Induces fever
	Macrophages	Enhances tumor destruction
		Causes anorexia
		Effects metabolism and can lead to cachexia
		Modulates immune function
		Activates neutrophils and macrophages

* Previously called B cell differentiation factor (BCDF).
† Previously called B cell growth factor (BCGF).

THE LYMPHORETICULAR (RETICULOENDOTHELIAL) SYSTEM

After being produced by the bone marrow, the cells of the immune system travel throughout the body in the blood. They leave the blood vessels through the endothelial junctions. In the interstitial spaces, they travel through the lymphatic vessels to the sites of inflammation or infection, or they reside in the lymphoreticular tissues until called upon as part of the body's defense system.

The term *defense system* designates collectively all organs, tissues cells, and functions that aid in maintaining a healthy body free from nonself organisms or molecules (Figure 43-4). The *lymphoreticular system* consists of all the cells and structures of the body's defense system associated with recognition of, response to, and memory of antigens. It extends throughout the body to cover all possible surfaces, routes, and avenues of possible attack by foreign agents. Included are lymphoid tissue, lymphatic cells,

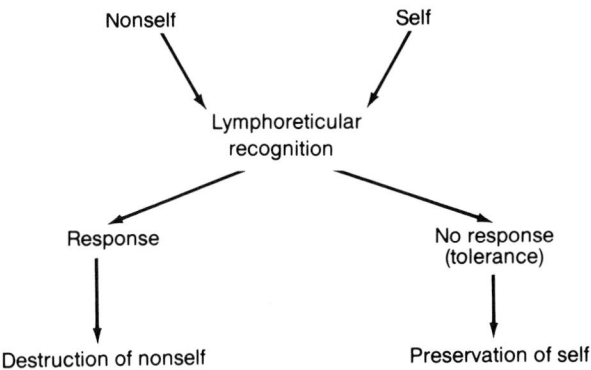

Figure 43-4 Preservation of the self by the lymphoreticular system.

and a network of phagocytic cells within the lymphatic system and other organs. Understanding of this system grew out of an earlier concept called the reticuloendothelial system, thought to consist mainly of a group of organs whose vascular sinuses were lined with phagocytic cells.

Thymus Gland

The thymus gland is an encapsulated, bilobate structure located in the anterior superior mediastinum immediately beneath the sternum. Most lymphoid structures are strategically located in the body to come into contact with foreign substances, but the location of the thymus protects it from such direct exposure. The thymus grows until puberty, after which it involutes into a small fatty structure that persists throughout adult life.

The main function of the thymus is the maturation and differentiation of the T cells. The thymus produces a hormone called *thymosin* that influences lymphopoiesis and the maturation and differentiation of the T cell subsets. The thymus seeds other lymphoid tissue as the T cells migrate to the peripheral structures.

Spleen

The spleen is a peripheral lymphoid organ located in the peritoneum and surrounded by a muscular fibrous capsule. It is filled with reticular connective tissue and venous sinuses lined with phagocytic cells. Portions of the reticular tissue are packed with lymphocytes called *white pulp*. The venous sinusoid areas are filled with blood instead of lymph and are collectively called the *red pulp*. The spleen is the largest lymphoid organ in the body.

During the circulation of blood, the spleen filters the blood to clear it of foreign material, dead or senescent cells, and debris. The spleen separates plasma from blood cells and stores the cells and platelets in the red pulp. The role of the spleen and its importance to the hematopoietic system is discussed in Chapter

40. The white pulp is a germinal center and important source for lymphocytes and plasma cells. It also helps to mediate immunological responses.

Immunologically, the spleen has a great capacity to clear the blood of foreign molecules (antigens), which it recognizes, traps, and processes. Resident T cells and B cells are activated to proliferate, differentiate, and destroy the antigen by producing antibodies and effector cells specific to it.

The spleen is an abdominal organ that may be injured by blunt trauma, necessitating splenectomy. It is not essential for life and may be removed. Other lymphoid organs can and usually do assume the functions of the spleen in its absence. However, survivors are at risk for overwhelming bacterial infection. This is particularly true for infants, children, and young adults.[4]

Liver

Among its many functions, the liver serves as a lymphoreticular organ. The blood returning from the small intestine (including absorbed nutrients and vitamins) is delivered to the liver via the portal vein. The blood then percolates through the sinusoids of the liver, which are lined with fixed macrophages called *Kupffer cells*. The Kupffer cells make up 60% of the reticuloendothelial cells of the body.[5]

The liver is an important phagocytic organ. It receives antigens from the intestine via the portal circulation and systemic antigens from the celiac artery. Hepatic phagocytes filter bacterial, food, or intestinal antigens and senescent RBCs and foreign matter from the circulation. The phagocytic Kupffer cells lining the sinusoids of the liver are so effective that virtually no bacteria reach the systemic circulation.[6] Immune complexes and endotoxin from the cell walls of gram-negative organisms are also cleared from the portal and systemic circulation by the liver.

Loss of phagocytic liver function may occur secondary to hepatic disease. The impaired filtration and phagocytic activity of the diseased liver allow immune complexes to accumulate, which may lead to immune complex disease. Blood levels of bacteria and endotoxin become elevated in liver disease.

Hepatic failure may lead to the development of portal hypertension. Obstruction of blood flow from the gut by the liver leads to splenic enlargement (splenomegaly) and overactivity (hypersplenism). In this condition, the spleen prematurely accelerates the destruction of all circulating blood cells. The resultant loss of WBCs contributes to an increased susceptibility to infection. Surgical shunting procedures may be performed to decrease the portal hypertension by redirecting blood flow from the intestine to bypass the liver. Although this surgery may reduce portal hypertension, effective filtration of the blood is lost because the blood returns to the systemic circulation without benefit of the hepatic phagocytosis. Patients surviving these shunting procedures are susceptible to bacterial infection.[6]

The liver is also the site where some of the immunologically active serum proteins called complement are synthesized. In liver disease, the production of these proteins diminishes, further impairing immune system function.

Complement

Collectively, *complement* is a group of 20 nonspecific noncellular proteins circulating in the blood in an inactive form. These proteins interact in a *cascade reaction* to enhance the immune process. Each protein activates the next in a step-wise sequence. The individual component is inactive until activated by the enzyme preceding it in the cascade. Complement activation, or fixation, generates enzymes that cause cell lysis of the invading organism. The proteins activated at different stages during the cascade reaction act as mediators of the inflammatory response, augmenting the immune system by enhancing phagocytosis.

The classic pathway for complement fixation is triggered when complement C1 encounters an antigen linked with an IgG or IgM antibody. This antigen–antibody complex guides the complement to attack the complex rather than other cells. As the cascade reaction continues, complements C5 through C9 are activated. They form a needlelike tube configuration that punctures the cell membrane of their target.[7] The internal cellular components leak out, causing lysis of the cell. Complement may also be activated by an alternate pathway: plasmin and proteases released by damaged cells or microorganisms during the inflammatory process can fix complement. The uncontrolled activation of complement is limited by the changing properties of the binding sites of the activated proteins and by the presence of other serum proteins that modulate and limit activity of the complement system.

Individual complement fragments produced during complement activation have been studied, and certain properties have been identified. Fragments C3a and C5a can stimulate the release of histamine and increase vascular permeability. C5a has been proposed as one of the mediators for the process of septic shock. A relationship has been demonstrated between increased levels of C5a and the reduced systemic vascular resistance seen in patients with septic shock.[8]

Lymphatic System

The system of lymph nodes, lymphatic vessels, and lymph is collectively called the *lymphatic system*. This system drains the interstitial spaces of the body. During the drainage process, the fluid is filtered and cleansed. The lymphatic system stores cells of the immune system until they are needed to attack foreign substances that have escaped other levels of defense.

Lymphatic capillaries arise in the interstitial spaces and drain fluid, protein, WBCs, and particulate matter from the tissues. The lymphatic fluid reflects a combination of these substances and the condition of the tissues from which it drains. Lymphatic vessels parallel the venous system and eventually drain into two large lymphatic ducts: the thoracic duct and the right lymphatic duct. These ducts drain into the central venous system at the junctions of the internal jugular and subclavian veins.

Lymph nodes are small, bean-shaped, encapsulated structures occurring in varying amounts throughout the body along the path of the lymphatic vessels. They frequently occur in groups or chains at the junctions of lymph vessels. They are multichanneled structures that receive lymph, percolate it through their internal sinuses, and return it to efferent lymphatic vessels.

While the lymph passes through the node it is exposed to a large supply of phagocytes and lymphocytes stored within the node. The WBCs come to the nodes through the lymphatic vessels and their vascular supply and are produced within the node when an immune response is triggered. White blood cells are able to process foreign substances and trap them within the node. Lymph nodes become enlarged and tender when they are actively involved in the immune response as lymphocytes proliferate in the nodes.

Other lymphoid tissues, or *nodules,* are present in the body. These tissues lack a connective-tissue capsule and are structured differently from a lymph node. Lymphoid tissue is strategically located in the submucosa of the respiratory, gastrointestinal, and genitourinary tracts close to potential sites of invasion by foreign substances. The tonsils at the opening of the respiratory–gastrointestinal tracts and Peyer's patches in the intestine are examples of this type of protective lymphoid tissue. Phagocytes and lymphocytes present within lymphoid tissue allow it to respond in both nonspecific and specific immune activity. Immunoglobins of the IgA and IgE categories are synthesized by lymphoid cells of the nodules, enhancing the protection of the mucosal surfaces against external environment pathogens.

CONCEPT OF HUMAN DEFENSE
Recognition of Self

Differences between individuals within a species, as well as those between species, start at the level of molecular structure. An individual's particular structure of proteins and other body materials is specified during genetic transcription of DNA. Although the proteins of one body within a species are similar in structure to those of all bodies of that species, there are small differences in composition and shape which give uniqueness to each individual. This uniqueness is what is meant by *biological self.*

The cells of the body's immune system work together to maintain the integrity of the biological self, or self. *Self* is determined genetically and is defined as anything synthesized by a person's own particular genetic blueprint or DNA code. In humans, a portion of chromosome 6 contains a group of genes that determine the *major histocompatibility (MHC) antigens* of the individual. These self antigens are called *human leukocyte antigens (HLA)* because they were first discovered on white blood cells. The self, or HLA, antigens appear on the surface of nucleated cells. Each individual inherits one set of self antigens from each parent in accordance with mendelian laws. Identical twins have an identical set of HLA antigens, whereas siblings or close relatives share some but not all of these antigens.

Under the auspices of the World Health Organization (WHO), the HLA Nomenclature Committee oversees periodic updates in nomenclature of the HLA system. The HLA complex has five genetic loci that are officially recognized. A *locus* is the position on the chromosome where a gene is found. These specific regions are designated HLA-A, HLA-B, HLA-C, HLA-D, and HLA-DR. Many different HLA antigens have been identified in these regions or categories.

The HLA antigens are further divided into two classes based on their tissue distribution and function of the antigens. *Class I antigens* are the HLA-A, HLA-B, and HLA-C antigens. They are found on virtually every human cell. Class I antigens serve as determinants for immune recognition of self. Class I antigens are those recognized by the host during a graft rejection. Class II antigens are the HLA-D and HLA-DR antigens. They are present only on the surfaces of immunocompetent cells. Monocytes/macrophages and B cells have class II antigens. These antigens act as communication receptors in the initiation and regulation of the immune response.

The HLA antigens were originally identified as antigens that evoked rejection of transplanted organs. They are now recognized as important in regulation of the immune response, as well as conferring resistance or susceptibility to a growing list of diseases.

Recognition of Nonself

The term *nonself* is used to describe that which is specified by a different set of chromosomes. Exogenous material such as microorganisms or transplanted cells or tissues is given its structure by an alien genetic code. Nonself substances are called "foreign" or "alien." Both self and nonself substances may carry antigens on their surfaces, but only nonself material evokes an immune response. An *antigen* can be defined as any substance with the ability to produce an immune response when introduced into the human body.[9]

Antigens are usually large molecules with a molecular weight of greater than 10,000. Smaller molecules are not ordinarily antigenic, but they may attach themselves to a naturally occurring body protein and thereby create a larger complex that will provoke an immune response. In this situation, the small molecule is called a *hapten,* the body protein is a carrier molecule, and the complex formed by the two together an antigen. Many drugs are haptens that in some people bring about an allergic response by the immune system.

Endogenous (self) material may become antigenic if there is a subtle error or change in its genetic code. Mutation of the genetic code or a physical change of its structure can cause native tissue to be perceived as foreign by the immune system. Still another situation of endogenous material becoming an antigen occurs when the native material is in an abnormal, or ectopic, location. The immune system may treat the molecules that are out of place as foreign.

NATURAL DEFENSES

Natural defense involves epithelial surface functions, inflammation, and nonspecific phagocytosis. These natural functions include preventing a nonself molecule from violating the human body or from destroying it. If a molecule gains entrance, it is quickly contained, destroyed, and removed by means of a vascular response (inflammation) and nonspecific phagocytosis. A cellular response then repairs any damage the invader may have caused. No specificity or memory is required, and therefore, no immunity follows.

Epithelial Surfaces: The First Line of Defense

The first concern in defense is to maintain the integrity of the body surfaces, which include: the skin; the oral, gastrointestinal, respiratory, and genitourinary epithelium; the lining of the external ear; and the conjunctivae and cornea of the eye. These epithelial surfaces prevent penetration by their anatomical structure as well as by their chemical secretions. Although all are epithelial in nature, their type and function vary from region to region. Table 43-3 summarizes the epithelial defense mechanisms. Investigators now recognize that epithelial cells have receptors for the attachment of certain antigenic determinants, thereby helping to maintain normal flora. The existence of these receptors explains the preferential

TABLE 43-3 Epithelial Barriers: The First Line of Defense

System	Defense Mechanisms
Skin	Protective barrier when intact
	Acid pH
	Exfoliation of outer surface
	Bacterial interference action of normal flora
	Sweat and sebaceous secretions
	Secretory IgA
Respiratory	Filtration by nasal hair and turbinates
	Escalatory flow of mucus by mucociliary membrane
	Sneeze, cough, and gag reflexes
	Secretory IgA
	Bacterial interference action of normal oral flora
	Lymphoid tissue (tonsils and adenoids)
	Alveolar macrophages
Gastrointestinal	Salivary secretions (lysozymes and secretory IgA)
	Acid pH of gastric secretions
	Mucosal epithelium when intact
	Bacterial interference of normal intestinal flora
	Lymphoid tissue (Peyer's patches)
	Intestinal motility and evacuation
Genitourinary	Flushing of urine
	Acid pH of urine
	Mucosal secretions, secretory IgA
	Phagocytic bladder mucosal cells
	Males: prostatic fluid
	Females: pH of vaginal secretions and bacterial interference of normal vaginal flora
Eyes	Cornea and conjunctivae when intact
	Flushing action of tears
	Lysozymes in tears
	Blink reflex
Ears	Lining of ear when intact
	Hairs in external auditory meatus
	Cerumen production

attachment of the normal flora of the skin and mucous membranes.

Many pathogens initiate infection by attaching to a receptor on an epithelial cell. The virulence of an infection may be determined by the organism's ability to attach to such a receptor, that is, its binding capacity. The host epithelium defends against pathogen binding by a number of nonspecific mechanisms, including pH, motility, the flow of mucus and other secretions, the movement of cilia, desquamation, and the preferential occupation of receptor sites by normal endogenous flora. It is now thought that the antibody

secretory IgA, present in most exocrine secretions and produced by local submucosal plasma cells, enhances these nonspecific activities by binding to antigens and, thereby, preventing their attachment to epithelial surfaces.

Skin and Its Appendages

The epidermal layer of skin is a stratified squamous epithelium with an acidic pH of about 5. It is dry; it constantly exfoliates its outer surface; and it continually regenerates its basal cell layer. Exfoliation will ultimately slough any bacteria or chemicals that penetrate the outer layers of intact skin. The normal flora that can exist in this acidic, dry, lipid environment are mainly staphylococci, corynebacteria, and propionibacteria. These particular organisms make survival of other microbes difficult by producing bacteriocidal fatty acids from the lipids of the skin. Mechanisms such as these keep the size of the inoculum of invading agents at a low level, and consequently other body defenses can destroy alien agents promptly when injury or a break in the epithelium occurs. However, these protective surface organisms can be dangerous to the body if they are introduced into the blood, as may occur during placement of an invasive vascular catheter.

Sweat glands, sebaceous (oil) glands, and mammary glands produce secretions whose flow, osmolality, pH, cellular components, and IgA protect against infection. Mammary secretions after childbirth contain many chemical and cellular components that not only defend the infant against infections and allergic reactions but also contribute to the maturation of the infant's intestinal mucosa and the immune system. This is a host defense maturation mechanism.

Respiratory Epithelium

The anatomical structure of the respiratory tract and its epithelium is crucial to maintaining healthy respiratory function. The ciliated, mucus-secreting epithelium lining the nose, sinuses, larynx, and trachea warm, moisturize, and cleanse the air before it reaches the functional level of the alveolar spaces where gas exchange occurs. The bony structure of the nasal cavity, with its turbinates (conchae), controls the flow patterns of air so that it swirls and deposits dust particles, microorganisms, or other foreign substances on the mucoid ciliated epithelium. They adhere to the mucus and are transported to the exterior of the body by ciliary movement.

The respiratory tract is usually sterile below the larynx. Ciliated simple columnar epithelium lines this area. Progressing toward the interior of the lung, the epithelium changes gradually to cuboidal and finally to squamous within the alveoli. Mucus is not secreted below the bronchioles. Cilia become progressively fewer from the trachea to the bronchioles and are not found in the alveolar areas. Mucociliary transport of inhaled particles toward the oropharynx, together with coughing and sneezing, helps to eliminate organisms from these areas. Deep breathing and proper coughing help prevent infection in a similar manner. Small quantities of microorganisms are usually aspirated during sleep but are physically removed by ciliary action. Phagocytosis by alveolar macrophages removes any remaining microorganisms that penetrate deep into the respiratory tract.

Gastrointestinal Mucosa

The oropharynx is lined with a squamous stratified epithelium that is similar anatomically to skin, but it does not produce keratin. Epithelial glands, which include the parotid, sublingual, and submandibular glands, produce saliva. This secretion contains water, lysozyme, mucus, secretory IgA, enzymes, and cells. Collectively these substances keep bacterial quantity in the mouth to a minimum and create a fluid flow that makes it difficult for chemical and foreign agents to be absorbed. The lining changes from squamous to cuboidal to columnar as it descends from the oral cavity to the esophagus to the stomach.

The epiglottis provides a structural barrier during the act of swallowing to protect the opening of the lower airway, thereby channeling secretions and food into the esophagus for passage into the stomach. The gastric mucosa produces hydrochloric acid, gastric juice, and mucus. Most microorganisms cannot survive the low pH of the gastric contents. The intestinal mucosa is lined with simple columnar epithelium and produces many intestinal fluids, enzymes, and hormones as well as secretory IgA, mucus, and other products.

The intestine has a large population of symbiotic bacteria that facilitate vital digestive assimilative functions and also compete with pathogenic organisms for epithelial receptors. Enteric bacteria consist of gram-negative species such as *Escherichia coli*, anaerobic bacteria, and *Clostridia*. Although helpful to the body when contained within the intestine, these organisms become potentially lethal if translocated into the blood during shock or spilled into the peritoneal cavity following intestinal trauma or surgery. Specific regional features, together with the epithelial receptor attachment of normal flora, normal peristaltic motility, and exfoliation, help eliminate millions of foreign agents daily by defecation.

Genitourinary Mucosa

Gender differences in anatomy exemplify the role of structure in susceptibility to infection by microorganisms. The male urethra is long and serves both the urinary and reproductive systems. Seminal fluid and urine maintain adequate flow through the system and add secretions that inhibit the survival of foreign substances. Prostatic secretions are antibacterial in much the same way as other glandular secretions. Infection of the bladder is rare in the male, even when the system is partially obstructed—unless catheterization has occurred. The female, in contrast, has a short urethra that serves only the urinary system. Bladder infections are more common in women than in men.

The urinary tracts of both sexes are lined with transitional epithelium which is capable of secreting mucus, lysozymes, secretory IgA, and other antimicrobial and antiviral substances. The peristaltic motility of the ureter, the acidity of the urine, and the reflexes of the bladder creating a unidirectional flow eliminate many microorganisms daily in the urine. The reproductive system of the female is defended by the acidity of its epithelial barrier as well as by its secretions.

Epithelium is an effective barrier between the body's internal and external environments. When epithelium is healthy, few microorganisms are able to reach the internal environment. Intact neurological reflexes such as cough, swallow, and blink assist the epithelial surfaces in mobilizing their protective secretions. Only when this first line of defense fails is there a need for others. (See Figure 43-5.)

Nonspecific Responses: The Second Line of Defense

If the first line of defense fails and foreign substances penetrate body tissues, an inflammatory re-

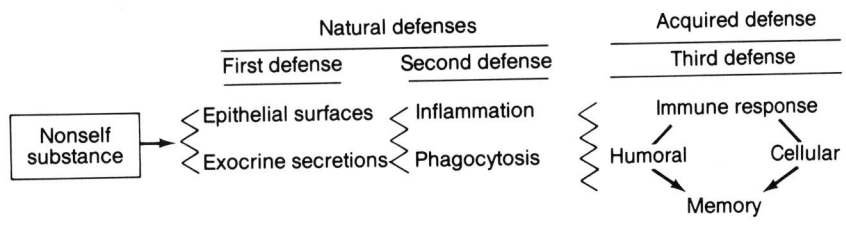

Figure 43-5 The concept of human defense.

sponse is evoked. The reaction to cellular injury is local vascular response characterized by increased blood flow, the release of chemotactic chemicals, migration of cells, and exudation. All these mechanisms are detrimental to the viability of the injurious agents.

Inflammation

Inflammation is nonspecific and is initiated by any cellular injury. Extrinsic causes of inflammation include trauma, burns, invasion by microorganisms, and surgical procedures. Examples of intrinsic conditions triggering inflammation are myocardial infarction, malignancy, and thrombosis. Damaged tissue may release histamine, serotonin, prostaglandins, lysosomal enzymes, clotting factors, kinins, complement fragments, and cytokines. These chemical substances are all mediators of the inflammatory process.

The localized signs and symptoms of inflammation are well known and universally experienced. The five classic signs (heat, pain, redness, swelling, and loss of function) occur as a result of functional changes in the flow of blood through the injured area. If the injury to the body is extensive, systemic evidence of inflammation occurs. Systemic evidence of inflammatory response includes leukocytosis, neutrophilia, fever, malaise, and weight loss. The local and systemic signs are the same for inflammation and infection. Inflammation can occur alone, but infection is always accompanied by inflammation.

The vascular changes that occur are attributed to the mediators that are released. Inflammation begins with a brief initial vasoconstriction and triggering of the clotting cascade in the blood vessels in the area of the injury. Red blood cells, platelets, and WBCs line the vessels. Histamine-induced vasodilatation produces redness and heat at the site. Capillary permeability is also induced by histamine, allowing plasma and cells to leak into the interstitial area to cause edema. Histamine is short acting, but prostaglandins and bradykinin are powerful and longer-acting substances that sustain the vascular effects. Complement activation at the site also contributes to the inflammatory process. Fragments C3a and C5a cause vascular permeability and also stimulate histamine release. The edema or inflammatory exudate causes swelling and pain at the site, which in turn restrict the function of the affected area. However, exudate has the beneficial effect of providing nutrients to the tissues for repair and carrying phagocytic cells to destroy invading organisms and to clean up the debris in the injured area.

Inflammation not only destroys injurious agents but also prepares the area for healing. Despite its importance in maintaining life, inflammation may also be destructive. Loss of homeostatic control of the process may lead to serious illness and death.

Phagocytosis

Chemotaxis is the chemical attraction of phagocytes to an injured area. Damaged cells, bacteria release, and mediators such as C5a act as chemotactants to bring phagocytes to the inflamed area. The bone marrow responds by releasing more leukocytes into the blood to increase the total number of circulating WBCs.

Phagocytosis is the nonspecific process by which injured cells, microorganisms, and cellular debris are removed from an area. Phagocytosis may occur before the inflammatory process or concurrently. It is increased by the inflammatory response and greatly enhanced by the immune response. Phagocytosis is not dependent on these processes and may occur independently.

Upon contact with the antigen or damaged cell, the phagocyte extends a pseudopod from its cell membrane to surround the invader within an envelope of the cell membrane, forming a *phagosome*. Lysosomes within the granules of the phagocyte fuse with the phagosome to create a *phagolysosome*. Digestive enzymes are released into the phagolysosome to destroy the invader.

Phagocytosis is enhanced by the presence of humoral substances called *opsonins*. Complement and antibodies are opsonins that coat the invader so that it adheres (binds) with the phagocyte.

Chemotaxis brings neutrophils to the site of inflammation within minutes. Once at the site of damage, neutrophils marginate along the vessel walls and move by the process of diapedesis into the interstitial space. For the first 24 hours after an injury, neutrophils predominate at the site of inflammation. Neutrophils and, to a lesser extent, eosinophils participate in phagocytoses of bacteria. During this time, other chemotactant substances recruit monocytes to the site.

Monocytes come to the site and are transformed into macrophages. At 48 to 72 hours, macrophages are the major phagocytes present. They are characterized by their ability to ingest debris as well as foreign materials and dead neutrophils. The macrophages release cytokines which are pyrogenic (producing fever).

Fever

Fever occurs when the body fails to maintain its normal range of temperature. Endogenous pyrogens elevate the body's hypothalamus setpoint. The cytokines IL-1, IL-6, and tumor necrosis factor (TNF) are endogenous pyrogens released during stimulation of macrophages. These cytokines initiate fever by causing release of arachidonic acid that is metabolized into prostaglandin E_2. Prostaglandin E_2 acts on temperature-sensitive neurons in the hypothalamus to raise the setpoint above the normal 37° C.

Fever is beneficial to the host in several ways. The cytokines activate production of lymphocytes to attack the invading organism. More phagocytic activity occurs at temperatures of 38° to 40° C. The production of virus-fighting interferon is increased at elevated temperatures.[9] Pyrogens induce a sleep pattern in the neurological system, thereby promoting conservation of energy for the defense against infection.

Detrimental effects of fever include increasing oxygen consumption, and tissue catabolism. To meet these demands, cardiac output, and therefore myocardial workload, increase. Respiratory rate and heart rate also rise. Dehydration from fever-induced tachypnea and sweating may occur. Persistent fever leads to weight loss, muscle wasting, and negative nitrogen balance from the increased catabolism. The resulting poor nutritional status can weaken the ability of the immune system to respond.[10]

When the foreign material is ingested by the macrophages, the material is recognized as nonself, processed, and presented to lymphocytes for destruction. This initiates the specific immune response.

Specific Acquired Immune Response: The Third Line of Defense

A specific acquired immune response is evoked when the natural defenses fail to eradicate the invading antigen from the body. This third line of defense is characterized by specificity and memory. *Specificity* in this sense means the ability of the lymphocyte upon exposure to an antigen to limit its response to that single antigen only. As lymphocytes develop, they acquire receptors for specific antigens that commit them to a single antigenic specificity for their life span.[11] Once exposed to an antigen, the lymphocytes produce antibodies and sensitized cells able to recognize, react with, and neutralize only the antigen for which they were designated. Immunological memory is the characteristic that allows lymphocytes the ability to "recall" exposure to a specific antigen. This memory promotes a faster response upon second or subsequent exposure.

Acquired immune response is said to be either active or passive. *Active acquired immunity* occurs when the body is exposed to an antigen and participates by manufacturing cells and antibody against the antigen. Administration of vaccine stimulates active acquired immunity. *Passive immunity* occurs when the antibody to an antigen is transferred from someone already immune to the antigen to a person lacking such immunity. The transfer of maternal antibody across the placenta to the fetus and the administration of gamma globulin via injection or intravenous infusion are examples of passive acquired immunity. It is passive in the sense that the immune system does not initiate production of antibody.

The specific immune response is comprised of both humoral and cellular components. Each type of immunity is mediated by different cells, produces different products, and works by a different method. Both mechanisms cooperate, interact, and are dependent on each other to provide normal immune protection to the host.

To understand the specific immune response it is useful to divide the immune response into two phases or limbs: the afferent limb and the efferent limb. The *afferent limb or phase* involves the recognition of the antigen by the lymphocyte and all events that are necessary to prepare an effective immune response to the antigen. This includes cellular cooperation, cloning, and differentiation of the lymphocyte into effector cells. *Cloning* refers to the production of a group of cells that descend from a single parent cell. The *efferent limb or phase* involves the functions performed by the fully differentiated lymphocytes and their products.

Afferent Limb

When an antigen penetrates the first line of defense, the nonspecific macrophage locates the antigen; identifies it as nonself; and ingests, destroys, and processes the antigen for presentation to a T4 lymphocyte. Antigen processing consists of enzyme modification of the antigen followed by reexpression of the processed antigen on the surface of the macrophage. The macrophage surface has the class II HLA-DR antigen, which acts as a communication link to initiate the immune response. At this time, the macrophage is also stimulated to produce the cytokine IL-1.

On its surface, the T4 cell has a receptor specific for the processed antigen and a receptor for the class II HLA-DR antigen. These receptors allow the T4 cell to bind with both the macrophage and the antigen. Both receptors must match for the binding to occur.

The effects of IL-1 and the binding process activate the T4 cell (Figure 43-6), which quickly clones itself into many similar cells, and the activated T4 cell begins to produce lymphokines. As already mentioned, lymphokines send powerful signals to other cells of the immune system. The lymphokine IL-2, produced by the activated T4 cell, enhances the proliferation

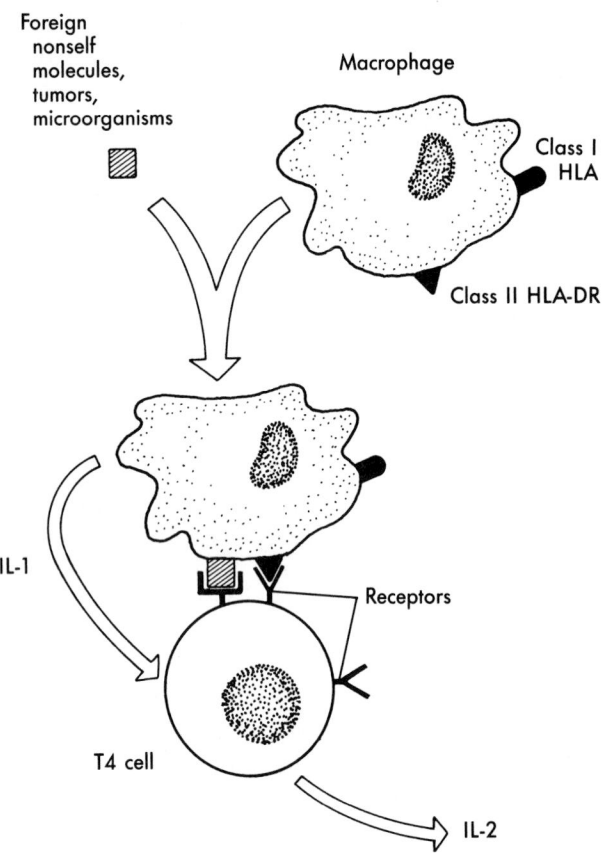

Figure 43-6 Activation of the T4 lymphocyte by the macrophage.

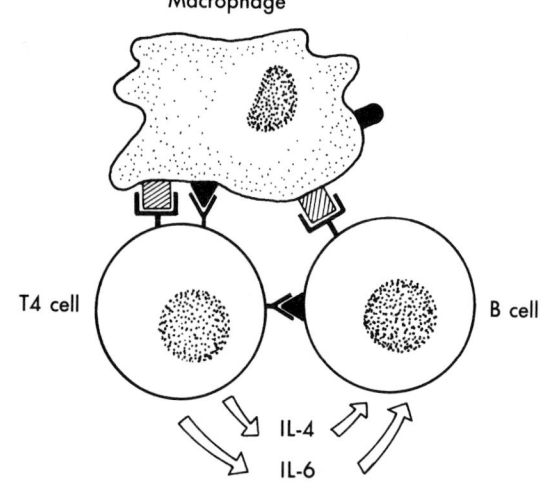

Figure 43-7 Activation of the B cell by the T4 cell and macrophage binding.

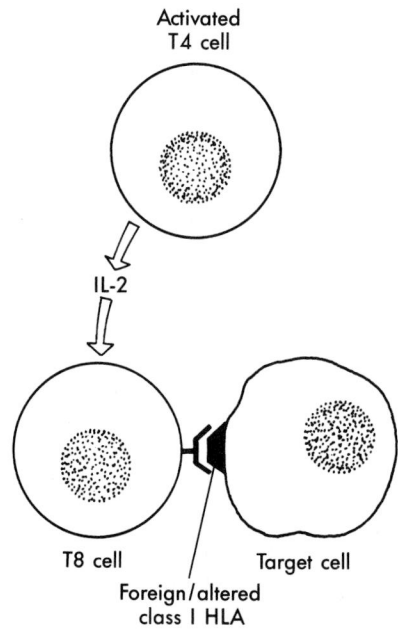

Figure 43-8 Cytotoxic T8 cell activation.

and differentiation of T4 cells. The T4 cell also develops a receptor for the IL-2 it produces. This receptor binds with the IL-2 and further enhances the proliferation and differentiation process of T4 cells.

The B cell also recognizes the processed antigen expressed on the surface of the macrophage that is already bound to the T4 cell. The B cell binds with the antigen on the macrophage and to the class II HLA-DR receptor on the T4 cell. This forms a complex of the three cells: macrophage, T4 cell, and B cell. The formation of this complex activates the B cell (Figure 43-7).

The activated B cell develops receptors for *B cell growth factor*, or *IL-4*, which is produced by the activated T4 cell. When the B cell binds with the IL-4, it is stimulated to proliferate. Some of the newly created B cells generate a different receptor that allows them to bind with another T4 lymphokine, *B cell differentiation factor*, or *IL-6*. Binding with IL-6 causes these B cells to differentiate into plasma cells that produce the immunoglobulin (antibody) specific for the antigen that initiated the specific immune response.

The cytotoxic T8 cell can recognize a foreign or altered class I HLA antigen on cell surfaces. For example, the T8 cell would recognize a transplanted tissue graft or a self cell whose class I antigen had been mutated (altered) by a viral infection. However, it appears that the T8 cell needs an induction signal (IL-2) from the activated T4 cell in order to function. Once binding to the target cell occurs, new receptors for IL-2 are generated by the T8 cell. Binding to IL-2 released by the T4 cell, T8 cells proliferate (Figure 43-8).

The activation of the afferent limb of the specific immune response requires sequential activity and cooperation among several cells: (1) The macrophage introduces the antigen to the lymphocytes; (2) the T4 cell produces lymphokines that (3) induce the B cells and (4) the T8 cells to clone themselves. An army of defensive cells then stands ready to respond to the foreign antigen.

Efferent Limb

The efferent limb of the specific immune response is characterized by a dual response to ensure destruction and removal of the offending antigen. The antigen can be destroyed by circulating antibody, by cytotoxic T cells, or by both. Interaction of T cells with B cells results in an antibody-mediated (humoral) response. Interaction between T cells culminates in a cell-mediated response. The efferent limb of the specific immune response includes antibody formation, lymphokine release, cytotoxicity, and immunoregulation.

Humoral Immunity. The humoral response is initiated by the binding of the macrophage, the T4 cell, and the B cell after the macrophage has processed the invading antigen. Binding leads to B cell activation, proliferative cloning, and the subsequent differentiation into antibody-producing plasma cells. The immunoglobin (antibody) produced is specific for the antigen stimulating the immune response. The response is humoral in that the plasma cells remain in lymphoid tissue, and only the antibody they produce circulates in the plasma and other body fluids. Hence, this type of immunity can be passively transferred in serum.

After initial exposure to and identification of the antigen, there is a delay of 4 to 10 days before there is evidence of primary antibody production. The initial antibody produced is of the IgM category. It does not reach a high level or persist unless a subsequent exposure to the antigen takes place. A second encounter causes a rapid (1- to 2-day) production of a much greater amount of antibody to the antigen. The level slowly decreases over months. The antibody produced in a secondary response is of the IgG category. Memory B cells retain a memory of the initial exposure to an antigen for months to years. This memory capability allows for the more rapid secondary response to the antigen.

When an antibody comes into contact with its specific antigen, it binds to that antigen at the Fab portion of the antibody molecule to form an *antigen–antibody complex* or *immune complex*. Subsequently, this complex is selectively destroyed by several processes. Some antibodies neutralize the antigen and render it harmless by interfering with its ability to attach to host cells and cause infection. Antibodies may act as an opsonin, coating the antigen and fa-

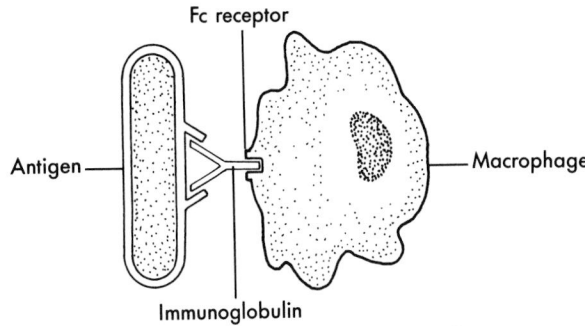

Figure 43-9   Antibody-dependent cellular cytotoxicity (ADCC).

cilitating nonspecific phagocytosis. Immune complexes may be removed from the blood. These processes create a solid, particulate lattice from soluble antibody and antigen that can be removed by precipitation or agglutination, phagocytosis, and degradation by activated macrophages.

Another means for elimination of immune complexes involves cells with Fc receptors. Macrophages, neutrophils, and NK cells have an abundance of Fc receptors. Cells with Fc receptors bind with the Fc portion of immunoglobin that is bound to the antigen (Figure 43-9). The cytotoxic cell is capable of antigen destruction and immune complex elimination. The term for this process is *antibody-dependent cellular cytotoxicity* (ADCC).

The B cells provide the body's primary protection against bacterial invasion. A deficiency of B cells results in an inability to produce antibody. Persons with this humoral immune deficiency are particularly susceptible to extracellular bacterial infections caused by *Hemophilus, Pneumococcus, Staphylococcus,* and *Streptococcus.* Antibodies provide one of the main mechanisms for defense against viruses. However, since viruses are intracellular organisms, cell-mediated immunity is more important in the eradication of established viral infections.

Cell-mediated Immunity. Cell-mediated immune functions are performed by cytotoxic cells at the site of the reaction. This type of immunity can be passively transferred from one person to another only by transferring T cells. The T lymphocyte recognizes the processed antigen on the surface of the macrophage and responds by enlarging and then proliferating a clone of sensitized T lymphocytes that migrate throughout the body and accumulate at the actual location of the antigen. These sensitized cells destroy the foreign antigen by secretion of lymphokines and activation of cytotoxic T8 cells. Unlike the antibody reaction, which is immediate, cell-mediated reaction is delayed. The delay allows time for the synthesis of cytokines and migration of cytotoxic cells.

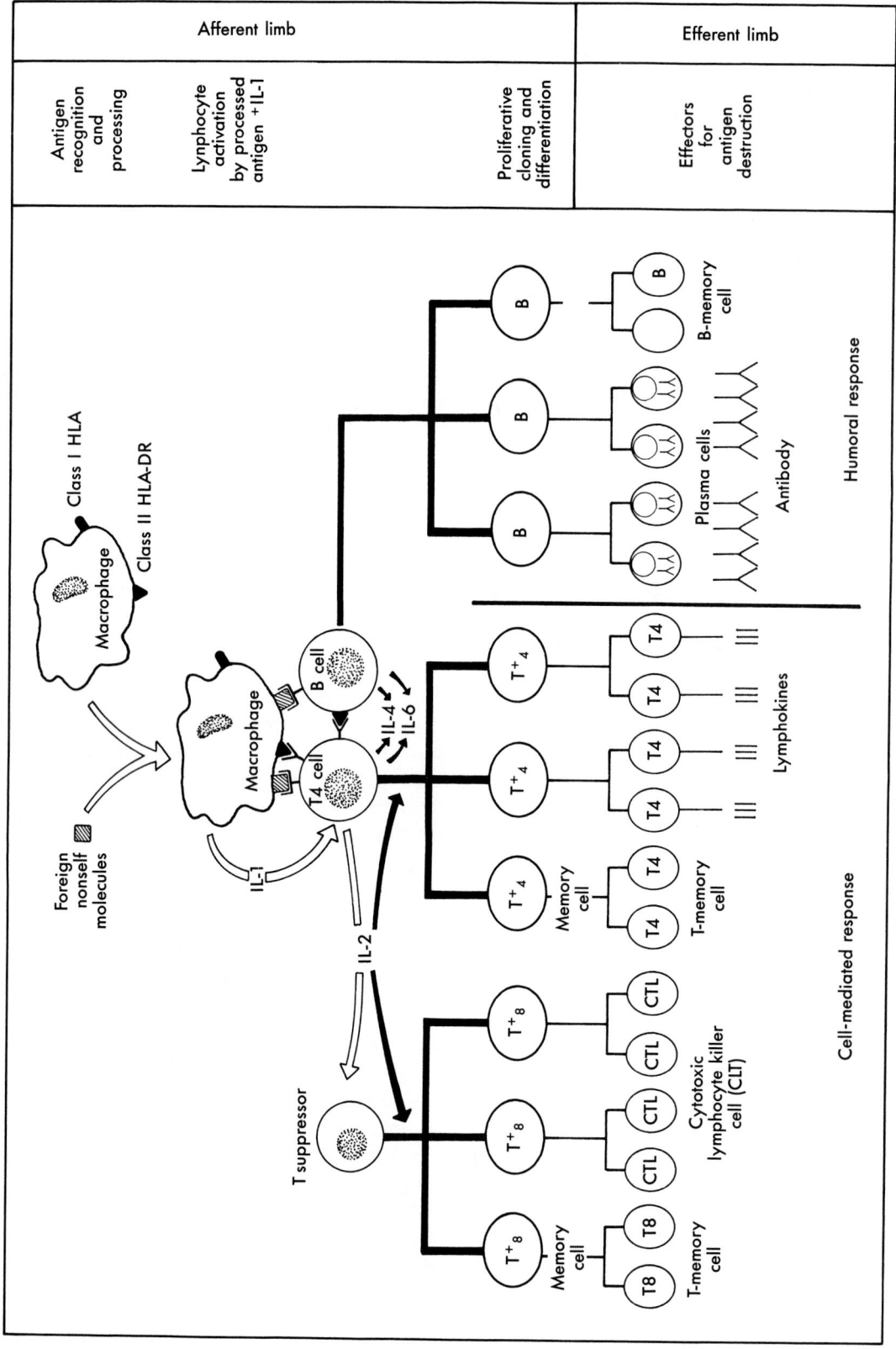

Figure 43-10   Summary of the specific immune response.

Cell-mediated immunity dominates in most cases of intracellular infection, in graft rejection, in graft-versus-host disease, and in immune defense against neoplasia. Defects in T lymphocytes cause recurrent infections of fungal, viral, and intracellular organisms.

The T4 cell has been called "the conductor of the immune system orchestra."[11] Without normal function of T4 cells, direction of all immune functions is abnormal. Release of lymphokines induce (1) growth and differentiation of T4 cells, (2) cytotoxicity of some T8 cells and suppression by other T8 cells, (3) activation of B cell humoral immunity, (4) activation of NK cells, and (5) stimulation of the actions of the nonspecific phagocytes.

Cytotoxicity, or the killing of the targeted antigen or cell, is accomplished by three mechanisms: NK cells, T8 cells, and the ADCC process already described. The NK cells are toxic to cells infected by a virus or to tumor cells. Their nonspecific, cell-mediated mechanism for destroying these cells has not yet been defined; however, it is known to be enhanced by the cytokines α-interferon, γ-interferon, and IL-2. The T8 cells can recognize and bind with nonself or mutated self class I HLA molecules. The release of IL-2 from activated T4 cells assists the T8 cell to proliferate a clone of T8 cells with specific cytotoxicity for the targeted cell.

A subset of T8 cells are called *T suppressor cells.* Their activity appears to turn off, or suppress, the activity of the B cells or humoral immunity. The mechanism for this immunoregulatory function has not been fully explained. The normal immune response reflects a T4/T8 ratio of approximately 2:1. Changes in this ratio alter the regulatory functions of these cells leading to immunopathological disorders.

T cells also produce memory T cells. As with the B memory cells, the T cells hold a memory of exposure to an antigen. During a subsequent exposure, the cell-mediated immune system is activated along with the humoral immune system to protect the host.

SUMMARY

Normal immune system function is a complex sequential interaction of many highly specialized cells (Figure 43-10). When an antigen penetrates the external barriers of defense and enters the body, the nonspecific response of inflammation, and phagocytosis is triggered. During phagocytosis, the macrophage distinguishes the antigen as nonself, processes the antigen, and expresses the antigen on its surface. The processed antigen is presented to the T4 lymphocyte. Activation of the T4 cell initiates both the humoral and cell-mediated specific immune re-

sponses. B cells are activated by the antigen–macrophage–T4 cell complex into plasma cells. Plasma cells become producers of antibody (immunoglobins) specific to the antigen. B memory cells are also produced. The T4 cell stimulates proliferation of T cells with helper, suppressor, killer, and memory functions.

Most antigens evoke the sensitization and proliferation of both T and B cells. However, in any given situation, one or the other type of immune response dominates as determined by the antigenic receptors on the lymphocytes. Antibodies and cytotoxic cells are assisted by complement and phagocytes in destroying the antigen. Several kinds of cytokines are produced that regulate the activity of the normal immune system. After the initial exposure to an antigen, a memory of the event is kept by memory B and T cells to facilitate future immune system response to the antigen to protect the body from disease.

REFERENCES

1. Alkire, K., & Collingwood, J. (1990). Physiology of blood and bone marrow. *Seminars in Oncology Nursing, 6,* 99-108.
2. Gurevich, I. (1985). The competent internal immune system. *Nursing Clinics of North America, 20,* 151-161.
3. Hays, K. (1990). Physiology of normal bone marrow. *Seminars in Oncology Nursing, 6,* 3-8.
4. Esperson, S. (1986). Nursing support of host defenses. *Critical Care Quarterly, 9,* 51-56.
5. Kaldor, P. K. (1988). Anatomy and physiology of the gastrointestinal system. In M. R. Kinney, D. R. Packa, & S. B. Dunbar (Eds.), *AACN's clinical reference for critical care nursing* (2nd ed.) (p. 1311). New York: McGraw-Hill.
6. Keith, J. S. (1985). Hepatic failure: Etiologies, manifestations, and management. *Critical Care Nurse, 5,* 60-86.
7. Alkire, K., & Groenwald, S. (1991). Relation of the immune system to cancer. In S. Groenwald, M. H. Frogge, M. Goodman, et al. (Eds.), *Cancer nursing principles and practice* (2nd ed.) (pp. 73-87). Boston: Jones & Bartlett.
8. Ognibene, F. P., Parker, M. M., Burch-Whitman, C., et al. (1988). Neutrophil aggregating activity and septic shock in humans: Neutrophil aggregation by a C5a-like material occurs more frequently than complement component depletion and correlates with depression of systemic vascular resistance. *Journal of Critical Care, 3,* 103-111.
9. Bruce, J. L., & Grove, S. K. (1992). Fever: Pathology and treatment. *Critical Care Nurse, 12,* 40-49.
10. Tribett, D. (1989). Immune system function implications for critical care nursing practice. *Critical Care Nursing Clinics of North America, 1,* 725-740.
11. Grady, C. (1988). Host defense mechanisms: An overview. *Seminars in Oncology Nursing, 4,* 86-94.

44

Immunological Data Acquisition

Debra Tribett

Accurate assessment of the immune system of critically ill patients is becoming increasingly important. Even if the patient enters the critical care unit with an intact immune system, the required procedures for diagnosis and treatment of serious illness pose risks for the development of nosocomial infection. However, an increasing number of patients present with an immune system that is already compromised. A life-threatening problem requiring critical care intervention may be due primarily to immune system impairment or may be secondary to immune dysfunction, therapeutic intervention, or both. Studies seeking the cause of many critical illnesses such as adult respiratory distress syndrome (ARDS) and septic shock have shown that the activation of normal immune mediators is frequently involved.[1] New therapies involving manipulation of the immune system in the critically ill patient are under clinical investigation. Therefore, baseline and ongoing assessments of immunological activity or compromise in today's critically ill patients are essential.

This chapter presents a framework for the critical care nurse to use in assessing the patient from an immunological perspective. It reviews risk factors that increase the likelihood of immune system compromise and relates physical assessment and laboratory data to the normal and impaired immune response. Knowledge in the field of immunology has expanded in recent years, and with it, so has the ability to identify disorders of excessive or inadequate immune system function.[2] Increasingly sophisticated techniques are used in the diagnostic process. This chapter focuses on the tests most often used in critically ill adults.

If the patient assessment reveals risk factors for impairment of normal immune system function (immunocompromise), nursing care can be planned to support normal immunological function and prevent the development of nosocomial infections. The nurs-

ing care interventions for these patients with such infections are presented in Chapter 45.

FACTORS INFLUENCING IMMUNE SYSTEM FUNCTION

The critically ill patient may present with many factors that are known to impair normal immune system function: age, malnutrition, use of certain medications, exposure to radiation, concomitant chronic disease, and stress. These factors should be assessed in all critically ill patients.

Age

The mean age of the general U.S. population has been increasing. Consequently, the age of patients seen in critical care is rising, too. Older patients often have many problems, one of which is the likelihood of impaired immune function. Compared with younger adults, elderly patients are more susceptible to infection and have a diminished capacity to destroy invading organisms.[3] Their normal protective mechanisms are diminished, and, coupled with increased immobility due to chronic or acute disorders, barriers that prevent microbial invasion are breached, allowing microorganisms to establish themselves in the body. Aspects of both cell-mediated and humoral immune mechanisms have been demonstrated to be impaired in elderly populations.[4] Additionally, elderly individuals are more likely to have chronic diseases that contribute to immune dysfunction.

Nutritional Status

Malnutrition is an escalating problem in the United States and throughout the world. Protein/calorie malnutrition has been associated with impairment of all aspects of immune system protection.[3] Malnutrition may be a preexisting problem, or it can result from the catabolic state associated with many critical illnesses. Muscle wasting, protein catabolism, negative nitrogen balance, and use of amino acids for energy needs have a detrimental effect on the immune system. Adequate energy sources and protein synthesis must be present to produce active immune components such as white blood cells (WBCs), complement, antibodies, and cytokines. Maintaining adequate nutrition in the critically ill patient may be made more difficult due to impaired gastrointestinal function or an inability to use the gastrointestinal tract, increased caloric requirements of the catabolic patient, and total parenteral nutrition fluid limitations in patients with cardiac or renal failure.[5]

A complete nutritional assessment should be performed for critically ill patients (see Chapter 11). The nurse should also be especially alert for poor nutrition status in patients who are elderly, homeless, alcoholic, or addicted to drugs, and in those who have eating disorders, gastrointestinal problems, or chronic renal failure.

Medication

Many therapeutic drugs can contribute to immunocompromise. A complete medication history of the patient may reveal one or more drugs that inhibit immune system function. Glucocorticoids are known to alter every aspect of immune defense. These drugs may (1) weaken the skin, making it more susceptible to trauma; (2) inhibit complement activity; (3) inhibit phagocytosis; (4) depress activity of B cells and immunoglobulins; and (5) decrease the quantity of T cells and impair their function.[6] Over-the-counter products containing aspirin and nonsteroidal antiinflammatory drugs such as ibuprofen impede the function of macrophages and the production of inflammatory mediators.[3] Antibiotics administered for an infection may also kill the normal protective flora on epithelial surfaces, leading to invasion and infection by pathogenic organisms. *Clostridium difficile* is an example of antibiotic-induced infection in the gastrointestinal tract of critically ill patients.[7]

General anesthetic agents such as halothane, nitrous oxide, or cyclopropane have been shown to reduce phagocytosis and inhibit T cell function. Patients treated with some antineoplastic agents develop bone marrow suppression leading to severe immunosuppression. The cytotoxic effects of these drugs on rapidly producing cells are nonspecific; therefore, they destroy the production site of immune system cells as well as the tumor. Patients who have undergone transplants are intentionally given immunosuppressive agents to prevent rejection of the organ. Patients receiving drugs such as azathioprine and cyclosporine A will definitely have an impaired immune response.

The patient's possible use of illegal drugs must also be evaluated. A history of intravenous (IV) drug abuse is a risk factor for human immunodeficiency virus (HIV) infection. HIV infection leads to immune system impairment by its destruction of T4 cells, which are the link between humoral and cell-mediated immune response.

Radiation Treatment

Exposure to or treatment with radiation is another factor leading to immune system impairment. Radiation is commonly used as a treatment for some forms of cancer. This therapy can destroy stem cells in the bone marrow, thereby impairing production of immune system cells. Radiation of the pelvis and sternum or any significant area of the body (with the exception of the head and neck) will affect the bone marrow.[8] Fractionated radiation results in a diminished, more transient decrease in WBC function.[8] However, in patients receiving total nodal radiation for lymphoma or total body radiation in preparation for bone marrow transplantation, effects on the immune system are extensive and prolonged.

In some patients receiving radiation treatment, skin breakdown may impair the natural or first line of normal immune defense. Tattoo markings are placed on the skin of patients receiving radiotherapy to guide precise delivery of therapy. Observation of these markers may prompt the nurse to clarify the type, amount, and date of the last treatment received by the patient.

Stress

Psychoneuroimmunology is the study of the complex interactions of the psychological, neurological, endocrine, and immune systems. The known physiological responses to stress include activation of the sympathetic nervous system and production of endogenous steroids. As described previously, steroids have a variety of immunosuppressive effects. Stress has been demonstrated to depress the immune system of healthy subjects.[9] Ongoing research is investigating the relationship of this depression with susceptibility to infection and disease.

The patient in a critical care unit is subjected to a variety of physiological and psychological stressors. Additionally, the patient may have experienced numerous stressors before being admitted to the hospital; these stressors may be related or unrelated to the illness that led to admission. The critical care nurse should assess the patient for the presence of perceived stressors and should evaluate the patient's coping ability. The patient's family or significant other may also provide insight into the patient's preadmission stress level.

Chronic Illness

A history of the patient's known chronic diseases is a routine part of admission assessment. Underlying disease states that may compromise immune system function are diabetes mellitus, renal failure, hepatic failure, and cancer. These conditions may be unrelated to the problem of bringing the patient into the critical care unit but will contribute to the individual's risk for immune system compromise.

Sexual Activity

Assessment of sexual activity is usually not a priority in critical care nursing. However, it does relate to risk factors for immune system dysfunction. Unprotected sexual intercourse with multiple heterosexual or homosexual partners or with IV drug abusers increases the likelihood of acquiring HIV infection, which leads to immunocompromise. The prevalence of HIV and AIDS is rapidly increasing. Obtaining a sexual history may provide additional data to identify certain patients at high risk for immune system impairment.

HISTORY OF INCREASED IMMUNE RESPONSE
Allergies

Besides identifying the factors that compromise immune system function, the critical care nurse must clarify any factor that could potentially trigger a hypersensitivity reaction in the patient. A complete history of allergies to medications, foods, or other substances must be obtained on admission to the hospital and reviewed upon admission to the critical care unit. The patient's response to these allergens must also be determined. The patient with only one allergy is at risk to develop another. Many new opportunities to develop an allergic reaction are provided to the patient during the administration of new medications employed in the management of critical illness.

Autoimmune Diseases

Autoimmune diseases are characterized by the production of antibodies to normal endogenous antigens. Diseases such as systemic lupus erythematosus, Hashimoto's thyroiditis, rheumatoid arthritis, scleroderma, and Goodpasture's syndrome are examples of autoimmune disorders. Autoimmune dysfunction may be related to genetic inheritance; therefore, both patient and family history are important when assessing this aspect of immune function.

IMMUNE SYSTEM CELLS AND STRUCTURES
WBC Count and Differential

The complete blood count (CBC) is one of the most frequently ordered screening tests that will provide information regarding the cells of the immune system.

The WBC count and differential WBC count are the two parts of the CBC pertinent to the immune system. The other aspects of the CBC are related to hemological function and are reviewed in Chapter 41.

WBC Count

The WBC count reflects the total number of circulating leukocytes (WBCs) in the body. The normal range for a WBC count is 5,000 to 10,000 cells per cubic millimeter (mm^3) of blood. This number does not reflect the total number of WBCs in the body because WBCs are marginated along capillary walls, circulating in the lymphatic system, and sequestered in lymph nodes and other body tissues. However, the leukocyte count indicates the severity of the disease process. Serial examinations are needed for diagnostic or prognostic value.

Leukocytosis. An elevation in WBC count is called *leukocytosis*. It is usually caused by an increase of only one type of WBC. Elevated counts rarely occur proportionally in all WBC types, but when this does occur, it is most likely a result of hemoconcentration.[10] Leukocytosis is most often associated with an infectious process. The degree of the increase depends on the severity of the infection and the patient's resistance, age, and bone marrow function. Patients with bone marrow suppression can have a severe infection without evidence of leukocytosis. Leukocytosis can be caused by inflammation, tissue necrosis, tissue trauma, hemorrhage, leukemia, administration of colony-stimulating factors, thyroid storm, or serum sickness. Leukocytosis may also be found in the absence of clinical disease. Any situation increasing blood flow can flush WBCs from the marginal pool, thereby raising the WBC count. Excitement, exercise, pain, heat, or cold may cause a transient leukocytosis.

Leukopenia. A level of WBCs below normal values is called *leukopenia*. It is associated with conditions that inhibit bone marrow production of WBCs. It also occurs when destruction of WBCs increases periods of infection. Leukopenia is seen during and following viral infections; in hypersplenism; in bone marrow depression due to drugs, heavy metals, or radiation; in primary bone marrow disorders such as aplastic anemia; or when bone marrow is occupied by malignancy or fungal infection.

WBC Differential

The WBC differential count is very important to the correct interpretation of the WBC count. The five different types of leukocytes produced by the bone marrow are reported as percentages of the total WBC count. The distribution of the type and number of cells is diagnostically significant. The percentage is the relative number of cells. The absolute number of

TABLE 44-1   **Normal White Blood Cell Values**

Cell Type	Differential, %	Absolute Number per mm³
Total WBC	*100*	*5,000-10,000*
Neutrophils	60-70	3,000-7,000
Segmented	56	2,800-5,600
Bands	3-6	150-600
Eosinophils	1-4	50-400
Basophils	0.5-1	25-100
Monocytes	2-8	100-800
Lymphocytes	20-40	1,000-4,000

each type of cell can be determined by multiplying its percentage by the total WBC count. The percentage of cells and the absolute number assess the ability of the bone marrow to produce the cells. An increase or decrease in the values of a specific type of WBC is indicative of different disease states or conditions. Table 44-1 lists the normal values of the WBC and differential.

Neutrophils. Mature (segmented) neutrophils are the effective phagocytes. They are the most numerous of the WBCs and constitute the initial response in the inflammatory process. The toxic enzymes produced by neutrophils during phagocytosis are nonspecific and can damage normal body tissues. *Bands* are the immature form of neutrophil released by the bone marrow.

Neutrophilia, an increased percentage of circulating neutrophils, is caused by the same situations as leukocytosis. When more phagocytes are needed, the bone marrow releases neutrophils in various stages of development. The term *left shift* is used to describe an increase in the percentage of bands. A left shift usually accompanies neutrophilia, but patients with recovering bone marrow following chemotherapy may show increased bands with a low or normal total WBC count. An increased proportion of mature neutrophils is referred to as a *right shift*. This is seen in association with chronic morphine addiction, in pernicious anemia, in hemolysis, and with tissue breakdown.

Although the terms left and right shift are commonly used in describing changes in the WBC differential, they have no physiological connection to the conditions they describe. Graphical representation of WBC categories on the traditional laboratory report had bands on the left and segmented neutrophils on the right side of the page.[11]

Neutropenia, a decrease in the number of neutrophils, is present in hematological malignancies, cytotoxic drug therapy, and aplastic anemia. Neutro-

penia occurs when an infection becomes overwhelming to the body and the host's resistance is exhausted. Neutropenia causes an increased risk for infection. A total neutrophil count of less than 1,000 per mm³ places the patient at risk for infection with gram-negative bacilli, *Staphylococcus aureus*, and fungal infections with *Candida* and *Aspergillus*.[12]

Eosinophils. Although eosinophils are phagocytic, their specific role is not known. They become active in the later stages of the inflammatory response and are thought to ingest immune complexes. Eosinophils are active in allergic reactions and parasitic infections. *Eosinophilia,* or an increased number of eosinophils, is seen during an allergic response. These cells may also be increased in parasitic infections, chronic skin infections, Addison's disease, and gastrointestinal diseases such as ulcerative colitis or Crohn's disease. *Eosinopenia,* a shortage of eosinophils, can result from adrenal steroid production in the stress response or may occur following ACTH administration, in Cushing's syndrome, in acute mononucleosis, and in other acute infections.

Basophils. A very small percentage of WBCs are basophils. Their exact function is not known. It is thought that they are involved in allergic reactions, during which they degranulate and release heparin and histamine. Basophilia is observed in some forms of leukemia and is associated less commonly with inflammation or allergy, postsplenectomy, and infections such as tuberculosis, influenza, and chicken pox. A decreased basophil count is associated with allergic reactions, hyperthyroidism, stress reactions, or prolonged corticosteroid therapy.

Monocytes. Monocytes participate in phagocytosis and activation of the specific immune response. They are scavenger cells that perform routine disposal of noninfectious materials. They are not as diagnostically significant as other subsets of WBCs measured in the differential count. Monocytosis can be detected in the recovery phase of infection and is a favorable sign. Increases may also be associated with viral, parasitic, and rickettsial infections; collagen diseases; and some hematological disorders. Decreases have no significant relationship to disease states but may be seen with prednisone therapy, rheumatoid disease, hairy cell leukemia, or HIV infection.

Lymphocytes. The total lymphocyte count is measured as part of the WBC differential. *Lymphocytosis,* or elevated lymphocyte count, is present in infectious mononucleosis and other vital infections, infectious hepatitis, some bacterial infections such as tuberculosis and syphilis, toxoplasmosis, Grave's disease, lymphocytic leukemias, and lymphoma. Lymphopenia is observed in many congenital immunodeficiency states, AIDS, aplastic anemia, after administration of ACTH or cortisone, in Cushing's disease, chronic uremia, and Hodgkin's disease. A decrease in the absolute number of lymphocytes to below 500 increases the susceptibility of the patient to infection, especially viral infection.[10]

More specific testing of lymphocytes can be done as part of assessment of the patient's immune function. Subsets of lymphocytes are identified and quantitated. These tests are discussed further in relation to the assessment of specific acquired immune response.

The critical care nurse must examine the total WBC count and compare it to earlier values, if available, to observe abnormal trends toward leukocytosis or leukopenia. The differential percentage should be reviewed and observed for the left shift commonly associated with inflammation or infection. The absolute count may or may not be provided by the laboratory. If not, it can be easily calculated using the following formula:

$$\text{Absolute value WBC/mm}^3 = \text{Relative value in \% } \times \text{ total WBC/mm}^3$$

This information must always be interpreted in light of the underlying condition of the patient. For example, a patient at the nadir of WBC count secondary to chemotherapy cannot mount an increase in WBCs or increase band production to respond to infection. Despite a WBC count showing leukopenia and neutropenia, such a patient may be experiencing severe sepsis. The laboratory data must always be correlated with patient assessment data for correct interpretation.

Status of Immune System Tissues

History

Patient history regarding diseases of or past problems involving the liver, spleen, or lymph nodes should be obtained as part of the assessment of immune system structures. Previous surgery to remove the spleen, thymus, or lymph nodes should be determined.

Physical Assessment

Physical assessment of the abdomen using palpation can reveal enlargement of the liver and spleen. Hepatomegaly or splenomegaly indicates dysfunction of the organ. Lymph nodes in the head; neck; axillae; and epitrochlear, inguinal, and popliteal areas can be palpated to assess the superficial nodes. The presence of lymphadenopathy can indicate infection or inflammation in the area drained by the nodes or may signify neoplasia. It is important to note whether the enlarged nodes are localized or generalized as an indicator of the extent of the infection or disease. Assessment of

the area drained by an enlarged chain may reveal evidence of impaired lymphatic drainage or inflammation. If the patient's tonsils have not been removed, these lymphatic structures may be directly observed for enlargement or inflammation.

Diagnostic Procedures

The critical care nurse may have data available from invasive diagnostic procedures that are pertinent to the cells and structures of the immune system. Bone marrow aspiration can provide information about the quantity and quality of immune cell precursors being produced or the presence of abnormal or tumor cells. Biopsy of the liver or lymph nodes may indicate abnormal function of these structures. Mediastinoscopy also may provide information about lymph nodes located deep within the chest. Lymphangiography is a specific procedure to study lymphatic flow and the condition of lymph nodes. Results of noninvasive tests such as nuclear medicine scans, computed tomography (CT scan), or magnetic resonance imaging (MRI) may show abnormal enlargement or tumor of the bone marrow, liver, spleen, or lymph nodes.

NATURAL DEFENSE STATUS

Once the basic assessment of cells and structures of the immune system is complete, the critical care nurse can begin to assess the status of the patient's natural defenses. The first-line, or natural, defenses of the patient may be breached as a result of the injury or problem bringing the patient to the hospital. More commonly, risk factors for impairment of natural defenses result from invasive therapies employed in critical care. The routine physical assessment of the critically ill patient will reveal risk factors for impairing natural defenses of each body system.

Skin

The epithelial surface of the skin is the largest first-line defensive structure of the immune system. The skin surface can be thoroughly assessed for actual or potential areas of impaired skin integrity during the patient's bath. Skin folds, axillae, groin, and perineal areas are frequent sites for moisture-related breakdown of the skin barrier. Fungal infections in these areas may also be detected. During routine oral care the patient's oral mucous membranes can be assessed for areas of breakdown. Organisms such as *Candida albicans* or the herpes simplex virus frequently superinfect the eroded oral mucosa in the immunosuppressed patient.[12] At the time of dressing change, known breaks in the skin at the site of intravascular catheters, chest tubes, surgical or traumatic wounds, orthopedic devices, or drains should be assessed. The condition of the skin and the presence, amount, and characteristics of any drainage are determined. Secondary damage to skin from tape or dressing materials may also be observed.

Neurological System

Neurological assessment may reveal deficits in motor and/or sensory function, cranial nerve function, or level of consciousness. Patients with stroke and those with head or spinal cord injury have varying degrees of mobility and sensation. Their inability to move or to sense pain places them at risk for developing trauma or skin breakdown while immobilized. Muscle weakness or paralysis of the intercostal muscles or diaphragm impedes deep breathing and coughing, thereby contributing to hypoventilation and interfering with mobilization of airway secretions. Loss of protective cranial nerve reflexes can lead to tissue damage or impair normal epithelial and mechanical protection. The corneal reflex may be impaired when the trigeminal nerve (cranial nerve V) is affected. Loss of blink protection leads to potential corneal abrasion and inflammation. When the hypoglossal (IX) and vagus (X) nerves are impaired, the gag, cough, and swallow reflexes may be absent or impaired. Aspiration of normal oral flora or other material into the normally sterile lower respiratory tract sets up the potential for infection of the respiratory system. Impaired level of consciousness due to injury, disease, or sedation limits the ability of the patient to change position, deep breathe, cough, and swallow. This impairment can contribute to skin breakdown or impaired airway protection and clearance.

Invasive monitoring of intracranial pressure carries with it the risk of infection. Any patient with an epidural, subarachnoid, or intraventricular access for drainage or monitoring must be closely observed for the development of infection. Epidural catheters are now being frequently used as a route for pain medication. Again, this invasive catheter provides direct access for microorganisms and must be added to the list of patient risk factors.

Respiratory System

The respiratory and the neurological systems are closely linked in regard to risk factors for impaired protective mechanisms. The ability of the patient to clear secretions effectively must be evaluated. The respiratory system is a common site for the development of nosocomial infection in critically ill patients.

Many patients managed in the ICU require an endotracheal tube. Intubation bypasses or impairs normal protective mucociliary clearance of the tracheobronchial tree. The epiglottis and vocal cords are held open, allowing aspiration of normal oral or gastric secretions to occur. Intubation facilitates the colonization of the usually sterile lower airway with organisms that may become pathogens. Ongoing evaluation of the nose or mouth and pharynx may reveal trauma caused by intubation to the protective mucous membranes in these areas. Prolonged nasotracheal intubation can impede drainage from the sinus cavity, leading to the development of sinusitis. The creation of a tracheostomy may restore some of the integrity of upper airway protection, but it brings additional risks. Not only does it break the integrity of the skin but creates an open wound leading directly into the lower respiratory tract. Even properly maintained airways traumatize the mucous membranes and interrupt normal secretion clearance.

Critically ill patients often require suctioning. This procedure can damage the mucous membranes and introduce organisms to the lower airway. Although necessary to maintain a patent airway, suctioning contributes to impairment of normal first-line defenses.

Cardiovascular System

Invasive cardiac monitoring devices create portals of entry for microorganisms into the internal environment from the skin and through the lumens of infusion catheters. The longer the catheter is in place, the higher the risk for a catheter-related infection. During dressing changes for intravenous catheters used for fluid administration, the condition of insertion sites should be monitored for signs of infection.

Hemodynamic data obtained from the monitoring devices provide information on the patient's ability to perfuse body tissues. Inadequate tissue perfusion can contribute to ischemia and eventual breakdown of protective epithelial surfaces throughout the body. Changes in vascular permeability and/or increased venous pressures can cause increased third-spacing of fluids. The resulting tissue edema contributes to organ dysfunction and epithelial barrier breakdown. Externally, evidence of inadequate perfusion is visible in the form of skin breakdown. Inadequate perfusion of the gastrointestinal mucosa leads to breakdown of the gut mucosal barrier that is not visible and contributes to the translocation of viable intestinal microorganisms into the circulatory system.[13]

A variety of vasoactive substances may be administered to manipulate cardiovascular function. Drugs with strong alpha-receptor activity such as high-dose dopamine, neosynephrine, or norepinephrine can shunt blood from the vascular beds of the skin and gastrointestinal tracts, contributing to ischemia and secondary impairment of protective epithelium in these areas. If these drugs infiltrate the skin, they lead to localized ischemia and necrosis. It is important to include the administration of these agents in the assessment of natural defenses.

Gastrointestinal System

During physical assessment of the abdomen, bowel sounds are auscultated. If decreased motility or ileus is present, retention of microorganism-laden intestinal contents increases the patient's normal risk posed by bacteria in the gut. The amount, consistency, and frequency of stools should be monitored as indicators of normal gastrointestinal natural defenses.

Critical illness often necessitates NPO status. It is important to determine how long the GI tract has not been used. Disuse of the gut contributes to impairment of the integrity of the gut mucosal barrier, thereby increasing the risk that intestinal organisms will be translocated into the circulation with consequent possible sepsis.[13]

Prolonged nasogastric intubation may lead to direct trauma to the skin of the nares where the tube is secured but may also injure the internal mucous membranes along the entire length of the tube. As with the nasotracheal tube, the nasogastric tube may contribute to the development of sinusitis.

The nasogastric tube may be connected to suction to decompress the stomach. Protective hydrochloric acid secretions are removed from the stomach during nasogastric suction. The tube may also be used to administer antacids to neutralize gastric acidity. The patient may be receiving intravenous administration of histamine-blocking agents to cause decreased gastric acid production. All of these interventions reduce the amount of acid in the stomach and, thereby, impede or eliminate its protective function of destroying bacteria that enter the stomach from the mouth. When checking gastric pH to assess for effectiveness of the medications administered, the nurse must remember the risk that is being placed on the natural defenses of this body system by a high gastric pH.

Genitourinary System

An obvious risk factor in critically ill patients is the indwelling bladder catheter. It not only provides a pathway for entrance of microorganisms into the bladder but can traumatize the epithelial surface of the bladder, urethra, and tissue surrounding the meatus, disrupting these barriers.

Low urine volume is also a concern for the immune system. Low urine flow deprives the bladder of bacteriostatic and flushing mechanisms.[12]

Characteristics of the urine should be assessed in determining whether protective defenses are intact. The normal acid pH may be altered if a patient has received intravenous sodium bicarbonate or if a hyperglycemic patient is spilling glucose into the urine. Although an alkaline pH may be desirable therapy in some clinical situations, it brings with it the risk of compromise to the natural defense in this system.

NONSPECIFIC DEFENSE STATUS

The second line of immune system defense, or the nonspecific defense, is assessed by monitoring for evidence of phagocytosis and the inflammatory response. Monitoring for activity or nonspecific defenses can identify localized or systemic signs and symptoms.

Localized Evidence of Inflammation

The classic signs of inflammation are redness, edema, warmth, and pain. These findings should be anticipated at sites of recent trauma or surgery. Obvious sites of inflammation should be assessed daily. The presence of purulent drainage at a site of injury provides evidence that phagocytosis is in progress. In a neutropenic patient, however, the ability to mount a nonspecific response is impaired. Classic signs may be absent or minimal due to the lack of neutrophils. Pain may be the only symptom detected.

Signs and symptoms of infection and inflammation may be identical. The only way to determine the presence of infection is by obtaining a culture from the suspected site. Growth of organisms and knowledge of the normal flora of the cultured area make the diagnosis of infection possible.

During a complete systems assessment, the critical care nurse may identify a suspected site of inflammation or infection. The critical care nurse must note the development of tachypnea, dyspnea, cough, changes in sputum, and/or the development of adventitious breath sounds. The chest x-ray may show the signs of pulmonary infiltrates, consolidation, or pleural effusion. Abdominal tenderness during palpation is suggestive of inflammation or infection. Pain, redness, or swelling around one or more joints should be noted. Characteristics of the pain and any effects on activities of daily living should be noted. Joint pain frequently is associated with autoimmune diseases such as rheumatoid arthritis or systemic lupus erythematosus. Changes in any body fluids and secretions from normal to a cloudy or purulent appearance should be reported to the physician and cultures obtained.

Systemic Evidence of Inflammation

When assessing the immune system the critical care nurse must pay attention to vague or nonspecific symptoms reported by the patient. There are no definitive signs and symptoms of underlying immune system disorders. Most patients with immune system problems report fatigue and weakness. Anorexia and unexplained weight loss may accompany fever, or these symptoms may be associated with immune system diseases. Elderly patients with infections often report generalized problems such as loss of appetite, weakness, change in mentation, or decline in ability to perform activities of daily living.[4]

Fever

The critical care nurse should be monitoring the patient's temperature for abnormal trends. Patient history of fever or previously recorded temperatures in the medical record may be available and should be analyzed for abnormal trends. Generally, 37° C ± 1° is considered normal body temperature.[14] Fever is defined as temperatures between 38° and 41° C.[14] Fever is an anticipated normal response to inflammation related to the release of pyrogens from phagocytes. Organisms causing infection and immunological disease processes also trigger increases in body temperature through the release of endogenous pyrogens. When fever is present, a search for infection should take place but a source may not be determined. The underlying patient condition must always be considered when evaluating fever. For example, the patient with a head injury may demonstrate fever, but its etiology may be due to damage to the hypothalamic temperature control center. The nurse must also remember that the elderly may not respond with fever even when infected.[15]

Over time, a pattern of fever can be identified, and this may assist in the diagnosis of its underlying cause. There are, however, many exceptions seen in clinical practice. Intermittent fever is defined as a return to normal or subnormal levels one or more times daily. It usually accompanies acute inflammation, bacteremia, or sepsis. With *remittent fever,* diurnal fluctuations are seen but normal temperature is never attained. Remittent fever is common with pulmonary infections, endocarditis, and *Salmonella* bacteremia. *Constant fever* is a persistent elevation in temperature with minor variation and without return to normal within a 24-hour period. Pneumococcal pneumonia, central nervous system infection, and rickettsial diseases are conditions that produce constant fever. A *relapsing fever* pattern shows fever periods for several days with spontaneous periods of normal temperature. Relapsing fever may occur with neoplasia.

Depending on the stage of fever, the patient may demonstrate additional signs and symptoms that accompany the elevated temperature. In the *cold stage* of fever, the temperature is rising steadily. The setpoint of the hypothalamus has been elevated, and the body is trying to generate heat to reach that higher level. The patient develops an increased metabolic rate leading to tachycardia, increased rate and depth of respirations, and a sense of thirst. Vasoconstriction causes the skin to be pale, cool, and dry; the nail beds are cyanotic. The patient complains of feeling cold and may demonstrate shivering and pilomotor reflex (goose flesh). In the *hot stage* of fever, the body has elevated to the higher setpoint. The patient's skin is flushed and warm. The patient complains of feeling hot. Increases in heart rate and respiratory rate persist. The patient may be drowsy or restless. Headache, photophobia, weakness, myalgias, and a loss of appetite may be reported. Finally, as the setpoint returns to normal, the patient experiences a *defervescence.* The skin is warm, flushed, and sweaty.

Systemic Inflammatory Response Syndrome

When monitoring patients in the critical care unit, the nurse must be ever vigilant for evidence of a systemic inflammatory response and the possible location of an infection. New criteria and terminology to describe the clinical manifestations of sepsis have been developed. A diffuse inflammatory response of unspecified origin has been termed *systemic inflammatory response syndrome* (SIRS). SIRS is characterized by the development of *two or more* of the following:[16]

- Temperature >38° C *or* temperature <36° C
- Heart rate >90/min
- Tachypnea (a respiratory rate >20/min) or hyperventilation indicated by a $PaCO_2$ <32 mmHg
- WBC count of >12,000/mm³, <4,000/mm³, *or* >10% bands

These physiological changes must represent an acute alteration from the patient's baseline unexplained by other known causes. The consensus definition of *sepsis* is the presence of SIRS with a confirmed infectious process.[16]

Severe Sepsis

The critical care nurse may receive a patient who is already in sepsis. The progression of the severity of the patient's signs and symptoms must be established. Using the above definition, *severe sepsis* is sepsis associated with organ dysfunction, hypoperfusion, or hypotension.[16] Evidence of hypoperfusion may include but is not limited to lactic acidosis (metabolic acidosis with an elevated serum lactate level); oliguria (<0.5 ml/kg/hr); or an acute alteration in mental status (decrease in total Glasgow Coma Score to <15 or a decrease by 1 in patient with an abnormal baseline).[16,17] Sepsis-induced hypotension is defined as systolic blood pressure <90 mmHg or its reduction by >40 mmHg, from the patient's baseline. In the absence of a known cause for the hypotension.[16]

Septic Shock

Severe sepsis may progress to septic shock. *Septic shock* is defined as severe sepsis with hypotension despite adequate fluid resuscitation, together with evidence of perfusion abnormalities as described for severe shock.[16] Patients who are receiving inotropic or vasopressive agents may not be hypotensive yet may manifest hypoperfusion. These patients would be included in the new definition of septic shock.[16] Patients with septic shock manifest tachycardia, hypotension, a normal or elevated cardiac output or cardiac index, and a decreased systemic vascular resistance.[18]

Laboratory and Microbiological Testing

Inflammatory/Phagocytic Response

Interpretation of the WBC count will provide evidence of the systemic response to inflammation. Leukocytosis, neutrophilia, and a left shift are the anticipated responses. As described earlier, the WBC count may drop in overwhelming infection or may remain normal with an increase in bands.

The erythrocyte sedimentation rate (ESR) is not considered diagnostic for any particular disorder. It is most often used to gauge the progress of an inflammatory disease. Different methods can be used, and normal values differ according to the type of test performed by the laboratory. An elevated ESR indicates the presence of inflammation or malignancy.

The C-reactive protein (CRP) test is a nonspecific method for evaluating the severity and course of inflammatory conditions. Normal value is less than 0.8 mg/dl.[10] The CRP tends to rise before the ESR and also fall sooner.[10] C-reactive protein is virtually absent in the healthy person and may be detected 18 to 24 hours after tissue damage.[10]

A Wright's stain of the peripheral blood may show morphological abnormalities such as Dole bodies or toxic granulations. These changes in the appearance of the WBC are evidence of severe infection.[2]

Phagocytic functions can also be assessed. Many laboratories perform peroxidase strain, which may permit the detection of myeloperoxidase deficiency of phagocytes.[2] More specialized tests of phagocyte function may be performed in more sophisticated centers. Testing for adherence, for chemotaxis by the Rebuck skin test, for phagocytosis of organisms and particles, and for oxidative metabolism by the nitroblue tertrazolium reduction test may be performed to assess different aspects of phagocytic function.[2]

Complement Assessment

The complement system may be evaluated to identify defects in this aspect of the immune system. Complement activity is part of the inflammatory and humoral immune responses. Total hemolytic complement (CH50) assesses the overall integrity of the complement system, normal values are 25 to 70 units/ml.[10] A normal response virtually excludes a complement deficiency.[2] Increased values are associated with most inflammatory responses.[10] Decreased levels provide no information about the cause of the abnormality; they may indicate a deficiency of a specific component or consumption by activation of the alternate pathway that occurs in infectious diseases or during autoimmune diseases.[2,10]

The individual complement components of C3 and C4 are easily measured. The C3 level indicates the status of the alternate pathway of complement activation; 75 to 150 mg/dl is normal. The C4 level indicates activity in the early components of the classic pathway; 10 to 30 mg/dl is normal.[2,10] Lower values may indicate a deficiency in that particular component. Interpretation of C3, C4, and CH50 must be integrated. Decreased C3 with a normal C4 level indicates alternative pathway activation.[2] Low C3, C4, and CH50 levels are observed with classic pathway activity.[2] Normal C3 and C4 with a low CH50 level indicates a deficiency in another of the complement components.[2] Specialized centers can test for levels of other complement components that are beyond the scope of this chapter.

Microbiological Specimens

Specimens of blood, wound exudate, urine, sputum, feces, genital secretions, cerebrospinal fluid, or tissue samples may also be collected. They may be processed by a smear, stain, culture, animal inoculation, or homogenizing and plating, to identify an organism causing infection. If an organism grows, sensitivity tests detect the amount of antibiotic or chemotherapeutic agent required to inhibit the growth of that particular organism.

Different stains are used to detect different organisms. The Gram stain is one of the most frequently ordered. This stain differentiates bacteria into two categories: gram-positive and gram-negative. The acid-fast stain is used to detect bacteria of the *Mycobacterium* genus (those causing tuberculosis). Orders for stain are based on the organism suspected of causing the infection.

Specific cultures may be done to detect bacteria, fungi, or viruses. Blood cultures are often performed in critical illness when sepsis is suspected. *Bacteremia* is the presence of viable bacteria in the blood.[16] The presence of viruses, fungi, or parasites should be described in a similar manner; viremia, fungemia, parasitemia.[16] In critical care, it is important to remember that blood cultures may be negative but that the patient may exhibit SIRS. Recent studies of clinically septic patients have shown that fewer than 50% have positive blood cultures and meet the criteria/definition of bacteremia.[17]

SPECIFIC ACQUIRED IMMUNE RESPONSE STATUS

To assess the patient for evidence of specific immune response, or third-line defenses, the critical care nurse must combine history of exposure to antigens with many laboratory tests. These tests assess the ability of the patient's immune system to recognize and process new antigens, recall previous antigen exposure, and produce competent lymphoreticular cells in normal amounts. Tests can be subdivided into those that assess the humoral immune response and those that assess the cell-mediated response.

Immune Response History

A complete history of specific immune responses includes a full disclosure of childhood communicable diseases and immunizations. Information about chronic infections such as genital herpes, can be important in the patient with compromised immune function. Foreign travel experiences and any recent immunizations received for international travel should be documented as well. In urban areas particularly, increasing numbers of patients from other countries are being seen in ICUs. The critical care nurse may need to learn more about diseases common in countries besides the United States.

Patients should be asked when they were last tested for tuberculosis by either skin testing or chest x-ray. The U.S. incidence of tuberculosis is rising. Patients with respiratory symptoms or HIV infection should definitely be queried about exposure and testing.

The patient's transfusion history should be obtained, since multiple transfusions may lead to difficulty with subsequent cross-matching. Additionally, their likelihood of exposure to transfusion-borne infections is greater. Hepatitis, cytomegalovirus, and HIV are viruses that can be spread via blood transfusion. The date of transfusion is also important. Blood transfused prior to March 1985 was not screened for HIV antibody. A patient whose transfusion(s) took place before that date is at greater risk for HIV infection.

Laboratory Studies: Humoral Immunity

B Cells

The total B lymphocyte or B cell count can be specifically determined. Generally, B cells comprise 3% to 21% of the total lymphocyte count. The absolute count of B cells is 92 to 392 cells per μl of blood (Table 44-2). B cells mature into plasma cells, the factory cells that produce antibodies (immunoglobulins). A decrease in B cells, therefore, affects im-

TABLE 44-2 **Subcategories of Lymphocytes**

	Total Lymphocyte Count, %	Absolute Counts, Cells/μl
B Cells	3-21	92-392
Total T Cells	60-88	644-2,201
T Helper	34-67	493-1,191
T Suppressor	10-42	182-785

Fischbach, F. T. (1992). *A manual of laboratory and diagnostic tests* (4th ed.). Philadelphia: Lippincott.

munoglobulin production. B cell deficiency is seen in X-linked hypogammaglobulinemia; selective deficiency of IgG, IgA, or IgM; lymphoma; nephrotic syndrome; and multiple myeloma.[10] B cells increase in active lupus erythematosus and chronic lymphocytic leukemia.[10]

Immunoglobulins

Protein electrophoresis may be performed on serum and urine to measure the gamma globulins (immunoglobulins of the IgG, IgA, IgM, IgD, and IgE categories) and other body proteins. Measurements disclose disorders such as dysproteinemias, hypogammaglobulinemias, and some inflammatory states.[10] Quantitative testing of the immunoglobulins IgG, IgA, and IgM can be performed. Normal adult values are presented in Table 44-3. Normal to low levels may exist in the patient whose immune system cannot mount a specific response.

If quantitative testing shows normal levels of immunoglobulins, the next step is to determine functional immunoglobulin. The clinical significance of functional testing is that the patient's immune system may be producing immunoglobulin that is ineffective against the antigen for which it was produced. More sophisticated determinations of humoral immunity can be performed in selected laboratories. Although B cell functions such as proliferation and antibody production can be assessed in vitro, these tests are primarily used for research purposes.[2]

Serological Testing

Specific serological testing can be performed to detect infectious diseases of bacterial, viral, fungal, and parasitic origin. These tests assay for the presence of antibody specific for a particular organism. The enzyme-linked immunoabsorbent assay (ELISA) is an example of such a test; it detects antibody to HIV and is used to screen blood and blood products for transfusion. It is also used to test persons exposed to HIV by risk behaviors, contaminated blood, or needlestick injury. If reactivity is found, the ELISA is re-

TABLE 44-3 **Quantitative Immunoglobulins***

IgG	700-1,500	mg/dl
IgA	60-400	mg/dl
IgM	60-300	mg/dl

*Normal values for males and females >18 years old.
Fischbach, F. T. (1992). *A manual of laboratory and diagnostic tests* (4th ed.). Philadelphia: Lippincott.

peated. If it is positive a second time, a Western blot, or indirect fluorescent antibody test is performed. These more specific tests are considered confirmatory for the presence of antibody to HIV. The presence of antibody is accepted as an indication that the patient is both infected and infectious to others. A negative test can occur during the period when the virus is present but antibody has not yet been produced in detectable quantities. An HIV antigen test may confirm HIV at this time. Because of policies that maintain confidentiality of HIV testing, the critical care nurse may not have access to the results of such tests.

Laboratory Studies: Cell-mediated Immunity

T Cells

The most simple quantitative test for T cells, the absolute lymphocyte count, has already been discussed. Refer to Table 44-2 for normal T cell values. Graves' disease can increase T cell counts. A decrease in this value is suggestive of a T cell deficiency. Low T cell counts are associated with DeGeorge's syndrome, Nezelof's syndrome, Hodgkin's disease or other malignant disease, and AIDS.[10] A transient decrease is seen in acute viral infection such as measles.

If the total lymphocyte count is abnormal, the subsets of T cells are assessed to identify an imbalance (see Table 44-2). Normally, the ratio of T helper to T suppressor cells is greater than 1:1. In AIDS, this ratio decreases because HIV destroys the T4 helper cell.

Skin Testing. Cell-mediated immunity can be studied in vitro through skin testing. Skin testing can also identify sensitivity to allergens, such as dust, mold, or pollen and to determine sensitivity to a microorganism suspected of causing disease; the tuberculin test is an example. Scratch, patch, or intradermal injection is used for skin testing.

Intradermal testing with *Candida albicans*, trichophyton, tetanus toxoid, mumps virus, and streptokinase-streptodornase (SKSD) is one way of determining cell-mediated immunity. Over 90% of normal adults will react to one of these antigens within 48 hours of administration.[2] A negative reaction (anergy) is indicative impaired cell-mediated immunity.

In vitro functional testing of cell-mediated im-

munity is available only in large institutions or laboratories. Blastogenesis testing examines the ability of purified patient mononuclear cells to respond to a variety of stimuli by proliferation.[19]

Combined Humoral and Cell-mediated Defects

When testing is performed to assess immune system function, a combined decrease in B and T cells may be detected. This finding indicates that both humoral and cell-mediated immune functions are defective. Combined defects are associated with congenital autosomal or sex-linked recessive disorders, such as Wiskott-Aldrich syndrome and immunodeficiency with ataxia and telangiectasis. It may be an aquired immunodeficiency caused by radiation or seen with aging.[11]

REFERENCES

1. Stroud, M., Swindell, B., Bernard, G. R. (1990). Cellular and humoral mediators of sepsis syndrome. *Critical Care Nursing Clinics of North America, 2,* 151-160.
2. Katz, P. (1985). Clinical and laboratory evaluation of the immune system. *Medical Clinics of North America, 69,* 453-463.
3. Beare, P. G., & Myers, J. L. (1990). *Principles and practice of adult health.* Philadelphia: Mosby.
4. Petrucci, K. E., Booth-Blaemire, E., & Watson, K. (1989). Aging, immunity, and critical care nursing. *Critical Care Nursing Clinics of North America, 1,* 787-795.
5. Tribett, D. (1989). Immune system function implications for critical care nursing practice. *Nursing Clinics of North America, 1,* 725-740.
6. Sheagren, J. N., & Young, M. J. (1987). Glucocorticoids. In J. E. Parrillo, & H. Masur (Eds.), *The critically ill immunosuppressed patient* (pp. 245-263). Rockville, MD: Aspen.
7. Adams, A. (1985). External barriers to infection. *Nursing Clinics of North America, 20,* 145-149.
8. Alkire, K., & Groenwald, S. L. (1990). Relation of the immune system to cancer. In S. L. Groenwald, M. H. Frogge, M. Goodman, et al. (Eds.), *Cancer nursing principles and practice* (2nd ed.) (pp. 72-87). Boston: Jones & Bartlett.
9. Locke, S. E. (1982). Stress, adaptation, and immunity: Studies in humans. *General Hospital Psychiatry, 4,* 49-58.
10. Fischbach, F. T. (1992). *A manual of laboratory and diagnostic tests* (4th ed.). Philadelphia: Lippincott.
11. Gurevich, I. (1985). The competent immune system. *Nursing Clinics of North America, 20,* 151-161.
12. Masur, H. (1987). Infections in critically ill immunosuppressed patients. In J. E. Parrillo, & H. Masur (Eds.), *The critically ill immunosuppressed patient* (pp. 215-242). Rockville, MD: Aspen.
13. Fink, M. (1991). Gastrointestinal mucosal injury in experimental models of shock, trauma, and sepsis. *Critical Care Medicine, 19,* 627-641.

14. Bruce, J. L., & Grove, S. K. (1992). Fever: Pathology and treatment. *Critical Care Nurse, 12,* 40-49.

15. Schimpff, S. C., De Jongh, C. A., & Caplan, E. S. (1989). Infections in the critical care patient. In W. C. Shoemaker, S. Ayres, A. Grenvik, et al. (Eds.), *Textbook of critical care* (2nd ed.). Philadelphia: Saunders.

16. Members of the American College of Chest Physicians/ Society of Critical Care Medicine Consensus Conference Committee. (1992). American College of Chest Physicians/Society of Critical Care Medicine Consensus Conference: Definitions for sepsis and organ failure and guidelines for the use of innovative therapies in sepsis. *Critical Care Medicine, 20,* 864-874.

17. Bone, R. C. (1991). Let's agree on terminology: Definitions of sepsis. *Critical Care Medicine, 19,* 973-976.

18. Parrillo, J. E., Parker, M. M., Natanson, C., et al. (1990). Septic shock in humans, advances in the understanding of pathogenesis, cardiovascular dysfunction, and therapy. *Annals of Internal Medicine, 113,* 227-242.

19. Golightly, M. G., & Dolan, J. T. (1991). Assessment of immunologic function. In J. T. Dolan (Ed.), *Critical care nursing clinical management through the nursing process* (pp. 1176-1180). Philadelphia: Davis.

45

Mechanisms for Immunological Injury

Debra Tribett

The immune response is a mechanism that normally protects the body against nonself antigens. The encounter between nonself and the host induces an immune response, and subsequent contact with the same antigen triggers a more rapid and intense immune response. This is the protective function of host resistance, or *immunity*. However, the immune response can be exaggerated beyond a purely protective effect, or it can be directed inappropriately toward a material that is not potentially harmful. Lewis Thomas, M.D., wrote the following in 1974: "Our arsenals for fighting off bacteria are so powerful and involve so many different defense mechanisms, that we are in more danger from them than from the invaders. We live in the midst of explosive devices: we are mined."[1] Almost 20 years later, we have begun to understand the role of the immune system and its potential danger for causing tissue injury.

The terms *allergy* and *hypersensitivity* have been used interchangeably to refer to the deleterious effects of the immune response. Allergy or hypersensitivity may be defined as the altered reactivity to an antigen that can result in pathological reactions upon the exposure of a sensitized host to that particular antigen.[2]

Inflammation, a nonspecific immune response, is involved with the immunological mechanisms in causing tissue injury. The mediators released during activation of phagocytes can generate the release of other mediators and can promote the release of themselves. The mediators overlap in their effects and ability to activate other cells such as platelets or the complement cascade. Inflammation precedes or is triggered by specific immunological injury.

The types of immunological injury can be classified in different ways. Because the efferent limb of the immune response has two pathways, humoral and cell-mediated, immunological injury can be described using these terms. The response can be described in

TABLE 45-1 Gell and Coombs' Classification of Hypersensitivity Reactions

Type	Manifestations
I	Immediate hypersensitivity
II	Antibody directed against cell or tissue
III	Toxic effects of antibody–antigen complexes
IV	Delayed cell-mediated hypersensitivity

relationship to the time it takes for the injury to manifest itself using the terms *immediate* or *delayed*. Over 20 years ago, Gell and Coombs developed a classification for the pathological mechanisms of hypersensitivity and called them types I, II, III, and IV (Table 45-1). As the understanding of the immune system has increased, types II and III from the Gell and Coombs' classification have been determined to be very closely related. Both involve formation of antigen–antibody complexes, but the site where this takes place is different. For the purposes of discussion, each mechanism of injury is presented separately in this chapter. Any given pathological process, however, may be comprised of more than one reaction. This intricate and interrelated pathophysiological process of immunological injury is still under study, and researchers are attempting not only to identify the mediators and mechanisms responsible for the injury but to devise therapies to block, neutralize, or eliminate their effects.

MEDIATORS OF INFLAMMATION
Activation of Phagocytes

The activation of phagocytes initiates the nonspecific inflammatory response. The substances produced by chemical reactions and liberated from the phagocytes are toxic to the offending antigen or abnormal tissue that initiated the response. As the term *non-specific* implies, the actions of these substances can also damage normal tissue in the immediate surrounding area or trigger the release of other substances that cause a generalized inflammatory response in the body. When the inflammatory response is stimulated by a major injury or if the response is prolonged, significant systemic damage can result.

In today's critical care patient population (excluding coronary care units), the leading cause of death is sepsis.[3] The term *sepsis* represents the systemic inflammatory response to the presence of infection.[4] Major research efforts are underway to describe the role of inflammatory mediators in the pathophysiological responses leading to adult respiratory distress syndrome (ARDS), sepsis, septic shock, and multiple organ dysfunction syndrome.

The term *septic cascade* has been used to describe the chain of events that follows activation of macrophages by gram-positive or gram-negative bacteria, fungi, viruses, or other microorganisms. The majority of cases of sepsis are caused by gram-negative bacteria. A lipopolysaccharide (LPS) called *endotoxin* is a part of the cell wall of gram-negative bacteria. It has been identified as an independent initiator of the septic cascade and may enter the blood in the absence of infection via gut wall injury or ischemia.[5]

Research continues to untangle the complex web of mediators and their overlapping pathways of interaction. Figure 45-1 attempts to clarify the mediators of the septic cascade. For purposes of discussion, each will be presented separately. In reality, the signs and symptoms seen in the patient no doubt result from an accumulation of many of these mediators.

Oxygen Free Radicals

Activation of neutrophils results in the respiratory burst and production of the parent toxic oxygen metabolite, superoxide anion (O_2^-). The O_2^- dismutates quickly into hydrogen peroxide (H_2O_2). Myeloperoxidase in the granules of the neutrophil catalyzes the reaction of Cl^- and H_2O_2 into hypochlorous acid or chlorine bleach, a very effective bactericidal agent.[6] The O_2^- and H_2O_2 also form two additional reactive substances, the hydroxyl radical and hydroxyl anion. These compounds are toxic to proteins, lipids, and nucleic acids (DNA and RNA). But because they are nonspecific, they can destroy a wide range of foreign antigens and normal host tissues, including neutrophils themselves.[6] Products released from the activated neutrophils are thought to be among the chief causes of endothelial damage in sepsis.[7]

A wide variety of agents that inhibit the products of the respiratory burst have been identified. However, most have been studied only in animal models. None have undergone large, multicenter clinical trials

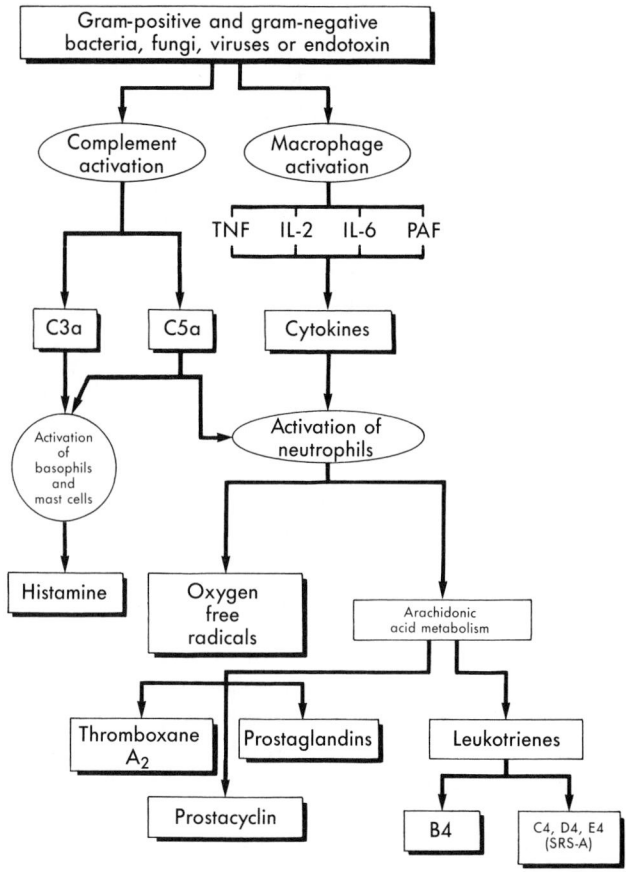

Figure 45-1   Summary of immune system mediators activated in response to invading organisms.

in patients with sepsis. Critical care nurses may be involved in research studies using agents targeted against the respiratory burst.

Naturally occurring cytokines interleukin-4 (IL-4) and interleukin-8 (IL-8) appear to inhibit adhesion of neutrophils to the vascular endothelium. Synthetic production of these substances for study may be feasible in the future. Drugs approved for other uses such as pentoxyfylline, adenosine, aminophylline, and terbutaline are all known to inhibit neutrophil function. Most have the effect of vasodilatation, which may prove to be beneficial to the patient with sepsis.[7] Antioxidant agents are able to scavenge O_2^- and H_2O_2. Some, such as superoxide dismutase and catalase, occur naturally. Allopurinol is a drug already approved for other uses that may be applied for this purpose. Oxygen radical scavengers such as N-acetylcysteine, vitamin E, and vitamin C may have some future role in protection of the patient from this mechanism of immune system injury.

Cytokines

Cytokines are protein substances normally produced by cells of the immune system. They provide chemical communication between cells of the immune system. Their beneficial properties include stimulation of antimicrobial function, healing of wounds, myelostimulation, and mobilization of substrate stores.[8] Exaggerated or prolonged secretion of these proteins may be detrimental for the host. Cytokines are implicated in the widespread endothelial destruction and increased membrane permeability seen in sepsis and septic shock.[7] The potential negative or injurious nature of cytokines is presented in this chapter. Refer to Chapter 43 for a discussion of these important mediators in the normal immune response.

Interleukin-1. Interleukin-1 (IL-1) is produced predominantly by monocytes, macrophages, and neutrophils. IL-1 can induce a rapid and sustained release of both mature and immature granulocytes from the bone marrow. It activates neutrophils in the blood. It brings granulocytes to the inflammatory site and increases the permeability of endothelial cells, allowing the WBCs to exit the blood vessels to the site of inflammation. When this action is excessive, margination of activated neutrophils into the pulmonary epithelium can lead to pulmonary failure.[8] Excessive IL-1 can also stimulate endothelial procoagulant activity, promoting the likelihood of disseminated intravascular coagulation.[8]

IL-1 is a pyrogen; it induces anorexia by direct action on the satiety center of the brain, and its metabolic effects cause skeletal muscle protein wasting.[8] These activities may be partially responsible for the cachexia seen in the critically ill patient. Currently, investigation of immunotherapeutic agents for sepsis includes phase II studies of IL-1 receptor antagonist and phase I study of soluble IL-1 receptor.[9,10]

Tumor Necrosis Factor Alpha (TNF-α). Within minutes of activation, the monocyte/macrophage can release *tumor necrosis factor alpha* (TNF-α). Synthesis of TNF-α is elicited by infectious or inflammatory stimuli. The cell wall–derived component lipopolysaccharide (LPS) is also a stimulus for TNF-α release.

Half-life levels of TNF-α are only 14 to 18 minutes in humans.[8] In this brief period, this cytokine has profound effects. It can release secondary cytokines and humoral factors that lead to localized and systemic responses.

Metabolic effects of TNF-α occur directly and indirectly. TNF-α is a pyrogen; it increases metabolic rate by causing an increase in body temperature. Directly it increases tissue utilization of glucose and glycogen, skeletal muscle protein degradation, and cellular lipolysis.[8] Catabolic effects of TNF-α are seen in patients with malignancy, parasitic disease, tuberculosis, AIDS, sepsis, and septic shock.

TNF-α stimulates neutrophil release from the bone marrow and initiates margination, activation, degranulation, and production of superoxides.[8] It also

induces activation of macrophages. Complement can be activated by TNF-α and intensifies the effects of neutrophils.[7] The activation of neutrophils produces the potential detrimental effects previously described.

TNF-α is a cytokine released early in the septic cascade (as is IL-1). It has been identified as one of the substances responsible for endothelial damage in sepsis and septic shock. Preliminary investigation of a soluble TNF-α receptor and an anti-TNF-α receptor antibody as immunotherapeutic agents for sepsis are underway.[9,10]

Interleukin-6. The cytokine interleukin-6 (IL-6) is rapidly released into the system by monocytes immediately after activation by microorganisms or injury. It is an endogenous pyrogen. It shares the ability to recruit and activate neutrophils with IL-1 and TNF-α. Elucidation of the exact role of this cytokine is incomplete, but it is suspected of being an integral part of the cascade of host mediators after inflammation or injury. It may not have direct negative effects on the cardiovascular system in sepsis as do IL-1 and TNF-α.[8]

Platelet Aggregating Factor. Platelet aggregating factor (PAF) is released from neutrophils, monocytes, and platelets. As its name implies, it is responsible for aggregation of platelets, but it is also a chemotactant for neutrophils. It is a strong promoter of arachidonic acid metabolism. Cardiovascular effects of PAF include increased microvascular permeability, negative inotropic effect on the heart, and lowered arterial blood pressure.[5] Pulmonary effects include bronchoconstriction, increased airway resistance, and pulmonary hypertension. Several platelet aggregating factor receptor antagonists have been identified and used in animal and preliminary human research.[7]

Eicosanoids/Arachidonic Acid Metabolites

The term *eicosanoids* refers to the products of metabolism of arachidonic acid. The eicosanoids are a group of chemical mediators released during the inflammatory/immunological response. Cell injury allows the enzyme phospholipase A_2 to release arachidonic acid from the cell membrane phospholipids (Figure 45-2). Arachidonic acid is then metabolized by two separate pathways into a variety of end products. The *cyclooxygenase pathway* leads to the formation of thromboxane A_2, prostacyclin, and prostaglandins. The leukotrienes are produced by arachidonic acid metabolism via the *lipoxygenase pathway*. All of these end products are mediators of inflammation by way of the septic cascade, and some may cause host injury.

Research has focused on the inhibition of phospholipase A_2 by using a monoclonal antibody to this enzyme. Such inhibition would limit the release of arachidonic acid and prevent the subsequent produc-

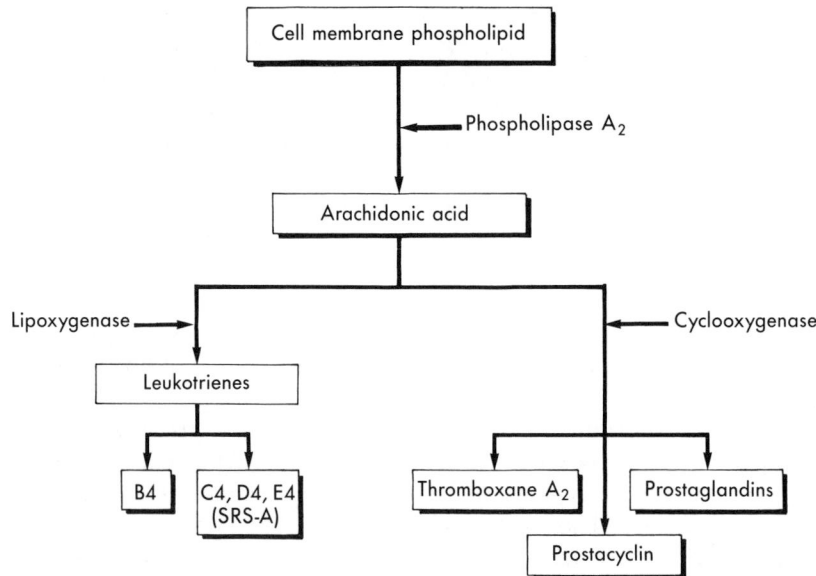

Figure 45-2   Arachidonic acid metabolism.

tion of its end products that act as mediators. In vivo trials have not been reported.[7]

Cyclooxygenase Pathway

Thromboxane A_2 induces platelet aggregation and neutrophil accumulation. Its vascular effects include increasing permeability and vasoconstriction of pulmonary, coronary, splanchnic, cerebral, and renal vascular beds. Pulmonary bronchoconstriction is another effect of this mediator. Thromboxane A_2 synthetase inhibitors and thromboxane blockers have been used in animal models with variable results in preventing the negative effects of this mediator. Human controlled trials have yet to be published.[11]

The prostaglandins and prostacyclin are vasodilators; they increase blood flow to the kidneys and increase the release of renin. Prostaglandins are potent inhibitors of gastric secretion and appear to exert a protective effect on gastric mucosa.[12] Prostaglandin E_1 and prostacyclin prevent platelet aggregation. Prostaglandin E_1 inhibits chemotaxis of neutrophils and release of free oxygen radicals. The prostaglandins are bronchodilators. It is not clear whether prostaglandins are protective or detrimental in sepsis. They seem to exert a beneficial effect on tissue perfusion, but their role in sepsis-associated hypotension has not been defined. Because prostaglandins and prostacyclin are considered beneficial in the septic cascade, research has focused on their therapeutic use. No conclusive studies have been done at this time.[7]

Researchers have tried to inhibit the cyclooxygenase pathway and, therefore, its mediators by using a variety of medications. Nonsteroidal antiinflammatory drugs (NSAIDs) have been used in animal models and in humans. Ibuprofen is the most widely studied and has shown encouraging responses in patients with sepsis and septic shock.[7] Further studies are needed to confirm initial results.

Lipoxygenase Pathway

The lipoxygenase pathway of arachidonic acid metabolism yields leukotrienes B4, C4, D4, and E4. Collectively, C4, D4, and E4 are known as the *slow reacting substance of anaphylaxis* (SRS-A). Leukotriene B4 is a potent leukocyte chemotaxin and aggregator.[12] The SRS-A increases vascular permeability and causes bronchoconstriction. The leukotrienes are much more potent than histamine in these capabilities. Increased levels of leukotrienes have been found in noncardiogenic pulmonary edema and ARDS.[7] Research has been conducted in animal models using inhibitors of the lipoxygenase pathway and an inhibitor to both cyclooxygenase and lipoxygenase pathways. No published studies have used these substances in humans with sepsis.[7]

Complement Activation

Complement activation by either the classic or the alternate pathway produces the complement fragments C3a and C5a. Both C3a and C5a are anaphylatoxins causing mast cells and basophils to release histamine. This release of histamine causes smooth muscle contraction and increased capillary permeability. C5a is a potent chemotactic factor and an aggregator of neutrophils. Migration and adhesion of neutrophils is also enhanced by C5a. When C5a attaches to neutrophils, it activates arachidonic acid metabolism.

An inhibitor of complement component C1 has been used to block the activation of the complement cascade in patients with septic shock. Preliminary reports of a small number of patients have been published.[7] In an animal model, an antibody specific for C5a has been used, but no use in humans has been published.[7]

Interacting Mediators

The complex interaction of mediators present during inflammation and sepsis has become increasingly clear. The ability of one substance to trigger another and the overlapping effects of multiple mediators lead to the assumption that the septic cascade may be self-perpetuating, independently of the original stimulus.[7] The end result of the systemic activation of immune system cytokines and mediators in the critically ill patient can lead to septic shock, ARDS, multiple organ dysfunction syndrome, and death.

In an attempt to prevent the activation of the septic cascade by gram-negative bacteria or endotoxin, another therapy has been under investigation. Monoclonal antibodies to endotoxin have been developed. E5 is a murine, and HA-1A is a human monoclonal antibody for endotoxin. Both have been shown to bind to endotoxin from a wide variety of gram-negative bacteria.[10] Both have been evaluated in randomized double-blind controlled studies in patients with sepsis and septic shock.

Because more than one mediator is involved, it is likely that the future therapy to block or inhibit these mediators will include multiple agents. This exciting area of clinical research is ongoing. The critical care nurse of today must be aware of the potential dangers to the patient's own immune system and possible therapies that may be tailored to the individual circumstances to modulate the patient's immune response. (See Chapter 56 for more information on care of the patient with sepsis.)

HUMORAL IMMUNE RESPONSE

The normal humoral immune response involves the production of antibodies, or immunoglobulins, by B lymphocyte plasma cells in response to exposure to a nonself antigen. Immunoglobulins are specific to the antigen and are classified into categories. Those in the IgE, IgG, and IgM categories are involved in the humoral hypersensitivity responses. The activation of complement and the recruitment of phagocytes to the site may additionally contribute to the injury seen in hypersensitivity responses.

Type I: Immediate Hypersensitivity Reactions

Following initial exposure to an antigen, antibody of the IgE category specific to the antigen is produced. The IgE antibody binds with mast cells and basophils in the body. The mast cells are found surrounding small veins in the submucosal and subcutaneous areas of the body that frequently encounter environmental antigens—the respiratory system, the gastrointestinal system, and the skin.

Type I reactions occur immediately after subsequent exposure to the antigen. The antigen binds with the variable portion, or Fab end, of the IgE antibody that is attached to the mast cell or basophil. The mast cell or basophil degranulates after this attachment. Histamine is immediately released from the mast cell. The effects are quick and not sustained. The damage to the cell wall also activates arachidonic acid metabolism described earlier. The production of leukotrienes known as SRS-A results. The synthesis of these mediators is begun by the interaction of antigen and antibody. The mediators are released after a delay, and their production continues over a longer period than the production of histamine. Also, the mediator *eosinophil chemotactic factor of anaphylaxis* (ECF-A) is released after the reaction of antigen with cell-bound IgE.[2] Eosinophils are recruited to the site to participate in the phagocytosis of antigen–antibody complexes and neutralization of the mediators present.

Atopy or Allergy

Many people are susceptible to natural sensitization by environmental antigens. These antigens include pollens, spores, animal dander, dust, and a variety of foods. Subsequent exposure to these antigens by inhalation, ingestion, or injection produces localized reactions. Conditions such as allergic rhinitis, asthma, urticaria (hives), angioneurotic edema, or diarrhea in food-induced reactions may result. There seems to be a genetic predisposition to this susceptibility. *Atopy* is the term used to describe this susceptibility. However, the term *allergy* is often used synonymously with atopy.

Anaphylaxis

Anaphylaxis is a potentially life-threatening allergic reaction. It is a systemic response elicited in a hypersensitive person within minutes of a second exposure to even a minute amount of antigen. An estimated 2,000 people die annually in the United States from anaphylaxis. The most common causes of severe reactions are penicillin, insect stings, and reaction to iodinated contrast media.[13]

The diagnosis of type I reactions is complicated by the fact that any stimulus that releases histamine mimics this type of immunological injury. The term *anaphylactoid reaction* is used to describe a non-IgE-mediated mast cell activation. Certain substances such as morphine and iodinated contrast media are examples of agents that release histamine from mast

TABLE 45-2 **Signs and Symptoms of Anaphylaxis**

System	Signs and Symptoms
Neurological	Uneasiness, apprehension, restlessness, faintness, syncope
Skin	Flushing, urticaria, pruritus, swelling of lips, tongue, eyes, hands, and feet
Respiratory	Dyspnea, stridor, air hunger, impaired phonation, hoarseness, increased mucous secretion, nasal congestion, laryngeal edema, laryngospasm, bronchoconstriction, wheezing, pulmonary edema
Cardiovascular	Tachycardia, palpitations, hypotension, shock, dysrhythmias
Gastrointestinal	Dysphagia, nausea, vomiting, diarrhea, abdominal distention, cramping, abdominal pain
Genitourinary	Urinary incontinence, vaginal bleeding

cells and may produce anaphylactoid reactions. Complement fragments C3a and C5a are also known as anaphylatoxins because of their ability to stimulate an anaphylactoid reaction. Anaphylactoid reactions occur in patients without previous exposure to the substance.

In either case, the patient manifests similar signs and symptoms. (See Table 45-2.) The clinical findings indicate the therapy required. The skin and the respiratory, gastrointestinal, and cardiovascular systems are target organs in anaphylaxis. During this type of reaction a continuum from localized signs to systemic reaction to distributive shock may be demonstrated in the patient. The onset and severity of the signs and symptoms depends on the route of antigen entry to the body, the amount of antigen absorbed, the rate of absorption, and the degree of the patient's hypersensitivity.

Histamine is the initial mediator released during anaphylaxis. The peak effect of histamine is in 1 to 2 minutes, and it persists for about 10 minutes. Histamine stimulates receptors identified as H_1 and H_2. Stimulation of H_1 receptors causes vasodilatation, increased capillary permeability, smooth muscle contraction, and increased secretion of mucus by goblet cells. Increased gastric acid production is a result of H_2 receptor stimulation.

Increased capillary permeability and vasodilatation lead to flushing and edema of the skin. The airways are affected by edema and smooth muscle contraction, leading to obstruction. Hypotension results from vasodilatation and generalized third spacing of fluid from leaky capillary beds. Smooth muscle con-

traction occurs in the intestinal tract, bladder, and uterus. The production of leukotrienes, prostaglandins, and PAF contributes to the effects on the vascular system and smooth muscle and to edema formation. The actions of each of these specific mediators has already been described.

Although the cutaneous manifestations may be the first clue of anaphylaxis, the upper airway obstruction and distributive shock are the causes of death.

Medical Management of Type I Reactions

Treatment of type I hypersensitivity reactions can occur at two levels: (1) active immunological intervention to desensitize the patient, or (2) treatment of the immunological response with medications to modify the release of mediators and their effects. The treatment of the patient will depend upon the unique situation. In a controlled instance, the critical care nurse may see the patient for desensitization therapy in order for a patient to receive a drug necessary to treat a specific condition. The critical care nurse must be ever ready to collaborate with physicians in the emergency management of a patient with an anaphylactic episode.

Desensitization. The most common form of desensitization is referred to as "allergy shots." In this form of active therapy, the patient receives a long series of injections of the allergen that would ordinarily produce symptoms. The allergen or antigen is given in gradually increasing doses. Patients may receive perennial therapy or preseasonal immunotherapy.

Rarely does this method eliminate the circulating level of IgE for the particular antigen.[14] Instead, it stimulates the production of IgG antibody specific for the antigen. Upon exposure to the antigen the IgG antibody binds to it, preventing the interaction with IgE and the subsequent allergic reaction.

The need to receive penicillin therapy in a patient with a known allergy to penicillin is an example of a situation where desensitization may be used. This type of desensitization therapy may be performed in the ICU setting to allow for close monitoring of the patient and quick intervention should complications arise.

The goal in this situation is to develop a short-term tolerance to the drug. The patient is pretreated with medications to minimize the allergic reaction; then tiny doses of the drug are given intravenously in increasing amounts to consume IgE antibody for the particular antigen. The continuing high level of drug administered intravenously will induce a state of tolerance that lasts only while the therapy is administered.[15] The antibody to the drug will return, and the patient will again be considered allergic.

Management of Anaphylaxis

The nurse may be the first observer of an allergic reaction in the patient. The initial priorities in this situation are to identify the likely cause of the reaction and to stop the administration if possible, to maintain a patent airway and support ventilation, and to support adequate tissue perfusion. However, the nurse must collaborate with the physician and respiratory therapist in accomplishing these goals in this potentially life-threatening situation. Calling for immediate emergency help is indicated. Depending on the severity of the reaction and the patient's response to therapy, some or all of the following interventions may be necessary to manage the patient with an anaphylactic reaction.

Limit Exposure to Provocative Agent. If possible, the provocative agent should be stopped from entering the circulation or its absorption retarded. However, time is of the essence, and the nurse should not delay initiation of respiratory and cardiovascular support if it is indicated by attempting to identify the offending agent.

If the stinger from an insect bite is present, it should be removed by scraping the stinger from the site with a dull object rather than trying to pull it out. Careful removal may prevent rupture of the venom sac and further release of the antigen.[16] A tourniquet or blood pressure cuff may be applied above the site to limit venous return and absorption of the antigen.

When intravenous (IV) administration of a drug is suspected as the cause of anaphylaxis, the infusion should be stopped immediately. The container and tubing should be removed from the IV catheter. Aspiration of the catheter can remove solution containing the drug from the IV line itself. This is of greater importance when a long IV catheter is used or when a tourniquet cannot be placed above the line, for example, when a subclavian or internal jugular infusion site is in use. For short peripheral IV sites or intramuscular (IM) injection, the application of a tourniquet above the site will aid in decreasing venous return and absorption of the antigen.

Epinephrine may be injected subcutaneously at the drug injection site or insect sting site. A 1:1,000 solution is used in doses of 0.1 to 0.2 ml. This is another technique to prevent further absorption.

Maintenance of Patent Airway and Ventilation. Assessment of the patient's ability to breathe, the presence of airway obstruction, and the level of consciousness determine the level of support required. The patient may be in some respiratory distress and may need to sit up and breathe humidified oxygen. Upper airway obstruction is a life-threatening event. If the patient is exhibiting signs of dysphagia, progressing to hoarseness and stridor, 0.3 ml of racemic

epinephrine in 3 ml of 0.9% saline may be given via nebulizer. Progressive airway obstruction may necessitate endotracheal intubation. If the patient has significant upper airway edema, a crycothyrotomy or an emergency tracheostomy may be indicated. Certainly the basics of cardiopulmonary resuscitation must be applied in the apneic patient until advanced cardiac life support techniques are available.

Epinephrine is the drug of choice for treating anaphylaxis because it can reverse vasodilatation, increased capillary permeability, and bronchospasm. These processes in the airways are treated with 0.3 to 0.5 ml epinephrine in the 1:1,000 solution administered subcutaneously. The dose may be repeated every 10 to 15 minutes.

Because of the effects of histamine, bronchorrhea and bronchospasm may be present. The antihistamine diphenhydramine is administered (25 to 50 mg IM or IV). If the antihistamine is not effective, 0.25 mg terbutaline or 0.25 mg metaproterenol diluted in 2 to 3 ml of 0.9% saline should be administered by nebulizer. Persistent or recurrent wheezing can be treated with IV aminophylline. A loading dose of 5 to 6 mg/kg is given IV over 20 minutes followed by an infusion of 0.2 to 0.9 mg per kg per hour.

Maintenance of Adequate Tissue Perfusion. Initial assessment of the patient's cardiovascular status should include pulse rate, pulse rhythm, and blood pressure. If the patient is hypotensive, placing him or her flat or in a modified Trendelenburg position may be indicated. Basic CPR must be initiated in the apneic or pulseless patient.

Establishing a usable IV access is essential to support the cardiovascular system. Depending on the situation, additional IV access may need to be obtained. If the patient's only IV is a peripheral site and the offending agent was given through the line, this line will be eliminated for use because a tourniquet is applied above the site. If the patient already has central venous access, removal of the provocative IV solution and tubing and aspiration of the line may restore this site for use in an emergency. Additional IV sites may be established according to the condition of the patient and whether cardiovascular collapse has occurred.

Epinephrine given to treat respiratory symptoms of anaphylaxis will also have cardiovascular effects. The alpha-receptor stimulation should elevate blood pressure by causing vasoconstriction. Beta-adrenergic properties increase heart rate and contractility. Additionally, epinephrine prevents progression of anaphylaxis by increasing intracellular cyclic AMP which inhibits the release of histamine by mast cells and basophils.[17] During administration of epinephrine, the patient's blood pressure should be monitored for the desired effect: increased systolic and mean arterial pressure. The critical care nurse must be aware of the development of negative effects of tachycardia, dysrhythmias, or chest pain.

Epinephrine is given IV when it is clear that the subcutaneous route is ineffective. Patients with poor perfusion, systolic blood pressure less than 70 to 80 mmHg, a decreased level of consciousness, and cyanosis are candidates for the IV or endotracheal administration of epinephrine.[17] The IV route of epinephrine uses a 1:10,000 solution at doses of 3 to 5 ml. Endotracheally, the dose should be diluted to a volume of 10 ml and injected via a catheter into the tube followed by vigorous manual ventilation.

It is important to note if the patient with anaphylaxis has previously received beta-adrenergic blocking drugs. These agents may inhibit the effects of epinephrine, the drug of choice for anaphylaxis, and necessitate prolonged and aggressive treatment.[16]

The H_1 blocker diphenhydramine has cardiovascular effects by limiting histamine release and the subsequent vasodilatation and capillary leakage. Receptors for H_2 may require blockade to minimize shock caused by histamine release. IV administration of 300 mg cimetidine or 50 mg ranitidine should be used in moderate to severe cases.[13]

Intravenous fluids should be administered to assist in maintaining an adequate intravascular volume. Isotonic solutions such as lactated Ringer's solution or 0.9% saline and/or colloid may be used. Hypotension unresponsive to epinephrine, H_1 and H_2 blockers, and fluids requires additional therapy.

Dopamine infusion of 5 to 20 μg per kg per minute may be used to increase blood pressure. In patients unresponsive to this agent, norepinephrine is started at 3 to 4 μg per minute and titrated to maintain an adequate mean arterial response pressure. Use of these agents is best carried out when the patient is monitored by ECG, intraarterial monitoring of blood pressure, and pulmonary artery catheter monitoring of cardiovascular function.

An additional therapy may be of benefit to the patient in anaphylaxis. Pneumatic pressure garments, also known as military or medical antishock trousers (MAST), have been shown effective in managing hypotension caused by vasodilatation and capillary leakage.[17] The trousers exert a counter pressure on the vascular bed, thereby decreasing capillary leakage and increasing systemic vascular resistance. The blood pressure can be increased using this device. An additional benefit is the engorgement of upper extremity superficial veins, which may aid in establishing a vascular access in the patient with anaphylaxis.[17]

Corticosteroids have no immediate effects on the symptoms of anaphylaxis.[13] Doses of 100 to 200 mg of cortisol may be given every 4 to 6 hours IV for 24 hours and then rapidly tapered.[18] Giving steroids may prevent prolonged or late sequelae.[13]

NURSING MANAGEMENT IN TYPE I REACTIONS

The critical care team must work closely together to successfully resuscitate the patient in anaphylaxis. After stabilization of the patient, the nurse must continue to monitor for signs of deterioration or response to the therapies that have been instituted.

The respiratory system must be assessed for evidence of airway obstruction and edema. The patient must be monitored for adequacy of ventilation and oxygenation. Additional nursing care measures may be instituted to manage any artificial airways in use or for the patient requiring mechanical ventilation.

The cardiovascular system must be monitored for side effects of the medications used to treat anaphylaxis. ECG monitoring for heart rate and rhythm and frequent measurements of blood pressure are indicated. Administration of IV fluids to correct hypovolemia may continue. If therapy has been effective, a decrease in capillary leakage and a remobilization of fluids from the third space should occur. It is important to monitor for potential fluid overload and adequate cardiac function. If invasive monitoring has been instituted, titration of vasoactive substances and fluids based on hemodynamic data must take place. Monitoring urinary output will also reflect perfusion to the kidneys and adequacy of intravascular volume.

The central nervous system must be monitored closely. The patient may be experiencing anxiety over the events that have occurred, but anxiety, tremor, and restlessness may also be side effects of the beta-adrenergic drugs used in the treatment of anaphylaxis. If the patient has lost consciousness during the anaphylactic episode or if CPR was instituted, close observation for any neurological deficits is important to determine any sequelae from hypoxia that may have occurred. Patients who are awake and alert will need support in understanding what they have experienced and assistance in adjusting to the critical care environment.

If this was the first anaphylactic episode experienced by the patient and his or her family, there will be a need for information, explanation, and patient and family education. Patient readiness and amount of patient education performed in the critical care unit will be determined individually. Unmet needs in this area must be referred to the nurses caring for the patient upon transfer from the critical care unit.

The patient with an allergy has the potential for injury from the immune response to the allergen and from future exposures to it. The nursing diagnosis potential for injury related to hypersensitivity may be used to summarize specific nursing actions related to the patient with an known or suspected allergy.

■ **NURSING DIAGNOSIS**

High risk for injury, related to hypersensitivity reaction.

OUTCOME STANDARD AND CRITERIA

Injury related to anaphylactic episode is prevented and likelihood of future episodes is minimized as evidenced by:

- Absence of injury associated with anaphylactic response
- Patient and family demonstration of knowledge related to prevention of exposure and emergency treatment

NURSING INTERVENTIONS

- Using hospital procedure, indicate known or suspected allergy on patient chart, identification bracelet, and nursing forms or records
- Maintain emergency equipment close to patient bedside
- Closely monitor patient when giving patient any medications known to cause histamine release (e.g., vancomycin, morphine)
- When administering new drugs to patient, monitor patient closely, particularly during second dose
- Prevent skin breakdown in patient who has manifested anaphylaxis
  Use topical agents to reduce itching.
  Remind patient not to scratch skin.
  Clip nails or mitt hands in patients with impaired level of consciousness.
  Use protective mattresses or devices to minimize pressure on edematous tissue.
- Begin patient and family education regarding offending agent, patient response, avoidance of exposure, and emergency treatment
  Assist patient or family in obtaining medical alert jewelry.
  If indicated, assist patient and family to obtain emergency kit and instruct in its use.

Type II: Cytotoxic Hypersensitivity

Cytotoxic hypersensitivity involves the combination of the Fab portion of IgG or IgM antibody with antigenic receptors on membranes of cells. Complement attaches to the Fc portion of the antibody and the classic pathway of complement activation occurs. The cell on which the antigen was expressed is lysed by complement. Complement activation produces C3a and C5a, which in turn recruit and activate neutrophils to aid in the phagocytosis of the target cell and possibly damage to surrounding tissues.

A similar situation may occur when, instead of activating complement, the antibody bound to the antigen on the cell activates a natural killer (NK) cell. The NK cell has a receptor for the Fc portion of the antibody. This cytotoxic cell is capable of destroying the immune complex and the cell to which it is attached. The term *antibody-dependent cellular cytotoxicity* (ADCC) is used to describe this process.

The target cell may be a red blood cell (RBC), white blood cell (WBC), or platelet. If the target cell is a circulating blood cell, destruction of the cell and clearance by the reticuloendothelial system result in a deficiency for that cell type. A hemolytic RBC transfusion reaction is an example of this type of hypersensitivity reaction.

A drug may become a hapten, bind with a body protein carrier molecule, and be recognized as an antigen against which the body will respond immunologically. Drugs such as alpha-methyldopa or quinidine bind to the surface of the RBC. They are then recognized by the antibody; it attaches, activates complement, and lyses the cell. The result is an immunologically induced anemia.

The antibody can react against antigen expressed on fixed tissues in numerous sites in the body. The glomerular basement membrane appears to be particularly vulnerable to this type of hypersensitivity reaction. Goodpasture's syndrome is an example of a cytotoxic reaction in the kidneys. In the disease myasthenia gravis, autoantibodies develop against the acetylcholine receptor and interfere with its function.

Type III: Immune Complex–Mediated Reaction

Normally, antigen and antibody form a circulating immune complex and activate complement. The antigen is destroyed by the combined reaction. This complex is ordinarily phagocytized by monocytes or macrophages and cleared by the reticuloendothelial system. When this does not happen, immune complex hypersensitivity occurs. Excessive amounts of complex or defective phagocytosis may be responsible for the lack of proper clearance. If, however, this complex becomes deposited in body tissues, complement activation and the activation of neutrophils at the site of deposition mediate an inflammatory reaction at that site. Release of the mediators previously described in this chapter (oxygen free radicals and arachidonic acid metabolites) causes an inflammatory reaction in the particular location of the deposit and may be destructive to the surrounding tissues.

There is usually no specificity for the tissue in which the complex localizes. The antigen is shed from the area of the original infection or pathological condition, complexed with antibody circulating in the blood, and physically deposited in an area as it circulates. Wherever the complex is trapped, the inflammatory reaction ensues. Complexes may form in blood vessels at bifurcations or sites of turbulence, or in the skin.

The usual resultant lesion is an ischemic necrosis of the area in which the complex has been deposited. When vessels are injured, either thrombosis or destruction of the vessel wall leads to impaired perfusion of the tissue served by that blood vessel. Loss of normal function of the tissue follows. The symptoms being manifested depend on the organ affected. In the case of the kidneys, glomerulonephritis may be seen; impaired circulation to the brain leads to neurological manifestations.

Arthus Reaction

The Arthus reaction is a typical immune complex–induced inflammatory reaction occurring in the skin. Within an hour of injection of antigen into a previously immunized host with circulating antibodies, a localized swelling, redness, and edema appear.[2] The lesion can become hemorrhagic and increase in intensity over the next few hours. The extent of the reaction depends on the quantity of antigen and antibody available. With a large amount of antigen–antibody complex, necrosis can occur. Over the next few days the reaction gradually diminishes and eventually disappears. An example of such a reaction occurs when a patient previously immunized for tetanus is given a tetanus toxoid injection.[2]

The pathophysiology of polyarteritis nodosa consists of typical Arthus reactions distributed in vessels throughout the body. Similar lesions have been demonstrated in the joints of patients with arthritis or in the kidneys of patients with glomerulonephritis. Arthus reactions are also responsible for hypersensitivity pneumonitis or alveolitis caused by inhaled organic dust.

Serum Sickness

When foreign serum has been injected into a patient, immune complexes form when antibodies are produced against the foreign serum proteins. This reaction, which became known as *serum sickness,* can result in vascular, cardiac, renal, cutaneous, or joint lesions.[2] Serum sickness may be caused by immune complex production in response to entry into the circulation by an infectious agent, passive transfer of antibody or antigen, or injection of preformed antigen–antibody complexes, or drugs. Serum sickness is now seen infrequently but may be seen with penicillin or sulfonamide administration or in patients who have received antilymphocyte serum to suppress rejection of transplanted tissue.

Manifestations of serum sickness include fever, malaise, urticarial and erythematous skin rashes, arthralgia, lymphadenopathy, and splenomegaly. They occur 3 days to 3 weeks after the injection of the foreign substance and usually subside within 1 to 2 weeks.

Immune Complex Disorders

Many diseases have been found to be associated with the chronic and persistent formation and deposition of intravascular immune complexes. They may be collectively termed *immune complex disorders.* Examples of immune complex disorders include acute poststreptococcal glomerulonephritis, subacute bacterial endocarditis, mycoplasmal pneumonia, syphilis, lepromatous leprosy, acute viral hepatitis, Guillain-Barré syndrome, systemic lupus erythematosus, rheumatoid arthritis, Crohn's disease, and ulcerative colitis. The deposition of the immune complexes leads to a wide variety of symptoms based on the tissues involved.

Autoimmune Disorders

Autoimmunity is a state in which the normal tolerance of self antigens ceases. This results in the immune system turning its normal defenses against self tissues. The exact mechanism causing this inappropriate immune response has not been identified. The damage caused by autoimmune disease results from all aspects of the immune system triggered by the autoantibody binding with the autoantigen. The formation of antigen–antibody complexes and their resulting damage is similar to that of type I and type II hypersensitivity reactions. The difference is that the antibody is specifically directed against self tissue antigens. The involvement of T cells in the autoimmune response also takes place, much as in type IV cell-mediated hypersensitivity.

Autoimmune disease may cause damage ranging from minor local effects to potentially life-threatening systemic disease. These diseases may be classified as organ specific or systemic. Examples of organ-specific autoimmune diseases are Hashimoto's thyroiditis, type I diabetes mellitus, and myasthenia gravis. Systemic autoimmune disorders include Goodpasture's syndrome, systemic lupus erythematosus, rheumatoid arthritis, and progressive sclerosis (scleroderma).

Nursing Management of Types II and III Reactions

In the critical care unit the patient is often exposed to blood transfusions and administration of multiple medications. This places the patient at risk of developing a type II reaction. The close monitoring instituted during transfusion administration and subsequent stopping of the infusion if a reaction occurs are nursing actions that may limit such a reaction. Observing side effects of medications in terms of physical signs and following trends in complete blood count values are other examples of monitoring for type II reactions performed by the critical care nurse. When a reaction is detected, stopping the offending agent is the primary treatment.

The critical care nurse may detect evidence of type III reactions during routine monitoring of the patient. However, it is more likely that the critical care nurse will be involved in the care of the patient after these reactions occur. The more serious organ or systemic involvement of the reaction may cause dysfunction or failure of one or more organ systems. Care of the patient in the ICU may be required if severe organ dysfunction or the multisystem effects of the organ failure are present. Plasmapheresis is another technique that may be performed in the ICU in an attempt to clear the patient's serum of the antibody that stimulates type II or III reactions.

CELL-MEDIATED IMMUNE RESPONSES

Cell-mediated immune (CMI) responses are carried out chiefly by sensitized T lymphocytes. These cells destroy antigen by direct or indirect means in the absence of complement or antibody. Direct destruction requires actual physical contact by sensitized T lymphocytes with the antigen. Indirect toxicity is accomplished by the production of lymphokine mediators and the recruitment of macrophages to the site. Macrophages participate in phagocytosis and release of mediators at the site.

Type IV: Delayed Hypersensitivity

The exact mechanism of delayed hypersensitivity is still uncertain. It is characterized by a response after one or more days at the site of exposure to the antigen. This delay in reaction presumably occurs because the reaction is mediated by cells that require time to migrate to the site.

The offending antigen is identified as nonself by the macrophage, but it is incompletely digested. The antigen must come into contact with previously sensitized T lymphocytes. For this to occur, the antigen must leak into the bloodstream, or lymphocytes migrating through tissue site encounter the antigen by chance. They react by releasing lymphokines that activate an inflammatory response at the site, attracting additional macrophages. The release of toxic substances by the macrophages leads to tissue damage.

Contact Dermatitis

Many contact allergies are type IV delayed hypersensitivity reactions. Poison ivy sensitivity is a classic example of this reaction, but cosmetics, tapes, alloys in jewelry, soaps, or rubber compounds in elastic may produce injury in the predisposed patient. These substances must be lipid soluble to penetrate the skin. They act as a hapten, combining with body proteins to become antigenic. In a previously exposed sensitive person, contact dermatitis develops from contact with the irritant.

Contact dermatitis is a skin condition manifested by redness, induration, vesiculation, and discomfort that develops 48 to 72 hours after contact with the antigen. It can be differentiated from an Arthus reaction because of the difference in time delay from exposure to symptoms.

Skin Testing

Skin testing, a useful clinical tool, is based on the type IV reaction. The most common example of delayed hypersensitivity testing is the *tuberculin skin test*. Intradermal injection of the tuberculosis bacillus produces erythema, induration, and possible necrosis of the area in approximately 24 to 48 hours in persons previously sensitized by the tuberculin antigen. Scratch or patch testing for allergies is another example of commonly used testing based on delayed hypersensitivity.

In persons with known previous exposure to antigens, the lack of a delayed hypersensitivity response when given skin tests with the antigen is considered anergy. This type of testing is incorporated into nutritional assessment and assessment for impaired immune response.

Transplant Rejection

Transplantation of organs from one person to another has become a commonplace situation. Rejection of transplanted tissue involves all aspects of the immune response but is primarily mediated by a type IV reaction. Sensitized T lymphocytes attach to the grafted tissue, causing rejection. This form of rejection takes place after the first 24 hours after transplantation.

To prevent or minimize rejection, the recipient and the donor are matched in blood type, histocompatibility antigens (HLA), and the presence of preformed antibodies to the donor HLA antigens. All recipients of transplanted organs must remain on an immunosuppressive regimen to prevent eventual rejection of the graft.

Nursing Management of Type IV Reactions

The critical care nurse must understand the mechanism behind the delayed hypersensitivity reaction. When skin tests are administered, this type of reaction may be induced to assess patients for exposure to diseases or in evaluating immune response. Additionally, contact hypersensitivity may be stimulated during care of the patient as solutions or tapes come into contact with the patient's skin. Assessment of these types of past reactions should be included when determining patient allergies.

Critical care nurses caring for organ transplant recipients must always be alert for the signs of transplant rejection. Often these signs are similar to those caused by infection. The medication-induced immunosuppressed state places the transplant patient at high risk for the development of sepsis as well. Close observation of the patient and collaboration with the physician are essential when providing care to patients who have received a transplant. (See Chapter 57.)

REFERENCES

1. Thomas, I. (1974). *The lives of a cell: Notes of a biology watcher* (p. 92). New York: Bantam.
2. Henson, P. M. (1985). Mechanisms of tissue injury produced by immunologic reactions. In J. A. Bellanti (Ed.), *Immunology III*. Philadelphia: Saunders.
3. Parrillo, J. E., et al. (1990). Septic shock: Advances in the understanding of pathogenesis, cardiovascular dysfunction, and therapy. *Annals of Internal Medicine, 113,* 227-242.
4. Members of the American College of Chest Physicians/Society of Critical Care Medicine Consensus Conference Committee. (1992). American College of Chest Physicians/Society of Critical Care Medicine Consensus Conference: Definitions for sepsis and organ failure and guidelines for the use of innovative therapies for sepsis. *Critical Care Medicine, 20,* 864-874.
5. Stroud, M., Swindell, B., & Bernard, G. R. (1990). Cellular and humoral mediators of sepsis syndrome. *Critical Care Nursing Clinics of North America, 2,* 151-160.
6. Zimmerman, J. J. (1989). Polymorphonuclear leukocytes—agents of host defense and autoinjury. In W. C. Shoemaker, S. Ayres, A. Grenvik, et al. (Eds.), *Textbook of critical care* (2nd ed.). Philadelphia: Saunders.
7. Bone, R. C. (1992). Inhibitors of complement and neutrophils: A critical evaluation of their role in the treatment of sepsis. *Critical Care Medicine, 20,* 891-898.
8. Fong, Y., Moldawer, L. L., Shires, T., et al. (1990). The biologic characteristics of cytokines and their implications in surgical injury. *Gynecology and Obstetrics, 170,* 363-378.
9. Cunnion, R. E. (1992). Clinical trials of immunotherapy for sepsis. *Critical Care Medicine, 20,* 721-723.
10. Bone, R. C. (1991). A critical evaluation of new agents for the treatment of sepsis. *Journal of the American Medical Association, 266,* 1686-1691.
11. Bone, R. C. (1992). Phospholipids and their inhibitors: A critical evaluation of their role in the treatment of sepsis. *Critical Care Medicine, 20,* 884-890.
12. Reines, H. D., & Halushka, P. V. (1989). Arachidonic acid metabolites—the eicosanoids. In W. C. Shoemaker, , S. Ayres, A. Grenvik, et al. (Eds.), *Textbook of critical care* (2nd ed.) (pp. 1028-1034). Philadelphia: Saunders.
13. Shelhamer, J. H., & Kaliner, M. A. (1987). Anaphylaxis and anaphylactic shock. In J. E. Parrillo (Ed.), *Current therapy in critical care medicine* (pp. 42-44). Philadelphia: Mosby.
14. Mosko, P. (1990). Hypersensitivity disorders: Four types. In B. Hodgson, K. Law, J. Lee, et al. (Eds.). *Immunologic problems* (pp. 46-47). Springhouse, PA: Springhouse.
15. Miller, F., & Habicht, G. (1991). Immune system: Underlying principles. In J. T. Dolan (Ed.), *Critical care nursing clinical management through the nursing process* (pp. 1155-1175). Philadelphia: Davis.
16. Dickerson, M. (1988). Anaphylaxis and anaphylactic shock. *Critical Care Nursing Quarterly, 11,* 68-74.
17. Thelan, L. A., Davie, J. K., & Urden, L. D. (1990). *Textbook of critical care nursing diagnosis and management* (pp. 808-815). Philadelphia: Mosby.
18. Haupt, M. T., & Carlson, R. W. (1989). Anaphylactic and anaphylactoid reactions. In W. C. Shoemaker, S. Ayres, A. Grenvik, et al. (Eds.), *Textbook of critical care* (2nd ed.) (pp. 993-1002). Philadelphia: Saunders.

46

The Immunocompromised Patient

Debra Tribett

Critically ill patients are compromised hosts; that is, their host defense mechanisms are inadequate because of age, disease, therapy, or stress, and they are likely to develop nosocomial infection. The term *immunocompromised* or *immunosuppressed* refers specifically to persons whose immunological defense mechanisms are less effective than normal.[1] These patients characteristically develop opportunistic infections. Immunocompromised patients are being seen in critical care units in increasing numbers, including organ transplant recipients who receive immunosuppressive drugs, patients with neoplastic disease receiving chemotherapy or radiation treatment, and individuals with acquired immunodeficiency syndrome (AIDS). In addition, some patients have congenital defects of the immune system. (AIDS is discussed separately in Chapter 47.)

The immune system protects the host from an environmental barrage of potentially dangerous microorganisms. Infection and the potential for sepsis occur when some or all of its components are compromised.

The occurrence of sepsis has more than doubled in the last decade.[2] *Sepsis* is defined as the systemic response to infection.[2] Sepsis is ranked 13th among causes of death in the United States[3] and is a potentially increasing problem for the national health care system and specifically for patients and personnel in intensive care. A large percentage of patients with sepsis progress to septic shock, which is the most common cause of death in ICU patients in the United States.[4]

CLASSIFICATION AND DETECTION

Generally, immunodeficiencies are classified into primary or secondary categories. *Primary immunodeficiencies* are those whose primary cause is within the immune system. This type of immunodeficiency is often congenital—associated with a genetic defect or malfunction. *Secondary,* or *acquired, immunodeficiencies* are more common than primary and more likely to be encountered in critically ill adults. They are caused by a variety of diseases, conditions, or treatments.

Deficiencies are additionally named according to the component of the immune system that is affected. Defects in *nonspecific* immune function include phagocytic defects and complement deficiencies. *Specific* immune response deficiencies may be due to dysfunction of B cells, T cells, or both.

Because the cells of the immune system interact, a defect in one component of the system can affect other cells that are in normal supply and have normal function. For example, lack of macrophages impairs phagocytosis but also limits the processing of antigen and the activation of T4 lymphocytes and the specific immune response. An insufficiency of T4 helper cells diminishes cellular immunity but secondarily affects B cell activation and the humoral response. Refer to Chapter 43 for a review of the immune response.

Immunodeficiency is suspected when an individual experiences chronic, recurrent infections that do not respond to treatment. Skin rash, chronic diarrhea, recurrent abscess, osteomyelitis, growth failure in infants and children, and hepatosplenomegaly further suggest immune system defects. A wide range of tests are available to assess each specific component of the immune system. Refer to Chapter 44 for information about these tests.

Additionally, a deficiency in a specific immune system component tends to be associated with the development of characteristic infections. This may aid in the initial detection and diagnosis of an immune deficiency disorder. Phagocytic disorders are associated with systemic infection by uncommon bacterial organisms of low virulence and superficial skin or systemic infection by pyogenic organisms. Complement deficiencies also are associated with recurrent pyogenic infection. With defective B cell/humoral immunity, recurrent bacterial sinopulmonary infections such as otitis media or pneumonia are seen. Cell-mediated immunodeficiency leads to fungal, viral, or protozoal infections of the skin, mucous membranes, lungs, or other organs. Although common patterns of infection occur in patients with a specific immunodeficiency, these do not preclude infection with other microorganisms.

The development of infection in the critically ill, immunocompromised patient depends on the status of the host defenses and the patient's endogenous and exogenous microbial environment.[1] The composition of critically ill patients' flora depends on the environmental and pharmacological history. Infections that develop while the patient is in the community are related to organisms encountered as a part of geographical location, during travel, or in the work environment. Infections that develop during hospitalization may be caused by an organism common to a particular hospital and introduced during treatment, or they may be caused by organisms spread from patient to patient by staff or inanimate objects.

CONGENITAL/PRIMARY IMMUNODEFICIENCIES

Primary congenital deficiencies are rare. They may affect specific and/or nonspecific human defenses. Congenital defects are usually recognized during the first 2 years of life. They are suspected when recurrent infections become apparent. Correct diagnosis is imperative because improper treatment can be fatal, whereas proper therapy may correct the defect (Table 46-1).

Phagocytic Defects

Patients with phagocytic defects have a susceptibility to infection ranging from mild recurrent skin infections to severe overwhelming fatal systemic infections from bacteria or fungi.[5] Characteristically, they have little difficulty with viral or protozoal infections.[5]

Chronic granulomatous disease (CGD) is inherited as an X-linked trait that generally manifests itself by age 2. The formation of oxygen-dependent superoxide and hydrogen peroxide by neutrophils and monocytes is impaired by an absence of enzymes necessary to the process. The immune system of affected children can phagocytize but not kill and degrade catalase-positive bacteria such as *Staphylococcus aureus, Klebsiella* species, *Pseudomonas aeruginosa,* and *Escherichia coli* nor fungi such as *Candida, Aspergillus,* and *Nocardia* species.

The primary intervention in CGD is the aggressive

TABLE 46-1   Primary Immunodeficiencies

Immune System Component Impaired	Name of Disease or Syndrome
Inflammatory response	Chediak-Higashi syndrome
	Job's syndrome
	Chronic granulomatous disease
Complement system	Deficiency of C1, C2, C3, C4, C5, C6, C7, C8, or C9
Antibody/B cell (Humoral)	Bruton's X-linked infantile agammaglobulinemia
	Common variable immunodeficiency
	Duncan's syndrome
	Selective IgM deficiency
	Selective IgA deficiency
Cell-mediated/T cell	DiGeorge syndrome (congenital thymic aplasia)
	Chronic mucocutaneous candidiasis
Combined B cell and T cell	Severe combined immunodeficiency disease (SCID)
	Nezelof's syndrome
	Immunodeficiency with ataxia-telangiectasia
	Wiskott-Aldrich syndrome
	Immunodeficiency with short-limbed dwarfism

diagnosis and treatment of infection, although transfusion of white blood cells and bone marrow transplantation have been attempted. Survival has improved with early diagnosis and aggressive therapy, but most children die by age 5.[6] Some cases of survival into the second decade and beyond have been documented.[5]

Chediak-Hagashi syndrome is a multisystem autosomal recessive disorder. Patients manifest recurrent bacterial infections with *Staphylococcus aureus, Streptococcus pyogenes,* and organisms similar to those seen in chronic granulomatous disease. Other symptoms include hepatosplenomegaly, partial albinism, central nervous system abnormalities, and a high incidence of lymphoreticular malignancies.[5] Chemotaxis is abnormal, and phagocytosis is delayed. There is no treatment except for antibiotic administration specific for the infection. Increased susceptibility to infection, progressive neurological deterioration, and development of malignancy cause most affected children to die by age 5. Survival into the second and third decades has been documented.[5,6]

Job's syndrome consists of recurrent staphylococcal abscesses of the skin, lymph nodes, or subcutaneous tissue. Few signs or symptoms of systemic inflammation are present.[5] The first patients described with the syndrome were female fair-skinned redheads of Italian descent.[5] Job's syndrome shares similar laboratory features with hyper-IgE syndrome and may be the same disorder.[5,6]

Complement Deficiencies

Deficiency in each of the complement components has been demonstrated, although they are quite rare. Complement opsonizes and kills bacteria and facilitates neutrophil chemotaxis. Therefore, defects in complement are usually associated with bacterial infections, particularly gram-positive organisms. Deficiencies in complement are also associated with the autoimmune disease systemic lupus erythematosus. Defects in C3 are associated with infections of *Staphylococcus aureus*, *Streptococcus pneumoniae*, *Pseudomonas* species, and *Proteus* species.[1] Patients with defects in C6, C7, and C8 are subject to recurrent *Neisseria meningitides* and gonorrheal infection.[1] Therapy is supportive, focusing on treatment of the infection.

Humoral Defects

Humoral immune defects are perhaps the most frequent of the congenital-primary defects. They are characterized by an inability to produce quantitatively and qualitatively functional antibodies. B cells are usually deficient or dysfunctional, allowing extracellular bacteria to infect tissues and cause uninhibited disease. Symptoms range from absent to severe. The more severe the deficit of antibody the earlier the defect will be detected. The onset of the defect may not be apparent until adulthood.

In *Bruton's X-linked infantile agammaglobulinemia*, immunoglobulin synthesis cannot occur because circulating B cells and plasma are deficient. Pre-B cells are found in the bone marrow and the blood, but serum immunoglobulins of all five classes are absent. Prevalence is approximately 1 in 100,000 males.[7] Infants with Bruton's agammaglobulinemia are asymptomatic until maternal passive immunity dissipates (about 5 to 6 months of age). Bacteria such as *Streptococcus pneumoniae*, *Hemophilus influenzae*, *Staphylococcus aureus*, and *Neisseria meningitides* then cause recurrent infections that are generally easily controlled with antibiotics. This may delay the diagnosis. Some children present with chronic conjunctivitis, abnormal dental decay, or malabsorption. Those with malabsorption are frequently found to be infested with *Giardia lamblia*. Growth retardation may be associated with severe malabsorption.

Because the cell-mediated immune system is intact, these patients may respond normally to common childhood viral disease.[5] However, poliomyelitis and progressive encephalopathy have been reported after

the administration of live virus vaccine to patients with Bruton's agammaglobulinemia.[5]

Survival into the second and third decade with this disease has been reported, but severe and chronic infection in infancy may cause irreversible damage. Chronic lung disease may develop in patients with pulmonary infection. Meningitis may leave residual neurological deficits.

Continuous administration of antibiotics may be necessary to prevent or treat infections. The main therapy for the underlying hypogammaglobulinemia is administration of commercially prepared gamma globulin, which contains mostly IgG. Fresh frozen plasma is given to some patients to provide IgG, IgM, and IgA antibodies. The use of plasma from a single donor to decrease the risk of blood-borne infection has been suggested.[5]

Common variable immunodeficiency (CVI) is an acquired hypogammaglobulinemia that can manifest itself at any age. Typically, the patient does not become symptomatic until age 15 to 35.[5] Both sexes are equally affected. The clinical presentation tends to be similar to that of Bruton's agammaglobulinemia. The syndrome is characterized by persistent diminished antibody production, which allows recurrent bacterial infections. The cause of this immunodeficiency is unknown. Most patients have adequate numbers of mature B cells circulating in the peripheral blood. The disorder may be a result of a diminished synthesis or release of immunoglobulin.[5] Additionally, these individuals have a higher than normal incidence of abnormal T cell immunity that shows progressive deterioration.[5] Autoimmune disease, leukemia, lymphoma, and gastric carcinoma can develop.[5] Chronic sinopulmonary infections and bacterial conjunctivitis are seen in CVI; malabsorption and giardiasis may occur. Physical assessment demonstrates splenomegaly and marked lymphadenopathy. Treatment of CVI is identical to that of Bruton's agammaglobulinemia.

Patients with CVI may live into the seventh or eighth decade, and women with CVI have delivered normal babies.[5] Chronic lung disease is a major complication of chronic infection. Malignancy may develop. If cell-mediated immunity is impaired, infections characteristic of both T and B cell deficiencies may develop.

Duncan's syndrome is an X-linked recessive trait leading to a lymphoproliferative state. It is associated with Epstein-Barr virus (EBV). Patients appear healthy until they contract EBV. The EBV infection (infectious mononucleosis) may cause death secondary to severe liver disease, hepatitis, or lymphoma. Immunodeficiency of acquired hypogammaglobulinemia may develop in patients with infectious mononucleosis who do not die from the EBV infection.

Some patients may lack antibody to EBV despite documented infection. Additional birth defects in the cardiovascular system or central nervous system and agranulocytosis have been documented.

Selective deficiency of IgA is the most common of all immunodeficiencies occurring approximately 1 in every 600 to 800 persons.[5] In IgA deficiency, serum IgA levels are less than 5 mg/dl. Secretory IgA is also absent in most patients. Cell-mediated immunity is usually normal. The etiology of the IgA disorder is not known. An arrest in the development of B cells associated with a decreased synthesis or release of IgA are postulated.[5] Acquired IgA deficiency may be secondary to the administration of phenytoin or penicillamine, in most cases returning to normal when the drug is stopped.

Most patients with this deficiency manifest symptoms by the age 10. Sinopulmonary bacterial or viral infections are most common. Recurrent or chronic right middle lobe pneumonia also is a presenting symptom. Some patients are almost entirely asymptomatic, but long-term follow-up indicates they may develop significant disease over time.[5]

For unknown reasons, IgA deficiency occurs more often in persons who have allergies. The role of IgA as a mucosal defense against foreign antigens may explain why those lacking it are prone to allergic reactions. Celiac disease, ulcerative colitis, and regional (Crohn's) enteritis are associated with IgA deficiency. Autoimmune diseases such as systemic lupus erythematosus and rheumatoid arthritis occur in a significant number of patients with IgA deficiency.[5] Reticulum cell sarcoma, squamous cell carcinoma of the esophagus and lung, and thymoma have been reported in association with IgA deficiency.[5]

Patients may live to the sixth or seventh decade without severe disease. Treatment of patients with IgA deficiency focuses on antimicrobial therapy. There is no means of replacing IgA antibody. The use of gamma globulin should be avoided because it may increase the risk for the development of anti-IgA antibodies and subsequent anaphylactoid reactions.[5]

Cell-mediated/T Cell Deficiencies

Pure T cell–mediated deficiencies without secondary effects on the humoral immune system are rare because the humoral and cell-mediated systems are interdependent. Patients with T cell deficiencies are susceptible to acute or chronic infections from viral, fungal, and protozoal microorganisms.

In *DiGeorge syndrome,* or *congenital thymic aplasia,* the thymus is absent, abnormally located, or extremely small. Consequently T cell immunity is absent at birth, as indicated by lymphopenia with variable T cell function. Other characteristics include visible facial abnormalities and hypoparathyroidism within 24 hours of birth causing hypocalcemia that is resistant to standard therapy. Congenital heart defects lead to congestive heart failure. Some infants also have renal abnormalities. Infants who survive the immediate neonatal period become susceptible to recurrent or chronic pneumonia, *Candida* infection of the mucous membranes, diarrhea, and failure to thrive.

Early diagnosis may allow successful restoration of immune function, correction of hypoparathyroidism, and surgical correction of the cardiac anomalies. Transplantation of fetal thymus tissue to restore cell-mediated immunity has reportedly prolonged survival.[5] Thymosin, a thymic hormone, has also been used. Calcium with vitamin D or parathyroid hormone is administered to reverse hypoparathyroidism. Immediate surgical intervention to correct the cardiovascular defects may be needed and may precede thymic transplant. Congestive heart failure may be so severe that the infant may not survive cardiac surgery.

Chronic mucocutaneous candidiasis (CMC) is associated with a selective defect in T cell immunity that causes susceptibility to chronic *Candida* infections. T cell numbers and function toward other antigens are normal. B cell immunity is intact with normal production of antibody to *Candida*. The disorder may be inherited as an autosomal recessive trait affecting both males and females. It may be apparent by age 1 or may not become evident until the second decade. Endocrinopathy is also associated with this disorder.

Chronic *Candida* infection or the appearance of idiopathic endocrinopathy may be the presenting symptom of CMC. If chronic *Candida* appears first, it may be years before the endocrine dysfunction is evident. Other patients present with an endocrine disorder, such as hypoparathyroidism or Addison's disease, then subsequently develop the chronic candidiasis.

Candida infections affect the mucous membranes, skin, nails, and, in older females, the vagina. Severe candidal infections of the skin develop in a "stocking–glove" pattern and form granulomatous lesions. *Candida* laryngitis and esophagitis are common.[6] Patients with CMC do not usually develop systemic *Candida* infections and rarely develop other fungal infections.

Hypoparathyroidism and complications from hypocalcemia and tetany are frequent. Addison's disease may develop suddenly and is the major cause of death in patients with CMC.[5] Hypothyroidism, diabetes mellitus, and ovarian dysfunction may develop.

Chronic *Candida* infection of the skin and mucous membranes is very difficult to treat. Topical application of antifungal agents may prove ineffective, and oral or intravenous administration may be required.

No treatment to prevent the development of endocrine dysfunction exists; when an endocrinopathy is present, it is treated by standard hormone replacement therapy. Patients who survive CMC to the second or third decades usually experience extensive morbidity. Those with severe chronic skin and mucous membrane involvement suffer significant psychological and emotional problems.[5]

Combined B Cell and T Cell Immunodeficiencies

Combined immunodeficiencies range from partial to complete B and T cell dysfunction. This type of immunodeficiency usually presents in infancy. Bacterial, viral, protozoal, and fungal microorganisms can cause recurrent infections.

Severe combined immunodeficiency disease (SCID), in which both humoral and cell-mediated immunity are absent, is the most extreme of all the immunodeficiency states. SCID is characterized by susceptibility to virtually any microorganism. It is inherited in either an X-linked recessive or an autosomal recessive form. Its exact incidence is not known because many patients die before the disorder is diagnosed.[5] The basic immunological defect in SCID is unknown. It is postulated that bone marrow stem cells may lack the ability to differentiate into B and T cells or that the thymus and bursa equivalent tissue fail to develop normally.[5]

During the first few months of life, maternal IgG transferred in utero may protect the infant. Failure to thrive, chronic diarrhea, persistent oral candidiasis, pneumonia, chronic otitis media, and sepsis then occur.[5] Cytomegalovirus, *Pneumocystis carinii*, and *Candida albicans* are common agents of infection. Most patients succumb to overwhelming infection by age 2.[5] Infants with SCID who are vaccinated with live attenuated vaccines may die from progressive viremia; therefore, they should not receive the usual childhood immunizations.

The total lack of cell-mediated immunity places the infant with SCID at risk for the development of graft-versus-host disease. Blood transfusion may trigger this response. If transfusion is required, irradiated cells should be used to eliminate viable white blood cells from the transfusion.

Aggressive management to diagnose and treat infection in the patient with SCID is necessary. Gamma globulin therapy has been used, but if the diagnosis is made early, transplantation with histocompatible bone marrow may be employed. Transplantation with fetal liver or thymus tissue have had varying success. Experimental gene therapy is still being investigated.

Nezelof's syndrome combines T cell dysfunction with abnormal immunoglobulin synthesis. No uniform clinical or laboratory presentation has been identified. T cell deficiencies and B cell immunodeficiency of varying degree may occur in combination. Nezelof's syndrome occurs in both males and females and has no definite genetic pattern. The primary defect may be in the thymus.[5]

During infancy the syndrome manifests itself with recurrent fungal, viral, protozoal, and bacterial infections. Marked lymphadenopathy and hepatosplenomegaly are present. Sites of infection include the lungs, skin, and urinary tract. Failure to thrive, oral candidiasis, and chronic diarrhea are seen. Gram-negative sepsis may also develop.

Continuous antibiotic coverage and gamma globulin may be used. To avoid complications, administration of attenuated live vaccines should be avoided, and only irradiated blood should be used in transfusions. Bone marrow transplantation has not proved effective in patients with Nezelof's syndrome.[5] Thymus transplantation and the use of thymus factors have been reported to restore T cell and some B cell immunity. Children with Nezelof's syndrome have reportedly survived until age 18.[5] Chronic lung disease, chronic fungal infection, and development of malignancy are long-term complications.

Immunodeficiency with ataxia-telangiectasia is a multisystemic, progressive autosomal recessive disorder. The immunodeficiency variably involves abnormalities in both humoral and cell-mediated immunity. The neurological, vascular, and endocrine systems also are affected. The pathogenesis of this disorder is unexplained. Onset occurs by age 2, but signs and symptoms vary in the order and timing of their presentation. Recurrent bacterial or viral sinopulmonary infections may develop early in life or as late as age 10 years. Evaluation of immune system function may reveal a variety of defects. Normal numbers of circulating B cells may be present, yet IgA is absent or decreased or IgE may be absent. The number of T cells may be normal or decreased. There may be no response to delayed hypersensitivity skin testing. With age, the immunodeficiency progressively worsens. Patients may also develop lymphoma or acute lymphocytic leukemia. Death from this syndrome is usually secondary to overwhelming infection or malignancy.

This syndrome was originally thought to be primarily neurological in origin.[5] Cerebellar ataxia or muscle incoordination may be evident as early as 9 to 12 months or as late as 4 to 6 years. With age, additional neurological symptoms such as dysconjugate gaze, choreoathetoid movements, and extrapyramidal and posterior column signs develop. Most patients eventually develop mental retardation.

Telangiectasia, or dilatation of capillaries producing an angioma, usually develops between ages 2 and

9 years. Lesions appear on the conjunctivae, bridge of the nose, ears, and the antecubital fossae. Endocrine dysfunction is not evident until puberty. Children fail to develop secondary sexual characteristics.

A variety of approaches may be used in treating patients with immunodeficiency with ataxia-telangiectasia. Recurrent sinopulmonary infection must be treated with the appropriate antibiotic therapy for the causative organism. Continuous broad-spectrum antibiotic coverage is sometimes helpful. Use of gamma globulin may reduce the number of acquired infections. Transplantation of bone marrow or fetal thymus tissue may be attempted if compatible donors are available. Treatment with thymus factors also has been attempted.

Patients have survived until the fifth decade, but most patients with this syndrome die in their twenties. Those surviving to this age have severe morbidity with chronic lung disease, mental retardation, and physical debility.

Wiskott-Aldrich syndrome (WAS) is a progressive X-linked disorder involving a triad of immunodeficiency, eczema, and thrombocytopenia. Its cause is unknown. The patient has normal numbers of B cells but is unable to produce adequate amounts IgM and produces increased IgA and IgE. T cell immunity is initially intact but declines with age.

Bleeding secondary to thrombocytopenia is the first abnormality detected, sometimes at birth. Bleeding usually increases when the patient becomes infected. The bleeding tendency becomes less severe as the child grows older. Recurrent infection develops after 6 months of age. The male infant with WAS is prone to infection with pneumococci, meningococci, and *Hemophilus influenzae*. Pneumonia, meningitis, otitis media, and sepsis from these organisms may develop. With age, the susceptibility increases to include recurrent infections by viruses and other organisms. By the age of 1, eczema develops and is often secondarily infected. Other allergic manifestations may be associated with the eczema.

Aggressive treatment has improved long-term survival. Antibiotic therapy appropriate for the organism is used to treat infection. Thrombocytopenia cannot be treated with corticosteroid therapy because this increases the risk of infection. Infusions of fresh frozen plasma and gamma globulin have been used for passive protection from infection. Successful bone marrow transplants have been performed.

Patients with WAS may succumb to complications associated with bleeding and infection. As they live, longer chronic inflammation of the cornea secondary to viral infection, central nervous system lymphoreticular malignancies, and myelogenous leukemia may be seen.

Short-limbed dwarfism may be associated with three different types of immunodeficiency. All varieties are characterized by short, pudgy hands and limbs with large joints. The head is of normal size but may exhibit extra skin folds around the neck. Type I is a combined T and B cell immunodeficiency identical to that of SCID. These children rarely survive past age 1. Their susceptibility to viral, bacterial, protozoal, and fungal infections and their symptoms are similar to those seen in children with SCID. The type II immunodeficiency is a lack of T cell immunity with an intact humoral component. These patients have delayed hypersensitivity skin testing. They are susceptible to recurrent sinopulmonary infection and varicella. A malabsorption syndrome may be present. The hair may be light, thin, and sparse. Type II patients have been known to survive until the fourth or fifth decade, succumbing to overwhelming varicella infection. Absent B cell immunity with intact T cell immunity is characteristic of the type III form of immunodeficiency with short-limbed dwarfism. Patients with this form of immunodeficiency have a course similar to that of X-linked hypogammaglobulinemia. Pyogenic microorganisms lead to infection in the form of pneumonia, otitis media, meningitis, and sepsis. These patients may live into the second or third decade. Treatment of all three groups includes the administration of the drug effective against the organism causing the infection. Therapy for the underlying immune system defect is similar to those previously described.

SECONDARY/ACQUIRED IMMUNODEFICIENCY

Secondary, or acquired, immunodeficiency is more common than primary/congenital immunodeficiency and is likely to be encountered in the critically ill adult patient population. Acquired immunodeficiency occurs when a person who once had normal immune function loses, either progressively or suddenly, the ability to recognize and respond to foreign antigens. An acquired immunodeficiency can be secondary to infection, aging, malnutrition, injury, certain disease states, and iatrogenic therapy. Secondary immunodeficiency may be persistent, or it may resolve if the underlying condition is corrected.

Infections

Microorganisms that grow intracellularly can disrupt the immune system. Cell-mediated immunity can be affected by viral infection of immune system cells. Measles, influenza-varicella, mumps, and type I polio vaccine can disrupt the delayed hypersensitivity reaction and cell-mediated immunity. Disseminated chronic intracellular infectious diseases such as lepromatous leprosy, miliary tuberculosis, and disseminated coccidioidomycosis are associated with suppression of cell-mediated immunity. The exact mechanism causing the immune system dysfunction is not known.

The human immunodeficiency virus (HIV) has the ability to cause a persistent immune system dysfunction. This virus infects and kills T4 lymphocytes, resulting in susceptibility to infections from viral, fungal, protozoal, and slow-growing bacteria. Lack of cell-mediated immunity places the patient with HIV infection at risk for the development of malignancies such as Kaposi's sarcoma and Burkitt's lymphoma. Infection with HIV is on the rise in the United States and throughout the world. This immunodeficiency and its complications are discussed in detail in Chapter 47.

Nutritional Status

Both malnutrition and excessive nutrition are associated with an increased incidence of infection and altered immune response.[8] Immune system cells such as the lymphocytes have a high metabolic rate and must have an adequate supply of nutrients to replenish cellular constituents. When nutritional status is altered, vitamin, mineral, and other nutrient deficiencies can affect the function of the immune system.

Protein-calorie malnutrition is widespread in non-hospitalized populations as well as those with chronic illness. In the past, the thymus was used as an indicator of nutritional status because it was known to atrophy during protein-calorie malnutrition. It is now known that all lymphoid organs become smaller.[8] Lymphopenia, decreased cutaneous hypersensitivity, and an absence of complement components are seen. Most B cells and immunoglobulins are normal, but secretory IgA levels are low. Macrophages and neutrophils are normal in quantity but have impaired killing ability.

A high incidence of infection, particularly with mycobacteria, viruses, and fungi, occurs with protein-calorie malnutrition. Additionally, immunization may be unsuccessful when administered during a period of protein-calorie malnutrition.

An excess of nutrients, particularly in the form of lipids and carbohydrates, has been shown to be detrimental to immune system function.[8] Diets high in polyunsaturated fats appear to be more immunosuppressive than those high in saturated fat for reasons that are not clear. Hypercholesterolemia has been associated with impaired function of lymphocytes and reticuloendothelial cells. Hyperglycemia is associated with impaired phagocyte and lymphocyte functions. This is demonstrated in the increased susceptibility of diabetic individuals to infection and their greater mor-

bidity when infection develops as compared with normal controls.[8]

Malignancy

One of the functions of the immune system is immunosurveillance for abnormal tissue (tumor cells) and their subsequent destruction by normal immune cells. When the immune system fails, more malignancies develop. However, tumor cells can circumvent a normal immune system through a variety of means, growing into a malignancy that causes immunodeficiency and the development of opportunistic infection. The association between malignancy and opportunistic infection is so strong that any patient presenting with opportunistic infection should be evaluated for the presence of a malignancy, particularly one involving cells of the immune system.[7]

Leukemias are malignancies characterized by the abnormal maturation and accumulation of white blood cells. Tumor invades the bone marrow, inhibiting production of normal cells and, thereby, predisposing the patient to the development of infection. *Lymphomas* are solid tumors of the immune system. Lymph nodes or the spleen may be directly invaded by tumor, interrupting lymph flow. If the blood supply is impaired, necrosis can develop.

B cell malignancies include Burkitt's lymphoma, most chronic lymphocytic leukemias, and multiple myeloma. Deficient or abnormal immunoglobulins are produced by the abnormal cells in patients with these diseases. T cell acute lymphocytic leukemia is characterized by variable defects in both the humoral and cell-mediated components of the immune system. Hodgkin's disease is a malignant lymphoma of mixed cell type that causes anergy to a variety of antigens and is associated with a predisposition to opportunistic intracellular infection, particularly with varicella zoster virus.

If a malignancy does not cause an immunodeficiency, the therapies used to treat it often do. Cancer chemotherapy and irradiation are both immunosuppressive. The patient who has escaped opportunistic infection before the tumor was treated is at high risk for its development during these treatments. (See Chapter 48 for a more detailed discussion.)

Immunosuppressive Drugs in Transplantation

A growing number of patients are undergoing transplantation of organs and tissues. The success of these procedures is dependent on the intentional suppression of the patient's immune system so as to prevent rejection of the transplanted tissue. Administration of immunosuppressive agents is begun a few days prior to the transplant procedure and is continued for the life of the graft.[9] Different centers performing transplantation use different drug protocols combining several agents that suppress different components of the immune system. There are two basic protocols; one is prophylactic therapy and the other is for actual rejection episodes.

Corticosteroids affect nonspecific and specific humoral and cell-mediated responses by mechanisms that are not clearly understood. Azathioprine, originally used as the cancer chemotherapeutic drug 6-mercaptopurine, has a greater action on T cells than on B cells. Suppression of the bone marrow may cause leukopenia, thrombocytopenia, and anemia. Cyclosporine has a selective action on production of interleukin 1 and 2, preventing macrophages and T4 helper cells from attacking the graft. Antilymphocyte globulin (ALG) or antithymocyte globulin (ATG) are polyclonal animal antibody preparations given to transplant patients to coat the patient's lymphocytes and render them ineffective. ATG acts more specifically against T cells than ALG, which coats all lymphocytes. A murine monoclonal IgG antibody called OKT3 is used to depress T cell function by binding to a surface antigen on T cells. Once coated by the antibody, the cells are removed by the reticuloendothelial system. OKT3 also may alter the ability of T cells to recognize antigen.

The risks of immunosuppressive therapy are the development of infection and the significant increase in the incidence of malignancies as a result of decreased immunosurveillance. Each individual drug has additional side effects that may cause serious complications for the patient.

Aging

It is generally accepted that immune function declines with age.[10] As with other body systems, not every elderly person displays the same declines in immune function. Inheritance and environmental factors influence the changes manifested in each individual.

Involution of the thymus and a decline in thymic hormones are universally associated with aging.[8] By ages 45 to 50, only 5% to 10% of the thymus mass remains. By age 60, no detectable level of thymic hormone can be found in the serum.[8] With the loss of this hormone and of functioning thymus tissue, differentiation of immature lymphocytes fails to occur. The rate of decline can be identified by the increasing proportion of immature lymphocytes in the peripheral blood, although the total number of T and B lymphocytes remains unchanged. However, the proportions of T lymphocytes does appear to change. T4 helper cells increase, and T8 suppressor cells decrease. Activity of the cells lines also may be altered. T cell function may be diminished by an impaired capacity to produce and bind with the cytokine interleukin-2. The decline in T8 cells may account for the emergence of autoantibody and autoimmune disease in the elderly.[11] Delayed hypersensitivity reactions to common skin tests such as mumps and *Candida albicans* is impaired in elderly persons, possibly reflecting an altered response to the antigen, loss of immunological memory, or both.[8] Overall, cell-mediated immunity is considered to be depressed.[10]

The absolute number of B cells in the peripheral blood does not appear to change with age. Impairment of the humoral response seems to be related to a decrease in T4 helper activity.[8] Serum concentrations of IgA and IgG rise, while the concentration of IgM falls.[8] More autoantibodies to self-antigens are produced, but the antibody response to foreign antigens appears to decline.[8]

The increased susceptibility of elderly people to infections and neoplastic disease may be a consequence of immunosenescence, as may predisposition to certain viruses and bacterial infections.[12] Reactivation of herpes zoster and reexpression of tuberculosis are examples of microorganisms that may reappear in the elderly.

Age-related changes in the structure and function of the natural barriers to infection may also contribute to an increased susceptibility to infection. Other acquired or secondary causes of immunodeficiency such as malnutrition and stress may contribute to the immunodeficiency associated with aging.

Stress

Physiological stress caused by hypoperfusion and tissue ischemia in critically ill patients is known to stimulate the adrenal cortex and activate the sympathetic nervous system. Release of glucocorticoids and catecholamines increases serum levels of these and other hormones and neuroendocrine factors.

Specific receptors for many neuroendocrine factors, such as ACTH, have been identified on the surfaces of monocytes and lymphocytes.[13] Activated lymphocytes and monocytes are capable of synthesizing and secreting the same messengers for which they bear receptors. Lymphocytes have been shown to produce ACTH and other hormones.[13] Cytokines produced by lymphocytes and monocytes, such as interleukin-2, have also been shown to increase circulating levels of ACTH and cortisol.[13] It is postulated that because the immune system and the neuroendocrine systems produce and bear receptors for similar substances, they could affect each other and communicate reciprocally.[13] The degree to which neuroendocrine–immune system interaction affects host defenses in the critically ill patient has not yet been clearly defined.

The effects of endogenous glucocorticoids on the immune system are known to inhibit the inflammatory response and specific immune system activity.

Although ACTH acts on the immune system in part through stimulation of the adrenal cortex to produce glucocorticoids, it may have some direct immunosuppressive actions on the immune system as well. ACTH has been shown to suppress both antibody formation and gamma-interferon production by T lymphocytes.[13]

The patient in a critical care unit is subjected to psychological as well as physiological stress. Research continues to elucidate the complex interaction of the psychological, neurological, endocrine, and immune systems. Normal subjects experiencing psychological stress have been shown to demonstrate immune system suppression.[14] The stress levels of patients in the critical care environment no doubt contribute to the level of immune system suppression caused by the release of endogenous steroids. Modulation of patient stress may be a method of promoting host defenses and preventing infection in the critically ill patient.

INFECTION

The critically ill patient with a compromised immune system is at tremendous risk for the development of infection. If infection develops, it can quickly progress to life-threatening severity. Fever in the critically ill immunosuppressed patient should be presumed to be a sign of infection until proven otherwise.[1]

Identification of Source

Evaluation to determine the location of infection may be hampered by the condition of the patient and the ICU environment. Altered mental status or intubation may prevent the patient from communicating symptoms. Physical examination may be impaired by mechanical devices or hemodynamic instability. Diagnostic procedures such as magnetic resonance imaging, easily performed in the ambulatory patient, may be impossible in the critically ill patient because of the limitations on equipment and observation imposed by this technique.

Intravascular lines in a febrile immunosuppressed patient must always be suspected as a source of infection. The results of blood cultures drawn from a suspected line and from a percutaneous venipuncture are likely to be all positive, all negative, or suspected of being contaminated during the sampling process.[1] The yield of positive blood cultures in patients identified as clinically septic is less than 50%.[15] The cost-effectiveness of Gram stain and culture of line tips remains controversial.[1] Strong consideration should be given to removing lines that have been in place for more than 72 hours in an immunosuppressed, febrile, hemodynamically stable patient.[1] If the patient is hemodynamically unstable or appears septic, all lines should be replaced using new sites.[1]

The *respiratory system* must be evaluated as a potential source of infection. Aspiration pneumonia is the leading cause of nosocomial infection acquired in the ICU.[1] The immunosuppressed patient is also at greater risk for the development of opportunistic pneumonia from organisms that would probably not cause an infection in a patient with a normal immune system. *Pneumocystis carinii* is an example of such an organism.

The upper respiratory system should not be overlooked. Mucosal lesions can produce localized sites of infection, particularly in the neutropenic patient. Sinus infection must be considered in patients with nasogastric or nasal endotracheal tubes in place. Radiography of the sinuses may be needed. Chest x-ray and sputum culture are performed to evaluate the lower airway for infection. A bronchoscopy with bronchoalveolar lavage and transbronchial biopsy may also be indicated in determining the source of pneumonia in the immunocompromised patient.[16] If a pleural effusion is detected, a thoracentesis should be a part of a routine fever evaluation if the effusion is accessible.[1]

The *gastrointestinal system* must be evaluated for a potential source of infection. Radiography or CT scan may be required to determine if viscus perforation has occurred. Diarrhea must be evaluated for the presence of *Clostridium difficile,* a common nosocomial infection in patients who have been receiving broad spectrum antibiotics.[1] Neutropenic patients must also be carefully examined for the presence of a perirectal abscess as the source of fever.

The *urinary tract* is a common source of infection in critically ill patients. Urine cultures and a physical examination of the genitourinary tract are indicated. If microorganisms are not found in culture, blockage of the ureter must also be considered.[1]

Neurological evaluation is often difficult in critically ill patients because of their level of consciousness and the use of medications causing sedation or skeletal muscle paralysis. CT scans are often useful to detect mass lesions prior to performance of a lumbar puncture. Abscesses of the brain occur more frequently than meningitis in the immunosuppressed patient population.

A *cardiac etiology* for fever in the immunocompromised patient can be endocarditis. Although unusual in the ICU, it does occur in patients with long IV catheters such as a pulmonary artery catheter. If the patient has a prosthetic heart valve, endocarditis is more likely. The incidence of bacterial endocarditis appears to be low in ICU patients, but fungal endocarditis is possible in patients who have received broad spectrum antibiotic coverage and whose intravascular lines have been infected with fungi.[1]

Medical Management

The effectiveness of therapy depends on the choice of a proper antimicrobial agent, drainage of any sites of purulent collections, and augmentation of host defense mechanisms.[1] The drug regimen must have in vitro activity against the proven or likely organism causing the infection. Empiric drug antimicrobial therapy depends on the likely site of infection and the patient's underlying disease.[1]

The pharmacokinetics and the tissue distribution of the drug should be considered by the physician making the selection. Many critically ill patients have impaired renal or hepatic function. It is particularly important to measure antibiotic drug levels. Biweekly assessment of peak and trough levels should be performed for any patient with unstable renal function and volume of distribution.[1] Selection of an antibiotic should also consider the cost of therapy, using agents that have comparable efficacy and toxicity and lower cost rather than a more expensive new drug with no additional clinical benefit to the patient.[1]

The correct selection of antibiotics by the physician is important to the treatment of infection, but it is the nursing administration of these drugs that delivers the treatment. Prompt administration of antibiotics to the infected patient is imperative. Even properly selected agents will not be effective for 24 to 48 hours. Precise timing of doses, complete administration of the drugs, and obtaining samples for drug level determination are often nursing responsibilities. These are key to the success of the antibiotic regimen.

Antibiotics alone may not improve the patient's status. Drainage or removal of the nidus of infection is necessary. The ability to do this is contingent upon finding such a source and the stability of the patient to withstand the procedure.

Augmentation of the patient's inflammatory and immunological defenses by withholding antiinflammatory or immunosuppressive therapy may or may not be possible due to the underlying condition of the patient. Transfusion with granulocytes has not been clearly demonstrated to improve the outcome in neutropenic patients.[1] Likewise, the use of lymphocyte transfusions has not been shown to reconstitute immunological function.[1] Bone marrow transplantation may restore immune function in some patients, but its availability and complexity limit its usefulness in management of acute situations. Intravenous gamma globulin or complement from fresh frozen plasma may improve the prognosis in patients with specific deficiencies or acute infection.

NURSING CARE MANAGEMENT

The potential for life-threatening infection is the major patient problem facing nurses caring for critically ill, immunocompromised patients. The patient's individual risk factors based on the underlying condition and immune system function, coupled with the risks for nosocomial infection from invasive therapies, challenges the nurse to plan and deliver care aimed toward preventing infection. Realistically, prevention of all infection in this patient population may be impossible. Therefore, the nurse must be as meticulous in patient assessment as in the performance of infection control procedures and aseptic technique. Recommended care for the patient with the potential for infection is presented below.

■ NURSING DIAGNOSIS

High risk for infection, related to a compromised immune system, due to:
- Impaired first-line of natural defenses (e.g., breaks in epithelium, skin, or mucous membranes; loss of normal flora; impaired or absent protective reflexes)
- Impaired second line of defense or nonspecific defenses (e.g., neutropenia, malnutrition, use of antiinflammatory agents)
- Impaired third line of defense of specific acquired immune response (e.g., congenital or acquired immune deficiencies in humoral or cellular immunity, HIV infection, use of immunosuppressive agents)
- Exposure to unusually virulent, invasive, or large inoculum of organisms (e.g., field trauma, development of resistant strain of organism)

OUTCOME STANDARD AND CRITERIA

Nosocomial infection is absent as evidenced by:
- Absence of signs and symptoms of localized infection (redness, tenderness, swelling, purulent drainage)
- Absence of signs and symptoms of systemic infection (fever, tachycardia, tachypnea, elevated or depressed WBC count with >10% bands)
- Early detection of systemic inflammatory response (SIRS), sepsis, and localized infection

NURSING INTERVENTIONS

- Monitor patient for signs and symptoms of inflammation or infection:

  Check temperature (avoiding rectal route in neutropenic patients) at regular intervals and monitor trend for elevation or hypothermia

  Interpret CBC with differential for elevations or decreases in WBC with left shift (increased percentage bands) neutropenia, and calculate absolute count for neutropenic patient

  Review trends in hemodynamic parameters; monitor for tachycardia, decreased blood pressure, decreased SVR, increased cardiac output/index

  Observe respiratory system for tachypnea, change in characteristics of sputum production, chest x-ray for infiltrations or consolidation, decreased $PaCO_2$, and hypoxemia

  Observe level of consciousness for changes or decreases in mental status or total Glasgow Coma Score

Assess for signs of impaired tissue perfusion such as urinary output <0.5 ml/kg/hr and increased lactic acid levels

Inspect insertion sites of all invasive devices used in care and monitoring of the patient for localized signs of inflammation, infection, or trauma to tissues at least once a day

Inspect skin folds, axillae, groin, and perineal areas for evidence of skin irritation, breakdown, or infections at least once a day

Inspect oral cavity for lesions at least once a day

Inspect any wounds or surgical incisions for signs of infection or changes in appearance of drainage at least once a day

Palpate cervical, axillary, and inguinal lymph nodes for enlargement or tenderness

Review results of any cultures taken from patient

Follow-up any patient complaint of pain with a full assessment and communicate findings to physician

Examine all secretions and excretions for suspicious changes

- Institute infection control measures to prevent nosocomial infection:

Enforce handwashing before patient contact for all health care workers, family, and other visitors

Screen all health care workers, family, and visitors for infectious illness before contact with patient. No one with fever, upper respiratory symptoms, diarrhea, open skin lesions, or recent exposure to contagious disease (e.g., childhood diseases) should care for or visit patient

If one-to-one nursing assignment is not feasible for patient, ensure nurse caring for patient is not caring for another patient with an infectious organism

Institute isolation appropriate for any patient infection

Protective or reverse isolation may be instituted by protocol in certain transplant recipients in the acute phase of treatment

Adhere to strict aseptic technique in all invasive procedures and care of invasive IVs, monitoring lines, etc.

Prohibit fresh flowers and plants from patient room to limit reservoirs for organism growth

Change fluids used in care of patient or IV infusions every 24 hours

Change tubings and dressings on invasive devices according to CDC recommendations or specific hospital policy

Collaborate with physicians and other health care workers to minimize invasive procedures and venipunctures and to avoid unnecessary procedures

Track all intravascular lines for site and length of time each has been inserted. Collaborate with physicians for line change and site rotations

Obtain cultures of any suspicious drainage or secretions

- Support adequate nutritional intake:

Collaborate with family and dietitian to maximize oral intake of diet appropriate for patient condition

In neutropenic patients, eliminate fresh uncooked fruits and vegetables from diet

If patient cannot eat, attempt enteral nutrition, even at very low flow rates (10 ml/hr) to attempt to prevent translocation of gut organisms into the circulation

Collaborate with physician to institute peripheral or total parenteral nutrition in patients whose GI tract cannot be used to supply adequate caloric intake

Monitor trend in daily weights

- Institute measures to support first-line or natural defenses

Maintain integrity of the skin:

Reposition patient every 2 hours using techniques to minimize friction and shearing forces

Lubricate and massage dry skin as needed

Use pressure-reducing devices (e.g., special mattress, specialized beds)

Use skin preparation before using tape

Use adhesive remover to facilitate dressing removal

Use skin barriers for incontinent patients

Provide perineal care, cleansing of axillae and other skin folds daily and as necessary; use blow dryer as needed to eliminate moisture after bathing

Use incontinence pads or briefs that absorb moisture and present a quick-drying surface to the skin

Use scissors, electric razors, or depilatory for hair removal

Avoid trauma to mucous membranes:

Provide frequent oral care to NPO patient and after meals to those able to eat; apply lubricant to lips as needed

Avoid alcohol-containing solutions for mouth care

Use chlorhexidine mouth rinses in neutropenic patients

Cleanse nares and secure any nasal tubes to prevent pressure necrosis

Reposition oral endotracheal tubes daily and secure to prevent pressure necrosis

Do not use rectal temperature probes, rectal tubes, or suppositories; avoid rectal digital examinations

Collaborate with physicians for administration of prophylaxis for gastric mucosa

Encourage pulmonary toilet:

Have nonintubated patient deep breathe and use incentive spirometer every 2 hours while awake and immobilized

Follow deep breathing with coughing to mobilize secretions

Maintain airway humidification with administration of oxygen

Encourage patient hydration

Maintain normal bowel and bladder elimination:

Implement individualized regimen to prevent constipation

Encourage high fluid intake unless contraindicated by other patient problems

Provide activity as appropriate to patient situation

Use condom catheters and frequent, scheduled offering of bedpan to incontinent patients rather than resorting to bladder catheterization

Minimize patient stress:

Administer pain medications and sedation to patient as necessary to control pain

Use other comfort measures—positioning, massage—to facilitate pain control

Use music, relaxation tapes, guided imagery, or other techniques to assist with patient stress reduction

Group activities and nursing care measures to provide uninterrupted rest periods during the day and at night for sleep

Administer medications to facilitate sleep at night as indicated

Eliminate ICU environmental stimuli as much as possible

- Provide patient and family with education appropriate to their level of understanding and situation, which may include:

Answering questions related to their lack of knowledge regarding disease and treatment

Explanation of risk factors for infection

Teaching signs and symptoms of infection

Providing rationale for interventions used in patient care

Practice performing specific self-care procedures, such as reading a thermometer or oral hygiene

Drug administration and side effects for immunosuppressant agents or antibiotics

REFERENCES

1. Masur, H. (1987). Infections in critically ill immunosuppressed patients. In J. E. Parrillo, & H. Masur (Eds.), *The critically ill immunosuppressed patient* (pp. 215-242). Rockville, MD: Aspen.
2. American College of Chest Physicians/Society of Critical Care Medicine Consensus Conference Committee. (1992). Definitions for sepsis and organ failure and guidelines for the use of innovative therapies in sepsis. *Critical Care Medicine, 20,* 864-874.
3. National Center for Health Statistics. (1989). *Annual summary of births, marriages, divorces, and deaths: United States, 1988.* Hyattsville, MD: U.S. Department of Health and Human Services.
4. Parrillo, J. E., Parker, M. M., Natanson, C., et al. (1990). Septic shock in humans: advances in the understanding of pathogenesis, cardiovascular dysfunction, and therapy. *Annals of Internal Medicine, 113,* 227-242.
5. Ammann, A. J. (1984). Immunodeficiency diseases. In D. P. Sites, J. D. Stobo, H. H. Fundenberg, et al. (Eds.), *Basic and clinical immunology* (pp. 384-422). Los Altos, CA: Lange.
6. Griffin, J. P. (1990). Primary and secondary immunodeficiency disorders: Preventing infection. In *Immunologic problems* (pp. 98-121). Springhouse, PA: Springhouse.
7. Golightly, M. (1990). Clinical application: Immunodeficiency disorders. In J. T. Dolan (Ed.), *Critical care nursing: Clinical management through the nursing process* (pp. 1213-1226). Philadelphia: Davis.
8. Lahita, R. G. (1984). Effects of sex hormones, nutrition and aging on the immune response. In D. P. Sites, J. D. Stobo, H. H. Fundenberg, et al. (Eds.), *Basic and clinical immunology* (pp. 288-311). Los Altos, CA: Lange.
9. Fedric, I. N. (1990). Immunosuppressive therapy in renal transplantation. *Critical Care Nursing Clinics of North America, 2,* 123-131.
10. Cohen, F. L. (1989). Immunologic impairment, infection, and AIDS in the aging patient. *Critical Care Nursing Quarterly, 12,* 38-45.
11. Petrucci, K. E., Booth-Blaemire, E., & Watson, K. (1989). Aging, immunity, and critical care nursing. *Critical Care Nursing Clinics of North America, 1,* 787-795.
12. Fulmer, T. T., & Walker, M. K. (1992). *Critical care nursing of the elderly* (pp. 32-47). New York: Springer.
13. Abraham, E. (1992). Physiologic stress and cellular ischemia: Relationship to immunosuppression and susceptibility to sepsis. *Critical Care Medicine, 19,* 613-618.
14. Locke, S. E. (1982). Stress, adaptation, and immunity: Studies in humans. *General Hospital Psychiatry, 4,* 49-58.
15. Bone, R. C. (1991). Let's agree on terminology: Definitions of sepsis. *Critical Care Medicine, 17,* 973-976.
16. Ognibene, F., Pass, H. I., Roth, J. A., et al. (1987). The diagnosis and therapy of respiratory disease in the immunosuppressed host. In J. E. Parrillo, & H. Masur (Eds.), *The critically ill immunosuppressed patient* (pp. 39-80). Rockville, MD: Aspen.

47

The Patient with Human Immunodeficiency Virus (HIV)

Debra Tribett

Since the first U.S. reports of unexplained immune system failure in adult males in 1981, the world has experienced an epidemic of infection by the deadly virus now known as human immunodeficiency virus (HIV). HIV is an equal opportunity disease, affecting young and old, men and women, heterosexuals, bisexuals, and homosexuals, the wealthy and the impoverished, and all races. The cell-mediated immune system eventually becomes suppressed, and the person with HIV develops a variety of opportunistic infections, malignancies, or both.

Knowledge about HIV has grown through clinical experience and research, yet many questions go unanswered, and no cure is available to those infected. However, therapies have been developed that slow the effects of the virus and offer treatment for the unusual infections that occur in the patient with HIV.

Critical care nurses were among the first in the nursing profession to be involved in the care of patients with HIV infection because many patients developed acute respiratory failure requiring intubation, mechanical ventilation, and a stay in the intensive care unit (ICU). Now the entire health care system today is involved in the prevention and care of HIV patients. Nurses practicing in all hospital specialties and in home care must be fully informed about HIV, how it is spread, and how to curtail transmission of the virus. As educators of patients, families, and neighbors, nurses can communicate current, factual information to the public.

This chapter provides information concerning HIV and its manifestations that was current at the time of writing. Discussion of medical therapy is limited to medications with FDA approval and does not attempt

to evaluate the multitude of research protocols underway. Nursing management and concerns unique to this patient population are presented. The immunocompromised patient with HIV is susceptible to the development of infection. Refer to Chapter 46 to review the nursing care related to the nursing diagnosis, potential for infection.

HUMAN IMMUNODEFICIENCY VIRUS (HIV)

Discovery

When acquired immunodeficiency syndrome (AIDS) was first being manifested in various parts of the world, researchers suspected a viral etiology. Many groups tried to isolate the cause of the syndrome. In May of 1983, Luc Montagnier and his team at the Pasteur Institute in Paris reported their discovery of the lymphadenopathy virus (LAV). In 1984, at the National Institutes of Health, Robert Gallo and his group announced the isolation of an organism they called human T cell lymphotropic virus III (HTLV-III). Other research groups used the term AIDS-related retrovirus (ARV). Controversy existed about who first identified the virus and whether the viruses discovered were the same. An international compromise was reached, and the virus causing AIDS was named human immunodeficiency virus type 1, or HIV-1. In May 1992, Montagnier and Gallo agreed that the viruses they had isolated were the same and that both had originally come from Montagnier's laboratory.[1]

Since 1985, a second variety of HIV, human immunodeficiency virus type 2 (HIV-2), has been identified.[2] It is most prevalent in Western Africa but has been reported in Central Africa, Western Europe, Canada, and Brazil. It is rare in the United States. The HIV-2 virus is also responsible for causing AIDS.

Structure

HIV has been identified as one of a category of viruses called *retroviruses*. The nucleus of a retrovirus has no DNA, only RNA. To replicate, it must use the DNA of the cell it infects. The virus uses the enzyme reverse transcriptase to "reverse transcribe" the viral RNA into DNA, which then integrates itself into the host cell's DNA.

The structure of HIV has been identified as two strands of RNA surrounded by a cylindrical inner protein core, or *capsid* (Figure 47-1). The molecular weight of this protein core is 24,000. It is referred to as p24, or the gag protein. The outer lipid envelope has balloonlike external surface glycoprotein antigens called gp120. The gp120 has an anchoring segment inside the cell wall, called gp41. The outer envelope region can create variants of HIV within the same individual over time.[3]

Replication

The HIV *virion*, or viral particle, can replicate only when it enters a cell and uses the reproductive apparatus of the cell to reproduce. When HIV enters the body, it preferentially infects cells with the CD4 surface molecule. The T4 helper lymphocyte is the predominant target, but the monocyte/macrophage and other cells may be infected (see upper box to the right).

The surface glycoprotein, gp120, of the HIV binds with the CD4 molecule. The CD4 molecule acts like a receptor for the virus, and the virus fuses to the cell. The virus is uncoated, and the viral RNA enters the cell. The enzyme reverse transcriptase transcribes the viral RNA into DNA. Some of this new DNA integrates itself into the DNA in the nucleus of the host cell, forming what is referred to as a *provirus*.[3] Some of the new DNA may remain in the cytoplasm of the target cell.

The provirus has a reprogrammed nucleus allowing for the production of more infected cells during cell replication. When the provirus cell divides during normal cell division, the proviral DNA is left in its progeny cells. This may explain why an individual with HIV infection is infected for life.[3]

Once infected, the target cell is infected for the lifetime of the cell. The provirus may remain latent for variable lengths of time before it is activated to produce new virus. The stimulus for the activation of HIV production is called a cofactor. Research has identified infection with other viruses and stimulation by endogenous cytokines as activators of HIV-in-

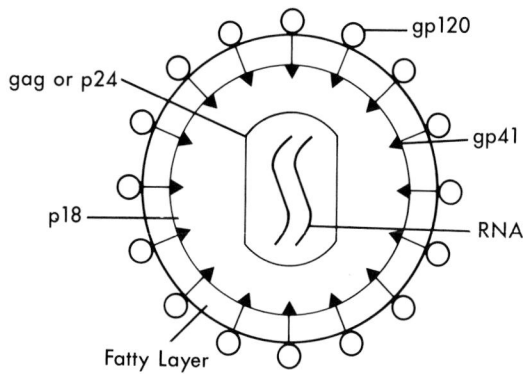

Figure 47-1   Structure of the human immunodeficiency virus (HIV).

Target Cells for HIV Infection

T4 lymphocytes
Monocytes/macrophages
Dendritic cells
Langerhans cells
Promyelocytic cell lines
Epstein-Barr virus–transformed B cells
Microglial cells

Cofactors for Activation of HIV Infected Cells

Herpes simplex virus (HSV)
Cytomegalovirus (CMV)
Epstein-Barr virus (EBV)
Hepatitis B virus (HBV)
Mycoplasma
Interleukin-6 (IL-6)
Tumor necrosis factor-α (TNF-α)
Granulocyte macrophage—colony-stimulating factor (GM-CSF)

---

fected cells into production of HIV virions. The microorganism *Mycoplasma* is suspected as a cofactor by Dr. Montagnier.[1] Many other exogenous and endogenous cofactors probably exist (see lower box above).

When the HIV-infected cell is activated, the cell nucleus transcribes messenger and genomic RNA, leading to the synthesis of new viral proteins. The viral proteins and RNA assemble on the cell surface and bud out as mature HIV virions. The budding out of the new HIV virus creates holes in the cell wall, allowing leakage of intracellular contents and leading to the death of the cell.[4]

HIV AND THE IMMUNE SYSTEM

HIV causes a syndrome characterized by a gradual, progressive, irreversible deterioration of the immune system. In infected individuals, HIV attacks the immune system before clinical signs and symptoms develop.

Cell-mediated Immune Function

The T4 lymphocyte with its CD4 surface molecule is the primary target of the virus. During the first few weeks after initial infection with HIV, the number of T4 cells drops significantly.[3] The T4 count then returns almost to preinfection levels, but subsequently a gradual destruction of T4 lymphocytes ensues. This rate of reduction in T4 cells increases as the disease progresses.

The decrease in lymphocytes can be detected as lymphopenia on the differential count of a complete blood count. Specific measurement of T4 lymphocytes gives more information about the effects of HIV on the immune system. Normal T4 counts range from 600 to 1,200 per mm³. When a patient's T4 cell count drops to 200/mm³, opportunistic infection is likely to occur. Patients with an advanced case of HIV infection may demonstrate a T4 count of less than 20/mm³. The loss of T4 lymphocytes reverses the normal 2 : 1 T4/T8 lymphocyte ratio.

It is ironic that the HIV virus attacks and destroys the very cell whose function (cell-mediated immunity) is to protect the body from viruses. The T4 cell's vital role is orchestration of the entire specific immune response. Loss of this important cell line further affects other aspects of the immune system.

The function of the remaining T4 cells is also impaired, and their ability to respond to antigen stimulation diminishes. Without antigen stimulation, the T4 cell does not produce lymphokine mediators that activate other immune system cell activity. This, in turn, affects the function of other components of the immune system and their ability to respond normally to antigens.

Anergy, or decreased delayed hypersensitivity reactions to common antigens, is seen in patients with HIV infection. Impairment of cell-mediated immunity leads to susceptibility to infections and diseases that are normally handled by this component of the specific immune response. Opportunistic infection with viruses, fungi, protozoa, and slow-growing bacteria develops in the HIV patient. Impaired immunosurveillance leads to the development of a variety of malignancies.

Humoral Immune Function

Another confusing aspect of the immune response in HIV-infected individuals involves the humoral activity of B cells. Impressive amounts of antibody to the HIV virus are produced, but it does not seem to inhibit the spread of HIV. Loss of the induction function of the T4 lymphocyte leads to a decreased ability to mount antibody response when exposed to new antigens. This places the HIV patient at risk of infection by antigens new to his or her immune system. When receiving immunizations such as for influenza, the HIV patient may not develop adequate immunity.

The regulatory effects of the T4 lymphocyte are also impaired. This malfunction allows the plasma cells to overproduce immunoglobulins, leading to a polyclonal hypergammaglobulinemia demonstrated serologically by elevated levels of total immunoglobulin, with increases in the IgG and IgA categories.[5] In most patients, this hyperactivity results in elevated levels immune complexes in the serum.[5] Clinical symptoms may be associated with these immune complexes; thrombocytopenia secondary to immune complex destruction of platelets is the most common problem.[6] Paradoxically, this hypergammaglobulinemia coexists with the inability to mount a humoral response to new antigens.

Monocyte/Macrophage Function

The monocytes/macrophages may be directly infected by the HIV virus. They are not destroyed by the virus as are the T4 lymphocytes; instead, they may act as a reservoir for the HIV virus in the body.[2] The function of monocytes/macrophages is affected in the patient with HIV. Abnormal functions include decreased chemotaxis, intracellular killing after phagocytosis, production of interleukin-1, and expression of class II HLA antigens.[6] Monocyte/macrophage dysfunction occur through a lack of lymphokine stimulation by the T4 cells or as a direct result of HIV infection of the cells. The loss of normal monocyte activity contributes to patient susceptibility to parasitic and other intracellular infections.[6]

TESTING FOR HIV

Today, the most common method of testing for HIV is based on the detection of HIV-specific antibody response to the virus. Detection of the antibody indicates that the individual (except neonates) has been directly exposed to the HIV virus and has produced an immune system response. Most people develop an antibody response within 6 weeks to 3 months after exposure, but in some cases, it may take 6 to 12 months for the antibody to be detected.

The *enzyme-linked immunoabsorbent assay* (ELISA) is the most widely used test to detect the presence of antibody to HIV. This test was first developed to screen blood and blood products prior to transfusion. It is still used for this purpose, but it is also used for screening, surveillance, and early diagnosis of HIV infection.

A normal result for the ELISA is nonreactive.[7] Because it was developed to screen blood, the ELISA is a very sensitive test. A false-positive, or reactive, ELISA can occur in multiparous women, recipients of multiple blood transfusions, or in other conditions causing increased presence of circulating antibody in the blood.

If a positive ELISA result is obtained, the test is repeated. If two or more ELISA tests on the same specimen are positive, the Western Blot or an immunofluorescence assay (IFA) is performed to confirm the ELISA test. A person with a positive ELISA confirmed by the Western Blot or IFA is considered positive for antibody to HIV. This means the patient is infected and is also infectious.

Because HIV-1 and HIV-2 are closely related, tests for antibody to one may cross-react with antibody to the other. The ELISA for HIV-1 has a sensitivity for HIV-2 of 60% to greater than 90%.[2]

A negative ELISA does not guarantee that the subject is not infected with HIV, especially if the exposure has been recent. During the window of time between exposure to the virus and antibody production to HIV, a nonreactive ELISA may be obtained. The person with HIV is infectious to others during this time, even though the screening test is negative.

Methods for detecting HIV other than the ELISA may be used. Detection of HIV by culture, through viral antigens in the blood (the p24 antigen assay), and by HIV gene amplification (polymerase chain reaction) are used mainly in clinical research. Most of these tests are still being developed, and their availability is limited.

Testing for HIV must be carried out after an *informed consent* has been obtained from the person to be tested. It should not be carried out without the prior knowledge of the person. It is essential that counseling precede and follow the test. The clinical and behavioral implications of the test results and the accuracy of the test results should be discussed with the patient. If necessary, the patient should be encouraged to make behavioral changes for the protection of self and others.

The person tested must also be informed who may have access to the test results. Precautions must be taken to maintain *confidentiality* and to prevent inappropriate disclosure of information. Positive test results must be reported to the state public health authorities according to the regulations established in each state.[7] Each hospital or testing facility has its own procedures for maintaining confidentiality of HIV testing information, and the nurse must be familiar with both hospital and state requirements.

THE SPREAD OF HIV INFECTION
Modes of Transmission

Although HIV infection is considered a global epidemic, it is not spread by casual contact. The HIV virus is transmitted during sexual intercourse via semen and vaginal secretions, by intravenous use of blood-contaminated needles, by transfusion of HIV-contaminated blood or blood products, or from mother to baby during the perinatal period or through breast milk. Although the HIV virus has been isolated from other body fluids such as saliva, tears, urine, cerebrospinal fluid, and amniotic fluid, there is no evidence of transmission via contact with these fluids. Transmission through organ and tissue transplantation has been reported.

The transmission of HIV caused by contaminated blood and blood products is fortunately declining. Since March 1985, all blood donations have been tested for HIV. Stringent assessment of donors for participation in high-risk behaviors and exclusion of donors from countries where AIDS is endemic have also been implemented.

High-risk Groups

In the United States, the first reported cases of AIDS were in homosexual males. High-risk groups in this country have been identified as homosexual or bisexual males; intravenous drug users; and those having unprotected heterosexual, bisexual, or homosexual intercourse with a known HIV-positive person or someone in a high-risk group.

Risks to Health Care Workers

Following the earliest reports of AIDS in the United States and before the HIV virus was identified, transmission of AIDS was likened to transmission of hepatitis B virus (HBV). Since health care workers were documented to be at significantly increased risk of occupational infection with HBV, the potential for occupational transmission of AIDS produced fear and anxiety among health care workers.[8] Subsequent identification of the HIV virus and clinical experience have demonstrated the risk of occupational transmission of HIV to be extremely small.[8]

The earliest patients with what is now known to be HIV infection were not treated with any special isolation precautions. Retrospective review of hospital records from that period has failed to demonstrate nosocomial transmission of HIV to health care workers or to other hospitalized patients.[8] Several large prospective longitudinal studies of health care workers with occupational exposure to HIV blood or body fluids through needle-stick injury or mucous membrane splash have been conducted. Although some seroconversions have occurred in health care workers following an exposure by needle stick or mucous membrane splash, the risk of acquiring HIV in health care–related activities is less than 1% at a 95% confidence level.[9]

Universal Precautions

Since 1982, the CDC has issued precautions for health care workers against what is now known as the HIV virus. In 1987, recommendations for the prevention of HIV transmission in health care settings described the use of universal precautions in the care of *all* patients.[10] The CDC emphasizes the need to consider all patients as potentially infected with HIV or other blood-borne pathogens and to adhere rigorously to infection control precautions for minimizing the risk of exposure to blood and body fluids of all patients[10] (see box below). In December 1991, the

Occupational Safety and Health Administration (OSHA) established a federal mandate regarding the prevention of occupational exposure to blood-borne pathogens.[11] The OSHA regulations are much more specific in their description of protective equipment and the responsibilities of the employer and the employee in following the prescribed regulations.

Implementation of universal precautions within the critical care unit is of utmost importance. Because of the unstable and unpredictable situations involving patient care faced by critical care nurses, almost any nursing activity can lead to contact with blood, body fluids, or both. Many invasive procedures are routinely performed during care of the critically ill. A collaborative effort among health care workers for the prevention of injury from contaminated needles or other sharp instruments during and after such pro-

---

Summary of Universal Precautions for Health Care Workers*

1. Appropriate barrier precautions to prevent skin and mucous membrane exposure from contact with blood or other potentially infectious materials must be used routinely. When differentiation of body fluids is difficult or impossible, all body fluids are considered potentially infectious material
   a. Gloves must be worn when it can be reasonably anticipated that the employee may have hand contact with blood, other infectious material, mucous membranes, nonintact skin; when performing vascular access procedures (some exceptions apply in volunteer blood donation centers); and when handling or touching contaminated surfaces.
   b. Masks in combination with eye protection devices, such as goggles or glasses with solid side shields or chin-length face shields, must be worn whenever splashes, spray, splatter, or droplets of blood or other potentially infectious materials may be generated and contamination of the eye, nose, or mouth can be reasonably anticipated.
   c. Gowns, aprons, and other appropriate protective body clothing shall be worn in occupational exposure situations. The type and characteristics will depend upon the task and the anticipated degree of exposure.
2. Handwashing
   a. Hands must be washed immediately after gloves are removed.
   b. Hands (or other skin surfaces) must be washed immediately and thoroughly if contaminated with blood or other infectious materials.
   c. Disposable single-use gloves shall not be washed or decontaminated for reuse.

3. All health care workers must take precautions to prevent injuries from contaminated needles and other sharps.
   a. Shearing or breaking of contaminated needles is prohibited.
   b. Bending, recapping, or removing contaminated needles or sharps shall not be performed unless no alternative is feasible or it is required by a medical procedure.
   c. Recapping a needle, if required, must be done with a one-handed technique or a mechanical device.
   d. As soon as possible after use, contaminated sharps are to be placed in easily accessible, closable, puncture resistant, leak-proof, appropriately labeled containers.
4. Mouthpieces, resuscitation bags, pocket masks, or other ventilation devices must be available for use when there is occupational exposure.
5. Health care workers who have exudative lesions or weeping dermatitis should refrain from direct patient care and from handling patient care equipment.
6. Pregnant health care workers are not known to be at greater risk of contracting HIV infection than nonpregnant health care workers. If a health care worker develops HIV infection during pregnancy, the infant is at risk for perinatal transmission of HIV. Therefore, pregnant health care workers should be familiar with and strictly adhere to precautions to minimize the risk of HIV transmission.

*This box summarizes key points from the CDC *Recommendations for Prevention of HIV Transmission in Health Care Settings* and OSHA regulations. Refer to these documents for more detailed specific information.

cedures is essential. Implementation of new equipment and technology designed to prevent such injury is desirable, but the cost of these items may delay their acquisition by some institutions.

THE SPECTRUM OF HIV INFECTION

The world learned first about AIDS, then about the HIV virus as the cause of the syndrome. Today, many people (health care workers included) use these terms interchangeably. Although all patients manifesting AIDS are infected with the HIV virus, all patients infected with HIV do not have AIDS. A spectrum exists between infection with the virus and the development of AIDS.

HIV Infection

Upon initial infection with the HIV virus, some individuals may experience an acute, self-limited mononucleosis-like illness within 3 weeks of exposure.[6] Symptoms may include fever, malaise, myalgias, and lymphadenopathy. Skin rash or aseptic meningitis is less common.[6] Seroconversion to HIV-positive usually occurs within 6 weeks to 3 months of initial contact with the virus but may take as long as 6 to 12 months.

A variable period of asymptomatic infection follows initial contact. The virus may lie dormant until activated by some cofactor. It is not known whether all infected people progress to demonstrate immunodeficiency or if some remain in an infectious but asymptomatic state. Currently, the median incubation time from HIV infection to the emergence of AIDS is thought to be 9 to 10 years.[13] It is crucial to identify HIV-positive individuals promptly. If they are kept under close observation, deterioration in the immune system can be detected early, and antiviral therapy can be instituted. Starting therapy before the patient develops AIDS may extend life expectancy.

Eventually, a state of persistent generalized lymphadenopathy may develop. At this time, the HIV patient is relatively healthy with no symptoms except persistent, palpable, enlargement of the lymph nodes at more than one extrainguinal site.

Diagnosis of AIDS

With testing available for determining the presence of HIV infection, and identification of a variety of indicator diseases known definitively or presumptively to indicate AIDS, the CDC has revised its original definition of AIDS to incorporate these criteria.[12] The development of opportunistic infections, malignancies, HIV wasting syndrome, or neurological changes establishes the diagnosis of AIDS. The box on this page lists the diseases indicative of AIDS in the HIV-positive patient.

Diseases Indicative of AIDS in HIV-positive Patients

Cryptosporidiosis
Cytomegalovirus
Isosporiasis
Kaposi's sarcoma
Lymphoma
Lymphoid pneumonia or hyperplasia
Pneumocystis carinii pneumonia
Progressive multifocal leukoencephalopathy
Toxoplasmosis
Candidiasis
Coccidioidomycosis
Cryptococcosis
Herpes simplex virus
Tuberculosis
Other mycobacterioses
Salmonellosis
Other bacterial infection
HIV encephalopathy (dementia)
HIV wasting syndrome

The deterioration of the immune system T4 cell count and the loss of protection and immune system regulation afforded by these cells leads to a wide range of problems manifested by the patient with AIDS. Once a diagnosis of AIDS has been made, over 80% of the patients die within 3 years.

As the experts on HIV infection and AIDS learn more about this disease and its manifestations, the defining characteristics of AIDS will continue to be modified. Currently, input is being solicited for the next revision of the CDC definition of AIDS. The use of T4 cell counts of less than 200/mm³ is one of the proposed criteria.

CLINICAL MANIFESTATIONS OF AIDS
Opportunistic Infections

The manifestation of opportunistic infection was the first encounter with AIDS for the health care system. Patients with no known reason for immunocompromise were developing opportunistic infections and seeking care for these problems. Subsequently, their impaired immune status was identified. Some of the infections were similar to those occurring in patients with known reasons for immunosuppression, such as patients receiving cancer chemotherapy or transplant patients receiving immunosuppressive agents. It soon became apparent that the opportunistic infections experienced by patients with AIDS were very diverse and behaved differently than those seen in other immunosuppressed patients. The AIDS-associated infections were predominately caused by intracellular organisms, the most common being the bacterial, fun-

Opportunistic Infections Seen in AIDS Patients

BACTERIAL
Mycobacterium tuberculosis (TB)
Mycobacterium avium complex disease (MAC)
Salmonella

FUNGAL
Candida albicans
Cryptococcus neoformans
Coccidioidomycosis

PROTOZOAL
*Pneumocystis carinii**
Toxoplasma gondii
Cryptosporidium
Isospora belli

VIRAL
Herpes simplex virus (HSV type 1 and type 2)
Cytomegalovirus (CMV)
Progressive multifocal leukoencephalopathy (PML)

* Classified by some as a fungal infection.

gal, viral, and protozoal microorganisms listed in the box above. The presence of these infections is now used in conjunction with HIV testing to make the diagnosis of AIDS.

Most of these microorganisms are ubiquitous in the environment and rarely cause disease in people with normal immune system function. The emergence of these infections in the immunodeficient patient may occur upon an initial contact with the microorganism or as the reactivation of a previously acquired pathogen. Although the infection may be localized, dissemination to several sites is common. Many opportunistic infections caused by many pathogens may coexist in the patients with AIDS.

Once an infection develops, it is nearly impossible to cure. The acute episode may be controlled, but long-term therapy to suppress recurrence is generally required. The organism may become resistant to the standard therapy, further complicating treatment. No drug may be available for some infections.

The patient with AIDS may develop other infections in addition to opportunistic infections. Normal body flora, particularly in the gastrointestinal tract, may cause serious infection. Exposure to environmental microorganisms also may cause infection in the immunocompromised patient. HIV causes defects in the humoral immune system that prevent the mounting of antibody response to new antigens. Hospitalized patients with AIDS are at high risk of developing nosocomial infections, especially when invasive techniques are employed. Adherence to aseptic technique and infection control measures is vital.

HIV Wasting Syndrome

Weight loss is an early symptom in HIV-infected patients, even though they report adequate caloric intake. HIV wasting syndrome is characterized by anorexia, fever, and diarrhea in addition to weight loss. The CDC diagnostic criteria for HIV wasting syndrome include a profound involuntary weight loss of greater than 10% of baseline body weight and either two or more loose stools per day *or* chronic weakness and documented intermittent or constant fever for more than 30 days.[12] Concurrent illness or conditions other than HIV that could explain the findings must be absent.

Patients with AIDS need a comprehensive nutritional and diet assessment to identify problem areas in providing an adequate dietary intake. Nursing plays an important role in the multidisciplinary team approach needed to deal with the multifactorial causes contributing to an inadequate intake of fluids and food.

When a patient with HIV or AIDS is admitted to the critical care unit for any reason, nutritional status must be a priority concern to prevent further weight loss associated with the hospitalization. Nutritional supplements; continuous enteric feedings; control of nausea, vomiting, and diarrhea; and/or total parenteral nutrition may be required, depending on the underlying condition of the patient.

Malignancies

Kaposi's Sarcoma

Early in the identification of the AIDS, Kaposi's sarcoma (KS) was seen in male homosexuals. It became one of the identifying diseases for the syndrome. Before AIDS was identified, KS was a rare form of indolent tumor seen mostly in elderly men of Mediterranean or Eastern European Jewish descent, in young adult equatorial African males, or in immunosuppressed organ transplant recipients. However, the classification of KS has been amended to describe its epidemiological occurrence and course.

The classification *epidemic or HIV-related Kaposi's sarcoma* is used to describe the incidence of this malignancy in patients with AIDS. When KS occurs in this group, it is fulminant and widely disseminated; survival is shorter than in other groups. In the United States, most early cases of AIDS involved male homosexuals, and the incidence of KS with AIDS was about 30%.[6] Today, with AIDS being diagnosed in larger numbers within other risk groups, the overall incidence of KS is about 10%.[6] It is thought that the predominance of KS in male homosexuals is related to an unidentified cofactor.

The first KS lesions develop subtly as subcutaneous, usually painless, violaceous, nonblanching, palpable tumors anywhere on the body. Cutaneous lesions often develop on the face, in the mouth, or on the trunk, arms, or legs. Lesions on the soles of the feet or in the mouth may be painful. Cutaneous distribution along lymphatic drainage channels is seen, and lymphedema may develop in the face or in the lower extremities.

Kaposi's sarcoma progresses cutaneously, and visceral KS lesions may develop in lymph nodes, the gastrointestinal (GI) tract, the lungs, or the heart. Kaposi's lesions may obstruct the GI tract or the upper airway, and pulmonary KS may mimic symptoms of pneumonia.

Visceral KS implies a poor prognosis.[13] Patients with a few small lesions and no opportunistic infection have a better prognosis.[13]

Isolated lesions that are causing obstruction to the airway or difficulty with swallowing, or lesions impairing ambulation, may be treated by radiation therapy, laser therapy, cryotherapy, or intralesion injection of vinblastine.[13] Rapidly progressing disease may be treated with single or combination agent chemotherapy. Drugs such as bleomycin, doxorubicin, vinblastine, vincristine, and etoposide have been used. No single protocol has proved superior. A major concern in using cytotoxic chemotherapy in patients with AIDS is the side effect of bone marrow suppression and the resulting impact on immune and hematological system functions. Therapy for epidemic KS, therefore, remains experimental and controversial.

Alpha-interferon therapy has also been used to treat patients with KS. This cytokine has both antitumor and anti-HIV activity. Its therapeutic success is dependent on the underlying state of the AIDS patient. A higher T4 cell count and no opportunistic infection are associated with a better response to this therapy and a better prognosis.[13]

The lesions of KS can be very disfiguring. Patients may require much psychosocial support in coping with their altered body image. Critical care nursing of patients with KS may be required when lesions become obstructive to the respiratory or GI tract.

Non-Hodgkin's Lymphoma

Lymphomas are cancers of the immune system. Non-Hodgkin's lymphomas are further classified by the lymphocyte cell line involved and the pathological findings. Most cases in patients with AIDS are from the B lymphocyte cell line. They are classified as intermediate or high grade lymphomas. The majority of the patients have widespread disease at the time of their diagnosis.

The tumor involves extranodal sites most often seen in the gastrointestinal tract, central nervous system, bone marrow, or liver. Tumors involving the heart and pericardium have been reported. Other un-

usual sites include the parotid glands, subcutaneous tissue, paranasal sinuses, and epidural space.[13]

Conventional protocols for the treatment of Hodgkin's and non-Hodgkin's lymphomas have been used in treating these diseases in patients with HIV. Drugs such as methotrexate, bleomycin, doxorubicin, cyclophosphamide, vincristine, and dexamethasone have been used in treatment regimens. An initial response to chemotherapy or radiation may occur, but most patients relapse, and overall survival is poor.[14]

All patients with AIDS are at high risk for opportunistic infection. The use of cytotoxic chemotherapy and the further immunosuppression it causes increase this risk. Unlike other oncology patients, patients with AIDS and cancer do not regain a normal immune function following chemotherapy. They continue to have HIV-related immunological defects and the potential for opportunistic infection.

Anecdotal reports of other cancers seen in AIDS patients have incuded testicular, cervical, oral, and rectal sites. At present, these malignancies are not considered diagnostic for AIDS.

Patients with lymphomas may be seen in the critical care unit for a variety of reasons. The space-occupying tumors may cause neurological deficits or GI obstruction or bleeding. After chemotherapy, patients with large tumor burdens may develop tumor lysis syndrome and require intensive fluid replacement and monitoring to prevent acute renal failure. The development of sepsis or septic shock secondary to infection following immunosuppressive chemotherapy is another potential cause for admission to a critical care unit. Care for the patient with AIDS and these problems includes the same therapies employed in treating patients with other etiologies for these conditions.

Neurological Involvement

An estimated 40% of persons with AIDS have neurological symptoms.[13,15] In approximately 10%, the neurological symptoms are the presentation of AIDS.[13,15] The incidence of neurological involvement with AIDS may be greater than these statistics indicate. Neurological abnormalities have been found at autopsy in 75% of AIDS patients.[14] Neurological manifestations of AIDS include HIV encephalopathy, opportunistic infection of the central nervous system (CNS), and CNS lymphomas.

HIV Encephalopathy

The monocyte/macrophage cells can be infected with HIV and may provide the route of entry for the virus to the CNS. HIV encephalopathy (also referred to as AIDS dementia or AIDS dementia complex) then develops. The precise mechanism by which the white matter and gray matter are destroyed is not known. Mild to moderate brain atrophy can be detected by computed tomography (CT) or magnetic resonance imaging (MRI).

Initially, the patient may have cognitive dysfunction displayed as mild memory loss, inability to concentrate, or slowness in thinking. Behavioral changes such as apathy, social withdrawal, or reduced spontaneity may be observed and misinterpreted as depression related to the illness. Neurological dysfunction becomes clearly evident when alterations in consciousness progress to frank confusion, disorientation, aphasia, psychotic behavior, or coma. Motor disturbances such as clumsiness, leg weakness, ataxia, paraparesis, and inability to walk may occur. In the final stages, patients with AIDS dementia complex may lie in bed unable to walk, with a vacant stare and little response to their environment, and become incontinent.

The CDC defines HIV encephalopathy as a clinical finding of disabling cognitive and or motor dysfunction interfering with occupation or activities of daily living in the absence of a concurrent illness or condition other than HIV that could explain the findings.[12] It is one of the diseases definitive for AIDS. The only treatment for this neurological condition is the anti-HIV drug zidovudine, which offers only temporary improvement.[13,15]

CNS Opportunistic Infections

Toxoplasma Gondii Encephalitis. The CNS opportunistic infection most common in AIDS patients is caused by *Toxoplasma gondii*. It is estimated that 28% of AIDS patients develop encephalitis from this protozoan.[15] Reactivation of a latent infection with *T. gondii* is almost always the source.

Symptoms may be vague and nonspecific, such as headache or lethargy. Altered mental status displayed as confusion, delusional behavior, psychosis, global cognitive impairment, or coma may be seen. Seizures are the presenting symptom in approximately one third of patients.[13] Motor deficits such as hemiparesis or ataxia may develop. Other neurological deficits may include aphasia, cranial nerve palsies, or loss of visual field.

A definitive diagnosis of *T. gondii* encephalitis requires a biopsy of brain lesions, which may be impossible due to the location of lesions and the risks the surgery would impose upon the patient. If CT scan or MRI has demonstrated lesions, empiric therapy is begun with the combination of sulfadiazine and pyrimethamine. Additional drugs may be prescribed: dexamethasone to reduce edema, phenytoin for seizures, and folinic acid to minimize bone marrow toxicity from pyrimethamine. Drug reactions may necessitate decreasing the dosages or discontinuing the drugs. Clindamycin may be used alone or in combination with pyrimethamine as an alternative

therapy. Long-term drug therapy to suppress the infection is needed because a cure is not possible for *Toxoplasma gondii* encephalitis in patients with AIDS.

Cryptococcal Meningitis. *Cryptococcus neoformans* is the fungal CNS infection most common in AIDS patients. Reactivation of a latent infection with this ubiquitous organism occurs in the patient as the immune system is destroyed.

Symptoms are insidious in their development and are not specific to differentiate this infection from other CNS infections. Classic signs of meningitis such as fever, nuchal rigidity, headache, or papilledema may not be present due to the impaired immune system function of the AIDS patient. Other symptoms such as malaise, nausea and vomiting, photophobia, altered mentation, focal deficits, or seizures may be seen.

A spinal tap to obtain cerebrospinal fluid (CSF) for visualization of cryptococci is used to diagnose this disease. Cryptococcal antigen titers may be detected in the blood or CSF. The organism may also be cultured from blood or CSF. CT scan may show focal lesions that may be cryptococcal but could also be toxoplasmosis or lymphoma.

Treatment of the initial episode of infection must be followed by long-term suppressive therapy in patients with AIDS. Intravenous amphotericin-B has been the drug of choice in treating cryptococcal meningitis. In resistant cases, 5-fluocytosine has been used with the amphotericin B for its synergistic effect; it has not been used alone due to the development of drug resistance. Until the recent approval of fluconazole in both oral and parenteral forms, no other agent besides amphotericin B was available for maintenance suppressive therapy.

Progressive Multifocal Leukoencephalopathy (PML). This opportunistic neurological infection is caused by the J.C. virus type of polyomavirus.[13] Reactivation of a latent infection leads to a subacute demyelinating CNS disease. The white matter of the brain develops multiple lesions. Sometimes the brainstem and cerebellum are involved.

Initial manifestations include extremity weakness and incoordination, ataxia, hemiparesis, cognitive dysfunction, personality changes, loss of vision, aphasia, headache, or seizures. A progressive irreversible course with worsening symptoms develops.

A definitive diagnosis of this disease can be made only by examination of brain tissue obtained via biopsy. A positive diagnosis rules out other CNS problems. However, no form of therapy for PML has been effective.

Cytomegalovirus (CMV) Retinitis. Cytomegalovirus is one of the family of herpesviruses. These viruses are opportunistic in that once the host has been infected, the virus can remain dormant in tissues to cause subsequent outbreaks of acute infection. Most people have been exposed to CMV at some time, and antibodies can be detected in the serum.

The patient with AIDS may have reactivation of this organism causing infection within the CNS, the lung, the GI tract, or the retina. Ocular infection can cause significant impairment of vision, leading to blindness.

Retinitis caused by CMV is usually painless. Partial loss of visual field, blurred vision, or unilateral or bilateral floaters prompt the patient to seek treatment. Impaired vision may also be the first sign of a disseminated CMV infection in the AIDS patient.[13] Positive cultures of tissue other than from the eye may yield the diagnosis of CMV when other sites are involved. In the eye, a presumptive diagnosis is based on progressive characteristic lesions found on ophthalmoscopic examination.[12]

Until recently, the only FDA-approved drug for CMV retinitis was the antiviral agent ganciclovir, which is given intravenously. This drug can suppress but not cure CMV infection. The major dose-limiting side effect of ganciclovir drug is neutropenia. This limits its use concomitantly with the anti-HIV agent, zidovudine, which is toxic to bone marrow. This drug is approved only for CMV infections of the retina. Treatment of other sites of CMV infections is still under investigation. The AIDS patient newly diagnosed with CMV retinitis has traditionally had to make a very difficult choice. If the patient had been taking zidovudine, concurrent use of ganciclovir was contraindicated. Patients had to choose between an improvement in vision with a shorter life span or possible blindness with fewer symptoms of HIV infection and a longer life. An alternative drug for treatment of CMV retinitis, foscarnet sodium, may allow the concurrent use of anti-HIV agents, thus eliminating this patient dilemma.

The critical care nurse may be called upon to give ganciclovir to maintain therapy for CMV retinitis while the patient is in the intensive care unit for other problems. When giving this drug, precautions for safe handling of antineoplastic agents must be followed to protect the health care worker from the toxic effects of this agent. Institutional protocols regarding these agents should be followed.

Foscarnet sodium is an IV antiviral agent currently used only for treating CMV retinitis. It cannot cure but may significantly alleviate CMV retinitis. It is not without toxicity. Renal impairment can occur, so close monitoring of renal function is essential. Foscarnet also alters electrolyte levels in the blood, contributing to the development of seizures. Close monitoring of serum calcium, phosphorus, potassium, and magnesium is necessary.

CNS Lymphoma

Primary B cell lymphomas are the most common neoplastic neurological complication in AIDS patients. Secondary lymphomas or Kaposi's sarcoma of the brain are seen less frequently. The clinical presentation of a CNS lymphoma may be similar to toxoplasmosis. Lethargy, confusion, dementia, or focal neurological dysfunction may be observed. The tumor lesions may be indistinguishable from toxoplasmosis on CT or MRI. A brain biopsy with its associated risks to obtain tissue for histological examination is the only way to definitively diagnose lymphoma.

Radiation therapy may be used alone or in combination with chemotherapy to reduce tumor size and manage symptoms. This disease in the AIDS patient is almost always fatal.[15]

The critical care nurse may be caring for an AIDS patient during the acute manifestation of focal neurological symptoms such as seizures or after diagnostic brain biopsy. During this time, close observation of mental status and motor and sensory ability may reveal individual patient needs for intervention to promote maximal independent function and safety.

Assessment of the patient's cognitive function is important when determining the patient's ability to participate in informed consent. A durable power of attorney for health care decisions or other advance directives may have been obtained if the patient's neurological status has been on a slow decline. A sudden event causing neurological impairment may necessitate the completion of such legal documents.

The patient, family, and significant others need support in dealing with the patient's deteriorating condition. Although the outcome of AIDS remains fatal, a combination of physical measures, occupational or speech therapy, and emotional support can improve the quality of the patient's remaining life.

Respiratory System

Pneumocystis carinii Pneumonia (PCP)

The first cases of what is now known to be AIDS were patients with a diagnosis of PCP. This opportunistic infection is the most common in HIV patients: An estimated 75% to 80% experience at least one episode.[16] During the 1980s, more effective measures for preventing and treating this opportunistic infection have been developed. Nevertheless, PCP can cause life-threatening respiratory failure requiring the intervention of critical care support.

Pneumocystis carinii is a ubiquitous microorganism. It is most often categorized as a protozoa, but some experts consider it to be a fungus. Whatever its classification, PCP is resident in the lungs of most people. In persons with AIDS, the previous infection is reactivated. The likelihood of infection increases as the T4 cell count drops below $200/mm^3$.

TABLE 47-1   **Standard Drug Therapies for *Pneumocystis Carinii* Pneumonia (PCP)**

Drug	Dosage	Side Effects
Trimethoprim/ Sulfamethoxazole	75-100 mg/kg/day 15-20 mg/kg/day	Rash, fever Nausea/vomiting, anorexia, leukopenia, thrombocytopenia, hyponatremia, abnormal liver function studies, Stevens-Johnson syndrome
Pentamidine Isethionate	4 mg/kg/day	Nausea/vomiting, metallic taste in mouth, anorexia, hypotension, dysrhythmias, azotemia, pancreatitis, hypoglycemia, diabetes mellitus

The *Pneumocystis* organism grows within the alveoli of the lung, filling them with organisms and proteinaceous fluid. Sites of infection outside the lung are rare. As the alveoli are filled, gas exchange is impaired, leading to ventilation/perfusion abnormalities. Interstitial inflammation leads to a reduction in lung compliance.[16]

Clinical symptoms have an insidious onset. Initially, they may be nonspecific. Fever, fatigue, and weight loss may precede respiratory symptoms by several weeks. Specific presenting respiratory symptoms are most often a dry, nonproductive cough progressing to become productive, and dyspnea on exertion progressing to dyspnea at rest. Physical examination of the patient may reveal tachypnea and crackles without evidence of consolidation.[16]

The chest films of the patient with PCP most often display diffuse bilateral perihilar interstitial infiltrates that progress to the peripheral lung fields. Between 5% and 10% of patients with PCP may be symptomatic with a normal chest x-ray.[13,16] Patients who have been receiving prophylactic inhalations of aerosolized pentamidine may develop infiltrates in the upper lobes, where the drug tends to be poorly distributed.[16]

Arterial blood gas studies demonstrate hypoxemia, hypocarbia, and an increased alveolar/arterial oxygen gradient, especially on exercise.[13] Pulmonary function studies may show a decreased lung capacity, decreased vital capacity, and a decreased single-breath diffusing capacity for carbon monoxide.[16] Gallium scans of the lung are sensitive for inflammation but are not specific for the presence of PCP.

To be definitively diagnosed, PCP must be cultured from the sputum or visualized from other lung fluids or tissue. The least invasive diagnostic method, the induced sputum procedure, is attempted first. A bronchoscopy with bronchoalveolar lavage and/or transbronchial biopsy may be needed. The open lung biopsy is reserved for situations where the other methods have not provided a diagnosis, the patient is being mechanically ventilated, there is progression of pul-

monary disease, or the patient has an uncorrectable coagulopathy.[16]

Drug treatment of an acute episode of PCP includes the use of trimethoprim/sulfamethoxazole (TMP-SMX) or pentamidine isethionate. Both drugs cause a high incidence of side effects in patients with AIDS. Table 47-1 lists the recommended dosages and the potential side effects of the standard PCP therapy. Five to seven days of therapy are required before evidence of improvement is seen. In fact, the patient may continue to deteriorate even though appropriate therapy has been instituted.

Administration of TMP-SMX by the IV route requires dilution in a large volume of 5% dextrose in water as compared to the volumes required by other antibiotic therapy. Doses are given every 6 to 8 hours for 14 to 21 days. An oral form of the drug is also available for less severe episodes of PCP when gastrointestinal absorption is normal and the patient is compliant. Over half the patients receiving this drug develop a rash, but stopping the drug is not always necessary.[16]

Pentamidine isethionate in one daily IV dose administered over 1 to 2 hours for 14 to 21 days is also an effective therapy for PCP. Originally, this drug was administered by a daily IM injection, and painful sterile abscesses were a common side effect. This drug is toxic to the beta islet cells of the pancreas.[16] Baseline blood glucose values must be determined before administration is started, and glucose must be monitored during and after a course of therapy. Concurrent therapy with pentamidine and dideoxyinosine (ddI) appears to increase the risk of pancreatitis.[13] Cardiovascular side effects such as hypotension and dysrhythmias including the development of torsades de pointe have been reported.

Aerosolized pentamidine and oral TMP-SMX are used prophylactically against PCP in patients with AIDS. These preventive therapies are discussed later in this chapter. Other drugs have been used to treat PCP in clinical trials: pyrimethamine-sulfadiazine, clindamycin and primaquine, dapsone, and trimetrexate.

Additional standard therapies are employed to treat AIDS patients with PCP. Oxygen is administered by nasal cannula or face mask, according to the patient's condition. Severe PCP can cause acute respiratory failure with a presentation similar to adult respiratory distress syndrome (ARDS). Intubation and mechanical ventilation may be required to deliver positive end-expiratory pressure (PEEP). Alternatively, continuous positive airway pressure (CPAP) may be administered via face mask. Because of its tight fit and the need to keep it on at all times, the CPAP face mask may be unsuitable for some patients. High-dose corticosteroids have been used effectively to reduce inflammatory response in some patients with PCP and acute respiratory failure. No controlled studies have been performed to prove the efficacy of this treatment.

Critical care admissions of patients with AIDS are most often the result of PCP-related acute respiratory failure. Early in the history of AIDS, open-lung biopsy was used in diagnosis, necessitating the use of intubation, chest tubes, and mechanical ventilation. These patients had almost 100% mortality. Much has been learned about AIDS and PCP since that time. Today, fewer patients with AIDS die of PCP-related respiratory failure, although mortality remains greater than 50%.

Many clinical and ethical issues surround the decision to use intubation and mechanical ventilation. The patient's wishes are primary. Advance directives may have stipulated the type of care the patient wishes to receive. In first episodes of PCP, if the patient is in relatively good general condition and desires the treatment, there is some consensus that assisted ventilation should be attempted.[16]

Caring for the mechanically ventilated patient with ARDS is a routine critical care nursing practice (see Chapters 29 and 30). The same principles of management are used for the AIDS patient with PCP and acute respiratory failure. Increasing PEEP to obtain the best oxygenation without causing pulmonary barotrauma or cardiovascular compromise is a critical care challenge. Management of fluid status to prevent pulmonary interstitial edema is also a concern. Universal precautions should be routinely and scrupulously observed.

Communication is often difficult for intubated patients. Hypoxemia, the use of sedatives, or skeletal muscle paralysis compounds the situation. Consequently, decisions about care are best made before the onset of critical illness when the patient is still competent to make legal decisions regarding health care. In reality, this may not transpire; therefore, the critical care nurse must serve as the advocate for the critically ill patient.

Mycobacterium tuberculosis

The incidence of *Mycobacterium tuberculosis* (TB) has been on the rise in the United States since the recognition of AIDS, and it has been identified as a sentinel disease. Patients with AIDS are at risk for the reactivation of a previous TB infection or the acquisition of a new, rapidly progressing infection. Nosocomial transmission of TB with multidrug resistance has been documented among outpatients and hospitalized patients with HIV infection.[17]

Tuberculosis is dangerous not only to patients with AIDS but also to health care workers. It is spread by inhalation of droplet nuclei that are aerosolized by coughing, sneezing, singing, or talking. Health care workers are at risk during procedures in which coughing is induced (sputum induction or aerosolized medication administration), and when performing endotracheal intubation, suctioning with mechanical ventilation, or bronchoscopy. Transmission of drug-resistant TB from patients to health care workers has been documented.[18] Many of the procedures associated with a high risk for transmission are conducted within the critical care unit, so awareness of the risk and observance of proper precautions are crucial when providing care to a patient with suspected or confirmed TB.

The CDC has issued guidelines for preventing the transmission of TB in health care settings with a special focus on the HIV patient population.[19] Presentation of TB may be atypical in the immunocompromised patient with AIDS, increasing the likelihood of an occupational exposure through omission of precautionary measures.

The more immunocompromised the patient, the less typical the clinical presentation.[13] A diagnosis of TB should be considered for any patient with persistent cough, weight loss, anorexia, night sweats, or fever. Dyspnea, chills, hemoptysis, and chest pain may occur with pulmonary TB. Patients with AIDS often have extrapulmonary TB in the GI tract, blood, urine, reticuloendothelial system, CNS, bones, or joints.

The Mantoux intradermal injection of purified protein derivative (PPD) is the only method currently available that demonstrates infection with TB in the absence of active disease.[19] Persons with AIDS may have a false-negative test, especially in the advanced stages of the disease.[19] Therefore, a negative PPD in a patient with AIDS does not rule out communicable TB. A previous positive PPD is a significant finding.

The chest x-ray in the HIV patient with TB may not show the classical cavitary lesions. Infiltrates may be seen in any area of the lung. Acid-fast bacillus

(AFB) smear and culture of three to five sputum specimens collected on different days is the main diagnostic procedure for pulmonary TB. Patients with AIDS may not have positive AFB smears because they have less cavitating lesions.[19] A definitive positive sputum culture can take 4 to 8 weeks to manifest.

A patient thought to have TB should be isolated until a satisfactory clinical and bacteriological response to drug therapy is achieved.[13] The time frame for isolation is variable. Patients who have received 2 to 3 weeks of drug therapy and have shown a reduction in cough, resolution of fever, and progressively less quantity of bacilli on smear are probably no longer infectious.[19] The box below summarizes tuberculosis (AFB) isolation precautions applicable to the critical care environment.

Drug therapy for the HIV patient with known or suspected TB includes a 2-month regimen of isoniazid, rifampin, an pyrazinamide. Ethambutal is added if CNS or disseminated infection is suspected or if resistance to isoniazid occurs.[13] Drug therapy with isoniazid and rifampin is then continued for a minimum of 9 months and at least 6 months after a culture-documented conversion.[13]

Summary of CDC Tuberculosis (AFB) Isolation Precautions for Critical Care Units*

1. Any patient suspected or known to have infectious TB should be placed in AFB precautions in a private room with the door shut.
2. The patient room should have six air exchanges per hour, with two outside air changes per hour. If the air is recirculated, it should be passed through a HEPA filter.
3. The direction of airflow should be negative pressure flow from the hall to the patient room.
4. Persons who enter the room should wear disposable personal respirators, especially during procedures such as bronchoscopy, endotracheal suctioning, sputum induction, or aerosolization of medication.
5. Patients should be instructed to cover their nose and mouth with a tissue when coughing or sneezing.
6. Patients who must be transported outside of the isolation room for a procedure should wear a properly fitting surgical mask or valveless personal respirator.
7. Installation of ultraviolet radiation lamps might be considered in ICUs.

*This box summarizes CDC recommendations pertinent to the critical care environment. Refer to the actual document for detailed recommendations.

Testing by PPD should be performed at least every 6 months in health care workers frequently exposed to patients with TB or involved with potentially high-risk procedures performed on patients who may have TB.[19] Annual testing is recommended for other health care workers. The risk for critical care nurses varies according to patient populations and types of procedures performed within different ICUs. The critical care nurse must be aware of the specific environmental risks and individual institutional policies.

Gastrointestinal System

Over 80% of patients with HIV develop some kind of gastrointestinal problem.[20] As already mentioned, HIV wasting syndrome with fever, anorexia, weight loss, and diarrhea is diagnostic for AIDS. Opportunistic infection, infection from normal GI flora, or contact with organisms such as *Salmonella* or *Giardia* may lead to significant GI dysfunction as the immune system deteriorates. Persistent GI dysfunction leads to malabsorption and malnutrition, contributing to further weight loss and the potential for severe dehydration. Malignant tumors and Kaposi's sarcoma lesions may obstruct the GI tract. Liver function may be impaired by infections such as hepatitis, by drug-induced hepatotoxicity, or by alcohol or drug abuse. Anorectal lesions and sexually transmitted infections may occur secondary to the patient's sexual practices and immune deficiency.

Candidiasis

Oral and esophageal candidiasis are common GI infections in patients with AIDS.[21] This fungus can also be present on the skin, nails, or vagina, or as a systemic infection. It may exist alone or may accompany other oral infections such as herpes simplex.

The most prevalent form of *Candida* in patients with HIV disease is oral *Candida,* or thrush. The tongue or buccal mucosa develops creamy, curdlike, yellowish patches that can be wiped off, leaving an erythematous base lesion that may bleed. Another form of oral *Candida* is candidal leukoplakia. These white oral lesions cannot be wiped off. The presence of these oral *Candida* lesions in patients with no known reason for immunocompromise is indicative of AIDS.[12]

Oral and esophageal *Candida* do not necessarily present concurrently.[13] Dysphagia, with a sensation of food sticking in the esophagus when attempting to swallow, is a common complaint with *Candida* esophagitis. Pain on swallowing and retrosternal pain are seen when esophagitis is caused by viral ulceration such as herpes simplex or CMV.[13]

Oral candidiasis is rarely cured in patients with AIDS. It is often chronic or recurrent. Antifungal agents available for treatment include oral nystatin suspension, clotrimazole troches, and ketoconazole. When ketoconazole is used, the patient's medication regimen should be carefully reviewed because absorption or metabolism of this agent may be affected by concurrently administered drugs. Long-term use of ketoconazole can lead to resistance of the organism. For skin lesions, topical clotrimazole or miconazole is available. Disseminated candidiasis requires IV administration of amphotericin B. Fluconazole is a newer antifungal agent available in both oral and IV forms for the treatment of oral, esophageal, or systemic candidiasis.

Nursing care of patients with or at risk for *Candida* infections requires close inspection of the oral cavity, skin folds, and perineal area for detection of lesions. Skin must be kept dry and exposed to air. Oral lesions may impede efforts to maintain adequate nutrition. Oral pain may be relieved by topical applications of agents such as lidocaine given in mouth rinses or swallowed in viscous form. Precautions to prevent aspiration because of numbness must be exercised. Routine oral care must avoid alcohol-containing mouthwashes or lemon-and-glycerine swabs, which cause pain and contribute to dryness of mucous membranes.

Cryptosporidium

Ingestion of the waterborne protozoan *Cryptosporidium* may cause infection in both patients with impaired immune function and immunologically intact individuals. The disease is self-limiting in a person with a normal immune system. In the patient with AIDS, profuse watery diarrhea, abdominal cramping, flatulence, weight loss, anorexia, fever, vomiting, myalgia, and malaise persist. Severe weight loss, dehydration, malabsorption, electrolyte imbalances, and voluminous diarrhea (10 to 15 L/day) usually result in the patient's death.

No effective treatment for cryptosporidiosis is available. Palliative medical therapy includes fluid and electrolyte replacement, parenteral nutrition, and antidiarrheal and antiperistaltic medications. This infection requires intensive nursing care. Maintaining the patient's dignity when severe explosive diarrhea and incontinence occur is important in helping the patient to cope. Keeping skin intact and preventing breakdown is another nursing challenge. Additionally, infection control measures must be instituted to prevent person-to-person or fomite transmission of *Cryptosporidium*. Handwashing, the use of gloves and gowns, and appropriate disposal of waste are essential.

Nutritional support for the patient with AIDS and diarrhea requires a collaborative team approach. Enteral feedings may not be tolerated because of malabsorption and diarrhea. Oral feedings may not be adequate to meet the patient's needs or may be contraindicated by concurrent conditions. The use of total parenteral nutrition must consider the patient's wishes in regard to aggressive therapies.

Isospora belli

The protozoan *Isospora belli* may be ingested in contaminated water. It is endemic in tropical climates. Infection of the small intestine causes malabsorption and nonbloody, watery diarrhea. Infection with this organism resembles the clinical features of cryptosporidiosis, but bowel movements are less frequent.

As with all infections in patients with AIDS, relapse and recurrence must be anticipated. In acute infection, administration of TMP-SMX for at least 10 days is recommended. Continued suppressive prophylaxis is necessary with TMP-SMX, sulfadoxine-pyrimethamine, or pyrimethamine alone in patients with a sulfa allergy. Although nosocomial transmission has not been documented, the use of infection control measures similar to those described for *Cryptosporidium* are considered prudent.

Renal System

The clinical incidence of renal complications appears to be low in patients with AIDS, but covert pathology has been detected upon autopsy.[22] As with other problems in patients with AIDS, it is postulated that as the disease progresses, so will renal complications. Renal complications of AIDS are of three general types: those resulting from hemodynamic instability, those associated with nephrotoxic agents, and AIDS-related glomerulopathy.[22]

Hemodynamic instability in patients with AIDS can be linked to dehydration and hypovolemia. Diarrhea and malabsorption from GI infections and vomiting as a side effect of medications cause dehydration, which leads to hypovolemia. A poor oral intake contributes to the fluid volume deficit. High fever and diaphoresis further dehydrate the patient. If the patient with AIDS develops sepsis and shock, the hemodynamic instability occurring may divert blood flow from the kidneys. Renal ischemia can occur alone or in addition to the toxic effects of drugs.

Most of the drugs used to treat opportunistic infection in AIDS have a potential for *nephrotoxicity*. AIDS patients require long courses of acute and suppressive therapy, increasing their chances of drug-related toxicity. Many concurrent infections are often present, and many toxic drugs may be administered concurrently to treat them. Drug-induced toxic effects on kidneys include alteration in renal circulation, decreased glomerular filtration, and tubular necrosis.[22]

An *idiopathic nephropathy* characterized by focal and segmental chronic, irreversible glomerulosclerosis has been documented in patients with AIDS. It has been called AIDS-related nephropathy and resembles heroin-induced nephropathy. It is most common in blacks, Haitians, and IV drug users with AIDS.[22] The kidneys appear normal or enlarged on ultrasound examination, and this is of diagnostic importance since the kidney usually atrophies from other causes of chronic renal failure.

The most common renal abnormalities seen in patients with AIDS include proteinuria, azotemia, and decreased creatinine clearance.[22] A nephrotic syndrome with proteinuria of greater than 3 g characterizes AIDS-related nephropathy. The peripheral edema and hypertension usually associated with heavy proteinuria do not appear; the reason is unknown.

Acute renal failure associated with hemodynamic instability, hypovolemia, or nephrotoxic drugs can be reversed by restoration of adequate fluid volume, a reduction in dosages of nephrotoxic drugs, or temporary dialysis. The majority of patients with chronic AIDS-related renal failure receiving maintenance dialysis die within 9 months.[22]

The fluid and electrolyte status of the patient with AIDS should be closely monitored. Accurate intake and output records, as well as close monitoring of electrolyte, BUN, and creatinine levels, is essential. Hemodynamic monitoring data can help to determine fluid volume status or to detect the presence of sepsis or shock.

Cardiovascular System

A variety of cardiac abnormalities can occur in patients with AIDS, including pericardial effusion with or without cardiac tamponade, congestive heart failure, dilated cardiomyopathy, myocarditis, KS of the pericardium or epicardium, lymphoma of the heart, and nonbacterial thrombotic endocarditis. Abnormal cardiac findings were first documented during autopsy in patients with AIDS who had no apparent antemortem clinical cardiac symptoms.[23] Subsequently, two-dimensional echocardiography studies have been used to evaluate the cardiac status of patients with AIDS, resulting in increased detection of abnormal cardiovascular findings in those without clinical evidence of cardiac dysfunction.

In most cases, the exact etiology of cardiovascular dysfunction is unknown. However, multiple infections with viruses including HIV itself, side effects of drugs used to treat HIV and opportunistic infection, malignancy, impaired immunological function, or lifestyle behaviors such as abuse of ETOH or IV drugs may individually or collectively contribute to the development of cardiovascular problems in the patient with AIDS.

When a patient with AIDS presents with the clinical symptoms of dyspnea and fatigue, congestive heart failure must be included in the differential diagnosis in addition to the likely pulmonary infections. If a cardiac abnormality is suspected, echocardiography should be performed to evaluate cardiac function and to detect pericardial effusion.

Patients with AIDS may be admitted to the ICU for emergency treatment of cardiac tamponade. Standard therapies are employed in treating this life-threatening condition.

Profound hypotension and circulatory collapse may bring a patient with AIDS to the ICU in a life-threatening condition. Sepsis, adrenal insufficiency secondary to adrenalitis, or drug side effects are likely causes for hemodynamic instability.[23] Supportive therapy with fluid resuscitation, use of vasopressors, and hemodynamic monitoring may be instituted to expand intravascular volume and restore an adequate mean arterial pressure.

Circulatory collapse may be seen as the terminal event in patients with AIDS who are dying of opportunistic infection. If the patient's underlying condition is severely debilitated and the infection is not responding to therapy, institution of critical care support may not be beneficial to the patient. Advance directives should be used to specify the patient's preferences before instituting aggressive life support measures.

PHARMACOLOGICAL MANAGEMENT

Before the HIV virus was identified, supportive therapy and administration of drugs to treat identified opportunistic infections were the only treatments for AIDS. No effective drugs were available for many of the opportunistic infections, particularly viral infections. Standard antiinfectious drug regimens were implemented, but nonresponse or quick relapse were the usual outcome. Even when HIV was identified, no effective antiviral agent was available.

During the 1980s, researchers sought means of combatting HIV, treating opportunistic infection and malignancies and restoring normal immune system function. Much progress has been made developing new antiviral and antifungal drugs, using biological response modifiers, and adapting chemotherapeutic agents for use in treating infection and tumors. The FDA has accelerated its approval process. Still, no cure exists for HIV or most of the AIDS-related opportunistic infections and malignancies. Early diagnosis and institution of anti-HIV therapy can slow the progress of the disease, but eventually, all current drugs become ineffective. Prophylactic therapy against PCP can be instituted. Acute infection with some viruses can be treated, but life-long suppressive therapy must be maintained. Significant side effects of drug therapy necessitate dosage modification, discontinuance of therapy, or the use of additional drug treatment. The new drugs are expensive, increasing the burden on the patient and often upon the health care system.

Research continues to develop new drugs, new dosage schedules, and new combinations of therapy to address the multitude of problems experienced by patients with AIDS. Drugs approved for use to treat specific opportunistic infections have already been mentioned. This section reviews currently approved anti-HIV agents and recommendations for PCP prophylaxis.

Zidovudine (AZT)

Zidovudine (also called AZT) was the first antiviral drug specific for HIV approved for use. It preferentially binds to reverse transcriptase, thereby preventing this enzyme from participating in the reverse transcription of RNA in HIV-infected cells. Initially, its use was approved for patients with advanced AIDS (T4 counts of less than 200 per mm^3). Its recommended use has been expanded to include HIV patients with T4 counts of less than 500 per mm.[3]

The oral dosage is 200 mg every 4 hours around the clock. To reduce toxicity while maintaining efficacy, the dosage may be lowered to 100 mg every four hours while awake for a total daily dose of 500 mg. An IV preparation is available. An IV dose of 1 mg per kg is approximately equivalent to the 100-mg oral dose. The IV dose of 1 to 2 mg per kg is delivered over 1 hour and given every 4 hours.[24]

The major dose-limiting toxicity of zidovudine is related to its adverse effects on the bone marrow. Hematological adverse effects include anemia, neutropenia, and thrombocytopenia either alone or in combination. Close monitoring of the patient's CBC is essential.

In the past, transfusion therapy was necessary to correct anemia. Now, zidovudine-induced anemia is treated with recombinant human erythropoietin. Patients with an abnormal serum erythropoietin level who are receiving more than 4,200 mg of zidovudine weekly are given this agent. A dose of 100 U per kg given intravenously or subcutaneously three times per week for 8 weeks reduces the transfusion requirements for patients taking zidovudine.[24]

The other major side effect of zidovudine is my-

opathy. Patients have developed muscle tenderness, weakness, and wasting. The legs are generally affected before the arms. Dosage modification may be required if the patient has these symptoms.

Dideoxyinosine (ddI)

In October 1991, the FDA approved dideoxyinosine (ddI). Like zidovudine, ddI interacts with reverse transcriptase to inhibit HIV replication. This agent is recommended for patients who are intolerant of zidovudine or who have shown immunological decline while receiving it. Its side effects include pancreatitis and peripheral neuropathy with complaints of distal numbness, tingling, or pain in the feet and hands.

It is taken in an oral form on an empty stomach twice a day. The drug contains a large sodium load as part of the buffers necessary to increase gastric pH to facilitate drug absorption.

Dideoxycytidine (ddC)

The drug most recently approved for treating HIV infection is ddC. It is recommended for use in combination with zidovudine in patients with advanced HIV infection who have T4 cell counts of less than 300 per mm^3 and have demonstrated clinical or immunological deterioration. A dose of 0.75 mg is given orally, together with 200 mg of zidovudine every 8 hours. The side effects of ddC include pancreatitis and moderate-to-severe peripheral neuropathy. Since the drug is given with zidovudine, the bone marrow side effects of this drug and possible impairment in renal function can also occur.

PCP Prophylaxis

In April 1992, the CDC issued recommendations for prophylaxis against PCP for adults and adolescents with HIV. The goal of this therapy is to reduce the frequency of both initial (primary) episodes of PCP and relapses or recurrent (secondary) episodes.

HIV-infected patients with T4 cell counts of less than 200 per mm^3 and those with constitutional symptoms regardless of cell counts should receive lifetime prophylaxis.[25] Any patient who has recovered from a documented episode of PCP should also receive prophylaxis.[25] Either of two prophylactic regimens is recommended, depending on the individual patient's physical condition and ability to comply with therapy:

1. TMP-SMX in one double-strength tablet taken once a day 7 days per week is suggested.[25] Side effects of pruritus, rash, cytopenias, or elevated transaminase levels may make this therapy intolerable.
2. Aerosolized pentamidine with the Respirgard II nebulizer using a dosage of 300 mg once a month

is recommended.[25] Use of the FisoNeb nebulizer requires an initial loading dose of five 60-mg doses over 2 weeks, followed by a 60-mg dose every 2 weeks.[25]

Aerosolized pentamidine is often administered by a respiratory therapist. However, the critical care nurse collaborates in providing patient care related to this treatment and must be aware of the required precautions. A baseline assessment of vital signs and breath sounds should be performed. The patient should be instructed to breathe in and out through the mouth during the procedure. Approximately every 20 seconds, the patient should exhale to residual volume before inhalation. An average treatment takes between 30 and 45 minutes. Patients should not be left unattended because complications may develop; the patient may need reminders about appropriate breathing, and airflow to the nebulizer must be controlled if the patient stops momentarily. Patients who are more debilitated may tire easily and need more assistance during pentamidine administration.

Bronchospasm with wheezing, dyspnea, tightness of the chest, and cyanosis can develop during a pentamidine treatment. These symptoms are most likely to occur in high-risk patients who have preexisting asthma or are heavy smokers. Allergic reaction is another potential side effect. Bronchodilators should be readily available. In patients with known allergy, pretreatment may prevent or minimize this reaction. Breath sounds should be auscultated prior to the treatment, 15 minutes into the procedure, and 30 minutes after the procedure to assess patient response.

Coughing related to aerosol deposition of pentamidine in the upper tracheobronchial tree should be anticipated during and after the treatment. When the patient stops the treatment to cough, the airflow to the nebulizer should be turned off to prevent loss of medication into the environment. The use of throat lozenges before and after the treatment may help with this problem.

A burning sensation in the back of the throat is a common complaint from patients receiving this therapy. Taking small sips of water during and after the treatment is recommended. A bitter taste in the mouth may occur. Using a mouth rinse of baking soda and saline or sucking on hard candy or licorice can minimize this sensation.

If the patient receiving pentamidine aerosolization has TB, strict adherence to AFB isolation precautions is necessary. Coughing induced during the procedure can spread TB from the patient to health care workers if appropriate precautions are not followed. Health care workers administering pentamidine to a patient with TB or who may be in the room during this ther-apy should wear particulate respirators.[25]

The long-term effects of inhalation of pentamidine on health care workers have not been conclusively determined. The short-term effects of inhaling pentamidine can be the same for a health care worker as a patient. Therefore, whenever the patient stops breathing through the mouthpiece of the nebulizer during therapy, the gas flow should be stopped to prevent environmental aerosolization and occupational exposure of the health care worker to this drug.

PSYCHOSOCIAL NEEDS OF THE HIV PATIENT

Patients with AIDS have complex physiological problems. Care during a physiological crisis may take precedence over other needs. No less complex are the psychosocial needs of the patient with HIV infection. Each patient responds differently to the diagnosis of HIV and its subsequent diseases. Culture, gender, age, socioeconomic factors, and physiological condition influence the patient's needs and ability to cope. Comprehensive nursing care of the critically ill patient includes the high-touch support of patients and families in addition to sophisticated technological support. Awareness of behavioral patterns common to many individuals with HIV allows the critical care nurse to anticipate needs of the patient, family, and significant others.

The patient's reactions and needs often follow the spectrum of the HIV infection. After initial diagnosis, patients are often fearful and anxious. Denial may be used as a coping mechanism. Guilt over past behaviors that led to the acquisition of the disease is common. Some individuals may contemplate suicide. Fear of transmission to others or fear that others will learn of the infection may lead patients to isolate themselves. A preoccupation with health and activities to maintain it has been described in asymptomatic persons with HIV.[20]

As the patient becomes symptomatic, illness may cause a loss of job, denial of insurance coverage, and impoverishment. Increasing physiological problems bring physical and emotional exhaustion. Intractable pain may develop. The patient may suffer from social isolation and rejection by friends and family as a result of the manifestations of HIV disease. Helplessness and worthlessness are commonly experienced symptoms of depression.

When the physiological condition worsens, the nurse may anticipate grieving. Anger may be directed at health care workers who cannot help the patient or who inflict pain during necessary procedures.[21] Patients become increasingly dependent on others for their basic needs and fear abandonment. Many patients want to attend to unfinished legal business. Spiritual needs may also be a priority. Relief of pain may be a major concern. If CNS involvement is extensive, cognitive function may be severely impaired and a wide range of behavioral patterns may be manifested.

Knowledge of problems faced by the patient with HIV can assist the critical care nurse in assessing the needs of the patient and incorporating individual approaches into the plan of care. When caring for terminally ill patients, the focus of the nurse's intervention may shift from the patient to supporting the surviving family or significant others.

REFERENCES

1. Gorman, C. (1992). Invincible AIDS. *Time, 140*(5), 30-34.
2. Centers for Disease Control. (1989). Human immunodeficiency virus—2. *Morbidity and Mortality Weekly Report, 38,* 572-574, 579-580.
3. Grady, C. (1992). HIV disease: Pathogenesis and treatment. In J. H. Flaskerud, & P. J. Ungvarski (Eds.), *HIV/AIDS: A guide to nursing care* (2nd ed.). Philadelphia: Saunders.
4. Pratt, R. (1991). *AIDS: A strategy for nursing care* (3rd ed.). London: Edward Arnold.
5. Fauci, A. S., Macher, A. M., Longo, D. L., et al. (1984). Acquired immunodeficiency syndrome: Epidemiologic, clinical, immunologic, and therapeutic considerations. *Annals of Internal Medicine, 110,* 92-106.
6. Grady, C. (1988). HIV: Epidemiology, immunopathogenesis and clinical considerations. *Nursing Clinics of North America, 23,* 685-695.
7. Fischbach, F. (1992). *A manual of laboratory and diagnostic tests* (4th ed.). Philadelphia: Lippincott.
8. Henderson, D. J. (1988). HIV infection: Risks to health care workers and infection control. *Nursing Clinics of North America, 23,* 767-777.
9. Gurevich, I. (1989). Acquired immunodeficiency syndrome: Realistic concerns and appropriate precautions. *Heart Lung, 18,* 107-112.
10. Centers for Disease Control. (1987). Recommendations for prevention of HIV transmission in health-care settings. *Morbidity and Mortality Weekly Report, 36*(3S), 3S-18S.
11. Federal Register. (1991). Occupational exposure to bloodborne pathogens: Final rule. 29 CFR. Part 1910.1030.
12. Centers for Disease Control. (1987). Revision of the CDC surveillance case definition for acquired immunodeficiency syndrome. *Morbidity and Mortality Weekly Report, 38S,* 3S-15S.
13. Flaskerud, J. H., & Ungvarski, P. J. (Eds.). (1992). *HIV/AIDS: A guide to nursing care* (2nd ed.). Philadelphia: Saunders.
14. Donehower, M. G. (1987). Malignant complications of AIDS. *Oncology Nursing Forum, 14,* 57-64.
15. Beckman, M. M. (1990). Neurologic manifestations of AIDS. *Critical Care Nursing Clinics of North America, 2,* 29-32.
16. Henry, S. B., & Holzemer, W. L. (1992). Critical care management of the patient with HIV infection who has *Pneumocystis carinii* pneumonia. *Heart Lung, 21,* 243-249.
17. Fischl, M. A., Uttamchandani, R. B., Daikos, G. L., et al. (1992). An outbreak of tuberculosis caused by multiple-drug-resistant tubercle bacilli among patients with HIV infection. *Annals of Internal Medicine, 117,* 177-182.
18. Pearson, M. L., Jereb, J. A., Frieden, T. R., et al. (1992). Nosocomial transmission of multidrug resistant *Mycobacterium tuberculosis* a risk to patients and health care workers. *Annals of Internal Medicine, 117,* 191-196.
19. Centers for Disease Control. (1990). Guidelines for preventing the transmission of tuberculosis in health-care settings, with special focus on HIV-related issues. *Morbidity and Mortality Weekly Report, 39,* RR-17.
20. Grimes, D. E., Grimes, R. M., & Hamelink, M. (1991). *Infectious diseases.* Baltimore: Mosby—Year Book.
21. Crocker, K. S. (1988). AIDS-related GI dysfunction: Rationale for nutrition support. *Critical Care Nurse, 8,* 43-45.
22. Pearlstein, G. (1990). Renal system complications in HIV infection. *Nursing Clinics of North America, 2,* 79-87.
23. Parrillo, J. E., & Masur, H. (Eds.). (1987). *The critically ill immunosuppressed patient: Diagnosis and management.* Rockville, MD: Aspen.
24. Gahart, B. L. (1992). *Intravenous medications* (8th ed.). St. Louis: Mosby—Year Book.
25. Centers for Disease Control. (1992). Recommendations for prophylaxis against *Pneumocystis carinii* pneumonia for adults and adolescents infected with human immunodeficiency virus. *Morbidity and Mortality Weekly Report, 41,* 1-11.

48

Acute Oncologic Disorders

Anne M. McCoy

Aline Mierzejewski

The concept of oncologic critical care as a specialty is receiving widespread recognition because of the unique and pressing complications that may arise from aggressive medical or surgical treatment of oncology patients. Nursing care of patients critically ill with oncologic disorders requires expanded theoretical knowledge as well as advanced technical and clinical skills. The advanced nursing skills required include invasive and noninvasive hemodynamic monitoring techniques to obtain data regarding possible neutropenic septic shock, complications related to chemotherapy or radiation treatment, electrolyte abnormalities, and postoperative fluid shifts. In-depth assessment and management of pain is often needed. New treatment protocols and the use of potentially highly toxic drugs influence the need for critical care nurses to assist the patient through possibly reversible complications. The nurse also needs to provide comprehensive psychosocial and emotional support interventions for the patient and significant other(s). Development of these skills is enhanced by a commitment to excellence in holistic care and professional accountability.

The diagnosis of cancer alone does not require admission to a critical care unit, but many patients in critical care units have cancer, particularly those having major thoracic, abdominal, urologic, gynecologic, hepatic, and head and neck operations. Most are admitted to the unit for management of single or multisystem organ failure, which may be related to treatment of their cancer or to a preexisting illness. Viability, prognosis, and meaningful recovery as defined by the patient must be considered when very sick patients are admitted to critical care units. For this reason, meeting the psychosocial needs of the patient is a high priority.

The critical care unit should not be regarded as a facility for prolonging the process of dying. As cancer treatment has become more successful in prolonging life, cancer is coming to be regarded as a chronic rather than a terminal illness. The prognosis for many patients with cancer has changed from one of hopelessness and impending death to one of expectation for a reasonable quality of life for as long as possible. Among the challenges to be met is that of containing the high morbidity that often accompanies massive corrective or palliative surgery and potentially toxic therapeutic methods.

CHEMOTHERAPY OVERVIEW

Chemotherapeutic agents destroy cancer cells by interfering with cellular function and replication. Because these agents act on rapidly dividing cells, some normal cells also are damaged, although the replication characteristics of the cancer cells make them more vulnerable. Chemotherapeutic agents are commonly classified according to the pharmacological properties of the drugs.[1] Table 48-1 lists the most commonly used agents. Some drugs cannot be classified because their mechanism of action is combined or not well understood.

Most chemotherapeutic regimens use these drugs or some combination of these drugs.[2] Drugs to be used in combined therapy are usually chosen from different classes to ensure a variety of action at the cellular level aiming for the maximal response while taking care not to overlap side effects.[3]

The therapeutic use of biological response modifiers (BRMs) has emerged as the fourth modality of cancer therapy along with surgery, radiation, and chemotherapy. BRMs are agents that directly or indirectly contribute to an antitumor response primarily through the use of the host's immune system.[4,5] Much research is currently being directed toward BRMs, which include the interferons, interleukins, colony-stimulating growth factors, monoclonal antibodies, and tumor necrosis factor.[6] Table 48-2 lists their actions and identified side effects.

TABLE 48-1 **Commonly Used Chemotherapy Agents**

Type	Effects	Nursing Implications
ALKYLATING AGENTS		
Nitrogen mustard Chlorambucil Busulfan Thiotepa	Cell cycle stage nonspecific; destroy resting and dividing cells; cause inability of DNA to replicate.	Major side effects related to rapidly dividing normal cells: hematopoietic, gastrointestinal, and reproductive. Nausea and vomiting common. Leukopenia reaches nadir in 7-14 days. Recovery in about 30 days.
NITROSOUREAS		
Carmustine (BCNU) Semustine Lomustine (CCNU) Streptozocin	Cell cycle nonspecific; affect DNA formation by inhibiting several enzymatic steps.	Cross the blood–brain barrier. Cause bone marrow suppression and gastrointestinal toxicities. Delayed nadir at 3-5 weeks. Thrombocytopenia common. Severe nausea and vomiting.
ANTIBIOTICS		
Actinomycin D Mitomycin C Doxorubicin Daunorubicin Bleomycin Mithramycin	Cell cycle stage nonspecific; interfere with nucleic acid synthesis and block DNA-directed RNA and DNA transcription.	Bone marrow suppression common, especially leukopenia and thrombocytopenia. Nadir occurs at 10-14 days with recovery in 21 days. Stomatitis and alopecia can be anticipated. Dose-related cardiotoxicity may be seen with doxorubicin and daunorubicin. Bleomycin may cause severe pulmonary toxicity.
ANTIMETABOLITES		
Methotrexate 5-Fluorouracil 6-Mercaptopurine Cytosine arabinoside (ARA-C) 6-Thioguanine (6-TG)	Cell cycle phase specific; inhibit DNA synthesis.	Bone marrow suppression common, nadir in 1-2 weeks. Alopecia, mucositis, nausea, vomiting, diarrhea common. Methotrexate can be lethal in high doses without leucovorin "rescue" of normal cells. Treatment with 6-MP and 6-TG can cause liver damage.
PLANT ALKALOIDS (Vinca Alkaloids)		
Vinblastine Vincristine	Cell cycle phase specific; destroy cells by crystallizing spindle proteins during metaphase, arresting mitosis.	Vinblastine causes myelosuppression with nadir in 4-10 days and recovery in 10-21 days. Vincristine may cause neurotoxicity often evidenced by peripheral neuropathy, cranial nerve palsies, vocal cord paralysis, and autonomic nervous system dysfunctional constipation.
HORMONES		
Estrogens Androgens Progestins Corticosteroids	Presence of specific receptor proteins inside cytoplasm of cell allows binding of hormone. Receptor proteins facilitate synthesis of mRNA. Using hormones antagonistic to process causes antitumor effects.	Side effects are directly related to normal action of hormone. Sex hormones: fluid retention and changes in secondary sexual characteristics can occur. Corticosteroids: Cushingoid state, peptic ulcer, hypertension, diabetes, osteoporosis.
MISCELLANEOUS		
Cell cycle phase specific: Hydroxyurea, procarbazine *Cell cycle phase nonspecific:* L-Asparaginase, hexamethylmelamine, cisplatin	Mechanisms are multiple or are not fully understood.	Profound nausea and vomiting common; may lead to electrolyte imbalance.

TABLE 48-2 **Biological Response Modifiers**

Agent	Action	Side Effects
Interferons (IFN) Alpha Beta Gamma	Proteins that enhance antiviral immunity, are capable of modifying immune responses, and enhance natural killer (NK) cell activity.	Flu-like syndrome: Fever, chills, malaise, fatigue, myalgias. CNS: Mild confusion and somnolence to seizure activity. GI: Nausea, vomiting, diarrhea, anorexia, weight loss. Hematological: Leukopenia, thrombocytopenia, anemia. Cardiovascular: Hypotension, tachycardia, dysrhythmias, myocardial ischemia.[7]
Interleukins (IL) Interleukin-2 (IL-2)	Peptides that signal between cells in the immune system; mediate expansion of T lymphocytes.	Flu-like syndrome: Fever, chills, headache. Cardiovascular/pulmonary: Capillary leak syndrome with resultant hypotension, decreased CVP, oliguria, peripheral edema. Renal: Proteinuria, hematuria, increased BUN and creatinine, azotemia. Neurological: Mental changes ranging from lethargy to psychosis. GI: Nausea, vomiting, diarrhea, mucositis. Hepatic: Liver function studies elevated. Integumentary: Erythematous rash to dry desquamation.[8]
Monoclonal antibodies	Antibodies produced by B lymphocytes targeted against tumor-cell antigen.	Potential for severe allergic reactions, fever, rigors, chills. Pulmonary: Dyspnea, respiratory stridor. Renal: Potential renal failure from tumor lysis.[9]
Tumor Necrosis Factor (TNF)	Soluble factor produced by macrophages; cytotoxic for some tumor cells and some parasites.	Flu-like syndrome: Fever, chills, headache, fatigue. Hematological: Leukopenia, thrombocytopenia. Hepatic: Triglyceride elevation, decreased cholesterol. Cardiovascular: Hypotension. Pulmonary: Dyspnea.[10]
Colony-stimulating factors (CSF) Granulocyte CSF (G-CSF) Granulocyte macrophage CSF (GM-CSF)	Naturally occurring glycoproteins that stimulate the growth of colonies of maturing blood cells from their hematopoietic precursors.	Flu-like syndrome: Fever, chills, rigors, myalgias, headache (GM-CSF mostly).[11]

TREATMENT TOXICITIES

Pulmonary System

Bleomycin chemotherapy injures the lungs by altering the normal alveolar cell mechanisms necessary for handling oxygen molecules. Lung parenchymal injury occurs by the direct effect of toxic oxygen molecules (free radicals) on the tissues resulting in irreversible pulmonary fibrosis. Both radiation therapy and oxygen therapy of greater than a 40% fraction of inspired oxygen (FiO_2) potentiate bleomycin toxicity and may cause clinical symptoms.[12] Dietary deficiencies of protein, vitamin E, copper, selenium, or unsaturated fatty acids also potentiate oxygen toxicities.

Clinical signs and symptoms of oxygen toxicity include bilateral interstitial infiltrates noted on chest x-rays, dyspnea at rest, and ensuing hypoxia. The forced vital capacity (FVC) is reduced as evidenced by pulmonary function tests.

Corticosteroid therapy is often prescribed, and the patient's response can be dramatic.[13] Fluid management is crucial in patients who have pulmonary toxicity because the interstitial pulmonary fibrosis obliterates lymph drainage from the lungs. These patients cannot handle crystalloid fluids and develop fluid overload and pulmonary edema easily. Early detection by hemodynamic monitoring and assessment of heart sounds for S_3 are important. Colloids are often used in patients with bleomycin pulmonary toxicity.

Pulmonary injury from radiation therapy, or *radiation pneumonitis*, consists of enlargement and degeneration of proliferating alveolar cells lining the alveolar sacs. These cells slough from the alveolar sac surface and become incorporated into a hyaline membrane. Thickening of alveolar septa may occur months after radiation treatment and may be mild, moderate, or severe depending upon the dose of radiation received. Injury occurs in 5% to 20% of patients.

Clinical signs and symptoms of radiation pneumonitis found on the chest x-ray range from ill-defined nonhomogeneous opacification to dense alveolar infiltrates. Diffusion capacity may be decreased resulting in hypoxia. The patient may experience dyspnea at rest or with minimal exertion. Related nursing diagnoses and interventions for these pulmonary problems are listed below.

■ NURSING DIAGNOSIS

Impaired gas exchange, related to pulmonary fibrosis secondary to bleomycin oxygen toxicity or radiation pneumonitis.

OUTCOME STANDARD AND CRITERIA

Hypoxemia is absent or reduced as evidenced by:
- $SaO_2 > 90\%$
- $PaO_2 > 65$ mmHg

NURSING INTERVENTIONS

- Maintain FiO_2 less than 40% or as low as possible to prevent O_2 toxicity
- Reduce oxygen demands through activity restriction and control of fever, pain, and shivering
- Provide adequate caloric intake through tube feedings or parenteral nutrition

■ NURSING DIAGNOSIS

Fluid volume excess, related to impaired lymph drainage from lungs.

OUTCOME STANDARD AND CRITERIA

Fluid volume is adequate as evidenced by:
- PAWP <18 mmHg
- Absence of pulmonary congestion
- Absence of S_3 heart sound

NURSING INTERVENTIONS

- Assess heart sounds for S_3
- Monitor intake/output and urine output
- Assess breath sounds for crackles
- Limit fluid intake at the prescribed level
- Provide adequte protein to maintain colloidal osmotic pressure

Cardiovascular System

Cardiomyopathy

The cardiomyopathies that occur in patients with cancer are related to the invasive nature of the disease or to the effects of therapy. They are usually irreversible. Invasion of the myocardium by tumor disrupts the arrangement of the contractile fibers. Weakening of the myocardium leads to dilatation of the muscle walls and, thereby, to congestive heart failure with reduced ejection fraction.

The hemodynamic profile usually reveals an arterial pressure in the normal range with a narrow pulse pressure reflecting the decreased stroke volume. Systemic vascular resistance (SVR) is usually elevated due to the peripheral vascular constriction that occurs to compensate for decreased cardiac output. Pulmonary vascular resistance (PVR) is slightly elevated. Preload indicators (right atrial pressure and pulmonary artery wedge pressure) are elevated, reflecting the degree of congestive heart failure that may be occurring. Contractility indicators (left and right ventricular stroke work index) usually are reduced, depending on the compensatory state of the patient.

Clinical symptoms of cardiomyopathy relate to the degree of functional impairment of the heart. Dyspnea on exertion progresses to orthopnea, paroxysmal nocturnal dyspnea, fatigue, weakness, and chest pain. Peripheral edema, enlargement of the liver, and ascites are late signs of severe disease. Heart sounds may reveal a summation gallop. Systolic murmurs of mitral and tricuspid regurgitation may occur with dilated cardiomyopathy. Breath sounds are clear to auscultation until clinically symptomatic pulmonary edema develops.

Care of the patient with cardiomyopathy is presented in Chapter 23. The oncology patient with cardiomyopathy presents several additional challenges related to treatment of the primary disease.

Doxorubicin Toxicity

Doxorubicin (Adriamycin) is highly effective in the treatment of malignant lymphoma, leukemia, and solid tumors such as sarcomas and carcinomas of the breast, lung, and thyroid. Repeated doses of doxorubicin and daunorubicin (a related drug) can cause cardiotoxicity. There is considerable individual variation in cardiac tolerance to this drug. Clinical expression of toxicity is often observed several months after the last dose of the agent.

Doxorubicin is a glycoside antibiotic from the family of anthracycline antineoplastic drugs. An important mechanism of action of doxorubicin is binding to cell membranes and receptor sites. This property of the drug causes alterations in sodium permeability and the metabolism of calcium by the cardiac tissue. Calcium overload occurs even with normal calcium levels. Calcium ions are critical to the regulation of myocardial contraction; thus, calcium accumulation in the myocardium coupled with a loss of myocytes may be partly responsible for the process of cardiomyopathy. Additionally, anthracyclines stimulate the release of histamine and catecholamines. Cardiomyopathic effects appear to be multifactorial, resulting from doxorubicin's multiple effects at cellular and subcellular levels.[14]

With acute cardiotoxicity from doxorubicin a pericarditis-myocarditis picture evolves. Left ventricular dysfunction, dysrhythmias, and rarely, myocardial infarction can be seen. Chronic cardiotoxicity is associated with persistent sinus tachycardia, pericardial effusions, left ventricular dysfunction, and low output

TABLE 48-3   **Dysrhythmias Associated with Cancer and Cancer Treatment**

Condition	Types of Dysrhythmias
Doxorubicin cardiotoxicity	Sinus and supraventricular tachycardia, ventricular dysrhythmias, rarely AV block, QRS voltage reduction of 30%
Multiple myeloma	First-, second-degree AV block (Mobitz type II), atrial fibrillation, complete AV block, right bundle branch block, or trifascicular block, left bundle branch block, atrial tachycardia with block, AV junctional rhythm, bradydysrhythmias, low QRS voltage, absence of or small R waves in right precordial leads
Leukemia	Nonspecific ST segment and T wave changes, sinus tachycardia, intraventricular conduction defect (IVCD), left axis deviation, atrial dysrhythmias, AV blocks
Pericardial effusions and tamponade	Tachycardia, electrical alternans, atrial flutter, atrial fibrillation, multifocal atrial tachycardia and nonsustained bursts of paroxysmal atrial tachycardia, decreased QRS voltage, T wave changes, and/or elevated ST segments
Pericarditis	Low voltage but normal QRS, ST elevation in precordial leads, inverted T waves after ST segment is isoelectric
Electrolyte imbalances Hypercalcemia	Short QT interval with covered ST segment, prolonged PR interval, lengthening QT interval, widening T wave
Hypokalemia	Prominent U wave, T wave inversion, TU fusion, depressed ST segment, atrial tachycardia, atrial flutter, PACs or PVCs
Hypomagnesemia	Prolonged PR and QT intervals; broad, flat T waves; PVCs; ventricular tachycardia; ventricular fibrillation
Hyperkalemia	Tall, thin T waves; prolonged PR interval; depressed ST segment; wide QRS; absent P waves; AV block; bradycardia; atrial standstill; ventricular fibrillation; cardiac arrest
Cardiac metastasis	Atrial fibrillation and atrial flutter, sick sinus syndrome, paroxysmal supraventricular tachycardia, PVCs, ECG may mimic myocardial infarction

heart failure often with a fatal outcome. Other dysrhythmias are listed in Table 48-3.

Multiple Myeloma

Amyloidosis features of multiple myeloma result from the infiltration of a proteinaceous, glassy, amorphous extracellular substance into the skin, kidney, heart, GI tract, liver, lungs, nerves, brain, bone marrow, joints, spleen, blood vessels, and eyes. Primary systemic amyloidosis is associated with multiple myeloma and usually results in cardiomyopathy. Corresponding cancers along with multiple myeloma include Hodgkin's disease, kidney, hairy cell leukemia, thyroid cancer, and all those treated with chemotherapy. Table 48-3 lists specific dysrhythmias associated with multiple myeloma.

Leukemia

Microscopic leukemic cell infiltrates of the heart often exist with accumulations of erythrocytes. These infiltrates are generally spotty and located in or immediately beneath the endocardium. The outflow tract and pericardium of the left ventricle are often the site of intense leukemic cell infiltration. Studies of leukemic cardiac metastasis have confirmed a significantly higher incidence of heart involvement by chronic lymphocytic leukemia cells than by cells in other types of leukemia.[15]

In addition to leukemic infiltrates, a major cause of cardiac morbidity and mortality is associated with the electrolyte and acid–base imbalances often triggered by the underlying disease and by treatment and supportive measures. Acute leukemia, even without coexisting septicemia, can lead to lactic acidosis and hyperkalemia. The cardiac abnormalities related to these alterations or to the effects of hyperkalemia, hyperphosphatemia, and reciprocal hypocalcemia have been implicated in the death of patients with leukemia. These chemical changes of the extracellular and intracellular compartments may initiate cardiac dysrhythmias and ECG changes as listed in Table 48-3.

Pericardial Effusions and Tamponade

Many factors contribute to the development of pericardial effusions and cardiac tamponade in the oncology patient. Tumor compression or infiltration may increase capillary pressure and obstruct lymphatic flow. Decreased plasma proteins in malnourished states and retention of fluids by the kidneys contribute in some cases. The tumor cells may secrete fluid that becomes trapped, leading to pleural effusions, pericardial effusions, and tamponade.

Compensatory tachycardia is seen with reduced cardiac output in an attempt to restore or maintain an adequate cardiac output. The filling of the pericardial sac with effusion fluid impairs ventricular filling and reduces stroke volume. In most cases, treatment is instituted to increase fluid volume to improve cardiac output until the effusion can be removed by pericardiocentesis or pericardial window.[16] These are temporary measures to relieve symptoms, not treat the disease.

Electrical alternans is the alternation in the configuration of the P wave and the RST complex seen on the ECG tracing with every other beat or every third beat. The mechanism for alternans in pericardial effusion appears to be unusually large variations in motion of the heart permitted by its suspension in a fluid medium. Proximity of the heart to the chest wall is associated with tall P and R waves, but with posterior movement the amplitude of P and R waves decreases. Dysrhythmias commonly seen with pericardial effusions are included in Table 48-3.

Pericarditis

Treatment for pericardial effusions may lead to pericarditis. As the fluid is removed, the pericardial sac rubs the myocardium and causes symptoms of pericarditis. Instillation of tetracycline or other sclerosing agents into the pericardial sac and tumor infiltration causing adhering lesions also may cause pericarditis and related dysrhythmias (see Table 48-3).

Electrolyte Imbalances

Hypercalcemia (serum calcium level of greater than 11 mg/dl) is the most common metabolic oncologic emergency. Hypercalcemia develops in 33% of patients with multiple myeloma and 5% of patients with solid tumors.[17] Over 80% of patients with hypercalcemia have bone metastases. Direct neoplastic bone resorption is considered to be the most common cause of hypercalcemia associated with cancer. Other causes include osteolytic humoral substances such as parathyroid hormone-like substances or prostaglandins thought to be secreted by tumor cells. Patients with squamous cell carcinomas of the head and neck, lung, and esophagus may develop a clinical syndrome suggestive of hyperparathyroidism, due to ectopic secretion of parathyroid hormone or parathyrotropic substances. When the patient is receiving digoxin therapy, even with a normal digoxin level, toxicity can be evident with any dysrhythmia, such as AV block or bradycardia.

Hypokalemia and hypomagnesemia occur as a result of treatment such as diuretic therapy, aggressive hydration treatment, or administration of amphotericin B. These agents increase the excretion of potassium by the kidneys and require monitoring and replacement therapy. Hypokalemia and hypomagnesemia produce ECG changes that are listed in Table 48-3.

Hyperkalemia occurs with tumor lysis syndrome, which is characterized by rapid cellular destruction and a shift of intracellular electrolytes into the serum. Serum potassium becomes elevated and causes ECG changes (see Table 48-3).

Cardiac Metastasis

When compared to other sites of metastasis such as the liver, lungs, or brain, metastases to the heart are less frequent and often clinically inapparent. Metastases to the heart occur 16 to 40 times more commonly than primary cardiac tumors, and usually occur with tumors of the lung and breast, as well as in melanoma, acute leukemia, and lymphoma. In large part, cardiac involvement is underestimated due to either the frequently silent nature of cardiac involvement by the tumor or the ability of the tumor to simulate coronary artery disease and valvular heart disease.

There are three possible mechanisms underlying cardiac metastases. Direct extension of the tumor may occur with intrathoracic tumors such as carcinomas of the lung or breast or from tumor growth within vessels. Implantation, largely to the pericardium, may result in studding, effusions, or a constrictive pericarditis. Blood-borne metastases and spread by the lymphatic system are probably the most frequent forms of cardiac metastases.

Dysrhythmias related to cardiac metastasis commonly include those listed in Table 48-3. Possible mechanisms responsible for these dysrhythmias are: (1) involvement of the atrial sympathetic fibers by the tumor, (2) invasion of a coronary artery by the tumor with production of an atrial infarction pattern, and (3) invasion of noninfarcted areas of atrial myocardium by the tumor. Another mechanism may involve invasion of the sinus node by the tumor and subsequent occurrence of sick sinus syndrome. Tumor metastasis to the heart may mimic an acute myocardial infarction or actually cause such an event. Q waves from electrical "dead zones" may be produced by tumor invasion of the myocardium.[18]

Renal System

Tumor Lysis Syndrome (TLS)

Rapid destruction of tumor cells by chemotherapy or radiation therapy may lead to tumor lysis syndrome. The rapid release of intracellular potassium, phosphorus, and uric acid as a result of tumor destruction causes metabolic imbalances. Serum calcium is also lowered secondary to the increase in phosphorus. TLS usually begins 1 to 5 days after the initiation of chemotherapy but may occur within 1 to 3 days depending on the type of tumor and the agents used. It occurs more frequently with liquid tumors (hematological malignancies) than with solid tumors. Bulky solid tumors with a high growth rate such as ovarian carcinoma are associated with an increased risk for the development of TLS.

Clinical signs and symptoms primarily emanate from the kidneys, which are affected by the increased metabolic load for excretion. Oliguria, anuria, urine crystals, flank pain, and hematuria may be seen. Electrolyte abnormalities (hyperkalemia, hyperphosphatemia, hypocalcemia, and hyperuria) cause cardiac dysrhythmias and neuromuscular cramps, tetany, and confusion. Diagnostic tests reveal elevated levels of serum BUN, creatinine, potassium, phosphorus, and uric acid and decreased levels of serum calcium.[19]

Obstructive Uropathy

Tumor lysis syndrome and the destruction of the tumor mass by radiation or chemotherapy may lead to obstructive uropathy. The rapid breakdown of tumor cells causes accumulation of metabolites. The purine bases that are generated when nuclear DNA is degraded are metabolized to uric acid. Urate is relatively insoluble at an acid pH; consequently, it crystallizes in the distal tubules of the nephron as the urine becomes more concentrated. Obstructive nephropathy and the resulting renal failure may worsen other metabolic abnormalities.

Urate nephropathy due to TLS is potentially fatal. Alkalinization of the urine to a pH greater than 7.0 should be protective against urate nephropathy and is best combined with a forced diuresis. Patients who present with oliguric renal failure and a high urate level may require dialysis but can often be treated by urinary alkalinization alone. Allopurinol, a drug that blocks the enzyme xanthine oxidase, reduces urate production. However, allopurinol cannot completely block the production of uric acid in patients with TLS.[20]

The majority of patients present with clinical signs of uremia, including nausea, vomiting, lethargy, and oliguria. Muscle twitching, clotting defects, hypertension, weight gain, edema, acidosis, pruritus, and anorexia may be seen. Progressive symptoms include pulmonary edema; proteinuria; and altered level of consciousness, usually lethargy, weakness, and fatigue. Laboratory results reveal hypernatremia; prolonged bleeding times; elevated levels of uric acid, BUN, creatinine, potassium, and phosphorus; and decreased creatinine clearance and calcium. The patient experiences oliguria and nausea or vomiting.

Nursing diagnoses and interventions for the renal problems of TLS and obstructive uropathy are listed in the following sections.

■ NURSING DIAGNOSIS

Altered fluid and electrolyte balance, related to renal insufficiency or failure.

OUTCOME STANDARD AND CRITERIA

Fluid and electrolyte balance is restored as evidenced by:

- Normal serum and urine electrolytes and osmolarity
- Normal filling pressures (CVP and PAWP)

NURSING INTERVENTIONS

- Administer intravenous fluids with sodium bicarbonate to increase diuresis and alkalinize the urine as prescribed
- Administer allopurinol and/or diuretics and monitor results to maintain adequate fluid volume as prescribed
- Monitor laboratory results for elevated uric acid, hypernatremia, prolonged bleeding times; increased BUN, creatinine, potassium and phosphorus; decreased creatinine clearance and calcium
- Monitor urine for occult blood and specific gravity

■ NURSING DIAGNOSIS

Self-care deficit, related to weakness from electrolyte imbalances.

OUTCOME STANDARD AND CRITERIA

Self-care is performed to maximal level of independence as evidenced by:[21]

- Bathing, feeding, and toileting appropriate to age and ability

NURSING INTERVENTIONS

- Assist with ADLs to conserve strength while maintaining hygiene needs
- Assist with feeding, nutritional support

COMPLICATIONS OF DISEASE OR TREATMENT

Neutropenic Sepsis

Neutropenia is a reduction in effective circulating white blood cells. With cancer treatment, these cells are often diminished in number and function because of myelosuppression (bone marrow suppression) from chemotherapy or radiation therapy.

The white blood cells most relevant to evaluation for neutropenia are the granulocytes, which are the most numerous and most important in function against infections. When the granulocyte count is less than 1,000/mm³, the patient is considered to be granulocytopenic or neutropenic, and the incidence of infection begins to rise. When the granulocyte count falls to 500/mm³, bacteremia dominates the clinical picture.[22] As the length of therapy and duration of granulocytopenia increase, so does the incidence of infections. Because of the short life span of granulocytes, counts are calculated daily. For each treatment that causes granulocytopenia, there is a period when the granulocyte counts are lowest; this period is called the *nadir*.

The use of cytotoxic drugs (chemotherapy) has direct and indirect effects on the bone marrow that reduce the number of effective white blood cells. Radiation therapy affects the marrow in the areas irradiated. In addition, the underlying disease process, such as bone marrow metastasis or primary bone marrow disease such as leukemia, may also reduce the number and function of granulocytes. The use of corticosteroids to treat the disease or the side effects of therapy further impairs the immune response.

Signs of infection or inflammation, such as purulence, erythema, or pain, may not occur, and fever may be the only reliable indicator that inflammation or infection is present. The only initial evidence of pneumonia may be crackles; cough or sputum production may not be present. The development of an infiltrate on chest x-ray may be delayed due to the lack of white blood cells.[23] The only symptom of a urinary tract infection may be frequency without dysuria. Life-threatening perianal infections may present only with pain on defecation; therefore, the skin must be examined carefully since a necrotic or gangrenous pustule can occur due to bacterial or fungal infection. In patients with skin breakdown, opportunistic fungal infections can occur and disseminate to the eyes. This is most common in patients with candidemia who have central venous catheters and indwelling urinary bladder catheters. Repeated fundoscopic examina-

tions should be performed in the neutropenic patient who has unexplained fever.

Fever may be caused either by the underlying cancer or by infection. It is often difficult to differentiate the cause. The mouth, sinuses, and teeth may harbor infection in neutropenic patients and should be inspected diligently. Acute periodonitis may be the cause of many febrile episodes. Abdominal distention or tenderness may be the only sign of an acute surgical abdomen caused by the underlying malignancy, cancer treatment, or more common abdominal problems, such as appendicitis and cholecystitis.[24]

The vast majority of infections originate from the patient's endogenous flora, and hospitalized patients may become colonized with more virulent pathogens.[25] It is of crucial importance in the febrile patient to obtain blood, urine, sputum, and other fluids (e.g., stool, pleural or peritoneal fluid, if available) for anaerobic and aerobic viral, fungal, and bacterial culture and Gram stain.[26] Table 48-4 lists the common causative organisms of infections.

Viral organisms include herpes simplex, varicellazoster, cytomegalovirus, Epstein-Barr virus, and viral hepatitis. Protozoa that cause infections in the neutropenic patient include *Pneumocystis carinii* and *Toxoplasma gondii*. Immunosuppressed patients are very susceptible to pneumonias that develop due to their inability to defend against inhaled or aspirated organisms and due to reactivation of past infections.

Toxoplasmosis is a disease caused by *Toxoplasma gondii*. There are two types: lymphandenopathic

TABLE 48-4   Neutropenic Sepsis Organisms

Organism	Source
GRAM-NEGATIVE	
Klebsiella	Widely distributed in nature, commonly found in intestinal tract. Frequent causes of endogenous and nosocomial infections in wounds, urinary and pulmonary systems.
Enterobacter	Widely distributed in nature, occurs in intestinal tract, may cause infections in neutropenic patients.
Serratia	Opportunistic pathogen, causes infections in endocardium, blood, wounds, urinary and pulmonary systems.
Pseudomonas species	Widely distributed in nature, cause severe, often fatal nosocomial infections.
GRAM-POSITIVE	
Staphylococcus species	Constantly present on skin and upper respiratory tract, most common cause of localized suppurating infections.
Corynebacteria species	Widely distributed in nature.
Clostridia species	Commonly found in feces, sewage, and soil. Cause gas gangrene.
Myobacteria (acid-fast bacteria)	Common inhabitants of vagina and cervix; cause infections of the male and female reproductive tracts as well as respiratory disease and pharyngitis.
FUNGI (anaerobes)	
Aspergillus	Found in the soil; endoparasitic and opportunistic pathogens.
Candida species	Yeastlike fungi; normal flora of the mouth, skin, intestinal tract, and vagina.
Cryptococcus	Yeastlike fungi; predilection for brain and meninges, also invade the skin, lungs, GI tract causing diarrhea.

toxoplasmosis, closely resembling mononucleosis, and disseminated toxoplasmosis, with lesions involving the lungs, liver, heart, skin, muscle, brain, and meninges.

Administration and monitoring of antibiotic therapy is of primary importance in the care of the neutropenic patient with sepsis. Antibiotics should be started within 1 hour after the onset of fever. Delay in administration of antibiotics increases mortality. Initial empiric treatment of septic shock generally should be aggressive and broad-spectrum, since failure to treat the true etiological agent is likely to result in death. Before treatment is instituted, blood and urine should be obtained for culture for bacteria and fungi.

■ **NURSING DIAGNOSIS**

Altered protection, related to neutropenia, infection, and therapy.

OUTCOME STANDARD AND CRITERIA

Protection is normal as evidenced by:
- Absence of infection
- Early detection and intervention for infection

NURSING INTERVENTIONS
- Assess effects of antibiotic therapy by specifically monitoring: electrolytes (magnesium and potassium with amphotericin B), antibiotic drug levels, organ toxicity (liver, renal, CNS), and culture and sensitivity tests.
- With aminoglycosides, also monitor BUN and creatinine
- With sulfonamides, also monitor liver function
- With gentamycin and tobramycin, monitor hearing loss as well as renal function

■ **NURSING DIAGNOSIS**

Impaired gas exchange, related to increased need, impaired utilization, and inadequate supply of oxygen.

OUTCOME STANDARD AND CRITERIA

Hypoxemia is absent or reduced as evidenced by:
- PaO_2 >65 mmHg
- SaO_2 >90%
- Respiratory rate, heart rate within tolerable limits
- Absence of cyanosis

NURSING INTERVENTIONS
- Monitor oxygenation via pulse oximetry and arterial blood gases
- Reduce oxygen demands by controlling fever, tachycardia, and instituting energy conservation measures

■ **NURSING DIAGNOSIS**

Altered nutrition, related to increased metabolic needs, inability to consume adequate calories.

OUTCOME STANDARD AND CRITERIA

Nutritional intake meets metabolic requirements as evidenced by:
- Positive nitrogen balance

- Adequate caloric intake

NURSING INTERVENTIONS
- Assess nutritional status, caloric and protein intake
- Administer enteral tube feedings and/or hyperalimentation
- Decrease metabolic needs by reducing fever, providing frequent rest periods, and limiting visitors when indicated

■ **NURSING DIAGNOSIS**

Altered tissue perfusion, related to septic syndrome, multisystem organ failure.

OUTCOME STANDARD AND CRITERIA

Tissue perfusion is adequate as evidenced by:
- Normal cardiac function
- Normal intravascular volume status

NURSING INTERVENTIONS
- Monitor preload (CVP and PAWP), afterload (SVR and PVR), and contractility indicators (VSWI and CI)
- Titrate IV fluid rate and vasoactive drugs to maintain adequate cardiac output and tissue perfusion

Typically, the hemodynamic picture is one of decreased preload (CVP and PAWP), decreased afterload (SVR and PVR), and initially, increased contractility (ventricular stroke work index and cardiac index), which progresses to decreased contractility as the septic syndrome progresses and the sequelae of multisystem organ failure follows. These values are used to determine fluid and vasoactive medication requirements.[27]

Titrated doses of vasoactive drugs can be administered to improve cardiac performance. Dobutamine, digoxin, or both can improve contractility. Dopamine is frequently used at low doses (less than 5 μg/kg/min) to maintain renal perfusion. Norepinephrine may be administered concurrently and titrated for vasopressor effects and increasing the SVR. These drugs are used in conjunction with fluid volume replacement. With sepsis, fluid shifts from the vascular compartment to the interstitial spaces. Total fluid volume may be increased to the extent of several liters, reflected in weight gain of 2 to 3 kg per day. The best indicators of vascular fluid volume status are the preload indicators (CVP and PAWP).

Complications of Blood and Blood Products Transfusion

Transfusions of blood and blood products occur frequently during treatment for cancer. This need may be related to the effects of the treatment or to the effects of the disease. Chemotherapy and radiation impair the ability of the bone marrow to produce the needed blood components at an adequate rate. Hematological tumors such as leukemias and lymphomas may be associated with anemia, thrombocytopenia, or both.

Indications for red blood cell transfusions in the critically ill oncology patient are: (1) hematocrit of less than 25% to 30%, (2) hemoglobin level below 10 g/dl, or (3) symptomatic manifestations (dyspnea, fatigue, orthostatic hypotension). Red blood cells are commonly prescribed. Each unit of packed cells has a hematocrit of 70% to 80% which can increase the patient's hematocrit by 3% and hemoglobin by 1 g.[28]

Patients with a platelet count of less than 20,000/mm³ are candidates for prophylactic platelet transfusion, and patients who are actively bleeding with a platelet count of 20,000 to 100,000/mm³ should also be recipients. Each unit of platelets transfused should produce an increase of 5,000 to 10,000/mm³ in the average adult.

Fresh frozen plasma and cryoprecipitate may be indicated for patients with coagulation deficiencies from disseminated disease or for patients with disseminated intravascular coagulopathy (DIC). Fresh frozen plasma and cryoprecipitate are useful in replacement of clotting factors and fibrinogen, respectively.

To reduce fatal infections in neutropenic patients, transfusions of granulocytes have been tried. Serious adverse reactions have been associated with these transfusions. In addition to the risks associated with transfusion of other blood products, granulocytes have been associated with lethal pulmonary reactions. Granulocyte transfusions should be considered only for patients with severe granulocytopenia in whom antibiotic therapy is failing but who indicate a potential for recovery.

The frequent transfusions required by the acutely ill oncology patient may result in one or more of the following adverse conditions:

Transfusion Reactions

Patients who receive multiple transfusions of any blood product are at risk for antigen–antibody reaction from leukocyte antigens on the surface of donor leukocytes and platelets. The blood can be treated in a variety of ways to reduce the likelihood of immunological reactions to leukocytes and platelets. The simplest and most cost-effective way is to filter the product using a special "leukocyte removal" filter. Other methods include radiation and washing red blood cell preparations or frozen deglycerolized red blood cells.

Engraftment

Patients with prolonged immunosuppression who receive multiple transfusions, particularly those patients undergoing bone marrow transplantation, are at risk for developing a graft-versus-host reaction if T lymphocytes are contained in the transfusion product and engraft in the recipient. Red blood cell preparations may be irradiated to inactivate lymphocytes that may remain in the products and, thus, reduce the risk of graft-versus-host disease due to transfusions.

Platelet Consumption Syndrome

Alloimmunization after repeated random donor platelet transfusions occurs in approximately half of patients who require extended transfusion support. This results in febrile reactions and a very short platelet life. These patients fail to achieve adequate platelet increments from regular platelet transfusions. Instead, they are often treated with HLA-matched platelets.

Malignant Effusions

Pleural Effusions

Malignant pleural effusions often have an insidious onset with relatively minor symptoms that gradually worsen over a period of months. Pleural effusions from nonmalignant causes typically have a more abrupt onset of symptoms.

Malignant pleural effusions most commonly result from primary tumors of the lung, breast, and hematopoietic system. The accumulation of fluid in the pleural space may be caused by increased hydrostatic pressure in the pulmonary microvascular circulation, decreased pressure in the pleural space, increased permeability of the pulmonary microvascular circulation, impaired lymphatic drainage from the pleural space, and/or movement of fluid from the peritoneal space.[29]

The most common cause of malignant pleural effusions in patients with solid tumors such as lung cancer is the migration of cancer cells into the pleural space, which leads to increased capillary permeability. Another cause is obstruction of pleural or pulmonary lymphatic channels, which prevents reabsorption of fluid. This is seen in lymphomas and breast cancers. Also, obstruction of pulmonary veins by tumor causes increased capillary hydrostatic pressure in the visceral pleura and movement of fluid from vascular to pleural space, as seen in lung cancers. Shedding of necrotic malignant cells into the pleural space increases the pleural colloid osmotic pressure and impairs the absorption of fluid into the pleural capillaries. In addition, obstruction and/or tearing of the thoracic lymphatic duct may cause lymphatic fluid to leak into the pleural space (chylous pleural effusion) as seen in lymphoma.[30]

Dyspnea, the most common symptom with pleural effusions, is caused by the collapse of a significant amount of lung tissue. The second most common symptom is chest pain caused by compression of the bronchial walls by fluid and by increased intrapleural or intraparenchymal pressure stimulating the sympathetic nerves. The presence of fever may be noted.

Assessment of the chest may reveal dullness to percussion, diminished or absent breath sounds, and egophony on the affected side. A pleural friction rub may be heard. Typically, 300 to 500 ml of fluid accumulates before abnormal physical findings can be detected. A chest x-ray including decubitus views will usually confirm the presence of fluid in the pleural cavity. Computed tomography (CT) can be useful in diagnosing effusions.

For small, symptomatic effusions such as those caused by lymphomas, leukemias, breast cancer, small cell lung cancer, or ovarian cancer, the first line of treatment is systemic chemotherapy or hormonal therapy. A thoracentesis may be performed if the patient is symptomatic. This alone may control the effusion for a time, but there will be a rapid reaccumulation of the fluid.

Placement of a thoracostomy tube for drainage may be indicated if the patient becomes symptomatic from reaccumulation of effusion fluid and if obliteration of the pleural space is desired. When the previous 24-hour drainage from the chest tube is about 100 ml, a sclerosing agent is instilled into the pleural space. Bleomycin and tetracycline are the most widely used sclerosing agents. These are instilled through the chest tube which is then clamped, usually for 45 to 60 minutes. The patient is instructed to lie in varying positions to allow the drug to come into contact with areas of the pleura where sclerosing needs to occur. This procedure causes considerable pain; therefore, lidocaine or other analgesics are injected into the pleural space before instillation of the sclerosing agent.

Surgical approaches to the management of malignant pleural effusions are pleural stripping, pericardial window, or placement of a pleuroperitoneal shunt. Radiation therapy has been used to control effusions due to mediastinal lymph node obstruction or metastasis from radiation sensitive tumors.

Ascites

Patients with ovarian, breast, gastric, pancreatic, hepatic, or colon cancers commonly develop malignant ascites. Patients with lymphoma, mesothelioma, testicular and lung cancers, sarcoma, multiple myeloma, and melanoma are also at risk for such development.

Malignant ascites results from a combination of subdiaphragmatic lymphatic obstruction and increased accumulation of intraperitoneal fluid. Damage to the capillary endothelium increases capillary permeability, thereby leading to increased peritoneal fluid accumulation. Ascites can also be caused by obstruction of the main thoracic duct or of the hepatic venous system. In diffuse hepatic metastases, ascites may be due to mechanical obstruction.

Symptoms of ascites include abdominal distention, weight gain, and indigestion. As the ascitic fluid accumulates, the diaphragm elevates and dyspnea, orthopnea, and tachypnea ensue. If the amount of ascites is large enough, intestinal obstruction may develop from increased intraabdominal pressure, resulting in nausea and vomiting.

Formation of malignant ascites is seen as an adverse prognostic sign and is often difficult to control. A paracentesis may be performed palliatively to improve comfort and decrease dyspnea. Intravenous infusion of colloids may be performed concurrently to prevent hypotension if large volumes of fluid are removed. Repeated paracentesis is not usually advisable since protein depletion and hypoalbuminemia can occur, resulting in the continued formation of ascites.

Systemic chemotherapy can reduce ascites formation, especially in ovarian cancer. Intraperitoneal instillation of drugs such as cisplatin and 5-fluorouracil may be considered with tumors that are resistant to chemotherapy. Instillation of sclerosing agents such as tetracycline has also been tried. These procedures are not without possible complications such as extensive peritoneal fibrosis, intestinal obstruction, bowel necrosis, infection, and fistula formation.

The most commonly used method for palliation of ascites is surgical implantation of a peritoneovenous shunt of either the LeVeen or Denver type. These shunts drain fluid from the peritoneal cavity into the superior vena cava. Potential complications from shunt placement are shunt occlusion, disseminated intravascular coagulation, pulmonary edema, and shunt-induced tumor embolization.

■ NURSING DIAGNOSIS
Altered fluid balance, related to fluid shifts.

OUTCOME STANDARD AND CRITERIA
Normal fluid balance evidenced by:
- Normal filling pressures (CVP and PAWP)

NURSING INTERVENTIONS
- Monitor CVP and PAWP, urine output
- Titrate IV fluid rate to maintain adequate urine output
- Assess for dyspnea, cardiac tamponade
- Administer diuretics with caution, monitor response

Superior Vena Cava Syndrome

Superior vena cava syndrome (SVCS) is an oncologic complication and potential emergency caused by the obstruction of the superior vena cava by external compression of the vessel by tumor or lymph nodes, direct invasion of the vessel wall by tumor, or thrombosis of the vessel. SVCS is most frequently caused by lung cancer (especially small cell) and lymphoma. It can also be caused by thrombus formation around an indwelling central venous catheter.[31]

Signs and symptoms of superior vena cava syndrome are caused by venous hypertension, delayed circulation time, and venous dilatation of collateral veins resulting from compression of the superior vena cava.[32] The most common symptoms include shortness of breath, facial edema, trunk and upper extremity edema, neck and chest vein distention, cough, hoarseness, and stridor. The patient may be dyspneic, cyanotic, or plethoric. Neurological symptoms are related to increased intracranial pressure and include headache, dizziness, visual disturbance, stupor, and convulsions.

Initial medical treatment is usually radiotherapy, but systemic chemotherapy may be used if the tumor is of a type responsive to chemotherapy. Diuretics may be administered to decrease venous pressure but should be used with caution because hypotension can occur. Corticosteroids may be used in respiratory compromise associated with inflammatory reactions. If symptoms do not resolve within 24 to 72 hours of initiation of radiation and/or chemotherapy treatment, a thrombus is suspected. Anticoagulant or fibrinolytic therapy may be initiated. In some cases, embolectomy may be attempted.

■ **NURSING DIAGNOSIS**

Ineffective breathing pattern, related to airway obstruction.

OUTCOME STANDARD AND CRITERIA

Breathing pattern is normal or improved as evidenced by:[21]

• Normal rate, volume, timing, and rhythm of respiration

NURSING INTERVENTIONS

• Support endotracheal intubation during radiation treatments
• Suction as needed
• Provide emotional support to patient and significant others

■ **NURSING DIAGNOSIS**

Alteration in cardiac output, related to decreased venous return.

OUTCOME STANDARD AND CRITERIA

Cardiac output is maintained at an adequate level as evidenced by:

• Normal blood pressure, filling pressures, and perfusion parameters

NURSING INTERVENTIONS

• Monitor intake and output
• Assess breath sounds
• Administer fluids cautiously according to hemodynamic parameters
• Assess response to diuretics to detect early signs of hypotension

BONE MARROW TRANSPLANTATION

Bone marrow transplantation is performed with curative intent for both malignant and nonmalignant diseases of bone marrow origin as well as for selected solid tumors. There are basically two types of bone marrow transplantation: allogeneic and autologous. *Allogeneic transplantation* involves matching the patient's human leukocyte antigen (HLA) identity as closely as possible to the donor in order to minimize rejection. *Autologous transplantation* uses the patient's own marrow or peripheral stem cells. Stem cells are noncommitted pluripotent cells that have the potential to reconstitute the hematopoietic system fully after infusion.[33] These are harvested from the patient's marrow or by apheresis with the use of a double-lumen hemodialysis catheter. Autologous transplantation follows high-dose, chemotherapy-induced myelosuppression; the purpose is to provide protection from infection and bleeding until the patient's marrow and circulating neutrophils and platelets regenerate.

Not all patients receiving bone marrow transplantation require critical care management. Two critical complications that may occur are acute graft-versus-host disease and hepatic venoocclusive disease.

Acute graft-versus-host disease (GVHD) occurs more frequently in allogeneic than in autologous transplants. Patients receiving autologous transplants may experience a mild acute reaction caused by an imbalance in the T4/T8 lymphocyte ratio or from leukocytes received in blood transfusions.

Patients receiving allogeneic transplants may develop acute GVHD within the first 100 days after bone marrow transplantation. This is associated with the rapid onset of skin rash, hepatic dysfunction, diarrhea, and immunological derangements. Three systems are assessed for the clinical stage of acute GVHD: the skin, liver, and gastrointestinal (GI) tract. The skin is assessed for the progression of maculopapular rash to generalized erythroderma to desquamation and bullae. Serum bilirubin is monitored, with elevation to 15 mg/dl indicating severe GVHD. GI involvement manifests with diarrhea from 500 to 1,500 ml/day resulting in electrolyte and metabolic imbalances, malabsorption, and protein deficiencies.

Hepatic venoocclusive disease (VOD) is a potentially fatal liver disorder that occurs in approximately 21% of bone marrow transplant patients.[34] It occurs most frequently in patients who have received high-dose chemotherapy or radiation. It involves partial or complete occlusion of the branches of the hepatic veins by endophlebitis and thrombosis. The diagnosis of VOD depends primarily on clinical signs: jaundice, hepatomegaly or right upper quadrant pain, and ascites or unexplained weight gain. A rising bilirubin level is one of the first signs of VOD; this occurs an average of 11 days after transplantation and reaches maximum values at day 17.

Critical care nursing management of acute GVHD

and VOD is described below. In addition, critical care management involves monitoring the patient's fluid volume status to evaluate the hemodynamic stability. Ascites or unexplained weight gain requires careful investigation. Spironolactone is useful to promote water and sodium excretion while conserving potassium. Assessment factors include daily weights, intake and output measurements, central venous pressure monitoring, and assessment of postural blood pressure changes to monitor fluid volume status. Nutrition is a critical management problem, and fluid and protein restrictions can often be handled with the use of concentrated parenteral nutrition solutions.

■ **NURSING DIAGNOSIS**

Impaired skin integrity, related to graft-versus-host disease.

OUTCOME STANDARD AND CRITERIA

Skin remains intact, and wound healing occurs as evidenced by:
- Tissue epithelialization/granulation
- Intact mucous membranes

NURSING INTERVENTIONS
- Use pressure-dispersing devices (special beds)
- Keep patient clean and dry
- Select adhesives that are least irritating to patient's skin
- Provide regular oral hygiene
- Maximize nutritional status
- Consult with clinical nurse specialist or enterostomal therapist for complex skin care needs

■ **NURSING DIAGNOSIS**

Altered fluid volume status, related to hepatic venoocclusive disease and/or diarrhea.

OUTCOME STANDARD AND CRITERIA

Fluid status is restored as evidenced by:
- Normal serum and urine electrolytes and osmolarity
- Normal filling pressure (CVP and PAWP)

NURSING INTERVENTIONS
- Provide adequate fluid intake and electrolyte balance by replacing fluid loss
- Maximize physiological function through titration of IV fluids, drug therapy
- Monitor effects of fluid and electrolyte replacement by CVP and PAWP
- Obtain daily weights

MAJOR ONCOLOGIC SURGERIES

Otolaryngology

Head and neck cancers of several types comprise approximately 5% of all cancers in the United States.[35] The prevalence of these cancers continues to increase, even though 90% of head and neck malignancies are related to lifestyle or environmental risk factors such as tobacco, alcohol use, and exposure to ultraviolet radiation or asbestos. Squamous cell carcinomas and their variants account for 80% of head and neck malignancies.

The goals of treatment are eradication of the cancer, maintenance of adequate physiological function in the areas of the special senses, mastication-deglutition, respiration, and speech; and achievement of socially acceptable cosmesis. Treatment methods are radiation therapy, chemotherapy, and surgery.

Radiation therapy can be curative or palliative. It is the treatment of choice for very early oropharyngeal and laryngeal carcinomas. A combined approach of radiation therapy and surgery may be necessary for advanced lesions. Conventional radiation is administered in divided doses over several weeks.

Chemotherapy has had limited success in patients with head and neck cancer. Several different chemotherapeutic agents and combinations have demonstrated improved response rates in previously untreated patients.[36] Chemotherapy given prior to surgery or irradiation may help to reduce the size of the tumor and may extend disease-free intervals. Long-term survival has not improved through the use of chemotherapy.

Surgical Procedures

The treatment of choice for head and neck cancers is surgery. Because of the postoperative edema associated with oropharyngeal head and neck surgical procedures, nursing care focuses on protection and preservation of the airway.[37] Often a tracheostomy, either temporary or permanent, is performed. Reconstructive microvascular surgery is performed for extensive defects, which has the advantages of function soon after surgery, reduced chances of infection, and a pleasing cosmetic effect.

Pharyngectomy. Lesions in the pharynx (oropharynx and hypopharynx) typically have an insidious onset. Pharyngectomy is often coupled with resection of the floor of the mouth and radical neck dissection because of the involvement of many structures. Laryngectomy may also be indicated. A myocutaneous flap is often needed to repair the defect. Surgical resections involving the pharyngeal constrictors interfere with swallowing.

Laryngectomy, Hemilaryngectomy. This type of surgical intervention for patients with cancer of the larynx depends on the size and location of the tumor. Patients with tumors in the supraglottic larynx may be treated with supraglottic laryngectomy, in which the area above the true vocal cords from the false vocal cords to the epiglottis is removed. Patients with small cancers involving only one vocal cord may be treated with laser excision or with hemilaryngectomy, in which one vocal cord or part of a vocal cord is removed. Tumors of the vocal cords with invasion or altered mobility are usually treated with total laryngectomy. This includes the removal of all laryngeal structures between and including the thyroid bone, thyroid cartilage, cricoid cartilage, and two to three tracheal rings. Managing copious secretions is a major postoperative concern because the patient is unable to swallow due to postoperative edema.

Mandibulectomy. This type of surgery is commonly performed when tumor invades the bone along with the floor of the mouth and the tongue. Glossectomy is indicated in cancer of the tongue. Partial glossectomy is used for limited lesions of the anterior tongue. Partial glossectomy results in resection of up to one third of the mobile tongue; hemiglossectomy involves resection of the anterior two thirds of the tongue. Glossectomy is often performed as part of a composite resection (excision of intraoral tumor along with a radical neck dissection and possible excision of portion of the mandible). Such extensive monobloc resections, which include one half or more of the tongue, floor of the mouth, adjacent lateral or hemimandible, and ipsilateral side of the neck, leave the patient with moderate impairment of swallowing.[38] Postoperative aspiration may occur. If prior irradiation has been performed, there is increased risk of fistula formation. Total glossectomy eliminates articulation of the oral phase of swallowing. Skin flaps are often used to provide laryngeal support and protection. If not previously performed, a laryngectomy may be necessary to prevent chronic aspiration and recurrent pneumonia.

A myocutaneous flap combines a muscle and the overlying skin along with an extensive blood supply (the major artery and vein).[39] This flap and its vascular pedicle are transposed to fit the defect. The pectoralis major flap is the most commonly used myocutaneous flap.

Classic Radical Neck Dissection. This procedure involves removal of the cervical lymphatics and lymph nodes from the level of the mandible superior to the inferior clavicle and from the midline anterior to the posterior border of the trapezius.[40] A modified neck dissection may spare the sternocleidomastoid muscle, the internal jugular vein, and the spinal accessory nerve, thereby minimizing functional deformity.

Surgical complications include muscle weakness and damage to the phrenic and vagus nerves. Respiratory complications, edema of the airways, infection, and fistula formation are all potential problems. Of particular concern is any fistula or infection that contaminates the carotid artery. Erosion of this vessel with resultant hemorrhage can lead to neurological insult or death and should be considered a surgical emergency. Related nursing diagnoses and interventions are listed in the following sections.

The patient will typically have wound drains connected to suction, which is vital the first 12 to 18 hours after surgery to prevent any collection of blood or fluids under the flap. The suction helps the surfaces of the wound to approximate and removes air from the space left by the tissue resection.

The most frequent source of graft failure is venous occlusion. Following surgery, both arterial and venous circulation of the flap should be assessed frequently for color and blanching. Hourly Doppler ultrasound determinations of a pulse in the flap will assess the presence of blood flow to the flap. Initial pallor and capillary refill slower than 2 seconds may indicate arterial occlusion, while initial cyanosis, engorged tissue, and capillary refill of more than 2 seconds may indicate venous occlusion.

■ **NURSING DIAGNOSIS**

Altered tissue perfusion, related to surgical flap.

OUTCOME STANDARD AND CRITERIA

Tissue perfusion is adequate as evidenced by:
- Absence of pallor and/or cyanosis on flap
- Presence of pulse on flap

NURSING INTERVENTIONS
- Assess circulation and oxygenation to the flap
- Monitor wound drainage for color and amount
- Maintain wound drainage suction to help approximate the wound surfaces

■ **NURSING DIAGNOSIS**

Ineffective breathing pattern, related to postoperative tracheostomy/laryngectomy.

OUTCOME STANDARD AND CRITERIA

Breathing patterns are effective, and hypoxemia is prevented as evidenced by:
- Absence of stridor
- Normal $PaCO_2$ and PaO_2

NURSING INTERVENTIONS
- Assess airway; suction frequently; monitor ABGs
- Administer humidified air or oxygen to maintain loose secretions
- Maintain patient in high Fowler's position to minimize edema and facilitate suctioning

■ **NURSING DIAGNOSIS**

High risk for decreased cardiac output, related to potential carotid artery hemorrhage.

OUTCOME STANDARD AND CRITERIA

Cardiac output is normal as evidenced by:
- Normal blood pressure and filling pressures
- Normal perfusion parameters

NURSING INTERVENTIONS
- Assess neck size and shape to detect carotid artery leakage
- Apply pressure and notify physician immediately if leakage is suspected
- Maintain RBCs on hold in blood bank

■ **NURSING DIAGNOSIS**

High risk for infection, related to surgical trauma.

OUTCOME STANDARD AND CRITERIA

Infection is absent as evidenced by:

- Absence of signs/symptoms of localized infection (redness, tenderness, swelling)

NURSING INTERVENTIONS
- Assess wound healing
- Cleanse frequently (every 8 hours) to reduce colonized bacteria at the suture lines
- Maximize nutrition for wound healing

Thoracic Surgeries

Indications for surgery: Since surgical treatment is usually limited to tumors identified as being completely resectable at the time of diagnosis, only cancers of the non-small-cell type are considered for surgical resection. Surgical resection is not associated with improved survival in small cell lung cancer. Only 2% of untreated individuals with lung cancer in a classic study survive beyond 5 years; virtually all patients who survived had been treated by surgery.[41]

Patients with stage I and II disease should be considered for possible surgical resection if warranted by their functional status. These tumors usually can be completely resected and are highly curable. Patients with clinical stage III disease usually have a much poorer prognosis and should be considered for surgery on a selective basis. Resections occasionally are considered for incomplete removal of the tumor to provide palliation of debilitating symptoms such as:

Infection and hemoptysis: Tumors that form abscesses or produce uncontrollable hemoptysis may necessitate resection, even though incomplete resection is anticipated. Other therapeutic interventions such as endoscopic laser therapy or radiation therapy can frequently afford similar symptom control.

Pain: Palliation of pain by incomplete resection of tumors invading the chest wall, combined with high-dose postoperative radiation therapy, may be of some benefit.

Debulking: At thoracotomy, a tumor may be found unresectable. It may be difficult for the surgeon to decide whether or not to attempt an incomplete resection. Postoperative adjuvant therapy may yield some relief of symptoms.

Surgical Procedures

At present, the *standard pneumonectomy* accounts for about 20% of pulmonary resections for lung cancer. Pneumonectomy may be required when a lung-conserving operation cannot remove all the tumor. A relatively large volume of functioning lung is removed, especially during right pneumonectomy, which may lead to the late development of pulmonary hypertension and chronic respiratory failure due to the strain on the smaller left lung.

Sleeve pneumonectomy involves the resection of the carina and mainstem bronchus. The lower bronchi are joined to upper bronchus structures, thus the name sleeve.

Lobectomy is the most commonly employed resection for lung cancer. Sleeve lobectomy has also become a standard and is applicable to tumors of the right upper lobe involving the right mainstem bronchus. *Segmentectomy* is usually reserved for patients with peripherally placed tumors and compromised pulmonary function.

Lesser resections in the treatment of lung cancer have been reserved for patients with extremely poor pulmonary function who could tolerate no more than a very limited resection because of their underlying medical condition or low pulmonary reserve. Two types of limited resections have been advocated: wedge excision and lumpectomy. *Wedge excision* in peripherally placed tumors has been successfully used in compromised patients. However, in most reported series, this operation has been a compromise with a higher incidence of local recurrence than lobectomy. *Lumpectomy* allows more proximal tumors to be widely excised, preserving the remaining lung in patients with severely compromised pulmonary function. If the procedure is performed with care, postoperative air leaks are minimal, and in selected high-risk patients, curative resections can be obtained.

A carcinoma involving the parietal pleura, intercostal muscle, and/or ribs may be totally resected for cure by *complete chest wall resection* of the involved structures. The survival rate is as high as 50% if only the parietal pleura is involved without lymph node disease.

■ NURSING DIAGNOSIS

Ineffective breathing pattern, related to postoperative incisional pain and chest tube(s).

OUTCOME STANDARD AND CRITERIA

Breathing pattern is normal as evidenced by:
- Respiratory rate and depth adequate to maintain ventilation

NURSING INTERVENTIONS
- Assess breathing patterns for adequate tidal volume
- Provide comfort measures to enhance normal respiratory excursion, lung volume via administration of pain medications
- Monitor effectiveness of interventions via ABGs
- Assess breath sounds; suction as needed
- Reposition for improved comfort and oxygenation

Esophagectomy

A postoperative mortality of 5% or less for resection of the esophagus has been achieved.[36] An attempt at a curative resection despite poor long-term survival rates may not only eradicate the esophageal tumor but may also restore swallowing, which is the primary goal of palliation.

Patients with esophageal carcinoma frequently present with a mean weight loss of 10%, dehydration, and blood volume deficits. These conditions should be corrected preoperatively. Patients should receive at least 5 days of total parenteral nutrition to reduce postoperative complications.

Preoperative assessment of pulmonary function is also important. Patients often have a long history of cigarette smoking, making preoperative instruction in the use of the incentive spirometer essential. The ability to learn effective use of the incentive spirometer may influence the decision to perform a thoracotomy. Cardiac and hepatic function should be carefully assessed preoperatively. Oral hygiene should be meticulous, and needed dental extractions should be performed preoperatively to prevent postoperative infections. Third-generation cephalosporins are often used prophylactically in the preoperative period.

The two most commonly used approaches to resection of esophageal tumors are a combined laparotomy and right thoracotomy or a left thoracoabdominal incision. When reconstruction is performed following resection, the stomach, colon, and jejunum have all been successfully used as conduits. The stomach is usually used because it is easily mobilized, has an excellent vascular supply, and has adequate length to reach the neck in most individuals. The colon is the most commonly used alternative to the stomach for replacement; jejunal loops have also been used.

Concern is often expressed about possible reflux due to resection of the cardiac sphincter when the stomach is used for replacement of the esophagus. Postoperatively, patients must be instructed not to recline during or immediately after eating and to sleep with the head of the bed elevated.

The major causes of morbidity are either pulmonary in origin or related to an anastomotic leak. Meticulous postoperative pulmonary care will prevent many complications. Patients have difficulty clearing their secretions and maintaining airway patency. Generally, patients will require a day or two of assisted ventilation. Septic complications related to anastomic leaks can occur, including empyema and mediastinitis. Most small intrathoracic leaks will heal with appropriate drainage, antibiotics, and hyperalimentation. Larger leaks can cause life-threatening mediastinitis and should be closed operatively.

Intraoperative placement of a nasogastric (NG) tube is critical to avoid gastric distension, which can compromise cardiac filling and/or disrupt the esophagogastric anastomosis. The NG tube should be connected to suction until bowel function returns to avoid tension on the suture line. Seven to ten days following surgery, a water-soluble contrast study is performed to assess integrity of the anastomosis.

Cardiac complications related to infarction or dysrhythmias are also frequent. These can be minimized through the maintenance of electrolyte balance and adequate oxygenation. Other frequently encountered complications include thrombophlebitis, pulmonary emboli, chylothorax, and recurrent nerve injury. Anastomotic strictures are a common late complication. Diarrhea and dumping syndrome may result following division of the vagus nerve and pyloroplasty.

■ NURSING DIAGNOSIS
High risk for infection, related to anastomotic leakage.

OUTCOME STANDARD AND CRITERIA
Normal wound healing occurs as evidenced by:
- Absence of signs or symptoms of systemic infection (fever, tachycardia)
- Nasogastric tube remains in place

NURSING INTERVENTIONS
- Perform meticulous postoperative pulmonary care
- Assess nasogastric tube placement, drainage, and patency
- Monitor for signs or symptoms of infection
- Observe for signs of gastric distention that may occur secondary to anesthesia administration and swallowing air

■ NURSING DIAGNOSIS
Altered fluid and electrolyte balance, related to large volumes of crystalloids administered during prolonged operative time.

OUTCOME STANDARD AND CRITERIA
Fluid balance is restored as evidenced by:
- Normal serum and urine electrolytes and osmolarity
- Normal filling pressures (CVP and PAWP)

NURSING INTERVENTIONS
- Assess breath sounds for crackles
- Monitor hemodynamic parameters, electrolytes
- Limit fluid at prescribed level

■ NURSING DIAGNOSIS
Ineffective airway clearance, related to endotracheal tube and ventilator.

OUTCOME STANDARD AND CRITERIA
Airway clearance is normal as evidenced by:
- Respiratory rate, volume, and rhythm adequate for ventilations and oxygenation

NURSING INTERVENTIONS
- Monitor for signs of airway obstruction (restlessness, inadequate chest expansion, stridor, noisy respirations, cyanosis, or dyspnea)
- Assess for signs of atelectasis secondary to airway obstruction (increased respiratory rate, pulse, and temperature; cyanosis; and diaphoresis)
- Monitor closed chest drainage system

- Observe for signs of pulmonary embolism (hemoptysis, right-sided heart failure, hypoxia, engorgement of neck veins, tachycardia, hypotension, apprehension, sense of impending doom, nausea, sweating)

■ **NURSING DIAGNOSIS**

Altered nutrition, related to inability to swallow postoperatively.

OUTCOME STANDARD AND CRITERIA

Nutritional intake adequate for caloric and protein needs as evidenced by:
- Adequate wound healing
- Adequate protein reserves
- Normal nitrogen balance

NURSING INTERVENTIONS
- Maintain nutritional intake adequate for caloric and protein needs
- Monitor electrolytes, albumin, and serum transferrin during hyperalimentation treatment
- Administer tube feedings via jejunostomy tube once bowel function has returned
- Begin oral feedings with liquids and advance as tolerated

Hepatic Surgeries

Indications for Surgery

Hepatic resection is currently the major potentially curative treatment for metastatic solid tumors of the liver. In colorectal metastases, hepatic resection has yielded 5-year survival rates of 20% to 40%; it has become an accepted treatment for this condition.[42] Sporadic reports of long-term survivors have appeared following hepatic resection of metastatic Wilms' tumor, melanoma, leiomyosarcoma, pancreatic carcinoma, hypernephroma, and adrenal carcinoma. In addition, resection has become an accepted palliative treatment with possible curative potential for endocrine tumors, particularly carcinoid tumor.

Factors that should be considered when determining the patient's prognosis with hepatic resection are: the stage of the primary tumor, the number of metastases, the disease-free interval, and the size of solitary lesions. The influence of these factors on survival is not strong enough, however, to be considered as contraindication for resection.

Surgical Procedures

The vascular anatomy of the liver dictates the type of resection possible. The hepatic artery, the portal vein, and the biliary tract divide to supply the right and left lobes of the liver. These segments are drained by the three hepatic veins: right, middle, and left. The right hepatic vein drains directly into the vena cava

and the middle hepatic vein drains into the left hepatic vein, which drains eventually into the vena cava.[43] Hepatic surgery can be divided into major and minor resections. The major resections include right lobectomy, left lobectomy, left lateral segmentectomy, right trisegmentectomy, and left trisegmentectomy. Minor resections, or wedge resections, involve removal of any portion of liver below the segmental level. A large wedge resection may produce more hemorrhage than a lobectomy because anatomical divisions are less well defined and hepatic tissue must be cauterized carefully to produce a hemostatic line.

■ **NURSING DIAGNOSIS/COLLABORATIVE PROBLEM**

High risk for bleeding, related to decreased clotting factors.

OUTCOME STANDARD AND CRITERIA

Bleeding and clotting studies will be within normal limits.

NURSING INTERVENTIONS
- Monitor bleeding times, hemoglobin, hematocrit, platelet count, partial prothrombin, and prothrombin time
- Administer blood replacement therapy as prescribed
- Protect patient from bruising, assess skin and mucous membranes for signs of bleeding
- Minimize trauma to the GI tract: use soft toothbrushes, minimize the use of nasogastric tube

■ **NURSING DIAGNOSIS**

Decreased cardiac output, related to fluid and electrolyte imbalance.

OUTCOME STANDARD AND CRITERIA

Cardiac output is adequate as evidenced by:
- Hemodynamic parameters within normal limits (CVP, PAWP, SVR, PVR, CI)
- Electrolytes within normal limits

NURSING INTERVENTIONS
- Monitor intake and output and electrolyte balance
- Administer fluids, electrolytes, and blood products
- Assess for evidence of fluid shifts by ascites and serum albumin level

The rate of complications seems to be proportional to blood loss.[44] Blood coagulation is often compromised and bleeding continues into the subhepatic space from the cut surface of the liver when there is extensive intraoperative blood loss. The loss of 4,000 ml of blood intraoperatively is not uncommon. Blood transfusions consist of packed red blood cells, fresh frozen plasma, and platelets as needed. The type and amount should be determined by blood coagulation studies.

Due to the fluid shifts from ascites collecting in the abdominal cavity and a low serum albumin level, nursing measures focus on monitoring fluid balance with pulmonary artery wedge and right atrial pressures, urine output, cardiac output, and blood pressure. Replacement of fluids and blood products is maintained per physician orders.

Postoperative hepatic failure is unlikely in patients with colorectal metastases presenting with normal liver function preoperatively, so long as the portion of liver that is removed is largely made up of tumor. A cirrhotic liver is at high risk for liver failure, especially if a high proportion of functioning liver parenchyma is removed. Patients with hepatomas (who usually have cirrhosis) may experience liver failure postoperatively.

Clinical presentation of liver failure includes altered mentation, flapping tremors, and incontinence. Bleeding studies may be abnormal and ammonia levels elevated. Bilirubin may be elevated if there is an obstructive component to the disease.

Nursing assessment includes the patient's level of orientation, assisting with activities of daily living, and providing emotional support to the patient and family with realistic expectations of the patient's condition. The patient should also be assessed for complications due to the potentiating effects of sedatives and hepatotoxic drugs.

Pelvic Exenteration

Indications for Surgery

Pelvic exenteration is a potentially curative treatment for selected cases of locally advanced pelvic malignancies such as colorectal, bladder, cervical, or vaginal lesions. Women with disease outside of the pelvis or with the triad of unilateral leg edema, sciatic pain, and ureteral obstruction are not candidates for pelvic exenteration.[45]

Surgical Procedures

A total pelvic exenteration involves removal of the rectum and distal sigmoid colon, the urinary bladder and distal portion of the ureters, and all the pelvic reproductive organs; and dissection of the pelvic lymph nodes and internal iliac vessels, as well as excision of the entire pelvic floor including the pelvic peritoneum, levator muscles, and perineum. A urinary conduit and colostomy are typically necessary. Vaginal reconstruction may be performed. An anterior exenteration preserves the rectum; a posterior exenteration preserves the bladder.[46]

Immediate postoperative problems include the potential for pulmonary embolism, cerebrovascular accident, or myocardial infarction due to manipulation of the inferior vena cava intraoperatively and postoperative immobility. Intraoperative hemorrhage and postoperative pulmonary edema necessitate the use

of a pulmonary artery catheter for determining fluid volume status and judicious replacement of colloid and crystalloid solutions. Use of a pulmonary artery catheter also allows interventions to improve cardiac contractility or modifications in peripheral vascular resistance.[47]

Infection and sepsis are great risks because the abdominal cavity is denuded of its peritoneum and is open to the outside through the perineum. Defenses against infection are compromised because of disrupted blood supply. Small bowel obstruction also is a potential complication because of manipulation of the bowel, the potential for adhesion formation, and the possibility of intestinal herniation through a perineal defect.[48]

Long-term problems include fistula formation related to possible rectosigmoid stump leakage,[49] urinary obstruction, and infection with the potential for development of sepsis from ureteroconduit or anastomosal leakage.

■ NURSING DIAGNOSIS

High risk for altered tissue perfusion, related to possible embolic event.

OUTCOME STANDARD AND CRITERIA

Normal tissue perfusion is maintained by:
- Early detection of embolic event and appropriate intervention

NURSING INTERVENTION

- Assess for possible pulmonary embolism, stroke, or myocardial infarction due to manipulation of the inferior vena cava intraoperatively and postoperative immobility

■ NURSING DIAGNOSIS

High risk for infection, related to loss of integrity of peritoneum.

OUTCOME STANDARD AND CRITERIA

Infection is absent as evidenced by:
- Absence of signs or symptoms of systemic infection (fever, tachycardia)

NURSING INTERVENTIONS

- Assess incisions for signs or symptoms of infection
- Monitor temperature and heart rate
- Assess for signs of peritonitis (firmness, pain on palpation, and changes in bowel sounds)

■ NURSING DIAGNOSIS

High risk for fluid volume deficit, related to preoperative blood loss and fluid shifts from intestinal edema.

OUTCOME STANDARD AND CRITERIA

Fluid status is maintained or restored as evidenced by:
- Filling pressures within normal limits (CVP, PAWP)
- Hematocrit and hemoglobin within acceptable limits

NURSING INTERVENTIONS

- Assess volume status via CVP and PAWP measurements
- Administer volume replacement as necessary (crystalloid, colloid, and blood)

Continent Urinary Diversion

Indications for Surgery

Construction of continent urinary reservoirs are frequently performed in patients undergoing radical cystectomy and radical cystoprostatectomy. These procedures can also be used as revisions in the patient presenting with ileal or colonic conduit, ureterosigmoidoscopy, or cutaneous ureterostomy.[50]

Surgical Procedures

A segment of intestine, part of the distal ileum, cecum, ascending, or transverse colon is folded and positioned in the right side of the abdomen. The capacity of the reservoir ranges from 550 to 1,200 ml. The intestine section is then opened, and the ureters are brought into the open reservoir for reimplantation. Three catheters (ureteral stents, Malecot and Robinson catheters) are brought out through separate openings in the reservoir and abdominal wall. Ureteral stents are inserted to ensure patency of the ureters while the postoperative edema is resolving. A Malecot catheter may be positioned in the low pressure reservoir for postoperative irrigation of clots and mucous that accumulate. A Robinson catheter may be inserted through the stoma to maintain its integrity and is left indwelling until postoperative edema has resolved. Wound catheter drains are placed in the abdominal cavity for drainage. These wound catheters will drain the urine and irrigation leakage from the pouch that occurs while the anastomosis heals.

Nursing Management

Patients with urinary diversions are at high risk for fluid volume deficit, related to preoperative blood loss and fluid shifts from intestinal edema. The outcome standards and criteria and nursing interventions have been described earlier. In addition, these patients need assessment and management for electrolyte and acid–base imbalance, related to reabsorption of acids from urine in the pouch. The nurse should monitor chloride levels and be alert for evidence of metabolic acidosis. The pouch should be irrigated every 6 hours to minimize the degree of imbalances.

A pulmonary artery catheter is typically used for accurate assessment of volume status. Both crystalloid and colloid replacement is often necessary. Elevated chloride levels and metabolic acidosis are frequently seen because some reabsorption of urine occurs from exposure to the intestinal pouch mucosa. Irrigation of the pouch with normal saline via the Malecot catheter every 6 hours minimizes the degree of imbalances. Monitoring of the serum creatinine is necessary to assess renal function. Measurement and recording of urine output from each ureteral stent is essential. If urine output from a stent decreases, the stent can be irrigated with a blunt-end needle, maintaining aseptic technique, to ensure patency. The reservoir is irrigated every 6 hours postoperatively to clear clots and mucous plugs from the pouch.

REFERENCES

1. Tenenbaum, L. (1989). *A reference guide: Cancer chemotherapy.* Philadelphia: Saunders.
2. Cunningham, M. (1990). Nonhematologic toxicities of selected chemotherapeutic agents used in the treatment of adult leukemia. *Seminars in Oncology Nursing, 6*(1), 67-75.
3. Brown, J. D., & Hogan, C. M. (1990). Chemotherapy. In S. L. Groenwald, M. H. Frogge, M. Goodman, et al. (Eds.), *Cancer nursing: Principles and practice* (2nd ed.) (pp. 230-283). Boston: Jones & Bartlett.
4. Skeel, R. T. (1987). The biologic and pharmacologic basis of cancer chemotherapy. In R. L. Skeel (Ed.), *Handbook of cancer chemotherapy* (2nd ed.) (pp. 3-14). Boston: Little, Brown.
5. Gilewski, T. A., & Golomb, H. M. (1990). Design of combination biotherapy studies: Future goals and challenges. *Seminars in Oncology 17*(Suppl. 1), 3-10.
6. Jassak, P. F. (1990). Biotherapy. In S. L. Groenwald, M. H. Frogge, M. Goodman, et al. (Eds.), *Cancer nursing: Principles and practice* (2nd ed.) (pp. 284-306). Boston: Jones & Bartlett.
7. Hahn, M. B., & Jassak, P. F. (1988). Nursing management of patients receiving interferon. *Seminars in Oncology Nursing, 4*(2), 95-101.
8. Padavic-Shaller, K. (1988). IL-2: Nursing applications in a developing science. *Seminars in Oncology Nursing, 4*(2), 142-150.
9. DiJulio, J. E. (1988). Treatment of B-cell and T-cell lymphomas with monoclonal antibodies. *Seminars in Oncology Nursing, 4*(2), 102-106.
10. Moldauer, N. P., & Figlin, R. A. (1988). Tumor necrosis factor: Current clinical status and implications for nursing management. *Seminars in Oncology Nursing 4*(2), 120-125.
11. Haluber, D. (1989). Recent advances in the management of biotherapy related side effects: Flu-like syndrome. *Oncology Nursing Forum, 16*(6), 35-41.
12. Wickham, R. (1986). Pulmonary toxicity secondary to cancer treatment. *Oncology Nursing Forum, 13*(5), 69-76.
13. Moseley, J. R. (1987). Nursing management of toxicities associated with chemotherapy for lung cancer. *Seminars in Oncology Nursing, 3*(3), 202-210.

14. Kapoor, A. S. (1986). Doxorubicin cardiotoxicity. In A. S. Kapoor, & R. D. Reynolds (Eds.), *Cancer and the heart* (pp. 227-231). New York: Springer-Verlag.

15. Khojasteh, A. (1986). Cardiac disorders in leukemias and plasma-cell dyscrasias. In A. S. Kapoor, & R. D. Reynolds (Eds.), *Cancer and the heart* (pp. 175-184) New York: Springer-Verlag.

16. Skelton, J. D., & Pizzo, P. A. (1987). Hematologic malignancy. In J. E. Parrillo, & H. Masur (Eds.), *The critically ill immunosuppressed patient* (pp. 433-479) Rockville, MD: Aspen.

17. Glover, D. J., & Glick, J. H. (1985). *Managing oncologic emergencies involving structural dysfunction* (vol. 35). New York: American Cancer Society.

18. Perry, M. C. (1986). Cardiac metastasis. In A. S. Kapoor, & R. D. Reynolds (Eds.), *Cancer and the heart* (pp. 76-81). New York: Springer-Verlag.

19. Findley, F. P. (1987). Nursing management of common oncologic emergencies. In C. R. Ziegfeld (Ed.), *Core curriculum for oncology nursing*. Philadelphia: Saunders.

20. O'Connor, N. T. J., Prentice, H. G., & Hoffbrand, A. V. (1989). Prevention of urate nephropathy in the tumour lysis syndrome. *Clinical and Laboratory Haematology, 11,* 97-100.

21. Kuhn, R., Ackerman, S., Barnsteiner, J., et al. (1990). *AACN outcome standards for nursing care of the critically ill.* Laguna Niguel, CA: American Association of Critical-Care Nurses.

22. Carlson, A. C. (1985). Infection prophylaxis in the patient with cancer. *Oncology Nursing Forum, 12*(3), 56-64.

23. Lazarus, H. M., Creger, R. J., & Gerson, S. L. (1989). Infectious emergencies in oncology patients. *Seminars in Oncology, 16*(6), 543-560.

24. Mower, W. J., Hawkins, J. A., & Nelson, E. W. (1986). Neutropenic enterocolitis in adults with acute leukemia. *Archives of Surgery, 121,* 571-574.

25. Morrison, V. A., Peterson, B. A., & Bloomfield, C. D. (1990). Nosocomial septicemia in the cancer patient: The influence of central venous access devices, neutropenia, and type of malignancy. *Medical and Pediatric Oncology, 18,* 209-216.

26. Wade, J. C. (1989). Antibiotic therapy for the febrile granulocytopenic cancer patient: Combination therapy vs. monotherapy. *Reviews of Infectious Diseases, 11*(Suppl. 7), 1572-1581.

27. Vincent, J. L., & VanDerLinden, P. (1990). Septic shock: Particular type of acute circulatory failure. *Critical Care Medicine, 18*(1), 71-74.

28. Erickson, J. M. (1990). Blood support for the myelosuppressed patient. *Seminars in Oncology Nursing, 6*(1), 61-66.

29. Varricchio, C. G., Miller, N., & Pazdur, M. (1990). Edema and effusions. In S. L. Groenwald, M. H. Frogge, M. Goodman, et al. (Eds.), *Cancer nursing: Principles and practice*. Boston: Jones & Bartlett.

30. Olopade, O. I., & Ultmann, J. E. (1991). Malignant effusions. *CA: A Cancer Journal for Clinicians, 41*(3), 166-177.

31. Rosen, N., Kaufman, D., & Young, R. C. (1987). Medical emergencies in patients with solid tumors. In J. E. Parrillo, & H. Masur (Eds.), *The critically ill immunosuppressed patient* (pp. 481-498). Rockville, MD: Aspen.

32. Sheppard, K. C. (1987). Superior vena cava syndrome: An oncologic complication. *Seminars in Oncology Nursing, 3*(3), 211-215.

33. Schryber, S., Lacasse, C. R., & Barton-Burke, M. (1987). Autologous bone marrow transplantation. *Oncology Nursing Forum, 14*(4), 74-80.

34. Grandt, N. C. (1989). Hepatic veno-occlusive disease following bone marrow transplantation. *Oncology Nursing Forum, 16*(6), 813-817.

35. Schleper, J. R. (1989). Prevention, detection, and diagnosis of head and neck cancers. *Seminars in Oncology Nursing, 5*(3), 139-149.

36. Roth, J. A., & Kelsen, D. P. (1989). Surgery and adjuvant chemotherapy for carcinoma of the esophagus. In J. A. Roth, J. C. Ruckdeschel, & T. H. Weisenburger (Eds.), *Thoracic oncology* (pp. 379-394). Philadelphia: Saunders.

37. Martin, L. K. (1989). Management of the altered airway in the head and neck cancer patient. *Seminars in Oncology Nursing, 5*(3), 182-190.

38. Goodman, M. (1990). Head and neck cancer. In S. L. Groenwald, M. H. Frogge, M. Goodman, et al. (Eds.), *Cancer nursing: Principles and practice* (2nd ed.) (pp. 889-929). Boston: Jones & Bartlett.

39. Mahon, S. M. (1987). Nursing interventions for the patient with a myocutaneous flap. *Cancer Nursing, 10*(1), 21-31.

40. Rook, J. L., & Rook, M. (1989). Head and neck cancer. *Journal of Post Anesthesia Nursing, 4*(6), 363-372.

41. Ginsberg, R. J., Goldberg, M., & Waters, P. F. (1989). Surgery for non-small cell lung cancer. In J. A. Roth, J. C. Ruckdeschel, & T. H. Weisenburger (Eds.), *Thoracic oncology* (pp. 177-199). Philadelphia: Saunders.

42. Hughes, S. K., & Sugarbaker, P. H. (1987). Resection of the liver for metastatic solid tumors. In S. A. Rosenberg (Ed.), *Surgical treatment of metastatic cancer* (pp. 125-164). Philadelphia: Lippincott.

43. Iwatsuki, S., Todo, S., & Starzl, T. E. (1990). Excisional therapy for benign hepatic lesions. *Surgery, Gynecology and Obstetrics, 171,* 240-246.

44. Delva, E., Camus, Y., Nordlinger, B., et al. (1989). Vascular occlusions for liver resections: Operative management and tolerance to hepatic ischemia: 142 cases. *Annals of Surgery, 209*(2), 211-218.

45. Morley, G. W., Hopkins, M. P., Lindenauer, S. M., et al. (1989). Pelvic exenteration, University of Michigan: 100 patients at 5 years. *Obstetrics and Gynecology, 74*(6), 934-942.

46. McKenzie, F. (1988). Sexuality after total pelvic exenteration. *Nursing Times, 18*(20), 27-30.

47. Lichtinger, M., Averette, H., Penalver, M., et al. (1986). Major surgical procedures for gynecologic malignancy in elderly women. *Southern Medical Journal, 79*(12), 1506-1510.

48. Jones, W. B. (1987). Surgical approaches for advanced or recurrent cancer of the cervix. *Cancer, 60,* 2094-2103.

49. Smith, D. B. (1989). Pelvic exenteration: A historical overview. *Journal of Enterostomal Therapy, 16,* 195-198.

50. Lockhart, J. L., Pow-Sang, J. M., Persky, L., et al. (1990). A continent colonic urinary reservoir: The Florida pouch. *Journal of Urology, 144,* 864-967.

PART ELEVEN

Gastrointestinal Patient Care Problems

49

Gastrointestinal Anatomy and Physiology

Joanne M. Krumberger

The gastrointestinal (GI) tract holds a unique position among body systems. Food and water are taken in, digested, and absorbed in an orderly and efficient sequence of physical and biochemical events. These processes depend upon intrinsic characteristics of the stomach, intestinal smooth muscle, visceral reflexes, and the actions of many gastrointestinal enzymes and hormones. The action of enzymes is assisted by hydrochloric acid secreted by the stomach and bile secreted by the liver. The actions of several key hormones are summarized in Table 49-1 for reference. In a coordinated response, the digestive secretions of the salivary glands, the pancreas, the liver, and the gallbladder contribute to the conversion of food and water into metabolic energy and substrates.[1,2,3,4]

This chapter is designed to follow and orderly anatomical course down the alimentary tract (Figure 49-1). Beginning at the mouth and terminating at the colon, the anatomy of each organ is discussed for its unique contribution to GI physiology. The GI acces-

sory organs, the pancreas, biliary system, and liver are discussed in the context of their digestive functions.

REGULATION OF HUNGER AND THIRST

Hunger

The desire or need for food is called *hunger*. It is a complex sensation involving many variables.

Two nuclei, or groups of cells, within the hypothalamus have been shown to mediate hunger and satiety. The ventromedial group, referred to as the feeding center, causes an increase in food intake when stimulated. The ventrolateral cell group, or satiety center, inhibits food ingestion when stimulated. Normally, these two centers interact. When a person is satiated, the ventrolateral nucleus inhibits the ventromedial nucleus; in a hunger state the reverse occurs. The net effect of this regulatory feedback loop in normal humans is an adjustment of food intake to match energy expenditures. Two major theories to

TABLE 49-1 Actions of Gastrointestinal Hormones

Action	Gastrin	Cholecystokinin (CCK)	Secretin	Gastric Inhibitory Peptide (GIP)
Acid secretion	S	S	I	I
Gastric motility	S	S	I	
Gastric emptying	I	I	I	I
Intestinal motility	S	S	I	
Mucosal growth	S	S	S	O
Pancreatic HCO_3^- secretion	S	S	S	O
Pancreatic enzyme secretion	S	S	S	O
Pancreatic growth hormone	S		S	S
Biliary HCO_3^- secretion	S	S	S	O
Gallbladder contraction	S	S	S	

Key: S = stimulates. I = inhibits. O = no effects. Blank = no information found or not yet tested.

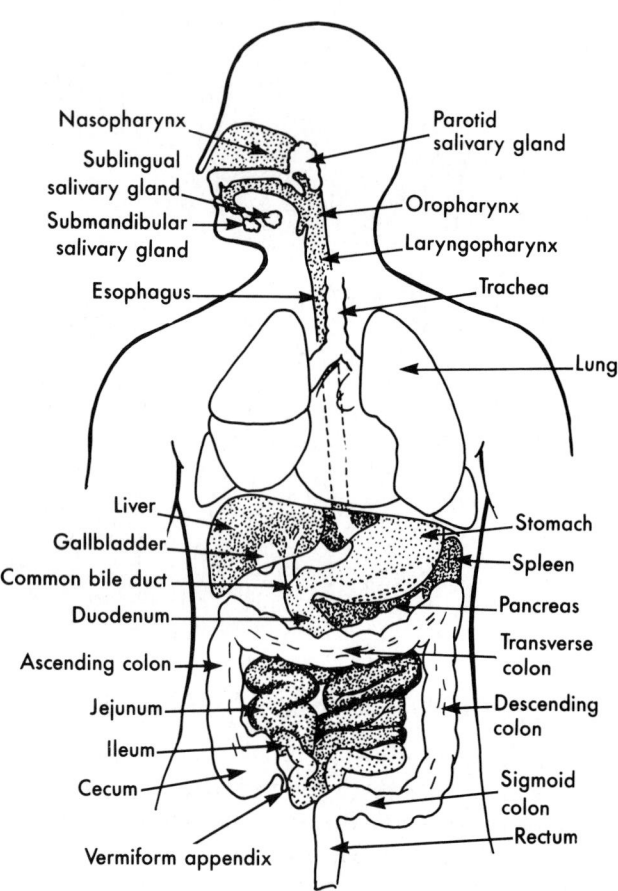

Figure 49-1   The gastrointestinal tract.

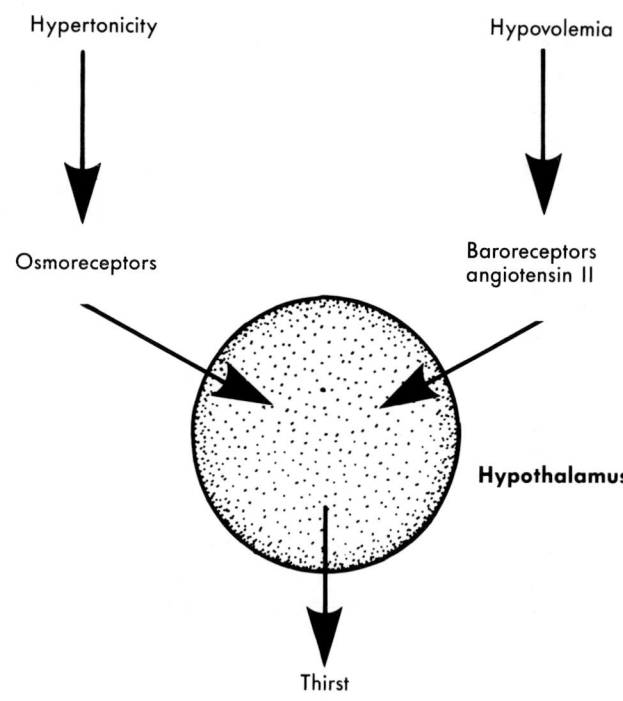

Figure 49-2   Factors regulating water intake.

explain the careful balance between these regulatory nuclei are proposed: blood glucose concentrations and hypothalamic temperature levels. Certain medications and hormones have also been implicated in hunger regulation, but all mechanisms of action are not completely understood. In humans, cultural factors, environment, and the senses associated with food also affect intake.[5,6]

Thirst

In a manner analogous to hunger, *thirst* can be defined as a need or desire for liquid. Interestingly, the sensation for thirst can be satisfied simply by moistening mucous membranes, even if no net change in body fluid occurs.

The kidney and hypothalamus are involved in the regulation and intake of water, more specifically by plasma osmolality and extracellular fluid (ECF) volume. Intake of water is increased with increases in plasma osmotic pressure (hypertonicity), and by decreases in ECF volume. These processes are mediated by volume, baroreceptors in the kidney, and osmoreceptors located in the anterior hypothalamus (Figure 49-2). The effect of decreased ECF volume on

thirst is mediated by the renin–angiotensin system with increased circulating angiotensin II. Angiotensin II stimulates neural receptors concerned with thirst.[2,4]

GASTROINTESTINAL SYSTEM OVERVIEW
Histological Layers

The structures that make up the wall of the GI tract from the pharynx to the anus are shown in Figure 49-3. The same histological structure is generally found in tubular structures of the alimentary canal with three layers of smooth muscle. The wall is lined by mucosa, except in the esophagus, which is covered by serosa. The histological layers of the digestive tube may be outlined as follows (proceeding from the innermost outward): (1) mucosa—epithelium, lamina propria, muscularis mucosae; (2) submucosa; (3) muscularis externa—inner circular fibers, outer longitudinal fibers; and (4) serosa or adventitia.

Mucosa

The mucosa is composed of three sublayers. From the inside outward they are the epithelial layer, the lamina propria, and muscularis mucosae. The *epithelium* varies throughout the tube. Squamous epithelium lines the mouth and anus, while columnar epithelium is found everywhere else. The cells in this layer are connected by tight junctions forming an effective barrier against large molecules and bacteria. Specific organs may have modified columnar epithe-

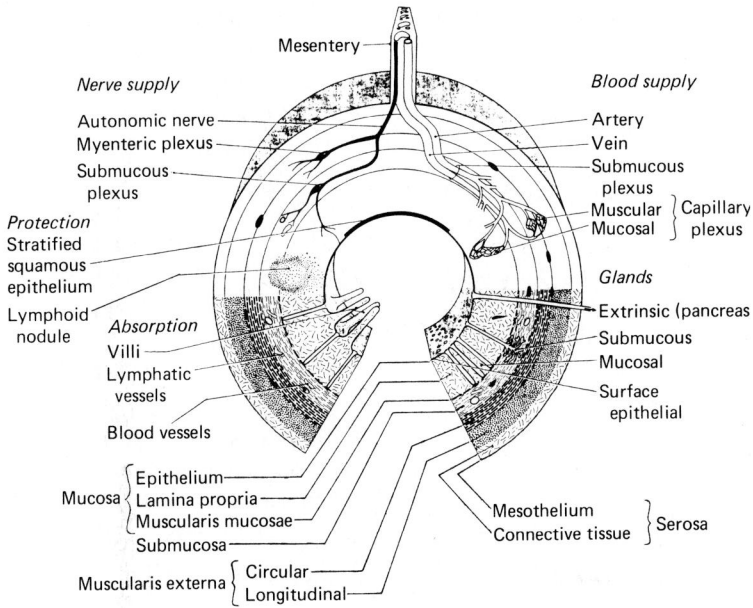

Figure 49-3 Histology of the GI tract.

lium that comprises what is known as the *gastric mucosal barrier*. Together with mucus and the inherent ability to rapidly regenerate cells, this physiological barrier is impermeable to hydrochloric acid (HCl). Interestingly, it is permeable to other substances such as salicylates, steroids, and bile salts. A disruption in this barrier is thought to be a major factor in ulcer development.[4,6] The *lamina propria* is loosely arranged connective tissue support, often rich in capillaries. The *muscularis mucosae* is smooth muscle only. It receives sympathetic innervation and is responsible for local mucosal foldings.

Submucosa

This second major layer of the gut wall contains dense connective tissue fibers, blood vessels, and nerve fibers. Meissner's plexus is a collection of parasympathetic nerves found in this layer. Fibers from this plexus stimulate the secretions of mucosal glands.[4,6,10]

Muscularis Externa

This is the major muscular layer of the wall. Normally, it is composed of smooth muscle, arranged as an inner circular layer and an outer longitudinal layer. The myenteric nerve plexus (Auerbach's plexus) is located between these two layers. It is responsible for muscular contractions of the wall and converts uncontrolled and purposeless motor and secretory activity into purposeful and coordinated intestinal activity. The esophagus, stomach, and colon have significant variations of the muscularis externa; they are discussed later.

Serosa or Adventitia

This is the outermost layer of the gut wall. It may be continuous with the surrounding connective tissue as in the adventitia, or it may be completely separate. If separate, it is named the *serosa*.

Blood Supply

Arterial Blood Supply

The arterial blood supply to the GI tract, also known as the splanchnic circulation, originates at the aorta and follows through the aortic arch, thoracic arch, and abdominal aorta to the celiac artery and the superior and inferior mesenteric arteries. Table 49-2 shows the branches of the celiac artery and mesenterics and areas they supply. Approximately one third of the cardiac output supplies these organs. This is an area for tremendous blood reserve in cases of increased need (e.g., increased metabolic demand or hemorrhage). Hypoperfusion can lead to mucosal necrosis and possibly necrosis. Necrosis of intestinal villi is known to destroy GI barriers to toxins and bacteria, which are then allowed to enter the bloodstream. This is called *bacterial translocation* and is thought to be an important factor in sepsis.[4,6,7]

Portal Vein System

All venous drainage from the GI tract and liver passes through the portal vein system. The main branches that bring blood to the portal vein include the gastric (returns blood from the stomach and esophagus), the splenic (returns blood from the stomach, esophagus, duodenum, pancreas, and gallblad-

TABLE 49-2 Arterial Blood Supply to the GI Tract

Artery	Area Supplied
Branch of Celiac	
Left gastric	Stomach
	Esophagus
Hepatic to right gastric	Stomach
Gastroduodenal	Stomach
	Duodenum
Cystic	Gallbladder
Splenic	Stomach
	Pancreas
	Spleen
Superior Mesenteric	
	Jejunum
	Ileum
	Cecum
	Ascending colon
	Part of transverse colon
Inferior Mesenteric	
	Transverse and descending colon
	Sigmoid colon
	Rectum

der), the superior mesenteric (returns blood from the small intestine and the ascending and transverse colon), and the inferior mesenteric (returns blood from the descending and sigmoid colon and rectum). The portal vein subdivides into liver sinusoids, which then unite with branches from the hepatic artery to form the hepatic vein, which empties into the inferior vena cava. The portal vein system is physiologically significant in that it delivers partially metabolized digestive products to the liver sinusoids for further metabolism. Liver dysfunction, then, can cause portal venous hypertension, resulting in ascites, varices, and incomplete metabolism of the products of digestion.

Innervation

Functions of the GI system are controlled by neural and hormonal factors. Hormonal effects are discussed in each section (see Table 49-1). The autonomic nervous system exerts multiple effects. The extrinsic nerves of this system are located outside the wall of the GI tract and contain parasympathetic (vagus and sacral) and sympathetic fibers. The sympathetic system consists of vertebral ganglia situated on either side of the vertebral trunk, terminating in all organs of the GI tract. Neurostimuli from postganglionic fibers include epinephrine, norepinephrine, and do-

pamine. Intrinsic nerves of the autonomic nervous system are located outside the wall of the GI tract and are extensions from the extrinsic nerves.

In general, parasympathetic cholinergic fibers or drugs are stimulatory to GI secretions and motility. Vagal influences are more prominent in the proximal portions (esophagus, stomach, and duodenum) than on the distal portions (small bowel and proximal colon). Conversely, sympathetic stimulation or adrenergic drugs inhibit GI processes.[6,7]

ORAL CAVITY AND PHARYNX

The alimentary tract begins with the mouth and oropharynx. The oral cavity includes the lips, cheeks, gums, palate, tongue, teeth, and salivary glands. Its main functions are ingestion, mastication, salivation, and the first stage of deglutition (swallowing).

Tongue

The tongue is a highly muscular organ. It is important for normal speech and for initiation of mastication and deglutition.

The lingual surface is covered with a specialized, durable squamous epithelium. This is further modified by visible clusters of cells called *papillae*. Within these papillae, specialized sensory cells, or *taste buds*, are found: the circumvallate, the foliate, and the fungiform papillae are mentioned by name because they contain the majority of the taste buds. Branches of the vagus nerve, along with two other cranial nerves, innervate the taste buds and mediate taste sensation.

Salivary Glands

A person secretes between 1,000 and 2,000 ml of saliva per day. Saliva keeps the mucous membranes moist. Its composition is 99% water and 1% glycoprotein (*mucin*) and amylase.

Salivary secretion is regulated by nervous innervation alone. Pressure receptors as well as chemoreceptors stimulate salivary secretion.

There are three major pairs of salivary glands in the mouth: the parotid, the submaxillary, and the sublingual (see Figure 49-1). Though histologically distinct, each pair of glands produces the substance saliva. This aqueous secretion facilitates the mixing of food early in the digestive process. Salivary glands are activated primarily by stimuli associated with food.

In addition, these glands synthesize an α-amylase. This enzymatic protein breaks down polysaccharides to disaccharides. Thus, even before carbohydrates reach the stomach or small intestine, their digestion has begun.

Normally, saliva has an alkaline pH of about 7.0. This keeps the saliva saturated with calcium and prevents loss of calcium from the teeth. In addition, saliva is rich in the secretory immunoglobulin IgA, which plays an important role in control of oral bacterial growth and again promotes healthy dentition.

Mastication and Deglutition

The mechanics of mastication involve biting off and chewing with the teeth; mixing the food bolus with mucins, amylase, and other glandular secretions, mainly by the actions of the tongue; and finally the backward propulsion of the bolus toward the oropharynx as deglutition or swallowing is initiated.

The reflex of deglutition requires 25 muscles, lasts 1 to 2 seconds, and begins as the food bolus reaches the oropharynx. The process can be thought of as an organized cascade of steps, each giving rise to the next (Figure 49-4):

Step 1: The backward propulsion of the food bolus stimulates pressure receptors in the wall of the oropharynx. These afferent signals go to the "swallowing center" in the medulla of the brain.

Step 2: The soft palate elevates to seal off the nasal cavity. This protects it from reflux.

Step 3: The central "swallowing center" inhibits respiration while the larynx elevates and the glottis closes.

Step 4: The central nervous system signals contraction of the upper esophageal sphincter, causing opening of the esophageal orifice. The food bolus then passes into the esophagus.

Step 5: Once in the esophagus, food passes into the stomach by peristaltic contractions. With swallowing, the lower esophageal sphincter relaxes, allowing passage. The tonic activity of the lower esophageal sphincter between meals prevents reflux into the esophagus.

Patients with neurological damage, those who have had resection of the oral cavity related to cancer, and patients with endotracheal tubes often have swallowing problems.[4,8]

ESOPHAGUS

The esophagus is a hollow tube extending from the pharynx to the stomach. It functions as a conduit for the passage of food and liquid from the mouth to the stomach. For the 25-cm length of the esophagus, no absorption takes place and only residual carbohydrate digestion from salivary amylase occurs.

Anatomy

The esophagus is located principally within the thoracic cavity. It is crossed anteriorly by the left bronchus. At the same level, it is also in close proximity to the aortic arch.

The esophagus obtains its blood supply from distinct branches of the thoracic descending aorta. Thus, the upper third, the middle third, and the lower third are independent.

Another outstanding anatomical feature of the esophagus is its venous drainage. The venous drainage also has three divisions. The upper third drains into the superior vena cava, the middle third to the azygos, and the lower third to the portal vein via the gastric veins.

The three systems come together below the diaphragm and merge with veins draining the stomach. Since the venous system of the stomach ultimately drains into the liver, the veins of the stomach and, therefore, the esophagus, are subject to increased pressure and flow if hepatic circulation is obstructed. Thus, if a patient develops portal hypertension (elevation of pressure in the portal vein secondary to obstructed flow), blood flow will be shunted to the

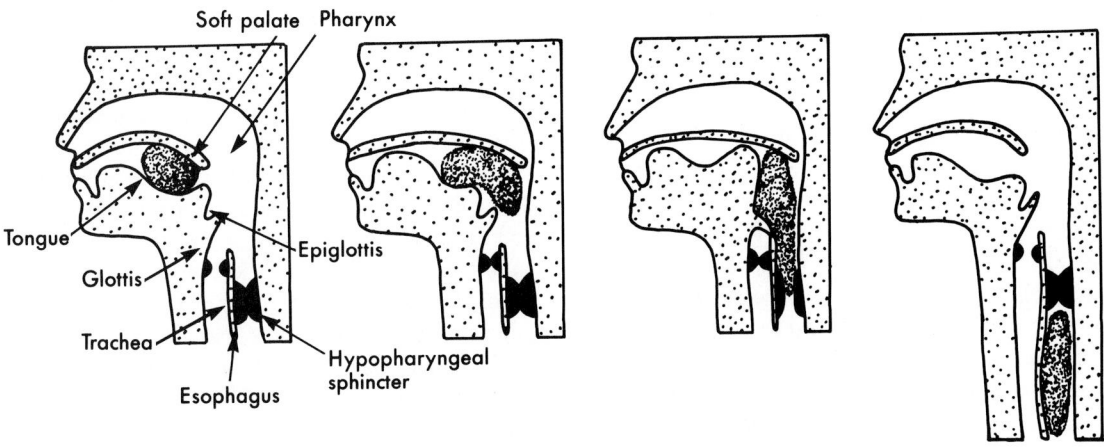

Figure 49-4   Mechanism of swallowing.

esophageal veins, causing massive dilatation of these vessels. These dilated veins, known as *esophageal varices*, carry tremendous quantities of blood under very elevated pressures. They are prone to rupture easily. Massive hemorrhage from ruptured esophageal varices is a major complication and a potential cause of death for patients with portal hypertension.

Histology

Histologically, the mucosa of the esophageal lumen contains squamous epithelium. It is poorly modified for food absorption and has only rare mucus-producing glands throughout its wall. No major digestive enzymes are secreted by the esophagus.

Unlike the other gastrointestinal organs, the upper third of the esophagus contains only striated muscle in the muscularis externa; the middle third has both striated and smooth muscle; the lower two thirds has only smooth muscle. The outer muscle layer of the esophagus runs longitudinally. This evolutionary change facilitates the voluntary aspect of swallowing.[6,9]

Motility

Along the esophagus, a series of rhythmic contractions called *peristaltic waves* propel the food bolus downward. A wave consists of a contracting and a relaxing phase. Each peristaltic movement lasts some 5 seconds and travels toward the stomach at about 3 cm/sec. Normal transit time from the top of the esophagus to the stomach is 9 to 10 seconds.[6]

The role of the upper esophageal sphincter (the hypopharyngeal sphincter) has already been discussed. This specialized muscular area of the esophagus contracts when stimulated by the central nervous system and permits relaxation of the esophageal opening.

Movement of the food down the esophagus is promoted by a pressure gradient and contraction or peristalsis of the esophageal wall. Governed by the myenteric plexus, vagal mediation helps propagate esophageal peristalsis and, therefore, passage of food into the stomach.

The lower esophageal sphincter (LES), also called the *gastroesophageal sphincter,* is not an anatomical sphincter but an area of high pressure that prevents acidic gastric contents from regurgitating into the esophagus. Normally, the LES is closed when swallowing is not occurring. Once the sphincter opens, food passes into the stomach, and the sphincter again contracts and closes.

Though anatomically most of the esophagus is in the thoracic cavity above the diaphragm, a small 3-cm portion is below the diaphragm. This special anatomical arrangement utilizes the pressure gradient

TABLE 49-3 Factors Affecting Lower Esophageal Pressure

Increased Pressure	Decreased Pressure
HORMONES	
Gastrin	Secretin
Motilin	CCK
	Glucagon
	Somatostatin
	Gastric inhibitory peptide (GIP)
	Vasoactive inhibitory peptide (VIP)
FOODS	
Meals high in protein	Meals high in fat
	Chocolate
	Peppermint
	Ethanol
	Caffeine
DRUGS	
Antacids	Theophylline
Metoclopramide	Serotonin
	Meperidine
	Morphine
	Dopamine
	Calcium channel blockers
	Diazepam
	Barbiturates
MISCELLANEOUS	
Increased intraabdominal pressure	Pregnancy

between the thoracic cavity and the abdominal cavity to further discourage gastric reflux. To prevent reflux into the esophagus, with possible mucosal damage from the acidity, the tone or pressure of the LES must increase and narrow the opening. The many factors that affect lower esophageal pressure are summarized in Table 49-3. Factors that decrease pressure promote reflux or treat functional obstruction of the esophagus. Conversely, factors that increase pressure have the opposite effects.[5,8]

Under normal circumstances, intraabdominal pressure exceeds intrathoracic pressure. The thoracic esophagus and the abdominal esophagus maintain the level of pressure within their respective anatomical cavities. Since the pressure at the gastroesophageal sphincter can and does increase with increases in intraabdominal pressure, sufficient tone can be generated at the LES to prevent reflux into the esophagus.

If, however, the LES is anatomically displaced by massive ascites or a growing fetus, then the distal esophagus, indeed the entire esophagus, is within the thoracic cavity. Corresponding increases in intraabdominal pressure are not transmitted to the lower esophagus. The LES is unable to generate sufficient pressure, and gastric reflux may occur.

Regulation

A complex series of mechanisms regulates the esophageal sphincters. Extrinsic control and coordination of esophageal motility is in the brainstem *swallowing center*. The upper sphincter opens and closes principally on signals from the central nervous system. Once the trachea is protected by closure of the glottis, the brain signals the upper sphincter to contract and, thus, permits entrance of food into the esophagus. Note that for the upper sphincter, contraction opens the entrance while relaxation closes it.

Unlike its upper counterpart, the lower esophageal sphincter is influenced by an enormous number of factors. The actual mechanism for many of these controls is still speculative. Two basic groups of controls are known. One is hormone mediated, and the other depends on neurological mechanisms.

The vagus is the primary nerve regulating lower esophageal sphincter tone and pressure. Though it is responsible, in part, for creating the normal resting tone of the sphincter, its major function is to relax the sphincter during swallowing.[2,5,7]

STOMACH

Unlike the esophagus, the stomach provides several major digestive functions in addition to mechanical mixing and transport of food. This organ produces important digestive secretions. It has a small but recognizable role in selected absorptive activities and provides a reservoir for partially digested food. *Chyme* (or food mixed with GI secretions) is retained in the stomach until it is sufficiently altered, both physically and chemically, to permit further digestion in the first part of the small intestine, the duodenum.

The stomach has a much greater secretory capacity than the esophagus. The hormones, acid, mucus, water, and electrolytes secreted by the stomach mix and interact while chyme is retained in the stomach.

In the stomach itself, little absorption of foodstuffs occurs. Most of the particles are large and ionically charged, making their diffusion across the cell membrane difficult. Because of the stomach's acid environment, substances that are weak acids convert to their noncharged, nonionic form. Under these conditions, they are easily absorbed. Thus, a weak acid, such as acetysalicylic acid (aspirin), is rapidly absorbed in the stomach. Though most alcohol absorption occurs in the small intestine, some occurs in the stomach as well.

Beyond its role in digestion, the stomach also has some antibacterial function. The acidity of the stomach is partially responsible for this phenomenon. This

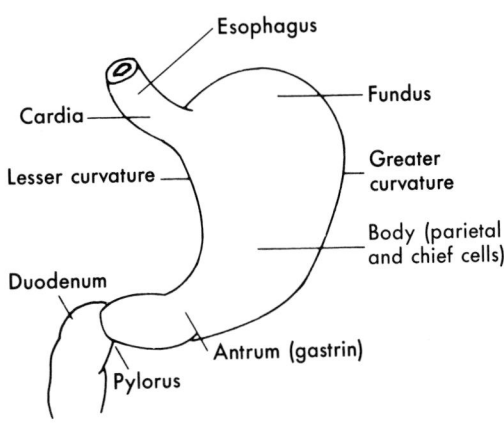

Figure 49-5 Gross anatomy of the stomach.

mild antibacterial control helps to keep the environment of the small intestine sterile.[10]

Anatomy

The stomach is located at the distal end of the esophagus. It is divided into five regions (Figure 49-5).
1. The *cardia* is the part adjacent to the esophagus.
2. The *fundus* rises above the cardia and merges with the main part of the stomach.
3. The major portion of the stomach is the *body*.
4. That area of the stomach immediately before the pylorus is the *antrum*.
5. The *pylorus* is the muscular sphincter between the stomach and the duodenum.

On gross inspection of the stomach, one finds muscular walls thrown into multiple folds, or *rugae*. These folds increase the actual surface area of the organ and, together with the muscular nature of the organ, allow for greater expansion of the stomach. The usual capacity is 1 to 1.5 L.

The major arterial blood supply of the stomach arises from the celiac artery directly off the aorta. Sympathetic nerve fibers from the celiac plexus and parasympathetic fibers, principally from the vagus nerve, innervate the stomach. Parasympathetic tone predominates.

Histology

Histologically, the mucosal surface of the stomach is lined with columnar epithelium. Most important, this surface itself is a continuous flow of involutions and convolutions forming deep gastric pits. The gastric pits are important because they increase the overall surface area and contain many secretory glands of the stomach. Note also that the muscularis externa of the stomach differs from other gastrointestinal organs. This third layer is arranged in an oblique fashion and forms the innermost fibers of the muscularis externa.

Gastric Secretions

Gastric Glands

There are some 15 million glands in the many glandular structures in the stomach wall. Grouped by location and function, they are the cardiac, the gastric (or fundic), and the pyloric glands. The cells of the gastric gland secrete about 2,500 ml of gastric juice daily. Gastric juice contains a variety of substances (see box below).

The *cardiac glands* are located near the cardia of the stomach. They are responsible for mucus secretion only.

At the distal end of the stomach the *pyloric glands* are found, just before the pyloric sphincter. Like their counterparts in the cardia, these glands are mucus secretors; however, the pyloric glands also synthesize the hormone gastrin.

The *gastric*, or *fundic, glands* located in the body of the stomach secrete many different substances (Figure 49-6). Their ability to produce more diversified products is a result of a more varied cell type in their epithelial layer. The *neck mucous cell* is found in the uppermost part of the gastric gland. It secretes mucus. The *parietal cell* is found in the middle of the gland. This cell secretes HCl and intrinsic factor, a substance necessary for the absorption of orally ingested vitamin B_{12}. The final cell type, located deepest within the gastric gland, is the *chief cell.* The specialization of this cell allows it to secrete other enzymes. The most well known of these is pepsinogen.

The secretory function of the stomach can be conceptualized as two fundamental groups: the acid and the nonacid secretions. Table 49-4 summarizes gastric secretions and their major regulator.

Acid Secretions

The parietal cells, located in the pit of the gastric gland, are solely responsible for secretion of HCl. The amount of HCl secreted is directly proportional to the parietal cell mass. Normally, almost 2 L of HCl is secreted per day.

The internal environment of each parietal cell is composed of normal cellular matrix and the various electrolytes—Na^+, K^+, Cl^-, and so on. Each cell is rich with large mitochondria that produce adenosine 5-triphosphate (ATP), thereby supplying the needed energy for HCl synthesis.

The secretion of the HCl requires active ionic transport of H^+ and Cl^-. As a consequence, large amounts of energy in the form of ATP are required. Appropriately, the parietal cells contain many large mito-

---

Contents of Gastric Juice

Water
Cations: Na^+, K^+, Mg^{2+}
Anions: Cl^-, HPO^{3-}, SO_4^-
Mucus
Intrinsic factor
Pepsins
Gelatinase

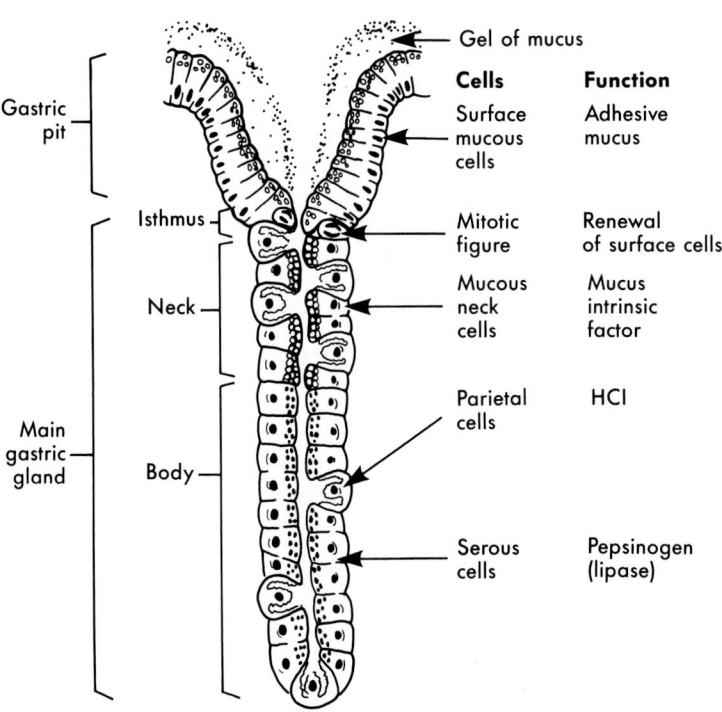

Figure 49-6   Histology of gastric glands.

TABLE 49-4 **Gastric Secretions and Their Regulators**

Gland/Cells of Origin	Secretion	Regulator
Cardiac gland	Mucus	Neural
Pyloric gland	Mucus	Neural
Fundic (gastric) gland		
Mucous neck cells	Mucus	Neural
Parietal cells	Water, HCl, Intrinsic factor	Hormonal
Chief cells	Pepsinogen, Mucus	Hormonal

chondria. The acidic environment of the stomach promotes the conversion of pepsinogen, a proteolytic enzyme secreted by gastric chief cells, to pepsin. Pepsin is effective only in an environment where the pH is less than 5; therefore, HCl secretion is essential for protein digestion. HCl also kills many ingested bacteria.

Despite years of study, many of the details surrounding HCl secretion are unclear. Several reactions occur concurrently within the parietal cell to generate and replenish the needed stores of ionic substrates.

The source of hydrogen ions (H^+) is believed to be the ionization of water (H_2O):

$$H_2O \rightleftarrows H^+ + OH^-$$

Coincidentally with this, an enzyme in the parietal cell, carbonic anhydrase, catalyzes the reaction of carbon dioxide (CO_2) and water (H_2O) to make carbonic acid (H_2CO_3):

$$CO_2 + H_2O \rightleftarrows H_2CO_3$$

The carbonic acid is further broken down into a bicarbonate ion (HCO_3^-) and a hydrogen ion (H^+):

$$H_2CO_3 \rightleftarrows H^+ + HCO_3^-$$

For each H^+ ion that is actively transported across the cell membrane into the stomach lumen, one HCO_3^- ion diffuses (not actively transported) back into the bloodstream. Since this is a 1:1 exchange, as the stomach contents become more acid, the venous blood leaving the stomach after a meal becomes more alkalotic.

Normally, body pH does not change significantly when food is ingested because the pancreas and duodenum secrete HCO_3^- into the intestinal lumen and neutralize the pH. An important point to keep in mind, however, is that measurable pH shifts can occur in patients who are vomiting profusely. With prolonged vomiting and, therefore, loss of H^+ greater than loss of HCO_3^-, patients may become alkalotic.

In summary, H^+ ions are derived from the ionization of H_2O. Both H^+ and Cl^- are actively transported across the cell membrane into the stomach lumen. For each H^+ ion that is transported into the lumen, one HCO_3^- ion diffuses back into the blood (Figure 49-7).[6,10]

Nonacid Secretion

Intrinsic Factor. Intrinsic factor is a glycoprotein, secreted by the parietal cells. It is necessary for the absorption of orally ingested vitamin B_{12}. Though the mechanism is incompletely understood, it is believed that cobalamine (vitamin B_{12}) binds to intrinsic factor. This complex travels to the distal ileum (third part of the small intestine) and binds to another receptor on the surface of the ileal mucosa. Once attached, the vitamin B_{12} is absorbed. With any surgical procedure or condition (e.g., gastrectomy, atrophic gastritis) that causes the loss of parietal cells, intrinsic factor will not be produced, and, therefore, vitamin B_{12} will not be absorbed. Vitamin B_{12} must be replaced parenterally. This vitamin is critical to formation of red blood cells, and absence of intrinsic factor can result in anemia. Resection of the distal ileum where absorption occurs also results in anemia.[5]

Signs and symptoms of vitamin B_{12} deficiency include neurological changes that may be confused with other neurological conditions, including Alzheimer's disease. These include parethesias involving the hands and feet, loss of position sense, disturbances of bowel and bladder function, and cerebral dysfunction.

Pepsinogen. Pepsinogen, a nonacid substance, is secreted by the chief cells of the gastric glands. In its initial form, this proteolytic enzyme is inactive. As described previously, it is activated only when the stomach pH becomes sufficiently acidic. In this acid

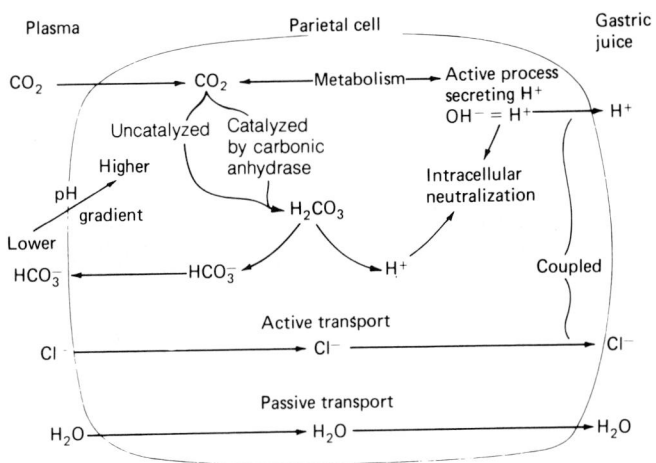

Figure 49-7 Acid secretion.

environment, part of the original molecule is hydro-lyzed, and the remaining active form, known as *pepsin,* cleaves amino acid bonds within protein chains. Maximal activity of pepsin occurs in a pH range between 1 and 3. Once the intestinal contents are neutralized by pancreatic and duodenal bicarbonate, pepsin loses its enzymatic activity.

Pepsin initiates the first major step in protein digestion. Whole proteins are broken down into small polypeptide fragments. As the digestive process continues, these newly formed fragments play a role in regulating gastric motility and secretion.[1,2,4,5,6,10]

Gastrin. The final major nonacid compound considered here is *gastrin.* This hormone has been intensively studied and is believed to be one of the major controlling factors in gastric acid secretion. Gastrin is secreted primarily by the cells of the pyloric glands in the antrum of the stomach. However, small amounts have also been found in the upper part of the duodenum and in certain cells of the pancreas. Structurally, gastrin is a peptide of 17 amino acids or, alternately, 34 amino acids. The four amino acids at the carboxyl terminal end are believed to be the active agents regulating acid control.

Gastrin's principal role is to stimulate secretion of HCl by parietal cells. This is accomplished through physical contact with a receptor on the parietal cell surface. Beyond its role as regulator of gastric acid, gastrin, in pharmacological doses, increases lower esophageal sphincter tone and also enhances gastric motility. The box below summarizes major actions of gastrin.[1,2,5,6,10]

Major Actions of Gastrin

GASTRIN STIMULATES
Growth of the gastric fundic mucosa
Secretion of pepsinogen
Secretion of gastric intrinsic factor
Secretion of pancreatic bicarbonate and pancreatic digestive enzymes
Insulin release from pancreatic islets
Secretion of bicarbonate from Brunner's glands in the duodenum
Hepatic secretion of biliary bicarbonate
Intestinal motility
Rhythmic contractions of the stomach and gallbladder

GASTRIN INHIBITS
Gastric emptying
Secretion of secretin
Gastric resting tone
Secretion of cholecystokinin
Sodium absorption from the ileum
Ileocecal valve resting tone

Regulation of Gastric Secretions

The regulation of gastric acid is as complex as the intricate molecular reactions responsible for HCl secretion. Like the control mechanisms for the lower esophageal sphincter, the regulation of acid secretion is both nerve and hormone mediated. The humoral and the neural mechanisms are so intermingled that it would be difficult to explore them separately, and this discussion treats them as one. Regulation of pepsinogen secretion virtually parallels HCl output and is included as well.[6,7]

The Cephalic Phase. The first phase of acid secretion, the cephalic phase, begins when one sees, smells, tastes, or even thinks about an appetizing meal. Thus, HCl is secreted even before food reaches the mouth. This phase of acid control is via parasympathetic input via the vagus nerve. In part, the vagus directly stimulates acid secretion by the gastric glands. In addition, the vagus increases gastrin production by the pyloric glands in the antrum. This added gastrin augments acid output. Note that antrectomy (removal of the antrum) does not totally obliterate acid secretion. This supports the evidence that the vagus stimulates the gastric glands directly; acid secretion is not mediated by gastrin alone.

Vagal impulses are increased by hunger, hypoglycemia, and anger, as well as by pleasant gustatory stimulation. Measurable reduction in vagal tone is found with hyperglycemia, an overdistended stomach, and certain drugs, especially the anticholinergic agents.

The Gastric Phase. The second phase of acid secretion, the gastric phase, occurs, as its name implies, when food reaches the stomach. Though vagal input is still present, the predominant regulatory factors during the gastric phase are humoral. Alcohol and coffee (because of peptides, not caffeine) have also been shown to increase HCl secretion during this phase.

The hormone of note in acid regulation is gastrin. Though gastrin increases pepsinogen secretion as well, it does so to a lesser degree. It should be remembered that during the cephalic phase, some gastrin is secreted; however, the gastric phase is responsible for the major outflow of this hormone. The secretion of gastrin is stimulated by antral distention, by polypeptide fragments in the antrum, and by an alkaline pH in the stomach. Simultaneous secretion of pepsinogen increases the amount of polypeptide fragments, thus adding indirectly to the stimulus for gastrin secretion.

Gastrin secretion is controlled by a feedback mechanism. As gastrin is secreted, HCl is poured out, lowering the pH of the gastric contents. When the pH becomes sufficiently low and, therefore, the H^+ ion concentration sufficiently high, gastrin secretion decreases.

The Intestinal Phase. The final step of acid control, the intestinal phase, begins as chyme enters the duodenum. When polypeptide fragments reach the antrum, gastric acid secretion increases. This mechanism remains operative even when the vagus nerve is not intact.

The intestinal phase has more inhibitory influence on gastric acid secretion than either of the earlier phases. If the pH within the duodenum is 2.5 or less, acid output markedly drops. Likewise, fat in the duodenum also decreases acid production. Cholecystokinin (CCK) and secretin, two duodenal hormones, exert an inhibitory effect on gastrin and, thereby, decrease acid output. Since CCK is stimulated by fat in the duodenum, there is some question as to the exact mechanism causing the acid reduction. Does fat directly inhibit acid? Or does CCK, stimulated by the presence of fat, inhibit acid? Or both?

In summary, control of gastric acid secretion has three major components: the cephalic phase, mediated principally by the vagus nerve; the gastric phase, influenced primarily by the hormonal effects of gastrin; and finally, the intestinal phase, mainly an inhibitory stage which reduces acid output as chyme leaves the stomach and enters the small intestine (Figure 49-8).

Gastric Motility

In the stomach, the physical and chemical breakdown of food continues. The partially digested food must be physically degraded into particles small enough to pass through the pyloric canal into the duodenum. Similarly, at the molecular level, gastric contents must be adequately mixed to ensure optimal enzyme exposure. Clearly, motility plays a central role in the stomach's contribution to digestion.

The movement of the stomach is both passive and active. Initially, as food enters the stomach, the passive phase of gastric motility, called *receptive relaxation*, occurs. It is a reflex initiated by earlier movements of the pharynx and the esophagus. As noted earlier, the usual reservoir capacity of the stomach is between 1 and 1.5 L. During receptive relaxation, volumes as high as 6 L have been recorded.

Active movements of the stomach, those which mix food and force it through the pylorus, combine peristaltic contractions across the body of the stomach with strong contractions of the terminal antral segment. These contractions are coordinated by the *gastric slow wave*, the pacemaker for peristalsis in the antrum and control of gastric emptying.

The trigger cells of the stomach's electrical pacemaker initiate electrical depolarization and subse-

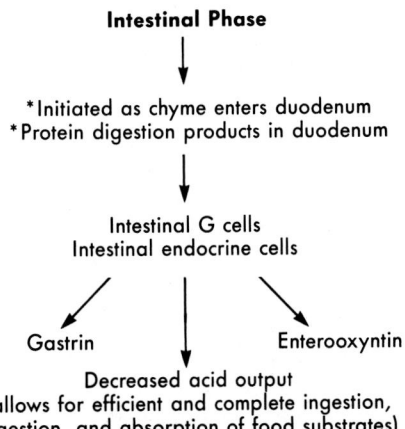

Figure 49-8 Phases of gastric acid secretion.

quent muscular peristalsis. Initially, the electrical and muscular activity travel in the outer muscle layer. Then they spread to the inner muscle layer and sweep across the body of the stomach toward the antrum. Normally, the frequency of contractions is three per minute. The initial rate of speed is only about 1 cm/sec. However, as the antrum is approached, the peristaltic waves travel faster and may reach speeds in the range of 3 to 4 cm/sec.

Slow, weak muscular contractions are the rule early in digestion. It is only after about 1 hour of digestive activity that the speed and intensity of the waves increase. When contractions reach the antrum, they have enough force to push small amounts of chyme ahead of them. Digested food accumulates in the antrum, and antral pressure rises and actually overcomes the pressure in the open pyloric canal. Small amounts of viscous chyme are then able to squeeze through into the duodenum.

However, the pylorus also contracts. While contracted, the pyloric canal is closed; chyme is not able to pass through. The antrum, contracting against a closed pylorus, cannot generate enough pressure to push food into the duodenum. Instead, the chyme is forced backward into the stomach. It is this retropulsion of chyme into the stomach when the pylorus is closed that accounts for the active mixing quality of gastric motion. After a vagotomy or resection of the stomach wall, peristalsis will become irregular because the gastric slow wave is disrupted.[5,6,8,11]

Regulation

Several factors control gastric motility, including mechanical, chemical, and neural influences. They all interact to produce optimal mixing of food in the stomach before it is passed to the small intestine for absorption.

Significant abnormalities of gastric motility often lead to malabsorptive states. Though food may reach its destined site of absorption in the small intestine, if it has been improperly or incompletely processed in the stomach, normal absorption will not occur.

Gastric processing of chyme also affects control mechanisms of gastric emptying. If chyme is adequately prepared, gastric motility increases, and chyme passes through the pylorus. When chyme is incompletely processed, the stomach detains emptying by decreasing gastric motility. If the duodenum is incapable of accepting more chyme, the stomach acts to delay further emptying.

Gastric Influences. The principal factors affecting gastric motility are gastrin and tension within the stomach wall. Tension builds within the stomach walls as the volume of food increases. To decrease wall tension, the rate of gastric emptying increases.

Gastrin, the hormone that causes increased secretion of hydrochloric acid, also enhances antral motility. Acid is for digestion, and mixing promotes digestion. It should be remembered also that the release of gastrin is related to increased pressure in the lower esophageal sphincter. Thus, during peak gastric motility, esophageal reflux is discouraged.

Intestinal Influences. Duodenal distension signals the stomach to slow gastric unloading. If the duodenum is unable to keep pace with the rate of emptying, incomplete interaction of hormones results, and chyme is inadequately prepared for transit further along in the small intestine. Similarly, if chyme reaching the duodenum is too acidic or too hypertonic, gastric emptying is inhibited. This checkpoint, called the *enterogastric reflex*, is partially mediated by the vagus nerve. Cutting the vagus nerves slows gastric emptying and may cause gastric atony and distention. Gastric inhibitory peptide and other hormones inhibit gastric motility.

The type of food ingested also affects the rate of stomach emptying. Fat in the duodenum stimulates the secretion of cholecystokinin, which in itself directly delays gastric motility. Fats leave the stomach more slowly than proteins and proteins more slowly than carbohydrates.

Receptors for HCl, fatty acids, and osmotic stimuli have been postulated to exist in the duodenum and jejunum. By unknown mechanisms, perhaps humoral or neural, these receptors affect gastric emptying. In summary, controls regulating gastric motility are designed to maximize the unique role of each organ along the gastrointestinal tract, allowing for efficient and complete ingestion, digestion, and absorption of food substrates.

The Vomiting Reflex

Vomiting is a reflex response integrated in the medulla of the brain. The partially digested food material in the stomach is forced back up through the esophagus into the mouth. Often the process is associated with common signs and symptoms of sympathetic nervous discharge (e.g., tachycardia and sweating). Salivation and nausea are also commonly associated.

Incoming signals to the medulla arise from various body sensory receptors. The more common emetic stimulants involve mechanical stimulation of the posterior oropharynx, increased intracranial pressure, overdistention of the stomach or duodenum, pain, or ingestion of certain chemical compounds. Vomiting can also be induced by psychogenic stimuli such as noxious experiences. Mechanically, five steps are involved:[2,3,8]

1. A deep inspiration is followed by closure of the glottis.
2. The soft palate rises.
3. The abdominal muscles contract and increase intraabdominal and intragastric pressure.
4. The gastroesophageal sphincter (LES) relaxes.
5. Respirations cease and the elevated intragastric pressure forces the food back through the esophagus, opens the upper esophageal sphincter, and forces food into the mouth.

The *vomiting center* in the reticular formation of the medulla controls these activities. Prolonged vomiting may lead to severe electrolyte and pH imbalances as well as dehydration. Drug therapy for nausea and vomiting acts centrally by decreasing afferent nerve impulses or peripherally by reducing stimuli.

PANCREAS AND BILIARY SYSTEM

Pancreas

Glands are considered *endocrine* if the hormones they synthesize are secreted directly into the blood. They are called *exocrine* if they secrete hormones into the nonvascular system of ducts. The pancreas has both endocrine functions (production of insulin and glucagon) and exocrine functions (production of digestive enzymes). The discussion focuses on its exocrine functions.

Anatomy

The pancreas is a long, slender organ, located retroperitoneally (posterior to the peritoneum) within the abdominal cavity. It is divided into a head, a body, and a tail. The head lies within the C-shaped portion of the duodenum. The body or main portion of the gland is posterior to the stomach. The tail extends to the spleen (Figure 49-9). Unlike the liver and the other abdominal organs, the pancreas has no defined pro-

tective external capsule. Inflammatory processes can, therefore, spread freely and affect the many surrounding organs.

The rich arterial supply of the pancreas comes principally from the celiac and superior mesenteric arteries. Sympathetic nerves from the celiac plexus and parasympathetic fibers from the vagus nerve innervate the organ.

Histology

The entire pancreas has a complex microscopic structure (Figure 49-10). The principal component is a system of lobules separated by connective tissue septa. Within this multilobulated structure, small grapelike structures called *acinar glands* are found. They are accompanied by a partner system of collecting ducts. These ducts branch into small ductules

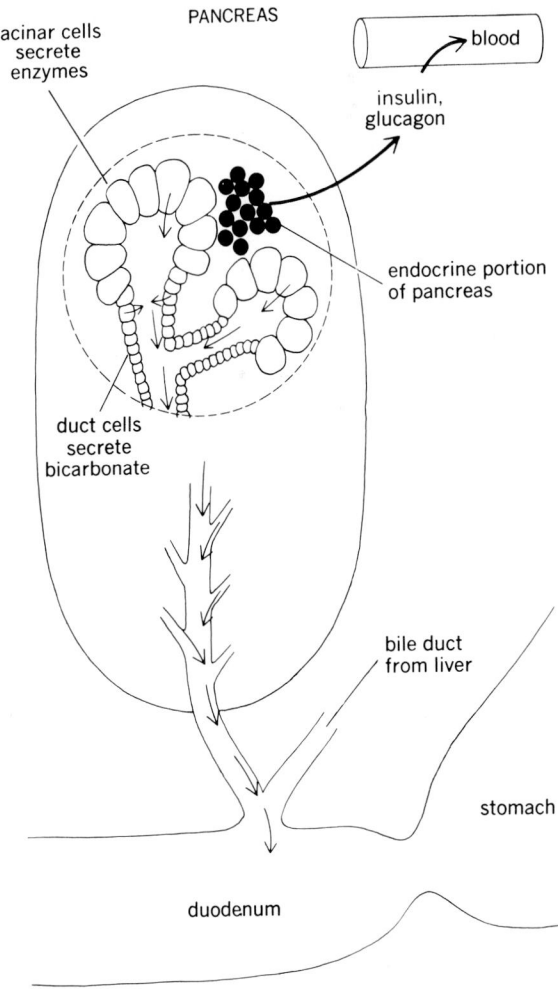

Figure 49-10   Endocrine and exocrine structure of the pancreas.

From Vander, A. J., Sherman, J. H., & Luciano, D. (1989). *Human physiology.* New York: McGraw-Hill.

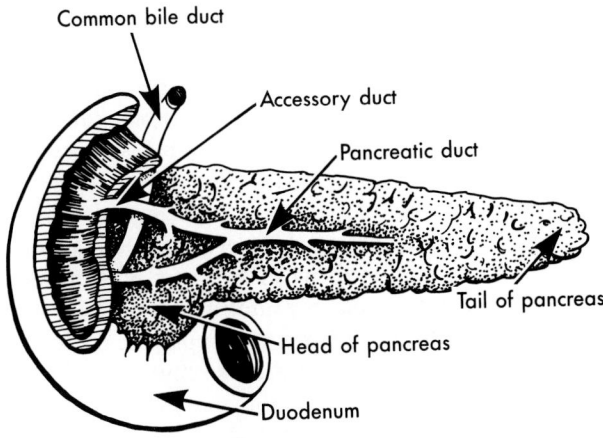

Figure 49-9   The pancreas.

which, in turn, merge to form larger ducts which eventually coalesce and form the major pancreatic duct of Wirsung. The duct of Wirsung then empties into the duodenum. In some individuals, there is an accessory pancreatic duct that enters the duodenum more proximally (duct of Santorini). Patients with gastric acid hypersecretion and duodenal ulcer are known to have a high incidence of nonpatency of this duct.[8]

Exocrine Secretions

Two major products are secreted by the exocrine pancreas: digestive enzymes and bicarbonate fluid. The acinar glands produce enzymes while the lining cells of the ducts secrete the bicarbonate-rich pancreatic juice. The combined output of enzymatic and bicarbonate secretions approaches 2 L per day. The actual proportion of the two components is determined by the nature of the food ingested.[4,6,10]

Bicarbonates. The ductal epithelium, or lining cells, of the pancreas produce a bicarbonate-rich fluid. Within the duct lumen, the alkaline secretion of the duct cells mixes with the enzymatic secretion of the acinar cells. What eventually reaches the major pancreatic duct and, therefore, the small intestine is a pancreatic juice rich in bicarbonate (HCO_3^-; pH approximately 8.0) and enzymes.

The mechanism of bicarbonate secretion by the exocrine pancreas is analogous to the secretion of hydrochloric acid by the stomach. However, in the case of the pancreas, it is bicarbonate and not hydrogen that is pumped into the intestinal lumen. Here, as in the stomach, and for similar reasons of unfavorable osmotic gradients, the process requires active transport, not simple diffusion. Just as the stomach acidifies venous blood during secretion of HCl, so the pancreas alkalinizes it because of secretion of bicarbonate.

Any condition that causes pancreatic ischemia is thought to contribute to the release of myocardial depressant factor (MDF). This factor depresses myocardial contractility and, therefore, affects cardiac output.[6,8]

Pancreatic Enzymes. The acinus, or glandular part, of the exocrine pancreas contains many secretory cells. These cells, rich in specialized intracellular organelles, are responsible for the enzyme synthesis and packaging. *Zymogen granules* are storage particles laden with digestive enzymes (Table 49-5).[10] The acinar cells secrete their enzymatic products into a central duct that travels the length of the pancreas. This duct connects with the common bile duct before it enters the duodenum.

The secretions of the acinar glands are a composite of enzymes, water, and salts. The successful digestion

TABLE 49-5   Pancreatic Enzymes

Enzyme	Action
Trypsin*	Digests protein
Chymotrypsin*	Digests protein
Carboxypolypeptidase*	Digests protein
Ribonuclease	Digests protein
Deoxyribonuclease	Digests protein
Pancreatic amylase	Digests carbohydrates
Pancreatic lipase	Digests fats
Cholesterol esterase	Digests fats

* Become activated only after they are secreted into the intestinal tract.

of fat, carbohydrate, and protein depends on the presence of these products. If the gland cannot produce sufficient enzymes because of disease, or if the enzymes cannot enter the small intestine because of anatomic obstruction, malabsorption in varying degrees may result. However, the pancreas has a tremendous reserve. Normal digestion can occur even if enzymatic secretion has been reduced to 10% of normal. Cholecystokinin (CCK) and secretin are the major endogenous substances that modulate pancreatic secretion.

The enzymes of the pancreas are secreted as inactive proenzymes. As the pancreatic juice enters the duodenum, trypsinogen is converted to trypsin, an active enzyme, by enteropeptidase. Trypsin converts other proenzymes into active enzymes. Pancreatic juice contains three basic groups of enzymes: amylytic (carbohydrate breakdown), proteolytic (protein breakdown), and lipolytic (fat breakdown).[1,6,10]

Amylytic. Of the amylytic group, α-amylase is the principal component. This enzyme, like salivary α-amylase, hydrolyzes carbohydrates. The principal end products are glucose and maltose, a disaccharide of two glucose molecules. Pancreatic amylase is active in its original form and, unlike salivary amylase, can digest raw as well as cooked starches.

Proteolytic. Trypsinogen, chymotrypsinogen, and procarboxypeptidase are the major proteolytic enzymes. Actually, these three substances are proenzymes: each must be altered before it becomes biochemically active.

Trypsinogen is converted to trypsin by the action of secretin. In addition, trypsin acts as a self-catalyst so that trypsin activates trypsinogen. Trypsin cleaves amino acid bonds in the interior of protein chains.

Chymotrypsinogen is activated to chymotrypsin by trypsin. Its biochemical function, like that of trypsin, is to cleave only interior amino acid bonds and, thus, add to the growing pool of small polypeptides and single amino acids in the intestine.

Procarboxypeptidase, unlike the other two proteolytic enzymes, cleaves terminal amino acids and produces amino acids with free carboxyl ends. Procarboxypeptidase is converted to its active form by secretin and probably by trypsin.

Lipolytic. The lipolytic enzymes, principally pancreatic lipase and phospholipase A, are important in early stages of fat digestion.

Lipase degrades triglycerides to free fatty acids and monoglycerides. Inactive in its original form, it requires the presence of bile salts to stabilize the fat–water interface of the intestinal contents. Phospholipase A hydrolyzes lecithin to lysolecithin. Phospholipase A has been implicated in the pathophysiology of acute pancreatitis, in which it causes necrosis of pancreatic tissue and fat when it is prematurely activated.

Two additional pancreatic enzymes, nuclease and deoxyribonuclease, do not fall into any of the groups described but deserve mention. As their names suggest, these enzymes are involved in the degradation of nucleotides within DNA and RNA molecules.

Endocrine Secretions

The islets of the pancreas have three main cell types, each responsible for secretion of specific products. The α cell produces glucagon. The polypeptide insulin is secreted by the β cells. The third cell type is the δ1 (delta) cell. Unlike the hormones of the exocrine pancreas, those of the endocrine pancreas, by definition, are secreted directly into the blood and not into a system of ducts. Table 49-6 summarizes actions of pancreatic hormones.

Biliary System

An understanding of fat digestion and absorption in the intestine requires knowledge of the biliary system. This vast network of connecting channels and ducts involves the gallbladder as well as the biliary passages of the liver (Figure 49-11). Among its many functions, the liver synthesizes and transports the bile salts and bile pigments needed for fat digestion.

From both an anatomical and a functional level, the liver is extremely complex. Only the biliary component of the liver is included in the present discussion. Other functions of the liver are presented later in this chapter.

Functional Anatomy

Bile is synthesized by the liver cells, or *hepatocytes.* Then it is secreted into *bile canaliculi,* or ductules, which lie adjacent to the liver cells. The bile canaliculi have many orders of branching and eventually merge to form the right and left hepatic ducts within the liver. After exiting from the liver, these two ducts join

TABLE 49-6　Pancreatic Enzyme Function

Secretory Cell Type	Enzyme	Physiological Actions
Alpha	Glucagon	Degradation of: Hepatic glycogen to glucose; Adipose tissue triglyceride; Gluconeogenesis from amino acids
Beta	Insulin	Stimulates glucose utilization by tissues (glucose and glycogen oxidation); Fat synthesis
Delta	Insulin-like growth factor (somatostatin)	Inhibits insulin, glucagon, and pancreatic growth hormone
PP cells	Polypeptides	Effects on humans not clearly understood; causes hypermotility and diarrhea in animals

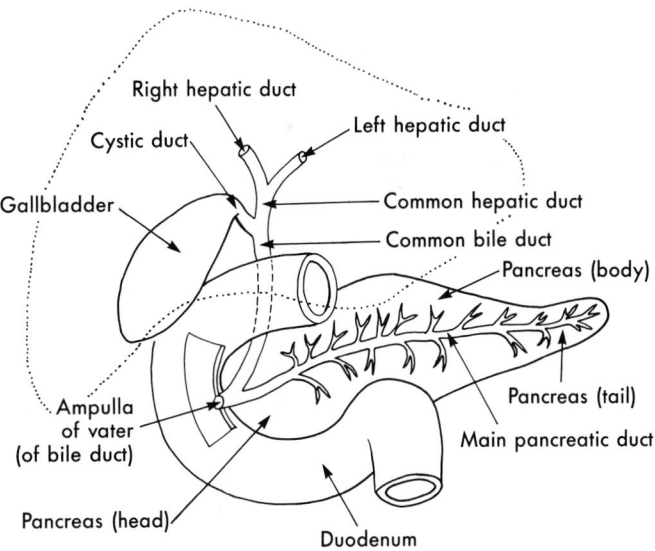

Figure 49-11　Ductal systems of the GI tract.

and become the common hepatic duct. The cystic duct, a continuation of the gallbladder, carries bile from the gallbladder; it joins the common hepatic duct to become the common bile duct. The common bile duct and the major pancreatic duct merge at the ampulla of Vater and enter the small intestine through the duodenal papilla (Figure 49-9).

The *gallbladder* stores and concentrates bile. It is

located on the undersurface of the right lobe of the liver. The adult gallbladder has a capacity of 30 to 50 ml. Between meals, bile reaches the gallbladder from the liver by way of the interconnecting duct system.

The common bile duct has a muscular sphincter surrounding its orifice. As the sphincter opens and closes, it determines the amount of bile that passes through from the gallbladder and liver. Note that, unlike the common bile duct, the pancreatic duct has no separate muscular sphincter. Hypothetically, this anatomical difference may make the pancreas more susceptible to bile reflux under certain circumstances. Reflux may cause pancreatitis.

The arterial blood supply of the gallbladder comes from the cystic artery. Most frequently, this is a branch off the right hepatic artery. Venous drainage is via the cystic vein into the portal vein.

In addition to the storage facility of the gallbladder, rapid absorption of water and certain electrolytes occurs there. Consequently, the bile found in the gallbladder is more concentrated than that found within the bile ducts of the liver. Occasionally, these shifts in bile concentration, coupled with other mechanisms, cause precipitation of bile components with resultant formation of gallstones (cholelithiasis). Acidification of bile is another function of the gallbladder.

Gallbladder secretions aid in digestion but are not essential. In patients who have undergone a cholecystectomy, nutrition is maintained by a slow but constant discharge of bile into the duodenum from the liver.[8]

Bile Metabolism and Function

The hepatocytes continually produce bile. After synthesis, bile is secreted into the canaliculi. The rate of synthesis approaches 0.6 ml per min in an average adult, with a total of 15 ml of bile being secreted for every kilogram of body weight. The rates of synthesis and secretion are controlled primarily by the amount of blood flow reaching the liver and the functional status of the liver.

The major constituents of bile include water (97%), bile acids and bile salts (principally sodium cholate and chenodeoxycholate), pigments (most notably bilirubin), cholesterol, phospholipids (especially lecithin), alkaline phosphatase, and electrolytes. About 500 ml is secreted per day.

Bile Salts. Bile salts are cholesterol derivatives. Together with lecithin they prevent the precipitation of cholesterol as cholesterol stones in the gallbladder. Bile salts are bipolar compounds; that is, they have a water-soluble and a fat-soluble end. Cholesterol and lecithin are fat-soluble molecules. In the gallbladder, bile salts interact with the water phase of the bile, leaving their fat-soluble end free to mix with choles-

terol and/or lecithin. The particles thus formed are called *micelles.* Eventually, the micelles become saturated with cholesterol. At this point of supersaturation, cholesterol precipitates out in the bile, and cholesterol stones are formed. The ratio of bile salts and lecithin to cholesterol is the basis of stone formation in the gallbladder. If the proportion of cholesterol in the bile increases (without a concurrent increase in bile salts or lecithin), stone formation is favored; likewise, if the bile concentration of salts and lecithin decreases, stones will form.

Bile salts are also important because of their role in fat digestion and absorption. Once in the small intestine, bile salts mix with fat. These water-stable complexes facilitate lipid (fat) absorption. In addition, bile salts are needed to activate pancreatic lipase, an enzyme needed for breakdown of triglycerides.

Normal fat digestion and absorption are not possible without bile salts. If obstruction or resection of the terminal ileum prevents the entrance of bile salts into the intestine, fat malabsorption and steatorrhea (fatty stools) result.[5,9]

Normally, bile salts are not lost in the stools. Instead, they are reabsorbed in the terminal part of the ileum (third part of the small intestine) and returned, via the venous system, to the liver, where they are taken up by the liver cells and used again. All but some 2% to 3% of bile salts is reutilized in this way.

Bile salts are recycled via the enterohepatic circulation. This vascular circuit, unique to the gastrointestinal tract, drains venous blood from all the alimentary organs and returns it to the liver. In passing through the liver, the venous blood meets a second set of capillaries. At the level of these specialized capillaries, the liver sequesters the substances it requires for synthetic and detoxifying functions and returns the blood to the heart. This type of anatomical "processing" is found only in the liver and in the vascular circuit of the anterior lobe of the pituitary gland.

Bile Pigments. Bilirubin and other bile pigments are products of hemoglobin degradation. Plasma bilirubin is bound to the protein albumin as it is delivered to the hepatocytes. However, only free bilirubin can enter the liver cell. Inside it binds to a hepatic protein carrier, thereby preventing escape back into the circulation. Bilirubin then reacts with two molecules of glucuronic acid via the enzyme glucuronyl transferase. The new water-soluble compound, bilirubin glucuronide, is then actively secreted into the bile canaliculi.

Once bile pigments are mixed in the bile and delivered to the small intestine, they are degraded by normal bowel flora. Pigments subsequently derived from the continued degradation are responsible for the normal color or stool. If extrahepatic biliary obstruction is present and no bile reaches the small intestine, stool color is gray—the *acholic* (without bile) *stool*.

In normal concentration, bile pigments do not form pigment stones. However, in disease states such as hemolytic anemias, in which an increased amount of bilirubin reaches the liver, the concentration of bile pigments increases and so-called pigment or bilirubinate stones precipitate out in the gallbladder. Most cases of cholelithiasis (90%) involve cholesterol stones. The remaining 10% of cases involve pigment stones.

Regulation. The regulation of bile secretion into the small intestine is a function of the neural and hormonal effects influencing the muscular sphincters of the biliary system and the contractility of the gallbladder.

In what might be called the cephalic phase of bile secretion, vagal stimulation received by the hepatocytes stimulates increased bile secretion and subsequent bile outflow. The sphincter of Oddi is normally in a partially opened state between meals. As a result, there is a constant trickle of bile into the small intestine. When food reaches the duodenum, however, a more active phase of bile regulation begins. As mentioned previously, fats and polypeptides are strong stimulants for secretion of cholecystokinin (CCK). In turn, CCK is the major hormonal stimulus for gallbladder contraction. When food is present within the stomach or duodenum, the sphincter of Oddi relaxes. As the gallbladder contracts, increased bile passes through the relaxed sphincter into the intestine. Between meals, when the stimulus for CCK decreases, the gallbladder does not contract. The sphincter remains contracted, and the bile, always in continuous flow, travels from the liver to the gallbladder. There it is stored and concentrated until the gallbladder is stimulated to empty.

Since there are no absolute stop valves on hepatic bile production, there is always a flow of hepatic bile arriving directly at the intestine. Hepatic bile contains more water and HCO_3^- than bile from the gallbladder. It is more alkaline and, therefore, important to the small intestine if a large acid load arrives at the duodenum. Precisely because of these differences, secretin (stimulated by increased acid) causes preferential stimulation of hepatic bile flow rather than contraction of the gallbladder. Likewise, gastrin, a strong stimulant of gastric acid, indirectly increases hepatic bile flow by enhancing the production of secretin. Furthermore, gastrin has its own direct effect on the liver and increases hepatic outflow of HCO_3^--rich bile.

SMALL INTESTINE

The small intestine comprises some 3 m of tubing coiled within the abdominal cavity. It extends from the stomach to the ileocecal valve, where the large intestine begins.

Together the three parts of the small intestine—the duodenum, the jejunum, and the ileum—perform most of the digestive and absorptive functions. The intestinal contents are combined with mucosal secretions and with pancreatic juice and bile. Almost all food types, as well as water and vitamins, are processed and absorbed before they reach the large intestine.

Mechanical transit of intestinal material, though less important than in other gastrointestinal organs, is still a specialized function of the small intestine. A mixing action predominates as the most important motor activity. Like other GI organs, the small intestine has a secretory role.

Anatomy

The first and the shortest segment of the small intestine is the duodenum. Normally about 20 cm long, the duodenum is critical because of its hormonal secretions; because of its anatomical proximity to the connecting ducts of the liver, gallbladder, and pancreas; and because of its unfortunate predisposition to ulcerative disease.

Continuing after the duodenum is the jejunum. Anatomically, the jejunum is defined as beginning at the ligament of Trietz.

The remainder of the small intestine, the ileum, terminates at the ileocecal valve. In addition to its role in routine nutrient absorption, the ileum also absorbs vitamin B_{12} and bile salts. Together the jejunum and the ileum usually measure 2 to 3 m in length.

Because of the important absorptive capacity of the small bowel, adequate blood supply to this organ is critical. As a result, even at rest, the small bowel has a blood flow of 1 L/min, or one fifth of the total resting cardiac output.[1,6]

The sole arterial blood supply of the ileum and jejunum is the superior mesenteric artery. The duodenum is supplied by several different vessels. Because of this anatomical difference, occlusion of the superior mesenteric artery may lead to infarction and cell death of the entire ileum and jejunum. However, the duodenum, with multiple blood sources, is less likely to suffer catastrophic necrosis if part of its arterial supply is cut off.

The venous drainage of the small intestine is noteworthy because, as mentioned before, it is part of the enterohepatic circulation. Venous blood leaves the intestine and undergoes hepatic processing before reaching the heart. In the liver, the hepatocytes extract what they need and detoxify noxious products. Venous blood then continues to the heart.

Both branches of the autonomic nervous system

innervate the small intestine. Extrinsic fibers meet in the various plexuses within the intestinal wall. Reflex pathways also contribute to overall functioning.[4,5,6]

The lymphatic system of the small bowel is important because of its central role in fat absorption. In the ileum, large collections of lymph nodules, called *Peyer's patches,* are grouped together within the intestinal wall.[6,12,13]

Histology

The microanatomy of the small bowel is specifically designed to maximize the absorptive functions of this organ. The inner surface of the entire intestine is folded, thus increasing the absorptive surface area. The surface of each fingerlike projection thus formed is itself covered with multiple small invaginations and projections called *villi,* further increasing surface area. Finally, each villus consists of epithelial cells, each of which is covered with thousands of hairlike projections called *microvilli,* further increasing the absorptive surface. This specialized histology increases the absorptive surface by 600-fold (Figure 49-12).

The villus is the main structural unit of the small bowel. It is constantly in motion, following the rhythmic contractions within the muscle layer of the wall. The contractions alter the length and, therefore, the

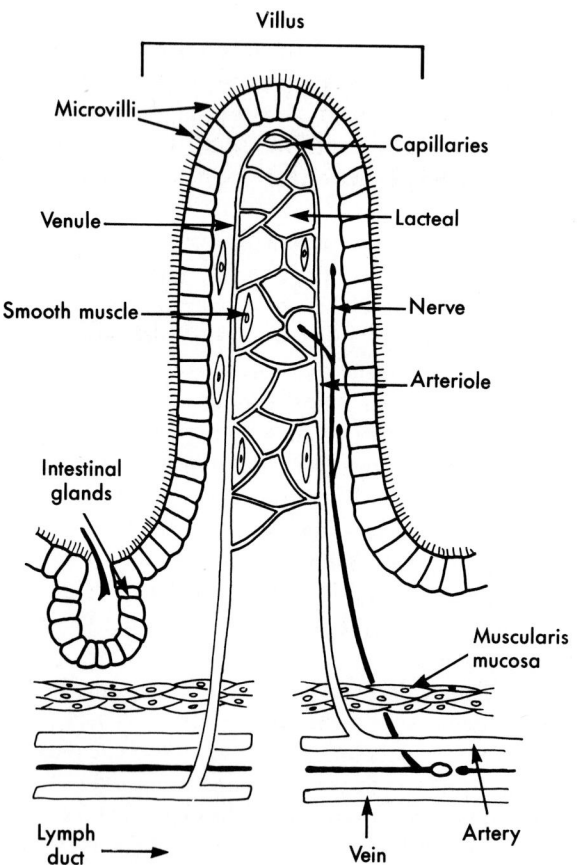

Figure 49-12   The small intestine villus.

surface area of the villus. Reflex pathways also contribute to overall functioning.

The microvilli contain certain enzymes needed for further nutrient digestion. In the center of the villus are found the artery, vein, nerve, and lymph vessel or lacteal. A *brush border* of many microvilli covers the surface of the mucosal cells in the small intestine (see Figure 49-12).[6,14]

The intestinal lining cells have one of the most rapid turnover rates in the body. New cells from the base of the villus and in the crypts of Lieberkuhn migrate up to the top to replace old, worn cells that are sloughed off into the intestinal lumen. The entire intestinal epithelium is replaced every 36 hours. This rapid epithelial turnover makes the small intestine particularly sensitive to radiation or chemotherapy, which interrupts cell division.[15]

Intestinal Function

Secretions

The brush border of the small intestine is rich in enzymes that hydrolyze carbohydrates and peptides. The lining epithelium of the small intestine is modified with numerous *goblet,* or mucus-producing, *cells.* Their mucous secretions and the CCK and secretin synthesized by the duodenal mucosa are the major secretory contributions of the small bowel. Note that CCK and secretin are synthesized by the duodenal mucosa, but they are secreted directly into the blood, not into the intestinal lumen.

The duodenal wall contains a collection of glands, *Brunner's glands,* which secrete fluid rich in bicarbonate (HCO_3^-). Like pancreatic HCO_3^-, the secretion of Brunner's glands helps to neutralize the acid contents and protect the duodenal mucosa. Secretion of HCO_3^- by Brunner's glands is stimulated by acid in the duodenum, by secretin, and by gastrin.[5,6,10,12]

Motility

Like each of the organs before it, the small intestine has its own specialized type of motility. The contractions of the small intestine are coordinated caudally by the *small bowel slow wave.* Since this organ is designed to digest and absorb chyme, it follows that the principal form of movement should promote mixing and facilitate contact with the absorbing surface. *Segmentation,* a unique ringlike type of contraction (Figure 49-13), achieves precisely these two objectives. When the intestinal wall is stretched, a peristaltic wave forms and contributes to the forward propulsion of chyme toward the colon. This is called the *myenteric reflex.*

In the duodenum, near the entrance of the common bile duct, intrinsic electrical pacemaker cells are found in the longitudinal muscle of the wall. The impulse travels from the duodenum to ileum. The strength, the frequency and the speed of the impulse *decrease* with distance from the duodenum, increasing the time available for digestion and absorption.

Segmentation contractions follow the intrinsic pacemaker rhythm but involve only rings of muscle around the small intestine. As one area relaxes, another contracts along the intestine, thus creating a sausage-link effect. This action mixes but does not propel intestinal contents. Since the small bowel must deliver the intestinal contents to the colon, a propulsive motion must exist as well. As chyme approaches the large intestine, ileal contractions *increase*. The ileocecal valve, normally in a closed position, relaxes and allows chyme to flow into the colon. This *gas-*

troileal reflex regulates the passage of chyme from the small intestine to the large intestine. Both segmentation and peristalsis require intact intrinsic (that is, within the intestinal wall) neural structures. For segmentation to occur, the duodenal pacemaker must transmit impulses. For peristalsis to occur, the pressure receptors and the nerve plexus in the intestinal wall must be intact in order to stimulate the myenteric reflex. Generally, sympathetic stimulation decreases intestinal motility whereas parasympathetic input increases activity. CCK promotes enhanced motility, but glucagon and secretin slow intestinal action.[5,6]

Absorption

Digestion and absorption occur primarily in the small intestine. Proteins, fats, and carbohydrates are broken down into absorbable parts (digestion), and products of digestion, vitamins, minerals and water cross the mucosa and enter the blood (absorption) (Figure 49-14). Because of the small bowel's large absorbing surface, almost 50% of the bowel may be removed without inducing clinical malabsorption.[8,12]

Carbohydrates. In the mouth, *salivary α-amylase* begins to digest carbohydrates. Some 50% of starches, mostly in the form of polysaccharides, are hydrolyzed to disaccharides. Hydrolization continues to a lesser degree as the food bolus moves down the esophagus. In the stomach, no significant starch digestion occurs, since the acid environment inactivates amylase. (The optimal pH for starch digestion is 6.7.)

Once in the small intestine, *pancreatic α-amylase* continues the process. The largest proportion of disaccharide formed is maltose. The microvilli of the

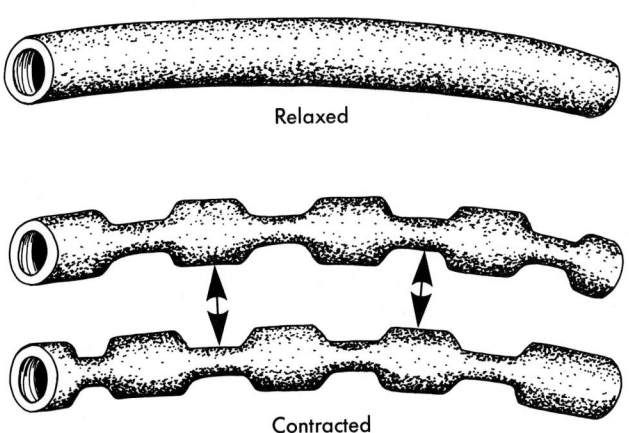

Figure 49-13 Segmentation contractions of the small intestine.

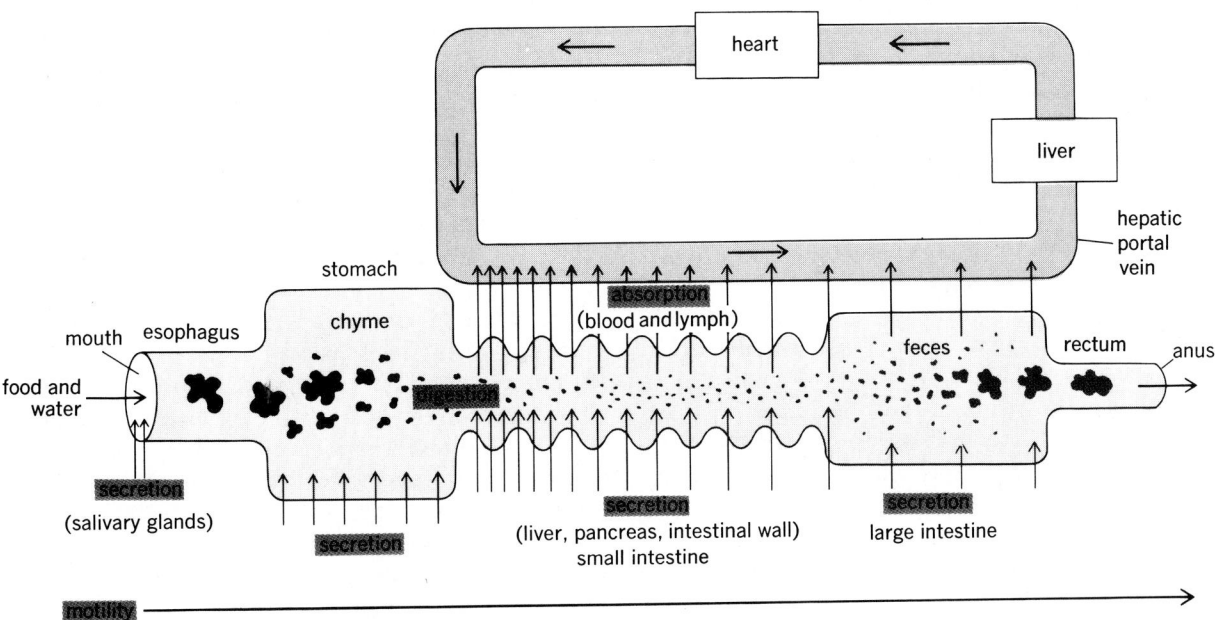

Figure 49-14 Summary of GI activity.

From Vander, A. J., Sherman, J. H., & Luciano, D. (1989). *Human physiology.* New York: McGraw-Hill.

small intestine contain special *sugar-splitting enzymes*—lactase, maltase, sucrase, and so on—which split the specific disaccharides into monosaccharides, or simple sugars. Lactose intolerance is a disease resulting from absence of the enzyme lactase. Consequently, patients with this disorder are unable to absorb lactose, and they experience diarrhea and abdominal disorders unless supplements are given.[2,6,8,12]

Once formed, the simple sugars—glucose, galactose, and fructose—are absorbed across the intestinal membrane by either active transport or by passive diffusion easily because of their smaller size. Most sugars are absorbed before reaching the terminal portion of the ileum. Both glucose and galactose require active transport across the intestinal membrane into the blood. Their absorption is, therefore, coupled to Na^+ transport and is directly proportional to the Na^+ concentration in the intestinal lumen. Fructose, however, passively diffuses through the membrane into the blood.

Once in the venous blood, the absorbed sugars are transported to the liver. In the specialized hepatic capillaries, the hepatocytes utilize the sugars either for immediate energy, for storage as glycogen, or as metabolic intermediates in other hepatic biochemical pathways.

Proteins. A daily protein intake of 45 to 55 g, under normal healthy conditions, is considered adequate for the average adult. This quantity provides the needed essential amino acids and meets the demands of ordinary protein synthesis and degradation. The diet of most adults in the United States averages about 200 g of protein per day.

Unlike the carbohydrate group, protein is not altered until it reaches the stomach. There the acid juices hydrolyze certain amino acid bonds, and gastric pepsin, activated by the acid, cleaves internal peptide bonds forming amino acid fragments (polypeptides).

In the duodenum, pepsin is inactivated because of the increased alkalinity. However, the pancreatic proteolytic enzymes trypsin and chymotrypsin (optimal pH 7.8) continue to cleave internal bonds. Carboxypeptidase, also from the pancreas, initiates removal of terminal amino acids. The protein pool is composed of peptide fragments and rare free amino acids.

Like the disaccharides of carbohydrate digestion, the polypeptide fragments are too large to be absorbed across the mucosal surface. Again, the intestinal microvilli supply specialized enzymes—dipeptidases, aminopeptidases, and so on—which split polypeptides into free amino acid components. Simple amino acids, like simple sugars, can be absorbed.

Amino acid absorption is highly specific, with unique mechanisms for neutral, acidic, and basic amino acids. The molecular structure of the compound determines, in part, whether active transport and Na^+ coupling or passive diffusion is needed for absorption. Most amino acid absorption occurs in the duodenum and the jejunum.

Like the products of starch metabolism, protein building blocks are returned to the liver. Once there, the amino acids are degraded by the liver into their two organic parts, carbon and nitrogen (ammonia). Free ammonia is toxic to the human body in abnormal amounts. Therefore, the liver uses the free ammonia to form the waste product urea. This urea then travels to the kidney and is excreted in the urine, thus disposing of a toxic product. If the liver has been significantly damaged and, therefore, cannot synthesize urea, free ammonia accumulates and reaches toxic levels. The liver's inability to handle a nitrogen (ammonia) load is, in part, the basis for *hepatic encephalopathy*, a condition associated with severe liver disease.

The series of metabolic events described above is the rationale for the protein-restricted diet in patients with hepatic encephalopathy. Likewise, gastrointestinal bleeding, which leads blood (composed of protein and, therefore, amino acids) to accumulate in the gut lumen, also predisposes some patients with liver disease to hepatic encephalopathy.

Fats. The fat content of the daily adult diet varies greatly. The biochemical form most commonly ingested is the triglyceride, but cholesterol and the complex phospholipids also add significantly to the daily lipid intake. Normally, stool contains only 5% of the daily dietary fat intake. Even this small proportion comes from bacterial metabolism rather than from dietary fats alone.

The overall digestion and absorption of lipids is more complex than the mechanisms involved in carbohydrate and protein metabolism. This is due to the size and solubility characteristics of the lipids.

No fat digestion occurs before the fat reaches the duodenum. Fat arrives at the duodenum mainly as triglycerides, cholesterol, and phospholipids. The enzyme *pancreatic lipase* carries out the first step of fat digestion.

Triglycerides are fat soluble. Enzymatic lipase is water soluble. Therefore, in an aqueous solution such as intestinal fluid, triglycerides lump together, forming large droplets. Because of their water insolubility, they will not mix with the water milieu. Lipase, being water soluble, can mix with the water. Bile salts are required to bring water-soluble lipase in contact with fat-soluble triglycerides.

Bile salts, coming from the liver but primarily from the gallbladder, enter the duodenum when a fatty stimulus is present. These salts contain both a water-soluble and a fat-soluble portion. As a result, they can bring together the two otherwise opposing elements.

The large lipid droplets, having been stabilized by the bile salts, now come in contact with lipase. The action of this enzyme, together with normal intestinal motility, causes mixing and breaking apart of the large fat droplets. This process, called *emulsification*, provides increased numbers of small fat particles and, thereby, increases the overall surface area on which lipase can act. Lipase is responsible for degrading triglycerides (TG) primarily to monoglycerides (MG) and free fatty acids (FFA).

Step 1: Emulsification.

$$\text{Triglycerides as large fat droplets} \xrightarrow[\text{lipase}]{\text{bile salts}}$$

$$\text{smaller droplets} \xrightarrow[\text{lipase}]{\text{bile salts}} \text{FFA} + \text{monoglycerides}$$

The FFA and monoglycerides thus formed combine with varying proportions of cholesterol and phospholipid and are again acted upon by bile salts. The new particle, now stabilized and water soluble, is called a *micelle*. It is from the micellar form that FFA and monoglycerides are absorbed across the intestinal mucosa.

Step 2: Micelle Formation.

FFA + MG + cholesterol

$$+ \text{ phospholipid} \xrightarrow{\text{bile salts}} \text{micelle}$$

When the micelle is close to the mucosal surface, passive absorption of the FFA occurs. Depending on the length of the FFA, absorption takes place directly into the blood (for FFA less than 10 to 12 carbons long), or, as is more often the case, the FFA (longer than 12 carbons) is resynthesized to a triglyceride within the intestinal cell (Figure 49-15).

Once resynthesized, the triglyceride is coated with cholesterol and phospholipid. This new complex, called a *chylomicron*, is then picked up by a lacteal (lymph vessel) of the intestinal villus and carried to sites of fat storage (adipose tissue) throughout the body. Thus, most free fatty acids travel as triglycerides in chylomicrons via the lymph, not via the blood.

Note that bile salts remain behind within the intestinal lumen when the free fatty acid diffuses into the intestinal cell. Reabsorption of these salts takes place in the terminal ileum. They are reabsorbed directly into the blood and are then recycled in the enterohepatic circulation. The greater part of the triglyceride absorption via lacteals takes place in the jejunum, not in the terminal ileum.

Water, Electrolytes, Vitamins, and Minerals. The water balance of the GI tract is summarized in Table 49-7. Ingested fluid accounts for 2,000 ml, while 8,000 ml is from the secretions of the GI tract and accessory glands. Reabsorption occurs in the jejunum,

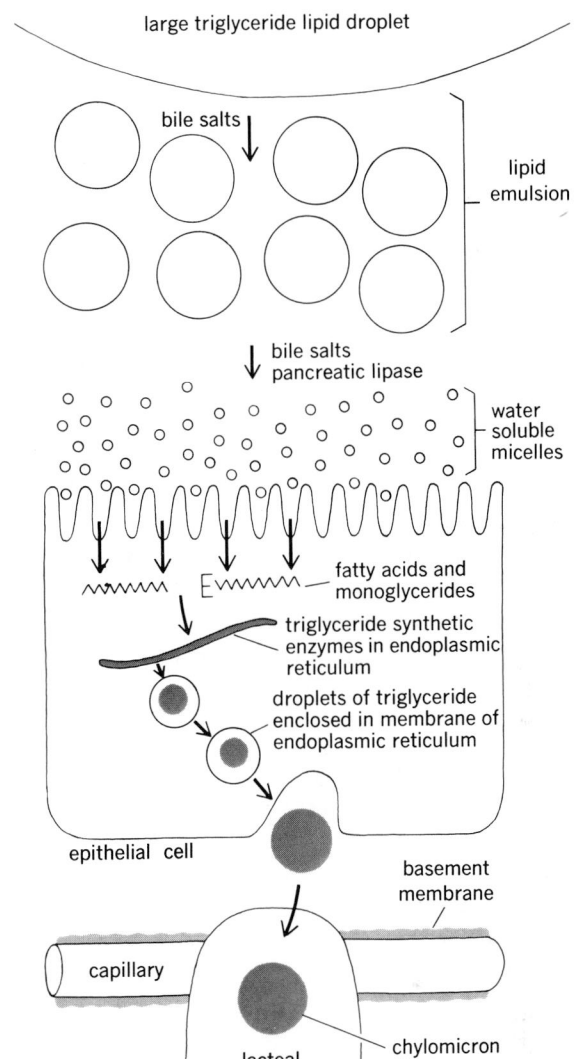

Figure 49-15 Summary of fat absorption across the walls of the small intestine.

From Vander, A. J., Sherman, J. H., & Luciano, D. (1989). *Human physiology.* New York: McGraw-Hill.

TABLE 49-7 **Water Absorption in the Small and Large Intestines**

Ingested	2,000		
GI Secretions			
Salivary	1,500	Reabsorbed	
Stomach	2,500	Jejunum	5,500
Bile	500	Ileum	2,000
Pancreas	1,500	Large intestine	1,300
Intestine	1,000	Total	8,800
Total	7,000	Balance in stool	200
	9,000		9,000

ileum, and colon (discussed in more detail later in the section). The usual volume lost in the stool is 100 to 200 ml per day.[6,12]

From the stomach to the large intestine, the mucosal surface is adapted for water reabsorption. Although the stomach contributes relatively little to volume control, the establishment of isotonicity with the plasma begins there. The duodenum, in contrast to the stomach, is a site of great fluid shifts. All contents leaving the duodenum are isotonic as they pass on to the jejunum. That implies absorption of osmotically active particles (sugars, amino acids) and/or secretion of buffering fluids to dilute intestinal contents.

Electrolyte shifts within the GI tract are important to overall function. Given the role of Na^+ ion in carbohydrate and protein metabolism, significant electrolyte imbalances may pose serious limitations on the normal absorptive functions of the bowel.[5,8] Normally, Na^+ is actively reabsorbed in the small intestine. Absorption is facilitated by aldosterone. Water passively follows. Active transport of Na^+ in the small intestine is important to the absorption of glucose and select amino acids. Chloride is absorbed in the ileum while HCO_3^- is secreted into the lumen in a one-to-one exchange. This accounts for the alkalinity of intestinal contents. Potassium is absorbed as well as secreted by colonic mucosa.

Between 30% and 80% of ingested calcium is absorbed. This occurs primarily in the upper small intestine by active transport and passive diffusion. Absorption of calcium is adjusted to body needs. Iron is important to the balance of hemoglobin synthesis and degradation. Iron is normally easily absorbed in the upper small intestine. It does, however, require active transport. Other minerals are absorbed by the GI tract, but it is beyond the scope of this chapter to further detail these processes.

Vitamins, with the exception of B_{12}, are absorbed in the upper part of the small bowel. The B_{12}–intrinsic factor complex is absorbed in the terminal ileum. Water-soluble vitamins do not require any special enzymes or mechanisms for absorption. The absorption of fat-soluble vitamins A, D, E, and K requires the presence of bile salts and the enzymes involved in routine fat absorption. If fat malabsorption occurs, the fat-soluble vitamins are not absorbed.

LARGE INTESTINE

Just as the mouth gives entrance to the gastrointestinal tract, the large intestine provides an exit. Some 150 cm long, it carries intestinal contents to the end of the gastrointestinal tract. Its major portion, the colon, together with its terminal portions, the rectum and anus, secrete mucus and absorb water and electrolytes. The large intestine contains natural bowel flora that are important to absorption and synthesis of vitamins and to particular metabolic pathways.

The function of the large intestine culminates in the production of stool. Normally, stool is one-quarter solid and three-quarters liquid. Its brown color is attributed to the products of hemoglobin degradation. Its characteristic odor results from certain bacterial metabolites, especially the amine compounds. The bulk of the stool is composed of cellulose and indigestible fibers, bacteria, degenerated cellular debris, fat, and inorganic material.

Anatomy

The large intestine begins just distal to the ileocecal valve. The cecum is a blind pouch which begins the colon. The vermiform appendix is a small outpouching off the cecum. The major part of the large intestine, the colon, is divided anatomically into four divisions: ascending, transverse, descending, and sigmoid, or S-shaped. Below the sigmoid colon are the rectum and the anus (Figure 49-16).[6,9]

The muscular ileocecal valve separates the small and large bowel. It projects into the cecum so that increases in colonic pressure close it, preventing reflux of colonic contents into the ileum. Each time a peristaltic wave reaches it, it opens briefly allowing ileal chyme to squirt into the cecum. At the distal end of the large bowel are two additional sphincters, the internal and the external anal sphincters, which regulate defecation.

The colon is a tube of wider diameter than the

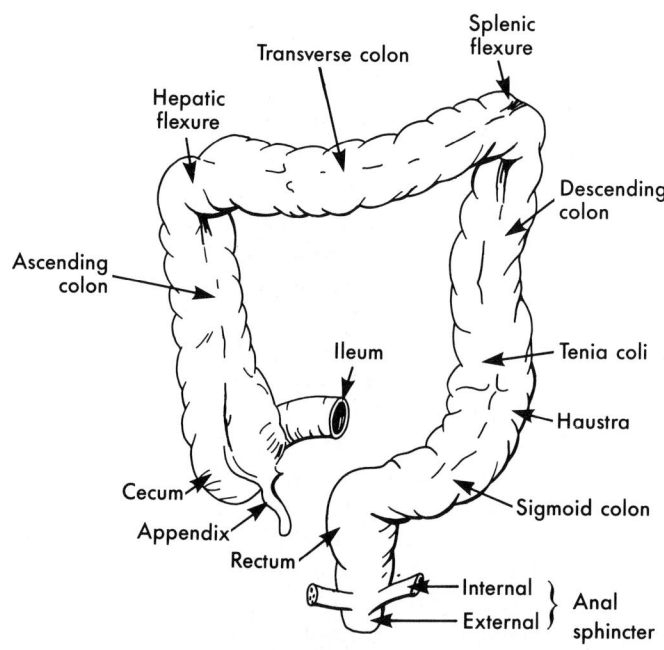

Figure 49-16 Anatomy of the colon.

small intestine. Inspection of the colon reveals an outer longitudinal muscle layer separated into three fiber tracts. The three muscular bundles eventually fan out at the rectum and form a complete muscle coat. These longitudinal bands, called *teniae coli*, are shorter than the colon itself. This difference in length, coupled with the contractions of the inner muscle layer, causes outpouchings of the colonic wall called *haustra*. The haustra and the teniae give the colon its unique anatomical appearance (see Figure 49-16).

The *internal anal sphincter* is a continuation of the inner muscle layer. It is under involuntary control. The *external sphincter* is a separate skeletal muscle. Unlike the internal sphincter, it is not an extension of the smooth muscle in the colonic wall. It extends the entire length of the anus and is under voluntary control.

The colonic blood supply originates from the superior and inferior mesenteric arteries. The venous system parallels the arterial system and is noteworthy because of the plexus of veins formed around the anus. This plexus, like the one at the base of the esophagus, may become tortuous and dilated. This condition, known as hemorrhoids, is common but is of special concern in patients with portal hypertension. Just as esophageal varices are prone to rupture when blood is shunted away from the liver, so too are the varices of the rectal plexus. The incidence of life-threatening hemorrhage from rectal varices is significantly lower than that from esophageal varices, however.[8]

The nervous innervation of the colon, like that of the other gastrointestinal organs, contains both parasympathetic and sympathetic fibers. Parasympathetic input has variable consequences, and its influences are not well understood. Sympathetic fibers apparently have more effect on colonic vasculature than on colonic muscle tone.

Histology

The microscopic anatomy of the large intestine is less detailed than that of the small intestine. There are relatively fewer foldings of the mucosa, and there are no villi or microvilli in the colon.

Columnar cells line the colonic mucosa, a more rugged stratified squamous epithelium covers the surface near the anus. Mucus-producing glands are found throughout the large intestine. Their viscous secretions are important lubricants for passage of fecal material.

Function

Motility

Unlike the small intestine, the large intestine does not move its contents along rapidly. Instead, its mo-

tions permit mixing and molding of stool followed by slow exit from the anus. Because the large intestine has a relatively small absorptive surface area, transit along its course is slowed to permit absorption of water and electrolytes.[4,7]

Chyme reaching the colon is in liquid form. Water must be absorbed in sufficient amounts to produce solid stools. It should be remembered that some 9 L of fluid enters the gastrointestinal tract each day. Of that total volume, 1 L reaches the colon. Since only 150 ml of fluid is lost in the stools each day, the colon must absorb between 800 and 900 ml of liquid daily.

The motion accountable for mixing and molding is segmentation. Like segmentation in the small intestine, colonic segmentation corresponds to contraction of the inner muscle layer and changes in the haustral configurations. Segmentation occurs concurrently in various parts of the bowel in a rather uncoordinated pattern. Again, this lack of coordination slows colonic motility and facilitates absorption.

Propulsive motions of the large intestine consist of weak peristaltic contractions occurring along its length. However, this relaxation and contraction of relatively short segments of bowel provides only minimal forward motion. Weak antiperistaltic waves may also be seen.

In each 24-hour period, the short, continual peristaltic waves are augmented by three or four stronger, more extensive peristaltic contractions. These peristaltic rushes are known as *mass movements* or *mass action* contractions. These contractions move material down the colon and into the rectum. Rectal distention stimulates the defecation reflex.

Defecation is initiated by increased tension in the rectal wall. If this pressor stimulus is not inhibited, the normal act of defecation occurs. The underlying mechanism of defecation involves contraction of the distal colon and rectum, shortening the rectum and increasing rectal pressure. As pressure mounts within the rectum, the involuntary internal anal sphincter and the voluntary external anal sphincter relax and stool is able to pass through.

If the urge to defecate is ignored, the walls of the rectum eventually relax and intraluminal pressure decreases. The desire to defecate subsides. When another mass movement delivers additional stool to the rectum, pressure again increases and the urge to defecate returns.

Humans are able to assist the basic mechanisms involved in evacuation by initiating the *Valsalva maneuver*. Deep inspiration, descent of the diaphragm, and closure of the glottis increase both intraabdominal and intrathoracic pressure. This greater pressure is transmitted to the intestine and aids in evacuation.

Although straining facilitates defecation, it has potentially dangerous consequences for cardiopulmonary function. As intrathoracic pressure increases, there is an initial abrupt rise in arterial blood pressure and peripheral venous pressure, leading to a marked decrease in cardiac output because of poor venous return to the heart. The decreased output causes a marked reduction in arterial blood pressure. Consequently, many patients, but especially those with cerebral vascular disease or coronary artery disease, are at greater risk for life-threatening events if allowed to strain during defecation.[4,6,8]

Diarrhea is abnormal evacuation from the colon, usually excessive in frequency and more liquid than solid. Many diseases and medications may induce diarrhea. Many theories on the underlying mechanisms have been offered. Some focus on colonic irritability and increased motility; others support defects of water and nutrient reabsorption. Excessive gut secretions mediated by cyclic adenosine 5-monophosphate (cAMP) have also been implicated. Diarrhea from whatever cause is clinically important because it may lead to dehydration, hypovolemia, hyponatremia, and hypokalemia. Acid–base imbalance may also occur.[4,8]

At the other end of the spectrum, *constipation,* or abnormally infrequent bowel movements, does not instigate the wide range of metabolic instability that is produced by diarrhea. Its major clinical significance is as a presenting symptom of possible underlying bowel disease such as carcinoma of the large intestine.

Secretion and Absorption

Unlike the stomach and small intestine, the large intestine does not produce an abundance of diversified secretions. The major secretory product in the large bowel is mucus. The goblet cells along the mucosal surface secrete a viscous fluid that mixes with the forming stool and assists its mechanical passage toward the anus.

The colon also secretes K^+ and HCO_3^- into the intestinal lumen. Potassium is secreted into a favorable electrochemical gradient, and active transport is not required. Serious shifts in K^+ and HCO_3^- are associated with altered colonic motility. Adequate K^+ replacement and careful management of pH changes are especially important in patients with severe diarrhea.

The major absorptive processes occurring in the large intestine are active Na^+ reabsorption accompanied by passive flow of water and active Cl^- absorption coupled to HCO_3^- secretion. Nearly 900 ml of fluid must be reabsorbed daily if body fluid balance is to be maintained. The highly absorptive capability of the large intestine provides a route for administration of many compounds including anesthetics, sed-

atives, corticosteroids, and tranquilizers. Anything that alters the normal motility of the large intestine or it mucosal surface threatens to alter its sodium–water regulation. Likewise, if chyme reaches the colon poorly processed because of abnormalities of the upper tract, the colon may be unable to handle the increased load. Thus, even a normal large intestine, if associated with a diseased small bowel or stomach or the effects of GI surgery, may not be able to complete the reabsorption process and adequately maintain body fluid balance.

Flora

The large intestine is a major storehouse for many types of bacteria. Its sluggish motility makes it a lush breeding ground for microorganisms. Enteral (intestinal) bacteria, especially *Escherichia coli* and *Enterobacter aerogenes,* are found in abundance. Other gram-negative rods, anaerobic species, and certain gas-producing organisms are present as well. When outside the intestinal tract, these can produce serious diseases (e.g., gas gangrene).

Certain of the large intestinal florae are responsible for vitamin production. Vitamin K, essential to hepatic synthesis of blood clotting factors II, VII, IX, and X, is produced by certain flora of the large bowel. In addition, several B vitamins and folic acid are derived from bacterial metabolism. Intestinal bacteria may also be involved in cholesterol metabolism.

Bacterial organisms are partially responsible for gas found in the intestine. Although 60% to 70% of flatus passed comes from swallowed air, the remaining portion is contributed by bacterial fermentation. At any given time, the normal large intestine contains as much as 100 cm^3 of gas.

As mentioned earlier, the large intestine produces and absorbs ammonia. When the liver is diseased, ammonia is not filtered from the blood and can cause neurological symptoms known as hepatic encephalopathy.[8,16]

LIVER

The liver, the largest gland in the human body, performs over 400 functions. To even begin to understand hepatic structure and function, one must focus on the detailed microscopic anatomy, the unique vascular circuits, and the continuous interconnecting channels found throughout the hepatic parenchyma. Certain salient features of the liver are presented here as they relate to unique hepatic functions. The box on p. 1125 summarizes the principal functions of the liver.[2,6,17]

In normal adults, the liver represents one fiftieth of total body weight. It has five interrelated yet anatomically definable functional components:
1. The parenchymal liver cells, or *hepatocytes,* per-

Major Functions of the Liver

VASCULAR FUNCTIONS
Blood storage
Blood filtration

SECRETORY FUNCTIONS
Formation of bile
Secretion of bilirubin
Conjugation of bilirubin
Formation of urea

METABOLIC FUNCTIONS
Carbohydrate metabolism
Fat metabolism
Protein metabolism
Synthesis of blood clotting components (factors II, VI, VII, VIII, IX, X)
Removal of activated clotting factors
Detoxification of drugs, hormones, and other substances
Reduction and conjugation of adrenocortical and gonadal steroid hormones
Synthesis of 25-hydroxycholecalciferol

STORAGE FUNCTIONS
Blood
Glucose
Vitamins (A, B_{12}, D, E, K)
Fat
Minerals (iron, magnesium)

---

form the major synthetic and storage functions of the organ.

2. A well-developed and extensive *reticuloendothelial system* throughout the liver provides an effective body defense against foreign intrusion. In fact, the defense system of the liver constitutes some 60% of the total body reticuloendothelial system.

3. The *hepatobiliary system* synthesizes and transports bile salts and pigments to the gallbladder as discussed in the section on fat digestion and absorption. The smallest branches of the biliary tree are the bile canaliculi. These extracellular areas are located between two or more adjacent hepatocytes. All biliary components formed within the liver or derived from the plasma must enter at the level of the bile canaliculi.

4. A vast *circulatory system* pervades the liver. One of the few organs with a dual blood supply, the liver must perfuse itself and must also process the metabolic end products of almost an entire GI system as well as the spleen.

5. The *connective tissue reticulum* of the liver provides the structural support for all the other components. A healthy hepatic reticulum promotes an environment for hepatocyte regeneration in cases of disease and injury. If the connective tissue

stroma is absent or damaged, the normal liver architecture cannot be sustained and hepatic function is impaired.

The biliary system has been discussed. Four areas of hepatic function remain for discussion: the vascular system, the hepatocytes, the reticuloendothelial system, and the connective tissue stroma. Before detailing the individual hepatic components, the gross and microscopic anatomy of the liver need to be considered.

Anatomy

The liver is located in the right upper quadrant of the abdomen. The entire organ is encapsulated by a thin connective tissue covering, the capsula fibrosa, called the Glisson's capsule.

The liver is attached to the diaphragm and moves with it. The porta hepatis is the point at which the hepatic artery, the portal vein, and the common bile duct emerge.

Histology

The basic functional unit of the liver is the lobule. It is a hexagonal prism of liver tissue, arranged in a series and demarcated by connective tissue. Blood flows past hepatic cells via *sinusoids*. These sinusoids form a rich intralobular vascular network that converges on the central vein (Figure 49-17).

Hepatocytes radiate from the central vein to the periphery. Blood from portal arterioles and venules empties into the sinusoid. The anatomical relation of the endothelium of the sinusoids facilitates close contact with each liver cell (Figure 49-18). There is one layer of hepatocytes between sinusoids, increasing the surface area. Lining the walls of the sinusoids are

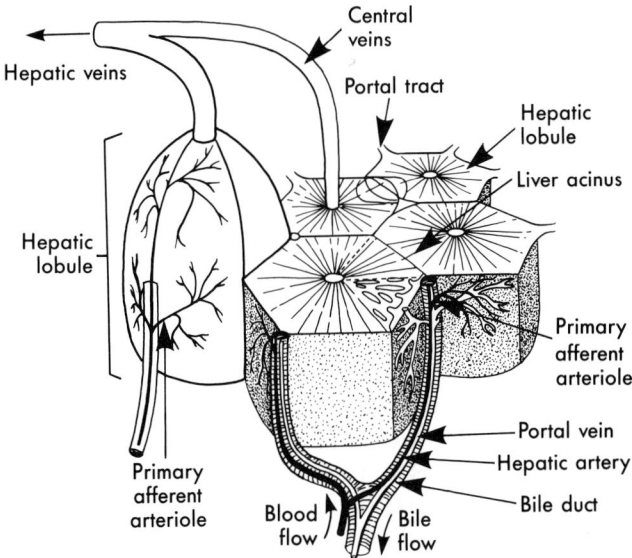

Figure 49-17   The hepatic lobule.

TABLE 50-3 Abdominal Findings and Related Disorders

Disorders	Inspection/Pain Characteristics	Percussion	Palpation	Auscultation
Peptic ulcer disease	Epigastric pain	Normal tympanic	May have abdominal tenderness	Hyperactive bowel sounds
Perforated ulcer	Sudden, severe, persistent pain; referred pain common. *Duodenal:* pain in RUQ		Boardlike	Absent bowel sounds within hours
Small-bowel obstruction	Cramping abdominal pain (periumbilical); abdominal distention			Bowel sounds increased then decreased
Large-bowel obstruction	Slow-onset, crampy abdominal pain; abdominal distention			Bowel sounds absent or hypoactive
Bowel infarction	Severe abdominal pain; abdominal distention	Hyperresonant, especially with paralytic ileus	General tenderness, guarding, rigidity	Bowel sounds absent or hypoactive
Peritonitis	Body posture and facial expression evidencing pain		Rebound tenderness; boardlike; rigid abdomen; guarding against palpation	
Ileus	Abdominal distention		Generalized tenderness, possibly localizing	Bowel sounds diminished or absent; when present may be high-pitched
Pancreatitis	Unrelenting abdominal pain in epigastrium and periumbilical regions; pain often radiating to chest and back; may have jaundice and abdominal distention; Grey Turner's sign and/or Cullen's sign with hemorrhagic pancreatitis	Dull over pancreas	May have poorly defined abdominal mass; rebound tenderness	Bowel sounds diminished or absent
Hepatic failure	Ascites	Enlarged liver; shifting dullness	Splenomegaly; hepatomegaly	Bowel sounds may be diminished
Gastric cancer	General abdominal pain	May have dullness in epigastrium	Hepatomegaly; splenomegaly; abdominal tenderness	Hyperactive or hypoactive bowel sounds
Cancer of the colon		Dullness at tumor site; liver may be enlarged	Palpable mass; abdominal tenderness	Hyperactive bowel sounds
Pancreatic cancer	Abdominal pain		Hepatomegaly; splenomegaly; distended gallbladder; may have palpable mass over epigastric area	Bowel sounds diminished or absent

Regional system

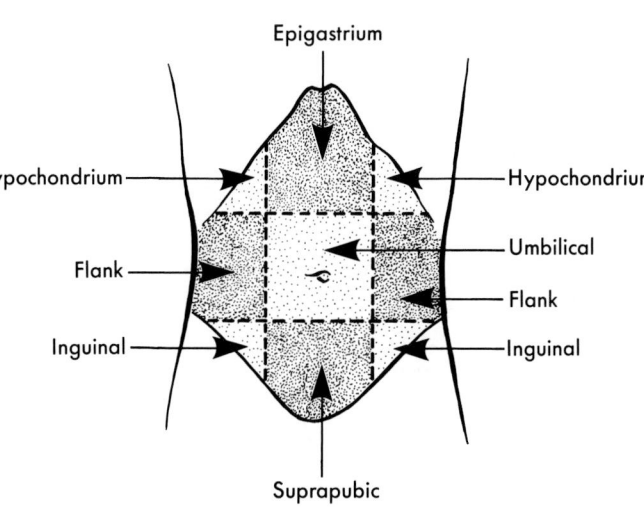

Four-quadrant system

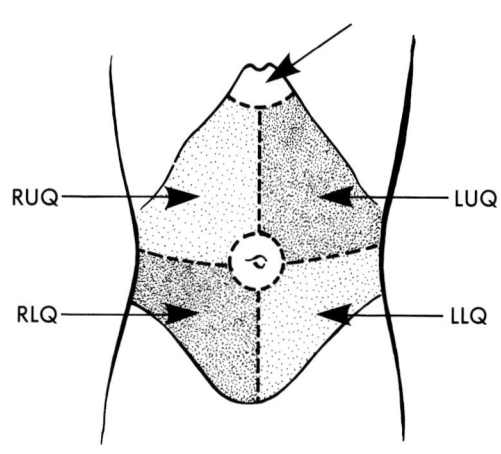

Figure 50-2 Anatomical mapping of the abdomen. The nine-region system: (1) Epigastric—pyloric end of stomach, duodenum, pancreas, portion of liver; (2) Umbilical—lower part of duodenum, omentum, mesentery, aorta, jejunum, and ileum; (3) Suprapubic (Hypogastric)—ileum, bladder, pregnant uterus; (4) Right Hypochondriac—gallbladder, right lobe of liver, portion of duodenum, hepatic flexure of colon, part of right kidney, right adrenal gland; (5) Left Hypochondriac—stomach, spleen, tail of pancreas, splenic flexure of colon, left adrenal gland, upper pole of left kidney; (6) Right Lumbar—ascending colon, lower half of right kidney, portion of duodenum, and jejunum; (7) Left Lumbar—descending colon, lower half of left kidney, portion of jejunum, and ileum; (8) Right Inguinal—cecum, appendix, lower end of ileum, right ovary or spermatic cord; and (9) Left Inguinal—sigmoid colon, left ureter, left ovary or spermatic cord.

Figure 50-3 Anatomical mapping of the abdomen. The four-quadrant system: RUQ (right upper quadrant)—liver and gallbladder, duodenum, pylorus, head of pancreas, portion of right kidney, right adrenal, hepatic flexure of colon, portions of ascending and transverse colon; LUQ (left upper quadrant)—left lobe of liver, spleen, stomach, body of pancreas, portion of left kidney, left adrenal, splenic flexure of colon, portions of transverse and descending colon; RLQ (right lower quadrant)—lower pole of right kidney, cecum and appendix, portion of ascending colon, bladder (if distended), ovary or right spermatic cord, uterus (if enlarged), right ureter; and LLQ (left lower quadrant)—lower pole of left kidney, sigmoid colon, portion of descending colon, bladder (if distended), ovary or left spermatic cord, uterus (if enlarged), right ureter.

TABLE 50-4 **Inspection Signs Associated with GI Disorder**

Name	Characteristics	Indication
Cullen's sign	Cyanotic or ecchymotic area around umbilicus	Free blood in peritoneal cavity
Grey Turner's sign	Cyanotic or ecchymotic area in flanks	Free blood in peritoneal cavity
Caput medusae	Circular pattern of distended veins around umbilicus	Portal hypertension
Sr. Mary Joseph's nodule	Metastatic lesion of navel	Cancer originating in abdomen, especially the stomach

bulence of partially obstructed arterial blood flow. Systolic bruits in the epigastric area are normal. Friction rubs are rare, but when present, they sound like rubbing sandpaper and are indicative of peritoneal irritation. Venous hums are also rare, but when heard, they present as a continuous humming sound and indicate increased collateral circulation between the portal and systemic venous systems.[3,7] Figure 50-4 indicates sources of diagnostic abdominal sounds that may be heard during auscultation of the abdomen and its blood supply.[8,9]

Percussion

Percussion is a useful technique for general orientation to the abdomen for identification of gas, air, and fluid in the abdominal cavity and/or organs, for identifying masses, and for measurement of the liver and spleen. This part of the examination begins with a general orientation to the abdomen by lightly per-

**Sources of diagnostic abdominal sounds
and blood supply**

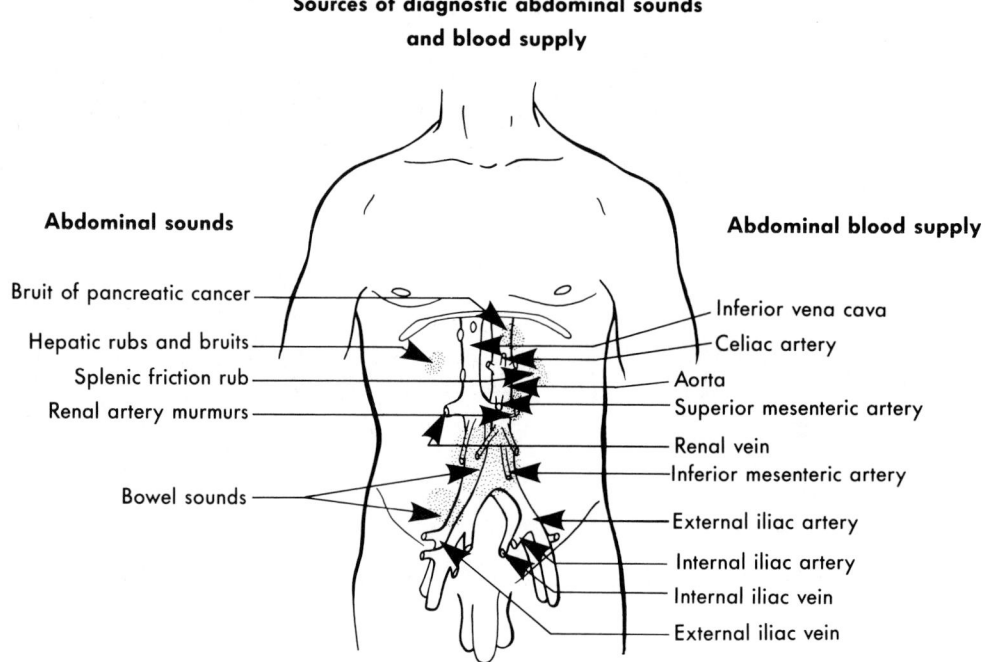

Abdominal sounds

Bruit of pancreatic cancer

Hepatic rubs and bruits

Splenic friction rub

Renal artery murmurs

Bowel sounds

Abdominal blood supply

Inferior vena cava

Celiac artery

Aorta

Superior mesenteric artery

Renal vein

Inferior mesenteric artery

External iliac artery

Internal iliac artery

Internal iliac vein

External iliac vein

Figure 50-4   Sources of abdominal sound and blood supply.

cussing all quadrants and determining the areas of tympany and dullness. Tympany is usually found over the stomach, gut, and any other air-filled viscera. Percussion in the left lower anterior rib cage area will reveal the gastric air bubble. Dullness is heard over the liver, spleen, a full bladder, or a pregnant uterus. Dullness is also heard over fluid, and therefore the technique of percussion is quite useful in determining the amount of free fluid present in the abdominal cavity. Percussion for shifting dullness is the technique used for detecting free fluid. For this purpose, with the patient initially supine, the examiner percusses from midline to first one side then the other. The point where dullness begins is marked on each side. The patient then is rolled to one side, then the other, and percussion is used in the same manner, with the line of dullness marked. The area between the two lines indicates the amount of free fluid (Figure 50-5). Patients with ascites or abdominal distention should also have abdominal girth measured.

Liver height, or vertical span, is used to estimate liver size and is determined through percussion as follows. The abdomen is percussed upward along the right midclavicular line from a point just below the umbilicus to determine the lower border of liver dullness, then downward on the midclavicular line from lung resonance to liver dullness. This identifies the upper border of the liver. The normal adult liver size is 6 to 12 cm (Figure 50-6). The span of liver dullness is increased with liver enlargement and decreased with liver atrophy. A cirrhotic liver seems square upon

percussion. There are, however, normal livers that extend as low as the right lower quadrant.[10]

Often, the spleen cannot be identified by percussion, but it is located near the 10th rib just posterior to the midaxillary line (see Figure 50-2). If the spleen is enlarged, it may be detected by percussing the lowest interspace in the left anterior axillary line. The normal sound in this area is tympanic. The examiner should have the patient take a deep breath before percussing. If the spleen is of normal size, the percussion sound will remain tympanic. If the spleen is enlarged, a dull note will be elicited on inspiration. This is termed a *positive percussion sign*.

Palpation

Light and deep palpation are most useful in detecting abdominal pathological conditions, identifying areas of muscular resistance or tenderness, and detecting abdominal masses and organ hypertrophy. Normal abdominal structures can be detected by palpation and should not be confused with disease (Table 50-5).

Before attempting deep palpation, the examiner should employ light palpation, using light, firm pressure, and moving smoothly to feel all quadrants. The technique of light palpation involves placing the entire palm and extended closed fingers of the hand on the surface of the abdomen and pressing gently with the fingertips to a depth of 1 cm (Figure 50-7). Areas of tenderness are elicited by this technique. Pain produced by light palpation suggests peritoneal inflam-

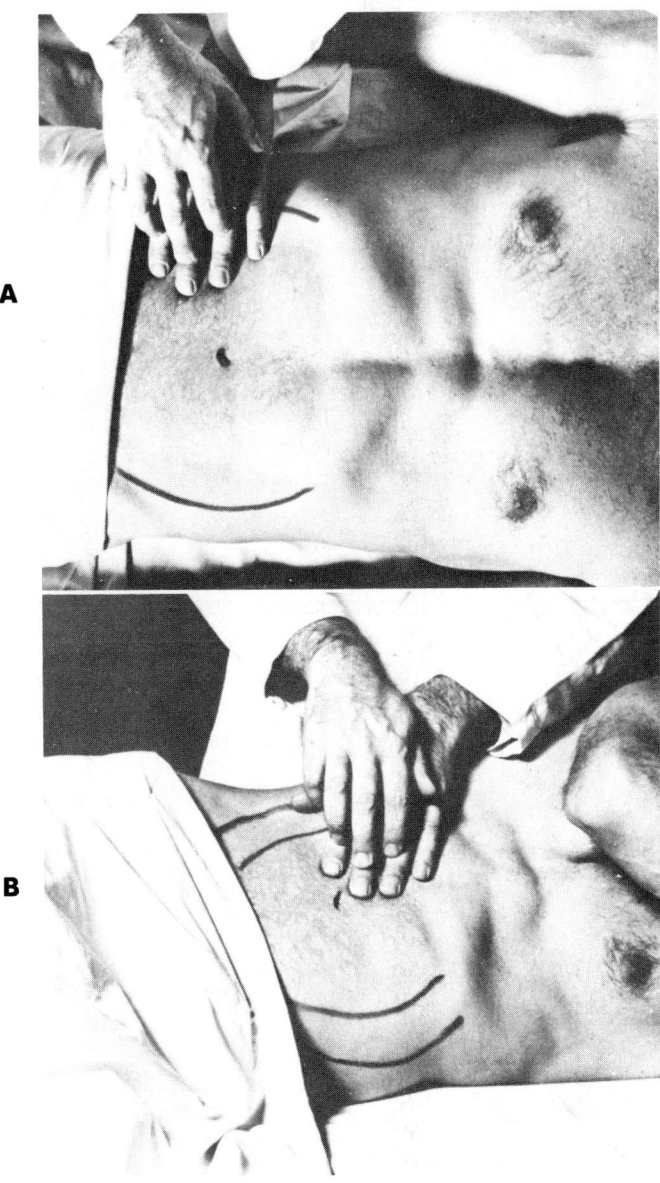

Figure 50-5 Technique for percussing shifting dullness. *A,* Patient on his back. *B,* Patient on his side.

From (1981). *GI series: Physical examination of the abdomen.* Richmond: A. H. Robins Co.

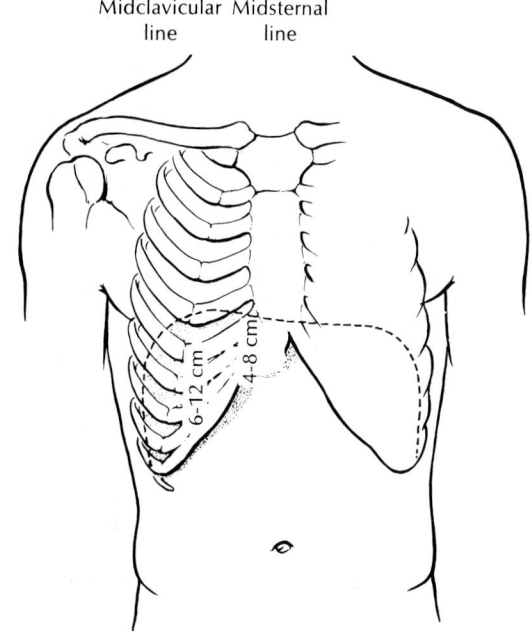

Figure 50-6 Normal liver span.

From Malasanos, L., Barkauskas, V., & Stoltenberg-Allen, K. (1990). *Health assessment* (4th ed.). Mosby–Year Book.

TABLE 50-5   Normal Findings on Abdominal Palpation

Area	Organ
LLQ	Sigmoid colon (firm, narrow tube); pulsation of left iliac artery
RLQ	Cecum
	Ascending colon
	Transverse and descending colon (firm, wider tube)
	Pulsation of right iliac artery
Below costal margin	Liver
RUQ	Lower pole of right kidney

mation and should be mapped accurately. Asking the patient to cough to determine where pain was produced also helps in localizing it. *Rebound tenderness* also suggests peritoneal inflammation and is elicited by pressing the fingers firmly into the abdomen and then quickly withdrawing them. Pain induced or exacerbated by the quick withdrawal is rebound tenderness (Figure 50-8).[4,5,11,12]

Deep palpation is used to determine the size of the liver, spleen, and kidneys, and to discover the presence of any abnormal intraabdominal masses. It should be performed carefully, especially if abdominal disease

or injury is present or suspected. Deep palpation is performed by pressing the entire palmar surface of the hand with approximated fingers into the abdomen to a depth of 4 to 5 cm. This may be done with only one hand or with the fingertips of the other hand pressing on the distal joint of the examining hand for increased tactile awareness of the examining fingers, as demonstrated in Figure 50-9. If a mass is felt on the initial deep palpation, the examiner should determine whether it is an intraabdominal mass or a mass in the abdominal wall. Having the supine patient raise the head during palpation will give the examiner this in-

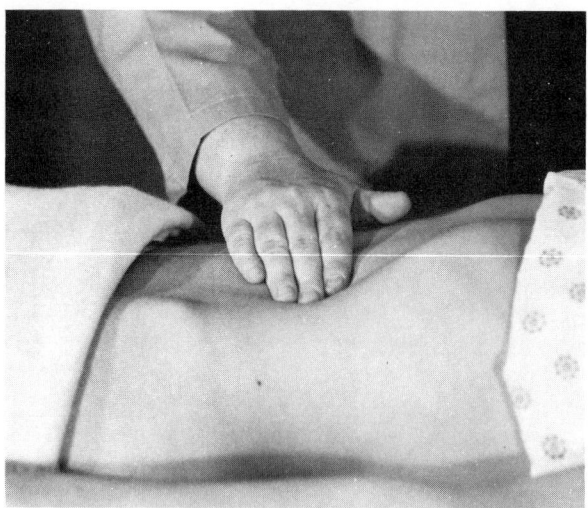

Figure 50-7   Light palpation.

From Malasanos, L., Barkauskas, V., & Stoltenberg-Allen, K. (1990). *Health assessment* (4th ed.). St. Louis: Mosby–Year Book.

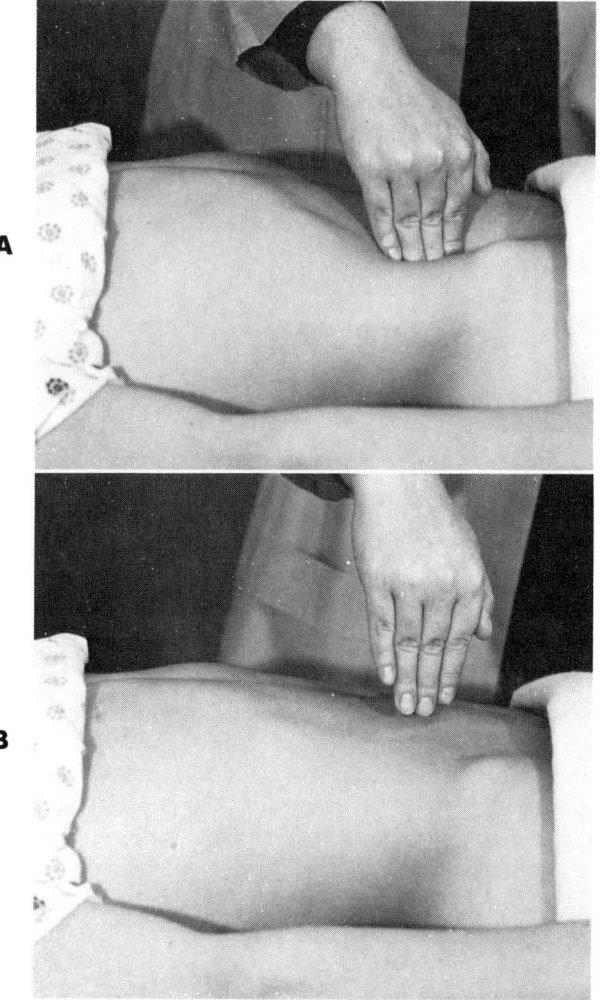

Figure 50-8   Rebound tenderness. Deep pressure is applied (*A*) and released (*B*).

From Malasanos, L., Barkauskas, V., & Stoltenberg-Allen, K. (1990). *Health assessment* (4th ed.). St. Louis: Mosby–Year Book.

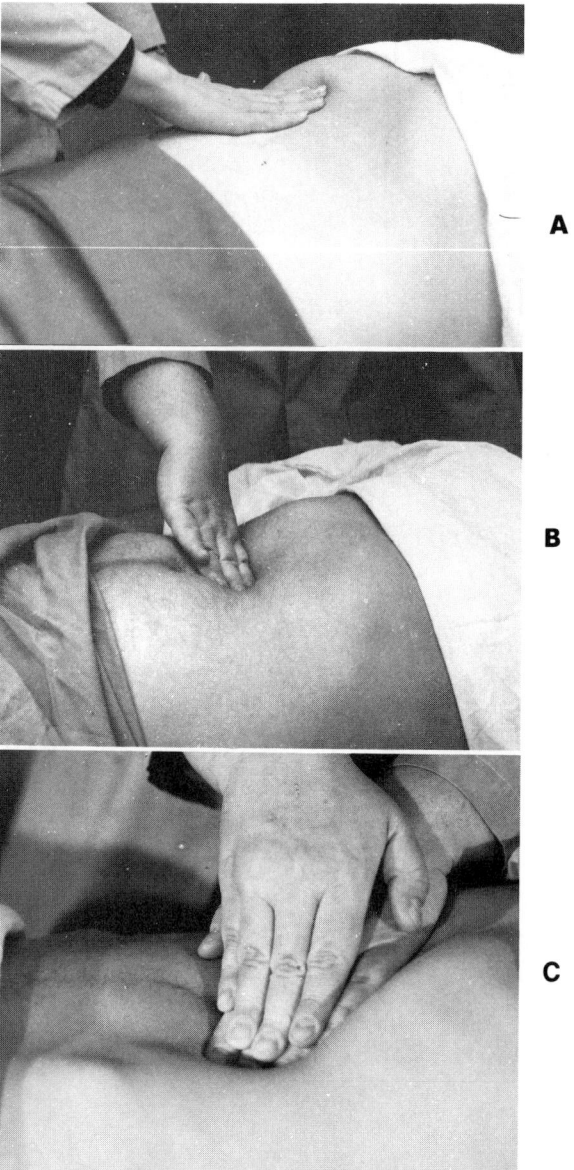

Figure 50-9   *A* and *B*, One-handed method of palpation. *C*, Two-handed method of palpation.

From Malasanos, L., Barkauskas, V., & Stoltenberg-Allen, K. (1990). *Health assessment* (4th ed.). St. Louis: Mosby–Year Book.

formation. An intraabdominal mass will move away from the examiner's hand, while a mass in the abdominal wall will be more readily palpable (Figure 50-10). Consistency, mobility, and movement with respiration of all abdominal masses should be noted. A pulsatile midline mass should not be palpated because it may be a dissecting aneurysm.[3]

The femoral arteries are palpated first. Diminished or absent femoral pulses could indicate common iliac artery thrombosis or dissecting aortic aneurysm.

The liver is located in the right upper quadrant. It is palpated by pushing up from the back with the left

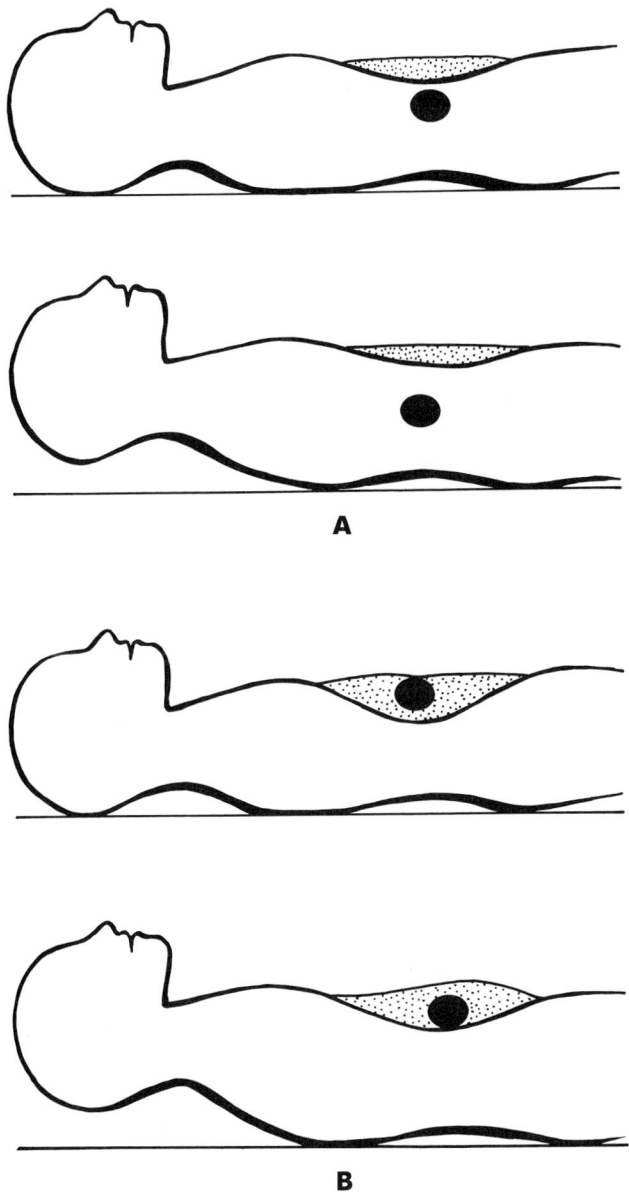

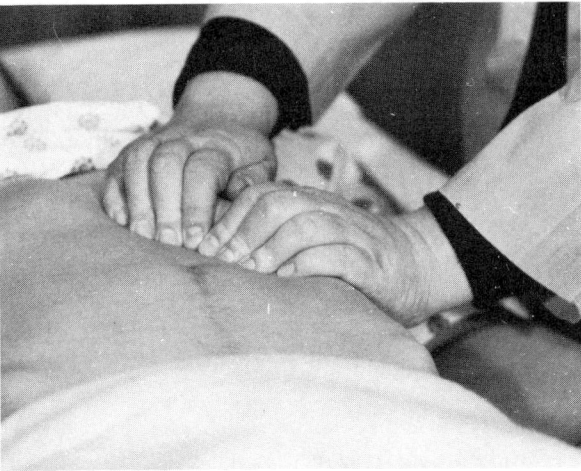

Figure 50-11 Bimanual palpation of the spleen.

From Malasanos, L., Barkauskas, V., & Stoltenberg-Allen, K. (1990). *Health assessment* (4th ed.). St. Louis: Mosby—Year Book.

Figure 50-10 Distinction between abdominal wall and intraabdominal masses. *A,* Intraabdominal mass. *B,* Intramural mass.

hand under the 11th to 12th rib. The right hand is placed on the patient's right abdomen with fingertips parallel to the right costal margin where the liver edge is anticipated while pressing gently up and in under the thorax as the patient inspires. The liver should be felt on deep inspiration. A normal liver edge is smooth and firm. A hard or lumpy liver may indicate carcinoma, whereas tenderness may suggest hepatitis.

A distended gallbladder may be palpated below the liver margin at the lateral border of the rectus muscle. An enlarged tender gallbladder may reflect obstruction of the common bile duct.

The left upper quadrant is palpated by standing on the patient's right side and reaching across the abdomen. The left lower rib cage is pulled up with the left hand while the right presses deeply toward the spleen (Figure 50-11). The spleen is not palpable unless enlarged; however, splenomegaly may be slight, moderate, or pronounced. Slight enlargement may result from lupus erythematosus, rheumatoid arthritis, or subacute bacterial endocarditis. Moderate enlargement may indicate cirrhosis, hepatitis, or infectious mononucleosis. A large spleen may suggest congenital syphilis or portal vein obstruction.

The kidneys are palpated by supporting the flank with the free hand and pressing deeply into the lower left or right quadrant with the examining hand (depending on which kidney is being examined). The lower pole of the kidney may be felt coming to the examiner's fingertips during deep inspirations. The right kidney is more easily felt because of its lower position. An enlarged kidney may be secondary to hydronephrosis, cysts, or neoplasm.

The aorta is palpated by pressing firmly deep into the upper abdomen and slightly left of the midline to identify aortic pulsation. The examiner may be able to feel the aorta between the thumb and fingers. Enlargement of the aorta may be indicative of an aneurysm. This component of the examination is another area where great caution is indicated, especially if problems (e.g., aneurysm) are suspected.

Rectum

The examination of the rectoanal region may be included in the assessment and is most effectively accomplished with the patient in the supine left lateral position. The index finger of the examining hand is lubricated. The perianal and sacrococcygeal areas are inspected for inflammation, lumps, lesions, excoriations, fistulas, or fissures. The patient is asked to bear down during inspection of the anus. Protruding tags of tissue are usually hemorrhoids. Digital rectal examination is used to detect polyps, low tumors, bowel obstruction, or impaction. To palpate the anal canal, the examiner has the patient relax and then slips the lubricated finger into the anal canal pointing toward the umbilicus. Sphincter tone, tenderness, and irregularities are noted. In the male, the prostate will be palpable on the anterior wall; in the female, the cervix is palpable on the anterior wall. The entire rectum is consistently and smoothly examined, and any material that adheres to the examining glove when it is withdrawn is inspected.

Examination of the rectum may need to be deferred if the patient is critically ill or has had a coronary thrombosis or occlusion, stroke, or injury to the area of the rectum. This is to avoid compounding existing damage or eliciting responses such as the Valsalva maneuver, which could induce a vasovagal response.

DIAGNOSTIC PROCEDURES

Diagnostic procedures used to detect gastrointestinal dysfunction include laboratory studies, radiographic procedures, and other special gastrointestinal procedures. An overview is presented here. Methods and parameters as they pertain to specific diseases are discussed in Chapter 51.

Laboratory Studies

Laboratory studies are used in the diagnosis and treatment of many diseases of the gastrointestinal system, but no one single test provides a complete picture of an individual organ's functional state. For example, more than 100 laboratory tests have been proposed for the study of the liver and biliary system alone. Tests commonly used in the critical care setting include measurement of serum bilirubin levels to assess the liver's function in metabolism and secretion of bilirubin. Serum proteins, serum albumin, immunoelectrophoresis, prothrombin time, partial thromboplastin time, and fibrinogen levels are evaluated to assess the liver's level of functioning in regard to protein synthesis (the formation of albumin and globulin and the production of clotting factors). Alkaline phosphatase, SGOT, and SGPT are indications of the amount of hepatic enzymes released into the bloodstream with hepatocyte necrosis.

Gastric content analyses may be used to determine pH, the presence of abnormalities, or hypersecretion

of hydrochloric acid by parietal cells in the stomach. Fecal analyses may also be done. Serum pancreatic enzymes are used to diagnose acute pancreatitis.[3,13,14,15]

Radiological Procedures

Radiological procedures may include a plain film of the chest, used to rule out thoracic diseases mimicking abdominal disease or esophageal foreign body. Ileus, obstruction, and perforation can be visualized on a flat plate of the abdomen. Further investigation to detect lesions in the esophagus, stomach, duodenum, or small bowel may include an upper gastrointestinal series with small-bowel visualization. A barium enema is used to detect lesions in the colon. A cholangiogram (increasingly replaced by use of an ultrasound) allows for visualization of the gallbladder and biliary tree. Table 50-6 summarizes common gastrointestinal radiological and other procedures and their clinical implications.[3,9,15]

Additional Procedures

An increasing variety of special procedures are used in diagnosing gastrointestinal problems. Many have become the "gold standard" for the diagnosis and treatment of certain disorders. Endoscopy allows for direct visualization of a specific site to ascertain the presence of bleeding, ulceration, or obstruction. It is also used in guiding treatment, as in esophageal variceal bleeding, for example.[16] Computed tomography (CT scanning), ultrasonography, and nuclear magnetic resonance imaging (MRI) are noninvasive procedures used for assessing many gastrointestinal organs and for defining tumors, masses, abscesses, or other space-occupying lesions.[17,18] Ultrasound is used to detect an pancreatic enlargement, aneursyms of the aorta, space-occupying lesions, ascites, portal dilatation, and gallstones. Radionuclide imaging of the liver and biliary tree is used in diagnosing many liver disorders. Angiography is the preferred method for diagnosing vascular abnormalities. Biopsy specimens may be taken for histological evaluation to detect the presence of malignant disease in the liver, rectum, esophagus, stomach, duodenum, and large and small bowel. *Paracentesis*, peritoneal tap with lavage of the peritoneal cavity, can identify gastrointestinal hemorrhage in cases of abdominal trauma. Table 50-6 summarizes common special procedures and clinical implications.[14]

TABLE 50-6 Diagnostic Procedures Commonly Used in GI Evaluation

Procedure	Clinical Implications
Radiological Procedures	
Plain films (without contrast medium)	
Abdominal plain film	Can visualize abnormal accumulation of gas/ascites within GI tract; visualizes size, shape, position of liver, spleen, and kidneys.
KUB (kidney, ureters, bladder)	Visualizes urinary tract.
Contrast studies	
Esophageal radiography; upper GI series	Visualizes position, patency of esophagus (also stomach, duodenum, and upper jejunum with upper GI series). Will show gastric diverticulitis, gastritis, gastric ulcer, cancer, and stomach polyps.
Radiography of small intestine (barium swallow)	Shows diseases of small bowel (e.g., ulcerative colitis, tumors, active bleeding obstruction).
Radiography of large intestine (barium enema)	Useful for diverticulitis, cancer, colitis, active bleeding, and obstruction.
Endoscopic Procedures	
Upper GI endoscopy	Uses fiberoptics to visualize lumen of GI tract. Used to detect cause of upper GI bleeding; may also be used to guide treatment bleeding (e.g., sclerotherapy, laser therapy).
Colonoscopy	Examination of large intestine for polyps, tumors, or areas of ulcerative colitis.
Proctoscopy	Visualizes rectum and part of sigmoid colon; primarily used for diagnosis of cancers, Crohn's disease, and ulcerative colitis.
Radionuclide scintigraphy	Imaging of liver and biliary tree by means of radioactive tracers.
CT scan/MRI	Visualize all GI organs.
Ultrasonography	Defines fluid, tumor, masses, stones, fistulas, pseudocyst, or abscess; diagnoses portal hypertension.

REFERENCES

1. Lang, C. E. (1987). Nutritional assessment in critical-care—the adult patient. In C. E. Lang (Ed.), *Nutritional support in critical care*. Rockville, MD: Aspen.

2. Smith, L. C. (1991). Nutritional assessment and indications for nutritional support. *Surgical Clinics of North America, 71*(3), 449-457.

3. Berk, E. J., et al. (1985). *Gastroenterology: Clinical approach to the patient*. Philadelphia: Saunders.

4. Buschiazzo, L., et al. (1986). Careful assessment of abdominal pain. *Journal of Emergency Nursing, 13,* 72.

5. Malasonos, L., Barkauskas, V., & Stoltenberg-Allen, K. (1990). *Health assessment* (4th ed.). St. Louis: Mosby–Year Book.

6. Bates, B. (1990). *A guide to physical examination* (4th ed.). Philadelphia: Lippincott.

7. Sleisenger, M. H., et al. (1989). *Gastrointestinal disease: Pathophysiology, diagnosis, management* (4th ed.). Philadelphia: Saunders.

8. Bongiovanni, G. (1988). *Clinical gastroenterology*. New York: McGraw-Hill.

9. O'Toole, M. T. (1990). Advanced assessment of the abdomen and gastrointestinal problems. *Nursing Clinics of North America, 25*(4), 771-775.

10. Thompson, J. M., McFarland, G. K., Hirsch, J. E., et al. (1989). *Mosby's manual of clinical nursing* (2nd ed.). St. Louis: Mosby–Year Book.

11. Munn, N. E. (1988). Acute abdomen. *Nursing 88, 9,* 34-41.

12. Sien, W. (1987). *Cope's early diagnosis of the acute abdomen* (17th ed.). New York: Oxford University Press.

13. Fischbach, F. (1988). *Laboratory diagnostic tests* (3rd ed.). Philadelphia: Lippincott.

14. Judge, R. D., et al. (1989). *Clinical diagnostics* (5th ed.). Boston: Little, Brown.

15. Lipper, B., et al. (1991). Radiographic manifestations of anomalies of the gastrointestinal tract. *Radiologic Clinics of North America, 29*(2), 335-349.

16. Schiller, K. (1988). Endoscopy in the management of upper gastrointestinal disease. *Postgraduate Medical Journal, 64*(Suppl. 1), 25-26.

17. Balthazar, E. J., et al. (1990). CT tomography in acute gastrointestinal disorders. *American Journal of Gastroenterology, 85*(11), 144-152.

18. Hahn, P. F. (1991). Advances in contrast-enhanced magnetic resonance imaging gastrointestinal contrast agents. *American Journal of Roentgenology, 156*(2), 6-18.

51

Gastrointestinal Disorders

Joanne M. Krumberger

This chapter presents an overview of common gastrointestinal disorders found in the critical care setting, including hepatic and pancreatic disorders. Gastrointestinal hemorrhage is presented first because it is encountered across the spectrum of gastrointestinal disorders.

CONDITIONS ASSOCIATED WITH ACUTE GASTROINTESTINAL HEMORRHAGE

Massive gastrointestinal hemorrhage may occur as a complication of peptic ulcer disease, stress ulceration, Zollinger-Ellison syndrome, Mallory-Weiss syndrome; in trauma; and with esophageal varices. Esophageal varices is discussed in a separate section. A brief overview of the pathophysiology of hemorrhagic shock is also presented.

Peptic Ulcer Disease

Peptic ulcer disease is characterized by a break in the mucosa of the duodenum or gastric area of the stomach extending through the muscularis mucosae.[1,2] The ulcer crater is surrounded by area of acute or chronic inflammation. *Gastritis* is an inflammation of the gastric mucosa. It may be erosive/hemorrhagic or nonerosive (not extending through the muscularis mucosae). Gastritis may be associated with peptic disease, smoking or ingestion of certain substances, or critical illness.

Many studies have addressed risk factors for the development of ulcer disease, diet, alcohol, drugs, and cigarette smoking. Although certain foods and spices cause dyspepsia, there are no conclusive data linking diet to the development of ulcer disease. Aspirin, other nonsteroidal antiinflammatory agents, and alcohol are toxic to the gastric mucosa and may cause dyspepsia and acute mucosal ulceration.[2,3] It is thought that these compounds damage the gastric mucosal barrier to hydrogen ions.[4] The effects of corticosteroids have also been studied widely, but findings are controversial. Cigarette smoking is associated with decreased biliary HCO_3^- secretion and increased duodenal gastric reflux; it increases the risk for both duodenal and gastric ulcers.

Heredity is strongly linked to the development of ulcer disease. An increased number of parietal cells and, therefore, acid hypersecretion; an increased meal-related and nocturnal secretory drive; and rapid gastric emptying have been associated with development of ulcer disease. Emotional factors and stressful events may also affect pepsin and mucous secretion and alter mucosal perfusion and motility of the stomach.[2]

Regardless of the etiology, the development of ulcers is dependent on acid and peptic activity as well as the normal mucosal defense mechanisms.[2,4] Increases in gastric acid secretion may be related to an excessive number of parietal cells, an increased sensitivity of parietal cells to the effects of secretagogues (gastrin, histamine, and acetylcholine), or an enhanced response to vagal stimulation. The rate at which gastric contents are emptied influences the rate of delivery of acid and pepsin to the duodenum and, thereby, affects duodenal pH. The tight junctions between surface epithelial cells, the mucus secreted, cell regeneration, mucosal blood flow, and mucosal bicarbonate secretion also protect the gastric mucosa from acidity. Defects in these mucosal defenses are an important factor in the pathogenesis of this disease. Decreased mucosal blood flow is believed to be the initial insult. Hypersecretion of acid which overcomes this natural mucosal defense, abnormal mucus, biliary reflux, increased mucosal permeability, and hypoperfusion of gut mucosa have been associated with altering host defense mechanisms. Mucosal infections have also been implicated. *Campylobacter pylori* (or *Helicobacter pylori*), a frequent inhabitant of the gastroduodenum, has been associated with peptic ulcer disease characterized by infection and inflammatory changes.[5] Patients who receive abdominal radiation and chemotherapy may develop gastrointestinal bleeding. Erosive gastritis or discrete ulcers may be found.

Stress Ulcer Syndrome

The condition known as *stress ulcer syndrome* is characterized by ulcer formation and upper gastrointestinal tract bleeding. The pathogenesis is not well understood, but is associated with major physiological stress. Stress may create an imbalance between mucosal barrier defense and factors that can lead to ulceration.[6,7,8,9]

Some studies suggest that 80% to 100% of severely ill ICU patients have gastric erosions within 72 hours of injury. Between 5% and 20% of patients with gastric erosion will have clinically apparent gastrointestinal bleeding.[6] Identification of patients at high risk is a priority so early treatment can be instituted and complications prevented (see the box below). The severity of illness and the development of acute gastrointestinal bleeding are related. Patients with multiple trauma, burns, hepatic failure, adult respiratory distress syndrome (ARDS), renal failure, and major surgical procedures are at high risk for gastrointestinal bleeding. The cardiovascular shock and tissue hypoxia related to these conditions are thought to decrease the quality and quantity of mucus secreted, increase the acidity of the gastric mucosa, cause back diffusion of HCl, and impair cell regeneration.[1,6,7,8,9] These factors contribute to the development of stress erosions through the pepsinogen activation and the release of histamine and serotonin. Mechanical ventilation for more than 5 days is associated with development of bleeding stress erosions. Patients with intracranial disease are known to hypersecrete gastric acid.

Stress ulcers are usually deep. They occur in the esophagus, stomach, and duodenum.[1,6,10] Patients with burns over 35% of their body have a high incidence of stress ulcers known as *Curling's ulcers*. Gram-negative sepsis causes gastric acid secretion and may lead to gastrointestinal bleeding. Clinically, the

---

Conditions Associated with a High Risk for Stress Ulcers

Adult respiratory distress syndrome (ARDS)
Mechanical ventilation >5 days
Shock
Acute renal failure
Acute liver failure
Burns >35% of body surface area
Head injury
Multiple trauma
Major operative procedures
Sepsis
Heart failure
Myocardial infarction

---

inability to maintain a gastric pH of less than 4.0 has been associated with sepsis.[11]

Zollinger-Ellison Syndrome

Zollinger-Ellison syndrome is characterized by a non-insulin-secreting tumor of the pancreas, hypergastremia, and multiple peptic ulcers. The non–beta cell adenoma (ulcerogenic tumor) of the pancreas increases the serum levels of the hormone gastrin, resulting in hypersecretion of gastric acids.[2]

The high gastric acid secretions in Zollinger-Ellison syndrome result in a massive amount of acids being poured into the upper small bowel, altering the pH of the duodenum, damaging the mucosa of the duodenum, increasing intestinal motility, and shifting fluid from extracellular volume into the bowel lumen.

In addition to ulcer disease, there also are abnormalities of the small intestine, including mucosaedema, hemorrhage, and multiple superficial erosions. These are usually located in the proximal jejunum.

Mallory-Weiss Syndrome

The Mallory-Weiss syndrome is a linear, nonperforating tear of the gastric mucosa near or at the gastroesophageal junction. A massive gastrointestinal hemorrhage may follow. The tear is a result of pressure changes in the stomach during vomiting. Alcohol abuse, hiatal hernias, gastritis, and esophagitis are associated with this syndrome.[2]

Hemorrhagic Shock

Regardless of the etiology, massive upper gastrointestinal hemorrhage that results in a sudden loss of blood volume decreases venous return to the heart, with a corresponding decrease in cardiac output. The lowered cardiac output leads to inadequate tissue perfusion. An understanding of this cycle of events, along with the compensatory mechanisms that come into action, is required for accurate assessment of an intervention in hypovolemic shock secondary to massive gastrointestinal bleeding (Figure 51-1).

Vasoconstriction, a vascular response to the decreased cardiac output and decreased right atrial pressure, shunts blood flow toward the cerebral and cardiopulmonary systems. If the vasoconstriction continues, the decreased blood flow to the kidneys may result in medullary tubular dysfunction or acute tubular necrosis (ATN). The urinary output is a good index of kidney perfusion and effectiveness of treatment.

The vasoconstriction phase with its associated decrease in tissue perfusion results in cellular dysfunction. The cells attempt to extract oxygen from the available blood, but as shock progresses, this mechanism is not adequate. The cells then shift to anaer-

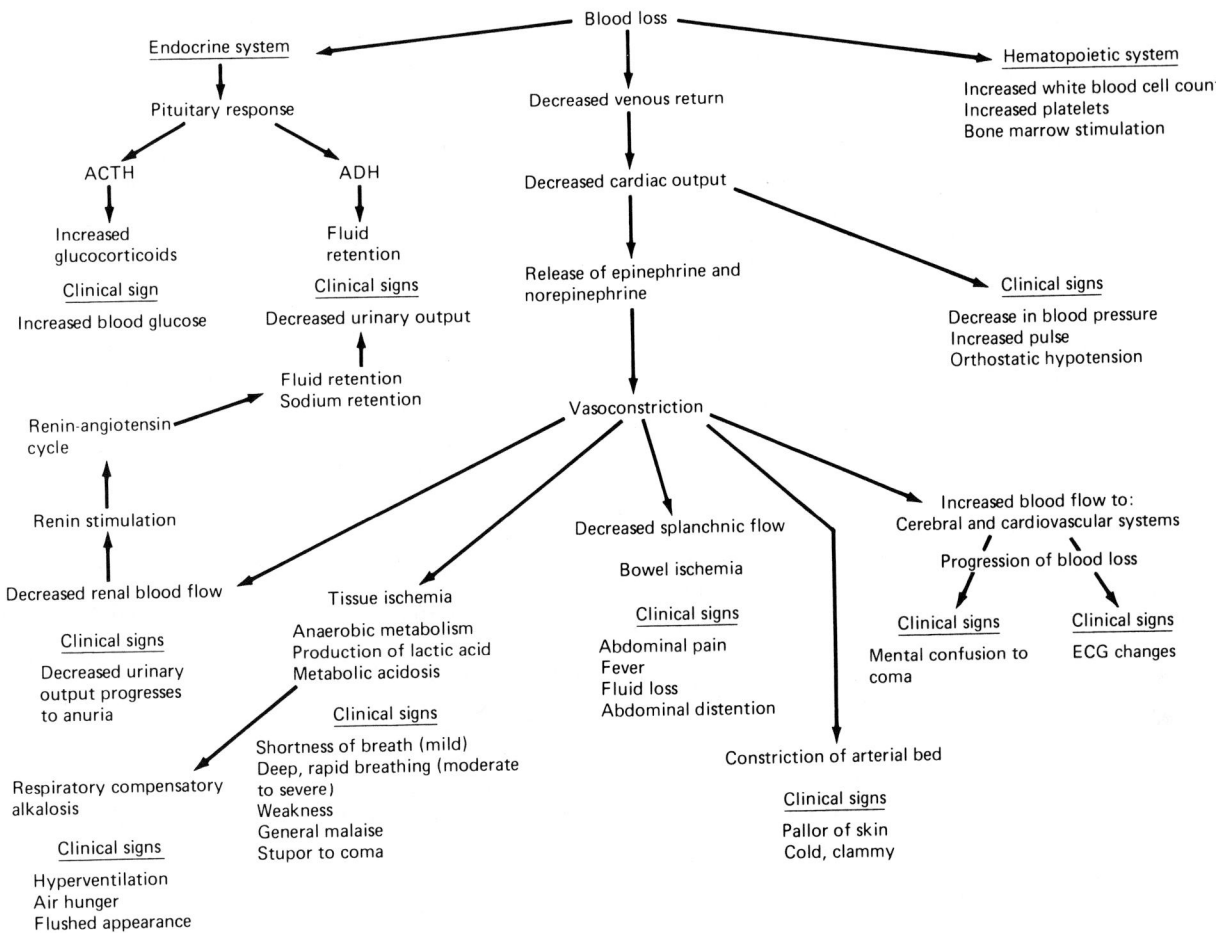

Figure 51-1   Hypovolemic hemorrhagic shock.

obic metabolism. Energy production is decreased, and large quantities of lactic acid are formed. The depressed blood flow to the hepatic and renal systems impairs the function of these systems in breaking down the lactic acid or removing it from the blood. As the lactic acid accumulates, a metabolic acidosis develops.

If the blood loss continues, cerebral flow becomes compromised. The patient may become confused, and mental changes will continue to worsen unless blood flow is increased. The occurrence of brain damage depends upon the duration of lowered tissue perfusion.

Coronary blood flow may also be compromised. A flattening of the T wave or a depression of the ST segment on the ECG denotes coronary blood flow insufficiency.

The body has two compensatory mechanisms that occur more gradually than does vasoconstriction. First, aldosterone and antidiuretic hormone (ADH) are released in response to blood loss. Stimulation by ADH and aldosterone leads to shifts of fluid from extravascular spaces to intravascular spaces. Second,

in the hematopoietic system, an increase in white blood cells and platelets occurs. The bone marrow is stimulated, with resultant increased red cell production and peripheral reticulocytosis. Correction of hemoglobin levels occurs over a period of weeks following the hemorrhage.

Data Acquisition

History

The clinical assessment integrates data gathered from the history, physical examination, and diagnostic tests. The history includes the signs and symptoms and precipitating factors. Blood loss from the gastrointestinal tract is evidenced in several ways. *Hematemesis* is either a brightened bloody vomitus that is associated with fresh bleeding, or coffee ground vomitus which indicates older blood that has been in contact with gastric juices for some time. Blood also may be passed via the colon. Melena is foul-smelling vomitus or stool with a black color that results from the degradation of blood by stomach acids or intestinal bacteria. Maroon or bright red blood also can be passed from the rectum. Gastrointestinal blood loss can also be occult, detected only by testing the stool with a chemical reagent (guaiac); however, gastrointestinal drainage can test positive for up to 10 days after an episode of bleeding and may not be a reliable tool to determine active bleeding.[1] Hematemesis, melena, or maroon stool indicate acute upper gastrointestinal bleeding. Lower gastrointestinal bleeding is noted by bright red blood from the rectum. It is rarely massive and is usually controlled with medical management.

If bleeding is gradual, faintness, fatigue, and pallor may be the only signs. If blood loss is greater than 30% of blood volume, the patient may exhibit shock-like symptoms, including hypotension; shallow, rapid respiration; and cold, clammy skin. Orthostatic hypotension and syncope also may be present. A change in blood pressure greater than 10 mmHg with a corresponding pulse rate increase of 20 beats per minute in a sitting or standing position indicates blood loss in excess of 1,000 ml (Table 51-1). As blood flow to the liver decreases, waste products accumulate in the blood and are noted by an increasing BUN. Urine output also is a very sensitive measure of tissue perfusion and blood flow.

The response of an individual patient to blood loss depends on the rate and amount of loss, the patient's age, preexisting conditions such as coagulopathy or liver disease, the degree of cardiovascular compensation, and rapidity of treatment. In ulcer disease, pain may be a presenting symptom; it is thought to arise from gastric acid bathing the ulcer crater. Diarrhea, melena, hematemesis, and pain unrelieved by medications are characteristic of Zollinger-Ellison syndrome. Data are needed regarding patterns of drug or alcohol intake, previous episodes of gastrointestinal bleeding, liver disease, or gastrointestinal pain. Concurrent diseases may influence the patient's response to the hemorrhage, to treatment. A psychosocial history may determine significant life events and patterns of coping that may be useful in assisting the patient/family in coping with ulcer disease.

Physical Assessment

Physical examination of the patient includes an abdominal examination to assess bowel sounds, with palpation for epigastric tenderness or muscle guarding. The abdomen may be soft or distended. Bowel sounds are most often hyperactive because the bowel is sensitive to blood. The patient may report epigastric tenderness, but this is an uncommon sign. The oropharyngeal area and skin should also be checked for pallor, an early sign of decreased perfusion to the skin.

Diagnostic Procedures

Laboratory Evaluation. The common laboratory studies ordered for a patient with acute gastrointestinal hemorrhage are listed in Table 51-2. The hematocrit does not change substantially during the first few hours after an episode of acute gastrointestinal bleeding.[1] Only when extravascular fluid enters the vascular space to restore volume does the hematocrit drop. Evaluation is further complicated by the therapeutic administration of fluid and blood. Platelet and white blood cell counts may be elevated, reflecting the body's attempt to restore homeostasis. Decreases in potassium and sodium are common due to the vomiting, but later, serum sodium may increase as intravascular volume is lost. Glucose is often elevated due to the stress response. An elevated BUN may result from absorption of blood products from the bowel. Liver function tests, a clotting profile, and serum ammonia are needed to rule out coexisting liver disease. Respiratory alkalosis is a common finding because perfusion to the lung is decreased, the sympathetic nervous system has been activated, and the patient is anxious. As hypovolemic shock progresses in severe bleeding, metabolic acidosis is a prominent result of anaerobic metabolism. Decreased circulating

---

TABLE 51-1   Physical Findings Related to Stages of Shock

	Early Shock	Late Shock
Physical findings	↓ Pulse pressure, ↑ diastolic pressure; restlessness, hyperventilation; pulse rapid and thready; skin cold, clammy, and pale; ascending cooling of the extremities; mucous membranes dry and pale; nail beds cyanotic upon pressure, with slow capillary refill	↓ Systolic pressure, ↓ urine volume, drowsiness, hypothermia, diaphoresis, pronounced tachypnea
Symptoms	Anxiety, apprehension, nervousness, thirst, perceived feeling of cold, nausea, perceived feeling of weakness	Pronounced confusion and lethargy
Laboratory findings	↓ Urine sodium concentration, ↑ urine osmolarity, respiratory alkalosis	Metabolic acidosis

TABLE 51-2 Laboratory Tests Used in Upper GI Bleeding

Measurements	Findings
COMPLETE BLOOD COUNT	
Hematocrit	May be normal, then decreased
Hemoglobin	May be normal, then decreased
White blood cell count	Elevated
Platelet count	Initially elevated, then decreased
ELECTROLYTE PANEL	
Serum potassium	Usually decreased with vomiting
Serum sodium	Elevated
Serum BUN	Elevated
Serum creatinine	Elevated
Serum glucose	Often elevated
Serum lactate	Elevated with severe bleeding
HEMATOLOGY PROFILE	
PT, PTT	Usually decreased
LIVER FUNCTION TESTS	
Enzymes	Elevated with liver disease
Ammonia	Elevated with liver disease
ARTERIAL BLOOD GASES	
Respiratory alkalosis	Early
Metabolic acidosis	With severe hypovolemic shock
Hypoxemia	
GASTRIC ASPIRATE FOR pH AND GUAIAC	
Guaiac positive	
Normal or acidotic pH	

TABLE 51-3 Comparative Gastric Analyses: 12-hour Nocturnal Results

Condition	Amount of HCl, mEq
Ulcer-free	18
Duodenal ulcer	60
Gastric ulcer	12
Zollinger-Ellison syndrome	>100

hemoglobin levels and a ventilation/perfusion mismatch may lead to hypoxemia. Gastric and fecal analyses may be done to rule out occult bleeding.

Elevated levels of gastric acid are associated with Zollinger-Ellison syndrome, which is diagnosed though gastric analysis, an augmented histamine test, and radioimmunoassays. Gastric analysis involves 12-hour overnight collection of gastric secretions through a nasogastric tube (Table 51-3). The *augmented histamine test* is begun after an overnight fast. A nasogastric tube is inserted and residual gastric contents are removed. Basal secretions are collected for 1 hour. Betazole is then injected subcutaneously, and gastric contents collected every 15 minutes for 2 hours. The presence of a non–beta cell adenoma is documented by the absence of a gastric response to betazole. When parietal cells are functioning at max-imum levels in response to serum gastrin, betazole does not increase cell response. Radioimmunoassay methods measure the serum gastrin level. The normal upper limit of serum gastrin is 200 picograms (pg) per milliliter of serum. In Zollinger-Ellison syndrome the serum gastrin level is more than 1,000 pg/ml.[2]

Endoscopic and Radiological Studies. The history, physical examination, and laboratory studies do not provide data for acute gastrointestinal bleeding because they do not define the lesion.

Endoscopy provides specific identification of gastrointestinal lesions through direct mucosal inspection with the use of a fiberoptic scope.[12,13] Unlike the earlier rigid technique, flexible endoscopy can be done at the bedside, which is a distinct advantage in a critical illness. This technique identifies the site and severity of the bleed and also determines whether the condition is generalized or localized. The diagnostic accuracy of endoscopy ranges from 60% to 90%.

Barium studies also may be done, although they are often inconclusive when there are clots in the stomach or when the bleeding is superficial. Angiography is used only when the source of bleeding is not accessible to the endoscope. Selective catheterization of the left gastric artery, usually via a femoral artery, may be done.

Medical Management

Management of acute gastrointestinal bleeding begins with hemodynamic stabilization, then to diagnosis. Specific and supportive therapies can then be based on the findings (Table 51-4).

Hemodynamic Stabilization

The patient in hemorrhagic shock requires immediate replacement of fluid volume and control of bleeding.[1,14] An intravenous line is inserted with a large-bore needle. Fluid replacement to prevent hypovolemia should begin using Ringer's lactate, normal saline, or D_5W. Vital signs are the best indicator of blood loss and should be monitored every 5 to 15 minutes during acute bleeding. An intraarterial line may be placed for constant monitoring and to obtain blood for laboratory analysis. As a rule, systolic pres-

TABLE 51-4   **Clinical Evaluation of a Patient with Hemorrhagic Shock**

Evaluation Item	Observation	Comment
Pulse	Weak, thready, rapid	Progression of shock
Blood pressure	Doppler flowmeter and intraarterial monitoring are more accurate than cuff blood pressure readings	Blood pressure fluctuation alone may not be significant; should be examined in conjunction with urinary output and respiratory function
ECG	Flattening of T waves; depression of ST segments	Continued loss of blood, with resultant decreased coronary blood flow
CVP and PAWP (Swan-Ganz catheter)	CVP less than 6 cmH$_2$O denotes fluid deficit. PAWP less than 10 mmHg suggests hypovolemia, more than 20 mmHg suggests pulmonary edema	CVP and PAWP readings must be evaluated in light of fluid challenge and not considered separately from other data
Respiration	Patent airway and blood gases. Decreased PaO$_2$ leads to respiratory alkalosis, hyperventilation, air hunger, flushed appearance. Check patient's nail beds and lips for cyanosis	A complication of shock is ARDS (wet-lung syndrome) from overhydration
Fluid balance	Check patient's color, mental status, temperature, skin (color, temperature), pulse, urinary output, daily weights, neck veins	Tissue perfusion. *Note:* The most important indicator of blood flow and tissue perfusion is urinary output. Hourly urine output should be 30 ml or more
Metabolic acidosis	Shortness of breath (mild); deep, rapid breathing (moderate to severe); weakness; general malaise; stupor, progressing to coma	A result of anaerobic metabolism
Laboratory data:		
BUN	240 mg/100 ml with normal serum creatinine	Blood loss reflected in BUN levels because of absorption of blood products in upper intestinal tract
Blood glucose	Elevated	ACTH secretion
Hct/Hb	Lowered	Should not be used alone for evaluating blood loss
Clotting factors	Prothrombin time; platelet count	If patient has lengthened prothrombin time (associated with liver disease), vitamin K is given parenterally

sure under 100 mmHg, or a postural drop of more than 10 mmHg reflects a blood loss of at least 1,000 ml or more than 25% of the total blood volume. Hemoglobin and hematocrit values often are difficult to interpret because the proportion of cells to fluids is rapidly changing.

The body has a normal reserve function that allows a specified loss of blood. Blood loss of less than 700 ml is usually well tolerated, and no fluid replacement is necessary. Blood loss of 700 to 1,500 ml should be replaced with fluids. Losses of greater than 1,500 ml require fluid and blood component therapy (Table 51-5). Packed red blood cells are usually used to reestablish oxygen-carrying capacity of the blood. One unit of packed red blood cells increases the hemoglobin by 1 g and the hematocrit by 2 to 3 g, but this outcome is influenced by the patient's intravascular volume and the presence of active bleeding. The physician also may prescribe colloids and crystalloids or

albumin depending on the initial data. Oxygen therapy also should be initiated. A Foley catheter is usually inserted for accurate evaluation of urinary output.

If the patient has known cardiovascular disease, a central venous pressure line or a pulmonary artery catheter may be inserted to monitor fluid status, especially if massive fluid replacement is anticipated. Auscultation of breath sounds during fluid administration is important in preventing fluid overload and pulmonary edema.

Maintenance of bed rest with the head of the bed elevated is an important supportive measure that helps to prevent further bleeding and to decrease the risk of aspiration. Exertion increases intraabdominal pressure and may thereby increase bleeding. Elevation of the head of the bed also prevents reflux of gastric contents into the esophagus. Prevention of aspiration is a nursing priority.

TABLE 51-5 Allowable Blood Loss

Blood Loss	Replacement
0-700 ml	None
700-1,500 ml	Fluid (1,000-2,000 ml) Colloid or crystalloids
>1,500 ml	Fluid (2,000-4,000 ml) Blood
>2,500 ml	Fluid (4,500-6,000 ml) Blood

Gastric Lavage

Gastric lavage may be ordered during acute bleeding episodes, but this treatment is controversial.[1,2,14,15] Some clinicians believe that it disrupts the normal body response to injury by dislodging clots which form over the bleeding site. Other clinicians claim it can help diagnose rate of bleeding, determine whether active bleeding is present, and clear the stomach in preparation for endoscopy. If lavage is ordered, 1,000 to 2,000 ml of room temperature normal saline is usually instilled via a nasogastric tube and then gently removed by manual or intermittent suction until secretions are clear. Ice lavage is not recommended because it may force hydrochloric acid to diffuse back into the submucosa and thereby increase bleeding.[15] Room temperature solution also helps prevent hypothermia and is better tolerated. After lavage, the nasogastric tube is usually removed because it may increase hydrochloric acid secretion.

Pharmacological Management

Pharmacological agents are used to decrease gastric acid secretion or to reduce acid effects on gastric mucosa. The most common agents are antacids, histamine antagonists, and mucosal barrier enhancers (Table 51-6).

Antacids act as a direct alkaline buffer to control the pH of the gastric mucosa.[12,14] Up to 90% of ulcers heal with antacid therapy alone. Antacids are usually given every 1 to 2 hours initially. If the nasogastric tube is left in place, antacids may be titrated to maintain a gastric pH above 5.0. The nurse is responsible for correctly aspirating gastric contents and obtaining gastric pH, for antacid administration, and for monitoring for side effects of the therapy. When antacids are given, it is important to irrigate the nasogastric tube with 10 to 15 ml of normal saline. The tube is clamped for 30 mintues, and suction is instituted for at least 30 minutes before a sample for pH analysis is obtained. Because a given pH value may not reflect the true gastric pH, trends should be used to guide therapy.[11] Antacids contain sodium, which should be considered when given to patients with heart failure,

TABLE 51-6 Management of Upper GI Bleeding

Therapy	Potential Complications
Antacids	Diarrhea, aspiration, hypermagnesemia, hypomagnesemia, hyponatremia, increased plasma albumin, CO_2 retention, metabolic alkalosis
Histamine blockers	
Cimetadine	CNS effects (confusion, lethargy), reversible bone marrow depression, hepatoxicity
Ranitidine	CNS effects, bradycardia, skin rash
Famotidine	Headache, constipation, hepatic dysfunction
Mucosal enhancers	
Prostaglandins	Nausea and vomiting, diarrhea
Sucralfate	Constipation
Colloidal bismuth	Constipation
Endoscopic sclerotherapy	Aspiration, reflux
Heater probe	Fever, bacteremial sepsis
Laser	Oozing from ulcer site, esophageal spasm/perforation, ARDS, bradycardia, allergic response to medications
Surgical interventions	Impaired wound healing, electrolyte imbalance, altered nutrition

hypertension, or liver failure. Complications of antacid therapy include diarrhea; electrolyte imbalances, such as magnesium imbalance, hypernatremia, and hypophosphatemia; and metabolic alkalosis. Antacids also may cause carbon dioxide retention.

Histamine is a potent stimulator of gastric acid secretion. Histamine blockers block parietal cell stimulation and secretion of hydrochloric acid. Common histamine blockers are cimetidine, ranitidine, and famotidine.[1,2,14,16,17,18,19] Omeprazole, a newer drug, suppresses gastric acid secretion by inhibiting the proton pump mechanism, thereby blocking the final step of acid secretion. It may be beneficial in patients resistant to histamine receptor antagonists.[19] The influence of pH elevation on the incidence of nosocomial pneumonia has been extensively studied.[6,8,14,20] Organisms gain access to the normally sterile tracheobronchial tree by way of colonized oropharyngeal gastric secretions. Medications that elevate the pH of gastric contents promote colonization and, therefore, may increase the incidence of nosocomial infection. For this reason, pharmacological intervention is begun only in patients who are actively hemorrhaging or are at high risk for hemorrhage. High gastric volume also may increase the risk of aspiration, and this risk must be considered in the administration of antacids.

Mucosal barrier agents act directly on the gastric mucosa to reduce the effects of acid secretion. The prostaglandin carbenoxolone improves the mucosal barrier and increases mucosal blood flow. Misoprostil, a prostaglandin E_1 analogue, effectively suppresses acid secretion for 3 to 5 hours. Side effects include nausea, vomiting, abdominal cramps, and diarrhea. Diphenoxylate (Lomotil) should not be used in treating patients with diarrhea due to gastrointestinal bleeding because the atropine in the medication enhances gastric secretion and gastric acidity. Sucralfate is used to treat duodenal ulcers by forming a protective barrier over the ulcer site. Colloidal bismuth binds to the ulcer base and also stimulates mucous secretion, which prevents further mucosal damage.

Endoscopic Therapies

The advantage of endoscopic therapies is that they can be applied at the time of diagnosis. *Sclerotherapy* involves injecting the bleeding ulcer with a necrotizing agent such as sodium moorheate or tetradecylsulfate.[1,2,7,8,13] These agents traumatize the endothelium, causing necrosis and eventual sclerosis of the bleeding vessel. Thermal methods of endoscopic tamponade include the heater probe, laser photocoagulation, and electrocoagulation. These therapies are usually performed at the bedside. Maintenance of a patent airway and breathing are a nursing priority. Placement of the patient in a left lateral reverse Trendelenburg position can help to prevent respiratory complications.[21] Other common complications of sclerotherapy include fever and oozing from the bleeding site. A more serious complication when sclerosing agents are used is the development of adult respiratory distress syndrome, which is thought to be related to the exposure of lung tissue to fatty substances liberated from the agent.

Surgical Intervention

Surgery is considered for patients who have massive bleeding that is immediately life-threatening, in patients who continue to bleed despite aggressive medical therapies, and in perforation or unremitting pyloric obstruction. Criteria for delayed surgery varies, but it is usually considered for patients who require more than 8 units of blood within a 24-hour period.[1,2]

Perforation of the gastric mucosa is a complication of peptic ulcer disease that requires immediate surgical intervention. The most common signs of this complications are an abrupt onset of abdominal pain followed rapidly by signs of peritonitis, including abdominal tenderness, abdominal rigidity, and an absence of bowel sounds. Presence of free air on the abdominal x-ray is also characteristic.

Surgical therapies for peptic ulcer disease or stress ulcers include gastric resections, such as antrectomy, gastrectomy, or gastroenterostomy; vagotomy; or combined surgeries, such as the Billroth I or Billroth II procedures to restore gastrointestinal continuity. An antrectomy may be performed for duodenal ulcers to decrease the acidity of the duodenum by removing the gastric acid–secreting cells in the antrum. A vagotomy decreases acid secretion in the stomach by dividing the vagus nerve along the esophagus. A pyloroplasty may be performed with a vagotomy to prevent stomach atony. A Billroth I procedure consists of a vagotomy and antrectomy with anastomosis of the stomach to the duodenum. A Billroth II consists of a vagotomy, a resection of the antrum, and anastomosis of the stomach to the jejunum (Figure 51-2). A perforation can be treated by simple closure with an omental patch to cover the gastric mucosal hole. Alternatively, the ulcer may be excised and the remaining ends sutured.

In Zollinger-Ellison syndrome, the recommended operative intervention is total gastrectomy with esophagojejunostomy, since any remaining gastric mucosa is capable of secreting large quantities of gastric acid that will cause recurrent ulceration and possible complications of intractable ulcer disease.[2,22] The pancreatic tumor is removed when possible. Early total gastrectomy for this syndrome carries a favorable prognosis.

Nursing Management

During initial management, the critical care nurse performs the nursing assessment and evaluates the

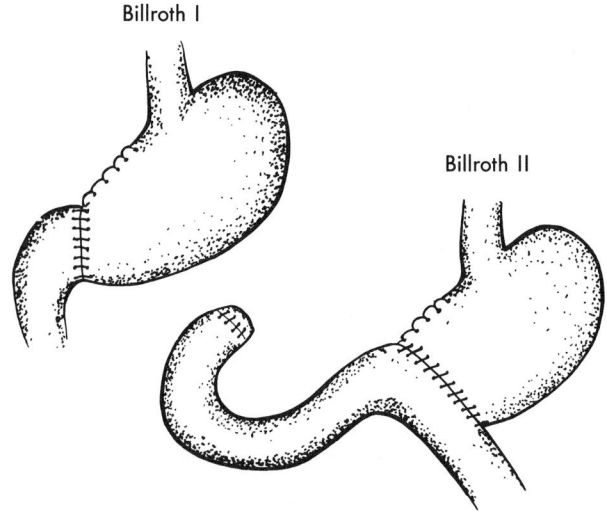

Figure 51-2   Billroth I and II.

diagnostic findings of laboratory studies, radiological studies, and other procedures (see Table 51-2). As treatment begins, the nurse assists in carrying out the prescribed medical and pharmacological regimens; monitors the patient response to interventions, including the development of complications; and provides supportive care. Teaching about diagnostic tests, monitoring procedures, and the critical care environment is adjusted to the individual needs of patient and family. Psychosocial responses to an acute episode of gastrointestinal bleeding are many and constitute a nursing priority.

Postoperative nursing care is focused on monitoring and the prevention of potential complications. Fluid and electrolyte imbalances are common because of intraoperative fluid loss and the drains left in place to decompress the stomach or to drain the surgical site.[23] Additionally, the gastrointestinal system may not function normally for some time, resulting in nausea, vomiting, and diarrhea. Provision of adequate nutrition is necessary for wound healing and to maintain anabolism. In cases of prolonged postoperative ileus, total parenteral nutrition may be considered.

ESOPHAGEAL DISORDERS

Esophageal Varices

Pathophysiology

In liver disease, especially cirrhosis, there is destruction of hepatocytes, hepatic tissue fibrosis, and disruption of hepatic vasculature. Venous and lymph vessels become compressed, and hepatic congestion results. Bands of connective scar tissue where liver cells are destroyed block blood flow in the sinusoids. As a result, portal pressure builds, and an elaborate system of collateral circulation develops which connects with systemic veins to shunt part of the portal venous blood to the systemic circulation, bypassing the liver and thereby decreasing portal pressure. These collateral channels are found at the esophagogastric junction, the anterior abdominal wall (gastric vein), and within the rectal vault the hemorrhoidal vein (Figure 51-3).[24,25] Splenomegaly also result. These vessels, which are called *varices*, contain little elastic tissue and become tortuous, distended, and fragile.

Acute upper gastrointestinal bleeding from ruptured esophageal or gastric varices is a serious complication of liver disease.[24,25,26] The bleeding is usually massive and clinically significant, causing the patient to seek prompt medical attention. The 5-year survival rate for a cirrhotic patient with esophageal varices is 5%. Hemorrhage recurs in 65% of these patients, contributing to the mortality. Other etiologies of portal hypotension and the development of varices include extrahepatic portal obstruction, hepatitis, trauma, and ingestion of toxic substances.

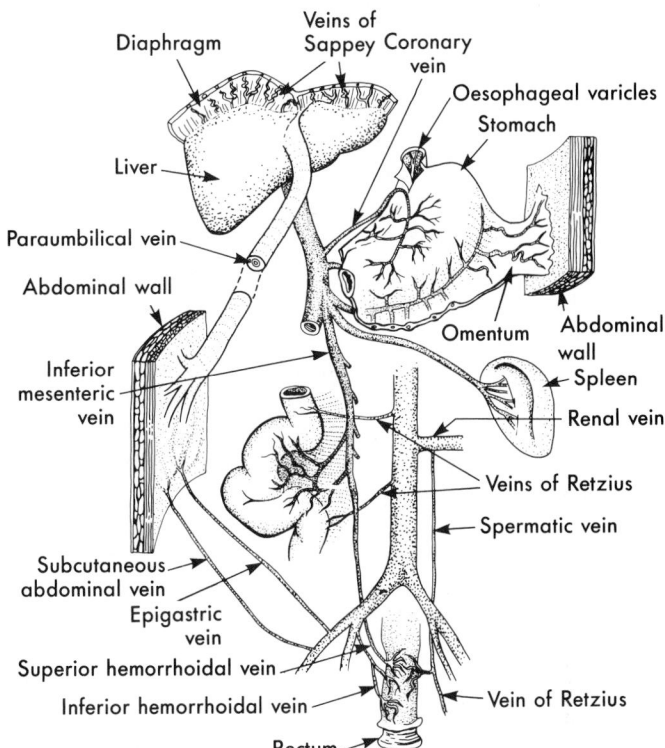

Figure 51-3   Collateral circulation in the liver.

Data Acquisition

History. During the acute phase of bleeding, a limited history focusing on patterns of alcohol ingestion and the presence of any preexisting liver disease or upper gastrointestinal bleeding is most appropriate. Cirrhosis may or may not have been diagnosed. Most patients underreport alcohol ingestion. Other signs of liver disease may need to be assessed for to make an accurate diagnosis of the cause of bleeding.

Physical Assessment. The patient with bleeding esophageal or gastric varices is not only hypovolemic but also has a dysfunctioning liver which cannot adequately perform metabolic, synthesizing, and detoxification functions. This liver dysfunction is a major factor in the patient's response to the treatment and the development of complications. The patient most commonly presents with a history of or active bright red emesis. Emesis is usually copious, and hypovolemic shock is likely to be present. The bleeding may have started after an innocuous episode of coughing or retching.

A patient with liver disease may also present with increased abdominal girth, jaundice, ascites, encephalopathy, splenomegaly, spider nevi, muscle atrophy, and anemia. The liver is usually nonpalpable because cirrhosis causes liver atrophy.

Diagnostic Procedures. Endoscopy allows for direct visualization of esophageal and gastric varices. Not all varices bleed. The size of the varix is assessed on a 1- to 4-point Likert-type scale.[13,27] The appearance of the varix has diagnostic significance. Telangiectasis or cherry red spots and bulges in the varix with a thin blue variceal wall are diagnostic for rupture. Wall tension also may be measured. Portal pressure greater than 12 mmHg is associated with an increased risk for hemorrhage. Prophylactic treatment of varices that are likely to rupture may reduce morbidity and mortality. Rupture of the varix is most commonly seen 5 cm above the esophagogastric junction.

Blood samples for assays of bilirubin, liver enzymes (SGOT, SGPT, LDH), and alkaline phosphatase may be drawn to determine hepatic excretory dysfunction and cellular integrity problems associated with liver disease. Parenchymal tests such as liver biopsy can differentiate the type of liver failure present by determining the architecture of the liver cells. Coagulation function tests are also commonly performed because they have direct implications for an actively bleeding patient.

Medical Management

Hemodynamic Stabilization. Hemodynamic stabilization and establishment of a patent airway are the first priorities (see section on Collaborative Management of Upper Gastrointestinal Bleeding). The patient with liver failure may be more difficult to stabilize because of limited circulatory compensatory mechanisms and the inability of the liver to synthesize the necessary clotting factors to maintain a stable clot.[24] Hypertension and aggressive fluid replacement should be avoided because some data suggest that increased intravascular volume and hypertension may increase variceal bleeding. Maintenance of a mean pressure of 60 is a realistic goal. Endoscopic evaluation to establish the etiology of the bleeding is the next priority so that definitive treatment for the varices can be undertaken.

Sclerotherapy. If the site of origin can be quickly identified, sclerotherapy is the treatment of choice for bleeding varices.[1,24,25,26,27] The sclerosing agent is injected into the varix and surrounding tissue. Usually, several applications are needed to decompress the bleeding varix. Nursing interventions include airway management and monitoring for complications. Potential complications include: esophageal ulceration, stricture, or perforation, retrosternal pain, dysphagia, or an allergic response to medications.

Vasopressin Administration. Vasopressin (Pitressin) is a synthetic antidiuretic hormone that acts directly on gastrointestinal smooth muscle as a vasoconstrictor. Vasoconstriction lowers portal venous pressure and decreases venous blood flow.[24,28,29] Ultimately, it decreases pressure and flow in the liver's

collateral circulation channels to decrease bleeding. Vasopressin is usually administered via an infusion pump in a dose of 0.2 to 0.6 units per minute. Because it is a vasoconstrictor, it should be infused via a central line. Vasopressin may be administered for up to 36 hours. Usually, the dosage is slowly reduced if no signs of rebleeding are seen. Beta-blockers, which decrease cardiac output, splanchnic flow, and portal pressure, may be used for the long-term treatment of portal hypertension.

The assessments performed by the critical care nurse are important during vasopressin administration because it has many potentially harmful systemic effects. Chest pain, dysrhythmias, and other symptoms of coronary ischemia are common side effects of this drug.[27,28] Intravenous nitroglycerin may be concurrently administered to combat these side effects. Cardiac dysrhythmias, most commonly bradycardia and torsades de point, also may occur. QT intervals should be measured on the patient's ECG, and class I antidysrhythmics, such as disopyramide phosphate (Norpace), procainamide (Procan), or quinidine, which are known to widen the QT interval, should not be given concurrently. Increased afterload from arteriolar vasoconstriction has also been reported. Vasopressin can also induce renal vasoconstriction, and fluid retention may be a serious complication. Strict intake and output, daily weights, and serum values need to be closely monitored. Concurrent liver failure and its associated fluid and hormonal imbalances further complicate the clinical presentation. Because vasopressin, being an antidiuretic hormone, induces water retention, ascites and edema associated with liver failure often worsen.

Glypressin is a newer drug that recently has been used in the clinical setting. It lowers splanchnic pressures within 1 hour of administration.[1,25,27,28]

Balloon Tamponade. A triple-lumen nasogastric tube may be inserted as a tampon to decrease azygous blood flow and to control bleeding.[1,24] The Sengstaken-Blakemore triple-lumen tube has two balloons and one lumen for gastric aspiration. It frequently is used to control hemorrhage from esophageal and gastric varices. Four major complications arise from the use of this tube: pulmonary problems secondary to aspiration, rupture of the esophagus, asphyxia, and erosion of the esophageal or gastric wall. The Linton tamponade tube has two aspiration lumens and a gastric balloon with a capacity of 800 ml. When filled, the balloon applies pressure on the intragastric veins. The two lumens of the Linton tube provide for gastric and esophageal aspiration. The advantage of the Linton tube is its capacity for esophageal aspiration and the large gastric balloon which alleviates the need for intraesophageal tamponade.

The procedure for insertion of the Sengstaken-Blakemore tube is similar to that for any nasogastric tube (Table 51-7). The balloons are checked prior to insertion, and tracheal suction is available during the actual insertion to prevent aspiration of vomitus. The gastric balloon is inflated and fitted snugly against the cardia of the stomach. Traction is then applied to the tube, and the tube is taped to a protective helmet worn by the patient.

If the gastric aspirate is bloody, the bleeding is from a gastric lesion. Additional air is inserted into the gastric balloon, and traction is continued. If the bleeding is from the esophageal varices, the esophageal balloon is inflated to a pressure of 20 to 25 mmHg. The patient should be observed closely while the Sengstaken-Blakemore tube is in place (Figure 51-4). Because swallowing is impossible with an inflated esophageal balloon, the patient will require frequent nasoesophageal suctioning to control saliva. Insertion of a Levin tube connected to intermittent suctioning above the esophageal balloon is recommended to prevent aspiration. If the gastric balloon ruptures, the entire tube will move upward and obstruct the patient's airway. The tube must be cut immediately across all three lumens and removed. A second Sengstaken-Blakemore tube should be available in the patient's room in case this should occur.

Surgical Intervention. Permanent decompression of portal hypertension can be achieved only through a surgical procedure called *portacaval shunts*, which diverts blood around the blocked portal system[27,30,31] (Figure 51-5). In these procedures, a connection is made between the portal vein and the inferior vena cava to divert blood flow into the vena cava thereby to reduce portal pressure. There are several variations of this procedure, including the end-to-side shunt and the side-to-side shunt. The end-to-side shunt is technically the easiest, but it diverts all blood from the gastrointestinal system directly into the systemic circulation before detoxification can occur. The most common complication of this procedure is portal encephalopathy.[30] The side-to-side shunt is intended to prevent this complication by allowing some of the portal blood to flow back into the liver for detoxification. The splenorenal shunt also provides some portal flow and is associated with a lower incidence of encephalopathy than the side-to-side shunt. Removal of the spleen eliminates hypersplenism but is associated with an increased rate of thrombosis.

Peptic ulcer formation is a complication of shunt procedures. The reasons for ulcer formation are unclear, but it may result from an increase in gastric acid secretions due to the shunt. Temporary increases in ascites may also occur after all of these procedures. Because of the many postoperative complications associated with shunt procedures, their use is being reevaluated.

NURSING MANAGEMENT

Nursing management of the patient with upper gastrointestinal bleeding from esophageal or gastric varices includes the assessment, goals, and interventions for any patient with acute hypovolemic shock. In addition, there is a potential for ineffective breathing pattern, related to aspiration of blood during acute bleeding episodes, or due to obstruction of the airway by the Sengstaken-Blakemore tube or other tamponade balloon.

■ NURSING DIAGNOSIS

Fluid volume deficit, related to decreased circulating blood volume, fluid and electrolyte imbalance.

OUTCOME STANDARD AND CRITERIA

Fluid volume is adequate as evidenced by:
- Vital signs within patients' normal limits
- Stable hematocrit/hemoglobin
- Preload indicators within normal limits
- Urine output greater than 30 ml/hr

NURSING INTERVENTIONS

- Monitor vital signs for hemodynamic instability, orthostatic hypotension
- Monitor ECG, skin, and urine output for signs of ischemia
- Monitor preload indicators if available
- Measure intake/output, correlate with weight changes; include fluid losses via emesis, gastric suction/lavage, and stools
- Maintain bed rest; administer oxygen
- Monitor response to fluid and blood replacement
- Monitor all laboratory reports
- Administer medications as indicated
- Prepare for/assist with endoscopy

■ NURSING DIAGNOSIS

Altered tissue perfusion, related to reduced hemoglobin, decreased cardiac output, vasoconstriction, and lactic acidosis.

OUTCOME STANDARD AND CRITERIA

Tissue perfusion is maintained as evidenced by:
- Stabilized vital signs
- Absence of mental status changes
- Warm skin
- Palpable peripheral pulses
- Urine output ≥30 ml/hr
- Arterial blood gas levels within normal limits

NURSING INTERVENTIONS

- Monitor for signs of hypoperfusion or hemodynamic instability:
  Vital signs every 15 minutes until stable
  Urine output
  ECG
  Mentation

TABLE 51-7   Nursing Responsibility with Use of Sengstaken-Blakemore Tube

Insertion of Tube

Activity	Rationale
Inflate both balloons of Sengstaken-Blakemore tube and hold them under water to observe for minute leaks	Any escaping air can be detected in water
Label all lumens carefully with waterproof marker	Prevents inflation and deflation of gastric balloon for esophageal balloon and vice versa
Have tracheal suctioning available in room	Vomiting often occurs during insertion, and aspiration is a hazard
Have rubber-shod hemostats available. Double clamp each balloon lumen. Place cotton disk around tube at patient's nares, then apply protective helmet. Tape tube securely to chin guard	Unprotected teeth or hemostats may cut into tubing, allowing air to leak. Double clamping assures occlusion of lumen. Traction applied to Sengstaken-Blakemore tube will create pressure necrosis if tube is taped to skin

Care of Patient

Possible Complications	Nursing Interventions	Rationale
Erosion and perforation of esophagus and/or gastric mucosa	Careful monitoring of vital signs, particularly blood pressure and respirations	Evaluation of response of bleeding to tamponade, complications, etc.
	Frequent (every 15-30 min) checks of mmHg pressure of esophageal balloon. Release pressure at intervals	Onset of back pain, upper abdominal pain, shock, and fluid in chest are signs of perforation; releasing pressure at intervals decreases incidence of tissue necrosis. Tube is removed after 48 hours because incidence of necrosis increases after this
Aspiration pneumonia	Mouth care; suctioning of nasoesophageal areas	Patient with inflated esophageal balloon is unable to swallow. Frequent mouth–esophageal suctioning is necessary to prevent aspiration. Option is insertion of nasogastric tube above esophageal balloon
	Irrigation of gastric tube; observe color, consistency, and odor of output and note changes	Patency of gastric tube. Color change in output indicates bleeding; change in amount indicates amount of fluid replacement needed
	Keep nostrils clean and well-lubricated; keep cotton disk in place between skin and Sengstaken-Blakemore tube	Patient comfort and prevention of pressure necrosis from traction
Pharyngeal obstruction (asphyxia)	Keep scissors and extra S-B tube readily available. Frequent observation of vital signs—particularly respiratory status. If patient becomes cyanotic, cut through three lumens simultaneously and remove tube	Patient begins gasping for air. Most likely cause is leaking or ruptured gastric balloon. Under traction, when balloon ruptures, tube is raised through esophagus and esophageal balloon obstructs airway. When tube is cut, both balloons are immediately deflated and tube can be removed without further trauma to mucosa. Also, when tube is cut, it can be removed without undoing tape

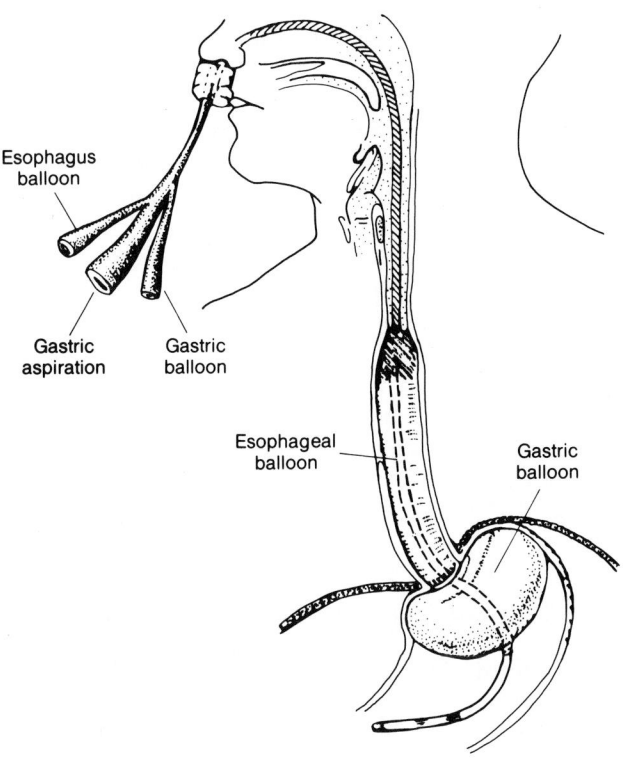

Figure 51-4 The Sengstaken-Blakemore tube in place with esophageal and gastric balloons inflated.

Preload indicators/cardiac output
Skin for perfusion
Auscultate bowel sounds
Bilirubin
• Administer fluids as indicated
■ **NURSING DIAGNOSIS**
   Fear and anxiety, related to bleeding, fear of dying, treatment regimen.
OUTCOME STANDARD AND CRITERIA
   Fear and anxiety are reduced or absent as evidenced by:
• Verbalization of understanding of cause of bleeding
• Demonstration or verbalization of decreased anxiety or fear with nursing interventions (e.g., explanations of environment or explanations of treatment regimen and goals)
NURSING INTERVENTIONS
• Assess level of anxiety
• Explain ICU environment and all procedures
• Provide reassurance to patient and family
• Approach family in a calm, concerned manner
• Structure environment to provide for rest; limit stimuli
• Anticipate treatments and procedures and provide explanations
• Provide for patient comfort

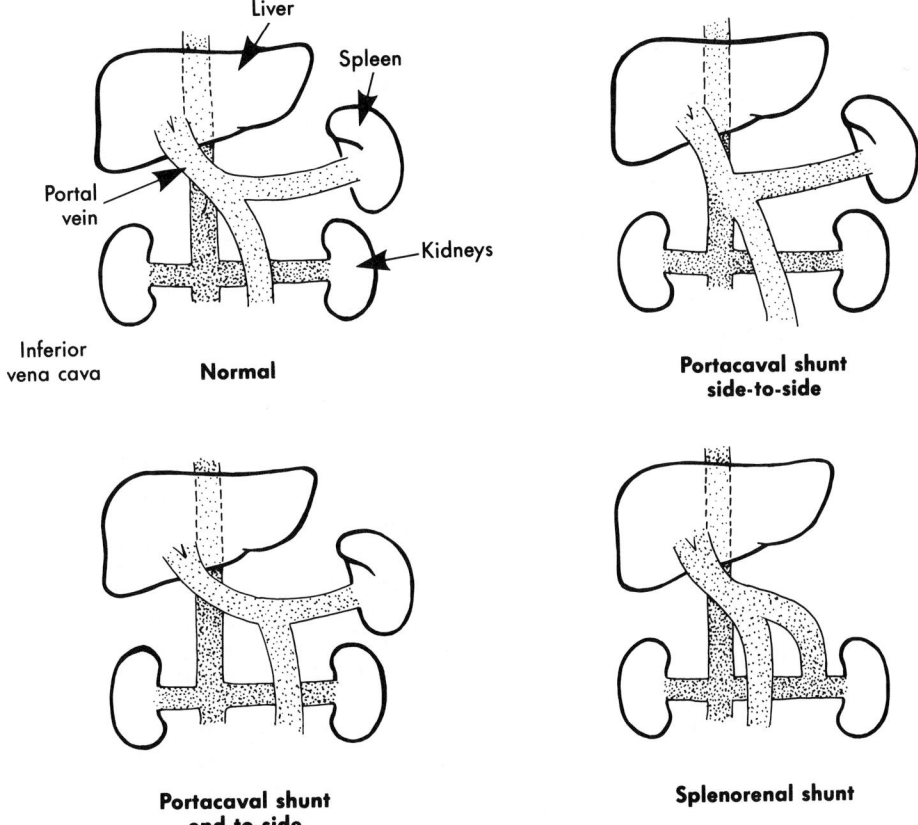

Figure 51-5 Normal portal system and portacaval shunts: end-to-side, side-to-side, and splenorenal.

- Involve patient and family in planning of care
- Encourage verbalization of fears or concerns

■ NURSING DIAGNOSIS

High risk for infection, related to contaminated surgical wound or translocation of bacteria into bloodstream.

OUTCOME STANDARD AND CRITERIA

Patient is free of infection as evidenced by:
- Absence of fever
- Normal WBC count
- Clean, dry wound without redness, swelling, erythema, pain, purulent drainage

NURSING INTERVENTIONS

- Monitor appearance of incision and surrounding tissue
- Document and report all wound drainage, color, amount of odor; complaints of pain or tenderness
- Culture any suspicious drainage
- Monitor WBC count and temperature trends

Esophageal Cancer

Pathophysiology

Of all cancer deaths in the United States, 2% to 4% are due to esophageal cancer.[32,33,34,35] The 5-year survival rate is less than 10%. Squamous cell cancers account for 98% of cases of carcinoma of the esophagus. Small cell carcinoma is rare. Microscopically, esophageal carcinoma is identical in appearance to small cell cancer of the lung. Tumors may involve the upper, middle, or lower third of the esophagus. The aggressive nature of this lesion is associated with rapid tumor growth and spread. Lesions most commonly spread to the lymph nodes of the surrounding area, with the liver and lungs the most commonly involved viscera.

Studies have not identified a common etiological factor. Certain lifestyle factors are associated with development of esophageal cancer including heavy alcohol intake and tobacco smoking. Patients with Barrett's esophagus are also at increased risk for this adenocarcinoma. Identification of high-risk groups is important. Until markers for early detection are known, the outcome for patients with esophageal cancer appears unlikely to be improved.

Data Acquisition

History. Major symptoms associated with esophageal cancer are listed in the box to the right.[32,33,34] Dysphagia is the classic sign, and it is progressive. The patient will most likely report a problem first with large boluses, then small boluses, and then liquids. The patient may describe a sensation of food lodged somewhere in the esophagus. For dysphagia to occur, the diameter of the esophagus must be occluded to less than 13 mm. Unfortunately, the lesion is far advanced by the time the patient notices this symptom. The patient may attribute problems in swallowing to some other cause such as poorly fitting dentures, which further delays seeking medical care. As the disease progresses, frequent expectoration or regurgitation may lead to recurrent aspiration pneumonia.

Pain can occur at the site or may be referred to the neck, jaw, or interscapular region. It may mimic chest pain. Substernal burning that the patient describes as heartburn also may be present. Anorexia, weight loss, and malaise are other common presenting symptoms. A complete nutrition history should be obtained. The patient may also report a history of hemoptysis or hematemesis.

Physical Assessment. Physical examination of the patient with carcinoma of the esophagus may be unrevealing except for the severity of malnutrition which may be present. A rancid odor may be evident from the necrotic tumor but is not common.

Diagnostic Procedures. A barium swallow with fluoroscopy is usually ordered to identify the obstructing lesion. An upper gastrointestinal endoscopy with biopsy is done to confirm the diagnosis.[13,33] Biopsy and cytological brushings determine the type of cancer involved. Magnetic resonance imaging, computed tomography, and ultrasonography may be used for staging and follow-up of local recurrence or for detection of metastases.

Complete blood tests will be done but are not diagnostic. Anemia is often present because of blood loss from the tumor. Hypoalbuminemia and negative nitrogen balance may indicate the severity of malnutrition present.

Medical Management

Treatment of esophageal cancer is controversial. No single treatment has proved to change mortality.

Signs and Symptoms of Esophageal Cancer

Dysphagia
Anorexia
Weight loss
Chest pain
Epigastric pain or burning
Hoarseness
Vomiting or regurgitation
Abdominal bloating
Palpable cervical nodes
Coughing and choking
Aspiration pneumonia
Hematemesis/hemoptysis

Endoscopic therapies, surgical resection, radiation, and chemotherapy have been used separately or in combination to attempt to cure or provide palliative care. In general, an approach is selected that offers the most comfort at the lowest risk.

Endoscopic Therapies. Endoscopic therapies are usually employed for palliative treatment of dysphagia. Endoscopic treatments for esophageal cancer include Nd:YAG laser ablation, photodynamic therapy, or bipolar or monopolar electrocoagulation. The major risk is esophageal perforation; bleeding is unusual. The procedure is uncomfortable for the patient, and safe methods of analgesia and sedation need to be considered.[36,37]

Endoscopy also can be used to insert a prosthesis. After the lesion is dilated, the prosthesis is pushed into position. Dilation is usually painful, and intravenous sedation is usually employed. After the procedure, a physical examination is carried out to look for air crepitation and a chest x-ray performed to look for evidence of perforation. Before the patient is allowed to drink, tube positioning is checked fluoroscopically with a water-soluble contrast medium. The patient is then allowed to eat and drink and can be discharged. It is essential to determine that the patient's chewing ability is adequate. Palliation can be achieved in over 90% of patients.

Surgical Therapies. Surgical resection of the lesion determines whether removal of growth is technically feasible. Surgical resection also is dependent on whether the patient can tolerate the procedure. The type of resection used, which include a blunt resection with or without anastomosis, lymph node dissection, and reconstruction procedures, depends mainly on the location of the tumor. The surgical approach for an esophagogastrectomy is via right or left thoracotomy. For lesions in the cervical esophagus, an extrathoracic esophagectomy is performed. A gastric drainage procedure such as pyloroplasty also is done. Attempts are made to avoid pulmonary complications by administering bronchodilators, mucolytic agents, and appropriate antibiotics. The patient may have a tracheostomy or endotracheal tube requiring careful monitoring for effectiveness of ventilation. Cardiovascular complications include dysrhythmias and hemorrhage. Anastomotic leaks are common and become apparent within 1 to 10 days after surgery.[38,39]

Chemotherapy and Radiotherapy. Adjunctive chemotherapy and radiotherapy have been used to control tumor growth and destroy metastases. Current research is focused on efficacious timing for these therapies. Combination therapies with surgical intervention seem to be the most promising. Trimetrexate, cisplatin/bleomycin, cisplatin/folinic acid, and 5-fluorouracil are the principal drugs being studied. Cis-

platin seems to be the most active single agent in the treatment of advanced cancer, although responses are short-lived. Irradiation is considered for patients who have disease of the upper third of the esophagus.[32,40]

NURSING MANAGEMENT

The major nursing concern for the patient with esophageal cancer is the alteration in nutrition that occurs because of dysphagia and other symptoms which interfere with oral intake.[41] Nursing interventions for the patient with this problem are listed below. Assisting the patient with the diagnosis and the prognosis are also important nursing concerns. A complete nursing assessment of patient and family coping patterns may help identify any psychosocial responses related to this catastrophic illness.

■ NURSING DIAGNOSIS

Altered nutrition, related to difficulty swallowing, frequent expectorations, and possible discomfort.

OUTCOME STANDARD AND CRITERIA

Nutritional intake meets metabolic requirements as evidenced by:
- Maintenance of present weight or gain until ideal weight is achieved
- Increase in oral intake
- Patient/family verbalization of knowledge of nutritional needs
- Fluid and electrolytes within normal limits
- Pink, moist mucous membranes and adequate skin turgor
- Positive nitrogen balance
- Adequate wound healing

NURSING INTERVENTIONS
- Complete a comprehensive nutritional assessment
- Monitor skin turgor, mucous membranes, and electrolytes to detect dehydration
- Maintain accurate intake and output record; daily weight
- Institute a calorie count
- Monitor results of laboratory studies, e.g., serum albumin, glucose, nitrogen balance
- Provide for frequent oral hygiene
- Provide comfort measures
- Provide for small frequent feedings using known diet preferences
- Elevate head of bed for meals and for 1 hour after meals
- Provide for rest before and after meals
- Monitor patient response to medical therapies to improve swallowing
- Instruct patient and family in specific nutritional needs and nutritional requirements after surgery if performed
- Document patient's tolerance to nutritional plan, nutritional supplements

INTESTINAL DISORDERS

Ischemic Disorders

Pathophysiology

Intestinal ischemia develops from a decrease in blood flow or decrease in tissue perfusion, producing an inadequate oxygen concentration to meet the requirements of the splanchnic bed.[1,2,42,43] Three major arterial trunks—the celiac axis, the superior mesenteric artery, and the inferior mesenteric artery—originate from the ventral aspect of the abdominal aorta and branch to form the vascular bed referred to as the *splanchnic circulation* (see Figure 51-6). These vessels interconnect to help protect against occlusive vascular disease. The splanchnic area receives approximately 20% of the cardiac output. Adequate splanchnic perfusion depends upon the patency of the major arteries, arteriolar resistance, perfusion pressure, arterial oxygen saturation, and the oxygen needs of the splanchnic bed. There are three broad categories of intestinal ischemia: acute occlusive mesenteric ischemia, chronic occlusive mesenteric ischemia, and nonocclusive mesenteric ischemia.

The box below summarizes factors that influence the splanchnic blood flow. Autoregulation, a physiological process by which changes in systemic arterial pressure are compensated for by a corresponding change in arterial tone, maintains a relatively stable capillary flow. The distribution of splanchnic blood flow within the intestinal wall and within the mucosa may be adjusted through the autoregulation process without altering the total splanchnic flow. Splanchnic blood flow is increased by the presence of food in the gastrointestinal tract. The process of digestion increases the oxygen requirement of the gastrointestinal organs, and the blood flow increases to meet the increased oxygen demand. The digestive hormones gastrin, secretin, and cholecystokinin increase the splanchnic flow when secreted during digestion.

Splanchnic blood flow is decreased when the cardiac output falls below a critical level and blood is shunted to the vital organs. Physical exercise, marked intraluminal pressure (abdominal distention), angiotensin II, alpha-stimulating sympathomimetic amines (epinephrine and norepinephrine), and cardiac glycosides (digitalis) result in arterial vasoconstriction, which decreases splanchnic flow.

The mucosal lining of the intestine is more sensitive to oxygen deprivation than the muscular and serosal layers. Changes occur in the absorptive cells within 5 to 10 minutes after occlusion of the blood flow. Necrosis, ulceration, and inflammatory cell infiltrate follow.[2,42] Inflammatory cell infiltrate is a response to the necrosis and the secondary bacterial invasion following ischemic episodes. The bacterial invasion occurs more commonly when the large colon (inferior mesenteric artery) is involved.

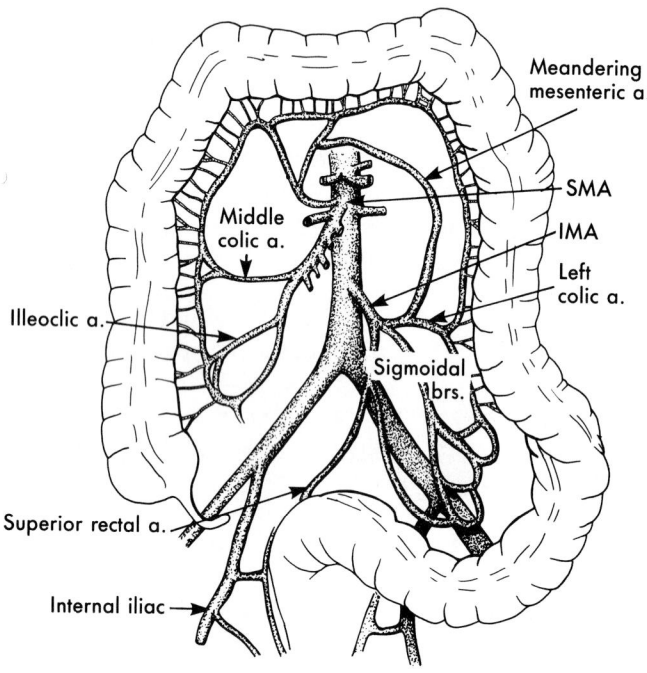

Figure 51-6   Splanchic circulation.

Splanchnic Blood Flow	
FACTORS INCREASING SPLANCHNIC BLOOD FLOW	**FACTORS DECREASING SPLANCHNIC BLOOD FLOW**
Presence of food	Physical activity
Digestive hormones: gastrin, secretin, cholecystokinin	Abdominal distention (marked increase in intraluminal pressure)
Metabolites produced during muscle activity	Angiotensin II
Beta-stimulating sympathomimetic amines (isoproterenol)	Alpha-stimulating sympathomimetic amines (epinephrine, norepinephrine)
	Cardiac glycosides (digitalis)
	Hypovolemia
	Decreased cardiac output

Acute Occlusive Mesenteric Ischemia. Acute occlusive mesenteric ischemia may be related to thrombosis or embolism. Acute mesenteric arterial thrombosis may be secondary to atherosclerosis, a dissecting aortic aneurysm, or systemic vasculitis. Acute mesenteric arterial embolism is commonly seen in elderly patients with a history of rheumatic heart disease, atherosclerotic heart disease with a mural thrombosis in the heart, or previous embolic episodes. It is also associated with oral contraceptive use. Occlusion by thrombus or embolus is generally seen in the superior mesenteric artery because of its small caliber and obliquity off the aorta. Occlusion of the superior mesenteric artery results in an intense spasm of the small intestine which is experienced by the patient as severe griping or colicky pain in the periumbilical area. The spasm relaxes, but the bowel is immobile. The immobility of the bowel results in a paralytic ileus. The abdomen becomes distended, and vomiting occurs. The abdominal distention and increased intraluminal pressure further decrease blood flow to the splanchnic bed. As the ischemia worsens, signs and symptoms intensify, and systemic signs as mediated by the autonomic nervous system occur.

The ischemic bowel loses protein, electrolytes, and fluid into the lumen and wall of the bowel. The third-space extracellular fluid loss decreases the circulating blood volume. Hypovolemia decreases cardiac output and arterial blood pressure and increases blood viscosity.

Chronic Occlusive Mesenteric Ischemia. The atherosclerotic changes in two of three of the major splanchnic vessels occuring over time are accompanied by the development of collateral blood flow. Under normal physiological functioning, the collateral flow minimizes and occasionally prevents intestinal ischemia. As the atherosclerosis progresses, the patient may develop intermittent transitory ischemia. After the ingestion of food, the oxygen requirement of the intestines increases. If blood flow cannot increase correspondingly with the increased need, intestinal ischemia occurs. The presenting symptom of chronic occlusive mesenteric ischemia is intestinal angina (intermittent midabdominal pain following eating). The intestinal angina may be compared to angina pectoris or coronary ischemia.

Nonocclusive Mesenteric Ischemia. Nonocclusive mesenteric ischemia is secondary to low blood flow to the mesenteric arteries without occlusion. Splanchnic vasoconstriction and atherosclerotic changes are predisposing factors. It is associated with severe hypoxemia, acute myocardial infarction, severe congestive heart failure, and shock. In the presence of lowered cardiac output and poor tissue perfusion, blood flow is redistributed to the vital organs. If vasocon-

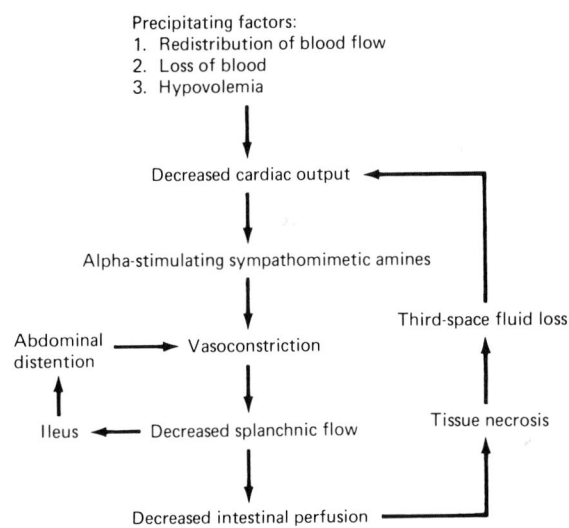

Figure 51-7   The self-sustaining cycle of nonocclusive mesenteric ischemia.

strictive drugs (e.g., alpha-adrenergics) are given to improve arterial pressure and cardiac output, the splanchnic blood flow is further decreased. If the ischemia continues because of atherosclerotic partial occlusions or the self-sustaining cycle of the temporary ischemia (Figure 51-7), transmural necrosis and frank infarction of the bowel may occur. The progression of ischemia has been previously described in the section on acute occlusive mesenteric ischemia above.

Ischemic Colitis. The reduction of blood flow to the inferior mesenteric artery is usually due to atherosclerotic disease, low flow states (hypovolemia), or interruption of the inferior mesenteric artery during abdominal surgery. The inferior mesenteric artery supplies the left colon and rectum.

Data Acquisition

History. Clinically, if the ischemic disorder is sudden or acute, the patient presents with an abrupt onset of severe abdominal pain, especially in the periumbilical area. Fluid loss, fever, and gastrointestinal bleeding may follow. Clinical signs of peritonitis and perforation, such as ileus, distention, and vomiting, are indications of the progression of the ischemia and the involvement of the muscular and serosal bowel layers. The clues to a diagnosis of nonocclusive mesenteric ischemia include (1) a history of atherosclerosis; (2) predisposing events of redistribution of blood flow, blood loss, and/or hypovolemia; and (3) abdominal pain of abrupt onset. The abdominal complaints may be severe, cramping periumbilical pain or, more commonly, diffuse, nonspecific abdominal pain. Dehydration, fever, an increased white blood cell count, and an elevated hematocrit may be present.

augments the progression to hypovolemic shock. In addition to the fluid loss, the toxins produced by the proliferation of bacteria cross the damaged intestinal membranes into the peritoneal cavity. The toxins are absorbed from the peritoneal cavity, and septicemia may result.[47,48,49,50]

Large Bowel Obstructions. Obstructions of the large intestine are most commonly related to neoplasms and volvulus of the sigmoid colon. The fluid and electrolyte loss is not as profound as in small bowel obstructions. The large bowel distends with gas and waste material and may perforate. When the ileocecal valve is competent, a colonic obstruction behaves like a closed-loop obstruction. Strangulation of the large bowel with the resulting sequelae may occur.

Data Acquisition

A review of clinical assessment findings found in bowel obstruction is presented in the box below.[47,48,49,50]

History. A patient with an intestinal obstruction may have a history of abdominal surgery that predisposes to the development of adhesions. Diverticulitis, a form of inflammatory bowel disease, also may lead to obstruction. The most common presenting symptoms of obstruction are crampy midabdominal pain, vomiting, abdominal distention, obstipation with failure to pass flatus or stool, and signs of fluid volume deficit. The crampy abdominal pain subsides as the intestinal motility decreases. Strangulation and peritonitis are suspected when the patient reports crampy pain followed by unrelenting severe abdominal pain. Vomiting is related to the location of the obstruction. Proximal obstructions are associated with profuse vomiting and minimal abdominal distention. In distal obstruction, abdominal distention is more pronounced. The vomitus in distal obstructions has a feculent odor, secondary to bacterial proliferation. Vomiting is not common in large bowel

obstruction when the ileocecal valve is competent. Abdominal distention is due to swallowed air. Systemic signs may also be seen with a superimposed infection including tachycardia, tachypnea, and fever.

Symptoms of bowel obstruction may be masked in elderly individuals in whom chronic constipation and fecal impaction are common. Misdiagnosis of abdominal distention can lead to delayed treatment. Abdominal pain may also be absent in elderly persons.[51]

Physical Assessment. In proximal bowel obstructions, auscultation of the abdomen reveals high-pitched, frequent bowel sounds known as *borborygmi*. The bowel sounds are slightly lower in pitch and last longer in the presence of distal obstructions. The changes in bowel sounds are related to the increased peristaltic contractions associated with early bowel obstruction. Bowel sounds usually decrease with vomiting and may disappear with complete obstruction. Rebound tenderness is also a common finding. Signs of peritonitis and shock may occur with a strangulated obstruction.

Diagnostic Procedures. Diagnosis of intestinal obstruction may be documented by abdominal x-rays including barium studies, which reveal abnormally large amounts of gas in the colon and the presence of dilated loops of bowel. In paralytic ileus, gaseous distention is more evenly distributed in the stomach and intestines.[13]

Abnormalites in electrolytes and renal function are common including depletion of sodium, chloride, and potassium and increased levels of BUN, creatinine, bicarbonate, and amylase. Elevated WBCs with a shift to the left are associated with sepsis the result of bacterial seeding from perforation and/or necrotic bowel produced by a strangulated obstruction. A decreased hematocrit may be seen if the patient has a strangulated obstruction with gastrointestinal bleeding.

Medical Management

The therapies used for intestinal obstruction are nasogastric decompression, fluid and electrolyte replacement, and surgery.[48,49,50] Treatment is initiated to prevent shock and restore fluid and electrolyte losses. Supportive therapy includes intravenous normal saline and nasogastric suctioning. A Foley catheter is inserted to obtain accurate measurement of urinary output. Normal saline is continued until renal blood flow is adequate as indicated by a urine output equal to or greater than 30 ml/hr. Electrolyte replacement is based on serum values. Potassium replacement needs to be carefully administered according to renal function.

Fluid assessments are crucial, and central venous pressure or pulmonary artery pressure monitoring

---

Common Signs and Symptoms of Bowel Obstruction
Abdominal pain (cramping; midabdominal)
Abdominal distention
Borborygmi with pain (early)
Decreased bowel sounds (after vomiting)
Muscle guarding and tenderness
Rebound tenderness
Obstipation
Peritonitis*
Hypotension*

* With strangulated obstruction.

may be used depending on the patient's cardiovascular status. If the patient is in hypovolemic shock (see section on gastrointestinal hemorrhage) or has a strangulated obstruction, blood and plasma are used with colloids or crystalloids to replace fluid volume.

Nasogastric intubation is used to decompress stomach contents, decrease edema, and relieve abdominal distention. Measurement of abdominal girths should be instituted early to monitor progress. Measures to ensure an effective breathing pattern also need to be started. Gastric decompression may be enough to restore peristalsis. Analgesics may be withheld because they mask the symptoms of bowel strangulation. The critical care nurse should institute general comfort measures and nursing interventions to assist the patient in coping with the pain. Nasogastric suction may help to relieve some of the discomfort.

Long, weighted gastrointestinal tubes such as the Miller-Abbott and cantor types are occasionally used for decompression. These tubes are inserted mechanically into the intestine after the balloon near the tip has been filled with mercury to weight the balloon. The tube passes by peristalsis through the pylorus into the duodenum. Advancement of longer segments may lead to kinking of the tube. Patency is maintained by irrigations. Accurate intake and output records of nasogastric or gastrointestinal output are mandatory. A patient may lose up to 3,000 ml or more via a nasogastric tube within 24 hours with intestinal obstructions, predisposing to further fluid and electrolyte problems.

Surgery is the usual treatment for intestinal obstruction.[49,52] The timing of surgery depends on the severity of fluid and electrolyte changes, the duration of the obstruction, the risk of strangulation, and changes in vital organ functioning. Many surgeons believe surgery is always indicated because strangulation may occur without signs and symptoms. A 2-day trial of nasogastric suction may be instituted. Radiological findings and symptoms are then evaluated to determine the need for surgery. Even if emergent surgery is performed on a strangulated bowel or bowel perforation, fluid and electrolytes are replaced before the procedure. Regimens vary, but broad-spectrum antibiotics often are used as prophylaxis against sepsis. Sepsis is thought to be associated with bacterial seeding from perforation or a necrotic bowel.

Different operative procedures are recommended for mechanical small obstructions according to their cause. Options include lysis of adhesions, reduction of hernias, bypass of obstructions, and excisions of obstructions or proximal enterocutaneous fistulas. Left colonic obstructions are generally treated in three stages. Initially, a proximal colostomy is performed to relieve distention and provide a fecal outlet. The

---

Nursing Diagnoses Applicable to Intestinal Obstruction

Fluid volume deficit, related to intraluminal fluid loop and hypovolemic shock

Altered comfort, related to bowel edema and distention

Potential for infection, related to bacterial seeding from perforation or necrotic bowel

Potential for ineffective breathing pattern, related to abdominal distention

---

diseased segment is then removed from the colon distal to the colostomy, with anastomosis of the distal segment. When the anastomosis has healed, the colostomy is closed.[52]

Nursing Management

The nursing plan of care is focused on reestablishing fluid balance and preventing infection. Nursing diagnoses applicable to this patient population are listed in the box above.[53,54,55]

Inflammatory Bowel Disease

The inflammatory bowel diseases, ulcerative colitis and Crohn's disease, are chronic disorders. *Diverticulitis* is a form of inflammatory bowel disease caused by perforation of one or more pouches of mucosa and submucosa (diverticula). These disorders have no known cure and are characterized by remissions and exacerbations. Patients with inflammatory bowel disease may be admitted to the critical care unit with acute exacerbations or complications.

Ulcerative colitis is an idiopathic inflammation involving the mucosa of the colon. *Crohn's disease* may occur in one or more areas involving any portion of the gastrointestinal system from the mouth to the anus. Intestinal and systemic manifestations of the disease, some of which may necessitate admission to the critical care unit, are common and affect almost all body organs (see the box on p. 1162).[56,57,58]

A brief review of the pathophysiology, clinical assessment, and medical management of Crohn's disease and ulcerative colitis are presented as they pertain to the critical care setting. Nursing management of the patient with an ileostomy is highlighted.

Crohn's Disease

Pathophysiology. Crohn's disease is an inflammatory disorder of the gastrointestinal tract sometimes referred to as regional enteritis, granulomatous colitis, granulomatous ileitis, or transmural disease. Crohn's disease may involve any part of the gastro-

---

Systemic Manifestations of Inflammatory Bowel Disease

ACUTE COMPLICATIONS
Toxic megacolon
Massive gastrointestinal hemorrhage
Perforation of the ileum
Bowel obstruction

CHRONIC MANIFESTATIONS
Rheumatoid arthritis
Ocular disease (iritis, scleritis)
Oral lesions
Fatty liver
Inflammation of the portal tract
Gallstones
Urinary tract calculi
Urethral obstruction
Iron deficiency anemia

TABLE 51-8 **Comparison of Crohn's Disease and Ulcerative Colitis**

Crohn's Disease	Ulcerative Colitis
Transmural	Mucosal
Segmental	Progressive, starting in the rectum and continuing proximally
Involves entire GI tract	Confined to the colon and rectum
Watery diarrhea	Bloody diarrhea
Partial intestinal obstruction	Hemorrhage
Fistulas, abscesses	Bowel perforation
Recurrence after surgical intervention	Cure with total proctocolectomy and ileostomy

intestinal tract, although the small bowel, particularly the terminal ileum, and the large intestine are the common sites. Bacterial, viral, allergic, autoimmune, and hereditary factors have been explored as possible causes of Crohn's disease, but the etiology remains unknown. The disease is pathologically different from ulcerative colitis even though the clinical signs are similar (Table 51-8).[2,56,59]

Data Acquisition

History and Physical Assessment. The initial clinical symptoms of Crohn's disease include crampy abdominal pain and diarrhea. Pain is most often associated with eating. The narrowing bowel lumen creates a partial bowel obstruction, leading to increased intestinal motility, watery unformed stools, and intestinal distention. The increased motility and distention exert pressure on the afferent visceral nervous system which is perceived as abdominal pain. Motility of the bowel is stimulated by the ingestion of food, increasing pain. These symptoms can progress to a self-inflicted nutritional deficiency when meals are omitted because of the associated pain. Weight loss can be severe. Gross bleeding is infrequent and perforation rare. The initial involvement in Crohn's disease is in the terminal portion of the ileum. The constant right-sided abdominal pain mimics appendicitis.

Several mechanisms are responsible for increased intestinal motility including partial intestinal obstruction, bacterial proliferation, lactose intolerance, and surgical loss of bowel. Increased fluid secretion in the bowel lumen and bowel motility associated with intestinal obstruction decrease the absorptive capacity in the diseased bowel. When the bowel contents stagnate behind the partial obstruction or after the surgical bypass of a loop of bowel, bacterial growth may proliferate and alter the pH of the bowel, thereby preventing the effective utilization and reabsorption of bile salts. Bile salts in the right colon have a cathartic effect and cause watery, frequent bowel movements.

Nutritional deficiency may develop in response to pain associated with eating, the effects of chronic water and electrolyte loss, or the decreased absorptive ability of the bowel. Loss of functioning of the terminal ileum results in malabsorption of vitamin B_{12} and fats and in fluid and electrolyte imbalances. Vitamin B_{12} must be replaced intramuscularly. Malabsorption of bile salts in the small intestine also occurs, altering the amount of circulating bile salts and fat absorption and causing steatorrhea.

Diagnostic Procedures. Clinical diagnosis of Crohn's disease is primarily done by sigmoidoscopy. Colonoscopic assessment is done to ascertain the extent of the colitis. Endoscopic evaluation usually reveals stenotic narrowing of the bowel lumen, longitudinal and transverse ulcers (cobblestoning), and fistulous tracts. The rectum is usually not involved. A rectal biopsy may help in the diagnosis.

Medical Management. Medical treatment of Crohn's disease focuses on symptomatic relief of diarrhea and abdominal pain. Analgesics including codeine, diphenoxylate hydrochloride with atropine (Lomotil), corticosteroids, and salicylazosulfapyridine (Azulfidine) are used. Cholestyramine (Questran) is given to bind bile salts when necessary, and anemia is treated with iron (intramuscularly), vitamin B_{12}, and folic acid. Corticosteroids may be given intravenously during an acute attack, progressing to oral tablets.

Nutritional support of the patient with inflammatory bowel disease is imperative. Most clinicians agree that bowel rest is important.[60] Use of central venous total parenteral nutrition provides bowel rest while achieving positive nitrogen balance and repletion of nutritional deficits (see Chapter 11). Remission rates of 60% to 80% have been achieved, surgical intervention has been avoided, and short bowel syndrome has been reduced.

Surgery is palliative and is generally performed only when medical therapy is ineffective and the disease process interferes with the patient's activities of daily living (intractable disease). Additional indications for surgery in Crohn's disease include partial or complete intestinal obstruction, internal or external fistulas, and massive hemorrhage.[61]

If the disease involves the distal stomach or duodenum, a bypass procedure (gastrojejunostomy) is sometimes necessary. When the disease involves the small bowel or segments of the large bowel, a segmental resection is employed. A bypass procedure is used only if an abscess is present. Resection of the diseased segment is also performed. If the entire large bowel is involved, total colectomy and ileostomy are necessary. An ileal stoma (ileostomy) may be created when Crohn's disease involves the entire colon or to treat ulcerative colitis (see Nursing Management).

Ulcerative Colitis

Pathophysiology. Ulcerative colitis is a disease of unknown etiology in which there is uniform inflammation of the mucosal lining of the colon and rectum. Pathological changes in the colon are usually confined to the mucosal and submucosal layers, generally beginning in the rectum and progressing proximally in the colon.

Toxic megacolon is associated with ulcerative colitis and is seen in fulminant disease. It occurs when the wall of the colon has been damaged by colitis. Contractility of the wall is lost, and massive dilatation of the large colon results.[58,59]

Data Acquisition

History and Physical Assessment. The presenting symptom of ulcerative colitis is bloody diarrhea, with as many as 30 stools a day. The rectal involvement creates a sensation of urgency with an immediate need to defecate when fecal material enters the rectum. The mucosa of the colon is very friable, and the first sign may be bright red blood in the stool. Signs and symptoms of orthostasis or hypovolemia may be present.

Additional symptoms observed in ulcerative colitis include abdominal pain, tenesmus, weight loss, vomiting, and fever. Extracolonic manifestations are common, including arthritis, iritis, skin lesions, and hepatic dysfunction. During exacerbation of the disease, extracolonic problems worsen, but with treatment, most improve. One exception is hepatic dysfunction.[57]

Diagnostic Procedures. Proctosigmoidoscopy reveals diffuse erythema, mucosal inflammation, and loss of the normal vascular network.[62] Bleeding may occur when the mucosa is gently touched with a cotton applicator. In advanced disease, ulcers and pseudopolyps may be seen. Radiography may show crypt abscesses, mucosal ulcerations, and shortening of the colon.

Medical Management. Medical management of ulcerative colitis is directed to treatment of symptoms. Antiinflammatory agents given intravenously (such as ACTH) are used initially; later, oral corticosteroids (prednisone) are used for maintenance therapy. Salicylazosulfapyridine (Azulfidine) and prednisone are most often used in managing ulcerative colitis.[63] Corticosteroid enemas may be used to treat symptoms.[64] Fluid and electrolyte replacement is based on the extent and duration of the disease. Weight loss is frequently observed, so dietary therapy is an important aspect of management.

In acute situations, the colon may be placed completely at rest with the use of elemental diets and clear liquids. Intravenous fluids and blood replacement may be necessary with symptoms of fluid volume deficit and rectal hemorrhages. Total parenteral nutrition may be used for severely debilitated patients to control symptoms such as abdominal pain and diarrhea. Bowel rest is thought to decrease the work of absorption, decrease mechanical trauma caused by passage of food, and decrease production of digestive secretions.

Diarrhea is treated by altering the contents of the bowel lumen. Metamucil, a bulk-forming agent, and aluminum hydroxide are used to thicken bowel contents. Opiates are not used as antidiarrheal agents because they may precipitate toxic megacolon.

When ulcerative colitis interferes with the patient's life, surgery, the only curative therapy, may be indicated. The usual procedures are general or subtotal colectomy and ileostomy.[61,65] Elective procedures may include a proctocolectomy and ileostomy, continent ileostomy, colectomy and ileorectal anastomosis, and ileoanal revision. These techniques preserve some intestinal continuity and anal sphincter continence. The incidence of colon cancer is higher in patients with a history of ulcerative colitis than in the general population. When cancer is suspected or diagnosed, the colon and rectum are surgically removed.

NURSING MANAGEMENT

Nursing in inflammatory bowel disease is primarily concerned with observation and monitoring of the patient, postoperative assessments and care if appropriate, and assisting with alterations in nutrition. If an ileostomy is planned or has been performed, this is an important aspect of care. The current discussion is confined to this topic, with emphasis on patient teaching.

For the patient undergoing ostomy surgery, rehabilitation begins before the surgical procedure and continues beyond the period of hospitalization. The nurse is involved in assessing the patient's needs and planning a rehabilitation program. This process may begin in the critical care area if the patient is physiologically stable and ready to learn. Initial assessments include the patient's and significant others' knowledge of the disease, the meaning of the ileostomy, and family dynamics. Patient teaching is a major nursing concern.

A confusing aspect of ileostomy care is distinguishing different surgical procedures and ostomy types. A *colostomy* is a fecal diversion procedure involving the large bowel; there are several types. An *ileal conduit* is a urinary diversion procedure. An *ileostomy* is a fecal diversion procedure employing the small bowel. Defecation cannot be regulated by diet or irrigations as in a colostomy. A pouch is worn at all times to collect fecal drainage. Bowel preparations are contraindicated because they precipitate severe fluid and electrolyte loss.

The stoma of an ileostomy is bright red and contains no nerve endings (Figure 51-8). Since there is no feeling in the stoma, close observation is necessary during pouch change for alteration in stomal color or the presence of small ulcers on the stoma. Change to a dusky color may indicate pressure on the vascular supply to the stoma. The presence of small ulcers may indicate recurrence of Crohn's disease. The stoma is

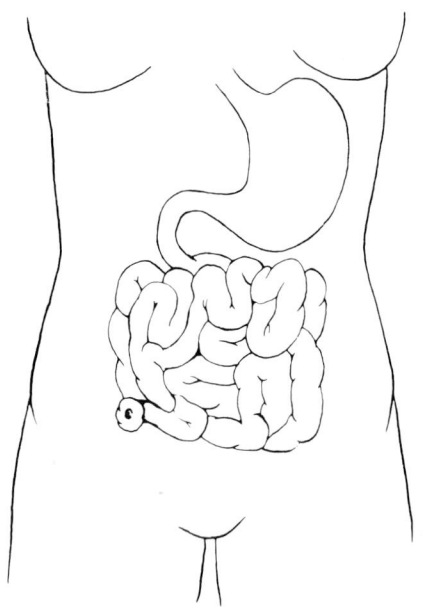

Figure 51-8 Ileal stoma.

a mucosal membrane and may bleed a small amount when cleansed.

The new ileostomate remains on a low-residue diet for approximately 6 weeks following surgery. This allows the bowel time to adjust. Then, one food is added each week from a list of high-fiber foods. The patient should be instructed to chew food thoroughly and to eat high-fiber foods only as part of a meal. High-fiber foods such as celery, nuts, corn, coleslaw, coconut, popcorn, dried fruits, and whole vegetables are not digested by the gastrointestinal tract. If a large mass of undigested food develops in the small bowel of an ileostomate, it could become lodged at a kink or narrowing in the bowel and create a food blockage. If the blocked food does not move forward, the result is complete intestinal obstruction. The cycle that follows intestinal obstruction begins with fluid and electrolyte accumulation in the bowel and progresses to shock.

The patient may recognize early signs of food obstruction (Table 51-9) by correlating changes in the ileostomy output with the diet. A food blockage may be relieved by the patient's getting into a knee-check position and cupping the hand gently under the stoma. Since tense abdominal muscles will prevent a blockage from moving out of the bowel, the ileostomate should relax in a hot tub or hot shower and then assume the knee-chest position. If the obstruction has been present for over 3 hours without relief or if the patient is nauseated or vomiting or no drainage is coming around the blockage, the physician should be notified. The physician may then prescribe mechanical removal of the blockage by irrigation.

The pouch opening may be too small because the stoma swells when the bowel becomes partially or totally obstructed. A disposable pouch with a larger stoma opening and a skin barrier should be applied and left on during the ileostomy irrigation. Careful recordings of intake and output are required so that adequate fluid replacement can be provided. The patient may experience diarrhea for several days following an obstruction.

The small bowel will absorb all the nutrients, fluid, and electrolytes an ileostomate requires. Immediately after surgery, the patient has a high fluid and electrolyte concentration in the ileostomy output. An ileostomy adaptation occurs approximately 3 to 6 months after surgery; the drainage becomes the consistency of toothpaste, and more fluid and electrolytes are reabsorbed. The ileostomate can lose more fluid and electrolytes faster than a person with a colon and should be taught to replace fluid losses immediately with products high in needed electrolytes. If the ileostomate cannot keep up with the fluid losses, the physician should be contacted.

TABLE 51-9   **Intestinal Obstruction from a Food Blockage with an Ileostomy**

Symptom	Cause
Discharge changes from semisolid to liquid	Food is blocked, but water passes around it—a partial intestinal obstruction
Total volume of output increases, and ileostomy functions constantly	Water is drawn from the extracellular fluid in an attempt to rid the body of the obstruction, and the intestines become hyperactive
Objectionable odor	Bacterial proliferation occurs at the site of obstruction and causes fermentation of the bowel content
Cramping, followed by increased watery output	Increased bowel activity to move blockage forward
Distended abdomen	The obstruction traps gas and liquids in the bowel lumen
Vomiting	Reverse peristalsis. The body's attempt to move the increased bowel contents in the direction of least resistance
No ileostomy output	Complete intestinal obstruction

Diarrhea in an ileostomate can be described as hot, watery stool that necessitates frequent (every 30 minutes) emptying of the pouch. Diarrhea may be associated with other medical problems or may be stimulated by specific foods in some persons. The amounts eaten at a given time also affect the amount of ileostomy output. Bananas, boiled milk, tapioca, and peanut butter are effective in thickening diarrheal stools.

The ileostomate with recurrent Crohn's disease or multiple small bowel resections may have chronic diarrhea associated with the *short bowel syndrome.* In the short bowel syndrome, the transit time is shortened, and absorption of fluid is limited. The result is watery stools. Absorption of vitamin B_{12} and fat may be affected if large amounts of terminal ileum have been resected. Steatorrhea may be noted with the ileostomy output.

The ileostomate cannot absorb hard tablets or enteric-coated tablets, and drugs formulated in this manner should not be prescribed. Timed-release and sustained-action capsules and tablets should also be avoided in patients with an ileostomy. The timed-release drugs may not remain in the bowel for 8 or 12 hours, so the dosage received by the patient cannot be ascertained. Lomotil tablets should be crushed, or the drug should be given in liquid form because it is not absorbed otherwise. Liquid medication is the best for ileostomates. If there is doubt about the absorbability of a tablet, it may be dropped into a glass without stirring and left undisturbed for 30 minutes. If the pill has begun to dissolve by that time, the patient should be able to obtain full benefit from the drug. Medications that promote potassium or sodium excretion (digoxin, diuretics) may create severe problems for an ileostomate because of the precise fluid and electrolyte balance the ileostomy patient maintains. Antibiotics will cause a flora change in the

ileum, resulting in diarrhea. Careful fluid replacement is necessary.

Sexuality is an important aspect of rehabilitation after ileostomy. The ileostomy should not alter the patient's sexual patterns. Preoperative sexual patterns should be assessed before nursing interventions are planned.

Odor is a major concern of many ileostomates. It can be controlled by the use of odor-proof pouches, oral preparations, or pouch deodorants. Bismuth subgallate (Devrom), oral preparation for odor control, may be purchased without a precription. The tablet is chewed before meals and will effectively control odor and thicken the stool. When the patient first starts taking bismuth subgallate, the tongue may turn black and the stool may become black. The discoloration is temporary. Bismuth subgallate is contraindicated in renal disease and with warfarin (coumadin) therapy. The drug should be omitted for 48 hours before radiography because it causes opaque areas on the films. Overdosage of bismuth subgallate or long-term misuse may result in metal toxicosis. The signs of metal toxicosis include myoclonic jerks, tremors, inability to walk, loss of balance, poor concentration, depression, insomnia, and confusion.

Dietary control of odors is also possible. Certain foods produce more odor, especially when eaten in large quantities. Fish, asparagus, eggs, onions, garlic, and some spices may be limited when odor is a concern. However, the use of odor-proof pouches is an effective method of controlling odor. Odor will be released when the pouch is emptied, but the patient can be reminded that people with rectums also have odor with bowel movements. Sprays and deodorizers are available for use when emptying the pouch.

A proper pouching system is important to prevent stool leakage. The stoma opening in the ileostomy pouch should be 1/8 inch larger than the stoma to

---

Basic Consideration in Choosing Disposable Pouches

1. Type of ostomy will indicate:
   a. Spout opening: drainable, urinary spout, closed
   b. Material of pouch: odor-proof, odor-resistant
   c. Skin protection: karaya, Stomahesive, Collyseels, HolliHesive
2. Parastomal skin area and stoma:
   a. Stoma size and shape: protruding, flushed, edematous
   b. Stoma drainage location
   c. Available space for faceplate
   d. Presence of abdominal folds, dimples, scars
   e. Stomal complications: prolapse, retraction, ulcerations
   f. Presence of a stomal support: rod, catheter, loop-lock
3. Physical abilities of patient:
   a. Arthritis, paralysis
   b. Poor eyesight, blindness
4. Mental abilities of patient
   a. Confusion, senility
   b. Emotional aspects: denial
5. Financial situation of patient
6. Patient sensitivities:
   a. Adhesives, tapes
   b. Plastics, vinyls, rubber
7. Pouches available in area:
   a. Starter openings helpful in hospital
   b. Pouch material: noise factors, odor-proof
   c. Drainable rather than closed-end for hospital use

---

allow peristaltic movements. The residual digestive enzymes in ileostomy output are very irritating to the skin, and severe skin denudation can develop with exposure to ileostomy output. A skin barrier is placed up to the base of the stoma to protect the exposed skin. There are many effective skin barriers on the market. Choosing an appropriate pouch, which should be odor-proof and drainable, is discussed in the box above. A consistent pouch application procedure should be used in teaching the patient.

■ **NURSING DIAGNOSES**

Nursing diagnoses most applicable to the patient with inflammatory bowel disease are *altered nutrition,* related to inadequate oral intake as a result of anorexia, taste alterations (resulting from side effects of medications used to treat inflammatory bowel disease), abdominal pain, diarrhea, and malabsorption; and *knowledge deficit,* related to ileostomy care.

OUTCOME STANDARDS AND CRITERIA

Expected outcomes for the patient with nutritional deficiencies include:

- Maintenance of weight, or weight gain
- Albumin, transferrin, and fibronectin levels within normal limits
- Positive nitrogen balance

Outcomes for the patient with a knowledge deficit should be tailored to the patient's individual situation and supportive of self-care needs. Significant others need to be included in the plan of care.

NURSING INTERVENTIONS

Nursing interventions are geared to nutrition assessments, body energy requirements, and evaluation of patient tolerance/response to the plan of care (see Chapter 11, Nutrition). Total parenteral solutions should be administered according to protocol. Monitoring for signs of hyperglycemia and line sepsis are important as they are the most frequent complications of this nutritional therapy.

Patient teaching should include self-care activities in anticipation of the patient's discharge. The foregoing section on ileostomy care discusses important teaching aspects.

PERITONEAL AND ABDOMINAL WALL DISORDERS

Peritonitis and cutaneous fistulas are common complications of gastrointestinal disorders. This section presents pathophysiology, clinical assessment, collaborative management, and appropriate nursing diagnoses.

Peritonitis

Peritonitis (inflammation of the peritoneum) may be primary or secondary. Approximately 1% of the cases of peritonitis result from primary infections of the peritoneum. Primary peritonitis may be idiopathic or tuberculous in origin. Secondary peritonitis occurs when the peritoneal cavity is contaminated as a result of a defect or alteration in the visceral wall. Perforated peptic ulcer, ruptured appendix, ischemic bowel disease, intestinal obstruction, trauma, pancreatitis, or perforated colon may progress to generalized peritonitis.[1,66]

Pathophysiology

The peritoneum is a semipermeable membrane that encloses the abdominal viscera and mesentery in a saclike structure open only in the female (at the fallopian tubes). A small amount of serous fluid is secreted by the peritoneum to prevent friction between the viscera during peristalsis. The surface area of the peritoneum is comparable to the skin. This large amount of absorption area and the bidirectional transfer of fluid, electrolytes, and other material play a role in the process of peritonitis.

As a defense mechanism, the peritoneum localizes,

or walls off, areas of contamination to prevent their spread. The local reaction of the peritoneum to contamination involves vascular dilatation and increased capillary permeability.[1,2] Large numbers of polymorphonuclear leukocytes pour into the peritoneal cavity. Phagocytosis of bacteria and any foreign material in the area is carried out by the polymorphonuclear leukocytes. Fibroplastic exudate is deposited on the peritoneum and plasters the adjacent bowel, mesentery, and omentum to the inflamed area, forming a watertight seal. This process is referred to as *localization,* or *walling-off,* of the inflammation, preventing diffuse peritonitis. Localization is not successful if the contamination is continuous or the original contamination is massive. In these instances, the peritoneal defense mechanism is overwhelmed.

The mechanism of peritoneal irritation in contamination from the stomach, pancreas, and upper small bowel is initially a chemical reaction from the spillage of potent digestive enzymes. Spillage from the lower portion of the small bowel and from the colon causes peritoneal inflammation from the entry of the bacterial content into the peritoneal cavity. The irritation stimulates vascular dilatation, hyperemia, and a fluid shift. The vascular dilatation and hyperemia lead to an increased number of polymorphonuclear leukocytes in the inflamed area. The absorption capacity of the peritoneum is also increased, facilitating the absorption of toxins and bacteria into the bloodstream and leading to septicemia and bacteremia. A fluid shift occurs from the extracellular fluid compartment into the free peritoneal space, into the loose connective tissue (as edema), and into the lumen of the atonic gastrointestinal tract. The translocation of water, electrolytes, and protein into this third-space compartment depletes the circulating blood volume. The rate of fluid loss from the circulating volume into the third-space compartment is proportional to the degree of peritoneal involvement.

Before treatment is instituted, the cardiovascular system response is based on hypovolemia secondary to the fluid shift. In hypovolemic shock, cardiac output falls, filling pressure is low, and tissue perfusion is diminished, with resultant tissue ischemia. If septicemia is associated with peritonitis, peripheral pooling with decreased venous return occurs, followed by a further decrease in cardiac output and a lower filling pressure. In septic shock there is failure of cardiac output, and preload should be sustained with volume replacement.

Catecholamines (epinephrine and norepinephrine) are released in response to the acute decrease in circulating volume, resulting in vasoconstriction, increased pulse rate, and diaphoresis (see Figure 51-1). Adrenocorticotropic hormone (ACTH) and aldosterone are released through a pituitary–adrenal axis response. This results in water and sodium retention and potassium loss, since the body attempts to conserve fluid. When the circulatory system is unable to maintain adequate tissue perfusion, metabolic acidosis develops secondary to anaerobic metabolism.

Primary Peritonitis. In primary idiopathic peritonitis the bacterial agent is thought to gain contact with the peritoneum through the vascular system or through the fallopian tubes.[66,67] The peritonitis is manifested by severe generalized, steady, burning abdominal pain; fever and chills; irritability; and diarrhea. The bowel sounds are either hypoactive or absent. Primary idiopathic peritonitis is seen more often in children than in adults and is associated with infection by the same organism elsewhere in the body.

Diagnostic findings include white blood cell counts in which there is an elevated number of leukocytes, primarily polymorphonuclear. Peritoneal aspiration is performed to distinguish between primary idiopathic peritonitis and a ruptured viscus. The aspirated fluid is evaluated by culture, sensitivity, and electrolyte studies.

Tuberculous peritonitis is associated with tuberculous invasion elsewhere in the body. There are two types of tuberculous peritonitis: wet and dry. Wet tuberculous peritonitis is associated with the presence of copious abdominal ascites. In dry tuberculous peritonitis, fibrinous adhesions are present and result in a matting effect in the intestines and omentum. The onset of tuberculous peritonitis is insidious, with development of dull, steady, generalized abdominal pain of varying intensity. Abdominal distention is seen in approximately half the subjects. General malaise, weakness, weight loss, low-grade fever, tachycardia, and a doughy abdomen are symptoms seen in tuberculous peritonitis. The slow onset of vague symtoms makes the diagnosis difficult. The diagnosis is based on evaluations of aspirated peritoneal fluid for specific gravity, albumin level, and white blood cell count. Less than half the patients have positive tuberculous cultures from the peritoneum. The drug treatment is isoniazid alone. *p*-Aminosalicylic acid and antibiotics are given if active tuberculosis is found elsewhere in the patient.

Secondary Peritonitis. Secondary acute peritonitis is the result of peritoneal contamination from various causes. Perforated peptic ulcer is the most common cause of peritonitis, followed by a ruptured appendix; gangrene of the bowel from strangulation, obstruction, or mesenteric ischemia; gonorrheal salpingitis (pelvic peritonitis); acute gangrenous cholecystitis; ruptured diverticulum; trauma; and surgery. In gangrene of the bowel, the rapid absorption of spilled toxins increases the severity of the process.[1] Penetrating trauma that ruptures a hollow viscus results in spillage contamination. Peritonitis may develop in the patient with penetrating abdominal trauma without visceral perforation because of the entry of foreign material, such as clothing or a bullet, into the peritoneal cavity, as well as the infection from the abdomen being open to the environment. Severe blunt trauma may lead to peritonitis by disrupting the abdominal viscera or separating the viscus from its blood supply. Peritonitis from surgery may occur if bile leakage develops, a localized infection spreads, or an anastomosis breaks down.[1,53,68]

Data Acquisition

History. The history obtained for a patient with peritonitis includes the possible sources of contamination and/or causes of infection of the peritoneum.

Physical Assessment. Presenting symptoms of peritonitis include pain with any movement, including respirations.[1,2] The pain is most intense at the site of advancing inflammation. If there is decreased intensity or decreased extent of pain, localization of the peritonitis is considered. The patient is very ill and may be found lying quietly in bed in the supine position with knees flexed. Since respiratory movements increase the pain, the patient's breathing is usually limited to shallow, rapid respirations. The respiratory system increases its effort to oxygenate the circulating blood to compensate for the metabolic acidosis. The increased respiratory activity creates an increase in the oxygen requirement of the muscles of respiration. Thus, there is an increased demand on the respiratory system at a time when painful respiratory movements limit the respiratory function. When the required workload exceeds the ability of the respiratory system, respiratory decompensation occurs, with resultant respiratory acidosis.

The pulse is rapid, weak, and thready, representing the cardiovascular changes that may be occurring, i.e., decreased cardiac output and decreased tissue perfusion. Rebound tenderness and muscle rigidity with voluntary guarding are also present in peritonitis. Additional clinical signs associated with peritonitis include anorexia, nausea, vomiting, fever with chills, decreased urinary output, abdominal distention, and absence of bowel sounds.

The workload of the kidneys is increased by the presence of circulating toxins, pigments, and necrotic tissue products in the bloodstream. Decreased cardiac output, vasoconstriction, and decreased renal perfusion affect the ability of the kidneys to excrete the metabolic waste products and toxins. Acute renal insufficiency is monitored by hourly observation of urine output and specific gravity measurements of the urine, and through periodic serum creatinine and BUN determinations.

Diagnostic Procedures. Diagnostic studies include white blood cell counts which demonstrate an elevated leukocyte level, especially polymorphonuclear cells. Serial white blood cell counts are made to evaluate the progress of the peritonitis. If the diagnosis is not clear-cut, the peritoneum may be aspirated. Abdominal x-rays demonstrate the amount of abdominal distention and inflammation and edema of the intestinal wall. Free air will be present on abdominal films in the event of a perforation.

Medical Management

Early detection of peritonitis and immediate intervention may inhibit its life-threatening cycle. The goals of therapy are fluid and electrolyte balance, control of infection, relief of pain and ileus, and maintenance of blood pressure.

The treatment of primary idiopathic peritonitis is conservative supportive therapy. Intravenous fluid replacement is monitored by CVP or PCWP blood pressure, and urinary output. Intravenous administration of broad-spectrum antibiotics is begun immediately. The antibiotics used may be changed after the causative organism has been isolated. The patient is maintained in a semi-Fowler's position to assist in localization of the infection. Nasogastric suctioning is instituted to prevent abdominal distention secondary to fluid and gas accumulation in the atonic bowel.

The treatment of secondary peritonitis is timely surgical intervention after supportive therapy has stabilized the patient's cardiac and pulmonary status. The supportive therapy includes insertion of an intravenous catheter to begin immediate fluid replacement, volume monitoring, a nasogastric tube for decompression, and an indwelling Foley catheter for urinary monitoring. The amount of fluid replacement is determined by the CVP and hourly urinary output. Plasma, albumin, Ringer's lactate, and D_5W may be given for fluid replacement. Antibiotics are started intravenously, and oxygen is used to augment the respiratory exchange. Analgesics are administered for pain relief. Patients with a history of heavy cigarette smoking, obesity, or debilitation may require mechanical respiratory assistance. Blood gas levels are determined to assess the patient's respiratory status. Early signs of respiratory decompensation include increased arteriovenous differentiation and decreased arterial carbon dioxide from hyperventilation. The pulse rate continues to be elevated, with a slight increase in blood pressure despite the restoration of blood volume. Clinically, the patient is flushed, restless, and anxious, with rapid, shallow, labored breathing.

The approach to operation includes control of contamination, removal of any foreign material, and drainage of any collected fluid. Contamination may be controlled by simple closure, excision, or exteriorization. Peritoneal irrigation during the surgical procedure decreases the mortality and morbidity from acute diffuse peritonitis. The type of contaminant and the age and general health of the patient influence the patient's prognosis.

After surgical intervention, some patients have an open wound, and intensive wound care is necessary. Continuous irrigation of the peritoneal cavity may be instituted. Two to four dialysis catheters may be placed in the peritoneal cavity during surgery. One to three catheters are used to instill antibiotic solution; one catheter is used for drainage. Accurate recording of the intake and output is essential.

The cause of the peritonitis determines the surgical procedure. Peritonitis secondary to perforation of the colon often necessitates diversion of the fecal stream by a colostomy. The care of the colostomy differs according to location of the stoma in the large intestine. The contents of the small bowel entering the ascending colon are liquid in consistency. The contents of the transverse colon are soft stool containing varying amounts of unabsorbed water. As the contents of the large colon move through the descending and sigmoid colon, the water is absorbed, and the stool becomes firm.

A general rule when caring for a new postoperative colostomy patient is to use a skin barrier and an open-end, drainable, odor-proof pouch. The skin barrier is placed on clean, dry skin at the base of the stoma. It is important that the barrier hug the stoma but not ride up onto the stoma. The opening cut in the pouch must be ⅛ inch larger than the stoma. The edema of the stoma decreases in the early postoperative days, and the opening in the pouch and the skin barrier are adjusted to these changes.

In a loop colostomy, a rod is placed under a loop of bowel to support the bowel until adhesions with the abdominal wall occur (Figure 51-9). The pouching procedure for a loop colostomy with a rod is made easier by keeping some simple facts in mind. It is almost impossible to place a skin barrier or pouch over a large stoma and not get mucus from the stoma onto the materials. Any mucus trapped under the skin barrier may irritate the skin and create a leakage in the pouch system. A washer is cut through one side and placed under the rod. The adhesive backing of the pouch is removed and cut into sections, then replaced over the adhesive. The adhesive is then protected as the pouch is placed on the patient's body. A pouch that is directed straight to the patient's side is often pulled off by the weight of the stool when the patient is up. The pouch should be angled toward the lateral aspect of the thigh as the patient's activities change (Figure 51-10). The pouch seal is often broken

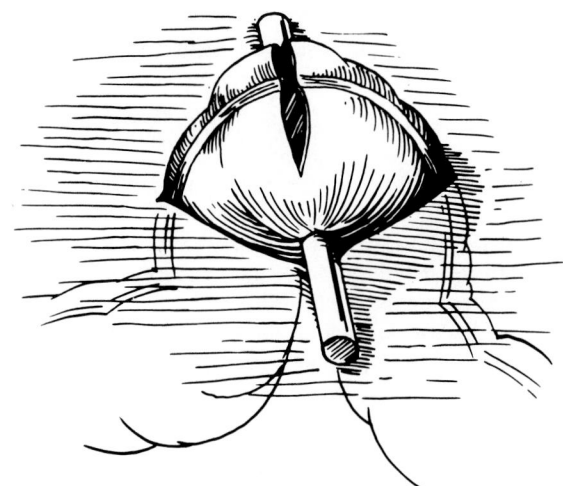

Figure 51-9   Loop ostomy rod procedure.

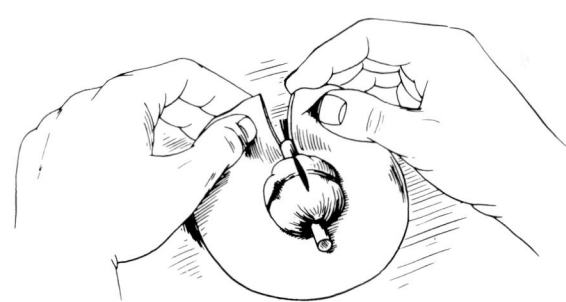

Figure 51-10   Application of a pouch on a stoma with a rod in place.

by the weight of the stool in an unemptied pouch or the tension from flatus trapped in the pouch. Pinholes for flatus work well for the nursing staff, but the patient suffers. Every time the covers are lifted or adjusted, the odor is present. This does not encourage a patient to accept the change in his or her body image. A fear of rejection because of the stoma and the odor is associated with colostomies.

A colostomy following peritonitis is often temporary; however, the duration of the need for the colostomy varies from patient to patient.

NURSING MANAGEMENT

Nursing diagnoses applicable to the patient are listed in the box on p. 1170. Patients who require diversion of the fecal stream are at high risk for disturbances of self-concept.

■ NURSING DIAGNOSIS

Disturbance in self-concept, related to altered elimination pattern.

OUTCOME STANDARD AND CRITERIA

Self-concept is positive as evidenced by:
• Identification of ways to cope with negative feelings

> ## Nursing Diagnoses Applicable to Peritonitis
>
> Fluid volume deficit, related to third-spacing fluid shifts from peritoneal inflammation
>
> High risk for infection of the peritoneum, related to secondary bacterial contamination
>
> High risk for ineffective breathing pattern, related to pain with respirations, compensatory pattern for lactic acidosis
>
> High risk for disturbances in self-concept, related to diversionary procedure

- Demonstration of self-care activities for management of ileostomy/colostomy system
- Exploration of feelings associated with perception of self
- Verbalization of strengths
- Identification of available resources
- Participation in social activities

NURSING INTERVENTIONS

- Explore patient's prior coping style
- Assess support system
- Encourage patient to identify and express feelings
- Encourage patient to set realistic goals
- Teach patient self-care activities
- Assist patient in accepting personal limitations
- Support and reinforce patient's accomplishments

Cutaneous Fistulas

Pathophysiology

A cutaneous fistula is a communication between an organ and the abdominal wall and is referred to as an *external fistula*. Most cutaneous fistulas are associated with surgical complications following intestinal, biliary, and pancreatic procedures. Drainage may be externalized through the surgical incisions, drain sites, or separate abdominal wall defects. Intestinal, biliary, and pancreatic fistulas require intensive medical and nursing care.[53,66,69,70]

Enterocutaneous (intestinal) fistulas may develop from anastomotic leaks, prolapse of the bowel into an abdominal or perineal wound, injury to the bowel when adhesions are divided or other surgical procedures performed, or injury to the bowel by wire mesh or retention sutures. Intestinal fistulas are more prone to develop in the presence of inflammatory lesions, neoplasms, or ischemic lesions. Fistulas most commonly appear in the ileum or jejunum, although they may affect any part of the bowel and may connect with any cavity in the abdomen. Postoperative external biliary fistulas may indicate operative injury to the bile duct or stricture of the common bile duct.

Proximal pancreatic resections involve anastomoses between the remaining portion of the pancreas and the upper jejunum, common bile duct, and stomach. Leakage may occur from any of the anastomoses.

Clinical Assessment

Diagnostic Procedures. Diagnosis of external fistulization may be established by *fistulogram* (radiographic delineation using injection of dye through the fistula). Small-bowel studies and intravenous cholangiograms may also be used in diagnosing fistulous tracts involving these structures.[13] The cause of the fistula determines the management: surgical or medical.

Medical Management

Conservative management of cutaneous fistulas involves fluid and electrolyte replacement, nutritional support, control of sepsis, drainage of associated abscess formations, and protection of skin from digestive enzymes. Surgical intervention may be necessary if the fistula does not close with conservative management. Conditions that adversely affect spontaneous closure include complete breakdown of an anastomosis, distal obstructions, and necrosis of segments of intestine.

The location of an intestinal fistula influences the amount and contents of the drainage. The higher in the small bowel a fistulous tract forms, the greater the fluid loss through the external communication. Intestinal fistula output contains digestive enzymes, sodium, chloride, and potassium. A patient may lose up to 3 L (3,000 ml) in a 24-hour period with a high-output jejunal fistula. Management of fluid and electrolyte loss from enterocutaneous fistulas is of crucial importance.[22] The fluid replacement is based on the patient's total output (milliliter for milliliter): fistulous, urinary, and insensible. Electrolyte replacements are calculated according to the contents of the fistula drainage and the results of laboratory blood studies. Biliary fistula electrolyte losses are predominantly of sodium chloride; pancreatic losses are of proteolytic enzymes and bicarbonate. Metabolic acidosis occurs when electrolyte and fluid equilibrium is not maintained.

Fistula drainage may be managed in three ways: by dressings, continuous suctioning, or pouching procedures. The location of the fistula and the amount and type of drainage should be considered in choosing an appropriate method. The low-output, nonirritating drainage may be effectively managed with dressings. Continuous sump drainage may be preferred with high-output fistulas. However, pouching of a fistula or a draining wound offers the greatest number of advantages. The cost of pouching a moderate- to high-volume fistula is less than the cost of the dressings necessary in a 24-hour period. Skin can be protected from the caustic drainage, which contains digestive enzymes. A small amount of drainage will often seep out around the sump tube and erode the skin. A pouch may be used in combination with a sump catheter. The sump catheter may open in the pouch or may come out through the bottom and connect to suction or to straight drainage. If the tube is left open in the pouch, the pouch should be connected to a bedside drainage bag or should be emptied for accurate measurements of the fistula output.

Many types of pouches are available, and choosing the appropriate equipment for the particular patient is essential. The first issue to examine is the need for sterility. Sterile pouches are available commercially, or pouches may be sterilized with ethylene oxide. External biliary fistulas are generally managed with sterile urinary equipment. Bile does not usually demonstrate bacterial growth, but the reflux of bile back to the fistula must be prevented and drainage into a collecting device (bedside drainage) facilitated. Urinary pouches used for control of liquid output are more effective than open-end ileostomy pouches. The urinary pouch can be disconnected from the bedside collecting device and the spout closed when the patient ambulates. In addition to biliary fistulas, surgically created drainage sites (i.e., the insertion of Penrose drains) are managed with aseptic techniques.

Jejunal and ileal (enterocutaneous) fistulas may develop through an operative incision. When wound dehiscence occurs, a fistulous tract may develop within the open wound. Clean, but not sterile, management of the drainage is indicated. An open-end drainable pouch is used for enterocutaneous fistulas. The shape and size of the wound or fistula to be contained will determine the pouch chosen. The pouch faceplate must be large enough to accommodate the wound with enough adhesive area retained to attach the pouch to the skin. The opening must be cut to avoid deep crevices, retention sutures, and fine wrinkles. In most cases, 1/8 to 1/4 inch of skin will be exposed between the fistula and pouch adhesive. This places the pouch seal on smooth skin away from the freely movable wound edges. If a pouch comes directly to the edge of the wound, patient activities including respirations, turning, and ambulation may lift up the inner edge of the pouch and create leakage.

The pouch may be attached directly to the skin; however, a skin barrier is recommended when pouching enterocutaneous fistulas. Sealant products in the form of sprays, gels, wipes, and liquids are available to coat the skin and prevent irritation from pouch adhesives. At the first indication of leakage, the pouch should be removed and a fresh pouching system applied.

Malnutrition is associated with external fistulas. The segment of intestine proximal to the fistula may be too short to ensure adequate nutritional support.[60,71] Food substances and digestive secretions may be excreted through the fistula before absorption can occur. Therefore, fluid and electrolyte loss may increase with oral feedings when an enterocutaneous fistula is present.

Bile is an emulsifying agent that facilitates the absorption of fats and fat-soluble vitamins. When bile is lost through an external biliary fistula, fats are not digested properly and malnutrition develops. In addition, fat-soluble vitamins are not available for absorption. Vitamin K loss is a potential threat, and prothrombin studies are used to evaluate the status of vitamin K. In addition, diarrhea may develop from the bile salts present in the large colon.

Total parenteral nutrition is recommended for the maintenance of a positive nitrogen balance (see Chapter 11). Adequate calories, amino acids, electrolytes, and minerals are supplied to meet the patient's daily requirement. Wound healing improves with positive nitrogen balance. TPN also places the bowel at complete mechanical rest and decreases the digestive secretions, thus lowering fluid loss via the fistula. TPN has been shown to increase the rate on spontaneous closures and to improve the outcome for patients who require operative closure.

Nursing Management

Potential nursing diagnoses for the patient with a cutaneous fistula include *fluid volume deficit,* related to high output fistula drainage with excessive loss of fluids, and *impaired skin integrity,* related to cutaneous fistula.

HEPATIC DYSFUNCTION

Hepatic dysfunction may present as an acute or a chronic disease process. *Hepatitis,* an acute inflammation of the entire liver, most often results from viral infection, although it may also be drug-induced or of toxic origin. In cirrhosis and advanced liver failure, liver cells are progressively destroyed as a result of alcohol ingestion, severe inflammation with necrosis, or biliary disease and are replaced with fibrotic tissue. Regardless of the cause of hepatic dysfunction, the effects on the patient are similar.

Hepatitis

Pathophysiology

In hepatitis, leukocytic-histiocytic reaction and infiltration causes necroses of hepatic cells. Bile duct proliferation is usual, with occasional damage. Fortunately, the reticuloendothelial framework is usually well preserved and facilitates cellular regeneration.

During the recovery phase, reticuloendothelial activity increases throughout the liver. Hepatitis may cause changes in other organs. Regional lymph node enlargement and hypoplastic bone marrow are noted. The brain shows acute nonspecific degeneration of ganglion cells. Occasionally, acute pancreatitis or myocarditis has been observed.[24]

Hepatitis is a viral process. Incubation periods vary from 7 to 60 days depending on the type of hepatitis (type A; type B; non-A, non-B type, sometimes referred to as type C; and hepatitis D).

In *Hepatitis A,* the most common type of hepatitis, a virus infects the liver and is eliminated by the feces. The virus is primarily spread through oral ingestion of food, water, and shellfish that have been infected by fecal contaminates. Hepatitis A was previously known as infectious hepatitis. The disease is usually mild in presentation, and individuals may be unaware of its occurrence.

Hepatitis B, a more serious form of hepatitis, is spread primarily by blood, blood products, and body fluids or secretions. The virus can spread percutaneously, through mucous membranes, or through contact with infected fluids. Health care providers are at risk for contracting this form of hepatitis. Hepatitis B can be dormant, a carrier state, and it can result in chronic hepatitis, cirrhosis, or cancer of the liver.

Hepatitis non-A, non-B, also called hepatitis C, is transmitted through blood, or blood products, or sexual contact. The virus can be mild and often the patient is asymptomatic. It rarely progresses to the fulminant form.

Hepatitis D relies on the presence of hepatitis B to spread. It is transmitted by the parenteral route.

Data Acquisition

History. The possible source of infection may be learned when the history is taken. The nurse should be aware that young, low-income persons who live in crowded facilities with minimal sanitation standards are most vulnerable to infection with the type A virus. An accurate health history is essential because in its preicteric phase diagnosis of type A cannot be made by a laboratory test. Exposure to persons known to have hepatitis, recent transfusions, needle pricks or needle sharing, ingestion of certain foods, and exposure to an infected person's blood or mucous membranes should be assessed in the health history.

Physical Assessment. Despite variations in etiology, the clinical course of all types of hepatitis is similar. Common signs and symptoms of hepatitis are reviewed in the box above.[2,24] The prodromal period before jaundice appears, 3 to 4 days or 2 to 3 weeks, is marked by nausea, vomiting, abdominal discomfort, and a low-grade fever. The patient reports fa-

> ### Signs and Symptoms of Hepatitis
> Brown urine
> Depression
> Loss of appetite
> Nausea and vomiting
> Fever
> Weakness/chills
> Headache
> Right upper quadrant discomfort or pain
> Clay-colored (alcoholic) feces
> Jaundice

tigue and malaise, and may note a weight loss. The liver becomes enlarged and tender. The urine darkens from bilirubin while the feces lighten and the skin becomes jaundiced. Transient pruritus may occur. The liver is palpable, with a smooth, tender edge, in 70% of the cases. During the icteric phase, the postcervical lymph nodes and spleen are enlarged.

Patients with the B type of hepatitis have a greater chance of developing fulminant hepatic failure, which is characterized by the sudden degeneration of the liver and the loss of all normal liver functions. An important clinical sign is a decrease in liver size. Other signs of impending fulminant failure include hyperexcitability, insomnia, irritability, vomiting, and alterations in level of consciousness.

Diagnostic Procedures. Diagnosis of non-A, non-B hepatitis is made when laboratory tests for hepatitis A and B are negative, yet clinical signs and symptoms of hepatitis are present, and liver function tests are abnormal. Common liver function tests and the findings most common in liver dysfunction are listed in Table 51-10. This virus has an incubation period of 2 weeks to 6 months.

Bile is usually present in the urine before jaundice is seen. Leukopenia, lymphopenia, and neutropenia also are evident in the preicteric phase.

Hepatitis A is diagnosed by the presence of hepatitis A antibodies, in the blood. These antibodies, also called immunoglobulins, occur within 2 to 6 weeks and remain in the serum indefinitely. Initially, antibodies are seen, indicating current infection. Later, these are replaced by the IgG class, indicating immunity to hepatitis A.

The diagnosis of hepatitis B is made through the presence of antigen–antibody systems in the blood. Hepatitis surface antigens (Ig) can be found 1 to 10 weeks following exposure to the virus. Patients are considered infectious as long as Ig is present. Several other antigen–antibody systems can be used to diagnose hepatitis B. These include HBeAG and HBcAG. These antibody complexes are detectable

TABLE 51-10 **Liver Function Tests**

Measurements	Alteration with Liver Dysfunction
SERUM OR PLASMA TESTS	
Albumin	↓
Ammonia	↑
Bile pigments	
Total bilirubin	↑
Direct or conjugated bilirubin	↑
Cholesterol	↑
Coagulation tests	
Prothrombin time (PT)	Prolonged
Partial thromboplastin time (PTT)	Prolonged
Enzymes	
Alkaline phosphatase	↑
Glutamic oxaloacetic transaminase (SGOT)	↑
Glutamic pyruvic transaminase (SGPT)	↑
URINE TESTS	
Bilirubin	↑
Urobilinogen	↑

throughout the acute stages of the illness. The incubation for hepatitis B can last from 6 weeks to 6 months.

Medical Management

There is no definitive treatment for hepatitis. Goals for medical and nursing care include provision of rest and assisting the patient in obtaining optimal nutrition.

Bed rest should be instituted immediately because it decreases metabolic demands on the liver. The nurse can assist the individual in spacing activities to ensure adequate rest. Medications to help the patient rest or decrease agitation may not be ordered because most require clearance by the liver, which is impaired during the acute phase.

Maintenance of nutritional status is a nursing priority. Loss of appetite, nausea, and vomiting may persist for weeks. A high-carbohydrate diet is usually recommended, and fatty, greasy foods should be avoided. Administration of antiemetics may be helpful, but all hepatotoxic drugs should be avoided. Small, frequent meals may be better tolerated. Evaluation of goals should be ongoing.

Special precautions must be implemented while caring for the patient to prevent self-contamination and spread of the virus. Enteric and blood precautions should be implemented, and all laboratory samples should be clearly marked. With the advent of jaun-

dice, the patient with hepatitis A is no longer infectious. As jaundice subsides, precautions may be suspended for hepatitis B patients, but blood precautions should continue as long as the patient is serum positive. Use of blood precautions for non-A, non-B hepatitis is usually advised. The use of universal precautions for all patients is the best policy. Prevention of infection is also important due to the loss of Kupffer cell activity during the acute phase.

Prophylactic measures against hepatitis A and hepatitis B viruses are available. Immune globulin can be administered to individuals both before and after exposure to the virus.

NURSING MANAGEMENT

■ NURSING DIAGNOSES

Nursing diagnoses associated with viral hepatitis include:

- *Activity intolerance,* related to fatigue, fever, and flu-like symptoms
- *Altered nutrition: less than body requirements,* related to loss of appetite, nausea, vomiting, and loss of liver metabolic functions
- *High risk for infection,* related to loss of liver cell function to phagocytize bacteria

OUTCOME STANDARDS AND CRITERIA

Resolution of hepatitis can be evaluated according to the following criteria:

- Ability to tolerate increasing levels of activity
- Absence of abdominal discomfort/pain
- Return of liver function tests to baseline
- Absence of active virus on serological test
- Maintenance of nutritional status
- Absence of infection

Hepatic Insufficiency and Failure

Pathophysiology

Hepatic insufficiency is the result of cirrhosis, which is the most common cause of liver failure. *Cirrhosis* is the third leading cause of death in U.S. males aged 35 to 54. In cirrhosis, the liver parenchymal cells are progressively destroyed and replaced with fibrotic (scar) tissue. Although some regeneration occurs, overgrowth causes irregularities in the shape of the hepatic lobules. Twisting and constriction of central sections of the lobules impede vascular flow, and portal hypertension results; lymphatic flow through the liver is also impeded. In addition, cirrhosis is characterized by fatty infiltration. Approximately three fourths of the liver may be destroyed without symptoms of impairment. Portal blood carrying unmetabolized substances enters the system and reaches the brain. These substances, of which ammonia is the most widely investigated, are toxic to the brain.[72] After long periods of damage and regeneration, necrosis and atrophy of the liver occur. An increased number of inflammatory cells is seen, as well as hepatomegaly. Scarring progresses and involves the ducts.

Hepatic failure is the inability of the liver to metabolize carbohydrates, fats, proteins, and vitamins and to conjugate ammonia.[24] In liver disease, the body is unable to maintain normal blood glucose levels and cellular nutrition. In addition, several vitamins are not stored. Moreover, the level of bile production is insufficient for absorption of the fat-soluble vitamins. Vitamin deficiencies result. Increased amounts of NH_3 with dissociation to NH_3 and H^+ (because of diarrhea, hypokalemia, and alkalosis) result in acidosis and elevated ammonia levels, which in turn result in interference with normal brain metabolism. Because almost all clotting factors are produced in the liver, the patient may have inadequate hemostasis. Because of decreased efficiency of the liver and splenic congestion, blood bacteria are often increased and the patient is more susceptible to infection.

There are four types of cirrhosis: alcoholic cirrhosis (Laënnec's), biliary cirrhosis, cardiac cirrhosis, and postnecrotic cirrhosis. Laënnec's cirrhosis, which results from chronic alcohol abuse, is the most common. Alcohol is known to be toxic to liver cells; however, not all alcoholics develop cirrhosis. Other alcohol-induced liver injuries include fatty liver and alcoholic hepatitis. Acetaldehyde, a toxic metabolite of alcohol, damages and kills liver cells. Fibrotic tissue replaces liver cells, and in the end stage, all functions of the liver are impaired.

Biliary cirrhosis is caused by a decrease in bile flow, most commonly due to long-term biliary duct obstruction. Cardiac cirrhosis is most commonly associated with severe, long-term right-sided congestive heart failure. Decreased oxygenation of liver cells and cell death characterize this disease.

Data Acquisition

History. Precipitating factors for liver failure may include chronic liver disease with superimposed stress such as excessive alcohol intake, toxic gastrointestinal bleeding, shock states, rapid diuresis, or sedatives. Other etiologies include viral hepatitis, gallbladder disease, drugs, or acute infectious processes.

Assessment should include the presence or absence of cirrhosis and any recent episodes of alcohol abuse. Acute hepatitis or drug abuse also need to be determined. The history should also include complete symptom assessment.

Physical Assessment. Initial clinical signs of hepatic failure may be vague: weakness, fatigue, loss of appetite, weight loss, abdominal discomfort, nausea and vomiting, and a change in bowel habits. As the destruction of the liver progresses, the systemic effects of the disease become apparent as liver function becomes impaired, affecting physical assessment and symptom findings. Systemic effects of hepatic insufficiency and failure include impaired bile formation and flow, reduced liver metabolic processes, and portal hypertension. Refer to the discussion of esophageal varices on p. 1149.[2,24,72]

The patient may appear jaundiced as a result of impaired bile formation and flow. Jaundice is associated with a bilirubin above 3.0 mg/dl.

Because of the complex metabolic functions of the liver, hepatic failure alters carbohydrate, fat, and protein metabolism. The patient is usually cachectic. Altered carbohydrate metabolism may result clinically in unstable blood sugars (cirrhotic diabetes). It may also diminish stress response. Altered fat metabolism causes fatty liver. All cells use fat for energy, and altered metabolism may cause fatigue and decreased activity tolerance. Alterations in skin integrity are common in patients with hepatic failure and are thought to be related to metabolic dysfunction. Inadequate production of bile salts leads to malabsorption in the small intestine and nutritional problems.

Protein metabolism also is decreased. The liver is the only organ that synthesizes albumin, the plasma protein that maintains colloid osmotic pressure in the blood vessels. An insufficiency of albumin can cause edema of the ankles and scrotum, ascites, and pleural effusion. Globulin is essential for transport of substances in the blood. Fibrinogen is necessary for normal clotting. The decreased metabolism of these proteins is coupled with decreased synthesis of clotting factors. Clinical signs and symptoms can range from bruising to nasal and gingival bleeding and frank hemorrhage. The development of disseminated intravascular coagulation is a complication. The liver also removes activated clotting factors from the circulation to prevent systemic clotting. Loss of this function predisposes the patient to the development of emboli.

Decreased metabolism and storage of vitamins, iron, and glucose exacerbates nutritional deficiencies. Detoxification of drugs, ammonia, and hormones also is lost. Because ammonia is not converted to urea, many of the neurological alterations are seen when ammonia enters the central nervous system. Neurological symptoms range from minor mentation changes to confusion or profound coma. *Asterixis,* a flapping tremor of the hands, is an early sign of encephalopathy associated with liver failure.

Hormonal imbalances are common in hepatic failure. Aldosterone and antidiuretic hormone (ADH) are not inactivated, with resultant fluid and electrolyte disturbances, sodium and water retention, and third-spacing of fluid from the intravascular space (ascites). Plasma volume decreases, compensatory mechanisms cause the release of ADH and aldosterone, and more sodium and water are retained. The renin–angiotensin system also causes systemic vasoconstriction to which the kidneys are particularly susceptible. Renal perfusion can be impaired and urine output decreased.

Sexual dysfunction is common because hormones are not effectively metabolized. Altered self-concept may ensue. Some patients have a dermatological lesion spider angioma, which is thought to be related to an endocrine imbalance. These spiderlike superficial vascular lesions may be venous or arterial and are most visible in the abdomen.

The inability of the liver to metabolize drugs is well known. Drug administration should be restricted. A fecal odor to the breath (fector hepaticus) is thought to be due to an accumulation of methyl mercaptan in the body.

Portal hypertension results from hyperdynamic circulation and the development of collateral circulation. Refer to the esophageal varices section on p. 1149. Liver cell destruction leads to shunting of blood and increased cardiac output. Vasodilatation is also present and leads to decreased perfusion to body organs. Clinical signs of hyperdynamic circulation are identical to heart failure and include jugular vein distention, crackles, and signs of decreased organ perfusion. Splenomegaly is also common. Initially, the patient may have hypertension, flushed skin, and bounding pulses. Blood pressure eventually falls, and dysrhythmias are common.

Clinical signs and symptoms of liver failure are reviewed in the box below.[1,27]

Diagnostic Procedures. Laboratory findings in patients with hepatic dysfunction are those associated with cell destruction (liver enzymes) or the effects of reduced metabolic processes. (Refer to Table 51-2.) Parenchymal tests such as a liver biopsy can be done to study cell architecture. The finding of an atrophied, small liver confirms the diagnosis. Ultrasonography may help to detect impaired bile flow. Tests of hepatic clearance of known substances may also be used to study liver function. Dyes are injected into the blood, and the clearance is measured at specific intervals.

Collaborative Management

Nursing and medical management of the patient with hepatic failure focus on supportive therapies and early recognition and treatment of complications, especially ascites. Hemodynamic instability and decreased organ perfusion may necessitate hemodynamic monitoring, although the benefits of invasive monitoring should be carefully weighed against the risk of infection due to decreased Kupffer cell activity in acute failure. Vasoactive drugs and fluid may be ordered to support blood pressure and organ perfusion.

Patients with liver failure also are at risk for bleeding complications because the synthesis of proteins and clotting factors is impaired. Patients with altered clotting profiles should be protected from injury. Padded siderails, needle-stick precautions, and therapeutic touch are common therapies. Blood products may be ordered in severe cases. The patient needs to be monitored for gastrointestinal bleeding due to stress ulcers.

Clinical Sequelae of Liver Disease

CARDIOVASCULAR
Portal hypertension
Hyperdynamic circulation
Dysrhythmias
Activity intolerance

FLUID AND ELECTROLYTE DISTURBANCES
Ascites
Edema
Decreased intravascular volume
Hypokalemia
Hyponatremia (dilutional)
Hypernatremia

INTEGUMENTARY
Jaundice
Spider angiomas
Pruritus

ENDOCRINE
Increased aldosterone secretion
Increased antidiuretic hormone secretion

GASTROINTESTINAL
Abdominal discomfort
Decreased appetite
Diarrhea
Bleeding
Malnutrition
Nausea and vomiting

HEMATOLOGICAL
Anemia
Impaired coagulation
Disseminated intravascular coagulation

NEUROLOGICAL
Hepatic encephalopathy

RENAL
Hepatorenal syndrome

Common complications of liver dysfunction include ascites, portal systemic encephalopathy, and hepatorenal syndrome. Early detection and treatment may improve patient outcomes.

Ascites. Impaired handling of salt and water by the kidneys and associated abnormalities of fluid homeostasis predispose the patient ascites, an accumulation of fluid in the peritoneum. The effects of pressure on the diaphagm impair the patient's breathing. Frequent nursing assessment of respiratory status and arterial blood gas determinations is critical. Measurement of abdominal girth alerts the nurse to small increases in fluid accumulation. Abdominal girth should be consistently measured at the umbilicus. Positioning the patient in a semi-Fowler's position allows for free diaphragmatic movement. Some patients may require elective intubation until control of ascites is accomplished.

Medical management of ascites includes bed rest, a low-sodium diet, fluid restriction, and diuretic therapy.[24,73,74] Diuresis should be limited to 2,000 ml per day to prevent rapid intravascular volume depletion and acute renal failure. Careful monitoring of electrolyte balance also is a priority. Paracentesis, or percutaneous needle aspiration of ascitic fluid, may also be done. Close monitoring of vital signs during this medical procedure is necessary. One to two liters is usually withdrawn at one time. Salt-poor albumin is usually administered to increase colloid osmotic pressure in the peritoneum and to prevent rapid reaccumulation of ascites.

Peritoneovenous shunts are surgical procedures used to relieve ascites that is resistant to medical management. A *LeVeen shunt* is inserted by placing the distal end of a tube under the peritoneum and tunneling the other end under the skin into the jugular vein or superior vena cava. A valve that opens and closes according to the pressure gradient allows ascitic fluid to flow into the vessel. Patient respirations trigger the valve. During inspiration, peritoneal pressure rises, and vena caval pressure falls, allowing fluid to flow from the peritoneum into the general circulation. Major complications of this shunt include clotting of the shunt and wound infection. A variation of this procedure is the *Denver shunt,* in which a pump is placed in addition to the peritoneal catheter. Ascites is allowed to flow through the pump at a uniform rate, or it can be "squeezed" to increase flow or to clear the catheter of any solid matter.

Portal Systemic Encephalopathy. The exact mechanism for portal systemic encephalopathy is unknown, but it is thought to be related to abnormal ammonia metabolism.[24,75] Elevated serum ammonia levels are thought to interfere with normal cerebral metabolism. Many conditions precipitate its development, including fluid and electrolyte disturbances, increased protein intake, shunts, blood transfusions, and drugs such as diuretics, narcotics, and sedatives.

Measures to decrease ammonia production are mainstays of treatment. Protein intake should be limited to 20 to 40 grams per day. Neomycin and lactulose can be administered to reduce bacterial breakdown of protein in the bowel. Neomycin is a broad-spectrum antibiotic that destroys normal gut flora and, thereby, decreases protein breakdown and ammonia production. Lactulose creates an acidic environment in the bowel, causing ammonia to leave the bloodstream and to enter the colon where it is trapped. Lactulose also has a laxative effect which allows for elimination. Nursing measures to protect the patient from injury are a priority during periods of altered mentation.

Hepatorenal syndrome. The mechanism for acute functional renal failure associated with hepatic failure is not well understood. It is seen in patients with end-stage liver disease, decreased albumin, and portal hypertension.[76] Decreased urine output and elevated serum creatinine develop acutely. The prognosis for the patient is poor because therapies to improve renal function are usually ineffective. Hepatotoxic drugs are discontinued. Hemodialysis is used to support renal function only if there is a chance for an improvement of liver function.

NURSING MANAGEMENT

■ NURSING DIAGNOSES

Actual and high-risk nursing diagnoses that can be derived from assessment data in the patient with hepatic insufficiency or failure are listed in the box below.

Nursing Diagnoses Related to Hepatic Insufficiency or Failure

Decreased activity tolerance, related to impaired liver metabolism and decreased nutritional intake

Fluid volume deficit, related to decreased effective vascular volume, bleeding from varices, or clotting dysfunction

Altered nutrition: less than body requirements, related to impaired nutrient metabolism, decreased intake, and impaired absorption of vitamins[74]

Ineffective breathing pattern, related to elevation of the diaphragm from ascites, impaired thought processes from impaired ammonia detoxification/or increased production

Altered thought processes, related to impaired handling of ammonia and drugs, protein intake, diuretic therapy, ascites; GI bleeding with increased protein load; dehydration and shock

OUTCOME STANDARDS AND CRITERIA

Hepatic function will be normal as evidenced by:
- Absence or resolution of active bleeding
- Coagulation function tests and blood counts returned to baseline
- Sufficient intake of protein for liver regeneration but not so much as to increase accumulation of nitrogen waste products
- Serum proteins returned to baseline
- Absence or control of ascites
- Effective breathing pattern
- Adequate oxygenation and ventilation
- Patient alert and oriented; or mentation returned to baseline
- Creatinine, BUN, urine output returned to baseline

NURSING INTERVENTIONS

Specific nursing interventions are discussed in the section Collaborative Management.

PANCREATIC DISORDERS

Acute Pancreatitis

Pathophysiology

Acute pancreatitis is an autodigestive disease in which the pancreas is damaged by the enzymes it produces. Normally, pancreatic juices including trypsin, phospholipase A chymotrypsin, elastase, and carboxypeptidase which are essential to normal carbohydrate, fat, and protein metabolism, are secreted into the duodenum. The etiological mechanism that initiates the autodigestive process has been widely sought, and several theories have emerged.[1,2,77,78,79]

One theory proposes that a toxic agent alters the way the pancreas secretes its enzymes, perhaps activating the enzymes prematurely. Drugs known to have the potential to induce acute pancreatitis when in toxic doses include thiazide diuretics, furosemide, estrogens, methyldopa, sulfonamides, tetracycline, and azathioprine. Alcohol ingestion also is associated with acute pancreatitis. Pancreatic inflammation from alcohol is precipitated by one or more of three mechanisms:

1. Alcohol stimulates secretion of gastric acid, which reaches the duodenum and stimulates cholecystokinin release from the antrum, where it intensely stimulates pancreatic secretion.
2. Alcohol increases pressure in the pancreatic ductal system, causing atony and edema of the sphincter of Oddi and, thereby, allowing reflux of duodenal contents with their activated enzymes.
3. Alcohol increases the pancreatic juice's content of trypsinogen, which is associated with the multisystem effects of this disease.

Duodenal reflux of activated enzymes into the pancreatic duct by an unknown mechanism has also been widely implicated. Obstruction of biliary ducts with hypertension of the pancreas is another theory. This increased pressure leads to rupture of the pancreatic duct and premature activation of enzymes, or reflux of bile and duodenal juice into the pancreas. Biliary obstruction also is thought to inhibit the release of trypsin inhibitor, which is normally secreted by pancreatic cells to prevent activation of proteolytic enzymes while in the pancreas. Regardless of the mechanism of enzymes activation, acute damage of acinar cells is the outcome (Figure 51-11).

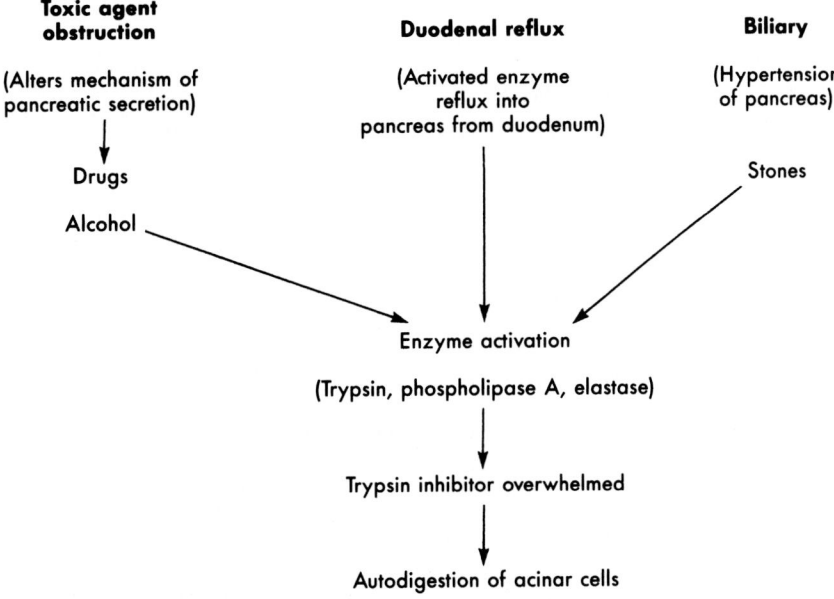

Figure 51-11 Pathogenesis of acute pancreatitis.

As pancreatic cells are damaged, more digestive enzymes are released, which in turn cause more pancreatic damage. Local effects include inflammation of pancreatic cells, inflammation of the peritoneum and fat around the pancreas, and accumulation of fluid in the peritoneal cavity.[77,78,80]

Acute pancreatitis is classified by the gradations of lesions found in the pancreas. The mild form is manifested by areas of fat necrosis around pancreatic cells with interstitial edema. With more severe forms, pancreatic cellular necrosis and hemorrhage into the pancreas occur. Endocrine and exocrine functions of the pancreas may be lost. Third-spacing of peritoneal fluid is also characteristic.

The systemic effects of acute pancreatitis have been widely studied.[80-86] The release of enzymes into the circulatory system is thought to be the mechanism of that causes vasodilatation, hypotension, and shock.[87] The release of trypsin is known to cause abnormalities in blood coagulation and clot lysis. The release of phospholipases is thought to cause the pulmonary complications associated with acute pancreatitis with acute respiratory failure and ARDS being the two most common.[80,85] Acute renal failure is thought to be a consequence of alterations in the renin–angiotensin mechanism.[82] Death during the first 2 weeks of acute pancreatitis usually results from pulmonary or renal complications. Metabolic complications include hypocalcemia and hyperlipidemia which are thought to be related to areas of fat necrosis around the inflamed pancreas. Various hormonal imbalances, particularly parathyroid hormone, have been implicated in the pathophysiology of these metabolic disturbances. Pancreatic complications include pseudocyst, a collection of inflammatory debris and pancreatic secretions that are part of the necrotizing process. (See the lower box below.[84])

Because the clinical presentation of patients with acute pancreatitis can range from mild to fulminating processes, criteria for determining the seriousness of the disease have been developed to predict mortality as well as to guide the aggressiveness of medical therapies. The upper box below lists the Ranson criteria, which are very commonly employed.

Data Acquisition

History. The exact etiology of acute pancreatitis is unknown. Precipitating factors include trauma, drugs (thiazides, steroids, isoniazid), infectious processes (mumps, scarlet fever, staphylococcus, food poisoning, viral hepatitis), hyperparathyroidism, hyperlipidemia, parasites, ingestion of a large meal (especially one high in fat), and alcohol ingestion.[68,78,79] Other causative factors may include a history of gallbladder or other biliary diseases, alcoholism, and he-

---

Ranson Criteria for Predicting Severity of Acute Pancreatitis

Age >55
Leukocyte count >1,600/μl
Glucose >200 mg/dl
Serum lactic dehydrogenase >350 IU/ml
Aspirate aminotransferase >250 IU/dl
Hematocrit decrease >10%
BUN >5 mg/dl
Serum calcium <8 mg/dl
Fluid sequestration >6 L
Arterial Pao$_2$ <60 mmHg

Systemic Complications of Acute Pancreatitis

PULMONARY
Hypoxemia
Atelectasis
Pneumonia
Pleural effusion
Adult respiratory distress syndrome (ARDS)

CARDIOVASCULAR
Hypovolemic shock
Myocardial depression (MDF)
Dysrhythmias

RENAL
Azotemia
Acute renal failure

HEMATOLOGICAL
Coagulation dysfunction
Disseminated extravascular coagulation

GASTROINTESTINAL
Gastrointestinal hemorrhage
Pancreatic pseudocyst
Pancreatic abscess

METABOLIC
Hypocalcemia
Hyperlipidemia
Hyperglycemia
Metabolic acidosis

NEUROLOGICAL
Pancreatic encephalopathy

reditary factors. The patient reports steatorrhea (foul-smelling grayish stools), as well as weight loss, nausea, vomiting, and abdominal distention. The history should include the location and duration of pain, the relation of the pain to meals and posture, alcohol ingestion, recent weight loss, nausea and vomiting, anorexia, and food intolerances. The urine should be observed for discoloration associated with obstructive jaundice. The characteristics and frequency of bowel movements should be observed. Fatty stools (steatorrhea) are associated with pancreatitis.

Physical Assessment. Signs and symptoms of acute pancreatitis vary according to the degree of functional alteration of the pancreas. There are two types of acute pancreatitis: interstitial and hemorrhagic. In interstitial acute pancreatitis, the pancreas is edematous. The pancreas may recover from mild attacks; however, if complications develop, it may become necrotic. The term *necrotic pancreatitis* is used interchangeably with *hemorrhagic pancreatitis*. The majority of patients with acute pancreatitis present with complaints of steady, severe abdominal pain. It is most often midepigastric but may be localized in the left upper quadrant.[78,79] The pain may be diminished by maintaining a sitting position or a fetal knee-chest position. Fever and chills are observed in acute pancreatitis. Vomiting due to reflux irritation from the inflamed pancreas does not relieve the epigastric pain and may be persistent. Dyspnea is due to diaphragmatic irritability which compromises pulmonary function. Slight jaundice may be present from obstruction due to edema of the pancreas.

Spillage of pancreatic enzymes into the peritoneal cavity may result in chemical peritonitis. Shock may develop from pooling of fluid and blood in the retroperitoneal area and peritoneal cavity. A bluish discoloration of the flanks (Grey Turner's sign) or around the umbilical area (Cullen's sign) results from the accumulation of blood in these areas and indicates hemorrhagic pancreatitis.[82] Diaphoresis, tachycardia, hypotension, and abdominal rigidity may be indicative of shock in acute pancreatitis. Bowel sounds are decreased, and there may be a paralytic ileus with its sequelae, including abdominal distention and loss of fluid into the bowel lumen. The physical examination may reveal upper abdominal tenderness.

Diagnostic Procedures. Serum and urinary amylase values are elevated in pancreatitis.[88] Serum amylase may return to normal within 2 to 3 days following an acute episode. Serum amylase levels are not used alone for diagnosing pancreatitis because increased serum amylase is observed also in acute cholecystitis, active alcoholism without pancreatitis, perforated peptic ulcer, intestinal obstruction, mesenteric thrombosis, ectopic pregnancy, renal failure, and

mumps and after the administration of meperidine (Demerol). Urinary amylase levels that are elevated for 5 to 7 days tend to reflect the amount of amylase secreted from the pancreas. Amylase values of pleural fluid and paracentesis drainage are used in diagnosing pancreatitis. Serum amylase measurement is more specific with elevated isoenzymes (isoamylase). The serum lipase level is elevated for 5 to 7 days. A lowered serum calcium level may be observed in necrotizing pancreatitis.

A glucose tolerance test is used to evaluate the endocrine function of the pancreas. The exocrine pancreatic function is assessed by a secretin stimulation study. Urinary amylase levels are obtained, and 72-hour stool samples are collected for measurement of fats.

The diagnosis of acute pancreatitis can be confirmed by computed tomography (CT scan) and magnetic resonance imaging (MRI). Mild edematous changes may not be identifiable, but pancreatic inflammation or biliary obstruction is usually identifiable. Gastrointestinal complications of acute pancreatitis such as pancreatic pseudocyst or abscess also are identifiable.

Common laboratory findings in addition to amylase abnormalities include an elevated white blood count due to the inflammatory process. Hypokalemia may occur because of associated vomiting. Hypocalcemia is common with fulminant disease and usually indicates pancreatic fat necrosis. Triglycerides may be extremely elevated and may be a causative factor in the development of the autodigestive process. Arterial blood gas analysis may show hypoxemia and retained carbon dioxide which indicate associated respiratory failure or effect of circulating pancreatic enzymes on lung tissue.

Medical Management

Priorities for the management of acute pancreatitis include fluid and electrolyte replacements, supportive therapies to decrease gastrin release from the stomach to the duodenum, nutritional support, analgesics for pain control, and monitoring and treatment of systemic complications.[78,79,88,89,90]

Fluid and Electrolyte Replacement. In all forms of acute pancreatitis, some fluid collects in the retroperitoneal cavity. Some patients may have sequestered up to 12 L of fluid. Hypovolemia and shock are major causes of death early in the disease process. Fluid rehydration may accomplished with colloid, Ringer's lactate, frozen plasma, or albumin. Fluid resuscitation also perfuses the pancreas, which is thought to slow the progression of the disease. Maintaining perfusion of the kidneys may prevent the development of acute renal failure.

Critical assessments to evaluate fluid replacement are discussed at the beginning of the chapter in the section on hypovolemic shock. Patients with more severe manifestations of the disease may need hemodynamic monitoring to assist in evaluating fluid status and responses to intervention. If the patient does not fail to respond to fluid therapy alone, medications to support blood pressure may be prescribed. Dopamine may be started at low doses. Patients with acute hemorrhagic pancreatitis may also need packed red blood cells to restore intravascular volume.

Hypocalcemia, a common electrolyte imbalance, is associated with a high mortality. It is thought to be related to decreased calcium binding with proteins in the plasma. The nurse is responsible for monitoring serum values and for monitoring patient responses. Calcium should be infused through a central line when possible because peripheral infiltration may cause tissue necrosis. Hypomagnesemia also may be present. Potassium may be low due to vomiting. Potassium is also abundant in pancreatic juices.

Resting the Pancreas. Nasogastric suction is generally used to suppress pancreatic exocrine secretion by preventing the release of secretin from the duodenum. Nausea, vomiting, and abdominal pain also may be decreased. Oral intake should not be started until the abdominal pain subsides and serum amylase levels have returned to normal. Premature oral feedings may induce further inflammation of the pancreas by stimulating the autodigestive process. They are also associated with increased risk of pancreatic abscess formation.

Nutritional Support. Patients with fulminant pancreatitis may be kept on prolonged NPO status with nasogastric suction because of paralytic ileus, persistent abdominal pain, or pancreatic complications. Total parenteral nutrition is recommended. Serum glucose must be particularly monitored since endocrine functions of the pancreas may be impaired. Lipids are also not recommended because they may increase triglycerides and exacerbate hyperlipidemia.[90]

Pain Management. Pain control is a nursing priority, not only to alleviate the patients' discomfort, but also because pain increases pancreatic secretions. The pain is due to edema and distention of the pancreatic capsule, biliary obstruction, and peritoneal inflammation from pancreatic enzymes. Careful pain assessment is needed, and analgesics should be administered. Morphine may exacerbate pain by causing spasm of the sphincter of Oddi, but hydromorphine (Dilaudid) has proven effective. A pain rating scale may be used to determine the amount of analgesia required and to evaluate effectiveness. Gastric decompression also may help relieve pain.

Pharmacological Interventions. Many pharmacological agents to induce pancreatic rest have been studied: anticholinergics, glucagon, somatostatin, cimetidine, and calcitonin. None has been shown to be effective. Histamine blockers and antacids are used to prevent stress ulcers. The effect of antibiotics on pancreatic inflammation has been studied, but none has proven effective. 5-Fluorouracil lowers the metabolic rate of pancreatic cells and production of enzymes and may be used in the acute phase. Bile salts may also be used to facilitate digestion and absorption of nutrients.

Peritoneal Lavage. Peritoneal lavage may used to remove vasoactive substances thought to be responsible for the systemic complications of acute pancreatitis. These include trypsinogen, kinins, histamines, and prostaglandins. An isotonic solution containing heparin, potassium, and antibiotics is infused and then drained by gravity. Some centers have been using peritoneal lavage every 1 to 2 hours for up to 7 days. These studies show a decrease in mortality early in the disease associated with a reduction in the late occurrence of pancreatic sepsis. If lavage is effective, hemodynamic effects are usually immediate.[85,91]

Surgical Interventions. A pancreatic resection may be performed to prevent systemic complications of acute necrotizing pancreatitis by removing necrotic or infected tissue.[92] In some cases, a pancreatectomy is performed. The indication for surgical intervention is clinical deterioration of the patient despite supportive therapies. Surgery may also be done to treat a pseudocyst by internal or external drainage or needle aspiration. Surgical intervention for pseudocyst is usually not done immediately because some resolve spontaneously. Immediate surgical intervention is required if the pseudocyst becomes infected or perforated. Another complication, abdominal abscess, requires surgery to drain because without surgery there is 100% mortality. Signs and symptoms of this problem include an elevated WBC count, fever, increasing abdominal pain, and vomiting. A CT scan provides a definitive diagnosis.

NURSING MANAGEMENT

Actual or high-risk nursing diagnoses and care associated with acute pancreatitis or complications of the disease are presented below.

■ NURSING DIAGNOSIS

Fluid volume deficit, related to loss fluid into peritoneal cavity, dehydration from nausea and vomiting/fever, gastric suction, bleeding into pancreas.

OUTCOME STANDARD AND CRITERIA

Fluid volume is adequate as evidenced by:
- Mean arterial pressure >60
- Preload indicators within normal limits
- Urine output ≥30 ml/hr
- Extremities warm, dry
- Stable blood count; absence of bleeding

NURSING INTERVENTIONS

- Monitor vital signs, hemodynamic parameters, peripheral circulation, urine output
- Administer fluid replacements, blood, or blood products and monitor patient responses
- Monitor for signs and symptoms of hemorrhage, Cullen's or Grey Turner's sign; measure abdominal girth

■ NURSING DIAGNOSIS

Pain, related to interruption of blood supply to the pancreas, edema and distention of the pancreas, peritoneal irritation.

OUTCOME STANDARD AND CRITERIA

Pain is absent or controlled as evidenced by:

- Verbalization that pain is relieved or manageable
- Absence of pain manifestations
- Relaxed body
- Normal respiratory rate, heart rate, and blood pressure

NURSING INTERVENTIONS

- Perform a pain assessment noting onset, duration, intensity, and location; differentiate from cardiac pain
- Control pain by administering prescribed analgesic; avoid morphine, which causes spasm of the sphincter of Oddi
- Maintain gastric suction
- Maintain bed rest; space activities

■ NURSING DIAGNOSIS

Altered nutrition, related to nausea and vomiting, pain, impaired nutrient metabolism due to pancreatic injury, and altered production of digestive enzymes.

OUTCOME STANDARD AND CRITERIA

Nutrition is adequate as evidenced by:

- Positive nitrogen balance
- Maintenance of weight
- Serum albumin within normal limits

NURSING INTERVENTIONS

- Assess nutritional status through clinical examination and laboratory analysis
- Calculate caloric needs and compare to intake
- Administer TPN according to protocol; maintain asepsis and monitor for signs of infection; monitor glucose; avoid lipid administration

■ NURSING DIAGNOSIS

Impaired gas exchange, related to atelectasis, pleural effusion, ARDS, splinting from pain.

OUTCOME STANDARD AND CRITERIA

Gas exchange is adequate as evidenced by:

- PaO_2 >60 on <50% oxygen
- $PaCO_2$ within normal limits or returned to baseline
- Pulmonary complications absent

NURSING INTERVENTIONS

- Monitor pulmonary status closely
- Administer vigorous pulmonary hygiene
- Note secretions

- Administer oxygen as prescribed; monitor arterial blood gases according to clinical status
- Administer analgesia to prevent pain due to splinting
- Reposition patient frequently to maximize ventilation perfusion and to prevent pooling of secretions
- Assist with peritoneal lavage as ordered

Pancreatic Tumors

Pathophysiology

Carcinoma of the pancreas is an insidious disease that characteristically progresses persistently and is almost always fatal. It is currently a major cause of death in the Western cultures.[1,2] The majority of tumors originate in the epithelium of the ductal system and are of the adenocarcinoma type. A small percentage of tumors arise from the islet cells and are manifested by the secretion of hormones. One endocrine tumor is known as *insulinoma*.

Adenocarcinoma. Adenocarcinoma of the pancreas is characterized by dense fibrotic tissue producing a compact mass in the retroperitoneum. Since the pancreas is not enclosed by an anatomical structure, the tumor often invades surrounding structures including the common bile duct, hepatic portal system, duodenum, stomach, and colon. The most common signs and symptoms of this tumor are those associated with encroachment on these organs.

Insulinomas. Insulinomas are the most common endocrine tumor of the pancreas.[23] They are usually discrete solitary masses and are usually benign. Insulinomas may also be associated with a syndrome called *multiple endocrine neoplasias* characterized by hyperplasia of two or more endocrine organs. Type I, Werner's syndrome, is associated with lesions of the pancreas, parathyroid, pituitary, adrenal cortex, and thyroid.

Clinical Assessment

History and Physical Assessment. Patients with *adenocarcinoma of the pancreas* typically report a history of vague, dull pain in the midepigastric area. Occasionally, it radiates to the back. Pain is related to invasion of the tumor into adjacent retroperitoneal organs or into the splanchnic nerves. Other insidious symptoms may be elicited from the history including weight loss, anorexia, diarrhea, weakness, and vomiting. Vomiting may signal invasion into the duodenum or gastric area with outlet obstruction. Occasionally, the patient may report an aversion to meats and a metallic taste in the mouth. A tumor in the head of the pancreas that obstructs the distal common bile duct will cause jaundice early in the disease. In carcinoma of the body or tail of the organ, jaundice may occur, but it will be a late sign and is associated with metastases.

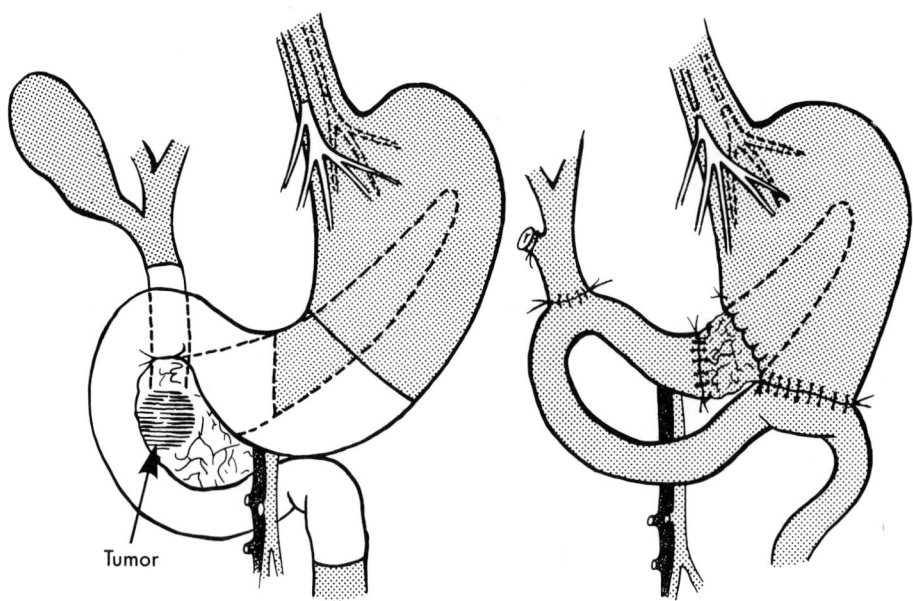

Figure 51-12   Whipple procedure.

The most characteristic symptoms of *insulinomas* are symptoms of insulin shock with fasting, a fasting blood sugar of less than 60, and relief of symptoms with infusion of glucose. The history may reveal minor symptoms of hypoglycemia including hunger, fatigue, nausea and vomiting, lightheadedness, and paresthesias. Dramatic symptoms are usually not reported because the patient often overeats to compensate for hypoglycemia.

Diagnostic Procedures

Adenocarcinoma. There is no single diagnostic test for pancreatic malignancy that is both highly specific to pancreatic cancer and sensitive enough to diagnose very small lesions. Early diagnosis is particularly important to defining resectable and, therefore, curable tumors. Tumor markers are not important in the diagnosis.

Imaging techniques are the "gold standard" for diagnosis of adenocarcinoma.[13] An upper gastrointestinal series may show abnormalities related to displacement of organs around the pancreas. Ultrasonography, a CT scan, and MRI allow for noninvasive visualization of the pancreas. Endoscopic retrograde cholangiopancreatography provides the only means of visualizing the entire pancreatic duct without surgery. Fine-needle aspiration biopsy or intraoperative transduodenal or wedge biopsy can provide definitive diagnosis by cytological examination.

Insulinoma. Diminished plasma glucose concentrations coupled with a fasting blood sugar of less than 60 are characteristic of insulinomas.[23] Radioimmunoassays for proinsulin and C-peptide also facilitate the diagnosis.

Medical Management

Adenocarcinoma. In general, few patients have pancreatic lesions that are resectable and potentially curable. The Whipple resection generally used for patients with small resectable carcinomas of the head of the pancreas (Figure 51-12).[1,2] A resection of the distal stomach, duodenum, common bile duct, and head of the pancreas containing the neoplasm is performed. In addition, a cholecystectomy and truncal vagotomy are done to minimize the chance of gallstones due to peptic ulceration in the jejunum and to stasis of bile in the gallbladder. Gastrointestinal continuity is restored by a pancreaticojejunostomy, a choledochojejunostomy, and a gastrojejunostomy. The major postoperative complication is anastomotic leakage and hemorrhage. Total pancreatectomy with resection of the entire pancreas, duodenum, spleen, and greater omentum together with subtotal gastrectomy and lymphadenectomy is used in many centers.

Palliative surgery for unresectable tumors is recommended to decompress the dilated biliary tree with its attendant symptoms of pruritus, fever, or jaundice. A cholecystojejunostomy is usually performed. Biliary stenting may also be done.

Chemotherapy has not been found to be effective for palliative care or improvement in survival. Pancreatic cancer is highly radioresistant and its retroperitoneal location makes it difficult to treat. Megavolt external beam radiation therapy appears the most promising.

Insulinoma. Surgical resection is the treatment of choice if a solitary lesion can be identified. Patients are generally given a trial dose of diazoxide, a drug that inhibits insulin release. If symptoms are controlled, a laparotomy is performed to identify whether there is a lesion. If a tumor is found, it is removed. If no tumor if found, the abdomen is closed, and transhepatic portal vein studies are done. If a tumor is demonstrated, another operation is performed to remove it. If no tumor is demonstrated, diazoxide therapy is continued.

Other drugs that may be used to control insulin secretion include phenytoin, diltiazem, verapamil, and mithramycin.

NURSING MANAGEMENT

Nursing care during the postoperative period is focused on interventions to maintain hemodynamic stability and prevent postoperative complications. Because most pancreatic tumors are not curable, nursing's unique focus is on patient and family responses to the medical diagnosis.

■ NURSING DIAGNOSIS

Anxiety, related to the threat of death.

OUTCOME STANDARD AND CRITERIA

Anxiety is absent or reduced as evidenced by:
- Verbalization of feelings
- Absence of anxiety manifestations

NURSING INTERVENTIONS
- Assess level of anxiety; look for nonverbal cues
- Note changes in vital signs with periods of anxiety
- Acknowledge the feelings expressed
- Evaluate patient and family coping mechanisms and review past patterns of coping
- Provide accurate information as appropriate
- Be available for listening and talking
- Provide for patient and family input into care decisions as possible
- Administer prescribed medications as needed

■ NURSING DIAGNOSIS

Patient and family powerlessness, related to the suddenness of the diagnosis and the nature of the potential outcome.

OUTCOME STANDARD AND CRITERIA

Sense of control is perceived as evidenced by:
- Involvement in aspects of care
- Expression of sense of control over some aspects of the situation
- Participation in activities of daily living
- Participation in decision making

NURSING INTERVENTIONS
- Identify locus of control (internal or external)
- Listen for statements of helplessness, hopelessness, fear, anger, depression, or withdrawal
- Be available for patient and family and show concern
- Acknowledge the reality of the feelings
- Help patient and family identify things they can do

or have control over in the current situation
- Provide explanations

■ NURSING DIAGNOSIS

Anticipatory grief, related to uncertainty of outcome of disease process.

OUTCOME STANDARD AND CRITERIA

Grief response is adaptive as evidenced by:
- Patient and family identification of ways to cope with loss
- Appropriate grief manifestations for setting
- Effective communication patterns
- Participation in decision making

NURSING INTERVENTIONS
- Identify how patient and/or family are dealing with the current situation
- Note verbal and nonverbal cues and verify meaning
- Provide opportunity to discuss meaning of potential loss
- Acknowledge feelings
- Assist individuals to identify control over what is happening
- Provide referrals as necessary to help patient and family deal with current situation and prepare them for the future

REFERENCES

1. Gitnick, G. (1987). *Handbook of gastrointestinal emergencies.* New York: Elsevier.
2. Sleisenger, M., & Fordtran, J. (1989). *Gastrointestinal disease* (4th ed.). Philadelphia: Saunders.
3. Taragin, M. I., et al. (1990). Gastrointestinal side effects of the nonsteroidal anti-inflammatory drugs. *Digestive Diseases, 8*(5), 269-280.
4. Turnberg, L. A. (1985). Gastric mucosal defense mechanisms. *Scandinavian Journal of Gastroenterology, 110,* 37-40.
5. Johan, G., et al. (1990). *Helicobacter pylori:* Infection of gastric mucin cell metaplasia: The duodenum revisited. *Journal of Pathology, 162*(3), 239-243.
6. Konopad, E., & Noseworthy, T. (1988). Stress ulceration: A serious complication in critically ill patients. *Heart Lung, 17*(4), 339-348.
7. Silen, W. (1987). The clinical problem of stress ulcers. *Clinical and Investigative Medicine, 10*(3), 270-274.
8. Durham, R. M., & Shapiro, M. J. (1991). Stress gastritis revisited. *Surgical Clinics of North America, 71*(4), 791-805.
9. Gottlieb, A. C., et al. (1986). Gastrointestinal complications in critically ill patients: The intensivist's overview. *American Journal of Gastroenterology, 81,* 227-238.
10. Reusser, P., et al. (1990). Prospective endoscopic study of stress erosions and ulcers in critically ill neurosurgery patients. *Critical Care Medicine, 18*(3), 270-274.
11. Eisenberg, P. (1991). Monitoring gastric pH to prevent stress ulcer syndrome. *Focus on Critical Care, 17*(4), 316-322.

12. Shoemaker, W. N., Ayers, C., Grenvik, A., et al. (Eds.). (1989). *Textbook of critical care* (2nd ed.). Philadelphia: Saunders.

13. Bender, T. M., et al. (1991). Radiographic manifestations of anomalies of the gastrointestinal tract. *Radiologic Clinics of North America, 29*(2), 335-349.

14. Cheung, L. Y. (1988). Pathogenesis, prophylaxis and treatment of stress gastritis. *American Journal of Surgery, 156,* 437-440.

15. Basuk, P. M., et al. (1990). Gastric lavage in patients with gastrointestinal hemorrhage. *Archives of Internal Medicine, 150*(7), 1379-1380.

16. Miller, T. A. (1990). Misoprostol: Another agent to prevent bleeding from stress gastritis. *Gastroenterology, 99,* 566-568.

17. Rovers, J. P., & Souney, P. F. (1989). A critical review of continuous infusion of H_2 receptor therapy. *Critical Care Medicine, 17,* 814-821.

18. Bhatt, B. D., et al. (1990). Survey of histamine 2 antagonist usage in acute upper gastrointestinal hemorrhage. *Journal of Clinical Gastroenterology, 12*(1), 14-16.

19. Buhl, K., et al. (1990). Omeprazole: A new approach to gastric acid suppression. *American Family Physician, 41*(4), 1225-1227.

20. Gentry, L. (1990). The influence of pH elevation on the incidence of nosocomial pneumonia. *Journal of Intensive Care Medicine, 5*(Suppl.), S17-S21.

21. Lipper, B., et al. (1991). Pulmonary aspiration during emergency endoscopy with patients with upper gastrointestinal hemorrhage. *Critical Care Medicine, 19*(3), 330-333.

22. Molell, E., et al. (1990). Functional endocrine tumors of the pancreas. *Current Problems in Surgery, 27*(6), 301-327.

23. McConnell, E. A. (1987). Fluid and electrolyte concerns in intestinal surgical procedures. *Nursing Clinics of North America, 22*(4), 853-869.

24. Keith, J. S. (1985). Hepatic failure: Etiologies, manifestations, and management. *Critical Care Nurse, 5*(1), 60-86.

25. Ricci, J. A. (1987). Alcohol-induced upper GI hemorrhage: Case studies and management. *Critical Care Nurse, 7*(1), 56-65.

26. Pierce, J. D., et al. (1990). Acute esophageal bleeding and endoscopic injection sclerotherapy. *Critical Care Nurse, 10*(9), 67-72.

27. Peck, S., & Griffith, D. (1988). Reducing portal hypertension and variceal bleeding. *Dimensions of Critical Care Nursing, 7*(5), 269-279.

28. Stump, D. L., et al. (1990). The use of vasopressin in the treatment of upper gastrointestinal hemorrhage. *Drugs, 39*(1), 38-53.

29. Nishiwaki, H., et al. (1990). Endoscopic measurement of mucosal blood flow with special reference to the effects of sclerotherapy in patients with liver cirrhosis. *American Journal of Gastroenterology, 85*(1), 34-37.

30. Maloney, J. (1986). Surgical intervention in the alcoholic patient with portal hypertension. *Critical Care Quarterly, 8*(4), 63-73.

31. Mitchell, R. L., et al. (1988). Distal splenorenal shunt: Standard procedure for elective and emergency treatment of bleeding esophageal varices. *American Journal of Surgery, 156,* 169-172.

32. Bruckstein, A. H. (1990). Carcinoma of the esophagus. *Postgraduate Medicine, 87*(6), 125-133.

33. Khoury, G. A. (1991). Squamous cell carcinoma of the oesophagus: 10 years on. *Annals of the Royal College of Surgeons of England, 73,* 4-7.

34. Mulder, L. D. (1991). Primary small cell carcinoma of the esophagus: Case presentation and review of the literature. *Gastrointestinal Radiology, 16,* 5.

35. Halvorsen, R. A., et al. (1991). Primary neoplasms of the hollow organs of the gastrointestinal tract. *Cancer, 67*(15), 1181-1188.

36. Fleischer, D. (1989). Endoscopic laser therapy for esophageal cancer. *Lasers in Surgery and Medicine, 9,* 6-16.

37. Tytgat, G. N. (1990). Endoscopic therapy of esophageal cancer: Possibilities and limitation. *Endoscopy, 22,* 263-267.

38. Kelesen, D. P., et al. (1990). Neoadjuvant chemotherapy and surgery of cancer of the esophagus. *Seminars in Surgical Oncology, 6,* 268-273.

39. Muller, J. M., et al. (1990). Surgical therapy of oesophageal carcinoma. *British Journal of Surgery, 77,* 845-857.

40. Hussein, A. (1990). Combination chemotherapy and radiotherapy for small-cell carcinoma of the esophagus. *American Journal of Clinical Oncology, 13*(5), 369-373.

41. Daly, J. M., et al. (1991). Nutritional support of patients with cancer of the gastrointestinal tract. *Surgical Clinics of North America, 71*(3), 523-535.

42. Sitges, S. A. (1988). Mesenteric infarction: An analysis of 83 patients with prognostic studies in 44 cases undergoing small bowel resection. *British Journal of Surgery, 75*(6), 544-548.

43. Sluzker, D. M. (1987). Small bowel infarction and death from primary mesenteric venous thrombosis. *American Journal of Emergency Medicine, 5*(2), 126-129.

44. Finucane, P. M. (1990). Acute mesenteric infarction in elderly patients. *Journal of the American Geriatrics Society, 37*(4), 355-358.

45. Smerud, M. J. (1990). Diagnosis of bowel infarction: A comparison of plain films and CT scans. *American Journal of Roentgenology, 154*(1), 99-103.

46. Martin, R. G. (1986). Malignant tumors of the small intestine. *Surgical Clinics of North America, 66*(4), 779-785.

47. Richards, W. O., & Williams, L. F. (1988). Obstruction of the large and small intestine. *Surgical Clinics of North America, 68*(2), 355-376.

48. Dalzell, T. (1989). Acute intestinal obstruction. *Nursing Times, 11*(85), 59-61.

49. McEntee, G., et al. (1987). Current spectrum of intestinal obstruction. *British Journal of Surgery, 74,* 976-980.

50. McConnell, E. A. (1987). Meeting the challenge of intestinal obstruction. *Nursing, 17*(7), 34-41.

51. Phillips, S. L., & Burns, G. P. (1988). Acute abdominal disease in the aged. *Medical Clinics of North America, 72*(5), 1213-1222.

52. Buechter, K. K. (1988). Surgical management of the acutely obstructed colon. *American Journal of Surgery, 156,* 163-168.

53. Flint, L. M. (1988). Early postoperative acute abdominal complications. *Surgical Clinics of North America, 68*(2), 445-455.

54. Frykberg, E. R., & Phillips, J. W. (1989). Obstruction of the small bowel in the early postoperative period. *Southern Medical Journal, 821,* 164-173.

55. Stewart, R. M., et al. (1987). The incidence and risk of early postoperative small bowel obstruction. *American Journal of Surgery, 154,* 643-646.

56. Reddy, B. S., & Jeejeebhoy, K. J. (1988). Acute complications of Crohn's disease. *Critical Care Medicine, 16*(5), 557-560.

57. Swartz, M. (1989). A nursing view of the extraintestinal manifestations of inflammatory bowel disease. *Gastroenterology Nursing, 12*(1), 3-9.

58. Rankin, G. B. (1990). Extraintestinal and systemic manifestations of inflammatory bowel disease. *Medical Clinics of North America, 74*(1), 39-50.

59. Garrett, J. W., & Drossman, D. A. (1990). Health status in inflammatory bowel disease. *Gastroenterology, 99,* 90-96.

60. Smith, L. C., & Mullen, J. L. (1991). Nutritional assessment and indications for nutritional support. *Surgical Clinics of North America, 71*(3), 449-457.

61. Dozois, R. R., & O'Rourke, J. S. (1988). Newer operations for ulcerative colitis and Crohn's disease. *Surgical Clinics of North America, 68*(6), 1339-1352.

62. Waye, J. D. (1990). Endoscopy in inflammatory bowel disease. *Medical Clinics of North America, 74*(1), 51-65.

63. Ruderman, W. B. (1990). Newer pharmacologic agents for the therapy of inflammatory bowel disease. *Medical Clinics of North America, 74*(1), 133-153.

64. Sutherland, L. R. (1990). Topical treatment of ulcerative colitis. *Medical Clinics of North America, 74*(1), 119-131.

65. Jagelman, D. G. (1990). Surgical alternatives for ulcerative colitis. *Medical Clinics of North America, 74*(1), 155-167.

66. Tally, F. P., & Ho, J. L. (1987). Management of patients with intraabdominal infection due to colonic perforation. *Current Clinical Topics in Infectious Diseases, 8,* 267-295.

67. Becerra, A. T. (1990). Natural history of peritonitis post-peritoneal dialysis. *Biomaterials, Artificial Cells, and Artificial Organs, 18*(1), 125-129.

68. Moore, E. E. (1991). *Trauma* (2nd ed.). Norwalk, CT: Appleton & Lange.

69. Goins, W. A. (1990). Intra-abdominal abscess after blunt abdominal trauma. *Annals of Surgery, 212*(1), 60-65.

70. Falcone, R. E., & Carey, L. C. (1988). Colorectal trauma. *Surgical Clinics of North America, 68*(6), 1307-1318.

71. Shikora, S. A., & Blackburn, G. L. (1991). Nutritional consequences of major gastrointestinal surgery. *Surgical Clinics of North America, 71*(3), 509-521.

72. Polio, J., & Groszmann, R. J. (1986). Hemodynamic factors involved in the development and rupture of esophageal varices. *Seminars in Liver Disease, 6*(4), 318-328.

73. Stassen, W., & McCullough, A. (1985). Management of ascites. *Seminars in Liver Disease, 5*(3), 291-304.

74. Latifi, R., et al. (1991). Nutritional support in liver failure. *Surgical Clinics of North America, 71*(3), 567-578.

75. Pappas, S. C., & Jones, E. A. (1983). Methods for assessing hepatic encephalopathy. *Seminars in Liver Disease, 3*(4), 298-305.

76. Davidson, E., & Dunn, M. (1987). Pathogenesis of hepatorenal syndrome. *Annual Review of Medicine, 38,* 361-372.

77. Jurkovich, G. J. (1990). Pancreatic trauma. *Surgical Clinics of North America, 71*(3), 575-593.

78. Fain, J. A., & Vealey, E. A. (1988). Acute pancreatitis: A gastrointestinal emergency. *Critical Care Nurse, 8*(5), 47-60.

79. Brown, A. (1991). Acute pancreatitis. *Focus on Critical Care, 18*(2), 121-130.

80. Patti, M. G. (1990). Gallstone pancreatitis. *Surgical Clinics of North America, 70*(6), 1277-1293.

81. Sabesin, S. (1987). Countering the dangers of acute pancreatitis. *Emergency Medicine, 19,* 15-96.

82. Jeffres, C. (1989). Complications of acute pancreatitis. *Critical Care Nurse, 9*(4), 38-48.

83. Greenstein, R., et al. (1987). Activation of the renin system in acute pancreatitis. *American Journal of Medicine, 82,* 401-404.

84. Vujic, I. (1989). Vascular complications of pancreatitis. *Radiologic Clinics of North America, 27*(1), 81-89.

85. Safrit, H. D., & Rice, R. P. (1989). Gastrointestinal complications of pancreatitis. *Radiologic Clinics of North America, 27*(1), 73-79.

86. Guice, K., et al. (1988). Pancreatitis-induced acute lung injury. *Annals of Surgery, 208*(1), 71-77.

87. Horton, J., & Burnweit, C. (1988). Hemodynamic function in acute pancreatitis. *Surgery, 103*(5), 538-546.

88. Agarwal, N., et al. (1990). Evaluating tests for acute pancreatitis. *American Journal of Gastroenterology, 85*(4), 356-365.

89. Jones, M. L., & Neoptolemos, J. (1990). Recent advances in the treatment of acute pancreatitis. *Surgery Annual, 22,* 235-261.

90. Latifi, R., et al. (1991). Nutritional management of acute and chronic pancreatitis. *Surgical Clinics of North America, 71*(3), 579-595.

91. Flaherty, J., et al. (1990). Pilot trial of selective decontamination for prevention of bacterial infection in an ICU. *Journal of Infectious Diseases, 162*(6), 1393-1397.

92. Ranson, J. H. (1990). The role of surgery in the management of acute pancreatitis. *Annals of Surgery, 211*(4), 382-391.

PART TWELVE

Integumentary Patient Care Problems

52

Integumentary Anatomy and Physiology

Nancy A. Stotts

The integumentary system is composed of the skin and its appendages. The skin, a complex structure of different tissues, is the largest organ in the body in weight and surface area. The hair, nails, and glands are the skin appendages. The skin and appendages interact to protect the body from external trauma and contamination; to regulate its temperature; and to participate in excretion, absorption, and sensation. The skin is critical to survival. This chapter presents the normal structure and function of the skin, including normal aging and differences in structure and function based on skin color.

ANATOMY

The skin consists of the epidermis and the dermis (Figure 52-1). The epidermis, the outer layer, is connected to the inner layer, or dermis, by the basement membrane. Below the dermis are the subcutaneous tissue, muscle, and the organs. Both the epidermis and the dermis are composed of layers of different types of cells that perform various functions (see box on p. 1190). These layers are not visible to the naked eye, so the only distinction that is made in clinical practice is between the dermis and epidermis.

Epidermis

The epidermis is composed of cells called *keratinocytes*. Their primary role is to produce keratin, a protein that protects the skin from external trauma and infection. Keratinocytes are produced in the deepest basal layer of the epidermis next to the basement membrane, migrate to the surface of the skin over a period of 28 to 45 days, die and are shed in a continual cycle. This ongoing replacement and loss of cells protects against infection. The epidermis is avascular and receives its nutrients from the blood vessels in the dermis and the subcutaneous tissue. Epidermal cells proliferate rapidly and arise from the edges of damaged tissue as well as from the skin appendages (hair

follicles and glands), so repair of damaged tissue proceeds rapidly. As individuals age, the rate of all cellular proliferation, including that of epidermal cells, slows down, increasing the individual's vulnerability to infection and external trauma.

Skin color is determined largely by melanocytes located in the epidermis. *Melanocytes* produce melanosomes, or pigment granules, and the number and size of the melanosomes are the primary determinants of skin color. Larger melanosomes produce darker color and are displaced more widely through the epidermal cells than are the smaller melanosomes produced by light-skinned individuals. Although researchers have explored the nature of the skin in dark- and light-skinned people, the only identifiable difference is in the pigmentation.

Chronic exposure to the sun stimulates the melanocytes to produce larger melanosomes, thereby temporarily changing the pattern of granules in the cells and causing the skin to be darker. Dark skin is protective against the sun's rays and diseases related to solar radiation. In pigment-related diseases of the skin, melanocytes often are implicated. For example, in *vitiligo*, melanocytes are destroyed, producing areas of whitening, whereas in albinism the number of melanocytes is normal, but they cannot synthesize pigment.

Skin color also is affected by carotene, oxyhemoglobin, and circulating substances in the plasma. Carotene is a yellow pigment located in subcutaneous fat and in the heavily keratinized areas of the palms of the hands and the soles of the feet. The amount of oxygen carried by the oxyhemoglobin molecule also affects the color of the skin. When the oxyhemoglobin molecules are well saturated, background skin color is pink; when oxyhemoglobin becomes desaturated, the color is more bluish. Substances carried in the plasma also affect skin color. For example, bilirubin in the bloodstream will cause tissues to turn yellow.

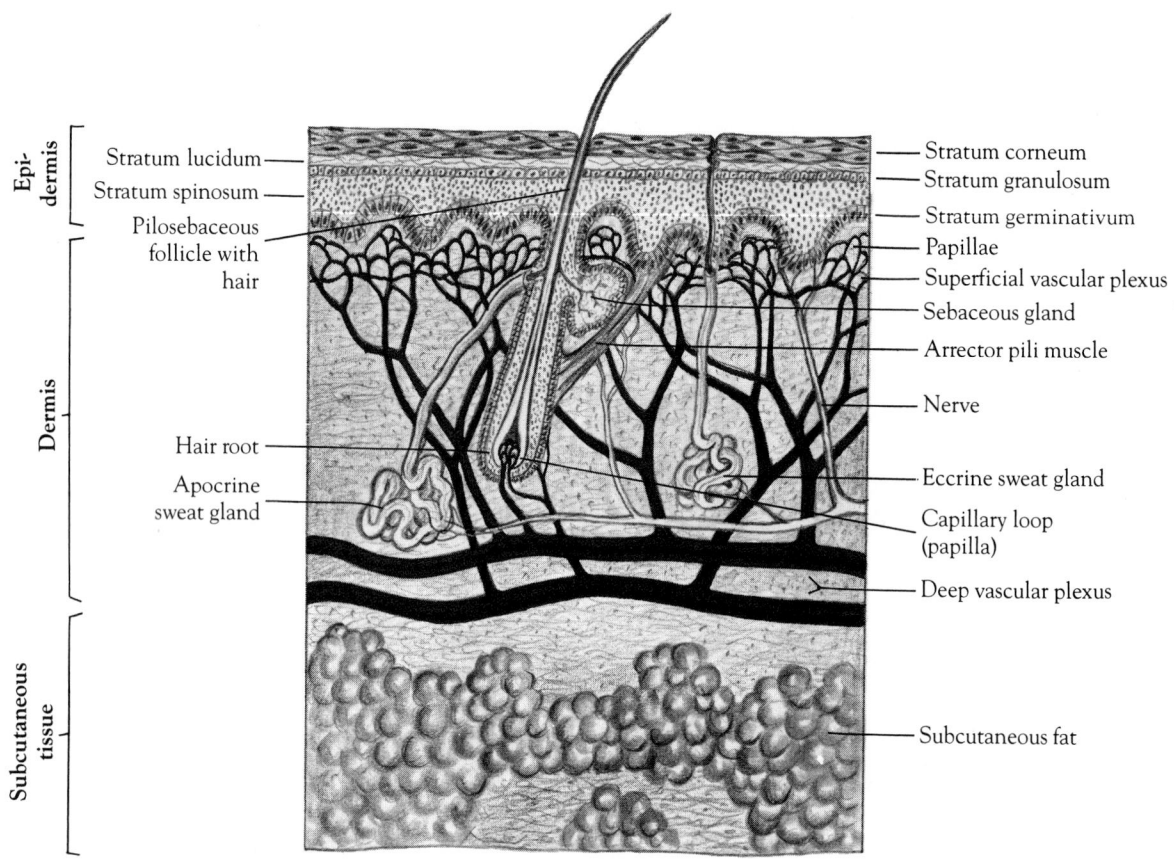

Figure 52-1   The skin.

Layers of the Epidermis

Stratum Corneum
Outermost layer of the epidermis. Consists of 25 to 30 rows of dead keratinocytes. Constantly shed and replaced.

Stratum Lucidum
Lower portion of stratum corneum on palms of hands and soles of feet. Consists of 3 or 4 rows of clear, flat dead cells.

Stratum Granulosum
Important in keratin formation.

Stratum Spinosum
Forms mechanical bulk of the epidermis. Consists of 8 to 10 rows of cells that have a prickly appearance. Together with the stratum basale forms the stratum germinativum where new cells are formed.

Stratum Basale
Anchors the epidermis to the dermis. Consists of columnar epithelium. Must be present for the epithelial cells to regenerate. Cells migrate to surface as they mature. Together with the stratum spinosum forms the stratum germinativum where new cells are formed.

The epidermis also has an immunological capacity that is a function of the Langerhans cells. *Langerhans cells* are macrophages that function primarily in delayed hypersensitivity reactions, especially contact dermatitis. They also produce interleukin-1, that aids in T-cell activation.

Merkel cells are located in the lower levels of the epidermis. This cell is thought to be a type of nerve cell that responds to mechanical stimulation and is sensed as touch.

Basement Membrane

The basement membrane holds the epidermis to the dermis, supports the epidermis, and allows materials to be transported between the epidermis and the dermis. Attachment of the epidermis to the dermis also is provided by the bases of the epidermal appendages, called rete pegs, that attach to deep fingerlike projections called *dermal papillae* and extend through the basement membrane.

Dermis

The dermis is connective tissue composed of collagen and elastic tissue. Collagen, which is produced

---

> ### Layers of the Dermis
>
> *Papillary Layer*
> Outermost layer of dermis. Attaches to the basement membrane. Large surface area due to presence of dermal papillae. Contains Meissner's corpuscles and pacinian corpuscles.
>
> *Reticular Layer*
> Innermost layer of dermis. Attaches to subcutaneous tissue. Consists of vasculature, collagen and fibrous tissue. Makes up the bulk of the dermis.

by fibroblasts, provides tissue with flexibility and resistance to stretch. This force is opposed by elastic tissue that allows for skin elasticity or stretch. The dermis contains the vascular supply to the epidermis (see Figure 52-1). It also houses a rich supply of nerves responsible for transmitting the sensations of touch, pressure, pain, temperature, and itch.

The dermis is divided into two layers, the papillary layer and the reticular layer (see box above). The upper papillary layer makes up approximately one fifth of the thickness of the total layer. The surface area is increased by projections called *dermal papillae,* which protrude into the epidermis and contain loops of capillaries. *Meissner's corpuscles,* nerve endings that are sensitive to light touch, are present in some dermal papillae. The papillary layer also contains pacinian corpuscles, nerve endings that are sensitive to deep pressure.

The inner reticular layer consists of dense, irregular, collagenous connective tissue. This layer also contains numerous blood vessels, as well as collagenous and elastic fibers that give toughness to the skin. The reticular layer is attached to the organs beneath it by the subcutaneous layer.

Circulation

Circulation to the skin is provided by two networks of vessels that perform distinct functions: nutrition of the cutaneous tissues and thermal regulation. Nutrition is provided by arteries, capillaries, and veins, while thermoregulation is provided by extensive subcutaneous venous plexuses capable of holding large amounts of blood and by arteriovenous anastomoses that link arteries and venous plexuses. Arteriovenous anastomoses are located in areas of the body exposed most often to extreme cold, such as the ears, nose, lips, and volar surfaces of the hands and feet.

Subcutaneous Fat

The dermis is separated from underlying structures by a layer of subcutaneous fat. The fat layer serves as insulation against extremes of temperature, provides physical padding, and acts as a storage site for energy. The subcutaneous fat layer is thin in cachexic persons and thick in the obese. Perfusion to subcutaneous tissue may be decreased during periods of stress, and this may result in compromised skin viability.

Epidermal Appendages

The hair, nails, and glands are the epidermal appendages. All three appendages developed from the embryonic epidermis and extend into the dermis. The base of each appendage forms epithelial cells, reducing the distance across which cells must migrate to repair injured tissue.

SKIN FLORA

Human skin contains a number of normal bacteria, but the number varies greatly. Sites that harbor larger numbers of bacteria include the perineum, groin, and axillae. Persons with oily skin harbor more bacteria than those with dry skin. Warm, humid weather also is more conducive to maintenance of skin bacteria than cold, dry weather. Gram-positive bacteria in contact with the apocrine glands in the axillae produce the odor characteristic of the axillae.

The normal pH of skin is 4.2 to 5.6. This pH helps to retard the growth of some bacteria. Leukocytes present in the epidermis are thought to defend against invasion of organisms.

AGING

Changes in the skin that occur with aging may alter each of the functions of the integumentary system. Skin turgor decreases significantly, and the skin takes on a transparent, tissuelike appearance. Secretions from the sebaceous and sudoriferous glands decrease significantly, causing dry skin, especially over the extremities. Hypopigmentation also tends to increase with age.

The amount of hair loss depends on several factors other than age, such as heredity and sex. Generally, by the mid-sixties hair loss is completed, and its distribution patterns are set. In most aging persons pigment cells fail, thus causing gray hair color. Reduction in hormonal levels causes a decrease in pubic and axillary hair.

In the older person the dermis loses its elasticity. Loss of collagen and elastic fibers causes shrinking of the dermis, which in turn causes wrinkling as the smaller dermal underbase that supports the dermis causes the dermis to fold.

Gravity pulls the skin down, causing marked facial changes such as jowls, drooping eyelids, and elongation of the earlobes. Bags under the eyes are herniations of fat into the subcutaneous layers. Nail growth may slow. Nails also change to a yellow or gray tone and become more brittle and thick.

Vascular changes and atrophy of the epidermis inhibit the function of skin sensory neurons. This in turn decreases the older person's ability to perceive sensations. The tactile sense is lost most frequently in the palms of the hands and the soles of the feet.

PHYSIOLOGY

Sensation

The function of the skin as an organ of sensation is extensive. It plays a major role in the collection of sensory information from the body through the *somatic senses*. The somatic senses are generally classified as the mechanoreceptive and thermoreceptive senses and the pain sense.

Mechanoreceptive Senses

Commonly referred to as the *tactile senses,* the mechanoreceptive senses include touch, pressure, vibration, tickle, and itch. Position sense is also included in this category.

The sensations of touch, pressure, and vibration, though classified independently, are closely interrelated. In fact, they are all detected by the same type of tactile receptor with only minor differences. (See box below.) Touch generally results from the stimulation of receptors found in the tissues just beneath the skin, whereas pressure is detected as a result of deeper tissue deformation. The sense of vibration results from rapid repetitive signals and uses the same receptors that detect touch and pressure.

Tactile Receptors in the Skin

Free Nerve Endings
Detect touch, pressure, tickle, and itch. Distributed throughout skin surface.
Meissner's Corpuscles
Detect touch. Found more frequently in lips and fingertips. Especially sensitive to light touch and low-frequency vibration.
Merkel's Disks
Detect touch. Help identify location of touch on body.
Hair End Organs
Detect movement of hair. Nerve located at base of each hair.
Ruffini End Organs
Detect touch and pressure. Located in deeper layers of skin and respond to heavy continuous touch and pressure.
Pacinian Corpuscles
Detect vibration. Stimulated by rapid movement.

Recent findings support the existence of specific free nerve endings that detect only the itch and tickle sensations. These nerve endings are found almost exclusively in the superficial layers of the skin, a site at which only these sensations can usually be elicited.

The sensation of itch is a response to weak, persistent stimulation leading to a response such as rubbing or scratching in an effort to remove or obtain relief from the irritant. If scratching is strong enough to cause pain, the itch sensation is thought to be inhibited or overridden by the sensation of pain.

The tickle sensation is also caused by persistent light stimulation, usually resulting in minor avoidance behavior such as jerking away from the source of stimulation.

Thermoreceptive Senses

The thermal receptors are capable of detecting heat and cold and discriminating between gradations of temperature. At least three types of sensory receptor play a role in this function: cold receptors, warmth receptors, and pain receptors.

Located just beneath the external surface of the skin, the cold and warmth receptors are positioned at specific but separate points. Each receptor has a stimulating diameter of approximately 1 mm. The areas of the body in which these receptors are located and the number within each area vary significantly. There are three to ten times as many cold receptors as warmth receptors. Specific areas of the body such as the lips contain 15 to 25 cold points per square centimeter as compared to the finger, which contains only 5 cold points per square centimeter. The number of warmth points is correspondingly fewer.

Specialized pain receptors are found throughout the superficial layers of the skin. Stimulation of these receptors occurs only in the presence of extreme degrees of heat and cold. The pain receptors along with the cold and warmth receptors are responsible for detecting "freezing cold" and "burning hot" sensations.

Pain Sense

The sensation of pain is a protective mechanism that is stimulated whenever tissue is being damaged. The response to this form of stimulation is an awareness of the abnormal stimulus and removal of the stimulus if possible.

Two major types of pain have been classified as acute pain and slow pain. *Acute pain* requires only about 0.1 second to be sensed. Also referred to as *sharp* or *fast pain,* this form of pain is generally sensed in the skin but not felt in most deeper tissues. *Slow pain,* on the other hand, is sensed only after a second or more has passed and increases slowly in its intensity over several more seconds or even minutes. *Throbbing, chronic,* and *aching pain* are additional terms used for slow pain. This form of pain can be sensed in both the skin and the internal tissues and is usually associated with tissue destruction.

The pain receptors also may be classified according to the type of stimulation necessary to excite the nerve ending. *Mechanosensitive pain receptors* are almost entirely excited by excessive mechanical stress or damage to the underlying tissues. Those receptors sensitive to heat and cold are referred to as *thermosensitive pain receptors.* A third type of receptor, called *chemosensitive receptors,* reacts to a variety of chemical substances such as bradykinin, serotonin, histamine, and prostaglandins. Even though there is receptor specificity, most receptors respond to more than one type of stimulus.

Pain receptors differ from most types of nerve endings in that they are nonadaptive. This lack of adaptation ensures that the subject remains cognizant of the damaging stimulus for as long as the pain persists.

Protection

Mechanical

The most well-known function of the skin is as a barrier to external environmental forces. The layers of the epidermis provide a relatively flexible and elastic supportive covering. Additional cushioning and bulk are provided by the dermis and subcutaneous fat. Thus, when mechanical manipulation of the skin is encountered, the skin gives but does not break. Once the manipulation has stopped, it can usually resume its normal position.

Protection from external radiation such as ultraviolet light, visible light, and ionizing radiation also is a function of the skin. Melanin plays a major role in shielding the body from the damaging effects of the sun.

Chemical

In addition to physical protection, the layers of the skin act as a barrier to the penetration and absorption of potentially harmful gases and liquids. The stratum corneum and free lipids provide the major barrier for their absorption. As a selectively permeable surface, the skin is more impermeable than permeable. The skin also protects the body from potentially harmful microorganisms, perhaps partly because of the low pH of the skin surface.

Temperature Regulation

A significant function of the skin is the regulation of body temperature. It is an essential component of the body's system for maintaining a constant internal or core body temperature despite variable environmental temperatures and metabolic activity.

Body temperature is regulated primarily by neural feedback mechanisms that operate through the perioptic area of the anterior hypothalamus and portions of the posterior hypothalamus. Stimulation of this area leads to activation of the autonomic nervous system via sympathetic nerve fibers found in the skin. Ambient temperature changes are relayed to the posterior hypothalamus via the peripheral thermosensitive receptors.

Heat Loss

Approximately 95% of the total body heat is dissipated by radiation, conduction, convection, and evaporation. *Radiation* is the transfer of infrared heat rays from one object to another. Therefore, if the body temperature is greater than that of surrounding objects such as the floor, ceiling, and furniture, body heat is reduced. However, if surrounding objects are at a higher temperature than the body, heat is absorbed by the body.

Conduction is the transfer of heat from the body to any object with which it comes in contact, such as clothing. Only minimal amounts of heat are lost through this method, because the object absorbing the heat soon approaches the temperature of the body. Once this occurs, the object becomes an insulator preventing more heat loss.

Convection is the conduction of heat to the air surrounding the body. When air makes contact with the skin, the heat of the body is conducted to the cooler air, which becomes warmed. Warmed air then is carried away by convection currents. The faster the air moves, the greater the loss of heat. Convection accounts for about 15% of body heat loss. A greater loss of heat via conduction and convection occurs in water because water absorbs much larger quantities of heat than air at moderate temperatures.

Evaporation is the conversion of a liquid to a vapor in which the evaporating substance removes heat from the body. Evaporation from the skin and lungs removes approximately 22% of normal body heat. A continuous diffusion of water through the skin and lungs results in an insensible water loss of approximately 600 ml per day. This is an uncontrollable evaporative process, making it an ineffective method of temperature regulation. There is, however, a very effective controlled method of evaporative heat loss through regulation of the sweat glands, which are controlled by the central nervous system in much the same way as the cutaneous vessels. Stimulation of the perioptic area of the hypothalamus by high external temperatures or an increased metabolic rate activates the sympathetic nerves in the skin throughout the body, and the sweat glands respond to the sympathetic innervation by producing perspiration at a rate equivalent to the strength of the stimulation. Approximately 4 L of perspiration per hour can be produced under extreme conditions.

Insulation

In addition to the temperature-regulating mechanisms mentioned above, the skin also provides the body with the capability of retaining internal body heat in an effort to maintain a constant core temperature. The outer layers of the skin, along with the subcutaneous fat, act as a thermal insulator. The fat tissue is particularly effective in preventing the escape of body heat because it conducts heat only one third as readily as other tissue. The thickness of the subcutaneous fat layer thus determines the degree of insulation possible.

Excretion and Absorption

Although they are not widely emphasized, the skin also has two other functions, excretion and absorption. The excretory function is limited, but profuse sweating can eliminate up to 1 g of nonprotein nitrogen per hour.

The absorption function is important in drug therapy. With percutaneous absorption, medication penetrates the epidermis through the strateum corneum or via the skin appendages and moves through the dermis to be absorbed by circulation.

Drugs are absorbed from the skin by passive diffusion and the lipid layer of the strateum corneum provides the greatest barrier to absorption. This barrier is a rate-limiting factor in absorption and allows drugs to be applied so absorption can occur at a constant rate over time.

The skin varies regionally in its ability to absorb substances. The forehead, scalp, and axillae have the greatest rate of absorption, while the forehead and palms have the slowest. In addition, age affects the rate of absorption. Preterm infants have markedly increased rates of absorption. Infants through adults have similar rates, and the elderly have decreased rates of absorption. However, because of their immature metabolic responses and large skin/surface area ratio, infants are at high risk for the systemic effects of topical agents.

The skin barrier can be changed by occlusion, altering the temperature, and manipulating the surface characteristics. Occlusion enhances hydration and so promotes absorption. Warmer temperatures increase blood flow and so enhance absorption. Changing the surface layer of the skin by removing oils with soap or alcohol also alters absorption. Thus, when medications are administered transdermally, the skin environment must be considered and maintain a consistent blood level of the drug.

The vehicle in which the substance is administered also may alter the rate of absorption. Knowledge of the vehicle in which a drug is administered is important to the nurse looking for a peak action and evaluating effectiveness of a drug. Changes merely in the drug's vehicle can significantly alter absorption and effects seen in patients.

Damage to the skin also can enhance the rate of absorption of drugs. Damage can be mechanical, chemical, or through radiation or disease.

Many factors at the skin level affect transdermal drug administration. Attention to the barrier function of the skin allows the nurse to manipulate the environment to maximize therapeutic effects.

BIBLIOGRAPHY

Arnold, H. L. (1990). *Andrew's diseases of the skin: Clinical dermatology* (8th ed.). Philadelphia: Saunders.

Berardesca, E., & Maibach, H. I. (1988). Skin occlusion: Treatment or drug-like device? *Skin Pharmacology, 1,* 207-215.

Bressler, R. S., & Bressler, C. H. (1989). Functional anatomy of the skin. *Clinics in Podiatric Medicine and Surgery, 6*(2), 229-246.

McDonald, C. J. (1988). Structure and function of the skin. Are there differences between black and white skin? *Dermatologic Clinics, 6*(3), 343-347.

Soter, N. A., & Baden, H. P. (1991). *Pathophysiology of dermatologic diseases* (2nd ed.). New York: McGraw-Hill.

53

Burns

James B. Winkler

Mary Ann DiMola

Jill A. Wooten

No one discipline can provide adequate burn care: A team approach must be developed, with each member providing his or her particular expertise in harmony with others. The nurse is a *pivotal* member for structuring an environment of recovery. Each nurse who endeavors to care for a critically burned patient must consider an approach to total coordination of therapy, incorporating basic nursing as well as specialty nursing skills. If measures or tasks are overlooked because they appear trivial, the resulting problems are soon compounded, often resulting in the unnecessary death of the patient. Thus, we see patients in whom initial shock has been successfully combatted by a meticulous fluid therapy program but who later die of pneumonia, which might have been controlled had vigorous preventive measures been instituted.

The routine essentials of nursing care are frequently neglected in the flurry of activity surrounding any critically ill patient. The practitioner may become distracted by intravenous infusions and medications, invasive monitoring, and respiratory therapy equipment, and may overlook the basic ingredients essential to recovery: comfort, rest, hygiene, nutrition, position change, deep breathing exercises, and infection control. These activities have traditionally been the nurse's domain and must never be neglected. Whenever possible, severely burned victims should be transferred to a facility with a specialized burn unit. Nurses should always initiate discussions regarding appropriateness of treatment versus transfer.

PATHOPHYSIOLOGY
Stages of Burn Injury

Based on the derangements that follow an appreciable full-thickness skin loss, burn care can be divided into three definable but overlapping periods,

each with well-defined principles on which care is planned. These are the emergent, the acute, and the rehabilitation periods. In the *emergent period,* the traumatic insult to the skin (the largest organ of the body) results in an immediate, dramatic, natural inflammatory response and massive shift of extracellular fluid from the bloodstream into the damaged tissues. The *acute period* deals with the loss of normal skin function, primarily necessitating protection against infection, and the body's attempt to heal the massive wound, creating a disposition to serious complications. During the *rehabilitation period,* the primary considerations are of the functional and cosmetic deficits caused by contracture and scar formation.

Emergent Period

The emergent period refers to the first 2 to 4 days after the burn injury, depending on the severity of the injury and when fluid resuscitation was begun. This generally is the period when the patient is admitted, the severity of the injury is determined, and first aid and wound care are initiated. The most important aspects of care involve determining and administering the required fluids, assessing respiratory status, and maintaining pulmonary function. The emergent period usually ends when initial fluid therapy is completed and the patient starts to lose some of the weight gained when large amounts of fluid were given intravenously.

Acute Period

The acute period of treatment begins at the end of the emergent period and lasts until all of the full-thickness wounds are covered with suitable, permanent skin covering. If the burn is only a partial-thickness injury, the acute period may be over within 10 to 20 days; healing is spontaneous, and grafts are not necessary. With larger burns encompassing a total burn surface area (TBSA) of more than 50%, 30 to 90 days to recover is not uncommon.

During the acute phase there are two main principles of management. The first is to remove the eschar (dead tissue) as soon as possible and to cover the wound with homografts (skin grafts from another person) or autografts (grafts of the patient's own skin). Tissue culture skin (cloned from the patient) and synthetic skin substitutes also are now being used as both temporary and permanent wound coverings. The second major task is to avoid the complications known to occur during this time. The most common complications are (1) infection leading to septicemia and pneumonia, (2) adult respiratory distress syndrome (ARDS), and (3) other multiorgan derangements. Some complications occur despite valiant attempts at prevention; therefore, it is necessary to detect these complications early and to treat them vigorously. It is very important to remember that the seriously burned patient is acutely ill for a long time. The patient is not in a chronic state, as this prolonged, difficult period would suggest, but rather is fighting to regain hemostasis and in serious danger of death from complications.

Only when the full-thickness wound is covered with permanent skin replacement is the patient considered to be recovering.

Rehabilitation Period

The rehabilitation phase is concerned with restoring the patient to his highest level of wellness. During this time the patient undergoes an intensive effort to regain or compensate for functions lost due to the burn. This stage may continue for many years. During this time, the point of care may shift from the nurse to other team members such as physical therapists, social workers, or occupational therapists.

Body Systems Alterations

Adverse effects from burn injury may be quite varied; some wounds heal without visible scarring, while others may result in death. The events that follow a major injury may progress to multiorgan failure and a devastating outcome. This progression is a complex and, in many cases, unexplained phenomenon. To better understand what is known about the body's response to heat, a systems approach is used.

Integumentary System

The skin is composed of three distinct layers: the epidermis, dermis, and subcutaneous layers. When heat is applied to the external surface of the skin, the

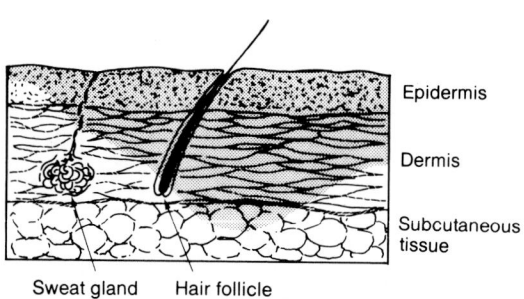

Figure 53-1   A smooth plane of burn can rarely be demarcated. More often, a combination of varying depth of burn occurs. The shaded area denotes damage due to burn. Other areas of skin section appear normal.

resultant damage is proportional to the degree of heat and the time of exposure.

Prolonged exposure to relatively low heat or short exposure to higher temperatures can cause cell destruction at progressively deepening levels. Tissue damage can occur at temperatures as low as 113° F (45° C) when the heat source is in contact with the skin for several hours. At 158° F (70° C), cellular destruction is so rapid that only brief periods of exposure are necessary for total destruction down to and including the subcutaneous layer.[1] Most large burn injuries cause damage at varying skin layers so that a smooth plane of burn cannot be demarcated (Figure 53-1). Once cell destruction has taken place, regardless of the cause of time frame, the physiological responses are similar.

In addition to changes in the skin, varying degrees of vascular destruction may occur. In full-thickness burns, complete cessation of blood flow to the burned area is common. This occurs as a result of thrombosis to the vessels in the injured area, a condition that can last for many weeks. Regardless of surgical or nonsurgical intervention, the healing process in full-thickness wounds needs to include the reestablishment of a vascular bed to the burned area. If the burn is of partial thickness, circulation to the affected area stops temporarily, resuming most often within 24 to 48 hours.

A point to be considered in tissue damage caused by heat is the thickness of the skin involved. It takes less heat and time to do similar damage in areas of the body covered with thin skin than in those areas where the skin is thicker. Skin is thickest over the back and thinnest around the medial arm and face. Skin is generally thinner in young children and in the elderly than in those in the prime of life. The elderly also have reduced layers of subcutaneous material and an overall decreased ability to respond to trauma.

Consequently, burns of similar size and degree often have a more serious effect in the young and the aged.

Immune System

Burn patients are susceptible to the invasion of pathogens because the injury has damaged the skin, thus destroying the body's natural first-line barrier. Yet these patients endure an even greater risk because of the dramatic immunological changes that occur. These changes involve such structures as the phagocytic system, the thymus, the lymphocytes, the plasma cells, and the immunoglobulins. The etiology of these changes is unknown; however, it is theorized that burned cells produce a "toxin" that alters the immune system's ability to respond in the normal fashion. The normal responses of cells associated with the immune system such as T helper/suppressor cells and natural killer cells are altered, and the patient with a major burn rapidly becomes immunosuppressed, much like a patient receiving chemotherapy or a person with AIDS. As a result, the infectious organisms that are now able to invade the body more easily also are less likely to be controlled by the impaired immune system. A phenomenon called *translocation* has also been discussed regarding the etiology of infection. Some researchers believe that microorganisms can migrate from one part of the body cavity such as the gut to the burn wound, causing an autoinfection. This theory has not been definitely proved. Sterilization of the gut immediately postburn has been performed in some burn units with moderate success.

Cardiovascular System

The most dramatic cardiovascular event seen after burn injury is burn shock. Until the 1930s and into the early 1940s, shock was the leading cause of death for all burn victims with greater than 35% TBSA. The patient who has suffered a severe burn experiences hemodynamic changes almost immediately following the injury.

A marked increase of capillary permeability occurs, possibly related to histamine release. In small burns (<20% to 25% TBSA), this permeability alteration is limited to the area burned; however, with a larger burn, this effect appears throughout the body. Fluid alterations quickly occur as large-diameter molecules such as plasma and albumin readily pass through capillary membrane pores, pulling fluid out of the vasculature. The mechanisms that cause alterations in fluid volume are not completely understood, and current research data have not provided conclusive evidence regarding the origin of this problem.

Increased capillary permeability presents a biphasic pattern. The initial peak occurs during the first

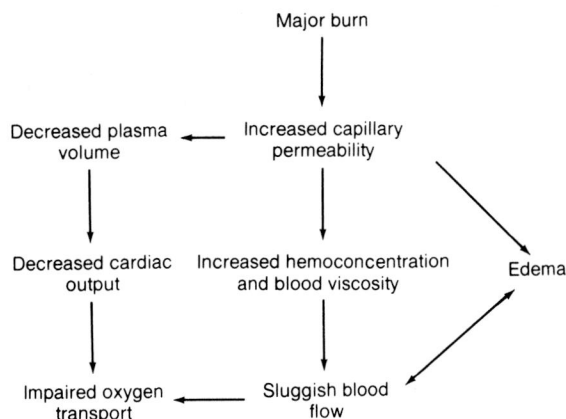

Figure 53-2 Following a major burn, capillary permeability increases, allowing plasma particles to leak from vascular to interstitial spaces. This results not only in massive edema and hemoconcentration but also in a decrease in cardiac output and impaired oxygen transport to vital organs.

2 hours postburn and then drops to within normal limits. Almost immediately, a very rapid rise is again noted and is of much longer duration. The second peak occurs 3 to 4 hours after the injury and slowly returns to normal over the subsequent 12 to 36 hours if the patient is to survive.[2]

The leakage of fluid from the capillary bed to the interstitium causes the lymphatic system to become overwhelmed, resulting in an excess of interstitial fluid and a deficit of intravascular plasma volume (Figure 53-2). This disruption in the Starling equilibrium causes edema, which is proportional to the size of the burn. Patients with large surface area burns often experience massive pitting systemic edema.

Beginning at approximately 48 hours postburn, the leaking of intravascular fluid to the interstitium subsides, and capillary permeability approaches normal. The lymphatics are now able to accommodate the fluid load, thus restoring the function of the Starling equilibrium. Excessive fluid in the interstitium is reabsorbed, and edema is diminished. Previous to this, most patients have received intravenous enhancement of the intravascular volume, and now circulatory overload can easily occur. The elderly and patients with a history of congestive heart failure are especially at risk.

The fluid volume deficit resulting from plasma loss can lead to irreversible shock because as much as 50% of the blood volume may leave the blood vessels in the form of a plasma leak. Cardiac output falls as a result of two mechanisms: hypovolemia and myocardial depressant factor (MDF).

Hypovolemic shock results from a loss of plasma

from the circulating blood volume. The patient experiences a devastating drop in circulating blood volume if not treated with adequate fluids. This drop in blood volume causes a decrease in both venous return and systemic blood pressure. The body compensates for the drop in cardiac output by shunting blood from the periphery to the vital organs and by increasing the heart rate. Fluid therapy must be prompt and adequate if shock is to be prevented.

In early stages of shock, myocardial deterioration is not severe despite poor coronary perfusion. However, if shock progresses, the myocardium deteriorates as a result of toxin factors in the circulation, especially MDF, lactic acid, and endotoxin. These factors weaken the myocardial reserve and can grossly exacerbate progressive shock.

Organ and tissue perfusion is impaired by a decreased cardiac output. This results from a combination of factors, which include decreased blood volume, poor myocardial function, and hemoconcentration (caused by the decreased plasma volume). Eventually, vital organs are not perfused, and death occurs if treatment is not efficient and effective. Other complications related to the alterations in plasma volume include changes in colloid osmotic pressure, hypoproteinemia, and electrolyte changes.

Respiratory System

Pulmonary function may be impaired as a result of direct pulmonary injury or secondary complications, and it may be minor or severe, depending on the circumstances of the burn injury. Four types of pulmonary injury are frequently seen in burn patients: (1) carbon monoxide poisoning, (2) upper airway thermal burns, (3) smoke poisoning, and (4) pulmonary parenchymal failure.

Carbon monoxide poisoning affects the lungs indirectly as a result of carbon monoxide toxicity. Carbon monoxide, a by-product of combustion, binds with the hemoglobin molecule, as does oxygen. The affinity of carbon monoxide for hemoglobin, however, is about 230 times as great as that of oxygen. As the resulting carboxyhemoglobin level increases, less oxygen is transported via the hemoglobin molecule, causing cardiopulmonary and central nervous system dysfunction. Figure 53-3 depicts some of the effects seen in the patient exposed to carbon monoxide.

Upper airway thermal burns occur when flame burns involve the upper chest, neck, or face or when superheated air from a heat source is inhaled. It is common for patients to suffer burns to the nasal mucosa, oral mucosa, and pharynx. The resulting edema

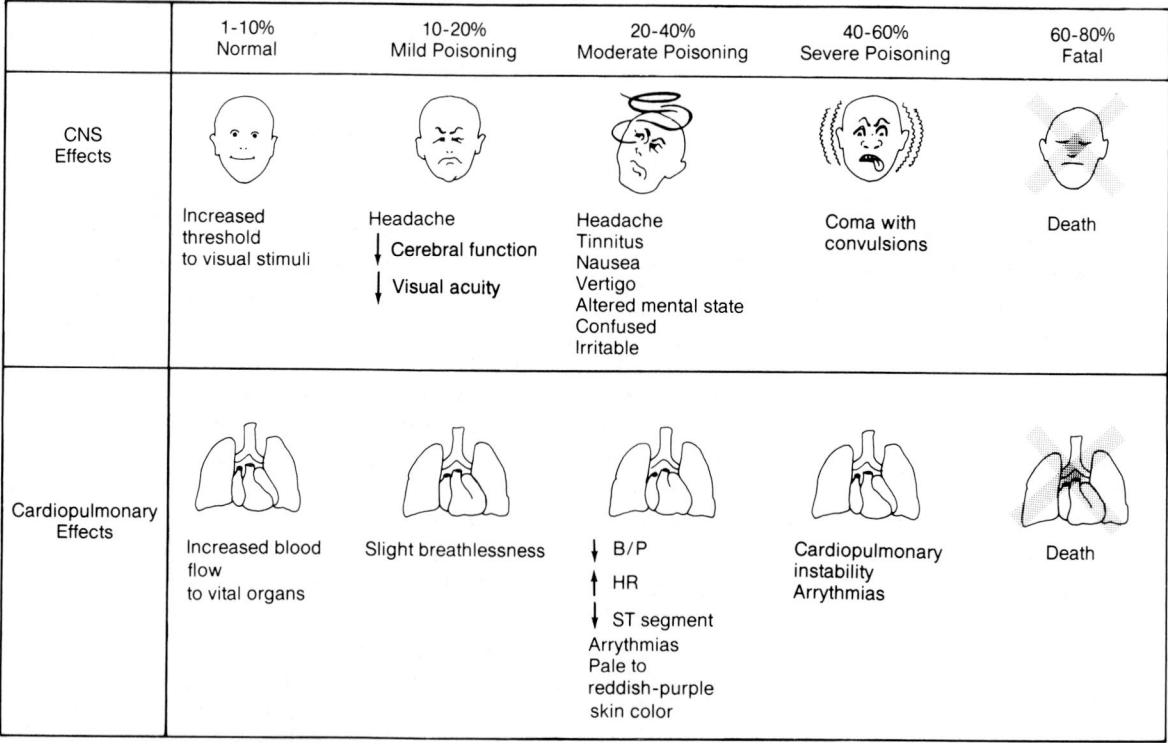

	1-10% Normal	10-20% Mild Poisoning	20-40% Moderate Poisoning	40-60% Severe Poisoning	60-80% Fatal
CNS Effects	Increased threshold to visual stimuli	Headache ↓ Cerebral function ↓ Visual acuity	Headache Tinnitus Nausea Vertigo Altered mental state Confused Irritable	Coma with convulsions	Death
Cardiopulmonary Effects	Increased blood flow to vital organs	Slight breathlessness	↓ B/P ↑ HR ↓ ST segment Arrythmias Pale to reddish-purple skin color	Cardiopulmonary instability Arrythmias	Death

Figure 53-3 Carbon monoxide effects. Progressive deterioration of the CNS and cardiopulmonary systems occurs as arterial levels of carbon monoxide increase.

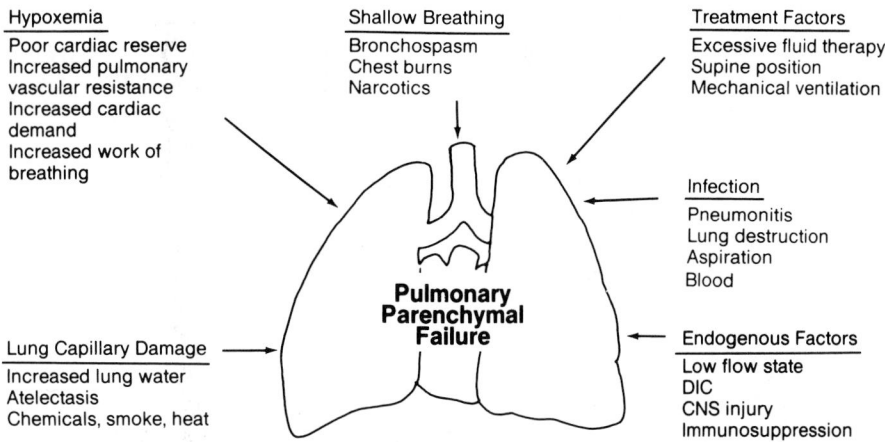

Figure 53-4   Factors contributing to respiratory failure in burn patients with pulmonary involvement.

in the local burn area, coupled with systemic changes in capillary permeability, often causes airway insufficiency or obstruction. Burns of the neck and chest may further complicate the problem if the forming eschar becomes noncompliant and the airway's correct anatomical position cannot be maintained.

Thermal damage from heat does not usually affect the lower respiratory tract because heat is quickly dissipated in upper airway structures. However, superheated steam often overcomes the capacity of the upper airway structures and reaches deeper levels of the lungs. Barring complication, upper airway edema resolves in 3 to 5 days once fluids are mobilized from the interstitium to the vasculature.

Smoke poisoning causes epithelial damage in the lower respiratory tract and is most frequently due to the presence of incomplete products of combustion; that is, oxides from sulfur, nitrogen, aldehydes, and hydrochloric acid. The effects of each agent on the lung may vary slightly, but overall effects can be generalized.[3]

The most significant effects of epithelial damage are atelectasis and pulmonary edema. A decrease in alveolar surfactant production and the immediate loss of bronchial epithelial cilia contribute to these events. Edema occurs as a result of changes in pulmonary capillary permeability and increased fluid loads. Tracheal and bronchial epithelial sloughing frequently occur within 72 hours after the injury, producing hemorrhagic bronchitis. The edema, first limited to small airways, intensifies, and the clinical picture referred to as ARDS may emerge.

Pulmonary parenchymal failure results when gas exchange in the alveoli becomes irreversibly impaired. Because smoke poisoning inhibits the function of pulmonary alveolar macrophages, an inflammatory exudate soon appears in the lungs. This, in conjunction with the edema caused by changes in pulmonary capillary permeability, large fluid loads, and immobility, can lead to bronchopneumonia. Patients experience pulmonary shunting, hypoxemia, alveolar air trapping, high airway resistance, and hypercarbia. The prognosis of patients in this late stage of respiratory failure is very grim (Figure 53-4).

Patients may suffer from a number of other pulmonary complications. The systemic capillary leak that occurs in patients with a significant burn (>25%), causes generalized body edema. Therefore, even those patients who have not sustained any specific pulmonary damage may experience significant loss of plasma from the pulmonary microcirculation into the lungs, which may result in inefficient exchanges of gases, an upper airway obstruction, or both.

Patients with circumferential third-degree burns to the chest and neck may develop problems with ventilatory excursion secondary to thick, leathery, nonelastic eschar surrounding the chest. It is essential in these patients to relieve the pressure so that pulmonary excursion can return to normal.

Renal System

Kidney damage may occur at any time during the patient's treatment and for any number of reasons. In the emergent phase, hypovolemic shock may result in a low-flow state in the renal tubules, leading to acute renal failure if the shock is not rapidly reversed. Renal damage may also occur early in the postburn period as a result of hemoglobinuria. The muscle destruction that may occur with deep dermal or electrical burns causes the destruction of red blood cells and the release of the pigment myoglobin. These particles can block renal tubules and contribute to severe renal dysfunction.

Other renal complications such as oliguria, anuria, or renal failure can occur at any time during the treatment phase due to local infection, trauma, sepsis, and drug therapy. It is imperative that the nurse recognize early signs of these conditions to ensure therapeutic intervention.

Gastrointestinal System

Although no direct insult to the gastrointestinal tract occurs in most thermal burns, alterations are seen in the function of the gastrointestinal tract. Metabolic imbalances may occur, causing tremendous changes in the patient's metabolic needs and indirectly affecting the gastrointestinal system.

In the initial postburn period, blood is shunted to the vital organs from the intestines and the spleen, which often results in a cessation of peristaltic function known as paralytic ileus. This condition can have serious consequences for the burn patient. Because oral fluids do not pass farther than the stomach, there is danger of aspiration. Over the long term, however, the presence of a paralytic ileus can hamper the body's ability to obtain calories. Paralytic ileus is most common during the first 24 to 48 hours in patients who have sustained burns of more than 25% TBSA. It is characterized by the absence of (1) signs of peristaltic function, (2) bowel sounds, and (3) passage of gas and feces along the digestive tract. Acute gastric dilatation can develop rapidly as a result of the functional disturbances in the gastrointestinal tract, such as decreased motility, distention, and decreased blood supply. Vomiting may occur, which can further exacerbate existing hypovolemia and electrolyte imbalances. Corrective action includes close assessment for gastric dilatation and passing a nasogastric tube.

Gastrointestinal ulcerations common in the burn patient are of two types: peptic ulcers and Curling's ulcers. Peptic ulcers are characterized by many small lesions found in the stomach, whereas Curling's ulcers are typically deep ulcerations in the duodenum (Figure 53-5). The etiology of both types of ulcers is thought to be related to the stress response in burn patients, which causes hypersecretion of acid in the gut, ischemia to the gastric mucosa, and decreased mucous production.

Metabolic System

The burn patient experiences many metabolic alterations that result from complex changes in circulating hormone levels. These effects occur to some extent in all burn patients, but they are far more pronounced in the patient whose burn exceeds 40% TBSA.

Several hormones are affected, and the alterations may persist for weeks following injury. The burn may stimulate an increased production of certain hormones (aldosterone and cortisol) while causing the

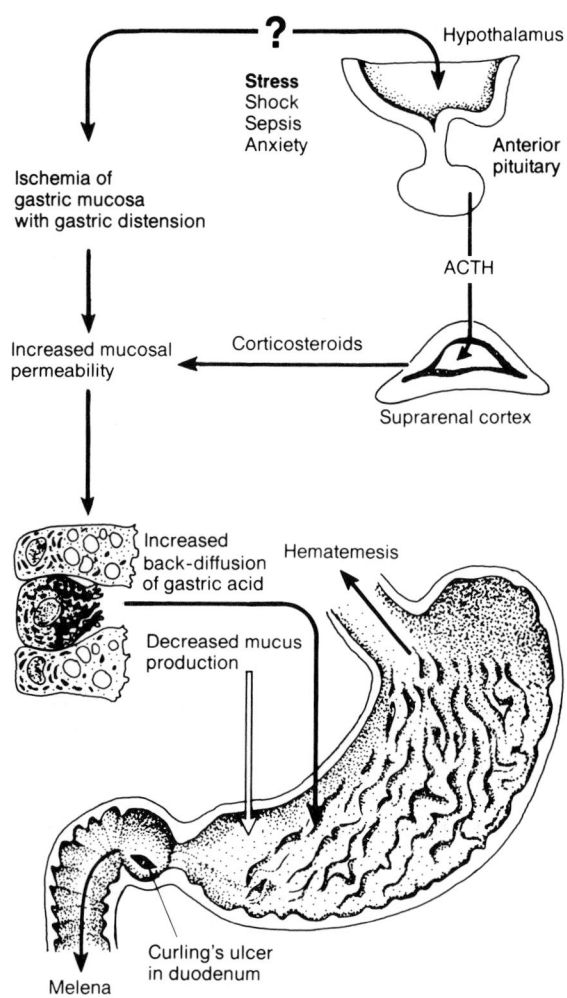

Figure 53-5 Factors predisposing burn patients to the development of Curling's ulcer.

suppression of others (thyroid and pituitary hormones). Table 53-1 summarizes the endocrine changes that occur in patients with major burns.

Increases in the burn patient's metabolic rate are greater than those seen in most other disease states. Patients with a 40% or greater burn may have a 100% increase in their normal metabolic rate at room temperature.

Energy requirements are tremendously increased due to hypermetabolism, energy deficits incurred from evaporative water losses through water-permeable eschar, and postburn catabolism. If energy requirements are not adequately met, the patient with a large burn (>40%) can lose 25% of his or her preburn weight within 3 weeks. In addition, inadequate nutrition leads to poor wound healing.

Hypermetabolism is affected to a certain extent by the ambient temperature. A response in the burn patient mediated by the hypothalamus causes a tem-

TABLE 53-1　Indicators of Endocrine Gland Response after Burn: Alterations (Frequency) during First Postburn Weeks

ACTH*	+ +	IRI†	+ + +
Cortisol†	+ + + +	Glucagon*‡	+ +
Aldosterone	+ + +	FSH	– – –
Catecholamines*‡	+ + + +	LH	+
Renin	+ + + +	PRL	+ +
Angiotensin II	+ + +	Testosterone (males)*	– – – –
ADH	+ + +	17β-Estradiol (males)*	+ + +
GH†	+ +	TSH	N
DHEA-S‡	– – –	T_3	– – – –
17-Ketosteroids	+ + +	rT_3*	+ +
17-Ketogenic steroids	+ + + +	T_4	– – –
17-Hydroxycorticosteroids in urine†	+ + + +	PTH*	+ +
		Calcitonin*	+ +

Semiquantitative evaluation from author's experience.
+ = increased; – = decreased; N = normal.
*Hormones closely related to such responses as immunological and inflammatory. Various data will probably change when more results are obtained.
‡Data obtained from various references.
From Dolocek, R. (1985). The endocrine response after burns. *Journal of Burn Care and Rehabilitation*, 6(3), 281-294.

perature reset to occur which increases core body temperature 1° to 2° C above normal. As ambient temperatures become cooler, patients strive to maintain their reset body temperature by shivering, further increasing the metabolic rate. Increasing the ambient temperature controls exacerbations of metabolic rate increases but does not prevent the process.

Other hypermetabolic effects caused by increases in catecholamine output results in aberrations in glucose kinetics. An increased glucose flow develops quickly and mimics the pattern seen in diabetes. New glucose formation in the liver, called *gluconeogenesis*, also occurs and is fueled from fat metabolism. Protein wasting and increases in oxygen consumption also occur.[4]

DATA ACQUISITION

A first consideration in planning care is the determination of the severity of the injury. Five major factors influence severity: (1) medical history, (2) extent of burn, (3) depth of injury, (4) age, and (5) distribution of the burn.

History

The history must be obtained immediately upon arrival in the health care facility because the patient is generally lucid and capable of providing pertinent information. If the interview is postponed, the nurse may find the patient intubated, sedated, or disoriented due to shock. It may be impossible to obtain an adequate history at a later time.

The burn victim may present with concomitant traumatic injuries, preexisting diseases or illnesses, or both. These may have in some way contributed to the circumstances causing the burn and may drastically affect morbidity. For example, a patient's diabetes may interfere with wound healing, and chronic congestive heart failure complicates fluid resuscitation. Emotional and physical stress may exacerbate an existing disease process and lead to increased mortality.

In taking a history from a patient who is burned, the nurse should keep in mind the complications associated with burn injury. Specific emphasis is placed on the history of the accident and should include the time of injury, source of heat, description of how the burn occurred, whether the influence of alcohol or drugs was a factor, the physical surroundings in the immediate area where the burn was sustained, the events occurring from the time of the burn to admission to the health care facility, and any other contributing events or circumstances.

In addition to the standard information obtained during the admission history, special emphasis is placed on the patient's preburn or "dry" weight. This value is of immediate importance because it is used to calculate fluid rates, energy requirements, and drug dosages. An admission weight should be taken as early in the course of treatment as possible.

Physical Assessment

Extent of Burn

The extent of the burn is expressed as a percentage of the total body surface area. There are two commonly used methods of determining burn extent. The *rule of nines* is "quick and dirty"; it does not require charts or diagrams and does not take into consideration proportional differences related to age. The body is divided into components of nine. The arms (from shoulder to fingertip) and the head are given a value of 9%. Each leg is valued at 18%, the anterior and posterior trunk areas are also valued at 18% each, and the perineum is given a 1% value, yielding a total of 100%.

A more accurate method developed by Berkow, Lund, and Browder requires the use of tables to calculate the changes in proportion of the head and lower extremities that occur with growth. For example, the head of an infant represents 19% of total body surface area, while in an adult the head accounts for only 7%. Use of this method is described in Figure 53-6.

Depth of Burn

It is difficult to accurately determine the depth of a burn. Certain signs and symptoms indicate the level of tissue damage, but only with demarcation, spontaneous healing, or the appearance of granulation tissue can the exact depth of injury be determined. Several burn centers are experimenting with Doppler flow analysis and magnetic resonance imaging techniques to assist with burn depth diagnosis, but to date, these techniques are inconclusive.

Burn depth is best described in terms of partial thickness or full thickness. These terms are anatomically descriptive and, therefore, are preferable to the popular references of "first- and second-degree" (partial-thickness) and "third-degree" (full-thickness) burns, which arose from visual impressions in a partial-thickness burn. In a *partial-thickness burn,* the tissue damage and destruction do not include the deeper dermal layer, which may regenerate (Figure 53-7A). All skin layers have been destroyed in a *full-thickness burn,* and there may be injury of subcutaneous tissues, muscle, and bone as well. These wounds require skin grafting to replace destroyed tissues (Figure 53-7B).

Certain classic signs and symptoms may be evident

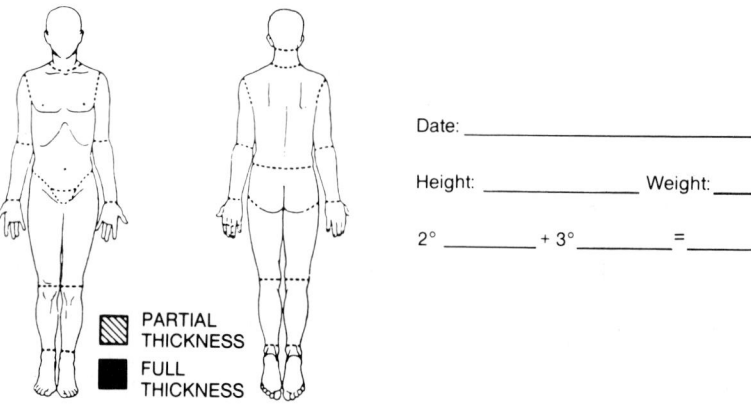

Date: _____

Height: _____ Weight: _____

2° _____ + 3° _____ = _____

PARTIAL THICKNESS

FULL THICKNESS

Percent Surface Area Burned
(Berkow Formula)

Area	0-1 YEAR	1-4 YEARS	5-9 YEARS	10-14 YEARS	15 YEARS	ADULT	2°	3°
Head	19	17	13	11	9	7		
Neck	2	2	2	2	2	2		
Ant. Trunk	13	13	13	13	13	13		
Post Trunk	13	13	13	13	13	13		
R. Buttock	2½	2½	2½	2½	2½	2½		
L. Buttock	2½	2½	2½	2½	2½	2½		
Genitalia	1	1	1	1	1	1		
R.U. Arm	4	4	4	4	4	4		
L.U. Arm	4	4	4	4	4	4		
R.L. Arm	3	3	3	3	3	3		
L.L. Arm	3	3	3	3	3	3		
R. Hand	2½	2½	2½	2½	2½	2½		
L. Hand	2½	2½	2½	2½	2½	2½		
R. Thigh	5½	6½	8	8½	9	9½		
L. Thigh	5½	6½	8	8½	9	9½		
R. Leg	5	5	5½	6	6½	7		
L. Leg	5	5	5½	6	6½	7		
R. Foot	3½	3½	3½	3½	3½	3½		
L. Foot	3½	3½	3½	3½	3½	3½		
TOTAL								

Figure 53-6 Berkow formula for calculating percentage of body surface burned.

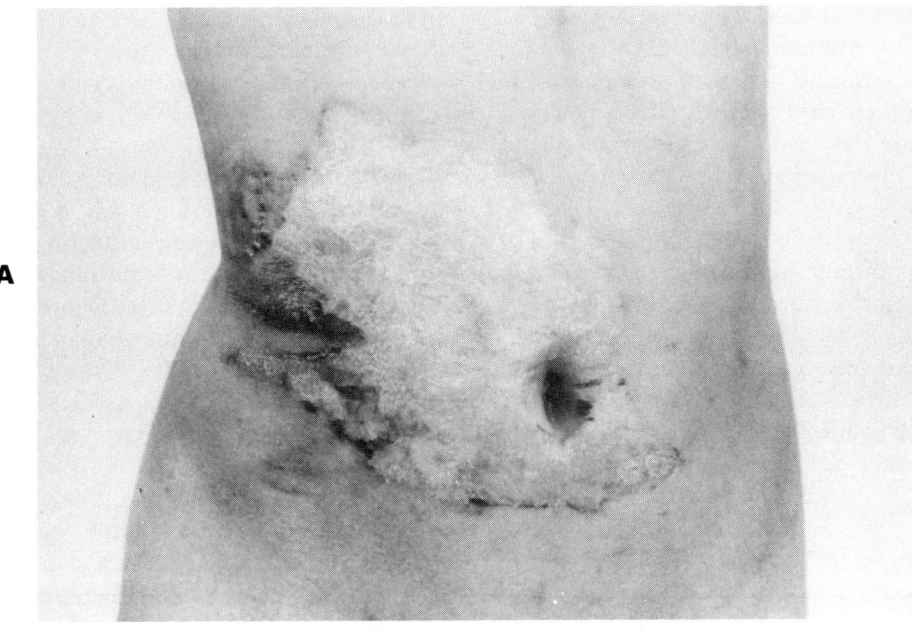

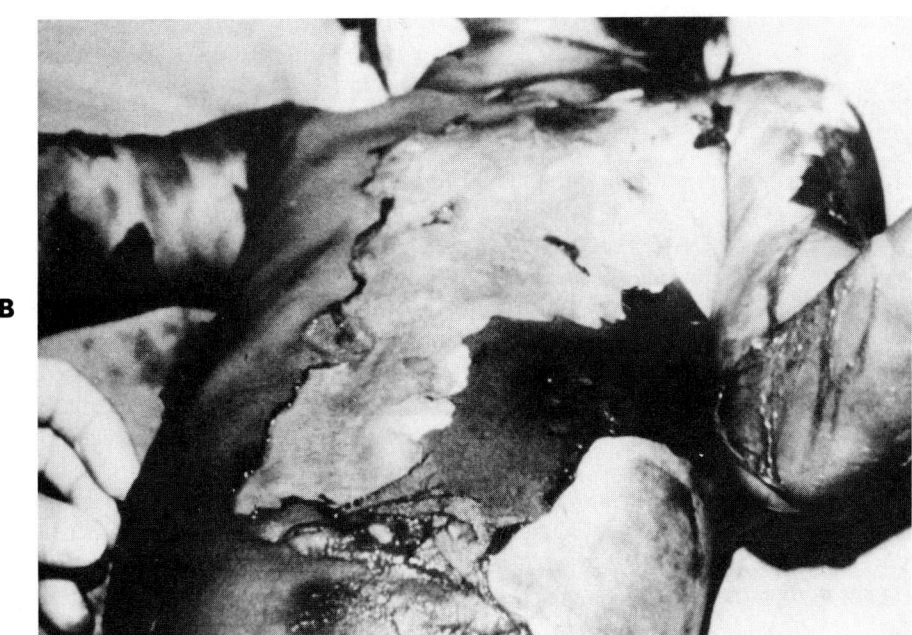

Figure 53-7   *A,* Partial-thickness burn to the abdomen. *B,* Full-thickness burn to the chest, flank, and arms.

and are helpful in differentiating depth of injury immediately after a burn injury. Erythematous areas that blanch with fingertip pressure and then refill are shallow partial-thickness burns; the erythema indicates tissue damage where viability remains. Vesicles that immediately increase in size usually represent a deeper partial-thickness injury.

Full-thickness burns are characterized by a leathery surface that may be white, tan, brown, red, gray, or black. Because of destruction of the dermis where

pain fibers terminate, there is no pain sensation. However, while deep partial-thickness burns may be anesthetic during the first few days, sensation returns as tissues recover. The patient's failure to react to stimuli such as a pinprick or the pulling out of a hair indicates full-thickness skin loss. Small vesicles caused by steam may be present in areas where intense heat destroyed all layers of the skin; these vesicles will not increase in size. Following a severe scald, there may be full-thickness skin loss, although the surface appears only red and discolored; however, this area will not blanch with pressure or refill.

In general, a painful erythematous surface with vesicles indicates a partial-thickness burn. When there is no complaint of pain and the surface is anesthetic, a full-thickness burn usually exists (Figure 53-7B).

Age

Age affects severity of injury on the extreme ends of the chronological spectrum. For example, a 40% TBSA burn is more likely to be fatal in the very young or in the elderly than in a healthy midlife adult. This is due to physiological factors such as the immature immune system in young children or the poor rate of reepithelialization in the elderly.

Distribution of Burn

Burns of the eyes, face, hands, and genitals, and all burns involving joints, are classified as *severe* by the American Burn Association. These burns require hospitalization for the special care that is needed for treatment of these areas, even if the total percentage of the burn is small.

Diagnostic Procedures

Serum Electrolytes

In the normal cell the ionic balance is maintained by the sodium–potassium pump and results in a high sodium concentration outside the cell. This active process of pumping sodium out of the cell in exchange for potassium into the cell becomes disrupted in the early postburn period. Following a burn injury, intracellular sodium concentration increases. This increase creates an osmotic pressure gradient that draws water into the cell. In exchange, potassium leaves the cell and is concentrated in the serum. This unusual shift of electrolytes contributes to the hyperkalemia frequently seen in the early hours after injury. Serum potassium levels are also increased when body tissues break down and cells such as red blood cells are hemolyzed.

Serum electrolyte values noted in burn patients can often be deceiving because of the dilutional effects seen in hemoconcentrated patients. This condition is present when serum electrolytes such as sodium and chloride are reported by the laboratory to be above the normally accepted limits. The number of sodium and chloride ions has not changed, but what has occurred is that the solute (water) has decreased, causing a disproportionate ratio.

Alterations in the ability of the skin to regulate the movement of electrolytes causes disruption in electrolyte balance as is evidenced by the amount of sodium sequestered in and lost through burn-injured tissues. In burn patients, chlorides are reabsorbed from the urine. This may cause an elevation in serum levels which can contribute to an existing acidosis.

Urinalysis

The kidneys perform a major role in regulating the electrolyte and fluid balance and in the excretion of waste products. Accurate measuring and testing of urine is crucial in assessing the patient's overall condition. Hourly testing of urine helps to determine the function of the kidney and the fluid and electrolyte balance of the body, as well as the systemic response to stress and therapy. Monitoring the urine during care provides another parameter by which to assess the patient's condition.

Specific Gravity (SG). Urine is composed of approximately 95% water and 5% wastes. Measuring the specific gravity indicates the amount of waste in relation to the water in the urine (the specific gravity of water is 1.000). This parameter is an indicator of metabolic changes and may signal either the need for or an excess of fluid therapy. The normal specific gravity of urine fluctuates between 1.002 and 1.035, depending on such factors as the amount of fluid intake or type of food eaten. A fixed specific gravity such as 1.008 to 1.012, regardless of intake, indicates kidney disease and demands treatment.

Protein. The amount of protein normally excreted by the kidneys is negligible; therefore, the test should be negative. If the body is burning tissue protein rather than food as in negative nitrogen balance, which recurs in the majority of severely burned patients, protein will be present in the urine. Protein in the urine may be considered normal when the patient is NPO for long periods. However, protein excretion is also seen in kidney diseases such as glomerulonephritis, and so should be reported when first noted.

pH. Testing the pH of the urine helps to monitor the acid–base balance of the body. Values greater than 7 or less than 6 should be reported and treated.

Glucose. Normally, urine contains no glucose; therefore, this test should be negative. A positive glucose test may indicate that the body is not utilizing ingested glucose or that there is a presence of diabetes or of pseudodiabetes, which is a symptom of stress sometimes seen in burn victims. A positive glucose result should be reported when it is first noted. Daily insulin may be necessary to compensate for the inability of the pancreas to meet the insulin needs of the burn patient during stress. Glucose intolerance is also one of the clinical signs of sepsis. Glycosuria should prompt a thorough examination of the patient.

Acetone. Acetone is not normally present in the urine. A positive reading may indicate that the body is burning its own fats and proteins because of starvation (NPO) or lack of proper dietary intake, or that the oxidation of fats is incomplete.

Color of Sediment. Normal urine is clear and yellow, or straw-colored. Discoloring may be due to drugs, and cloudiness is not necessarily abnormal, but both should be recorded and reported. When brown urine is seen on admission, massive hemolysis and kidney damage are likely and should be reported immediately because an osmotic diuretic is indicated to flush the tubules. Any abnormal color or sediment should be reported when first noted and if it continues to be present.

Blood. Red blood cells are not normally present in the urine. A positive reading in the burn patient may indicate hemolysis from initial injury or from septic shock.

Output. During the period immediately following the burn injury, urinary output is an effective guide to replacement fluid therapy.[5] Throughout the acute period, urinary output reflects the patient's general systemic response to the injury and to therapy. An indwelling catheter is inserted when the burn exceeds 20% of TBSA or when there are complications or problems in the medical history. Keep in mind that an indwelling urinary catheter penetrates an anatomical barrier; aseptic technique is essential.

Volume. The amount of urine output varies with such factors as intake, condition of the cardiovascular system, and kidney function. An output of 50 to 100 ml per hour indicates adequate renal perfusion in patients in the emergent period. During the acute burn phase, an output of 30 ml per hour is generally considered acceptable. A daily output of 1,200 ml is considered average. An output of less than 400 ml in 24 hours indicates oliguria and possible renal failure; more than 2,000 ml daily (polyuria) may indicate high-output renal failure. Intervention should take place before anuria occurs because this indicates a grave prognosis. As a general rule during fluid resuscitation, 1 ml of urine per kg of preburn body weight per hour is considered a positive sign of successful fluid replacement.

Arterial Blood Gases

The fluid disturbances and electrolyte imbalances that occur in the postburn period cause acid–base alterations. After an extensive burn, metabolic acidosis develops. This problem is best corrected by rapid fluid resuscitation and restoration of the normal cardiac output. Metabolic acidosis may also occur if the topical application of mafenide acetate (Sulfamylon) covers a large surface of body (>20% TBSA). Removal of all or a portion of the Sulfamylon usually corrects the problem.

Acid–base derangements also occur secondarily to other complications such as pulmonary insufficiency or acute renal failure. These acid–base changes can further interfere with the balance of electrolytes if not corrected.

Frequent blood gas analysis is mandatory in assessing pulmonary function and acid–base status. Blood gases are analyzed to determine the effectiveness of gas exchange and arterial oxygen tension (PaO_2) in the lungs and to evaluate the acid–base status of the patient through measurement of the hydrogen ion concentration (pH) and bicarbonate (HCO_3^-) concentration level.

Arterial blood gas (ABG) analysis is indicated when there is suspicion of respiratory involvement on admission or any change in the patient's condition (such as hypotension, unusual cardiac dysrhythmias, restlessness, or agitation). For patients receiving mechanical ventilation, blood gases are analyzed 20 minutes after any ventilator setting changes that would alter measurements such as rate, FiO_2, tidal volume, and PEEP, and during the weaning period. Arterial blood gases also are a good way to monitor fluid resuscitation. In assessing blood gas values it is important to indicate the inspired oxygen concentration, or FiO_2, the mode of ventilation, and the patient's temperature. If the patient is being mechanically ventilated when blood gases are drawn, the setting of flow rates, percentage of oxygen, and tidal volume when blood gases are drawn should be recorded to aid in evaluation. Arterial blood gas samples may be considered as emergency specimens.

Complete Blood Count

Alterations in hematological parameters (RBC, WBC, platelets) occur in response to burn injury. A small amount of red cell destruction (<10%) occurs as a result of local heat damage to the burned area; hematopoietic function is also affected. The half-life of erythrocytes in burn patients, as compared to those of nonburn patients, is markedly decreased.[6] Patients with extensive burns experience an increase in the hematocrit initially, due to loss of plasma volume and resultant hemoconcentration. Hematocrit values are used to determine hemoconcentration and are repeated every 6 hours during the first day and as often as indicated thereafter. The hematocrit rises immediately after an extensive burn injury. Circulation is decreased due to increased viscosity of blood and increased peripheral resistance, leading to formation of thrombi. Anemia results as a progressive destruction of RBCs (hemolysis) occurs over the course of the acute phase of hospitalization.

Leukocytosis occurs in the immediate postburn period, with values falling to 20,000 to 30,000 white blood cells per cubic milliliter. However, persistent leukocytosis is an indicator of possible infection. A transient and reversible leukopenia has been reported as a side effect of silver sulfadiazine,[7] a common topical wound therapy, but it is not necessarily an indication for cessation of the drug. Thrombocytopenia may be evident during the first 48 to 72 hours postburn. The platelet count then returns to above normal levels. The temporary drop in the platelet count may result from microvascular thrombosis and some degree of disseminated intravascular coagulation (DIC). As the patient responds to fluid therapy, the hemoconcentration dilutes to normal and then falls below normal as a result of hemolysis and anemia.

Admission Laboratory Tests

Values of the laboratory tests listed in the box to the right should be assessed on admission and monitored throughout recovery.

The need for baseline values is paramount. The rationale for some of the above tests, their baseline values, and postburn variations are outlined in Table 53-2.

In addition to routine laboratory tests and examinations, tests are needed for specific organs involved. For example, in patients with suspected eye burns, ophthalmic evaluation must be done. Fluorescein strips can be used to detect corneal damage. If trauma

---

Laboratory Tests for Assessment on Admission and Subsequent Monitoring

Arterial blood gases
Carbon monoxide level (if pulmonary involvement is suspected)
Serum electrolytes
Serum osmolality
Serum glucose
BUN/creatinine
Complete blood count (CBC) with differential and platelets
Drug screen or alcohol (ETOH) level (if suspicious)
Sickle cell preparation (for black patients)
Urinalysis
Urine culture/sensitivity
Chest x-ray
Liver enzymes
Total protein, albumin, and globulin
Prothrombin time/partial prothrombin time (PT/PPT)
Type and cross-match
VDRL
Electrocardiogram
Pregnancy
HIV status

TABLE 53-2 **Baseline Laboratory Values and Postburn Variations**

Laboratory Test	Normal Baseline Value	Postburn Variation	Rationale
Hemoglobin	12-16 g/dl	Elevated	Fluid volume loss
Hematocrit	40% to 50%	Elevated	Fluid volume loss
Urea nitrogen	8-20 mg/dl	Elevated	Fluid volume loss
Glucose	60-120 mg/dl	Elevated	Stress response
Serum electrolytes		Elevated	Fluid volume loss and disruption of sodium–potassium pump.
Sodium	136-145 mEq/L		
Potassium	3.6-5.0 mEq/L	Elevated	Disruption of sodium–potassium pump, tissue destruction, and red blood cell hemolysis
Chlorides	95-106 mEq/L	Elevated	Fluid volume loss and reabsorption of chlorides in urine
ARTERIAL BLOOD GAS STUDIES			
P_{O_2}	85-100 mmHg	Normal	
P_{CO_2}	35-45 mmHg		
pH	7.35-7.45	Low	Metabolic acidosis
Carboxyhemoglobin	0	Elevated	Inhalation of smoke and carbon monoxide
Total proteins	6.0-7.8/dl	Low	Loss of protein exudate through wound
Albumin	3.5-5 g/dl	Low	Loss of protein through wounds and through vascular membranes due to increased permeability

is suspected in organs such as the kidneys, brain, or lungs, an intravenous pyelogram, computed tomograpy (CT) scan, or bronchoscopy may need to be performed.

MEDICAL MANAGEMENT

Emergent and Acute Periods

Chemical Burns

Burns caused by chemical agents are usually progressive. Damage to the skin is attributable to the heat of the chemical reaction and changes caused by the chemical reacting with the protein in the skin. Generally, the result is a deep cutaneous injury; however, the chemical may also damage the eyes or digestive tract (if swallowed) and, if inhaled, may cause an inhalation injury.

Initial treatment of chemical burns varies with the specific chemicals causing the damage. Early treatment should include copious water lavages initially and every 4 to 6 hours to neutralize the chemical while removing the heat of reaction. In the case of dry chemicals, the chemical substance should be brushed off before beginning water lavage of the wound.

Electrical Burns

An electrical injury causes tissue destruction as the current flows through the body from the point of contact to the point of grounding (Figure 53-8). Electrical injuries are often marked by healthy, viable surface tissue because the greatest damage generally occurs close to the bone in the deep muscle compartment. Signs of deep muscle injury include myoglobinuria and compartment syndrome.

Electric current can also cause cardiac changes. It is advisable to monitor the patient's ECG for up to 96 hours after injury. Emergency treatment in the case of electrical injury begins with the stabilization of the cardiopulmonary system. Treatment should include a thorough examination of all body parts including the skeletal system for long-bone dislocations and fractures.

Radiation Burns

Radiation injuries occur from exposure to high doses of radioactive material. Damage occurs at the cellular level where altered function causes cell death and, consequently, organ failure. Survivors of radiation exposure experience varying degrees of damage, from minor erythema to absolute bone marrow suppression. Skin destruction sometimes occurs; it is treated similarly to other burn injuries.

Victims of radiation burns must undergo decontamination. Staff members who are decontaminating patients should be careful to wear appropriate iso-

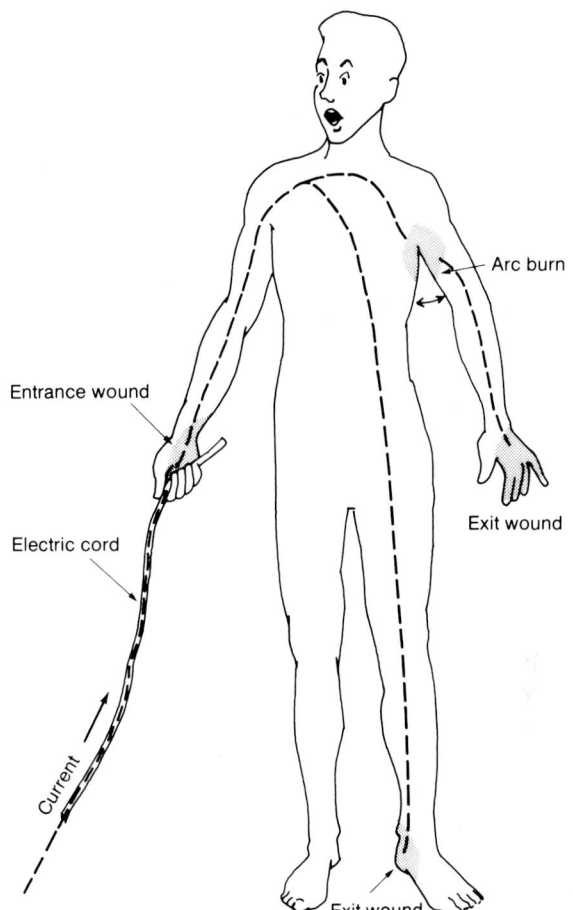

Figure 53-8 Pathway of current in an electrical injury from the point of contact to the point of grounding. *Note:* Current travels along the path of least resistance; nerves being the least resistant tissue followed by blood vessels, skin, muscle, and bone.

lation clothing including cap, mask, plastic shoe covers, and waterproof cover gowns. Double gloving is recommended when handling contaminated equipment.

Emergency Care

When administering emergency care to any seriously injured patient, breathing, bleeding, and shock are paramount considerations, usually in the order presented. Aseptic technique is essential to all phases of management. All clothing and dressings should be removed for a satisfactory appraisal of the extent of the burn and possible associated injuries.

The burned patient is likely to have respiratory difficulties. The history of the accident is a good indicator of imminent respiratory difficulty. If the patient was burned in an enclosed space and forced to breathe smoke and other products of combustion, there is strong likelihood of immediate airway involvement. Blackened oral and nasal mucous membranes, singed nasal hairs, and burn injury including the face and neck indicate the probability of impending airway obstruction. Carbon monoxide poisoning may also be present and should be watched for.

Hemorrhage, internal as well as external, may be due to associated trauma at the time of injury and should be carefully evaluated and treated as indicated. The burn injury itself causes no external bleeding; however, as much as 10% of the red blood cell volume may be destroyed by the hemolysis from deep thermal injury.

Shock may be neurogenic initially but later is due to extensive and rapid fluid shifts. The goal of fluid therapy for severely burned patients is to avoid hypovolemic shock during the first few days of therapy and to prevent hypervolemic complications.

Analgesics may be required if the patient is in pain and are always given intravenously. Subcutaneous or intramuscular injections pool locally because of hypotension and are suddenly released when normal systemic circulation returns, resulting in high blood levels from accumulated doses.

After immediate emergent matters and preliminary evaluation have been attended to, the patient and family should receive reassurance and explanation of the problems.

Pharmacological Management

Oxygen Therapy

Poor oxygenation can occur due to carbon monoxide poisoning, adult respiratory distress syndrome, pneumonia, pneumothorax, inhalation injury, or other respiratory insults. Treatment involves giving humidified oxygen via face mask, cannula, or mist. If necessary, intubation is performed and mechanical ventilation is instituted. Oxygen toxicity is associated with tissue fibrosis and central nervous system deterioration. In some cases, paralytic agents such as vecurium (Norcuron) may need to be used when the patient's activity severely compromises respiratory function.

Diuretics

Mannitol is used only when hematuria or hemoglobinuria (black urine), which indicate impending acute tubular necrosis, are evident in a urine specimen obtained by catheterization. Usually, this occurs in patients who have sustained electrical burns or deep muscle damage. Mannitol is given intravenously, and it is rarely necessary to repeat the dose.

Furosemide is rarely used in the emergent phase; however, it is frequently used during the acute phase of treatment for restoring fluid equilibrium. Of course, serum electrolytes must be carefully moni-tored when using any diuretics. The nurse should also be attentive to interactions of the many drugs burn patients can be receiving. For instance, it is believed that furosemide may increase the propensity for hearing loss caused by aminoglycoside therapy.

Antibiotic Therapy

Tetanus toxoid or antitoxin is administered routinely, the choice being dependent upon previous immunizations. Tetanus immune human globulin (Hyper-Tet) is given as additional passive coverage. Prophylactic antibiotic therapy is controversial; however, antibiotics often are used in this way during the perioperative period. If pneumonia or other infection is suspected, antibiotics are recommended for all patients with positive sputum, urine, or wound cultures. Antibiotics, therefore, are used extensively, especially the aminoglycosides which include amikacin, gentamicin, and tobramycin. These drugs, although helpful in combatting severe infections, are associated with a wide range of adverse effects. The most significant of these effects are ototoxicity and nephrotoxicity. Peak and trough serum levels of these drugs are monitored because burn patients often require a higher than normal dosage of these drugs to maintain therapeutic serum levels. The nurse must carefully monitor patients treated with aminoglycosides and agents such as amphotericin B for signs of renal failure and hearing impairment.[8] Dosages of antibiotics also may need to be altered.

While waiting for wound closure, especially if using the conservative treatment approach, topical antibiotics are often applied. The primary goal of topical antibiotics, called *topical antimicrobial therapy*, is to keep bacterial proliferation in the burn wound to a minimum. Most topical antimicrobial agents can be used prior to and following eschar separation. Topical antimicrobial therapy can be accomplished by the closed or open technique. A summary of commonly used topical antimicrobial agents is presented in Table 53-3. Further discussion of wound healing is in Chapter 54.

Analgesics

Narcotic and nonnarcotic analgesics are given with relative frequency for the duration of hospitalization. These drugs, however, rarely offer more than moderate relief during acutely painful procedures. Many nurses are reluctant to administer analgesics for fear of diminishing respirations and bowel motility. The dilemma relates to the need to maintain the integrity of respiratory function and the delivery of adequate nutrition while reducing pain.

Anesthetic agents such as ketamine (Ketalar), sodium pentobarbital (Nembutal), and nitrous oxide

TABLE 53-3   **Topical Burn Therapy**

	Description	Actions	Advantages	Disadvantages	Nursing Considerations
ANTIBIOTICS					
Nitrofurazone (Furacin)	Antibiotic available as cream, solution, and water-soluble powder.	Wide-spectrum antibacterial.	Is effective against *Staphylococcus aureus* and some antibiotic-resistant organisms. Causes neither pain nor maceration. Available in a wide assortment of forms.	May cause contact dermatitis (rare). Is messy to apply in cream form. May cause renal problems if used in patients with extensive burns.	Observe patient carefully for signs of allergic reaction and for evidence of a superinfection.
Gentamicin sulfate (Garamycin)	Wide-spectrum antibiotic, available as a cream or solution for topical use.	Exerts antibiotic action against many organisms that do not respond to other topical antibiotics.	Effective against many organisms, including *Pseudomonas*. Does not cause pain.	May cause ototoxicity and nephrotoxicity. Organisms may become resistant.	Use with caution in patients with decreased renal function because of possible nephrotoxicity. Order serum creatinine and urine creatinine clearance studies before treatment and weekly during treatment to monitor renal function.
Neomycin sulfate	Wide-spectrum antibiotic in 0.1% to 0.5% aqueous solution.	Bactericide used to decrease organisms before debriding and grafting.	Effectively combats most organisms. Can be applied easily. Is inexpensive.	May cause ototoxicity and nephrotoxicity. Is absorbed systemically.	Remove from wound after 24 hours to decrease systemic absorption. Monitor patient's temperature after application of cold solution. Order serum and urine creatinine tests to watch for signs of nephrotoxicity.
Bacitracin with Polymyxin B	Combination bactericidal ointment effective on small burn areas.	Bactericidal for gram-positive and gram-negative organisms.	Is capable of minimal systemic absorption. Is aesthetically suitable for use on the face. Does not cause pain.	May cause itching, burning, or inflammation. Cannot be used for full-thickness burns.	Observe patient closely for signs of sensitivity, i.e., rash. Wash ointment off and reapply it every 8 hours.

Adapted from Gaston, S. F., & Schumann, L. L. (1980). Burn wound management. *Critical Care Update*, October, 5–17.

Continued.

TABLE 53-3   Topical Burn Therapy—cont'd

	Description	Actions	Advantages	Disadvantages	Nursing Considerations
ENZYMATIC DEBRIDING AGENTS					
Sutilains ointment (Travase)	Proteolytic enzymes developed from *Bacillus subtilis* in a petroleum base.	Digests necrotic tissue, aiding escharotomies and debridement.	Aids initial debridement before patient can tolerate surgical debridement. Can be easily applied.	Increases fluid loss. Requires refrigeration. May cause bleeding. Irritates wound and sometimes surrounding skin. Is not bactericidal.	Patient must be stable enough for surgery after a few days so that digested wounds can be covered with membranes or grafted. Use with Silvadene, Sulfamylon, bacitracin. Neomycin, or Garamycin. Do not use with hexachlorophene, iodine, Furacin, or silver nitrate. Observe for infection. Change every 18 hours. Use on no more than 15% total burn surface at one time.
Fibrinolysin and desoxyribonuclease, combined (bovine) (Elase)	Two lytic enzymes combined in a petroleum base.	Digests necrotic tissue, aiding escharotomies and debridement.	Does not require refrigeration. Has long shelf life.	Causes sensitivity in patients allergic to bovine materials. Causes itching and burning. Requires preparation immediately before application.	Wait for physician to remove any thick, dry eschar before applying Elase. Observe for infection. Change dressings daily.
MISCELLANEOUS					
Silver sulfadiazine	A nontoxic salt of silver sulfadiazine in water-based cream.	Binds to bacterial cell membranes and interferes with DNA.	Does not cause hypochloremia, hyponatremia, electrolyte imbalance, or kidney disease. Has a wide-spectrum antimicrobial action against both gram-negative and gram-positive organisms. Has a long shelf life. Delays eschar separation less than many other topicals.	Absorbed into eschar less than mafenide acetate (Sulfamylon). May cause rash, pruritus, and burning. Not consistently effective for burns covering more than 60% of patient's body or against some bacteria and yeasts. Depresses granulocyte formation.	Watch for signs of infection such as soupiness. Watch for allergic reaction causing drop in white blood cell counts.

TABLE 53-3 **Topical Burn Therapy—cont'd**

	Description	Actions	Advantages	Disadvantages	Nursing Considerations
MISCELLANEOUS—cont'd					
Mafenide acetate	A soft, white, nonstaining water-based cream.	Exerts a bacteriostatic action against many gram-negative and gram-positive organisms.	Effective against *Pseudomonas*. Long shelf life. Excellent for treating electrical burns. Penetrates thick eschar. Very effective against *Pseudomonas*.	May lead to superinfection. May cause metabolic acidosis, hyperpnea, and rash. Causes pain when applied. (Pain usually lasts 30-40 minutes.) Slows eschar separation.	Premedicate patient for pain before application. Monitor blood gases and serum electrolytes if patient develops hyperpnea in response to metabolic acidosis. Do not use in cases of sulfa drug allergy or respiratory or kidney disease.
Sodium hypochlorite solution	An aqueous sodium hypochlorite solution.	Bactericidal.	Helps dry wounds that have become soupy. Aids debridement.	Dissolves blood clots and may inhibit clotting. May irritate skin. May cause electrolyte imbalances.	Change dressings every 4 to 12 hours. Observe site carefully for signs of irritation. Keep dressings moist.
Povidone-iodine (Betadine)	Iodine complex. Available as a solution, ointment, and foam.	Microbicidal against gram-positive and gram-negative organisms.	Is effective against many infections not well controlled by Silvadene. Is available in a wide assortment of forms.	May cause metabolic acidosis and elevated serum iodine levels. May form crusts if burns are not cleansed properly. Causes rash and burning with some patients. Stains clothing and linen. Deactivated by wound proteins.	Check serum electrolytes and serum iodine levels frequently.
Silver nitrate	10% silver salt solution, diluted to 0.5% for application.	Antimicrobial.	Is inexpensive. Applies easily.	Penetrates wound only 1-2 mm, so it acts only on surface organisms. Stains and stings. May cause hyponatremia, hypochloremia, and hypocalcemia. Must be applied as constant soaks.	Keep dressings wet with solution. Check serum electrolytes daily.

Continued.

TABLE 53-3 Topical Burn Therapy—cont'd

	Description	Actions	Advantages	Disadvantages	Nursing Considerations
MISCELLANEOUS—cont'd					
Bismuth tri-brom-phenate (Xeroform)	A yellow substance gauze.	Debrides and protects donor sites and grafts.	Conforms to wound. Nontoxic and nonsensitizing. Has a long shelf life.	Sticks to wound so that removal is painful. Neither antiseptic nor antibacterial.	Apply carefully so that sheets do not overlap. Observe for signs of infection.
Scarlet red	A red dye in an oil base on gauze.	Promotes healing of wound, but has antiseptic effect.	Protects donor site. Long shelf life. Promotes reepithelialization.	Stains clothing and temporarily stains skin. Irritates skin. Causes pain when patient moves.	Apply to donor sites at time of harvest. Leave until site heals and scarlet red gauze sloughs. Observe for infection beneath gauze. If needed, use heat lamp for a few minutes every hour to dry site.
"Thirds" solution	Solution of ⅓ 5% hydrogen peroxide, ⅓ 0.25% acetic acid, and ⅓ normal saline.	Inhibits bacterial growth by oxidizing pH. Effervescence cleans wound.	Provides good cleansing action. Causes no known side effects. Is inexpensive.	Decomposes quickly and is short-acting. Exerts limited antimicrobial action.	Add new solution to the dressing or change dressing every 4 to 6 hours.
Merbromin (Mercurochrome)	Organic mercurial compound available as a solution or tincture.	Acts as a desiccating agent which promotes epithelialization.	Is not expensive. Aids epithelialization of small areas. Dries wound.	Causes stains. Is not antibacterial or antiseptic.	Cover wound with nonadherent dressing to prevent sticking.

have been effectively used. Extreme caution is necessary in their administration, and the presence of an anesthesiologist or nurse anesthetist is required. Diazepam (Valium) is also an effective sedative for the burned patient. Other medications commonly used for burns are listed in the box to the right.

Fluid and Electrolyte Replacement

Each patient should be given the quantity and type of fluid required to compensate for losses sustained during the first few days. To meet fluid therapy objectives, it is important to determine which patients require fluid therapy and the type and amount of fluid to be given. Formulas attempt to predict specific volume requirements for each patient; however, calculated rates require adjustment based on clinical indicators such as blood pressure and urine output.

Not all burned patients require fluid therapy. If the burn involves less than 20% of TBSA, intravenous therapy may not be necessary. Generally, fluid therapy is indicated when the total area burned is greater

---

Medications Commonly Used for Burns

Pain control
  Morphine IV prn for pain on admission; dose by body weight; alternate weekly with equivalent dose of meperidine
Prevent Curling's ulcer
  Maalox 60 ml via NG tube 12 hours; alternate with Amphogel
Heart action
  Digoxin (Lanoxin) when necessary
Vitamin and mineral supplements
  Multivitamins, 1 ampule IV, PB or 1 tablet PO daily
Vitamin B_{12} weekly
Vitamin C daily
Folic acid, 1 mg IV daily (adult)
Sedation and sleep
  Pentobarbital sodium (Nembutal) IM, HS, prn
  Chlordiazepoxide (Librium), diazepam (Valium), or meprobamate (Miltown) for sedation prn

than 20% of TBSA, or there are individual considerations such as dehydration, past medical problems, or concurrent injuries.

Most of the fluid lost from the bloodstream into the tissues is plasma. It is necessary, therefore, to replace this fluid with plasma or a plasmalike substitute. A variety of fluids have been advocated, but a balanced salt solution with plasma or protein added is generally used. Hartmann's (lactated Ringer's) solution is good because it contains electrolytes in concentrations approximating those in the blood. Serum albumin (25 to 50 g per L) may be added to supply the protein to make a plasmalike solution. Plasma may also be used, but it is extremely expensive. The use of hypertonic saline, blood, or other solutions remains controversial. The amount of fluid required for replacement varies, depending on extent and depth of burn, the patient's age, and medical history. Each patient requires individual consideration. The correct amount of fluid is that which achieves maintenance of normal blood pressure and urinary output without overlooking the vascular system.

There are many formulas for calculating the amount of fluids needed after a severe burn (Table 53-4). Electrolyte solutions vary in resuscitation based on the particular formulas employed. The most popular resuscitation formula, the Parkland formula, uses Ringer's lactate and indicates that one half of the calculated fluid (4 ml × % burn × weight in kg) is given in the first 8 hours following the burn. The other half is then administered over the next 16-hour period for a total of 24 hours. Colloids such as albumin may be given in the third or fourth 8-hour period postburn if indicated in the clinical assessment. The Parkland formula also recommends the practice of "catching up" on fluids. If, for example, a client were burned at 8:00 A.M. but admitted to the hospital at 10:00 A.M., his or her first 8-hour period would end at 4:00 P.M., or 8 hours following the *time of injury*. Thus, if resuscitation were delayed until admission, calculated fluids would need to be administered over a 6-hour rather than an 8-hour period. In the second 24-hour period, 5% dextrose in water replaces lactated Ringer's as the crystalloid solution of choice.[9]

Frequent, accurate adjustments of hourly flow rates may be necessary to maintain perfusion in the optimal ranges. Signs of adequate resuscitation include clear mentation and adequate blood pressure, central venous pressure, pulse, and urine output. These parameters are indicators of tissue perfusion to

TABLE 53-4 **Formula for Calculation of Fluid Requirements**

	Electrolyte	Colloid	Glucose in Water
FIRST 24 HOURS			
Evans	Normal saline 1.0 ml/kg/% burn	1.0 ml/kg/% burn	2,000 ml
Brooke	Lactated Ringer's solution 1.5 ml/kg/% burn	0.5 ml/kg/% burn	2,000 ml
Modified Brooke	Lactated Ringer's solution 2 ml/kg/% burn		
Parkland (Baxter)	Lactated Ringer's solution 4 ml/kg/% burn		
Hypertonic sodium solution (2 amps NaHCO₃ in 1 L Ringer's lactate)	Volume to maintain urine output at 30 ml/hr (fluid contains 250 mEq Na/L). Approximately 2 ml/kg/% burn		
SECOND 24 HOURS			
Evans	½ of 1st 24-hour requirement	½ of 1st 24-hour requirement	2,000 ml
Brooke	½ to ¾ of 1st 24-hour requirement	½ to ¾ of 1st 24-hour requirement	
Modified Brooke		0.3-0.5 ml/kg/% burn	To maintain adequate urinary output
Parkland (Baxter)		20% to 60% of calculated plasma volume	2,000 ml
Hypertonic sodium solution	⅓ isotonic salt solution orally up to 3,500 ml limit		

From Nicosia, J. E., & Petro, J. A. (1983). *Manual of burn care*. New York: Raven.

the brain, heart, and kidneys, respectively. During resuscitation, the waning of any one of these parameters usually suggests a decrease in tissue perfusion in that organ. Indirectly, this signals a deficit in fluid volume and a diminished cardiac output. One of the best indicators of adequate cardiac output in the absence of renal disease is urine output.

The hourly urine output indicates whether the fluid volume replacement is adequate to perfuse all organ systems and, thereby, combat hypovolemia and prevent shock. During the emergent period, intravenous fluids may need to be titrated to maintain urinary output at 1 ml/kg of preburn weight per hour. For the aged, and in patients with respiratory or renal problems or congestive heart failure, close titration is very important since fluid overload is often seen.

Maintaining urine output greater than these recommended amounts risks fluid overload, increased interstitial edema, congestive heart failure, wet-lung syndrome, and renal failure. Too much urine output is as serious a clinical sign as too little.

Other parameters that indicate the status of the cardiovascular system are blood pressure, pulse, central venous pressure (CVP), and pulmonary artery pressure (PAP). These measurements are recorded hourly.

Recording the preburn weight and accurate daily nude weights also serves as a useful indicator of cardiovascular status. Each liter of fluid retained results in a weight gain of 2.2 lb. The total weight gained in the first few days of fluid therapy should not exceed 10% to 15% of the patient's total body weight.

Once the patient has been successfully resuscitated and capillary permeability returns to normal, fluids return to the intravascular spaces, and profuse diuresis occurs, which signals the end of the emergent period. At this time, the rate of fluid administration is reduced, and fluids are changed to glucose in water to compensate for the fluid, sodium, and other electrolytes that are returning to the vascular space.

During the acute period of care, after resuscitation, the adult patient with a large ungrafted wound requires a large-bore cannula with an average infusion rate of 1,000 to 1,500 ml per 24 hours. The types and amounts of fluids that patients require depend on their metabolic balance. It is the responsibility of the nurse to monitor the electrolytes and request appropriate adjustments of fluid administration.

Blood and blood products are administered as needed. Whole blood, which is approximately 45% cellular and 55% plasma, is required to replace losses from bleeding during wound debridement, from hemolysis due to the burn injury or sepsis, or as a result of coagulopathies and hemorrhage. Burned patients should always receive fresh blood that is not more than 3 days old because (1) the clotting factors are more effective in fresh blood, (2) older blood may contain a higher potassium concentration due to hemolysis, and (3) the oxygen-carrying efficiency is decreased in older blood.

Packed cells obtained by centrifuging whole blood to draw off plasma (plasmapheresis) are given to replace red blood cell loss in anemia, to replace red blood cells lost through marrow depression, or when there is danger of circulatory overload from whole-blood therapy; for example, in the patient with congestive heart failure.

Imbalances of electrolytes must be modified. Sodium is lost from the serum and deposited in the burn wound. Additionally, the defect in the efficiency of the sodium–potassium pump (as described previously) causes sodium concentrations within the cells to rise. Both of these factors can markedly decrease serum sodium. Initially, hyponatremia is usually resolved by the administration of sodium in IV fluids. The clinician must be aware that a dilutional hyponatremia may be seen in cases of overaggressive resuscitation with hypotonic solutions.

Serum potassium rises because of defects in the sodium–potassium pump and the release of potassium from injured tissues and red blood cells. Hyperkalemia is rarely treated in the initial resuscitation phase unless acute tubular necrosis is present because it often converts to hypokalemia in a few days. In the acute period, sodium and potassium replacement is the rule rather than the exception. Careful monitoring of these electrolytes is essential. In addition to sodium and potassium, calcium, chlorides, and phosphate may need to be supplemented.

As one would expect in patients undergoing such vast fluid shifts, strict documentation of 24-hour *intake and output* is essential. Daily fluid replacements are calculated and based on body surface area burned and insensible water loss. In general, hourly fluid intake rates are adhered to strictly so that fluid balance can be carefully controlled. All fluids given through the GI tract and IV route must be included in intake and output calculations.

Astute comparisons of intake to output are made hourly and daily. In addition to the differences in daily intake and output values, a change in daily weight as well as clinical observations of fluid overload or dehydration must be considered. Diuretic therapy may also be indicated to clarify the sometimes hazy picture of fluid status.

INFECTION PREVENTION
Infection Control Principles

The interactions of patients, staff, equipment and supplies, air conditioning, and housekeeping methods contribute to both the spread and the control of infection. Traditionally, nurses have been responsible for monitoring and controlling infection. Today, however, this responsibility is multifaceted and must be shared by many. Infection prevention is one of the primary goals of burn care.

Infection is one of the most devastating complications a burned patient faces. Of all burned patients who die, 50% do so because of infection. Infection has numerous consequences such as pain and nutritional imbalance. Bacterial invasion may cause partial-thickness wounds to become full-thickness wounds or may result in graft rejection, both of which necessitate additional operative procedures. Infection can also result in delayed healing, scars, contracture, and prolonged hospitalization. Septicemia and death are even more costly consequences. Complications of infection result not only in a drain on the patient's metabolic and emotional resources but also in a greater cost to the patient and family in terms of time, financial strain, and chronic problems after discharge from the hospital. For the health team, these complications necessitate long hours of detailed care and follow-up. The tangible effects can be measured in time and money spent on medications, treatments, and procedures. The intangible consequences, such as pain, worry, and apathy which add to the emotional stress of the patient and all those concerned with the patient's care, are of even greater relevance in the assessment of the need for an infection control program.

As important as elimination of infection may be, both to the recovery of the patient and to the preservation of energy among the health team, a sterile environment can never be achieved. The struggle is more precisely defined as a campaign to decrease the risk of infection that demands constant caution and refinement of technique in all aspects of burn care.

The principles of controlling infection are (1) the elimination of reservoirs of infection, (2) suppression of infection transfer channels, (3) support of the patient's natural immunity, and (4) judicious use of antimicrobials.

Elimination of Infection Reservoirs

The elimination of reservoirs of infection begins with the patient, who is autocontaminated by the bacteria in the gastrointestinal (GI) and upper respiratory tract, on the unburned skin, and in the hairy areas of the body. In addition, the burn wound provides an ideal medium for bacterial growth; it offers bacteria nourishment, warm climate, and moisture. In addition to the patient's bodily environment, hospitals and, especially, intensive care units have a host of resident bacteria that can be extremely virulent and

transferrable to the already immunosuppressed burn patient. Many studies have been done regarding the prevention of burn wound infection using various methods of cleaning and cohorting. In the past, room fogging, positive and negative room pressure gradients, isolettes, and even laminar flow have been attempted. To date, none of these extraordinary methods have proven to be better than routine and common infection control practices. Thorough and diligent wound care, basic hygiene, careful housekeeping, using a good antiseptic solution, and personnel awareness are still the indispensable methods of preventing infection.

Suppression of Infection Transfer Channels

Cross-contamination—the transfer of pathogens from an infection source or reservoir to the patient—is probably the greatest threat to the infection control program. Cubicle isolation and aseptic technique are time-tested methods of preventing contamination. Handwashing remains the single most effective method of preventing the spread of infection. The Centers for Disease Control (CDC) recommendations for infection control of treating burn patients are a good guide to follow (Table 53-5).

Support of Natural Immunity

Support of the patient's immune mechanisms involves reinforcement of the patient's natural and acquired immunity. This may be accomplished by basic nursing care measures concerning diet, rest, hygiene, positioning, and emotional support, and by vaccines, serums, and globulins that may be specific or nonspecific for particular organisms.

Judicious Use of Antimicrobials

The judicious use of topical and systemic antimicrobials (antibiotics and chemotherapeutics) is one of the most important factors in assisting the body's resistance to invasive infection. These agents are effective when properly used because they are harmful in one way or another to microbes but less harmful to viable tissues. Disinfectants, which may be bacteriostatic or bactericidal, are also toxic to the body. Use of antimicrobials requires consideration of the interaction that will occur between the host, the microbes, and the antibiotic. Experience, team discussions, including a clinical pharmacist, and dialogue are essential to any good treatment program.

Infection Control Methods

While discussing the different procedures for the controlling infection, it is worthwhile to consider the environment in which these procedures are to be accomplished. No effective infection control program

TABLE 53-5 Isolation Precautions

Disease	Precautions Indicated Private Room?	Masks?	Gowns?	Gloves?	Infective Material	Apply Precautions How Long?	Comments
Skin, wound, or burn infection — Major	Yes	No	Yes, if soiling is likely	Yes, for touching infective material	Pus	Duration of illness	Major = draining and not covered by dressing, or dressing does not adequately contain the pus.
Minor or limited	No	No	Yes, if soiling is likely	Yes, for touching infective material	Pus	Duration of illness	Minor or limited = dressing covers and adequately contains the pus, or infected area is very small.
Staphylococcal disease (S. aureus) — Major	Yes	No	Yes, if soiling is likely	Yes, for touching infective material	Pus	Duration of illness	Major = draining and not covered by dressing, or dressing does not adequately contain the pus.
Minor or limited	No	No	Yes, if soiling is likely	Yes, for touching infective material	Pus	Duration of illness	Minor or limited = dressing covers and adequately contains the pus, or infected area is very small.
Streptococcal disease (group A Streptococcus)	Yes	No	Yes, if soiling is likely	Yes, for touching infective material	Pus	For 24 hours after start of effective therapy	Major = draining and not covered by dressing, or dressing does not adequately contain the pus.
Multiply-resistant organisms,* infection or colonization†	Yes	No	Yes, if soiling is likely	Yes, for touching infective material	Pus and possibly feces	Until off antimicrobials and culture-negative	In outbreaks, cohorting of infected and colonized patients may be indicated if private rooms are not available.

* The following multiply-resistant organisms are included:
1. Gram-negative bacilli resistant to all aminoglycosides that are tested. (In general, such organisms should be resistant to gentamicin, tobramycin, and amikacin for these special precautions to be indicated.)
2. Staphylococcus aureus resistant to methicillin (or nafcillin or oxacillin if they are used instead of methicillin for testing).
3. Pneumococcus resistant to penicillin.
4. Haemophilus influenzae resistant to ampicillin (beta-lactamase positive) and chloramphenicol.
5. Other resistant bacteria may be included if they are judged by the infection control team to be of special clinical and epidemiological significance.

†Colonization may involve more than one site.

CDC guidelines for isolation precautions in hospitals. (1983). Atlanta, GA.

can take place in a chaotic or poorly planned environment, nor can apathetic or uneducated personnel be expected to be responsible for the effectiveness of infection control. Maintaining this environment once it has been established requires constant vigilance and is the responsibility of all involved in patient care.

The patient's life depends on the actions of all those involved in care; therefore, all personnel coming into contact with the patient or the patient care area are responsible for maintaining and monitoring the principles and practices of infection control. It is the responsibility of physicians, nurses, and ancillary services to enforce the infection control program.

An initial training program in infection control is essential for all personnel, including environmental services and medical staff, as well as for visitors. Staff members must be trained in the principles of infection control before they can be expected to follow the principles. A continuous reinforcement program is also essential.

The nursing staff shoulder the greatest burden of infection control because they provide continuous care and are the "gate keepers" to the patient. Through education, practice, and example, infection control should become a habitual part of the thinking process for all involved. Infection control is one aspect of burn care philosophy that demands that each person develop a surgical conscience; that is, a strong sense of what is correct and necessary to maximize each patient's chance of survival.

Wound Infection and Clinical Sepsis

The battle against invasive infection begins when the severely burned patient is admitted. The burning agent has produced an avascular area composed of nonviable material called *eschar*. The permeability of blood vessels in this area has been altered, and edema forms. Potential pathogens are in the patient's normal flora and in the hospital environment. There is a great likelihood that these pathogens will be transferred from their reservoirs to the burn wound, which provides an ideal climate for bacterial growth, the outcomes of which may be wound infection, septicemia, pneumonia, and eventually, death. In addition, research has shown the effectiveness of white blood cells is decreased in burned individuals.[10] Protein is used for wound healing, and if proper basic supportive care is not provided, the patient is further debilitated.

The burn wound cannot be completely sterile; some degree of colonization is expected. However, once bacterial growth in the wound exceeds 100,000 organisms per gram of wound tissue, the patient is said to have a wound infection. An infected wound does not look clean: purulence, debris, and odor are present.

The methods of isolation used in burn care are varied and controversial. In some cases, virtually no isolation is practiced, and in others, total sterile conditions prevail. As previously mentioned, in most cases, the recommendations of the Centers for Disease Control (CDC) in Atlanta, Georgia, are followed.[11] As such, isolation for the patient with burns centers on handwashing as the most effective weapon against transmission of infection. In addition, patients are isolated according to the specific disease or microorganism involved. The suggested precautions for common burn unit pathogens are outlined in Table 53-5.

As previously discussed, burn patients are immunologically suppressed. Because of this condition, a patient can often develop infections that warrant isolation techniques different from those used for burn injury alone. The use of antibiotics both topically and systemically can often lead to the development of bacteria and viruses that are panresistant. Other highly contagious pathogens such as herpes and varicella viruses are common in burn patients. Any time the foregoing conditions are reported in the burn patient, the most stringent techniques recommended by the CDC should be used. For instance, if a patient develops an infection caused by a panresistant organism, total isolation to the extent of separate staffs and geographic locations may be warranted. Cases such as these should be referred to the hospital's infection control committee. *Handwashing cannot be stressed too much, and, in fact, if handwashing were performed consistently and perfectly, there would be virtually no cross-contamination in burn patients.*

In addition to isolation precautions, use of sterile gloves is recommended for all contact with open wounds. Gloves also should be changed between handling of wounds on different areas of the body.

Patients in a burn unit should not share equipment. Disposables such as pillows, syringes, and dishes are used as much as possible. Equipment used in daily routine care, such as thermometers, blood pressure cuffs, and stethoscopes, should be assigned to each patient.

Thorough cleaning and housekeeping are essential to environmental infection control. All equipment must be cleaned and disinfected after use with one patient and before use with another. Because *Pseudomonas* has been shown to sequester in plants, these are prohibited. Rugs and upholstered articles are difficult to clean and may harbor organisms and, therefore, should be prohibited in the burn unit.

Careful monitoring of the burn wound is done every day. Wounds are examined by the nurse for signs of infection, which include a pervasive odor, color changes in the wound, change in wound texture, pus, exudate, and redness at wound edges. Laboratory cultures and biopsies are recommended. Quantitative biopsies of the eschar and granulation tissue should be done three times a week to monitor proliferation of organisms. Clinical signs of burn wound sepsis may be present. Nurses must take an active role in evaluating each of these parameters, assimilating the information and relaying their assessments to the health team.

Medical Management of Wound Infection

Treatment of an established wound infection can be summarized as follows:

1. Culture the involved areas to identify the organisms.
2. Reduce the number of organisms by cleansing the infected wound areas aggressively; debride the eschar, open subeschar pockets of infection, and change dressings more frequently.
3. Apply an appropriate topical agent as indicated by culture and sensitivity studies.
4. Provide basic nursing care (adequate diet, rest, hygiene, positioning) and encourage the patient to turn, cough, and deep breathe regularly to prevent pneumonia.

Further discussion of wound care can be found in Chapter 54.

Pharmacological Management. Antibiotics are used extensively, especially the aminoglycoside class, which includes amikacin, gentamicin, and tobramycin. These drugs, although helpful in combatting severe infections, are associated with a wide range of adverse effects. Ototoxicity and nephrotoxicity are the most significant of these effects. Peak and trough serum levels of drugs must be monitored. Burn patients require a higher than normal dosage of these drugs to maintain therapeutic serum levels. The nurse must be careful to monitor patients treated with aminoglycosides and other agents such as amphotericin B for signs of renal failure and hearing impairment. Dosages of antibiotics may need to be altered.

Clostridium tetani grows on necrotic tissue and is a strict anaerobe. In the burn patient, wound conditions favor the growth of this organism. Tetanus toxoid is given to produce immunity or resistance to *Clostridium tetani*. The administration of tetanus immune human globulin (Hyper-Tet) is recommended when the history of immunizations is questionable. Tetanus toxoid, 0.5 ml, is given on admission or shortly thereafter and is usually the only drug that is given via the intramuscular route during the emergent period.

Surgical Management. In addition to pharmacological treatment, surgical intervention may be indicated. Infected burn wounds whose colony counts are at or approaching 10^5 organisms per gram of tissue are life-threatening. Even with antibiotic therapy, loss of control of infection can occur, followed by sepsis

and death. Surgical intervention may be the only treatment option available. Aggressive surgical debridement or excision of the burn wound may be necessary. Some burn surgeons today are advocating early surgical debridement as a method to improve survival. This technique is still controversial but is gaining general acceptance.

Wound Sepsis

If a wound infection is not controlled, bacteria will begin to seep into the bloodstream via the lymphatic system. This condition is first termed *transient* and then *persistent* (or *breakthrough*) *bacteremia*. The patient will begin to show signs of an impending sepsis. If the infection is not stopped at this level, the patient will soon develop septicemia, which has a poor prognosis.

Once large numbers of microbes are in circulation, the patient is at the last line of defense, the systemic filters. If the pathogens are particularly virulent, the body's defenses are soon taxed, and the patient will succumb to septicemia. Detecting subtle signs and symptoms of impending burn wound sepsis allows early initiation of therapies that may prevent or better control a life-threatening septicemia or fungemia (see box below).

Clinical signs of impending systemic sepsis are a temperature greater than 101° F or less than 98.6° F, an increase in pulse or respiratory rate, an insidious decrease in blood pressure or urinary output, glucose intolerance, thrombocytopenia, and a white blood cell count that either plummets or rises with a shift to the left.[12] General signs of sepsis include mild confusion, headache, chills, general malaise, cyanosis, and swollen regional lymph nodes.

Late symptoms of sepsis (septic shock) that are seen as septicemia becomes overwhelming include a drop in temperature to below 98° F, a decrease in WBC

Diagnosis of Burn Wound Sepsis
Intense periburn erythema
Rapid sudden separation of eschar
Breakdown in areas of healing burns or skin graft
Conversion of partial to full-thickness injury
Pus beneath eschar
Black or red hemorrhagic areas in eschar and in unburned adjacent skin
Histological evidence of bacteria or fungi in deep tissues, especially the perivascular lymphatics seen either on frozen or permanent section histology
Quantitative bacterial counts of 10^5 per gram of tissue

From Nicosia, J. T., & Petro, J. A. (1983). *Manual of burn care* (p. 32). New York: Raven.

count to less than 10,000/ml, an ileus from septic shock, an enlarged liver and spleen, metastatic lesions, necrotic granulation tissue, and pneumonia. If irreversible shock occurs, the patient will die. The nurse should be alert! When it seems that "something just doesn't seem right about the patient," all parameters should be reviewed to rule out or treat bacteremia before it becomes septicemia.

Fungemia

Monilial septicemia, a severe infectious complication usually caused by *Candida albicans*, mimics the clinical response to gram-negative sepsis except that the course is much more insidious. The temperature and WBC count respond slowly to the invasive organisms, continuing to rise despite broad-spectrum antibiotic coverage. Debilitation and long-term broad-spectrum antibiotic therapy set the stage for fungemia.

The diagnosis of systemic moniliasis should be suspected in the debilitated patient who is on antibiotics but not responding to treatment. If this patient also has *C. albicans* organisms in the urine, treatment should be started (see treatment for septicemia).

PULMONARY COMPLICATION PREVENTION

More than 90% of severely burned patients require some form of respiratory therapy. Therefore, burn care includes an awareness of the principles and procedures required for effective ventilation and a working knowledge of pulmonary function, of ventilators, and of other equipment. It is important to remember that new developments in the field of pulmonary therapy do not replace basic nursing care.

Pulmonary complications may be grouped into those that occur within the first 24 to 48 hours as a result of the accident, and those that occur any time after that. Immediate complications include upper airway obstruction secondary to edema of the face, neck, mouth, pharynx, and larynx; and primary pulmonary damage from forced inhalation of products of combustion, such as smoke, gases, and noxious chemicals. The second group of complications includes pulmonary insufficiency secondary to shock, trauma, and increased lung water due to overhydration or secondary to extensive injury characterized by alveolar collapse. Other complications include pneumonia and pulmonary embolism. These complications may occur anytime after a burn injury. Embolism, if seen, is usually a late occurrence.

Treatment of these complications ranges from basic nursing care measures to maintenance of respirations through an artificial upper airway by a mechanical ventilator. The basic principle of respiratory therapy is to assist or support the patient's ventilation, without causing additional complications, until the patient has resumed effective spontaneous ventilation.

Types of Complications

Respiratory complications resulting directly from the accident are either upper airway obstruction or primary pulmonary damage. Little can be done to prevent immediate respiratory distress. However, merely "observing" the patient for signs and symptoms, or "watchful waiting," can be fatal.

Definitive signs and symptoms may not be apparent during the first several hours after a burn or until edema forms. Stridor is a fairly late symptom of obstruction. Early chest x-rays frequently show no abnormality, and arterial hypoxemia may be the first sign of pulmonary insufficiency.

The following signs indicate probable respiratory involvement; the presence of one or more indicates the need for immediate action:

- A history of forced inhalation of products of combustion (such as occurs in house fire or explosion)
- Burns of the face, especially around the nose and mouth, or of the neck and upper chest
- Singed nasal hairs
- Darkened oral and nasal mucous membranes
- Coughing up of darkened sputum

Medical Management

The principles of care are to ensure a patent airway and to maintain adequate ventilation. This may be accomplished by providing humidified oxygen with a face mask, or it may require an artificial airway such as an endotracheal tube for severe upper airway obstruction or a tracheostomy for primary pulmonary damage. If the trauma has affected the alveoli, treatment is difficult. Antibiotics and bronchodilators may also be indicated.

The steps discussed here may be taken to decrease the seriousness of respiratory involvement and pave the way for proper clinical management. If one or more of the signs of respiratory involvement are present, elevate the patient's head and torso (if systolic blood pressure is not less than 100 mmHg) to ensure a patent airway; set up intratracheal suction at the bedside; place a laryngoscope, endotracheal tube, and supplies near the bedside; and have a tracheostomy tray and tubes on hand. Start measured humidified oxygen and obtain specimens for arterial blood gas analysis. Instruct the patient to cough and deep breathe every 20 minutes. Begin an hourly turning schedule from side to back to side. Begin chest physiotherapy, if indicated. Watch for any signs of cerebral depression and keep narcotics at a minimum to prevent a decrease in cerebral response. Observe for tight chest or neck eschar and perform an escharotomy as soon as indicated. Monitor resuscitation fluids, respirations, and other vital signs closely. Begin pulmonary artery pressure monitoring if necessary.

Upper airway obstruction decreases as edema subsides and trauma to tissues of the upper airway resolves. With proper management, this problem will not require long-term care. Deep lung damage, however, cannot be resolved as quickly and may prove fatal. The symptoms of primary pulmonary damage are similar to those of respiratory distress and failure, and treatment is similar. The following principles of care provide a basis for management of all pulmonary complications.

The burned patient is predisposed to pulmonary complications (which occur other than as a direct result of the accident) from a number of factors that may not be obviously related to pulmonary problems. If these factors are recognized and controlled, the incidence of pulmonary complications can be reduced. The predisposing factors are:
- Hypovolemic shock and fluid therapy, which, if not properly managed or if combined with primary pulmonary damage, lead to overhydration and stiff, wet lungs due to pulmonary interstitial edema
- Lowered resistance to infection due to decreased immunity, nutritional imbalance, protein loss, and continuous wound infections
- Stasis of secretions due to prolonged bed rest, infrequent turning and positioning, and limited activity

The following general principles of care underlie prevention as well as management of early and late pulmonary complications. These measures alone may be inadequate to maintain oxygenation, ventilation, and acid–base balance; an artificial upper airway and mechanical respiratory support also may be required.

The clinical signs and symptoms of pulmonary involvement and possible insufficiency also are noted with many other problems. Subtle changes may be the first indications of insufficiency. The nurse should be especially alert to insidious changes in respiratory rate and volume, noting tachypnea or bradypnea; irregular breathing patterns; dyspnea; or apnea. Chest pain or a change in the amount, color, or consistency of sputum may indicate a problem. A change in pulse rate or blood pressure may be significant, and anxiety or restlessness should be noted. Peripheral cyanosis and stridor are crude guides to oxygenation status because they are late signs of a problem. Therefore, frequent blood gas analysis is mandatory at the first suspicion of pulmonary insufficiency.

Extravascular water can accumulate in the lungs for a variety of reasons. If there has been significant inhalation of noxious gases at the time of injury, there will be pulmonary interstitial edema. Toxins released from injured burn tissue also are thought to contribute to wet lungs. In addition, fluids required for initial resuscitation increase interstitial edema. Overhydration results in stiff, wet lungs. Use of colloids such as salt-poor albumin and plasma for initial resuscitation, however, tends to decrease lung water extravasation. Ultrasonic nebulization can also contribute to wet lungs and consideration of this factor should dictate use of the device. Extravascular lung water (EVLW) measurements can be done hourly to evaluate a patient's status. The technique uses a dye injectate and can indicate signs of pulmonary failure.[13] Treatment includes frequent turning.

Intravenous fluid administration should be carefully monitored. Whenever regulating fluid balance, the possibility of circulatory overload and pulmonary insufficiency should not be overlooked.

WOUND CARE
Principles of Burn Management

Current methods of burn wound management include the conservative method and the early excision method, or some combination thereof. *Conservative treatment* is that method which allows for separation of eschar over time through the process of autolysis. *Autolysis* is the spontaneous disintegration of tissues by the action of their own enzymes. The eschar is debrided daily during hydrotherapy treatments, and skin grafting is done on third-degree burns when a healthy granulation bed is exposed.

Hydrotherapy is performed daily to debride necrotic tissue and visualize wounds. In addition, topical agents are removed, and remaining eschar is softened. Showering the patient on a table and immersing the patient in a tub are two currently used methods of hydrotherapy. Showering enhances visualization of wounds and allows water temperature to be kept constant. Immersion of the burn patient in large tubs of water or antiseptic solutions has been associated with autocontamination and increased losses of sodium through the burn wound. Figure 53-9 depicts a shower table used in hydrotherapy.

The *early excision method*[14] exemplifies the recent trend toward operative management of the wound. Patients are taken to the operating room as early after injury as possible. The burn wound is excised by either a tangential or fascial excision technique. A skin graft or other temporary covering is placed over the excised wound. Operative debridement and grafting procedures, if necessary, are done every 5 to 7 days until complete, permanent coverage is achieved.

Permanent skin coverage is achieved only through the application of an autograft or another suitable permanent wound cover such as tissue cultured skin or the self-healing of partial-thickness injuries. Skin

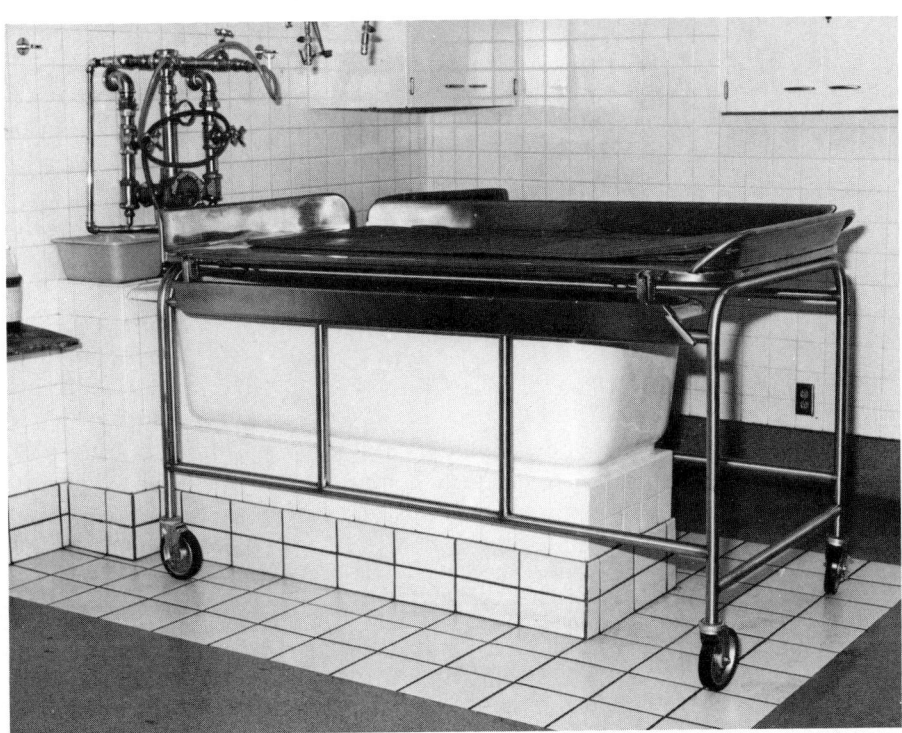

Figure 53-9   Shower table used for daily hydrotherapy, debridement, and hygiene.

grafts are generally of split thickness (0.015 inch) and are placed either on a clean granulation bed or an excised area of burn. Generally, grafts are meshed to increase the area of coverage at ratios from 1:1.5 to 1:3. In large percentage burns, skin can be meshed and expanded at ratios from 1:6 to 1:9. In areas where cosmesis is a concern, such as the face or breast area, skin is not meshed, and sheet grafts are applied. Once applied, mesh grafts are sutured or stapled in place and covered with fine-mesh gauze impregnated with an antibiotic ointment such as polysporin or gentamicin. This limits bacterial invasion of open-meshed areas in the graft (interstices), thus limiting graft loss due to infection. Because infection is the leading cause of graft failure, perioperative antibiotics are prescribed. Thick gauze padding and pressure bandages are then applied over the grafted areas to prevent graft loss due to manual dislocation of the graft. Skin grafts become attached to the body through the establishment of capillary networks from the graft to the body. Destruction of these bonds occurs when the graft is moved or traumatized. The development of hematomas or seromas under the graft also can inhibit the formation of circulatory bonding patterns and be detrimental to grafts.

Body image is a primary concern and must be considered in wound management therapy from the time the burn occurs. Cosmetic and/or functional surgical procedures are often performed for many years fol-lowing the initial insult. The use of microvascular free flaps, pedicle flaps, or rotation flaps can greatly improve tissue survival, save a questionable extremity, or improve function and appearance in deformed areas (see Chapter 54).

The nurse must be vigilant in observing for the development of clots or seromas beneath the graft surface. The surgeon should be promptly notified and the obstruction removed. (See Chapter 54 for discussion of postoperative wound healing.)

Skin Grafting

Full-thickness wounds require autografting to obtain permanent skin coverage and to achieve the natural immunity of the intact anatomical barrier of the skin destroyed by the burn injury. With good care, the body can heal a partial-thickness wound through the process of reepithelialization.

Types of Grafts

The four types of grafts are autograft, tissue culture grafts, homografts, and heterografts. These grafts can be applied as either full-thickness grafts, in which the full thickness of the dermis is cropped, or as split-thickness grafts, in which approximately 0.015 inch of dermis is taken. Once taken, the skin can be applied as a sheet graft or can be meshed to increase the surface area of the skin (Figure 53-10). Artificial skin may prove useful in covering patients with large sur-

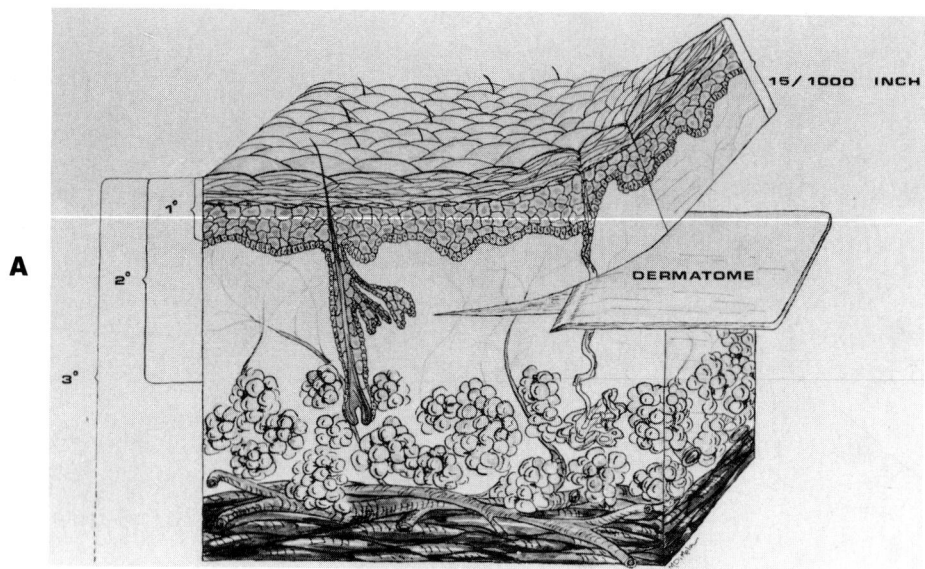

Figure 53-10 *A,* Split-thickness skin grafts are harvested at a depth of 0.015 inch.

Continued.

face area burns. Its use, however, is still under investigation.[15]

In burn care, homografts (usually cadaver skin) are applied to provide temporary coverage. Homografts are used as a biological cover to decrease infection, to protect nerve endings, and to prevent heat and fluid loss. Homografts may be used on partial-thickness wounds to protect them while healing takes place, or on full-thickness wounds until the patient can tolerate the autografting procedure or has donor areas available. Homografts also may be used to prepare an area for autografting.

Donor Site

The donor site (the area of the body from which the autograft is taken) represents a partial-thickness wound that temporarily increases the total wound area. Meticulous care is required to heal the donor site as rapidly as possible and, thereby, decrease the total size of the wound. The principles of donor site care are (1) to keep the area free from infection, (2) to dry and heal the area, and (3) to provide patient comfort.

PAIN CONTROL AND SEDATION

Burn pain is both chronic and acute. It is a biopsychosocial process with many factors contributing to its severity. If not controlled, excessive pain can contribute to intensive care unit psychosis, complications in sleep–wake cycles, and personality disorders.

When the patient's condition permits, pharmacological pain management can be beneficial in reducing stress during painful procedures. Morphine is the most commonly used narcotic; however, codeine, me-

perdine, levorphanol, and propoxyphen have been used effectively. Methods of delivery of pharmacological agents can also affect the level of relief experienced by the patient. For example, patient-controlled analgesia, a system by which the patient can self-administer analgesics as pain increases, has been beneficial in decreasing the amount of drugs needed for pain relief and in increasing the patient's sense of well-being. Also, the timely and prompt administration of analgesics by the nurse offers the patient reassurance that prolonged periods of pain will not occur. Effective analgesic administration requires that drugs be given in advance of painful procedures.

Nonpharmacological pain relief measures include acupuncture, transcutaneous electrical nerve stimulation (TENS), acupressure, relaxation therapy, music therapy, and distraction. The degree of pain relief depends on the type of procedure being performed and the individual patient's response.

Sedatives and tranquilizers help reduce anxiety associated with pain and offer assistance in the promotion of adequate sleep patterns. Although these pharmacological agents do not themselves reduce burn or procedural pain, they reduce the behavioral responses that often contribute to the pain mechanism.

NUTRITIONAL SUPPORT

Because metabolic requirements double in the client with severe burns,[16] body wasting, delayed wound healing, and, in some cases, death will occur if energy needs are not met. Nutritional intake must meet the body's requirements. Further discussion of nutritional needs and management of the burn patient are discussed in Chapter 11.

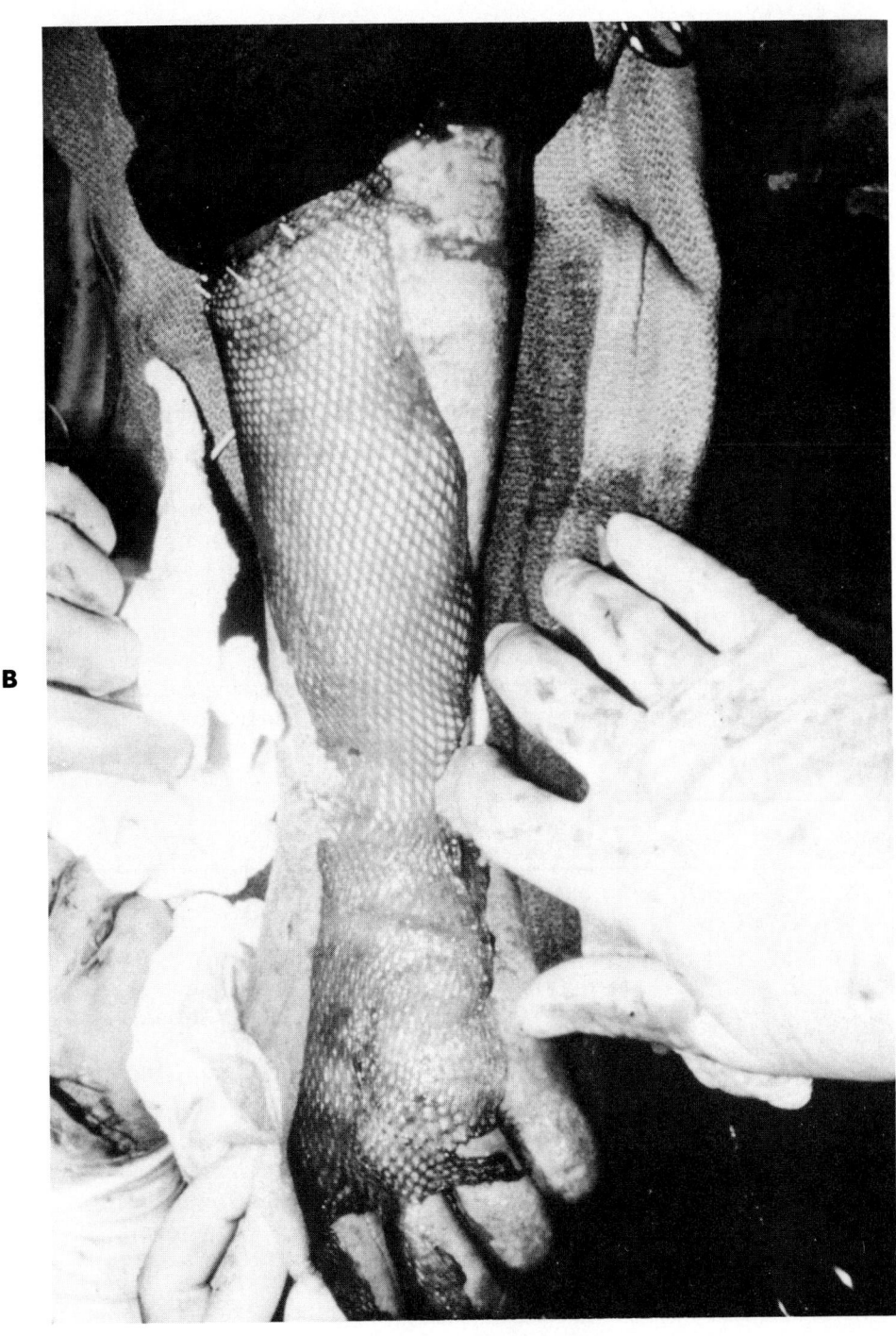

B

Figure 53-10, cont'd. *B,* Grafts are meshed and placed on a healthy granulation bed.
Continued.

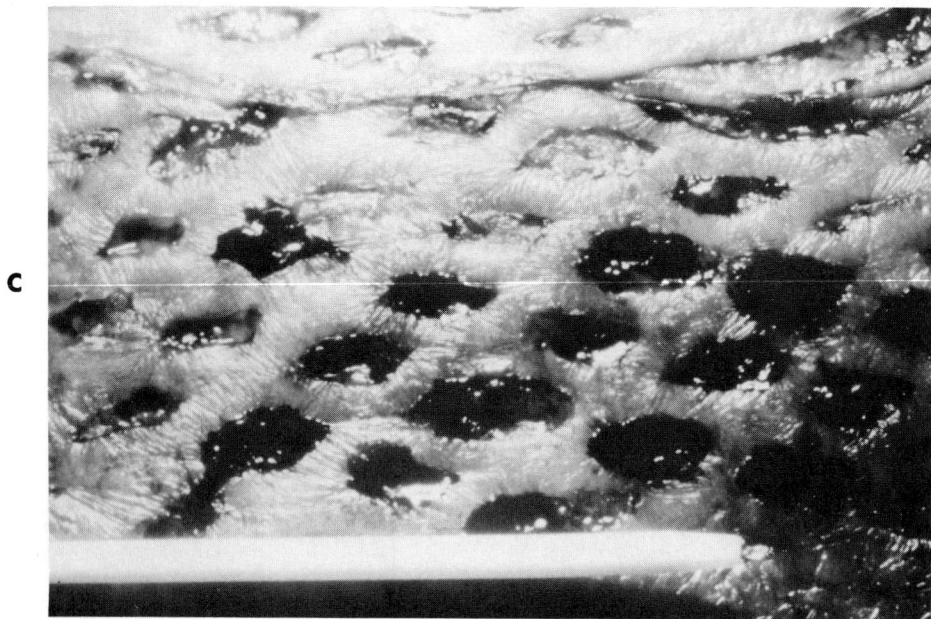

Figure 53-10, cont'd. C, Interstices heal within 7 days.

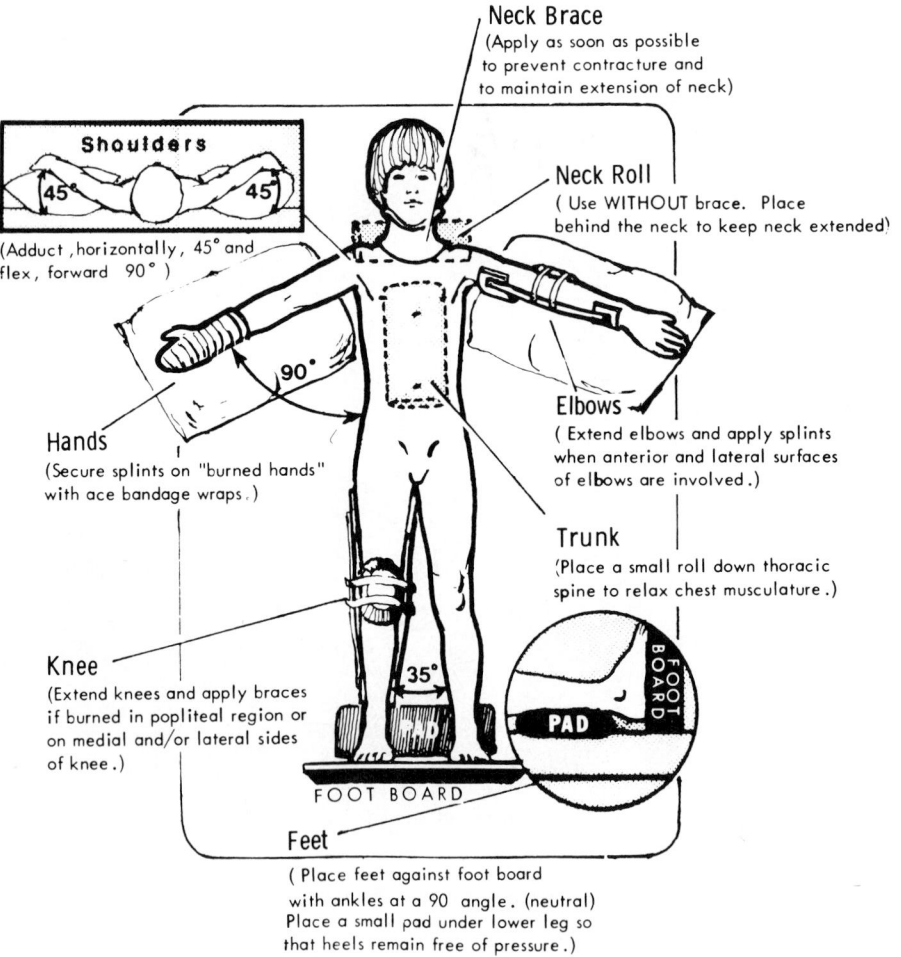

Neck Brace
(Apply as soon as possible
to prevent contracture and
to maintain extension of neck)

Shoulders
45° 45°

(Adduct, horizontally, 45° and
flex, forward 90°)

Neck Roll
(Use WITHOUT brace. Place
behind the neck to keep neck extended)

90°

Hands
(Secure splints on "burned hands"
with ace bandage wraps.)

Elbows
(Extend elbows and apply splints
when anterior and lateral surfaces
of elbows are involved.)

Trunk
(Place a small roll down thoracic
spine to relax chest musculature.)

Knee
(Extend knees and apply braces
if burned in popliteal region or
on medial and/or lateral sides
of knee.)

35°

FOOT BOARD
PAD

FOOT BOARD

Feet
(Place feet against foot board
with ankles at a 90 angle. (neutral)
Place a small pad under lower leg so
that heels remain free of pressure.)

Figure 53-11 *A,* Supine positioning of the burn patient to prevent contracture formation.

POSITIONING, CONTRACTURE CONTROL, EXERCISE, AND SPLINTING

Positioning

A position the patient considers comfortable is seldom one that will control contracture formation. However, if proper positioning is initiated early in care, explained frequently, and continued, the patient will accept these positions as comforting. Attempting to correct established contractures later in burn care is far more time-consuming and painful. The nurse must make the patient as comfortable as possible while maintaining a position of contracture control. The nonfetal position is generally desired. It is easier to flex an extended tendon than to extend a tendon in a fixed position.

Position change and proper body alignment are an essential part of nursing any severely ill patient. The objectives of positioning may be any of the following: to reduce the workload of the heart; to prevent or reduce contracture formation (Figure 53-11); to reduce the incidence of phlebitis, thrombi, and emboli; to promote lung expansion and drainage of pulmonary secretions; to reduce the incidence of pneumonia; to prevent decubiti; or to provide patient comfort.

Range of Motion Exercises

Exercises that take the joints (burned or unburned) through the full range of motion are done at least once daily. However, joints should not be pushed beyond free range of motion unless this is prescribed by a physician or therapist. Bed rest, decreased protein, altered fluids and electrolytes, and poor circulation serve to decrease joint function and to encourage heterotopic bone formation and contracture. Exercising is best done while the patient is in the hydrotherapy tub. Active and passive range of motion may be combined, depending on the patient's capabilities. The physiatrist and physical therapist (PT) are skilled in providing these exercises; a nurse, however, can conduct them. Exercising should not be neglected because of lack of PT coverage. Active range

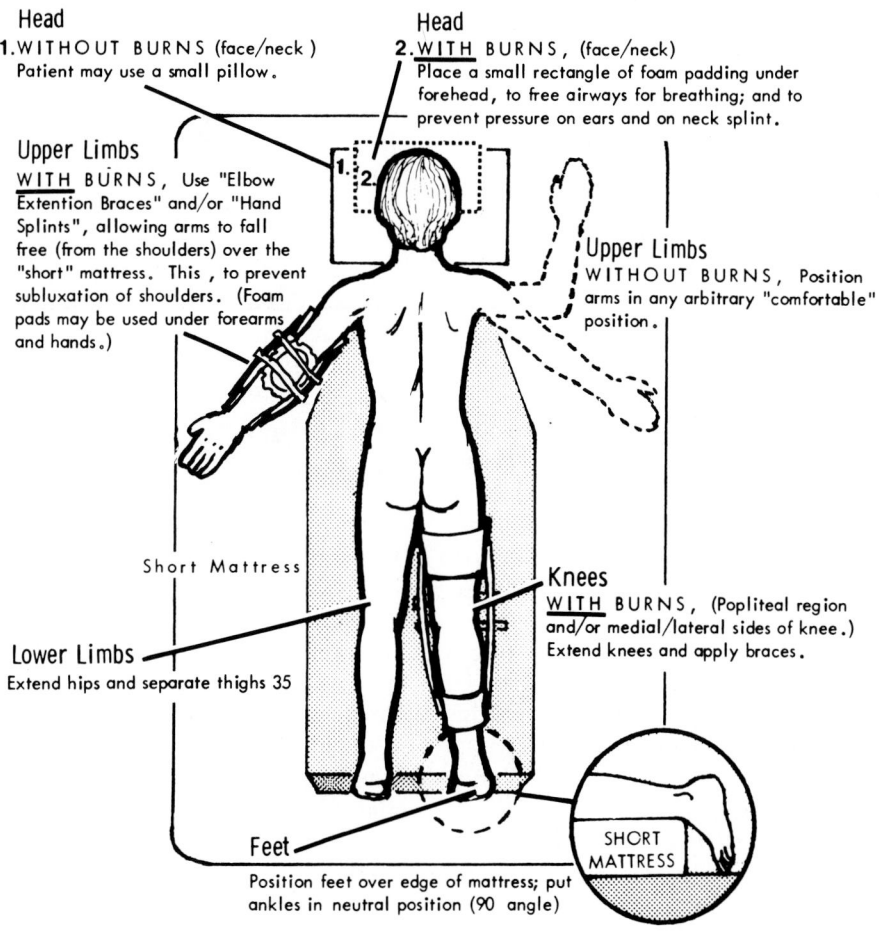

Figure 53-11, cont'd.   *B,* Prone positioning of the burn patient to reduce contracture formation.
Courtesy Shriners Burns Institute, Galveston, Texas.

of motion requires that the patient exercise voluntarily. Full range of motion as well as increased self-care is encouraged; for example, brushing teeth, combing hair, and feeding. Many devices may be provided by the occupational or physical therapist to increase or enhance this type of exercise.

Passive range of motion requires that the patient be taken through range of motion exercises by another individual. The exercises are best done in hydrotherapy or immediately after tubbing. If done at the bedside, a pain medication may be useful prior to exercising.

Splinting

The principle of splinting any area of the body is to place the area in a position that will preserve or restore function. Splinting may be employed throughout burn care. If contractures continue after discharge, which may be the case regardless of preventive measures, corrective splinting is necessary. Custom-made splints, those fashioned for a particular area of a particular patient, are ideal. However, custom-made splints are not always available or necessary. Ingenuity may substitute for them. An elbow or knee joint may be maintained in proper position by use of a padded IV board. Contracture of the Achilles tendon, which causes foot drop, may be prevented by use of sandbags, towels, or pillows. The preservation of function is always the primary guide in the use of splints.

Dorsal and Total Hand Burn

The objectives in treating burns of the hand are to prevent deeply damaged tissues from becoming infected and to maintain a position that will preserve function. Because severe consequences result when hand function is damaged or lost, special or custom-made splints are desirable. Because the tendons of the dorsum (back) of the hand have little fatty padding and protection, they require special care. If the hand has sustained either a deep partial-thickness or a full-thickness burn, contractures may be expected. However, much can be done to minimize these contractures, and in some instances, they can be avoided.

Exercising or using the hand without splinting is excellent; however, use must be consistent to prevent contractures. The splinting method recommended is one that maintains most of the joints of the hand in an extended position (Figure 55-12). This splinting method can be very effective, provided that the splints are correctly applied immediately after the burn injury and are checked frequently to see that they are maintained in proper position.

Initially, the extent and depth of a burn often cannot be accurately determined, and hand splints may be applied as a precautionary measure; they can be

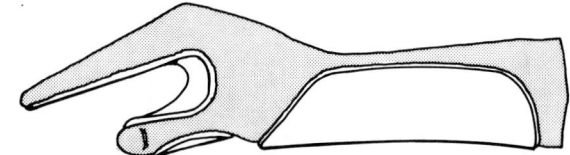

Figure 53-12 Splint applied to burned hand. *Note:* The splint maintains wrist and hand position to prevent contractures.

removed later if not required. Hand splints are continued until the major healing process has been completed in a partial-thickness burn or until grafting is completed in a full-thickness injury. After grafting, splints are removed, and full use of the hand is encouraged.

Palmar Burns

Full-thickness burns limited to the palm of the hand may be less deforming than dorsal burns because the flexor tendons are protected by thick palmar fascia and fat. Palmar burns are usually treated by splinting in a position with the fingers extended and the thumb in abduction.

Pressure Dressings

Pressure dressings, in the form of elastic wraps or specialized pressure garments called *Jobst garments,* are believed to reduce the amount of scar tissue that forms over burned areas of the body. Once wounds are closed, custom-fitted Jobst garments are worn over all areas of the body affected. These garments are worn for 23 hours a day, then every day for 1 to 2 years, or until the scar tissue is mature. Figure 53-13 illustrates the types of Jobst garments available. Temporary measures of applying pressure to healed wounds include the use of elastic wraps or other pressure bandages.

REHABILITATION

Once released from the care of the burn team, the patient and family must deal with wound care, dressing changes, ambulation, eating, sweating, itching, pressure garments, and a host of other aspects of physical care. Psychologically, the prospect of going home may be an uplifting thought to the patient; however, once at home, the difficulties and stress encountered may alter feelings of excitement. The burn team must anticipate problems the patient will face and take measures to intervene when possible. Occasionally, problems are numerous, or the coping mechanisms of the family are inadequate, and referral of a patient to a rehabilitation facility is indicated. The family must be evaluated in terms of its support, reliability, cooperation, and ability to perform the necessary care. Referral to a visiting nurse service in

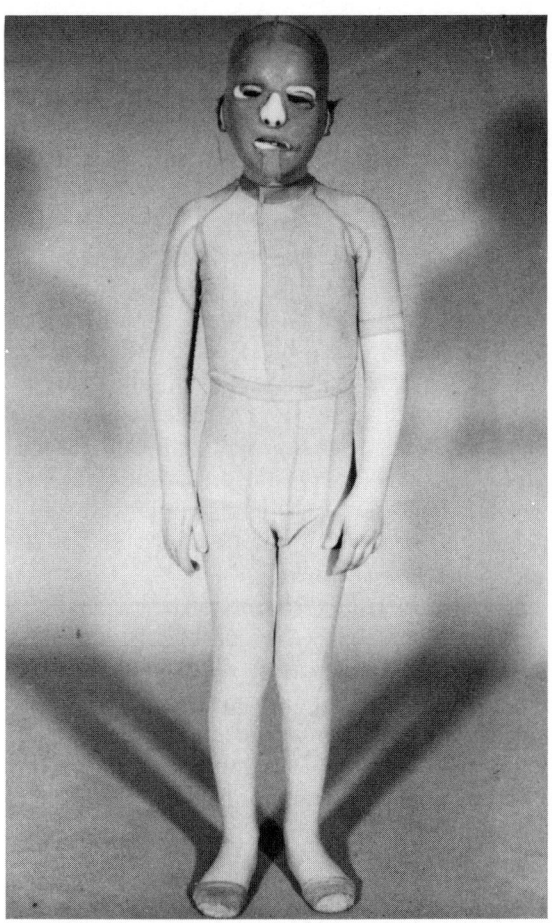

Figure 53-13 Patient in full Jobst garments.

the community is often made, and the frequency of home visits depends on the level of care the family is able to deliver.

Referrals are often made to community agency health team members such as physical or occupational therapists, social workers, schools, psychiatrists, family counselors, or others. Often, the need for equipment arises, and a route for acquisition must be established.

Home arrangements are detailed, complex, and extremely time-consuming. For this reason, home care planning and community referrals are begun on admission to the burn unit. Failure to follow this process leads to problems when the patient returns home.

Reconstructive and cosmetic surgery is performed for many years following burn injury. Restoration of function and improvement of cosmetic appearance through surgical techniques may greatly improve the patient's body image and feelings of self-worth. As with acute skin grafting procedures, the nurse must caution the patient about graft or cosmetic outcomes. Patients may expect grafted skin or reconstructed areas to appear equal in quality and looks to their previous state. This is never the case, and proper ed-

ucation can help prevent shock and depression following surgery. The patient who has developed contractures, keloids, microstomia, or other conditions that limit movement frequently requires surgical intervention to restore function.

Plastic surgery involves the use of classic techniques; however, some new approaches are being studied. Use of tissue expanders is one example of a relatively new area of burn surgery. Contracture releases are most commonly performed on the neck, axillae, or elbow area. Surgical procedures to improve movement are many, varied, and individualized to each client.

Nursing care involves postoperative care of grafts or suture lines. Bolster dressings are often used to limit movement. The position of the client can have a direct effect on the success of the procedure. The nurse also must assure long-term success of the surgical procedure. Patients must be taught about the need to use splints or assistive devices.

Rehabilitation may last for many years. Often, reentry into society is difficult in terms of relationships, lifestyle, and vocation.[17] The burn team must understand the process of rehabilitation and offer support to the patient to assist a successful transition.

INTEGUMENT DISORDERS NOT RELATED TO HEAT

Three specific nonburn conditions are often referred to burn centers for treatment: scalded skin syndrome (SSS), Stephens-Johnson syndrome (SJS), and toxic epidermal necrosis. These disorders present the medical team with many of the same derangements seen in burn patients. Most often, large areas of skin have sloughed off the body, leaving the patient in need of infection control protocols and other immune system support.

The least lethal of these disorders, *scalded skin syndrome,* is most often caused by a staphylococcal infection. This disease is most often present in children and is manifested by superficial layers of the epidermis sloughing and exposing as much as 80% of the body surface area. Diagnosis is based on clinical manifestations and positive laboratory findings of staphylococci. Presenting symptoms are fever, severe malaise, and anorexia. Recovery usually occurs rapidly, between 5 and 7 days, when the client is treated appropriately with systemic antibiotics. Palliative care includes topical antimicrobial therapy, placement in an air-fluidized bed, and strict infection control practices. Pharmacological treatment can include sedation with diazepam or pain control with appropriate analgesics.

The more complicated disorders of Stephens-Johnson syndrome (erythema multiforme major) and toxic epidermal necrosis are less responsive to drug therapy and more dependent on the body's natural healing process. Stevens-Johnson syndrome, a severe form of erythema multiforme, is characterized by target lesions present over large portions of the body. Also, lesions are often present within external compartments such as the mouth and vaginal cavity. Causes of this disorder remain unknown, but it is often associated with antecedent infections such as *streptococcus*, herpes simplex, or pneumonias. Drug hypersensitivity has also been implicated as a cause. Recovery usually takes between 3 and 6 weeks and treatment is primarily supportive. Mortality rate for SJS is between 5% and 25%, and as with scaled skin syndrome, infection control and topical antimicrobial treatment are indicated. Attention should also be paid to the patient's eyes for possible lesion formation in the eyelid which could lead to severely decreased ocular function.

Toxic epidermal necrosis, the most lethal of the three disorders, is characterized by large epidermal slough, mucosal inflammation, and severe ulceration. This is a life-threatening skin disease in which the epithelium peels off in large sheets, leaving widespread denuded areas that must be covered by reepithelialization or by artificial means. Toxic epidermal necrosis is most often seen in adults, and most commonly in females. All known cases are considered drug induced or idiopathic. Many different drugs have been implicated in cases of toxic epidermal necrosis, but sulfonamides, anticonvulsants, and nonsteroidal antiinflammatory drugs are most often blamed. Studies also suggest that a generic propensity may exist.

It is often difficult to differentiate toxic epidermal necrosis from Stevens-Johnson syndrome. It has been suggested that denudation of greater than 10% TBSA be considered diagnostic for toxic epidermal necrosis, with less than 10% involvement being diagnosed as Stevens-Johnson syndrome. Other clinicians look for severe involvement of mucous membranes as characteristic of Stevens-Johnson syndrome.

Toxic epidermal necrosis has more serious prognosis with severe morbidity and mortality (60% to 70%). Sepsis is the primary cause of death. Hypovolemia and gastrointestinal hemorrhage also are severe complications of both diseases.

Treatment for all three disorders includes (1) control of infection and bacterial invasion, (2) monitoring of fluid and electrolyte imbalances, (3) correction of thermal disturbances, (4) control of pain and discomfort, and (5) promotion of wound healing. Frequent ophthalmological examinations are essential, and comfort measures surrounding the eyes and mouth should be taken. Probably the most controversial development involving these maladies is the condemnation of the use of systemic corticosteroids. Corticosteroids had been routinely prescribed for their antiinflammatory characteristic. Studies have now associated corticosteroid use with longer hospitalizations, increased time for healing injured skin, and increased mortality. They also mask infection. Antibiotics are not routinely used except in the presence of sepsis.

NURSING MANAGEMENT OF THE CARDIOVASCULAR SYSTEM

Problems related to the cardiovascular system include tachycardia; pallor; cool, clammy skin; weak, thready pulse; hypotension; disorientation or poor mentation; low urine output; ileus; loss of peripheral pulses; falling, hemodynamic pressures (CVP, PWP); low cardiac output; and dysrhythmias. Nursing diagnoses related to the cardiovascular system follow.

■ NURSING DIAGNOSES
- Alteration in cardiac output (decreased), related to increased capillary permeability
- Fluid volume deficit and electrolyte imbalance, related to loss of plasma volume from the vascular space
- Alteration in tissue perfusion: cerebral, cardiopulmonary, renal, gastrointestinal, peripheral, related to decreased cardiac output and generalized edema

OUTCOME STANDARD AND CRITERIA
Cardiac output is maintained by increasing intravascular fluid volume to a level which provides adequate perfusion to vital organs as evidenced by:
- Positive pulses in all extremities
- Absence of acute tubular necrosis (ATN)
- Clear sensorium
- Heart rate, blood pressure, and cardiac rhythm within normal limits
- Fluid and electrolyte status within normal limits
- Urine output >30 to 50 ml/hr

NURSING INTERVENTIONS
- Administer fluid according to the Parkland formula
- Insert Foley catheter and monitor urine output hourly
- Obtain daily nude weights
- Monitor mentation, heart rate, blood pressure, CVP, and PWP every 15 minutes to hourly
- Monitor temperature and cardiac output hourly
- Monitor peripheral pulses every 15 minutes to hourly
- Provide pre- and postoperative escharotomy care
- Titrate fluids
- Administer medication intravenously or orally as prescribed

NURSING MANAGEMENT OF THE RESPIRATORY SYSTEM

Problems related to the respiratory system include drowsiness; stupor; coma; elevated carboxyhemoglobin; hypoxia; respiratory distress; upper airway edema; blisters and soot in mouth, nose, pharynx; burns of the face, head, and neck; singed nares, eyebrows, and eyelids; progressive hoarseness; dyspnea; stridor; cyanosis; coughing; and circumferential chest burns. Related nursing diagnosis follows.

■ NURSING DIAGNOSIS

Ineffective breathing pattern, related to respiratory distress from inhalation injury, airway obstruction, or pneumonia.

OUTCOME STANDARD AND CRITERIA

Breathing pattern is normal or improved as evidenced by:
- Absence of obstruction (edema, secretions)
- Patent airway (physiological, endotracheal tube, or tracheostomy)
- Respiratory rate within normal limits
- Absence of stridor, dyspnea, cyanosis
- Skin/eschar about chest expanding (escharotomies done)
- Adequate perfusion in lungs
- Arterial blood gases within normal limits
- Absence of acidosis/alkalosis
- Absence of pulmonary edema
- No ventilatory assistance required
- Incentive spirometry used
- Cough reflex intact
- Tidal volume, inspiratory force, and minute volume within normal limits

NURSING INTERVENTIONS
- Perform chin lift/head tilt maneuver in unconscious victim
- Prepare for and assist with nasal or oral intubation or tracheostomy
- Suction as necessary
- Perform chest physiotherapy
- Observe ventilator for proper mechanical function
- Monitor gas exchange through laboratory tests: ABG, VBG, carboxyhemoglobin levels
- Administer antibiotics as indicated
- Turn patient frequently
- Administer vigorous chest physiotherapy
- Evaluate fluid balance
- Administer sedative and paralytic agents when indicated
- Monitor lung water measurements when indicated
- Monitor pulmonary artery and wedge pressure when indicated
- Monitor central venous pressures
- Administer oxygen
- Encourage incentive spirometry
- Encourage coughing and deep breathing exercises
- Assist with weaning from mechanical ventilator

NURSING MANAGEMENT OF PAIN

Manifestations of pain include: crying, verbal expressions, complaints, irritability, lethargy, depression, facial grimacing and tensing, increased heart rate and blood pressure, abnormal sleep–wake patterns, withdrawal of body part when touched, poor mobility, poor joint range, inflammation or redness of area, and edema.

■ NURSING DIAGNOSIS

Pain, related to exposed nerve endings found in the damaged dermis.

OUTCOME STANDARD AND CRITERIA

Pain is reduced or alleviated as evidenced by:
- Decreased crying, moaning, or verbal expressions of pain
- Decreased facial grimacing and tensing
- Decreased heart rate
- Increase in sleep and rest periods
- Ability to ambulate and move body parts (ROM)
- Increased ability to tolerate painful procedures

NURSING INTERVENTIONS
- Administer analgesics promptly
- Administer medications as indicated, especially 30 to 45 minutes prior to painful procedures
- Teach patient relaxation techniques and meditative breathing
- Use techniques of guided imagery, music therapy, hypnosis, therapeutic touch, acupressure when appropriate
- Allow sleep and rest time to prevent ICU psychosis
- Change position frequently
- Maintain ambient temperature at 85° to 90° F to decrease shivering and trigger relaxation response
- Establish a contract with the patient to enhance his or her feeling of control over pain
- Explain all procedures

NURSING MANAGEMENT OF THE INTEGUMENTARY SYSTEM AND INFECTION

Problems related to the integumentary system and infection include positive wound sputum, blood, or urine cultures, or an increase in colony counts; hypo- or hyperthermia; positive burn wound biopsies; pus and/or purulent wound drainage; foul-smelling odors from wounds; glucose intolerance; increased WBC count with a shift to the left; thrombocytopenia; change in mentation; redness surrounding wounds; redness or maceration of healthy skin; areas of burn that do not heal; autograft loss; poor "take" of skin substitutes or autograft; eschar on donor sites; wound detritus; and change in wound texture. Related nursing diagnoses follow.

■ NURSING DIAGNOSIS

Impaired skin integrity, related to cell loss caused by heat or chemicals.

OUTCOME STANDARD AND CRITERIA

Skin is intact, or integrity is improved as evidenced by:

- Absence of areas of redness due to pressure or immobility
- Absence of cellulitis
- Absence of maceration of healthy skin near areas of burn
- Absence of tissue breakdown secondary to tube placement (e.g., breakdown of nares with long-term use of nasogastric tube)
- Absence of open areas
- Absence of temporary skin substitutes
- Adherence of all skin grafts
- Absence of infection in newly grafted skin
- Healing of donor sites

NURSING INTERVENTIONS

- Perform hydrotherapy and debridement of burn wounds
- Give postoperative care to autograft, skin substitutes, and donor sites
- Position patient to prevent pressure on grafted or donor areas
- Use low-pressure mattresses or beds (i.e., air-fluidized therapy)
- Roll sheet grafts hourly
- Observe for development of clots, seromas, or bleeding beneath the surface of grafts postoperatively
- Apply heat lamps to donor sites
- Give skin care daily to healthy skin
- Use assistive devices to prevent decubiti

■ NURSING DIAGNOSIS

High risk for infection, related to varying depths of damage to dermal and epidermal cells.

OUTCOME STANDARDS AND CRITERIA

Infection is absent as evidenced by:

- Negative cultures from wound, sputum, blood, and urine
- Absence of temperature spikes
- Negative burn wound biopsies
- Absence of clinical signs of sepsis
- Absence of foul-smelling wounds
- Absence of pus and purulent wound exudate

In the presence of infection, the patient will not experience a spread, and the degree of infection will be reduced as evidenced by:

- A decrease in wound colony counts
- Improvement in wound appearance or odor
- Decrease in wound exudate or pus
- Improvement in clinical signs of sepsis
- Temperature within normal limits

NURSING INTERVENTIONS

- Implement isolation precautions when indicated
- Perform thorough handwashing procedures

- Procure wound, blood, sputum, and urine cultures
- Procure burn wound biopsies
- Monitor wound, blood, sputum, and urine cultures and burn wound biopsies
- Observe for signs of sepsis
- Take temperature hourly
- Administer appropriate antibiotics
- Administer tetanus toxoid on admission
- Apply topical antimicrobials

NURSING MANAGEMENT OF THE METABOLIC SYSTEM

Problems related to metabolism include increased metabolic rate, heart rate, and core temperature; anorexia; paralytic ileus; diarrhea; weight loss; and poor wound healing.

■ NURSING DIAGNOSIS

Altered nutrition: less than body requirements, related to increases in metabolic rate.

OUTCOME STANDARD AND CRITERIA

Nutrition is adequate as evidenced by:

- Adequate protein reserves
- Progressive wound healing
- Absence of paralytic ileus
- Weight loss <10% of preburn weight

NURSING INTERVENTIONS

- Provide high-protein, high-calorie diet
- Monitor bowel sounds
- Encourage feeding
- Administer tube feedings or TPN when indicated
- Monitor intake and output
- Monitor calories by the use of a calorie count sheet
- Weigh patient daily
- Offer high-calorie, high-protein snacks between meals

NURSING MANAGEMENT OF PHYSICAL MOBILITY

Problems related to physical mobility include loss of function; poor range of motion in burns that involve a joint; inability to ambulate independently; development of scar tissue causing contractures in areas, especially joints, that have been burned; hypertrophic scar tissue formation; and inability to perform activities of daily living.

■ NURSING DIAGNOSIS

Impaired physical mobility, related to open burn wounds, scar and contracture formation, and poor joint range of motion.

OUTCOME STANDARD AND CRITERIA

Mobility is maintained or increased as evidenced by:

- Increased range of motion in involved joints
- Increased function in specific area involved
- Independent ambulation
- Flattening of hypertrophic scars

- Reduction in extent of contracture
- Performance of activities of daily living

NURSING INTERVENTIONS

- Assist in range of motion exercises as indicated
- Apply splints and conformers appropriately
- Position the patient for contracture prevention
- Apply pressure garments when wounds heal
- Ambulate patient frequently
- Encourage self-assistance with activities of daily living
- Administer postoperative care following reconstructive surgery

NURSING MANAGEMENT OF SELF-ESTEEM AND SUPPORT SYSTEMS

Manifestations of problems related to self-esteem and underutilization of support system may include crying, anger, apathy, evidence of abuse, inability to identify support systems, and dependence. Adjustment may be affected by cultural mores, demographics (sex, age), and previous problems with self-concept.

■ NURSING DIAGNOSIS

Self-esteem disturbance, related to change in physical appearance.

OUTCOME STANDARD AND CRITERIA

Self-esteem is maintained or improved as evidenced by:

- Expression of feelings and thoughts
- Increased decision-making
- Establishment of new role function
- Appropriate movement through stages of grieving, denial, anger, bargaining, depression, and acceptance
- Asking for assistance of family or other previously successful support systems
- Cooperation with hospital-based social service or nursing supports
- Keeping scheduled appointments
- Verbalization of problems and working toward solutions
- Increase in self-ambulation
- Increase in independent activities of daily living such as eating, bathing, dressing
- Input into daily plan of care
- Improved role mastery
- Improved interpersonal relations

NURSING INTERVENTIONS

- Reassure patient that feelings of grief and loss are normal
- Accept the patient physically and psychologically
- Conduct counseling sessions for patient and family
- Identify support systems for patient to use
- Foster independence and decision-making in the patient

- Make provisions for community health assistance after discharge
- Explain reconstructive and cosmetic surgical procedures that can be done in future

REFERENCES

1. Artz, C. P., Moncrief, J. A., & Pruitt, B. A. (1979). *Burns: A team approach* (p. 25). Philadelphia: Saunders.
2. Artz, C. P., Moncrief, J. A., & Pruitt, B. A. (1979). *Burns: A team approach* (pp. 170-171). Philadelphia: Saunders.
3. Heimbach, D. (1983). Smoke inhalation: Current concepts. In T. Wachtel, V. Kahn, & H. Frank (Eds.), *Current topics in burn care*. Rockville, MD: Aspen.
4. Wilmore, D. W., Aulick, L. H., Mason, A. D., Jr., et al. (1977). Influence of the burn wound on local and systemic responses to injury. *Annals of Surgery, 186,* 444-458.
5. Baxter, C. R. (1971). Fluid volume and electrolyte changes of the early post-burn period. *Clinics in Plastic Surgery, 1*(4), 693-709.
6. Loebl, E. C., Marvin, J. A., Curreri, P. W., et al. (1974). Erythrocyte survival following thermal injury. *Journal of Surgical Research, 16,* 96-101.
7. Chan, C. K., Jarrett, F., & Moylan, J. A. (1976). Acute leukopenia as an allergic reaction to silver sulfadiazine in burn patients. *Journal of Trauma, 16*(5), 395-396.
8. Hall, J. W., Winkler, J. B., Herndon, D. N., et al. (1987). Auditory brainstem response in auditory assessment of acute severely burned children. *Journal of Burn Care and Rehabilitation, 8*(3), 195-198.
9. Curreri, P. W. (1979). Burns. In S. I. Schwartz, G. T. Shires, F. C. Spencer, et al. (Eds.), *Principles of surgery* (3rd ed.). New York: McGraw-Hill.
10. Ninniman, J. L. (1983). The effect of thermal injury of host immunologic defenses. In T. Wachtel, V. Kahn, & H. Frank (Eds.), *Current topics in burn care*. Rockville, MD: Aspen.
11. Garner, J. S., & Simmons, B. P. (1983). Guidelines for isolation precautions in hospitals. *Infection Control, 4*(4), 245-349.
12. Guyton, A. C. (1986). *Textbook of medical physiology* (7th ed.). Philadelphia: Saunders.
13. Allison, R. C., Carlile, P. V., & Gray, B. W. (1985). Thermodilution measurement of lung water. *Clinics in Chest Medicine, 6*(3), 439-457.
14. Herndon, D. N., Thompson, P. B., Desai, M. H., et al. (1985). Treatment of burns in children. *Pediatric Clinics of North America, 32*(5), 1311-1331.
15. Burke, J. F., et al. (1981). Successful use of a physiologically acceptable artificial skin in the treatment of extensive burn injury. *Annals of Surgery, 194*(4), 413-428.
16. Wilmore, D. W. (1974). Nutrition and metabolism following thermal injury. *Clinics in Plastic Surgery, 1,* 603-619.
17. Herndon, D. N., et al. (1986). The quality of like after major thermal injury in children: An analysis of 12 survivors with 80% total body, 70% third degree burns. *Journal of Trauma, 26,* 609-619.

54

Wound Healing

Nancy A. Stotts

Wound healing, restoration of tissue integrity, is an integral part of critical care nursing. Recent advances in the field have revolutionized wound care. Scientifically based clinical practice requires an understanding of current knowledge about wound healing.[1]

TYPES OF HEALING

Normal healing progresses in an orderly fashion regardless of the etiology of injury. Generally, tissue damage is divided into partial- and full-thickness injury: Partial-thickness injury involves only the epidermis, and full-thickness injury extends to the dermis and subcutaneous tissues.

In partial-thickness injury, epithelial cells are stimulated to migrate across denuded areas. New epithelial cells move from the wound edges and up skin appendages (the hair follicles and glands). When epithelial cells come into contact with other epithelial cells, they cease migration and begin to build layers of new cells until tissue damage has been repaired. Because the skin appendages are widely distributed throughout the skin, the distance that epithelial cells must migrate is small, and so partial-thickness injuries heal rapidly. The stimulus for epithelial migration is not entirely understood but includes a molecule called epidermal migration factor.

Healing of full-thickness injury involves the formation of new vessels to perfuse the area, the production of collagen to fill the tissue defect that has occurred, and epithelialization to cover the tissue defect. Wound contraction, the process of the wound area getting smaller, also occurs in full-thickness injuries that are left open to heal. Full-thickness injuries are said to heal by primary, secondary, or tertiary intention.[2,3]

Healing by primary intention occurs when there has been little or no tissue loss, a low level of contamination is present, and tissue edges can be readily approximated. Surgical incisions usually heal by primary intention.

Healing by secondary intention occurs when a wound is left open to heal. In this situation, there may be either substantial tissue loss or a high level of contamination. Traumatic wounds, grade III or IV pressure ulcers, and full-thickness burns are examples of wounds healing by secondary intention.

Healing by tertiary intention, frequently called *delayed primary closure,* occurs when a wound with a high bacterial content is left open through the subcutaneous tissue at the time of surgery. It is dressed using sterile technique at the time of surgery and the dressing left untouched. If there are no signs of infection, the surgeon closes the wound on about day 4 to 6. These wounds do not appear to begin the healing process with their closure but rather proceed along the healing trajectory counting day 1 as the day of the original surgery. Examples of wounds that may be closed by delayed primary closure are incisions of a ruptured appendectomy repair and some penetrating stab wounds.

THE HEALING PROCESS

The process of healing involves many complex processes that overlap. For the sake of understanding the process, healing has been divided into three phases: inflammatory, proliferative, and remodeling.

Inflammatory Phase

The inflammatory phase begins at the moment of injury and lasts until approximately day 3 or 4 after injury. Activities that take place in this phase are protection of the organism from blood loss, isolation of the wound from the rest of the body, and development of inflammation.

The series of events that begins with wounding is followed immediately by coagulation. As platelets enter the wound site, they release serotonin-containing granules; this leads to a brief period (approximately 10 minutes) of vasoconstriction of the vessels in that area and the contraction of the vascular smooth muscles adjacent to the wound site. This combination of vasoconstriction and muscle contraction leads to a slowing or cessation of blood flow in the wounded area. Concurrently, the platelets adhere to collagen exposed at the site of injury and release thromboplastin. In the presence of thromboplastin, plasma prothrombin is converted to thrombin, which in turn converts fibrinogen to fibrin. Ultimately, fibrin forms a loose matrix, trapping other platelets and blood cells, and a hemostatic plug or clot is formed. This initial vasoconstrictive activity serves to wall off the wound from other areas in the body and to reduce the potential for invasion by bacteria. In addition, however, the platelets that enter the wound area are activated and secrete growth factors.

The growth factors released include platelet-derived growth factor (PDGF), platelet-derived angiogenesis factor (PDAF), platelet-derived epidermal growth factor (PDEGF), platelet factor-4 (PF-4), and transforming growth factor-beta (TGF-β). These are patient chemotactic and mitogenic factors that stimulate all phases of healing.[4,5,6]

Vasodilatation follows the initial brief period of vasoconstriction. Cells that have adhered to the endothelium of the injured vessels move out into the tissues. The fluid that accompanies them creates a local edema.

Lymphocytes follow neutrophils, aiding in phagocytosis and playing a significant role in both humoral and cell-mediated immunity. Sensitized T lymphocytes destroy foreign antigens, while B lymphocytes, or circulating antibodies, attack invading microorganisms.

Approximately 24 hours after the neutrophils reach their peak activity in the uncomplicated wound, there is an influx of monocytes, which modulate to become macrophages. Macrophages move toward the leading edge of the severed vessel where the pH is low, the CO_2 is elevated, and the oxygen content is low. From this point, the macrophages, with a minimal backup vascular supply of nutrients, move out from the leading edge of the vessel and secrete growth factors that stimulate angiogenesis and collagen synthesis.[7,8,9,10] Wounds deficient in macrophages do not heal normally.[7]

The other major cells to exhibit some activity during this initial phase of wound healing are the epithelial cells. These cells, which lie over the dermis, migrate toward one another until they meet other epithelial cells. The point at which these like cells meet and cease to migrate is known as the *contact inhibition point*. The reasons underlying this regulatory phenomenon have yet to be elucidated. Once the cells have ceased migrating, further mitosis occurs until the five layers of epithelium are restored. In a full-thickness wound, the ancillary structures are absent,

so epithelial cells must migrate from the edges of the wound. In wounds healing by primary intention, this distance is short, so healing occurs rapidly. With wounds healing by secondary intention, epithelial closure takes longer because of the greater area that needs to be covered.

Proliferative Phase

The proliferative phase begins about 4 days after wounding and continues until the wound is about 3 weeks old. Critical to the proliferative phase of healing are endothelial cells and fibroblasts. Endothelial cells are stimulated by growth factors and the hypoxic, acidotic, lactate-rich environment that is created when blood flow is disrupted with injury. They elongate and move into the hypoxic environment and begin to develop the new vasculature. Vessels grow in what appears to be a random fashion and attach to other capillaries that are developing in the injured tissue. Angiogenesis, new vessel formation, ceases when the hypoxic stimulus abates as blood flow through the new vessels brings fresh oxygen to the area and carries away the lactate-laden, acidotic wound fluid.[11]

The new vasculature provides a base across which fibroblasts travel to the wound edge and release collagen. The collagen provides the tensile strength of the wound and protects against dehiscence and disruption of the skin. The formation of collagen through the hydroxylation of proline requires vitamin C (ascorbic acid); oxygen; amino acids; and the minerals zinc, iron, and copper.[12]

Tensile strength at the wound site rises sharply. Though no tissue surface once interrupted ever achieves its original strength, most wounds heal to as much as 80% of their original tensile strength.[2]

The cell most responsible for increasing the strength of the wound is the fibroblast. The fibroblast is triggered to action by injury and initially stimulated to divide in mild hypoxia and an environment rich in ascorbate; like other cells, it functions best in optimal conditions. In an open wound, the results of this phase of healing can be observed. The healthy wound shows beefy, red, shiny tissue commonly termed *granulation tissue*.

Remodeling Phase

The final phase of healing begins approximately 3 weeks after wounding and ends 1 to 2 years later. During this remodeling phase, maximum tensile strength is achieved. Tensile strength increases 30% over that achieved during the fibroblastic phase. The dynamic interaction between collagen synthesis and lysis of collagen lysis by collagenase and other lytic enzymes causes the wound to become more malleable.

This final phase of wound healing is characterized not by the presence of any "new" or particular cell but rather by the activity of lysosomal enzymes, which cleave collagen extracellularly.

RISK FACTORS

A variety of factors have been associated with impaired healing. Alterations in oxygenation, perfusion, and nutritional status are frequently associated with disrupted healing. Other significant risk factors include impaired acid–base balance, age, obesity, stress, and various metabolic events.

Oxygenation is important to support of normal wound healing. Oxygen is critical for collagen formation.[13] It lowers infection rates, minimizes lesion size, facilitates angiogenesis, and stabilizes cell structure.[14,15] Cellular function is decreased in the presence of hypoxia, affecting *all* aspects of healing.[16]

Perfusion must be adequate for normal healing to occur and oxygen to be transported to the tissues. In fact, tissue oxygenation has been used as an indicator of perfusion.[17] Yet alterations in perfusion may be quite subtle; it has been shown to be depressed in the presence of normal vital signs and normal urine output in postsurgical patients.[18] This suggests that tissue oxygenation may be jeopardized at a time when available clinical indicators are unable to detect it. In addition, invasive measures of PaO_2 do not correlate well with tissue oxygenation, indicating that the critical care nurse cannot conclude that tissue oxygenation for wound healing is adequate because PaO_2 is within an acceptable range for major organ function.[16,17]

Also, as the majority of oxygen content is bound to the hemoglobin, *anemia* has been implicated in impaired healing. Data show that the hematocrit must be less than 20 g/dl before healing is impaired, but the combination of less severe anemia with hypovolemia may impair healing.[18,19] This situation is seen frequently in critical care, and consideration needs to be given to the wound under these conditions.

Acid–base balance mediates the availability of oxygen for wound healing, and so with imbalance, wound healing may be affected. Acidosis is accompanied by increased release of oxygen from hemoglobin; however, the available oxygen often does not approach requirements in acidosis because tissue demand for oxygen often is increased in these conditions. On the other hand, with alkalosis the oxygen is bound more tightly to hemoglobin, making it unavailable for support of wound healing.

Nutrition also is critical to all phases of healing. Lack of sufficient protein, fat, carbohydrate, vitamins, and minerals contributes to impaired healing, seen most often as impaired collagen formation, delayed development of wound tensile strength and an increased incidence of infection.[12,20,21,22]

Nutrient needs in the critically ill are not unique to healing but are required for healing to take place. Healthy patients can survive brief periods of starvation without deleterious effects, but impaired nutritional status has been linked with less hydroxyproline accumulation when depleted patients were compared with normally nourished individuals.[20,23] This suggests that a history of impaired nutritional intake or depressed levels of acute phase proteins are signs of substantial deficiencies, and these patients need to be referred for evaluation early in their critical care stay. If deficiencies are found, aggressive nutritional support must be considered.

Other factors may predispose the patient to impaired healing.[2] For example, *age* is a risk factor for impaired healing. The very young and the very old are especially vulnerable populations. *Obesity* also is a risk factor because poor subcutaneous perfusion is present in fat tissue.

Patients with *high levels of stress* also are at risk for altered healing.[24] Stress results in high levels of catecholamines, and vasoconstriction may cause ischemia to the subcutaneous tissue. In addition, high levels of circulating catecholamines are associated with high glucose levels, insulin resistance, and depleted levels of intracellular glucose. Although studies documenting deleterious clinical consequences are lacking, logic indicates that psychological stress, pain, cold, and hypovolemia are frequent events in critical care and may be implicated in impaired healing.

Metabolic events also may contribute to impaired healing.[25] Situations that predispose to delayed or altered healing include poor perfusion seen in patients with cardiovascular disease, high glucose levels seen in patients with diabetes, inadequate oxygenation seen in various forms of shock, inadequate substrate availability in malnutrition, and lack of immune response seen in immunocompromised and infected patients. The use of medications also may alter wound healing. Corticosteroids are the most notorious for delaying healing and impair all phases of healing. Many drugs may alter metabolic pathways important to healing, including antiinflammatory agents and anticoagulants.

WOUND ASSESSMENT

Assessment of the wound and the support system for healing of the wound is an essential step in care of the injured patient. Although valid and reliable clinical tools have not yet been developed for assessment,[26] a thorough and consistent evaluation will provide the best possible base for subsequent therapy.

Wounds must be assessed with dressings removed and in a well-lighted environment. It is more important to describe the nature of the injured tissue than it is the dressing that has been applied. Separate assessment is proposed for partial-thickness injuries and for full-thickness injuries healing by primary and secondary intention. Full-thickness injuries closed by delayed primary closure are initially evaluated as wounds healing by secondary intention and after being closed are assessed as those healing by primary intention.

Normal healing in partial-thickness injury involves the development of a new epithelium that usually is pink and is fragile. This process is slowed when a scab is present, and significant disruption is present when exudate develops at the site of injury.

In wounds healing by primary intention, the size of the wound is usually recorded only with traumatic wounds or multiple wounds or where the nature of the injury suggests that healing will be complicated. Under these circumstances, the length and location of each wound is noted. The appearance of the wound then is evaluated. In wounds healing by primary intention, normal healing is manifested by a well-approximated incision line with redness, pain and induration lasting 3 to 4 days, and a healing ridge of collagen appearing by postinjury day 7 to 9 (Table 54-1).

Impairment in this process is apparent if (1) edges are not well approximated, (2) inflammation does not appear by day 3 or 4 or is prolonged more than 4 to 5 days, (3) a healing ridge does not develop by postinjury day 7 to 9, or (4) there is drainage along the incision line after 72 hours in a patient who does not have a drain in place. Usually, epithelialization is expected to be completed within 24 to 72 hours after injury, but actually visualizing the epithelial cells on the incision line is difficult because it is a narrow line and a scab often has been allowed to form.

The nurse must understand the manifestations and their meaning. Wound edges that are well approximated reflect a small wound space across which healing must occur. Those edges that are not as well approximated suggest a difficult closure or the presence of concurrent problems that have led to disruption, for example, excessive edema or infection. The inflammation seen in the early postinjury period reflects the events of the inflammatory phase of healing, and these are critical to normal healing. Lack of an inflammatory response may be seen in patients who are immunosuppressed and indicates there may be a delay in all phases of healing or disruption in those processes. On the other hand, continued inflammation after day 4 of injury suggests that some stimulus remains at the wound site that is continuing inflammation. Usually, this stimulus is a high bacterial count, but it may be another process taking place, such as the development of fistula.

A *healing ridge*, a palpable ridge reflective of the development of collagen and wound tensile strength, is present by day 7 to 9 in all surgical procedures except cosmetic surgery. When a healing ridge is not present, the patient is at risk for wound dehiscence and evisceration. Epithelialization of the wound is expected within 24 to 72 hours of injury, thus sealing the wound from external contamination and stopping drainage coming from inside the wound. Continued drainage indicates that the expected wound approximation has not occurred and that epithelialization also is not complete.

In wounds healing by secondary intention, wound size and location are first measured and recorded. The tissue response to healing needs to be appraised (Table 54-2). Early after injury, the new wound left

TABLE 54-1 **Assessment of Wounds Healing by Primary Intention**

Normal Findings	Abnormal Findings
Wound edges well approximated	Wound edges not well approximated
Inflammation present for first 3 to 4 days after injury	Inflammation not present by day 4 or prolonged for more than 4 to 5 days
Healing ridge present by postinjury day 7 to 9	Healing ridge not present by postinjury day 7 to 9
	Drainage at incision site that persists more than 72 hours postinjury

TABLE 54-2 **Assessment of Wounds Healing by Secondary Intention**

Normal Findings	Abnormal Findings
Granulation tissue initially is avascular, progresses to pink and then to beefy red	Granulation tissue does not develop in a timely manner; fistula or tract present
Wound is moist	Wound is dry or excessively moist
No exudate present	Exudate present; may be serosanguinous, yellow-green, or brown
No necrotic tissue visible	Necrotic tissue present
No distinctive odor of wound	Wound odor present or has changed
Epithelial edge progressively covers wound	Epithelial edge does not surround the wound or is not moving to cover the open wound

to heal by secondary intention is rather avascular. It moves to a pink and then to a beefy red as the new vasculature builds in the wound and red blood cells begin to traverse the new vessels. The wound is moist but not excessively wet. No exudate or necrotic tissue is present, and the dressings do not have a distinctive odor. The edges of the wound are surrounded by epithelial tissue that progressively moves over the wound edge into the wound bed.

Abnormal findings reflect delay in the process or multiplication of bacteria in the wound. Granulation tissue may be delayed in developing in the absence of a healthy vasculature. At times fistular tracts develop, and these need to be noted so that they can be treated. The wound may be dry or excessively moist; either condition inhibits cellular proliferation. When the bacteria count in the wound rises, exudate develops. Its color and odor need to be noted and recorded. Specific organisms have characteristic color and odor (e.g., *Pseudomonas*). The diagnosis usually is made with a wound culture, but recording subjective signs provides baseline data for subsequent comparison. Necrotic tissue is dead and is usually black or gray. Because it is a nidus for infection, necrotic tissue may develop an odor as bacteria multiply. Also, epithelial tissue migration may be delayed or disrupted around the wound edge.

Often special assessment considerations based on the etiology of the wound need to be taken into account. For example, patients with a pressure ulcer need to have the depth of the wound evaluated using a grading system, and those with mediastinal wounds that extend through the viscera need the nature of the underlying organ assessed.

WOUND-RELATED PARAMETERS

Patients with wounds need to have a thorough evaluation that allows the nurse to determine whether the patient has systemic ability to support healing. Parameters that routinely need to be considered in relation to wound healing include tissue oxygenation, nutritional status, immunological status, glucose control, and factors related to the etiology of the wound. For example, if the patient has pressure ulcers, the risk of impaired mobility or incontinence needs to be considered. If the injured patient has peripheral vascular disease, a branchial–ankle index may need to be added to the evaluation as a measure of perfusion.

NURSING MANAGEMENT

Both local and systemic factors are important to healing in the patient with a wound. With partial-thickness injuries and wounds healing by primary intention, local care is designed to maintain a physiological environment and protect the wound from disruption. With wounds healing by secondary intention, local care of wounds is planned to minimize contamination and debris in the wound and to keep the tissue moist. Systemic care is aimed at providing the environment needed for healing.

Local Care

Dressings are designed to provide an optimal environment for healing.[27] Until recently, most dressings were made of cotton gauze. Gauze absorbs in its threads or interstices and removes exudate from direct contact with the injured tissue. It is subsequently removed from the wound with the dressing change.

In the last 30 years, a wide array of dressings have been introduced to supplement gauze.[27,28,29] The development of these dressings was based on research that showed that wound healing progressed most rapidly in a moist environment. Specific benefits of moist healing are more rapid epithelialization, augmented angiogenesis, more rapid granulation tissue formation, and enhanced collagen metabolism.[27,28,29]

Initially, the beneficial effects of moist wound healing were questioned. The prevailing belief was that a dry environment was more beneficial for wound healing because it inhibited the growth of organisms and helped to prevent infection.[30,31] These beliefs were supported by early studies that showed that moist healing was associated with an increased number of organisms present in the wound site.[32] Subsequent work clarified the issue and showed that although there was greater colonization, it was not associated with increased rate of infection.[33,34]

Dressing materials include gauze, hydrocolloids, hydrogels, polyurethane films, and foams (Table 54-3).[28,29,30,35] These dressings can be used with partial-thickness injuries healing by primary intention and in shallow full-thickness injuries. The manufacturer's recommendations need to be followed so that maximal therapeutic effects can be actualized. Lack of therapeutic effect may be due to not using the dressing as intended; for example, if the films are intact but changed daily, they may disrupt healthy skin.

When there is a full-thickness injury that has a large wound space, gauze remains the mainstay of treatment. It is placed in the wound moistened and acts to keep tissues moist and separated so healing can progress from the bottom of the wound upward. This approach prevents abscess formation. In the past, gauze dressings often were removed from the wound dry to debride foreign material and exudate that adhered to the dressing as it dried. Bleeding of tissue consistently accompanied removal of dry gauze from the wound. Today, it is recognized that removal of gauze dressing from the wound dry disrupts the new capillary bed and places an added burden on the

TABLE 54-3   **Topical Agents Frequently Used on Open Wounds**

Normal saline	"Gold standard"
	Isotonic solution
	No bactericidal properties
Hydrogen peroxide	Oxidizing agent—renders organic material inert
	Mild germicide
	Cannot be used in a closed cavity
	Causes pain
Povidone-iodine (Betadine)	Broad-spectrum germicide
	Systemically absorbed resulting in increased iodine levels; implicated in renal failure, acid–base disorders
	Most effective in dilute solutions
Sodium hypochlorite (Dakin's solution)	Germicide
	Dissolves necrotic material and may dissolve clots leading to bleeding
	Disrupts healthy skin
	May cause pain

injured tissue. If a wound is excessively exudative or full of debris, another approach needs to be taken to remove those substances: more frequent dressing changes, a different dressing, or high-pressure irrigation.

Germicidal agents often are used in heavily contaminated wounds. There is controversy over whether a solution should be used and the type of solution to use,[36] but these solutions remain an integral part of wound care. It is important to appreciate the therapeutic and iatrogenic effects of these solutions so the effects of the treatment can be appraised.[37-42]

In addition to dressings, local care also often involves cleansing of the wound. This may be done with dressings or with high-pressure irrigation. High-pressure irrigation consists of mechanically removing foreign substances using a pressure greater than 8 lb/in². [43,44,45,46] The pressure is created by elevating a solution to take advantage of the force of gravity, using a syringe with a large-bore (#18) catheter attached, or using a machine such as a dental irrigation device that generates high pressure. Large volumes of fluid are applied under pressure, and debris is loosened and removed. Low-pressure irrigation as is produced with a bulb syringe is not effective in wound irrigation.

Absorptive products also have been designed to remove debris from wound. Hydrophyllic beads, powders, and gels are effective in removing massive exudate from wounds.[47,48,49] Examples are Debrisan

Beads and Bard powder. These products have a limited but important role in containing major drainage from wounds; their principal disadvantage is the cost.

Systemic Support

The entire body can influence the healing process. Oxygenation, perfusion, and nutrition are consistently seen as critical factors in facilitating healing. Research to date does not provide direction for providing data-based interventions aimed specifically at supporting oxygen and perfusion to the wound.[16,50] It is recommended that (1) patients be assessed for volume status, (2) a pulmonary hygiene plan be established, and (3) an activity regimen be instituted. Individuals at high risk should receive supplemental oxygen.[16,50] Nutrition should include protein, fats, and carbohydrates; in addition, vitamin C, iron, zinc, and copper are critical to the production of collagen. Epithelial proliferation requires vitamin A, and in general, multivitamins probably are indicated because of their role in cellular function.[12,51] If patients are managed with appropriate nutritional support,[52,53] in the majority of patients wound healing needs are met. Research is needed to determine whether such interventions produce a measurable difference in wound healing.

Control of diabetes,[54] approaches to mitigate stress, pain, and noise,[24,55,56,57] all are important in care of the patient with a wound. Significant research remains to be undertaken in a number of areas to establish the specific role of the different treatments in support of wound healing in critically ill patients.

REFERENCES

1. Stotts, N. A. (1990). Wound care: Preface. *AACN Clinical Issues in Critical-Care Nursing, 1,* 543.
2. Norris, S. O., Provo, B., & Stotts, N. A. (1990). Physiology of wound healing and factors that impede the healing process. *AACN Clinical Issues in Critical-Care Nursing, 1,* 545-552.
3. Orgill, D., & Demiling, R. H. (1988). Current concepts and approaches to wound healing. *Critical Care Medicine, 16,* 899-908.
4. Brown, G. L., Nanny, L. B., Griffen, J., et al. (1989). Enhancement of wound healing by topical treatment with epidermal growth factor. *New England Journal of Medicine, 321*(2), 76-79.
5. Knighton, D. R., Siegel, V. D., Doucette, M. M., et al. (1989). The use of typically applied platelet growth factors in chronic nonhealing wounds: A review. *Wounds, 1,* 72-78.
6. Jackson, D. S., & Rovee, D. T. (1988). Current concepts in wound healing: Research and theory. *Journal of Enterostomal Therapy, 15,* 133-137.
7. Simpson, D., & Ross, R. (1972). The neutrophilic leukocyte in wound repair: A study with antineutrophil serum. *Journal of Clinical Investigation, 51,* 2009.

8. Stein, J., & Levenson, S. (1980). Effect of the inflammatory reaction on subsequent wound healing. *Plastic Surgery, 31,* 484-485.

9. Banda, M., Knighton, D., Hunt, T., et al. (1982). Isolation of a nonmitogenic angiogenesis factor from wound fluid. *Proceedings of the National Academy of Science, 79,* 7773-7777.

10. Niinikoski, J. (1977). Oxygen and wound healing. *Clinics in Plastic Surgery, 4,* 361-374.

11. Knighton, D., Silver, I., & Hunt, T. (1981). Regulation of wound angiogenesis—effect of oxygen gradients and inspired oxygen concentrations. *Surgery, 90,* 262-270.

12. Levenson, S., Seifer, E., & Van Winkle, W., Jr. (1979). Nutrition. In T. K. Hunt (Ed.), *Fundamentals of wound management* (pp. 286-363). New York: Appleton-Century-Crofts.

13. Hunt, T. K., & Pai, M. P. (1972). The effect of varying ambient oxygen tensions on wound management and collagen synthesis. *Surgery, Gynecology and Obstetrics, 135,* 561-567.

14. Pai, M. P., & Hunt, T. K. (1972). Effect of varying oxygen tensions on healing of open wounds. *Surgery, Gynecology and Obstetrics, 135,* 756-758.

15. Hunt, T. K., Linsey, M., Grislis, G., et al. (1975). The effect of differing ambient oxygen tensions on wound infection. *Annals of Surgery, 181,* 35-39.

16. Whitney, J. D. (1989). Physiologic effects of tissue oxygenation on wound healing. *Heart Lung, 18,* 466-474.

17. Gottrup, F., Gellett, S., Kirkegaard, L., et al. (1988). Continuous monitoring of tissue oxygen tension during hyperoxia and hypoxia: Relation of subcutaneous, transcutaneous, and conjunctival oxygen tension to hemodynamic variables. *Critical Care Medicine, 16*(12), 1229-1234.

18. Heughan, C., Chir, B., Grislis, G., et al. (1974). The effect of anemia on wound healing. *Annals of Surgery, 174,* 163-167.

19. Hunt, T. K., Zederfeldt, B. H., Goldstick, T. K., et al. (1967). Tissue oxygen tension during controlled hemorrhage, *Surgical Forum, 18,* 3-4.

20. Modolin, M., Bevilacqua, R. G., Margarido, N. F., et al. (1985). Effects of protein depletion and repletion on experimental open wound contraction. *Annals of Plastic Surgery, 15*(2), 123-126.

21. Greenhalgh, D. G., & Gamelli, R. L. (1987). Is impaired wound healing caused by infection or nutritional depletion? *Surgery, 102*(2), 306-312.

22. Irvin, T. T. (1978). Effects of malnutrition and hyperalimentation on wound healing. *Surgery, Gynecology and Obstetrics, 146,* 33-37.

23. Haydock, D. A., & Hill, G. L. (1987). Improved wound healing response in surgical patients receiving intravenous nutrition. *British Journal of Surgery, 74,* 320-323.

24. West, J. M. (1990). Wound healing in the surgical patient: Influence of perioperative stress response on perfusion. *AACN Clinical Issues in Critical-Care Nursing, 1,* 595-601.

25. Dimick, A. R. (1988). Delayed wound closure: Indications and techniques. *Annals of Emergency Medicine, 17,* 1303-1304.

26. Cooper, D. M. (1990). Human wound assessment: Status report and implications for clinicians. *AACN Clinical Issues in Critical-Care Nursing, 1,* 553-565.

27. Alvarez, O., Rozint, J., & Meehan, M. (1990). Principles of moist wound healing: Indications for chronic wounds. In D. Krasner (Ed.), *Chronic wound care: A clinical source book for health care professionals* (pp. 266-281). King of Prussia, PA: Health Management Publications.

28. Cuzzell, J. Z. (1990). Choosing a wound dressing: A systematic approach. *AACN Clinical Issues in Critical-Care Nursing, 1,* 566-577.

29. Hutchinson, J. J., & McGuckin, M. (1990). Occlusive dressings: A microbial and clinical review. *American Journal of Infection Control, 18,* 257-268.

30. Katz, S., McGinley, K., & Leydon J. J. (1986). Semipermeable occlusive dressings: Effects on growth of pathogenic bacteria and reepithelialization of superficial wounds. *Archives of Dermatology, 122,* 58-62.

31. Bennett, R. G. (1982). The debatable benefit of occlusive dressings for wounds. *Journal of Dermatologic Surgical Oncology, 8,* 166-167.

32. Bibel, D. J., & LeBrum, J. R. (1975). Changes in cutaneous flora after wet occlusion. *Canadian Journal of Microbiology, 21,* 496-500.

33. Eaglestein, W. H. (1985). Experiences with biosynthetic dressings. *Journal of the American Academy of Dermatology, 12,* 434-440.

34. Falanga, V. (1988). Occlusive wound dressings. *Archives of Dermatology, 124,* 872-877.

35. Hutchinson, J. J., & Lawrence, J. C. (1991). Wound infection under occlusive dressings. *Journal of Hospital Infection, 17,* 83-94.

36. Rodeheaver, G. T. (1990). Controversies in topical wound management: Wound cleansing and wound disinfection. In D. Krasner (Ed.), *Chronic wound care: A clinical source book for health care professionals* (pp. 282-289). King of Prussia, PA: Health Management Publications.

37. Lineaweaver, W., Howard, R., Soucy, D., et al. (1985). Topical antimicrobial toxicity. *Archives of Surgery, 120,* 267-270.

38. Gruber, R. P., Vistnes, L., & Pardoe, R. (1975). The effect of commonly used antiseptic on wound healing. *Plastic and Reconstructive Surgery, 55,* 472-476.

39. Viljanto, J. (1980). Disinfection of surgical wound without inhibition of normal wound healing. *Archives of Surgery, 115,* 253-256.

40. Lammers, R. L., Fourre, M., Callaham, M. L., et al. (1990). Effect of povidone-iodine and saline soaking on bacterial counts in acute, traumatic, contaminated wounds. *Annals of Emergency Medicine, 19*(6), 709-714.

41. Bassan, M., Dudai, M., & Shalev, O. (1982). Near-fatal systemic oxygen embolism due to wound irrigation with hydrogen peroxide. *Postgraduate Medical Journal, 58,* 448-450.

42. Berkelman, R., Holland, B., & Anderson, R. (1982). Increased bactericidal activity of dilute preparations of povidone-iodine solutions. *Journal of Clinical Microbiology, 15,* 635-639.

43. Rodeheaver, G. T., Petty, D., Thacker, J. G., et al. (1975). Wound cleansing by high pressure irrigation. *Surgery, Gynecology and Obstetrics, 141,* 357-362.

44. Hamer, M. L., Robson, M. C., Krizek, T. J., et al. (1975). Quantitative bacterial analysis of comparative wound irrigations. *Annals of Surgery, 181,* 819-822.

45. Brown, L. L., Shelton, H. T., Bornside, G. H., et al. (1978). Evaluation of wound irrigation by pulsatile jet and conventional methods. *Annals of Surgery, 187,* 170-173.

46. Wheeler, C. B., Rodeheaver, G. T., Thacker, J. G., et al. (1976). Side-effects of high pressure irrigation. *Surgery, Gynecology and Obstetrics, 143,* 775-778.

47. Floden, C. H., & Wikstrom, K. (1978). Controlled clinical trial with dextranomer (Debrisan) on venous leg ulcers. *Current Therapeutic Research, 24,* 753-760.

48. Jacobson, S., Rothman, U., Arturson, G., et al. (1976). A new principle for the cleansing of infected wounds. *Scandinavian Journal of Plastic Reconstructive Surgery, 10,* 65-72.

49. Pace, W. E. (1978). Beads of a dextran polymer for the local treatment of cutaneous ulcers. *Journal of Dermatologic Surgery and Oncology, 4,* 678-682.

50. LaVan, F. B., & Hunt, T. K. (1990). Oxygen and wound healing. *Clinics in Plastic Surgery, 17,* 463-472.

51. Lee, K. A., & Stotts, N. A. (1990). Support of the growth hormone-somatomedin system to facilitate wound healing. *Heart Lung, 19,* 157-163.

52. Berger, R., & Adams, L. (1989). Nutritional support in the critical care setting: Part 1. *Chest, 96,* 139-150.

53. Berger, R., & Adams, L. (1989). Nutritional support in the critical care setting: Part 2. *Chest, 96*(2), 372-380.

54. Rosenberg, C. S. (1990). Wound healing in the patient with diabetes. *Nursing Clinics of North America, 25,* 247-262.

55. Hargreaves, A., & Lander, J. (1989). Use of transcutaneous electrical nerve stimulation for postoperative pain. *Nursing Research, 38*(3), 159-161.

56. Angus, J. E., & Faux, S. (1989). The effect of music on adult postoperative patients' pain during a nursing procedure. In S. G. Funk, E. M. Tournquist, M. T. Champagne, et al. (Eds.), *Key aspects of recovery: Management of pain, fatigue and nausea* (pp. 166-172). New York: Springer.

57. Wysocki, A. B. (1986). The effect of intermittent noise exposure on the rate of wound healing in albino rats. Unpublished dissertation, University of Texas at Austin.

PART THIRTEEN

Selected Multisystem Patient Care Problems

55

Trauma

Alice E. Davis

TRAUMA AS A PUBLIC HEALTH PROBLEM

Injury is a public health problem affecting Americans of every socioeconomic level, ethnicity and race, age group, and community.[1] Trauma is not a new problem; physical injury is well documented throughout history. However, injuries from vocational and recreational activities have steadily increased since the Industrial Revolution. In 1966, the National Academy of Sciences, National Research Council (NASNRC) published a landmark paper, *Accidental Death and Disability: The Neglected Disease of Modern Society*.[2] This government report validated the magnitude of the injury problem, identified inefficiencies in the health care delivery system contributing to the problem, and offered recommendations for the development of a comprehensive emergency medical care system. Today, 25 years after this document was published, traumatic injury continues to be a major health problem exceeded only by cardiovascular disease and cancer as the leading cause of death in the United States.[1,3,4] Injury is responsible for over 140,000 deaths each year and remains the leading cause of death for Americans under the age of 40. Even more alarming is the fact that for every fatal injury that occurs, there are three nonfatal injuries requiring hospitalization.[4]

Injury permanently disables over 80,000 Americans each year. As the leading cause of short-term and long-term disability, traumatic injury is responsible for the loss of over 4 million years of future worklife annually. The cost to society each year has been estimated between $75 and $100 billion.[1,4]

In *Healthy People 2000*, the U.S. Public Health Service formulated health promotion and disease prevention objectives for unintentional and violent injuries, confirming the seriousness of traumatic injury as a public health problem.[5] Although the magnitude of traumatic injuries of all types has been recognized, research in the area of injury control has been poorly funded, and investigations have been fragmented.[1] The lack of support for trauma research may be due to three misconceptions about injury: that traumatic injury is an "accident," implying that injuries result from random events that cannot be predicted and, thus, prevented; that an injury-producing event is an isolated occurrence with a single cause; and that human behavior that is highly related to injury cannot be changed.[1]

These misconceptions underscore a lack of understanding, even in public health circles, about the multifaceted nature of traumatic injury. Public health experts have not reached consensus on the best approach to preventing injuries. Some experts believe that protecting people from injury is the best solution (passive protection such as automatic seat belts, air bags, better road and vehicle designs), while others argue for educational approaches aimed at reduction of individual risk (active protection such as risk assessment; trauma education at the primary and secondary grade school levels; drinking, drugs, and driving programs).[6]

Although not sufficient to reduce the magnitude of the problem, some progress toward understanding trauma has been made. In a model of trauma (Figure 55-1) proposed by Haddon, the interrelatedness of injury phases and factors associated with trauma is described.[7] Haddon identifies the injury phases as (1) preinjury (activity or event that may lead to injury), (2) injury (activity or event that causes the injury), and (3) postinjury (activity or event that occurs following the injury). In a cross-table design, Haddon matched the injury phases with the factors associated with injury. These included (1) human factors, (2) energy sources, and (3) environment. As an example, ingestion of alcohol when riding a motorcycle may be the antecedent to injury. An environmental factor may be a slick roadway after a rainstorm. Injury occurs when the drunk motorcyclist crashes into a guardrail at 60 miles per hour. During the postinjury phase, resuscitation and recuperation of the injured motorcyclist occur.

Through the use of Haddon's model, injury phe-

	Human factors (host)	Energy sources (agents)	Physical-sociocultural (environment)
Preevent phase			
Event phase			
Postevent phase			

Preevent   Those events and factors before the injury. It is the interaction of these factors that leads to the injury.

Event   During the injury process. It is the physical response, the intensity of the energy, and the environment mental situation.

Postevent   Following the injury. The body's response to the energy source, the final energy dose, and the emergency care are provided by those in the environment.

Figure 55-1   Injury model.
Adapted from Haddon, W. (1972). A logical framework for categorizing highway safety phenomenon and activity. *Journal of Trauma, 12,* 193.

nomena have been systematically classified and reviewed and prevention strategies identified. Research in the areas of epidemiology, sociology, psychology, and medicine has focused on human factors, energy sources, and the environments related to the preinjury and injury phases. As a result, high-risk populations have been identified,[8,9] appropriate surgical interventions have been delineated,[10] and protective measures have been recommended.[1] The majority of the work using Haddon's model has focused on the energy sources and environment associated with motor vehicle injury (blunt injury). Less information is available on injury phases and factors associated with gunshot or stabbing (penetrating) injuries. For injuries of this nature, research-generated knowledge has contributed to an understanding of demographics, socioeconomic status, substance abuse, and violence.[1,11,12] Death and disability due to penetrating injury have not been substantially reduced, and the need for research in penetrating injury is well documented.[13]

Research focusing on the human factors associated with blunt and penetrating injury has used psychological and sociological models. These studies have explored personality traits, psychopathology, and sociopathic behaviors in all phases of injury.[14,15,16] For the most part, psychological and sociological studies of the human factors related to traumatic injury in the preevent and event phases have virtually been abandoned. Research emphasis, at least for motor vehicle collisions (MVC), has been on automatic protection rather than on attempts to understand or change behavior.[17] Definitive care of the injured has focused primarily on trauma resuscitation and surgical intervention. The value of early rehabilitation

services and successful community integration following injury has been recognized, but further investigation is needed. Unfortunately, recidivism (repeated injury) is prevalent in the trauma population, and strategies to reduce recurrence of injury have not been well formulated.

Useful or productive return of the injured individual to the community is the ultimate goal of trauma care, with trauma best described as a cycle. Persons from the community are injured; prehospital, emergency care, critical care, acute care, and rehabilitation are provided; and the person returns to the community.

Although no clear-cut methods to eliminate traumatic injury in the near future are available, nurses clearly have a role in trauma care and trauma prevention. As health care providers, nurses participate directly or indirectly in all phases of trauma care. Nurses must realize that recognizing the antecedents of injury and intervening to prevent future injury is as much a part of trauma care as is trauma resuscitation. With knowledge of Haddon's model, the trauma cycle, and current research findings, nurses can optimize care for the injured patient and focus on trauma prevention strategies simultaneously.

Historical Perspectives

Current models of systematic care for the critically injured emerged from battlefield experience. As early as the Napoleonic Wars, triage was used to sort war casualties for treatment. Successful treatment of wounded soldiers during the American Civil War was impeded by lack of knowledge related to trauma physiology as well as by crowded hospitals and unsanitary conditions. Significant improvements in care were noted during World War II and further refined during the Korean and Vietnam wars. With each conflict, scientific knowledge related to the physiological response to injury grew. This knowledge, coupled with rapid evacuation of casualties to definitive care, improved the chances of survival.[3,18]

Although civilian injury was occurring concurrently with wartime injury, military models of injury care were not used for civilian populations until the late 1960s. The NASNRC paper was the catalyst for the development of a more efficient civilian emergency medical system. In addition to identifying injury as the neglected disease of modern society, the paper outlined recommendations for improvement in care. A major focus of the paper was the need for categorization of facilities to improve the quality of care and to provide more cost-efficient avenues for the delivery of care. Categorization of care was defined as horizontal (the ability of a community hospital to deliver emergency care), vertical (the ability of the hospital to provide definitive care in seven emergency categories including trauma), and circular or regional (the ability to provide emergency care on a regional or areawide basis).[19] Improvements targeted for delivery of care were ambulance services (transport of injury victims was being carried out by funeral parlor services in some areas) and radio communication between ambulances and hospitals. The early framework for what is now the nation's emergency medical services (EMS) system stemmed from the NASNRC document.

By the early 1970s, appropriate and timely care of the sick and injured was being delivered in the prehospital setting by emergency medical technicians (EMTs). Rapid transport and definitive care in the field improved the chances of survival of injured patients from the scene to the emergency department. Unfortunately, hospital emergency care has not significantly changed to correspond to the improved status of prehospital care. Studies have shown that critically injured adults, brought to the emergency room alive, die unnecessarily.[19,20,21] The causes of death were related to errors in management and treatment. These and other studies clearly explicated the need not only for rapid transport of injured individuals to emergency care but the need for well-trained emergency department staffs. Through the years, it became evident to trauma care advocates that a well-trained staff and a well-defined categorization system were necessary to provide optimal care for trauma patients.

In 1976, the American College of Surgeons' (ACS) Committee on Trauma published a document that encouraged hospitals to commit resources, facilities, and personnel to address the special needs of injured

persons.[10] As a result, highly specialized hospitals (trauma centers), geared to the immediate needs of injured persons, began to emerge. Despite advances in EMS services and attempts at categorization of trauma facilities, little progress had been made since the publication of the NASNRC paper in 1966. A second report of the National Academy of Sciences National Research Council, *Injury in America,*[1] outlined the deficiencies in trauma care related to epidemiology, prevention, prehospital care, hospital care, biomechanics, and rehabilitation.

The ACS Committee on Trauma published guidelines for optimal care of the injured patient in 1986.[22] The guidelines, revised in 1990, form the basis for categorization of regionalized trauma systems and outline the requirements for trauma center designation that have been adopted by many state trauma systems.[23] The four components stressed in the ACS document were access to care, prehospital care, hospital care, and rehabilitation. Commitment was determined to be the most essential factor for success of a trauma system. For hospital administrators, commitment included providing capable personnel; use of sophisticated equipment and services; and priority use of diagnostic laboratories, radiological equipment, surgical suites, and critical care units. Commitment for medical staff included prompt availability, education, and quality assurance. Levels of care that were intended to utilize the resources of a community in the best possible manner were also outlined in this document.

Classification

Injuries have been classified as severe, urgent, and nonurgent. Classifying injuries in this manner assists trauma care providers to triage injured persons, thereby assuring the best possible care based on the severity of the injury. *Severe injuries* account for 5% of total injuries, but because of their immediately life-threatening nature, they are responsible for 50% of all trauma deaths. *Urgent deaths* comprise 10% to 15% of all injuries. Although they are not immediately life-threatening, they may progress to life-threatening if improperly attended, and they carry significant risk for long-term disability. The *nonurgent injury* classification accounts for the largest volume of injury at 80%. These injuries are not immediately life-threatening and carry little risk for permanent disability.[23]

Death from traumatic injury has a trimodal distribution (Figure 55-2). The first death peak occurs within seconds or minutes following injury. Generally, these individuals die from lacerations of the brain, brainstem, upper spinal cord, aorta, or other large vessel. In many cases, these patients cannot be

Trimodal Death Patterns

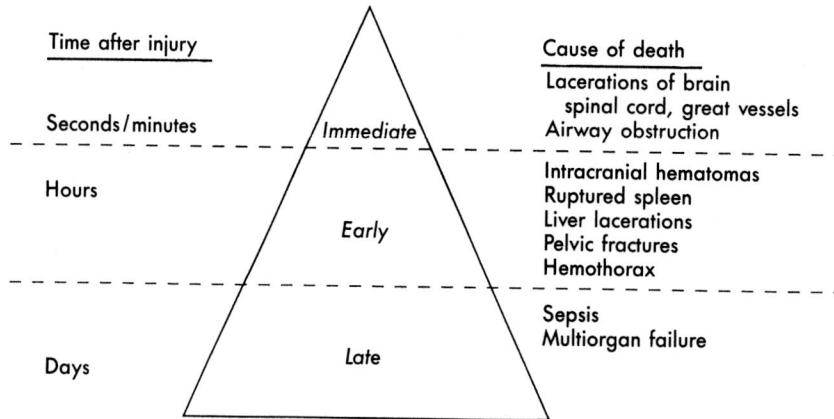

Figure 55-2 Trimodal death patterns.
Adapted from Committee on Trauma. (1990). *Resources for optimal care of the injured patient.* Chicago: American College of Surgeons.

saved. However, survival has occurred in urban areas with rapid transport systems.[23]

The second death peak occurs within the first 2 hours after injury. These critically injured patients generally die from intracerebral, subdural, or epidural hematoma; hemopneumothorax; ruptured spleen; lacerations of the liver; fractured femur; or multiple injuries associated with hypovolemia. Time is a critical factor for survival in these patients. This is the group who will benefit most from a regionalized trauma system. Favorable outcomes in this group have been directly related to time from injury to definitive care. It is well documented that survival rates have increased when definitive treatment is provided within the first hour after injury. Thus, the "golden hour" is of major importance to survival.[23]

The third death peak in trauma patients occurs days or weeks after injury. Cause of death is attributed to sepsis or multiorgan failure. Because of their complex needs, this patient group will benefit from the collaborative expertise available at a trauma center.[23]

Based on the categories of injury and the trimodal distribution of trauma deaths, the ACS developed a stratified trauma care system that optimizes care of the traumatically injured.[23] Level I and Level II trauma centers have surgeons and other members of a trauma team immediately available. Therefore, Level I and Level II centers can provide care to the severely and urgently injured at a moment's notice. The primary difference between a Level I and a Level II center is in commitment to training and research in trauma. For a Level I center, research and training is an *essential* characteristic. These activities are considered *desirable* characteristics for Level II centers. The Level III center reflects a maximum commitment

to trauma care based on available resources. Because many of these Level III centers are located in remote settings or small communities, prompt availability of surgeons and support staff is more realistic than the availability of an in-house staff. The primary goal for Level III centers is stabilization (prevent death from immediately life-threatening injuries if resources are available) and transfer to a Level I or II center for further treatment.[23]

Quality Assurance

Since the immediate goal of trauma care is to save lives and prevent morbidity, development of a trauma care program that ensures quality trauma care is imperative. Systematic evaluation of trauma mortality and morbidity is a requirement of all designated trauma centers. In some trauma systems, this evaluation process is extended to the regional or state level.

Typical quality assurance activities at a trauma center consist of monthly reviews of selected trauma cases. This review is performed by a committee that is responsible for the evaluation of trauma care. Members of the committee may include the trauma director; trauma surgeons; neurosurgeons; emergency physicians; anesthesiologists; pathologists; trauma nurse coordinators; hospital administrators; head nurses from the emergency department, operating room, and intensive care unit (ICU); and EMS personnel serving the trauma center. Mortality and morbidity are the focus of committee discussion. All trauma deaths are reviewed as are the records of patients requiring complex care. Patients whose expected outcome differs from actual outcome (persons who died but should have survived and persons who survived but had been expected to die) are also reviewed.

Trauma registries are also used to assist in the evaluation process. *Trauma registries* are a source of information about patients who receive hospital care for injuries. Data on trauma patients are entered into the registry according to standard case criteria. A core set of data elements is collected and entered into the registry data bank once the patient is determined to be eligible for the trauma registry. Minimum data collected on registry admissions should consist of demographics, mechanism of injury, types of injuries, prehospital care, emergency room care, surgical interventions, complications, rehabilitative care, discharge information, and cost of care. With concurrent data collection and timely evaluation of data, trauma registries provide ongoing surveillance.[24] Additional uses for trauma registry data include programs for injury research, prevention, and education.

In addition to monthly evaluation of trauma outcomes, concurrent evaluation of patient needs must also be considered. Once admitted to the hospital, trauma patients are followed throughout their hospitalization by a trauma nurse coordinator, trauma clinical nurse specialist, or both, who monitor care and intervene through medical or nursing pathways to ensure optimal care.

Administrative Considerations

Hospitals providing trauma care must develop an operational plan. Organizational analysis of existing information systems, personnel resources, equipment, and support systems must be ongoing. Management and structure of the trauma program must be outlined and lines of authority for care and support services delineated. Policies and procedures must be written, coordination of services addressed, and roles and responsibilities clearly stated. To become a designated trauma center, the hospital must meet the criteria of the trauma system organized by the state or local government agency to which it applies.

The care of injured patients requires a coordinated effort of administrators, nurses, physicians, and other health care providers: the *trauma team*. Roles and responsibilities of personnel depend on the time in the trauma cycle services are provided.

Trauma care services are under the direction of a surgeon who is responsible for implementing and maintaining operational aspects of care. A collaborative relationship exists between the hospital administrator and the physician-director. This relationship provides an avenue for decision making related to hospital policies and augmentation of support services. The emergency department physician also plays a collaborative role. Although the emergency department physician may be responsible for the overall care in the emergency department, the trauma surgeon is usually the team leader during trauma resuscitations.

Nurses play a vital role in all phases of the trauma cycle. Not only do they provide direct care, they also facilitate and coordinate trauma services. There is a direct link between the trauma director and nursing service administrators.

The *trauma nurse coordinator* (TNC) plays a crucial role in trauma care. Within the trauma center, the TNC is in a pivotal role, communicating between nursing service and trauma service. Primary responsibilities are the coordination of trauma care services including patient care management, trauma quality assurance, and nursing education; maintaining the registry; and supervision of trauma registry personnel. The TNC may interact directly with hospital administrators, support service department heads, nurse administrators, and physicians. Community involvement is another major aspect of the role. As the trauma center liaison to the community, the TNC may plan trauma prevention programs, interact with law enforcement agencies and other trauma centers and hospitals, and communicate with prehospital agencies.

The *trauma clinical nurse specialist* (TCNS) is responsible for the clinical management of trauma patients. Priority responsibilities in this role are management of complex trauma patients, implementation of standards of care, coordination of support services, education of staff, and conduct of trauma research studies. It is not uncommon for the TCNS to consult with other clinical nurse specialists when special needs arise, for example, elderly, pregnant, neonatal, or pediatric patients. Family support and education may also be a major responsibility of the TCNS. In these roles as case manager and coordinator of care, the TCNS and the TNC should be highly interactive.

The *staff nurse* caring for trauma patients provides direct care and has the support of the TNC and TCNS. In some states, trauma center designation requires all nurses caring for trauma patients to have completed a trauma course and to be certified in the speciality where they work (e.g., CCRN for critical care areas, CEN for emergency care).

Other personnel who play an integral role in trauma care are mental health clinical nurse specialists, social workers, chaplains, respiratory therapists, physical therapists, occupational therapists, speech therapists, and nutritionists. Participative interaction among all members of the trauma team ensures optimal care from admission to discharge.

CONCEPTS OF INJURY

A traumatic wound or injury results from exposure of the body to destructive energy. Types of destructive energy include kinetic (crash, fall, or missile), chemical, thermal, electrical, or radiation. A lack of vital substances, such as oxygen in drownings or heat in frostbite, can also cause injury. Injuries are characterized by a change in physical structure or physiological balance when the energy is released into the bone or tissue. The nature and severity of the injury is determined largely by the amount of energy imparted and by the body's ability to tolerate the energy (tissue response). Depending upon the age, gender, and underlying medical problems of the injured individual, injuries may seem unique. However, specific patterns of injury have emerged which allow the astute clinician to make judgments based on a high "index of suspicion." Understanding mechanisms of injury and their associated patterns of injury increases accuracy of emergency and critical care treatment. Knowledge of mechanisms and patterns of injury also increases the ability to identify common injury combinations as well as predict patient outcomes.[25,26]

Injury Patterns

A variety of factors influence patterns of injury. These include age, gender, substance abuse, season, and geographic location.

Age

Injury occurs in all age groups. However, individuals between the ages of 15 and 24 years are at highest risk for injury and death. Although the elderly have less exposure to trauma and the total number of injuries is lower, they suffer the highest mortality.[26] This mortality may be due in part to their decreased resilience, limited organ reserve, underlying health problems, and anatomical changes. These factors are not as significant in children, adolescents, or young adults.

Gender

Gender differences are clearly evident in traumatic injury, with males sustaining injury at rates three to four times higher than females. The number of exposures to potentially injurious events is the most obvious reason for this gender difference. Although the anatomical structure of males and females is significantly different, there has been little effort to relate anatomical differences to type and severity of injury. For instance, there is evidence that front seat female passengers suffer more severe maxillofacial injuries[27,28] than male front seat passengers. This information seems contradictory in that males generally weigh more than females and when exposed to impact forces should sustain more severe injury. On the other hand, the heavier skeleton and greater muscular development in the male should provide more protection for some types of injuries.[26] Increased understanding of these contradictory concepts and how they relate to type and severity of injuries between males and females may lead to the development of

different evaluation methods or different indices of suspicion based on gender.

Substance Abuse

Substance abuse is a well-known factor associated with all types of injury. Alcohol-related injuries are particularly well documented.[1] However, the contribution of marijuana, heroin, and cocaine to injuries is not well documented. Although the effect of alcohol use on the severity of injury, the response to resuscitation, and the final outcome is controversial, it remains clear that alcohol use has serious physiological effects that must be kept in mind when caring for the trauma patient.

Alcohol does not require digestion and is absorbed directly into the tissues. The brain absorbs greater amounts of alcohol than other tissue; thus, evaluation of intoxicated individuals is difficult. Resuscitation of injured persons under the influence of alcohol may be impeded by an alcohol-associated vasodilatation resulting in hypotension. Control of hemorrhage may be related to the effects of alcohol on platelet function and formation. Chronic alcoholism may lead to cardiomegaly and a decreased cardiac reserve as well as an altered defense response to infection.[26]

Studies evaluating the outcomes of injured persons using alcohol and those not using alcohol have reported that anatomical distribution of injuries is similar except that head injuries are more common in the alcohol group. Survivors in the alcohol group have tended to have higher injury severity scores (ISS) but a lower mortality than the nonalcohol group. Examinations of patterns of injury, ISS, and hospital course in alcohol and nonalcohol groups have not revealed any differences related to blood alcohol levels at admission.

Life Crisis Trauma Profile

A trauma personality or profile has been described by trauma care providers and researchers. Lifestyle patterns frequently ascribed to trauma patients include unstable home environment, undereducation, poor work history, and propensity toward risk taking. Personality traits such as low self-esteem and aggressiveness have also been identified in the trauma population.[16,29] Life crises may also influence traumatic injury. Trauma patients have been found to have 50% more life crises in the 6 months prior to injury than a noninjured control group. Recent unemployment, change in residence, and incarceration were the three life crises most frequently reported.[30]

Injury Mechanism

A variety of biomechanical factors influence injury, including motion, force, velocity, mass, and object shape. (Burns are discussed in Chapter 53.) Motion is a concept explained by physical laws. Newton's first law of motion states that a body at rest or a body in motion will remain in that state until another outside force acts upon it.[31] Force, which changes motion, is another physical factor. Force is calculated by the following equation:

$$Force = mass \times acceleration$$

As is evident in the equation, mass and acceleration (change in velocity) will greatly influence the amount of force that is created. The force also changes motion. The duration, direction, magnitude, and application of the force must be considered when estimating injury. The rate of onset (the speed by which the force is applied) and the extent of surface area upon which the force is applied alter the effect of the force. A force applied slowly releases energy slowly, resulting in less tissue deformation than if the force were applied rapidly. When force is applied to a larger surface area, the energy is dissipated over a wider area, resulting in less tissue damage than if the force were applied to a smaller area.[25]

Four types of force have been described related to traumatic injury: (1) acceleration, (2) deceleration, (3) shearing, and (4) compression. Acceleration forces change the rate of speed or velocity of a body. Deceleration forces are forces that stop or slow the velocity of a moving object. Shearing forces occur as energy is applied across a plane and structures slip relative to each other. Compressive forces are those which squeeze or exert inward pressure on an object.[25]

Tissue has the ability to withstand forces because of characteristics inherent to its structure. These characteristics are tensile strength, compressive strength, viscosity, and elasticity. *Tensile strength* is the amount of tension a tissue can withstand and its ability to resist stretching forces. *Compressive strength* is the ability of a tissue or structure to resist squeezing forces or inward pressure. *Viscosity* is the tissue's ability to resist change in shape during motion. *Elasticity* is the ability of tissue to resume its original shape after stretch.[26]

Damage to tissue or body structures occurs when forces being exerted on the body exceed the limits of its inherent ability to resist change. Change in tissue or structure as a result of force is known as *strain*. Tensile and shear strain are two common types of strain. *Tensile strain* occurs when tissue stretches beyond its normal length, resulting in varying degrees of tissue tear or a complete transection. Injuries of this type can be seen in arteries, bones, and organs. *Shear strain* occurs when parts of a tissue or a structure are moved in opposite directions. Twisting or rotational movements can result in shearing strain injuries in which organs, arteries, or bones are forced

in opposite directions. Examples of shear strain include the forcing of the upper part of the torso to the right while the lower part of the torso is forced to the left or movement of the brain when the brainstem remains fixed or moves in the opposite direction. *Compression* strain occurs when tissue, arteries, or bones are squeezed or crushed beyond their ability to resist the force. Contusion, fracture, and rupture are injuries that occur as a result of crushing forces.[25,26]

Anatomical Considerations

The design of the skeleton and tissue provides some protection against impact forces. Some of the organs are protected from blunt force by the skeleton. The thick muscular cover in the trunk region serves as a shock absorber, protecting the enclosed organs from blunt and penetrating forces. Although anatomical design may assist in modifying certain types of injury, it is important to consider that anatomical design may actually contribute to injury.

The spleen is a mobile organ which lies posterior to the peritoneal cavity. It is protetcted by the 9th, 10th, and 11th ribs. Because of its maneuverability, it is the most commonly injured organ. Frequently, it is punctured or lacerated by the very ribs that afford it protection.[26]

The brain floats in cerebrospinal fluid (CSF) and is protected by the cranial vault. With deceleration injuries, the cranial vault is halted by the stationary object, but the brain continues to move. This action results in a secondary impact when the brain finally comes to rest against the vault. Focal brain lesions, such as contusions, lacerations, or vessel tears, may occur as a result of contact impact. The rotational impact of these forces may stretch the spinal cord and rotate and stretch the brainstem.[25,26,32]

Skeletal injuries, especially to the first and second ribs, sternum, scapula, and femur, suggest considerable force was involved in the injury event. Since these skeletal structures are the strongest in the body, their injury produces a high index of suspicion for associated injuries.[26]

The first rib is the strongest of all the ribs. Fractures of the first rib are associated with injuries to the chest, head, and abdomen.[33] Investigators have reported an 89% mortality in persons with a first-rib fracture and an 80% mortality in those with a second-rib fracture.[34] In addition, local structures such as the brachial plexus, sympathetic chain, and subclavian artery are also at risk for injury.

Fractures of the sternum, although uncommon, occur with impact injuries. A driver is most often injured from the impact of the chest on the steering wheel. Cardiac contusion, cardiac rupture, or transection of the descending aorta are associated injuries.[35,36]

Scapula fractures are also indicators of thoracic

injury. The scapula is protected on both sides by muscles. Pulmonary contusions and rib fractures on the same side as the scapular fracture are common. Arteries of the ipsilateral upper extremity can also be damaged with injuries to the scapula.

The femur is described as the longest and strongest bone in the body.[26] Considerable impact forces to the lower extremity are necessary to fracture the femur. This type of injury is commonly seen in front passengers involved in a motor vehicle collision (MVC). Associated injuries to the patella, knee ligaments, and acetabulum must be suspected when the femur is fractured.[37]

The attachment of body parts to fixed structures in the body is of concern in traumatic injury. Since these structures are tethered, acceleration and deceleration forces can cause injury as the tethered structure moves forward and the fixed structure remains stationary.

In the thorax, the descending thoracic aorta is attached at or distal to the ligamentum arteriosum, the diaphragm, and the aortic valve. As the forward motion of the chest is stopped, the aorta continues to move. The resultant shear or tensile strain may cause partial or complete laceration of the aorta at the point of the ligamentum arteriosum.[25,32] During a fall, the heart may actually be torn away from the aorta, resulting in an aortic tear.[25,32]

Fixation of body parts is also of concern when decelerating forces are exerted on the abdominal cavity. It is postulated that tensile and shear forces are applied at points of fixation, especially to organs attached to the mesentery such as the kidneys, small intestine (particularly the jejunum), cecum, ascending colon, and spleen. Liver injuries are postulated to occur when the liver's forward motion hits the ligamentum teres which traverses from the umbilicus to the liver. In the case of a down-and-under deceleration event, the liver impacts the ligamentum teres with such force that the organ splits down the middle.

Blunt Trauma

Injuries that result from blunt impact are generally described as having no outside communication with the environment. This description is accurate for the most part, since injuries related to blunt trauma are frequently unobservable. This is not true, however, when blunt forces impact skeletal structures and cause open fractures.

Common causes of blunt trauma are motor vehicle collisions (MVCs), motorcycle collisions, pedestrian collisions, falls, assaults, and contact sports. Direct impact (when the body meets the injuring agent without a buffering substance) causes the greatest injury. This type of injury may occur in falls, contact sports,

assaults, and ejection injuries since the body is in contact with the injury force directly. Indirect impact is the result of the body's meeting some object that is between the injury force and the body. Energy is transmitted internally from the object to the body.[25] This buffering effect may occur when an automobile hits a tree and buffers some of the forces before the body hits the steering wheel.

Motor Vehicle Collisions. Motor vehicle collisions include all types of vehicles, not only automobiles; they account for more fatal injuries and permanent disabilities than all other injury mechanisms.[1] Although automobile collisions are the most common MVC-related cause of death and disability, motorcycle, pedestrian, bicycle, and train collisions must also be considered. Factors that influence MVCs are road design, seatbelt use, substance abuse, car design, and speed limits. All of these factors are prime targets for prevention campaigns.

For a moving body to be brought to rest (deceleration force), the energy of its motion must be transferred to another object. In an MVC, the forward energy of the automobile may be partially absorbed by impedances in its path such as a guardrail, a tree, or another car. Within the car, the occupants are also in motion. This motion is halted when the body meets a stationary object, usually the car, which has just stopped. Likewise, body organs are also moving and abruptly stop when they hit a stationary object (the stopped body). Since deceleration of the three objects (car, body, or organ) is not occurring simultaneously, there are three separate collisions.[25,26,32] In attempting to predict or diagnose injuries associated with MVCs, it is important to remember the three-collision concept.

The severity and patterns of injuries associated with automobile collisions are numerous. Car size, occupant's position inside the car, type of collision, and use of restraints are all important considerations in injury outcome. Knowledge of these factors assists in predicting and diagnosing injuries and aids in maintaining a high index of suspicion for associated injuries.

Car Size, Occupant Position, and Restraints. Smaller cars are involved in more crashes per miles traveled than larger cars, and there is a higher incidence of death and injury in a smaller car.[25,26]

Position of occupants provides valuable information about the potential injuries sustained. Information related to occupant position after the collision also provides information about the movement of the occupant and the forces imparted to the vehicle. Identifying whether restraints were used and the type of restraints is necessary because movement within the car produces injuries. Types of restraints are lap only, shoulder only, or the three-point restraint (shoulder-lap combination). Information pertaining to the inflation of air bags is also necessary because it provides clues to the type of collision and may explain injuries that are related to the inflation of the air bag.

Types of Collisions. Front impact, side impact (sideswipe, lateral), rear impact, and rollover are the four types of collisions described. Force is a major factor in all types of collisions. The importance of the concept of force during a collision is clearly illustrated in the following example. If a man weighing 180 pounds is involved in a low-speed collision (20-30 miles/hr) at an acceleration of 30 G (gravitational acceleration), the force exerted is 5,400 pounds. If unobstructed, the person will hit the stationary object with 5,400 pounds of force. From this perspective, the argument for not wearing a seatbelt is absurd.

Head-on Collision. The unrestrained driver in a head-on collision will follow one of three pathways on impact: down-and-under, up-and-over, or ejection. In the down-and-under pathway, the driver is pushed under the steering wheel where the knees will impact with the dashboard. This action brings the lower body to a rapid stop. The upper part of the body continues in motion until it is stopped by the steering column. The head may or may not come into contact with the windshield. Potential injuries associated with this pathway are dislocation of the knees, fracture of the femur, fracture-dislocation of the posterior hip, or a combination of these injuries. Chest and head injuries may also occur.

In the up-and-over pathway, the body of the unrestrained driver is hurtled forward over the steering wheel. The first impact is the head hitting the windshield. Because the head is a strong dome-shaped structure, it may resist serious injury, depending upon the strength of the force applied. However, as the trunk continues to move against the stationary head, the cervical spine may hyperflex, hyperextend, or be crushed. Ultimately, the forward movement of the trunk is stopped by the steering wheel. This deceleration force may be equated to standing against a wall and having a pole rammed into the chest at 30 miles per hour (mph).[32] Injury to the chest and abdomen is inevitable.

If the occupant is ejected, any combination of events may occur. Injuries may result from hitting the automobile doors or a windshield, a guardrail, or the road surface.

Survivors of head-on collisions have the potential for serious injury combinations. Common injuries to the head and neck are lacerations of the face and scalp, skull or brain injury, fractures of facial bones including the jaw, crushed larynx, whiplash, or fractured cervical (C) spine. Chest injuries include pulmonary and cardiac contusions, rib fractures, cardiac rupture, and transection of the descending thoracic aorta. Spleen and liver lacerations are common abdominal injuries. Fractures of the tibia, fibula, patella, femur, and pelvis are expected. Disruption of knee ligaments and posterior dislocation of the hip should also be suspected.

If the driver is restrained with a lap belt, major head injuries are less likely to occur. However, with the lap belt, forward motion in the thoracolumbar area will stop first while upper trunk and lower extremities continue to move. The force of this deceleration pattern may result in hyperflexion of the spine from T12 through L2, resulting in an anterior compression fracture of the spine. If the lap belt is loosely fitted over the abdomen, the belt will stop motion in the abdominal region, and all the deceleration forces will be directed posteriorly into the abdominal organs. Gastrointestinal injuries and aortic disruption may result. Since the upper torso is not restrained, the chest will collide with the steering column. If the belt is properly placed over the pelvis, it is possible that injuries to the face and neck will occur as a result of forward and rotational movement of the trunk. In such movement, the occupant can hit the rear-view mirror, the A column (column that separates the windshield from the front side window), or other objects, including passengers.

When the diagonal strap is used with the lap restraint (three-point restraint), the neck is still at risk for injury since the range of neck motion is not impaired. Although less common, intrathoracic and intraabdominal injuries may occur with a three-point restraint and are related to the magnitude of the deceleration force. Rotational forces or twisting of the restrained torso may also occur. Injuries to the thorax below the shoulder should always be suspected in any deceleration injury.[26,32,38] Use of a shoulder restraint alone has been associated with serious neck and decapitation injuries. Clearly this type of restraint should be avoided.

Side Impact. The side-impact or lateral collision occurs when a vehicle moving forward is struck from the side. Initially, the unrestrained occupant in the struck vehicle will continue in forward motion until the body is forced to move laterally. This lateral movement may be caused by the movement of another unrestrained occupant or the crushed door moving inward. The first impact results in chest and abdominal injuries such as rib fractures, pulmonary contusions, and lacerations to the spleen, liver, or kidney. If the trochanter absorbs the side impact force, the head of the femur moves laterally, resulting in a pelvic fracture, or the impact may force the femoral head into the retroperitoneal space. Head injuries occur if the head collides with the side window, and neck injuries occur as the supporting ligamental structures in the neck are stretched.

Sideswipe and side-impact injuries are similar. In the sideswipe collision, the side of the car that is hit stops but the remainder of the car continues to move around the stationary point. This rotational force moves the occupant forward and laterally.

Rear Impact. In rear-impact collisions, it is usually a slow moving or stopped vehicle that is hit from behind. When the vehicle is struck, a forward transfer of energy occurs to all parts of the body in contact with the car. Therefore, if the headrest is in an upright (high) position, the entire body moves forward toward the steering column or dashboard. If the headrest is lowered and the head is not in contact with it, the body moves forward and the head lags behind. As the head snaps back across the headrest, energy is transferred to the C-spine. This whiplash injury causes strains and sprains to the cervical ligaments. Generally, serious injuries do not occur with this type of collision, but there are always exceptions.

Rollover. In the rollover collision, injuries cannot be predicted, especially if the driver and passengers are unrestrained. Moving bodies, interior objects, intrusion or collapse of the car, and ejection all have the potential to cause injury.

Occupant Position. The incidence of cranial injuries is higher in unrestrained front passengers during a head-on collision. If the front seat passenger is restrained, the incidence of head injury is similar to that of the driver. Although the front seat passenger is not afforded any protection from the windshield (by the steering wheel), there is a lower incidence of chest and abdominal injuries when compared with drivers. If the passenger is restrained with a loosely fitted lap belt, injuries may occur as the head hits the dashboard or windshield. As the forward motion of the middle trunk is stopped by the belt, injuries to the bladder, lumbar spine, bowel, and pelvis can occur. Injuries associated with side-impact collisions are similar to driver injuries but with an increased incidence of liver injury since the liver is positioned on the right side of the body.[26,32,38]

Rear seat passengers, if unrestrained, suffer injuries similar in type and severity to unrestrained front seat passengers. The deceleration forces actually move these passengers from their original positions inside the car. They can be found in the front seat floorboard area, invading front seat passenger space, or ejected through the windshield or other windows. It is important to note that the risk of injury doubles for the front seat passengers if there is an unrestrained passenger in the rear seat. Although the loosely fitting lap belt will keep the rear seat passenger in place, there is a high incidence of abdominal, pelvic, and gastrointestinal injuries associated with improperly placed lap belts.[26,32,38]

Motorcycle Collisions. The motorcyclist is unprotected from the energy forces associated with deceleration injuries since none of the impact forces are absorbed by an external object. Some protection is afforded by protective clothing such as boots, leather jackets, and helmets. The helmet is designed much like the cranial vault with a dome-shaped hard exterior and a soft interior. This design aids in the absorption of energy and does decrease the incidence of skull, brain, and facial injury. The risk of head and face injury increases 30% to 50% if no helmet is worn. Head-on or side-impact collisions are commonly seen with motorcycles. In addition, slick roadways or impact with debris on the roadway may actually cause the motorcycle to move out from under the cyclist. In any type of collision, the bike may fall onto the driver or the driver may be ejected from the bike.

The center of gravity on the motorcycle is above the axle. The center of gravity for the driver is at the iliac crest. In a head-on collision, the bike tilts upward and the driver is thrust forward into the handlebars. Contact with the head, chest, or abdomen is possible. If the feet remain stationary, the femur absorbs most of the forward impact. In an angular collision, the bike tends to fall onto the driver, crushing the lower legs. With ejection, injuries can be sustained to any part of the body as it hits a car, pole, or roadway. Any combination of injuries can be seen including facial fractures and injuries to the head, spine, chest, abdomen, and pelvis. Multiple fractures of the extremities are very common.

Pedestrian Collisions. Pedestrians sustain injuries from moving vehicles for a variety of reasons. Often, pedestrians are not clearly seen by motorists because of poor lighting or because pedestrians enter roadways between parked cars. Alcohol intoxication is often implicated in these collisions, and either pedestrians or drivers may be intoxicated. An injury triad (Waddell's triad) associated with adult pedestrian collisions has been identified. The pedestrian can actually be struck at three different times. The automobile bumper will impact initially at the lower extremity, causing fractures to the tibia and fibula. The pedestrian is then thrown forward onto the car or into the air. The deceleration forces against the car or roadway cause injury to the trunk. Finally, as the brakes of the vehicle are applied, the pedestrian may slide off the car onto the roadway, sustaining injuries to the head and upper extremities. In some cases, crushing forces are applied if the car runs over the pedestrian. The triad of injuries related to pedestrian accidents is consistent; therefore, a high index of suspicion should be operant when examining a pedestrian struck by a motor vehicle.[32,38]

Falls. Injuries related to falls are variable and depend upon the distance of the fall and how the body lands. In suspecting injury, one must account for the vertical deceleration forces, the application of the forces, and the tissue cohesion at the time of impact. Injury forces at impact may produce compression, stretching, and shearing. These forces may occur singly or in combination. Individuals may land on their feet or heels, back, or buttocks. Skeletal injuries, especially to the lower extremities, are common. Fracture-dislocations, wedge fractures, and compression fractures of the vertebrae are also common. Pelvic fractures and abdominal, chest, and head injuries may be present. Aortic tears also are noted in this injury population.[25,38]

Assaults. Blunt injuries may occur during altercations or beatings and are often produced by acceleration forces. Whether the victim is hit with a foreign object, punched, or kicked, serious injury to head, chest, or abdomen can occur. External bruises such as lacerations and contusions should provide a high index of suspicion for organ injury below. Most commonly injured are the head, kidneys, spleen, liver, and ribs.

Contact Sports. As with falls and assaults, a variety of injury combinations can be seen in sports-related injuries. In attempting to diagnose extent of injuries, one must keep in mind the type of sport, the objective of the sport, and the playing position of the injured person. If the head is used in football ramming maneuvers, C-spine or head injuries can result. Concussions, lacerations, contusions, and hemorrhage may occur in boxing. Spinal cord injuries are frequently associated with swimming and diving.

Penetrating Trauma

Injuries that occur as a result of piercing objects are classified as penetrating trauma. The piercing object may be set in motion with a weapon or human force, or the injury may be the result of being struck by or thrown onto an object. Gunshots, stabbings, and impalements are the major categories of penetrating injury.

Energy is created by the moving object and is dissipated into the surrounding tissue. Extent of injury can be determined only by evaluating the characteristics of the injurious object (type, shape, and speed), the distance from discharge point to target, energy release capabilities, and tissue characteristics. All penetrating wounds must be considered serious until proven otherwise by diagnostic data or exploration.

Ballistics. Predicting the extent of wounds and determining care of wounds associated with firearms is best accomplished with some knowledge of the kinetic energy of missiles and their ability to cause tissue damage. The following equation demonstrates the mathematical relationship between energy, mass, and velocity:

$$\text{Energy} = \text{mass} \times \text{velocity}^2/2 \times G$$

In the above equation, energy can be doubled if the mass is doubled. Energy is quadrupled if the velocity is doubled. Therefore, the wounding capability of a missile is based on its weight (mass) and its speed (velocity) at discharge (muzzle velocity).

Knowledge of the muzzle velocity is essential in understanding the wounding capabilities of a weapon. *Muzzle velocity* is the speed at which a missile leaves the barrel of the weapon. The extent of cavitation (tissue displacement by the missile) and tissue deformation is estimated using the muzzle velocity. A low-velocity missile travels less than 1,000 feet per second (ft/sec). Cavitation effect and blast effect (injury to tissues as energy moves through the tissue) are minimal with low-velocity weapons. A .22 caliber handgun is a type of low-velocity weapon. The muzzle velocity of this weapon is approximately 950 ft/sec. This type of missile causes some cavitation.[25,26,39,40] The entrance wound is small and the exit wound will be small if the missile exits. Often, this type of missile takes a meandering course once inside the body, bouncing off bony structures and changing direction. Extent of injury will depend on the type and number of organs or structures hit. As many as 30 enterotomies have been identified in patients shot with a .22 caliber handgun.

Medium-velocity missiles travel 1,000 to 2,000 ft/sec. These missiles produce larger cavitations, and they damage tissue by blast effect. Penetration of bone may occur, and bone fragments may become secondary missiles. Wounding from these secondary missiles is highly likely.[25,26,39,40]

High-velocity missiles travel at speeds greater than 2,000 to 3,000 ft/sec. Rifles and military weapons such as the M16 are well known for their wounding capabilities. Cavitation and blast injury are extensive with these weapons. The cavitation tract may be 30 to 40 times larger than the missile and is created as the missile compresses tissue and moves it away from the missile pathway. Contamination and devitalization of tissue occur along the cavitation tract. Debridement and subsequent repair of wounded tissue and organs is required.[25,26,39,40] A small entrance wound is usually seen with this type of weapon. Exit wounds will vary depending on the specific characteristics of the missile and the thickness of the target. For example, the exit wound of a high-velocity missile may be jagged and wide if it strikes the arm but small if it transverses the abdominal cavity.[41]

Impact velocity is of considerable importance when determining wounding patterns related to missiles. *Impact velocity* is the actual speed of the missile at the time of penetration and is dependent on muzzle velocity, distance from assailant to victim, influence of air friction, and drag of the missile. In most civilian shootings, victim and assailant are relatively close to one another (less than 7 yards). Thus, the impact velocity and muzzle velocity are similar. Impact velocity must be at least 150 ft/sec to penetrate the skin and 195 ft/sec to penetrate bone.[25,26,39,40] Injury patterns associated with specific tissue areas or organs are determined by their density, elasticity, and viscosity much the same as in blunt trauma. Severe injuries associated with major blood loss are possible from gunshot wounds, depending on the underlying structures damaged.[38] Gunshot wounds to the abdomen may carry a high morbidity and mortality if the peritoneum is contaminated.

Knowledge of wound ballistics is becoming more and more complex. A variety of projectiles are manufactured, and the type of projectile can alter the wounding capabilities of weapons. Weapons can be customized in many ways, thereby changing the wounding capabilities of standard weapons. Readers are referred to other sources for a greater understanding of ballistics.

Shotgun Injuries. Shotguns are considered separately from other weapons because their wounding capabilities are unique. At close range, shotguns can inflict lethal wounds destroying massive amounts of tissue, while insignificant wounds may occur at longer ranges.

Shotguns, designed for hunting birds and fast-moving animals, shoot multiple pellets instead of a single bullet. A shotgun shell holds the pellets, which vary in number according to their size. Within the shell, the pellets are separated from the explosive powder by a cardboard or plastic wad. When the pellets leave the barrel of the shotgun, they are bunched tightly together, but they spread out in flight. The degree of spread is determined by the choke on the barrel, which can be altered to allow maximum pellet spread. At short range (within 4 feet), the pellets stay together and act as one mass with a muzzle velocity of 1,300 ft/sec. The wound is a single hole with the wadding embedded deeply in the cavity. If the shell is discharged through glass, wood, or clothing, this material is also found in the wound. At intermediate range (4-12 feet), the entrance wound is 2 inches in diameter with separate holes at the borders of the wound from pellet spread. Wadding and other material are in the wound but closer to the surface. At long ranges (beyond 12 feet), the pellet spread depends on choke, barrel length, and type of ammunition used.[39,40] The sawed-off shotgun, which has no choke, is capable of hitting several targets with one shot.

Stab Wounds and Impalements. Stab wounds and impalements are considered low-velocity, low-energy injuries. Predictions of injury to underlying structures can usually be based on the type of weapon or object used, its length and trajectory, and the location of penetration. Although these wounds tend to have more local damage, deeper organs and multiple cavities can be penetrated. This is especially true if the wound is in the thoracolumbar area where diaphragmatic excursion can alter the thorax and abdominal cavities. Often, multiple stab wounds are seen. If the offending weapon does not remain in place, or even if the weapon is available but not in place, the wound cannot be dismissed as superficial. Exploration of the wound and observation of the patient are important. At one time, knowing the gender of the assailant was thought to be helpful in determining the direction of the stab. It was thought that women tend to stab downward and men to stab upward, but this may be more myth than fact. Therefore, a thorough exploration of the penetrating wound should not be deferred. Handedness has significance when investigating the contact between assailant and victim. A high index of suspicion should be operant when the victim suffers a stab wound to the chest and the assailant is right-handed. Because the heart lies left of the median plane and extends into the left chest, right-handed assailants will tend to stab in the left chest area. The right ventricle lies more anterior in the chest and for this reason it is the most commonly injured chamber of the heart.[26] Hemothorax, pneumothorax, cardiac tamponade, and aortic laceration can also occur. Stab wounds to the neck require special attention due to the proximity of the trachea, esophagus, and carotid vessels. Blood loss can be severe with stab injuries, causing rapid deterioration.[38]

Impalement injuries are more prevalent with falls and ejection. If possible, impaled objects should remain in place until diagnostic and definitive care can be provided. Often, impaled objects may occlude or tamponade vessels or organs, thereby preventing deterioration from hemorrhage. Regardless of the cause of penetrating injury, contamination of the wound tract is frequent. Judicious exploration and debridement of wounds should be a priority.

Trauma Scoring

The need for data on the physiological status of the injured patient and data that can predict patient outcome prompted the development of scales for scoring traumatic injuries. The trauma score (TS) (see the box to the right), the revised trauma score (RTS) (Table 55-1), and the injury severity score (ISS) are discussed in this section.

Trauma Score

The TS and RTS are used to assess the physiological status of the injured person. The trauma score was revised to increase the ease and usefulness of the tool for triage, emphasize the importance of coma, and improve quality care assessment methods.[22] The RTS consists of the Glasgow Coma Score (GCS) (see Table 33-5 in Chapter 33), systolic blood pressure (SBP) and respiratory rate (RR). Each variable (GCS, SBP, and RR) is assigned a coded value based on patient responses. Scores for each variable are added for a total trauma score. For example, a GCS of 10 (coded value 3) plus an SBP of 90 (coded value 4) plus an RR of 29 (coded value 3) equals a trauma score of 10. A score less than 11 indicates that a patient should be transported to a trauma center.[23] The TS, which assesses respiratory expansion and capillary refill in addition to GCS, SBP, and RR, is included for comparative purposes.

Injury Severity Score

The injury severity score (ISS) provides data for triaging and treating patients, allocating resources, assessing quality care, and conducting studies related to mortality and morbidity.[42] The ISS is a calculated score based on the site and severity of anatomical injury. Injuries from six body regions—head and neck, face, chest, abdominal and pelvic contents, extremities and pelvic girdle, and external (skin)—are classified from minor to severe and assigned a number from 1 to 5 using the Abbreviated Injury Scale (AIS) directory. Scores from the three most severely injured body regions are squared then added to obtain the ISS.[43] For a patient with an epidural hematoma (AIS = 4), a unilateral pulmonary contusion (AIS = 3), a perforated colon (AIS = 3), and a lacerated arm (AIS = 1) the ISS is 34 (16 + 9 + 9 = 34). The laceration is not included in the calculation because the three most severely injured body areas are the head, chest, and abdomen. If injury to only one body part occurs, the ISS is calculated on that injury alone.

An ISS of more than 15 indicates serious injury, and an ISS of 75 (maximum score) is probably not survivable. The ISS is helpful to those who are responsible for resource allocation, patient placement, or patient care assignments, and to the nurse in planning an appropriate atmosphere for clinical management.[44]

The TRISS (trauma/ISS) method takes trauma

Trauma Score

PARAMETER	POINT SCORE
Respiratory rate:	
36/min or more	4
25-35/min	3
10-24/min	2
0-9/min	1
No respiration	0
Respiratory expansion:	
Normal	1
Shallow	0
None or retraction	0
Systolic blood pressure; mmHg:	
90 or more	4
70-89	3
50-69	2
0-49 or less	1
No pulse	0
Capillary fill:	
Normal	2
Delayed	1
None	0
Eye opening:	
Spontaneous	4
To voice	3
To pain	2
None	1
Verbal response:	
Oriented	5
Confused	4
Inappropriate words	3
Incomprehensible words	2
None	1
Motor response:	
Obeys command	6
Localizes pain	5
Withdrawal (pain)	4
Flexion (pain)	3
Extension (pain)	2
None	1

Note: The last three items, constituting the Glasgow Coma Score (GCS), may be scored separately and then added to the trauma score as follows: GCS score of 14-15 = 5, 11-13 = 4, 8-10 = 3, 5-7 = 2, 3-4 = 1, making a possible total trauma score ranging from 1-16
From Champion, H. R., Sacco, W. J., Carnazzo, A. J., et al. (1981). Trauma score. *Critical Care Medicine, 9*(9), 672-676.

scoring one step further. TRISS was developed to better define probability of survival.[23] Using age, ISS, RTS, and mechanism of injury (blunt or penetrating) as predictor variables, the probability of survival can be calculated. A low probability of survival (high ISS and low trauma score) indicates severe injury that can be fatal. A high probability of survival (low ISS and high trauma score) indicates a good chance of recovery. For quality assurance purposes, probability of

TABLE 55-1 Revised Trauma Score

Parameter	Coded Value	
GLASGOW COMA SCORE (GCS)		
13-15	4	
9-12	3	
6-8	2	
4-5	1	
3	0	Patient score = _____
SYSTOLIC BP (SBP) (mmHg)		
>90	4	
70-89	3	
50-69	2	
0-49	1	
No pulse	0	Patient score = _____
RESPIRATORY RATE (RR) (BREATHS/MINUTE)		
20-24	4	
25-35	3	
>36	2	
1-9	1	
None	0	Patient score = _____
		Trauma Score = GCS + SBP + RR = _____

survival is a key issue. Care of patients who are outliers on either side of the probability curve should be reviewed. Problems or innovative approaches to care should be discussed so that appropriate changes in care can be instituted and shared with other trauma centers.

ASSESSMENT AND MANAGEMENT OF INJURY

Understanding injury patterns and mechanisms provides the astute clinician with the necessary knowledge to initiate treatment and manage the critically injured patient. After being injured, the patient moves into the next phase of the trauma cycle, which is assessment and management. The treatment phases included in this portion of the cycle are prehospital care, emergency care, critical care, acute care, and rehabilitation. Each phase of the cycle has unique characteristics, and knowledge of one phase provides important data for subsequent phases.

Prehospital Care

Successful outcomes for patients with traumatic injury begin in the prehospital phase. It is in this early stage of the "golden hour" that triage and preliminary stabilization are accomplished. Assessment, extrication, initial resuscitation, and rapid transport are the hallmarks of this phase. A "scoop and run" philosophy has been advocated for transporting these patients because life-threatening injuries are ultimately stabilized in the emergency department or surgical suite. On-scene times should be as brief as possible unless problems associated with extrication hinder transport.[23]

Prehospital personnel provide treatment based on preestablished protocols as well as through radio medical control. Priority care given by paramedics consists of a primary survey focusing on the ABCs (Airway, Breathing and Circulation). Initially, the C-spine is immobilized, an airway is established, and ventilation is maintained. Circulatory status is evaluated, intravenous lines are started, and external hemorrhage is controlled. Administration of oxygen and infusion of a balanced salt solution will also begin at the scene. Transport should not be delayed to perform any of the above procedures.

The initial resuscitation effort is followed by a systematic head-to-toe assessment. This survey is done rapidly to identify other injuries and to assist paramedics in determining the triage status of the patient. All assessment data are recorded on the prehospital record or "trip sheet." These data should include serial vital signs, Glasgow Coma Score, TS or RTS, medical history, interventions, and overt injuries. The trip sheet should also contain details related to the mechanism of injury, status of other persons involved, extrication information, and damage to the vehicle.

Review of the trip sheet data will assist nurses in the emergency department and the ICU to identify immediate and long-term needs of the patient. Often, these data are predictive of long-term survival and future complications. For instance, hypotension at the scene may be a precursor to multiorgan failure.

Prehospital clinical assessment is also essential for determining the destination of the patient. Persons who have life-threatening injuries should be transported to a level I or II trauma center if available. Patients should be transported to a trauma center according to the triage decision schema recommended by the American College of Surgeons, Committee on Trauma (Figure 55-3).[23]

Emergency Department Care

Upon arrival of the patient to the emergency department, the trauma team begins the resuscitation phase of the trauma cycle using a predetermined systematic plan. This phase consists of the primary assessment, actual resuscitation, secondary assessment, and definitive care.

Primary Survey and Resuscitation

The primary survey of the patient is repeated in the emergency department to determine if any change in patient status occurred during transport. The trauma score calculated upon arrival should be compared to the field trauma score. The primary survey in the emergency department should be performed within 60 seconds and should focus on the ABCDEFs of trauma care. Using the ABCDEFs of trauma care, the life-threatening problems should be prevented and the work of stabilizing the patient initiated.

Resuscitation is an ongoing process that technically begins the moment the patient is brought to the emergency department. Resuscitative efforts in the emergency department should not continue for longer than 1 hour. Patients with refractory hypotension, cardiac tamponade, cardiac penetration, and in some cases cardiac arrest require surgical intervention. If surgical interventions cannot be performed adequately in the emergency department, these patients should be transported to the surgical suite immediately.

Trauma ABCDEFs

A: Airway. Since airway obstruction is recognized as the most rapidly fatal problem and the one most easily correctable in the emergency department, priority care consists of securing an airway and minimizing tissue hypoxia.[45,46] If apnea or airway obstruction is present, the oral cavity must be inspected for debris. Removal of the foreign body (teeth, etc.) may be accomplished with suction or by manual removal. Oral intubation may be required to maintain the airway. An oral-pharyngeal airway may be useful in the comatose patient to prevent further obstruction by the tongue. If maxillofacial injuries are present, bleeding is profuse, anatomical distortion exists, or foreign bodies cannot be removed, cricothyroidotomy should be performed to secure the airway. Tracheostomies are not advocated.[46]

Cricothyroidotomy is accomplished by making a 2- to 3-cm transverse incision directly over the cricothyroid membrane. An appropriately sized tracheostomy tube is then inserted, and the cuff is inflated.[45,46] Extreme care must be taken to protect the C-spine when establishing an airway.

B: Breathing. Once the airway has been established, respiratory effort is assessed. Injuries that may impair ventilation almost as rapidly as obstruction are pneumothorax, tension pneumothorax, and flail chest. Initial respiratory assessment includes (1) respiratory rate, depth, and effort; (2) length of inspiratory—expiratory cycle; (3) air exchange at mouth, nose, or tube; (4) respiratory noise; (5) symmetry of chest movement; and (6) evidence of paradoxical chest movement, splinting, and aspiration. Surface markings on the chest, use of accessory or abdominal muscles, and attempts by the patient to maximize ventilation by positioning must also be noted.[46] If indicated, high-flow oxygen via face mask should be administered or mechanical ventilation initiated.

If respiratory distress persists after the airway has been established and mechanical ventilation initiated, further investigation is necessary. Palpation of the trachea for deviation, of the chest for crepitus, and of the chest wall for stability, as well as ascultation for breath sounds may provide clues to the etiology of the respiratory distress. In severe respiratory distress, bilateral chest tubes may be indicated. These should be inserted immediately without waiting for radiographic verification of pathology.[46] Head injury and substance abuse must also be considered as possible causes for hypoxia and agitation.

C: Circulation. Circulatory status is assessed to determine the degree of shock, estimate intravascular volume needs, and determine the size and type of intravenous (IV) catheter required.[46] A minimum of two large-bore IV catheters should be inserted. If injury to the upper extremities prevents insertion of the IV catheter in the arms or if great vessel injury is suspected, the catheter may be inserted in the lower extremity or groin. Use of central venous catheters is recommended by some sources for best access.[35]

In cases of cardiac arrest, establishing circulation is of primary importance. Attempts to identify and control hemorrhage may be occurring while cardiopulmonary resuscitation (CPR) is in progress. Thoracotomy with cross-clamping of the aorta may be performed. However, the role of emergency department thoracotomy is a controversial issue. Some experts believe that thoracotomy should be reserved for

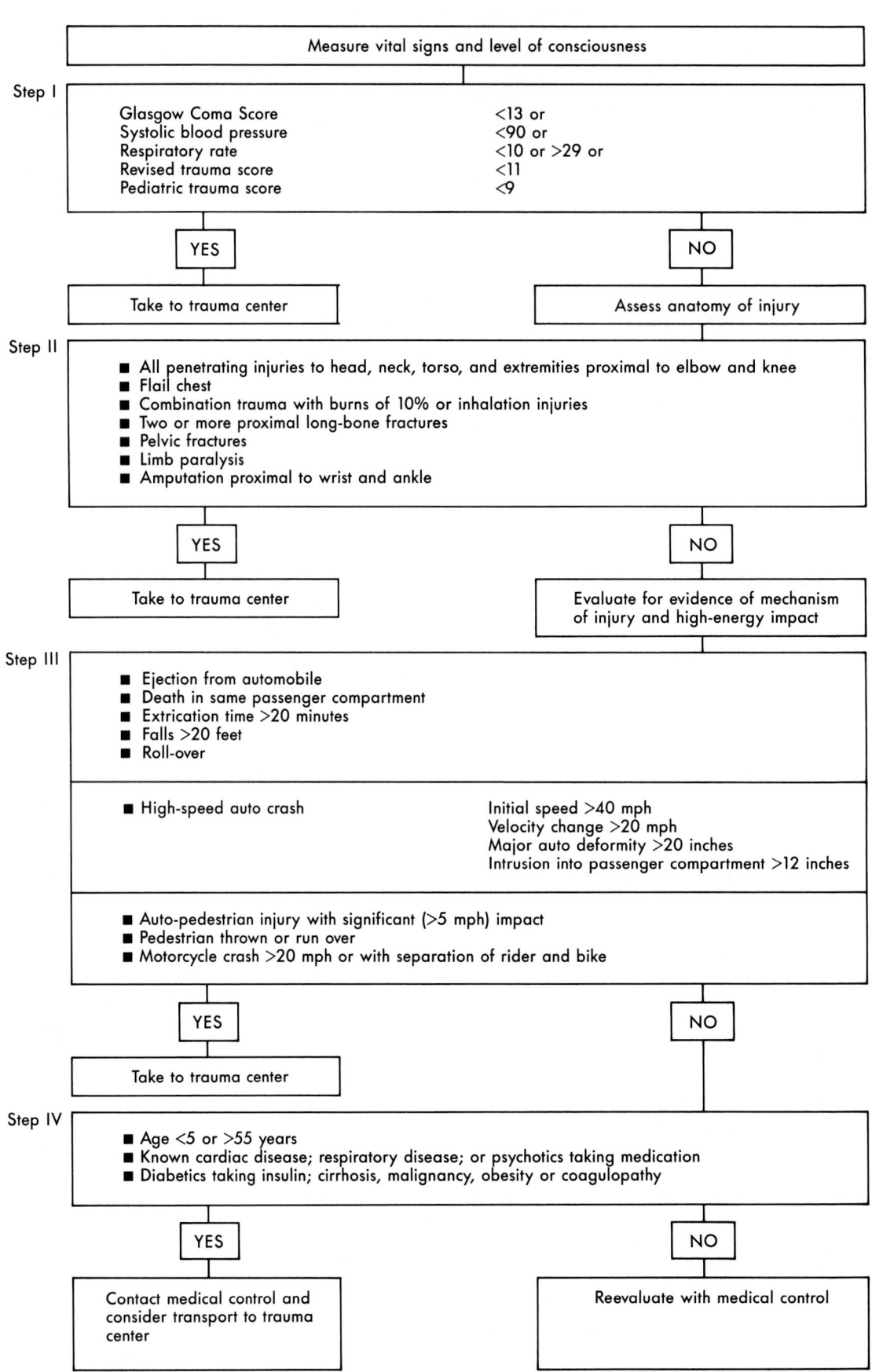

Measure vital signs and level of consciousness

Step I

Glasgow Coma Score	<13 or
Systolic blood pressure	<90 or
Respiratory rate	<10 or >29 or
Revised trauma score	<11
Pediatric trauma score	<9

YES → Take to trauma center

NO → Assess anatomy of injury

Step II

- All penetrating injuries to head, neck, torso, and extremities proximal to elbow and knee
- Flail chest
- Combination trauma with burns of 10% or inhalation injuries
- Two or more proximal long-bone fractures
- Pelvic fractures
- Limb paralysis
- Amputation proximal to wrist and ankle

YES → Take to trauma center

NO → Evaluate for evidence of mechanism of injury and high-energy impact

Step III

- Ejection from automobile
- Death in same passenger compartment
- Extrication time >20 minutes
- Falls >20 feet
- Roll-over

- High-speed auto crash
  - Initial speed >40 mph
  - Velocity change >20 mph
  - Major auto deformity >20 inches
  - Intrusion into passenger compartment >12 inches

- Auto-pedestrian injury with significant (>5 mph) impact
- Pedestrian thrown or run over
- Motorcycle crash >20 mph or with separation of rider and bike

YES → Take to trauma center

NO →

Step IV

- Age <5 or >55 years
- Known cardiac disease; respiratory disease; or psychotics taking medication
- Diabetics taking insulin; cirrhosis, malignancy, obesity or coagulopathy

YES → Contact medical control and consider transport to trauma center

NO → Reevaluate with medical control

WHEN IN DOUBT TAKE TO A TRAUMA CENTER

Figure 55-3 Triage decision schema.

the surgical suite where sophisticated equipment and trained personnel are immediately available. Others believe that emergency department thoracotomies are useful. Regardless of where the thoracotomy is performed, patients with penetrating injuries have better outcomes when thoracotomies are performed during cardiac arrest because an isolated injury may be responsible for the hemorrhage. With blunt injury, cardiac arrest carries a high mortality even with emergency department thoracotomy because extent and location of injuries are not well defined.

The circulatory status can be quickly assessed through a variety of noninvasive mechanisms. The pulse is a rapid and sensitive indicator of volume status. A strong radial pulse indicates a blood pressure of approximately 80 to 90 mmHg. Presence of a femoral pulse indicates a blood pressure of 60 to 70 mmHg, while a carotid pulse indicates a pressure of 40 mmHg. A pulse rate above 120 beats per minute is an indication of hypovolemia even in the presence of pain, anxiety, fear, and catecholamine release. In young patients, heart rate may accelerate up to 160 beats per minute with hypovolemia. Older patients rarely sustain rates greater than 140 beats per minute.[46]

Change in blood pressure is not a sensitive indicator of volume loss because of compensatory mechanisms activated by the stress response. No significant changes in blood pressure will be clinically apparent until 15% to 20% of blood volume is lost. A blood pressure in the 60 to 80 mmHg range indicates a blood loss of 30%. A 40% blood loss is suspected when the blood pressure drops into the 30 to 50 mmHg range. Elderly patients may have difficulty maintaining or initiating the compensatory response and may demonstrate clinical signs of hypovolemia with a 15% blood loss. It should be noted that head injury is not an etiology for hypotension. If hypotension exists in a head-injured patient the cause of hemorrhage must be found. Hypotension is present with spinal cord injuries; however, this hypotension should respond to volume replacement.

Skin changes are also important indicators of hypovolemia. Cool, pale, moist skin develops rapidly as epinepherine and norepinepherine are released and vasoconstriction occurs. Lower extremities below the knees are first to manifest skin changes, which should be considered early warning signs of impending shock in all age groups.[46]

Urine output should be monitored every 15 minutes during the resuscitation. Urine output of less than 30 ml/hr indicates activation of the compensatory mechanisms. Fluid administration should be initiated rapidly to ensure adequate urine volume. Diuretics should not be used to increase urine output because they will further deplete volume.

Central venous pressure (CVP) is not a precise measure of volume status. The normal CVP range is 3 to 8 mmHg, which overlaps with the hypovolemic range of 0 to 5 mmHg. The importance of CVP lies in its usefulness in differentiating hypovolemic from cardiogenic shock. Cardiogenic shock may occur if compensatory mechanisms have failed or if cardiac tamponade, tension pneumothorax, or cardiac contusion is present. The injured patient in hypovolemic shock will have a CVP less than 5 mmHg. A CVP of 25 mmHg is required to produce a similar degree of cardiogenic shock.[46]

Circulatory instability, once recognized, necessitates infusion of adequate fluid volume and restoration of oxygen-carrying capacity. Fluid resuscitation begins with infusion of crystalloids such as Ringer's lactate (RL) or normal saline. Rapid volume infusers can administer up to 1,500 ml/min without high pressure and maintain the fluid temperature at 37° C.[47] The amount of fluid administered is based on the clinical manifestations of shock and the patient's response. Return of stable vital signs (BP >100 mmHg; HR <110 beats per minute; urine output >50 ml/hr) indicates resolution of hypovolemia. The volume of fluids can then be decreased, but observation for return of shock should continue.[48,49]

The *three-for-one fluid replacement rule* serves as a guideline for fluid requirements. Most patients in hemorrhagic shock require 300 ml of electrolyte solution for each 100 ml of blood loss.[48] Administration of crystalloids alone may cause hemodilution. If more than 1,000 to 1,500 ml is needed for stabilization, packed red blood cells (RBCs) should be administered if further resuscitation is necessary. A basic rule of thumb is 1 unit of packed RBCs should be administered for every 3 L of crystalloids. Maintaining the hematocrit at 30% is desired. Type O Rh-positive blood can be given to all patients until typing and cross-matching are completed. The use of packed RBCs is preferred over whole blood. Clotting factors and platelets, which are essential to trauma patients, are available in fresh whole blood, but they are lost when whole blood is stored. Therefore, separate administration of packed RBCs, platelets, and fresh frozen plasma is recommended over administration of stored whole blood.[49,50] These blood products are administered according to the clinical status of the patient and laboratory results. They are most frequently given in the operating room and critical care unit. The use of shed blood from the thorax (autotransfusion) has increased over the last few years because it protects the patient from the complications associated with banked blood. Blood may be reinfused up to 4 hours after it has been collected.[50] Autotransfusion should be performed on the basis of an approved protocol that specifically delineates candidates for the procedure. Patients with known or suspected contamination of the chest should not receive auto-transfusions.

Arguments about the administration of colloids or crystalloids continue. The merits of crystalloids include low cost, nonallergenic properties, reduction of viscosity; repletion of interstitial and intravascular volume; and lower renal, pulmonary, and third-spacing complications. Crystalloids do, however, dilute plasma and RBCs and move out of the intravascular space quickly. Colloids are favored because of their oncotic properties. Volume for volume, colloids are more effective in reversing signs of shock.[48] In addition to maintaining circulatory status via volume infusion, control of external hemorrhage by direct pressure must also be initiated.

D: Deficits, Deformities, and Drainage. Prompt assessment for deficits and deformities provides information about the neurological and musculoskeletal status of the patient. Abnormal drainage increases the index of suspicion for injury. The Glasgow Coma Score (GCS), which is part of the TS and RTS, is the recommended tool for assessing neurological status. Intubated patients cannot verbally respond, so the score is calculated using a T to indicate intubation. If there is severe bilateral eye swelling and the eyes cannot open, the best eye-opening response is scored with an S for swelling. With both intubation and eye swelling, the remaining parameters should be scored. Changes in neurological status occur rapidly; therefore, continuous evaluation is imperative. If the GCS drops 1 point from the previous evaluation, further investigation is essential. This change in neurological status may indicate brain swelling or hematoma formation. The pupil size, shape, and response to light should be assessed frequently. Development of a fixed dilated pupil on one or both sides is an emergent problem and must be treated immediately. It is important to note that substance use (alcohol and drugs) and hypoxia also may alter the neurological status of the patient.

Once neurological status has been assessed, the patient should be quickly scanned for deformities of the chest, abdomen, or extremities. Changes in a thigh from a cylinder shape to a ball shape may indicate a closed femur fracture. Such an injury can accommodate up to 1,000 ml of blood. Drainage from the mouth, nose, ears, penis, or urethral meatus necessitates further investigation.

E: Exposure, Entrance and Exit, ECG. No thorough evaluation of a trauma patient can be accomplished without removal of clothing. Careful inspection of the anterior and posterior surfaces of the body provides information about injuries. Entrance and exit wounds should be identified. Cardiac monitoring should also be instituted at this time.

F: Fluids, Foley. Although rapid evaluation and stabilization is the purpose of the primary survey, many resuscitative activities are being performed concurrently. Analysis of fluids is an essential component of diagnosis and treatment for the trauma patient. Blood studies include arterial blood gases (ABGs), hematocrit, hemoglobin, white blood count, platelet count, prothrombin and partial thromboplastin, type and cross-match, electrolytes, alcohol level, cardiac isoenzymes (if cardiac injury is suspected), and general admission blood studies.

Care must be taken when inserting a Foley catheter in a patient with obvious injury to the pelvis or with bleeding from the penis or urethral meatus. In some cases, a suprapubic catheter will have to be placed. After the insertion of a Foley catheter, the following urine studies should be requested: urinalysis, drug screen, urine human chorionic gonadotrophin (HCG) for women of childbearing age, and myoglobin.

Nasogastric fluid should also be evaluated in this phase. Gastric contents may be tested for occult blood. Insertion of a nasogastric tube (sump) attached to low suction will empty and decompress the stomach and will decrease the risk of aspiration. Although the nasogastric (NG) tube is important, it should be the last tube inserted if maxillofacial or basilar skull injury is suspected. For the patient with a maxillofacial injury, care must be taken that airway and breathing are not compromised when the tube is inserted. For the patient with a basilar skull fracture, oral insertion of the NG tube is imperative to eliminate the potential of inserting the tube through the cranial vault and into the brain. Later, the NG tube is useful for monitoring stomach acidity and absorption capabilities.

Secondary Survey

The purpose of the secondary survey is to evaluate the injured patient systematically for injuries and to provide diagnostic and definitive care. However, unstable patients should not be held in the emergency department for definitive treatment.

History and Physical Assessment. The secondary survey is done using a systems review. A medical history from the patient, if possible, or from a family member should be obtained at this time. This section addresses the diagnostic activities performed during the secondary survey. Definitive care of specific injuries is addressed in the critical care section. Refer to other sources for an extensive review of the assessment activities associated with the secondary survey (see reference 46).

Diagnostic Procedures

Radiographic Studies. Patients who are stable but require further evaluation may undergo radiographic studies in the emergency department or ICU. Diagnostic studies not available in the emergency department may be performed en route to the operating room or the ICU. In the absence of clinical deterioration from increased intracranial pressure, skull films may be obtained to determine fractures of the cranial vault or extent of penetrating wounds. Computed tomography (CT scan) is the preferred diagnostic tool for patients with suspected brain injury.

Lateral C-spine films (C1 to T1) are taken to rule out vertebral fracture and to identify movement of vertebral bodies into the spinal canal. To prevent iatrogenic spinal injury, the patient's neck must remain immobilized until the C-spine films are evaluated and the integrity of C1 through T1 is confirmed.

Chest x-rays are obtained to identify pathological changes and to verify placement of endotracheal and chest tubes. An upright anterior-posterior view is optimal but may not be possible if the patient cannot be moved. The chest x-ray should be examined for evidence of pneumothorax, hemothorax, pneumohemothorax, fractures, mediastinal shift, integrity of the aortic arch, position of the diaphragm, air or blood in the chest cavity, and presence of foreign bodies.

If an abdominal injury is suspected and the patient is stable, a flat plate abdominal film or an abdominal CT scan with contrast may be obtained to verify blood, air, or foreign bodies in the peritoneal cavity. Peritoneal lavage, which is discussed in the following section, may also be considered. If genitourinary (GU) trauma is suspected, a single intravenous pyelogram (IVP) may be obtained. A single film of the lower abdomen is obtained 5 to 10 minutes after the contrast dye is injected.

Pelvic x-rays may be indicated if there is pelvic pain or pelvic rocking. Radiographic studies of deformed or painful extremities may also be performed.

Penetrating injuries to the neck require special attention. Patients with neck injuries from penetrating wounds (gunshots, stabbings) should have an angiogram and barium swallow to rule out vessel injury and esophageal injury.

Diagnostic Peritoneal Lavage. In patients with blunt abdominal trauma, diagnostic peritoneal lavage may be performed to identify the presence of blood in the peritoneum. If the tap is negative, exploratory laparotomy is deferred. The trend toward conservative management and use of abdominal CT scans has led to controversy over the efficacy of peritoneal lavage. In rural hospitals where CT scans are not readily available, however, it may be used.

The indications for performing diagnostic peritoneal lavage are painful or tender abdomen, unexplained hypotension with a falling hematocrit, hyperesthesia from a spinal cord injury, fractures of the lumbar or thoracic spine, pelvic fractures, head injury, or decreased level of consciousness from alcohol or drug use.[45] A small incision that penetrates the peritoneum is made above or below the umbilicus. A trocar is inserted into the peritoneal space, and the contents of the cavity are aspirated for blood or fluid. If there is no fluid aspirated, 1 L of a balanced salt solution is infused, allowed to circulate, and drained. The drained fluid is sent to the laboratory for evaluation. The test is considered positive if the RBC count is more than $100,000/mm^3$; the WBC count is more than $500/mm^3$; amylase is elevated; or there is evidence of bile, bacteria, or vegetable fiber in the fluid. Persons with a positive tap must undergo an exploratory laparotomy.[45,51]

Critical Care

Traumatic injury is no longer considered simply as physical injury to tissue or organs resulting from energy forces. Rather, clinical and laboratory research in progress provides support for the complex physiological and pathophysiological responses associated with injury. For the most part, these complex events unfold in the critical care unit. Sophisticated monitoring techniques assist critical care nurses in rapidly identifying changes in the critically ill trauma patient. An understanding of the pathophysiology assists the nurse in making critical decisions.

Monitoring Physiological Trends

Fluid volume loss and translocation is a serious problem for the severely injured trauma patient. The pulmonary artery (PA) catheter provides valuable information about the fluid status of the patient. In addition, the PA catheter allows for repeated measurements of cardiac output, central venous pressure, and mixed venous blood. Use of the PA catheter is indicated for patients with the potental for circulatory instability or sepsis. Hourly monitoring of PA pressures and the frequent calculation of cardiac output and systemic and pulmonary vascular resistance allows the nurse to titrate fluids and vasoactive drugs. Trends in PA pressures lead to identification of insidious changes in patient status.

Recently, the value of monitoring mixed venous saturation ($S\bar{v}O_2$) has been reported. The $S\bar{v}O_2$ catheter, a variation of the simple PA catheter, provides valuable information about the overall utilization of oxygen by the tissues. Increases or decreases from the normal range (60% to 80%) are early signs of cardiorespiratory problems or tissue perfusion problems.

Arterial pressure lines are especially useful in caring for the severely injured patient. Monitoring trends in blood pressure provides ongoing assessment of the compensatory response as well as responses to fluid and drug therapies. Samples for arterial blood gas studies can be drawn via the line and respiratory status monitored. Pragmatically, the line serves as an access for drawing blood samples for the numerous laboratory studies necessary for evaluating fluid and electrolyte status. Arterial pressure monitoring is especially important in patients with head injuries. Mean arterial pressure (MAP) is a primary determinant of cerebral perfusion pressure (CPP). Data to calculate CPP are easily obtainable with an arterial pressure monitor.

Continuous intracranial pressure monitoring may also be performed in the ICU. Intracranial pressure (ICP) can be monitored using an intraventricular catheter, epidural sensor, subarachnoid bolt, or intraparenchymal catheter. These devices may be inserted in the operating room or at the bedside. Normal ICP is less than 15 mmHg. Since CPP is a key concept in understanding intracranial pressure dynamics, CPP should also be monitored. CPP is a calculated value based on MAP and ICP (CPP = MAP − ICP). MAP can be calculated (MAP = systolic − diastolic/ 3 + diastolic) or determined from the arterial pressure monitor. An optimal CPP is greater than 60 mmHg. For greater detail on intracranial pressure and hemodynamic monitoring, the reader is referred to Chapter 4.

Use of the pulse oximeter with trauma patients has steadily increased. This simple device provides continuous information about the oxygen saturation level of the patient. End-tidal carbon dioxide (CO_2) monitors are also useful in monitoring respiratory status of the injured patient.

Trauma Physiology

Physiological Responses. A cascade of events aimed at survival is activated following traumatic injury. Physiological compensatory mechanisms are derived from the complex interactions of the nervous, endocrine, and immune systems. The paradox in trauma care is that the systems that arise to support the injured person through the initial injury have the potential for creating lethal complications. Although there are no clear explanations for this "self-destructive" pathological response, understanding the normal response to stress and the evolution of traumatic shock may provide some guidelines for care. (See Chapter 56.)

Traumatic Shock. Shock is defined as circulatory failure characterized by inadequate tissue perfusion. Shock leads to alterations in tissue metabolism, structure, and function at the subcellular, cellular, and system levels. An extensive review of shock pathophysiology is provided elsewhere in this text (see Chapter 56). However, a general review of hypovolemic (traumatic) shock as it relates to the injured person is presented.

The most common cause of shock in the injured person is hypovolemia resulting from acute blood loss which may be external or internal. Acute blood loss from external injuries such as lacerations, amputations, fractures, or penetrating wounds, although obvious, may be miscalculated. Internal blood loss, which is less obvious, must be estimated according to a high index of suspicion. Internal blood loss is usually concealed in body cavities such as the chest, abdomen, retroperitoneal space, femur, and pelvis. Such injuries may account for 2 to 6 L of blood loss.

Fluids other than blood may be lost and account for hypovolemia, especially with soft tissue injuries and burns. Fluid translocation into the interstitial space can account for life-threatening fluid losses.[48,49]

Shock is manifested clinically by inadequate tissue perfusion. Unfortunately, the clinical picture of shock is evident much later than the cellular response to shock. Although assessment of vital signs may indicate shock, this is not an early revelation. Change in oxygen consumption at the tissue level is the earliest predictor of impending circulatory failure. Unfortunately, cellular oxygen consumption is not as easily measured as are vital signs. Knowledge of the clinical indicators of volume loss may assist clinicians in predicting impending failure. The four classes of hemorrhage provide baseline information for predicting failure.

- *Class I Hemorrhage:* With up to 15% (750 ml) of total blood volume lost, the clinical manifestations of shock are not observable by monitoring vital signs. At this time, the volume deficit is compensated. Patients have normal vital signs and adequate urine output but may demonstrate some anxiety. Crystalloids are used for fluid replacement.[48,49]

- *Class II Hemorrhage:* Fluid loss between 15% and 30% (750-1,500 ml) of total blood volume results in multiple physiological responses. Anxiety, agitation, or restlessness may be due to catecholamine release or to hypoxia. Heart rate should rise, and peripheral vasoconstriction should occur as catecholamines are released. A decline in systolic blood pressure indicates that at least 20% of volume has been lost. Orthostatic changes in blood pressure are manifested when 25% of volume is lost. The skin becomes cool and wet due to peripheral vasoconstriction. Capillary refill is delayed, and muscle fatigue and weakness may be evident as the body shifts toward an anaerobic metabolism. Crystalloid replacement using the "three-to-one" rule is indicated.[48,49]

- *Class III Hemorrhage:* Compensatory mechanisms are inadequate when 30% to 40% of circulating blood volume is lost. Alterations in tissue perfusion are evident. The patient is confused because cerebral hypoperfusion, hypoxia, and acidosis affect level of consciousness. Tachycardia is present, and systolic blood pressure is decreased to 50 to 60 mmHg. Metabolic acidosis occurs as the oxygen-driven metabolism is shut down, resulting in tachypnea and deep, rapid respirations. Urine output is poor, and cutaneous circulation is severely impaired.[48,49] Fluid replacement should include blood products as well as crystalloids based on the "three-to-one" rule.[48]

- *Class IV Hemorrhage:* Compensatory mechanisms are exhausted, and symptoms of profound shock are evident with blood losses of 40% or more (>2,000 ml). The patient is stuporous, lethargic, or unconscious; pupils may be dilated, and the heart rate is faster than 140 beats per minute and irregular. Severe hypotension with a decreased pulse pressure occurs. Urine output is minimal. No capillary refill is noted, and skin is cold and clammy. Rapid administration of crystalloids and blood products is imperative, and surgical intervention may be immediately required.[48,49]

Since blood loss and shock are interrelated, knowledge of hemorrhage classifications provides the basis for determining the stage of shock.

- *Stage I—Nonprogressive Shock:* Tissue perfusion is altered, but the compensatory mechanisms are adequate to prevent cardiovascular deterioration. This stage is reversible. Class I and early class II hemorrhage may be categorized in the nonprogressive stage of shock.
- *Stage II—Progressive Shock:* Cardiac collapse due to inadequate compensatory mechanisms characterizes stage II. Without control of hemorrhage or adequate resuscitation, tissue perfusion will diminish, and death will result. Late class II and class III hemorrhage fall into this category.
- *Stage III—Irreversible Shock:* Shock is refractory to blood replacement and other forms of therapy. Cardiovascular collapse is irreversible. Patients with class IV hemorrhage who are not treated aggressively will ultimately move to irreversible shock.

Metabolic Response to Hemorrhage and Shock. Metabolic responses in trauma have been well documented, and two phases of metabolic activity have been described. The ebb phase occurs early after injury and the flow phase occurs days after the initial injury.

The *ebb phase* encompasses the time between injury and physiological stabilization and is initiated as the body prepares to provide substrates for energy needs. This phase is characterized by the mobilization of large stores of glycogen, amino acids, and triglycerides. Because skeletal muscle is catabolized in this phase, it has been called the *hypercatabolic phase*. With activation of the sympathetic nervous system and subsequent release of catecholamines, blood pressure, heart rate, and respiratory rate are increased, and blood volume is centralized. Hyperglycemia results as all available stores of glucose are mobilized and new glucose is made. Stabilization of the cell membrane and protection of peripheral cells is attempted through the release of glucocorticoids.

Normally, the *flow phase* is the body's attempt to achieve a steady state. For the trauma patient, this phase is characterized by increases in oxygen consumption and carbon dioxide production. The hypermetabolic nature of this phase can be equated to autocannibalism. Even in the face of hyperglycemia, the body continues to mobilize glucose stores. Fat is utilized as the primary energy substrate, and the muscles use fat even if sufficient supplies of glucose are available. Protein catabolism occurs with an increase in nitrogen losses and is most severe between days 4 and 8. Decreases in plasma albumin, transferrin, and lipoprotein are also seen.[52,53] This state of negative nitrogen balance results in malnutrition which potentiates the vicious cycle of increased oxygen consumption, muscle wasting, and delayed wound healing. With the immune system already blunted, the inflammatory response causing mircoaggregation in the blood vessels, and the body mass being used as the primary energy source, the patient is a prime candidate for sepsis and multiorgan failure.

Nursing Management

Mental/Emotional Responses. Support of the patient's psychological and emotional status is extremely important in any critical care environment. The psychological disruption may be intensified after traumatic injury. Many factors contribute to the fear and anxiety experienced by trauma patients. The injury event was sudden and unexpected. Knowledge of the events may be fragmented and unclear to the patient. The event itself may have been frightening. Status of relatives and friends involved in the event may not be known. Treatment interventions during resuscitation and in the ICU are painful, invasive, and embarrassing. These actions are often carried out without permission or explanation. Injuries may involve loss of limb, loss of motion, and severe disfigurement. Plans for the future may be shattered and the future now unknown.

In addition to the psychological events the patient experiences, the critical care milieu imposes other burdens. Communication may be impaired by an endotracheal tube, stabilization device, or a language barrier. Sleep deprivation is common as is isolation from family and friends; time orientation is lost. Depression, powerlessness, loneliness, anger, guilt, loss of self-esteem, alteration in body image, and posttraumatic distress syndrome can all be experienced by the trauma patient. Prompt recognition and support by the critical care nurse is important. Appropriate consultation with other members of the health care team is advocated.

Nutrition. Nutritional support cannot be delayed for the trauma patient, who rapidly utilizes stored fat and muscle as primary energy sources. The critical care nurse should collaborate with the trauma physician and the nutrition support team in assessing the nutritional needs of the patient. Once the assessment has been completed, nutritional goals for the patient should be developed and implemented.

The nutritional needs of the trauma patient can be determined in a variety of ways. Anthropometric measurements are used to determine the adipose tissue stores and the muscle protein compartment. Evaluation of visceral proteins should be done routinely. Visceral protein deficiency is confirmed if serum albumin is less than 3.0 g/dl, serum transferrin level is below 150 μg/ml, and total lymphocyte count is less than 1,500/mm^3. Protein requirements for the trauma patient are at least 1 g per kg per day. Caloric requirements must also be calculated. Depending upon the extent of injury, caloric requirements for the trauma patient may exceed 20 kcal per kg per day. Caloric requirements are calculated using the basal metabolic rate, physical activity, and the metabolism of substrates. Assessment of the nitrogen balance indicates whether the patient is in a state of anabolism or catabolism. Clinically, the 24-hour urea nitrogen excreted is compared to the nitrogen intake.[54,55]

Indirect calorimetry determines energy needs of the trauma patient through the quantification of gas exchange. The calculation is based on the relationships among oxygen consumption, carbon dioxide production, and nitrogen excretion. Calorimetry measurements can be taken for a short period (20 minutes) and the results used to estimate the projected caloric needs for the next 24 hours.[53]

Nutritional support should be initiated within 48 to 72 hours after injury. Both enteral and parenteral feeding methods are used. Absence of bowel sounds is no longer considered an indication to defer nutritional support. The optimal nutritional program should avoid high glucose loads since the patient is already hyperglycemic. Fat emulsions and branch chain amino acids should provide a substantial part of the caloric needs.

Nutritional support may not shift the patient from a negative to positive nitrogen balance overnight. However, continued evaluation and revision of nutritional supplements will move the patient toward an anabolic state. Since nutrition is an integral requirement for wound healing, readers are directed to the chapter on wound healing for greater detail (see Chapter 54).

Postoperative Fluid Management. The postoperative management of fluids is an important consideration in trauma care. Fluid derangements identified in trauma patients can be accounted for by overt losses due to hemorrhage, covert losses due to translocation of fluid, injuries to fluid-regulating organs such as the brain and kidneys, and discrepancies in intake and output during resuscitation.

Volume abnormalities are seen in the trauma patient immediately after surgery and later in the clinical course.[56] Postoperative circulatory instability is recognized first, with changes in other body systems occurring hours later. Extracellular fluid depletion occurs postoperatively due to the continued loss of fluid into the injury or surgical site. Over a period of hours, several liters of extracellular fluid can be sequestered and are functionally lost. The extent of loss is not always quantifiable, but continued volume deficiency produces clinical manifestations. After surgery, blood pressure of less than 90/60 mmHg or heart rate greater than 120 beats per minute should be considered a clinical indication of circulatory insufficiency. Readers are referred to Chapters 8 and 9 for a comprehensive review of normal fluid and electrolyte regulation and acid–base balance.

Overview of Anatomical Injuries

Head Injuries. Although advances in technology provide valuable diagnostic data, the neurological assessment continues to be the keystone of care for the brain-injured patient. Upon admission to the ICU, a baseline neurological assessment should be performed. To evaluate the ongoing status of the patient, this baseline assessment should be compared to the prehospital and emergency department neurological assessments. The neurological assessment should be as comprehensive as possible. Because the type of injury and the patient's ability to follow commands affect the assessment, the comatose patient is assessed somewhat differently from a patient who is able to follow commands. For a comprehensive review of the neurological assessment, refer to Chapter 32.

The neurological assessment should be performed at least every hour and more often, if indicated. The assessment should include GCS, pupillary response to light, diameter of pupils, conjugate gaze, visual ability, motor movement of the face, and reflexes (gag, cough, blink, corneal). An extensive mental/emotional examination may not be possible, but observing the coherence and relevance of speech is important. Orientation to person, place, and time should be elicited. Asking the patient to show two fingers is an excellent way to test comprehension and motor ability. If the patient is unable to follow commands, an extensive motor examination may not be possible. Hemiparesis may be assessed even if the patient is not able to follow commands. Often extremities on one side of the body will use antigravity muscles during movements and the other side will have only lateral movements (dragging leg or arm across the bed). Patients who do not use antigravity muscles (flexion of the arm or knee) may have a hemiparesis. If this observation is new, it should be reported because it may indicate increased ICP from edema or a developing hematoma. Sensory evaluation is often difficult with the brain-injured patient since most of the tests require a patient response. Testing deep tendon reflexes may be useful for comparative purposes. Pathological responses such as Babinski's sign, absence of the occulocephalic reflex (doll's eyes), or a dilated unresponsive pupil should be reported immediately.

Injuries to the head can occur from blunt or penetrating forces. Injuries to the brain or skull are diagnosed primarily by CT scans, but skull x-rays may also be useful. Three types of injuries must be considered. The first type is *extracranial:* scalp lacerations, soft tissue swelling, and injuries to vessels such as the carotid artery, which may lead to brain anoxia or ischemia. Cleansing, debriding, and suturing of scalp lacerations should be performed after priority care has been given.

The second type of injury is *fracture of the cranial vault,* most commonly linear, basilar, closed depressed, open depressed, or comminuted. Linear skull fractures are frequently associated with epidural hematomas, which are secondary injuries. The epidural hematoma arises from the laceration of an artery or vein that was damaged by the bone as it fractured. Arterial bleeding is common, and change in patient status occurs rapidly; immediate surgical intervention is essential for survival. Basilar skull fractures are easily recognized by periorbital (racoon's eyes) and mastoid (Battle's sign) ecchymosis. The dura also may be torn with this type of injury; therefore, leaking of cerebrospinal fluid (CSF) from the nose or ear is common. Since bleeding and CSF leaks may occur simultaneously, it is difficult to determine with a glucose stick if drainage from the ears and nose is actually CSF. The fluid should be tested for the halo or ring sign. CSF dries in rings and looks much like a bull's eye pattern when placed on a white surface. Because the ethmoid and orbital sinuses are fractured along with the base of the skull, there is the potential for communication directly to the brain. Nasogastric and endotracheal tubes must be inserted orally.

Depressed skull fractures are either open or closed; therefore, lacerations should be explored to rule out open fractures. The dura remains intact with a closed depressed skull fracture in which there is no opening from the brain to the outside environment. These fractures may or may not be associated with brain injury. The need for surgical elevation of the depression will depend upon the depth of the depression and the clinical status of the patient. Open depressed skull fractures are the result of either penetrating or blunt forces. Tracts of injury can be created by the missile and bone fragments. Local injury to the surrounding brain tissue is common. Since the brain is exposed to the outside environment, the chance for contamination is great. These injuries require surgical debridement and meningitis and seizures are common complications.

The third type of injury, classified as *primary brain injury,* results from acceleration, deceleration, and compression forces. A variety of injuries ranging from mild to severe can occur in the cortex and brainstem and may or may not be associated with skull fractures. Lacerations, contusions, and diffuse axonal injury are common. Surgical intervention for these injuries may not be possible. Definitive care for these patients includes ICP monitoring and medical therapeutics.

Secondary injury results from the primary injuries, with the most lethal being cerebral edema. Intracranial, intracerebral, epidural, subdural, and subarachnoid hemorrhage can also occur. Surgical intervention for most epidural and subdural hematomas is imperative but may not be possible for intracerebral or subarachnoid hemorrhage.

Intracranial hypertension is a threat for all head-injured patients. Surgical and nonsurgical patients must be observed for changes in intracranial pressure dynamics. An initial treatment for increased ICP is hyperventilation with the $PaCO_2$ maintained between 25 and 30 mmHg. Controlled ventilation (10-12 breaths per minute), moderately high tidal volumes, and a high FiO_2 may be required. Arterial blood gases must be monitored and respiratory alkalosis treated. Osmotic diuresis, a hallmark of ICP management, is achieved using mannitol combined with furosemide. In addition to the osmotic effects of these agents, the secondary benefit is an increase in intravascular volume that temporarily raises mean arterial pressure. The dehydrating effects of osmotic diuresis must be carefully observed. Increases in serum osmolality and serum sodium levels and decreases in potassium must be reported. Supplemental potassium may be necessary, and aggressive diuresis may be supplemented with an hourly urine output/IV replacement protocol. Fluids, once withheld from patients with head injury, are being given to maintain CPP. Albumin and other volume expanders may be used. In addition, vasopressors such as dopamine hydrochloride are being given to support MAP and increase CPP.

Sedation, also previously withheld, is being used widely to reduce the metabolic demands of the brain. Morphine sulfate and other narcotics are being given as continuous drips or on an as-needed basis. Drugs such as diazepam and midazolam are also used. Barbiturates are given to induce the *Barbiturate coma* and are used extensively in some centers to control ICP. These medications limit the usefulness of the neurological assessment. Therefore, patients must have ventilatory support and an ICP monitor to detect changes in ICP status. At this time, the efficacy of corticosteroids is questionable. The use of dexamethisone is no longer a hallmark of care. However, research related to cerebral ischemia may lead to new drugs that are effective in reducing cell destruction and cerebral edema.

Nursing care of the head-injured patient should be individually planned. Position changes in head-injured patients are not contraindicated. Rather, authorities advocate careful observation of the patient after a position change. The neck should be carefully aligned without flexion, and 90° angles of the hip should be avoided. Head of bed elevation should be adjusted to maximize CPP and minimize ICP. Not all patients can tolerate an elevation of 30°. Nursing care activities should not be clustered (several activities performed in succession) since these activities may cause sustained increases in ICP well above the patient's baseline ICP. Rather, activities should be performed separately, allowing time for the ICP to return to baseline.[57,58,59,60]

Sensory stimulation can affect intracranial pressure dynamics. Touch has been demonstrated to reduce ICP, while negative conversations increase ICP. Sensory stimulation programs have also been useful in the care of comatose head-injured patients.[61] Rehabilitation consultation should be initiated immediately to ascertain the patient's short-term and long-term needs. Complications frequently associated with head injuries include stress ulcers, diabetes insipidus, syndrome of inappropriate antidiuretic hormone (SIADH), hydrocephalus, and severe cognitive and physical disabilities. Family needs during the critical stage of injury are tremendous. The critical care nurse must be aware of their need to be with the patient, their desire for information, and their need to know the patient is getting the best possible care.[62] For further information on the needs of the critically ill patient's family, refer to Chapter 17.

Maxillofacial Injuries. Blunt and penetrating forces can cause devastating cosmetic and structural injuries to the face. Injuries to the face may include muscle and soft tissue damage, laceration of facial arteries, transection of cranial nerves, and fractures. The primary concern with serious injuries to the face is patency of the airway. Foreign bodies and tooth fragments may contribute to airway problems. In cases of severe injury, surgical intervention to establish the airway may be required. Internal and external hemorrhage may result in aspiration and impairment of respiratory status. Lacerations, contusions, abrasions, and arterial disruption may contribute to severe blood loss and may lead to disseminated intravascular coagulation (DIC). Cardiorespiratory stabilization is the immediate concern and not the cleansing and suturing of facial lacerations. Tissue injuries that may require surgical management include parotid gland or duct injury, facial nerve injuries, nasolacrimal injuries, and avulsion injuries.[63]

Eye injuries are also a serious concern in patients with facial trauma. Injuries to the ocular globe may require enucleation. These injuries may be evident in the immediate operative stage when cleansing and debriding are accomplished or later in the course of convalescence. Patches may be used to protect the injured eye until surgery can be performed. Simple vision testing such as holding up fingers or objects for identification will provide assessment data. Loss of vision should be documented. Cortical vision loss may occur in brain-injured patients and should not be confused with peripheral vision loss.

Facial fractures may be identified initially by palpating for the presence of crepitus, tenderness, and irregularity of facial structures. Observation of the face for symmetry and dental occlusion is also helpful. An intraoral examination may also be performed. CT scan and facial x-rays (Water's view, Towne's view, lateral, anterior-posterior skull, and mandible) confirm fractures. Nasal fractures are the most common injuries. Zygoma and orbital floor fractures may occur separately or in combination. Loss of upward eye movement may be noted if the inferior rectus muscle is entrapped. Mandibular fractures occur either to the body of the mandible or at the condylar–subcondylar region. Pain on jaw movement and dental malocclusion are common.

There are three classifications of maxillary fractures (Figure 55-4). *LeFort I* is a transverse or horizontal fracture separating the maxillary alveolus from the upper facial skeleton. The *LeFort II* is a pyramid-shaped fracture that separates the nasomaxillary segment from the zygomatic and orbital sections of the facial skeleton. In the *LeFort III* fracture, there is craniofacial dysjunction with actual separation of the facial bones from the cranium. CSF leaks may occur with LeFort II and III fractures, indicating extension of the fracture through the cribriform plate.

Immediate surgery for a LeFort III fracture is recommended to achieve the best results. However, frequently the surgical repair of facial fractures may be

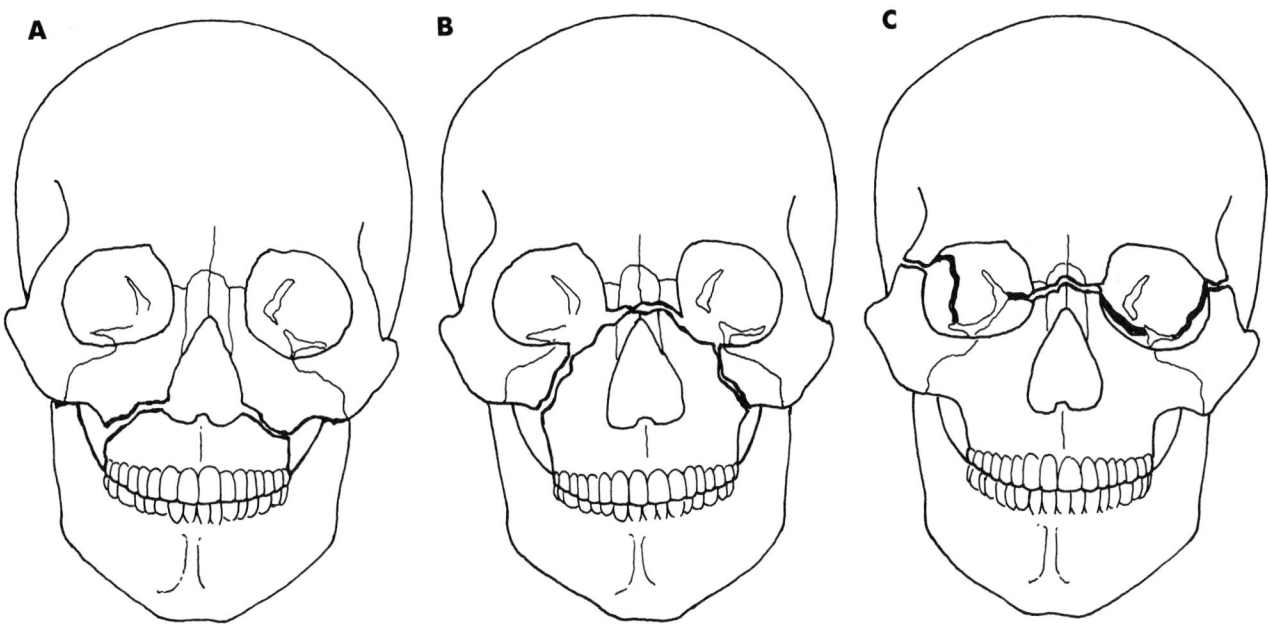

Figure 55-4   Injuries to the midface. *A,* LeFort I. *B,* LeFort II. *C,* LeFort III.

delayed until the patient is stable. The type of surgery performed depends on the injury. Common surgical procedures include closed reductions with arch bars, intermaxillary fixation, external fixation, internal wiring, bone grafting, and complex reconstruction.

The primary focus of the critical care nurse for the patient awaiting surgery or in the postoperative period is maintaining the airway. Before repair, facial fractures are extremely painful. Eating may be compromised due to dental malocclusion, deformities, or pain.

Neck Injuries. The complex anatomy of the neck makes it susceptible to a variety of injuries from blunt and penetrating forces. The trachea, esophagus, arteries, veins, nerves, and cervical spine are potential sites of injury. Missile injuries that cross the midline or blunt forces that increase airway pressure against a closed glottis should alert the nurse to potential injury to the organs and vessels of the neck. Neck swelling, crepitus, dyspnea, hoarseness, cervical tenderness, pain, oral or nasogastric blood, hemoptysis, resistance to passive motion, difficult intubation, and inadequate ventilation despite intubation raise the index of suspicion for injuries to the neck.

The most common *tracheobronchial injury* is to the mainstem bronchus above the carina. Longitudinal and circumferential tears as well as avulsions of the bronchi have been reported. With penetrating injury, esophageal, carotid, and jugular vein trauma may also occur. Clinical manifestations may develop early with persistent pneumothorax, mediastinal air, and subcutaneous emphysema. Alternatively, the in-

jury may become clinically evident several days later when the patient develops subcutaneous emphysema and pneumothorax. A persistent air leak in an existing chest tube may also signal tracheal injury. A covert manifestation of tracheal injury is the development of early and sustained atelectasis due to the occlusion of the bronchi by blood and secretions.[64,65] Diagnosis is confirmed by tracheobronchoscopy or emergency surgical exploration.

Surgical anastomosis may be required for large tears while conservative management may be the preferred approach for smaller injuries. Ventilation is supported by intubation or tracheostomy. In some cases, independent lung ventilation may be considered. Extreme care must be taken with the airway to prevent dislodging or repositioning of the tube prior to and after surgical repair. Frequent assessment of the chest for changes in breathing patterns, breath sounds, or subcutaneous air is important. Continuous air leaks in the pleural chest tube should be reported. Sudden rises in airway pressure can compromise the surgical repair and should be avoided.

Early detection of *esophageal perforation* is important because tissue corrosion by digestive juices and bacteria can occur. Massive fluid loss can lead to pulmonary distress. Fever, dysphagia, and pain may be clinical signs of esophageal tears. Diagnosis is made by esophagoscopy or esophagography. Surgical repair may be a layered closure with drainage or temporary closure of the esophagus and creation of a gastrostomy. Nasogastric intubation, antibiotics, and drainage of the wound are essential.[51,64] Meticulous skin care must be provided because esophageal enzymes can cause erosion of the skin. A bag made from enterostomal products and attached to the neck is ideal for drainage and skin protection. Jejunal feedings or parenteral nutrition must be considered as alternative methods for providing caloric needs. Mediastinitis, esophageal abscess, fistulas, empyema, and peritonitis are potential complications.

Vascular injuries may involve the carotid or vertebral arteries or the jugular veins. Acute or delayed rupture of the carotid or vertebral vessels may present as a rapid change in level of consciousness or as cardiac arrest. Because of the importance of these vessels to cerebral perfusion, anoxic brain injury is likely to occur. Treatment of the brain injury is the same as previously described. The vessel should be repaired immediately. Proximal arteries are repaired by direct suture but distal arteries may require extracranial–intracranial anastomosis.[45] Postoperatively, care must be taken to protect the suture site. The patient should be observed for neck swelling and tongue deviation which may indicate leaking at the surgical site. Outcomes for these patients who may have suffered severe brain anoxia are variable; rehabilitation must be initiated early.

Spinal Cord Injuries. Blunt and penetrating forces are responsible for injuries to the vertebral bodies and the spinal cord. These injuries result from hyperflexion, hyperextension, rotation, or compression. Injuries occur most frequently at the cervical (C-spine) level followed by the lumbar and thoracic levels. Fractures, dislocations, and subluxations occur to vertebral bodies. Concussions, contusions, lacerations, hematomas, and transections are common injuries to the spinal cord. Vertebral and spinal cord injuries can occur alone or in combination. Spinal cord injuries (SCI) are diagnosed by clinical evaluation, C-spine x-rays, and CT scan. The clinical manifestations of injury depend on the level of the cord involved and the physiological damage to sensory and motor tracts. Complete physiological transection of the cord results in complete sensory and motor loss below the level of the lesion. In cervical injuries, quadraplegia results; injuries below T1 produce paraplegia. Incomplete lesions produce a variety of sensory and motor deficits.

The admission neurological assessment establishes a baseline that can be compared to the prehospital and emergency department assessments. Changes in sensory and motor status should be reported immediately. Patients with spinal cord injuries may also have a head injury. With patients in coma, an extensive motor and sensory examination cannot be performed.

Early definitive care of the spinal cord injury centers on stabilization of the spine, which is accomplished for cervical injuries by Gardner-Wells tongs or halo traction. Traction of the cervical spine is achieved by the use of weights which freely swing from the traction apparatus. Usually 10 pounds of weight is sufficient to realign the spine. For lower back injuries, Harrington rods or other stabilizing devices are used. Until recently, pharmacological interventions were not used extensively for SCI. However, large doses of methylprednisolone have been shown to improve motor function, pinprick sensation, and touch if initiated within 8 hours of injury. The initial dose of methylprednisolone given as a bolus is 30 mg per kg over 1 hour, and this is followed by a continuous infusion of 5.4 mg per kg per hour over 23 hours.[66]

The timing of surgical intervention for patients with SCI remains controversial since early intervention has not been associated with better outcomes. Immediate surgical intervention has been recommended if there is an open wound with a CSF leak or if there is spinal canal infringement from bone fragments or moving vertebrae. Cervical fusion or wiring of vertebrae is necessary for neck stability and head control and is done when the patient is stable.

Following SCI, reflex activity below the lesion is suppressed. This condition, known as *spinal shock*, is characterized by flaccid paralysis, hypotension, hypothermia, and bradycardia. Spinal shock may last days to weeks following injury. The sympathetic pathways are impaired in SCI; therefore, patients with SCI have an unopposed parasympathetic response. Persistent bradycardia is best treated with 0.6 mg atropine given intravenously. Vasodilatation and subsequent hypotension should respond to fluid administration. Vasoactive drugs may be used but may not be effective since they target sympathetic pathways.

In planning care, the critical care nurse must consider the myriad of problems associated with SCI. Monitoring ECG and blood pressure is necessary since the parasympathetic nervous system is unopposed. Autonomic dysreflexia is a life-threatening event and should be treated immediately. The inability to vasoconstrict predisposes SCI patients to deep venous thrombosis and pulmonary emboli. Ascending edema of the cervical cord may cause respiratory compromise and arrest if not recognized and treated quickly. Loss of intercostal muscles deceases intrathoracic pressure, so coughing is ineffective. Paralytic ileus may further compromise respiratory status by moving the abdomen into the thoracic space. Bowel and bladder function are impaired, and normal evacuation processes no longer function. Early removal of the Foley catheter and replacement by intermittent catheterization will decrease the potential for urinary tract infections and begin the process of training the bladder for reflex voiding. A bowel regimen should be initiated early. The SCI patient cannot shiver or sweat below the level of the lesion; therefore, body temperature cannot be adjusted. Critical care nurses caring for SCI patients are confronted with frightened and immobilized individuals. Recognition of the losses the SCI patient faces will assist the nurse to develop a plan of care that supports the patient's needs.[67]

Lung and Thoracic Injuries. All injuries to the chest have the potential to be life-threatening. However, prompt recognition of these injuries and rapid intervention can decrease morbidity and mortality. Changes in patient status can be detected by physical examination; evaluation of laboratory studies, such as ABGs; and changes in ventilator parameters. Results of diagnostic studies performed prior to admission to the ICU such as chest x-rays, arteriograms, bronchoscopy, ECG, and CT scans will also be useful in assessing the changing status of the patient. Knowledge of the mechanism of injury provides a high index of suspicion for the evolution of potential life-threatening injuries.

Development of a *tension pneumothorax* may be acute or delayed. It may develop from the injury event, from a therapeutic intervention such as covering a sucking chest wound, or from barotrauma. Barotrauma is an iatrogenic complication caused by excessive amounts of positive end-expiratory pressure (PEEP). The tolerable limits of PEEP may be individualized at levels below 20 cmH$_2$O. However, with high levels of PEEP, barotrauma should be anticipated.

A tension pneumothorax occurs when there is an injury to the pleura that allows air from the lung to escape into the pleural space during inspiration. A flap of tissue or some other obstruction acts as a one-way valve preventing the escape of air during exhalation. Consequently, with each inspiration there is a buildup of air, and pressure inside the pleural cavity increases. This pressure prevents the injured lung from expanding and pushes the thoracic structures to the opposite side of the chest. Compression of the noninjured lung, great vessels, and heart occurs. Respiratory effort is decreased and cardiac output is compromised. Clinical manifestations include tracheal deviation to the unaffected side, agitation and restlessness, neck vein distention, and cyanosis. Tension pneumothorax is an emergent problem and must be treated quickly. Insertion of a large-gauge needle into the second intercostal space at the midclavicular line on the affected side will relieve the pressure. Creating a simple pneumothorax should ameliorate respiratory distress. Insertion of a chest tube should follow any temporary measures used to relieve the pressure.

When covering an open sucking chest wound, complete occlusion of the wound can predispose the patient to a tension pneumothorax. Allowing one side of the dressing to remain open prevents the development of a one-way valve.

A moderate to large *hemothorax* may occur with blunt or penetrating wounds to the heart or great vessels. Injury to pulmonary or systemic vessels such as the intercostal artery or branches of the aorta may also produce hemothorax. As large amounts of blood fill the pleural space, lung compression occurs, followed by a mediastinal shift, impairment of venous return, and respiratory distress. The amount of blood filling the pleural space is not well visualized in a supine x-ray since large amounts of blood will collect in the posterior gutters. Insertion of a chest tube with connection to suction is necessary. The goal is to evacuate the blood completely from the pleural space and restore respirations to normal. Observation of the patient for respiratory distress, changes in chest tube drainage, and air leaks are important activities for the critical care nurse. Indications for an exploratory thoracotomy are:

- Persistent drainage greater than 200 ml/hr for 3 to 4 hours
- Increased bleeding over 3 to 5 hours
- Drainage greater than 500 ml over 2 hours
- Large clotted hemothorax

A decrease in chest tube drainage should also be investigated. Causes for decreased drainage are cessation of bleeding, occlusion of the chest tube, or thrombus formation. Reinsertion of the tube or exploratory thoracotomy may be required.

Flail chest is common with blunt trauma, especially MVCs, and is characterized by paradoxical movement of the chest and tachypnea. The flail is created by double fractures of several ribs or the presence of sternal and rib fractures. Pulmonary contusion may be an associated injury. Mechanical ventilation with PEEP stabilizes the flail segments. Chest wall pain may be alleviated by analgesics or intercostal nerve blocks.[45,64]

Pulmonary contusions occur more frequently from blunt trauma but may be seen in penetrating injury. Rib fractures with or without a flail chest are associated injuries. Chest wall abrasions or ecchymosis may be present. Bloody secretions may be suctioned from the trachea. Respiratory distress develops secondary to interstitial edema and alveolar hemorrhage. A pulmonary shunt is created, and hypoxia ensues. Although chest x-rays may demonstrate nonsegmental infiltrates, the extent of pulmonary contusions is usually underestimated by the chest x-ray. The best clinical indicators of a pulmonary contusion are decreased lung compliance and a PaO$_2$/FiO$_2$ ratio less than 300 on supplemental oxygen.[45,64] Intubation and PEEP are the recommended treatments. These patients have the potential to develop pneumonia, pulmonary edema, and adult respiratory distress syndrome (ARDS). Refer to Chapter 29 for further information.

Heart Injuries. *Cardiac tamponade* frequently occurs in penetrating chest wounds but is not as common in blunt injuries. Direct perforation of the pericardial sac, the heart, or coronary vessels results in pericardial tamponade. The classic symptoms of tamponade are decreased blood pressure, distended neck veins, increased CVP, paradoxical pulse, electromechanical dissociation, and muffled heart sounds (rare). Restlessness and agitation are seen if the patient is conscious. These symptoms occur as the pericardium fills with blood and the ability of the heart to contract is restricted. Stroke volume is decreased and cardiac output is compromised. The emergent treatment for tamponade is pericardiocentesis. Surgical exploration of the chest and repair of injuries are required. Often, a pericardial window is created to prevent further episodes of tamponade. Surgical repair of vessels or lacerations to the right ventricle may also be indicated.

Myocardial contusion must be suspected with blunt injuries to the chest. Ecchymosis, chest wall pain, and abrasions suggest underlying injury to the heart. Dysrhythmias, conduction blocks, and myocardial ischemia may be present. Hypotension that is refractory to fluid resuscitation is a strong indicator of myocardial injury. A definitive diagnosis may require serial ECGs and evaluation of isoenzymes. A CPK-MB/total CPK greater than or equal to 5% or elevated LDH1 and LDH2 confirm cardiac contusion. Treatment for cardiac contusion is the same as the treatment for myocardial infarction.[45,64]

Aortic disruption can be a rapidly fatal injury, or it may be an insidious killer. Sudden deceleration injuries (occurring more frequently with ejection) may disrupt the thoracic aorta at the takeoff of the subclavian artery. Almost 85% of individuals with this injury die at the scene. Of the survivors, 20% die within 6 hours after injury and 72% die within the first week.[45] Clinical manifestations of aortic disruption are not always overt. Intrascapular pain, dysphagia (secondary to compression of the esophagus), hoarseness, dyspnea, and upper extremity hypertension (acute coarctation) may be present. The initial chest x-ray may appear normal. Abnormalities in the chest x-ray that increase suspicion include ill-defined aortic knob, superior mediastinal widening, depression of the mainstem bronchus, tracheal deviation to the right, and deviation of the nasogastric tube to the right. Aortography will confirm the diagnosis.[45] Sur-

gical repair should be accomplished as quickly as possible. Comparison of upper and lower extremity blood pressures is not routinely done in the emergency department or ICU. In patients who have sustained severe deceleration injuries, however, upper and lower blood pressure checks should be standard care.

Injuries to the diaphragm may be caused by blunt or penetrating forces. These injuries are frequently associated with intraperitoneal injuries. Injuries to the left diaphragm occur most frequently with blunt trauma. Clinical manifestation of a diaphragmatic disruption include respiratory distress, shock, hyperresonance to percussion, and bowel sounds in the lower chest. An x-ray of the chest may reveal a NG tube in the left thorax, visceral herniation as evidenced by air bubbles in the left chest, or mediastinal shift. Danger of bowel obstruction or strangulation is significant since the bowel will herniate through the diaphragmatic opening. Surgical repair should be performed as soon as possible.

Abdominal and Pelvic Injuries. Injuries to the abdomen and pelvis from blunt or penetrating forces may result in significant lesions. Successful management requires rapid detection of vascular and visceral injuries and control of hemorrhage. In some cases, abdominal injury is latent; therefore, changes in the abdominal examination, referred pain, fever, or circulatory instability must not be overlooked.

When caring for a patient with suspected or diagnosed injury to the abdomen, it is important to remember the locations, types, and functions of the organs. Hollow organs can rupture if intraabdominal pressures are high, as in the case of blunt forces, or hollow organs can be penetrated in the case of gunshots or stabbings. Contamination occurs when the contents of these organs (urine, feces, food particles, and digestive enzymes) spill into the peritoneal cavity. Injury to solid organs can result in massive hemorrhage and abscesses. Pelvic fractures can cause serious injury to genitourinary structures and hemorrhage into the retroperitoneal space. In the female patient of childbearing age, the possibility of pregnancy must be considered.

The abdominal examination when performed on admission to the ICU should be compared to abdominal findings during the prehospital and emergency department phases. Frequent abdominal assessments are crucial whether the patient is being treated conservatively (observation without surgery) or has had surgery. Review of the intraoperative record and physician's postoperative notes provides a foundation for care. Knowledge of fluids administered intraoperatively, type of anesthesia, and surgical procedure assists the nurse to create an appropriate management plan.

Special attention should be directed to pain, not only for management of pain but because development of pain may be an indication of latent or overlooked injury. Incision sites, colostomies, and drains must be inspected frequently. Output from the NG tube, drains, and wound dressings should be recorded and excessive drainage reported. Persistent oozing of blood should arouse concern. Creative use of enterostomal products provides protection to the skin from draining wounds and fistulas. Careful review of fluid and electrolyte balance will alert the nurse to fluid volume deficits or electrolyte abnormalities. Coagulation studies, hemoglobin, hematocrit, and arterial blood gas studies should be evaluated frequently. Feeding alternatives must be considered early. Signs of infection must be investigated immediately and antibiotics administered as prescribed.

Gastrointestinal Injuries. *Gastric injury* is most often caused by penetrating forces but can also occur from blunt forces. Blood in NG aspirate in a patient with a penetrating wound indicates injury to the stomach but may also indicate swallowed blood in a patient with multiple injuries. An upright chest x-ray may reveal a pneumoperitoneum indicative of stomach perforation. Peritoneal lavage is positive for red blood cells. Exploratory laporatomy is performed to decrease contamination, debride devitalized tissue, and close the defect.[45] Postoperatively, the patient should receive antibiotics and retain an NG tube for gastric decompression.

Injuries to the *duodenum* may result from either penetrating or blunt trauma. Significant morbidity and mortality are associated with duodenal injuries. Clinical indicators of injury are abdominal tenderness in the right upper quadrant and vomiting. Fever may occur within hours of injury. Pneumoperitoneum or right upper quadrant gas bubbles may be visualized on x-ray. Surgery is performed to close the defect, debride tissue, and decrease contamination. An NG tube for decompression and administration of antibiotics are common postoperative therapies. A feeding jejunostomy may be inserted at the time of surgery so that enteral feedings can be started postoperatively.[45,68]

Injuries to the *small bowel* are common in both blunt and penetrating trauma. Abdominal pain and peritoneal irritation are clinical signs of injury. Pneumoperitoneum may not be present on x-ray. Peritoneal lavage may be positive for bile, and the white cell count may be elevated. Injury to the small bowel is not confined to perforation alone. Frequently, contusions of the small bowel are present and pose a hazard because necrosis and perforation may occur later. Surgery is directed toward repair of the enterotomies and may be accomplished by simple over-

sewing or resection with anastomosis. A primary closure may be done. Postoperatively patients will have an NG tube and require antibiotics. Parenteral feeding may be initiated. Complications following surgery include abscess formation and disruption of the anastomosis.[45]

Because of high bacterial count in the *large bowel*, injuries to this area carry a high morbidity and mortality. Injuries in this area are the result of blunt and penetrating forces. Abdominal pain and peritoneal irritation may be present. Peritoneal lavage may be positive for vegetable fiber and demonstrate an elevated white count. Surgical treatment varies, depending on the extent of injury to the colon. Small lacerations may be sutured. If severe contusions or large or multiple lacerations are present, resection may be required. Exteriorization of the bowel is common, as are loop colostomies. Nasogastric tubes and antibiotics are standard therapy. Peritonitis and sepsis are primary complications in this group of patients.[45]

Liver and Biliary Tract Injuries. Liver injuries, occurring from blunt and penetrating forces, range from mild to severe. Hemorrhage is a major complication, followed by intraabdominal abscess. Shock, right hemithorax injury, right upper quadrant ecchymosis, and pain are manifestations of liver injury. Diagnosis is made by exploratory laparotomy, liver scan, CT scan, or angiography. Associated injuries to hepatic vasculature and the biliary drainage system increase morbidity and mortality. Surgical goals are hemostasis, debridement, and drainage. Extent of surgery depends on the amount of bleeding. Minimal bleeding may be handled by local control and drainage; moderate bleeding may require suture of the lacerations, ligation of vessels, or embolization; severe bleeding may be complicated by hypothermia and coagulopathies. If bleeding cannot be controlled in the operating room, the abdomen may be packed with laparotomy pads and the patient taken to the ICU. Removal of the laparotomy pads and surgical repair is usually performed 1 to 2 days later when hemostasis is achieved and bleeding has subsided. Debridement of small sections of devitalized tissue is recommended unless the liver is severely pulped. Pulped injuries of the liver require a lobectomy.[45] Caring for the patient with liver injuries is a challenge. Achieving hemostasis in the face of coagulopathy requires continuous evaluation of patient status and laboratory studies and the administration of numerous blood products.

The *spleen* is the solid organ most commonly injured from blunt trauma. Splenic injuries are rarely seen from penetrating forces. Because of the highly vascular composition of the spleen, massive hemorrhage is possible. Abdominal pain localized to the left upper quadrant, left lower rib fracture, distended abdomen, and pain in the left shoulder in Trendelenberg position are clinical manifestations of splenic injury. Radiological studies may show displacement of the stomach or the splenic flexure of the colon. Peritoneal lavage is positive for red blood cells if the capsule has been penetrated. Delayed splenic rupture is possible from an undiagnosed injury or dissolution of a clot. Left upper quadrant pain and symptoms of shock may appear 7 to 14 days after initial injury.[45] Surgical intervention is directed toward controlling hemorrhage and salvaging splenic tissue. Splenectomy may be performed if severe damage is present, the patient is unstable, or coagulopathy develops. The spleen is thought to have a role in immune function; therefore, splenorrhaphy is the procedure of choice, since the spleen is not removed and its role in immune function is preserved.

Pancreatic injury is more common in penetrating trauma and more easily detected. Injury following blunt trauma can be very deceptive, increasing morbidity and mortality. Injuries can occur to the head, tail, or body of the pancreas. Control of hemorrhage, debridement of devitalized tissue, and external drainage are the major operative considerations. Early clinical manifestations following blunt trauma include upper abdominal pain or tenderness. Rising amylase levels suggest pancreatic injury. Epigastric pain, guarding, cardiovascular instability, respiratory insufficiency, or sepsis are later signs. External injury to the abdomen such as ecchymosis, spinal fractures of T11-T12, and lower rib fractures produce an index of suspicion for pancreatic injury. Small lacerations of the pancreas are sutured, but larger wounds may require a distal pancreatectomy. Drainage of the pancreas is imperative. Fistulas, pseudocysts, abscesses, pancreatitis, and delayed hemorrhage are complications of pancreatic injury.

Urinary Tract Injuries. Injury to the urinary tract should be suspected with blunt trauma to the back and flank areas. Any penetrating injury has the potential to damage the urinary tract. Abdominal, back, or flank pain and inability to void are general manifestations of injury. Urinary tract injury must be ruled out in patients with hypotension, evidence of pelvic trauma, lower rib fractures, hematuria, blood at the urethral meatus, absence of urine after catheterization, or difficulty passing a urethral catheter. Diagnostic studies performed are CT scan, IVP, and renal angiography.

Kidney injuries are classifed by severity. Class I is most severe, may be associated with massive bleeding, and requires surgery. Class II is considered a moderate injury involving transcortical lacerations and subscapular hematomas. Surgery may be delayed for this group. Class III is a minor injury such as a renal contusion and requires no surgery.[45] Renal arteries and veins may also be injured. Ligation of the artery may be necessary to control hemorrhage. Infection, renovascular hypertension, fistulas, and ureteral obstruction are complications of kidney injury.

Bladder perforations can lead to significant mortality and morbidity if not detected early. Bladder injuries are confirmed by cystography and are described as intraperitoneal or retroperitoneal. An intraperitoneal injury is commonly seen when the full bladder is perforated. Retroperitoneal injuries are associated with anterior pelvic fractures. Bladder rupture requires surgical repair with debridement and bladder decompression. Foley catheters are used for decompression for all patients and suprapubic cystostomy is recommended in males.[45]

Injuries to the posterior *urethra* are associated with pelvic fractures. Cystography reveals an elevated bladder. This injury is suspected in males if the prostate feels soft, is high riding, or is absent on the rectal examination. Catheterization should not be attempted in these patients. Suprapubic cystostomy is recommended. Surgery to repair the defect is delayed until pelvic hematomas have resolved. Trauma to the anterior urethra is suspected in straddle injuries and penile lacerations. These patients should not void because voiding will cause massive extravasation of urine. Small lacerations can be repaired promptly. Suprapubic cystostomy is reserved for larger injuries.[45]

Skeletal Injuries. The prevalence of musculoskeletal injuries related to trauma is high. In the face of life-threatening injury, skeletal injuries seem to be given secondary status, but prudent care of these injuries prevents early complications and long-term disabilities. Fractures are classifed as closed (simple) or open (compound). When the skin overlying the fracture remains intact, the fracture is considered closed. The fracture is open when the skin overlying the fracture is disrupted. Open fractures are graded according to the severity of injury. A grade I open fracture has a small wound with little soft tissue damage. Grade II fractures are associated with contusions to the skin and muscle. Moderate or massive wounds and trauma to muscle, blood vessels, and nerves are classified as grade III fractures.

The classic signs of musculoskeletal trauma include deformity, swelling, pain, pallor, diminished or absent pulses, paresthesia, paresis, and paralysis. The length of the extremity is palpated to determine displacement, crepitus, pain, and pulses. Joints above and below the fracture are checked for associated ligamentous and meniscal injuries. Loss of full range of motion in a limb should be noted. Pelvic stability is evaluated by pushing down on the iliac wings.

The amount of bleeding associated with multiple fractures can be overlooked. It is important to monitor serial hematocrits during and after the resuscitation phase. Frequently, a crystalloid resuscitation is adequate to raise blood pressure. As bleeding continues, however, patients may develop metabolic acidosis. Administration of red blood cells and cardiorespiratory support may be warranted. If the pulse is compromised or ischemic changes occur in the limb distal to the fracture, angiography with subsequent vascular repair may be necessary.

Treatment for fractures is reduction. Open fractures should be surgically debrided and reduced within 18 hours of injury. Complications such as infection and nonunion increase with intervention delays. Closed reduction occurs when good alignment can be obtained with plaster cast or splint. Continuous reduction (skeletal traction) is achieved by a system of weights and counterweights that realign the extremity. External skeletal traction achieves internal bone alignment using internal pins and external bars. Pins are surgically placed in proximal and distal bone fragments, then connected to a series of bars which are strategically connected to the pins to assure alignment. Visualization of the fracture and repair requires open reduction and internal fixation. Reduction of fractures should reduce pain. Unrelieved pain or new pain should be investigated. Serial neuromuscular checks should be considered standard care for patients with extremity injuries.

Injuries to the *pelvis* range from simple fractures requiring bed rest to open fractures carrying a high mortality. Pelvic fractures are associated with massive bleeding and organ injuries. Retroperitoneal bleeding is common, and the source of the bleeding is difficult to isolate. Often blood extravasates into the perineum, scrotum, and buttocks. Reabsorption of blood and clot dissolution may be physiologically overwhelming tasks leading to abscess formation. Unstable fractures are treated with external fixation. Infection of the pin sites, pelvic wound, and pelvic bones is possible.

Large blood losses also are associated with femoral fractures. Reduction of the fracture can be achieved using the classic Steinmann pins for skeletal traction, closed reduction and internal fixation by intermedullary nailing, open reduction and internal fixation by intermedullary nailing, or open reduction and internal fixation by plating.[45] Weight-bearing restrictions range from days to months. The method of femur repair and the imposed immobility can affect respiratory status.

Complications associated with fractures have been recognized. *Fat embolism* can occur with fractures of the long bone. If restlessness, dyspnea, disorientation, and truncal petechiae occur, fat embolism should be considered. *Compartment syndrome* develops when fluid accumulates in the muscle compartments secondary to bleeding or fluid extravasation. The tight fascial covering prevents expansion of the muscle, resulting in compression of nerves and muscles in the compartment. Pain is a hallmark of compartment syndrome and should not be ignored. Fasciotomy is the treatment of choice. *Crush syndrome* is a systemic response to prolonged pressure or compression of an extremity and is characterized by hypovolemia, rhabdomyolysis, acute tubular necrosis, and compartment syndrome. Acid–base balance and fluid and electrolyte balance are disrupted, and cardiac dysrhythmias occur. A high index of suspicion and early detection of events leading to crush syndrome may limit mortality and morbidity.

REHABILITATION

Rehabilitation is a dynamic process whereby abilities are maximized.[69] It begins the moment the patient is admitted to the hospital. The trauma patient may require a number of rehabilitation services such as cognitive, physical, vocational, social, and psychological. Although many of these services cannot be provided in the critical care unit, recognizing the need for rehabilitation care and planning for it is a short-term goal with long-term impact.

Rehabilitation is a team effort. The team should include the primary nurse, trauma physician, physiatrist, physical therapist, occupational therapist, speech therapist, social worker, psychologist, nutritionist, and other designated health care providers.

Trauma rehabilitation should be implemented in three phases. *Phase one* is the critical care phase. A rehabilitation consultation should be obtained within the first 24 to 48 hours after admission. A preliminary plan should be developed that addresses the immediate needs of the patient and the long-term goals. Since recovery from injury is a dynamic process, the plan should be flexible and easily revised. The patient's progress toward stabilization should be monitored closely by the primary nurse. When the patient emerges from the life-threatening stage of injury, rehabilitation should begin. Initially, the patient may be a passive participant in the rehabilitation process. Passive range of motion exercises, sensory stimulation programs, or splinting may be provided for a comatose patient. Most often, a rehabilitation specialist will be seeing the patient in the unit. Active participation by the patient may not begin until much later in the recovery process. Communication between team members is an integral part of the implementation of the plan. If possible, weekly staff meetings should be held to evaluate the patient's progress and update the plan.

Phase two of the rehabilitation process begins when the patient is transferred to a step-down unit or general nursing unit. In this phase, the patient may be taken to the rehabilitation department where more sophisticated interventions and treatments can be provided. The patient may now be an active participant. Family visitation is less restricted in this area and involvement of family members in rehabilitation is encouraged. Identification of resources for continuation of rehabilitation services after discharge is essential. Insurance coverage, if available, may be limited. Communication with a rehabilitation center for inpatient or outpatient services should be initiated early. The rehabilitation evaluation for the center should be scheduled early so that alternative centers can be found if the patient is not eligible. The family should be encouraged to visit the center or communicate with personnel from the center as soon as possible.

The *third phase* of rehabilitation is either in a rehabilitation center or at home. Education of family members should prepare them for this phase. Refer to other sources for detailed information on rehabilitation services and interventions.

ORGAN DONATION

The balance between life and death is often fragile for the trauma patient. No one understands this better than the critical care nurse who directs much energy to saving the patient's life. The critical care nurse may be the first to confront the sensitive issue of brain death. For this reason, knowledge of the process of organ donation is essential for the nurse caring for trauma patients.

Organ donation or procurement involves the retrieval of viable organs for the purpose of transplantation from an individual who has been declared brain dead. Organs suitable for donation are kidney, liver, pancreas, heart, lung, cornea, bone marrow, bones, and skin.

Persons who die from traumatic injury are generally young and healthy. For this reason, they are major contributors to organ donor programs. Up to 24,000 persons are declared brain dead annually. Unfortunately, the actual number who donate organs is small. In some states, laws have been passed that require physicians to request organs from family members of brain dead patients. Although the law forces action on the issue, the emotional connection between the patient and the family at such a stressful time is an obstacle. Familes are often distraught and know very little about brain death. They are often reluctant to make the decision to donate. Critical care nurses are key figures in educating families about organ donation. The relationship between the nurse and the family is established quickly in the trauma setting. Family members are comfortable asking the nurse questions about patient status. Often, discussions with the family about brain death, the organ retrieval

---

Criteria for Organ Donation

CRITERIA FOR ACCEPTABILITY

- Brain death from brain damage in a previously healthy person *and*
- Suitable physiological age (age requirements vary depending on the organ donated) *and*
- Satisfactory blood pressure, physical examination, and history (requirements depend on organ donated)

CRITERIA FOR NONACCEPTABILITY

- Prolonged ischemia due to profound hypotension or asystole *or*
- Trauma or disease of the organ to be donated *or*
- Selected malignant diseases *or*
- History of diabetes mellitus, hypertension, cardiovascular disease, or peripheral vascular disease[71] *or*
- History of substance abuse, especially IV drug abuse, as evaluated on an individual basis *or*
- History or clinical evidence of infectious diseases such as hepatitis or HIV

---

process, and the potential good that can come from donation will assist the family to make an informed decision about donation.

Organ procurement occurs under the direction of a donor coordinator who is a member of an organ procurement agency such as Life Link or Kidney One. Organ procurement agencies are organized within a regional system for the purpose of timely procurement and matching of donors and recipients. When a potential donor is identified, the agency is notified. The coordinator is responsible for validating the eligibility of the donor, obtaining signed consents, determining the organs to be donated, and overseeing the pretrieval organ viability interventions. The coordinators are available to the family at all times. Criteria for organ donors are listed in the box above.

Once consent has been obtained for donation, the critical care nurse receives direction from the coordinator. Matching the donor with an eligible recipient is an immediate concern. Laboratory studies are sent, and results are reported to the donor agency. A computer search of potential recipients is done, and the organ retrieval team is notified. The time between locating a recipient and arrival of the retrieval team may be hours; therefore, the viability of the organs must be assured. This is especially important because the brain no longer has control of the fluid and electrolyte balance of the body. Previous therapies are terminated, and interventions to protect the viability of the organs are initiated.

The nurse and the family need to be supported through this final phase. Protecting the viability of the organs may be an intensive process; therefore, it is a very busy time for the nurse. The nurse may also experience feelings of loss for the patient. At the same time, the nurse is continuing to support the family. If organ retrieval occurs frequently, a support group for the nurses who are involved in donation should be considered.

DISASTER MANAGEMENT

A disaster is a community or regional event that disrupts normal community function and raises concerns about the well-being of the people and property of the community.[70] This definition is consistent with the World Health Organization's view that a disaster is a sudden ecological phenomenon of sufficient magnitude to require external resources.[71] Disasters are classifed as natural (earthquakes, floods, hurricanes, tornadoes, volcanic eruptions, fires, blizzards, and landslides) and man-made (airplane crashes, train wrecks, explosions, fires, collapsed buildings, terrorist activities, and release of hazardous material).

Disasters are complex events that cannot be handled when the victims arrive at the hospital doorstep; therefore, a well-prepared community plan that involves hospitals, emergency services, and community organizations is essential.[70] The goal of disaster management is to reduce morbidity and mortality in a situation with limited supplies and personnel.[63] Coordinated disaster planning was mandated by the 1973 Emergency Medical Services Act. Therefore, management of a local disaster may be under the disaster policy of a city or a state. The state health planners for disaster and the local emergency management agencies work together so that personnel and resources are available during a disaster.[72] A community disaster committee sets the standards and reviews the disaster policy to meet community needs. Each hospital in the community interfaces with the external or community-wide disaster plan. In addition, the hospital has an internal disaster plan that includes policies and operational guidelines for a disaster. Each department in the hospital has a disaster plan that outlines the responsibilities of the department and the roles of department members. The plan is activated when the hospital is notified of an actual or potential disaster.

Disasters typically produce three types of patients: those with surgical problems (physical injury), medical problems (inhalation or system toxicity), or psychiatric problems. A patient flow line is established from the point of injury to the hospital. This flow or movement of patients through the health care system should be well planned and communicated. A field command post is set up at the disaster site. Two objectives should be operant at this level. The first objective is to identify, treat, and transport the victims and the second objective is to notify the hospitals of the type and number of victims that may be sent. Triage of patients by EMS personnel occurs at this location. Priority care is given to persons who will survive. These victims are transported by ground or air ambulance to the hospital emergency department. It is important to note that other victims may also be arriving. These are victims who may have been brought by bystanders or who come on their own. Arrival of this ambulatory group may be the first notification to the hospital that a disaster has occurred.

If the hospital has advance notice, the internal disaster plan should be underway. Admission and discharge of patients occurs simultaneously, and resources are mobilized to the emergency department, operating room, and ICU. Once in the emergency department, patients are again triaged. Four traiage categories are used in disasters:

Category I patients require minimal treatment.

Category II patients require immediate treatment for survival.

Category III patients can tolerate delayed treatment with good survival.

Category IV patients have multiple injuries and have a poor chance of survival.

When the status of the patient has been determined, the patient is transferred to the location where the best care can be provided. Patients will be directly admitted to the operating room, ICU, general nursing unit, or mental health units. The coordinated effort of all hospital personnel will make disaster and mass casualty situations less chaotic. Periodic review of the internal disaster plan and participation in community-wide disaster drills are important factors in evaluating the "ready" status of the hospital.

CASE STUDY: PENETRATING TRAUMA

A 22-year-old female is brought to the trauma center with a gunshot wound to the left upper quandrant of the abdomen. Mechanism of injury is a penetrating wound from a .22 caliber handgun. The weapon was discharged approximately 3 feet from the victim. At the scene, the woman was found lying on the floor awake but lethargic. Paramedics estimated a 200-ml blood loss at the scene.

Prehospital
Assessment:

Glasgow Coma Score = 14
Blood pressure = 86/60 mmHg
Heart rate = 130 beats per minute
Respiratory rate = 30/min
RTS = 10

One liter lactated Ringer's (LR) solution infused via a 16-gauge IV line. Second liter hung as patient was brought into the emergency department. Oxygen administration via face mask at 10 L/min. Abdominal dressing applied now saturated with blood.

Emergency Department
Primary Survey

Airway clear, respirations rapid and shallow. Respiratory rate is 30/min. Decreased breath sounds on the left side. Oxygen via face mask at 10 L/min. Femoral pulse present. Blood pressure is 90/60 mmHg after 2 L of LR. Second IV line started and infusing LR. GCS 14, opens eyes to verbal stimuli, follows commands; speech clear and comprehensible. RTS increased to 11 after crystalloid infusion. Blood is oozing from the abdominal wound. ECG shows sinus tachycardia at 120 beats per minute. Entrance wound noted left upper quandrant. No exit wound identified. Foley catheter is inserted. Urine output is 300 ml. Urine output maintained at 15 ml every 15 minutes. Nasogastric tube inserted, and drainage is Hematest negative.

Laboratory Studies

ABG   = pH 7.41, P_{O_2} 91, P_{CO_2} 38,
                  Bicarb 27, Sat. 94%
Hematocrit   = 28%
WBC   = 12,400
Urine HCG   = Positive
Blood alcohol   = 0.00 mg/dl
Urine drug study = Negative

Secondary Survey

Abdomen painful, distended, and dull to percussion over all quadrants. Blood found in rectum. No bowel sounds heard. Free air in left upper chest seen on chest x-ray. No other injuries identified. Blood pressure decreased to 82/64 mmHg. Diagnostic peritoneal lavage deferred. Patient given tetanus toxoid and antibiotics. Discharged to OR at 0230.

Index of Suspicion

1. Injury to colon, small bowel, possibly stomach. *Rationale:* Low-velocity weapon discharged at close range. Muzzle velocity similar to impact velocity. Left upper quadrant injury, suspect transverse colon or splenic injury. Meandering nature of low-velocity weapons without exit wound suggests presence of other injuries. Rule out stomach perforation. Elevated WBC count suggests contamination.

2. Injury to diaphragm. *Rationale:* Upper left quadrant injury. With diaphragmatic excursion missile can penetrate the chest cavity. Air on the chest film suggests movement of abdominal contents into the chest. Absence of breath sounds on the left may indicate air or fluid inhibiting lung expansion.

3. Class II hemorrhage with hypovolemic shock. Painful, distended abdomen and rectal blood suggest internal bleeding. Hypotension with elevated heart rate indicates volume loss of greater than 750 ml. Recurrent hypotension following fluid resuscitation indicates continued bleeding. Hematocrit of 28% suggests bleeding.

4. Contaminated peritoneum. WBC count elevated. Gunshot wound with clothing or other debris entering wound is possible. With potential penetration of large and small bowel and stomach, must always consider contamination.

5. Pregnancy. In women of childbearing age, pregnancy should be ruled out. Patient has a positive HCG.

Medical Management

Exploratory laparotomy with repair of diaphragmatic laceration, multiple small bowel enterotomies, and left transverse colostomy. No injury to stomach or spleen. Intraoperative blood loss estimated at 1,800 ml. Five liters LR and 1 unit packed red cells administered. Intraoperative hematocrit 30%. Arterial line inserted. Discharged from the operating room with an endotracheal tube in place and mechanically ventilated with 6 intermittent mandatory ventilations (IMV) per minute. ABGs within normal limits. Blood pressure was 90/56 mmHg and heart rate was 110 beats per minute. Intraoperative urine output was 400 ml.

NURSING MANAGEMENT: CASE STUDY

■ NURSING DIAGNOSIS

Altered tissue perfusion, related to hypovolemic shock that began at the scene.

OUTCOME STANDARD AND CRITERIA

Respiration and nutrition at the cellular level is supported as evidenced by:
- Stable hemodynamic parameters
- Absence of hemorrhage

NURSING INTERVENTIONS

- Administer crystalloid and colloid solutions to maintain systolic blood pressure >90 mm Hg
- Investigate continued hemodynamic instability for possible untreated or unrecognized injuries
- Prepare patient for possible surgery
- Administer vasoactive drugs as prescribed to achieve and maintain hemodynamic stability
- Support respiratory status by administration of oxygen, intubation, and mechanical ventilation
- Monitor hemodynamic parameters including $S\bar{v}_{O_2}$; level of consciousness; vital signs; fluid and electrolyte status; hematocrit and hemoglobin (H&H); and prothrombin, partial thromboplastin, and platelets[74]

HIGH-RISK NURSING DIAGNOSES

Activity intolerance, altered body temperature, ineffective breathing, decreased cardiac output, fluid volume deficit, or impaired gas exchange,[73] related to multiorgan failure, sepsis, DIC, renal failure, ARDS, and liver failure.

■ NURSING DIAGNOSIS

Potential for infection, related to contaminated wound.

OUTCOME STANDARD AND CRITERIA

Local or systemic infection is absent as evidenced by:
- Absence of signs and symptoms of localized infection (redness, tenderness, swelling, purulent drainage, odor)[74]
- Absence of signs and symptoms of systemic infection (fever, tachycardia)[74]

NURSING INTERVENTIONS

- Perform dressing changes as needed

- Establish routine infection control measures
- Administer antibiotics, antifungal medications as prescribed
- Observe status of wound for healing, signs of infection
- Obtain blood cultures as needed
- Monitor fevers of unknown origin, changes in level of consciousness, central and peripheral line insertion sites, status of immune response (WBCs), skin integrity, and nutritional status

HIGH-RISK NURSING DIAGNOSES

Impaired skin integrity, impaired mobility, alteration in nutrition: less than body requirements, or pain,[73] related to sepsis and peritonitis.

COLLABORATIVE DIAGNOSIS

High risk for spontaneous abortion, related to injury while pregnant.

OUTCOME STANDARD AND CRITERIA

Pregnancy is maintained as evidenced by:
- Fetus is not aborted *or*
- Spontaneous abortion is recognized, and therapeutic interventions are initiated to protect mother from untoward complications

NURSING INTERVENTIONS

- Validate pregnancy and determine gestational age of fetus
- Collaborate with other health care professionals in establishing a plan of care to support pregnancy and minimize risk of spontaneous abortion
- Maintain hemodynamic stability of mother
- Assure safety of fetus from invasive and noninvasive procedures whenever possible
- Select medications with known effects on pregnancy if possible
- Provide patient and family with spiritual and emotional support as needed or requested
- Monitor fetal heart tones; vaginal bleeding; fundal height; abdominal pain, cramping, or uterine contractions; endocrine and metabolic changes consistent with pregnancy; and nutritional status

■ NURSING DIAGNOSES

Anxiety, impaired coping, altered growth and development, or altered tissue perfusion,[73] related to incomplete abortion, hemorrhage, and uterine injury.

■ NURSING DIAGNOSIS

Altered elimination, related to colostomy

OUTCOME STANDARD AND CRITERIA

Bowel function reestablished and consistent with site of colostomy as evidenced by:
- Stoma healing
- Intact skin surrounding stoma
- Initiation of colostomy care and teaching
- Patient's demonstration of interest in care of colostomy

NURSING INTERVENTIONS

- Initiate stoma care
- Consult an enterostomal therapist for colostomy care and teaching
- Explain procedures to patient
- Encourage open and honest communication regarding the colostomy
- Initiate nutritional support
- Evaluate effects of nutritional support on elimination patterns
- Encourage patient and family participation in colostomy care when they demonstrate interest
- Institute hygiene measures that respect patient's privacy and body image concerns
- Monitor gastrointestinal motility; passing of flatus; abdominal distention; color, odor, consistency of stool; integrity of stoma; skin integrity surrounding stoma; and fluid and electrolyte balance

HIGH-RISK NURSING DIAGNOSES

Impaired skin integrity or altered body image,[73] related to colonic impaction and wound infection.

■ NURSING DIAGNOSIS

Altered body image, related to colostomy.

OUTCOME STANDARD AND CRITERIA

Verbal or nonverbal acknowledgment of colostomy as evidenced by:
- Seeking information about colostomy
- Inspection of colostomy site by patient

NURSING INTERVENTIONS

- Answer patient's question related to surgery openly and honestly
- Assess meaning of loss for patient and family
- Encourage ventilation of feelings and grieving
- Support and intervene in responses of loss, anger, depression, and denial as possible
- Encourage communication of feelings between patient and family
- Encourage viewing of site and participation in care
- Respect need for privacy
- Consult psychiatric clinical nurse specialist as needed
- Monitor verbal and nonverbal expressions, related to colostomy; grieving stage; and interactions with others

HIGH-RISK NURSING DIAGNOSES

Alteration in elimination, sexual dysfunction, anxiety, altered self-concept,[73] related to posttraumatic distress syndrome.

■ NURSING DIAGNOSIS

Altered nutrition: less than body requirements,[73] related to pregnancy.

OUTCOME STANDARD AND CRITERIA

Nutritional requirements are met for age, gender, and metabolic demand as evidenced by:
- Maintenance of normal weight
- Progressive wound healing
- Absence of Kwashiorkor-type malnutrition
- Maintenance of fluid and electrolyte balance

- Adequate protein reserves
- Equal or positive nitrogen balance[53,74]

NURSING INTERVENTIONS

- Initiate enteral or parenteral feedings within 72 hours of injury
- Determine energy needs and expenditures using the Harris-Benedict equation or indirect calorimetry[53]
- Obtain anthropometric measurements to note changing trends in nutritional status[53]
- Estimate nitrogen losses
- Estimate protein stores
- Provide adequate nutrients required for catabolic and anabolic phases (fat, carbohydrates, protein, vitamins and trace elements)
- Consult nutrition support specialist
- Administer prescribed diet
- Regulate feedings based on patient tolerance
- Perform meticulous mouth care
- Monitor enteral feeding method (tube placements if enteral feeding, tube feeding tolerance, gastric residuals, elimination patterns), parenteral feeding method (infusion site, glucose tolerance, metabolic acidosis), and general considerations (weight, intake and output, respiratory status, wound healing, and fluid and electrolyte balance)

HIGH-RISK NURSING DIAGNOSES

Altered nutrition: more than body requirements, high risk for aspiration, diarrhea, high risk for infection, impaired skin integrity, activity intolerance, or altered fluid volume,[73] related to sepsis, aspiration pneumonia, and kwashiorkor.

CASE STUDY: BLUNT TRAUMA

A 19-year-old male is brought to the trauma center after a high-speed motor vehicle collision. He was the unrestrained driver in a single-vehicle collision. The car struck a telephone pole head-on, and he was found pinned between the mangled steering wheel and front seat. One-foot intrusion of dashboard into front seat was reported, and starburst pattern on driver's side window was noted. No other passengers were in the vehicle.

Prehospital
Assessment:

Glasgow Coma Score	= 8
Blood pressure	= 100/72 mmHg
Heart rate	= 110 beats per minute
Respiratory rate	= 8/min
RTS	= 7

Ringer's lactate (LR) solution infused via 16-gauge IV line at 50 ml/min. Patient was unresponsive with shallow respirations. Intubated en route with positive pressure ventilation at 10 breaths per minute. C-spine was immobilized. Extrication was difficult and took 35 minutes.

Emergency Department
Primary Survey

Intubated and requiring mechanical ventilation at 10 IMV/min with an FiO_2 of 50%. Vesicular breath sounds

bilaterally. Femoral pulse present. Blood pressure 108/74 mmHg. Second IV line started infusing LR to keep vein open. GCS 9, opens eyes to painful stimuli, localizes to pain, intubated. Right pupil sluggish and 3 mm, and left pupil nonreactive and 5 mm. RTS remains 7. Blood oozing from open left tibia/fibula fracture. ECG shows sinus tachycardia at 110 beats per minute. Foley catheter inserted with urine output of 500 ml. Urine output maintained at 20 ml every 15 minutes. NG tube inserted. Drainage Hematest negative.

Laboratory Studies

ABG	= pH 7.40, PO_2 98, PCO_2 38, Bicarb 26, Sat. 98%
Hematocrit	= 32%
WBC	= 5,000
Blood alcohol	= 180 mg/dl
Urine drug study	= Negative

Secondary Survey

Closed depressed skull fracture left frontal parietal area. Circular ecchymotic patterns noted at midchest level. Respiratory excursion symmetrical. Chest x-ray shows bilateral pulmonary contusions. Abdomen flat with bowel sounds present. Pelvis stable. Left femur distended. Left forearm deformed. X-ray confirms femur, radius and tibia/fibula fractures. C-spine cleared to T1. CT scan of the head shows left parietal contusion with local swelling. Serial 12-lead ECGs initiated. Isoenzymes sent to the laboratory. No rectal blood noted. Diagnostic peritoneal lavage is positive. Patient given tetanus toxoid and antibiotics. Osmotic diuresis initiated. Discharged to operating room for insertion of intracranial pressure monitoring device; exploratory laparotomy; and reduction and fixation of radius, femur, and tibia/fibula fractures.

Index of Suspicion

1. Injury to the head. *Rationale:* Unrestrained driver. Starburst pattern on driver's side window. High-speed MVC. GCS 9. Potential for secondary brain injuries.
2. Pulmonary contusion and possible injury to the thoracic aorta, cardiac valves, cardiac contusion, fracture of sternum. *Rationale:* Driver with circular pattern on midchest.
3. Femur fracture, pelvic fracture, posterior hip dislocation, tibia/fibula fracture. Potential for associated injury to the GU or GI tracts. *Rationale:* Head-on collision, down-and-under pathway. Invasion of passenger space by dashboard.
4. Injury to spleen. *Rationale:* Common injury in blunt trauma because of its mobility. Deceleration forces hit body on left side.

Medical Management

Insertion of intracranial pressure monitoring device. Exploratory laparotomy with splenorrhaphy. No other abdominal injuries. Intraoperative blood loss estimated at 1,000 ml. Three liters LR infused. Intraoperative hematocrit 34%. Arterial line inserted. Reduction and fixation of radius and femur fractures. Debridement and reduction of tibia/fibula fracture. Discharged from OR with an endotracheal tube in place mechanically ventilated at 10 IMV/min. ICP was 12 mmHG. ABGs within normal limits. Blood pressure 110/68 mmHg and heart rate was 104 beats per minute. Intraoperative urine output was 800 ml.

NURSING MANAGEMENT: CASE STUDY

■ NURSING DIAGNOSIS
Altered tissue perfusion, related to brain injury.
OUTCOME STANDARD AND CRITERIA
Cerebral perfusion is adequate or improved as evidenced by:
- Cerebral perfusion pressure of less than 60 mmHg
- Intracranial pressure of less than 15 mmHg

NURSING INTERVENTIONS
- Maintain head and neck in neutral midline position at all times
- Avoid hip flexions of 90°
- Elevate head of bed to maintain maximum CPP and minimum ICP
- Suction endotracheal tube only as needed using no more than two passes
- Hyperventilate with 100% oxygen prior to suctioning
- Turn patient side to side based on patient's tolerance, noting adverse changes in CPP and ICP
- Avoid adverse environmental stimuli based on patient's responses
- Calculate CPP with each set of vital signs or more frequently based on patient's status
- Space nursing care activities to coordinate with return of ICP to baseline
- Administer medications as prescribed for maintenance of CPP and reduction of ICP
- Monitor effects of interventions, CPP and ICP, Glasgow Coma Score, motor and sensory status, ICP waveform, respiratory pattern and rate, fluid and electrolyte status, arterial blood gases, urine output, and cardiovascular status

HIGH-RISK NURSING DIAGNOSES
Activity intolerance, impaired airway clearance, impaired breathing pattern, or impaired physical mobility,[73] related to cerebral edema, seizures, intracranial hypertension, meningitis, and acute hydrocephalus.

■ NURSING DIAGNOSIS
Altered tissue perfusion, related to cardiac injury.
OUTCOME STANDARD AND CRITERIA
Myocardial tissue perfusion is adequate or improved[74] as evidenced by:
- Absence or reduction in ECG manifestations of myocardial ischemia[74]
- Hemodynamic parameters within normal limits

NURSING INTERVENTIONS
- Limit activities that increase cardiac demand
- Administer oxygen as prescribed
- Administer vasoactive medications to maintain or improve hemodynamic stability
- Administer medications to minimize pain
- Monitor ECG characteristics, chest pain, hemodynamic parameters, arterial oxygenation, cardiovascular status, myocardial enzymes, level of consciousness, pulse pressure changes, upper and lower extremity blood pressures, and paradoxical pulses

HIGH-RISK NURSING DIAGNOSES
Activity intolerance, alteration in comfort, or anxiety,[73] related to myocardial contusion, myocardial infarction, great vessel injury, flail chest, and cardiac tamponade.

■ NURSING DIAGNOSIS
Impaired gas exchange, related to pulmonary injuries.
OUTCOME STANDARD AND CRITERIA
Hypercapnia and hypoxemia are absent or reduced as evidenced by:
- Normal breathing pattern with or without ventilator support
- Normal arterial oxygenation and saturation for age and preexisting diseases
- Maintenance of arterial CO levels between 40 and 45 mmHg (P_{CO_2} levels may be maintained between 25 and 30 mmHg for the first 72 hours to treat head injury)
- Arterial pH within normal range FiO_2 <0.50 if patient is mechanically ventilated

NURSING INTERVENTIONS
- Support ventilation with intubation and mechanical ventilation
- Maintain oxygenation by using adjunct therapies (e.g., PEEP, positive pressure support, independent lung ventilation, jet ventilation, CPAP)
- Adjust ventilator parameters to maintain normal arterial blood gases
- Suction only as needed using no more than two passes and hyperventilate before and after each pass
- Monitor pulmonary status, pain, mechanical obstruction, level of consciousness, and arterial blood gases

HIGH-RISK NURSING DIAGNOSES
Aspiration, activity intolerance, impaired communication, anxiety, or altered tissue perfusion,[73] related to ARDS, atelectasis, pneumonia, tension pneumothorax, hemothorax, pneumothorax, and flail chest.

■ NURSING DIAGNOSIS
High risk for fluid volume deficit, related to blood loss and head injury.
OUTCOME STANDARD AND CRITERIA
Fluid volume is normal as evidenced by:
- Absence of dehydration
- Absence of postural hypotension
- Normal filling pressures
- Fluid and electrolytes within normal range

- Hemoglobin and hematocrit within normal range
- Urine output >30 ml/hr
- Balanced intake and output
- Moist mucous membranes

NURSING INTERVENTIONS

- Replace fluid based on the amount and type of fluid lost
- Warm fluids when replacing large volumes
- Provide nutritional supplements as soon as possible
- Monitor hemodynamic parameters, wound drainage, serum electrolytes, serum osmolality, urine specific gravity, urine osmolality, urine output, hemoglobin and hematocrit, gastrointestinal losses, and weight daily

HIGH-RISK NURSING DIAGNOSES

Altered tissue perfusion, potential for fluid volume excess, ineffective breathing pattern, or impaired skin integrity,[73] related to diabetes insipidus, SIADH, hemorrhage, and hypovolemic shock.

■ **NURSING DIAGNOSIS**

Altered nutrition: less than body requirements,[73] related to head injury and hypermetabolic state. Refer to p. 1264 for discussion of this diagnosis.

■ **NURSING DIAGNOSIS**

High-risk for infection, related to open tibia/fibula fracture and ICP monitor.[73]

OUTCOME STANDARD AND CRITERIA

Infection is absent as evidenced by:

- Absence of signs and symptoms of localized infection at fracture sites or ICP monitor insertion sites (redness, tenderness, swelling, purulent drainage, odor)[74]
- Absence of signs and symptoms of systemic infection (fever, tachycardia)[74]

NURSING INTERVENTIONS

- Institute routine infection control measures
- Perform dressing changes as needed
- Administer antibiotics as scheduled
- Observe wounds for evidence of healing
- Obtain wound and blood cultures as needed
- Observe for signs and symptoms of localized and systemic infections
- Observe ICP insertion site for drainage
- Change cerebrospinal fluid drainage bags (if used) following sterile technique
- Monitor febrile states, level of consciousness, and immune response (WBCs)

HIGH-RISK NURSING DIAGNOSES

Impaired skin integrity or alteration in tissue perfusion,[73] related to sepsis, meningitis, and osteomyelitis.

REFERENCES

1. National Academy of Sciences, Committee on Trauma. (1985). *Injury in America: A continuing public health problem.* Washington, DC: National Academy Press.

2. National Academy of Sciences, National Research Council. (1966). *Accidental death and disability: The neglected disease of modern society.* Washington, DC: U.S. Government Printing Office.

3. Boyd, D. (1980). Trauma—a controlled disease in the 1980's. Stone lecture, American Trauma Society. *Journal of Trauma, 20,* 14-24.

4. Congressional Record—Senate (1987). Senate bill 10. January 6, 1987, pp. 211-217.

5. U.S. Department of Health and Human Services, Public Health Service. (1990). *Healthy People 2000, National health promotion and disease prevention objectives.* DHHS Publication # (PHS) 91-5012. Washington, DC: U.S. Government Printing Office.

6. Tolsma, D. (1984). Health promotion approaches to occupant protection: An epidemiological framework. *Health Education Quarterly, 11,* 133-140.

7. Haddon, W. (1972). A logical framework for categorizing highway safety phenomenon and activity. *Journal of Trauma, 12,* 193-207.

8. Baker, S. (1975). Determinants of injury and opportunities for intervention. *American Journal of Epidemiology, 101,* 98-102.

9. Baker, S., O'Neill, B., & Karpf, A. (1984). *The injury fact book.* Lexington, MA: Lexington Books.

10. American College of Surgeons, Committee on Trauma. (1976). Optimal hospital resources for care of the seriously injured. *Bulletin American College of Surgeons, 61,* 15-22.

11. Guliad, J., Onwuachi-Saunders, E., Sacks, J., et al. (1988). Differences in death rates due to injury among blacks and whites, 1984. *Journal of the American Medical Association, 261,* 215-216.

12. Jagger, J., & Dietz, P. (1986). Death and injury by firearms: Who cares? *Journal of the American Medical Association, 255,* 3143-3144.

13. Prothrow-Smith, D. (1987). Violence prevention. *Injury in American Conference, 102,* 615-616.

14. Mattsson, E. (1975). Psychological aspects of severe physical injury and its treatment. *Journal of Trauma, 15,* 217-234.

15. Weiss, M., & Boyd, D. (1972). Psyche-trauma-psyche: Surgeons' observations of psychiatric conditions in trauma patients. *Israel Annals of Psychiatry and Related Disabilities, 11,* 91-98.

16. Titchner, J. (1970). Management and study of psychological response to trauma. *Journal of Trauma, 10,* 974-980.

17. Baker, S. (1987). Injuries: The neglected epidemic. Stone lecture, American Trauma Society. *Journal of Trauma, 27,* 343-348.

18. Veise-Berry, S. (1988). Evolution of the trauma cycle. In V. Cardona (Ed.), *Trauma nursing from resuscitation through rehabilitation* (pp. 3-15). Philadelphia: Saunders.

19. Trunkey, D., Boyd, D., Keller, M., et al. (1981). Panel: Current status of emergency medical services. *Journal of Trauma, 21,* 196-203.

20. Von Wagner, F. (1961). Died in hospital: A three year study of deaths following trauma. *Journal of Trauma, 1,* 401-408.

21. West, J., Trunkey, D., Lim, R., et al. (1979). Systems of trauma care: A study of two counties. *Archives of Surgery, 114,* 455-460.

22. American College of Surgeons, Committee on Trauma. (1986). Caring for the injured patient. *Bulletin of the American College of Surgeons, 71,* 1-56.

23. American College of Surgeons, Committee on Trauma. (1990). *Resources for optimal care of the injured patient.* Chicago: American College of Surgeons.

24. Pollack, D., & McLain, P. (1989). Report from the 1988 trauma registry workshop, including recommendations for hospital based trauma registries. *Journal of Trauma, 29,* 827-829.

25. Weigelt, J., & McCormick, A. (1988). Mechanism of injury. In V. Cardona (Ed.), *Trauma nursing from resuscitation through rehabilitation* (pp. 105-126). Philadelphia: Saunders.

26. Feliciano, D., & Whall, M. (1991). Patterns of injury. In E. Moore, K. Mattox, & D. Feliciano (Eds.), *Trauma* (2nd ed.). Norwalk, CT: Appleton & Lange.

27. McFarland, R., Ryan, G., & Dingman, R. (1968). Etiology of motor-vehicle accidents with special reference to the mechanisms of injury. *New England Journal of Medicine, 278,* 1383.

28. Nahum, A. (1975). The biomechanics of maxillofacial trauma. *Clinical Plastic Surgery, 2,* 59.

29. Tsuang, M., Boor, M., & Fleming, J. (1985). Psychiatric aspects of traffic accidents. *American Journal of Psychiatry, 142,* 538-546.

30. Davis, A. (1989). The relationship between the phenomenon of traumatic injury and the patterns of power, human field motion, esteem and risk taking. Dissertation abstracts.

31. Weaver, J. (1987). *The world of physics.* New York: Simon and Schuster.

32. McSwain, N. (1987). Mechanisms of injury in blunt trauma. In N. McSwain, Jr., & M. Kerstein (Eds.), *Evaluation and management of trauma* (pp. 1-24). Norwalk, CT: Appleton-Century-Crofts.

33. Richardson, J., McElvein, R., & Trinkle, J. (1975). First rib fracture: Hallmark of severe trauma. *Annals of Surgery, 3,* 251.

34. Wilson, J., Thomas, A., & Goodman, P. (1978). Severe chest trauma. Morbidity implications of first and second rib fracture in 120 patients. *Archives of Surgery, 113,* 846.

35. Crowley, R., & Dunham, M. (1982). *Shock trauma/critical care manual: Initial assessment and management.* Baltimore: University Park Press.

36. Harley, D., & Mena, I. (1986). Cardiac and vascular sequelae of sternal fractures. *Journal of Trauma, 26,* 553.

37. Kaufer, H. (1983). Expressway syndrome. *Infections in Surgery, 2,* 412.

38. Beaver, B. (1990). Care of the multiple trauma victim, the first hour. *Nursing Clinics of North America, 25,* 11-20.

39. Barach, E., Tomlanovich, M., & Nowak, R. (1986). Ballistics: A pathophysiologic examination of the wounding mechanisms of firearms: Part 1. *Journal of Trauma, 26,* 225-235.

40. Barach, E., Tomlanovich, M., & Nowak, R. (1986). Ballistics: A pathophysiologic examination of the wounding mechanisms of firearms: Part 2. *Journal of Trauma, 26,* 374-383.

41. Swan, K., & Swan, R. (1989). *Gunshot wounds: Pathophysiology and management* (2nd ed.). St. Louis: Mosby–Year Book.

42. Baker, S., O'Neill, B., & Haddon, W. (1974). The injury severity score: A method for describing patients with multiple injuries and evaluating medical care. *Journal of Trauma, 14,* 187-196.

43. Champion, H., Sacco, W., Lepper, R., et al. (1980). An anatomical index of severity. *Journal of Trauma, 20,* 197-202.

44. Morgan, T., Civil, I., & Schwab, C. (1988). Injury severity scoring: Influence of timing on nursing practice. *Heart Lung, 17,* 256-261.

45. Dunham, M., & Crowley, J. (1986). *Shock trauma/critical care handbook.* Rockville, MD: Aspen.

46. Lewis, F. (1991). Primary assessment. In D. Trunkey, & F. Lewis (Eds.), *Current therapy of trauma* (3rd ed.) (pp. 135-139). St. Louis: Mosby–Year Book.

47. Smith, L., & Glowac, B. (1989). New frontiers in the management of the multiply injured patient. *Critical Care Clinics of North America, 1,* 1-9.

48. American College of Surgeons. (1989). *Advanced trauma life support course.* Chicago: American College of Surgeons.

49. McQuillian, K., & Wiles, C. (1988). Initial management of traumatic shock. In V. Cardona (Ed.), *Trauma nursing from resuscitation through rehabilitation* (pp. 160-183). Philadelphia: Saunders.

50. Drury, T. (1991). Blood administration. In M. Mancini, & J. Klein (Eds.), *Decision making in trauma management: A multidisciplinary approach* (pp. 40-42). Philadelphia: Decker.

51. Mason, P. (1988). Abdominal trauma. In V. Cardona (Ed.), *Trauma nursing from resuscitation through rehabilitation* (pp. 491-524). Philadelphia: Saunders.

52. Klein, D. (1990). Physiologic response to traumatic shock. *AACN Clinical Issues, 1,* 505-521.

53. Stanek, G. (1988). Metabolic and management of the trauma patient. In V. Cardona (Ed.), *Trauma nursing from resuscitation through rehabilitation* (pp. 284-315). Philadelphia: Saunders.

54. Hoppe, C. (1983). Nutritional management of the trauma patient. *Critical Care Quarterly, 6,* 1-16.

55. Huggins, B. (1990). Trauma physiology. *Nursing Clinics of North America, 25,* 1-10.

56. Shires, T. (1985). Postoperative fluid management. In T. Shires (Ed.). *Principles of trauma care* (3rd ed.) (pp. 477-487). New York: McGraw-Hill.

57. Mitchell, P., & Mauss, N. (1978). Relationship of patient–nurse activity to intracranial pressure variations: A pilot study. *Nursing Research, 27,* 4-10.

58. Mitchell, P. (1986). Intracranial hypertension: Influence of nursing care activities. *Nursing Clinics of North America, 21,* 563-574.

59. Mitchell, P., Ozuna, J., & Lipe, H. (1981). Moving patients in bed: Effects on intracranial pressure. *Nursing Research, 30,* 212-218.

60. Parsons, C., & Wilson, M. (1984). Cerebrovascular status of severe closed head injury patients following passive position changes. *Nursing Research, 33,* 68-75.

61. Kater, K. (1989). Response of head-injured patients to sensory stimulation. *Western Journal of Nursing Research, 11,* 20-33.

62. Mathis, M. (1984). Personal needs of family members of critically ill patients with and without brain injury. *Journal of Neuroscience Nursing, 16,* 36-44.

63. Boggs, R. (1987). Multiple trauma. In M. Kinney, D. Packa, & S. Dunbar (Eds.), *AACN's clinical reference for critical-care nursing* (2nd ed.) (pp. 1485-1518). New York: McGraw-Hill.

64. Hammond, S. (1990). Chest injuries in the trauma patient. *Nursing Clinics of North America, 25,* 35-43.

65. Hurn, P. (1988). Thoracic injuries. In V. Cardona (Ed.), *Trauma nursing from resuscitation through rehabilitation* (pp. 127-159). Philadelphia: Saunders.

66. Bracken, M., Shepard, M., Collins, W., et al. (1990). A randomized, controlled trial of methylprednisolone or naloxone in the treatment of acute spinal cord injury. *New England Journal of Medicine, 332,* 1405-1411.

67. Davis, A. (1991). Acute-care management of patients with spinal cord injury: Part 1. *Critical Care Nursing Currents, 9,* 1-4.

68. Wagner, M. (1990). The patient with abdominal injuries. *Nursing Clinics of North America, 25,* 45-55.

69. Klender, K. (1988). The demand for trauma rehabilitation. In V. Cardona (Ed.), *Trauma nursing from resuscitation through rehabilitation* (pp. 449-490). Philadelphia: Saunders.

70. Leonard, R., & Teitelman, U. (1991). Manmade disasters. *Critical Care Clinics, 7,* 293-320.

71. Noji, E. (1991). Natural disasters. *Critical Care Clinics, 7,* 271-292.

72. Dow A., Clark, W., Farmer, C., et al. (1991). Organizations and academic perspective. *Critical Care Clinics, 7,* 271-292.

73. Carpenito, L. (1989). *Nursing diagnosis, application to clinical practice.* Philadelphia: Lippincott.

74. Kuhn, R. (Ed.). (1990). *AACN outcome standards for nursing care of the critically ill.* Laguna Niguel, CA: American Association of Critical-Care Nurses.

56

Multisystem Organ Failure

Maurene A. Harvey

Multisystem organ failure related to sepsis or septiclike syndromes is the most common cause of death in critical care units. It is estimated that the U.S. incidence increased during the 1980s from 70,000 cases annually to between 300,000 and 500,000 cases annually. The mortality is about 10% to 40% when one organ system fails, 40% to 60% when two fail, and 80% to 100% when three fail.

Ironically, the increasing incidence of multisystem organ failure is attributed to knowledge gained in the first three decades of critical care, a fairly young subspecialty. In the 1960s, we learned to better use blood gases and ventilators to support patients with respiratory failure. In the 1970s, we learned to use hemodynamic monitoring to support patients with perfusion failure. In the 1980s, we learned to monitor and meet the nutritional requirements of the critically ill. With these and many other advances, seriously ill patients can be brought through more acute insults, surviving long enough to develop sepsis-driven multisystem organ failure.

In the 1990s, we are learning to intervene in this syndrome. It is imperative that critical care nurses have a thorough understanding of the pathophysiology involved if they are to achieve prevention, early recognition, and skillful application of new treatment modalities.

As is often the case, new and rapidly developing knowledge fields suffer from a lack of standardization of terms. Sepsis, septic syndrome, multisystem organ failure, septic shock, and hypermetabolic syndrome all have a variety of overlapping definitions that make following the literature and communicating at the bedside difficult. Accordingly, a consensus conference was convened to standardize terminology as well as to set priorities for patient management and research. The results were published simultaneously in the June 1992 issues of *Chest* and *Critical Care Medicine*. The recommended definitions will be used in this chapter and are as follows:

Systemic inflammatory response syndrome (SIRS):
The systemic inflammatory response to a variety of severe clinical insults, including infection, trauma, immune-mediated injury, and ischemia

Sepsis: The systemic response to infection

Septic shock: Sepsis with hypotension despite adequate fluid resuscitation along with the presence of perfusion abnormalities

Multiple organ dysfunction syndrome (MODS): Presence of altered organ function in an acutely ill patient such that homeostasis cannot be maintained without intervention

LOCAL RESPONSE TO INJURY

Immune System

The immune system is designed to recognize and control foreign antigens and injured or diseased tissue. The components involved include the phagocytes, the lymphocytes, and the complement cascade (see Chapter 43).

Phagocytes

The most abundant circulating pool of phagocytes are the granulocytes, specifically neutrophils. They are produced only in the bone marrow which normally also contains a reserve supply for times of high demand. This supply is about three times the circulating number. Once released, they circulate in the bloodstream for 6 to 8 hours and then are either lost from the body or gather in tissue beds in need of phagocytes.

Monocytes are also produced primarily in the bone marrow and, like neutrophils, once released into the bloodstream, circulate for only 6 to 8 hours. The difference is that monocytes do not gather only in abnormal tissue but also migrate into normal tissues. Within hours, monocytes change into macrophages, the largest and most potent phagocytes, and become part of the important first line of defense against infection. When stimulated, they can divide and release substrates. These mediators attract other cells such as lymphocytes, granulocytes and platelets, stimulate the bone marrow to release more neutrophils into the circulation, and trigger the hypothalamus to increase body temperature.

Phagocytes are able to identify antigens and abnormal cells, engulf, and then destroy them. This process requires what has been called *respiratory burst*, a 20-fold increase in oxygen combustion. Substances produced during phagocytosis include proteolytic enzymes, hydrogen peroxide, oxygen radicals, and acids. The phagocytes themselves are destroyed in the process.

Lymphocytes

Lymphocytes are white cells that accumulate and circulate in the lymphoid tissues as well as in the bloodstream. They develop into two important types which, in response to antigen invasion, can be stimulated to clone large numbers of lymphocytes sensitized to that particular invader. This response occurs more quickly after the first exposure.

B cell lymphocytes are involved in humoral immunity in that they produce antibodies and activate complement, the two main humors or substances required for an immune response. The spleen and lymph nodes are major sites of lymphocyte cloning and antibody synthesis. There are at least 50,000 types of lymphocytes, each capable of producing antibodies against a specific antigen.

The antigen–antibody reaction is one of the most important aspects of defense. Antibodies attach to the antigen, thus inactivating it and allowing better recognition by other immune cells. This reaction also promotes agglutination.

T cell lymphocytes are responsible for regulatory cellular immune response. Unlike B cells, from which only the antibody is released, antigen exposure causes the entire sensitized T cell line to be produced and released from lymphoid tissue to travel to the site of invasion.

The three major subsets of T cells are killer, helper, and suppressor T cells. Killer T cells contain lymphotoxins that can degrade organic matter. Helper T (CD4) cells release factors that attract more lymphocytes and phagocytes to the site. Suppressor T (CD8) cells mitigate the response once the antigen is controlled. This last step is an important method of keeping the response to injury appropriately confined, of preventing the immune system from attacking normal tissue.

Substances released by one white cell to affect another are called *interleukins*, and, to date, 22 have been identified (IL-1 through IL-22). Other groups of substances are named by taking the root of the cells that produce them and adding the suffix "-trein" or "kine."

Complement Cascade

Complement formation is the result of a cascade of reactions between normally inactive proteins, labeled C1 through C9, some with subsets a-c. Complement is stimulated by the presence of an antigen–antibody reaction. The complement then enhances many aspects of the immune response and inflammation. It promotes antigen–antibody fixation, acts as a chemotactic or attracting factor for appropriate white cells, increases vessel and platelet reactivity, and weakens walls of cells needing degradation.

Response to Pathogens and Antigens

The body is defended from injury by endogenous and exogenous pathogens and antigens through a complex and highly interactive process. A disturbance in any one of these components can threaten the effectiveness of the whole immune system (Figure 56-1).

The antigen is first processed by the tissue macrophage, the primary line of defense. Interleukin-1

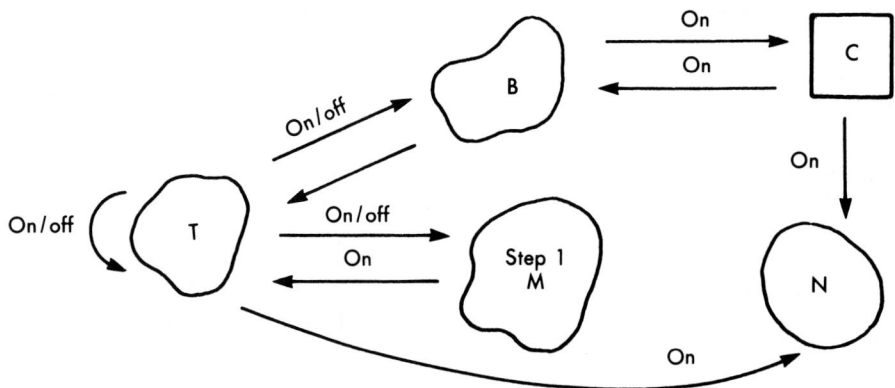

Figure 56-1 Interactions between the components of immunity. T cells (T), B cells (B), macrophages (M), neutrophils (N), and complement (C). Process starts in macrophages (step 1).
From Harvey, M. H. (1992). *Study guide for the core curriculum for critical care nursing* (2nd ed.). Philadelphia: Saunders.

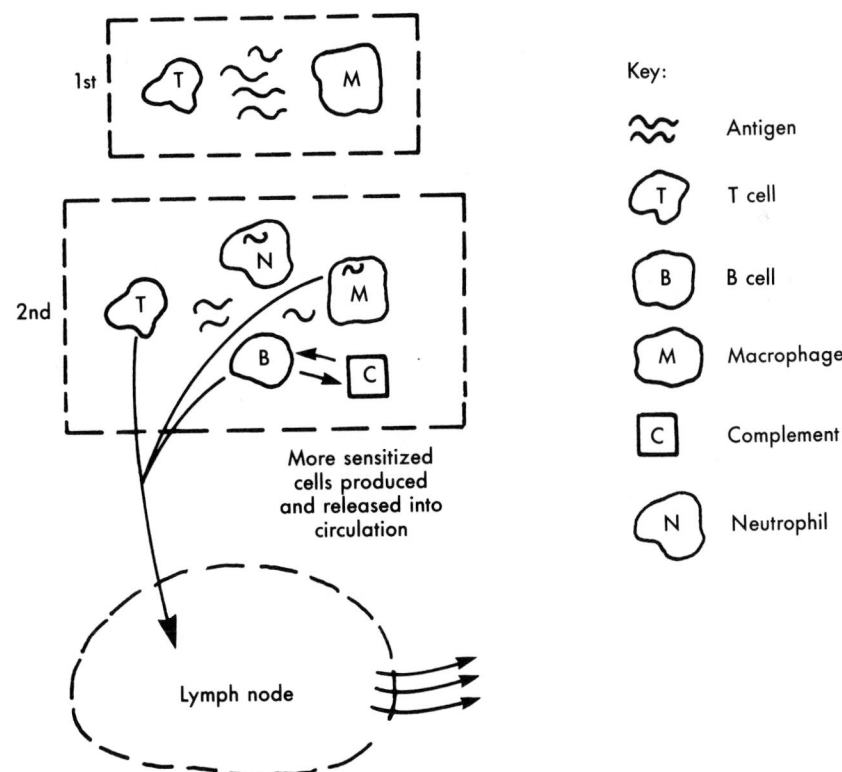

Figure 56-2   Summary of phases of anti-antigen defense.
From Harvey, M. H. (1992). *Study guide for the core curriculum for critical care nursing* (2nd ed.). Philadelphia: Saunders.

and a portion of the antigen are displayed on the macrophage membrane surface, activating the helper T cell which amplifies the immune response. Inflammation and phagocytosis result. Suppressor T cells dominate once the threat has subsided (Figures 56-1 and 56-2).

Hyperactivity of the Immune System

There are two types of abnormal reactions of the immune system (see Chapter 45). The first, called *autoimmune disease*, is caused by activation of various components of the immune system against normal tissue. It can involve almost any part of the body. Examples include Guillain-Barré syndrome, myasthenia gravis, systemic lupus erythematosus, and rheumatoid arthritis, as well as some forms of renal failure, thyroid disorders, fibrotic lung disease, and inflammatory bowel disease.

The second, *hypersensitivity reactions*, are exaggerated responses to antigens. The rapidity and severity with which sensitivity reactions occur vary according to the degree of reactivity, the amount of sensitization, and the type of immune components involved.

There are three types of reactions. *Immediate* hypersensitivity reactions occur within seconds to minutes of exposure to the antigen and are primarily mediated by antibodies. Cytotoxic transfusion reactions and anaphylaxis are two examples. *Subacute* hypersensitivity reactions take minutes to hours because they involve both antibodies and phagocytes. Examples include serum sickness and Arthus reaction. *Delayed* hypersensitivity reactions take hours to days to manifest because they are caused primarily by T cells. Chronic graft rejection, skin tests, and many subcutaneous reactions are examples.

Some of the sensitivity reactions involve the release of a particular type of antibody, IgE. This immunoglobulin stimulates the release of histamine and other similar substances. Effects can include anaphylaxis, urticaria, or asthma.

Immunosuppression

The longer a person remains critically ill, the more likely he is to become significantly immunosuppressed (see Chapter 46). Common contributing factors, with examples, are listed in the box on p. 1288.

Evaluation of the Immune System

Quantifying the function of the immune system is difficult in critically ill patients (see Chapter 45). Since malnutrition and immunosuppression often coexist, however, evaluation of the patient's nutritional status is sometimes revealing. Anthropometric measure-

Factors Contributing to Immunosuppression

FACTORS	EXAMPLES
Bypassed skin and irritated mucous membranes	Endotracheal tubes Vascular catheters Foley catheters Nasogastric tubes Surgical procedures Endoscopy
Altered protective mechanisms	Endotracheal tubes that bypass nares, prevent epiglottis function, and inhibit cough Drugs that raise gastric pH above bactericidal levels
Altered nutrition	Metabolic demands may be hard to estimate or meet. Stressed patients tend to use nutrients given for catabolic or acute phase reactions rather than for anabolic needs. They may particularly have difficulty metabolizing glucose calories. Poor GI motility may preclude using the tract, thereby potentially further insulting its mucosal integrity.
Sequential infections	In response to the first infection, the patient's bone marrow is capable of dramatically increasing the white count by using fully mature cells. It takes time to rebuild reserves to that point and to respond to a second infection as effectively.
Drugs that can cause immunosuppression	Bone marrow–depressing agents Steroids Antibiotics Anesthetics Analgesics
Age and associated diseases	Very old or very young age Chronic disease or stress Splenectomy Infection with human immunodeficiency virus (HIV) Diabetes mellitus Renal failure Hepatic failure Chronic malnutrition Prosthetic heart valves Small-bowel resection

ments and anergy tests can be misleading, so laboratory values are more commonly followed. When the serum albumin is below 2.5 g/dl, the transferrin is below 160 g/dl, and when the lymphocyte count is under 900, the nutritional status and, thereby, the immune function is severely compromised. Values that move toward and away from these levels can reflect trends in immune status.

Inflammation

The process of inflammation is the substance-mediated tissue response to injury (see Chapter 43). The goal is to allow the cells and substrates required for defense and repair into the appropriate areas. Several phases are involved (Figure 56-3). The vascular reaction, mediated in part by histamine, prostaglandins, and bradykinin, causes both increased flow and in-creased permeability to fluid and protein. The early cellular reaction involves neutrophils and macrophages which are attracted to the area and begin phagocytosis. The response of the bone marrow is increased production and release of phagocytes into the bloodstream. This process is mediated by factors released by the white cells (leukocytes) and by the injured tissue. The formation of pus occurs when larger areas of inflammation and infection cause accumulations of white cells, edema, and debris.

Hemostatic Mechanisms

Tissue and vessel injury stimulate white cell reactions and inflammation. In addition, the hemostatic mechanism, which is designed to reduce the risk of blood loss, may be activated.

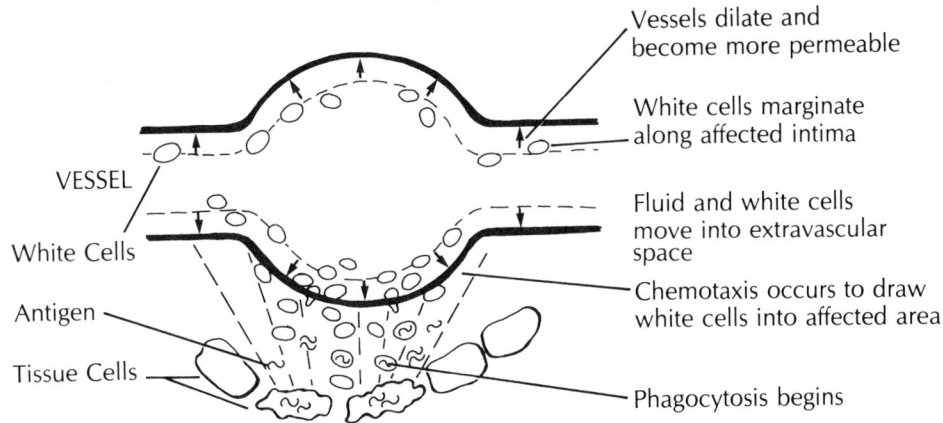

Figure 56-3 Major early stages of inflammation.
From Harvey, M. H. (1992). *Study guide for the core curriculum for critical care nursing* (2nd ed.). Philadelphia: Saunders.

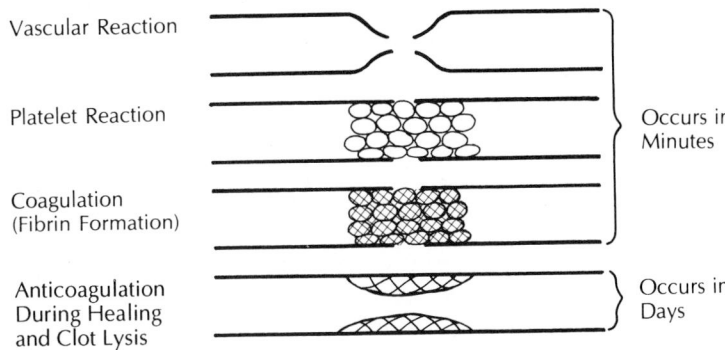

Figure 56-4 Major mechanisms involved in hemostasis.
From Harvey, M. H. (1992). *Study guide for the core curriculum for critical care nursing* (2nd ed.). Philadelphia: Saunders.

Coagulation

The hemostatic mechanism involves four steps (see Chapter 40). The first three take minutes; the last usually occurs over several days (Figure 56-4).

The first step is the vascular reaction. A damaged vessel immediately constricts, thereby decreasing blood loss. The second step is the platelet cellular reaction. Damaged vessels cause platelets to aggregate, agglutinate, and secrete substances. The resulting plug is soft but will stop the bleeding. The substances secreted are important triggers for the next step of hemostasis. If the damage is limited, the vascular and platelet response is also limited. They may subside and dissipate without triggering the third step, fibrin formation.

To produce a firm clot, fibrinogen, a circulating protein, is bound into fibrin strands, becoming a structural mesh for platelets and other cells. The trigger required for this conversion is thrombin, and there are two pathways to its production (Figure 56-5). The intrinsic pathway begins with factors activated in the

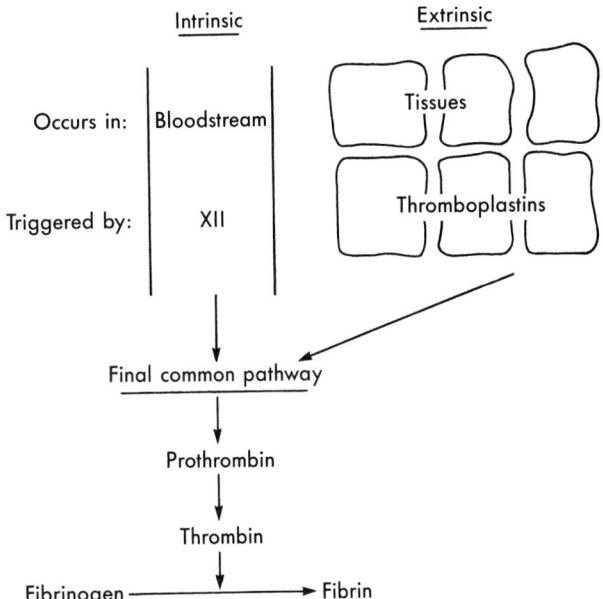

Figure 56-5 Intrinsic and extrinsic pathways of fibrin formation.
From Harvey, M. H. (1992). *Study guide for the core curriculum for critical care nursing* (2nd ed.). Philadelphia: Saunders.

bloodstream; the extrinsic begins with factors activated outside the blood itself in injured tissues. Over the next 30 to 60 minutes, the clot retracts to extrude fluid and pull the vessels in.

The fourth step is fibrinolysis. Slowly, as the vessel heals, fibrin is lysed, and the clot dissolves. Fibrinolysis is triggered by the continual activation of plasminogen into plasmin, a proteolytic enzyme found incorporated into the clot itself.

Anticoagulation

The hemostatic mechanism must be balanced so that the coagulation system does not become overreactive causing clots to continually re-form during the process of fibrinolysis. Several balancing factors prevent this from happening. Antithrombin absorbs excessive amounts of thrombin to prevent triggering of fibrin formation elsewhere. Heparin is produced primarily by mast cells and further anticoagulates by greatly potentiating the effect of antithrombin. The fibrin degradation products also act as local anticoagulants and are constantly released from dissolving clots to prevent a vicious cycle of reclotting.

Evaluation of Hemostatic Mechanisms

Evaluation of the hemostatic mechanisms involves a wide variety of tests, some fairly specific to certain disorders (see Chapter 41). There are a few general tests commonly done in critical care.

Bleeding time evaluates the first three steps leading to clot formation and is, therefore, fairly nonspecific. Since it is most affected by platelet number and effectiveness, it can sometimes be helpful in diagnosing decreased platelet activity. When the platelet count, the prothrombin time (PT), and the partial thromboplastin time (PTT) are normal but the bleeding time is long, decreased platelet activity should be suspected.

Clotting time also evaluates the first three phases and can be used as a general assessment tool.

The PT is designed to evaluate the extrinsic pathway and is, therefore, affected by many clotting factors. Coumadin affects the extrinsic factors and is, therefore, assessed by the PT. The PTT is designed to evaluate factors involved in the intrinsic pathway where heparin acts. It can be used to assess heparin therapy.

Bleeding

The critically ill patient is also at high risk for bleeding diathesis (see Chapter 42). Several of the risk factors and related causes may be present in a single patient (see the box on p. 1289).

Two conditions listed in the box deserve further emphasis: liver failure and heparin. *Liver failure* can cause bleeding diatheses by several mechanisms. These include thrombocytopenia via platelet destruction or splenomegaly when portal hypertension is present, platelet inhibition, decreased clotting factor production, and inability to metabolize drugs and factors involved.

Heparin can potentially cause three hemostatic defects. Of patients receiving heparin, 1% to 2% develop significant bleeding, 1% to 2% develop significant thrombosis, and 30% develop thrombocytopenia. Bleeding and clotting phenomena as well as platelet counts should be monitored. The platelet count may drop gradually over days in patients receiving therapeutic doses of heparin (pure thrombocytopenia). It can drop suddenly from even minimal doses of heparin in flush solutions (arterial lines, pulmonary artery catheters) in patients developing a risk of thrombotic episodes. This phenomenon is known as heparin–platelet/thrombotic–thrombocytopenia syndrome, heparin–platelet aggregation syndrome, or *white clot syndrome*. Patients in whom this syndrome is suspected should have a heparin–platelet aggregation study done and all heparin discontinued if the study is positive.

Thrombotic Events

As with other physiological responses, hemostatic mechanisms may be under- or overactive. Critically ill patients are at risk for both.

Several aspects of routine nursing care of the acutely ill involve the prevention of thrombotic or embolic events (see Chapter 42). Again, many patients may have multiple risk factors, which can be categorized according to *Virchow's triad* (see the box on p. 1290).

The treatment of thrombotic events depends on the site but may include treatment of the cause, prevention of further clotting by nursing measures and anticoagulation, and lysis of the clot with thrombolytic agents.

The Arachidonic Acid Cascade

Cell membranes contain phospholipids which, when triggered by injury, initiate a complex reaction called the *arachidonic acid cascade*. This cascade involves dozens of active metabolites and enzymes, many with competing effects which, when properly timed, promote protection. Three important mediators produced are prostacyclin, thromboxane, and the prostaglandins. These mediators help regulate the immune response, inflammation, and coagulation in the area of injury. Other effects include modulation of pain, fever, and alteration of bronchial and vascular tone.

Prostaglandin inhibitors such as aspirin, ibuprofen,

Factors Affecting Risk of Bleeding Diathesis

RISK FACTORS	CAUSES
Disrupted vessels	Surgery
	Trauma
	Invasive procedures
Thrombocytopenia	Massive transfusion therapy (washout phenomenon)
	Massive fluid resuscitation (dilution phenomenon)
	Trauma, sepsis, DIC, and ARDS (sequestering phenomenon)
	Drug-induced via:
	Heparin
	Antibiotics, sulfonamides
	Antidysrhythmics
	Digoxin
	Phenytoin
	Bone marrow depression
	Prosthetic devices (valves, intraaortic balloon pump, extracorporeal circuits)
	Splenomegaly
Platelet inhibition	Drug-induced via fairly strong inhibitors such as ASA, quinidine, or ETOH
	Drug-induced via more moderate inhibitors such as beta blockers, calcium channel blockers, anesthetics, antihistamines, antibiotics, tricyclic antidepressants, and colloids (especially dextran)
	Disorders such as renal failure, liver failure, viral infections, and hypothermia
Interference with thrombin formation	Massive transfusion therapy (washout phenomenon)
	Diseases such as liver failure, DIC, and congenital factor deficits such as hemophilia and von Willebrand's disease
	Vitamin K deficiencies caused by malnutrition or antibiotic therapy that decrease the GI flora that produce vitamin K
	Decreased fibrinogen levels due to disease or drugs such as thrombolytic agents
Enhanced clot lysis	Thrombolytic agents such as streptokinase, urokinase, and tissue plasminogen activators
	Increased circulating endogenous anticoagulants

and other nonsteroidal antiinflammatory agents (NSAIDs) have long been available and widely used in a variety of settings. Several prostaglandins are now also being administered to subsets of critically ill patients, primarily as vasodilators. They are being used for patients with pulmonary hypertension, for postoperative cardiovascular surgical patients, and after liver transplant. In the next decade, more will be learned about how to alter aspects of the arachidonic acid cascade to the patient's benefit.

Oxygen Radicals

Oxygen radicals are by-products of oxygen metabolism, including hydroxyl radicals and oxygen singlets. Three main sources of oxygen radicals play a role in septic syndrome. The radicals are produced by activated neutrophils and macrophages during phagocytosis. Because they kill organisms and degrade organic matter, they are an appropriate aspect of the body's defense system.

Oxygen radicals can also be formed during reperfusion of ischemic tissues. All cells use xanthine oxidase in the process of using oxygen. This enzyme increases in hypoxic cells. When reperfusion makes oxygen available again, xanthine oxidase triggers the formation of a high concentration of free radicals. This reaction is thought to be a primary contributor to reperfusion injury. Oxygen radicals can damage DNA, inactivate intracellular proteins, increase other intracellular metabolic by-products, damage cell

Virchow's Triad and Contributing Factors

RISK FACTOR	CONTRIBUTING FACTORS
Stasis or reduced blood flow rates	Decreased cardiac output
	Heart failure
	Vasoconstriction
	Vascular obstruction by external compression
	Increased blood viscosity via polycythemia, hyperproteinemia, or dehydration
Vessel damage	Preexisting atherosclerosis
	Trauma or surgery
	Intravascular procedures, studies, or lines
	Irritation by drugs, inflammatory processes, or septic syndrome
Hypercoagulability	Heparin–platelet aggregation (white clot) syndrome
	Stress
	Catecholamines
	Third trimester pregnancy
	Drugs such as desmopressin acetate (DDAVP)
	Red blood cell or platelet disorders
	Smoking
	Immediately postoperative in splenectomy due to thrombocytosis

membranes, and trigger the arachidonic acid cascade.

The third source of O_2 radicals is the injured pneumocytes presented with high concentrations of inspired oxygen. Normal alveolar cells can metabolize extra oxygen to water. A damaged pneumocyte may not be able to complete the process, which requires the production of several enzymes. The intermediate breakdown products that may result are oxgyen radicals. In patients with ARDS, widespread pneumocyte injury coupled with oxygen radicals produced by phagocytes may overwhelm the enzyme systems that metabolize them.

Healing Phase

Healing begins early but may take weeks depending on the type of tissue, extent of damage, the continued presence of injury processes, and factors that may inhibit healing.

White cells present due to the inflammatory process and the immune response are also responsible for wound healing (see Chapter 55). Macrophages seem to be a critical factor. They, along with platelets and endothelial cells, produce growth factors that stimulate proliferation of angioblasts to generate new vessel growth and fibroblasts to cause collagen and scar formation. Later, the area is remodeled into appropriate tissue. The original tensile strength is never regained.

Healing requires adequate tissue perfusion, a normal immune system, good nutrition, and an infection-free environment. All may be compromised in the critically ill. Early laboratory evidence suggests that noise, sleep deprivation, and pain may also inhibit healing.

Additional Reactions

Several additional cellular responses are under investigation. One area of particular interest is heat shock proteins released by many stressed cells and bacteria. They seem to stimulate immunity and serve to preserve intracellular functions.

A second area of interest is opsonins. These are substances such as fibronectin, a circulating protein, and the complement and antibodies previously discussed, which attach to the antigen surface. They enhance the step that leads to phagocytosis. Opsonizing means literally "prepare to eat." Many of these substances are found in fresh frozen plasma and cryoprecipitate.

These proteins as well as others that mediate immunity and inflammation, and those which result from injury, such as oxygen radicals, are metabolized by enzymes or offset by other mediators. These neutralizing systems may be taxed in widespread injury.

Many factors released by bacteria also have localized and systemic effects. The most widely studied is endotoxin released from the membranes of gram-negative bacteria. It appears to be a potent trigger for the response to injury. It may also uncouple oxidative phosphorylation and, thereby, inhibit ATP synthesis.

Endotoxin is also one of the strongest stimuli for the release of cachectin or tumor necrosis factor (TNF) from macrophages. Since it may be an important second messenger responsible for much of the systemic response in septic patients, it too has been widely studied. Injection of either endotoxin or TNF has been shown to cause vasodilation and increased cardiac output and to mimic the clinical presentations of septic syndrome.

SYSTEMIC INFLAMMATORY RESPONSE SYNDROME

Systemic inflammatory response syndrome (SIRS), or septic syndrome, results when the local response to injury becomes systemic. Tissue injury triggers systemic vascular inflammation. Vessels dilate, lowering systemic vascular resistance and, thereby, causing a reflex increase in cardiac output, heart rate, and respiratory rate. Platelets and granulocytes aggregate along vessel walls. The immune system is activated. Monokines and cytokines trigger fever, neutrophilia, and lymphocytosis. Heat shock proteins are released by injured and white cells.

Phagocytes, proteins, and fluid enter tissues. When stimulated, phagocytes increase oxygen combustion to produce proteins, hydrogen peroxide, oxygen radicals, and acids. The arachidonic acid cascade cycles to produce prostaglandins, thromboxane A_2, and leukotrienes. Eventually, tissues distant from the original injury are damaged.

SIRS, then, is a host response triggered by a local insult. The macrophage-derived factor appears to be a major driving force with the granulocytes being a primary target. Activated complement potentiates the response. Paradoxically, lymphocytes seem to be overwhelmed and dysfunctional, contributing to co-existing generalized immunosuppression.

Triggers

The most common trigger for SIRS is a nidus of infection. The site and causative agent vary widely. The majority of patients have bacterial infections, gram-positive bacilli being more common in infections not hospital acquired and gram-negative in those that are. Gram-negative infections have become increasingly common over the years. Other infecting organisms include fungi, mycobacteria, mycoplasmas, and viruses.

Important sites of nosocomial infections are well known. They include lungs, bladder, invasive lines, wounds, and sinuses. The patient's clinical signs and risks often suggest the most likely cause.

The ability of a colonizing organism to cause infection depends on the host's immune defense system as well as characteristics of the organism. These include the colony count, its virulence, the toxins it produces, and its resistance to antibiotic therapy. Although the battle of normal flora competing for substrates and bonding sites is usually protective, some combinations of bacteria seem to be synergistic, allowing each to flourish in the other's presence. It is well documented that the presence of a foreign body such as a catheter, suture, or tube allows infection to occur with one third as many organisms present.

Infection is not the only cause of SIRS. The concept of the septic syndrome was developed to describe patients who behave clinically as though they are septic and have negative cultures. These patients may have either occult infections or other triggers of the systemic response. Although many studies suggest that infection is the most common, autopsy study of patients with SIRS has revealed that one third are made septic by a local infection, one third are infection free, and one third develop infection after developing the syndrome.

Other potential triggers include a persistent area of necrosis, inflammation or trauma, or persistent hypoxic states. These triggers activate the same local response to injury. Areas of necrosis include retained fetus, bowel infarcts, and occlusive peripheral vascular disease. Areas of inflammation include aspiration pneumonitis, pancreatitis, and hematomas. In spaces with hemorrhage, red blood cells are broken down into iron and bilirubin, which are highly inflammatory. Trauma may be induced by accidents and thermal injury but also by major surgical intervention. Even localized trauma is known to cause observable histological changes indicative of a systemic injury response within hours of the event. Episodes of prolonged hemorrhagic and cardiogenic shock can trigger a septic syndrome or may aggravate and potentiate the ongoing response to prior insults.

A major remaining question is why some patients exposed to similar triggers develop SIRS and others do not. Those who do are at risk of dying from the response, not the trigger. It may turn out that those who are likely to have a fulminant response can be identified and treated prophylactically.

Systemic Responses

Cardiovascular System

Systemic vascular inflammation leads to generalized vasodilation and, in patients with adequate cardiac reserves, an increased cardiac output. This response is recognized clinically as episodes of hypotension and tachycardia with warm skin. Patients with pulmonary artery catheters in place demonstrate cardiac outputs two to four times normal with low systemic vascular resistance. Those with mixed venous oxygen staturation ($S\bar{v}O_2$) monitoring show $S\bar{v}O_2$

values above normal. Echocardiograms reveal large end-diastolic volumes and low ejection fractions for both ventricles.

These episodes may last minutes or days. In patients with poor cardiovascular function, the response is blunted and may not be clinically evident. It may also be missed in patients whose concurrent disease or drug therapy masks the response. In each of these situations, the noncardiovascular systemic manifestations become even more important clinical clues.

Increased vascular permeability is a second response to systemic inflammation. Over time, skin edema is clinically obvious. Other effects of edema are more insiduous. It may contribute to increased intracranial pressure, pulmonary insufficiencies, cellular hypoxia, gut hypomotility, and poor wound healing.

Endocrine System

In describing the response of the endocrine system to stress, it is easier to list the hormones that do *not* increase: those responsible for fertility and reproduction, and thyroid-stimulating hormone. The first few hours or days are dominated by a very high level of catecholamine release. They decrease but still remain fairly high for several days during which ACTH, cortisol, and glucagon levels are also elevated.

Catecholamines have renowned effects on every organ system through α- and β-receptors by regulating blood flow. The organs that have "luxury" perfusion (blood flow proportionately well above oxygen demands) during nonstressed periods are the skin, the gut, and the kidneys. Catecholamines decrease perfusion to these areas to provide for increased oxygen demand of other organs, such as the heart, and to protect cerebral blood flow. They also contribute to hyperglycemia via glycogenolysis and gluconeogenesis.

Increased ACTH and cortisol are important in that they suppress local white cell mediators in inflammation and also cause lymphocytopenia. Cortisol stimulates glycogenolysis and gluconeogenesis which contribute to hyperglycemia. It dramatically enhances the actions of other stress hormones, including catecholamines, and, as a result, orchestrates the stress response.

Increased levels of cortisol, catecholamines, and glucagon, in addition to increasing glucose formation, also inhibit insulin activity. Blood sugar rises despite normal or even elevated insulin levels.

Increased ADH causes water retention in the kidneys, potentially causing vasoconstriction, especially in the grastrointestinal vessels. Aldosterone causes sodium retention with secondary water retention and potassium secretion. Both hormones contribute to oliguria.

Metabolic Response

The metabolic response can be divided into two phases. The first is the acute phase, which occurs during the first hours to days and often begins with shock and resuscitation. Catecholamines and other hormones act to stimulate glycogenolysis and gluconeogenesis. Under normal circumstances, stress-induced glycogenesis alone can maintain high blood glucose levels for 12 to 18 hours. In septic patients, hyperglycemia can become a significant problem that may be unresponsive to insulin therapy.

Although energy expenditure is increased, often to over twice resting levels, it is usually effectively met by these hormone-mediated alterations in metabolism. Not only are proteins catabolized to produce glucose (gluconeogenesis), but they also become an important primary source of energy, providing 40% of calories consumed. The lipolytic pathway of gluconeogenesis leads to an increase in fatty acids and glycerol, which can enter the Krebs cycle to produce energy. Ketones are also formed in the process and may build up if not properly metabolized. Lipolysis provides 30% of the calories used; glucose provides the remaining 30%. These mechanisms depend on adequate liver function and may not occur in patients with hepatic impairment.

The second phase may last as long as 3 weeks. The endocrine, autonomic, and immune responses mobilize protein for survival and wound repair. Somatic proteins are metabolized for energy and to subsidize acute phase reactions involving visceral proteins. The net nitrogen balance is negative; that is, more protein catabolism than synthesis occurs. For this reason patients with septic syndrome have been called obligatory cannibals.

Specific metabolic changes occur in several organs. The immune cells utilize increased amounts of glucose and glutamines for energy. Muscles such as the heart continue to need free fatty acids, their preferred fuel. These are made available by hormone-driven alterations in liver function. In the process, skeletal-muscle branch chain amino acids are metabolized, as well as other amino acids from connective tissue and the gut.

Cellular Response to Hypoxia

Even though the cardiac output may be elevated, there is evidence of tissue hypoxia in septic patients. Supportive findings include elevated lactate levels, elevated $S\bar{v}O_2$ values, and histological studies.

One important contributing factor is thought to be a maldistribution of blood flow to the point that areas of hyper- and hypoperfusion coexist. Although some areas may be vasodilated and have increased perfusion, others have decreased perfusion. Decreased flow may occur in areas of vasoconstriction as a result of increased α-adrenergic tone, of vascular obstruction from white cells and platelets, or of peri-vascular edema. In addition, the intra- and extracellular edema may decrease oxygen diffusion. Enzymes or metabolites required for synthesis of AMP, ADP, and ATP are thought to become depleted. Endotoxin and possibly other cytokines may interfere with the mitochondrial uptake of oxygen.

These potential causes of decreased oxygen supply occur in the face of increased oxygen demand. The results of cellular hypoxia include decreased ATPase and energy to maintain normal electrolyte gradients across the cell membrane. The extracellular potassium increases while the intracellular sodium and calcium increase. Secondarily, the shift of fluid into the cell with sodium and calcium has cytotoxic effects. Further depletion of adenosine substrates leads to anaerobic metabolism, lactic acidosis, and production of other abnormal metabolites. Ischemic injury leads to increased oxygen radicals, degradation of cell membranes, and activation of the arachidonic acid cascade.

The end result is dysfunction and eventually death of cells. When the cells of a particular organ are sufficiently disrupted, that system dysfunctions, and the patient progresses to multiple organ dysfunction syndrome (MODS).

Interactions

Continuing investigations reveal a variety of interactions between the components of the response to injury among the immune, neurological, and the endocrine systems. These findings have given rise to a new subspeciality—neuroimmunoendocrinology. Many interactions between immunity, inflammation, phagocytosis, and platelet complement activity were detailed in the section on the local response to injury. Examples from the field of neuroimmunoendocrinology include:

1. Immune cells have receptors for many hormones such as ACTH; catecholamines; acetylcholine; endomorphin; growth hormone; prolactin; and substance P, a neurotransmitter involved in the transmission of pain.
2. Activated monocytes and lymphocytes can produce hormones and neurotransmitters, including most of those listed in item 1.
3. Interleukins stimulate the nervous and the endocrine systems.
4. Catecholamines are proinflammatory, but both catecholamines and cortisol seem to decrease lymphocyte proliferation.
5. Microbes produce substances similar to such hormones as insulin, endorphins, ACTH, and somatostatin.

The clinical implications of these findings have yet to be defined, but two issues are clear. Unraveling the interrelationships among these complex systems will take years of research. Drugs that modulate any one of these three systems are likely to have effects on the other two. This interaction increases the difficulty of developing target-specific interventions with single effects. Furthermore, what drugs do in a test tube or even in an animal model cannot be assumed to be as simple or straightforward in human subjects, despite the importance of these research methods.

Diagnosis

Until reliable laboratory markers become available, sepsis and SIRS will remain a clinical diagnosis. The manifestations are usually overt and numerous. The patient's temperature may go up or down. Typically, the blood pressure drops while the heart rate and respiratory rate rise. The patient's skin may feel warm and look flushed. Shaking and chills may occur, and the level of consciousness often declines. A complete blood count reveals leukocytosis and thrombocytopenia.

These findings in a patient with a known risk for SIRS make the diagnosis. Patients likely to develop occult sepsis include those with diminished cardiovascular, neurological, and immune function, and those in whom the episode is so transient it may be unappreciated. In these diagnostically problematic patients, the first suspicion of septic syndrome comes much later as successive organ systems fail.

It is imperative that critical care nurses recognize these episodes and communicate them promptly to physicians. The diagnosis of SIRS will set into motion several actions to diagnose and treat sources of infection, to prevent organ dysfunction, and to support failing systems. As methods of pharmacological intervention become available, the situation becomes analogous to patients with myocardial infarction presenting in the emergency department. The faster diagnosis is made and thrombolytic therapy is administered to appropriate patients, the better the outcome.

Medical Management

The management of patients with SIRS includes (1) eliminating or treating the focus or the cause of injury, (2) modifying the systemic response to it, (3) protecting the target organs from dysfunction, and (4) supportive care. The first two general areas are addressed here. The second two are discussed subsequently.

Treating the Cause

Often the nidus of injury is known. Many studies have examined methods of reducing the insult caused by different triggers. Examples include debridement of wounds, early surgical repair of areas of trauma and necrosis, removal of extravascular blood in areas of hemorrhage and hematomas, and drainage or removal of abscesses.

Even when a potential noninfectious cause is known, secondary infections must be suspected. Blood cultures are frequently requested even though it is well known they may be intermittently negative in patients with systemic infections or may be positive with skin contaminants. Still, identification of organisms is very helpful in directing therapy.

Gram stains and cultures are also commonly done on urine, sputum, and wounds. Invasive lines that have been in place too long or are no longer needed may be replaced or removed and cultured. The longer these lines are left in place, the higher the risk they may become contaminated. An estimated 250,000 cases per year of device-related septicemia currently occur in the United States.

Antibiotic therapy may be initiated once a quick Gram stain has been reported as positive. The empiric administration of antibiotics to patients with negative studies, covering organisms most likely to be involved, is controversial. The dilemma comes from data indicating that some culture-negative patients may have occult areas of infections. If these infections go untreated, the patient is less likely to survive. Patients who are treated but have no infection unnecessarily incur the cost and risks of antibiotic therapy including potential superinfection or nosocomial infection.

Autopsy studies have shown that in medical patients, occult infections are most often in the lung; in surgical patients, they are most often in the abdomen. Many useful noninvasive and invasive diagnostic tests have been developed over the years. Each must be evaluated by the physician in terms of the risk/benefit ratio. Is the cost of the study and the risk of the procedure or transport warranted for *this* patient? The important nursing implication is the need to assess patients for signs of occult areas of injury and to report any unusual findings.

Modifying the Systemic Response

The goal of new treatments is to eliminate detrimental host reactions while leaving the required defense systems intact. Much of the ongoing research in SIRS and MODS has been focused on these aspects. Clinically applicable interventions are beginning to emerge.

One of the first such developments is the use of *human monoclonal antibody* to endotoxin. Endotoxins stimulate inflammation, clotting, phagocytosis, and systemic immune reactions. Clinical trials have shown that monoclonal antibody to endotoxin, when given early, improves survival (about 15% to 20%)

in specific subsets of patients with SIRS. One major trial showed a benefit to those with gram-negative bacteremia without shock, but a second major trial showed a benefit only to those in shock. Although further investigation is required, this technique is now known to be safe but expensive.

Corticosteroids are one of the oldest drug categories with a potential role in septic syndrome. They block neutrophils, lysosomes, the arachidonic acid and complement cascades, interleukins, and inflammation. Although these effects seem desirable, well-designed clinical trials have so far failed to demonstrate any improvement in morbidity or mortality. Indeed, corticosteroids may actually increase morbidity in some patient subsets and, therefore, cannot be recommended at present unless adrenal insufficiency is suspected.

Arachidonic acid and *prostaglandin inhibitors* also are under widespread investigation because of their potential for mitigating the local and systemic response to injury. Their drawbacks include renal failure and bronchospasm.

Tumor necrosis factor (TNF), or cachectin, has long been incriminated as an early and potent mediator of the septic syndrome. Monoclonal antibodies to TNF have been developed. It is hoped that they will be even more effective than those against endotoxin, in part because their benefit would not be limited to gram-negative bacteremia.

Antioxidants targeted against oxygen radicals and metabolites are another important area under study. They include superoxide dismutase (SOD), allopurinol, mannitol, and other specific proteins.

Other fertile areas of pharmacological research include antibodies to various interleukins, endorphin blockers such as nalaxone and thyroid-releasing factor, splanchnic vasodilators such as vasopressin inhibitors, local anesthetics such as lidocaine, healing agonists such as growth hormone, energy substrates such as ATP, opsonants such as fibronectin, and anticlotting drugs such as heparin and thrombolytic agents.

The primary mechanical therapies investigated in the treatment of septic syndrome are continuous arterial-venous hemofiltration and hemodialysis (CAVH and CAVD). The primary aim is to remove metabolites mediating the systemic reaction as well as the waste products of the hypermetabolic state. A secondary effect is the removal of fluid to allow tolerance of the volume from therapeutic intravenous infusions required by some patients. Conflicting results of studies reported to date have stimulated continuation of clinical trials.

The remainder of the management involves the prevention and treatment of resultant organ system failure, and general supportive care. A discussion of each follows.

PATHOPHYSIOLOGY OF MULTIPLE ORGAN DYSFUNCTION SYNDROME

Cellular organ damage in patients who develop MODS begins with the onset of local injury. Damage is thought to be compounded not only by mediators from the initiating event but also by those arising from subsequent episodes of hypotension, hypoxemia, or secondary infections. Endogenous flora and toxins normally confined to the gastrointestinal tract may translocate and continue to drive the systemic response.

The target systems of SIRS seem to be those in which significant numbers of phagocytes are normally found and those systems with the lowest reserve. As each system fails, loss of its function causes further insults.

In patients without preexisting organ dysfunction, ARDS may develop within 1 to 3 days, putting the patient at risk for further tissue hypoxia. Over the next several days, renal failure, hepatic failure, gastrointestinal failure, and coagulopathy may occur. These processes add uremic toxins, hepatic toxins, more gut toxins, bleeding, and clotting to the list of systemic insults. The majority of patients respond to therapy and remain in a hyperdynamic state. The 40% who do not respond develop septic shock and have added ischemic injury.

The overall mortality from MODS is approximately 50% to 60% in those with two systems involved, and 80% to 100% in those with three or more involved. The primary goal, then, is to identify SIRS and sequential organ involvement early, in order to institute appropriate protective and therapeutic measures.

Septic Shock

Pathophysiology

As previously stated, patients with normal cardiovascular function respond to widespread inflammatory vasodilation with increased cardiac output. The early hemodynamic profile, therefore, is decreased systemic vascular resistance (SVR), high cardiac output (CO), and tachycardia. The ventricles dilate to high end-diastolic volumes with stroke volumes maintained at normal levels and with low ejection fractions. As time goes by, the CO can become primarily a function of increased heart rate.

The cause of ventricular dilation is not clearly understood. The specific mediator that has been most widely studied is myocardial depressant factor, which is probably released from the pancreas early in the septic syndrome. Endotoxin and TNF have also been

shown to have negative inotropic effects. Autopsy studies, however, have revealed subendocardial hemorrhage and necrosis in patients who died of SIRS. Many other factors may be involved. Those who survive SIRS and septic shock normalize their ejection fraction soon after the shock subsides, suggesting a chemical rather than a structural defect.

Diagnosis

Usually the diagnosis of shock can be made clinically in a matter of seconds to minutes (see Chapter 7). The exception is septic shock. Cold, clammy skin may not occur in septic shock because peripheral vasodilation masks the condition. The definition of shock is inadequate tissue oxygenation. This usually occurs because of decreased cardiac output. However, in septic shock, evidence of tissue hypoxia occurs long before the patient's cardiac output falls below normal, because it is due not to low overall flow but to maldistribution of blood flow and decreased oxygen extraction in the face of increased oxygen demand.

The presence of oxygenation deficits must be inferred in septic patients by evidence of ischemia and anaerobic metabolism. A marker that works reasonably well is the lactate level. Not only does this marker indicate the degree of anaerobic metabolism, but serial lactate values can guide treatment. It has been shown that lactate levels decrease 5% per hour once oxygen demands are met. This information can be very helpful in treatment since optimal cardiac output end points can be hard to identify. A patient with a lactate level of 6 mg/dl should have a level below 4 mg/dl 7 hours after an adequate level of hemodynamic support has been reached. Lactate levels have also been shown to be helpful prognostic indicators. Patients with values below 2 mg/dl have a 90% survival, whereas those with values above 10 mg/dl have a 90% mortality. The major problem with monitoring lactate levels is that lactate is produced primarily by muscle and red blood cells and utilized by the liver and kidneys. In some clinical situations, lactate levels do not correlate well with anaerobic metabolism.

Two other parameters are being evaluated for their potential contribution to hemodynamic monitoring in the septic patient. The first is mixed venous hemoglobin oxygen saturation ($S\bar{v}O_2$) as measured by pulmonary catheters equipped with oximetry fiberoptics. The $S\bar{v}O_2$ reflects the interaction in overall oxygen supply and demand dynamics (see Chapter 7). The problem in patients with septic syndrome is that many factors that alter $S\bar{v}O_2$ can occur coincidentally, making interpretation of changes very difficult. The cardiac output may be rising or falling, causing the $S\bar{v}O_2$ to increase or decrease, respectively. The demand increases, and $S\bar{v}O_2$ falls in patients who shiver, convulse, or struggle to breathe or move. The $S\bar{v}O_2$ will increase again as these phenomena subside. Furthermore, the overall $S\bar{v}O_2$ will be misleading when maldistribution of blood flow leads to areas of hypo- and hyperperfusion. Accordingly, the time that the $S\bar{v}O_2$ may be the most helpful in patients with septic shock is at the onset of the hyperdynamic phase. In patients in whom other clinical manifestations are subtle or masked, a rise in $S\bar{v}O_2$ from the 70s to the 80s may herald a septic episode.

The second parameter is cardiac ejection fraction. The right ventricular ejection fraction (RVEF) can now be monitored with devices built into pulmonary artery catheters. Whether or not this will be helpful in monitoring septic patients has yet to be determined.

Much of the work in assessing the adequacy of tissue oxygenation in the last decade has been in the relationship between oxygen delivery and oxygen consumption. This relationship is reviewed in the section on supportive care.

Medical Management

The primary therapeutic intervention used to support cardiovascular function in septic patients is fluid administration. When shock or hypotension occurs or hyperdynamic status begin to wane, fluid administration improves outcome because vasodilation and shifting of fluid from the intravascular to interstitial or intracellular space are part of the pathophysiology.

Fluid administration is guided by the wedge or pulmonary artery occlusion pressure (PAOP) and cardiac output. Although the optimum PAOP for each patient should be individually determined, it is usually 12 to 15 mmHg. This range takes advantage of the Frank-Starling law without raising the risk of pulmonary edema in patients with a potential for acute lung injury and ARDS.

Either extracellular crystalloids or colloids can be used; little difference in morbidity or mortality has been demonstrated. When crystalloids such as normal saline or Ringer's lactate are used, three quarters of the volume accumulates in the interstitial space. Colloids, in contrast, remain in the bloodstream and draw interstitial fluid toward them. In other words, crystalloids cause edema, and colloids reverse it. Colloids are more expensive than crystalloids but can be used in smaller quantity. Combinations of crystalloid and colloid solutions are often used.

Patients with low hemoglobin levels also may benefit from packed red blood cells. Although there are risks involved in transfusion therapy, the benefits are increased oxygen content and delivery. The benefit of anemia associated with hemodilution is decreased blood viscosity and resistance to flow. Optimal hemoglobin levels are difficult to identify, but many authors and clinicians have recommended a minimum of 10 to 11 g/dl.

If fluid therapy alone does not increase CO to desired levels, an inotropic agent such as digitalis, dobutamine, or dopamine is added. Digitalis is often effective, but its effect cannot be titrated. Dobutamine has been shown to increase CO significantly, but it has a mild vasodilating effect. Vasodilation can cause a relative hypovolemia, decrease preload, and decrease stroke volume. Fluid resuscitation, therefore, must be established first and then reassessed after dobutamine administration. Dopamine may also be appropriate, but its α-adrenergic effect begins with dosages as low as 3 to 5 μg per kg in some individuals. Although increased SVR can contribute to the maldistribution of blood flow, it may be desirable in patients with a very low diastolic pressure. The renal effects of low-dose dopamine are reviewed in the section on renal failure.

Other inotropes include epinephrine and norepinephrine, both of which have a peripheral α-adrenergic effect. Although few data regarding combination therapy are yet available, patients who do not respond adequately to a single agent may do well on two or more similar agents. The drug and dose response variability is thought to be due to the down-regulation of β-receptors. Over time, endogenous and exogenous catecholamines may deplete cell membrane receptor sites faster than the cell can reproduce and replace them. The patient's response capability diminishes, or is down-regulated. Increasing the administration rate will not increase efficacy in such circumstances, but changing or adding agents may.

Corticosteroids have been shown to modulate adrenergic receptors. Therefore, a second potential explanation for failure to respond to catecholamine administration is a corticosteroid deficiency. It is important to consider this often occult phenomenon since steroid replacement therapy can be life-saving in these patients.

Many inotropic agents are in various stages of clinical investigation. Some act on β-adrenergic receptors and others through alternative membrane or intracellular mechanisms. They have the potential for becoming important primary or secondary therapies, but also of undergoing down-regulation.

Similarly, peripheral α-receptors may also become down-regulated. Because of this phenomenon and the vasodilatory effect of some of the septic metabolites, most patients with septic syndrome sustain a low SVR throughout their course. When SVR is critically low and mean arterial pressure is unacceptable, vasopressor therapy may be initiated. Often, these drugs are ineffective from the start or become so in time. Agents that do not act on α-receptors, such as angiotensin II, are under investigation.

A few patients develop an increased SVR. Such cases are usually managed with the addition of direct vasodilators such as nitroprusside. Even though receptor sites are not involved in their action, enzymes are involved, and these agents are also prone to loss of efficacy over time.

Optimal therapeutic endpoints in the manipulation of hemodynamic parameters are difficult to identify in patients with septic syndrome. Much of the work reported to date has shown that a cardiac index greater than 4.5 L/min/m^2 and an oxygen delivery ($\dot{D}o_2$) of over 600 ml/min/m^2 are associated with a better outcome. The question becomes even more complex when the pulmonary and metabolic factors that contribute to tissue oxygenation are considered. They interact dynamically with the cardiovascular component and are discussed more fully in the section on supportive care.

Impact on MODS

When cardiovascular function is inadequate to meet tissue oxygenation requirements and therapeutic interventions fail, systemic ischemic injury results. This ischemic injury may occur episodically or for prolonged periods, causing further cellular dysfunction. Specifically, the occurrence of myocardial ischemia or infarction can be devastating.

Adult Respiratory Distress Syndrome

Pathophysiology

Adult respiratory distress syndrome (ARDS) is a common early development in MODS, occurring in 25% to 40% of patients (see Chapter 29). The lung has little reserve, and, although studies have shown that the injury process begins almost immediately in the patient with SIRS, the clinical hallmarks of the disease take 1 to 3 days to develop. With better understanding of this sequential pathology and pathogenesis has come a change in terminology. Although the nursing literature tends to retain the term ARDS, much of the medical literature has adopted the term acute lung injury (ALI).

Circulating mediators cause neutrophils and platelets to aggregate in the pulmonary microcirculation. This aggregation, coupled with increased vascular permeability, damages both the capillary and alveolar membranes and activates alveolar macrophages. There is widespread damage to the type 1, or typical, alveolar epithelial cells, followed by loss of the type 2 cells. Type 2 cells are unique, highly metabolic pneumocytes which secrete substances such as surfactant.

Eventually, loss of surfactant leads to alveolar collapse.

The other metabolic functions of the type 2 cells are difficult to quantify. It is known that the lungs are responsible for activating some substrates such as angiotensin I to angiotensin II. They are also thought to deactivate substances such as bradykinins and norepinephrine. The role that this loss might play in the pathogenesis of ARDS and multiorgan failure is not yet clear.

Diagnosis

The earlist clinical manifestations of ARDS are due to microvascular changes: cellular aggregations and increased permeability. Patients develop high pulmonary vascular resistance and, therefore, high pulmonary artery pressures along with a noncardiogenic pulmonary edema. Although not easily or often done, measurements of pulmonary lymphatic flow show dramatic increases. Despite this attempt to compensate, interstitial edema develops.

The consequences of pulmonary edema are a decrease in both oxygen diffusion and pulmonary compliance. This type of hypoxemia is responsive to increased doses of inspired oxygen. Decreased compliance causes increased work of breathing in spontaneously breathing patients and increased static or plateau pressures in patients undergoing mechanical ventilation.

As the injury process continues, there is widespread alveolar collapse, causing more dramatic problems with oxygenation and pulmonary compliance. At this point, the patient's hypoxemia becomes refractory to oxygen therapy because collapsed alveolar do not benefit from higher fractions of inspired oxygen (Fio_2).

One clue that ARDS is developing is noting that a patient has broken one of the "50-50" rules. Since most other causes of hypoxemia are responsive to oxygen therapy, the arterial oxygen tension (Pao_2) will usually reach the 50s with an Fio_2 of 0.50. Patients who break this rule have refractory hypoxemia, which is usually caused by conditions that lead to alveolar consolidation or collapse. Alveolar consolidation may be widespread in pneumonia, alveolar collapse in ARDS. If pneumonia can be ruled out, the presence of ARDS must be considered.

The hallmarks, then, of ARDS are decreased compliance, progressively refractory hypoxemia, and pulmonary edema as seen by chest radiographs. The associated findings are dyspnea and tachypnea. Other early laboratory findings include respiratory alkalosis or hyperventilation due to the microatelectasis, and increased intrapulmonary shunting. Shunts often measure over 50% in patients with late ARDS. Dead space is also increased due to increased PVR and hyperventilation. Both of these responses lead to ventilation in excess of perfusion, the classic definition of dead space (see Chapter 27).

The diagnosis is more difficult in patients with confounding cardiac or pulmonary disease. Distinguishing ARDS from cardiogenic pulmonary edema involves documenting the absence of other signs of heart failure, such as crackles, a high wedge pressure, or an enlarged heart. Distinguishing ARDS from pneumonia involves evaluation of sputum cultures and other signs of infection. ARDS can be very difficult to diagnose in either situation in patients who have septic syndrome since the cardiovascular and immune system function may both be altered. While the search continues for an early specific diagnostic marker for acute lung injury, it pays to have a high index of suspicion to aid in early recognition.

Medical Management

The primary therapeutic goal in ARDS is to prevent further lung damage while maintaining adequate tissue oxygenation. The fall in PaO_2 and hemoglobin saturation (SaO_2) must be treated without decreasing overall oxygen delivery ($\dot{D}O_2$). Two potential interventions are increased FiO_2 and positive end-expiratory pressure (PEEP).

Increasing the FiO_2 has two main drawbacks. First, late ARDS is refractory to oxygen therapy, and doses above 50% may not have much impact on the patient's PaO_2. Second, high-dose oxygen can lead to the formation of added oxygen radicals in the already injured lung. Type 2 cells contain enzymes that normally metabolize excess oxygen into water. Type 2 cell dysfunction in ARDS patients may lead to incomplete oxygen metabolism and the accumulation of intermediate breakdown products, oxygen radicals, and hydrogen peroxide.

The alternative method for treating hypoxemia is PEEP. Although low-dose PEEP of 5 cmH_2O or less can be used in a wide variety of settings, therapeutic PEEP at levels of 10 cmH_2O and above is reserved primarily for patients with ARDS. PEEP increases the functional residual capacity toward normal by reinflating partially or totally collapsed alveoli. Once collapsed alveoli are reopened, they become responsive to oxygen therapy.

PEEP trials can be used to help confirm the diagnosis of ARDS. In patients with refractory hypoxemia due to consolidating processes, PEEP does not reverse the hypoxemia. In patients with refractory hypoxemia due to ARDS, PEEP will increase the arterial PaO_2.

Titrating PEEP therapy is best done by monitoring changes in the intrapulmonary shunt and $\dot{D}O_2$. Both are important since the desired outcome is increased $\dot{D}O_2$ or tissue oxygenation. Although PEEP can increase the oxygen content, increasing the intrathoracic pressure can decrease venous return and cardiac output. Since the two variables that affect $\dot{D}O_2$ are oxygen content and cardiac output, increasing one while decreasing the other will not benefit the patient.

In patients with pulmonary artery catheters, PEEP therapy can be rationally applied by following the percentage of intrapulmonary shunting and the $\dot{D}O_2$. When a level is reached that has decreased the shunt and decreased the $\dot{D}O_2$, cardiac output should be supported. Patients usually respond to fluid therapy since the cause of decreased cardiac output is decreased venous return. If fluid therapy is ineffective, inotropes may be considered. Decreased cardiac output must be supported since it not only decreases $\dot{D}O_2$ but also leads to increased extraction and decreased $S\bar{v}O_2$. The $S\bar{v}O_2$ indicates the degree of desaturation of the blood that is shunted to the left heart. The lower the $S\bar{v}O_2$, the lower the SaO_2 in patients with significant intrapulmonary shunting.

The second major complication from PEEP therapy is barotrauma. Increased intrathoracic pressure in diseased lungs can lead to pneumothorax, pneumomediastinum, and subcutaneous emphysema. It is very important that nurses caring for patients receiving PEEP therapy know how to recognize signs of barotrauma quickly. Although barotrauma can often be managed with chest tubes, it further compromises the patient's pulmonary status. Moreover, the presence of chest tubes adds significantly to patient discomfort.

In the vast majority of patients with ARDS, an adequate PaO_2 (60 mmHg or greater) and SaO_2 (90% or greater) are reached using a combination of increased FiO_2 and PEEP. In patients who do not respond to conventional therapy, intravascular devices that support gas exchange (IVOX) are undergoing clinical trials. Extracorporeal membrane oxygenation (ECMO) has been studied repeatedly since the 1960s. Both require further investigation before they can be recommended.

Many alternative modes of mechanical ventilation to improve oxygenation and decrease the risk of impaired cardiac output and barotrauma in patients with ARDS have been studied. Thus far, none has been associated with improved morbidity or mortality.

Patients with ARDS often require mechanical ventilation, not usually because they are hypoventilating but because the increased work of breathing is too costly. Typically, their minute ventilation is two to three times normal, and their lungs are half as compliant. The metabolic cost of breathing becomes too high, and mechanical support is instituted. The other benefit derived from mechanical support of ventilation is diminished diaphragm perfusion. Resting the diaphragm may allow a portion of the cardiac output to be diverted to other organs.

Impact on MODS

Critical care nurses play a pivotal role in the early diagnosis and management of patients with ARDS. The hallmarks are often first clinically recognized by the nurse with a high index of suspicion caring for a high-risk patient.

Once diagnosed, the hypoxemia must be managed without increasing lung injury or compromising DO_2 by using the appropriate combinations of oxygen, PEEP, and cardiovascular support. Intubation and mechanical ventilation also carry risks which can further compromise patient outcome and require skilled nursing management (see Chapter 30).

It is more difficult to recognize the loss of metabolic functions in Type 2 cells. Like the liver, the lung may have important responsibilities for detoxification of circulating metabolites. None of the interventions as yet in place address this issue.

Renal Failure

Pathophysiology

Renal failure develops in 15% to 40% of patients with septic syndrome (see Chapter 36). Since the kidneys have a large reserve, failure usually is not manifested until after several days.

The factors involved include the mediators described, activated granulocytes and ischemic injury. The kidney produces several vasodilating and vasoconstricting agents used for autoregulation and the response to stress. These agents have been implicated in the perpetuation of dysfunction. Further insults include shock episodes and nephrotoxic agents such as antibiotics or contrast media. Other patients may have circulating hepatotoxins, myoglobin, and hemoglobin. All of these substances are known to cause renal failure in the form of acute tubular necrosis (ATN). Occasionally, glomerular nephritis occurs as a result of immune complexes.

Diagnosis

It is important to differentiate prerenal failure from parenchymal or intrarenal failure since the first is less serious and usually responds to adequate cardiovascular support. If left undertreated, however, prerenal failure may progress to acute tubular necrosis, a form of intrarenal failure.

The differential diagnosis includes serum and urine laboratory indices. The BUN can be very misleading in critically ill patients since it is elevated in patients who are catabolic, are receiving corticosteroids or some amino acids, have gastrointestinal bleeding, or have prerenal failure. These causes of elevation are associated with a BUN/serum creatinine ratio above 20:1. With intrarenal failure, the BUN and creatinine both rise together, and the normal 10:1 ratio is more likely to be maintained.

It is important to obtain a baseline serum creatinine since the creatinine often doubles when intrarenal failure develops. In a patient with an admission creatinine of 0.6 mg/dl, a rise to 1.2 mg/dl is significant yet remains within the normal range. Patients with preexisting renal dysfunction can also be identified by an admission creatinine test, and measures to protect them may be considered.

The urinalysis can be helpful in the differential diagnosis. The urine is free from abnormal sediment or casts in prerenal but not in intrarenal failure. The urine osmolality is above 500 mosm in prerenal and below 350 mosm in intrarenal failure. The urine sodium is below 20 mEq/L in prerenal and above 40 mEq/L in intrarenal failure. The fractional extraction of sodium (FeNa) is under 1% in prerenal and above 3% in ATN. The problem with the last three tests is that they are invalid if the patient has received diuretics or is receiving dopamine. Since both are often the case, the urine microscopic examination becomes even more important.

Another fairly accurate way of monitoring renal function is the creatinine clearance. It may differentiate prerenal from intrarenal failure, trend the course of the disease, and help determine appropriate dosages of drugs excreted by the kidney.

Oliguria can be a helpful indicator of the presence and reversal of prerenal failure. Decreased urinary output can be a sign of decreased renal blood flow, which should normalize with adequate support of cardiac output. Urinary output can be misleading in patients with intrarenal failure. Although most patients with ATN become oliguric, the incidence of nonoliguric failure is increasing.

Medical Management

One of the treatment goals in renal failure is to maintain adequate urinary output. When support of cardiovascular function is not sufficient and oliguric intrarenal failure is thought to be present, low-dose dopamine, diuretic therapy, or both are considered. It is clear that oliguric renal failure carries a much higher mortality than nonoliguric, but it is not certain whether or not therapeutic interventions that convert oliguria to nonoliguria affect overall outcome. Although the available data are difficult to interpret, many clinicians try to reverse oliguria. In addition to potentially improving chances of survival, increasing the urinary output makes the patient's management easier. These patients often require multiple intravenous medications which, when added to enteral or parenteral nutrition, may amount to several hundred ml per day. Patients need an adequate output to allow for this intake of solution.

The second management goal is to protect the patient's kidneys from further insults. Each episode of hypotension and each dose of nephrotoxic agent may cause further damage. It is important for critical care nurses to recognize hypotension and rapidly intervene if it occurs and to question nephrotoxic agents in patients at high risk.

Adjustments also need to be made in nonnephrotoxic drugs, which are eliminated by the kidneys. Digitalis is a well-known example. More controversial are the adjustments that should be made in the patient's nutrition. Although patients with renal failure do not tolerate protein well, meeting protein and caloric needs is important in patients with septic syndrome. As will be discussed in the section on nutritional support, meeting nutritional needs may require instituting or increasing dialysis therapy.

Many physicians initiate dialysis when the serum creatinine is above 8 mg, the BUN is above 100 mg, or serious complications such as life-threatening electrolyte imbalances, gastrointestinal hemorrhage, or pericarditis are present. The dialysis treatment options include standard hemodialysis (HD), peritoneal dialysis (PD), and continuous arterial–venous hemofiltration (CAVH) or CAVH with hemodialysis (CAVHD) (see Chapter 36). These options vary in their capabilities, limitations, complications, and technological problems. They are under investigation for their role in patients with MODS and renal failure. It may be that methods can be identified that not only treat renal failure but also remove some of the detrimental mediators of the septic syndrome.

One concern regarding the use of hemodialysis techniques is the occurrence of hypotensive episodes and the potential for decreased renal blood flow which may further the ischemic insults of prerenal failure and increase the likelihood of developing ATN. The risk/benefit ratio is weighed for each individual patient, taking into account the options available.

Newer pharmacological agents are also under investigation, primarily for their role in augmenting renal blood flow and metabolism. They inlcude calcium channel blockers, prostaglandins, atriopeptin, and ATP-MgCl. All have systemic as well as renal effects

that must be elucidated before any recommendations can be made.

Impact on MODS

When MOF involves renal failure, the mortality is 70% to 80%. This high mortality was not appreciated before the mid-1980s. Since then, clinicians have become much more careful about renal protection. Loss of renal function causes further multisystem dysfunction related to uremic toxins, fluid and electrolyte imbalances, and acid–base imbalances. In septic syndrome patients, mediators must be metabolized or excreted as well.

These patients present many clinical dilemmas and represent many clinical trade-offs. Should diuretics be administered to oliguric patients even though some of them are potentially nephrotoxic? Should nutritional needs be met, thereby increasing dialysis needs? Should antibiotic therapy emphasize agents less likely to damage the kidneys but also less likely to cover the pathogens? The answers should become clearer over the next few years.

Hepatic Failure

Pathophysiology

Hepatic failure develops in 10% to 40% of patients with SIRS. Like the kidneys, the normal liver has a large reserve capacity. Failure usually does not occur until several days after the onset of the syndrome. The liver contains Kupffer cells, which represent about 90% of the total tissue macrophages. They are triggered by septic mediators. The inflammation and phagocytic activity cause intrahepatic block to bile flow and microthrombosis, resulting in secondary damage to the hepatocytes.

The other potential trigger for hepatic failure is ischemic injury. The liver is exquisitely sensitive to decreased blood flow. It has been observed that the serum SGOT and SGPT spike to very high levels after episodes of shock but decrease again once perfusion is reestablished. Hepatotoxic agents and certain protein and lipid nutrients may also play a role.

The liver is strategically placed between the gastrointestinal tract and the lungs. When the liver loses its detoxification functions, toxins from the gastrointestinal tract as well as other septic mediators may not be adequately phagocytized or metabolized. It is not clear how much this loss of liver function and increase in circulatory toxins contributes to ARDS.

Hepatic failure leads to the loss of other functions as well. Hepatocyte dysfunction leads to release of false neurotransmitters with central as well as peripheral effects. Encephalopathy, myopathy, and polyneuropathy may ensue. Amino acid clearance and protein synthesis decrease. Albumin levels drop early, and antibody levels drop late. Ureagenesis increases, making the BUN an even poorer marker of renal function in patients with liver failure. There is decreased production of clotting factors, which may potentiate bleeding tendencies. Gluconeogenesis is spared, making hypoglycemia a late and ominous development.

On the positive side, the liver also has a tremendous ability to regenerate. Patients who recover from MOF also usually recover adequate liver function.

Diagnosis

Due in part to the large reserves it possesses and in part to the lack of sensitive and specific markers, liver failure is not recognized until late in the course of MOF. An elevated bilirubin is often one of the first signs but can also occur in hemolytic anemias, with infectious agents that destroy red blood cells, and in cholelithiasis. Alkaline phosphatase and transaminases may also rise. SGOT and SGPT elevate for short periods after episodes of shock. They rise in a more sustained fashion along with the LDH with hepatocellular dysfunction. Prolongation of the prothrombin time (PT) occurs when coagulation factors have dropped by one third. Elevation of the PT to two to three times normal for more than 2 days is considered a grave prognostic sign.

Medical Management

No direct interventions for hepatic failure are currently available. The principal goals are to limit further damage, to decrease the demands placed on the liver, and to manage complications.

Limiting further damage entails preventing hypotensive episodes and removing potentially hepatotoxic agents. As with all other organ systems involved in septic syndrome, treating the cause and controlling the response to mediators should also reduce the amount of liver dysfunction that occurs.

To decrease the demands placed on the liver, two other areas are being addressed. The detoxification requirements for the liver may be reduced by decontamination of the gastrointestinal tract to limit the quantity of toxins brought to the liver by the portal circulation. The second method is high-quality nutrition. The closer nutrients administered are to a metabolically useful form, the less the manipulation required by the liver.

Liver failure causes the aromatic amino acids to rise, and they may contribute to encephalopathy. On the other hand, branch chain amino acids fall and, thus, contribute to the loss of lean muscle mass. Overall, liver failure results in a hypercatabolic state that may double the amino acid requirements. Ongoing clinical studies are attempting to determine the optimum nutritional prescription for this patient subset.

Another area of ongoing research is the development of mechanical devices that support or replace lost hepatic function. The design problems are numerous, but some systems in clinical use for liver transplant patients may someday play a role in septic syndrome.

Impact on MODS

The impact of liver failure is similar to that of renal failure. Loss of the metabolic and detoxification functions not only increases the levels of circulatory offending mediators of the septic process but also adds toxic by-products of normal metabolism that would otherwise have been eliminated by the liver. When patients with MODS develop severe liver impairment as reflected by a bilirubin over 8 mg/dl, the mortality is over 90%.

Gastrointestinal Failure

Critical illness causes many disruptions in gastrointestinal (GI) physiology and function, including alterations in perfusion, secretion, motility, regeneration, and protection. Each may contribute to the pathophysiology of multisystem organ failure. In fact, the GI tract has been called the motor that drives the septic process.

Hypotension and stress activate endogenous catecholamines. The α-adrenergic compromise causes mesenteric vasoconstriction. Exogenous catecholamines and digitalis may cause further constriction of GI vessels. The physiological response to acute stress is well designed, since the GI tract is one organ with luxury perfusion (supply in excess of oxygen demands). However, mucosal ischemia may occur in critically ill patients with a prolonged clinical course. Nasogastric tubes equipped with tonometry to monitor gastric mucosal pH may become important to the identification of GI ischemia. These devices monitor the pH of the lining, not the solutions in the GI tract, and the mucosal pH drops when blood flow no longer meets oxygen demands.

Sympathetic responses also decrease GI secretion and motility. The decrease in secretion of mucus may significantly impair mucosal protection and contribute to the development of stress ulcers.

Another important role of the intestine is the absorption of nutrients. Unlike the rest of the body, the GI transports nutrients into the bloodstream rather than receiving nutrients received from it. The substrates used for regeneration of the mucosal membranes, which normally occurs every 36 hours, are derived from enteral nutrition. The process is stimulated by some of the digestive enzymes released when stimulated by the intake of food. Glutamine is the preferred fuel used for regeneration, especially in the time of stress. It is not administered in pareteral nutrition because it is an aromatic amino acid that forms ammonia when added to intravenous solutions. When patients are NPO and the GI tract is underperfused, the lack of both nutrients and oxygen impairs the ability to regenerate.

Last, the GI tract normally protects the rest of the body from its bacterial flora, toxins, and digestive enzymes. This type of immune function requires adequate lymphocyte activity, IgA production, digestive enzyme actions, Peyer's patch function, and competition for attachment to receptors between bacteria and nutrient substrates. All are diminished when patients are NPO. The height of intestinal villi has also been shown to decrease dramatically.

Consequences

In patients with SIRS, the insults described above are coupled with the injury caused by mediators and activated granulocytes. When the GI barrier becomes more permeable, bacterial endotoxin and other toxins gain access to the circulation. This translocation may continuously fuel the systemic septic response or may cause secondary infections. Ernest Moore summarizes the impact by reminding us that the GI tract is metabolically active, immunologically important, and bacteriologically critical in stressed patients.

A second consequence of these alterations in GI function is the risk of stress ulcers. Endoscopic studies have shown almost universal irritation of the gastric lining in severely ill patients unprotected by standard prophylactic measures. Upper GI bleeding has dramatically decreased since the institution of widespread routine prophylaxis, but the incidence is still estimated at 3% to 25%.

Medical Management

The current literature is replete with studies examining methods to preserve GI integrity in patients with SIRS. Areas of interest include (1) the use of enteral nutrition as early as possible, (2) the administration of agents that promote regeneration and perfusion, and (3) selective decontamination of the GI tract by nonabsorbable enteral antibiotics.

There is also ongoing research in balancing the need for stress ulcer prophylaxis with the potential risks of increasing GI flora and, thereby, infection. Flora are normally controlled in large part by the low pH created by the secretion of gastric acid, which is bacteriocidal. Although the use of antacids and H_2 antagonists has proved effective in preventing stress ulcers, these measures also increase GI flora. The concern is that increased flora can become a source of secondary infection. Organisms may migrate up the nasogastric tubes to colonize the mouth, sinuses, or lungs. They may also translocate across the permeable

intestinal mucosa. Although enteral feeding and sucralfate protect against stress ulcers, it is not clear whether they alone are effective enough in seriously ill patients.

Several additional questions remain unanswered. If H_2 blockers are used, which ones have the best risk/benefit ratio? Cimetidine is now given to critically ill patients less frequently than other H_2 blockers because of this issue. If H_2 blockers are used, should they be given continuously or intermittently? What is the optimal pH for titrating antacid or H_2-blocker therapy? Are combinations of prophylactic measures capable of preventing stress ulcers without increasing the risk of infection? Since small volumes of gastric contents are aspirated intermittently by most intubated and even unintubated patients, what are the pulmonary consequences of the aspiration of various types and amounts of particulate matter? Some have even questioned if prophylaxis is still worth the potential risk. Given the impact on cost and patient outcome, the answers will be very important to the practice of critical care.

If upper GI bleeding does occur, it is important to document the cause. Endoscopy can be both diagnostic and therapeutic. The gastric fundus must be visualized because it is not only technically the most difficult to see but the most common site of bleeding. Most episodes can be treated with medical interventions, but about 10% of patients require surgical intervention to control bleeding.

Another potential GI complication is acalculous cholelithiasis. The incidence is significant, and the exact mechanisms are unclear. Decreased GI motility, ischemia, and morphine have all been implicated. It is worth having a high index of suspicion for development of cholelithiasis in septic patients. Its presence can be masked in those who cannot complain of abdominal pain and already have high bilirubin levels from liver dysfunction. The diagnosis is made by noninvasive studies, but the treatment is cholecystectomy or cholecystotomy. Undiagnosed, it is life-threatening.

Patients may also develop pancreatitis, prolonged ileus, and diarrhea. Each may result from the septic injury process or be a complication of medical or surgical interventions. These conditions are easier to diagnose and, therefore, missed less often than cholecystitis. However, they represent major management challenges and have their own impact on outcome.

Impact on MODS

Although the advent of GI failure, short of bleeding, is difficult to diagnose, the assumption is made that the GI tract becomes more involved over time. When coupled with hepatic failure, loss of GI integrity may allow bacteria, endotoxins, and other noxious substrates normally removed by the liver to circulate systemically. Measures to protect against further injury are instituted according to the best research currently available. The impact of loss of GI integrity or stress ulcers is increased morbidity and mortality.

Disseminated Intravascular Coagulopathy

Pathophysiology

Disseminated intravascular coagulopathy (DIC) is an exaggeration of a normal response to tissue or vessel wall injury. It is obvious why it can occur in patients with SIRS: Widespread tissue injury causes platelet aggregation and activation. When enough stimulation occurs, the intrinsic and/or extrinsic pathways to thrombin formation trigger fibrin formation. A soft white clot composed of platelets becomes a firm red clot containing primarily erythrocytes. Obstruction of microscopic vessels adds to the ischemic injury and the progression of MODS.

To the purist, DIC is not present unless inappropriate clotting is accompanied by a bleeding tendency. This tendency results from a consumption of the coagulation factors, which are normally limited. It can occur earlier in patients who have additional risk factors such as liver involvement or the washout phenomenon. The latter is the process seen in patients who suffer massive blood loss and receive several units of blood components for replacement. Standard replacement therapy does not reestablish normal blood components.

Spontaneous bleeding occurs most frequently in the GI tract, the lungs, and the skin. Other significant sites include the adrenal gland and the central nervous system.

As DIC develops, patients develop secondary reasons for both clotting and bleeding. Clotting is aggravated by the concomittant consumption of antithrombin factors primarily made by the liver. Bleeding is enhanced because clot dissolution and fibrin breakdown results in the formation of fibrin breakdown products (FDPs). These FDPs are normal endogenous anticoagulants meant to limit local clot reformation during healing and thrombolysis. Thromboplastin plays a role in both coagulation and fibrinolysis and may play a pivotal role in DIC.

The clinical presentation can range from a moderate smoldering course to an acute life-threatening bleeding diathesis. There does not seem to be a sex or age of vulnerability. It is difficult to determine why some patients with seemingly similar levels of risk and injury develop DIC and others do not.

Diagnosis

The clotting aspects of DIC are observed insidiously as the progression of MODS and overtly as

acrocyanosis. The bleeding aspects are usually obvious, but the diagnosis of DIC is often still clouded by the presence of other potential causes. Bleeding in critically ill patients can also be related to trauma and surgical lesions, severe thrombocytopenia, liver failure, washout phenomenon, and anticoagulant or fibrinolytic therapy.

Laboratory studies are more diagnostic in late rather than early DIC. The earlier findings include thrombocytopenia, prolonged clotting times, and decreased levels of clotting factors such as fibrinogen. Many critically ill patients develop these changes from other causes and do not go on to develop DIC.

The measurement of clotting factors is important in patients with MODS if liver involvement is possible. Liver failure alone can cause a low-grade DIC. When it is the cause, factor VIII will be normal, while other factors are decreased. Factor VIII is the only major clotting factor not produced by the liver.

When bleeding develops in the later stages, coagulation studies can help with the differential diagnoses. One of the goals of diagnosis is documenting clotting in the presence of bleeding. Laboratory signs of widespread clotting include increased fibrin degradation products or D-dimers, a positive protamine sulfate test, schistocytes, and bilirubinemia. The latter two are manifestations of the damage and breakdown of red blood cells that have been involved in clot formation and then released. At this point, serial hemoglobin assays and platelet counts may help monitor the course of the syndrome as well as the efficacy of therapy.

It is very important to get a coagulation panel drawn as soon as the possibility of DIC is entertained. Many patients receive multiple transfusions and blood component therapy. Waiting until after several units have been received is more reflective of the pooled coagulation status of banked blood than of the patient. Neglecting to get early studies means losing an important piece of the diagnostic puzzle.

Medical Management

The primary therapy of DIC, as with all the other forms of MODS, is directed at the triggering insults. Today, in patients with SIRS, the injury processes are very difficult to control. Management of aggravating factors is advisable but often difficult to achieve. Ischemia, acidemia, uremia, hepatotoxins, and niduses of infection, inflammation or necrosis should be managed to the extent possible. These principles are not necessarily specific to DIC.

The other therapeutic intervention is supportive care. Massively bleeding patients need aggressive resuscitation to survive the hypovolemic shock. The question is what combination of replacement solutions to use. The alternatives include packed red blood cells; platelets; crystalloids; colloids; cryoprecipitate; and fresh frozen plasma, which contains all the important clotting factors. Endpoints for hemoglobin, platelets, and coagulation studies have not been agreed upon and must be individually determined.

There is even more controversy over whether heparin should be administered to patients with DIC. Heparin has several potentially therapeutic actions including inhibition of the Hageman factor and thrombin formation. A problem arises because, although clotting precedes bleeding in the pathological sequence, patients with DIC are usually bleeding at the time the diagnosis is made. Giving anticoagulants to bleeding patients is more difficult to rationalize. In addition, the proper dosage and timing have not been agreed upon.

Many agents that affect coagulation or fibrinolysis are being investigated for the treatment of DIC. Some are combination agents that affect both.

Impact on MODS

The incidence and mortality of DIC are difficult to determine, in part because of a lack of a consensus in published studies on how DIC is defined. When full-blown DIC occurs in the setting of MODS, it has a tremendous impact on outcome. Ischemic injury becomes more pronounced due to microembolic and generalized hypoperfusion. DIC limits the patient's tolerance for invasive procedures which may otherwise be indicated. Massive transfusion therapy carries both acute and long-term risks.

Dysfunctions in Other Systems

Central Nervous System Dysfunction

Alterations in central and peripheral nervous system function are very common in patients with septic syndrome, as they are in critically ill patients in general. The general etiologies overlap with those specific to septic syndrome, and, thus, it is difficult to differentiate one from the other.

Autopsy studies of patients who have died of sepsis reveal soft edematous neural tissue with micronecrosis and loss of glial cells. These are probably consequences of the same injury process that leads to dysfunction in other organ systems. Increased permeability of the blood–brain barrier may lead to edema and subsequent alteration in neurotransmitters and other metabolic proteins. Local and systemic hypoperfusion can result in ischemia and contribute to cerebral edema. The central nervous system is more sensitive to hypoxic episodes than other tissues, in part because it can take up glucose without the action of insulin. This is normally a protective mechanism. The brain glucose usually reaches 60% of the blood

glucose, and, therefore, it can become quite high in hyperglycemic patients. There is building concern for whether increased glucose in the presence of hypoxia and anaerobic metabolism causes increased lactic acid formation and acidosis in the brain. It is not yet clear whether this influences outcome in the patient with septic syndrome.

Encephalopathy may also result from altered metabolism. Some septic patients have alterations in protein metabolism similar to those of patients with hepatic encephalopathy. Both develop increases in aromatic amino acids and decreases in branch chain amino acids. In patients with septic syndrome, this is thought to occur as a result of the hypermetabolic state driven by the stress hormones. Faced with decreased insulin effect for glucose utilization and lack of availability of free fatty acids, muscles metabolize their own protein stores. Proteins are also being mobilized by hormones for liver gluconeogenesis. Muscles, however, can metabolize only branch chain amino acids, and they release the aromatic amino acids into the circulation. If the patient also has liver dysfunction, the level of circulating false neurotransmitters that contribute to encephalopathy also increases.

Some septic patients develop intracranial hypertension which can further alter neurological function. Vasogenic and cytotoxic causes are thought to contribute to the development of cerebral edema and increased intracranial pressure (see Chapter 33). What remains unclear is whether treating the increased pressure influences outcome. It is known that in some patients, increased pressure leads to herniation and death, but the point at which intervention should begin and what should be done is under investigation. For decades, brain resuscitation research has been examining the issue of preserving neurological function in the face of injury and ischemia. What investigators learn should be very helpful in the management of the neurological consequences of SIRS.

Peripheral neuropathy that impairs sensory and motor function as well as myopathy occurs in 50% of patients who remain in septic syndrome for more than 2 weeks. Although they slowly recover these functions, the ongoing deficits may contribute to occult causes of failure to wean from mechanical ventilation.

Metabolic Changes

Three additional specific metabolic alterations are worth mentioning: metabolic acidosis, hypocalcemia, and hypoglycemia.

Metabolic acidosis is common in patients with SIRS and septic shock. It is sometimes difficult to control and may potentiate cellular injury and organ failure. The resulting compensatory respiratory alkalosis along with that related to ARDS and septic encephalopathy may increase the work of breathing. The causes of metabolic acidosis in these patients include lactic acidosis and renal failure. Studies have demonstrated that significant levels of other unknown acids may be involved. Studies of the anion gap reveal that half of the anion gap cannot be explained by the measurement of all the known causes of increased circulatory anions. The unknown anions contribute significantly to acidemia in these patients. Discovering the specific acids involved should improve this aspect of patient management.

Hypocalcemia is also very common in patients with SIRS. The causes include hypoalbuminemia, transfusion therapy, diuretics, endocrinopathy, GI dysfunction, and renal failure. Hypocalcemia is of concern because it can affect myocardial contractility and neuromuscular irritability. On the other hand, calcium is cytotoxic and may enter the injured and ischemic cells when the membrane ATPase pumps fail. Furthermore, serum calcium values are not as significant as ionized calcium levels. Although most clinicians realize this and try to calculate the ionized value from the serum calcium and protein, this technique does not correlate well with measured ionized calcium in the critically ill.

The third metabolic alteration is *hypoglycemia.* Hyperglycemia is the rule in a typical patient with septic syndrome. Hypoglycemia, on the other hand, is considered to be a late finding correlating with a very poor prognosis. It is thought to reflect severe liver or endocrine failure. When hypoglycemia occurs, it is important to rule out more reversible causes like overzealous insulin administration and adrenal insufficiency.

MANAGEMENT OF MODS

The initial care of patients with SIRS revolves around early recognition, prompt treatment, and control the systemic response to injury by modulation of medications. The next focus is the prevention, early recognition, and management of sequential or individual organ system dysfunction. The other important aspects involve good general supportive care such as maintaining adequate tissue oxygenation, providing adequate nutritional support, and preventing secondary infection. The ultimate decision in many patients is when and whether to withhold or withdraw support.

Providing Adequate Tissue Oxygenation

Despite our skill at treating frank shock in most patient populations, providing adequate tissue oxygenation in patients with SIRS is still a major problem.

The issue here is not simply treating low cardiac output states, but supporting cardiac output to appropriate levels in these hyperdynamic patients. Supportive care goes beyond evaluating and manipulating the cardiovascular contribution to tissue hypoxia. There are also pulmonary and metabolic contributions, and all three of these factors interact in a complicated fashion (see Chapter 7).

Pulmonary Component

The pulmonary contribution to tissue oxygenation deficits is most reliably assessed by the intrapulmonary shunt. Measuring the percent shunt (Q_{sp}) requires drawing simultaneous arterial and venous blood samples for calculation of both bound and dissolved portions of their oxygen content (CaO_2 and CvO_2). The third oxygen content required is the content of an ideal or perfect pulmonary alveolar–capillary unit (CcO_2). The formulas used are:

$$CaO_2 = (Hb \times 1.34\ ml \times SaO_2) + (PaO_2 \times 0.0031ml)$$
$$CvO_2 = (Hb \times 1.34\ ml \times S\bar{v}O_2) + (PvO_2 \times 0.0031ml)$$
$$CcO_2 = (Hb \times 1.34\ ml \times 0.98) + (PaO_2 \times 0.0031ml)$$

In normal CaO_2 and CcO_2, there are about 20 ml of oxygen per 100 ml of whole blood, and the normal CvO_2 is about 15 ml.

The Q_{sp} measures the percentage of blood flow that does not perfectly exchange and equilibrate with alveolar gas. The normal value is less than 10%. Attempts to estimate the intrapulmonary shunt using oxygen tension indices have been shown to be unreliable and potentially misleading in critically ill patients.

Cardiovascular Component

The cardiovascular contribution to tissue oxygenation can be assessed by examining oxygen delivery, oxygen extraction, or oxygen extraction ratios. Oxygen delivery ($\dot{D}O_2$) quantifies the amount of oxygen transported to the tissues per minute:

$$\dot{D}O_2 = (CaO_2)\ 10 \times CO$$

Oxygen extraction ($Ca - vO_2$) measures the amount of oxygen the tissues extract per 100 ml of blood by comparing two simultaneously drawn samples:

$$Ca - vO_2 = CaO_2 - CvO_2$$

The normal $Ca - vO_2$ is 5 ml/100 ml of blood. Critically ill patients with good cardiovascular reserves will increase oxygen delivery and, thereby, decrease extraction to 3 to 4 ml. As mentioned in the section on septic shock, the goal in patients with septic shock is a cardiac index of 4.5 L/min/m² and a $\dot{D}O_2$ over

600 ml/min/m^2. These values are well above resting normal values of 3.0 L and 500 ml, respectively.

Metabolic Component

Metabolic carts can noninvasively and accurately measure the amount of oxygen consumed ($\dot{V}o_2$) and carbon dioxide produced per minute. $\dot{V}o_2$ can also be derived from the formula:

$$\dot{V}o_2 = (Ca - o_2)\ 10 \times CO$$

The more difficult question to answer, however, is: Is the amount of oxygen consumed enough? Is it meeting the patient's oxygen demand? Formulas used to estimate oxygen or energy requirements are not reliable in the critical care population. Clinical manifestations of inadequate tissue oxygenation are too late, too insensitive, and too nonspecific to be of value in titrating therapy. Lactic acidosis is also a late manifestation, although it is more sensitive and specific.

One area under current investigation is whether we can assume that the body extracts only the oxygen it demands and, therefore, whether delivery should be increased until extractions plateau. There is accumulating evidence to indicate that many septic syndrome patients reach a $\dot{V}o_2$ plateau at some point when $\dot{D}o_2$ is progressively increased. However, these manuevers are clinically tedious, and there are other related questions. When can we assume that a plateau reflects a met need and not a limited extraction capability? What are the regional demands, and are they being met?

Another important aspect of care is reducing the oxygen demand whenever oxygen supply is taxed. This involves controlling fever, shivering, and seizures; eliminating detrimental work of breathing; and minimizing useless struggling activities.

Monitoring the Components

Monitoring of the pulmonary, cardiovascular and metabolic components involves measuring the following variables: Pao_2, Pvo_2, Sao_2, $S\overline{v}o_2$, Hb, and CO. Thus far, the Pao_2 is the only single variable for which reliable noninvasive technology exists for use in this patient population. The transcutaneous Po_2 electrode can monitor the Pao_2 accurately but requires user attention to detail and does not offer enough information when considered alone. Blood samples are required to measure the oxygen saturations and the hemoglobin. Although pulse oximetry is attractive because of its noninvasive continuous nature, the potential percentage of error is unacceptable for these calculations. The same is true of the reliability of the available pulmonary artery catheters with mixed venous oximetry capability. The weakest link in all available monitors for this list of variables is the cardiac output. The Fick formula is probably the best way to measure CO, but it requires simultaneous blood gas sampling.

When invasive technology is required for patient management, three additional questions must be answered to maximize the risk/benefit ratio:

1. Is every effort being made to collect and record accurate data?
2. Is there something else this device can tell me that would be of value in this patient's care?
3. Are attempts being made to minimize and monitor for potential complications?

All are important aspects of skilled nursing care for patients with multisystem organ failure.

Providing Adequate Nutritional Support

There is a substantial body of convincing evidence that providing adequate nutrition decreases morbidity and mortality in the critically ill generally, and in the patient with SIRS specifically. Nutrition is an important aspect of supportive patient care.

Effects of Malnutrition

Malnutrition impairs muscle function, including that of the heart and diaphragm. Five days of semi-starvation blunts the respiratory center's response to Po_2 and Pco_2 changes. Malnutrition decreases the numbers and the function of neutrophils and lymphocytes. Helper T cell lymphocytes are especially depressed. GI villous height is decreased. Wound healing is retarded. The last four factors contribute to immunosuppression and increase the risk of secondary infection. These conceerns constitute a major reason for meeting nutritional needs of the critically ill patients.

Timing and Nutrients Supplied

Although the standard practice is to provide adequate nutrition within the first 3 to 4 days of intensive care whenever possible, research indicates that hours are probably a more useful measure than days. One study of trauma patients showed that those with nutritional support started in 5 days had an incidence of septic syndrome three times that of those in whom it was begun within 12 hours.

As already mentioned, specific metabolic demands are difficult to predict or measure in patients with SIRS. The availability of nutritional teams who keep up with developments in this rapidly changing field can be of tremendous help to the management of critically ill patients.

It is important to meet both total caloric and protein needs. A typical patient can be started at 24 to 35 kcal per kg per day consisting of 1.5 g protein per kg per day with fat providing fewer than half of the remaining calories. Once the nutritional prescription is agreed upon, it can be implemented and altered according to the patient's response. Nitrogen balance studies reveal whether metabolic needs are being met, whereas metabolic studies of the respiratory quotient can evaluate what substrates are being utilized.

Potassium, magnesium, and phosphate move to the intracellular compartment during refeeding and can be added to the solutions as necessary. These electrolytes are monitored along with serum albumin and glucose. Trace elements and vitamins are also routinely added, but copper is of particular concern in patients with cholestasis since it can worsen their condition.

It is now clear that nutritional substrates have metabolic effects; therefore, it is important to select the appropriate types of amino acids and fats. There are dozens of proteins and amino acids and thousands of fats from which to select. A growing body of evidence suggests that in the patient with septic syndrome:

- The amino acid glutamine is important to immune, GI, and muscle function
- Branch chain amino acids may decrease encephalopathy and increase retention of muscle mass
- The lipid linoleic acid (omega 6) stimulates prostaglandin E_2, which in turn inhibits the immune system
- The lipid omega 3, on the other hand, inhibits prostaglandin E_2
- Lipids may lead to high levels of free fatty acids and to pancreatitis
- Metabolically active fiber may be better than inactive fiber

Currently, only omega 6 is widely available, and glutamine can be given only by enteral routes because it forms ammonia in parenteral solutions.

SIRS dramatically alters the patient's metabolism. As knowledge increases, nutritional support is becoming a metabolic intervention that can alter the patient's physiological response in addition to meeting the nutritional needs.

TPN and TEN

Total parenteral nutrition (TPN) gained popularity in critical care in the 1970s and 1980s. Since then, it has become clear that total enteral nutrition (TEN) has many advantages over TPN. TEN improves GI, liver, and immune function; protects GI barrier integrity; prevents stress ulcers; and lowers infection, morbidity, and mortality rates.

Because of these advantages, the enteral route is used today in patients for whom it was previously contraindicated: those with decreased GI motility or diarrhea. Although many patients have hypoactive bowel sounds, most bowel sounds are created by the

stomach, and loss of gastric motility often occurs without loss of intestinal motility. In fact, many critically ill patients have a hypoactive stomach and a hyperactive small intestine. Even when GI function is decreased, the GI tract may still produce and absorb 6 to 8 L of solution per day.

The stomach can be bypassed by the placement of nasoduodenal, gastroenteral, or jejunostomy tubes. Tubes are often necessary because the goal is to feed patients as early as possible and because the enteral route is preferred. Elemental substrates must be used if feedings are delivered directly to the jejunum. Nasogastric tubes may also be necessary to reduce the risk of aspiration.

Parenteral routes include peripheral, central, and peripherally inserted central catheters. Selection depends on the type and concentration of substrates needed as well as patient tolerance and length of delivery expected.

Delivery of TPN and TEN

Concentration and delivery rate begin well below the patient's total requirement and are increased as patient tolerance is monitored. Primary complications include aspiration, diarrhea, hyperglycemia, fluid and electrolyte imbalance, and overfeeding. Aspiration of minute volumes may occur almost continuously or in bolus fashion. The use of duodenal tubes for feeding along with nasogastric tubes for gastric emptying, the placement of tracheal tubes with inflated cuffs, the elevation of the head of the bed, and the addition of metoclopramide (Reglan) to enteral solutions have all been advocated to reduce the risk.

The incidence of diarrhea has ranged from rare to frequent, depending on the institution and patient population studied. Diarrhea almost always occurs when the albumin is below 2.5 g/dl. Lactose or fat intolerance is also thought to be a common cause. It is important to rule out causes unrelated to the tube feedings such as antibiotic therapy, medication, GI infection, and electrolyte imbalances. Diarrhea is managed with several strategies, the most important of which is to treat the cause.

The concentration or rate of infusion is often decreased inappropriately, leading to episodes when the patient is underfed and malnourished. When other causes are ruled out, patient tolerance can be enhanced by adding to the solutions Kaolin pectate, paregoric, lactobacilli, or soluble fiber.

Patients receiving either TPN or TEN are routinely monitored for hyperglycemia and fluid and electrolyte imbalances. Hyperglycemia is treated with insulin administration. Fluid and electrolyte imbalances are treated by altering the amounts infused.

Overfeeding is another very common complication

of TEN or TPN. Too much glucose can contribute to increased CO_2 production, hepatic stenosis, fluid and electrolyte disorders, vitamin B_1 deficiency, and decreased phagocyte function.

Prevention of Secondary Infection

The prevention of secondary infection is an important aspect of critical care nursing. Most severely ill or injured patients should be assumed to be immunosuppressed until proven otherwise. Not only are they physiologically immunosuppressed, but their normal protective barriers are bypassed with incisions, drains, tubes, and lines. Critical care units have established strict protocols according to CDC guidelines on how long these devices can remain in place, when the paraphernalia attached to these devices should be changed, and how the entry site should be managed. Nurses are becoming experts at evaluating wound and entry sites and devising individual care plans based on their observations. Nurses understand that infections may go beyond these local sites to phlebitis, endocarditis, meningitis, sinusitis, abscesses, pneumonia, and septicemia.

The prophylactic use of antibiotics in patients with SIRS who are at very high risk of secondary infection is very controversial. In general, the practice is becoming less common because of the concern for antibiotic toxicity, the development of more resistant strains of bacteria, and the rise in circulating endotoxin levels that occurs after antibiotic administration.

The second dilemma is how to handle septic episodes. When a patient has fever, chills, and leukocytosis and the site of infection is not known, what is the proper approach? Many physicians request appropriate cultures and the removal and culture of suspicious lines, and then initiate or alter antibiotic therapy. The change is based on analysis of where the infection is likely to be and which organisms are involved. Nurses contribute valuable information when they notice changes in assessment parameters and help determine the site. What is desperately needed are laboratory studies that qualify and quantify organisms in minutes rather than days.

Withdrawal of Support

Despite all the advances in our understanding of the SIRS and MODS, the mortality remains high. Because of advances in the ability to support dysfunctional systems, the patient's length of stay and suffering can be prolonged yet result in death. It is difficult to determine at what point efforts become futile.

The discussion of when to withdraw or withhold support is often initiated by the nurse. This is especially true when the medical care is accomplished by several teams of specialists rather than one internist who looks at the whole picture. Critical care nurses, physicians, and the patient and/or family all need to contribute to the discussion. Both nurses and physicians are developing a strong knowledge base in the ethical aspects of critical care. In addition, the nurse has become a specialist in this patient's clinical course and response to septic syndrome. The physician has the best understanding of the implications or prognosis. The patient and/or family are the ultimate source of information about the patient's values and beliefs and what the patient would want in this particular situation.

It is important that nurses begin these discussions with physicians early. It may take days to achieve group discussion. Although these discussions should never be rushed, beginning them early increases the likelihood of the patient's desires being determined. It also allows the family and patient time to work through their feelings. The nursing focus during this period is to facilitate higher quality discussions among family, nurses, physicians, and other team members. These discussions may take place in large organized groups or in small one-on-one routine conversations.

Once the decision is made to withdraw or withhold care, the nursing role may become more intense, not less. Attention now turns to providing a high-quality death. Since 70% of Americans can expect to die in institutions, we need to be as good at providing the patient with the best possible experience of dying as we are with offering the chance of surviving. The primary goals are the patient's physical and emotional comfort and dignity. Everything done to and for the patient must be guided by the question: Is this prolonging suffering or promoting comfort? The secondary goal is the family's well-being and their ability to spend the amount of time they need with the patient.

BIBLIOGRAPHY

Abraham, E. (1991). Physiologic stress and cellular ischemia: Relationship to immunosuppression and susceptibility to sepsis. *Critical Care Medicine, 19,* 613-618.

Ahmed, A. J., Kruse, J. A., Haupt, M. T., et al. (1991). Hemodynamic responses to gram-negative sepsis in critically ill patients with and without circulatory shock. *Critical Care Medicine, 19,* 1520-1525.

Barron, P. T., Watters, J. M., & Wesley-James, T. (1987). Perforated ulcers in critical illness. *Critical Care Medicine, 15,* 584-586.

Barton, R., & Cerra, F. B. (1989). The hypermetabolism multiple organ failure syndrome. *Chest, 96,* 1153-1160.

Bihari, D. J., & Cerra, F. B. (1989). *New horizons—multiple organ failure.* Fullerton, CA: Society of Critical Care Medicine.

Bone, R. C. (1991). Let's agree on terminology: Definitions of sepsis. *Critical Care Medicine, 19,* 973-976.

Bone, R. C., Fisher, C. J., Clemmer, T. P., et al. (1987). A controlled clinical trial of high-dose methylprednisolone in the treatment of severe sepsis and septic shock. *New England Journal of Medicine, 317,* 653-658.

Boyd, J., Stanford, G. G., & Chernow, B. (1989). The pharmacotherapy of septic shock. *Critical Care Clinics, 5,* 133-147.

Cain, S. M., & Curtis, J. F. (1991). Experimental models of pathologic oxygen supply dependency. *Critical Care Medicine, 19,* 603-611.

Chwals, W. J., & Bistrian, B. R. (1991). Role of exogenous growth hormone and insulin-like growth factor I in malnutrition and acute metabolic stress: A hypothesis. *Critical Care Medicine, 19,* 1317-1322.

Clarke, C., Edwards, J. D., Nightingale, P., et al. (1991). Persistence of supply dependency of oxygen uptake at high levels of delivery in ARDS. *Critical Care Medicine, 19,* 497-502.

Cunnion, R. E., & Parrillo, J. E. (1989). Myocardial dysfunction in sepsis. *Critical Care Clinics, 5,* 99-118.

Engelhardt, H. T. (1991). Ethics in critical care medicine: Mortality in the fact of finitude. *Critical Care: State of the Art, 12,* 103-120.

Field, B. E., Devich, L. E., & Carlson, R. W. (1989). Impact of a comprehensive supportive care team on management of hopelessly ill patients with multiple organ failure. *Chest, 96,* 353-356.

Filkins, J. P. (1991). Cytokines: Mediators of the septic syndrome and septic shock. *Critical Care: State of the Art, 12,* 351-373.

Fink, M. P. (1991). Gastrointestinal mucosal injury in experimental models of shock trauma and sepsis. *Critical Care Medicine, 19,* 627-640.

Gentry, L. O. (1990). The influence of pH elevation on the incidence of nosocomial pneumonia. *Journal of Intensive Care Medicine, 5*(Suppl.), S17-S20.

Gregory, J. S., Bonfiglio, M. F., Dasta, J. F., et al. (1991). Experience with phenylephrine as a component of the pharmacological support of septic shock. *Critical Care Medicine, 19,* 1395-1406.

Gutierrez, G. (1991). Cellular energy metabolism during hypoxia. *Critical Care Medicine, 19,* 619-626.

Haupt, M. T., Jastremski, M. S., Clemmer, T. P., et al. (1991). Effect of ibuprofen in patients with severe sepsis. *Critical Care Medicine, 19,* 1339-1347.

Heyman, S. I., & Rinaldo, J. E. (1989). Multiple system organ failure in the adult respiratory distress syndrome. *Journal of Intensive Care Medicine, 4,* 192-200.

Hinshaw, L. B., Peduzzi, P., Young, E., et al. (1987). Effect of high-dose glucocortical therapy on mortality in patients with clinical signs of systemic sepsis. *New England Journal of Medicine, 317,* 659-665.

Horn, J. K., & Lewis, F. R. (1991). Acute lung injury: Pathophysiology and diagnosis. *Critical Care: State of the Art, 12,* 1-30.

Iberti, T. J. (1990). The hemodynamic effects of H₂ antagonists in intensive care unit patients. *Journal of Intensive Care Medicine, 5*(Suppl.), S42-S43.

Jacobs, R. F., & Tabor, D. R. (1989). Immune cellular interactions during sepsis and septic injury. *Critical Care Clinics, 5,* 9-26.

Kruse, J. A., Haupt, M. T., Puri, V. K., et al. (1990). Lactate levels as predictors of the relationship between oxygen delivery and consumption in ARDS. *Chest, 98,* 959-964.

Layon, A. J., Florete, O. G., Jr., Day, A. L., et al. (1991). The effect of duodenojejunal alimentation on gastric pH and hormones in intensive care unit patients. *Chest, 99,* 695-701.

Lister, G. (1991). Oxygen supply/demand in the critically ill. *Critical Care: State of the Art, 12,* 311-350.

McEver, R. P. (1991). Role of the endothelium in the inflammatory response. *Critical Care: State of the Art, 12,* 121-141.

Meakins, J. L. (1991). Diagnosis and mechanisms of occult sepsis. *Critical Care: State of the Art, 12,* 41-156.

Moore, E., & Moore, F. A. (1991). Immediate enteral nutrition following multisystem trauma—a decade of experience. *Journal of the American College of Nutrition, 10,* 633.

Natanson, C., & Parillo, J. E. (1988). Septic shock. *Anesthesiology Clinics of North America, 6,* 73-85.

Peitzman, A. B., Udekwu, A. O., Ochoa, J., et al. (1991). Bacterial translocation in trauma patients. *Journal of Trauma, 31,* 1083-1087.

Sprung, C. I., Cerra, F. B., Freund, H. R., et al. (1991). Amino acid alterations and encephalopathy in the sepsis syndrome. *Critical Care Medicine, 19,* 753-756.

Stahl, W. M. (1987). Acute phase protein response to tissue injury. *Critical Care Medicine, 19,* 613-618.

Strong, A. G. (1991). Case management of a patient with multisystem failure. *Critical Care Nurse, 11,* 10-18.

Tracey, K. J., Lowry, S. M., & Cerami, A. (1988). Cachetin/TNF-alpha in septic shock and septic adult respiratory distress syndrome. *American Review of Respiratory Disease, 138,* 1377-1379.

Tryba, M. (1991). Sucralfate versus antacids or H₂ antagonists for stress ulcer prophylaxis: A meta-analysis on efficacy and pneumonia rate. *Critical Care Medicine, 19,* 942-949.

Tuchschmidt, J., Oblitas, D., & Fried, J. C. (1991). Oxygen consumption in sepsis and septic shock. *Critical Care Medicine, 19,* 664-671.

Weg, J. G. (1991). Oxygen transport in ARDS and other acute circulatory problems: Relationships of oxygen delivery and oxygen consumption. *Critical Care Medicine, 19,* 650-657.

Ziegler, E. J. (1991). Treatment of gram-negative bacteremia and septic shock with HA-IA human monoclonal antibody against endotoxins. *New England Journal of Medicine, 324,* 429-436.

Zobel, G., Kuttnig, M., Grubbauer, H. M., et al. (1991). Reduction of colonization and infection rate during pediatric intensive care by selective decontamination of the digestive tract. *Critical Care Medicine, 19,* 1242-1246.

57

Transplantation

Susan L. Smith

The field of organ transplantation has expanded since its early beginnings to include the possibilities of using cadaver or live donor organs and tissues to replace the majority of bodily organs and tissues that have become irreparably diseased or injured. The advances made in transplantation are largely due to advances in biomedical technology and immunobiology. As people live longer and overcome, with the help of modern medicine, conditions that once were considered hopeless, more critical care nurses are likely to be caring for patients with end-stage organ disease who are potential transplant candidates. The critical care nurse, therefore, plays an important role not only in care of the transplant recipient but also in identification of potential organ donors and the care of critically ill patients waiting for a transplant.

HISTORICAL PERSPECTIVE

Although blood transfusions were administered as early as the 17th century, the era of modern transplantation began in the 18th century with the replacement of a human tooth by John Hunter.[1] However, despite numerous attempts at replacing lost limbs and substituting body parts from one person or animal to another, solid organ transplantation was not successful until 1902, when Alexis Carrel developed the techniques for surgical suturing and vascular anastomosis.[2] Much of the work in the field of transplantation in the 19th century focused on biological and immunological problems. It was not until the early 1900s, though, that ABO and Rh blood group antigens were discovered.[3] This discovery laid the foundations for later development of histocompatibility testing procedures that are critical to successful kidney transplantation today. In 1937, the histocompatibility antigen (major histocompatibility complex or MHC) in humans was discovered by Gorer,[1] and in 1943, Medawar described the immune response of acute rejection.[4] In 1964, Terasaki and colleagues developed techniques for histocompatibility testing,[5] and by the 1970s, the disparity between donor and

recipient MHC was recognized as the basis for allograft rejection.

Although there were many attempts at experimental kidney transplantation in the early 1900s, it was not until 1954 that Merrill and Murray performed the first successful kidney transplant between identical twin brothers. In 1990, 9,560 kidney transplants (cadaveric and living) and 549 pancreas transplants were performed in the United States.[6] Experimental attempts at heart transplantation also took place in the early 1900s, but it was not until the 1960s that human heart transplantation was performed, first in 1964 when Hardy transplanted the heart of a chimpanzee (xenograft) into a 68-year-old man[1] and then in 1967 when Barnard performed the first human-to-human (allograft) heart transplant.[7] In 1990, 2,085 heart transplants, 50 heart–lung transplants, and 262 lung transplants were performed in the United States.[6] Experimental liver transplantation began in the 1950s, and in 1963, Starzl performed the first human liver transplant.[8] It was not until 1967, however, that the first successful liver transplant was performed, also by Starzl. In 1990, 2,655 liver transplants were performed in the United States.[6]

With current success rates and survival statistics, these procedures are no longer considered experimental but are therapeutic options for some patients with end-stage kidney, liver, heart, and lung disease. Although by no means the sole factor, the drug cyclosporine is largely responsible for improving the long-term success of organ transplants. Before the advent of cyclosporine immunosuppression, 1-year survival for kidney, liver, and heart transplants was 30%, 25%, and 63%, respectively.[9] Currently, 1-year patient survival rates are: kidney, 92% (cadaveric kidney) and 97% (living related donor); pancreas, 89%; liver, 76%; heart, 83%; heart and lung, 57%; and lung, 48%.

Other factors in the improved status of transplantation include advances in surgical techniques, a better understanding of immunological aspects of transplantation, development of more effective cadaver organ and tissue preservation techniques, and a legal redefinition of death to include brain death. With the promise of an extended and better quality of life, organ and tissue transplantation has generated numerous complex economic, social, and ethical issues related to allocation of scarce and costly health care resources. The average costs for the procedure and the first year of posttransplant care are: kidney, $25,000 to $50,000; heart, $95,000 to $148,000; and liver, $130,000 to $320,000.[10] The Social Security Act was amended in 1972 to cover the cost of dialysis and transplantation for end-stage renal disease, which now exceeds $2 billion annually. Although private insurers, HMO, and Medicare/Medicaid coverages have increased for heart and liver transplantation, the high cost of these procedures remains a major factor in the decision to transplant.

The shortage of cadaver donor organs is the most significant factor limiting transplantation for treating end-stage organ disease. There are not enough organs donated for the thousands of patients with terminal kidney, heart, and liver disease who need transplants. Volunteerism has not been a successful solution. Although required-request or -referral and presumed consent programs are being implemented to increase organ donation, the major focus for the future will be on efforts to increase the donor organ supply.

Redefining death to include cerebral death (chronic vegetative state) and anencephaly is a partial solution. Equally controversial is the research in xenografting (transplanting organs from one species to another), and live extrarenal organ donors. A more realistic and less controversial approach is to accept organs, especially livers, from donors over the age of 65. Other future perspectives include the cultivation of human cell cultures, transplantation of human fetal tissue, development of artificial organs, and development of new pharmacological agents for immunosuppression.

NURSING MANAGEMENT IN END-STAGE ORGAN DISEASE

An often ignored component of transplant nursing is the care of the patient with end-stage organ disease who is in need of and waiting for transplant. More than 80,000 people in the United States die each year from end-stage renal disease.[11] Of these, approximately 25,000 are on chronic hemodialysis, and 8,500 are waiting for a transplant.[12] Approximately 12,000 persons are diagnosed each year in the United States with insulin-dependent diabetes mellitus (IDDM).[13] IDDM affects morbidity and mortality through secondary complications including retinopathy, nephropathy, and atherosclerosis. Many of the

yearly cardiovascular deaths are potentially treatable by heart transplantation.[14] Cirrhosis is the fourth leading cause of death in adults and the third leading cause of death in males 40 to 55, accounting for more than 26,000 deaths annually.[15] The estimated annual need for liver transplants is 5,000 to 10,000.[12]

The patient with end-stage organ disease may or may not be a candidate for an organ transplant. Understanding the indications and contraindications for transplantation is essential when caring for these patients. A comprehensive physical and psychosocial assessment must be done as a basis for developing a complete list of medical, surgical, and nursing diagnoses to guide care before, during, and after transplant surgery.

Some transplant candidates may be well enough to stay out of the hospital until they are admitted for the surgery. More often, intermittent or constant acute hospital care is required. Approximately 30% of adult candidates die while waiting for a transplant.[9] The attendant psychosocial issues for the patient experiencing life-threatening events such as infections that also may delay a transplant are numerous. Expert nursing skills in the area of psychosocial support are required.

Waiting for a transplant is perhaps the most stressful time for patients and families as they try to cope with terminal illness, altered lifestyles, financial strain, the necessity for the death of another person for organ donation to occur, impending major surgery, and the reality of a lifetime of immunosuppressant therapy. Patients waiting for transplant may suffer from anxiety, depression, fear of the unknown, and fear of death. They may also experience helplessness or hopelessness, dependency, regression, organic brain syndrome, psychotic states, cognitive dysfunction, and, occasionally, suicidal ideations.[16]

Adaptive defense mechanisms or coping responses commonly used by patients waiting for transplant include denial, minimization, isolation of effect, and reaction formation.[16] *Denial*, a way of dealing with ambivalent feelings, is the most common. It occurs primarily in the early stages of transplant evaluation. When adaptive, it prevents depression. If denial is used excessively, the patient becomes noncompliant. *Minimization* is distortion of the severity or prognosis of an illness or complication. When minimization is adaptive, realistic insight is gained over time. With excessive use, the patient becomes noncompliant. *Isolation of effect* is obsession with technical aspects such as laboratory values or statistics. Those who use this mechanism intellectualize situations and often read the medical literature on the subject obsessively. When adaptive, the patient eventually expresses true emotions related to the transplant. With excessive use, the patient becomes overwhelmed by the information. *Reaction formation* is doing or saying the opposite of what one wants to do or say. The patient who is angry at the medical staff but showers them with compliments and praise is using reaction formation. Conflicts over death of a donor also trigger this response when the patient actually feels guilty but jokes about the chances of more fatal automobile accidents on New Year's Eve. When adaptive, the patient eventually expresses true emotions related to the transplant. Excessive use leads to anxiety and guilt. Among the nursing diagnoses in the pretransplant period is knowledge deficit.

■ **NURSING DIAGNOSIS**

Knowledge deficit, related to end-stage organ disease, impending surgery, and expectations after transplantation.

OUTCOME STANDARD AND CRITERIA

Knowledge will be adequate as evidenced by:

• Demonstration of an understanding of the natural history of the disease process
• Verbalization knowledge of the information needed during the waiting period while searching for a donor organ
• Demonstration of an understanding of posttransplant expectations

NURSING INTERVENTIONS

• Use written materials for preoperative transplant teaching if available
• Explain tests and procedures needed during the transplant evaluation process
• Introduce patient to an organ transplant recipient
• Teach patient about the natural history of the disease (organ-specific):
  Need to conserve energy
  Dietary concerns
  Report signs of worsening organ failure
  Difficulty concentrating
• Educate patient on how to wait for a donor:
  Telephone numbers
  Beeper
  Transportation
  Stressful time
  Clinic visits
• Explain sequence of events on day of surgery:
  Notification
  Nothing by mouth
  Admission to hospital
  Surgery preparation
  Waiting room for significant others
• Provide emotional support and answer questions

PATIENT SELECTION

Careful patient selection is a major factor in successful transplantation. A primary responsibility of

the transplant team is, to the extent possible, to transplant organs into those with the best chance for a successful outcome, meaning both long-term graft function and satisfactory quality of life. Evaluation of patients for organ transplantation is a complex, multidisciplinary process. The goals of evaluation are to:

1. Determine the medical necessity for and proper timing of transplantation.
2. Determine the technical feasibility of the procedure.
3. Identify any precluding conditions, systemic diseases, or risk factors.
4. Determine physiological and psychosocial suitability.
5. Identify organ systems that may require treatment to bring the patient to optimal health before transplantation.
6. Assess immunological and histocompatibility status.

General contraindications to transplantation, regardless of type, are listed in the box below. In addition, morbid obesity places the patient at high risk for pulmonary compromise and infection after transplantation and is associated with a higher operative mortality.

Optimally, the transplant candidate has the benefit of time to establish a trust relationship with the transplant team, to participate in a meaningful educational experience, and to grasp the realities of life after transplant. An important point is that transplantation is not a panacea for life problems. Instead, transplantation usually means trading one set of problems for another, which may be significant. The problems associated with end-stage organ disease may be re-

---

General Contraindications to Organ Transplantation

Presence of active systemic infection (bacteremia, fungemia, viremia)

Malignant disease (except skin cancer and some primary tumors of the diseased organs)

Active peptic ulcer disease

Active abuse of alcohol or other substances

Severe damage to organ system(s) other than that to be transplanted (such as severe cardiovascular dysfunction in the potential liver transplant recipient)

Severe psychiatric disease

Demonstration of past or current inability to comply with a prescribed medical regimen

Lack of a functional social support system

Lack of sufficient financial resources to pay for surgery, hospitalization, medications, and follow-up care

solved, but new problems occur which are associated primarily with chronic immunosuppressant therapy, such as drug side effects and infection. In addition, the financial burden of posttransplant care can be overwhelming.

ORGAN DONATION AND RECOVERY

Gifts of tissue and organ donation are vital to transplantation. Beginning in 1968 with the Uniform Anatomical Gift Act, several legislative initiatives aimed at increasing volunteer organ donation have become law. The National Organ Transplant Act of 1984 and the Omnibus Reconciliation Act of 1986 addressed many of the complex issues of impeding organ donation.

The National Organ Transplant Act established a task force that studied the medical, legal, ethical, social, and economic issues of organ donation, recovery, and transplantation.[17] In addition, a National Organ Sharing System, the National Organ Procurement and Transplant Network (OPTN), was established to cre-

ate a national patient registry and coordinate donor organ allocation and distribution. Currently, the United Network for Organ Sharing (UNOS) is under contract from the U.S. Department of Health and Human Services to operate the OPTN. The Omnibus Reconciliation Act of 1986 tied Medicare and Medicaid reimbursement to hospitals to compliance with required-request or -referral legislation, and required transplant centers and organ procurement organizations (OPOs) to be members of the OPTN.[18]

OPOs are either independent or hospital based. They must meet certification criteria mandated by the Health Care Financing Administration. In addition to coordination of organ recovery, OPOs provide many important services including public and professional education, assistance to hospitals with potential donor evaluation, and family counseling.

Role of the Critical Care Nurse

The critical care nurse plays an extremely important part in organ donation beginning with early iden-

TABLE 57-1 **Criteria for Vascular Organ Donors**

Organ or Tissue	Age	Cause of Death	Specific Criteria	General Criteria
Kidney	6 months to 65 years	Brain death	No preexisting renal disease or injury	
Heart	Term newborn to 55 years	Brain death	No preexisting cardiac disease or injury	
Liver		Brain death	No preexisting hepatic disease or injury	
Pancreas	Term newborn to 55 years	Brain death	No preexisting pancreatic disease or injury	**All organs**
Lung		Brain death	No preexisting pulmonary disease or injury; no smoking history; no chest tubes	No sepsis, transmittable diseases, extracranial malignancy, IV drug abuse, or death of unknown etiology
Heart–lung	1 to 60 years / 12 to 55 years / Term newborn to 65 years	Brain death	No preexisting cardiac or pulmonary disease or injury; no smoking history; no chest tubes	
Bone	15 to 65 years	Brain death or cardiac death	Documented time of death	**All tissues**
Fascia	Term newborn to 55 years			No malignancy, uncontrolled infections, death of unknown etiology, tissue radiation, transmittable diseases, chronic steroid therapy, IV drug abuse, history of homosexuality, active hepatitis or AIDS, viral encephalitis, Creutzfelt-Jakob disease, rabies, or death of unknown etiology
Connective tissues				
Bone marrow	No age limit	Brain death or cardiac death		
Heart valves				
Eye				

Adapted from Hawke, D., Kraft, J., & Smith, S. L. (1990). Tissue and organ donation and recovery. In S. L. Smith (Ed.), *Tissue and organ transplantation: Implications for professional nursing practice.* St. Louis: Mosby–Year Book.

tification of potential donors, in making the initial referral to the OPO, and in assisting with the management of the brain dead organ donor. This role was clearly delineated by the American Association of Critical-care Nurses (AACN) in two position statements.

The ideal organ donor is the brain dead individual who has suffered a fatal brain injury (usually a severe closed head injury or penetrating head injury), has been previously healthy, has intact cardiovascular function, and is free of contagious or neoplastic (except primary brain tumor) disease.[19] Specific criteria for vascular organ donors are listed in Table 57-1. Initiation of the organ donation process should proceed according to hospital policy. Crucial roles of the critical care nurse are to participate in providing the option of donation to the family and to provide emotional support. The critical care nurse should be familiar with and supported in the implementation of this policy.

The goal of potential organ donor management is maintenance of optimal conditions that will ensure functional, intact, and infection-free organs. This is accomplished by careful management of hydration and tissue perfusion, oxygenation, diuresis, infection control, and temperature control. Hypotension and shock, electrolyte imbalances, pulmonary compromise, loss of thermoregulation, and infection are commonly encountered problems. Ideal clinical parameters are listed in Table 57-2. Organ recovery occurs in the operating room only after a series of important events takes place: timely recognition of a potential donor, notification of an OPO, diagnosis of brain death, family consent, and optimal donor management.[19]

Multiple Organ Recovery

Multiple organ recovery, or recovery of more than one type of organ from a single cadaver donor, is routine. As many as four separate surgical teams may be operating for this purpose in the same surgical field to recover the kidneys, heart (or heart–lung or lung), pancreas, and liver. Generally, after a standard midline incision is made from xiphoid to pubis, multiple organ recovery proceeds in the following order. First, the kidneys and liver are dissected but left intact and cannulated for cold flushing. Second, the inferior vena cava and the aorta are cross-clamped, cardioplegia is begun, and the heart is recovered. Last, the liver and then the kidneys are recovered. The organs are preserved via cold storage in either Euro-Collins solution or Viaspan (see Table 57-3). Euro-Collins solution is a balanced electrolyte solution, and Viaspan is an electrolyte solution that also contains hydroxylethyl starch which meets the cellular metabolic needs and allows for prolonged cold storage.

KIDNEY TRANSPLANTATION

The potential kidney transplant recipient has end-stage renal disease, most frequently due to hypertension, glomerulonephritis, diabetic nephropathy, a he-

TABLE 57-2 **Ideal Clinical Parameters for Organ Donors**

Parameter	Optimal Value
Systolic blood pressure	90-160 mmHg
Mean arterial blood pressure	>70 mmHg
Central venous pressure	6-12 cmH$_2$O
Urine output	>1.0 ml/kg/hr
Heart rate	60-120 beats/min
Arterial blood gases	Pao$_2$ ≥80 torr
	Paco$_2$ 35-45 torr
	pH 7.35-7.45
	S$\bar{a}$o$_2$ ≥90%
Body temperature	36.1°-38.9° C

Adapted from Hawke, D., Kraft, J., & Smith, S. L. (1990). Tissue and organ donation and recovery. In S. L. Smith (Ed.), *Tissue and organ transplantation: Implications for professional nursing practice.* St. Louis: Mosby–Year Book.

TABLE 57-3 **Tissue and Organ Recovery Times**

Organ/Tissue	Maximum Recovery Time	Maximum Preservation Time	Preservation Medium
Bone	24 hours	2 hours indefinite	Fresh frozen, sterilized in ethylene oxide or irradiated
Bone marrow	6 hours	Indefinite	Frozen in liquid nitrogen
Cornea	6 hours	7 days	Cold gentamicin with pH buffer
Heart	Immediate	3-5 hours	Cold normal saline
Kidney	Immediate	48 hours	Cold Euro-Collins, Viaspan
Liver	Immediate	24 hours	Cold Euro-Collins, Viaspan
Pancreas	Immediate	8 hours	Cold Euro-Collins, Viaspan

Adapted from Hawke, D., Kraft, J., & Smith, S. L. (1990). Tissue and organ donation and recovery. In S. L. Smith (Ed.), *Tissue and organ transplantation: Implications for professional nursing practice.* St. Louis: Mosby–Year Book.

reditary or congenital disorder, or systemic lupus erythematosus.[11] In general, the kidney transplant candidate has been maintained on chronic hemodialysis and significant dietary restrictions and is hypertensive, anemic, and fatigued. Specific contraindications to transplantation include active vasculitis or glomerulonephritis (systemic lupus erythematosus, Wegener's granulomatosis, Goodpasture's syndrome) and a positive T lymphocyte cross-match with the potential donor.

Unlike the patient waiting for a heart, liver, or pancreas transplant, the patient with end-stage renal disease has two potential organ donor sources, a cadaver and a living donor (either related or nonrelated). Approximately 80% of kidney transplants are from cadaver donors. The graft survival rate for living kidney donor transplantation is 10% to 15%, greater than for cadaver renal transplant.[11]

More extensive histocompatibility testing is required for kidney transplantation than for heart or liver transplantation. ABO and human leukocyte antigen (HLA) typing are done for cadaver renal transplantation, as well as white cell cross-match and mixed lymphocyte cross-match tests. For a living related renal transplant, a mixed leukocyte culture is also done.

Another difference between kidney transplantation and heart or liver transplantation is that the native diseased kidneys are not removed as they are with orthotopic heart or liver transplants. The standard placement of the donor kidney is extraperitoneally, usually in the right iliac fossa but sometimes in the left iliac fossa. The surgical incision is made between the pubis and the iliac crest. The renal vein of the donor kidney is anastomosed end-to-side to the recipient's external iliac vein, and the donor renal artery is anastomosed end-to-end to the recipient's internal iliac artery. Revascularization takes approximately 30 minutes. Next, the graft ureteral anastomosis, most commonly via a ureteroneocystostomy (donor ureter passed through the posterior bladder wall and anastomosed to the bladder mucosa to create an opening into the bladder), is completed. Two nursing diagnoses for the transplant recipient follow.

NURSING MANAGEMENT

■ NURSING DIAGNOSIS

Knowledge deficit, related to posttransplant regimen.

OUTCOME STANDARD AND CRITERIA

Knowledge will be adequate as evidenced by:
- Demonstration of knowledge and understanding of routine postoperative course

NURSING INTERVENTIONS
- Assess patient's readiness to learn
- Provide written teaching booklet along with oral instructions
- Utilize resources: pharmacist, dietitian, physical therapist, social worker, clergy
- Reinforce teaching throughout immediate hospital stay in the following areas (these should be organ-specific):
  Signs and symptoms of rejection
  Signs and symptoms of infection
  Diet
  Medications
  Vital signs (how to take blood pressure, pulse, temperature)
  Physical activity
  Signs and symptoms
  Instruction on diabetic monitoring, wound care if indicated

■ NURSING DIAGNOSIS

Pain, related to transplant surgery.

OUTCOME STANDARD AND CRITERIA

Pain is absent or controlled as evidenced by:
- Statement that pain is relieved or manageable
- Absence of pain manifestations
- Relaxed body

NURSING INTERVENTIONS
- Assess recipient's pain tolerance level
- Provide comfort measures
- Encourage deep breathing and relaxation
- Administer pain medication as prescribed

■ NURSING DIAGNOSIS

High risk for ineffective coping after transplantation, related to increased stress, anxiety, potential dependency, fear of rejection and/or death, body image disturbance, and lifestyle changes.

OUTCOME STANDARD AND CRITERIA

Coping is effective as evidenced by:
- Freedom from anxiety
- Ability to perform activities of daily living
- Participation in decisions regarding health
- Acceptance of support from social network
- Acknowledgment of physical limitations

NURSING INTERVENTIONS
- Offer emotional support
- Establish rapport with significant others
- Assess recipient's level of anxiety
- Explain tests and procedures; provide a plan of care with choices
- Consult social worker, clergy, or psychologist if indicated
- Reinforce postoperative teaching throughout hospital stay
- Provide ways to deal with body image changes (hair remover, diet, exercises)
- Set priorities and goals with recipient
- Encourage recipient to return home and establish a normal routine

PANCREAS AND KIDNEY–PANCREAS TRANSPLANTATION

Like kidney transplantation, pancreas or simultaneous kidney–pancreas transplantation is not an immediate life-saving operation. Pancreas transplantation is indicated for the restoration of normal glucose metabolism in the patient with IDDM and secondary complications, specifically end-stage renal disease due to glomerulopathy. Although a single-organ (pancreas) transplant may be performed, a simultaneous kidney–pancreas transplant is the most common approach. Contraindications are the same as those for kidney transplantation.

There are three surgical techniques: (1) grafting of the entire pancreas with or without the duodenal cuff, (2) segmental grafting (body and tail of the pancreas), and (3) grafting of islet cells, which is experimental and will not be discussed further. In the whole-pancreas and segmental-pancreas procedures, the native pancreas is left in situ to maintain normal exocrine function, which is not affected by IDDM, and drainage.

When the pancreas is transplanted alone (without a simultaneous kidney transplant) and an extraperitoneal approach is used, the graft is placed in the right iliac fossa. When a simultaneous kidney–pancreas transplant is done, the kidney graft is placed in the right iliac fossa, and the pancreas graft is placed in the left iliac fossa. The pancreas graft may also be placed intraperitoneally, although the risk of fistula formation and peritonitis is greater with this approach. Donor-pancreas venous drainage is anastomosed to the common iliac vein, and arterial supply is from a donor splenic artery with an aortic Carrel patch.

Exocrine drainage (secretion of proteolytic and lipolytic enzymes) of the donor pancreas graft continues after transplantation and is the greatest technical challenge in pancreas transplantation.[20] There are three surgical approaches to the management of this problem: (1) ductal occlusion or injection into the main pancreatic duct of a polymer substance that hardens and occludes the duct; (2) enteric drainage or pancreaticojejunostomy, which involves anastomosing the graft to a Roux-en-Y loop of recipient jejunum; and (3) urinary diversion or pancreaticoduodenocystostomy, which involves anastomosing the pancreas to the recipient's bladder, most often via a donor duodenal cuff. Ductal occlusion was the most commonly used method in early pancreas transplantation but has been abandoned because of complications of graft fibrosis and failure. Enteric drainage provides the most physiological means of exocrine drainage but is associated with delayed healing of the anastomosis, fistula formation, and sepsis. Urinary

diversion is advantageous in that exocrine function of the graft (urine amylase levels), which is an early index of graft rejection, can be directly assessed.[21] Complications associated with this approach are metabolic acidosis due to urinary bicarbonate loss, ulceration and bleeding of the duodenal cuff, and cystitis.[22]

HEART TRANSPLANTATION

The most common indications for heart transplantation are cardiomyopathy and coronary artery disease. Less common indications include congenital heart disease, valvular disease, myocarditis, and graft rejection requiring retransplantation.[23] Candidates for a heart transplant must be refractory to the myriad of medical and surgical treatments for cardiovascular disease and must meet the New York Heart Association Class III or IV criteria. In other words, the heart transplant candidate has decreased functional ability, a severely decreased left ventricular ejection fraction, and/or life-threatening dysrhythmias. Specific contraindications include pulmonary hypertension, unresolved pulmonary infarction, and IDDM.

The heart transplant procedure can be either orthotopic (excision of the native recipient heart and replacement of it with a donor heart) or heterotopic (anastamosis of the donor heart in the right side of the chest next to the native recipient heart which is left in situ). Heterotopic heart transplantation, also referred to as a "piggyback" transplant, is done when the pulmonary vascular resistance is increased or when the donor heart size is significantly smaller than the recipient's. Orthotopic heart transplantation is the more common procedure.

For orthotopic heart transplantation, the chest is opened through a median sternotomy, and cardiopulmonary bypass is begun. The native heart is excised at the midatrial level, leaving the atrial cuffs intact above the atrioventricular groove. After the four major anastamoses between the donor and recipient atrial cuffs, aorta, and pulmonary artery and veins, and at the interatrial septum are completed, the patient is weaned from cardiopulmonary bypass.

HEART–LUNG TRANSPLANTATION

The first heart–lung transplant was performed in 1968. After many advances in this field were made in the 1970s, Stanford University began the first heart–lung transplant program in 1981. The candidate for a heart–lung transplant has pulmonary-induced right ventricular failure, usually secondary to pulmonary hypertension (primary, secondary or the Eisenmenger complex), chronic lung disease (emphysema, alpha-$_1$-antitrypsin deficiency, chronic bronchitis, pulmonary fibrosis), patent foramen ovale, or cystic fibrosis.[24] Specific contraindications include previous thoracotomy because of pleural adhesions, and current steroid usage, which prohibits healing of the tracheal anastamosis.

For heart–lung transplantation, the chest is opened through a median sternotomy and a pericardectomy. The heart and lungs are dissected out, and the trachea is transected above the carina. The donor heart–lung bloc is sewn in with three anastamoses: tracheal, right atrial, and aortic. The omentum may be brought up and wrapped around the trachea to assist in its vascularization. An interesting note is that the patient needing a heart–lung transplant who has a normal right ventricle can donate her or his excised heart to someone in need of a heart transplant.

LUNG TRANSPLANTATION

The first lung transplant was performed in 1963. Only since 1983, however, largely through the efforts of the Toronto Lung Transplant Group, has the procedure become a viable therapeutic option for some patients with severe end-stage restrictive or obstructive lung disease. Lung transplantation can be single or double. Preoperatively, the lung transplant candidate has a severe alteration in gas exchange resulting in hypoxemia, hypercarbia, and acidosis. Regardless of whether a single- or double-lung transplant is indicated, intensive preoperative and postoperative nursing and rehabilitative care are required to optimize pulmonary function.

Indications for single-lung transplant are idiopathic interstitial pulmonary fibrosis, sarcoidosis, primary pulmonary hypertension, and emphysema. A single-lung transplant can be done on either side but is technically easier on the left.[25] A standard posterolateral thoracotomy is performed through the bed of the excised fifth rib. A midline laparotomy is performed to tunnel the omentum beneath the sternum for use in aiding in vascularization of the airway anastamosis. Specific contraindications to lung transplantation include steroid dependency, cardiac insufficiency, a right ventricular ejection fraction less than 20%, a left ventricular ejection fraction less than 40%, and dependence on mechanical ventilation, and presence of a nonrehabilitative pulmonary disability.[25]

Indications for double-lung transplant include emphysema, alpha₁-antitrypsin deficiency, eosinophilic granuloma, lymphangiolyomyomatosis, and cystic fibrosis. A single-lung transplant may be indicated in the patient with emphysema who exceeds the age limit for double-lung transplantation. Double-lung transplantation is usually performed as a double-lung bloc through a median sternotomy and after initiation of cardiopulmonary bypass. Double-lung transplant may also be performed as two single-lung transplants as described above.

LIVER TRANSPLANTATION

Indications for liver transplantation include advanced cirrhosis secondary to cholestatic syndromes or hepatitic disease, hepatocellular diseases, metabolic liver disease, unresectable malignancies, and acute fulminant hepatic failure.[26] In adults, the most frequent indications are cirrhosis secondary to chronic active hepatitis, cryptogenic cirrhosis, primary biliary cirrhosis, and primary sclerosing cholangitis.[26] Other indications include Budd-Chiari syndrome and acute life-threatening and refractory variceal bleeding. Specific contraindications to liver transplantation may, but do not necessarily, include active hepatitis (positive serology for HBsAG or HBeAg), active alcohol or drug abuse, hepatic malignancy, and portal vein thrombosis.

According to a panel of experts at the 1990 Conference on Liver Transplantation sponsored by the National Digestive Diseases Advisory Board, "The clinical conditions that warrant transplantation should not be based on an etiologic diagnosis of the disease; rather, the decision to proceed with transplantation should be based on the presence of irreversible organ failure and the likelihood that transplantation will improve significantly the health of the individual in question."[27] Patient evaluation, then, takes into account technical feasibility, physiological and psychological suitability, and factors related to optimal timing of the surgery.

Specific evaluative procedures for the potential liver transplant candidate include esophagogastric duodenoscopy, liver biopsy, quantitative measures of liver function such as the galactose elimination capacity and galactose clearance, calculated measurement of liver and spleen volumes, venous and arterial phase superior mesenteric artery arteriography, electroencephalography, and measurements of liver hemodynamics (portal and liver blood flow).[28] Specific psychosocial evaluative factors include a thorough evaluation of the patient's support system and a committment to sobriety in the alcoholic patient. Evaluation of the patient with alcoholic liver disease is often complex, and at present, there is no single criterion to predict a successful outcome in this patient population.

The liver transplant has been called the most complex surgical procedure performed. Like the heart transplant, the liver transplant can be either heterotopic or orthotopic. The orthotopic procedure involves four major vascular anastamoses (suprahepatic inferior vena cava, infrahepatic inferior vena cava, portal vein, and hepatic artery) and a biliary anastamosis and typically takes 8 to 10 hours to complete.

The recipient hepatectomy begins with opening the abdomen via a bilateral subcostal and midline incision extending up to the xiphoid. This can be the most difficult phase of the surgery because of the effects of chronic liver disease (portal hypertension, portal-systemic collateral vessel formation, coagulopathy, and a hyperdynamic circulation) on the systemic vasculature and the hepatic system.[26] During this phase, the patient is at high risk for significant hemorrhage. For this reason, 50 to 100 units of packed red blood cells, 20 to 30 units of fresh frozen plasma, and 10 to 20 units of cryoprecipitate are typically made available for the patient before the surgery is begun. The use of the autologous transfuser or cell saver device significantly decreases the amount of donor red blood cells that are used. The use of a rapid infusion device is sometimes necessary and life-saving when a patient is hemorrhaging profusely.

Prior to removal of the native liver, the patient is placed on heparinless venovenous bypass so that venous return to the heart will be maintained when the vena cavae below and above the liver are clamped and transected. Blood is drained from the infrahepatic vena cava and the portal vein to a centrifugal pump that returns blood to the ipsilateral axillary and internal jugular vein.

The surgical anastamoses are completed in the order given above. The biliary anastamosis can be done via a choledochocholedochostomy (end-to-end donor to recipient) or a choledochojejunostomy (end-to-side donor common bile duct to Roux-en-Y limb of recipient jejunum). A choledochocholedochostomy is stented with a T tube, and the choledochojejunostomy is not usually stented but may be. Three Jackson-Pratt drains are typically placed in the right and left subphrenic spaces and in the area of the liver hilum, and the abdomen is closed.

Reduced-size Liver Transplantation

Reduced-size liver transplantation is now performed mainly in pediatric patients or to reduce pretransplant mortality secondary to prolonged waiting for suitable donors for very small adults or those adults with very small liver volume. The procedure is a left lobe graft from a live donor, or a left lobe graft or left lateral segmental graft from a cadaver donor. The success with this procedure is comparable to whole-liver allografting. Another procedure called split grafting is done to donate two halves of a cadaver donor liver to two recipients. Split grafting is used when a left lateral segment graft is too large for a pediatric patient. Split graft survival is not as good as reduced-size graft survival.[29]

CARE OF THE TRANSPLANT RECIPIENT

Care of the transplant recipient is challenging in that the disease processes that necessitate transplant are physiologically and sometimes psychologically devastating, the surgical procedures are physiologically stressful and contribute to many alterations in homeostasis in the postoperative period, the pharmacological regimens necessary after transplant are associated with many significant side effects, and the psychodynamics of the entire transplantation process are complex.

Caring for the transplant recipient is a multidisciplinary effort that assigns the critical care nurse three important roles: (1) as the primary care provider and patient advocate in the immediate postoperative period, (2) as a direct collaborator with the primary physician, and (3) as a liaison and coordinator with the other members of the transplant team. General principles of care of the surgical patient apply to the transplant recipient as well: recovery from anesthesia, fluid shifts and electrolyte imbalances, immobility predisposing to pulmonary stasis and skin breakdown, wound and surgical drain management, and prevention of infection. Knowledge of the normal course after transplantation and the problems that may occur is fundamental to this process. Refer to *Tissue and Organ Transplantation: Implications for Professional Nursing Practice*[30] for a detailed discussion of care of the transplant recipient. The two most common problems after transplantation, rejection and infection, are discussed below.

Rejection

Transplantation of allografts (organs or tissue between genetically different individuals of the same species) elicits a powerful immune response called *rejection*. Antigens present on the cells of transplanted tissue are recognized by the recipient's immune system as foreign, and a series of events occurs involving the recognition and attempted destruction of the antigen-bearing cells and, therefore, the allograft.

All cells except mature erythrocytes express human leukocyte antigens (HLAs) that are determined by the major histocompatibility complex (MHC), a gene cluster located on chromosome 6. HLAs are divided into two classes (class I and class II) based on their structure, tissue distribution, function, and specificity. Class I antigens function as surface recognition molecules for the receptors of cytotoxic T lymphocytes. Exposure to class I antigens can occur through pregnancy, blood transfusions and previous transplants, resulting in the development of preformed circulating cytotoxic antibodies to those antigens. Class II antigens are surface recognition molecules for the receptors on B lymphocytes and helper and suppressor T lymphocytes.

HLAs are the genetic basis (inherited) for self and the recognition by the immune system of nonself. Human T and B lymphocytes have surface receptors that can recognize antigens expressed on other cell surfaces. The recognition of foreign HLA by recipient lymphocytes is the beginning of the rejection response.

These receptors, like the HLAs, are genetically determined and are specific and unique to each individual. There are five HLA loci: HLA-A, HLA-B, HLA-C, HLA-D, and HLA-DR, each containing many alleles designated by numbers following the locus symbol, for example, HLA-B5. Because human chromosomes exist in pairs (half of the total HLA identity from each parent), a total of 10 HLAs can be identified in each individual.

Rejection is classified into four types: hyperacute, acute, accelerated, and chronic. *Hyperacute rejection* occurs within minutes to hours of vascularization of the allograft. It is caused by the presence in the recipient of preformed circulating cytotoxic antibodies. A humoral or antibody-mediated (B lymphocyte) response to class I antigens on vascular endothelium of the graft results in immediate graft thrombosis and necrosis. There is no treatment for hyperacute rejection. If it occurs in the kidney or kidney–pancreas transplant, the recipient must return to dialysis. If it occurs in an extrarenal organ, the recipient must receive retransplantation. Fortunately, the majority of hyperacute rejection episodes can be prevented by histocompatibility testing and matching.

Acute rejection begins within about 1 week of transplantation. It is caused by the cellular immune response mediated by T lymphocytes against class II antigens on donor organ cells. Diagnosis of acute rejection is generally based on clinical, laboratory, and invasive diagnostic evidence, such as biopsy findings, of graft alteration and dysfunction. Patient responses to acute rejection vary, depending on the organ, the degree of rejection, and response to immunosuppressant therapies. Acute rejection has great clinical significance for the transplant team because, unlike hyperacute and chronic rejection, it can be suppressed and treated by powerful pharmacological agents. The critical care nurse must be familiar with the indications for, mechanisms of action of, dosages, routes of administration, and side effects of the drugs used for the prevention and treatment of rejection.

Accelerated rejection is thought to be a cellular response that occurs earlier than classic acute rejection and is diagnosed and treated in the same manner as acute rejection.

Chronic rejection usually occurs after 3 months posttransplantation and is mediated by T and B lymphocytes. Chronic rejection takes the course of progressive loss of vital components, graft function and graft failure, and cannot be treated. The kidney or kidney–pancreas transplant recipient again has the option of dialysis, and the extrarenal transplant recipient requires retransplantation.

An armamentarium of immunosuppressants are currently used to alter immune responses so as to prevent and treat acute rejection. These drugs include corticosteroids (methylprednisolone, prednisone), azathioprine (Imuran), cyclosporine (Sandimmune), antilymphocyte globulin (ALG), antithymocyte globulin (ATG), and the monoclonal antibody OKT3.[31] A wide range of immunosuppressant protocols exist, employing different combinations of prophylactic and maintenance use of these drugs. It is important to remember that, while these drugs singly and in combination may allow the recipient to tolerate a foreign organ, they are powerful drugs with numerous important side effects. The goals of immunosuppression then are to prevent (1) graft destruction and (2) toxic drug side effects and complications. Finding this precarious balance is not easy. It often requires extensive monitoring of parameters of organ function and rejection and blood levels of cyclosporine.

Infection

Infection is the most common cause of morbidity and mortality after transplantation.[32] Many factors contribute to the development of infection in this patient population (see the box on p. 1321). The most important factor is the necessary use of powerful drugs that alter natural and acquired host defense mechanisms, rendering the patient susceptible to a variety of internal and external potentially pathogenic organisms. The net state of immunosuppression consists of the (1) total dose of the drugs used in the immunosuppressant regimen, (2) types of drugs and duration of use, (3) degree of granulocytopenia induced, (4) presence of mucocutaneous injury, (5) metabolic factors, and (6) nutritional status. This net state determines the patient's risk of infection.[32] "Infection is a unique and persistent challenge" in the transplant population.[33]

Most infections that occur in transplant patients are opportunistic in that they are caused by organisms that are ubiquitous in the environment but rarely cause disease in the immunocompetent person. Infections seen in transplant patients are related to specific mechanisms (cellular, humoral, phagocytic, combined mechanisms) of pharmacological suppression or alteration of immune defenses.

Suppression of the T lymphocyte response (cellular immunity) is desirable in the transplant recipient because the acute rejection response is mediated principally by T lymphocytes. Specifically, T helper cells mediate clonal proliferation of antigen-sensitized cytotoxic T cells.[34] The drug cyclosporine (Sandimmune) is very effective in inhibiting this mechanism, and it is the mainstay of most posttransplant immunosuppressant regimens. Cytolytic drugs such as antilymphocyte globulins (the polyclonal antibodies ALG or ATG) and the monoclonal antibody OKT3 (Orthoclone) kill and deplete circulating lymphocytes. Because T lymphocytes provide specific protection against viral and fungal infections, long-term administration of these drugs is associated with a high incidence of viral and fungal infections. Antilymphocyte antibodies also contribute to viral infections by reactivating latent or dormant herpesvirus infections.

B lymphocytes provide humoral or antibody-mediated immunity which provides protection against pyrogenic bacterial infections such as pneumococcal, streptococcal, and meningococcal infections. Because the major secondary lymphoid organ for B lymphocytes is the spleen, which also produces opsonins and immunoglobulin and functions as a major reticuloendothelial organ through the filtering action of sinus macrophages, the splenectomized patient is at great risk for pyrogenic bacterial infections. Patients who are splenectomized must receive a prophylactic pneumococcal vaccine (Pneumovax) and may be placed on a regimen of low-dose antibiotic therapy indefinitely. Otherwise, they are at risk for fatal infections such as pneumococcal or meningococcal meningitis.

Phagocytosis by granulocytes, primarily neutrophils and tissue macrophages, is the first line of immune defense and is necessary for the initiation of protective cellular and humoral immune responses. Granulocytopenia occurs as a result of immunosuppression with corticosteroids, azathioprine (Imuran), and antilymphocyte globulin. Corticosteroids profoundly decrease serum levels of lymphocytes and monocytes by redistributing them from the peripheral circulation, and in high doses, they inhibit serum IgG levels.[31] The exact mechanism of action of azathioprine is unknown, but its primary immunosuppressive effect is thought to be inhibition of RNA and DNA synthesis in immune cells in the bone marrow.[31] Total body irradiation used primarily in bone marrow transplantation and experimentally in some solid organ transplant programs is associated with severe granulocytopenia and lymphocytopenia, and the suppression of immunoglobulin production.

The time frame in which infections occur after transplantation can be used as a guideline for early diagnosis of the general type of infection.[32] Infections that occur within 1 month after transplantation are usually caused by organisms that were present in the donor organ prior to transplant, or are routine bacterial infections of the surgical wound, lungs, urinary bladder catheter, or intravascular catheters. Infections that occur between 1 and 6 months after transplant are opportunistic bacterial, viral, fungal, and parasitic infections and are related to the type, intensity, duration, and temporal sequence of immunosuppressant regimens.[32] Infections that occur more than 6 months after transplant are usually progressive viral infections that do not respond to decreasing the immunosuppression regimen or antiviral drug therapy and are associated with poor prognoses.[32]

Bacterial Infections

The majority of bacterial infections in transplant patients are caused by gram-negative bacteria that were previously colonizing the patient at sites of mucosal and integumentary damage, ciliary dysfunction, or loss of mucosal protection. The gastrointestinal tract serves as a primary reservoir of potentially pathogenic bacteria in the transplant patient.

Prophylactic broad-spectrum antibiotic therapy is usually given in the perioperative and immediate postoperative periods, and organism-specific, organism-sensitive antibiotics are used when infection occurs. Antibiotic therapy carries the risk of eliminating protective normal flora from the oral pharynx and the vagina, and subsequent fungal overgrowth, otherwise called *thrush*. Oral antifungal therapy and antifungal vaginal suppositories beginning immediately after surgery can prevent this problem. Frequent assessment of the skin and mucous membranes, wounds, and bodily secretions and excretions for local infection, and of the white blood cell count, temperature, and hemodynamics for systemic infection are necessary.

Viral Infections

The family of herpesviruses are responsible for the majority of viral infections in transplant patients.[32] The herpesviruses include herpes simplex virus (HSV) 1 and HSV2, varicella zoster virus, cytomegalovirus (CMV), and Epstein-Barr virus. Other viral infections that occur in the posttransplant period include hepatitis B, C, and non-A, non-B, presumably from blood transfusions and donor organs. The development of a viral infection after transplantation is associated with significant morbidity and mortality related to its contribution to the net state of immunosuppression, its potentiating effect on malignant disease, and, paradoxically, its potentiating effect on rejection.

Viruses are entirely dependent on host cells for survival because synthesis of viral proteins takes place within the nucleus of the host's cells. Transmission patterns of viral infection include primary infection, secondary or reactivation infection, and superinfection.[35] A *primary infection* occurs in the recipient who was seronegative for that virus prior to receiving an organ from a donor seropositive for that virus. Seropositivity most often means that there was a previous exposure and the host has established long-term immunity, or it may mean active infection. Primary active infections in immunosuppressed patients are generally more severe than primary infections in the general population. *Secondary* infections occur in recipients who at some time had a primary infection and were seropositive prior to transplantation. After the primary infection, the virus establishes a latent and permanent residence in either the lymphocyte or monocyte pool (CMV) or the sensory ganglia (HSV) of the host. Reactivation of viral replication occurs in immunosuppressed states and, in the transplant patient population, is associated with immunosuppressant regimens consisting of lymphotoxic drugs such as cyclosporine and the antilymphocyte globulins that are known to trigger reactivation. Secondary infections are not generally as severe as primary or superinfections. *Superinfection* occurs in the seropositive recipient who receives an organ from a donor seropositive for a (presumably) different viral strain.

Early recognition of viral lesions on the skin and mucous membranes and knowledge of appropriate therapies is important. In the immunosuppressed patient, tiny lesions left untreated can grow to overwhelming size and incur significant tissue damage in just 1 to 2 days.

Herpesvirus. HSV1 infections manifest most often as painful oropharyngeal ulcerations associated with gingivitis, stomatitis, or pharyngitis. Corneal infection with the herpesvirus can lead to blindness. HSV2 infections most often manifest as painful clusters of vesicular lesions on the penis, vulva, vaginal mucosa, or cervix. HSV2 infections are associated with fever, general malaise, lymphadenopathy, and neuralgias of the lower extremities. Associated complications include aseptic meningitis, transverse myelitis, urethral stricture, and secondary bacterial and fungal infections.[36] HSV infections are treated with acyclovir and by decreasing the net state of immunosuppression.

Cytomegalovirus. CMV is a common viral cause of morbidity in transplant patients, with peak activity between 1 and 4 months after transplantation.[32] An individual can become infected by more than one strain of CMV. Prior antibody protection from one strain, therefore, will not be protective against another. It is this situation that constitutes superinfection in the transplant patient.

Typically, the patient will present with leukopenia, lymphocytosis, thrombocytopenia, increased respiratory rate, and pneumonitis on chest x-ray.[32] CMV infections can disseminate and cause multisystem disease of the retina, lungs, liver, pancreas, stomach, intestines, kidneys, brain, and nervous system and can lead to death.[37] CMV infection impairs alveolar macrophage function and is associated with the development of *Pneumocystis carinii* pneumonia.[32] CMV infections are treated with gancyclovir and by decreasing the net state of immunosuppression.

Currently, prophylactic regimens of acyclovir, gancyclovir, and immunoglobulin for the prevention of CMV infections are being investigated. Prophylactic treatment is desirable because of the high incidence of CMV infections in transplant patients and the associated morbidity and mortality and may be efficacious because of the delay in onset after transplant of these infections.

Epstein-Barr Virus. Epstein-Barr viral infections are more difficult than others to diagnose and, therefore, may be more prevalent than previously thought. Like CMV, Epstein-Barr infection potentiates immunosuppression. Its particular importance to the transplant patient, however, is its association with lymphoproliferative disease, namely B cell lymphomas.[32] Unfortunately, these lymphomas do not respond to radiation therapy, but some cases will respond to decreasing the dosages of immunosuppressants.

Fungal Infections

The combined factors of prolonged hospitalization, broad-spectrum antibiotic therapy, corticosteroid therapy, invasive vascular accesses, hyperalimentation, abdominal surgery, and ulceration of the gastrointestinal tract place transplant patients at high risk for fungal infections. The most common fungal pathogens are of the *Candida* species: *C. albicans, C. glabrata,* and *C. tropicalis*. Other problematic fungi include *Aspergillis fumigatas, Cryptococcus neoformans,* and *Coccidioides immitis*.

The most common *Candida* infections are vaginal candidiasis and oropharyngeal candidiasis.[34] Early recognition of viral lesions on the skin and mucous membranes is, therefore, important. Vaginal candidiasis does not usually progress to disseminated disease, but oropharyngeal infection can if not recognized and treated promptly. More severe *Candida* infections can also occur as disseminated disease in the form of septicemia, pneumonia, esophagitis, duodenitis, hepatitis, encephalitis, retinitis, cystitis, myocarditis, myositis, and dermatitis. Prophylactic oral (and vaginal in females) antifungal therapy is necessary to prevent oropharyngeal and vaginal *Candida* infections in the immediate posttransplant period when the risks are greatest. This therapy may be necessary for prolonged periods. Fungal infections are treated with amphotericin B and fluconazole and by decreasing the net state of immunosuppression.

Parasitic Infections

Pneymocystis carinii and *Toxoplasma gondii* are the two most common parasitic infections in transplant patients. *P. carinii* is an extracellular ameboid organism that is ubiquitous in the environment. *P. carinii* affects the lungs, causing pneumonia that initially manifests clinically as dyspnea and tachypnea at rest, hypoxia, cyanosis, fever, and a nonspecific cough.[38] Bilateral alveolar infiltrates are seen on chest x-ray, and a definitive diagnosis is made with bronchoalveolar lavage. Treatment is with trimethoprim sulfamethoxazole, pentamidine isethionate, or Bactrim. *T. gondii* is an intracellular protozoan parasite that is also ubiquitous in the environment. *T. gondii* affects multiple organ systems, most notably the central nervous system and musculoskeletal system, and manifests clinically as a mononucleosis-like syndrome. Treatment is with pyrimethamine and sulfadiazine.

Management of Opportunistic Infection

Definitive antimicrobial therapy for the several opportunistic organisms has been described. Although these agents are life-saving in many cases, attempts at prevention must precede these interventions. Recognizing the implications of host–environment interactions provides the basis for protecting, to the extent possible, the transplant recipient from potentially pathogenic and fatal organisms. The hospital environment where personnel frequently come in contact with blood, pulmonary secretions, surgical wounds and drainage, feces, and urine is potentially hostile to the patient with alterations in natural and acquired immune defenses.

The traditional approach to protecting the patient from infection, protective or reverse isolation, has not proved efficacious and is costly in terms of time and supplies. Since the 1850s, handwashing has been identified as the most effective measure for decreasing the transmission of infection.[39] Pathogens acquired through direct and indirect contact with colonized or infected patients are responsible for the majority of nosocomial infections. Handwashing removes these organisms mechanically and chemically from the hands.

Infection control protocols for transplant patients vary widely among the hundreds of transplant programs in the United States. The recognition that many opportunistic infections are caused by latent or other internal organisms has helped to refocus protocols to keeping the environment clean but not sterile, maintaining patent skin and mucous membranes, limiting the number and duration of invasive devices and procedures, providing adequate nutritional support, keeping net immunosuppression to a minimum, and emphasizing handwashing.

REFERENCES

1. Flye, M. W. (Ed.). (1989). History of transplantation. In *Principles of organ transplantation*. Philadelphia: Saunders.
2. Guthrie, C. C. (Ed.). (1912). Applications of blood vessel surgery. In *Blood vessel surgery*. New York: Longmans, Green.
3. Landsteiner, K. (1928). Cell antigens and individual specificity. *Journal of Immunology, 15,* 589-600.
4. Medawar, P. B. (1945). A second study of the behavior and fate of skin homografts in rabbits. A report to the War Wounds Committee of the Medical Research Council. *Journal of Anatomy, 69,* 157-176.

5. Terasaki, P. I., Marchioro, P. L., & Starzl, T. E. (1965). *Histocompatibility testing.* Washington, DC: National Academy of Sciences.

6. Cate, F. H., & Laudicina, S. S. (1991). Transplantation white paper. Current statistical information about transplantation in America. Washington, DC: Annenberg Washington Program, Communications Policy Studies, Northwestern University.

7. Barnard, C. N. (1967). A human cardiac transplant. *South African Medical Journal, 41,* 1271-1274.

8. Starzl, T. E., Marchioro, T. I, Von Kulla, K. N., et al. (1963). Homotransplantation of the liver in humans. *Surgery, Gynecology and Obstetrics, 117,* 659-676.

9. Cosimi, A. B. (1989). Transplantation. *American College of Surgeons Bulletin, 74*(1), 41-47.

10. Swerdlow, J. L. (1989). Matching needs, saving lives. Washington, DC: Annenberg Washington Program.

11. Perryman, J. P., & Stillerman, P. U. (1990). Kidney transplantation. In S. L. Smith (Ed.) *Tissue and organ transplantation: Implications for professional nursing practice.* St. Louis: Mosby–Year Book.

12. Baily, M. A. (1988). Economic issues in organ substitution technology. In D. Mathieu (Ed.), *Organ substitution technology: Ethical, legal and public policy issues.* Boulder, CO: Westview.

13. Southerland, D. E. R., Moudry, K., & Najarian, J. (1988). Pancreas transplantation. In G. J. Cerilli (Ed.), *Organ transplantation and replacement.* Philadelphia: Lippincott.

14. Overcast, T. D., & Merriken, K. (1988). The patient and entitlement to benefits. In D. Mathieu (Ed.), *Organ substitution technology: Ethical, legal and public policy issues.* Boulder, CO: Westview.

15. Galambos, J. T. (1979). *Cirrhosis: Major problems in internal medicine* (Vol. 17). Philadelphia: Saunders.

16. Reither, A. M. (1990). Psychiatric aspects of transplantation. In S. L. Smith (Ed.), *Tissue and organ transplantation: Implications for professional nursing practice.* St. Louis: Mosby–Year Book.

17. Task Force on Organ Transplantation. (1986). *Organ transplantation: Issues and recommendations.* (NTIS No. HRP-0906976). Rockville, MD: Health Resources and Services Administration.

18. Office of Organ Transplantation. (1987). *The status of organ donation and coordination services: Report to Congress for fiscal year 1987.* Washington, DC: U.S. Department of Health and Human Services.

19. Hawke, D., Kraft, J., & Smith, S. L. (1990). Tissue and organ donation and recovery. In S. L. Smith (Ed.), *Tissue and organ transplantation: Implications for professional nursing practice.* St. Louis: Mosby–Year Book.

20. Wills, B. G., & Post, L. C. (1990). Pancreas transplantation. In S. L. Smith (Ed.), *Tissue and organ transplantation: Implications for professional nursing practice.* St. Louis: Mosby–Year Book.

21. Corry, R. J. (1987). University of Iowa experience in pancreatic transplantation. *Transplantation Proceedings, 19*(4S), 37-39.

22. Corry, R. J., Wright, F. H., & Smith, J. L. (1988). Whole organ pancreas transplantation. *Transplantation Proceedings, 20*(3S), 420-425.

23. Macdonald, S. N., & Naucke, N. A. (1990). Heart transplantation. In S. L. Smith (Ed.), *Tissue and organ transplantation: Implications for professional nursing practice.* St. Louis: Mosby–Year Book.

24. Ahrens, T. S., & Powers, C. (1990). Heart–lung transplantation. In S. L. Smith (Ed.), *Tissue and organ transplantation: Implications for professional nursing practice.* St. Louis: Mosby–Year Book.

25. Boychuk, J. E., & Malen, J. F. (1990). Lung transplantation. In S. L. Smith (Ed.), *Tissue and organ transplantation: Implications for professional nursing practice.* St. Louis: Mosby–Year Book.

26. Smith, S. L. (Ed.). (1990). Liver transplantation. In *Tissue and organ transplantation: Implications for professional nursing practice.* St. Louis: Mosby–Year Book.

27. The National Digestive Diseases Advisory Board. (1990). Conference on Liver Transplantation, Arlington, VA: February 11-12, 1990.

28. Millikan, W. J., Henderson, J. M., Stewart, M. T., et al. (1988). Orthotopic liver transplantation. *Emory University Journal of Medicine, 2*(3), 192-198.

29. Thistlethwaite, J. R., Emond, J. C., Woodle, P., et al. (1990). Increased utilization of organ donors: Transplantation of two recipients from single donor livers. *Transplantation Proceedings, 22,* 1485-1486.

30. Smith, S. L. (Ed.). (1990). *Tissue and organ transplantation: Implications for professional nursing practice.* St. Louis: Mosby–Year Book.

31. Hooks, M. A. (1990). Immunosuppressive agents used in transplantation. In S. L. Smith (Ed.), *Tissue and organ transplantation: Implications for professional nursing practice.* St. Louis: Mosby–Year Book.

32. Rubin, R. H. (1988). Infectious disease problems. In W. C. Maddrey (Ed.), *Transplantation of the liver.* New York: Elsevier.

33. Schweizer, R. T. (1989). Infection control and the transplant patient. *ASEPSIS: The Infection Control Forum, 11*(1), 2-5.

34. Smith, S. L. (Ed.). (1990). Immunologic aspects of transplantation. In *Tissue and organ transplantation: Implications for professional nursing practice.* St. Louis: Mosby–Year Book.

35. Ciferni, M., & Kelley, A. (1990). Cytomegalovirus infection in the liver transplant patient: A case study. *Critical Care Nurse, 10,* 10-21.

36. Wong, K. K., & Hirsch, M. S. (1984). Herpes virus infections in patients with neoplastic disease. Diagnosis and therapy. *American Journal of Medicine, 76,* 464-468.

37. Schumann, D. (1987). Cytomegalic virus infection in renal allograft recipients. Indicators for intervention in the surgical intensive care unit. *Focus on Critical Care, 14*(3), 40-47.

38. Ruskin, J. (1981). Parasitic diseases in the compromised host. In R. H. Rubin, & L. S. Young (Eds.), *Clinical approach to infection in the compromised host.* New York: Plenum.

39. Hempel, C. G. (1966). *Philosophy of natural science.* Englewood Cliffs, NJ: Prentice-Hall.

58

Poisoning

Deborah L. Scherger

Kathleen M. Wruk

In 1990, 8,811,333 human poison exposures were reported to the American Association of Poison Control Centers' (AAPCC) National Data Collection System.[1] These exposures included accidental childhood ingestions, intentional overdoses, therapeutic misadventures, use and abuse of recreational drugs, and chronic exposures in the home and work settings.

A *poison* is a substance absorbed by the ocular, dermal, oral, or parenteral routes that causes illness or death. *Poisoning* implies the presence of clinical symptoms and an accidental exposure. An intentional toxic exposure is described as an overdose. Ingestion of a substance may not be a poisoning unless symptoms develop. Poison centers provide information regarding management of poisoned patients and interface with emergency departments and critical care units to give advice on patient management.

Determining if a poisoning has occurred may be difficult. A complete history and patient assessment can provide essential information. A poisoning or overdose is suspected in (1) a psychiatric patient; (2) a trauma patient (especially if young); (3) a comatose patient with unknown etiology; (4) cardiac dysrhythmia; (5) a child with unexplained lethargy or any puzzling presentation; (6) a patient with multiple symptom presentation, either chronically or acutely; (7) a patient with seizures of unknown etiology; (8) a patient with cyanosis that is unresponsive to oxygen; (9) elevated anion gap acidosis; or (10) hyperthermia.[2]

Management of the poisoned patient involves specific interventions including stabilization of vital signs, prevention of absorption, enhancement of toxin excretion, and administration of antidotes if applicable. The most important aspect of care is to *focus on the clinical presentation of the patient, not the poison ingested by history.*

POISONED PATIENT: CASE STUDY

A young adult man called an emergency operator from a public pay phone booth, saying he had ingested a bottle of pills about 1 hour before calling. He complained of drowsiness, and his speech was slurred. An ambulance was dispatched.

He was comatose on arrival in the emergency department, with spontaneous respirations at 10 per minute. His blood pressure was 80/50, and his pulse was 130. His skin and mucous membranes were dry, his face was flushed, and his pupils were dilated. On auscultation, bowel sounds were decreased. Paramedics reported the patient had a generalized seizure in the ambulance. His serum pH was 7.32, and an ECG showed a widened QRS. No pills were found on the patient or at the site of exposure.

Data Acquisition

Although a thorough history is essential, the nurse's priority is to identify life-threatening symptoms that necessitate treatment. Once the ABC's are assessed and stabilized, the data needed to provide ongoing management of the patient are determined.[3]

The initial history includes name of the poison, route of exposure, current symptoms, amount ingested, age, time of exposure, and length of exposure. Clarification of the amount involved, circumstances surrounding the poisoning, and whether the exposure was accidental or intentional is also established.[3] It may be necessary to send someone to the exposure site to look for open or empty containers, chemical spills, or other evidence.

A general health history, which includes recent or chronic illnesses, current medications, and known allergies, is obtained. Exposures to other substances and concomitant exposure of other persons at the site are ruled out. Any first aid treatment already initiated is also determined. Examples of inappropriate first aid

Four Common Poisoning Syndromes

ANTICHOLINERGIC

Substances causing anticholinergic symptoms include antihistamines, some antipsychotic drugs, antidepressants, over-the-counter (OTC) sleep medications, cold medications, chemicals, and plants. Symptoms include:

- Dry flushed skin
- Dry mucous membranes
- Decreased or absent bowel sounds
- Confusion, hallucinations, hyperactivity, and seizures
- Tachycardia, hypertension, and dysrhythmias which may be delayed
- Mydriasis
- Urinary retention

SYMPATHOMIMETIC

Substances causing sympathomimetic symptoms include drugs such as ephedrine, phenylpropanolamine, phenylephrine, pseudoephedrine, metaproterenol, albuterol, and terbutaline. These drugs are commonly found in oral nasal decongestants, OTC diet pills, street drugs, and prescription medications. Symptoms include:

- Nausea and vomiting
- Anxiety, restlessness, hyperactive reflexes, irritability, and seizures
- Tachycardia, hypertension, and dysrhythmias

NARCOTIC SYNDROME

Narcotics are available in both oral and parenteral forms. Propoxyphene may be found alone or with other analgesic drugs such as acetaminophen or aspirin. Dextromethorphan is an ingredient in many OTC cough preparations and may have a narcotic effect. Clonidine may cause similar symptoms in overdosage. Symptoms include:

- Coma, areflexia, and seizures
- Miosis or mydriasis
- Hypotension and bradycardia
- Respiratory depression or apnea
- Pulmonary edema

CHOLINERGIC SYNDROME

Substances that may cause these symptoms include pesticides, certain mushrooms, physostigmine, and drugs used to treat myasthenia gravis such as pyridostigmine, neostigmine, or ambenonium chloride. Symptoms include:

- Increased secretions (a mnemonic that may be helpful in remembering symptoms is SLUDGE):

Salivation	S
Lacrimation	L
Urination	U
Defecation	D
Gastrointestinal cramping	G
Emesis	E

- Muscle fasciculations and seizures
- Miosis
- Bradycardia
- Diaphoresis
- Bronchorrhea

Adapted from Hall, A. H., Kulig, K. W., & Rumack, B. H. (1985). Management of acute poisonings and overdose. Unpublished manuscript. Rocky Mountain Poison and Drug Center, Denver, CO.

interventions are tourniquets with snake envenomations, neutralization of bases and acids, administration of substances other than ipecac for emesis induction, and use of emetics in caustic exposures.

MEDICAL AND NURSING MANAGEMENT

Nursing and medical roles are interdependent in this phase. The nurse needs to know the common toxic syndromes to anticipate needed care. Analysis of these syndromes may help in determining the causative agent (see the box above). In addition, certain symptoms or symptom groups provide clues that may be useful: for example, if a patient presents with coma and hypotension, suspected agents include sedatives, benzodiazepines, and ethanol (see the box on p. 1327).

■ NURSING DIAGNOSIS

Possible nursing diagnoses are listed in the box on p. 1328.

OUTCOME STANDARDS AND CRITERIA

- Respiratory function
  Maintain adequate respiratory function and oxygenation.
  Maintain hemodynamic stability.
  Maintain cerebral blood flow.
  Maintain adequate respiration and oxygenation.
- Cardiovascular function
  Maintain stable vital signs.
  Maintain warm extremities.
  Maintain normal hemodynamic pressures.
  Maintain normal temperature.
  Maintain normal sinus rhythm as evidenced by:
    Atrial rate 60-100 beats per minute
    Constant PR interval 0.12-0.20 second
    Constant QRS interval 0.06-0.10 second
- Neurological function
  Remain seizure-free.

Diagnostic Clues to Toxins

Coma, hypotension
- Sedatives, hypnotics, narcotics
- Benzodiazepines
- Ethanol
- Isopropanol
- Methanol
- Ethylene glycol
- Carbon monoxide

Pulmonary edema (noncardiogenic)
- Sedatives, hypnotics (especially Placidyl)
- Narcotics
- Salicylates
- Carbon monoxide
- Cyclic antidepressants

Metabolic acidosis
- Salicylates
- Methanol
- Ethylene glycol
- Isoniazid (with seizures)
- Iron
- Ethanol

Cyanosis unresponsive to oxygen (methemoglobinemia)
- Chemicals such as nitrites; nitrates; aniline; phenols; local anesthetics; nitrobenzene; and drugs such as phenacetin, phenazopyridine (Pyridium), and antimalarials
- Sulfones (Dapsone)

Cardiac dysrhythmias
- Tricyclic antidepressants
- Theophylline
- Caffeine
- Arsenic
- Cyanide
- Hydrogen sulfide
- Anticholinergies
- Beta blockers
- Calcium channel blockers
- Digitalis and related compounds

Psychosis/Hallucinations
- Hallucinogens
- Cocaine
- Amphetamines
- Anticholinergics
- Sympathomimetics
- LSD
- Toluene (glue sniffing)
- Phencyclidine (PCP)
- Heavy metals (chronic)
- Certain mushrooms
- Ethanol

Seizures
- Aspirin
- Amphetamines
- Anticholinergic substances
- Camphor
- Carbon monoxide
- Cyanide
- Cocaine
- Propoxyphene
- Phencyclidine
- Strychnine
- Isoniazid
- MAO inhibitors
- Tegretal
- Heavy metals
- Herbicides
- Insecticides
- Lithium
- Nicotine
- Salicylates
- Sympathomimetics
- Theophylline
- Antidepressants
- Caffeine

Radiopaque drugs*
- Potassium chloride
- Ferrous sulfate
- Calcium carbonate

Extrapyramidal (dystonic reaction or oculogyric crisis)
- Phenothiazine derivatives (Thorazine, Compazine)

Butyrophene (Haldol, Inapsine)

Adapted from Hall, A. H., Kulig, K. W., & Rumack, B. H. (1985). Management of acute poisoning and overdose. Unpublished manuscript. Rocky Mountain Poison and Drug Center, Denver, CO.
*Savitt, D. L. (1987). The radiopacity of ingested medications. *Annals of Emergency Medicine, 16,* 331.

Respond appropriately to verbal and tactile stimuli and be oriented to person, place, and time.
- Psychosocial function
Verbalize and acknowledge unresolved problems and concerns.
Develop appropriate mechanisms for dealing with stress.
Be injury-free while in hospital.
- Gastrointestinal function

Maintain normal bowel function.
Maintain hydration.

NURSING INTERVENTIONS
- Respiratory function
Maintain airway, breathing, and circulation through basic and advanced life-support measures.
Prevent absorption of poison through gastrointestinal decontamination.

Nursing Diagnoses That May Be Used in Toxicology

Altered bowel elimination: constipation, diarrhea, incontinence
Altered oral mucous membranes
Altered tissue perfusion: cerebral, cardiopulmonary, renal, gastrointestinal, peripheral
Anxiety
Decreased cardiac output
Disturbance in self-esteem
Fear
High risk for altered parenting
High risk for fluid volume deficit
High risk for poisoning
High risk for self-directed violence
Impaired gas exchange
Ineffective airway clearance
Ineffective breathing pattern
Ineffective family coping: compromised
Ineffective individual coping
Knowledge deficit
Noncompliance
Pain
Potential for impaired skin integrity
Powerlessness
Social isolation

Adapted from Novotny-Dinsdale, V. (1985). Implementation of nursing diagnosis in one emergency department. *Journal of Emergency Nursing, 11,* 140-144.

Perform or assist with gastric lavage with large-bore orogastric tube and normal saline solution until clear

After assessing that bowel sounds are present, administer 60 to 100 g of activated charcoal and 30 g magnesium citrate via gastric tube as ordered by physician

Obtain blood and urine for toxicology tests.

Assess respiratory rate and depth.

Auscultate breath sounds for clarity, resonance, and depth.

Assess peripheral circulation for good color, warmth, and brisk capillary refill.

Maintain patent airway.

Assess need for endotracheal intubation and mechanical ventilation.

Administer oxygen as indicated by patient's condition and as ordered by physician.

Obtain arterial blood gases (ABGs) in accordance with hospital policy.

• Cardiovascular function

Assess blood pressure, heart rate, peripheral circulation, and body temperature.

Perform hemodynamic monitoring if indicated by physical means; i.e., intraarterial and central venous pressure lines.

Administer IV fluids; put patient in Trendelenburg position; administer vasopressors as indicated for decreased blood pressure as ordered by the physician.

Provide continuous cardiac monitoring.

Monitor for conduction abnormalities and dysrhythmias. Measure PR and QRS intervals as needed. Report any widening of PR or QRS interval or ectopy to physician.

Maintain physiological pH (7.40-7.45) for optimal cardiac conduction. Administer sodium bicarbonate as needed and ordered by physician.

Obtain 12-lead ECG.

• Neurological function

Assess neurological function and perform neurological checks every 4 hours as indicated by patient's condition.

Maintain adequate oxygenation, manifested by PaO_2 80 to 100 mmHg.

Administer anticonvulsant medications, e.g., as indicated and ordered by physician.

Protect patient from harm related to sensorium change.

Side rails should be up at all times; pad rails prn
Wrist, ankle, Posey restraints prn

• Psychosocial function

Speak warmly and openly to patient.

Provide unhurried atmosphere to encourage verbalization of concerns.

Allow patient private time with family and significant others.

In addition to psychiatric intervention, other appropriate interventions include social service: social worker, financial counseling, and chaplain.

Maintain suicide precautions while patient is in depressed state:

There should be no sharp objects (needles, metal silverware) in room
Monitor objects brought into room by visitors
Keep curtains or blinds open to observe patient when possible

• Gastrointestinal function

Assess presence of bowel sounds in all four quadrants before administering charcoal and cathartic.

Monitor for increase in abdominal girth, distention, and firmness.

Maintain adequate fluid volume if diarrhea ensues.

Report absence of bowel sounds and suspicion of paralytic ileus to physician as indicated.

After the patient's vital signs are stable, a complete physical examination is performed. If the patient's clinical condition warrants cardiac monitoring or there is a history of an exposure to a potentially cardiotoxic substance, cardiac monitoring and a 12-lead ECG are initiated if needed. Electrolytes and ABGs are monitored for the presence of acidosis. An elevated anion gap (greater than 12 to 16 mEq/L) is also indicative of acidosis. To calculate the anion gap, the serum bicarbonate and chloride values are subtracted from the sodium value:

$$Na^+ - (HCO_3^- + Cl^-)$$

A chest x-ray rules out noncardiogenic pulmonary edema, infiltrates, and trauma. Toxicology screening of blood and urine also may assist in the patient's assessment.[2] Rarely are gastric contents analyzed. A list of symptoms and suspected ingestants is sent to the laboratory with the toxicology specimen. Some substances are more easily identified if the possibility of their presence is noted.

Specific nursing considerations for common therapies following a poisoning are noted below.

- Naloxone and $D_{50}W$ are routinely given to comatose patients. If prepackaged boluses are unavailable, check the concentration of the ampule or multidose vial. Adults are given thiamine prior to, or along with $D_{50}W$ to avoid precipitation of Wernicke's encephalopathy.
- If ipecac is indicated, administration is followed by 200 to 300 ml of fluids in adults, and the patient should be given a large receptacle for emesis. Observe the patient at all times.
- Because of its appearance, some clinicians administer charcoal in an opaque cup with an opaque straw. Avoid letting the patient see the charcoal and administer it in a positive manner. Charcoal will transiently discolor the skin.
- Cathartics are often given with activated charcoal. Be prepared to manage resultant diarrhea. If the patient is discharged soon after cathartic administration, advise the patient to expect black diarrhea.[3]

Psychosocial Considerations

The psychosocial needs of the patient are assessed to aid in prevention of repeated poisonings. Consider the circumstances of the exposure: Was it intentional or accidental? Ingestions of potentially toxic substances should be investigated for possible suicide ideation.

Self-directed Violence

- *Assessment:* Frequently assess the potential for suicide. Even a non-life-threatenting gesture indicates a potential for a more serious attempt. Signs of suicide potential include suicide threats, a previous suicide attempt, history of prolonged depression, marked changes in behavior or personality, or the making of final arrangements.
- *Intervention:* Follow suicide precautions as outlined in the institution to provide a safe environment and prevent injury. Place the patient in a central area, preferably near the nurses' station. Avoid having the patient near exits, stairwells, or elevators. Windows should be locked. Remove sharp or dangerous objects from the patient's environment. Use restraints if necessary. Check the patient frequently at irregular intervals and when there is a decrease in staffing. Assist family members in understanding restrictions the patient must observe.
- *Evaluation:* Patient is protected from further injury.

Disturbance in Self-concept

- *Assessment:* Patients may have a sense of worthlessness and powerlessness or be socially isolated.
- *Intervention:* Always call the patient by name. Explain suicide precautions. Tell the patient you are willing to discuss emotions, feelings, and actions. Involve the patient in care and encourage talk about self, family, work, or other activities that have provided identification for life. Allow time for visits with appropriate significant others. Ensure that mental health counseling is available to the patient. Caretakers should convey a caring attitude for the patient and family.
- *Evaluation:* The patient will discuss feelings, behaviors, and actions and develop insight and a more positive self-image.

Therapeutic Misadventure

- *Assessment:* Does the patient have the resources (sight, knowledge, memory) to self-medicate?
- *Intervention:* Instruct patient about medication administration, focusing on importance of adhering to schedule and explaining side effects. Involve significant others to assist.
- *Evaluation:* The patient will not be readmitted with an accidental drug overdose and will achieve therapeutic results from the medication.

Evaluation

Evaluation assesses the nursing care received and the overall quality of care given. Ongoing reassessment of vital signs and systems review according to outcome standards will evaluate the patient's response to therapy.

GENERAL MANAGEMENT OF THE POISONED PATIENT
Primary Management

The primary interventions for a poisoned patient are stabilization of vital signs and supportive therapy. An intravenous line may be started and appropriate fluids given, depending on the status of the patient. Adults who present in a comatose state require intravenous (IV) naloxone hydrochloride and glucose. Thiamine, 100 mg IV, is also recommended when there is a history of alcoholism.

Prevention of Absorption

The six common routes of exposure to a toxic substance include ingestion, dermal, ocular, inhalation, parenteral, and envenomation. Ingestion is most common. To prevent or limit toxic effects of the poison, initial management includes considering the removal of some of the unabsorbed substance. Prevention of absorption from the gastrointestinal tract may be accomplished with gastric emptying and administration of activated charcoal with or without a cathartic.[2] After a dermal or ocular exposure, the skin or eye is copiously irrigated for at least 15 to 20 minutes with lukewarm water or saline. Following caustic exposures, the skin may need to be irrigated longer depending on the concentration, amount, and duration of exposure to the chemical. Ocular exposures to caustics should be irrigated with sterile saline for at least 1 hour or until the superior and inferior cul-de-sacs have been examined for particles and returned to a neutral pH. This can be determined by touching pH paper to the lower cul-de-sac.[4] Patients exposed to insecticides require a more thorough decontamination by removing their clothing and performing three soap and water washings which include all potentially exposed areas including the scalp, groin, beneath nails, and the navel.[4]

After an inhalation exposure, the patient is moved into fresh air. First aid manuals and container labels may recommend neutralization of a substance; *this is an inappropriate first aid measure that may increase damage.* When a substance is neutralized following an oral, dermal, or ocular exposure, the chemical reaction releases heat, which may cause more deleterious effects than the initial exposure.

Dilution with milk or water is recommended in all conscious patients who have ingested household products or potentially irritant or caustic chemicals.[2] Milk is preferred in caustic ingestions because it is a demulcent and its high protein content provides a substrate for the products. The recommended amount of fluids is 15 ml/kg in a child and up to 250 ml in a 16-kg or larger patient.[4] Excessive amounts of milk or water may cause vomiting which is contraindicated in a caustic ingestion as it can reexpose the esophagus to the caustic agent and promote burns and subsequent stricture formation. Dilution is not recommended for medication ingestions because placing the drug into solution may increase the rate of absorption.

Two methods of gastric emptying are ipecac syrup–induced emesis and gastric lavage. Spontaneous emesis following an ingestion may not adequately empty the stomach. Induction of emesis by gagging with a finger or blunt object is ineffective, and the throat or finger may be injured. Administra-

tion of copper sulfate, dishwashing liquid, or a saltwater solution to induce emesis is no longer recommended because copper sulfate may cause renal and hepatic failure, dishwashing liquid may be aspirated into the lungs, and a saltwater solution may cause hypernatremia and seizures.[2] Dry mustard powder or soap solutions are ineffective and are no longer used. Soap solutions may also produce gastrointestinal irritation. Apomorphine, used as an emetic in veterinary medicine, produces emesis rapidly, but it is not available in a sterile preparation for parenteral administration and is no longer used in humans because it produces central nervous system depression.[2]

Ipecac

Ipecac syrup is an emetic widely used. Its popularity can be attributed to its effectiveness in inducing emesis. Ipecac is derived from the dried root of *Cephaëlis ipecacuanha* or *C. acuminata*. Emetine and cephaeline are the alkaloids contained in ipecac which cause the emetic response. Emesis with ipecac generally occurs within 20 to 30 minutes after its administration. The early vomiting is due to the direct irritant effects on the gastrointestinal tract. Vomiting that occurs after 30 minutes is a result of centrally induced action on the chemoreceptors of the medulla after systemic absorption.

The recommended dose of syrup of ipecac is 30 ml for teenagers and adults. If emesis does not occur within 30 minutes, the dose may be repeated once. The administration of fluids does not hasten the induction of emesis.[5] Data indicate that the efficacy of ipecac in removing a portion of the ingested poison decreases if the time of administration is delayed more than 30 minutes from the time of ingestion.[6] Other studies demonstrate that even when given immediately after ingestion, the percentage of ingestant recovered is small.[7,8] Studies have also shown that most patients do no better clinically when given ipecac syrup and activated charcoal instead of activated charcoal alone.[9] In two studies, ipecac-induced emesis delayed the administration of charcoal, prolonged the emergency department stay, and was associated with more complications.[9]

Protracted vomiting, abdominal cramping, diarrhea, and mild CNS depression have been reported following administration of ipecac.[9] Fluid extract of ipecac, 14 times as potent as ipecac syrup, is no longer generally available and should not be used. Cephaeline is more locally irritating than emetine and produces more nausea and vomiting. Emetine appears to increase intestinal peristalsis, thereby causing diarrhea. Emetine is also more toxic to the heart and may cause tachycardia or dysrhythmias in larger doses. Some isolated cases of side effects following ipecac syrup administration have been reported, which incude Mallory-Weiss tears of the esophagus, cerebral vascular accident in the elderly, pneumomediastinum and retropneumoperitoneum, and aspiration pneumonitis.[9,10,11,12] The deaths of two children, one from gastric rupture during prolonged vomiting and one from herniation of the stomach through a preexisting diaphragmatic hernia, have also been reported.[9] Individuals with eating disorders who chronically abuse syrup of ipecac may develop significant toxicity; some deaths have occurred. A "Munchausen's syndrome by proxy" has been seen, in which infants have recurrent vomiting due to repeated administration of ipecac syrup.[9]

Administration of ipecac syrup is contraindicated for patients who are comatose, have lost their gag reflex, exhibit seizure activity, or have ingested a corrosive substance. It is also not recommended when substances are ingested that produce central nervous system depression, respiratory depression, or seizures within the first 30 minutes of ingestion. Examples include camphor, strychnine, propoxyphene, tricyclic antidepressants, narcotics, and cyanide. Use of ipecac syrup following a hydrocarbon exposure is controversial and depends on the specific type of hydrocarbon, the amount ingested, and the other ingredients in the products, such as pesticides.

Gastric Lavage

The preferred method of gastric emptying is controversial. Early animal studies indicate that lavage is the least effective method regardless of when the procedure is performed after the ingestion.[13] Studies in children revealed similar data with a significant amount of ingestion recovered by ipecac-induced emesis even when lavage had been performed before ipecac administration.[14] In a simulated overdose, gastric lavage with a 34 Fr. orogastric tube and ipecac was significantly less effective than activated charcoal when treatment was initiated 60 minutes after the ingestion of 5 g of ampicillin by human volunteers.[15]

When deciding which method of gastric emptying to use, aspects to consider include the time since the ingestion, the type of exposure, and the efficacy of activated charcoal in adsorbing the substance. If the patient presents to the emergency department more than 30 minutes postexposure, gastric lavage is the preferred procedure because it will not delay activated charcoal administration.[16] Gastric lavage is also recommended in ingestions in which ipecac syrup is contraindicated. However, the most recent studies indicate that in the emergency department, gastric lavage does not lead to an improved clinical outcome, increases the duration of the emergency department stay, and may delay administration of activated char-

coal. It is best reserved for patients who present within 1 hour of ingestion of a substance known not to be well adsorbed by activated charcoal.[9]

Gastric lavage is performed with a large-bore orogastric hose. Endotracheal intubation is indicated for airway protection only in patients who are comatose or have no gag reflex. Gastric lavage should be conducted with the patient in a side-lying, head-down position. Suction must be readily available.[9] Gastric lavage is contraindicated in patients who have ingested caustics or are convulsing. Some potential side effects seen with gastric lavage include esophageal perforation and aspiration pneumonitis.[9]

Activated Charcoal

Activated charcoal decreases toxicity by adsorbing drugs and chemicals to its surface. Its efficacy in acute poisonings is dependent on timing of administration and the amount of charcoal administered. It is most effective when given within 30 minutes of the exposure. In ingestions of drugs with delayed absorption, the charcoal may be effective for up to 24 hours after the exposure. To ensure maximum adsorption of drug, an activated charcoal drug ratio of 10:1 is recommended.[9] Because the patient rarely provides an accurate history of the amount of drug ingested, the recommended dose is 30 to 100 g for adults and 15 to 30 g for children (1 to 2 g/kg as a rough guideline). The abdomen is auscultated for bowel sounds. Activated charcoal is not given in the presence of ileus.

Charcoal is effective only in its activated form. Activated charcoal is obtained by treating charcoal with substances such as steam and air at high temperatures, which increases its adsorptive capabilities. Most commercially prepared activated charcoal products come premixed in a water suspension, ready for administration, or in solution with either flavoring or cathartic doses of sorbitol. Especially in multiple-dose regimen, it is imperative to know whether cathartic doses of sorbitol are present in activated charcoal preparations. Significant cathartic overdose with severe side effects may occur if the wrong preparation is inadvertently used. Attempts have been made to make charcoal more palatable by adding lubricants, flavoring, and sweetening agents; however, these additives may be adsorbed, diminishing the adsorptive capacity of the activated charcoal. It is also not recommended to mix activated charcoal with pudding, ice cream, or other substances that may decrease its efficacy.

Several factors influence the adsorptive capacity of charcoal: pH, amount and type of gastric contents, and the charcoal/drug ratio. Weak acids and bases are adsorbed more effectively when they are in the nonionized form. For example, aspirin is more effectively adsorbed at a pH of 1 rather than at a neutral or alkaline pH. Food in the stomach may decrease the absorptive capacity of activated charcoal. The adsorption of drugs to charcoal is a reversible process, and if inadequate amounts of charcoal are given, desorption will occur. *Desorption* is defined as removing an adsorbed material by a chemical or physical process, thus causing free drug to be released from the drug–charcoal complex. Ethanol, acids, methanol, arsenic, boric acid, bromide, DDT, ethylene glycol, heavy metals, iron, iodide, lithium, potassium, tobramycin, and alkalis are not adsorbed by charcoal in clinically significant amounts.[9] Most drugs are well adsorbed by activated charcoal.

In certain ingestions, multiple doses of activated charcaol are indicated to increase the clearance of systemically absorbed drugs. Drugs may reenter the gastrointestinal tract from the vascular system through diffusion, active secretion, or enterohepatic circulation. If unbound activated charcoal is present in the gastrointestinal tract, a drug concentration gradient between blood and intestinal contents is formed which favors diffusion from the vascular system to the intestinal lumen. This process is referred to as gastrointestinal dialysis.[17]

Multiple-dose charcoal is effective in theophylline, phenobarbital, carbamazepine, and phenylbutazone overdoses. It has also been demonstrated to increase clearance for the drugs listed in the box below. After the initial dose of activated charcoal, recommended doses are 25 g every 2 hours to 50 g every 4 to 6 hours until plasma levels of the drug are within the therapeutic range and the patient is asymptomatic. Optimal doses have not yet been determined. A cathartic is administered as needed to maintain bowel motility but is generally given with only the first dose.

Cathartics

Cathartics are frequently administered with activated charcoal to hasten the elimination of the drug/chemical–charcoal complex. The efficacy of cathartics in preventing absorption of poisons has not been clinically demonstrated.[9]

Cathartics routinely administered include magnesium sulfate, sodium sulfate, magensium citrate, and 70% sorbitol. The recommended doses of magnesium or sodium sulfate are 30 g, for an adult, and of magnesium citrate 4 ml/kg, up to 300 ml a dose. Oil cathartics are not used because of the possibility of serious lipoid pneumonia if aspirated.[9] Cathartics are administered cautiously to patients with recent bowel surgery and to patients with absent bowel sounds. Sodium cathartics are avoided in patients with congestive heart failure and hypertension, as are magnesium cathartics in patients with renal failure. Repeat doses of magnesium cathartics should be used cautiously because of reported toxicity in individuals who received multiple doses.[18,19] Sorbitol is used cautiously in the very young or very old and during multiple-dose charcoal administration because there is a higher incidence of dehydration associated with its use.

Whole-bowel irrigation has recently been recommended as an efficient and rapid means to evacuate the bowel. A nonabsorbable, osmotically active solution—polyethylene glycol lavage electrolyte solution (PEG-ELS), Golytely, Colyte—is administered orally or through a nasogastric tube. The dose, 2 L/hr for adults, is given 4 to 6 hours until the patient is having clear stools. Vomiting may occur and may be related to fluid administration rate. Contraindications to whole-bowel irrigation include significant gastrointestinal pathology or dysfunction such as ileus, perforation, or obstruction.[2,3] Whole-bowel irrigation may be effective in overdoses involving sustained-release drugs, drugs not adsorbed by charcoal, and drug packets.

Advanced Management

Enhancement of the excretion of certain absorbed poisons may be accomplished by diuresis, charcoal hemoperfusion, hemodialysis, and plasma exchange or exchange blood transfusion. The therapy depends on the characteristics of the specific poison, any underlying medical conditions, and the clinical status of the patient.

Supportive therapy is the most important treatment for all poisoned patients. Maintenance of respiration, circulation, and other vital functions take precedence. The indiscriminate use of drugs, anti-

---

Drugs for Which Clearance Is Improved by Multidose Activated Charcoal[7]

Dextropropoxyphene	Sotalol	Nortriptyline	Proscillaridin
Disopyramide	Digoxin	Atrazine	Quinine
Phenytoin	Digitoxin	Chlorpropamide	Piroxicam
Methotrexate	Amitriptyline	Cyclosporine	Salicylates
Benzodiazepine	Doxepin	Dapsone	Sedative/hypnotics
Nadolol	Imipramine	Porphyrins	

dotes, or procedures in patients exposed to toxic substances should be avoided.

Diuresis can take several forms. Neutral diuresis is seldom used in poisoned patients. Although acid diuresis has been shown to increase the elimination of phencyclidine and amphetamines, it is no longer recommended because it may lead to myoglobinuric renal failure in the presence of rhabdomyolysis.[4] Alkaline diuresis is used in salicylate and phenobarbital overdose.[4] Alkalinization of the urine ionizes weak acids, thus preventing passive reabsorption of molecules and increasing elimination.[2] The urine pH must remain between 7 to 8 for the procedure to be beneficial. The urine pH is maintained by adjusting sodium bicarbonate administration. Serum potassium (K^+) is monitored closely because alkaline diuresis cannot be effectively achieved with hypokalemia present. Potassium is added to the IV solution as needed to maintain a normal serum K^+. Hypocalcemia can also occur during alkaline diuresis with sodium bicarbonate; the serum calcium should be monitored. Bicarbonate presents a significant sodium and osmotic load to the body.

Diuretics such as furosemide or mannitol may be administered to maintain diuresis. Diuretic therapy is potentially dangerous because it may lead to noncardiogenic pulmonary edema. Contraindications to diuretic therapy are cerebral edema, pulmonary edema, and renal failure.[4]

Hemodialysis and *hemoperfusion* are extracorporeal procedures that can remove certain absorbed drugs from the body. Their use in the poisoned patient is limited because they are costly and have inherent risks. Water-soluble, low-molecular-weight drugs are more easily removed by hemodialysis than are fat-soluble, high-molecular-weight drugs. Drugs or their metabolites that are highly protein bound, have a large volume of distribution (the larger the volume of distribution, the less amount of total drug found in the plasma), and have a long distribution phase are poorly dialyzable.

Patients who can be managed with supportive care do not require hemodialysis. Indications for hemodialysis include (1) progressive clinical deterioration despite standard treatment measures; (2) a removal rate of poison by dialysis greater than physiological clearance; (3) an impaired elimination system in the patient; (4) poisoning by substances with metabolic and/or delayed effects (such as ethylene glycol or methanol); and (5) depression of midbrain functions producing hypothermia, hypoventilation, and hypotension. Side effects of hemodialysis include hypotension, thrombosis, and, infrequently, hepatitis and infection.[4]

Hemoperfusion with charcoal or resin columns may increase the extraction of certain medications from the body by the passing of anticoagulated blood through a column containing absorbent particles. The extraction ratio of most drugs from the serum is higher for hemoperfusion than for hemodialysis. The efficacy of hemoperfusion is dependent on the drug's volume of distribution, plasma clearance, elimination half-life, and affinity for the absorbent material. Side effects include bleeding, pyrogenic reactions, thrombocytopenia, leukopenia, charcoal embolization, hypotension, hypocalcemia, early saturation of the charcoal column, hypothermia, hypoglycemia, and noncardiogenic pulmonary edema.[4]

When considering these procedures, several factors need to be addressed: the clinical presentation of the patient, the efficacy of the procedure in removing the drug ingested, the side effects of the procedure, and whether supportive care alone is sufficient for recovery (see boxes on pp. 1334 and 1335).

Plasma exchange or *plasma phoresis* removes plasma from a patient by using centrifugal or filtration devices and substituting it with fresh plasma. Exchange blood transfusion removes a specific quantity of blood from a patient and replaces it with fresh whole blood. Both techniques have been used infrequently in poisoning overdose, and their effectiveness is unclear.[2]

Antidotes

Only a few poisons have specific antidotes. Stabilization of vital signs, prevention of absorption, and enhancement of excretion of the poison are the foci of care in most poisonings. For those substances that have a specific antidote, it is important to manage the patient's clinical symptoms initially, not just to administer the antidote (Table 58-1).

COMMON POISONINGS

Acetaminophen

Acetaminophen in therapeutic doses results in antipyretic and analgesic effects mediated through the central nervous system. Because of its wide availability as a nonprescription medication, the incidence of acetaminophen overdose has increased. Overdose amounts can cause acute, transient hepatotoxicity. Prompt, appropriate treatment can avert hepatic damage.

Pathophysiology

The metabolism and kinetics of acetaminophen are well known. After ingestion, 94% of the dose is converted to nontoxic metabolites in the liver, and 2% is excreted unchanged in the urine. The remaining 4% is metabolized via the cytochrome P450 pathway in the hepatocytes. Acetaminophen is metabolized to

Agents for Which Hemodialysis May Be Effective

Acetaminophen/Par-acetamol	Chloral hydrate	Heroin	Penicillin
Acetone	Chloramphenicol	Iodide	Pentobarbital
Acetophencitidin	Chlordiazepoxide	Iron	Phenelzine
Acetophenetidine	Chloride	Isocarboxazid	Phenobarbital
Acetylsalicylic acid	Chloroquine	Isoniazid	Phosphate
Alkyl phosphate	Chlorpropamide	Isopropanol	Polymyxin
Amanita phalloides	Chromic acid	Kanamycin	Potassium
Amanitin	Cimetidine	Lead	Potassium chlorate
Amikacin	Colchicine	Lithium	Potassium dichromate
Ammonia	Colistin	Magnesium	Practolol
Amobarbital	Copper	Mannitol	Primidone
Amphetamine	Cyclobarbital	Meprobamate	Procainamide
Ampicillin	Cyclophosphamide	Mercury	Propoxyphene
Aniline	Cycloserine	Methamphetamine	Propranolol
Aprobarbital	Demeton-S-methyl-sulfoxide	Methanol	Quinalbital
Arsenic	Dextropropoxyphene	Methaqualone	Quinine
Atenolol	Diethyl pentenamide	Methotrexate	Salicylic acid
Azathioprine	Digoxin	Methyl Mercury Com-plex	Secobarbital
Azlocillin	Dimethoate	Methyldopa	Snake bite
Bacitracin	Dinitro-ortho-cresol	Methylprednisolone	Sodium chlorate
Barbital	Dinitrophenol	Methylsalicylate	Sodium citrate
Borates	Diphenhydramine	Methypyrlon	Sotalol
Boric acid	Diphenylhydantoin	Monoamine Oxidase Inhibitors	Streptomycin
Bromide	Diquat	Nafcillin	Strontium
Butabarbital	Ergoramine	Neomycin	Sulfonamides
Butalbital	Ethanol	N-Acetylprocainamide	Tetracycline
Calcium	Ethchlorvynol	Nitrates	Thallium
Camphor	Ethinamate	Nitrite	Thiocyanate
Carbamazepine	Ethylene glycol	Nitrofurantoin	Thiols
Carbenicillin	Eucalyptus oil	Ouabain	Tobramycin
Carbon monoxide	Flucytosine	Oxalate	Trancylpromine
Carbon tetrachloride	Fluoridem chlorate	Oxalic acid	Tranylcypromine
Carbromal	Fostomycin	Paraidehyde	Trichlorethylene
Cefamandole	Gallamine triethiodide	Paraquat	Tricyclic secondary amines
Cephaloridine	Gentamicin	Pargyline	Tricyclic tertiary amines
Cephalothin	Glutethimide		Vancomycin

Adapted, with permission, from POISINDEX Information System: Micromedex, Inc. (1974-1992). Denver, CO.

a toxic metabolite, conjugates with the enzyme glutathione, and is excreted as two nontoxic metabolites, mercapturic acid and cysteine.[4]

In therapeutic doses, acetaminophen is easily conjugated to glutathione. In large overdoses, glutathione is rapidly depleted. When levels fall below 70% of normal, unbound amounts of the toxic metabolite accumulate. Toxicity results when the metabolite covalently binds with hepatic macromolecules, resulting in liver cell necrosis. The larger the amount of acetaminophen ingested, the greater the amount of toxic metabolite produced and the greater the potential hepatic damage.[4]

Acetaminophen overdose causes hepatotoxicity. A latent period of 24 to 36 hours can occur between the time of exposure and the onset of symptoms.

Right-sided abdominal pain and tenderness, hypoglycemia, and abnormal clotting can follow. Nausea, vomiting, and anorexia can develop 2 to 14 hours after ingestion. Coma and metabolic acidosis rarely occur; all such patients had extremely high acetaminophen levels (>800 μg/ml) and symptoms begun within 3 to 4 hours of ingestion. Renal damage and, very rarely, pancreatitis also may occur.[4,20]

Patients who eventually die, whether treated late with NAC or not all, continue to have high serum liver enzyme levels after 72 to 96 hours.[2]

Medical Management

Treatment guidelines are based on the patient's history of the amount of acetaminophen ingested. In adults, an ingestion of greater than 7.5 g has potential

---

Agents for Which Hemoperfusion May Be Effective	
Amanita mushrooms	Methotrexate
Amobarbital	Methsuximide
Carbromal	N-Acetylprocainamide
Carbon tetrachloride	Oxycholordone
Chloral hydrate	Paraquat
Colchicine	Phenobarbital
Cortinarius mushrooms	Phenothiazines
Digitoxin	Phenytoin
Digoxin	Primidone
Diquat	Procainamide
Ethchlorvynol	Quinidine
Glutethimide	Secobarbital
Gyromitra mushrooms	Theophylline
Hexobarbital	Thallium
Lidocaine	Trichloroethanol
Meprobamate	Tricyclics (resin)
Methaqualone	

Adapted, with permission, from POISINDEX Information System: Micromedex, Inc. (1974-1992). Denver, CO.

for hepatotoxicity. General management principles for gastric emptying apply to acetaminophen ingestions. Gastric lavage is preferable to ipecac-induced emesis when gastric emptying is desired because ipecac syrup may enhance or prolong the emesis associated with acetaminophen overdose and delay the time to initiation of N-acetylcysteine (NAC) therapy.[3] Toxicity is determined with the Rumack-Matthew nomogram (Figure 58-1). Peak plasma levels with therapeutic doses are seen in 70 to 160 minutes. In overdose situations, peak plasma levels may not be seen until 4 hours after ingestion when absorption is completed.[4] Blood samples for testing of acetaminophen levels should be drawn at 4 hours or more after acute ingestion. At 4 hours after exposure, plasma levels of 150 μg/ml or greater are considered potentially hepatotoxic, and NAC treatment is mandated.

NAC therapy should be started within 8 hours of ingestion when possible. The efficacy of NAC decreases 8 to 16 hours after ingestion[21] but may be of some benefit for up to 24 hours.[4] If levels cannot be obtained within 6 to 8 hours after ingestion and the history indicates a potentially toxic dose, treatment should be initiated and continued until plasma levels are available.[2]

N-acetylcysteine is the best available prophylactic antidote for prevention of acetaminophen-induced hepatotoxicity.[2] The NAC derivative of the naturally occurring amino acid L-cysteine constitutes the central portion of the glutathione molecule. The antidotal mechanism for NAC is not completely understood, although it is known that NAC is metabolized to cysteine, a glutathione precursor. One possible mechanism of action is that the administration of NAC maintains protective levels of glutathione so that the reactive metabolite of acetaminophen will be detoxified by conjugation. NAC may stabilize cell constituents, avoiding the deleterious effects of covalent binding between the hepatocytes and the toxic acetaminophen metabolites.[2]

The NAC regimen in common use in the United States is an oral loading dose of 140 mg/kg followed by 17 oral maintenance doses of 70 mg/kg given at 4-hour intervals.[2] If a patient vomits within 1 hour of any dose, that dose must be repeated. If emesis occurs more than 1 hour after dosing, the next dose should be administered as scheduled. NAC is commercially available in 10% and 20% solutions containing 100 mg or 200 mg NAC per milliliter, respectively.

Currently, oral administration is the only method approved by the Federal Drug Administration (FDA) for NAC administration. When administering NAC, it is diluted to a 5% mixture. Mix one part NAC to one part diluent for 10% NAC and one part NAC to three parts diluent for 20% NAC. To make NAC more palatable, it can be mixed with soda or fruit juice and served over ice in a covered container. If patients are comatose or unable to tolerate the medication by mouth due to vomiting, it may be given by nasogastric tube or a weighted jejunal tube such as a cantor or Miller-Abbott tube. For nasogastric administration, NAC need not be mixed with a diluent and can be given by slow nasogastric drip. Reported side effects of NAC are primarily nausea and vomiting.[4] For persistent vomiting, 1 mg per kg metoclopramide (Reglan) may be given IV or IM 30 minutes before the NAC dose, or 1.25 to 2.0 mg droperidol (Inapsine) may be given IV in adults 60 minutes before the NAC dose. Metoclopramide may cause extrapyramidal side effects.[4]

The use of NAC concomitantly with activated charcoal is controversial. Current recommendations are to avoid the use of NAC within 1 hour of charcoal administration.[22]

Many patients experience vomiting as a consequence of acetaminophen overdose or as a side effect of NAC, and health care providers often wish to use an intravenous NAC preparation. Intravenous administration of NAC is permissible in the United States only under an Investigational New Drug (IND) protocol. A pyrogen-free preparation is available at poison centers throughout the country participating in a multicenter clinical trial. The location of the nearest participating center can be obtained by calling 1-800-525-6115. Information about oral administration is also available at this number.

As both mother and fetus are at risk for hepatotoxicity following an acetaminophen overdose during

TABLE 58-1 Antidotes

Antidote	Toxic Agent	Dose and Techniques for Administering	Comments
N-Acetylcysteine (NAC)	Acetaminophen	Oral loading dose: 140 mg/kg. Oral maintenance dose: 70 mg/kg every 4 hr × 17 doses.	Most effective if given within 8 hours; questionable effectiveness after 24 hours.
Physostigmine	Anticholinergics	Therapeutical trial: 2 mg IV slow over 5 minutes. Second dose of 1-2 mg IV slow may be done in 20 minutes if no symptom reversal. Therapeutic dose: 1-4 mg IV slow over 5-10 minutes. Do not give continuous IV infusion.	Possible indications: convulsions, severe hallucinations, hypertension, and dysrrhythmias not responding to standard measures. Side effects: convulsions, bradycardia, asystole. Use cautiously.
Oxygen	Carbon monoxide	100% oxygen until CO level less than 5%.	Side effects: patients on 100% oxygen for more than 24 hours may develop oxygen toxicity.
Cyanide antidote kit: Amyl nitrite, sodium nitrite, and sodium thiosulfate	Cyanide Hydrogen sulfide	Amyl nitrite inhalant: Every 30 seconds until sodium nitrite administered. A new ampule is used every 3 minutes. Sodium nitrite: Adult 300 mg IV over no less than 5 minutes. Sodium thiosulfate: 12.5 g IV after sodium nitrite.	Side effects: hypotension and methemoglobinemia. Sodium thiosulfate is inefficacious in hydrogen sulfide poisoning.
Methylene blue	Methemoglobinemia-inducing agents: Nitrites and related compounds available in fertilizers; aniline dyes; gunpowder; well water; and drugs such as phenacetin, Pyridium, antimalarials, and dapsone	0.1-0.2 ml/kg (1-2 mg/kg) 1% methylene blue slowly IV to reverse methemoglobinemia. May need to be repeated.	May consider its use in the cyanotic patient unresponsive to O_2 therapy.
Atropine	Organophosphates (malathion, parathion) and carbamate insecticides (Sevin, etc.)	Adults: 2-5 mg slow IV. Repeat every 10-30 minutes as needed to obtain full atropinization.	Atropinization best indicated by clearing of bronchial and pulmonary secretions, not pupillary dilation.
2-PAM (Pralidoximine)	Organophosphate and carbamate (except carbaryl) insecticides	Adults: 1 g IV at 0.5 g/min or infused in 250 ml saline over 30 minutes. Doses may be repeated 1 hour after initial dose and every 6-12 hours if muscle or diaphragmatic weakness is not relieved.	Indicated for nicotinic and central effects as coma, convulsions, fasciculations, and profound muscle weakness. Give only after atropine. Early administration is probably more efficacious.

Adapted, with permission, from POISINDEX Information System: Micromedex, Inc. (1974-1992). Denver, CO; and Wruk, K. (1982). Administering emergency antidotes to the acutely poisoned patient. *Dimensions of Critical Care Nursing, 1,* 206-211.

TABLE 58-1 Antidotes—cont'd

Antidote	Toxic Agent	Dose and Techniques for Administering	Comments
Naloxone	Opiates, Darvon, Lomotil	Adults and children: Initial dose of 0.4-2 mg every 2-3 minutes. If no response after 10 mg given, diagnosis of opioid toxicity should be questioned.	Since the half-life of naloxone is shorter than that of the opiate, it should be repeated when opiate symptoms reappear.
Digibind	Digitalis	Dose according to total body burden on package insert.	Should be used only in cases of serious overdose.

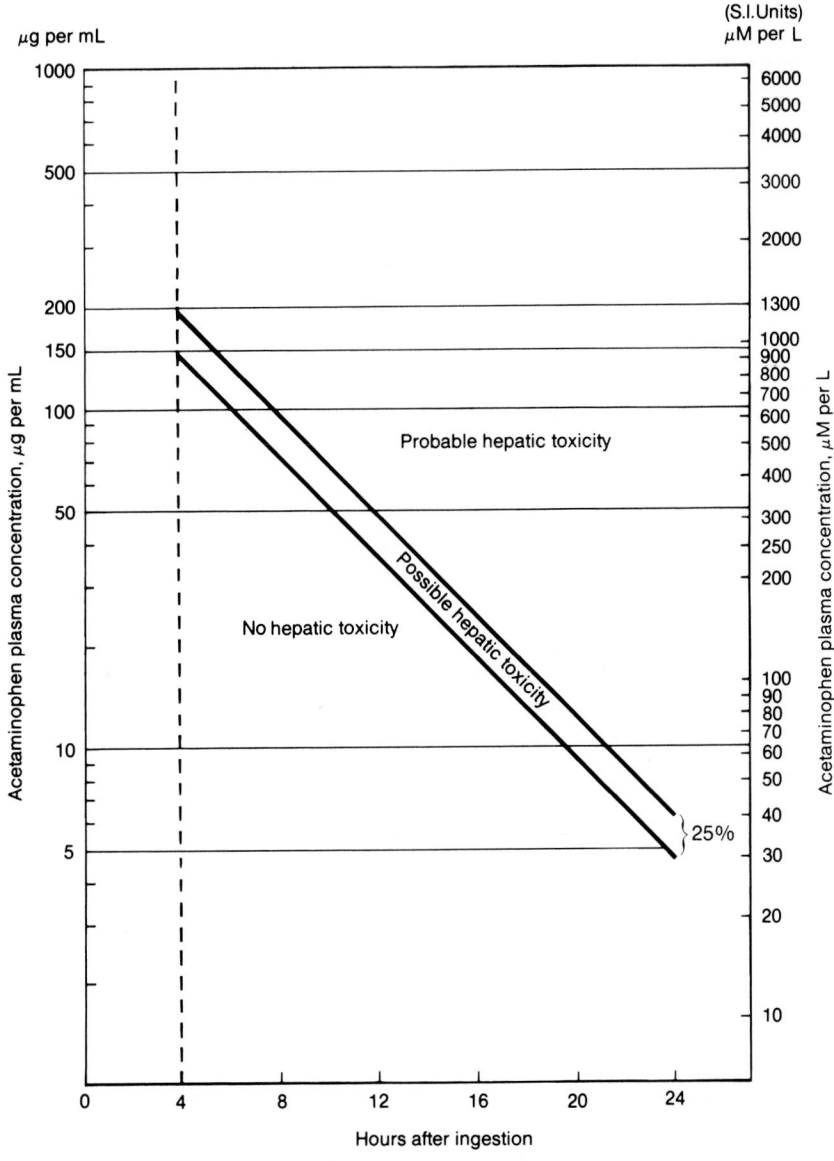

Figure 58-1 Rumack-Matthew nomogram for acetaminophen poisoning.
Copyright Micromedex, Inc. 1974-1992. Adapted from *Pediatrics*, 1975; 55:871-876.

pregnancy, NAC therapy is administered as it would be to nonpregnant patients. Early delivery of the fetus is not recommended. It is easier and probably more effective to treat the fetus in utero with NAC than after the birth.[23]

Evaluation

If the first acetaminophen level reveals toxicity, NAC must be continued even if subsequent levels are plotted as nontoxic on the nomogram.[5] NAC effectiveness is judged best by serial determinations of liver function tests, including an SGOT, SGPT, total bilirubin, and prothrombin time. Elevations seen within 48 to 72 hours of the overdose should begin to decline within 96 hours. Patients whose treatment with NAC was delayed or who were not treated may develop hepatotoxicity with a greater increase in liver enzymes. Plasma levels will remain elevated for long periods of time. The PT and total bilirubin are good indicators of outcome when patients develop excessive hepatotoxicity. A total bilirubin of greater than 4 or PT twice normal indicates the possibility for a worse outcome. Death is rare from acetaminophen-induced hepatotoxicity. Survivors' liver function usually returns to normal on subsequent evaluations.

Alcohols

Methanol, Ethylene Glycol

Methanol, also known as methyl or wood alcohol, is used commercially as a solvent, antifreeze, windshield washer fluid, and canned fuel (Sterno).[4] Ethylene glycol is a colorless, odorless, sweet-tasting, water-soluble liquid. It is in such commercial products as detergents, paints, cosmetics, and solar collection systems, and most commonly is used as a deicer and antifreeze.[4] Deicers and antifreeze may contain from 70% to 95% ethylene glycol. Methanol and ethylene glycol may be accidentally ingested by children or intentionally ingested by adults in suicide attempts or as a substitute for alcoholic beverages.

The formation of toxic metabolites causes the type of toxicity most often seen in ethylene glycol and methanol posioning. Management of ethylene glycol or methanol intoxication focuses on halting production of toxic metabolites.

Pathophysiology of Methanol Toxicity. Methanol is readily absorbed by the gastrointestinal tract and distributed throughout the tissues. Toxicity from skin and lung absorption has been reported, but ingestion is usually the main route of exposure.[24,25]

Methanol is slowly metabolized in the liver by the enzyme alcohol dehydrogenase via formaldehyde to formic acid. The oxidation of methanol proceeds independently of the plasma concentration at a rate one fifth that of ethanol.[4] Complete oxidation and excretion may take several days. The approximate half-life of methanol in the body is about 8 hours.[26] Between 3% and 5% of ingested methanol is excreted unchanged by the kidneys, and a small amount is excreted by the lungs.[2,4]

Formaldehyde and formic acid, the metabolites of methanol, are highly toxic and account for the metabolic acidosis, ocular symptoms, and other effects seen following ingestion. The local production of formaldehyde in the retina was once thought to be responsible for optic papillitis and retinal edema with subsequent blindness; however, newer findings indicate that ocular injury is directly correlated with the methanol dose, degree of metabolic acidosis, and formate concentration.[4] Blindness has occurred following ingestion of 4 ml of absolute methanol. In one patient, death occurred after ingestion of 15 ml of a 40% solution, whereas another patient survived after 500 ml of the same mixture.[4]

Clinical Manifestations of Methanol Toxicity. The onset of symptoms occurs between 40 minutes and 72 hours; a coingestion of alcohol may delay symptoms with a latent period of 12 to 24 hours.[27]

Toxicity includes three major symptoms: central nervous system depression, severe anion gap metabolic acidosis, and a number of reversible or irreversible optic changes.[4] The toxicity is related to the degree of metabolic acidosis and, therefore, to the time between exposure and treatment.

After methanol ingestion, neurological symptoms mimic an ethanol hangover and include malaise, headache, dizziness, vertigo, and weakness. Profound coma and seizures can occur in severe exposures. Elevated anion gap metabolic acidosis is one of the most significant clinical findings. Other symptoms include gastrointestinal distress, dyspnea, tachypnea, and tachycardia.[4]

Visual abnormalities seen in methanol poisoning include blurred or double vision, constricted visual fields, spots in the eyes ("snowfield" effect), and reduced visual acuity. These ocular abnormalities are often delayed for 12 to 24 hours after ingestion. Funduscopic examination may show peripapillary edema, hyperemia of the optic disk, or retinal edema. Permanent blindness frequently occurs, although blindness has occasionally resolved.[4]

Pathophysiology of Ethylene Glycol Toxicity. Ethylene glycol is rapidly absorbed by the gastrointestinal tract, whereas topical and dermal absorption are thought to be minimal. Toxicity from inhalation is unlikely to occur except at high temperatures. Ethylene glycol is metabolized by alcohol dehydrogenase into several toxic organic acids (Figure 58-2). These metabolites (especially glycolic acid and oxalic acid)

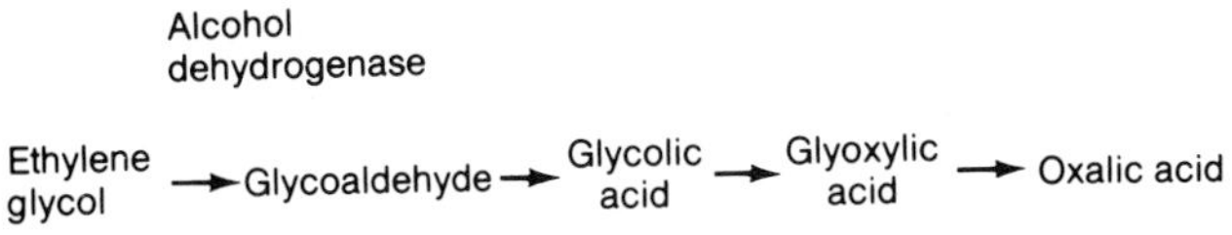

Alcohol
dehydrogenase

Ethylene $\longrightarrow$ Glycoaldehyde $\longrightarrow$ Glycolic $\longrightarrow$ Glyoxylic $\longrightarrow$ Oxalic acid
glycol   acid   acid

Figure 58-2   Ethylene glycol metabolism.

Adapted, with permission, from POISINDEX Information System: Micromedex, Inc. (1974-1992). Denver, CO.

are responsible for the central nervous system, metabolic, cardiopulmonary, and renal symptoms following ethylene glycol ingestion.

Toxicity from ethylene glycol ingestion is caused by tissue destruction from deposition of calcium oxalate crystals and the production of severe acidosis due to organic acid accumulation. As a consequence of the oxalic acid deposition in the kidneys and other tissues, calcium ions are chelated forming calcium oxalate, and hypocalcemia may occur.[2] Oxalic acid may also precipitate in the urine as calcium oxalate crystals. These crystals may assume many shapes, including octahedral (envelope-like), prismatic (spindles), or dumbbell shapes. Because only 3% to 10% of ethylene glycol is converted to oxalic acid, renal toxicity is not entirely explained by the formation of this metabolite. Glycolic aldehyde, glycolic acid, and glyoxylic acid may also cause significant renal tubular damage and may account for renal insufficiency occurring in the absence of renal oxalosis.

The central nervous system depression associated with ethylene glycol ingestion may be caused by unchanged ethylene glycol or the aldehyde metabolite concentration (glycoaldehyde). Glycoaldehyde is at its highest concentration 6 to 12 hours after ethylene glycol ingestion when central nervous system symptoms are most severe.[2]

The minimal toxic or lethal dose of ethylene glycol is not well defined but has been approximated at 1.4 ml per kg or about 100 ml for a 70-kg adult. Death has been reported from as little as 60 ml, while ingestion of 240 ml has been survived.[4]

Clinical Manifestations of Ethylene Glycol Toxicity. Ethylene glycol intoxication characteristically occurs in three stages: (1) central nervous system depression and metabolic acidosis, (2) cardiopulmonary complications, and (3) renal failure. The initial phase occurs between 30 minutes and 12 hours after ingestion. Symptoms include ataxia, slurred speech, somnolence, nausea, and vomiting. Coma, convulsions, and death may result after large ingestions. The central nervous system findings resemble those of ethanol inebriation but without ethanol breath odor, unless ethanol has been concurrently ingested. Metabolic acidosis usually accompanies central nervous system depression but may develop later. Low levels

of serum bicarbonate, decreased CO_2, increased anion gap (12 to 16 mEq or more) and tachypnea with Kussmaul's respirations are characteristic of metabolic acidosis with respiratory compensation. Calcium hyperoxaluria, hematuria, and proteinuria are frequent findings. Since oxalate crystals are not invariably seen, their absence does not rule out ethylene glycol poisoning.[4]

Stage 2 usually occurs 12 to 36 hours after ingestion and is characterized by progressive respiratory distress and pulmonary edema secondary to congestive heart failure. Death occurs most frequently in this stage.

If the patient survives the first two stages, the clinical course proceeds to stage 3. This usually occurs 2 or 3 days after ingestion and is characterized by renal insufficiency. Flank pain and tenderness with oliguria, proteinuria, and anuria are common. Timing of occurrence of the phases is delayed if ethanol is concurrently ingested with ethylene glycol.

Medical Management. Medical management of a patient who has ingested methanol or ethylene glycol begins with stabilization and prevention of further absorption. Gastric decontamination with lavage may be helpful if the patient presents within 2 hours of exposure and may be helpful up to 4 hours after ingestion if coma or coingested drugs reduce gastrointestinal motility.[4] Charcoal and cathartics are probably not effective for decreasing the absorption of ethylene glycol and methanol.

Arterial blood gases, serum electrolytes, and bicarbonate provide data useful in determining the severity of the poisoning. A pH of less than 7.0 and bicarbonate less than 7 mEq/L are common following severe intoxication. Methanol or ethylene glycol levels greater than 50 mg/dl indicate a serious exposure. Methanol and ethylene glycol (as well as ethanol and isopropyl alcohol) are osmotically active and may cause a disparity between measured and calculated plasma osmolality. Determination of the osmolar gap is especially valuable when methanol or ethylene glycol levels are not readily available.[4] To determine the calculated osmolality, the following formula is used:

$$2 \times \text{Na} + \frac{\text{Glucose}}{18} + \frac{\text{BUN}}{2.8} + \frac{\text{ETOH}}{4.6}$$

Ethanol therapy prolongs the half-life of ethylene glycol and methanol and, thereby, prevents their breakdown (Table 58-2). Alcohol dehydrogenase (ADH) has approximately 20 times as much affinity of ethanol as methanol, and, therefore, administering ethanol effectively inhibits oxidation of methanol to formaldehyde and formic acid.[4] ADH has a similar affinity for ethanol compared to ethylene glycol. Eth-

***TABLE 58-2* Ethanol Therapy for Methanol/ Ethylene Glycol Poisoning**

Loading dose: 7.6-10 ml/kg IV of 10% ETOH in D_5W over 1 hour
Maintenance dose: Volume of 10% ETOH needed IV

Average	1.40 ml/kg/hr
Chronic drinker	1.96 ml/kg/hr
Nondrinker	0.83 ml/kg/hr

Note: A 5% alcohol solution for intravenous infusion is commercially available; however, excessive volumes of fluids are required to maintain adequate blood alcohol levels.
Adapted, with permission, from POISINDEX Information System: Micromedex, Inc. (1974-1992). Denver, CO.

anol competitively inhibits ADH from metabolizing ethylene glycol to its toxic metabolites.[4]

Ethanol therapy is indicated in any patient with a plasma level between 20 and 50 mg/dl and any symptomatic patient with a history of methanol or ethylene glycol ingestion. The blood ethanol level is maintained between 100 and 130 mg/dl during therapy. Ethanol may cause hypoglycemia.[4] The blood glucose needs to be monitored closely. Patients who have concurrently ingested methanol or ethylene glycol along with ethanol may have a normal acid–base status despite extremely elevated levels. With these patients, ethanol therapy should be considered until methanol or ethylene glycol levels can be determined.[4] Ethanol should be administered cautiously in patients taking disulfiram while assessing for the antidote reaction (flushing, sweating, severe hypotension, and dysrhythmias).[4]

Hemodialysis is effective in removing methanol or ethylene glycol from the plasma.[26,28] Indications for its use include a blood methanol or ethylene glycol level greater than 50 mg/dl, a severe acid–base or fluid and electrolyte disturbance despite conventional therapy, ocular symptoms in patients who are methanol poisoned, and renal failure. The ethanol infusion is continued during hemodialysis and increased as needed to maintain the blood ethanol level at 100 to 130 mg/dl. If ethanol is not added to the dialysate, the maintenance IV infusion during dialysis is an additional 91 mg/hr of 10% ETOH solution.[26]

In methanol poisoning, formic acid is metabolized to carbon monoxide and water via a folate-dependent system. Administration of folic acid or leucovorin (an active metabolite of folic acid) may enhance formic acid elimination. After ethylene glycol metabolism, the excessive amount of glyoxylate may deplete body stores of pyridoxine. Pyridoxine is administered because it is essential for the conversion of glyoxylate to nontoxic glycine. Thiamine administration may also be necessary because it converts glyoxylate to the nontoxic metabolite, alpha-hydroxy-beta-ketoadipate.[4]

Evaluation. To evaluate the effectiveness of therapy in patients poisoned by methanol or ethylene glycol, assessment includes vital signs, orientation, acid–base status, and methanol or ethylene glycol blood levels. When evaluating management outcomes specifically, assessment also includes visual fields in methanol poisoning, and renal function in ethylene glycol poisoning.

Ethanol, Isopropyl Alcohol

Ethanol (ethyl alcohol) and isopropyl alcohol are central nervous system depressants. Ethanol is found in alcoholic beverages and medicines, and special denatured ethanol is found in colognes, perfumes, aftershaves, other cosmetics, and rubbing alcohol. Isopropyl alcohol is a common ingredient in rubbing alcohol (70% isopropyl alcohol) and cleaning agents. Ethanol may be accidentally or intentionally ingested by adults in suicide attempts, alone or with other medications. Toxicity is frequently seen when ethanol is ingested as a recreational beverage. Isopropyl alcohol, ingested accidentally or intentionally, may also be consumed as a substitute for an alcoholic beverage.

Pathophysiology of Ethanol Toxicity. Ethanol is rapidly absorbed from the gastrointestinal tract. Vaporized ethanol may be absorbed via the lungs, whereas absorption through the skin is negligible. Several factors may delay absorption of ethanol from the stomach, including the presence of food, the concentration of ethanol, and the time period in which ethanol is consumed. Absorption from the small intestine is rapid and complete and is independent of the presence of food. Peak blood ethanol concentrations may be achieved 30 minutes after ingestion.[4,20]

Ethanol is metabolized in the liver by alcohol dehydrogenase to acetaldehyde.[29] Only 2% to 10% of ingested ethanol is eliminated unchanged by the lungs and kidneys.[4] The rate of oxidation is constant with time and increases little with increased concentration in the blood (zero order kinetics).[30] The amount of ethanol oxidized is proportional to body weight and liver weight. This slow and constant rate of metabolism limits the amount of ethanol that can be consumed over time without intoxication due to ethanol accumulation.

Ethanol is not generally considered a seriously toxic agent but may have serious effects. Each ounce of whiskey, glass of wine, or bottle of beer can raise the blood ethanol concentration approximately 25 mg/dl. Blood ethanol levels below 50 mg/dl rarely produce marked sensory or motor impairment.[4] Concentrations of 150 to 300 mg/dl are generally associated with mental confusion, ataxia, exaggerated emotional status, and muscular incoordination.[4] Most fatalities from ethanol occur with levels greater than 400 mg/dl.[4] The lethal dose of ethanol for adults is 5 to 8 mg/kg. Alcoholics are more tolerant of higher ethanol levels than abstainers.

Clinical Manifestations of Ethanol Toxicity. Ethanol poisoning may produce nausea, vomiting, central nervous system depression, acid–base disturbances, hypoglycemia, and respiratory depression. Central nervous system depression and peripheral vasodilation may lead to hypothermia. Deep tendon reflexes also may be absent. Hypoglycemia resulting in convulsions is a serious complication of acute ethanol intoxication, especially in children and chronic alcoholics. Moderate metabolic acidosis may occur from increased production of lactate and fatty acids. Few cases will progress to frank ketoacidosis. Death usually results from respiratory failure.[4,29]

Pathophysiology of Isopropyl Alcohol Toxicity. Isopropyl alcohol causes greater central nervous system depression than ethanol at similar blood levels.[2] It may produce toxic symptoms following ingestion, inhalation, or dermal exposures. Isopropyl alcohol is oxidized to acetone which is then metabolized to acetate and CO_2. The acetone may contribute to central nervous system depression.[4] The metabolism of isopropyl alcohol is much slower than ethanol.[2]

Toxic effects from isopropyl alcohol are usually seen at blood levels between 50 and 100 mg/dl. Levels of 150 mg/dl are associated with deep coma, and levels greater than 200 mg/dl have been reported to cause death. Ingestion of 3 ounces of 70% isopropyl alcohol by a 70-kg person may produce a blood level of 100 mg/dl.[4]

Clinical Manifestations of Isopropyl Alcohol Toxicity. The signs and symptoms of isopropyl alcohol ingestion are similar to those of ethanol ingestion. Within hours, lethargy, hypothermia, and coma occur. Areflexia, deep coma, hypotension, and respiratory failure may follow severe intoxication. Isopropyl alcohol has a stronger irritant effect on the stomach than ethanol, which can result in hemorrhagic gastritis and an associated decreased hematocrit. Although hypoglycemia is uncommon, the blood glucose needs to be monitored closely. Hyperglycemia has been reported in adults.[2,4]

Medical Management. Basic life support and prevention of absorption are instituted after ingestion of ethanol and isopropyl alcohol. Because ethanol and isopropyl alcohol are rapidly absorbed liquids, emesis or lavage and administration of activated charcoal and a cathartic are most effective within 2 hours after ingestion. However, the absorption of ethanol is not decreased appreciably by the administration of activated charcoal, and it is currently not known how well charcoal binds isopropyl alcohol.[4] To avoid aspiration of vomitus, the patient is placed in a semi-lateral decubitus position with the head forward and mouth down. Suction should always be readily available. If significant central nervous system or respiratory depression is present, induction of emesis is contraindicated.

In ethanol or isopropyl alcohol ingestion, management is primarily directed at supportive care. The patient should be assessed for hypotension, and the blood pressure should be maintained with IV fluids, semi-Trendelenberg position, and vasopressors as needed. In severe intoxication, the patient's respiratory functions are closely monitored by assessing respiratory rate, tissue perfusion, and arterial blood gases.

In ethanol ingestion, the blood glucose needs to be monitored frequently because hypoglycemia may be delayed for several hours.[4] Glucose may be administered IV as needed. Monitoring blood ethanol and isopropyl alcohol concentrations closely may indicate the seriousness of the exposure. Concurrent ingestion of additional sedatives or tranquilizers may precipitate symptoms at substantially lower blood ethanol concentrations.[4] Following isopropyl alcohol ingestion, the blood and urine can be checked for acetone.[4] Because both ethanol and isopropyl alcohol ingestions may result in acidosis, the acid–base status is monitored closely. Sodium bicarbonate is administered as indicated.

Hemodialysis may be effective for patients with excessive blood ethanol or isopropyl alcohol levels, impaired hepatic function, and those unresponsive to standard therapy.[2,4] It is unusual for a patient to require hemodialysis in ethanol poisoning.

Because the patient's sensorium may be altered following an ethanol or isopropyl alcohol ingestion, it is important to protect the patient from self-harm. Side rails need to be kept up and patients should be located in a room close to the nurses' station. Mental status is assessed frequently to guide appropriate interventions.

Evaluation. The patient is evaluated for response to medical and nursing interventions following ethanol or isopropyl alcohol exposure. The patient should be assessed for normal pulse, blood pressure, and respiratory function, blood ethanol or isopropyl levels below 50 mg/dl, improved mental status, and normal electrolytes and acid–base status.

Carbon Monoxide

Carbon monoxide (CO) is an insidious poison because it has no odor or taste and is nonirritating. It is produced during incomplete combustion of a carbon-containing fuel. Four common sources of CO are automobile exhaust fumes, burning charcoal, poorly ventilated wood or coal stoves, and malfunctioning furnaces. Carbon monoxide is present in all fires and may be a hazard to firefighters. Natural gas does not contain CO, but it may be produced if the gas is burned without sufficient oxygen. Methylene chloride and methylene iodide are metabolized in vivo to CO.[31] An adequate history of the exposure may help to confirm the diagnosis: where the patient was found, activity at the time of exposure, if any combustible fuels were being used, and if there was adequate ventilation.

Pathophysiology

CO binds rapidly, specifically, and avidly with hemoglobin in erythrocytes to form carboxyhemoglobin (COHB). The affinity of hemoglobin for CO is over 200 times that for oxygen. The COHB reduces the carrying capacity of hemoglobin for oxygen and, in a minor fashion, impairs cellular utilization of oxygen by binding to the cytochrome oxidase system.[2] The result of CO inhalation is hypoxia. Because the brain and the heart are most dependent on oxygen, the major toxic symptoms are noted in these organs. Tissue hypoxia may, however, be seen in all organ systems.[4]

Carbon monoxide is absorbed and eliminated by the lungs. Its half-life when inhaled in room air is 5 to 6 hours. With 100% supplemental oxygen, the half-life can be reduced to 40 to 90 minutes. Hyperbaric oxygen decreases the half-life to less than 30 minutes and increases the delivery of oxygen to hypoxic tissues, thus diminishing the severity of cerebral edema and other central nervous system sequelae.[2] Carbon monoxide crosses the placenta, and the fetal concentration may be 10% to 15% greater than the CO concentration of the mother. The fetal CO elimination half-life is approximately five times longer than that of the mother's.[4]

Clinical Manifestations

Symptoms reported following CO poisoning include headache, nausea, vomiting, dizziness, weakness, decreased exercise tolerance, visual disturbance, and irritability. Acute signs are tachycardia, tachypnea, fever, confusion, hypotension, dysrhythmias, seizures, coma, pulmonary and cerebral edema, and respiratory failure.[2] Cardiac effects may include ECG changes such as ST segment depression, T wave abnormalities, atrial fibrillation, and intraventricular conduction block.[4] COHB causes earlier onset of angina and decreased exercise tolerance in patients with coronary artery disease because myocardial oxygen supply is already reduced.[2] Retinal hemorrhages, decreased visual acuity, and transient hearing loss have

been reported. Other signs of COHB poisoning include hyperglycemia, albuminuria, cutaneous lesions from erythema and edema to blister and bullae formation, and alopecia. Residual or delayed neurological effects include masklike facies, mental deterioration, abnormal reflexes, incontinence, hypertonicity, and gait disturbances. Neuropsychiatric sequelae such as personality changes and memory impairment may be noted.[4]

Medical Management

After CO exposure, the patient is moved immediately from the contaminated atmosphere, and basic life support is begun. One hundred percent oxygen is administered by a tightly fitting face mask or endotracheal tube.

Arterial blood gases are closely monitored. If the patient has been comatose but has regained consciousness, he or she is managed as a severe exposure regardless of the COHB level.[4]

A carboxyhemoglobin level is obtained immediately and repeated 2 to 4 hours after initiation of treatment. The COHB may not represent the peak level because oxygen has often been administered for sometime before the sample was drawn. If the patient is having seizure activity, IV diazepam may be administered. The ECG is monitored for signs of myocardial ischemia and dysrhythmias.[4] Acidosis is treated with sodium bicarbonate. Patients who have or have had neurological signs or symptoms, an abnormal ECG, acidosis, or a COHB level above 30% should be admitted to an intensive care unit (ICU) and considered for hyperbaric oxygen (HBO) therapy. Hyperbaric oxygen increases the concentration of oxygen in the plasma and displaces CO from the hemoglobin.[4]

Indications for hyperbaric oxygen include coma at any time during the exposure; seizures; syncope; any neurological deficits (abnormal psychometric testing, mental disorientation, confusion, irritability, or aggressive behavior); severe metabolic acidosis; cardiovascular involvement such as hypotension, shock, angina, or ECG evidence of ischemia; or a COHB level higher than 30%. Determining need for HBO is difficult, in that CO levels often do not correlate with symptoms. The need for hyperbaric oxygen is controversial in patients with COHB levels above 30% with minimal or no symptoms.[4] When assessing whether HBO treatment is efficacious, a specialist at a hyperbaric facility may be consulted by contacting a poison center for referral.

A history of cardiovascular disease necessitates admission to an ICU with a COHB level of 15% or greater. Complications of CO exposure include cerebral edema and noncardiogenic pulmonary edema.[4]

The physician should be notified if the patient has

signs of increased intracranial pressure. It may be necessary to hyperventilate the patient with 100% oxygen via an endotracheal tube to keep the $PaCO_2$ level at 25 to 30 mmHg. Parenteral fluids need to be limited to two thirds to three fourths of normal maintenance for the patient's weight.[4]

If pulmonary edema develops arterial blood gases should be closely monitored. Positive end-expiratory pressure (PEEP) in intubated patients or continuous positive airway pressure (CPAP) in nonintubated patients may be necessary if the PO_2 cannot be maintained above 50 mmHg with inspiration of 60% oxygen by face mask or by mechanical ventilation. A central venous line or Swan-Ganz catheter is used to monitor status. Fluids must be administered carefully to avoid a net positive fluid balance.[4]

If the patient is pregnant, a fetal monitor is used. Oxygen administration is continued even after the COHB level is zero because oxygen is needed about five times as long in the fetal circulation to assure elimination of carbon monoxide.[4] The decision to use HBO for a pregnant patient is based on the maternal need for HBO, the proven fetotoxicity of CO, the theoretical fetotoxicity of HBO, and the absence of clearly demonstrated efficacy of HBO to prevent CO fetotoxicity.[4]

In accidental exposures, the patient must not be released until the causative factor has been corrected. For intentional exposures, mental health counseling should be arranged.

Evaluation

Efficacy of treatment may be assessed by noting improvement in the level of consciousness, cessation of seizures, normalization of blood gases, stabilization of vital signs, and a COHB level that subsequently becomes undetectable.

Cyanide

Few poisons are more lethal than cyanide. Death may occur within minutes of an inhalation exposure. Successful management of severe cyanide poisoning requires accurate assessment of the clinical symptoms, patient decontamination, basic and advanced life support, and prompt administration of the antidote kit.

Pathophysiology

Hydrocyanic acid (HCN, hydrogen cyanide) is one of the most toxic forms of cyanide.[2] It is used in industry as a fumigant and rodenticide and is liberated when products containing carbon, hydrogen, oxygen, and nitrogen are burned. Wool, silk, nylon, polyacrylonitrile, and polyurethane are all combustible materials that liberate HCN by pyrolysis.[32] The soluble salts of HCN (potassium or sodium cyanide) react with acids to release HCN gas.

Small amounts of cyanide normally enter the body in foods and tobacco smoke. Most severe poisonings occur with an exposure to sodium or potassium cyanide and are usually associated with a suicide or homicide attempt. Accidental exposures to cyanide may occur in the workplace and be seen in electroplaters, metal polishers, and firefighters. Accidental exposure may also occur from eating cyanide-containing food products such as amygdalin found in bitter almonds and in apricot and peach seeds, and from drugs containing cyanide such as Laetrile and nitroprusside.[32]

Cyanide may be absorbed by inhalation of dust or fumes, by ingestion, or, possibly, by eye contact. Death may occur within minutes after inhalation of a sufficient concentration of HCN gas.[2,32] Tissues are unable to utilize the oxygen present, causing venous blood to remain bright red. Since cytochrome oxidase is present in most cells, many organs are affected.

Rhodanase is a naturally occurring enzyme that detoxifies cyanide by complexing it with sulfur from sulfane pools to form much less toxic thiocyanate. Thiocyanate is excreted in the urine. Rhodanase is found in the mitochondria of the liver, and, to a lesser extent, in the kidneys and plasma. Because rhodanase is abundant in the body, it is the limited availability of sulfur that determines the amount of cyanide that can be detoxified. When large amounts of cyanide are absorbed, the metabolism of cyanide depletes the sulfur pool, allowing unmetabolized cyanide to bind to cytochrome oxidase.[33]

Cyanide poisoning may result from high-dose sodium nitroprusside administration. Adverse effects include those due to its hemodynamic effects as well as symptoms associated with cyanide intoxication.

Amygdalin is found in Laetrile and some fruit pits, plants, and berries. If sufficient quantities are ingested, symptoms of cyanide intoxication may ensue. Breakdown of the amygdalin to cyanide depends on the enzyme emulsin, contained in the fruit pit, or beta glucosidase, an enzyme found in the gastrointestinal tract. There may be a delay of symptoms after ingestion of amygdalin-containing products because emulsin does not maximally hydrolyze amygdalin until it enters the alkaline environment of the small intestine.[34]

The toxic or lethal dose of cyanide is not well defined. The lethal dose has been reported to be 50 mg of absolute cyanide acid, 200 to 300 mg potassium sodium salt, and 200 to 300 ppm of HCN gas.[2,4,32]

Clinical Manifestations

Rapid progression of symptoms is usually seen in patients after cyanide inhalation or injection, or sometimes after oral administration of cyanide-containing liquids. With ingestion of the solid forms of cyanide, crystals or capsules, death may occur within 30 minutes or be delayed for several hours.[32]

Initial symptoms of cyanide exposure include giddiness, headache, palpitations, and dyspnea, which may progress to agitation, stupor, apnea, convulsions, and death. Vomiting and abdominal pain also may occur. An odor of almonds may be noted on the breath or in vomitus, although 30% to 50% of the population are incapable of detecting this.[2,4,32]

Cyanide directly affects the respiratory center in the medulla, causing an early increase in the rate and depth of respirations, which later become slow and labored. This may progress to apnea. Noncardiogenic pulmonary edema also has been reported.[4,32] There is an initial rise in the blood pressure with a reflex bradycardia which may be followed by hypotension and tachycardia. The ECG may show marked ST segment elevation or depression, and cardiac dysrhythmias secondary to hypoxia may ensue.[4]

A high anion gap metabolic acidosis (lactic acid) is frequently present following cyanide exposure. A markedly reduced $A-Vo_2$ difference may be present in simultaneously drawn arterial and central venous blood samples. On funduscopic examination, equally red retinal arteries and veins may be noted. Death usually results from respiratory arrest. Antidotal therapy may be effective so long as there is a heartbeat.[4]

Symptoms of chronic cyanide poisoning are characterized by hoarseness, conjunctivitis, anorexia, weight loss, weakness, and altered mental status. Tobacco amblyopia and various ataxic neuropathies have also been attributed to chronic cyanide exposures.[35,36,37,38] Sodium nitroprusside–induced toxicity is characterized by metabolic acidosis, tachycardia, dyspnea, vomiting, dizziness, headache, ataxia, and loss of consciousness. An increased tolerance to the pharmacological effects of the drug may be noted despite an increase in the dose.[39]

Medical Management

Emergency medical treatment of cyanide poisoning includes basic life support, administration of 100% oxygen, and administration of the cyanide antidote kit. The Lilly cyanide antidote kit contains amyl nitrite, sodium nitrite, and sodium thiosulfate. The theoretical mechanism of action of the cyanide antidote kit is based on the fact that cyanide has a high affinity for ferric ions (Fe^3). The largest store of iron in the body is in the hemoglobin in the ferrous state (Fe^2). When hemoglobin (Fe^2) is converted to methemoglobin (Fe^3), the methemoglobin (Fe^3) competes for the cyanide ion to form cyanmethemoglobin, sparing the essential enzyme system cytochrome oxidase.[2] This mechanism has, however, been called into question by animal research.[40] The conversion is accomplished

pharmacologically by administering the first two drugs in the cyanide antidote kit: amyl nitrite pellets by inhalation, and sodium nitrite intravenously. The third medication in the antidote kit, sodium thiosulfate, is administered to provide adequate amounts of sulfur for rhodanase to detoxify the cyanide to thiocyanate.

The amyl nitrite pellets are given by inhalation 30 seconds of every minute while an intravenous line is established. A new amyl nitrite pellet must be used every 3 minutes. Sodium nitrite in an adult dose of 300 mg is administered intravenously over no less than 5 minutes to avoid severe hypotension from its vasodilating effects. The sodium nitrite is followed by intravenous administration of 12.5 g of sodium thiosulfate. If symptoms persist, sodium nitrite may be repeated at one half the initial dose after 30 minutes. While the nitrites are administered, the patient is closely monitored for hypotension and excessive methemoglobinemia. Nitrite-induced methemoglobin does not carry oxygen. Levels of 30% to 40% are potentially harmful, while levels greater than 60% cause tissue hypoxia.[34] Use of proper doses of nitrites prevents excessive methemoglobinemia. Slow intravenous administration with careful blood pressure monitoring precludes development of hypotension. Newer antidotes such as hydroxycobalamin and dicobalt EDTA (Kelocyanor) are not currently available in the United States.[4,32] Hydroxycobalamin has been shown to be effective in preventing nitroprusside-induced cyanide toxicity by forming the compound cyanocobalamin (vitamin B_{12}) which is then excreted in the urine.[39]

To prevent self-poisoning, health care workers should avoid direct contact with cyanide-contaminated emesis, clothes, or skin. Decontaminants should follow antidote therapy. Gastric lavage, charcoal, and cathartics should be considered if less than 2 hours has passed since ingestion.

Hyperbaric oxygen therapy (HBO) may improve the clinical outcome of cyanide poisoning victims who fail to respond to other therapy. HBO may also be indicated for those patients poisoned by both cyanide and carbon monoxide from smoke inhalation.[4,41]

Important laboratory evaluation after cyanide poisoning includes monitoring arterial and venous blood gases, electrolytes, serum lactate levels, and whole blood cyanide levels. When the cyanide antidote kit is administered, methemoglobin levels should be monitored closely. For excessive methemoglobinemia, methylene blue has been used successfully without worsening the course of the poisoning.[4] Cyanide levels may be measured, but the results take too long for guidance of initial therapy.

Interpretation of the patient's arterial and venous

blood gases, electrolytes, and percentage of O_2 saturation is important in assessment. Laboratory values suggestive of cyanide poisoning are:

Arterial PO_2: Normal

Central venous measured % O_2 saturation: Elevated (>70% approaches arterial % O_2 saturation)

Arterial pH: Low (acidotic)

Electrolytes: Anion gap present (greater than 12 to 16)

Peripheral venous PO_2 or measured % of saturation: Elevated (venous PO_2 >40 mmHg)

Lactic acid level: Elevated (>1.8 mEq/L)

To prevent cyanide poisoning during nitroprusside therapy, excessive doses and high rates of administration of the drug are avoided.[39] The patient is closely monitored for symptoms of nitroprusside-induced cyanide poisoning such as an increase in aerobic metabolism evidenced as base deficits, increased serum lactate, or other evidence of metabolic acidosis.

Evaluation

Appropriate interventions following cyanide exposure are indicated by the following parameters: stable vital signs, improved mental status, normal cardiac rhythm, normal electrolytes, and acid–base balance. The effectiveness of the cyanide antidote kit is based on the cessation of symptoms due to cyanide toxicity.

Cyclic Antidepressants

Since the introduction of tricyclic antidepressants (TCAs) for the treatment of depressive illnesses in the late 1950s, the incidence of overdose with these drugs has steadily increased. Because of the toxic effects of the original TCAs, newer agents have been developed that are safer but as effective for treating depressive illnesses. The four newer drugs marketed in the United States are trazadone, amoxapine, maprotiline, and fluoxetine.

Pathophysiology

Clinical manifestations of overdoses of TCAs stem from four pharmacological mechanisms of action. TCAs have anticholinergic properties that increase heart rate and blood pressure due to competitive acetylcholine blockade at cholinergic receptors. This mechanism results in sinus tachycardia, which is usually seen early and may be the only manifestation of cardiac involvement.[42] The effects of the anticholinergic properties have little influence on later symptoms of cardiotoxicity because cholinergic innervation to the ventricles is sparse. Other abnormalities seen with TCA overdose such as choreoathetoid movements and seizures are probably the result of anticholinergic action.[43] Because anticholinergic ef-

fects result in delayed gastric emptying, drug absorption may be retarded, and manifestations of toxicity may be delayed.[44]

TCAs also block norepinephrine at the cellular membrane of adrenergic nerve fibers, which results in increased levels of the neurotransmitter at the receptor site.[42] Because norepinephrine cannot return to the presynaptic neuron for reuse and its remanufacture is delayed, eventually the action potential threshold is delayed. Norepinephrine excess contributes to hypertension and tachycardia seen in the early stages of overdose. As norepinephrine is metabolized and depleted, hypotension and bradycardia ensue.

The most probable cause for cardiotoxic effects of TCAs are quinidine-like or membrane-stabilizing effects on the myocardium.[42] TCAs also affect intraventricular conduction. This action may be due to an inhibition of adenosine triphosphate, resulting in abnormalities in sodium–potassium pump action. This mechanism may also be responsible for induction of reentrant dysrhythmias associated with unidirectional blocks because of the TCA ability to increase antegrade conduction.[45,46]

TCAs exert a direct peripheral α-adrenergic blockade, causing a decrease in peripheral vascular resistance with resultant hypotension. Data regarding the role of this mechanism are inconclusive, and the exact action needs clarification.[42]

Clinical Manifestations

Because TCAs have the greatest affinity for the brain, heart, lung, circulatory, and nervous systems, these organ systems are principally affected.[47] Symptoms of TCA toxicity range from sinus tachycardia, hypotension, and lethargy to cardiac conduction disturbances, ventricular dysrhythmias, seizures, coma, and cardiac arrest.[48,49,50]

Patients may present in an alert and lucid state but deteriorate rapidly to unconsciousness. Choreoathetoid movements, involuntary muscle twitching, and grand mal seizures may precede unconsciousness. Impaired levels of consciousness are common, ranging from stupor and lethargy to coma. Many patients demonstrate quasi-purposeful movements involving all extremities in response to noxious stimuli. Seizures occur less frequently than other manifestations of toxicity and appear early.[51] Alterations in consciousness may be influenced by concomitant ingestions of sedative or hypnotic drugs that impair neurological response.

Cardiovascular abnormalities are more indicative of TCA toxicity than those involving the CNS. Cardiac disturbances include sinus tachycardia, atrioventricular and intraventricular conduction defects, ST and T wave abnormalities, supraventricular tachycardia, ventricular dysrhythmias, bradycardia, and asystole.[52] Sinus tachycardia typically occurs with prolongation of PR and QRS intervals and ST and T wave changes, causing difficulty in differentiating between sinus rhythm with atrioventricular and intraventricular conduction abnormalities and supraventricular or ventricular tachycardia.[53]

Medical Management

Because of individual variations in TCA metabolism, it is difficult to predict the severity of an acute ingestion based on the amount ingested. Since responses to TCA ingestions are unpredictable, recommendations for treatment are based on the patient's clinical status rather than the amount ingested. Any TCA ingestion should be considered significant initially.

The usual methods of gastrointestinal decontamination—lavage, charcoal, and cathartics—should be used for all suspected ingestions. Ipecac syrup should be avoided because of the ability of TCAs to cause central nervous system changes and seizures. Because the tricylic antidepressants undergo enterohepatic circulation, multiple-dose activated charcoal therapy is also recommended, but multiple doses of cathartics are avoided.

An accurate history of the time of ingestion, other medications ingested or taken chronically, and the amount of drug taken are essential. The information may be obtained upon initial contact with the patient. After vital signs have been measured, cardiac monitoring should be initiated. Serial measurements of QRS and PR intervals and heart rate help to assess the severity of toxicity. A QRS duration greater than 0.10 second may be the best indication of a severe overdose. Prolonged PR and QT intervals are also indications of potentially severe toxicity.

Manifestations of anticholinergic toxicity include decreased gastrointestinal motility, decreased mucosal secretions, and urinary retention. To avoid complications due to these side effects, bowel sounds should be checked before each charcoal dose to detect ileus development. Frequent urine output measurements help to assess bladder competency. Humidified oxygen prevents patient discomfort related to administration of oxygen alone.

Sodium bicarbonate ($NaHCO_3$) is an effective treatment for drug-induced cardiac dysrhythmias. Its exact mechanism of action is controversial. Because TCAs are pharmacologically inactive when protein bound and have an increased affinity to plasma protein in alkaline media, it is postulated that in alkaline serum a decreased amount of active drug is available to produce symptoms. Case studies report modification or reversal of dysrhythmias after sodium bicar-

bonate administration or mechanical hyperventilation resulting in an increased serum pH. Serum potassium and calcium must be monitored frequently if bicarbonate therapy is undertaken, as it may cause significant hypokalemia or hypocalcemia.

If $NaHCO_3$ therapy is used to manage dysrhythmias, serum pH assays are needed. Intravenous $NaHCO_3$ is given at doses of 1 to 2 mEq/kg as needed to keep the serum pH at 7.4 to 7.5.[4] Induction of respiratory alkalosis by mechanical ventilation may also be effective for pH adjustments.[54] However, frequent arterial blood gas determinations are needed to avoid a pH greater than 7.5 and Pco_2 levels less than 20.

Phenytoin therapy is based on electrocardiographic changes with an increase in QRS width being most definitive. Measurements greater than 0.10 are considered significant and may be used as the basis for treatment. Administration of phenytoin should begin with a loading dose of 15 mg/kg up to 1 g IV, not to exceed a rate of 0.5 mg/kg/min with continuous cardiac monitoring. Because intravenous phenytoin may be irritating to the skin and blood vessels, IV insertion sites should be checked frequently to prevent extravasation and necrosis. If the patient complains of pain or burning during the infusion, the rate may be slowed.

Quinidine, disopyramide, and procainamide are contraindicated for the treatment of TCA-induced cardiac dysrhythmias because their effects on myocardial conductivity are similar to those of the TCAs. Lidocaine and bretylium in standard doses may be used effectively.

Seizures usually respond to intravenous diazepam, but the newer antidepressants (amoxapine and maprotiline) appear to cause an increased incidence of seizures, some of which are refractory to standard anticonvulsants. In these situations, neuromuscular blockade and induced pentobarbital coma with continued EEG monitoring may be necessary.

Hypotension often responds to intravenous fluid administration. Hypotension unresponsive to fluid administration may indicate the need for a vasopressor. Because norepinephrine is depleted due to its blocked retake and decreased manufacture, levoterenol (Levophed) is usually used.

In the past, physostigmine was widely recommended as the antidote for TCA intoxication. Studies report exacerbations of cardiac and CNS symptoms after physostigmine administration and associate its use with seizures, hypotension, bradycardia, heart block, and asystole.[55,56] Although physostigmine may produce a transient improvement in consciousness, its use puts the patient at greater risk for seizures and cardiac deterioration. Current recommendations do not include routine use of physostigmine for TCA toxicity.

Because of the large volume of distribution and extensive tissue binding to TCAs, diuretic therapy and peritoneal or hemodialysis are of no benefit in treatment. Hemoperfusion with either a charcoal or resin filter has been used for TCA overdose. Controlled studies revealed that the percentage of drug removed with this method was small and that significant numbers of patients demonstrated rebound effects and the return of symptoms.[57]

All patients with a history of TCA ingestion must be observed for a minimum of 6 hours. If symptoms develop, admission to an intensive care unit is required and the patient must remain asymptomatic and dysrhythmia-free for 24 hours before discharge.[4]

Evaluation

Continuous ECG monitoring with measurements of atrio- and intraventricular conduction times and frequent blood pressure checks and neurological examinations allow assessment of the degree of toxicity and effectiveness of treatment.

Organophosphates

Ten percent of all poisoning deaths are due to exposures to insecticides and commercial sprays found in the home.[58] Because of their effectiveness for pest control, organophosphate use is increasing. Exposures are most frequent in farmers and unskilled laborers; however, children frequently ingest these products accidentally. Pesticides also have been used for intentional suicide attempts. The carbamate pesticides produce symptoms similar to those of the organophosphates; however, their duration of action is shorter, and the severity of toxicity is often lower.[58]

Pathophysiology

Understanding the pathophysiology of organophosphates requires a basic knowledge of neurotransmission. Acetylcholine is one of four neurotransmitters at synaptic junctions in the autonomic nervous system and is present at postganglionic parasympathetic nerve endings, at preganglionic nerves to parasympathetic and sympathetic ganglia, at somatic motor nerve endings to striated muscle, and at certain synapses in the central nervous system. With its release, action is potentiated at neuroreceptor sites. The enzyme acetylcholinesterase metabolizes acetylcholine. If its availability were continuous, repetitive action potentials would occur at neuroreceptor sites.

Organophosphates act as powerful inhibitors of acetylcholinesterase by irreversibly binding to active sites, forming a phosphorylated enzyme. Organophosphates act as antiacetylcholinesterases, thereby preventing the breakdown of acetylcholine.[58] With enzyme inhibition, acetylcholine accumulates at synaptic junctions, and cholinergic overdrive occurs. Overabundance of acetylcholine initially excites, then paralyzes transmission of cholinergic synapses. Organophosphate binding with acetylcholinesterase is considered irreversible because, although enzyme reactivation can occur, it is too slow to be of clinical value.[58]

Clinical Manifestations

Organophosphates are well absorbed by all routes of exposure. The time between exposure and onset of symptoms is dependent on many variables, including exposure, route, particular compound, and dose, but symptoms almost always occur within 24 hours.[2]

Individual organophosphates can be classified into those with high toxicity, such as those used in agriculture (TEPP, parathion); intermediate toxicity, such as those used in animal husbandry (chlorpyrifos ronnel); and low toxicity, such as those used for household pest control (diazinon, malathion).[2] However, significant poisoning can be caused by "low toxicity" organophosphates if the dose and duration of exposure are sufficient.

If the route of exposure is inhalation, respiratory symptoms occur initially, whereas if the product is ingested, gastrointestinal symptoms appear first. An early sign of ocular exposure is miosis. Onset is most rapid after organophosphate inhalation and slowest with dermal exposures.[58]

Symptoms are categorized as muscarinic, nicotinic, or central, but all relate to excessive amounts of acetylcholine. *Muscarinic* effects related to parasympathetic stimulation are sweating, increased lacrimation, excessive salivation, vomiting, diarrhea, and urinary incontinence. Effects on the cardiovascular system are inhibitory and are evidenced by bradycardia and hypotension. Increased secretions in the respiratory tract result in wheezing and may progress to pulmonary edema.

The mnemonic SLUDGE is used to recall the common muscarinic symptoms seen with organophosphate poisoning (see the box on p. 1326). Pancreatitis, although rare, has been reported recently along with hyperamylasema and hyperglycemia.[2]

Nicotinic effects are due to the stimulating action of acetylcholine on sympathetic ganglia and striated muscle. These include fasciculations, cramps, weakness, and paralysis. Nicotinic cardiovascular effects include tachycardia and hypertension.

Organophosphates have diverse effects on the central nervous system, causing anxiety, restlessness, ataxia, coma, and circulatory and respiratory depression. Death usually occurs from bronchorrhea, bronchospasm, diaphragmatic paralysis, and inability of the central nervous system to control respirations.[58] Delayed peripheral neurotoxicity of the motor or sensorimotor type may occur 6 to 21 days after acute exposure by ingestion, inhalation and, with some of the organophosphates, the dermal route.[2]

Medical Management

Baseline patient status is assessed with a complete physical examination, an ECG, chest x-ray, and arterial blood studies. Metabolic products of organophosphates can be found in the urine but are not routinely assayed. Red blood cell cholinesterase and serum pseudocholinesterase levels can be used to help confirm the diagnosis but are not useful for management. A depression of red blood cell cholinesterase by 25% or greater is indicative of significant exposure. Symptomatic patients usually show a depression in red blood count cholinesterase in excess of 50%. Red blood cell cholinesterase levels will not return to preexposure levels for several days and possibly not for up to 4 months.[2]

General management principles for absorption prevention apply if the route of exposure to organophosphates is oral. Ipecac is contraindicated because of the early onset of respiratory depression and seizures[4] with the risk of pulmonary aspiration of gastric contents, especially as many organophosphates are formulated with a hydrocarbon base.

For dermal exposure, the skin is decontaminated with three soap and water washings.[4] Tincture of green soap, which contains ethanol, may be more effective for removal of organophosphates, especially parathion, from the skin. Personnel can protect themselves from exposure by wearing gloves, gowns, and masks during the procedure. Leather must be disposed of by burning. Laundering may not completely remove organophosphates from contaminated clothing. It should be disposed of in accordance with state and federal regulations for disposal of hazardous materials.[4]

Because atropine blocks the action of excessive acetylcholine at receptor sites, it is the drug of choice for initial treatment of muscarinic symptoms.[2] However, nicotinic effects are relatively refractory to atropine administration. Pralidoxime chloride (2-PAM) is recommended for reversal of nicotinic effects because it binds to the phosphate group of the organophosphate and frees acetylcholinesterase to metabolize acetylcholine. Use of 2-PAM is recommended if the red blood count cholinesterase level is less than 25%; however, its use is based primarily on the presence of nicotinic symptoms.[58] A combination of atropine and 2-PAM is probably the most effective treatment. Judicious suctioning prevents respiratory distress

from excessive salivary and bronchial secretions. Because atropine may precipitate ventricular fibrillation in a poorly oxygenated patient, adequate ventilation must be assured.[58] Administration of humidified oxygen helps to keep mucous membranes moist during atropine use.

Organophosphate-poisoned patients are generally tolerant to the toxic effects of atropine (dry mouth, tachycardia, and dilated pupils). If these findings occur after a diagnostic administration, the patient probably is not seriously poisoned. A diagnostic dosage of atropine is 1 to 2 mg IV for adults. To attain therapeutic effects, for severly poisoned patients, large doses of atropine may be needed (up to 100 mg or more over a few hours).[5] The dosage is individually based on the exposure and the patient's response.[4] Suggested doses are 2 to 5 mg IV repeated every 10 to 30 minutes to attain full atropinization.[4]

If 2-PAM is ordered, 1 to 2 g is mixed in 250 ml of normal saline and is infused over 30 minutes. It can also be given with 0.5 g pushed IV per minute.[4] Doses may be repeated at 1 hour after the initial dose and every 6 to 12 hours thereafter if muscular and central nervous system involvement does not subside.[4] Pralidoxime is most effective if given within 24 to 48 hours of exposure.[2] In therapeutic doses, toxicity is minimal with some reports of mild weakness, blurred vision, headache, and nausea. Because 2-PAM is excreted in the urine and may accumulate to toxic levels in the presence of renal dysfunction, accurate urine output measurements are necessary.

Evaluation

Pupillary dilation and rapid heart rate are unreliable signs when assessing the effectiveness of atropine. The most reliable sign of atropinization is drying of excessive secretions, especially pulmonary. If the effects of atropine are not evidenced, the dosage is insufficient. With organophosphate toxicity, the risks of underdosage outweigh those of overdosage. Continued administration of 2-PAM is based on disappearance of skeletal muscle and central nervous system manifestations of toxicity.

Salicylates

Salicylates commonly used by consumers and health care professionals include acetylsalicylic acid (aspirin), sodium salicylate, and salicylic acid. Aspirin is frequently combined with other drugs such as caffeine, codeine, and acetaminophen. Other salicylates are found in a variety of topical preparations and teething gels.

Salicylate poisoning may occur in several ways. Accidental ingestion of salicylates is a common childhood poisoning, usually involving 1- to 5-year-old children. Children also are frequently poisoned when parents inadvertently overdose them during febrile illnesses. Because of the accessibility of aspirin and aspirin-containing products, intentional ingestion by adults in suicide attempts is common. Chronic therapeutic salicylate intoxication in adults may also occur. Since salicylates readily cross the placenta, a newborn may develop salicylate poisoning if the mother has ingested large quantities of aspirin preceding the delivery.[2]

Pathophysiology

In therapeutic doses, aspirin is rapidly absorbed from the stomach and small intestine. In an overdose, absorption occurs more slowly and symptoms of toxicity may be delayed, resulting in rising serum levels for up to 12 hours.[4] The delayed absorption of aspirin occurs because of the inhibitory effects of aspirin on gastric emptying and because tablets adhere, forming a bolus that dissolves slowly. Absorption is also delayed after an ingestion of enteric-coated aspirin. Topical application of salicylates may produce systemic toxicity, while rectal absorption is slow and incomplete.

Aspirin is rapidly hydrolyzed by the liver to salicylic acid and distributes into most body tissues and water. A small amount of salicylic acid is excreted unchanged in the urine while the majority of aspirin is eliminated through the formation of the inactive metabolites salicyluric acid and salicyl phenolic and acyl glucuronides, which are then excreted in the urine. The pathways that form the inactive metabolites are saturable. The time for a given fraction of a dose of salicylate to be eliminated increases with increasing doses. Salicylates can accumulate, and repeated small doses may profoundly increase body stores and blood levels.[2] As these metabolic pathways become saturated, more salicylate needs to be renally excreted.[59]

In overdoses, salicylates stimulate respirations directly and indirectly. They directly stimulate the respiratory center in the medulla to increase both the rate and depth of respirations.[60] Salicylates also uncouple mitochondrial oxidative phosphorylation, increasing oxygen consumption and carbon dioxide production. This rise in carbon dioxide levels stimulates respirations and accounts for the indirect effect of salicylates on respirations. With compensatory tachypnea, the PCO_2 decreases, resulting in a respiratory alkalosis with a decreased PCO_2 and a rise in arterial pH.[4] Bicarbonate, accompanied by sodium, potassium, and water, is excreted by the kidneys in an attempt to normalize the arterial pH.[59] This results in dehydration and hypokalemia. The increased bicarbonate excretion diminishes the buffering capacity

of the body and allows acidosis to develop more easily. With very high concentrations of salicylates, the respiratory center may be depressed.

The major toxic effects of salicylate ingestion result from the adverse effects on cellular metabolism. Salicylates not only uncouple mitochondrial oxidative phosphorylation but also inhibit specific Krebs cycle dehydrogenases and aminotransferases and increase the metabolism and peripheral demand for glucose. This results in hyperthermia and an increased production, accumulation, and excretion of organic acids with an elevated anion gap metabolic acidosis.[4]

Salicylates penetrate the central nervous system rapidly, especially during acidemia, and produce a decrease in mental alertness. Convulsions and cerebral edema may occur in severe intoxications. Although the exact etiology of the seizures is unclear, it is thought to be excessive accumulation of carbon dioxide in the central nervous system, decreased brain glucose concentration, or a direct toxic effect.[4]

Salicylates may decrease prothrombin formation, factor VII production, platelet adhesiveness, and platelet levels, and increase capillary fragility. Despite coagulation abnormalities, hemorrhage is not a common clinical manifestation of salicylate toxicity.[59]

Gastrointestinal distress following salicylate intoxication is produced by local gastric irritation and stimulation of the medullary chemoreceptor trigger zone. Tinnitus and hearing loss frequently experienced are due to increased pressure in the labyrinth of the auditory apparatus. Tinnitus is associated with serum levels greater than 30 mg/dl (Figure 58-3).[4]

Single oral doses greater than 300 mg of salicylate per kilogram of body weight may produce severe poisoning. Chronic ingestion greater than 100 mg per kilogram of body weight every 24 hours over two or more days is associated with toxicity. Greater morbidity in adults and children is seen with chronic salicylism.[4]

Salicylate levels are plotted on the Done nomogram.[61] The nomogram predicts the clinical severity of the poison based on the serum level and time since a single acute ingestion. The nomogram cannot be used to predict severity of symptoms in a chronic salicylate overdose. The salicylate level should be drawn at least 6 hours after ingestion, and two or more levels should be obtained to assure that peak serum concentration has occurred. It may be useful to obtain a 2-hour level following acute ingestion of methyl salicylate due to rapid absorption. Large amounts of ingested aspirin may form a concretion in the stomach, delaying absorption for up to 24 hours.[62] With ingestion of sustained-released preparations (Verin, Zorprin), absorption may be prolonged, and the serum salicylate level may be persis-

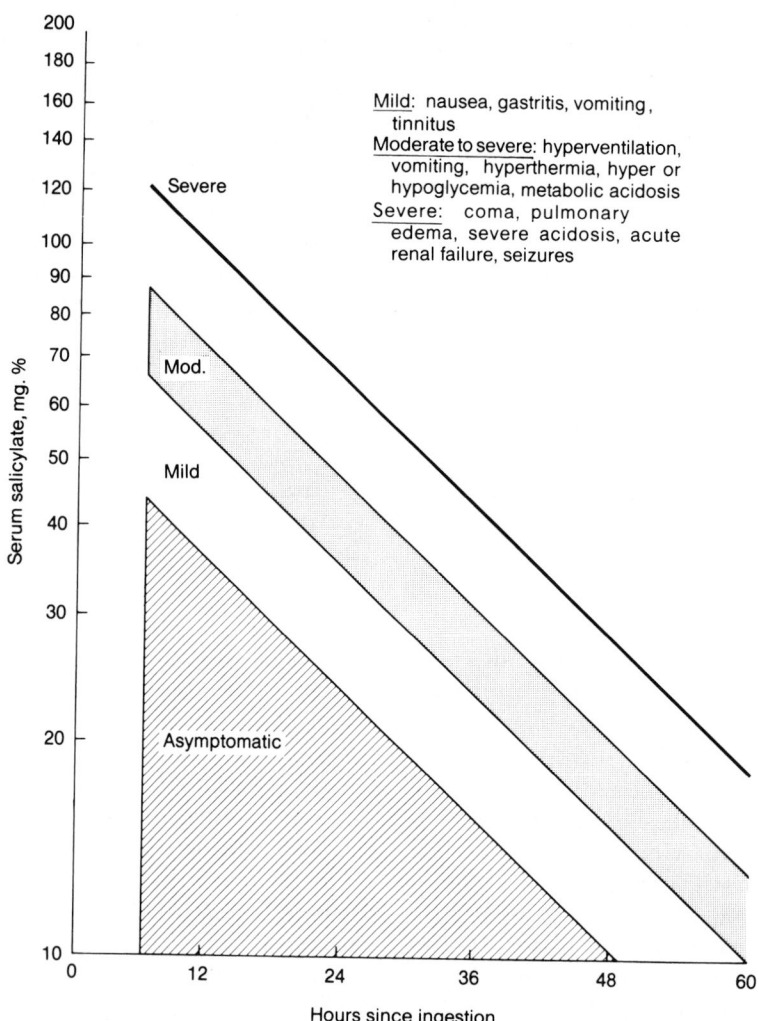

Figure 58-3 Salicylate nomogram with inset.
Adapted, with permission, from POISINDEX Information System: Micromedex, Inc. (1974-1992). Denver, CO.

tently elevated. Using the Done nomogram for ingestion of sustained-released preparations is of questionable value.

Clinical Manifestations

Most patients with significant salicylate toxicity experience nausea, vomiting, tinnitus, and hearing loss. Other early clinical signs include profuse sweating, flushing, hyperpyrexia, hyperpnea, and hyperventilation.

In serious poisonings, severe acid–base imbalance (elevated anion gap, metabolic acidosis) and dehydration occur. The metabolic symptoms seen following acute salicylate poisoning may be divided into three stages (Table 58-3). In the first stage, hyperventilation from direct and indirect respiratory center stimulation produces respiratory alkalosis. To normalize the arterial pH, bicarbonate is excreted by the

TABLE 58-3 Metabolic Stages of Acute Salicylate Toxicity

Stage	Plasma*	Urine†
1	Alkaline	Alkaline
2	Alkaline	Acid
3	Acid	Acid

* A normal plasma pH 7.36-7.46.
† "Alkaline" urine is pH 6 or greater; "acid" urine is pH less than 6.
Adapted from Temple, A. R. (1978). Pathophysiology of aspirin overdosage toxicity with implications for management. *Pediatrics, 62,* 873-876; and Temple, A. R. (1981). Acute and chronic effects of aspirin toxicity and their treatment. *Archives of Internal Medicine, 14,* 364-368.

kidney, resulting in an alkaline urine (a pH of 6 or greater). In the second stage, the serum pH remains alkaline with a compensated metabolic acidosis, while the urine becomes more acidotic from the excretion of organic acids. In the third stage, both serum and urine are acidotic.[60,63,64]

Following severe salicylate poisoning, symptoms may progress to confusion, coma, and seizures. Noncardiogenic pulmonary edema and cerebral edema may also occur. Hypoglycemia in children and hyperglycemia in adults may be noted. An increased bleeding time may also occur.

Medical Management

Treatment of salicylate poisoning includes stabilization, gastrointestinal decontamination, enhancement of elimination, and reduction of toxic effects of salicylates. Because large ingestions of aspirin delay gastric emptying, emesis or gastric lavage may be effective up to several hours after exposure. Multiple doses of activated charcoal may enhance the elimination of salicylates already absorbed, but multiple doses of cathartics, should be avoided. Alkalinization of the urine effectively enhances salicylate excretion. Alkalinization alone is at least as effective or more effective than forced alkaline diuresis in enhancing salicylate removal.[65] When the urine is alkaline, the ionized salicylic acid molecules are "trapped," thus preventing reabsorption into the renal tubules. A change of the urine pH from 5 to 8 increases the urine excretion of salicylic acid greater than 20-fold.[4] To alkalinize the urine, a solution with two to three ampules of sodium bicarbonate and 30 mEq of potassium chloride in each liter of D_5W solution is administered at a rate of 2 to 3 ml per kg per hour to produce a urine flow of 2 to 3 ml per kg per hour. The urine pH is checked hourly, and additional sodium bicarbonate is given as needed to maintain a pH of 7 to 8. Some patients with severe intoxications may be difficult to alkalinize.

Careful evaluation of the fluid and electrolyte status, especially the potassium level, is important since hypokalemia, a common problem in salicylate overdose, may cause difficulty in achieving alkalinization. Significant hypocalcemia may occur during bicarbonate therapy; serum calcium should be monitored. Sodium bicarbonate also presents a significant osmotic and sodium load to the body. Other important laboratory values include serum salicylate levels, arterial blood gases, electrolytes, glucose, and prothrombin time.

Hemodialysis effectively increases salicylate clearance and improves fluid and electrolyte balance. Hemodialysis may be considered when the patient is not responding to other therapy, and is probably the treatment of choice with cerebral or pulmonary edema or renal failure.[2,4]

Evaluation

Efficacy of the therapeutic interventions administered during salicylate poisoning can be assessed throughout the clinical course of the patient's treatment. Indicators of appropriate nursing and medical treatment include stable vital signs, appropriate mental status, normal electrolytes and acid–base balance, normal renal function, and decreasing serum salicylate levels. In chronic salicylate poisoning, the serum salicylate level is of less value in assessing the efficacy of medical and nursing interventions.

Snake Envenomation

About 120 species of snakes are found in the United States. Nearly 20 of these species are venomous.[66] Bites by nonvenomous snakes are much more common and are treated as simple puncture wounds. Venomous snakes include pit vipers (Crotalidae—cottonmouths, copperheads, rattlesnakes) and coral snakes (Elapidae). Efforts should be made to identify the species of snake, although this may be difficult.

Pathophysiology

Snake venoms are complex mixtures of toxins consisting mainly of proteins with enzymatic activity. Certain peptides and proteins found in venoms have a relatively low molecular weight and may produce the most deleterious effects. It has been common practice to divide snake venoms into groups such as neurotoxins, hemotoxins, and cardiotoxins. Such grouping may be misleading because all snake envenomations present as multiple poisonings with toxic reactions and pharmacological changes occurring simultaneously or consecutively. The severity of poisoning following snake envenomation is related to the location and severity of the bite, the species and size of the snake, the amount of venom injected, the age and size of the victim, and sensitivity of the victim to antivenin.[2]

Clinical Manifestations

Edema and pain may begin within 5 minutes in a Crotalidae envenomation. Edema usually progresses slowly over 8 to 36 hours. However, in severe envenomations, an entire extremity may be affected within an hour. Weakness, faintness, nausea, and sweating are common symptoms. Tingling or numbness of the tongue, mouth, or scalp may be accompanied by a metallic taste. Muscle fasciculations sometimes occur.

Venoms of pit vipers (Crotalidae) may cause severe

local tissue effects, coagulopathies, and changes in blood cells. The hematocrit may fall rapidly, and platelets may nearly disappear. In severe poisoning, pulmonary edema occurs, and there may be bleeding in the lungs, peritoneum, kidneys, and heart, resulting in alterations in cardiac dynamics and renal function.[4]

Most North American Crotalidae venoms cause minimal change in neuromuscular transmission. An exception is the venom of the Mojave rattlesnake *(C. scatalatas),* whose bite is generally associated with less tissue destruction.[4]

The venom of coral snakes (Elapidae) produces more changes in neuromuscular transmission and nerve conduction than do pit viper venoms, resulting in weakness, muscle fasciculations, and a type of bulbar paralysis that may occur within 90 minutes.[66] The immediate cause of death is respiratory paralysis.[4] The local reaction may be minimal, and it is common to lack major clinical findings early in the clinical course even following a severe envenomation. Other symptoms of coral snake envenomation include drowsiness, weakness, dysphoria, diplopia, headache, and respiratory distress.[4] Neurological symptoms may be delayed for 12 hours. In patients bitten by a positively identified coral snake, antivenin should be administered early and early endotracheal intubation considered.[4]

Medical Management

Before treating a snake bite, it is important to distinguish whether the snake was venomous or if the injury was caused by an animal bite or plant thorn injury. After establishing the possibility of snake envenomation, proper management includes repeated hourly assessment, noting any progression of signs or symptoms, use of antivenin therapy when appropriate, and observation and supportive therapy.[2]

Pit viper envenomation is graded to determine the seriousness of the bite (see box above). The circumference of the extremity is measured frequently, and the measurement sites are marked on the skin. Use of a tourniquet is not recommended because it may impede circulation. If a tourniquet has been placed, a less constricting band should be applied proximal to the tourniquet, making certain that it only impedes lymphatic flow. An IV infusion of a crystalloid solution is started, and the tourniquet is slowly removed. Incision and suction are helpful only if done in the first 30 minutes following the bite and should be done only by trained personnel to avoid damage to deep structures. A commercially available first aid device, the Sawyer Extractor, can be safely used by nonprofessionals and has been shown to remove some venom from the bite site.[4] The wound is cleansed, the affected part immobilized at heart level and a func-

---

> ### Grading Envenomation from Pit Viper Bites
>
> *Trivial envenomation:* Signs and symptoms are confined to the bite area. There are no systemic symptoms or laboratory derangements.
> *Minimal envenomation:* Signs and symptoms confined to bite area, with minimal edema and erythema immediately beyond. Perioral paresthesias are the only systemic symptoms present. No laboratory derangements.
> *Moderate envenomation:* Significant systemic symptoms and signs. Edema extends beyond the immediate bite area. Moderate laboratory derangements are seen (hemoconcentration, decreased fibrinogen, platelets, prolonged PT, and hematuria).
> *Severe envenomation:* Swelling involves entire extremity or part. There are serious systemic signs and symptoms and severe laboratory derangements. All signs, symptoms, and laboratory values should be considered in grading envenomation. Edema and swelling may be absent in some severe bites.

Adapted, with permission, from POISINDEX Information System: Micromedex, Inc. (1974-1992). Denver, CO.

tional position, and the patient kept at rest. The injured part must not be placed in ice because this may freeze the tissues. Excision of the bite and fasciotomy also are not routinely recommended.

Fasciotomy may be necessary in those infrequent cases when patients first present for treatment with a compartment syndrome days after the bite and where insufficient antivenin was administered early in the course of the poisoning.[4] About 90% of pit viper bites are in subcutaneous tissue. The tissue necrosis is caused by the action of the venom, not by pressure from edema.[66]

It is important to give pit viper antivenin early because it is most efficacious if given within 4 hours of the bite.[4] It is less effective if the administration is delayed for 8 hours and the effects are questionable if given after 26 hours.[4] Use of antivenin is advised up to 30 hours after the bite in all cases of severe pit viper envenomation.[4]

If it is determined that antivenin is needed, the skin is tested with the material in the antivenin package or with a diluted aliquot of the antivenin itself. The skin test should not be done until it is certain that the antivenin will be needed because the material in the skin test may sensitize the patient to horse serum. If the patient has an allergy to horse serum, diphenhydramine (Benadryl) may be given intravenously before the antivenin treatment.

In pit viper envenomation, antivenin (Crotalidae)

polyvalent IV is administered initially at a slow rate, then faster (15 to 20 minutes per vial) if no reaction occurs. The amount of antivenin is determined by the grade of envenomation (see the box on p. 1352). For minimal envenomation, 5 to 8 vials are given. For moderate envenomation 8 to 12 vials are given, and for severe envenomation 13 to 30 vials or more may be used.[4] Antivenin is not indicated in trivial envenomations. Each vial is diluted to 50 to 200 ml (e.g., 5 vials in 250 to 1,000 ml diluent) and given by continuous intravenous infusion. The total dosage is given during the first 4 to 6 hours.[66]

If a reaction to the antivenin occurs, the infusion is stopped for 5 minutes, diphenhydramine is given intravenously, and the infusion is resumed at a slower rate with close observation and resuscitative equipment at hand. If the reaction recurs, the antivenin is discontinued and consultation sought.[4] Antivenin may be administered more than 24 hours after envenomation to reverse coagulopathies. The circumference of the extremity 10 and 20 cm proximal to the bite is measured every 15 minutes during antivenin administration and 1 to 2 hours thereafter.

Antivenin is never given intramuscularly unless it is absolutely impossible to give intravenously, and it is never injected into a toe or finger. Emergency equipment should be at the bedside while giving antivenin.

Intake and output is monitored closely, and all urine is checked for the presence of red blood cells and for hemoglobin. Once the patient is stable, analgesics may be administered for pain control.

Because of the possibility of shock, bleeding, and coagulopathies, the patient's blood type and cross-matching are done. Complete blood count, hematocrit, platelet count, bleeding and clotting times, and prothrombin time need to be followed closely. These may need to be done several times a day in cases of severe envenomation. Because of the multisystem effects of envenomation, arterial blood gases and electrolytes are evaluated. Other tests that may be useful include serum protein, fibrinogen titer, and partial thromboplastin time. Baseline renal function tests should be ordered, and all urine samples should be checked for the presence of red blood cells and hemoglobin.

Fluid administration is generally sufficient to treat the hypotension which may result from snake envenomation. Antihistamines may be needed to treat allergic reactions to the antivenin. There have been no clinical trials to indicate that corticosteroids are useful. Corticosteroids are not recommended in the acute phase of poisoning unless needed for shock or severe allergic reactions.

The wound may need to be debrided on the third through the tenth day.[4] A physical therapy evaluation may be done on about the third day. If antivenin was given, the patient needs to be informed that symptoms of serum sickness may occur in 10 to 14 days.

Victims of a coral snake envenomation should be kept at rest with the injured area lightly immobilized in a functional position and kept just below heart level. With any signs of bulbar paralysis, endotracheal intubation is recommended. North American coral snake antivenin should be administered in all cases of confirmed coral snake bite. Skin testing with antivenin may not be reliable in predicting which patients will have a reaction.[4]

As signs and symptoms can occur rapidly, North American coral snake antivenin is administered intravenously by diluting 3 to 5 vials of antivenin in 250 to 500 ml of sodium chloride for injection as soon as possible if the skin test is negative. If signs and symptoms of envenomation such as drowsiness, weakness, dysphoria, diplopia, headache, or respiratory distress occur, an additional 3 to 5 vials may be given.[66] Narcotics are not recommended.[4] All individuals bitten by a "positively identified" coral snake need to be hospitalized and carefully observed for 24 hours.[4]

Most patients bitten by a venomous snake become very anxious and need reassurance. The patient may be relieved to know that death or the loss of an extremity from a snake bite is rare. A thorough explanation of the treatment and of expected lessening of the symptoms is also reassuring. All cases of snakebites should be observed a minimum of 6 hours.[4]

Evaluation

Local and systemic signs and symptoms are monitored closely. A close review of laboratory studies is needed to rule out worsening of coagulopathies. If signs or symptoms worsen, more antivenin may be needed. Data are gathered regarding the adequacy of analgesia and whether the level of anxiety has decreased.

Theophylline

Theophylline toxicity occurs frequently as a result of accidental or intentional overdose. Oral and intravenous preparations of theophylline are used for the therapy of acute and chronic airway obstruction in conditions such as asthma, COPD, pulmonary edema, and apnea. Patients may accidentally overdose by misunderstanding the prescribed dosage or from increasing the dosage if symptoms do not improve.

Pathophysiology

Theophylline stimulates the central nervous system, acts on the kidneys to produce diuresis, stimulates cardiac muscle, and relaxes smooth (particularly bronchial) muscle. It also may stimulate the medullary respiratory centers.[4]

Nonsustained release preparations of theophylline are absorbed rapidly when administered orally. With sustained-release preparations absorption may be erratic and peak concentrations may occur 4 to 6 hours after ingestion or later.[4] The rate of elimination varies greatly in normal individuals and is primarily controlled by the rate of hepatic metabolism. The average half-life of therapeutic doses of theophylline in adults is 2 to 16 hours. Clearance and half-life may be quite variable and are affected by factors including age, smoking, liver disease, and concomitant administration of other drugs.[2] Cimetidine decreases theophylline clearance and phenobarbital, phenytoin, and carbamazepine increase clearance.[4]

Clinical Manifestations

Therapeutic serum levels of theophylline range from 10 to 20 μg/ml.[4] Toxic symptoms may occur at any level above 20 μg/ml. Because the toxic level is so close to the therapeutic level, a small overdose may cause toxicity. Overdoses with sustained release preparations may cause severe and prolonged central nervous system and cardiovascular toxicity with delayed onset. Toxic effects may be seen in patients who have used ephedrine-theophylline preparations in which the theophylline serum concentration is not considered toxic.[4]

Symptoms of theophylline toxicity include nausea, vomiting, and diarrhea. In severe intoxication, bloody emesis may be seen. The patient may become dehydrated and hypokalemic from the vomiting, diarrhea, and diuretic effect of theophylline.[2] Tachycardia is seen in almost all intoxicated patients, and dysrhythmias such as atrial fibrillation, ventricular tachycardia, and cardiac arrest may also occur. Neurological symptoms include nervousness, irritability, and headache. In severe intoxications, restlessness, agitation, and seizures are seen. Seizures may not respond to standard anticonvulsant therapy. There is no predictable progression of symptoms.[2] Whether an ingestion is acute (suicidal intent) or chronic (excessive therapy) also determines the severity of symptoms.[2]

Medical Management

Following oral ingestion of theophylline, gastric emptying with lavage is recommended. Gastric lavage is performed with a large-bore tube and the airway is protected. Subsequent treatment measures are the same whether the exposure was oral or parenteral.

Seizures are treated initially with IV diazepam. For seizures unresponsive to diazepam, phenytoin is administered IV with the ECG being monitored for dysrhythmias. For refractory seizures, further therapy such as neuromuscular blockade and pentobarbital-induced coma with continuous EEG monitoring may be necessary in severe poisonings. A serum sample for theophylline is obtained. Additional levels are obtained every 2 hours until the peak is passed and then every 4 hours until the level is in the therapeutic range. A single theophylline measurement may be inadequate following sustained-release preparation overdoses, as levels can increase over the next hours and may not peak until 12 to 24 hours. If hypotension develops, dopamine or norepinephrine may be given.[67] Repeated oral doses of activated charcoal have been shown to increase the clearance of theophylline in both oral and IV exposures.[68] Administration of multidose activated charcoal is recommended until the serum theophylline level is therapeutic and/or signs and symptoms resolve. Multiple doses of cathartics, however, are not recommended. In severe overdoses, persistent vomiting may occur, which prevents charcoal administration. When emesis is unresponsive to antiemetic therapy such as metoclopramide or droperidol, the H$_2$ blocker ranitidine may be useful.[4] The patient needs careful cardiac monitoring, and electrolytes (particularly potassium) are monitored closely.

Although theophylline is about 58% protein-bound at therapeutic serum concentrations, high levels in the toxic patient indicate that a large amount of the drug is in the plasma and may be removed by hemodialysis or charcoal hemoperfusion. Hemodialysis or hemoperfusion may be considered when theophylline serum concentrations are greater than 60 μg/ml or in patients with severe symptoms (cardiac dysrhythmias, hemodynamic instability, or seizures not responsive to anticonvulsant therapy).[2] Chronic theophylline toxicity may cause more severe symptoms at lower serum theophylline levels.[4]

Evaluation

Evaluation includes assessing the efficacy of therapy. Decreased tachycardia, cessation of seizures, stability of intake and output, a theophylline serum level in the therapeutic range, and evidence of charcoal stools indicate successful therapy. The patient's level of understanding of the use of this medication is also assessed.

REFERENCES

1. Litovitz, T. (1991). *1990 annual report of the data collection system.* American Association of Poison Control Centers.
2. Haddad, L. M., & Winchester, J.F. (1990). *Clinical management of poisoning and drug overdose* (2nd ed.). Philadelphia: Saunders.
3. Goldfrank, L. R., Flomenbaum, N. E., Lewin, N. A., et al. (1990). *Toxicologic emergencies* (4th ed.). Norwalk, CT: Appleton & Lange.

4. POISINDEX Information System: Micromedex, Inc., Denver, CO. Copyright from 1974 through current year.

5. Grande, G., & Ling, L. (1987). The effect of fluid volume on sympotipeial emesis time. *Journal of Toxicology and Clinical Toxicology, 25,* 473-481.

6. Neuvonen, P. J., Vartiainen, M., & Tokola, O. (1983). Comparison of activated charcoal and ipecac syrup in prevention of drug absorption. *European Journal of Clinical Pharmacology, 24,* 557-562.

7. Corby, D. J., Lisciandro, R. C., & Lehman, R. H. (1967). The efficacy of methods used to evaluate the stomach after acute ingestions. *Pediatrics, 40,* 5.

8. Corby, D. J., & Decker, W. J. (1968). Management of acute poisoning with activated charcoal. *Pediatrics, 42,* 361-364.

9. Hall, A. H., & Krenzelok, E. (1991). Gastrointestinal decontamination: Sifting through supportive therapeutic options. *Emergency Medicine Reports, 12,* 171-178.

10. Tandberg, D., Liechty, E. J., & Fishbein, D. (1981). Mallory-Weiss syndrome: An unusual complication of ipecac induced emesis. *Annals of Emergency Medicine, 10,* 521-523.

11. Klein-Schwartz, W., Gorman, R. L., & Oderda, G. M. (1984). Ipecac use in the elderly: The unanswered question. *Annals of Emergency Medicine, 13,* 1152-1154.

12. Wolowdiuk, O. J., McMicken, D. B., & O'Brien, P. (1984). Pneumomediastinum and retropneumoperitoneum: An unusual complication of syrup of ipecac-induced emesis. *Annals of Emergency Medicine, 13,* 1148-1151.

13. Abdallah, A. H., & Tye, A. (1967). A comparison of the efficacy of emetic drugs and stomach lavage. *American Journal of Diseases of Children, 113,* 571-575.

14. Boxer, L., Anderson, F. P., & Rowe, D. S. (1969). Comparison of ipecac-induced emesis with gastric lavage in the treatment of acute salicylate ingestion. *Journal of Pediatrics, 74,* 800-803.

15. Tenenbein, M., Cohen, S., & Sitar, D. S. (1985). Efficacy of ipecac-induced emesis, orogastric lavage and activated charcoal for acute drug overdose. *Veterinary and Human Toxicology, 27,* 321.

16. Kulig, K., Bar-or, D., & Cantrill, S. (1985). Management of acutely poisoned patients without gastric emptying. *Annals of Emergency Medicine, 14,* 562-567.

17. Donovan, J. W. (1987). Activated charcoal in management of poisoning: A revitalized antidote. *Postgraduate Medicine, 82,* 52-59.

18. Jones, J., Heiselman, D., & Dougherty, J. (1986). Cathartic-induced magnesium toxicity during overdose management. *Annals of Emergency Medicine, 15,* 121-125.

19. Smilkstein, M., Smolinske, S., & Kulig, K. (1986). Severe hypermagnesemia due to multiple-dose cathartic therapy. *Veterinary and Human Toxicology, 28,* 494. (Abstract)

20. Caldarola, V., Harsett, J. M., Hall, A. H., et al. (1986). Hemorrhagic pancreatitis associated with acetaminophen overdose. *American Journal of Gastroenterology, 81,* 579-582.

21. Smilkstein, M. J., Knapp, G. L., Kulig, K. W., et al. (1988). Efficacy of oral N-acetylcysteine in the treatment of acetaminophen overdose: Analysis of the national multicenter study (1976-1985). *New England Journal of Medicine 319,* 1557-1562.

22. Hall, A. H., & Rumack, B. H. (1991). Prevention of absorption in overdose. In M. L. Callaham (Ed.), *Current practice of emergency medicine* (pp. 1142-1145). (2nd ed.). Philadelphia: Decker.

23. Riggs, B. S., Bronstein, A. C., Kulig, K., et al. (1989). Acute acetaminophen overdose during pregnancy. *Obstetrics and Gynecology, 74,* 247-253.

24. Demey, H., Daelemaens, R., DeBroe, M. E., et al. (1984). Propylene glycol intoxication due to intravenous nitroglycerin. *Lancet, 1,* 1360.

25. Glasgow, A. M., Boeck, R. L., Miller, M. K., et al. (1983). Hyperosmolality in small infants due to propylene glycol. *Pediatrics, 72,* 353-355.

26. Ellenhorn, M. J., & Barceloux, D. G. (1988). *Medical toxicology: Diagnosis and treatment of human poisoning.* New York: Elsevier.

27. McCoy, H. G. (1979). Severe methanol poisoning: Application of a pharmacokinetic model for ethanol therapy and hemodialysis. *American Journal of Medicine, 67,* 804-807.

28. Peterson, C. D., Collins, A. J., & Himes, J. M. (1981). Ethylene glycol poisoning. Pharmacokinetics during therapy with ethanol and hemodialysis. *New England Journal of Medicine, 304,* 21-23.

29. Massachusetts Poison Control Systems. (1981). Ethanol intoxication. *Clinical Toxicology Review, 41,* 1-2.

30. Wilkinson, P. K. (1980). Pharmacokinetics of ethanol: A review. *Alcoholism Clinical and Experimental Research, 4,* 6-21.

31. Finkel, A. J. (1983). *Hamilton & Hardy's industrial toxicology* (4th ed.). Boston: Wright-PSG.

32. Wood, G. C. (1982). Acute cyanide intoxication: Diagnosis and management. *Clinical Toxicology Consultant, 4,* 140-149.

33. Cohen, M. (1984). Treatment of cyanide poisoning. *Veterinary and Human Toxicology, 26,* 503-504.

34. Beamer, W., Shealy, R., & Prough, D. (1983). Acute cyanide poisoning from Laetrile ingestion. *Annals of Emergency Medicine, 12,* 449-451.

35. Wilson, J. (1983). Cyanide in human disease: A review of clinical and laboratory evidence. *Fundamental and Applied Toxicology, 3,* 647-649.

36. Osuntokun, B. O., Monekessa, G., & Wilson, J. (1968). Plasma amino acids in the Nigerian nutritional ataxia neuropathy. *British Medical Journal, 3,* 647-649.

37. Osuntokun, B. O., Monekessa, G., & Wilson, J. (1968). Relationship of a degenerated tropical neuropathy to diet: Report of a field survey. *British Medical Journal, 1,* 547-550.

38. Montgomery, R. D. (1965). The medical significance of cyanogen in plant foodstuffs. *American Journal of Clinical Nutrition, 17,* 103-113.

39. Drew, R. (1983). The use of hydroxycobalamin in the prophylaxis and treatment of nitroprusside-induced

cyanide toxicity. *Veterinary and Human Toxicology, 25,* 5.

40. Way, J. L., Sylvester, D., & Morgan, R. L. (1984). Recent perspectives on the toxicodynamic basis of cyanide antagonism. *Fundamental and Applied Toxicology, 4,* S231-S239.

41. Litovitz, T. L., Larkin, R. F., & Myers, R. A. (1983). Cyanide poisoning treated with hyperbaric oxygen. *American Journal of Emergency Medicine, 1,* 94-101.

42. Callahan, M. (1979). Tricyclic antidepressant overdose. *Journal of American College of Emergency Physicians, 8,* 413-415.

43. Burks, J., Walker, J., & Rumack, B. (1974). Tricyclic antidepressant poisoning: Reversal of coma, choreoathetosis and myoclonus by physostigmine. *Journal of the American Medical Association, 230*(10), 1405-1407.

44. Marshal, J., & Forker, A. (1982). Cardiovascular effects of tricyclic antidepressant drugs: Therapeutic usage, overdose, and management of complications. *American Heart Journal, 103*(3), 401-414.

45. Gilman, A., Goodman, L., & Gilman, A. (1980). *The pharmacologic basis of therapeutics.* New York: Macmillan.

46. Cantrill, S. V. (1983). Prophylactic phenytoin in tricyclic overdose. *Journal of Emergency Medicine, 1,* 169-177.

47. Cassano, G. B., Sjostrana, S. E., & Hansson, E. (1965). Distribution and fate of C^{14}-amitriptyline in mice and rats. *Psychopharmacologia, 8,* 1.

48. Noble, J., & Matthews, H. (1969). Acute poisoning by tricyclic antidepressants: Clinical features and management of 100 patients. *Clinical Toxicology, 2*(4), 403-421.

49. Woodhead, R. (1979). Cardiac rhythm in tricyclic antidepressant poisoning. *Clinical Toxicology, 14*(5), 499-505.

50. Fasoli, R., & Glauser, F. (1981). Cardiac arrhythmias and ECG abnormalities in tricyclic antidepressant overdose. *Clinical Toxicology, 18*(2), 155-163.

51. Starkey, I. R., & Lawson, A. H. (1980). Poisoning with tricyclic and related antidepressants—a ten year review. *Quarterly Journal of Medicine, 193,* 33-49.

52. Burrows, G. D., Bohra, J., & Hunt, D. (1976). Cardiac effects of different tricyclic antidepressant drugs. *British Journal of Psychiatry, 129,* 335-341.

53. Crome, P. (1982). Antidepressant overdose. *Drugs, 23,* 431-461.

54. Kingston, M. E. (1979). Hyperventilation in tricyclic antidepressant poisoning. *Critical Care Medicine, 7,* 550-551.

55. Vance, M. A., Ross, S. M., & Millington, W. R. (1977). Potentiation of tricyclic antidepressant toxicity by physostigmine in mice. *Clinical Toxicology, 11*(4), 413-421.

56. Lum, B., Follmer, C., & Lockwood, R. (1982). Experimental studies on the effects of physostigmine and isoproterenol on toxicity produced by tricyclic antidepressant agents. *Journal of Toxicology and Clinical Toxicology, 19*(1), 51-65.

57. Heath, A., Wickstrom, I., & Martensson, E. (1982). Treatment of antidepressant overdose with resin hemoperfusion. *Human Toxicology, 1,* 361-371.

58. Kline, S., & Bayer, M. (1983). Insecticide poisoning. In B. Rumack, & M. Mayer (Eds.), *Poisoning and overdose.* Baltimore: Aspen.

59. Vale, J. A., & Meredith, T. J. (1981). *Poisoning: Diagnosis and treatment.* London: Update Books.

60. Temple, A. R. (1981). Acute and chronic effects of aspirin toxicity and their treatments. *Archives of Internal Medicine, 141,* 364-369.

61. Done, A. K. (1960). Salicylate intoxication: Significance of measurements of salicylates in blood in cases of acute ingestion. *Pediatrics, 26,* 800-807.

62. Done, A. K., & Temple, A. R. (1971). Treatment of salicylate poisoning. *Modern Treatment, 8,* 528-551.

63. Temple, A. R. (1978). Pathophysiology of aspirin overdosage toxicity with implications for management. *Pediatrics, 62,* 873-876.

64. Snodgrass, W., Rumack, B. H., & Peterson, R. G. (1981). Salicylate toxicity following therapeutic doses in young children. *Clinical Toxicology, 18,* 247-259.

65. Prescott, L. F., Critchley, J. A. J. H., Proudfoot, A. T. (1983). Diuresis or urinary alkalinization for salicylate poisoning? *British Medical Journal, 286,* 147.

66. Russell, F. H. (1980). *Snake venom poisoning.* Philadelphia: Lippincott.

67. Berlinger, W. G., Regroed, S., & Goldberg, M. J. (1983). Enhancement of theophylline clearance by oral activated charcoal. *Clinical Pharmacology and Therapeutics, 33,* 351-354.

68. Sessler, C. N., Glauser, F. L., & Cooper, K. R. (1985). Treatment of theophylline toxicity with oral activated charcoal. *Chest, 87,* 325-329.

59

Chemical Dependency

Mary Ann House-Fancher

Substance abuse and chemical dependency have become two of the nation's leading health care concerns. New designer drugs, changing methods and patterns of use, increased availability, and decreased costs have raised the nation's awareness of the acute and chronic effects of abuse and dependency. Issues beyond physical abuse and addiction surround drug use in U.S. society. Increasing crime statistics and violence, work-related concerns, mandatory and random urine drug testing legislation, and an increasing number of newborns addicted to or affected by drugs ingested by their mothers and possibly their fathers are but a few of these issues.

Patients with chemical dependency or abuse problems may be admitted to the intensive care unit for one problem, such as intestinal ischemia, hypertension, or motor vehicle accident, while being intoxicated or having illicit drugs in their systems. Their drug dependency may increase the potential for major complications, such as adult respiratory distress syndrome, thereby increasing their risk of death. Therefore, observing for drug abuse during assessment is a habit that all nurses should adopt.

Drug abuse has always been surrounded by myths and misinformation. The classic image of a "drug addict" was a poverty-stricken, immoral, needle-addicted person who murdered to obtain drugs. These images of the addict and of addictive substances have faded. Users of illicit drugs are of all ages, come from all social and economic classes, and cross all socioeconomic boundaries. Although the public recognizes that street drugs today are more powerful, more potent, and different from the drugs of the 1960s, the notion has persisted that some drugs are "recreational" and can be used safely and for "fun." Consequently, we are well into the third decade of a nationwide epidemic of addiction to drugs and alcohol.

The facts about addiction in the United States today are encouraging when they apply to the number of people who have recognized a problem and are doing something about it, but distressing when they indicate the immensity of the national fix. Membership in Alcoholics Anonymous grew from 96,000 in 1950 to some 775,000 in 1989. The number of Narcotics Anonymous groups has increased sevenfold—from 2,000 in 1982 to 14,000 in 1988. The National Council on Alcoholism estimates that 10.5 million Americans are currently alcoholics, and the National Institute on Drug Abuse says that nearly 6 million Americans are regular cocaine users.[1]

INCIDENCE OF CHEMICAL DEPENDENCY

Dr. Mark Gold, a leading authority concerning alcohol and illicit drug use and abuse, has reported the incidence of abuse and addiction in U. S. society in the last few years. Alcohol is still the number one abused drug in the United States.[2] It has been estimated that 67% of all motor vehicle accidents in which a death has occurred are secondary to alcohol.[3] The health of countless others is ruined by alcohol-related disease, and alcohol-related deaths account for 10% of all U.S. deaths every year.[2]

Marijuana remains the drug used most commonly, with more than 18 million people using it at least once a month.[2] The marijuana that is on the street today is a potent drug, more powerful than hashish, and is an addictive drug with complications of use and abuse.

Cocaine is the second drug of use in the United States, with well over 2.2 million people addicted to its stimulant effects. Incidence of use of other drugs, in order of use, include analgesics, inhalants, other stimulants, tranquilizers, sedatives, hallucinogens, and heroin (Figure 59-1).

More than 60% of persons between the ages of 18 and 35 have tried an illegal drug. Almost 30% of those aged 12 to 17 responded on questioning that they, too, had used an illegal drug at least once.[2] However, drug abuse is not only a problem of teens; it includes all age groups. Each year, more people die

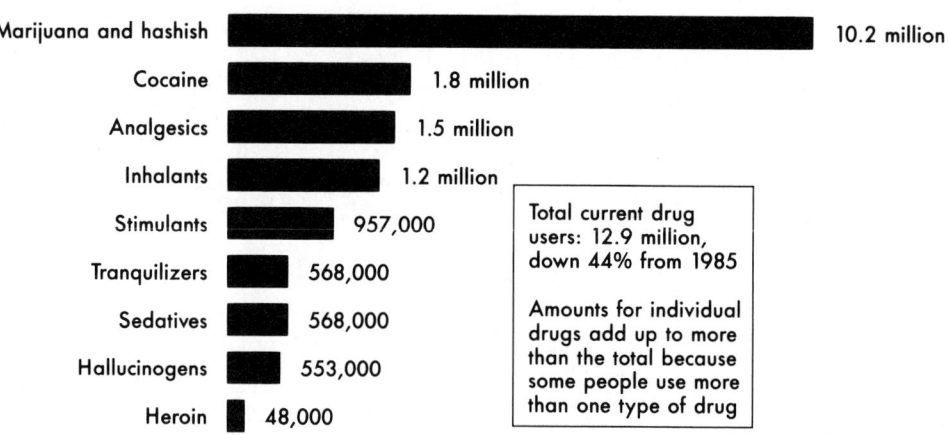

*Figure for cocaine includes 494,000 users of crack cocaine

Figure 59-1 Current users of individual drugs: 1990. Persons age 12 and older who have used a drug within the last month.

From the National Institute on Drug Abuse. (1990).

from prescription drugs, obtained legally but used improperly, than from all illegal substances combined.[2] These statistics and incidence reports indicate that drug use and dependency is a problem of enormous proportion and should be recognized by all health care providers.

DEFINITIONS

Numerous terms are used in the literature regarding chemical dependency and abuse. *Drug abuse* indicates use of any drug, to the extent that the use seriously interferes with the health, economic status, or social functioning of the drug user or others affected by the drug user's behavior. Drug abuse may be a single event but generally is a series of events that form a pattern. Abuse may or may not lead to addiction, depending on other factors such as craving, drug tolerance, and profound physical and psychological alterations.

One myth about drug abuse suggests that the use of legal drugs does not lead to illegal drug use. Users of drugs, whether legal or illegal, are much more likely than nonusers to be users of other forms of drugs. In the past, this "domino theory" of drug abuse was more of a social notion, but a statistical correlation between using cigarettes and alcohol and illegal substances has now been identified.[2] This sequence of involvement with drugs progresses from the use of at least one legal drug, alcohol or cigarettes, to marijuana, and from marijuana to other illicit drugs or psychoactive drugs.

Drug dependency is an adverse effect of all drugs. Anyone can become dependent on any drug taken too long or at a high dose. Some people have a higher dependency potential than others to certain drugs

based on genetic history. Dependency may be physical or physiological, when the body must have a drug to function without withdrawal symptoms. Or the drug can produce a psychological dependency—a preference of the intoxicated state with variable degrees of obsessive need for the drug.

Dependency usually occurs when *tolerance* to a drug is present. Tolerance to a drug develops when the dose must be increased to produce the same effects. This may be the first sign that the user is dependent upon the drug. Tolerance is almost always present when the user is addicted. Switching drugs does not relieve the tolerance, since cross-tolerance occurs with drugs of the same class. People who use heroin often take a "heroin holiday," or a period of abstinence so that their dosage of heroin can be reduced.

Another important sign of drug dependence is *withdrawal syndrome,* or the presence of a physical reaction to the sudden cessation of the drug. Withdrawal syndrome has been associated with opiates or drugs that depress the central nervous system (CNS); however, signs of withdrawal have been observed more recently with stimulants such as cocaine.

The entire relationship of tolerance and dependency and addiction is controversial. There are many drugs that produce addiction, in which tolerance and dependency are difficult to measure. Both alcohol and marijuana fit into this category. It also appears that in some cases as tolerance increases, dependency decreases. Alcoholics, for example, have a great tolerance level and may have few withdrawal symptoms.[2]

Chemical dependency, then, is the frequent repetitive use of mood-altering substances that significantly impair, or are detrimental to, the individual's health,

Substance Abuse Terms and Definitions

Alcoholism: A chronic behavioral disorder manifested by repeated drinking of alcoholic beverages in excess of dietary and social uses of the community and to an extent that interferes with the drinker's health or social or economic function

Alcohol dependency: The use of alcohol to the point of impairment of social or occupational functioning, but with the presence of tolerance or withdrawal symptoms

Psychological dependency: Variable degrees of obsessive preoccupation with drugs, preference for the intoxicated state, and chronic or recurrent abuse

Physical dependency: An altered physiological state produced by repeated drug use and requiring continued drug use to prevent the emergence of withdrawal symptoms

Withdrawal: Physical signs or symptoms associated with discontinuation of drug use after the development of tolerance

Addiction: A person's pattern of drug use that is characterized by compulsive drug use, overwhelming involvement in the use and procurement of its supply, and relapse into use after a period of abstinence

family relationships, employment, or other areas of physical, mental, or social functioning.[4] This impairment is further defined by compulsion, loss of control, and continued repeated use despite adverse consequences.

The definition of addiction also includes an irresistible compulsion to use a drug at increasing dosage and frequency, despite knowing the serious physical or psychological side effects and the extreme disruption of the user's personal relationships and system of values. Anyone who uses any chemical in this manner is suffering from addictive disease. Chemical addiction also includes preoccupation with the acquisition of a drug. When obtaining a drug plays a central role in a person's life, addiction may be present or near. Addicts rank finding their drugs as more important than satisfying basic needs (e.g., hunger, sex, and survival; see the box above).

The use and abuse of drugs often leads to a sequence of violence, accidents, and death. This syndrome may be summarized as: use leads to tolerance, which leads to abuse, which leads to chemical dependency and addiction.

ALCOHOL ABUSE

Definitions and Incidence

With more than 10.5 million alcoholics in the United States, plus countless others who are social drinkers, it is no surprise that alcohol abuse is one of the most commonly seen problems in the hospital setting, emergency department, and critical care areas. Approximately 50% of all patients in an acute care setting have problems related to alcohol.[5]

There is no single "correct" definition of alcoholism, since it is so subtle in progression. The point where heavy drinking becomes alcoholism is often unclear, so applying an overall definition of addiction—compulsive use and continued abuse in spite of adverse consequences—is helpful in explaining alcohol abuse. Alcohol is an addiction primarily since it contains three crucial elements seen in addiction to all drugs: preoccupation with acquisition, compulsive use, and relapse.

As a progressive disease, alcoholism is characterized by gradual and increasingly impaired functioning in one or more aspects of an individual's life. The impairment occurs in an individual's social, mental, physical, and spiritual life and is related to increasing loss of control over the amount, time, and manner of consumption of alcohol. Although the exact etiology of alcoholism remains unknown, genetic, psychological, developmental, and social factors are relevant.

The American Psychiatric Association[6] categorizes alcoholism as either alcohol abuse or dependency. *Alcohol abuse* is characterized by the need for daily or frequent intake of alcohol for adequate functioning, the inability to reduce consumption, and the failure of attempts at abstinence. Binges, or remaining intoxicated for at least 2 days, occasional consumption of a fifth of spirits or its equivalent in 1 day, blackouts, and continued use despite problems are additional signs.

Alcohol dependency includes the same signs and symptoms as abuse, with the addition of tolerance or signs of withdrawal. The primary differences between abuse and dependency are the signs of physical addiction: withdrawal and tolerance. In clinical use, however, the differentiation is less important then evaluating the impact that drinking has on the individual's health and ability to function productively.

Signs of Alcohol Dependency

It is easy to recognize the patient who is admitted for acute alcohol intoxication or who is in withdrawal. It is also not difficult to identify those patients with traditional alcohol-associated illnesses, such as hepatic cirrhosis, upper gastrointestinal bleeds, acute pancreatitis, or delirium tremens.

Several other illnesses that are associated with alcoholism may not be as easy to identify. These include pneumonia, tuberculosis, cellulitis, ulcers, peripheral neuropathy, cardiomyopathy, uncontrolled diabetes, anemia, cerebellar degeneration, depression, suicide attempts, injuries from accidents or victimization, and malnutrition.[5]

Patients who are not as easily identified as having problems with alcohol may be those with a low pain threshold and a high tolerance for pain medication or those who require an unusual amount of anesthesia or who are particularly sensitive to small amounts of anesthesia.[5] Additional subtle signs of alcoholism include illness or infection that responds poorly to treatment, scars or bruises on the extremities from accidents and injuries, evidence of frequent falling, or "accident prone" behavior.

Alcohol Metabolism

Alcohol abuse produces four major categories of effects: acute intoxication, dependency (addiction), withdrawal, and complications such as gastritis and liver failure.

Historically, alcohol was viewed primarily as a psychoactive compound. However, it has been recognized more recently that the metabolism of ethanol plays a major pathogenic role in several diseases associated with alcohol abuse. It was believed that liver disease and other major associated organic complications were due exclusively to the malnutrition that commonly complicates alcoholism. It has now been demonstrated that much of the pathology can be explained by some direct toxicity of alcohol.[6]

Ethanol is soluble in water and is distributed throughout the body by simple diffusion. Ethanol is metabolized in the liver where it is converted to acetaldehyde. First, ethanol is transformed into acetate, which is one of the most important precursors of the Krebs cycle. Thus, ethanol serves as an alternative source of energy. The oxidation of alcohol in the hepatocytes proceeds at a constant rate, whether or not the body requires the energy produced. The amount of acetate produced invariably exceeds the liver's capacity to metabolize it. This oversupply of acetate is added to the acetate pool and consequently saturates metabolic pathways, diverting available coenzymes from the metabolism of other foodstuffs.[6] The result is an inhibition of fatty acid metabolism, which is further complicated by the fact that ingestion of alcohol stimulates the release of fatty acids from adipose tissue, which contributes to fatty infiltration of liver tissue.[7] Alcohol also inhibits the metabolism of glucose, via the citric acid cycle, in a similar fashion as the acetate. Therefore, glucose levels are abnormal, causing hypoglycemia and further metabolic dysfunction.

Alcohol Withdrawal

Alcohol withdrawal is a common emergency that can encompass a wide range of symptoms, ranging from nausea and vomiting to hallucinations and complex seizure activity. Four stages of withdrawal have been identified with symptoms and treatment protocols developed to maintain patient stability and improve outcome. Although patients may not progress from stage to stage in order, the classification is helpful in determining triage and treatment modalities.

Stage 1: The first stage usually occurs within 8 hours of decreased alcohol intake and reflects adrenergic hyperactivity, including symptoms such as anorexia, nausea, anxiety, insomnia, diaphoresis, and tremor. Patients in this stage usually do not seek medical help and try to alleviate their symptoms by drinking more alcohol.

Stage 2: Between 8 and 72 hours after a decrease in alcohol intake, the symptoms of stage 1 worsen. The patient may now experience illusions which may progress to frank hallucinations. Symptoms are not usually relieved by the increased consumption of alcohol, and patients may seek medical help due to severe nausea and vomiting.

Stage 3 withdrawal is characterized by major motor seizures. These seizures do not occur when the patient has had alcohol intake, only with sudden cessation of intake. Seizures occur within 48 hours of cessation, and approximately 40% of patients have only a single seizure.[6] Data suggest that repeated withdrawals are an important variable in the predisposition to further seizures because of cumulative central nervous system dysfunction.[8]

Stage 4 is characterized by delirium tremens. This occurs 3 to 5 days after ethanol ingestion. This stage may be absent, but when it occurs, there is a 5% to 15% mortality. The patient may have a flushed face, oral temperature is elevated, and autonomic activity increases: heart rate increases (130 to 150 beats/min), blood pressure rises, and peripheral vasoconstriction may occur. Nausea and vomiting as well as diarrhea and diaphoresis are sufficient to cause significant fluid and electrolyte loss.

Treatment for patients in alcohol withdrawal has four primary goals: (1) to prevent worsening of symptoms, (2) to relieve current symptoms, (3) to treat any underlying medical or surgical disorder, and (4) to provide proper support or rehabilitation and follow-up care.

In the early stages of withdrawal, hydration may be necessary with correction of metabolic disorders such as hypokalemia and hypomagnesemia. Assessment for and treatment of alcoholic ketoacidosis should be included. If a patient has severe acidosis and an anion gap that is markedly increased, the nurse should assess for methanol or ethylene glycol ingestion (see Chapter 58). Glucose should also be monitored.[6]

For the treatment of anxiety and tremors, sedatives such as diazepam and chlordiazepoxide are appropriate. To sedate adequately a patient without allowing toxic amounts of active metabolites to accumulate, large doses of a benzodiazepine may be used in the earlier stages of withdrawal. Dosage can be tapered over 4 to 5 days.[6]

Multiple seizures are more common than single episodes, but status epilepticus is uncommon in withdrawal. Medical therapy for the seizure patient is directed at determining the cause of the seizure and controlling seizure activity. Phenytoin is used for patients with underlying seizure disorders and prophylactically for patients who have not yet seized. The drug of choice for the seizure patient is diazepam given IV in an amount sufficient to control seizure activity. Occasionally, patients may require chemically induced paralysis to control status epilepticus.[8]

Nursing care of this complex patient requires frequent assessment, monitoring, and reevaluation of therapy. Airway maintenance, oxygen saturation monitoring, prevention of aspiration pneumonia, blood pressure support, and hemodynamic monitoring are essential in the care of the patient in withdrawal. Observing for coagulation disorders and liver failure also is important in providing nursing care of the alcoholic patient.

The patient's family and/or friends should be included in the care of the alcoholic patient. After the withdrawal syndrome is complete, crisis intervention may be needed for the patient and the family members. A major nursing responsibility is to make appropriate referrals for long-term treatment and rehabilitation. After ethanol ingestion has stopped, it can take up to 1 year before normal sleep patterns, memory, and judgment return.

HALLUCINOGENS

Substances that produce hallucinations and illusions have been used in many contexts by human beings for thousands of years. They first captured the American public's imagination and concern in the early to mid-1960s during the age of psychedelic experiences. With proponents such as Timothy Leary, a whole culture grew up surrounding psychedelic or hallucinogenic substances such as lysergic acid diethylamide (LSD), mescaline, and psilocybin.

The incidence of hallucinogenics is difficult to ascertain. Surveys used to examine and document drug use define the age groups and agents differently and may represent a limited geographic area. Many studies include adolescents in school, but the serious users are not usually in school.

The epidemiology of drug abuse suffers from lack of documentation. Drug assays for hallucinogens are frequently inconclusive. The small molecules of hallucinogen taken in small dosages distribute widely; thus, the drug is generally undetectable even when the patient is clinically intoxicated.[9]

The definition of a *hallucinogen* is a drug that produces a distortion of perceived reality and does not produce hallucinations. The following substances are termed hallucinogenic: LSD, mescaline, psilocybin, PCP, morning glory, nutmeg, and jimson weed.

Cannabis

Marijuana is a $10 million industry in the United States. More marijuana, or pot, is grown than soybeans, grapes, lettuce, tomatoes, and other cash crops. It has become the third leading commodity in the United States. Despite some minimal penalties for possession in some states, it remains a Class I and II drug, which is highly restricted.[2]

Kinetics and Metabolism

The cannabis plant is the source of a number of different compounds known collectively as cannabinoids. The major cannabinoid is delta-9-tetrahydrocannabinol (THC). In general, the concentration of THC in marijuana is 1% to 2%, while in hashish it is 5% to 15%, and in hashish oil it is 11% to 28%.[10]

THC is inhaled in smoke or ingested in a plant product or resin. The bioavailability of THC appears to be reduced when the substance is ingested. Hepatic enzymes metabolize 99% of absorbed compounds first to several psychoactive intermediates, then to inactive compounds that are excreted in the urine and feces. The half-life of elimination of THC from the plasma is estimated to be 28 hours for chronic marijuana users and 56 hours for naive users. The half-life of elimination from fatty tissues is estimated to be 8 days.[10]

Inhaled THC produces effects within 5 minutes, reaches a peak within 20 minutes, and may last as long as 2 hours. This time sequence is delayed if the drug is ingested: onset occurs in 30 to 60 minutes; effects reach a maximum by 2 to 3 hours and last for 5 hours. The severity of psychological and physical effects appears to be dose related, with higher doses producing more severe symptoms. A lethal dose has not been determined.[10]

Clinical Effects

Central nervous system effects include mild euphoria characterized by relaxation, increased auditory and visual sensations, and altered perception. Short-term memory, learning ability, and psychomotor performance may be impaired. Other effects that may be observed in usual doses include ataxia and a decrease in hand steadiness and muscle strength. Larger doses may produce confusion, delirium, and hallucinations. Acute anxiety states occur more commonly in inexperienced users, although higher doses may produce this state in experienced individuals. Very large doses may result in disorientation, depersonalization, and paranoia.[10]

The most common cardiovascular effect of THC is sinus tachycardia. Blood pressure is not altered significantly. ECG alterations (ST and T wave changes) may imply a risk of cardiac dysfunction for those with underlying cardiac disease. The primary acute pulmonary effect is bronchodilation. The results of chronic marijuana or hashish smoking are not clear, but there have been reports that chronic marijuana smoking may produce more lung disease than cigarette smoking due to the toxic effects of the drug itself.[10]

Management

There is no antidote for intoxication of marijuana, and medical and nursing treatment of the patient with symptoms of intoxication or overdose is supportive. Removal of large amounts of ingested cannabis may be helpful in reducing potential morbidity in children with accidental ingestion. Adolescents or adults usually arrive in the emergency department already suffering from the effects of absorbed THC, and GI decontamination is not beneficial. Generally, treatment is supportive of the usual benign symptoms.

Phencyclidine (PCP)

PCP is a schedule II controlled substance. It was first synthesized by Parke Davis Laboratories in 1956 and was directed into three areas of clinical use: as a surgical anesthetic for humans, as an experimental drug in producing model psychoses, and as a veterinary tranquilizer.[11]

As an illicit street drug, PCP was first reported in Los Angeles in 1965. Today, the drug is illegally sold under an array of street names, such as amoeba, angel dust, CJ, cadillac, crystal, crystal joints, cyclones, Mr. Lovely, and windowpane, to name a few. PCP is one of the most widely used and most widely available psychoactive drugs in the United States. The heaviest incidence of PCP use is in males in their late teens and early twenties. Several studies of adolescent PCP use have found that the average age of first use is 14 years.[11]

PCP appears in many forms: as a crystalline powder and as tablets and capsules in a variety of colors, shapes, and sizes. It is often used to adulterate such drugs as LSD, MDA, STP, psilocybin, and, most commonly, THC. PCP is taken for its euphoric effects, pseudohallucinogenic potential, ability to decrease inhibitions, and ability to instill feeings of power and eliminate pain.

Clinical Effects

In most cases, the effects of PCP begin within 1 hour if the drug is orally ingested or within 5 minutes if the drug is smoked, insufflated, or injected. PCP also may be taken rectally or in eye drops, but the most popular method is smoking. The typical high from PCP lasts 4 to 6 hours and is followed by a "come down" which may last 6 to 24 hours. Depending on the chronicity of use, it may take up to 4 weeks for the person once again to feel normal.[11]

A dose of 1 to 5 mg of PCP normally produces feelings of euphoria and numbness. The user can best be described as being in a giddy, drunken state that resembles ethyl alcohol intoxication. Disinhibition and emotional lability are also regularly observed at low doses. A moderate dose, 5 to 10 mg, often results in an excited, confused intoxication marked by ataxia and dysarthria. Other clinical manifestations include depersonalization, repetitive motor movements, myoclonus, vomiting, flushing, diaphoresis, fever, decreased peripheral sensation, and horizontal and vertical nystagmus. Psychotic reactions in the form of stuporous catatonia, excited catatonia, or paranoid schizophrenia may emerge at both moderate and high doses.[11]

With pharmacological overdose, the primary cause of death is respiratory depression caused by seizure activity. In rare cases, extreme hypertension or uncontrollable increases in body temperature may occur. Prolonged coma, seizure activity, and death may result from 20 or more mg of PCP.[11]

Treatment

The effects of PCP on the user are unpredictable. One aspect of care remains essential: the user may be extremely dangerous, and safety of the patient and staff should be paramount. This includes reducing sensory stimulation by isolating the patient in a quiet room with reduced lighting, if possible.

Treatment of PCP overdose requires intensive nursing and medical management of the physical effects of the drug, such as hypertensive crisis, seizures, coma, and respiratory depression. Full life support measures and ACLS protocols may be instituted. In addition to supportive measures, gastric lavage may be necessary if the patient had taken PCP orally. Hydrating the patient, then promoting a diuresis with furosemide may enhance excretion of the drug. There is no antidote for PCP.

Haldol is commonly used as a tranquilizer for the patient with PCP agitation or psychosis. This does not shorten the drug-induced psychosis but may help manage the behavior of the patient while hospitalized.

STIMULANT ABUSE

Stimulant abuse is the nation's second leading illicit drug problem, after marijuana. Stimulants include nicotine, caffeine, amphetamines, methamphetamine, and cocaine. The two major stimulants discussed here are cocaine and methamphetamine (MAP).

Cocaine

Cocaine abuse has increased steadily despite vigorous efforts to curtail the drug's entry into the United States. It is estimated that more than 2 million Americans are addicted to some form of cocaine.[12] Recently, use has shifted from the upper middle and working classes to lower socioeconomic levels. First-time drug users are now younger, as evidenced by studies investigating high school seniors' patterns of use. Addiction rates have increased.[13]

Studies indicate that cocaine addiction continues to climb despite the large number of rehabilitation programs available. According to the Drug Enforcement Administration (DEA), cocaine-related emergency department visits in 1989 were up 200% from those in 1985.[14] In 1991, more than 75 of every 1,000 deaths were related to cocaine. These deaths may be from drug overdose, effects of abuse, violence, and vehicular and job-related accidents.[15]

Chemical Action and Metabolism

Cocaine is a tropane alkaloid of the evergreen shrub *Exythroxylon coca,* which is cultivated mainly in Bolivia, Columbia, Peru, and Brazil. About 80% of that harvest is smuggled into the United States.[16] Cocaine is classified as a local anesthetic because it interferes with the cellular sodium permeability during electrical stimulation or depolarization and, therefore, causes a neurological blockade of impulses. A sympathomimetic-like drug, cocaine causes a rapid increase in serum catecholamines, producing the "flight or fight" systemic response of the sympathetic nervous system (see the box to the right).

In the brain, cocaine blocks the normal synaptic reuptake of the neurotransmitters norepinephrine and dopamine. In early cocaine use, this action potentiates sympathetic stimulation and produces the stimulant effect. Acting first at the cortical level, cocaine then affects the mesocortical and limbic areas to produce the pleasure response and euphoria. With chronic cocaine abuse, the blockade of neurotransmitter reuptake causes a depletion of norepinephrine and dopamine in the original cell. This depletion and hyperstimulation may cause an intense physiological craving for cocaine and cause addition.[17]

Cocaine absorption is related to dosage and route of administration. It can be absorbed through all mucous membranes, but its vasoconstricting effects somewhat limit or prolong its absorption through subcutaneous tissue and muscle. Minimal absorption occurs in the gastrointestinal tract until the substance passes from the acidotic stomach to the more alkaline intestine, so cocaine is not often taken orally.

Cocaine is metabolized by liver and serum pseudocholinesterase and is largely excreted in the urine as the water-soluble metabolite benzoylecogonine (BE). Individuals with liver disease or pseudocholinesterase deficiency, therefore, may experience prolonged or more toxic effects with cocaine use. BE may be detected in urine 24 to 48 hours after cocaine use, in the blood 72 to 96 hours after use, and in the hair possibly up to 6 months after use.

Depending on the urine acidity (more excretion occurs with a decreased urine pH), 10% to 20% of the cocaine dosage is excreted unchanged.[18] Accurate toxicology screening for cocaine is difficult because BE is unstable in urine and blood and may dissipate before analysis is complete, leading to a false-negative result.

Administration

Cocaine is usually sold as a water-soluble hydrochloride salt or powder. It can be used for snorting

---

Systemic Findings Associated with Stimulant Use

CARDIOVASCULAR

↑ Heart rate
↑ Force of contraction
↑ Blood pressure (systolic)
Peripheral vasoconstriction
Atrial and ventricular dysrhythmias

PULMONARY

↑ Respiratory rate
Dyspnea

NEUROLOGICAL

Dilated pupils
↑ Deep tendon reflexes
Manic behavior
Tremors
Seizures

Compiled from Gold, M. S., Washtom, A. M., & Dackis, C. A. (1985). Cocaine abuse: Neurochemistry, phenomenology, and treatment. *National Institute of Drug Abuse Research Monograph Service, 61,* 130-150; and Gawin, F. H., & Kleber, H. D. (1985). Cocaine use in a treatment population: Patterns and diagnostic distinctions. *National Institute of Drug Abuse Research Monograph Service, 61,* 182-192.

(insufflation) or intravenously (IV). When snorted, cocaine reaches peak serum levels in approximately 90 seconds and lasts approximately 60 to 90 minutes, depending upon the dosage. When heated or mixed with water, cocaine powder melts easily and is used for IV injection or the skin "popping" (subcutaneous injection). Intravenous cocaine produces a rapid 30- to 60-second rise in serum level which lasts approximately 30 minutes.

Cocaine hydrochloride is not suitable for smoking because it does not vaporize when heated. For smoking, its form is changed via a "free base" process to make cocaine alkaloid that vaporizes when heated. Most commonly, powder cocaine is mixed with equal parts of water and sodium bicarbonate (baking soda) to form a cocaine base which is then heated, cooled, and cut into "rocks" of cocaine. Another method of forming a vaporizing crystal involves mixing powder cocaine with ammonia. This mixture hardens into the crystal form to produce "rocks" of crack.

When "free-base" cocaine is vaporized and inhaled, serum levels rapidly rise and fall, peaking in 3 to 5 seconds and dissipating in 5 to 10 minutes. Rocks may be smoked in many ways: in a pipe, with a marijuana cigarette, in a water pipe, or in a collapsed soft drink can. When the rocks are lit, an initial flash appears, followed by a cracking sound: thus the name "crack" cocaine.

Large doses and rapid routes of administration lead to high plasma concentrations that produce an extreme sense of euphoria. Once experienced, such euphoria shifts the patterns of stimulant abuse toward high-dose "binges."[19] The rapid decline in the drug's effect, often within minutes, combines with the immediate memory of the intense euphoric state to create an extreme desire to re-create the experience by readministering the drug. Up to 90% of abusers in treatment are former daily users who progressed to this type of intensive bingeing activity.[20]

Methamphetamine

Methamphetamine (MAP) abuse has waxed and waned, but with the new smokeable form ("ice"), its popularity has again increased. MAP was a common form of "speed" in the 1960s and 1970s. It was used by a wide variety of people for its stimulant effects of decreased sleep needs, increased alertness and energy, increased physical activity, and promotion of a sense of well-being. In the 1970s, the magazine *Rolling Stone* published an article explaining how to make MAP, or crank as it was known.

Pharmacology of Amphetamines

Some sources attribute the discovery of amphetamines to a German scientist in 1887, others to a Japanese scientist in 1919. Pharmaceutical researchers determined how to synthesize a naturally occurring substance released by the brain in response to stress. Amphetamines are the copies of that natural substance.[21]

In 1932, Smith, Kline, and French marketed a Benzedrine inhaler for the treatment of pulmonary congestion, asthma, colds, and hay fever. As people realized the euphoric effects of Benzedrine, the first abuse of the drug began. By breaking open the inhaler and pouring a soft drink over the drug-impregnated filter paper inside, users could extract the basic amphetamine.[21] Over the next decade, despite isolated instances of abuse, amphetamines became known as a type of universal tonic. The drugs were promoted as nonaddictive, and amphetamine derivatives such as MAP were developed in both oral and IV preparations. A warning was included with the drug, indicating that doses higher than recommended might cause restlessness and sleeplessness.

World War II saw heavy use of amphetamines. According to the National Institute for Drug Abuse (1990), 200 million amphetamine tablets were distributed to the United States troops to increase activity and to decrease hunger and sleep needs.

In 1970, the FDA permitted the use of amphetamines in three areas: short-term weight reduction, narcolepsy, and attention deficit disorder. When amphetamines or related drugs such as phenmetrazine (Preludin) are given to obese patients, they exert an anorectic effect. This is a specific CNS effect; however, tolerance develops within a few weeks, and weight loss stops. Amphetamines and related stimulants increase vigilance and impulse control as well as improving attention; these drugs can effectively treat narcolepsy and attention deficit disorder.[22]

Peripherally, the amphetamines exert both alpha and beta effects. Their effects on the cardiovascular system include increased heart rate, elevated systolic and diastolic blood pressure, and increased force of contraction. Smooth muscle response to amphetamines results in a slight relaxation of the bronchial tree, a slight increase in uterine tone, and generally unpredictable effects on the gastrointestinal (GI) tract, the most common being a slowing of GI motility. The urinary bladder sphincter smooth muscle responds to amphetamines with marked contractibility, often leading to difficulty in voiding.[22,23]

Centrally, amphetamines produce restlessness, agitation, tremor, and insomnia, probably due to their stimulant effect on the reticular activating system and the cortex. The effects on the psyche include increased wakefulness, alertness, concentration, and production of speech, as well as enhanced physical performance. There is a false sense of well-being and an elevated mood. Sleep is suppressed by the amphetamines, with REM being markedly depressed. After discontinuation of use, total sleep increases, and REM rebound occurs. Two to three months may elapse before sleep patterns return to normal after chronic use.[22,23,24]

Methamphetamine (MAP) is a N-methyl homologue of amphetamine and closely resembles its pharmacology. Legal forms of the drug consist of a white, odorless, crystalline, bitter powder soluble in water or alcohol.[23] MAP is detoxified in the liver and kidneys. The long serum half-life of MAP and subsequent prolonged clinical effects can be attributed to the lack of an enzyme (such as cholinesterase) to detoxify it. In some cases, there is a delay, possibly up to 1 hour, between intake of MAP and its appearance in urine screens; therefore, repeat toxicology screens may be warranted.[23] Concomitant use of alcohol or tricyclics increases MAP blood levels and brain levels, respectively.[25,26] After MAP use, urine toxicology screens may be positive for either MAP or its metabolite amphetamine. Urine screens may be inconclusive because decongestant cold remedies may mask the metabolites and, therefore, interfere with testing results.

At the molecular level, MAP has two chemical structural configurations which are identified by the D and L stereoisomers. The slight difference in these stereoisomers is clinically significant. The D-form isomer has greater effects on the CNS and is considered to have a more potent sympathetic effect than does the L-form isomer, which acts peripherally.[23,27] The D-form isomer is produced when the drug is changed from the MAP powder to the crystalline form ("ice"), which vaporizes easily for smoking.

Administration

MAP is commonly available as a white or brown powder. In this form, MAP can be used intranasally, mixed in liquid and taken orally, or melted and injected intravenously. Another form of MAP that has recently grown in popularity is a smokeable form that vaporizes when heated and is inhaled. The powder form of MAP is referred to as "MAP" or "crank," and the smokeable form is known as "ice."

MAP powder is extremely versatile in administration. The powder can be used intranasally, or it can be liquified either by heating or mixing in water for injection intravenously. The powder is often mixed into a drink (commonly coffee or tea) and taken orally. Onset of effect is 15 to 30 minutes when taken orally, 3 to 5 minutes intranasally, and 30 to 60 seconds IV. In contrast, when "ice" is inhaled, it has an onset of effect in 5 to 10 seconds.

"Ice" crystals are placed in a glass pipe, a heat source is applied to the bowl of the pipe, the ice vaporizes, and it is inhaled. Rapid onset and its convenience make smoking popular. Intravenous use of MAP is associated with a dramatic "rush" of euphoria seconds after injection. No other routes of administration are associated with this rush.

The duration of action of MAP is 4 to 8 hours, according to the route and amount of tolerance developed. Because tolerance develops, continuing use necessitates increasing doses at more frequent intervals to obtain the same euphoria. The process of using increased doses is referred to as "amping."

Systemic Effects of Stimulants

The effect of stimulants on the body of the user as well as abuser are primarily due to dopaminergic, alpha-, and beta-adrenergic stimulation. This results in a pronounced systemic sympathetic response with changes in myocardial, pulmonary, neurological, renal, and GI function. Cocaine and MAP have essentially the same clinical effects and are discussed together. The cardiovascular system is the major organ affected by stimulant abuse with high mortality and morbidity.

Cardiovascular Effects

The stimulant-induced alpha- and beta-adrenergic stimulation causes arterial and venous constriction. The beta-adrenergic stimulation has positive chronotropic, inotropic, and dromotropic effects on the myocardium. These effects increase afterload, systemic vascular resistance, heart rate, and contractility, thus greatly increasing myocardial oxygen consumption (MVO_2).

Although the clinical manifestations of stimulant abuse are dose related, changes in cardiovascular function may occur with very small doses and with first time use (Table 59-1). Nursing assessment must focus on the clinical presentation and patient response to initial therapy because stimulants may produce varied individual reactions.

Dysrhythmias. The sympathetic response to both cocaine and MAP causes a variety of dysrhythmias including sinus tachycardia, paradoxical atrial tachycardia, atrial fibrillation, flutter, ventricular tachycardia or fibrillation, and asystole.[28] An increase in catecholamines increases heart rate by directly stimulating the sinoatrial node and the atrial and ventricular tissue. Increases in sympathetic discharge may lead to atrial and ventricular tachycardia, as well as systematic vasoconstriction causing increased afterload and MVO_2. Increases in MVO_2 in excess of myocardial oxygen supply may cause ischemia, another cause of dysrhythmias—with or without underlying coronary artery disease.

Treatment of the dysrhythmia is regulated by the

TABLE 59-1 Dose Related Clinical Effects of Stimulants

Dose	Behavioral Findings	Physical Findings		
5-mg single dose	Excited	↑ BP		↑ Muscle tone
	Euphoric	↑ HR		Pupils dilated
		↑ RR		
Multiple doses	Restless	BP change		Twitches
Repeated dosing/ bingeing	Dizziness	↑ HR		Tremors
	Paranoia	↑ HR		↑ Deep tendon reflexes
	Visual disturbances	↑ Temperature		
	Hallucinations			
	Disorientation			
Intoxication	Agitation	PVCs		Seizures
		Acute		Focal neurological findings
	Confusion	Cardiopulmonary arrest		
		Cerebrovascular accident		
		Hypertension		
Overdose	Coma	Respiratory arrest		Flaccid
		Ventricular tachycardia or fibrillation		Dilated pupils

BP = blood pressure.
HR = heart rate.
RR = respiratory rate.
PVCs = premature ventricular contractions.
From Gay, G. R. (1982). Clinical management of acute and chronic cocaine poisoning. *Annals of Emergency Medicine, 11*, 562-572.

patient's hemodynamic response, according to the Advanced Life Support protocol. The beta-blocker propranolol hydrochloride is effective in treating cocaine- and MAP-induced tachycardias (and hypertension), as is Esmolol.[29] Propranolol blunts the stimulating effect of cocaine on the heart, decreasing contractility and heart rate. A decrease in blood pressure may follow. The use of propranolol has been opposed because the combination of alpha-adrenergic stimulation (vasoconstriction) and beta-adrenergic medicated vasoconstriction seen in stimulant ingestion may aggravate existing hypertension. A paroxysmal increase in blood pressure after treatment of cocaine intoxication with propranolol has been documented.[30] These observations imply that propranolol should be administered with caution in patients experiencing hypertension, or should be reserved only for management of tachydysrhythmias.

Acute Myocardial Infarction. Numerous case studies have documented the association between cocaine abuse and myocardial ischemia and infarction.[31,32] Although the direct etiology of acute myocardial infarction (AMI) from stimulant use remains unclear, two major theories have been suggested. An increase in MVO_2 secondary to increased sympathetic stimulation is thought to contribute to the development of prolonged ischemia.[33] Cocaine and MAP may cause coronary vasospasm and vasoconstriction through the same mechanism of catecholamine-induced injury. In addition, constriction of small arteries is known to occur after cocaine administration.

Focal endothelial injury resulting from vasospasm or vasoconstriction may lead to increase platelet aggregability and adherence, increased thromboxane production, and decreased endothelial prostacycline release. This potential predisposition to clotting may explain the in situ formation of coronary thrombi in patients with normal coronary arteries.

Acute myocardial infarction may occur after cocaine use in patients with either normal or diseased coronary arteries. Patients presenting with chest pain after using cocaine or MAP should be promptly and thoroughly evaluated to exclude myocardial ischemia and infarction. When AMI is documented, thrombolytic therapy may be considered for patients who meet standard criteria and who do not quickly respond to coronary vasodilator therapy such as sublingual nefidipine or intravenous nitroglycerin. Further treatment after vasodilator therapy should include the standard medical and nursing interventions for the AMI patient. Since there is no antidote for cocaine or MAP, management of patient symptoms and early recognition of complications remains foremost in treatment.

Myocarditis. Although the cause of myocarditis in cocaine users is unknown, infectious agents are a possible primary or contributory factor. Chronic administration of cocaine in animals markedly increases the concentration of norepinephrine in the left ventricle, which may cause myocyte necrosis with accompanying inflammatory infiltrate. Infectious agents and the toxic effect of cocaine itself may lead to isolated myocyte necrosis, either by causing vasospasm or by direct damage of myocytes through local catecholamine release.[34]

Clinical presentation of the patient with cocaine-induced myocarditis may include:

- Pleuritic chest pain or atypical chest pain, which may be the first sign of impending congestive failure
- Congestive heart failure due to left ventricular failure with clinical findings of left sided heart failure
- ST and T wave abnormalities
- Dysrhythmias

Ventricular tachycardia and fibrillation are rare in the presence of myocarditis alone but may be seen clinically in cocaine-induced myocarditis. Diagnosis of suspected myocarditis is confirmed by clinical manifestations and myocardial biopsy.

Treatment includes correction of dysrhythmias and the treatment of heart failure with inotropes, diuretics, and vasodilation therapy. Corticosteroids may be used to reduce inflammation and in patients with worsening heart failure, but few data are available to support routine use.

Cardiomyopathy. The mechanism of cocaine cardiotoxicity is not well understood, but the end result appears to be a recognizable lesion consisting of contraction band necrosis and inflammatory infiltrates. In animals, chronic cocaine use increases norepinephrine levels in the left ventricle.[35] In humans, chronic exposure to elevated norepinephrine levels, as in long-standing pheochromocytoma, is associated with contraction band necrosis, inflammatory infiltrates, and eventual scarring.[35]

Other factors possibly contributing to the development of cardiotoxicity include contaminants in street drugs and coronary artery vasospasm. Drug contaminants may initiate an immunological reaction causing inflammation or eosinophilic myocarditis and leading to cardiomyopathy.[35] Findings in several reported case studies suggest ischemic stunning of the myocardium, secondary to coronary artery vasospasm, could cause clinically significant left ventricular dysfunction.[36,37,38]

Stimulant-induced cardiomyopathy presents as a dilated, congestive cardiomyopathy. Initial examination may elicit typical complaints of progressive fatigue, dyspnea, edema, orthopnea, and exertional chest pain. Physical findings may include underlying tachycardia, normal or low blood pressure, and possible S_3 and jugular venous distention. The lungs may be clear or congested as evidenced by crackles.

Diagnosis is made in the routine manner with chest x-ray, ECG, echocardiography, and cardiac catheterization. Myocardial biopsy offers a definitive diagnosis. Viral serologies may be used during the acute and convalescent stages of the illness to rule out a viral etiology. Most cocaine abusers also use alcohol, which has cardiotoxic effects that may add to the effects of cocaine on the myocardium.

Treatment follows the standard management for congestive cardiomyopathy. Absolute abstinence from cocaine, MAP, and alcohol is essential. Withdrawal from the drugs may actually reverse the left ventricular dysfunction with improvement in cardiac function. Transplantation may not be offered to patients who continue to abuse illicit drugs.

Sudden Death. Sudden cardiac death (SCD) associated with the use of cocaine has frequently been attributed to underlying cardiac disease or massive drug overdose. Coronary artery disease (CAD), cerebral aneurysm or atrioventricular malformation, and pseudocholinesterase deficiency have been mentioned as factors contributing to SCD.[39] Cutting agents, including procaine, phencyclidine (angel dust), amphetamines, quinine, talc, and strychnine, and the concurrent use of other drugs such as heroin also have been cited as precipitating causes of SCD.[40]

Mash,[41] at the University of Miami, is studying SCD in cocaine users. Preliminary data indicate that mixing cocaine with alcohol, a common combination, produces a third chemical, cocaethylene, which increases and prolongs the euphoria but also raises the risk of SCD. Further, mixing cocaine with alcohol raises the risk of SCD to 20 times that of nonusers with CAD.[41]

Congestive Heart Failure. Stimulant abuse may result in congestive heart failure (CHF) secondary to the precipitous onset of increased MVO_2, severe ischemia, myocardial infarction, and/or dysrhythmias. Treatment goals are aimed at the etiology of the CHF. If symptomatic hypertension develops, inotropic support with a combination of dopamine and dobutamine may be indicated. Pulmonary congestion or edema should be treated with diuretics, vasodilators, or both.

Another potential etiology of CHF is acute renal failure. Several reports in the literature[22,25,42] describe a scenario of MAP or cocaine use, severe hyperthermia (up to 111° F), rhabdomyolysis, and finally, acute renal failure with pulmonary congestion. Treatment includes aggressive hypothermia (cool baths), intravenous fluids for hydration, and possible emergency dialysis.

Pulmonary Effects

Smoking crack and ice has resulted in numerous problems with pulmonary congestion, shortness of breath, chronic cough, cough with sputum production, and ill-defined chest pain. These symptoms are secondary to drug-induced vasoconstriction within the pulmonary bed and toxicity to the alveoli.

Inhalation of cocaine or MAP vapors involves a deep, prolonged inspiratory effort, often followed by a Valsalva maneuver and violent coughing which can cause spontaneous pneumomediastinum or pneumothorax. An increase in intralveolar pressure causes rupture of alveoli, with escape of air into the interstitial tissues. The air may dissect centrally along the bronchovascular sheaths into the mediastinum and to the planes of the neck.[43]

Smoke and its toxic combustion products reduce mucociliary clearance and cause bronchiolar damage in both laboratory animals and humans.[44] Atelectasis ensues from accumulation of secretions in bronchioles narrowed by mucosal swelling. Respiratory excursion may be limited by pain, also contributing to atelectasis. Damage to the alveolar capillary membrane by smoke and other noxious gases may be followed by the transudation of fluid, with resulting diffuse or localized areas of pulmonary edema.[43]

Diffuse alveolar hemorrhage was found at open lung biopsy of several patients who had smoked crack cocaine. This hemorrhage was thought to be due to vasoconstriction resulting in anoxic cell damage or to a direct toxic effect of cocaine on the alveolar lining cells, with subsequent involvement of the basement membrane.[45]

Lung damage from the inhalation of the superheated gases of cocaine and MAP may result in upper airway burns and produce a marked reduction of lung's capacity to diffuse carbon monoxide. This diffusion abnormality may result in abnormal blood gases, with or without underlying chest trauma or disease.[46] For patients entering the hospital as a result of trauma or other diagnosis, pulmonary examination of the stimulant smoker is mandatory.

Due to these underlying abnormalities, smoke inhalation, diffusion abnormalities, burns, and toxic drug effects, patients may have varied presentations. Between 25% and 50% of persons who chronically smoke crack and ice complain of dyspnea on exertion, cough, cough with a characteristic black or brown sputum, and ill-defined chest pain.[46] One common complication for the individual with a history of stimulant inhalation is adult respiratory distress syndrome (ARDS). It may occur in conjunction with other primary illnesses, as with trauma or surgery, or may occur with the abuse pattern of bingeing. The increased incidence of ARDS also is associated with increased mortality. Nurses caring for individuals who inhale stimulants must first identify them as having a high risk for complications and then carefully monitor arterial blood gases, pulmonary function tests, and pulmonary assessment data.

Neurological Effects

Neurological complications of stimulant use include ischemic stroke, headaches similar to migraines, subarachnoid hemorrhage, tonic-clonic seizures, and extraparenchymal hemorrhage. Partial seizures, quadriplegia from anterior spinal artery syndrome, and ischemic attacks have also been reported.[47] These events may result from underlying vascular abnormalities exacerbated by cocaine or MAP, but stroke and hemorrhage have occurred in patients whose vessels were normal on angiography.[47] In addition, cocaine and MAP intoxication can cause acute confusion, paranoid ideation, and assaultive behavior, as well as decreased appetite and sleep disorders. As already noted, stimulant abuse can cause sudden increases in blood pressure and vasoconstriction which can lead to vascular rupture, embolus formation, and hypoxia. These may lead to an embolic or hemorrhagic stroke, even without underlying disease.

Seizures are a common complication of stimulant abuse. All types of seizures have been documented, but grand mal seizures have the highest incidence. Seizures may be treated with diazepam as the first line of therapy, although some clinicians are using Ativan with good results. Phenytoin is less effective in stimulant abusers and should not be used. If the patient continues to have seizures, general anesthesia may be employed. Oxygen therapy and pressure support also must be carefully maintained. The patient should be treated as any patient with increased intracranial pressure, with nursing interventions focused on the restoration of normal cerebral blood flow.[47]

Hyperthermia

Cocaine and MAP have pyrogenic properties. Stimulant administration may lead to increased body temperature by resetting of the hypothalamic heat regulating centers, by vasoconstriction, and possibly by increased muscle contractions (manic activity or seizure activity). Peripheral heat loss capacity is diminished, and core temperatures rise. Combative behavior with extreme skeletal muscle activity contributes to the hyperthermia and may present with the clinical picture of heat stroke, with typical acid–base disturbances, rhabdomyolysis, hyperuricemia, and myoglobinuric renal failure. This syndrome may be life-threatening. Hyperthermia may escalate to temperatures above 108° F, causing further neurological, cardiac, and pulmonary dysfunction; it may also precipitate DIC.[48]

Therapy for drug-related hyperthermia requires

prompt recognition and rapid cooling of the patient. Evaporative cooling methods should be initiated in the field and continued in the hospital. Hypothermia blankets and iced water baths may be helpful. Direct external cooling by immersion in ice water or packing may be effective but is potentially dangerous. This condition differs from malignant hyperthermia in that direct pharmacological intervention is of secondary importance. Chlorpromazine may prevent shivering during cooling, but antipyretics have not proved useful in treating drug-induced hyperthermia.[48]

Stimulant Addiction

Addiction to cocaine or MAP is a complex physiological and psychological entity that requires astute physical assessment and intervention skills. Acute complications from stimulant use include cardiovascular effects, cerebral infarction, seizure activity, renal failure, rhabdomyolysis, gastritis, alterations in immune response, and pulmonary dysfunction. Chronic manifestations may include continued sore throat, cough with sputum, dyspnea with exertion, ill-defined chest pain, insomnia, impotence, weight loss, and depression (Table 59-2).

TABLE 59-2 **Physical Assessment, Symptoms, and Findings in the Stimulant Abuser**

	Physical Findings	Symptoms
General	Weight loss Manic behavior Depression/paranoia Nosebleeds	Insomnia
Cardiovascular	Heart rate changes Blood pressure changes (systolic hypertension) Angina/ischemia Congestive heart failure/cardiomyopathy Myocarditis Acute myocardial infarction	Palpitations Headaches/blurred vision Chest pains Shortness of breath/fatigue Diaphoresis, nausea, vomiting
Pulmonary	Dyspnea Inhalation injury (superheated gas) Sputum production black/brown Chronic bronchiolitis (unresponsive to therapy) New patchy infiltrates Altered diffusion capacity	Chronic inflamed sore throat Chronic cough Ill-defined chest pain Pallor/cyanosis
Neurological	Change in mental status Change in locus of control Paranoid behavior ↑ Deep tendon reflexes Dysarthria Seizure activity Focal neurological findings: paresthesias	Confusion Headaches Blurred vision Verbosity Twitching
Otolaryngological	Inflamed throat Sinusitis Nasal ulcerations Dilated pupils Rhinitis Facial burns/eyebrows/eyelashes Buccal mucosal color change/teeth discolored	Chronic sore throat Facial pain Running nose Watery eyes
Sexual	↑ Incidence STD ↓ Libido/bizarre sexual behavior	↓ Libido impotency
Gastrointestinal	Peptic ulcer findings Bowel obstruction (mules) Bowel ischemia with ↑ WBC	Stomach pain Abdominal pain Pain
Renal	Renal failure Electrolyte abnormalities Ca^{2+}, K^+, Cl^- Edema (periorbital)	↓ Urinary output Uremic signs and symptoms

Compiled from Moody, C. K. (1988). Neurologic complications of cocaine abuse. *Nephrology, 387,* 1189-1193; Gold, M. S., Washtom, A. M., & Dackis, C. A. (1985). Cocaine abuse: Neurochemistry, phenomenology, and treatment. *National Institute of Drug Abuse Research Monograph Service, 61,* 130-150; and Menashe, P. I., & Gottlieb, J. E. (1988). Hyperthermia, rhabdomyolysis, and myoglobinuric renal failure after recreational use of cocaine. *Southern Medical Journal, 81,* 379-380.

Medical Management of Stimulant Intoxication

Management of the patient with stimulant intoxication is based on an understanding of the drug's manifestations, and the patient's phase of presentation: from an early reaction to more advanced toxicity or overdose. Patients "wired" on sympathomimetics can resemble one another regardless of the agent used (e.g., cocaine, crack, crank, ice, or phenylpropanolamine). Without a complete history and a drug toxicology screen, the health care provider may have difficulty distinguishing stimulant abuse from abuse of anticholinergics such as jimson weed or belladonna, an antiparkinsonian agent such as cogentin, or, more commonly, an antihistamine.

A person overdosed on an anticholinergic agent also has tachycardia, delusions, paranoia, hyperpyrexia, mydriasis, and hypertension. A major physical finding is that diaphoresis is present with the sympathomimetic overdose and absent in the anticholinergic overdose.[17] Acute and chronic stimulant use may lead to a variety of altered physical findings on examination and symptoms described by the user. Patients presenting with symptoms of early stimulation characteristic of the stimulant reaction should be approached calmly, since they are highly stimulated. Presentation of a young, previously healthy person with headache, seizures, or chest pain should raise the suspicion of stimulant abuse. Vital signs should be monitored frequently until they have returned to a normal range. Once the patient is symptom-free, he or she may be discharged. Serum levels of stimulants, if metabolism occurs normally, should be returning to baseline within 12 to 24 hours.

If the patient is admitted in a more advanced, stimulated state, initial nursing management should focus on the fundamental ABC's. The basic approach to a potential drug overdose is a combination of thiamine, 50% dextrose, and naloxone, along with gastric lavage and administration of charcoal and a cathartic agent.[49]

Evaluation of pulmonary status may include the need for oxygen by nasal cannula or face mask to correct hypoxia. Respiratory depression or severe hypoxia may necessitate intubation and mechanical assistance. Circulatory management involves starting intravenous lines, monitoring, and managing hypertension and dysrhythmias according to ACLS guidelines.

There is no antidote for stimulant overdose, but propranolol hydrochloride and Esmolol can lower heart rate and blood pressure in these patients. Careful administration is necessary to prevent further decreases in myocardial contractility.

For seizure activity, 2.5 to 5.0 mg of diazepam is usually given.[18] Seizures not uncontrolled by diazepam may be treated by secobarbitol or general anesthesia. Seizures may be secondary to a neurological focus or to hyperthermia. Preventive measures against hypoxia, hyper- or hypotension, and hypercapnia should be instituted to avert further increases in intracerebral pressure. If congestive heart failure also is present, positive inotropics, diruetics, and vasodilators may improve left ventricular function. Intravenous nitroglycerin may reduce preload and increase oxygen supply to the myocardium, also improving function.

Persons who abuse MAP are recognized as being among the most violent of drug abusers. MAP psychosis is seen in the majority of patients seeking treatment; paranoia often is seen.[23] Haloperidol is the drug of choice for treatment of psychosis. A primary concern of the nurse should be protection of the patient and staff. Ensuring a safe environment and providing continual observation of the patient are necessary.

Persons using stimulants are often polydrug abusers. Synergistic effects may complicate the clinical picture, making it difficult to identify the drug(s) and to formulate a plan of care. Initial management of the drug abuser is symptomatic, since there are no antidotes for many drugs used today. Physical assessment and monitoring of the patient's response to treatment are of paramount importance. Once care has been planned, early evaluation and adjustment of the plan of care are essential.

NARCOTICS

By definition, *narcotic* means an agent that causes sleep, although some clinicians refer to narcotics as opiates. Narcotics are analgesics but also are used for other conditions, such as cough suppression and diarrhea. The class includes the opium derivatives as well as purely synthetic agents. For the purpose of this chapter, the narcotics addressed are the opiate agonist and opiate partial agonists. (See the box on p. 1371.)

Pharmacology

Most narcotic agents can produce analgesia without loss of consciousness, although with some degree of drowsiness. Most opiate derivates exert their effect on the CNS and intestines at specific opiate-receptor binding sites. All of these agents produce some degree of respiratory depression, mood changes (euphoria or dysphoria), mental clouding, and nausea and vomiting.

Possibly the most dangerous complication of narcotic abuse is respiratory depression caused by direct suppression of the respiratory centers in the brainstem, which reduces sensitivity and responsiveness to increased serum carbon dioxide tension. These agents probably obtund the voluntary control of respiration

Classification of Opiate Drugs

OPIOID AGONISTS
Natural opium derivatives
   Morphine
   Codeine
Semisynthetic opioids
   Heroin
   Hydromorphone (Dilaudid)
   Oxymorphone (Numorphan)
   Oxycodone (Percodan, Percocet)
Synthetic opioids
   Meperidine (Demerol)
   Methadone (Dolophine)
   Levorphanol tartrate (Levo-Dromoran)
   Paregoric (Parepectolin, tincture of opium)
   Diphenoxylate (Lomotil)
   Fentanyl (Sublimaze)
   Propoxyphene (Darvon)

AGONISTS/ANTAGONISTS
Nalorphine (Nalline)
Levallorphan (Lorfan)
Pentazocine (Talwin)
Butorphanol (Stadol)
Nalbuphine (Nubain)
Cyclazocine
Propiram
Profadol

PURE OPIOID ANTAGONISTS
Naloxone (Narcan)
Naltrexone (Trexan)

as well as the CNS centers that regulate respiratory rhythm.[50]

With the exception of mild orthostatic hypotension, narcotics have little effect on the cardiovascular system. The opiates appear to have more of an effect on peripheral vasodilation than do the nonopiate narcotics. Large doses of opiates, especially when used intravenously, induce bradycardia. All of the narcotics cross the placental barrier so that infants born to physically addicted mothers usually demonstrate withdrawal from 1 to 4 days after birth.[51]

Heroin

Until 1972, most opium was grown in India, Russia, and Turkey with Iran producing very little. Today Iran, Afghanistan, and Pakistan are major sources of opium for the United States. The opium is changed into morphine, which reduces the bulk without loss of potency. The morphine is delivered to another laboratory to be converted into heroin, which is three times more potent than morphine. Brown heroin is transported to the United States from Mexico in larger amounts than ever before. Three additional areas in Asia also produce opium: Laos, Burma, and Thailand.[51]

Heroin's role as the best-known street drug and one of the most addictive of all known drugs has been diminished by crack and other new drugs. A new form of heroin called "black tar" or "tootsie roll" first appeared in the southwest. Mexican or Asian forms of heroin have a purity level of 2% to 5%, but black tar has a reported purity between 60% and 85%.

Heroin is liquified from powder, cooked down, and injected. It is sometimes sniffed, and a smokeable form of heroin is now produced. The technique of smoking is called "smoking the dragon." The intravenous route of use is still the most popular and is the quickest way to become addicted. Once in the body, heroin acts like any other opiate, binding to the opiate receptor sites. However, it stimulates the mood-regulating centers of the brain, such as the hypothalamus, to produce euphoria. It depresses the CNS and regulates the perception of pain.[2]

Like other drugs, heroin fills the addictive model of repeated, compulsive use, preoccupation with the drug, and relapse after treatment. In addition, a tolerance to heroin is quickly built. Addicts often withdraw from the drug or lower their dose for a heroin "holiday," then resume their habit at a lower dose (see the box on p. 1372).

Heroin users are prone to concomitant illness such as malnutrition, numerous forms of hepatitis, vascular problems, tuberculosis, and sexually transmitted diseases. Users of intravenous heroin are the fastest-growing AIDS-infected population. Overdose is not the only medical danger of heroin use. The medical complications may be due to adulterants used to cut the heroin. In a study of heroin addicts with nephrotic syndrome, heroin use was highly correlated with sclerosing glomerulonephritis and end-stage renal disease. Glomerulonephritis in adolescents addicted to heroin also has been reported.[51] Other complications of heroin use include skin lesions, abscesses, cellulitis, fever, infections due to unsterile conditions, and subacute bacterial endocarditis. In addition, there are respiratory problems with cough, dyspnea, and chest pain. Pneumonia is common, as well as liver dysfunction.

Medical and nursing care of the patient with a narcotic overdose is treated according to symptoms. Narcan may be administered as an opiate antagonist, but symptoms may not decrease with Narcan alone. Continuous monitoring of vital signs, with close observation of respiratory status, is necessary.

DRUG TESTING

According to the U.S. Chamber of Commerce, 65% of individuals who enter the full-time work force

Clinical Manifestations of Opioid Withdrawal

EARLY (4-10 HOURS)
Yawning
Lacrimation
Rhinorrhea
Sneezing
Sweating

INTERMEDIATE (12-18 HOURS)
Restless sleep
Piloerection
Restlessness
Irritability
Anorexia
Flushing
Tachycardia
Tremor
Hyperthermia

LATE (>24 HOURS)
Fever
Nausea
Vomiting
Abdominal pain
Diarrhea
Difficulty sleeping
Muscle spasm
Joint pain
Involuntary ejaculation
Suicidal ideation

TABLE 59-3   Approximate Retention Times of Drugs in Urine

Drugs or Drug Class	Approximate Retention Times
Amphetamines	1-2 days
Barbiturates	Short-acting (e.g., secobarbitol), 1-3 days
	Long-acting (e.g., phenobarbitol), 1-3 days
Benzodiazepines	1-14 days
Cannabinoids	Occasional use, 1-7 days
	Chronic use, 1-4 weeks
Cocaine metabolites	12-48 hours
Methadone	1-3 days
Methaqualone	1-7 days
Opiates	1-3 days
Phencyclidine (PCP)	Occasional use, 1-8 days
	Chronic use, up to 30 days

for the first time have used drugs illegally. More than $110 billion is grossed annually from the illegal sales of drugs in the United States. Other sources indicate that substance abuse costs U.S. society in excess of $135 billion annually. These and other data reveal that the United States has the highest rate of drug abuse among the world's industrialized nations.

These facts have prompted employers to become concerned about employees' use and abuse of illicit drugs and alcohol and has led to the development of drug testing in the workplace. Five types of substance abuse testing programs are available: preemployment, random, for cause, postaccident, and periodic testing.

For many reasons, drug testing is not always accurate. Some drugs such as cocaine do not have a long period for detection: 24 to 48 hours in the urine. Marijuana has a long half-life and may be detected in the urine up to 30 days after ingestion. Metabolites of specific drugs also may be masked by the presence of other drugs, such as nonprescription antihistamines or cold remedies (Table 59-3).

Nursing Management

Drug testing and toxicology screens for the patient admitted to the hospital can become the nurse's guide for the care of the patient. However, repeated testing may be required to identify all drugs that may be present. The patient's initial care does not change with the results of a toxicology screen. Assessments and interventions are made according to patient presentation and response to therapy. There are no common protocols for the treatment of drug intoxication and overdose; supportive and individual care are priorities.

Critical care nurses continue to see the effects of the drug's action on the body and the results of violence surrounding the drug culture, including trauma from accidents while intoxicated or from a result of another's intoxication. The box on p. 1373 outlines appropriate assessment and interventions when drug intoxication or use is suspected.

Nursing Assessment and Interventions Related to Possible Drug Intoxication or Use

ASSESSMENT

Patient Information

History
- Initial presentation
- Chief complaint
- ETOH abuse
- Drug abuse

Physical examination
- General survey
  Possibility of drug use
  Burns on face and/or facial hair
  Needle tracks
  Needle marks
  Behavior: stimulated/depressed
  Pupil size and reaction
  Smell: ETOH, etc.
- Cardiac
- Pulmonary
- Neurological
- Gastrointestinal
- Renal
- Hematological

Family History
- Possibility of patient's drug use
- ETOH use
- Accident history

Toxicology Results
- Serum and urine screens
- Initially drawn at scene or in the ED
- Redrawn 4-6 hours after initial screen

INTERVENTIONS
- ABC's
- Fluid replacement
  IVs, D_5W
  Possible thiamine
  Naloxone
  Possible D_{50}
- Gastric lavage
- Activated charcoal
- Cardiovascular response
  Monitor rate, rhythm
  BP
    Hypertension: Nipride
    Hypotension: Fluids, vasopressors
  Dysrhythmias: ACLS protocol
  CHF: Diuretics, inotropes, vasodilators
- Pulmonary
  Oximetry
  Oxygen therapy
  ABGs/chest x-ray for diagnosis
  Airway protection and maintenance
  Mechanical ventilation
- Neurological
  CNS stimulation/depression: Calm, quiet environment
  Seizure activity: Diazepam, airway protection
- Hyperthermia
  Ice bath
  Ice lavage

REFERENCES

1. Editors. (1989). Addiction in America. *Addiction*, January/February, 59.
2. Gold, M. S. (1988). *The facts about drugs and alcohol.* New York: Bantam.
3. Lindenbaum, et al. (1989). Patterns of alcohol and drug abuse in an urban trauma center: The increasing role of cocaine abuse. *Journal of Trauma, 29*(12), 1654-1658.
4. American Psychiatric Association. (1978). *Diagnostic and statistical manual of mental disorders* (Vol. 3). Washington, DC: Author.
5. Zahourek, R. P. (1986). Identification of the alcoholic in the acute care setting. *Critical Care Quarterly, 8*(4), 1-10.
6. Madden, J. F. (April 15, 1990). Calming the storms of alcohol withdrawal. *Emergency Medicine,* 23-28.
7. Kelly, F. M. (1986). Caring for the patient in acute alcohol withdrawal. *Critical Care Quarterly, 8*(4), 11-19.
8. Ripley, J. B. (1990). Case review: Fatal alcohol withdrawal. *Journal of Emergency Nursing, 16*(2), 67-69.
9. Brown, R. T., & Braden, N. J. (1987). Hallucinogens. *Pediatric Clinics of North America, 34*(2), 341-347.
10. McGuigan, M. A. (1984). Toxicology of drug abuse. *Emergency Medicine Clinics of North America, 2*(1), 87-101.
11. Young, T., Lawson, G. W., & Gacono, C. B. (1987). Clinical aspects of phencyclidine (PCP). *International Journal of the Addictions, 22*(1), 1-5.
12. U.S. Drug Enforcement Administration. (1990). *Yearly reports.* Washington, DC: U.S. Government Printing Office.
13. Partnership for a Drug-Free America. (1989). Report. December.
14. U.S. Drug Enforcement Administration. (1989). *Statistical report.* Personal communication.
15. U.S. Drug Enforcement Administration. (1990). *Statistical report.* Personal communication.
16. Gawin, F. H., & Kleber, H. D. (1985). Cocaine use in a treatment population: Patterns and diagnostic distinctions. *National Institute of Drug Abuse Research Monograph Service, 61,* 182-192.
17. Gold, M. S., Washtom, A. M., & Dackis, C. A. (1985).

Cocaine abuse: Neurochemistry, phenomenology, and treatment. *National Institute of Drug Abuse Research Monograph Service, 61,* 130-150.

18. Gay, G. R. (1982). Clinical management of acute and chronic cocaine poisoning. *Annals of Emergency Medicine, 11,* 562-572.

19. Gawin, F. H., & Kleber, H. D. (1986). Abstinence symptomatology and psychiatric diagnosis in cocaine abusers. *Archives of General Psychiatry, 43,* 107-113.

20. Rappolt, R. T., Gay, G. R., & Inaba, D. S. (1976). Properties in the treatment of cardiopulmonary effects of cocaine. *New England Journal of Medicine, 295*(8), 488.

21. Sager, M. (February 8, 1990). The ice age. *Rolling Stone Magazine,* 53-56, 110-114.

22. Mack, R. B. (1990). The ice man cometh and killeth: Smokeable methamphetamine. *North Carolina Medical Journal, 51*(6), 276-278.

23. Moser, L. (1990). *Crack, cocaine, methamphetamine, and ice.* Texas: Multi Media Production.

24. Woolverton, W., et al. (1989). Long term effects of chronic methamphetamine administration in rhesus monkeys. *Brain Research, 486,* 73-78.

25. McMullen, M. J. (1988). Stimulants. In P. Rosen (Ed.), *Emergency medicine concepts and clinical practice* (2nd ed.). St. Louis: Mosby.

26. Elliott, R. H., & Rees, G. B. (1990). Amphetamine ingestion presenting as eclampsia. *Canadian Journal of Anaesthesia, 37*(1), 130-133.

27. King, P., & Coleman, J. (1987). Stimulants and narcotic drugs. *Pediatric Clinics of North America, 34*(2), 349-363.

28. Tazellar, H. D., et al. (1987). Cocaine and the heart. *Human Pathology, 83,* 601.

29. DeRlet, R. W. (1989). Cocaine intoxication. *Postgraduate Medicine, 86*(5), 245-253.

30. Romoska, E. (1985). Propranolol-induced hypertension in treatment of cocaine intoxication. *Annals of Emergency Medicine, 14,* 1112-1113.

31. Smith, H., et al. (1987). Acute myocardial infarction temporally related to cocaine use. *American College of Physicians, 107,* 13-18.

32. Simpson, R. W., & Edwards, W. D. (1986). Pathogenesis of cocaine-induced ischemic heart disease. *Archives of Pathology and Laboratory Medicine, 110,* 479-484.

33. Ascher, E. K., Stauffer, J. C. E., & Gaasch, W. H. (1988). Coronary artery spasm, cardiac arrest, transient electrocardiographic Q waves and stunned myocardium in cocaine-associated acute myocardial infarction. *American Journal of Cardiology, 61,* 939-941.

34. Karch, S. B., & Billingham, M. E. (1986). Myocardial contraction bands revisited. *Human Pathology, 17,* 9.

35. Hogya, P., & Wolfson, A. (1990). Chronic cocaine abuse associated with dilated cardiomyopathy. *American Journal of Emergency Medicine, 8,* 203-204.

36. Isner, J. M., Estes, N. M., Thompson, P. D., et al. (1986). Acute cardiac events temporally related to cocaine abuse. *New England Journal of Medicine, 315,* 1438-1443.

37. Hannan, D. J., & Adler, A. G. (1990). Crack cocaine: Do you know enough about it? *Postgraduate Medicine, 88,* 141-139.

38. Wiener, R. S., Lockhart, J. T., & Schwartz, R. G. (1986). Dilated cardiomyopathy. *American Journal of Medicine, 81,* 699-701.

39. Cregler, L. L., & Mark, H. (1986). Medical complications of cocaine abuse. *New England Journal of Medicine, 315,* 1495-1500.

40. Mittleman, R. E., & Wetli, C. V. (1984). Death caused by recreational cocaine use: An update. *Journal of the American Medical Association, 252,* 1889-1893.

41. Staff. (1991). *Monday morning report.* Newsletter published by the Jacksonville Partnership for a Drug-Free America.

42. Manoguerra, A. (1990). The highs and lows of cocaine and amphetamine use. Emergency Nurses Association, Scientific Assembly, Chicago.

43. Eurman, D. W., et al. (1989). Chest pain and dyspnea related to "crack" cocaine smoking: Value of chest radiography. *Radiology, 172*(2), 459-462.

44. Alvert, R. E., Lippmann, M., & Briscoe, W. (1969). The characteristics of bronchial clearance in humans and the effects of cigarette smoking. *Archives of Environmental Health, 18,* 738-755.

45. Murray, R. J., et al. (1988). Diffuse alveolar hemorrhage temporally related to cocaine smoking. *Chest, 93,* 427-429.

46. Itkonen, J., Schnoll, S., & Glassroth, J. (1984). Pulmonary dysfunction in "freebase" cocaine users. *Archives of Internal Medicine, 144,* 2195-2197.

47. Moody, C. K., Miller, B. L., McIntyre, H. B., et al. (1988). Neurologic complications of cocaine abuse. *Neurology, 38*(8), 1189-1193.

48. Menashe, P. I., & Gottlieb, J. E. (1988). Hyperthermia, rhabdomyolysis, and myoglobinuric renal failure after recreational use of cocaine. *Southern Medical Journal, 81*(3), 379-380.

49. Goldfrank, L. R. (1986). *Goldfrank's toxicologic emergencies* (3rd ed.). Norwalk, CT: Appleton-Century-Crofts.

50. Sternbach, G., Moran, J., & Eliastom, M. (1980). Heroin addiction: Acute presentation of medical complications. *Annals of Emergency Medicine, 9,* 143.

51. King, P., & Coleman, J. H. (1987). Stimulant and narcotic drugs. *Pediatric Clinics of North America, 34*(2), 349-362.

Drug Appendix

Ruth Stanley

ANALGESICS

Nonsteroidal Antiinflammatory Agents (NSAIDs)

Pharmacology

These agents possess analgesic, antiinflammatory, and antipyretic properties. Their exact mechanism of action is not clearly established. All agents inhibit the enzyme cyclooxygenase, which leads to a reduction in prostaglandin biosynthesis. Prostaglandins, both peripherally and centrally, are involved in the regulation of body temperature, the sensitization of pain receptors, and the inflammatory response to injury. The differences in potency and pharmacological effects among these agents are secondary to a differential sensitivity of enzymes in various tissues to the individual agents.

Uses

As analgesics, these agents are effective for low to moderate intensity pain. They are effective for short-term use as antipyretics. Their chief clinical application is as antiinflammatory agents in the treatment of musculoskeletal disorders.

Dosing and Administration (See Table 1)

- All agents should be given with food, milk, or antacids to reduce gastric upset.
- These agents are contraindicated in pregnancy and in patients with a history of hypersensitivity to aspirin or other nonsteroidal antiinflammatory agents.
- Avoid the use of aspirin in children with influenza or chicken pox because of an increased risk for Reye's syndrome.
- Aspirin possesses greater antiplatelet effects than the other nonsteroidal antiinflammatory agents and may be used for transient ischemic attacks (325 mg qd) or myocardial infarction risk reduction (325 mg qd). See antiplatelet section on p. 1415.
- Monitor occult blood loss, visual changes, and weight gain.

Adverse Effects

- Renal dysfunction is common, especially in patients who depend on renal vasodilatory prostaglandins to maintain renal blood flow. Predispositions to NSAID-induced renal dysfunction are hypovolemia, hypotension, cirrhosis, diabetes mellitus, heart failure, glomerular disease, renal ischemia, chronic pyelonephritis, autoimmune disease, mild renal insufficiency, age greater than 60 years, and diuretic use. Manifestations include increased serum creatinine and BUN, sodium and water retention, hyponatremia, edema, and possible hypertension. The onset varies from 1 day to 2 months, most often occurring within the first 2 weeks. A history of previous tolerance to NSAIDs does not exclude the diagnosis; all agents have nephrotoxic potential in predisposed patients. The drug should be discontinued if patients experience significant impairment of renal function.
- Dyspepsia, heartburn, epigastric distress, nausea, and vomiting occur in 2% to 30% of patients. Occult gastrointestinal bleeding is dose related, painless, minimal (<10 ml/day), and greater with aspirin than with other NSAIDs. Acute hemorrhage from gastric erosion is rare.
- Other adverse effects include tinnitus, hypoprothrombinemia, hepatotoxicity, skin rash, visual changes, edema, and hematological effects.

Drug Interactions

- NSAIDs may enhance the hypoprothrombinemic effects of warfarin and heparin.
- NSAIDs may enhance the hypoglycemic effect of the sulfonylureas.
- Concurrent use with uricosurics, alcohol, lithium, or ulcerogenic drugs should be carefully monitored.

TABLE 1 **Nonsteroidal Antiinflammatory Agents (NSAIDs)**

Drug	Trade Name	Adult Dosage	Comments
Aspirin	Various	325-650 mg q4h PO (2.6-5.2 g/day)	Long safety record; increased GI effects with higher dosages; side effects include tinnitus
Indomethacin	Indocin	25-50 mg PO tid	Higher incidence of GI, CNS, and renal side effects; potent agent
Sulindac	Clinoril	150-200 mg PO bid	bid dosing; long half-life
Ibuprofen	Motrin, Advil	200-800 mg PO tid or qid	Long safety record; lower incidence of GI side effects
Naproxen	Naprosyn, Anaprox	250-500 mg PO q12h	Long acting; good safety profile; easily tolerated
Piroxicam	Feldene	10-20 mg PO qd	Dosages greater than 20 mg qd increase risk for GI bleeding
Ketorolac	Toradol	Loading dose: 30-60 mg IM, then one half loading dose q6h IM (max 120 mg/day) Oral dose: 10 mg q4-6h up to 40 mg maximum total daily dose	Only parenteral NSAID available; for short-term use only

- NSAIDs may reduce the antihypertensive effect of ACE inhibitors, diuretics, and calcium channel blockers in some patients.

Narcotic Analgesics

Pharmacology

The narcotic analgesics exhibit a wide range of activity and produce their main pharmacological effects by interacting with stereospecific opiate receptors in the central nervous system and other tissues. They are the most effective analgesics available and relieve pain by interfering with pain impulses at the subcortical level of the brain. Other CNS effects include medullary depression of respiration, stimulation of the chemoreceptor trigger zone, constriction of the pupils, and depression of the cough reflex. Gastrointestinal effects include an increase in smooth muscle tone and a decrease in propulsive movements and emptying time. Butorphanol and pentazocine are partial agonists with weak antagonist activity; both of these agents increase the cardiac workload and should be used cautiously in patients with cardiac disease.

Uses

These agents are indicated for moderate to severe pain. Morphine can be used to relieve the dyspnea of acute left ventricular failure and pulmonary edema.

Dosing and Administration (See Tables 2 and 3)

- Administration of these agents should be on a scheduled rather than a prn basis in patients with chronic debilitating pain (e.g., cancer) and in the first 24 to 48 hours postoperatively. Prevention of pain recurrence results in less suffering, slower tolerance development, easier dosage adjustment, less pain behavior, and usually lower narcotic requirements.
- The steady state effects of methadone, morphine, and levorphanol on CNS and respiratory depression may not occur for several days. To avoid accumulation, the dosages should be increased in small increments at weekly intervals when possible in patients receiving long-term therapy.
- Oxycodone and hydrocodone are available as combination products with acetaminophen.
- These agents should not be given by rapid IV push.
- Unpreserved solutions of morphine should be used for epidural or intrathecal analgesia.
- Fentanyl transdermal patches can be substituted for morphine in the management of chronic pain. A dosage of 60 mg IM per day or 360 mg PO per day of morphine is equivalent to a 10 mg (100 µg/hr) fentanyl transdermal patch. Most patients can be maintained by replacing the patches every 72 hours, but 48-hour intervals may be necessary in some patients. Supplemental opiates will be necessary in the first 24 hours of patch therapy.
- Initial dosages should be low and titrated up slowly. Reduce initial doses in elderly or debilitated patients. Some patients may require very high dosages if tolerance has developed with chronic use. These patients typically tolerate these dosages with minimal complications.
- Naloxone can be used to antagonize narcotic overdosage. Initial adult dosage is 0.4 mg (IM, IV, SC),

TABLE 2   Narcotic Analgesic Comparison

Drug	Analgesic	Antitussive	Sedative	Emetic	Constipative	Respiratory Depressive	Addictive
Codeine	+	+ + +	+	+	+	+ +	+ +
Fentanyl	+ + +	0	+ +	+	+	+ + +	+ + +
Hydromorphone	+ + +	+ +	+	+	+	+ + +	+ + +
Levorphanol	+ +	+ +	+ +	+	?	+ +	+ + +
Meperidine	+ + +	0	+	+	+	+ + +	+ + +
Methadone	+ + +	+ +	+	+	+	+ + +	+ +
Morphine	+ + +	+ +	+ +	+ +	+ +	+ + +	+ + +
Oxycodone	+ +	+ + +	+ +	+ +	+ +	+ + +	+ + +
Butorphanol	+	0	+ + +	+	?	+	+
Pentazocine	+	0	+	+	?	+	+

0 = no effect.
+ = mild effect.
+ + = moderate effect.
+ + + = significant effect.
? = unknown.

repeated at intervals of 2 to 3 minutes as needed. Monitor respiratory and circulatory depression.

Adverse Effects

- Respiratory and circulatory depression are the major adverse effects of the narcotic analgesics. These effects are dose related and may be seen with therapeutic dosing. Manifestations include miosis, drowsiness, decreased rate and depth of respiration, bradycardia, and hypotension. Rapid IV administration increases the risk for serious adverse effects.
- Other adverse effects include dizziness, sedation, nausea, vomiting, sweating, euphoria, dysphoria, dry mouth, and urinary retention. Skin rashes may occur with administration; allergic reactions are very rare.
- Meperidine has an active metabolite, normeperidine, which may precipitate tremors, myoclonus, or seizures. Predisposing factors include renal failure, history of seizures, and dosages greater than 100 mg every 2 hours for 24 hours or more.
- Use of concomitant CNS depressants should be cautiously monitored.
- All patients should be monitored for the development of constipation with continued dosing. The elderly and patients receiving high dosages are more prone to this adverse effect.
- All of the pure narcotic analgesics have high addiction potentials. Lowest possible dosages given over a short duration of therapy are recommended for the treatment of acute pain syndromes.

Acetaminophen (Tylenol, Various)

Pharmacology

Acetaminophen raises the pain threshold and affects the hypothalamic heat-regulating center. The drug inhibits prostaglandin synthesis in the central nervous system (CNS) through a peripheral action by blocking pain impulse generation. The peripheral action may also be related to inhibition of the synthesis or actions of other substances that sensitize pain receptors to mechanical or chemical stimulation. Acetaminophen may act predominantly on the CNS. The drug has the same analgesic activity as aspirin but lacks equivalent antiinflammatory and uricosuric activity.

Uses

Acetaminophen is used for mild to moderate pain and as an antipyretic.

Dosing and Administration

- The usual adult oral dose is 325 to 1,000 mg every 4 to 6 hours. Do not exceed a total daily dose of 4 g/day.

Adverse Effects

- Potentially fatal hepatic necrosis may occur with acute overdosage. Management of overdosage includes emesis, gastric lavage, and acetylcysteine if less than 24 hours have elapsed since ingestion. Activated charcoal should not be administered because it may interfere with the absorption of acetylcysteine. Plasma concentrations greater than 200 $\mu g/ml$ at 4 hours postingestion are associated with severe hepatic damage; toxicity is uncommon with plasma levels less than 150 $\mu g/ml$. Acetylcysteine administered within 10 to 16 hours of overdosage may minimize hepatotoxicity and can be given as a 140 mg/kg load followed by 70 mg/kg every 4 hours for 17 doses. Acetylcysteine should be diluted 1:3 in cola, grapefruit juice, soft drinks, or water.

TABLE 3 **Narcotic Analgesics**

Drug	Trade Name	Use	Adult Dosage	Route	Duration of Action (hr)	Equianalgesic Oral Dose* (mg)	Equianalgesic IM Dose* (mg)	Comments
Codeine	Various	Analgesia Anti-tussive	15-60 mg q4-6h 10-20 mg q4-6h	PO, SC, IM, IV PO, SC	3-6	200	120	Excellent antitussive agent
Fentanyl	Sublimaze	Analgesia	2.5-10 mg q48-72h	Transdermal patch	48-72		0.1	Used more commonly as an anesthetic; may be given epidurally or intrathecally for pain using parenteral solution
Hydro-morphone	Dilaudid	Analgesia Anti-tussive	2-4 mg q4h 3-6 mg q6-8h 1 mg q3-4h	PO, IV, IM PR PO	3-5	7.5	1.5	Higher doses may be used in terminally ill patients who exhibit tolerance
Levorphanol	Levo-dromo-ran	Analgesia	2-4 mg q6h	PO	4-6	4	2	May be used as a supplement to anesthesia; optimum dosage unclear
Meperidine	Demerol	Analgesia	50-150 mg q3-4h	PO, SC, IM, IV	2-4	150-200	75	Oral doses half as effective as parenteral doses; reduce dose when using with phenothiazine
Methadone	Dolo-phine	Analgesia	5-15 mg q4-6h 2.5-10 mg q3-4h	PO, SC IM	4-8	20	10	May be used for detoxification treatment

Drug	Brand	Indication	Dose	Route				Comments
Morphine	Various	Analgesia	8-20 mg q4h	PO	4-6	60	10	Intrathecal dose one tenth of epidural dose; some patients with chronic pain may require doses greater than 100 mg/hr for relief
			30-60 mg q8-12h	SR				
			2-15 mg q4h	SC, IM, IV				
			10-20 mg q4h	PR				
			1-10 mg/hr	IV infusion Epidural				
			Loading dose: 5 mg, then 1-2 mg max prn (max 10 mg/day)					
			1 mg per activation with 6-10-minute lockout	PCA				
Oxycodone	Various	Analgesia	5 mg q6h	PO	3-6	30	15	Most often used in combination with acetaminophen or aspirin
Butorphanol	Stadol	Analgesia	1-4 mg q4h	IM	3-4		2	Partial agonist
			0.5-2 mg q4h	IV				
Pentazocine	Talwin	Analgesia	50-100 mg q3-4h	PO	3-4	120	40	Partial agonist
			30-60 mg q3-4h	SC, IM, IV				

* Doses considered equivalent to 10 mg IM morphine and 60 mg PO morphine.

PO = oral.
SR = sustained release.
SC = subcutaneous.
IM = intramuscular.
IV = intravenous.
PR = rectal.
PCA = patient-controlled analgesia.

- Other uncommon adverse effects include anemia, pancytopenia, leukopenia, urticaria, and rare instances of methemoglobinemia and hemolytic anemia.
- Toxic hepatitis has been reported with chronic ingestion of greater than 5 g/day for several weeks or 3 g/day for a year.

Drug Interactions

- Concurrent use with anticoagulants may increase the anticoagulant effect.
- Use with alcohol or hepatic enzyme–inducing agents increases the risk of hepatotoxicity.

ANTIANGINAL AGENTS

Beta Blockers

Pharmacology

Beta-adrenergic blockers competitively inhibit adrenergic neuronal and hormonal action at the beta receptor. Beta$_1$-receptor inhibition results in decreased heart rate, electrical conduction, and contractility. Beta$_2$-receptor inhibition results in bronchoconstriction and peripheral vasoconstriction. Beta blockers are classified by their pharmacological actions such as cardioselective (beta$_1$-receptor antagonist with little beta$_2$), intrinsic sympathomimetic activity (some agonist properties), or lipophilicity (relative lipid solubility). At equipotent doses, most beta blockers exert the same effect on cardiac and vascular smooth muscle tissue.

Uses

Beta blockers are used for a myriad of disease states. The primary critical care uses of these agents are for acute myocardial infarction, dysrhythmias, hypertension, and angina.

Dosing and Administration (See Table 4)

- Metoprolol and atenolol can be used IV for the treatment of early acute myocardial infarction. These agents are excellent adjunct therapy to thrombolytics and aspirin. Oral therapy should be instituted after IV loading as follows: Metoprolol 50 mg every 6 hours for 48 hours, followed by 50 to 100 mg twice daily, and atenolol 50 mg every 12 hours for 48 hours, followed by 50 to 100 mg daily thereafter. Maintenance dosages should keep the heart rate between 50 and 60 beats per minute.
- Nadolol and atenolol dosages should be reduced in patients with a creatinine clearance less than 30 ml/min.
- Abrupt cessation of therapy should be avoided to prevent rebound hypertension or withdrawal. Taper the dosage gradually over 2 weeks.

- These agents are contraindicated in patients with severe bradycardia, third-degree heart block, overt left ventricular heart failure, peripheral vascular disease, Raynaud's phenomenon, poorly controlled diabetes mellitus, severe depression, and severe asthma or bronchospasm.
- These agents should be used cautiously in the elderly or in patients with diabetes mellitus, renal failure, liver disease, pregnancy, hypertension, hyperlipidemia, and COPD.
- These agents should be avoided in Prinzmetal's variant angina because they may worsen coronary spasm.
- These agents are effective in combination with nitrates and calcium blockers for the treatment of unstable angina.
- Vasodilatory beta blockers are selective beta$_1$ antagonists and beta$_2$ agonists. These properties allow for the beneficial effects of beta blockers for angina or hypertension while having the advantages of preventing adverse effects on pulmonary function and peripheral circulation. Celiprolol is the prototype for these agents.

Adverse Effects

- The major adverse effects of beta blockers are bronchospasm, cold extremities, bradycardia, heart block, excessive negative inotropic effects, insomnia, depression, and fatigue.
- These agents reduce exercise tolerance, elevate LDL lipoproteins, and reduce the quality of life. Vasodilative beta blockers, cardioselective beta blockers, and agents with intrinsic sympathomimetic activity may lessen these adverse effects.
- Beta blockers mask hypoglycemic symptoms that are mediated through the adrenergic system. These agents may also delay the recovery time to euglycemia.
- Other adverse effects include dizziness, weakness, nightmares, vivid dreams, and headache. These effects may be lessened by reductions in dosage or use of more hydrophilic agents.
- Impotence, nausea, rash, and hypotension may also occur with these agents.

Drug Interactions

- Concurrent use with oral diltiazem or verapamil may result in additive effects, especially when given in high doses.
- Concurrent use with digitalis glycosides may result in excessive bradycardia with possible heart block.
- Concurrent use with epinephrine, phenylephrine, or phenylpropanolamine may result in significant hypertension with excessive bradycardia or possible heart block.

TABLE 4 Beta Blockers

Agent	Trade Name	Adult Oral Dosage	Adult IV Dosage	Cardio Selective	Intrinsic Sympathomimetic Activity	Hydrophilic
Propranolol	Inderal	40-160 mg bid-qid	0.1-0.15 mg/kg given in 1-mg increments q5min	−	−	−
Metoprolol	Lopressor	50-100 mg bid	5 mg q5min × 3 doses	+	−	−
Atenolol	Tenormin	50-100 mg qd	5 mg q5min × 2 doses	+	−	+
Nadolol	Corgard	40-160 mg qd		−	−	+
Timolol	Blocadren	10-20 mg bid		−	−	−
Pindolol	Visken	5-30 mg bid		−	+	−
Dilevalol	Unicard	100-800 mg qd		−	+	−
Acebutolol	Sectral	200-600 mg bid		+	+	+
Betaxolol	Kerlone	10-40 mg qd		+	−	+
Esmolol	Brevibloc		500 µg/kg/min × 1 min, then 50 µg/kg/min titrated up by 50 µg/kg/min q5min; maximum dose: 300 µg/kg/min	+	−	−
Labetalol*	Normodyne Trandate	100-400 mg bid	IV push: 20 mg, then 40-80 mg q10-15min; maintenance infusion: 1-2 mg/min	−	+	−
Oxprenolol	Trasicor	80-240 mg bid or tid		−	+	−
Penbutalol	Levatol	10-20 mg qd		−	+	−
Carteolol*	Cartrol	2.5-10 mg qd		−	+	+
Celiprolol*	Selecor	400 mg qd		+	+	+
Bisoprolol	Monocor	5-10 mg qd		+	−	−

* Vasodilatory beta blockers.
+ = present.
− = absent.

- Concurrent use with isoproterenol may result in mutual inhibition of therapeutic effects.

Calcium Channel Blockers

Pharmacology

Calcium channel blockers inhibit the influx of extracellular calcium ions across the membranes of myocardial and smooth muscle cells. There are three classes of calcium blockers: papavarine derivatives (verapamil), benzothiazine derivatives (diltiazem), and dihydropyridine (DHP) derivatives (nifedipine, nicardipine, nitrendipine, nimodipine). Verapamil and diltiazem depress AV nodal tissue as well as vasodilate vascular tissue. The dihydropyridines such as nifedipine have no effect on nodal tissue and are primarily vasodilators. Bepridil is a unique agent with antianginal and class I antidysrhythmic properties. It is structurally unrelated to the three other classes of calcium channel blockers but inhibits transmembrane calcium influx significantly.

Uses

These agents are all equally effective in the treatment of coronary artery spasm, angina, and hypertension. Verapamil and diltiazem may be used for supraventricular dysrhythmias. Bepridil is only indicated for the treatment of unstable angina in patients who have failed to respond to other antianginal therapy.

Dosing and Administration (See Tables 5 and 6)

- Verapamil is the only calcium blocker for IV use in supraventricular tachycardia. IV verapamil can be given as a bolus 5 to 10 mg (0.1 to 0.15 mg/kg) over 1 minute and repeated 10 minutes later. If there is risk for hypotension, pretreat the patient with 1 g (90 mg elemental calcium) of calcium gluconate. An infusion of 0.0001 to 0.005 mg/kg/min can be titrated against ventricular response.
- Diltiazem and verapamil should be used cautiously in combination with beta blockers or other antidysrhythmics.
- Nimodipine is approved for use in subarachnoid hemorrhage only.
- Diltiazem and verapamil are contraindicated in patients with bradycardia, sick sinus syndrome, third-degree AV block, and significant left ventricular failure.
- The newer agents are DHP derivatives and have pharmacological actions similar to nifedipine. These agents are more selective for vascular smooth muscle and coronary vasculature. These properties may improve efficacy and reduce reflex-mediated adverse effects. These agents have significantly less negative inotropic effects than the first-generation agents.

- These agents do not affect the lipid profile and are safe for patients with hyperlipidemia. These agents improve quality of life and exercise tolerance.

Adverse Effects

- Verapamil: constipation, hypotension, bradycardia, headache, and dizziness.
- Diltiazem: rash, hypotension, bradycardia, headache.
- Nifedipine (and similar agents): dizziness, reflex tachycardia, flushing, headache, edema, nausea, hypotension, syncope, and rash.

Drug Interactions

- An additive effect may occur if diltiazem or verapamil are given with beta-adrenergic blocking agents. This additive effect may prolong AV conduction, which may lead to severe hypotension, bradycardia, and cardiac failure. This is especially true in patients with impaired ventricular function or abnormal cardiac conduction.
- Verapamil increases digoxin serum levels.
- Diltiazem increases cyclosporine serum levels.

Nitrates

Pharmacology

Nitrates relax smooth muscle in small blood vessels and dilate arteries and capillaries, especially in coronary circulation. Myocardial ischemia is reduced secondary to a reduction in left ventricular preload and afterload and a more efficient distribution of blood flow within the myocardium.

Uses

Nitrates are used for the treatment of angina, hypertension, and acute myocardial infarction.

Dosing and Administration (See Table 7)

- Tolerance develops with continued use of nitrates. Nitrate-free intervals of 8 to 16 hours are recommended to restore sulfhydryl groups, which are necessary for the peripheral metabolism of nitrates. Tolerance develops less rapidly in patients with poor left ventricular function. Transdermal patches are discouraged unless used intermittently. A daily schedule of 8 A.M. and 2 P.M. for twice-daily dosing is recommended.
- Sublingual tablets should cause a burning sensation when placed under the tongue.
- Nitroglycerin for injection should be diluted and placed in glass containers if possible. The IV drip should be titrated to relieve pain and keep the systolic blood pressure above 90 mmHg. Avoid concentrating the drip more than 150 mg per 250 ml of IV fluid.

TABLE 5 **Calcium Channel Blockers**

| Agent | Trade Name | Route | Onset (min) | Peak (hr) | Duration (hr) | Dosage (mg) | Cardiovascular Actions | | | | | |
| | | | | | | | Vasodilatation | | | Contractility | Heart Rate | AV Nodal Conduction |
							Peripheral	Coronary	Cerebral			
Diltiazem	Cardizem	Oral	30-90	0.5-1	6-10	30-120 q6-8h	+	+++	+	0, ↓	0, ↓	↓
		SR	Gradual	6-11	12-24	120-480 q12-24h						
		IV	2-5	0.25	1-2	0.25-0.35 mg/kg initially as bolus followed by 10- to 15-mg/hr infusion up to 24 hours						
Verapamil	Isoptin, Calan	Oral	30	0.5-1	6-8	40-120 q6-8h	++	+	+	↓↓	0, ↓	↓
		SR	Gradual	5-7	12-24	120-480 q12-24h						
		IV	1-5	0.25-0.5	2-4	5-10 mg IV bolus followed by 5-mg/hr infusion						
Nifedipine	Procardia, Adalat	Oral	30-90	0.5-2	4-8	10-30 q6-8h	+++	++	++	↓, Reflex ↑	0, Reflex ↑	0
		SR	Gradual		24	30-90 q24h						
		SL	10-30	0.5-1	3-4	10-20 prn						
Nicardipine	Cardene	Oral	20-30	0.5-2	6-8	20-40 q8h	+++	++	++	↓, Reflex ↑	0, Reflex ↑	0
Nitrendipine	Baypress	Oral	30-90	1-2	8-24	10-40 q12-24h						
Nimodipine	Nimotop	Oral		0.5-1	4-6	60 q4h for 21 days	+	+	+++	0	0	0

Adapted from Kinney, M. R., Packa, D. R., Andreoli, K. G., et al. (1991). *Comprehensive cardiac care* (7th ed.). St. Louis: Mosby–Year Book.

SR = sustained release.
SL = sublingual.
↑ = increase.
0 = no change.
↓ = decrease.
+ = mild.
+ + = moderate.
+ + + = potent.

TABLE 6   **Second-generation Calcium Antagonists*****

Drug	Trade Name	Adult Oral Dosage	Negative Inotropic Effects	Systemic Vasodilation	Vasodilatory Side Effects	Adverse Effects	Comments
Amlodipine	Norvasc	2.5-10 mg qd	0	+ +	+	Peripheral edema; dizziness; flushing; tachycardia and headache less than with other DHPs	Long-acting once-daily therapy
Felodipine	Plendil	5-10 mg qd	+	+ +	+ +	Peripheral edema; headache; dizziness; flushing; fatigue	Higher doses poorly tolerated; twice-daily therapy usually necessary
Isradipine	DynaCirc	2.5-10 mg bid	0	+ +	+ +	Ankle edema; fatigue; facial flushing; arthralgias; headache	Doses for angina are 2.5-7.5 mg tid; increased ADR with higher doses
Nisoldipine	Baymycard	10 mg qd or bid	0	+ +	+ +	Ankle edema; flushing; headache; dizziness	May be better tolerated

* All are dihydropyridine (DHP) derivatives with more selectivity for vascular smooth muscle.
   0 = no effect.
   + = minimal effect.
   + + = maximal effect.
ADR = adverse drug reactions.

TABLE 7 Nitrates

Agent	Onset (min)	Peak (hr)	Duration (hr)	Dose
ISOSORBIDE DINITRATE				
Sublingual	5-20	0.5-1.0	1-3	2.5-10 mg prn
Oral tablet	15-45	1-2	4-6	10-100 mg q3-6h
Sustained release	30-180	1-2	6-12	20-80 mg q6-12h
NITROGLYCERIN				
Sublingual	2-5		0.25-0.5	0.2-0.6 mg prn
Buccal	1-2	0.5	4-6	1-3 mg q4-6h
Spray	2-5		0.25-0.5	1 or 2 sprays prn
Topical paste	30-60	2-3	3-6	0.5-3 inches q3-6h
Transdermal patch	30-60	2-3	12-24	2.5-15 mg daily
Tablet	20-45	1-2	3-6	6.5-19.5 mg q4-6h
Intravenous	<1		0.25-0.5	10-300 µg/min
Sustained release	20-45	1-2	8-12	2.6-9 mg q8-12h
ISOSORBIDE MONONITRATE				
Oral tablet	30-60	1-2	4-6	20 mg given 7 hours apart

Adapted from Kinney, M. R., Packa, D. R., Andreoli, K. G., et al. (1991). *Comprehensive cardiac care* (7th ed.). St. Louis: Mosby–Year Book.

Adverse Effects

- Common adverse effects are hypotension, syncope, dizziness, headache, flushing, tachycardia, and nausea. These effects are dose related and may be alleviated by reducing the dosage. Tolerance will usually develop in 1 to 2 weeks with stable therapy. Acetaminophen will relieve headache symptoms. If symptoms continue after 1 to 2 weeks, the dosage should be reduced.
- Rashes are common in patients treated with patches or ointment. The site of placement should be rotated daily to prevent sensitivity reactions.
- Methemoglobinemia and bradycardia may occur rarely with excessive dosing.

ANTIDYSRHYTHMICS

Class IA Agents

Pharmacology (See Table 8)

These agents block the sodium channel with moderate affinity, thus prolonging the repolarization time and action potential duration. The effective refractory period/action potential duration ratio (ERP/APD) is increased. Quinidine has mild vagolytic effects, which may facilitate AV conduction and increase the ventricular rate in atrial flutter or fibrillation. Disopyramide is forty times more potent as an inhibitor of muscarinic receptors. This inhibition results in significant anticholinergic side effects and a reflex sympathetic response that blocks the depressant effects of disopyramide on nodal and conduction tissue. Quinidine and procainamide are ganglionic blockers and may produce hypotension with IV administration. Moricizine acts slightly differently in ventricular tissue and shortens the action potential duration.

Uses

These agents are used for the treatment of ventricular dysrhythmias. Quinidine, disopyramide, and procainamide are also useful in treating atrial fibrillation, atrial flutter, and supraventricular dysrhythmias.

Dosing and Administration (See Table 9)

- The dosages of all these agents should be reduced in patients with creatinine clearance less than or equal to 30 ml/min. The typical starting dose is half the recommended dose or the usual dose at twice the recommended interval.
- Trough levels should be measured for all these agents. Steady state levels are usually achieved within 36 hours with most of these agents. With the use of regular release procainamide capsules, steady state is achieved within 16 hours.
- Procainamide has an active metabolite, N-acetylprocainamide (NAPA), which is eliminated renally and has class III antidysrhythmic properties. NAPA may accumulate in patients with renal impairment and should be monitored. Normal levels are 10 to 20 µg/ml.
- Oral loading doses of these agents are discouraged because of poor GI tolerance.

TABLE 8 Electrophysiological Effects of Antidysrhythmic Agents*

Agent	Sinus Rate	PR	QRS	QT	A-H	H-V	ERP: AV Node	ERP: His-Purkinje	ERP: Atrium	ERP: Ventricle
Disopyramide	0, ↑	0, ↑	↑	↑	↑, →	0, ↑	↑, →	0, ↑	↑	↑
Procainamide	0	0, ↑	↑	↑	0, ↑	0, ↑	0, ↑	0, ↑	↑	↑
Quinidine	0, ↑	0, ↑	↑	↑	↑, →	0, ↑	↑, →	0, ↑	↑	↑
Lidocaine	0	0	0	0	0, ↑, →	0, ↑	↑, →	0, ↓	0	0
Mexiletine	0	0	0	0	0	0	↑, →	0, ↑	0	→
Tocainide	0	0	0	0, →	0	0	→	0	0	0
Phenytoin	0	0	0	0, ↓	0	0	0, →	→	→	→
Flecainide	0	↑	↑	0	↑	↑	0	0, ↑	0, ↑	0
Propafenone	0	↑	↑	↑	↑	↑	↑	↑	↑	↑
Indecainide	0	↑	↑	0	↑	0	↑	0	0	0
Propranolol	↓	0, ↑	0	0, ↓	0, ↑	0	↑	0	0	0
Amiodarone	↓	↑	0, ↑	↑	↑	0, ↑	↑	0	0, ↑	↑, →
Bretylium	0, ↑	0	0	0	0	0	→, ↑	0	↑, →	0, ↑
Verapamil	0, ↓	0, ↑	0	0	0, ↑	0	↑	0	0, →	0

From Kinney, M. R., Packa, D. R., Andreoli, K. G., et al. (1991). *Comprehensive cardiac care* (7th ed.). St. Louis: Mosby–Year Book.
* See Tables 9 through 12 for trade names and classes of dysrhythmic agents.
↑ = increase.
↓ = decrease.
0 = no change.
ERP = effective refractory period.

TABLE 9 **Class IA Antidysrhythmics**

Drug	Trade Name	Adult Dosage	Route	Plasma Concentration (µg/ml)	Half-life (hr)	Adverse Effects	Comments
Disopyra-mide	Norpace	100-300 mg q6h 150-300 mg q12h	PO SR	4-8	3-8	Dry mouth; urinary retention; CHF; QRS-QT prolongation; prominent vagolytic and negative inotropic effects	Weakest agent of class; high incidence of ADR
Moricizine	Ethmozine	200-300 mg q8h	PO	2-4		Dysrhythmias; dizziness; nausea; headache; fatigue; dyspnea; palpitations	Unique agent; lowest incidence of non-cardiac adverse effects
Procainamide	Procan, various	Loading dose: 10-15 mg/kg at 20-50 mg/min, then 1- to 4-mg/min infusion 250-1,000 mg q3-4h 500-2,000 mg q6h	IV PO SR	4-8	3-4 3-4 6-8	Hypotension (IV use only); torsades de pointes; lupuslike syndrome; arthralgias; rash; positive antinuclear antibodies (ANA); nausea; prodysrhythmic; neutropenia	Give IV no faster than 50 mg/min; IM therapy painful and absorption variable; reduce dosage in renal failure
Quinidine	Quinaglute, various	IV load: 5-8 mg/kg at 0.3 mg/kg/min 200-600 mg q6-8h 324-648 mg q6-12h	IV PO SR	2-5	6-11 6-12	Nausea; diarrhea; abdominal cramps; vomiting; cinchonism; prodysrhythmic; thrombocytopenia; leukopenia; hepatotoxicity; torsades de pointes	Avoid IM administration; concomitant use with digoxin increases digoxin levels

SR = sustained release.
ADR = adverse drug reactions.
CHF = congestive heart failure.

- Patients with atrial fibrillation or flutter should be digitalized before receiving quinidine.
- Monitor blood levels, ECG, CBC.

Adverse Effects (See Table 9)

- The most common adverse effects of disopyramide are anticholinergic and can be alleviated by reducing the dosage. Exacerbation of heart failure develops in 15% of patients with no history of congestive heart failure and 80% of patients with a positive history.
- Nausea, vomiting, and anorexia are common with these agents, especially procainamide and quinidine. These agents may be given with food or antacid to reduce GI irritation.
- Diarrhea is most common with quinidine, and tolerance usually develops in 1 to 2 weeks. Giving quinidine with food or antacids, changing to the gluconate salt preparation, or temporary use of antidiarrheal agents usually alleviates these effects.

Class IB Agents

Pharmacology (See Table 8)

These agents block fast sodium channels with less potency than the class IA agents. These actions result in a shortening of the action potential duration and the repolarization time. The ERP/APD ratio is increased with these agents. Class IB agents are selective for diseased tissue where they bind to inactive sodium channels and interrupt reentry circuits. These drugs have affinity for ventricular tissue only.

Uses

These agents are used in the treatment of ventricular dysrhythmias.

Dosing and Administration (See Table 10)

- Lidocaine is available for parenteral use only. The clearance of lidocaine decreases with continued therapy; thus, serum levels should be monitored. Steady state levels are achieved in 6 hours.
- The dosages of all these agents should be adjusted in renal failure.
- Dosages greater than 1,200 mg/day of mexiletine or tocainide are associated with a higher incidence of toxicity. Steady state serum levels are achieved 36 to 48 hours after initiation of therapy. Trough levels should be drawn.
- These agents may be used in combination with other antidysrhythmics for complex, life-threatening ventricular dysrhythmias.

Adverse Effects (See Table 10)

- Mexiletine and tocainide may be given with food to reduce GI upset.

- Most CNS and GI adverse effects are dose related and may be alleviated by reducing the dosage.

Class IC Agents

Pharmacology (See Table 8)

The class IC antidysrhythmics are potent inhibitors of the sodium channel. They primarily slow conduction through the His-Purkinje system and prolong refractory periods with little effect on action potential duration and increase the ERP/APD ratio. These agents are the most potent antidysrhythmics of this class and the most prodysrhythmic.

Uses

These agents are used in the treatment of life-threatening ventricular dysrhythmias.

Dosing and Administration (See Table 11)

- Titrate doses slowly with increments of 3 to 5 days between changes in dose. More rapid escalation of dosages may result in serious toxicity.
- Trough levels are useful with flecainide or indecainide therapy. Steady state is achieved in 3 to 5 days.
- These agents should be monitored closely because of their prodysrhythmic potential.

Adverse Effects (See Table 11)

- Most adverse effects are dose related and may be alleviated by reducing the dosage. GI side effects may be minimized by giving the agent with food or antacid.
- Flecainide possesses significant negative inotropic effects. Heart failure may be exacerbated in patients with serum levels greater than 1 mg/ml, ejection fractions less than 35%, and complex ventricular dysrhythmias.
- All these agents are prodysrhythmic in 10% to 15% of patients.

Class III Agents

Pharmacology (See Table 8)

Class III agents lengthen the action potential duration and refractory period. These agents increase the ERP/APD ratio. The class III agents vary in structure and exact mechanism of action.

Uses

These agents are used for ventricular dysrhythmias. Amiodarone can also be used for atrial dysrhythmias or supraventricular dysrhythmias.

Dosing and Administration (See Table 12)

- Amiodarone distributes extensively into tissues, and the half-life is approximately 40 to 80 days. Serum

TABLE 10 Class IB Antidysrhythmics

Drug	Trade Name	Adult Dose	Route	Plasma Concentration (µg/ml)	Half-life (hr)	Adverse Effects	Comments
Lidocaine	Xylocaine, various	Loading dose: 1-2 mg/kg, then 1- to 4-mg/min infusion	IV	1.5-6	1.5	Headache; drowsiness; dizziness; disorientation; confusion; light-headedness; hypersensitivity	Side effects are dose related and mild
Mexiletine	Mexitil	150-400 mg q8h	PO	0.5-2	12	Tremor; dizziness; light-headedness; parathesias; confusion; nausea; vomiting; anorexia; rash	Give doses with meals or snacks; often used in combination with IA agents
Phenytoin	Dilantin, various	IV load: 10-15 mg/kg at 20-50 mg/min; 100-200 mg q8h	IV; PO, IV	10-20	24	Nystagmus; sedation; confusion; gingival hyperplasia; hypotension; rash; fever; leukopenia; folate deficiency	Rarely used as an antidysrhythmic; oral sustained release capsules can be given as a daily dose rather than q8h
Tocainide	Tonocard	400-800 mg q8h	PO	4-10	12	Blood dyscrasias; lung fibrosis; tremor; dizziness; lethargy; seizure; psychosis; nausea; vomiting; anorexia	Precise role unclear; more toxic than mexiletine

TABLE 11 Class IC Antidysrhythmics

Drug	Trade Name	Adult Dosage	Route	Plasma Concentration (µg/ml)	Half-life (hr)	Adverse Effects	Comments
Encainide*	Enkaid	25-50 mg q6-8h	PO		3-4	Dizziness; light-headedness; visual disturbances; headache; prodysrhythmic; metallic taste; tremor	Two long-acting metabolites that are more potent than encainide; may increase risk of lethal dysrhythmias
Flecainide	Tambocor	50-200 mg q12h	PO	0.2-1.0	16-20	Negative inotrope; CHF; prodysrhythmic; anorexia; nausea; vomiting; visual disturbances; dizziness	Adverse effects seen in 10% to 30% of patients; avoid in CHF patients
Indecainide	Decabid	50-200 mg q12h	PO	300-900	15	Dizziness; headache; nausea; prodysrhythmic	Reduce dosage in renal impairment
Propafenone	Rhythmol	150-300 mg q8h	PO		3-6	Dizziness; headache; altered taste; nausea; constipation; negative inotrope; CHF	Saturable first-pass absorption; may increase prothrombinemic effect of warfarin

*Removed from commercial sales in 12/91; available for compassionate use only.
CHF = congestive heart failure.

TABLE 12 **Class III Antidysrhythmics**

Drug	Trade Name	Adult Dosage	Route	Adverse Effects	Comments
Amiodarone	Cordarone	800-1,600 mg/day for 7-10 days, then 200-600 mg qd	PO	Pulmonary fibrosis; hyperthyroidism; torsades de pointes; metallic taste; bradycardia; tremor; anorexia; headache; hypothyroidism; myopathy; nausea; corneal microdeposits; photosensitivity; increased liver function tests	Increased digoxin levels; increased prothrombinemic effect of warfarin
Bretylium	Bretylol	Loading dose: 5-10 mg/kg, then 1- to 4-mg/min infusion	IV	Hypotension; nausea and vomiting with rapid IV administration in conscious patients	Loading doses can be repeated up to a total of 15 mg/kg administered
Sotalol	Sotacor	160-480 mg q12h	PO	Bradycardia; worsened CHF; torsades de pointes; similar ADR as other beta blockers	Contraindications usually seen with other beta blockers

CHF = congestive heart failure.
ADR = adverse drug reactions.

levels are a poor indicator of efficacy and are not recommended.
- Avoid rapid IV push of bretylium.
- Amiodarone should be loaded orally over 7 to 10 days, then the dose reduced to the lowest effective dosage. It may take weeks to months to achieve steady state.

Adverse Effects (See Table 12)
- Amiodarone causes adverse effects in 100% of patients receiving the drug. Most side effects are seen at dosages greater than 400 mg/day.
- Patients should be carefully monitored while receiving amiodarone with periodic evaluations of the eye, thyroid function, pulmonary function, hepatic function, cardiac function, and neurological function.

Miscellaneous (Adenosine, Atropine)

Pharmacology

Adenosine vasodilates coronary arteries, reduces atrial contractility, depresses SA and AV nodal activity, and inhibits the stimulating effect of catecholamines on the myocardium. Atropine is used to antagonize the effects of increased vagal tone.

Uses

Adenosine is used for the conversion of paroxysmal supraventricular tachycardia to normal sinus rhythm.

Dosing and Administration
- Adenosine is available IV only and given as a 6 mg rapid IV bolus over 1 to 2 seconds and repeated in 1 to 2 minutes if needed. Doses of 12 mg may be used for the repeated dosages.
- Atropine should be given as a 0.5 to 1 mg rapid bolus and repeated until a total dose of 2 mg is reached. This agent may be administered through the endotracheal tube if necessary.

Adverse Effects
- The major adverse effects of adenosine are facial flushing, dyspnea, retrosternal chest pressure, and dysrhythmias. Most side effects are transient and last less than 1 minute.
- Usual side effects of atropine are urinary retention, dryness of the skin and mucous membranes, blurred vision, tachycardia, and mydriasis. Dosages greater than 5 mg may produce speech disturbances, swallowing difficulties, ataxia, confusion, and delirium.

ANTICONVULSANTS

Phenobarbital

Pharmacology

Barbiturates act as nonselective depressants of the central nervous system, capable of producing all levels of CNS mood alteration from excitation to mild sedation, hypnosis, and deep coma. Recent studies suggest that the sedative-hypnotic and anticonvulsant effects of barbiturates may be related to their ability to enhance and/or mimic the inhibitory synaptic action of gamma-aminobutyric acid (GABA). Barbiturates produce their sedative-hypnotic effect by depressing the sensory cortex, decreasing motor activity, and altering cerebral function, which produces drowsiness, sedation, or hypnosis. The barbiturates appear to act at the level of the thalamus, where they inhibit ascending conduction in the reticular formation, thus interfering with the transmission of impulses to the cortex. Barbiturates are believed to act as anticonvulsants by depressing monosynaptic and polysynaptic transmission in the CNS. They also increase the threshold for electrical stimulation of the motor cortex.

Uses

Phenobarbital is used as an anticonvulsant, anxiolytic, or sedative-hypnotic.

Dosing and Administration

- For status epilepticus, give 250 mg IV at a rate no greater than 60 mg/min. Dose may be repeated every 30 minutes up to a maximum of 20 mg/kg until seizures are controlled.
- For epilepsy, give 30 mg PO or IM two or three times daily initially and increase in increments of 60 mg/day every 5 days to effective dosage. IM injections should be administered deep into large muscles.
- Subcutaneous injections of the commercially available parenteral solutions should be avoided because of tissue irritation and possible necrosis. Treatment of subcutaneous irritation or extravasation involves the application of moist heat and the injection of 0.5% procaine hydrochloride to the immediate area.
- Phenobarbital should be withdrawn gradually to avoid precipitation of withdrawal seizures.
- Monitor trough levels of phenobarbital. Steady state is usually achieved in 14 to 21 days if no loading dose is given. Normal therapeutic range is 15 to 40 μg/ml. Toxicity develops at levels greater than 40 μg/ml and is manifested by ataxia, dysarthria, and nystagmus. Stupor and coma may develop with levels above 70 μg/ml.
- Monitor blood levels, CBC, and liver function tests.

Adverse Effects

- Dose-related sedation is the most common side effect; tolerance usually develops with continued administration. Paradoxical excitement may occur in children or elderly patients.
- Other side effects include confusion, nausea, dizziness, diplopia, skin rashes, hepatitis, exfoliative dermatitis, folate deficiency, and respiratory depres-

sion. Respiratory depression is more common with IV use, particularly when the drug is infused faster than 60 mg/min.

Drug Interactions

- Phenobarbital levels may be increased in the elderly or in patients receiving valproic acid or phenytoin.
- Phenobarbital levels may be decreased in children or in patients with alkaline urine.
- Concomitant use of alcohol, anesthetics, or other CNS depressants may increase the CNS depressant effects of phenobarbital.

Phenytoin

Pharmacology

Phenytoin's anticonvulsant action is not completely known, but it is believed to stabilize neuronal membranes and limit the spread of seizure activity by either increasing the efflux or decreasing the influx of sodium ions across cell membranes during generation of nerve impulses.

Uses

Phenytoin is used in treating seizures and ventricular dysrhythmias. It is the drug of choice for generalized tonic=clonic seizures.

Dosing and Administration

- An IV loading dose of 15 to 18 mg/kg given at a rate no greater than 50 mg/min produces therapeutic plasma levels for up to 18 to 24 hours in most patients. IM administration is painful and not recommended because of slow absorption and phenytoin crystal deposition in the muscle. Oral maintenance therapy should be initiated within 12 hours of the loading dose.
- Therapy may be initiated with an oral loading dose by giving 1,000 mg divided into 3 doses (i.e., 400 mg, 300 mg, 300 mg) over a 4-hour period. An alternative regimen is 19 mg/kg total dose divided over 6 to 12 hours.
- Oral maintenance dosages range from 300 to 500 mg/day or 4 to 7 mg/kg/day. Phenytoin undergoes dose-dependent metabolism, and small increases in dosage may result in disproportionately large increases in plasma levels. Therefore, dosages should be increased cautiously and serum levels followed closely. Dosages should be individualized to therapeutic response and blood levels.
- Serum levels should be monitored closely. The usual therapeutic range is 10 to 20 μg/ml for both adults and children. Serum levels may be drawn 2 to 4 hours after an intravenous loading dose, and serum trough levels measured periodically after initiating therapy. Peak concentrations are most useful for detecting toxicity. Serum concentrations should be

interpreted in conjunction with the patient's clinical response, concurrent drug therapy, and desired therapeutic endpoint.

- When anticonvulsants are to be discontinued, dosages should be reduced gradually to prevent possible seizures.
- Phenytoin is an alkaline solution and should be diluted for IV use in ½ normal saline or normal saline only. It should not be mixed with other medications or fluids as precipitation may occur.
- Concurrent use of a benzodiazepine is recommended for status epilepticus because phenytoin's anticonvulsant effects are not evident for 20 to 30 minutes after the start of infusion.
- Monitor blood levels, CNS effects, seizure activity, CBC, and liver function tests.

Adverse Effects

- Most adverse effects are dose related and begin to develop with concentrations in excess of 20 μg/ml. CNS effects include dizziness, nystagmus (15 to 30 μg/ml), blurred vision, ataxia (>30 μg/ml), confusion, dysarthria, drowsiness, and coma (>40 μg/ml).
- Bradycardia and hypotension are common with rapid IV administration, and slowing the rate of administration should alleviate these complications. The IV rate of administration should never exceed 50 mg/min.
- Hypersensitivity reactions are uncommon and usually occur within 2 months. Such reactions include fever, elevated liver function tests, lymphoid hyperplasia, eosinophilia, erythema multiforme, leukopenia, exfoliative dermatitis, thrombocytopenia, and serum sickness.
- Chronic, long-term administration of phenytoin may lead to hypertrichosis, gingival hyperplasia, folate deficiency, and coarsening of facial features.
- Reduced albumin concentration leads to increased free levels of phenytoin. Therefore, therapeutic effects may be seen with "low" plasma levels and toxicity with "normal" plasma levels.

Drug Interactions

- The following factors may increase phenytoin serum concentrations: hepatic immaturity (preterm infants); chronic liver disease; and concomitant drug therapy with barbiturates, chloramphenicol, disulfiram, isoniazid, warfarin, cimetidine, amiodarone, sulfonamides, valproic acid, and trimethoprim.
- The following factors may decrease phenytoin serum concentrations: age (0 to 12 weeks); pregnancy; renal disease; mononucleosis; acute hepatitis; alcohol; and concomitant drug therapy with barbiturates, carbamazepine, folic acid, antineo-

plastic agents, diazoxide, rifampin, and sucralfate.
- Phenytoin decreases the therapeutic effects of calciferol, dexamethasone, doxycycline, and levodopa.
- Concurrent use of phenytoin with oral contraceptives may result in reduced contraceptive reliability and/or loss of seizure control.
- Concurrent use of phenytoin with antidysrhythmics can produce additive cardiac depressant effects.

ANTIDEPRESSANTS AND ANXIOLYTICS

Antidepressants

Pharmacology

Heterocyclic and related antidepressants block, in varying degrees, the reuptake of various neurotransmitters at the neuronal membrane. These agents potentiate the effects of norepinephrine and serotonin. The tricyclic antidepressants produce strong anticholinergic activity, direct quinidine-like cardiotoxic properties, and various degrees of sedation in normal patients. Therapeutic dosages of these agents do not affect respiration, but overdosage results in respiratory depression.

Uses

These agents are primarily used in depressive affective (mood) disorders.

Dosing and Administration (See Table 13)

- The initial dose should be reduced in geriatric patients or in patients with cardiovascular or hepatic disease.
- Symptoms of depression (e.g., insomnia, anorexia, decreased energy) should improve after 1 week, while mood (e.g., pessimism, hopelessness) may require 2 to 4 weeks.
- Moderate to severe toxicity occurs with antidepressant doses of 10 to 20 mg/kg, while doses greater than 30 to 40 mg/kg are often fatal. Treatment of overdosage involves symptomatic and supportive care.

Adverse Effects

- Sedation, postural hypotension, and anticholinergic side effects are the most common adverse effects.
- Antidepressants may lower the seizure threshold and should be used cautiously in patients with a history of seizure disorder.
- These agents are contraindicated in the initial recovery phase after myocardial infarction.

Drug Interactions

- Antidepressants may potentiate or be additive to other CNS depressants such as hypnotics, sedatives, anxiolytics, and alcohol.

TABLE 13 Commonly Used Antidepressants

Drug	Trade Name	Adult Oral Dosages*	Biochemical Effects		Sedation	Anticholinergic
			S	N		
Amitriptyline	Elavil, various	75-150 mg/day	++++	++	++++	++++
Desipramine	Norpramin, various	75-150 mg/day	0	++++	++	++
Doxepin	Sinequan, various	75-150 mg/day	++	+	++++	+++
Imipramine	Tofranil, various	75-150 mg/day	+++	++	+++	+++
Nortriptyline	Pamelor, Aventil	75-150 mg/day	+++	++	+++	++
Trazodone	Desyrel, various	100-400 mg/day	+++	0	++	+
Fluoxetine	Prozac	20-40 mg/day	+++	0	0	+
Buproprion†	Wellbutrin	200-400 mg/day	0	0	0	0
Sertraline	Zoloft	50-200 mg/day	+++	0	0/+	0

* Maintenance dosages listed; acute dosages may be higher in severe depression.
† Affects dopamine only.

    0 = none.
    + = slight.
  + + = moderate.
 + + + = high.
+ + + + = very high.
    S = serotonin uptake blocked.
    N = norepinephrine uptake blocked.

- These agents may block the antihypertensive effect of clonidine and guanethidine.

Anxiolytics (Benzodiazepines)

Pharmacology

The exact mechanism of action of the benzodiazepines is unclear, and the differences in individual agents is probably a result of different specific mechanisms of sites of action. All agents exert their action in the CNS and potentiate the neural inhibition that is mediated by gamma-aminobutyric acid (GABA). There are many GABA binding sites at all levels of the neuraxis that lead to varying degrees of sedation, hypnosis, muscle relaxation, anticonvulsant activity, and anxiolytic activity.

Uses

Benzodiazepines may be used as anxiolytics, sedative-hypnotics, anticonvulsants, muscle relaxants, preoperative anesthetics, or for the prevention of alcohol withdrawal.

Dosage and Administration (See Table 14)

- IM doses should be injected deeply and slowly into a large muscle mass.
- Diazepam is poorly compatible with most IV fluids and adsorbs to the plastic of most intravenous infusion bags and tubing. The drug should be given by slow direct intravenous injection when possible.
- Higher initial doses of chlordiazepoxide, diazepam, oxazepam, and lorazepam may be necessary when used for alcohol withdrawal. Doses may be reduced after the first day and titrated off within 5 days in most instances. Benzodiazepines are preferred over other anxiolytics for alcohol withdrawal because of equal efficacy, superior anticonvulsant activity, and less toxicity. No evidence suggests that one benzodiazepine is superior.
- Elderly patients or those with hepatic disease may exhibit enhanced CNS sensitivity to these agents. Initial dosages should be reduced in these populations.
- Abrupt discontinuation of these agents may lead to withdrawal. The drug should be gradually tapered (10% reductions at weekly intervals) in those patients who are psychologically or physically dependent on these agents. This is particularly important in patients with seizure disorders to prevent recurrence of seizure activity.

Adverse Effects

- The most frequent adverse effects include drowsiness, dizziness, ataxia, fatigue, vertigo, syncope, and confusion. These effects are usually seen with initiation of therapy and may dissipate with con-

tinued therapy or dose reductions.
- Paradoxical CNS stimulation manifested by talkativeness, restlessness, euphoria, anxiety, and excitement may occur. These behaviors are more commonly seen in children and psychiatric patients. The drug should be discontinued if CNS stimulation occurs.
- Other adverse effects include headache, nausea, weight changes, metallic taste, amnesia, and behavioral effects.
- Bradycardia, hypotension, apnea, and cardiac arrest have occurred with rapid parenteral administration of benzodiazepines.

Drug Interactions

- Avoid concurrent use with monoamine oxidase inhibitors.
- Concurrent use with CNS depressants produces additive depression.
- Increased pharmacological effects of benzodiazepines may be seen with concomitant drug therapy including cimetidine, oral contraceptives, disulfiram, and omeprazole.

ANTIEMETICS

Pharmacology and Uses

Prochlorperazine, promethazine, and thiethylperazine are phenothiazine neuroleptics that are primarily used for their antiemetic properties. These agents suppress the chemoreceptor trigger zone (CTZ) in the CNS. They are poorly effective for motion sickness or vertigo.

Diphenhydramine and hydroxyzine are antihistamines that have CNS depressant, anticholinergic, antiemetic, antihistaminic, and local anesthetic effects. The antiemetic effect is secondary to inhibition of vestibular stimulation. These agents are weak antiemetics and are primarily used for motion sickness or vertigo.

Metoclopramide is a unique agent that blocks dopamine receptors in the CTZ and promotes gastric emptying. It is primarily used as an antiemetic.

Ondansetron is a serotonin antagonist that is highly selective for serotonin with no effect on dopamine receptors. It is indicated for chemotherapy prophylaxis only.

Dosing and Administration (See Table 15)

- None of these agents is indicated for subcutaneous administration.

Adverse Effects

- Adverse effects common to all these agents are drowsiness, dizziness, dry mouth, hypotension, and urinary retention.

TABLE 14 **Commonly Used Benzodiazepines**

Drug	Trade Name	Adult Dosage	Route	Active Metabolite	Half-life (hr)	Major Indications	Comments
Chlordiazepoxide	Librium, various	15-100 mg/day 50 mg initially, 25-50 mg q6-8h	PO IV, IM	Yes	5-30	Anxiety, alcohol withdrawal	Efficacy of long-term use not established (24 months); available in combination products; for IM administration, use manufacturer's diluent only
Diazepam	Valium, various	6-40 mg/day 2-10 mg initially and repeated q3-4h prn	PO IV, IM	Yes	20-50	Anxiety, muscle relaxation, status epilepticus, alcohol withdrawal	For status epilepticus — 10 mg IV stat and repeat q10-15min up to a total dose of 30 mg; do not exceed IV rate of 5 mg/min; drug may precipitate when diluted; do not mix with other IV solutions; avoid extravasation; administer directly into large veins when possible
Alprazolam	Xanax	0.75-4 mg/day	PO	Yes	12-19	Anxiety, depression	Effective in the treatment of panic disorders using dosages up to 16 mg/day; more effective than diazepam in mixed anxiety/depression
Lorazepam	Ativan, various	1-10 mg/day 1-4 mg q8-12h 0.25-0.5 mg/hr	PO IM, IV IV infusion	No	10-20	Anxiety, alcohol withdrawal	Can be used preoperatively to lessen anxiety; useful for ventilator-dependent patients who need an effective sedative/anxiolytic
Oxazepam	Serax, various	30-120 mg/day	PO	No	5-10	Anxiety, alcohol withdrawal	Effective for short-term oral maintenance in alcohol withdrawal protocols; useful in patients with hepatic disease who require benzodiazepines

Drug	Trade name	Dosage	Route		Half-life	Indication	Comments
Flurazepam	Dalmane, various	15-60 mg/day	PO	Yes		Insomnia	Rapidly and completely metabolized to active metabolite; unwanted morning hangover or drowsiness common in up to 40% of patients, especially the elderly
Midazolam	Versed	0.5-2.5 mg initially and repeat at intervals of 2-3 min up to a total dose of 100-150 µg/kg, then repeat as needed for sedation	IV, IM	No	1-2	Sedation, anxiety	Reduce dosage by 25% with concomitant opiates or in geriatric patients; initial dosages greater than 2.5 mg should be avoided; total dose of 5 mg is usually adequate for conscious sedation in healthy adults
Temazepam	Restoril, various	15-30 mg/day	PO	No	9-12	Insomnia	Shorter acting than flurazepam but longer acting than triazolam; gradually taper when discontinuing agent
Triazolam	Halcion	0.125-0.5 mg/day	PO	Yes	2-4	Insomnia	Rapid onset and short half-life; questionable efficacy with long-term use; potential rebound insomnia; best agent for insomnia in the elderly

TABLE 15 Commonly Used Antiemetics

Drug	Trade Name	Adult Dosage	Route	Cancer Chemotherapy Prophylaxis	Route	Onset (min)	Duration (hr)
Prochlor-perazine	Compazine, various	5-10 mg q6-8h 10-25 mg q6-12h	PO, IM, IV PR	10-20 mg	IV	30-40 (PO) 10-20 (IM) 60 (PR)	3-4
Promethazine	Phenergan, various	12.5-25 mg q4h	PO, IV, IM, PR			20 (IM, PO, PR)	2-8
Thiethyl-perazine	Torecan	10 mg q8-24h	IM, PR, PO			3-5 (IV) 30	4
Diphen-hydramine	Benadryl, various	25-50 mg q6-8h	IM, PO, IV			15	3-6
Hydroxyzine	Vistaril, various	25-100 mg q6h	IM, PO			15-30	4-6
Metoclo-pramide	Reglan	10-20 mg q4-6h	IM, PO, IV	1-2 mg/kg initially and q2-3h × 3 doses	IV	1-3 (IV); 10-15 (IM); 30-60 (PO)	1-2
Trime-thobenza-mide	Tigan, various	250 mg q6-8h 200 mg q6-8h	PO PR, IM			10-40	3-4
Ondansetron	Zofran			0.15 mg/kg initially and q4h × 2 doses	IV	30	4

- Extrapyramidal reactions, especially dystonias or dyskinesias, may occur with the use of prochlorperazine, promethazine, thiethylperazine, or metoclopramide.
- High dosages of metoclopramide may cause diarrhea.

ANTIHEMORRHAGIC AGENTS

Aminocaproic Acid (Amicar)

Pharmacology

Aminocaproic acid controls bleeding by competitive inhibition of plasminogen activator substances and, to a lesser degree, by noncompetitive inhibition of plasmin (fibrinolysin) activity. It is ineffective in bleeding caused by loss of vascular integrity. Therefore, a definite clinical or laboratory diagnosis of hyperfibrinolysis is needed before initiation of therapy.

Uses

Aminocaproic acid is indicated for fibrinolysis-induced hemorrhage, hemorrhage following cardiovascular surgery, subarachnoid hemorrhage, and urinary fibrinolysis.

Dosing and Administration

- The usual oral adult dose is 5 g the first hour, followed by 1 or 1.25 g every hour to sustain plasma concentrations of 130 μg/ml. No more than 30 g/day is recommended.
- The usual adult parenteral dose is intravenous infusion of 4 to 5 g administered over a period of 1 hour followed by continuous infusion at the rate of 1 g per hour for approximately 8 hours or until the desired response is obtained.
- When the bleeding tendency is chronic, 5 to 30 g/day administered at intervals of 3 to 6 hours has been recommended.
- Aminocaproic acid can be used as an antidote to thrombolytic agents.
- Rapid IV injection may cause bradycardia, hypotension, and/or dysrhythmias.
- The drug should be diluted before administration. It is compatible with most IV fluids.

Adverse Effects

- Nausea, cramping, diarrhea, dizziness, tinnitus, malaise, nasal stuffiness, headache, and rash may occur with aminocaproic acid use. These effects are usually mild and disappear when the drug is discontinued.
- Other adverse effects include myopathy, seizures, psychotic reactions, and prolongation of menstruation.

Desmopressin (DDAVP)

Pharmacology

Desmopressin is a synthetic posterior pituitary hormone. It produces antidiuretic activity by increasing water reabsorption in the collecting duct of the nephron. Desmopressin increases clotting factor VIII activity, which reduces bleeding.

Uses

Desmopressin is used primarily as an antihemorrhagic in the critical care unit but can also be used as an antidiuretic for diabetes insipidus.

Dosing and Administration

- Desmopressin can be administered intranasally for neurogenic diabetes insipidus at dosages of 10 to 40 μg/day in 1 to 3 divided doses. The dose should be adjusted according to the patient's response; morning and evening doses may be adjusted separately for adequate control.
- The antihemorrhagic dosage is 0.3 μg/kg given by slow IV infusion over 15 to 30 minutes daily. The dose should be diluted in 10 to 50 ml of normal saline and given 30 minutes before any procedure (e.g., dialysis).

Adverse Effects

- Side effects are rare with intranasal administration. Nasal congestion, sore throat, headache, and conjunctivitis may occur.
- Parenteral administration may lead to thrombotic events, transient headaches, nausea, abdominal cramping, and slight fluctuations in blood pressure. Large IV doses may produce tachycardia, hypotension, and facial flushing.

Drug Interactions

- The following agents may decrease the effect of desmopressin: lithium, epinephrine, demeclocycline, heparin, and alcohol.
- Chlorpropamide, urea, or fludrocortisone may potentiate the antidiuretic response to desmopressin.

Vasopressin (Pitressin)

Pharmacology

The primary physiological role of vasopressin (antidiuretic hormone, or ADH) is to maintain serum osmolality within a normal range. In doses greater than those used for antidiuretic effects, vasopressin directly stimulates contraction of smooth muscle, particularly the capillaries and small arterioles. These effects cause a reduction in blood flow to the splanchnic, coronary, GI, pancreatic, skin, and muscular systems.

Uses

Vasopressin may be used to control or prevent polydipsia, polyuria, and dehydration associated with neurohypophyseal diabetes insipidus. It may also be used in the management of acute massive hemorrhages caused by esophageal varices, peptic ulcer disease, esophageal lacerations, or intestinal perforations. The use of this agent in GI hemorrhage is as an adjunct and should not preclude the use of other treatments when indicated.

Dosing and Administration

- Vasopressin may be given by IM or IV injection. The injection may be used subcutaneously or applied topically to the nasal mucosa. The injection form should not be inhaled.
- The dosage for antidiuresis is patient dependent and should be adjusted according to patient response. For diabetes insipidus, the usual adult dosage is 5 to 10 units IM or SC every 6 to 12 hours. The dosage may range from 5 to 60 units/day.
- For GI hemorrhage, vasopressin should be diluted to a concentration of 0.1 to 1 unit/ml and given by continuous IV infusion at a rate of 0.2 to 0.4 unit/min. The dosage should be individualized; doses greater than 0.9 unit/min offer little additional benefit. After 24 hours, the infusion should be tapered if possible by 0.1 unit/min every 6 to 12 hours. These recommendations are for adults only.

Adverse Effects

- Adverse effects with low dosages of vasopressin are uncommon when fluid intake is not excessive. Higher dosages may produce sweating, tremor, nausea, abdominal cramps, and headache.
- In large doses, such as with intravenous use, vasopressin may produce increased blood pressure, bradycardia, myocardial infarction, vascular collapse, coronary insufficiency, heart block, or dysrhythmias. Coronary vasodilators (e.g., nitroglycerin) may be used concomitantly with vasopressin to reduce the incidence of coronary vasoconstriction.
- Other adverse effects include hypersensitivity reactions, bronchoconstriction, urticaria, and ischemic colitis.

Drug Interactions

- Lithium, epinephrine, demeclocycline, heparin, and alcohol may block the antidiuretic effect of vasopressin.
- Chlorpropamide, carbamazepine, clofibrate, tricyclic antidepressants, phenformin, urea, and fludrocortisone may potentiate the effects of vasopressin.

ANTIINFECTIVES (See Table 16)

Aminoglycosides

Pharmacology

Aminoglycosides are actively transported across the bacterial cell membrane, and then bind irreversibly to one or more specific receptor proteins, and interfere with an initiation complex between RNA and the 30 S subunit. Aminoglycosides are bactericidal.

Uses

Aminoglycosides are used for the treatment of serious infections caused by susceptible strains of gram-negative bacteria or mycobacteria. Aminoglycosides are active against the following gram-negative aerobic bacteria: *Acinetobacter*, *Citrobacter*, *Enterobacter*, *Escherichia coli*, *Klebsiella*, *Proteus*, *Providencia*, *Pseudomonas*, *Salmonella*, *Serratia*, and *Shigella*. Aminoglocysides are active against most strains of *Staphylococcus aureus* and *S. epidermidis*, as well as most strains of mycobacteria.

Dosing and Administration

- Aminoglycosides are poorly absorbed from the GI tract and available for parenteral use only.
- Aminoglycosides diffuse poorly into the CSF following IV or IM administration, and concentrations are usually low. Gentamicin (special formulation) may be used intrathecally or intraventricularly to supplement IV or IM dosing for the treatment of CNS infections caused by susceptible *Pseudomonas* bacteria.
- Aminoglycosides are widely distributed to other tissues and body fluids and may be used for bone and joint infections, skin and soft tissue infections, respiratory tract infections, septicemia, and intraabdominal infections.
- Aminoglycosides appear to be synergistic with the cephalosporins and extended spectrum penicillins (mezlocillin, piperacillin, and ticarcillin) and can be used in combination for the treatment of serious gram-negative infections. The drugs should be administered separately to avoid in vitro inactivation.
- Penicillins appear to be additive with aminoglycosides for the treatment of enterococcal infections, particularly enterococcal endocarditis.
- Gentamicin and tobramycin may be given as aerosols for long-term prophylaxis of acute exacerbations of bronchopulmonary *Pseudomonas* infections in cystic fibrosis patients.
- Patients with renal dysfunction should be carefully monitored while receiving aminoglycosides. The following guidelines should be used for initiating

TABLE 16 Commonly Used Antiinfectives

Drug Class	Individual Agents	Adult Dosages	Route	Dosing Interval (hr)	Peak (µg/ml)	Trough (µg/ml)	Hepatic Metabolism	Dosage Adjustment in Renal Failure	Supplement After Dialysis (P)	(H)
Aminoglycoside	Amikacin	Loading dose: 5-7.5 mg/kg, then 15-20 mg/kg/day	IV, IM	8-24	20-35	<10	No	Yes	Yes	Yes
	Gentamicin	Loading dose: 1.5-2.0 mg/kg, then 3-6 mg/kg/day	IV, IM	8-24	4-10	<2	No	Yes	Yes	Yes
	Tobramycin	4-8 mg/day	IT	24						
		Loading dose: 1.5-2.0 mg/kg, then 3-6 mg/kg/day	IV, IM	8-24	4-10	<2	No	Yes	Yes	Yes
Beta-lactam	Aztreonam	2-8 gm/day	IV, IM	6-12	—	—	Yes	Yes	Yes	Yes
	Imipenem	1-4 g/day	IV	6-8	—	—	No	Yes	—	Yes
	Cefazolin	2-8 g/day	IV, IM	6-8	—	—	Yes	No	No	Yes
Cephalosporins	Cephalothin	2-12 g/day	IV, IM	4-6	—	—	Yes	Yes	Yes	Yes
	Cefamandole	4-12 g/day	IV, IM	4-8	—	—	Yes	Yes	No	No
	Cefonocid	0.5-2 g/day	IV, IM	24	—	—	No	Yes	No	No
	Ceforanide	1-4 g/day	IV, IM	12	—	—	No	Yes	—	Yes
	Cefotetan	1-4 g/day	IV, IM	12	—	—	No	Yes	No	Yes
	Cefoxitin	4-12 g/day	IV, IM	6-8	—	—	Yes	Yes	—	Yes
	Cefuroxime	2.25-6 g/day	IV, IM	6-8	—	—	No	Yes	—	Yes
	Cefoperazone	2-6 g/day	IV, IM	6-12	—	—	Yes	No	No	No
	Cefotaxime	4-12 g/day	IV, IM	6-8	—	—	Yes	No	No	No

Continued.

Note: Dashes indicate not applicable.
IT = intrathecal.
P = peritoneal.
H = hemodialysis.

TABLE 16 Commonly Used Antiinfectives — cont'd

Drug Class	Individual Agents	Adult Dosages	Route	Dosing Interval (hr)	Therapeutic Plasma Levels Peak (µg/ml)	Trough (µg/ml)	Hepatic Metabolism	Dosage Adjustment in Renal Failure	Supplement After Dialysis (P)	(H)
	Ceftazidime	3-8 g/day	IV, IM	6-8	—	—	No	Yes	Yes	Yes
	Ceftizoxime	3-12 g/day	IV, IM	8-12	—	—	No	Yes	No	No
	Ceftriaxone	1-4 g/day	IV, IM	12	—	—	Yes	No	No	No
	Moxalactam	2-12 g/day	IV, IM	8-12	—	—	No	Yes	No	Yes
Penicillin	Penicillin G	1-20 million units/day	IV, IM	4-6	—	—	No	Yes	No	No
	Oxacillin	4-8 g/day	IV, IM	4-6	—	—	No	No	No	No
	Nafcillin	4-8 g/day	IV, IM	4	—	—	Yes	No	No	No
	Methicillin	6-12 g/day	IV, IM	4-6	—	—	No	No	No	No
	Ampicillin	4-12 g/day	IV, IM	4-6	—	—	Yes	Yes	No	Yes
	Ticarcillin	4-16 g/day	IV	4-6	—	—	Yes	Yes	No	Yes
	Mezlocillin	6-24 g/day	IV	4-6	—	—	No	Yes	—	Yes
	Piperacillin	6-24 g/day	IV	4-6	—	—	Yes	Yes	Yes	Yes
	Ticarcillin/ Clavulanate	9.3-18.6 g/day	IV	4-8	—	—	Yes	Yes	Yes	Yes
Chloramphenicol		50-100 mg/kg/ day	IV	6	25	10	Yes	No	No	No
	Clindamycin	0.6-2.7 g/day	IV	6	—	—	Yes	No	No	No
	Erythromycin	1-4 g/day	IV	6	—	—	Yes	No	No	No
	Metronidazole	1-4 g/day	IV	6	—	—	Yes	No	No	Yes
Quinolone	Ciprofloxacin	400-800 mg/day	IV	12	—	—	Yes	Yes	No	Yes

Class	Drug	Dose	Route	Interval (h)						
Sulfonamide	Sulfamethoxazole/Trimethoprim	40-75 mg/kg/day SMX and 8-15 mg/kg/day TMP	IV	6-12	—	—	Yes	Yes	—	Yes
Vancomycin	Vancomycin	0.75-2.5 g/day	IV	6-48	20-40	<10	No	No	No	No
Antifungal	Amphotericin	0.25-0.7 mg/kg/day	IV	24	—	—	No	No	No	No
	Fluconazole	200-800 mg/day	IV	24	—	—	No	Yes	—	Yes
	Flucytosine	25-50 mg/kg/day	PO	6	—	—	No	Yes	—	No
	Ketoconazole	200-400 mg/day	PO	24	—	—	—	—	No	No
	Itraconazole	200-400 mg/day	PO	12-24	—	—	Yes	No	No	No
Antiprotozoal	Pentamidine	4 mg/kg/day	IV	24	—	—	Yes	No	No	No
	Pyrimethamine	25 mg/day	PO	24	—	—	No	—	—	—
	Sulfadiazine	2-4 g/day	PO	6	—	—	Yes	Yes	Yes	Yes
Antituberculosis	Ethambutol	15-25 mg/kg/day	PO	24	—	—	No	Yes	—	—
	Isoniazid	300 mg/day	PO, IM	24	—	—	Yes	No	—	No
	Pyrazinamide	20-35 mg/kg/day	PO	6-8	—	—	—	—	—	—
	Rifampin	600 mg/day	PO, IV	24	—	—	Yes	No	No	No
Antiviral	Acyclovir	15-30 mg/kg/day	IV	8	—	—	No	—	—	Yes
	Ganciclovir	10 mg/kg/day	IV	12	—	—	Yes	Yes	—	Yes
	Zidovudine	0.4-1.2 g/day	PO	4	—	—	Yes	Yes	—	—
		6-12 mg/kg/day	IV	6	—	—	Yes	—	—	—

amikacin (4.25 to 6.5 mg/kg/dose) and gentamicin and tobramycin (1.0 to 1.5 mg/kg/dose):

Cl$_{cr}$ (ml/min)	Dosing Interval (hr)
>60	8
40-60	12
20-30	18-24
10-20	24-48
<10	Follow serum levels and dose accordingly

- Peak and trough levels may be drawn after the third dose. The trough level should be drawn immediately before the dose. The dose should be infused over 30 minutes; after an additional 30 minutes, the peak level may be drawn such that 1 hour has elapsed between the initiation of the dose and the blood level measurement. Dosages should be adjusted on the basis of serum level measurements to provide a therapeutic peak level and an acceptable trough level.
- Loading doses and maintenance doses are based on ideal body weight once daily dosing has been used in special circumstances.
- Use cautiously with other nephrotoxic, neurotoxic, or ototoxic drugs.
- Monitor renal function tests (every 2 to 3 days) and blood levels.

Adverse Effects

- Ototoxicity and nephrotoxicity are the most serious adverse effects and most often occur in geriatric or dehydrated patients, patients with renal insufficiency, patients receiving other ototoxic or nephrotoxic agents, and patients receiving high dosages for long periods.
- Ototoxicity is infrequent but often permanent. Vestibular damage may be manifested by dizziness, nystagmus, vertigo, tinnitus, ataxis, or varying degrees of hearing impairment. No aminoglycoside appears to be less ototoxic than another.
- Nephrotoxicity occurs frequently and is usually reversible following discontinuation of the drug. Manifestations include an increase in serum creatinine and BUN, increased trough concentrations, and the appearance of renal tubular casts, enzymes, and beta$_2$-microglobulin. The initial phase of nephrotoxicity is usually a nonoliguric azotemia, which progressively worsens. All aminoglycosides appear to be equally nephrotoxic.
- Aminoglycosides may produce neuromuscular blockade or sensitivity reactions.

Beta-lactam

Pharmacology

These agents inhibit mucopeptide synthesis in the bacterial cell wall. Aztreonam has a high binding af-finity for penicillin-binding protein 3 (PBP3) of susceptible gram-negative bacteria. Imipenem binds to multiple penicillin-binding proteins but has greatest affinity for PBP2 and the lowest for PBP3. Both these agents are bactericidal.

Uses

Aztreonam is used for the treatment of infections secondary to susceptible gram-negative aerobic bacteria. Aztreonam has a narrow spectrum of activity and should not be used alone for empiric therapy in seriously ill patients. The drug has little or no activity against gram-positive aerobic bacteria, anaerobic bacteria, mycoplasma, or viruses. Imipenem has a broader spectrum of activity and is active against most gram-positive and gram-negative aerobic and anaerobic bacteria. The drug also has some activity against mycobacterium but none against mycoplasma, fungi, or viruses. Imipenem is used for the treatment of polymicrobial bacterial infections and for some mixed nosocomial infections. Imipenem should not be used for the treatment of monobacterial infections when an antimicrobial with a more narrow spectrum can be used.

Dosing and Administration

- Aztreonam is administered by IV injection or deep IM injection. The IM route of administration should be avoided in patients with septicemia, intraabdominal abscess, peritonitis, and severe infections.
- The dose of aztreonam should be adjusted in patients with a creatinine clearance less than 30 ml/min. Patients with a creatinine clearance of 10 to 30 ml/min should receive an initial loading dose of 1 to 2 g followed by half the usual dose given at the usual intervals. Patients with creatinine clearance less than 10 ml/min should receive a loading dose of 1 to 2 g followed by a maintenance dose of one quarter the usual dose given at the usual intervals. Supplemental doses may be given after dialysis.
- Imipenem is administered by intermittent IV injection only. The commercial preparation contains an equal amount of cilastin sodium, which has an antimicrobial activity but prevents imipenem's metabolism by proximal tubular kidney cells. The combination of cilastin with imipenem increases urinary imipenem concentrations and possibly prevents nephrotoxicity.
- The dose of imipenem should be decreased in patients with a creatinine clearance less than 70 ml/min. For clearances of 30 to 70 ml/min, the usual dose is 500 mg every 6 to 8 hours. If the creatinine clearance is 20 to 30 ml/min, the dosage should be

500 mg every 8 to 12 hours and lowered to 250 mg every 12 hours for creatinine clearances less than 20 ml/min. The manufacturer recommends that imipenem not be used in patients with a creatinine clearance less than 5 ml/min unless hemodialysis is instituted within 48 hours.

Adverse Effects

- Aztreonam is well tolerated, with less than 7% of patients reporting adverse effects. Adverse effects include diarrhea, nausea, abdominal cramps, rash, eosinophilia, pruritus, leukopenia, thrombocytopenia, transient increases in liver function tests, phlebitis, and transient increases in serum creatinine and/or BUN.
- Adverse CNS effects including seizures and myoclonus have been reported with imipenem. Patients predisposed to the CNS effects are those with preexisting CNS disorders, those with renal impairment receiving high dosages of the drug, those receiving ganciclovir, and the elderly. The drug should be discontinued if seizures occur.
- Nausea, vomiting, pseudomembranous colitis, eosinophilia, rash, phlebitis, and hypotension have also been reported with imipenem use.
- Cross-sensitivity has been rarely reported with imipenem use in patients allergic to penicillin.

Cephalosporins

Pharmacology

The cephalosporins are bactericidal. They inhibit bacterial septum and cell wall synthesis, probably by acylation of membrane-bound transpeptidase enzymes. Cell division and growth are inhibited, and lysis and elongation of susceptible bacteria frequently occur. Rapidly dividing bacteria are those most susceptible to cephalosporins. The first-generation cephalosporins are effective against gram-positive cocci and some gram-negative rods. The second-generation cephalosporins are effective against *Enterobacter*, *Haemophilus influenzae*, *Neisseria gonorrhea*, *Salmonella*, and *Shigella* as well as those listed for first-generation agents. The third-generation cephalosporins are more active against gram-negative bacteria with less activity against gram-positive cocci. Some of the third-generation cephalosporins are effective against *Pseudomonas*, *Serratia*, and *Proteus*.

Uses

Cephalosporins are used in the treatment of serious respiratory tract infections, skin and skin structure infections, urinary tract infections, septicemia, and bone and joint infections. Selected cephalosporins may be used for endocarditis, intraabdominal infections, CNS infections, and *N. gonorrhea* infections.

Dosing and Administration

- Cephalosporins may be administered orally or IV, or by deep IM injection. Below is a chart listing the current agents and available dosage forms.

First-generation cephalosporins:

Drug	Trade Name	Dosage Forms
Cefadroxil	Duricef	Oral
Cefazolin	Ancef, Kefzol, various	Parenteral
Cephalexin	Keflex, various	Oral
Cephalothin	Keflin, various	Parenteral
Cephapirin	Cefadyl, various	Parenteral
Cephradine	Anspor, Velosef, various	Oral, parenteral

Second-generation cephalosporins:

Drug	Trade Name	Dosage Forms
Cefaclor	Ceclor	Oral
Cefamandole	Mandol	Parenteral
Cefonicid	Monocid	Parenteral
Ceforanide	Precef	Parenteral
Cefotetan	Cefotan	Parenteral
Cefoxitin	Mefoxin	Parenteral
Cefuroxime	Zinacef	Parenteral
Cefmetazole	Zefazone	Parenteral
Cefuroxime, Axetil	Ceftin	Oral

Third-generation cephalosporins:

Drug	Trade Name	Dosage Forms
Cefixime	Suprax	Oral
Cefoperazone	Cefobid	Parenteral
Ceftizoxime	Cefizox	Parenteral
Ceftriaxone	Rocephin	Parenteral
Moxalactam	Moxam	Parenteral
Cefotaxime	Claforan	Parenteral
Ceftazidime	Fortaz, Tazidime, Tazicef	Parenteral

- Patients with renal dysfunction (creatinine clearance <50 ml/min) require decreases in dose and/or frequency with many of these agents. Ceftriaxone and cefoperazone are notable exceptions. The dosage adjustment should be based on the degree of renal dysfunction, severity of infection, and susceptibility of the causative organism. Guidelines are provided by the manufacturer for each agent.

Adverse Effects

- Hypersensitivity reactions occur in approximately 10% of patients known to be allergic to penicillins. These agents should be avoided in patients with a history of an immediate reaction to penicillin.
- Rash, pruritus, urticaria, eosinophilia, angioedema, erythema, and exfoliative dermatitis may occur in up to 5% of patients receiving cephalosporins. Signs and symptoms occur within several days of initia-

tion of therapy and subside within a few days after discontinuation. Antihistamines and topical corticosteroids are effective palliative therapy.

- Cefamandole, cefonicid, cefoperazone, cefotetan, and moxalactam may be associated with an increased risk of disulfiram-like reactions and hypoprothrombinemia. Prophylactic administration of vitamin K is indicated in geriatric, debilitated, or vitamin K–deficient patients to reduce the incidence of bleeding. Moxalactam may further impair hemostasis through an antiplatelet effect; periodic evaluation for bleeding is suggested with this agent.

- The most frequent adverse effects are nausea, vomiting, and diarrhea with orally administered agents. Pseudomembranous colitis is a rare complication of cephalosporin therapy.

- Other adverse effects include phlebitis; transient increases in BUN, serum creatinine, and liver function tests; and a positive Coombs test.

Penicillins

Pharmacology

The natural penicillins (the penicillin-G group) are bactericidal. Their potency depends on their ability to reach and bind penicillin-binding proteins located in bacterial cytoplasmic membranes. These agents inhibit bacterial septum and cell wall synthesis, cell division, and growth. Lysis and elongation of susceptible bacteria occur. Penicillinase resistant penicillins are derivatives that prevent attachment of the staphylococcal penicillinases to the beta-lactam ring. The aminopenicillins are derivatives with enhanced activity against gram-negative bacteria. Finally, the extended spectrum penicillins, a group of semisynthetic penicillins, have the widest spectrum of activity against gram-negative bacteria.

Uses

The natural penicillins are used principally for the treatment of infections caused by gram-positive aerobic cocci, gram-negative aerobic cocci (except *N. gonorrhea*), gram-positive aerobic bacilli, gram-positive anaerobic bacteria, and spirochetes. Penicillinase-resistant penicillins are used to treat infections caused by penicillinase-producing staphylococci. Aminopenicillins are used for infections caused by gram-negative aerobic cocci and gram-negative aerobic bacilli. Extended spectrum penicillins are used for infections caused by gram-negative aerobic bacilli and for mixed aerobic–anaerobic bacterial infections.

Dosing and Administration

- Penicillins may be administered orally, IV, or by deep IM injection. Below is a chart listing the current agents and available dosage forms.

Natural Penicillins	Trade Name	Route
Penicillin-G Benzathine	Bicillin	IM only
Penicillin-G Potassium/Sodium	Various	Oral, parenteral
Penicillin-G Procaine	Wycillin	IM only
Penicillin-V Potassium	Various	Oral

Penicillinase-resistant Penicillins	Trade Name	Route
Cloxacillin	Cloxapen	Oral
Dicloxacillin	Dynapen	Oral
Methicillin	Staphcillin	Parenteral
Nafcillin	Various	Oral, parenteral
Oxacillin	Various	Oral, parenteral

Aminopenicillins	Trade Name	Route
Amoxicillin	Amoxil	Oral
Ampicillin	Omnipen	Oral, parenteral
Bacampicillin	Spectrobid	Oral
Cyclacillin	Cyclacillin	Oral
Amoxicillin/Clavulanate	Augmentin	Oral

Extended Spectrum Penicillins	Trade Name	Route
Carbenicillin	Geocillin	Oral
Ticarcillin	Ticar	Parenteral
Mezlocillin	Mezlin	Parenteral
Piperacillin	Pipracil	Parenteral
Ticarcillin/Clavulanate	Timentin	Parenteral

- The extended spectrum penicillins and aminopenicillins may be synergistic with aminoglycoside antibiotics.

- Some penicillin preparations may contain high amounts of sodium and/or potassium, which could lead to electrolyte disturbances. Patients with renal failure or heart failure are particularly susceptible to these effects.

Adverse Effects

- Hypersensitivity reactions are frequently seen with penicillins. These reactions range from mild pruritic rashes to anaphylaxis. The most common reactions are dermatological, consisting of urticarial, erythematous, or morbilliform rashes with pruritus. Exfoliative dermatitis occurs rarely. Rash is more common with the aminopenicillins and appears to be nonimmunological in most cases. Side effects also include fever, eosinophilia, and serum sickness. These reactions resolve quickly with discontinuation of the drug. The most serious reaction is anaphylaxis, which occurs in 0.05% of patients. Anaphylaxis is most common with the natural penicillins and generally takes place within the first 30 minutes after the drug is administered. If anaphylaxis occurs, the drug should be stopped immedi-

ately and the patient given appropriate therapy.
- Other adverse effects of penicillins include neutropenia, leukopenia, thrombocytopenia, nausea, vomiting, pseudomembranous colitis, interstitial nephritis, phlebitis, and CNS effects.

Chloramphenicol (Various)

Pharmacology

The bacteriostatic activity is due to inhibition of ribosomal protein synthesis in susceptible microorganisms.

Uses

The toxicity of chloramphenicol restricts its use to serious infections when less toxic antibiotics are ineffective or contraindicated. Not all species or strains of a particular organism may be susceptible to chloramphenicol. It is a broad spectrum antibiotic active against *Haemophilus influenzae, Salmonella,* most anaerobic species, and some gram-positive organisms.

Dosing and Administration

- The usual adult oral or IV dosage is 50 to 100 mg/kg/day divided into 4 equal doses. This drug should not be given by IM injection.
- Oral doses should be administered with a full glass of water on an empty stomach.
- Blood levels over 25 μg/ml are associated with bone marrow depression, and levels greater than 50 μg/ml with gray baby syndrome. Therapeutic levels are 10 to 25 μg/ml.
- Monitor blood levels, CBC, platelets, and liver and renal function.

Adverse Effects

The most serious adverse effect is bone marrow depression. Reversible bone marrow depression most often follows large-dose parenteral therapy of prolonged duration. Complete recovery from bone marrow depression usually occurs within 1 to 2 weeks after discontinuation. Irreversible bone marrow depression leading to fatal aplastic anemia can appear weeks or months after therapy. Aplastic anemia is rare (1 in 40,000) but often fatal and is unrelated to dosage or duration of therapy.

Drug Interactions

- Chloramphenicol is an enzyme inhibitor and can affect the metabolism of oral anticoagulants, sulfonylureas, and phenytoin.
- Concurrent use with other bone marrow–depression drugs should be avoided.
- Chloramphenicol can antagonize the bactericidal effects of the penicillins and cephalosporins.
- Chloramphenicol may decrease the effects of vitamin B_{12}, folic acid, and iron preparations in anemic patients.

Clindamycin (Various)

Pharmacology

Clindamycin inhibits ribosomal protein synthesis in susceptible microorganisms. Although usually considered bacteriostatic, clindamycin may be bactericidal in high concentrations or when used against highly susceptible organisms.

Uses

Clindamycin can produce severe and sometimes fatal colitis and should be reserved for serious infections where less toxic antibiotics (especially the penicillins and erythromycins) are ineffective or contraindicated. Clindamycin is active against most gram-positive organisms except enterococci and *Clostridium difficile.* Gram-negative aerobes are highly resistant, but gram-negative anaerobes are very sensitive.

Dosing and Administration

- The usual oral adult dosage is 150 to 300 mg every 6 hours. The adult dosage for more severe infections is 300 to 450 mg every 6 hours.
- The usual adult parenteral dosage is 600 to 2,700 mg/day in 2 to 4 equal doses. Severe infections may require up to 4,800 mg/day.
- Clindamycin must be given on an empty stomach with a full glass of water 1 to 2 hours before meals, and no food should be ingested for at least 1 hour after administration.
- Single IM doses greater than 600 mg are not recommended.
- Infuse intravenous solutions no faster than 30 mg/min.
- Clindamycin is physically incompatible with ampicillin, phenytoin, barbiturates, aminophylline, calcium gluconate, and magnesium sulfate.

Adverse Effects

- Anorexia, nausea, vomiting, cramps, and diarrhea may occur with oral therapy. Oral and parenteral therapy may cause severe pseudomembranous colitis. Symptoms appear 2 to 9 days after initiation of therapy. Therapy should be stopped immediately and the condition managed with oral metronidazole or vancomycin as appropriate.
- Other adverse effects include rash, urticaria, anaphylaxis, erythema multiforme, agranulocytosis, and thrombocytopenia.

Drug Interactions

- Kaolin and pectin suspensions greatly reduce the oral absorption of clindamycin.

- Antibiotic antagonism can exist between clindamycin and chloramphenicol, the erythromycins, the penicillins, and the cephalosporins when used concurrently.
- Concurrent administration with anesthetics or neuromuscular blocking agents may result in skeletal muscle weakness and respiratory depression or paralysis.

Erythromycin (Various)

Pharmacology

Erythromycin is bacteriostatic in normal concentrations and bactericidal in high concentrations. It is effective only against actively dividing organisms. Erythromycin has a spectrum similar to penicillin G but is also active against mycoplasma and *Legionella*.

Uses

Often used in lieu of penicillin for patients allergic to penicillin, erythromycin is also useful for certain other specific diseases, such as Legionnaire's disease and mycoplasma infections.

Dosing and Administration

- There are several salt forms of erythromycin available commercially. Only the lactobionate and gluceptate salts are available for IV injection. The ethylsuccinate salt is for IM injection only.
- The adult IV and oral dosage is 1 to 4 g/day divided into 4 doses. The IM dosage is 100 mg IM every 4 to 8 hours.
- IM administration is painful and may produce sterile abscesses. IV administration frequently produces pain, irritation, and phlebitis. Intravenous solutions should be diluted and given by slow infusion.
- Oral forms should be taken with a full glass of water and food or antacid.

Adverse Effects

- Nausea, vomiting, abdominal cramps, and diarrhea are frequent adverse effects of oral therapy. The drug may be given with food or antacids to lessen the discomfort.
- Reversible intrahepatic cholestatic jaundice may be seen rarely with the estolate and ethylsuccinate salts. Usually occurring within the first 2 weeks of therapy, the syndrome is manifested by malaise, fever, vomiting, nausea, and abdominal pain. Symptoms will resolve after 1 to 2 weeks when the drug is discontinued.

Metronidazole (Flagyl, Various)

Pharmacology

Metronidazole is a potent bactericidal, amebicidal, and trichomonacidal agent. The exact mechanism of action is poorly understood, but the drug is equally effective against both dividing and nondividing cells. Metronidazole is inactive against aerobic and microaerophilic bacteria but bactericidal against most anaerobic bacteria.

Uses

Metronidazole is used for the treatment of trichomoniasis, amebiasis, giardiasis, rosacea, antibiotic-associated diarrhea and colitis, and anaerobic bacterial infections. Metronidazole should be combined with other antimicrobials if mixed aerobic–anaerobic infections are suspected.

Dosing and Administration

- Metronidazole may be given orally or by IV infusion. When taken orally, it may be given with food to minimize stomach upset. Metronidazole is available commercially as a ready-to-use solution and as a powder for reconstitution. Care must be taken to follow the manufacturer's recommendations for reconstitution of the powder so that the solution is properly neutralized.
- The adult oral dosage for antibiotic-associated colitis is 250 to 500 mg 3 or 4 times daily for 7 to 10 days.
- The adult IV dosage for anaerobic infections is a 15 mg/kg load then 7.5 mg/kg every 6 hours up to a maximum of 4 g/day. Each dose should be infused over 1 hour.
- Patients with severe hepatic impairment may require lower doses of metronidazole. There are currently no guidelines available.

Adverse Effects

- High dosages of metronidazole may produce nausea, headache, and anorexia; a dry mouth; and an unpleasant metallic taste. A harmless discoloration of the urine may also occur.
- Dizziness, vertigo, and peripheral neuropathy have been reported with both oral and parenteral therapy. The drug should be discontinued if these effects are manifested.
- Other adverse effects include leukopenia, thrombocytopenia, urticaria, rash, and phlebitis.

Ciprofloxacin (Cipro)

Pharmacology

Ciprofloxacin is a fluroquinolone antibiotic that inhibits bacterial DNA-gyrase. It is bactericidal and active against Enterobacteriaceae, *Pseudomonas,* and other gram-negative aerobic bacteria. Ciprofloxacin has good activity against many gram-positive aerobic bacteria with the exception of most streptococci. It is poorly active against most anaerobic bacteria.

Uses

Ciprofloxacin is used to treat infections caused by susceptible organisms. It should not be used alone for mixed aerobic–anaerobic infections.

Dosing and Administration

- The intravenous solution should be infused over 60 minutes. The usual adult dosage is 200 to 400 mg IV every 12 hours. Do not mix the parenteral injection with other medications.
- The dosage adjustment for patients with a creatinine clearance less than 30 ml/min is 200 to 400 mg IV every 18 to 24 hours. Patients receiving hemodialysis should be dosed immediately after dialysis.
- The usual oral dosage is 500 to 750 mg every 12 hours. Patients with creatinine clearance of 30 to 50 ml/min should receive 250 to 500 mg every 12 hours, and those with a creatinine clearance less than 30 ml/min may receive 250 to 500 mg PO every 18 hours.

Adverse Effects

- Adverse effects are seen in 5% to 14% of patients receiving ciprofloxacin. The most common are nausea, diarrhea, abdominal pain, headache, and restlessness.
- Other adverse effects include rash, eosinophilia, tremor, dizziness, joint pain, elevated serum creatinine and BUN, and elevated liver function tests.

Drug Interactions

- Ciprofloxacin increases theophylline serum levels and may precipitate theophylline toxicity.
- Antacids, sucralfate, and tube-feeding formula may decrease the absorption of oral ciprofloxacin.

Sulfamethoxazole-trimethoprim (Bactrim, Septra, Various)

Pharmacology

Sulfamethoxazole-trimethoprim (SMX-TMP) is bacteriostatic and inhibits folic acid synthesis. Sulfamethoxazole is a competitive antagonist of p-aminobenzoic acid, while trimethoprim inhibits the enzyme dihydrofolate reductase. Consequently, two successive steps in the biosynthesis of folic acid are blocked, resulting in enhanced antimicrobial activity in susceptible organisms.

Uses

Sulfamethoxazole-trimethoprim (SMX-TMP) is indicated for the treatment of urinary tract infections, respiratory tract infections, and soft tissue infections caused by susceptible strains of *Enterobacter* spp., *Escherichia coli*, *Klebsiella* spp., *Proteus mirabilis*, *Proteus morganii*, and *Proteus vulgaris*. It can be used as an alternative for treating otitis media caused by susceptible strains of *Haemophilus influenzae* or *Streptococcus pneumoniae*. SMX-TMP is also used to treat infections caused by *Shigella* and *Pneumocystic carinii*.

Dosing and Administration

- The intravenous adult dosage for severe gram-negative infection is 40 to 50 mg/kg/day SMX and 8 to 10 mg/kg/day TMP in 2 to 4 equally divided doses.
- The adult oral or intravenous dosage for *Pneumocystis carinii* pneumonia is 100 (PO) or 75 (IV) mg/kg/day of SMX and 20 (PO) or 15 (IV) mg/kg/day of TMP given in 2 to 4 divided doses. For oral prophylaxis, the dosage is 20 mg/kg/day SMX and 4 mg/kg/day TMP in 2 equally divided doses.
- The dosage should be reduced in patients with severe renal impairment (creatinine clearance <30 ml/min). The dosage should be halved for patients with a creatinine clearance of 10 to 30 ml/min and reduced by one quarter to one half in patients with a creatinine clearance less than 10 ml/min. The drug is not recommended for patients with a creatinine clearance less than 10 ml/min because of unpredictable blood levels and potential toxicity.
- SMX-TMP should never be given by IM injection. Each 5 ml of SMX-TMP can be diluted with 75 to 125 ml of D_5W and infused over 60 to 90 minutes. Rapid or direct IV injections should be avoided.
- Oral doses should be administered with a full glass of water on an empty stomach. The patient should be encouraged to drink additional glasses of water throughout the day when possible.
- Monitor CBC and renal function.

Adverse Effects

- Nausea, vomiting, anorexia, rash, and urticaria are the most common adverse effects of SMX-TMP. Rashes are usually erythematous, maculopapular, morbilliform, and/or pruritic. Patients who are HIV-positive are at greater risk for developing moderately severe rashes. The drug should be discontinued if a rash appears.
- SMX-TMP may induce aplastic anemia, agranulocytosis, leukopenia, neutropenia, eosinophilia, or hemolytic anemia. Those at greatest risk are the elderly; those who are malnourished, alcoholic, or debilitated; or those with renal insufficiency.
- Other adverse effects include headache, exfoliative dermatitis, phlebitis, muscle weakness, fever, Stevens-Johnson syndrome, photosensitization, peripheral neuritis, hepatitis, and lupus erythematosus phenomenon.

Drug Interaction

- Concurrent use with paraaminobenzoic acid (PABA) may cause antagonism of the bacteriostatic effects of the sulfonamides.
- Anticoagulants, hypoglycemics, methotrexate, phenytoin, and thiopental may be displaced from protein-binding sites, and/or metabolism may be inhibited by sulfonamides.
- Concurrent use with penicillins is not recommended because of possible interference with its bactericidal effects.

Vancomycin (Various)

Pharmacology

Vancomycin binds to the bacterial cell wall and blocks glycopeptide polymerization. This action inhibits cell wall synthesis and damages the cytoplasmic membrane. The agent is bactericidal against most gram-positive organisms but is inactive against gram-negative organisms.

Uses

Vancomycin is used in the treatment of serious infections caused by susceptible gram-positive organisms. It is principally used for staphylococcal or streptococcal infections, including methicillin-resistant strains for which it is the drug of choice. Vancomycin may be used orally for the treatment of antibiotic-associated pseudomembranous colitis caused by *Clostridium difficile*. Oral therapy is not effective for systemic infections.

Dosing and Administration

- The adult oral dosage for antibiotic-associated colitis is 125 to 500 mg every 6 hours.
- The intravenous adult dosage is 20 to 30 mg/kg/day (usually 2 g/day) in 2 to 4 divided doses. The intravenous solution should be diluted (500 mg/100 ml IVF) and infused over 30 to 60 minutes. Rapid infusion may result in fever, chills, phlebitis, hypotension, erythema, pruritus, or localized edema ("red man" syndrome). This will not occur with subsequent doses if the infusion rate is slowed.
- The dosage of vancomycin should be adjusted in patients with renal insufficiency. A maintenance dosage of 17.5 mg/kg (total body weight) can be given at the following intervals based on creatinine clearance after an initial 20 mg/kg loading dose:

Cl_{cr} (ml/min)	Interval (hr)
65-85	18
50-65	24
40-50	30
35-40	36
25-35	48
16-25	72

Patients with a creatinine clearance less than 15 ml/min should be monitored closely and require dosing at 5- to 7-day intervals. Patients requiring hemodialysis may be dosed once weekly as may those with end-stage renal disease. Vancomycin is not substantially removed by hemodialysis or peritoneal dialysis, and supplemental dosing is not necessary.

- Serum peak and trough levels should be monitored. Peak levels are 25 to 35 μg/ml and troughs should be kept below 10 μg/ml. Patients with endocarditis occasionally require higher trough levels up to 15 μg/ml. The trough level should be drawn immediately before the dose and the peak level 1 hour after a 1-hour infusion.
- Monitor renal function and serum levels
- Do not give by IM injection.

Adverse Effects

- Vancomycin is irritating to tissues and may cause necrosis when given IM. Pain and thrombophlebitis may occur with IV administration.
- Ototoxicity may occur and is related to excessive peak levels (>80 μg/ml). Vertigo, dizziness, and tinnitus may mark the onset of deafness.
- Nephrotoxicity occurs more often in patients with preexisting renal impairment, those with high trough levels (>15 μg/ml), and those receiving other nephrotoxic agents. Vancomycin-induced nephrotoxicity may be manifested by transient elevations in BUN or serum creatinine and the appearance of granular casts and albumin in the urine.
- Other adverse effects include leukopenia, eosinophilia, hypersensitivity reactions, and nausea.

ANTIFUNGAL AGENTS

Amphotericin B (Fungizone)

Pharmacology

Amphotericin is fungistatic in normal concentrations and fungicidal in high concentrations. Amphotericin binds to the sterols in fungal cell membranes and effectively destroys the cell. Amphotericin is active against most fungi and some protozoa. It has no activity against bacteria or viruses.

Uses

Amphotericin is indicated for the treatment of infections caused by susceptible strains of *Aspergillus* spp., *Blastomyces* spp., *Candida* spp., *Coccidioides* spp., *Cryptococcus* spp., *Histoplasmosis* spp., *Mucor mucedo*, and *Sporotrichum schenckii*.

Dosing and Administration

- Amphotericin is available for intravenous use only. A 1-mg test dose should be given in 10 to 100 ml of D_5W over 1 hour. If tolerated, the dosage may be increased by 5 to 10 mg each day (or doubled) as tolerated up to a dosage of 0.5 to 0.7 mg/kg/day. For fulminant infections, patients may receive 0.25 mg/kg of amphotericin after the initial test dose and 0.3 to 0.5 mg/kg the following day depending on the severity of infection and tolerance of the previous dosage.

- Heparin (500 to 1,000 units) may be added to solutions infused peripherally to reduce thrombophlebitis.
- Hydrocortisone (25 to 50 mg) may be added to solutions except in those patients already receiving steroids.
- Amphotericin should be diluted in D_5W only and administered at a concentration no greater than 0.1 mg/ml. All patients should be pretreated with acetaminophen and diphenhydramine before daily administration of amphotericin. The drug should be infused over a period of 4 to 6 hours.
- Monitor electrolytes, renal function, and CBC.

Adverse Effects

- The most common adverse effects are shaking, fever, chills, headache, nausea, and pain at injection site during the intravenous infusion. This reaction may be reduced by diluting the solution, lengthening the infusion time, adding heparin and hydrocortisone to the infusion, and premedicating with acetaminophen and diphenhydramine. Narcotics may be used if the patient still complains of reactions after the above interventions have been attempted.
- Nephrotoxicity is common in more than 80% of patients. If the renal function deteriorates by 20% to 60% of normal, the drug may be stopped for 2 to 5 days and reinstituted at the previous dosage when renal function stabilizes. Sodium loading may prevent or reduce nephrotoxicity. If renal failure occurs, the dosage should be reduced or the drug discontinued if possible.
- Potassium and magnesium wasting usually occurs with amphotericin use. These electrolytes should be monitored and appropriately supplemented.
- Other adverse effects include normochromic, normocytic anemia, hypotension, rash, and eosinophilia.
- Intrathecal administration may produce peripheral nerve pain, paresthesias, nerve palsies, paraplegia, and seizures.

Fluconazole (Diflucan)

Pharmacology

Fluconazole inhibits fungal cytochrome P450 sterol C14 alpha-demethylation. This agent is fungistatic.

Uses

Fluconazole is indicated for the treatment of serious candidal infections and cryptococcal meningitis.

Dosing and Administration

- The oral and intravenous doses of fluconazole are equivalent. Fluconazole cannot be given by IM administration.
- The recommended adult dosage for cryptococcal meningitis or systemic candidiasis is 400 mg on the first day followed by 200 mg every day. Dosages of 400 mg/day may be used in cryptococcal meningitis depending on the patient's response to therapy.
- Cryptococcal prophylaxis or suppression requires dosages of 200 mg/day.
- Do not add any other medications to the intravenous injections; infuse the solution by itself at a rate no greater than 200 mg/hr.
- The dosage should be reduced in renal impairment. The manufacturer recommends 50% of the usual dosage for patients with a creatinine clearance of 20 to 50 ml/min and 25% of the usual dosage for a creatinine clearance of 10 to 20 ml/min. Patients receiving dialysis should receive the usual recommended dose after each dialysis.

Adverse Effects

- Adverse effects are reported more frequently in HIV-positive patients. The most common adverse effects are nausea, headache, skin rash, abdominal pain, and diarrhea.
- Other adverse effects include exfoliative skin disorders and elevation of liver function tests.

Drug Interactions

- Fluconazole may increase the prothrombinemic effect of warfarin.
- Fluconazole may increase cyclosporine and phenytoin blood levels.
- Rifampin may enhance the metabolism of fluconazole.

Flucytosine (Ancobon)

Pharmacology

Flucytosine penetrates fungal cells and interferes with pyrimidine metabolism. Nucleic acid and protein synthesis are disturbed. The compound is selectively toxic against fungi.

Uses

Flucytosine is indicated for the treatment of infections caused by susceptible strains of *Cryptococcus* and *Candida*.

Dosing and Administration

- Flucytosine is available as an oral agent only.
- The oral dosage is 50 to 150 mg/kg/day in 4 divided doses.
- The dosage should be reduced in patients with a creatinine clearance of less than 40 ml/min. The following dosing intervals are recommended for a 12.5- to 37.5-mg/kg dose:

Cl_{cr} (ml/min)	Interval (hr)
20-40	12
10-20	24
<10	48

- Patients receiving regular dialysis may receive a 20- to 50-mg/kg dose after each dialysis.
- Flucytosine is commonly used as an adjunt to amphotericin.

Adverse Effects

Nausea, vomiting, diarrhea, bone marrow depression, and elevated liver function tests occur most commonly.

ANTIPROTOZOAL AGENTS (PENTAMIDINE)

Pharmacology

The exact mechanism of action of pentamidine is unclear and may involve many mechanisms that vary among the different protozoa. Pentamidine is active against a variety of protozoa and *Pneumocystis carinii*.

Uses

The primary use of pentamidine is for treating *Pneumocystis carinii* pneumonia. Other uses include the treatment of trypanosomiasis and leishmaniasis infections.

Dosing and Administration

- Pentamidine may be administered by IM, IV, or inhalational routes.
- When given IV, the drug should be administered over a period of 60 minutes.
- The adult parenteral dosage for the treatment of *P. carinii* is 4 mg/kg/day given once daily.
- The inhalational dosage is 300 mg given once every 4 weeks for prophylaxis of *P. carinii*.

Adverse effects

- Nephrotoxicity occurs in up to 24% of patients and hypoglycemia in 5% to 10%. Other adverse effects include pancreatitis, fever, rash, leukopenia, and elevated liver function tests.
- The IM injection produces pain and abscess formation at the injection site.

- The IV injection produces hypotension if given too rapidly.
- Cough and bronchospasms occur frequently with inhalational therapy.

ANTITUBERCULOSIS AGENTS

Pharmacology

The antituberculosis agents are used to treat tuberculosis and other disorders caused by the genus *Mycobacterium*. Those most frequently used are isoniazid, rifampin, ethambutol, pyrazinamide, and streptomycin. These agents inhibit the synthesis of various cell substrates and arrest multiplication.

Uses

These agents are used in combination for the treatment of tuberculosis.

Dosing and Administration

- All these agents are available orally. Rifampin may be given by IV infusion (not IM), and isoniazid may be given by IM injection only. The parenteral and oral dosages are identical for both agents.
- Administer 25 to 50 mg of pyridoxine daily with isoniazid.

Adverse Effects

- Ethambutol: optic neuritis, hyperuricemia, headache.
- Isoniazid: pyridoxine responsive peripheral neuropathy, hepatitis, elevated liver function tests, hypersensitivity reactions, and hematological effects.
- Pyrazinamide: elevated liver function tests, hyperuricemia, rash, and hepatotoxicity.
- Rifampin: GI upset, headache, drowsiness, dizziness, hepatic dysfunction, hypersensitivity reactions, elevated liver function tests, hematological disorders, and discoloration of urine and feces (red-orange). Rifampin is a potent hepatic enzyme inducer and should be used cautiously with other agents that are metabolized in the liver.

Drug Interactions (Rifampin)

- Concurrent use may require dosage adjustment for corticosteroids, dapsone, digitalis glycosides, methadone maintenance, oral anticoagulants, and oral hypoglycemics.
- Oral contraceptives may lose significant activity during rifampin therapy.
- Concurrent use with alcohol or isoniazid may result in increased incidence of rifampin-induced hepatotoxicity.
- Concurrent use with methadone may decrease the effects of this medication.

ANTIVIRAL AGENTS

Acyclovir (Zovirax)

Pharmacology

Acyclovir intereferes with DNA synthesis and inhibits viral replication. It is active against herpes simplex virus types 1 and 2, varicella-zoster virus, Epstein-Barr virus, *Herpesvirus simiae*, and cytomegalovirus.

Uses

Acyclovir is used to treat viral infections caused by susceptible viruses.

Dosing and Administration

- Acyclovir may be administered orally or by IV infusion. Acyclovir should never be given by IM injection.
- The usual adult IV dosage is 5 mg/kg every 8 hours for most infections and 10 mg/kg every 8 hours for viral encephalitis. Infusions should be given over 30 minutes.
- The oral dosage is 1 g/day in 5 divided doses.
- Dosage adjustments are necessary for patients with a creatinine clearance of less than 50 ml/min. The following dosage intervals are suggested for a parenteral dose of 5 to 10 mg/kg:

Cl_{cr} (ml/min)	Interval (hr)
>50	8
25-50	12
10-25	24

If the clearance is less than 10 ml/min, the dose should be halved and given every 24 hours.

Adverse Effects

- Phlebitis, local irritation, and pain are common with IV administration. Nausea, vomiting, and headache are common with oral administration.
- Nephrotoxicity occurs in up to 10% of patients and may be related to rapid infusion rates.
- Other adverse effects include rash, lethargy, tremors, seizures, and alopecia.

Ganciclovir (Cytovene)

Pharmacology

The mechanism is similar to that of acyclovir. Ganciclovir's principal use is for cytomegalovirus (CMV), but it also has limited activity against other viruses.

Uses

Ganciclovir is used to treat cytomegalovirus in immunocompromised patients and CMV retinitis.

Dosing and Administration

- Ganciclovir is administered by slow IV infusion. The drug should not be given by IM or SC administration.
- The usual adult dosage is 5 mg/kg every 12 hours for 14 to 21 days followed by 5 mg/kg/day given once daily.
- The dose should be reduced in renal impairment as follows:

Cl_{cr} (ml/min)	Dose (mg/kg)	Interval (hr)
50-79	2.5	12
25-50	2.5	24
<25	1.25	24

Doses should be administered after dialysis.

Adverse Effects

- Most adverse effects are dose related and reversible.
- The most common adverse reactions are hematological and occur in 25% to 50% of patients. Neutropenia is the most common and develops within 2 weeks of therapy. Reductions in drug-free intervals or dosage may reverse the neutropenia. Thrombocytopenia may also occur.
- Other adverse effects include ocular damage, central nervous system effects, liver dysfunction, phlebitis, and nausea.

Zidovudine (Retrovir)

Pharmacology

Zidovudine (AZT) inhibits in vitro replication of retroviruses, including the human immunodeficiency virus (HIV). AZT exerts a virustatic effect against retroviruses by acting as a reverse transcriptase inhibitor.

Uses

AZT is used for the management of HIV infections.

Dosing and Administration

- The adult oral dosage is 100 to 200 mg every 4 hours. The drug should be taken on an empty stomach with a full glass of water. Less toxicity is seen with dosages of 300 to 400 mg/day; the minimal therapeutic dosage is 300 mg/day.
- The adult parenteral dosage is 1 to 2 mg/kg every 4 hours given over 60 minutes.
- An IV dose of 1 mg/kg is equivalent to 100 mg PO.
- Regimens may change pending ongoing trial results for AZT use.

Adverse Effects

- The most common adverse effects are hematological. AZT causes bone marrow depression resulting in severe anemia and/or granulocytopenia. These effects are directly related to dose and duration of therapy.
- Other adverse effects include headache, vertigo,

nausea, vomiting, myalgia, increases in liver function tests, and pigmentation.

ANTITHROMBOTIC AGENTS

Anticoagulants

Pharmacology

Heparin acts indirectly at multiple sites in both the intrinsic and extrinsic blood clotting systems to potentiate the inhibitory action of antithrombin III (heparin cofactor) on several activated coagulation factors. Heparin forms a complex and induces a conformational change in the antithrombin III molecule. Inhibition of activated factor X interferes with thrombin generation and, thereby, inhibits the various actions of thrombin in coagulation. Heparin also accelerates the formation of an antithrombin III–thrombin complex, thereby inactivating thrombin and preventing the conversion of fibrinogen to fibrin; this action prevents extension of existing thrombi.

Warfarin prevents the formation of active precoagulation factors II, VII, IX, and X in the liver by inhibiting the vitamin K–mediated gamma-carboxylation of precursor proteins. All therapeutic action is delayed until circulating coagulation factors are removed by normal catabolism, which usually takes 3 to 7 days. This agent has no direct thrombolytic effect, although it may limit extension of existing thrombi.

Uses

Heparin is used for a variety of conditions including prophylaxis and treatment of pulmonary embolism, venous thrombosis, atrial fibrillation with embolization, acute and chronic consumption coagulopathies, peripheral arterial embolism, coronary embolism, and reocclusion immediately after angioplasty. Heparin is also used as an anticoagulant to prevent clotting during open heart surgery, arterial surgery, blood transfusions, extracorporeal circulation, dialysis, and collection of blood samples.

Warfarin is used in the treatment and prophylaxis of pulmonary thrombosis, venous thrombosis, and atrial fibrillation with embolization. Warfarin has been used after myocardial infarction to prevent reinfarction and for mural thrombi.

Dosing and Administration

- Heparin is available for parenteral administration only; IV and subcutaneous routes are preferred over IM therapy, which produces local hemorrhages.
- Anticoagulant doses for heparin are determined by clotting times or APTT, both of which are maintained at 1.5 to 2.5 times control values. Continuous infusions are recommended over intermittent injections so that a continuous anticoagulant effect is maintained. Patients should be given a loading dose of 5,000 to 10,000 units as an IV bolus, followed by a continuous drip at 1,000 units/hr (or 10-25 U/kg/hr). The APTT should be checked 6 to 8 hours after the initiation of the drip or any change in the infusion rate. The following is a suggested guideline for maintaining the APTT at 1.5 to 2.5 times control:

APTT	Change in Heparin Dose
<1.2	Bolus 50 U/kg, increase infusion by 200 U/hr
1.2-1.3	Bolus 25 U/kg, increase infusion by 100 U/hr
1.3-1.5	Increase infusion by 100 U/hr
1.5-2.5	No change
>2.5	Hold infusion 1-2 hours; decrease infusion rate by 100-200 U/hr

After the patient has been stabilized, the APTT may be drawn daily.

- For the prevention of stasis thrombosis, heparin may be given as 5,000 units subcutaneously every 12 hours.
- Warfarin is available in oral form only. Therapy may usually be initiated with 10 mg nightly for 3 consecutive nights, followed by a maintenance dose of 2.5 to 10 mg nightly. Maintenance doses should be individualized on the basis of prothrombin time, which should be 1.2 to 1.5 times the normal value depending on the disease state being treated. Lower prothrombin times are equally efficacious for some disease states and are associated with a significantly lower incidence of bleeding complications. Five to seven days are usually required to see the maximal effects of a given regimen for warfarin. Doses should be slowly titrated to prevent bleeding complications. Daily prothrombin times are required until steady state is achieved.
- The anticoagulant effects of warfarin can be reversed by the use of vitamin K given as 10 to 20 mg either IV, IM, or SC. Heparin activity is reversed by protamine sulfate; 1.0 to 1.5 mg of protamine sulfate will antagonize 100 units of heparin.

Adverse Effects

- Hemorrhage is the predominant side effect of heparin and warfarin. These agents are contraindicated in the presence of active bleeding or hemorrhagic tendencies. Minor bleeding and bruising are normal with most patients and should not preclude the use of these agents.
- Thrombocytopenia occurs in 5% to 15% of patients receiving heparin, especially the bovine-derived products. Thrombocytopenia usually develops within the first week of therapy, and heparin should be discontinued if the platelet counts fall below 100,000/mm^3.
- Other adverse effects of heparin include alopecia, osteoporosis, neuropathy, and priapism.
- Adverse effects of warfarin include nausea, vomit-

ing, diarrhea, jaundice, urticaria, leukopenia, skin necrosis, crystalluria, purple toe syndrome, and anemia.

Drug Interactions

- The following drugs may increase the prothrombinemic effect of warfarin: amiodarone, androgens, cephalosporin antibiotics, chloral hydrate, chloramphenicol, clofibrate, dextrothyroxine, disulfiram, erythromycin, glucagon, cimetidine, metronidazole, nalidixic acid, quinidine, salicylates, sulfamethoxazole-trimethoprim, sulfinpyrazone, and vitamin E.
- The following drugs may decrease the prothrombinemic effect of warfarin: aminoglutethimide, barbiturates, carbamazepine, cholestyramine, ethchlorvynol, glutethimide, griseofulvin, rifampin, and vitamin K.

Antiplatelet Agents

Pharmacology

Antiplatelet drugs interfere with the metabolism of prostaglandins and thromboxane, resulting in reduced aggregability of platelets. Aspirin is an irreversible inhibitor of cyclooxygenase; dipyridamiole increases cyclic adenosine monophosphate (cAMP). Both these agents decrease platelet aggregation but do not affect platelet adhesion. Aspirin is the most efficacious agent both alone and in combination with other agents, while dipyridamole is ineffective when used alone and useful only when combined with aspirin.

Uses

See Table 17.

Dosing and Administration (See Table 17)

- "Baby" aspirin (81 mg) may be used in patients who cannot tolerate 325-mg doses. The ideal dose of aspirin remains controversial. Low dosages (81

mg daily) may be clinically ineffective in some patients, while higher dosages (1,000 mg or more daily) offer no greater benefit but increase the incidence of side effects. The currently recommended dosages are those that have been used in the clinical trials for these indications.

Adverse Effects

- Aspirin side effects include nausea, abdominal pain, anorexia, GI bleeding, tinnitus, hepatotoxicity, rash, anemia, and hypersensitivity.
- Adverse effects with dipyridamole include headache, dizziness, nausea, peripheral dilatation, flushing, weakness, rash, pruritus, and anginal pain.

Thrombolytic Agents

Pharmacology

These agents lyse formed thrombi by converting plasminogen to plasmin through various mechanisms. Streptokinase, urokinase, and APSAC (an anisoylated streptokinase complex) bind directly to circulating plasminogen, prompting the conversion to plasmin. Tissue plasminogen activator (TPA) binds specifically to fibrin in the thrombus and converts entrapped plasminogen to plasmin. TPA is more clot-specific than the other agents. At this time, no one agent appears superior when comparing morbidity and mortality if used within 6 hours of the onset of pain in acute myocardial infarction.

Uses

These agents are used for thrombolysis in acute myocardial infarction, deep vein thrombosis, and pulmonary embolism. Urokinase may be used to clear occluded catheters.

Dosing and Administration (See Table 18)

- Heparin therapy should be initiated 3 to 6 hours after the completion of streptokinase or APSAC infusions and immediately after the completion of

---

TABLE 17 **Antiplatelet Agents**

Indication	Aspirin Dosage (mg)	Aspirin (mg) + Dipyridamole (mg)
Acute myocardial infarction	325 qd or tid	325 tid + 75 tid
Unstable angina	325 qd, tid, or qid	
AV shunts	325 qd	
Coronary artery bypass	325 qd	325 tid + 75 tid
Heart valves	325 tid	325 tid + 75 tid
CVA and TIA	325 qid	
Angioplasty	325 qd or tid	

From Kinney, M. R., Packa, D. R., Andreoli, K. G., et al. (1991). *Comprehensive cardiac care* (7th ed.). St. Louis: Mosby–Year Book.
  AV = arteriovenous.
  CVA = cerebrovascular accident.
  TIA = transient ischemic attack.

TABLE 18 **Thrombolytic Agents**

Agent	Trade Name	Dose (after MI)	Dosage (DVT/PTE)	Reocclusion (%)	Reperfusion (%)	Clot Specificity	Bleeding Complications	Expense
Streptokinase	Streptase, Kabikinase	1.5 million IU over 1 hr	250,000 IU over 30 min, then 100,000 IU/ hr for 24-72 hr	20	65	+	+ + + +	+
Tissue plasminogen activator (TPA)	Activase	60 mg over 1 hr (6-10 mg in the first 1-2 min), then 20 mg/hr for 2 hr for total dose of 100 mg		20	70	+ + +	+ + + +	+ + + +
Urokinase	Abbokinase		Loading dose: 4,400 IU/kg IV over 10 min, then 4,400 IU/kg/ hr for 12 hr	<10	66	+ +	+ + + +	+ + +
APSAC	Eminase	30 units IV over 3-5 min		<10	68	+ +	+ + + +	+ +

From Kinney, M. R., Packa, D. R., Andreoli, K. G., et al. (1991). *Comprehensive cardiac care* (7th ed.). St. Louis: Mosby–Year Book.

MI = myocardial infarction.
IU = international units.
DVT/PTE = deep vein thrombosis/pulmonary thromboembolism.
+ = weakly positive.
+ + = positive.
+ + + = strongly positive.
+ + + + = very strongly positive.

TPA infusions. The APTT should be kept at two times the control value.

- Aspirin therapy should be initiated within 24 hours of admission for acute myocardial infarction patients. Aspirin has been shown to reduce mortality and reocclusion when used in combination with thrombolytic agents. There is no significant increase in the risk of bleeding with dosages of 81 to 325 mg.
- Contraindications to thrombolytic therapy include active internal bleeding, intracranial neoplasm, severe hypertension (systolic >180 mmHg or diastolic >110 mmHg), recent cerebrovascular event (within 2 months), recent surgery (within 10 days), trauma, recent organ biopsy, prolonged cardiopulmonary resuscitation, or hemostatic defects.
- Known allergy to streptokinase or APSAC or exposure within the last 6 months precludes the use of either agent.
- When diluting these agents, gently roll the vial between your hands to mix. Do not shake vials.

Adverse Effect

- Hemorrhage requiring cryoprecipitate, fresh frozen plasma, packed red blood cells, or whole blood occurs in 3% to 10% of patients. Patients should be typed and cross-matched on admission. Cryoprecipitate is the best blood product for correction of the lytic state after thrombolytic therapy. Ten units of cryoprecipitate will raise the fibrinogin level by 0.7 g/L and factor VIII by 30%. Antifibrinolytic therapy is seldom necessary.
- Intracranial hemorrhage occurs in 0.5% to 1.5% of patients.
- Most patients experience minor bleeding at catheter and venipuncture sites, which can be controlled by pressure application and minimal manipulation of arterial lines.
- Allergic reactions may occur with streptokinase or APSAC. Premedication with diphenhydramine or

steroids before administration prevents this reaction.

- Hypotension may occur with the use of these agents and can be corrected with volume replacement. Hypotension resulting from streptokinase may respond to IV atropine 0.5 to 1.0 mg in addition to volume replacement. Transient reperfusion dysrhythmias may also occur.

BRONCHODILATORS

Theophylline (Various)

Pharmacology

Theophylline competitively inhibits phosphodiesterase, resulting in increased concentrations of cyclic adenosine monophosphate (cAMP). Increased concentrations of cAMP lead to bronchodilation and pulmonary vasodilation. Other pharmacological actions include diuresis, coronary vasodilation, cardiac stimulation, cerebral stimulation, and improved diaphragmatic contractility.

Uses

Theophylline is used in the treatment of various pulmonary diseases including asthma, COPD, periodic apnea, and pulmonary edema.

Dosing and Administration (See Table 19)

- Theophylline can be administered orally, rectally, or parenterally. IM and PR administration are not preferred routes of administration.
- The recommendations in Table 19 provide guidelines only. Theophylline has a narrow therapeutic index and should be carefully monitored to avoid toxicity. The usual therapeutic range is 10 to 20 µg/ml. Levels above 20 µg/ml are associated with toxicity, while levels below 5 µg/ml are considered ineffective. Dosages resulting in serum levels of 20 to 25 µg/ml should be reduced by 10% and levels rechecked after 3 days. Dosages resulting in levels

---

TABLE 19 **Theophylline***

Patient Population	Aminophylline Loading Dose (IV)	Theophylline Loading Dose (IV)	Oral Theophylline (mg/kg/day)	Initial IV Aminophylline† (mg/kg/hr)	Initial IV Theophylline‡ (mg/kg/hr)
Healthy adult smokers	6 mg/kg	5 mg/kg	13-20	0.8	0.65
Healthy adult nonsmokers	6 mg/kg	5 mg/kg	10-13	0.5	0.4
Cardiac decompensation, cor pulmonale, liver dysfunction, elderly	6 mg/kg	5 mg/kg	5†	0.25	0.2

*Dosages are estimates to achieve plasma levels of 10-20 µg/ml; adjust dosage to serum level, toxicity, and therapeutic response.
†Caution should be used for doses >400 mg/day.
‡Represents initial IV maintenance dose; obtain serum level after 4 to 6 hours and adjust infusion rate accordingly.

of 25 to 30 µg/ml should be held for one dose and then reduced by 25%. Dosages resulting in levels greater than 30 µg/ml should be held for 2 doses and then reduced by 50%. For subtherapeutic or low serum levels, dosages may be increased by 25% in 3-day increments with repeated serum level monitoring.

- Intravenous administration should be no greater than 25 mg/min. Each 1 mg/kg of theophylline (1.25 mg/kg aminophylline) results in an approximate 2-µg/ml increase in serum concentrations.
- Patients should be switched to extended release preparations when possible. The sustained release formation should not be crushed or chewed. Contents of sustained release capsules that contain beads may be sprinkled on food if necessary.
- Oral preparations may be given with food or antacids to reduce GI upset.
- Steady state levels are reached within 2 days in most patients. Trough levels are preferred. Oral dosing should be initiated when the IV infusion is discontinued.
- Monitor serum levels and adverse effects.

Adverse Effects

- Theophylline produces GI irritation including nausea, vomiting, epigastric pain, abdominal cramps, anorexia, and diarrhea. These are more frequently seen with serum levels above 20 µg/ml but may occur with "therapeutic" levels. Reductions in dosage usually alleviate these symptoms.
- Adverse CNS effects include headache, irritability, restlessness, nervousness, insomnia, dizziness, and seizures. Serious CNS effects usually occur with levels greater than 35 µg/ml. These effects are dose related and are minimized with reduced dosages.
- Other adverse effects include palpitations, sinus tachycardia, increased heart rate, flushing, hypotension, dysrhythmias, and circulatory failure. These cardiovascular effects are usually associated with rapid IV administration or excessive serum levels.

Drug Interactions

- The following drugs may increase theophylline serum levels: cimetidine, ciprofloxacin, oral contraceptives, disulfiram, erythromycin, and calcium channel blockers.
- The following may decrease theophylline serum levels: food, barbiturates, phenytoin, and rifampin.

Beta Agonists/Anticholinergics

Pharmacology

These agents stimulate beta-adrenergic receptors and have little or no effect on alpha-receptors. This stimulation relaxes bronchial and vascular smooth muscle and inhibits mast cell release.

The anticholinergic agents competitively inhibit the effects of acetylcholine on muscarinic receptors, leading to bronchodilation and decreased tracheobronchial secretions.

Uses

These agents are used for the symptomatic treatment of asthma and bronchospasm.

Dosing and Administration (See Table 20)

- See Table 20 for commonly used bronchodilators.
- The metered dose inhalers (MDI) should be shaken well before use and the mouthpiece placed in the mouth with the lips tightly closed around it. The patient should exhale through the nose as completely as possible and then inhale deeply while actuating the inhaler. The patient should hold his/her breath for a few seconds and then exhale slowly.
- These agents may be diluted with normal saline for nebulization.

Adverse Effects

- The most common adverse effects of beta agonists are tachycardia, tremor, palpitations, hypertension, ECG changes, nervousness, headache, fatigue, dizziness, nausea, throat irritation, and cough. These effects can be minimized by appropriate dosing and administration. The beta$_2$ selective agents tend to cause fewer cardiovascular adverse effects.
- The major adverse effects of the anticholinergic agents are dryness of mouth and eyes, flushing, light-headedness, and tachycardia. These effects are generally mild and are minimized by careful administration of the dose.

COLLOID PLASMA VOLUME EXPANDERS

Pharmacology and Use

The three primary colloid solutions available are albumin, hetastarch, and dextran. All of these are used for plasma volume expansion in hypovolemic shock associated with hemorrhage, trauma, sepsis, or burns. They may also be used as pump primers and volume expanders in cardiopulmonary bypass. These agents should be used cautiously during the "leaky phase" of adult respiratory distress syndrome (ARDS).

Dosing and Administration/Adverse Effects (See Table 21)

- These agents should be used in conjunction with crystalloids and blood products where appropriate. Patients should be monitored closely to prevent volume overload. Invasive hemodynamic monitoring is preferred when possible.

TABLE 20 Commonly Used Inhalational Bronchodilators

Pharmacological Class	Drug	Trade Name	Adult Dosage	Route	Receptor B₁	Receptor B₂	Onset (min)	Peak (min)	Duration (hr)
Beta Agonist	Isoproterenol	Isuprel, various	1-2 inhalations up to 5 times daily	MDI	++++	++++	2	3-5	2-3
			2.5 ml of 0.1% solution q1-2h prn	NEB			2	3-5	1-2
	Isoetharine	Bronkosol, various	1-2 inhalations q4-6h	MDI	++	+++	2	15-30	2-3
			5-10 mg q2-4h	NEB			2	15-30	2-3
	Metaproterenol	Alupent, Metaprel, various	1-3 inhalations q4-6h	MDI	++	++	2	30-60	2-3
			15 mg q2-4h	NEB			5	30-60	2-3
			20 mg q4-6h	PO			15	30-60	4-6
	Albuterol	Proventil, Ventolin	1-2 inhalations q4-6h	MDI	+/0	++++	5	15-60	2-6
			2.5-5 mg q4-6h	NEB			5	15-60	2-6
	Terbutaline	Brethine, various	2-4 mg q6-8h	PO			30	120-180	4-8
			1-3 inhalations q4-6h	MDI	+/0	++++	5	15-30	2-6
			5-7 mg q4-6h	NEB			5	15-30	2-6
			0.25-0.5 mg q2-6h	SC			5	30	2-4
	Fenoterol	Berotec	5 mg q6-8h	PO	+	++++	30-60	120-180	4-8
			1-2 inhalations q4-6h	MDI			5	15-30	2-6
Anticholinergic	Atropine	Various	5-10 mg q6-8h	PO	0	0	30-60	120-180	4-8
			0.4-1 mg	NEB			5-15	30-120	3-5
	Ipratropium	Atrovent	1-2 inhalations q4-8h	MDI	0	0	3-30	90-120	3-8

MDI = metered dose inhaler.
NEB = nebulization.
PO = orally.
SC = subcutaneous.
0 = no effect.
+ = mild.
++ = moderate.
+++ = high.
++++ = very high.

TABLE 21 **Colloid Plasma Volume Expanders**

Agent	Sodium Content (mEq/L)	Plasma Volume Expansion per 500 ml (ml)	Duration of Expansion (hr)	Dosing Limitations	Adverse Effects	Comments
Albumin 25%	130-160	1,700	≤24	125 g/day maximum; rate should not exceed 1 ml/min	Allergic reactions; fluid overload; pulmonary edema; hypocalcemia	Expensive; $110-150/25 g
Albumin 5%	130-160	500	≤24	125 g/day maximum; rate should not exceed 4 ml/min	Same as for 25% albumin	$110-150/25 g
Dextran 40 (NS) (D₅W)	154 0	500-1,000 500-1,000	1-6	2 g/kg/day maximum for first 24 hours, then 1 g/kg/day up to 5 days	Renal failure; osmotic diuresis; anaphylaxis; interference with blood crossmatching; hemorrhage	$60-90/500 ml
Dextran 70 (NS) (D₅W)	154 0	500-700 500-700	≤24	1.2 g/kg/day maximum for first 24 hours, then 600 mg/kg/day up to 5 days	Same as for dextran 40	$60-90/500 ml
Hetastarch 6%	154	500-700	≤36	1,500 ml/day maximum	Coagulopathy; pulmonary edema; anaphylaxis; hyperamylasemia	$50-60/500 ml

DIURETICS

Pharmacology

Diuretic agents increase the elimination of salt and water by the kidney and are classified by their mechanism of action. The loop diuretics (furosemide, bumetanide, ethacrynic acid) promote the excretion of water, sodium, chloride, and other electrolytes by inhibiting tubular reabsorption in the medullary and cortical portions of the ascending loop of Henle. The thiazide diuretics inhibit sodium reabsorption in the early distal tubule portion of the nephron. The potassium-sparing diuretics are weak agents that work in the collecting duct to promote sodium excretion and potassium retention.

Uses

Diuretics are indicated for hypertension, chronic and acute heart failure, edema or fluid overload, and renal insufficiency.

Dosing and Administration (See Table 22)

- Loop diuretics are the most potent and may be given alone or in combination with other diuretics. These agents are preferred over thiazides as initial therapy in patients with renal insufficiency or pulmonary congestion. For acute pulmonary edema, the dose of furosemide is 0.5 to 1 mg/kg initially. Bumetanide is 40 times more potent than furosemide, and many patients respond well to alternating loop diuretics if they appear tolerant with chronic use.
- Thiazide diuretics are moderately potent and are preferred for the initial management of hypertension. Except for metolazone, these agents are useless in patients with a creatinine clearance less than 30 ml/min. Dosages of hydrochlorothiazide greater than 100 mg/day (or 1,000 mg/day chlorothiazide) are usually ineffective, and patients should be changed to loop diuretics.
- Patients with poor renal function or low albumin or sodium levels respond better to larger doses of loop diuretics given once daily rather than smaller doses given at multiple intervals. Combinations of loop and thiazide diuretics may be necessary in patients who fail to respond to high doses of loop diuretics alone.
- Potassium-sparing diuretics are weak and ineffective when used alone; they are most useful when combined with other diuretics.

Adverse Effects

- Hypokalemia is the most common and serious adverse effect of diuretic therapy. These agents may reduce serum potassium by 0.5 to 1 mEq/L, depending on the preexisting potassium levels and diuretic dose.
- Potassium-sparing diuretics may cause hyperkalemia, especially in patients with renal impairment. These agents should be cautiously used in patients receiving potassium supplements or ACE inhibitors.
- Loop diuretics may cause ototoxicity if given parenterally in high doses over short periods. The risk is greatest with ethacrynic acid and least with

TABLE 22 **Commonly Used Diuretics**

Agent	Trade Name	Route	Onset (min)	Peak (hr)	Duration (hr)	Dose (mg/day)
THIAZIDES						
Chlorothiazide	Diuril	Oral	60-120	3-6	6-12	500-1,000
		IV	15	0.5	2	250-1,000
Hydrochloro-thiazide	Hydrodiuril	Oral	60-120	3-6	6-12	12.5-100
Metolazone	Zaroxolyn	Oral	60-120	3-6	12-24	5-20
LOOP DIURETICS						
Ethacrynic acid	Edecrin	IV	30	2	6-12	50-400
Furosemide	Lasix	Oral	30-60	1-2	6-8	40-1,500
		IV	5-10	0.5-1.0	2	40-1,000
Bumetanide	Bumex	Oral	30-60	1-2	4-6	1-10
		IV	5-10	0.5-1.0	2-3	1-10
POTASSIUM-SPARING DIURETICS						
Amiloride	Midamor	Oral	120	10	24	5-10
Spironolactone	Aldactone	Oral	Gradual	72	48-72	25-200
Triamterene	Dyrenium	Oral	120-240	6	9-24	100-300
CARBONIC ANHYDRASE INHIBITORS						
Acetazolamide	Diamox	Oral	60	2-4	8	250-500

From Kinney, M. R., Packa, D. R., Andreoli, K. G., et al. (1991). *Comprehensive cardiac care* (7th ed.). St. Louis: Mosby–Year Book.

bumetanide. Doses should not be given faster than 40 mg/min for furosemide, 1.0 mg/min for bumetanide, or 2.5 mg/min for ethacrynic acid.
- Thiazide diuretics may produce glucose intolerance and lipid abnormalities.
- Other adverse effects of diuretics are hyponatremia, hypomagnesemia, abnormalities in uric acid and calcium, fatigue, exercise intolerance, hypovolemia, and metabolic alkalosis. Most are dose related and can be minimized by dose reduction or electrolyte replacement.

ELECTROLYTE REPLACEMENT

Calcium (Various)

Pharmacology

The presence of free ionic calcium in body fluids is required for many complex physiological processes such as blood clot formation, muscle contraction, and nerve impulse transmission.

Uses

Calcium is used in the treatment of cardiac resuscitation, hypocalcemia, hyperkalemia, and hypermagnesemia.

Dosing and Administration
- The usual adult parenteral dose is 0.5 to 1 g calcium chloride given slow IV push or 1 to 2 g of calcium gluceptate or gluconate given slow IV push. One gram of calcium chloride has 13.6 mEq/L of elemental calcium, while 1 g of either calcium gluceptate or gluconate has only 4.5 mEq of elemental calcium.
- Extravasation of calcium chloride can cause tissue necrosis or sloughing.
- A continuous monitoring of cardiac function should accompany the use of intravenous calcium.
- Patients should be constantly monitored for signs of additional electrolyte imbalance.

Adverse Effects
- Calcium salts may cause bradycardia, cardiac arrest, diarrhea, irregular heartbeat, loss of appetite, mental depression, and fatigue.

Drug Interactions
- Administration of intravenous calcium preparations to patients who are also receiving calcium-ion influx inhibitors may diminish the effect of calcium-ion influx inhibitors.
- Administration of intravenous calcium to patients who are also receiving digitalis glycosides or who have been digitalized may cause severe cardiac dys-

rhythmias; some may be fatal.
- Hypercalcemia may occur in patients receiving vitamin D and calcium preparations concurrently during long-term therapy.
- Concurrent use with magnesium sulfate may neutralize effects.
- Use with tetracyclines may decrease absorption of tetracycline.

Magnesium

Pharmacology

Magnesium is the second most common intracellular cation and is essential in many metabolic pathways. The average daily amount required to maintain magnesium balance is 0.3 to 0.4 mEq/kg/day. In excessive doses, magnesium has anticonvulsant and cathartic actions. The anticonvulsant activity is caused by inhibition of peripheral neuromuscular transmission. Cathartic activity may be related to the hyperosmotic effect of the magnesium ion.

Uses

Magnesium is used as an anticonvulsant for seizures associated with eclampsia and as a saline laxative, and for the treatment of magnesium deficiency.

Dosing and Administration
- Asymptomatic magnesium deficiency may be treated with normal doses of magnesium-containing antacids. Symptomatic magnesium deficiency is best treated by IV infusion of 10 g the first day (6 g over 4 hours, then 4 g over the remainder of the day) and 5 g IV daily thereafter for 1 to 4 days. For life-threatening magnesium deficiency, 2 to 4 g given IV over 2 to 4 minutes followed by 10 g over the remaining 24 hours is given on day 1 and 5 g daily thereafter for 1 to 4 days. All these dosages are for adults and assume normal renal function. IV infusions should be diluted in 250 to 500 ml of IV fluid and infused over 4 to 6 hours.
- For the treatment of eclampsia, a loading dose of 4 to 5 g (20% solution) should be given over 4 to 5 minutes followed by an IV infusion of 1 to 2 g/hr. The infusion should maintain a therapeutic magnesium level of 4 to 7 mEq/ml. Magnesium should be continued for 24 hours after the delivery.
- Magnesium may be given by IM injection using a 50% solution for adults.
- The adult IM dose for symptomatic magnesium deficiency is 2 g every 4 hours for 6 doses on day 1 followed by 1 g every 4 hours for 6 doses on day 2. If continued replacement is necessary, 1 g IM every 6 hours can be given for an additional 3 days.
- Replacement therapy should be carried out over 4

to 7 days to allow intracellular stores to be replenished.

Adverse Effects

- Use of magnesium salts in patients with renal impairment may lead to hypermagnesemia.
- Adverse effects are primarily due to hypermagnesemia and include flushing, sweating, hypotension, CNS depression, electrolyte disturbances, respiratory difficulties, and circulatory collapse.
- Dehydration may occur if taken with insufficient fluids.

Phosphorus

Pharmacology

Phosphorus is the major intracellular anion and essential for a large variety of biochemical processes. The adult body contains 700 to 800 g of phosphorus, and normal serum levels are 2.7 to 4.5 mg/dl for adults. Normal oral requirements are 30 to 90 mmol/day.

Uses

Phosphorus is used to treat hypophosphatemia or as a cathartic.

Dosing and Administration

- For treatment of profound hypophosphatemia (<1 g/dl) or symptomatic hypophosphatemia, intravenous therapy is recommended. The usual adult dosage is 1 to 1.5 mmol/kg given over 24 hours. Serum levels should be checked every 6 to 12 hours until the level has stabilized.
- For the treatment of simple hypophosphatemia (serum PO_4 >1 mg/dl), the adult IV dosage is 0.08 to 0.5 mmol/kg given over 4 to 6 hours. Parenteral phosphorus must be discontinued when serum levels are above 2 mg/dl; repletion should be continued with oral therapy. It may take several days of oral therapy to replace intracellular stores.
- Large oral doses of phosphate liquid preparations induce diarrhea and can be used as laxatives or bowel preps. When used for phosphorus replacement, these solutions should be adequately diluted to prevent diarrhea.
- Phosphorus precipitates in the presence of calcium salts, and no more than 40 mmol should be added to 5 mEq calcium per liter of fluid.

Adverse Effects

- The most frequent adverse effects are diarrhea and upset stomach with oral dosing.
- Hyperphosphatemia, metastatic calcium deposition, dehydration, hypotension, hypomagnesemia,

and hyperkalemia or hypernatremia may also occur.
- Use cautiously in patients with renal dysfunction.

Potassium

Pharmacology

Potassium is the predominant cation within cells, while sodium content is relatively low. In extracellular fluid, sodium predominates, and the potassium content is low. A membrane-bound enzyme, sodium/potassium–activated adenosine triphosphatase, actively transports or pumps sodium out of and potassium into cells to maintain these concentration gradients. The gradients are necessary to conduct nerve impulses in such tissues as the heart, brain, and skeletal muscle, and to maintain normal renal function and acid–base balance. High intracellular potassium concentrations are necessary for numerous metabolic processes.

Uses

Potassium is used for the treatment of hypokalemia.

Dosing and Administration

- The adult dosage is variable and must be adjusted on the basis of the needs of the individual. The following guidelines are considered rough estimates of potassium deficit. A serum level of 3 mEq/L represents a deficit of approximately 100 to 300 mEq, and each additional 1 mEq/L fall in serum potassium represents an additional deficit of 200 to 400 mEq.
- The average maximum recommended concentration of potassium in IV fluid is 80 mEq/L. Any concentration greater than 30 mEq/L may result in pain and phlebitis. Rates of infusion should not exceed 20 mEq/hr, and maximum daily amounts of replacement should be limited to 200 mEq in patients with normal renal function.
- Oral solutions should be diluted before administration either orally or enterally.
- Serum levels should be closely monitored throughout replacement therapy.

Adverse Effects

- Bad taste, nausea, vomiting, diarrhea, and abdominal pain are frequent with oral preparations. Esophageal and small bowel ulcerations have occurred with enteric coated tablets.
- Local tissue necrosis has occurred with extravasation of the IV solution. The addition of lidocaine to IV solutions is not recommended.
- Use cautiously in patients with renal impairment.

GI AGENTS

H$_2$ Antagonists

Pharmacology

These agents inhibit basal and nocturnal gastric acid secretion by competitive inhibition of the action of histamine at the histamine H$_2$-receptors of the parietal cells and inhibit gastric acid secretion stimulated by food, pentagastrin, caffeine, and insulin.

Uses

These agents are used to treat duodenal and gastric ulcers, hypersecretory conditions, and gastroesophageal reflux, and for stress ulcer prophylaxis.

Dosing and Administration/Adverse Effects (See Table 23)

- The efficacy of these agents may be reduced by cigarette smoking.
- Rapid IV administration is not recommended with any of these agents because of the risk of cardiac dysrhythmias and hypotension.
- Antacids may be administered with any of these agents as adjunct agents to reduce both pain and gastric secretion.
- These agents may be given IM or by IV intermittent or IV continuous infusion or added to total parenteral nutrition infusions for daily IV administration.

Drug Interactions

- Cimetidine reduces the metabolism of the following drugs: warfarin, phenytoin, benzodiazepines, lidocaine, metronidazole, and theophylline.
- Famotidine and nizatidine do not appear to significantly inhibit the metabolism of drugs by the crytochrome P450 enzyme system.
- Ranitidine has less of an effect on hepatic metabolism than does cimetidine and does not appear to influence drug metabolism significantly in most patients. However, patients should be monitored closely when initiating concurrent therapy with any of the following agents: warfarin, theophylline, benzodiazepines, or nifedipine.

Omeprazole (Prilosec)

Pharmacology

Omeprazole inhibits basal and stimulated gastric acid secretion by specific inhibition of an ATPase enzyme system at the secretory surface of the gastric parietal cell. The degree of inhibition is dose related.

Uses

Omeprazole is used to treat gastric and duodenal ulcers, gastroesophageal reflux, severe erosion esophagitis, and hypersecretory disease.

Dosing and Administration

- The recommended adult oral dosage is 20 mg daily for 4 to 8 weeks. If omeprazole is used for hypersecretory conditions, the starting dosage should be 60 mg daily and adjustments should be made as needed up to a maximum dosage of 120 mg PO three times daily.
- The drug is available in a sustained release formula only and should not be opened, crushed, or chewed.
- The concomitant use of antacids is safe, but concurrent use of anticholinergics and H$_2$ antagonists should be avoided.
- Dosage adjustments are not necessary in renal or hepatic dysfunction.

Adverse Effects

- The most common adverse effects are headache, diarrhea, nausea, abdominal pain, dizziness, constipation, rash, and asthenia.
- Gastric carcinoids and mucosal hypertrophy have occurred in patients being treated for hypersecretory disease. Short-term use of omeprazole appears to represent no carcinogenic risk, but long-term use remains questionable.

Sucralfate (Carafate)

Pharmacology

Sucralfate binds to the surface of gastric and duodenal ulcers, with a greater affinity for duodenal ulcers than for gastric. Sucralfate also binds to drug-induced gastric erosions. This binding results in a barrier that protects the mucosa from further damage and allows it to heal.

Uses

Sucralfate is used to treat gastric and duodenal ulcers.

Dosing and Administration

- Sucralfate is available orally only. It should be taken on an empty stomach 1 hour before meals and at bedtime.
- Sucralfate administration should be separated from administration of antacids and other medications by 30 to 60 minutes.
- The adult dosage is 1 g four times daily or 2 g twice daily.
- A slurry can be made by dissolving the tablet in 20 ml of water for 5 minutes.

Adverse Effects

- Sucralfate is well tolerated. The most frequent adverse effect is constipation. Other adverse effects include diarrhea, nausea, flatulence, dry mouth, rash, and headache.

TABLE 23 **Histamine H$_2$-receptor Antagonists**

Agent	Trade Name	Adult Oral Dosage*	Adult IV Dosage	Adjust Dosage (Cl$_{cr}$<50 ml/min)	Duration of Action (hr)	Adverse Effects
Cimetidine	Tagamet	300 mg qid; 400 mg bid; 800 mg qhs	300 mg q6-8h	Yes	4-6	Dizziness; confusion; rash; hypotension (IV); bone marrow suppression; gynecomastia; arthralgias
Famotidine	Pepcid	40 mg qhs; 20 mg bid	20 mg q12h	Yes	10-18	Headache; diarrhea; dizziness; constipation
Nizatidine	Axid	150 mg bid; 300 mg qhs		Yes	10-12	Fatigue; urticaria; sweating; hyperuricemia
Ranitidine	Zantac	150 mg bid; 300 mg qhs	50 mg q6-8h	Yes	6-8 (IV) 10-12 (PO)	Headache; rash; dizziness; diarrhea; constipation; confusion; hepatotoxicity; increased liver function tests; thrombocytopenia

* Regimen will depend on diagnosis (i.e., ulcer type, acute treatment *vs.* chronic prophylaxis, stress ulcer prophylaxis).
Cl$_{cr}$ = creatinine clearance.

IMMUNOSUPPRESSIVES

Antibodies

Pharmacology

This group of agents includes antithymocyte globulin (ATG) and monoclonal antibodies of the CD3 complex (OKT3). These agents inhibit cell-mediated immune responses such as allograft rejection and delayed hypersensitivity reactions. ATG interacts with lymphoid cells leading to their destruction, while OKT3 specifically blocks their function.

Uses

These agents are used to prevent and treat acute episodes of rejection in recipients of transplanted organs. These agents may also be used in bone marrow allotransplantation.

Dosing and Administration (See Table 24)

- ATG concentrate for injection should be diluted before use with half normal saline or normal saline to yield a solution no greater than 1 mg/ml. The ATG concentrate should be injected directly into the fluid for dilution, allowing no contact with air inside the container. The solution can be mixed by rotating the bag or bottle. Do not shake. Do not use after 12 hours, and refrigerate until use.
- OKT3 is available as a 1 mg/ml solution for injection. The dose should be filtered and then bolused.
- Both these agents require premedication with methylprednisolone (1 mg/kg) or hydrocortisone (25-100 mg), acetaminophen (650 mg orally or rectally), and/or diphenhydramine (25 to 50 mg orally or parenterally). Patients should be monitored closely for signs of hypersensitivity reactions.
- Skin testing for ATG before the initial dose is recommended. An intradermal injection of 0.1 ml of a 1:1,000 dilution of ATG with a control of normal saline should be used. A positive skin test reaction consists of a wheal and/or area of erythema 10 mm or more in diameter.

Adverse Effects/Drug Interactions (See Table 24)

- The concomitant use of other immunosuppressants with these agents should be monitored closely. Doses of corticosteroids and azathioprine may need to be reduced, and cyclosporine therapy may need to be reduced or temporarily discontinued.

Corticosteroids

Pharmacology

The pharmacological effects of the corticosteroids are numerous and widespread. Adrenocorticoids diffuse across cell membranes and join with cytoplasmic receptors. These complexes then enter the cell nucleus, bind to DNA, and stimulate transcription of mRNA. Subsequently, various enzymes are synthesized that are responsible for glucocorticoid and mineralocorticoid effects. The glucocorticoid effects include antiinflammatory, immunosuppressive (prevention or suppression of cell-mediated immune reactions), and metabolic (decreased peripheral use of glucose, increased glycogen storage in the liver, increased blood glucose concentrations and insulin resistance). The mineralocorticoid effects cause sodium reabsorption, potassium and hydrogen excretion, and subsequent water retention.

Uses

Because of their widespread effects, these agents are used for many disorders other than adrenocortical replacement therapy. Some of these uses include treatment of arthritis, renal disease, collagen and skin disorders, allergic disease, asthma, COPD, ocular disease, cerebral edema, inflammatory disease of the GI tract, malignancy, organ transplantation, and liver disease. Clinically, these drugs are used primarily for their antiinflammatory and immunosuppressive effects.

Dosing and Administration (See Table 25)

- The dosage of corticosteroids varies depending on the disease state being treated and individual patient responses. Administration of shorter acting preparations in the early morning produces fewer side effects and less pituitary–adrenal suppression. More frequent dosing and use of longer acting preparations promotes hypothalamic–pituitary axis suppression.
- Patients who have received more than 40 mg of prednisone daily (or an equivalent) for more than 1 to 2 weeks must be carefully withdrawn from corticosteroid therapy to prevent withdrawal. Protocols are dependent on dosage, corticosteroid preparation, duration of therapy, and the disease state being treated.
- Corticosteroids may also be administered by joint and soft tissue injection as well as by intralesional, topical, ophthalmic, and rectal administration.
- The dosage of corticosteroid used should be the lowest possible to maintain good therapeutic response with minimal adverse effects.
- Patients under stress usually require higher than normal doses of corticosteroids during the stressful period. Patients with Addison's disease typically require as much as 200 to 400 mg of hydrocortisone daily.

Adverse Effects

- Prolonged therapy may lead to suppression of pituitary–adrenal function resulting in acute adrenal insufficiency if therapy is abruptly discontinued.

TABLE 24 **Immunosuppressive Agents**

Drug Class	Agent	Trade Name	Adult Dose for Transplantation*	Route	How Supplied	Comments	Clinical Toxicity
Cyclic polypeptide	Cyclosporine	Sandimmune	15 mg/kg/day for 1-2 wks, then 3-10 mg/kg/day maintenance	PO	Oral: 100 mg/ml	Store IV solutions in glass; do not use tubing with polyvinyl chloride; give IV as slow infusion over 2-6 hr; give oral solution in milk or orange juice	Nephrotoxicity (25% to 75%); hypertension (>30%); neurological toxicity; elevated hepatic enzymes; infection; hirsutism; gingival hyperplasia; leukopenia
Cytotoxic agents	Azathioprine	Imuran	2-6 mg/kg/day given bid or tid	IV	Injection: 50 mg/ml	Protect IV solutions from light; give IV over 30-60 min	Myelosuppression; mucositis; nausea; cholestatic liver toxicity; restrictive lung disease; rash; malignancy
			3-5 mg/kg/day for 1-2 days before transplant, then 1-3 mg/kg/day	PO	Tablet: 50 mg		
Antibodies	Antithymocyte globulin (ATG)	Atgam	3-5 mg/kg initially, then 1-3 mg/kg/day	IV	Injection: 100 mg	Skin test recommended; give by slow IV infusion over 4-6 hours and premedicate; use in-line filter	Febrile reactions; myelosuppression; hypersensitivity; serum sickness; rash; dermatological reactions; headache; hypotension; dizziness; fatigue; malaise; dyspnea
			15 mg/kg/day for 14 days, then qod for 14 days	IV	Injection: 50 mg		
	Monoclonal antibody	Orthoclone OKT3	5 mg/day for 10-14 days	IV	Injection: 1 mg/ml	Give undiluted over 1 min; premedicate; filter before use	

* Represents guidelines and may vary significantly.

TABLE 25   Adrenal Corticosteroid Comparison

Drug	Relative Antiinflammatory Potency*	Equivalent Doses (mg)	Relative Mineralocorticoid Activity*	Daily Dosage (mg) Above Which Pituitary Suppression Normally Occurs†		Biological Activity (hr)
				Male	Female	
Cortisone	0.8	25	0.8	25-35	20-30	8-12
Hydrocortisone	1	20	1	20-30	15-25	8-12
Methylprednisolone	5	4	0.5	7.5-10	7.5	12-36
Prednisolone	4	5	0.8	7.5-10	7.5	12-36
Prednisone	3.5	5	0.8	7.5-10	7.5	12-36
Triamcinolone	5	4	0	7.5-10	7.5	12-36
Betamethasone	25	0.6	0	1-1.5	1-1.5	36-54
Dexamethasone	30	0.75	0	1-1.5	1-1.5	36-54

*Based on hydrocortisone as the standard.
†Provided as estimate only; will vary with individual patients.

Symptoms of adrenal insufficiency include fever, myalgia, arthralgia, malaise, hypotension, and confusion. Abrupt withdrawal may also exacerbate the disease state for which the patient is being treated.
- Other adverse effects include fluid and electrolyte disturbances, hypertension, hypoglycemia, glycosuria, infection, peptic ulcers, osteoporosis, myopathy, menstrual irregularities, behavioral disturbances, leukocytosis, poor wound healing, ocular cataracts, glaucoma, and Cushing's syndrome.
- These effects are reduced by smaller dosages of shorter acting agents given at longer intervals.

Drug Interactions

- Severe hypokalemia can occur with concurrent use of acetazolamide, chlorthalidone, ethacrynic acid, furosemide, metolazone, and thiazides.
- Concurrent use with indomethacin and other ulcerogenic drugs can produce GI erosions.
- Corticosteroids antagonize the effects of the oral anticoagulants.
- Concurrent use with antidiabetic agents may require higher doses of the antidiabetic drugs.
- Concurrent use with cardiac glycosides may enhance the possibility of dysrhythmias or digitalis toxicity associated with hypokalemia.

Cyclosporine (Sandimmune)

Pharmacology

The exact mechanism of action is unknown but seems to be related to selective and reversible inhibition of the T helper lymphocytes, which play a major role in both cellular and humoral immune responses. Cyclosporine does not affect nonspecific myelosuppression.

Uses

Cyclosporine is used to treat and prevent organ rejection.

Dosing and Administration (See Table 24)

- Cyclosporine blood concentration monitoring is recommended for all patients receiving the drug. Therapeutic trough levels of 150 ng/ml (high-pressure liquid chromatography, whole blood) for the first 2 months post–renal transplant and then 50 to 100 ng/ml thereafter have been associated with less nephrotoxicity. Levels above 300 ng/ml may lead to nephrotoxicity. Other blood concentration methods may be used, and the following are acceptable ranges for radioimmune assay: whole blood—250 to 800 ng/ml; and plasma—100 to 250 ng/ml. Lower blood levels of cyclosporine may be associated with increased risk of rejection, while higher blood levels may lead to excessive immunosuppression and nephrotoxicity.
- Cyclosporine therapy should be initiated 4 to 12 hours before transplantation and continued at 15 mg/kg/day for 1 to 2 weeks. Dosages may be tapered by 5% weekly to an eventual maintenance dosage of 3 to 10 mg/kg/day.
- The parenteral dosage of cyclosporine is one third that of the oral dosage.
- Rapid IV dosing may cause acute nephrotoxicity.
- Monitor blood levels and renal function.

Adverse Effects (See Table 24)

- Dose dependent nephrotoxicity occurs in over 35% of patients receiving cyclosporine. Nephrotoxicity is manifested by increased serum creatinine and BUN, fluid retention, dependent edema, hypertension, and metabolic acidosis. The risk for nephrotoxicity is increased with the use of other nephrotoxic agents. The dosage of cyclosporine should be gradually reduced.
- Hypertension occurs in approximately 25% to 40% of patients receiving cyclosporine. There is a rise in both systolic and diastolic pressures that occurs gradually in the initial weeks of therapy. Most pa-

tients respond to dosage reduction and/or antihypertensive therapy.

- Central nervous system effects occur in as many as 50%; manifestations include tremor, headache, seizures, paresthesias, flushing, and confusion.

Drug Interactions

- The following may decrease cyclosporine blood levels: loperamide, cholestyramine, somatostatin, phenobarbital, phenytoin, carbamazepine, rifampin, corticosteroids, and cigarettes.
- The following drugs may increase cyclosporine concentrations: metoclopramide, chenodeoxycholic acid, ketoconazole, dilitazem, and nicardipine.
- Concurrent use with other immunosuppressive agents increases the risk of infection and development of lymphoproliferative disorders.
- Concurrent use with other nephrotoxic agents (amphotericin B, aminoglycosides) may result in enhanced nephrotoxicity.

Cytotoxic Agents (Azathioprine)

Pharmacology

Azathioprine (Imuran) is a purine analogue that is converted to mercaptopurine in the body, which inhibits RNA and DNA synthesis. Azathioprine primarily suppresses cell-mediated hypersensitivity and may alter antibody formation.

Uses

Azathioprine is used as an adjunct in preventing the rejection of transplanted organs. It is also used for rheumatoid arthritis.

Dosing and Administration/Adverse Effects (See Table 24)

- The principal effect of azathioprine is bone marrow suppression manifested by leukopenia, macrocytic anemia, pancytopenia, and thrombocytopenia.
- The dosage of azathioprine should be reduced by 25% to 30% when used concomitantly with allopurinol.

INOTROPES (See Tables 26 and 27)

Digitalis Glycosides

Pharmacology

The digitalis glycosides increase the force of myocardial contraction by enhancing calcium influx and augmenting the release of free calcium ions within the myocardial cells. Digitalis glycosides increase the refractory period of the atrioventricular and sinoatrial nodes and decrease the conductivity of the bundle of His and the heart rate. These actions result from a direct effect on the myocardium and reflex vagal stimulation.

Uses

Digoxin is the most widely used digitalis glycoside. Digoxin is used primarily for the treatment of congestive heart failure, atrial fibrillation, atrial flutter, and paroxysmal tachycardia.

Dosing and Administration

- The serum half-life of digoxin is 36 hours in patients with normal renal function. The half-life increases as renal function declines, so less frequent dosing is necessary in patients with renal impairment. Patients with normal renal function require 0.125 to 0.5 mg/day to achieve serum levels of 0.5 to 2.0 ng/ml. In patients with a creatinine clearance less than 30 ml/min, starting maintenance dosages should be no greater than 0.125 mg/day and serum levels closely monitored to adjust the dosage. Anephric patients typically require every other day (qod) dosing but may occasionally require special regimens to maintain therapeutic serum levels.
- Loading doses are necessary when treating dysrhythmias but are seldom indicated when treating heart failure. A total dose of 10 to 15 μg/kg or 1 to 1.5 mg can be given as 0.25 mg IV or orally every 6 hours over 24 hours to load the patient. Serum levels should be monitored closely, and trough levels are preferred. Digoxin levels drawn within 6 to 8 hours of the administered dose are generally higher than the actual serum level because of the distribution of digoxin in the body.
- A daily maintenance dosage can be estimated as follows: (loading dose) $\times$ (% lost daily) = daily maintenance dose, where loading dose = 10 μg/kg and % lost = 14 + Cl_{cr}/5 expressed as %. For example, an 80-kg patient with a creatinine clearance of 80 ml/min would require 0.25 mg daily to initiate therapy.
- Generic preparations of digoxin may not have absorption and bioavailability equivalent to the more established Lanoxin product. Caution should be exercised when switching product preparations.
- Digoxin antibodies (Digibind) are available for the treatment of life-threatening digoxin toxicity. Each vial of Digibind binds approximately 0.6 mg of digoxin. Refer to the package insert for dose calculations. Digibind may be given as an IV bolus or infused over 30 minutes.
- The following conditions may increase myocardial sensitivity to digoxin: severe congestive heart failure, hypothyroidism, hypokalemia, hypomagnesemia, hypercalcemia, pulmonary heart disease, myocardial ischemia, myocardial infarction, myocarditis, cardiomyopathies, and valvular lesions.
- The following diseases may increase serum digoxin levels: renal impairment, hepatic disease, and severe congestive heart failure.

TABLE 26 **Sympathomimetic Pharmacology**

Drug	Adult Dose	Receptor Binding Strength Alpha	Beta₁	Beta₂	Dopamine	Relative Receptor Affinity (%) Alpha	Beta	HR	CO	TPR
Epinephrine	1-4 µg/min	+ + + +	+ + + +	+ + + +	0	50	50	↑↑	↑/↓	↑/↓
Norepinephrine	8-24 µg/min	+ + + +	+ +	0	0	90	10	↑↑	0/↓	↑↑
Isoproterenol	2-20 µg/min	0	+ + + +	+ + + +	0	0	100	↑↑	↑↑	↓
Dopamine	0.2-2 µg/kg/min	+	0	0	+ + + +	*	*	↑	↑	0/↓
	2-10 µg/kg/min	+ +	+	+	+ + + +			↑	↑	0/↑
	>10 µg/kg/min	+ + + +	+ +	+ +	+ + + +			↑	↑	↑
Dobutamine	2.5-20 µg/kg/min	+ +	+ + + +	+ +	0	0	100	↑	↑↑	↑/↓
Phenylephrine	0.04-0.2 mg/min	+ + + +	0	0	0	100	0	0	↓	↑↑

*Varies with dosage and individual patients.

  0 = no effect.
  + = minimal effect.
  + + = significant effect.
  + + + = strong effect.
  + + + + = strongest effect.
  HR = heart rate.
  CO = cardiac output.
  TPR = total peripheral resistance.
  ↑ = increased.
  ↑↑ = greatly increased.
  ↓ = decreased.

TABLE 27 **Newer Inotropic Agents**

Drug	Trade Name	Pharmacological Action	Dosage	Comments
Xamoterol	Corwin	Beta blocker with pronounced intrinsic sympathomimetic activity	200 bid PO	Contraindicated in severe CHF; may be of benefit in class I, II, or III; place in therapy unclear
Enoximone	Perfan	Phosphodiesterase inhibitor	90 μg/kg/min over 10-30 min	May worsen mortality in some patients; place in therapy unclear
Pimobendan		Phosphodiesterase inhibitor	2.5 mg bid PO	Benzimidazole derivative
Fenoldopam		Dopaminergic vasodilator		May be useful as adjunct agent; vasodilator with no inotropic activity
Ibopamine	Inopamil	Dopaminergic and beta-adrenergic agonist	50-200 mg bid or tid PO	May see some alteration of response with chronic therapy; early studies show benefit to class II, III CHF patients
Dopexamine		Dopaminergic with limited beta agonist activity		Vasodilator with inotropic activity

- Digoxin toxic patients are sensitive to electrical countershocks and may develop ventricular tachycardia or fibrillation if they receive electrical cardioversion.
- Electrolyte levels should be closely monitored. Hypokalemia or hypomagnesemia may worsen dysrhythmias.

Adverse Effects

- Digoxin side effects are common in a large percentage of patients because the drug has a narrow therapeutic range; overlap exists between therapeutic serum levels and toxicity.
- Cardiac toxicity may be evident in up to 90% of patients. Manifestations include ventricular tachycardia, premature ventricular contractions, AV junctional tachycardia, AV block, bradycardia, and atrial tachycardia.
- Neurological adverse effects may occur in up to 25% of patients and include personality changes, abnormal visual changes, headache, vertigo, peripheral neuritis, and generalized muscular weakness.
- Gastrointestinal adverse effects occur more often in the elderly population and may be seen in up to

75% of patients. Manifestations include anorexia, nausea, vomiting, and diarrhea.
- All these effects are more common with toxic or high serum blood levels. Most can be minimized or alleviated by decreasing the dosage of digoxin. If the toxicity is not life-threatening, hold the digoxin dose and reinstitute therapy at a lower dosage.

Drug Interactions

- The following drugs may increase digoxin levels: quinidine, verapamil, amiodarone, spironolactone.
- The following drugs may decrease digoxin levels: antacids, kaolin–pectin preparations, and bile acid–binding resins.

Sympathomimetics

Pharmacology

These agents stimulate the adrenergic nervous system to different degrees depending on the affinity and strength of binding to the adrenoreceptors (see Table 26). Epinephrine is a direct acting sympathomimetic agent that stimulates both alpha- and beta-adrenoreceptors, resulting in increased cardiac output, heart rate, conductivity, and total peripheral resistance. At low doses, epinephrine elicits greater $beta_2$-agonist effects, and vascular resistance or diastolic blood pressures may fall. The systolic pressure is maintained if there is adequate blood volume for the cardiac output. Alpha-receptor stimulation dominates at doses greater than 0.02 µg/kg/min, resulting in vasoconstriction and increased total peripheral resistance. Epinephrine significantly increases myocardial oxygen consumption, which limits its use as an inotropic agent.

Norepinephrine stimulates primarily alpha-adrenergic receptors. Very low doses of norepinephrine may produce $beta_1$-adrenergic effects leading to increased chronotropic, inotropic, and dromotropic effects. In the dosages used most often clinically, norepinephrine exerts a greater effect on alpha-receptors resulting in increased peripheral vascular resistance and mean arterial pressure. Cardiac output is usually unchanged or slightly decreased because of the increased afterload and reflex vagal effects.

Isoproterenol is a pure beta-adrenergic agonist and acts on both $beta_1$- and $beta_2$-receptors. Isoproterenol relaxes bronchial smooth muscle, skeletal muscle vasculature, and the alimentary tract. Clinically, isoproterenol increases the rate, contractility, and conductivity of the heart while lowering peripheral vascular resistance and diastolic blood pressure. Although this drug increases the cardiac output significantly, it also greatly increases myocardial oxygen consumption.

Dopamine acts on both adrenergic and dopaminergic receptors. At low dosages, dopamine stimulates primarily dopaminergic receptors, resulting in increased mesentery and renal blood flow. At moderate dosages, dopamine stimulates beta-adrenergic receptors as well, manifested as an increase in cardiac output and a fall in preload. These effects are more pronounced in patients with good left ventricular function. Those patients with poor left ventricular function may not benefit as greatly from moderate dosages of dopamine but typically respond best at low dosages. At higher dosages, all patients manifest primarily alpha-adrenergic effects with an increased mean arterial pressure and total peripheral resistance. It is important to note that as much as 50% of dopamine's hemodynamic actions may be produced by norepinephrine release.

Dobutamine is a synthetic catecholamine designed to exert positive inotropic effects with very little chronotropic, dromotropic, or alpha-adrenergic effects. It is a selective $beta_1$ agonist that increases contractility while lowering preload and renovascular resistance. Dobutamine has no dose dependent effects. It affects cardiac output consistently while affecting myocardial oxygen demands minimally. Dobutamine

is the preferred agent for inotropic support in most clinical situations.

Phenylephrine is a synthetic alpha agonist. The primary clinical manifestations are those seen with norepinephrine. This agent is very potent and induces a reflex vagal response. Phenylephrine has no direct effect on cardiac output but decreases it indirectly because of the increase in afterload.

Uses

Dobutamine and dopamine are used as inotropes in the management of low output syndromes. Dopamine, norepinephrine, epinephrine, and phenylephrine are used to treat cardiogenic shock, cardiac arrest, and hypotension. Isoproterenol is used primarily to enhance pacemaker activity and improve AV nodal conduction.

Dosing and Administration (See Table 26)

- All these agents are given by intravenous administration. Epinephrine and isoproterenol may be given by endotracheal routes when IV access is not possible.
- Dopamine, norepinephrine, and phenylephrine drips should be carefully monitored for extravasation. If local extravasation occurs, tissue necrosis is possible. Treat the area immediately with small intradermal injections of phentolamine for a total dose of 5 to 10 mg. Phentolamine is maximally effective if used within 6 hours of extravasation and useless after 24 hours.
- Dosages of these agents should be adjusted on the basis of invasive hemodynamic monitoring when possible. Monitor CO, ECG, PCWP, MAP, SVR, blood pressure, heart rate, renal function, electrolyte levels, and signs and symptoms of perfusion.
- These agents have additive effects when used in combination. Individual agents should be maximized before other agents are added to the regimen. The smallest dosage of the fewest possible agents should be used.
- An adequate circulating blood volume must be maintained for vasopressor agents. Hypovolemic patients will not respond to large vasopressor doses, and continued high dosages may worsen cardiac function.
- These agents can be easily titrated. Remember that the final hemodynamic response depends on the action of the drug and the response of the patient to those drug actions. Dosage adjustments may be made every 15 to 30 minutes in most patients. Many patients exhibit a threshold response and will not respond to higher dosages; combination therapy is indicated in these patients.

- All these agents are inactivated in alkaline solutions.
- Dobutamine may develop a pink discoloration with time. No significant potency is lost if used within 24 hours. Discoloration of any of the other agents is unacceptable, and they should be discarded.
- Tolerance to these agents may develop with time and can be overcome by increasing the dosage or altering concomitant therapy.
- Prediluted syringes of 1:10,000 of epinephrine are used for cardiac arrest while 1:1,000 dilutions are used for anaphylaxis. Accidental use of 1:1,000 dilutions given IV push (IVP) could result in cerebral hemorrhage or vascular collapse in some patients.
- Norepinephrine may be added to gastric lavage solution to treat acute gastrointestinal bleeding. The dose is 16 mg in 200 ml of iced saline.
- Dobutamine may be used intermittently in some patients with congestive heart failure. Dosages of 1.5 to 15 µg/kg/min for 4 to 72 hours weekly have been used beneficially in some patients.

Adverse Effects

- The most serious adverse effect of these agents is genesis or exacerbation of dysrhythmias. Cardiac rhythm should be monitored while administering these agents, especially when many agents are employed simultaneously.
- These agents increase the myocardial oxygen demand and may further myocardial ischemia in the presence of coronary artery disease.
- Other adverse effects include agitation, nausea, vomiting, headache, restlessness, and tremor.
- Low-dose dopamine may cause hypotension in some patients, especially when titrating the patient off the drug. Hypotension that develops with dosages lower than 2 µg/kg/min can be corrected by stopping the drug or administering fluids.

Phosphodiesterase Inhibitors

Pharmacology

These agents increase myocardial contractility by inhibiting myocardial cellular phosphodiesterase, thereby increasing the availability of calcium in the myocardium. They are also vasodilators and reduce systemic vascular resistance by an unknown mechanism. The inotropic effects of these agents are comparable to those of dobutamine, and both amrinone and milrinone are additive when used in combination with other inotropes. Although these agents are potent and effective, they remain second-line agents because of their toxicity. Oral use is associated with increased mortality and adverse effects; there is some speculation that long-term IV use may be detrimental.

Uses

These agents are indicated for the short-term management of low-output syndromes.

Dosing and Administration

- These agents are available for IV use only.
- These agents are compatible in half normal saline or normal saline only. Amrinone is light sensitive and should be covered after dilution. Dilutions greater than 3 mg/ml are not recommended for amrinone.
- Loading dose: (1) amrinone—0.75 mg/kg IV bolus over 5 to 30 minutes. The bolus may be repeated in 30 minutes if necessary; (2) milrinone—50 µg/kg over 10 minutes.
- Maintenance dose: (1) amrinone—5 to 20 µg/kg/min; (2) milrinone—0.375 to 0.75 µg/kg/min.
- Invasive monitoring is recommended when these agents are used. Monitor CO, ECG, PCWP, MAP, SVR, heart rate, electrolyte levels, and signs and symptoms of perfusion.
- Intermittent amrinone therapy has been used in patients with end-stage congestive heart failure.
- The duration of hemodynamic effects is 60 to 90 minutes with both agents and potentially longer in some patients with severe congestive heart failure. Titration of these agents is more difficult than with the sympathomimetic agents. Amrinone should be titrated 1 to 2.5 µg/kg/min every 1 to 3 hours and milrinone 0.025 to 0.1 µg/kg/min every 1 to 3 hours. Titration is more difficult in patients with a low CO and high PCWP. Never abruptly stop these agents; patients may decompensate and suffer cardiovascular collapse. It may take 24 to 72 hours to titrate these drugs in some patients. Lower increments at prolonged intervals may be necessary for patients who have received the drugs for more than 7 days.

Adverse Effects

- Amrinone produces a dose-dependent thrombocytopenia in up to 4% of patients treated. The frequency of this adverse effect increases with dosages greater than 18 mg/kg/day. Platelet counts will normalize in 2 to 7 days with reduction in dosage or discontinuation of the drug. The drug may be continued if necessary and platelet transfusions used when needed. Milrinone induces thrombocytopenia in only 1% of patients.
- Milrinone exacerbates dysrhythmias in 12% of patients. Milrinone increases AV nodal conduction. The drug should be discontinued in patients who develop changes in rhythm.
- Other adverse effects include nausea, headache, an-

gina, hypotension, increased liver function tests, and worsened heart failure with prolonged use.

SKELETAL MUSCLE RELAXANTS

Pharmacology

These agents cause skeletal muscle relaxation by competitively blocking the effects of acetylcholine at the neuromuscular junction. Analgesia is not provided by skeletal muscle relaxants.

Uses

These agents are primarily used to promote skeletal muscle relaxation and to facilitate the management of mechanical respiration.

Dosing and Administration (See Table 28)

- The dosages in Table 28 are those used for assisting in muscle relaxation for mechanical ventilation. Refer to the manufacturer's recommendation for other indications.
- The actions of these agents can be reversed by the administration of cholinesterase inhibitors such as neostigmine, pyridostigmine, or edrophonium.

Adverse Effects

- The major adverse effects of atracurium are mild and occur in less than 5% of patients. Skin flush, erythema, pruritus, and urticaria occur most commonly and are usually seen with low dosages rather than high dosages.
- Pancuronium may cause dose-related increases in blood pressure and occasional rashes and wheezing.
- Vecuronium is well tolerated, and most adverse effects are related to histamine release (e.g., flushing, redness, hypotension).

SYNTHETIC HORMONES

Cosyntropin (Cortrosyn)

Pharmacology

Cosyntropin elicits the same pharmacological responses produced by endogenous corticotropin. In patients with normal adrenocortical function, cosyntropin stimulates the adrenal cortex to secrete hydrocortisone (cortisol), corticosterone, some androgens, and small amounts of aldosterone.

Uses

Cosyntropin is used diagnostically to evaluate adrenocortical insufficiency.

Dosage and Administration

- Cosyntropin may be given by IV or IM administration as a 0.25-mg dose. IV doses are infused over 2 minutes. Plasma cortisol levels should be drawn

immediately before cosyntropin administration and then 30 or 60 minutes after the injection. Plasma cortisol levels drawn at 30 minutes should increase at least 7 μg/ml over the previous baseline value, and levels at 60 minutes should be greater than 11 μg/ml over the baseline value. These responses indicate normal adrenocortical function.

- Cosyntropin may also be administered over 6 hours at a rate of 0.04 mg/hr when a greater stimulus to the adrenal cortex is desired. The adrenal response is measured by plasma cortisol concentrations or urinary metabolite measurements.
- The powder should be reconstituted with 1 ml of normal saline.

Adverse Effects

- The use of cosyntropin as a diagnostic agent is not associated with any significant adverse effects. Hypersensitivity is a rare complication of therapy.

Glucagon (Various)

Pharmacology

Glucagon promotes hepatic glycogenolysis and gluconeogenesis. It stimulates adenylate cyclase to produce increased cAMP, which is involved in a complicated series of enzymatic activities. The results are an increased concentration of plasma glucose, a relaxation of smooth musculature, and an inotropic myocardial effect. Hepatic stores of glycogen are necessary for glucagon to elicit an antihypoglycemic effect.

Uses

Glucagon is used for the emergency treatment of severe hypoglycemia in patients with diabetes mellitus and in psychiatric patients with insulin shock.

Dosing and Administration

- Glucagon may be given by subcutaneous, IV, or IM injection. The powder should be diluted with diluent provided by the manufacturer. If the diluent is unavailable, sterile water for injection may be substituted.
- As an antihypoglycemic: intramuscular, intravenous, or subcutaneous doses of 0.5 to 1 USP unit (0.5 to 1 mg) of glucagon repeated every 20 minutes as needed.
- As a diagnostic aid: glucagon can be given IM or IV as the equivalent of 0.25 to 2 USP units (0.25 to 2 mg) of glucagon; the dose is dependent on the time of onset of action and the duration of effect required for the specific examination.
- Glucagon is effective in correcting hypoglycemia only in those patients having available liver glycogen. Intravenous glucose must be given if the patient

TABLE 28 Commonly Used Skeletal Muscle Relaxants

Drug	Trade Name	Onset (min)	Duration (min)	Recovery from Complete Block (min)	Accumulation	Cardiac Toxicity	Dosage*
Atracurium besylate	Tracrium	4-6	15-20	30-40	No	No	Loading dose: 0.4-0.5 mg/kg followed by infusion of 0.4-1.0 mg/kg/hr
Pancuronium	Pavulon	3-4	60-120	>60	Yes	Yes	0.01-0.2 mg/kg prn for agitation
Vecuronium	Norcuron	4-6	15-30	30-40	No	No	0.1-0.2 mg/kg qh or 0.05- to 0.1-mg/kg/hr infusion

* Dosage for use as a skeletal muscle relaxant to assist mechanical ventilation in the critically ill.

fails to respond to glucagon. Supplemental sugar (glucose or sucrose) must be given to prevent secondary hypoglycemia after the patient has revived sufficiently to receive oral administration.

Adverse Effects

• Glucagon is well tolerated, and adverse effects are rare. Dose-related nausea and vomiting may occur and may be associated with hypoglycemia rather than drug therapy.

Insulin (Various)

Pharmacology

Insulin is a hormonal factor that controls the storage and metabolism of carbohydrates, protein, and fats. Such activity occurs primarily in liver, muscle, and adipose tissues subsequent to attachment of insulin molecules to receptor sites on cellular plasma membranes. Although the mechanisms of molecular actions in the cellular area are still being explored, it is known that cell membrane transport characteristics, cellular growth, enzyme activation and inhibition, and alterations in protein metabolism are all influenced by insulin.

Uses

Insulin is used to control hyperglycemia of various causes.

Dosing and Administration (See Table 29)

• The dosage and administration of insulin varies greatly and must, therefore, be determined for each individual patient. Blood and urine glucose determinations must be used to individualize the regimen.

• Insulin resistance is usually due to obesity, stress,

TABLE 29   Insulin Preparations*

Type of Insulin	Common Name	Trade Name	Species	Onset (hr)	Peak (hr)	Duration (hr)
Rapid-acting	Regular insulin injection	Iletin	Beef or pork	0.5-1	2-3	5-7
		Novo-Nordisk	Pork	0.5-1	2-3	5-7
		Iletin II	Beef or pork	0.5-1	2-3	5-7
		Purified Novo-Nordisk	Pork	0.5-1	2-3	5-7
		Humulin-R	Human	0.5	2-4	5-7
		Novolin-R	Human	0.5	2.5-5	6-8
	Prompt insulin–zinc suspension	Semilente	Beef or pork	0.5-1	4-7	12-16
Intermediate-acting	NPH	Iletin	Beef or pork	1-2	8-12	18-24
		Novo-Nordisk	Beef	1-2	8-12	18-24
		Iletin II	Beef or pork	1-2	8-12	18-24
		Purified Novo Nordisk	Pork	1-2	8-12	18-24
		Humulin-N	Human	1-2	6-12	18-24
		Novolin-N	Human	1-2	6-12	18-24
	Insulin–zinc suspension	Lente	Beef or pork	1-2	8-12	18-24
			Human	2.5	7-15	22
Long-acting	Protamine zinc suspension	Iletin	Beef or pork	4-8	14-20	36
	Extended insulin–zinc suspension	Ultralente	Beef or pork	4-8	16-18	36
			Human	4-6	8-20	24-28

*Eli Lilly has discontinued animal-source insulins effective December 1992.

or exogenous steroid administration. Some patients may require in excess of 200 units/day due to a decrease in insulin action at the receptor site.

- Because of its rapid onset and ability to be administered IV, regular insulin is the insulin preparation of choice in the treatment of emergency situations.
- For the treatment of diabetic ketoacidosis, regular insulin can be given as an initial bolus of 0.1 U/kg followed by an IV infusion of regular insulin at a rate of 0.1 to 0.15 U/kg/hr. The dose should be titrated in accordance with the glucose level. If the serum glucose is unchanged at 2 hours, the infusion rate may be doubled. Some adults have required as much as 1,000 units in the first 24 hours, whereas patients with insulin resistance may require doses as high as 20,000 units in rare instances. The blood glucose should be drawn hourly until stable.
- Insulin binds to plastic tubing and linings; therefore, IV tubing should be flushed with the insulin solution before administration.
- Insulin requirements may change when switching from one source of insulin to another.
- The usual initiating maintenance dose of insulin is 0.5 U/kg/day. This dose can be given as two thirds of total dose in the morning and one third of total dose in the evening. Regular insulin may be given, with a longer acting preparation for maintenance therapy. The usual dosage of regular insulin is one third to one half of the total dosage to be given and should be adjusted on the basis of several glucose determinations (e.g., 0700, 1100, 1600, 2100).
- As a general rule, regular insulin should be drawn first, as the supply of regular insulin may become cloudy because of the inadvertent contamination with the other insulin. Regular insulin may be mixed with NPH insulin in any proportion without loss of the characteristics of the individual insulins. It is generally recommended that the resulting mixture be used within 5 minutes unless the manufacturer's literature states otherwise.
- Regular insulin mixed with insulin zinc preparations may not give predictable clinical results. Lente, Semilente, and Ultralente insulins may be mixed in any proportion without loss of the characteristics of the individual insulins.
- Most brands of regular insulin may be mixed with PZI insulin, but the excess free protamine in the PZI combines with the regular insulin to give various durations of action.
- Insulin commercially available in the United States is a mixture of beef and pork insulin or, if it is from a single source, appropriately marked "beef," "pork," or "human" insulin.
- Human insulin is the least antigenic and the insulin of choice for newly diagnosed patients or those with insulin resistance or allergy.

Adverse Effects

- Hypoglycemia is the most common adverse effect and is dose related.
- Allergic reactions occur because of insulin impurities and are least common with human or purified pork insulins. Manifestations include local irritation, lipoatrophy, and insulin resistance.
- Lipohypertrophy at the injection site may occur and can be minimized by rotating the site of injection.

Drug Interactions

- Adrenocorticoids, danazol, dextrothyroxine, epinephrine, ethacrynic acid, furosemide, oral contraceptives, phenytoin, sympathomimetics, thyroid, and thiazide diuretics may increase blood glucose concentrations and enhance the possibility of hyperglycemia.
- Alcohol, anabolic steroids, oral hypoglycemics, MAO inhibitors, large doses of salicylates, disopyramide, or guanethidine may enhance the hypoglycemic effect.

VASODILATORS

(See antianginal section for nitrates and calcium channel blockers.)

ACE Inhibitors

Pharmacology

The angiotensin-converting enzyme (ACE) inhibitors block the conversion of angiotensin I to angiotensin II. All of the agents currently available are equally effective at equipotent doses. By lowering the production of angiotensin I, a potent endogenous vasopressor, these agents produce balanced arterial and venodilatation. Mild reductions in aldosterone result in limited diuresis and reduced volume expansion.

Uses

These agents are indicated for the treatment of hypertension and heart failure.

Dosing and Administration (See Table 30)

- Dosages should be low at initiation and gradually titrated upward to the desired response. Patients with low serum sodium, recent diuresis, or long-standing heart failure may be sensitive to these agents, and initial therapy should be carefully monitored to prevent hypotension or renal insufficiency.
- Diuretic dosages may need to be lowered with concomitant ACE inhibitor therapy. These agents may worsen cardiac and renal function in hypovolemic patients.
- Cautiously use with potassium-sparing diuretics or potassium supplementation. Patients may develop hyperkalemia with chronic use of these agents concurrently.

Index

Page numbers in *italics* designate figures. Page numbers followed by the letter *t* designate tables or boxes.